Respiratory Care

Respiratory Care

A Guide to Clinical Practice

FOURTH EDITION

Edited by

George G. Burton, MD

Medical Director, Respiratory Services, Kettering Medical Center, Kettering, OH
Clinical Professor of Medicine, Wright State University School of Medicine, Dayton, OH

John E. Hodgkin, MD

Clinical Professor of Medicine, University of California, Davis
Medical Director, Respiratory Care and Pulmonary Rehabilitation, St. Helena Hospital, Deer Park, CA

Jeffrey J. Ward, MEd, RRT

Program Director, Rochester Community College / Mayo, Respiratory Therapy Program,
Assistant Professor, Mayo Medical School, Department of Anesthesia, Rochester, MN

Associate Editors

Dean R. Hess, PhD, RRT
Assistant Director, Respiratory Care
Massachusetts General Hospital
Boston, MA

Susan P. Pilbeam, MEd, RRT
Assistant Dean, Allied Health
Respiratory Care
Greenville Technical College
Greenville, SC

Judy A Tietsort, RN, RRT
Respiratory Management Consultants
Arvada, CO

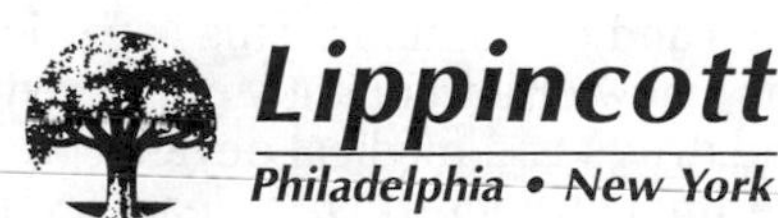

Acquisitions Editor: Lawrence McGrew
Editorial Assistant: Holly Collins
Project Editor: Barbara Ryalls
Production Manager: Helen Ewan
Production Coordinator: Kathryn Rule
Design Coordinator: Doug Smock
Indexer: Kathleen Pitcoff

Edition 4

9 8 7 6 5 4 3 2 1

Library of Congress Cataloging in Publications Data

Respiratory care : a guide to clinical practice / edited by George G. Burton, John E. Hodgkin, Jeffrey J. Ward ; associate editors, Dean R. Hess, Susan P. Pilbeam, Judy A. Tietsort. — 4th ed.
p. cm.
Includes bibliographical references and index.
ISBN 0-397-55165-7 (alk. paper)
1. Respiratory therapy. I. Burton, George G., 1934– . II. Hodgkin, John E. (John Elliott), 1939– . III. Ward, Jeffrey J.
[DNLM: 1. Respiratory Tract Diseases—therapy. 2. Respiratory Therapy. WF 145 R434 1997]
RC735.I5R47 1997
616.2′0046—dc21
DNLM/DLC
for Library of Congress

96-40216
CIP

Care has been taken to confirm the accuracy of the information presented and to describe generally accepted practices. However, the authors, editors, and publisher are not responsible for errors or omissions or for any consequences from application of the information in this book and make no warranty, express or implied, with respect to the contents of the publication.

The authors, editors and publisher have exerted every effort to ensure that drug selection and dosage set forth in this text are in accordance with current recommendations and practice at the time of publication. However, in view of ongoing research, changes in government regulations, and the constant flow of information relating to drug therapy and drug reactions, the reader is urged to check the package insert for each drug for any change in indications and dosage and for added warnings and precautions. This is particularly important when the recommended agent is a new or infrequently employed drug.

Some drugs and medical devices presented in this publication have Food and Drug Administration (FDA) clearance for limited use in restricted research settings. It is the responsibility of the health care provider to ascertain the FDA status of each drug or device planned for use in their clinical practice.

This book is dedicated to our long-suffering wives and to our children. Their patience and understanding have made this work possible. They continue to bring joy to the hours and days of our lives.

Jean Burton, Jean Hodgkin, and Julie Ward

Joan Rubino; David, Kevin, and Jon Burton; Janelle Rasi; Steven, Jonathan, and Jamie Hodgkin; Carolyn Bakland and Kathyrn Glendrange; Caryn Ward

Contributors

Timothy E. Albertson, MD, PhD
Division of Pulmonary and Critical Care Medicine
University of California, Davis, School of Medicine
Sacramento, CA

Donna L. Arand, PhD
Sleep Disorders Center
Kettering Medical Center
Kettering, OH

Thomas A. Barnes, EdD, RRT
Director
Respiratory Therapy Program
Northeastern University
Boston, MA

Michael H. Bonnett, PhD
Sleep Disorders Center
Kettering Medical Center
Kettering, OH

Karen M. Boudin, MA, RRT
Educator
Respiratory Care Department
Stanford University Hospital
Stanford, CA

Richard D. Branson, RRT
Assistant Professor of Surgery
Division of Trauma and Critical Care
Department of Surgery
University of Cincinnati Medical Center
Cincinnati, OH

W. Mark Brutinel, MD
Assistant Professor of Medicine
Division of Pulmonary Medicine
Mayo Medical Center
Rochester, MN

A. Janelle Burton-Rasi
Resident in Radiology
University of Cincinnati Medical Center
Cincinnati, OH

George G. Burton, MD
Medical Director
Respiratory Services
Kettering Medical Center
Kettering, OH

Robert S. Campbell, RRT
Senior Research Associate
Division of Trauma and Critical Care
Department of Surgery
University of Cincinnati Medical Center
Cincinnati, OH

Gerilynn L. Connors, RCP, RRT, BS
Director
Pulmonary Rehabilitation Program
Clinical Coordinator
Nicotine Intervention Program
St. Helena Hospital
Deer Park, CA

Dennis A. Cortese, MD
Professor of Medicine
Mayo Medical Center
Rochester, MN

Thomas J. DeKornfeld, MD
Professor of Anesthesiology (Emeritus)
University of Michigan Medical School
Ann Arbor, MI

Terry Des Jardins, MEd, RRT
Department of Respiratory Care
Parkland College
Champaign, IL

David A. Desaultels, MPA, RRT
Respiratory Therapy Department
St. Joseph's Hospital
Tampa, FL

F. Herbert Douce, MS, RRT
Assistant Professor and Director
School of Allied Health Professions
Respiratory Therapy Division
Ohio State University
Columbus, OH

Paul L. Enright, MD
Respiratory Sciences Center
University of Arizona
Tucson, AZ

John M. Fiascone, MD
Assistant Neonatologist
Division of Newborn Medicine
Floating Hospital for Children
New England Medical Center
Boston, MA

James B. Fink, RRT
Respiratory Therapy Department
Hines Veteran Administration Hospital
Hines, IL

William J. Fulkerson, MD
Professor of Medicine
Division of Pulmonary Medicine
Duke University Medical Center
Durham, NC

Douglas R. Gracey, MD
Chairman
Division of Thoracic Disease
Mayo Medical Center
Rochester MN

Timothy Hatfield, PhD
Professor
Department of Counselor Education
Winona State University
Winona, MN

H.F. Helmholz, Jr., MD
Emeritus Staff
Mayo Medical Center
Rochester, MN

Dean R. Hess, PhD, RRT
Assistant Director
Respiratory Care
Massachusetts General Hospital
Boston, MA

Lana Hilling, CRT, RCP
Mt. Diablo Medical Center
Concord, CA

Oleh W. Hnatiuk, MD
Pulmonary and Critical Care Service
Walter Reed Army Medical Center
Washington, DC

John E. Hodgkin, MD
Clinical Professor of Medicine
University of California, Davis
Medical Director, Respiratory Care & Pulmonary Rehabilitation
St. Helena Hospital
Deer Park, CA

James M. Hurst, MD, FACS
Professor of Surgery and Anesthesiology
Vice Chairman and Chief of Clinical Operations
Department of Surgery
University of Cincinnati Medical Center
Cincinnati, OH

James T.C. Li, MD
Assistant Professor of Medicine
Division of Allergy/Outpatient Infectious Diseases
Mayo Medical Center
Rochester, MN

Glen A. Lillington, MD
Professor of Medicine
Pulmonary Section
University of California, Davis, School of Medicine
Sacramento, CA

Jackie L. Long-Goding, RRT
Respiratory Care Program
Massachusetts Bay Community College
Wellesley Hills, MA

Neil R. MacIntyre, MD
Associate Professor of Medicine
Medical Director, Respiratory Care Services
Duke University Medical Center
Durham, NC

John J. Mahoney
Researcher and Developer
LifeScan, Inc.
Milpitas, CA

Susan L. McInturff, RCP, RRT
Staff Therapist
Farrell's Home Health
Bremerton, WA

Elizabeth Moore, MD
Assistant Professor of Radiology
University of California, Davis
Sacramento, CA

Walter J. O'Donohue, Jr., MD
Chairman
Department of Medicine
Creighton University School of Medicine
Omaha, NE

F. Ross Payne, RRT
Program Director
Respiratory Care
Arkansas Vocational Technical College
Fort Smith, AR

Steven G. Peters, MD
Division of Thoracic Disease
Mayo Medical Center
Rochester, MN

Col. Yancey Y. Philips, MD
Chief
Dept. of Internal Medicine
Walter Reed Army Medical Center
Washington, DC

Susan P. Pilbeam, MS, RRT
Assistant Dean, Allied Health
Respiratory Care
Greenville Technical College
Greenville, SC

David J. Plevak, MD
Department of Anesthesiology
Mayo Medical Center
Rochester, MN

Alan L. Plummer, MD
Medical Director
Respiratory Care Department
Associate Professor of Medicine
Pulmonary Disease and Critical Care Medicine
Emory University Hospital
Atlanta, GA

Udaya B.B. Prakash, MD, FRCP, FACP, FCCP
Consultant in Pulmonary, Critical Care and Internal Medicine
Director of Bronchoscopy
Mayo Medical Center
Professor of Medicine, Mayo Medical School
Rochester, MN

Charles E. Reed, MD
Assistant Professor of Medicine
Allergy Research
Mayo Medical Center
Rochester, MN

Susan Rickey-Hatfield, PhD
Associate Professor
Speech Communication
Winona State University
Winona, MN

John S. Sabo, MS, RRT
Director
Respiratory Care
St. Luke's Episcopal Hospital
Houston, TX

Dennis C. Sobush, MA, PT
Associate Professor
Marquette University
Walter Schroeder Complex
Milwaukee, WI

Peter A. Southorn, MD
Department of Anesthesiology
Mayo Medical Center
Rochester, MN

Judy A. Tietsort, RN, RRT
Respiratory Management Consultants
Arvadea, CO

Kenneth Torrington, MD
Pulmonary and Critical Care Service
Walter Reed Army Medical Center
Washington, DC

Brent Van Hoozen, MD
Division of Pulmonary and Critical Care Medicine
University of California, Davis, School of Medicine
Sacramento, CA

Antonius L. Van Kessel, MD
Director
Respiratory Care Services, Emeritus
Stanford University Hospital
Stanford, CA

Jeffrey J. Ward, MEd, RRT
Respiratory Therapy Program
Mayo Medical Center
Rochester, MN

John A. Washington, MD
Chairman
Department of Microbiology
The Cleveland Clinic Foundation
Cleveland, OH

John T. Wheeler, RT
Respiratory Therapist
Supervisor of Respiratory Therapy
Mayo Medical Center
Rochester, MN

Irwin Ziment, MD
Medical Director
Olive View Medical Center
University of California, Los Angeles
Sylmar, CA

Preface to the Fourth Edition

More than 2 decades have elapsed since the first edition of *Respiratory Care: A Guide to Clinical Practice* was first published. Each subsequent edition has allowed us an opportunity to process the contributions of dozens of educators into a volume that sets out a current review of the knowledge and skills base for the practice of respiratory care. Description of the practice domain of respiratory care practitioners (RCPs) has always been the reason for this volume; a rapidly evolving data base has required subsequent editions over the years.

The interval between publication of the 3rd and 4th editions has been outstanding in the paradigm shifts that have accompanied it. As we predicted in the Preface to the 3rd edition, not only have RCPs increasingly found themselves working in criterion-referenced, therapist-driven protocol (TDP) environments, but also in functions far removed from the traditional acute-care hospital settings. No longer do "entry-level job openings exist in nearly every (acute care) hospital in the country." However, new graduates are now finding employment in other loci in the seamless health care model, including skilled nursing facilities, outpatient rehabilitation facilities, physician offices, homecare organizations, and hospice services.

Where, in the past, only respiratory care *educators* were much concerned with outcomes, now each new RCP is indoctrinated with such an orientation—"Did what I do make a difference?" In all these settings, the basic competencies implicit in the TDP paradigm seem to apply, ie, assessment and treatment selection skills, along with technologic competence.

The competitive job market has forced RCPs not only to have specialized knowledge and skills, but to have them in sufficient "value-added" measure to justify their existence. Let us illustrate this with lessons that have been learned from the "Patient-Focused Care" movement, which has suggested that economies can be achieved by extensive cross-training of health care workers. In many parts of the country, this movement has been responsible for the decentralization of respiratory care departments, and transfer of responsibility for the performance of respiratory care procedures away from RCPs to other allied health care givers.

Add to this, the increasing reliance on patients and nonskilled caregivers to assess and treat *themselves.* This is nowhere more evident than in the case of the mandates implicit in the NHLBI Asthma Education Program (NAEPP) Guidelines, which suggest that such individuals should assess (eg, symptom diary), measure (eg, peak expiratory flow measurements), diagnose severity (green? yellow? red?), select and perform treatment (eg, more bronchodilator medication? start/taper steroids? go to the Emergency Department?), and re-evaluate the effects thereof.

These two powerful forces have necessitated a whole reappraisal of the role and function of the RCP in modern health care. Clearly, his or her technical competence must be outstanding, particularly in the "high-tech, high-touch" procedures attendant to the pulmonary diagnostic laboratory and intensive care unit. However, it is in the sophistication of the answers to the "What's going on here?" and "What can I do about it?" questions that the RCPs' real value will (or will not, depending on their preparation) be seen.

To meet these challenges, the format of the Fourth Edition has been completely re-engineered. The section dealing with patient assessment has been considerably strengthened, while chapters dealing with respiratory care modalities and equipment have been based almost entirely on the new *AARC Clinical Practice Guidelines* (CPGs) and accepted TDP therapy strategies.

We have been aided in our efforts by new associates: Dean Hess has added his expertise in integrating CPGs throughout the volume; Sue Pilbeam has skillfully upgraded the section dealing with respiratory care equipment and has contributed an entirely new chapter on mechanical ventilation; and Judy Tietsort has edited much of the volume with an eye to use of respiratory care modalities in the protocol environment. New pedagogic approaches have been used in the forms of Key Concept emphasis, listings of both technical and nontechnical skills in keeping with current NBRC examination matrices and the addition of an extensive glossary of key terms.

Our appreciation is again extended to our secretaries, Flossie Hodgson and Carolyn Wilson at Kettering and Patricia Jones at St. Helena, who tolerated (again) our forays into the ordered world of their word processors to allow us to revise, re-word, re-arrange, and otherwise wreak havoc with their already busy lives.

In this edition, we are indebted to 48 contributors for their sharing of wisdom. We thank our editors at Lippincott-Raven Publishers for their encouragement and patience as this volume has been in development and production. Andrew Allen, Holly Collins, and Barbara Ryalls have been particularly patient and helpful.

And, lastly, we thank the respiratory care profession for being what it is, in these challenging times.

Contents

Respiratory Care

SECTION

I

THE RESPIRATORY CARE PROFESSION: PAST, PRESENT, AND FUTURE

1 Roots of the Respiratory Care Profession

Jeffrey J. Ward
H.F. Helmholz, Jr.

PROFESSIONAL SKILLS

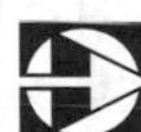

Upon completion of this chapter, the reader will:

- Identify early philosophers, scientists, and medical personnel whose discoveries and inventions led to the evolution of medicine
- Describe the work of scientists and inventors which led to the development of clinical applications of oxygen therapy and mechanical ventilation
- Recount the transition from conceptual respiratory care to a scientific basis for its implementation
- Denote the development of Clinical Practice Guidelines and Therapist-Driven Protocols
- Trace the evolution of the professional, credentialing, and school accreditation organizations involved in maintaining the quality of the respiratory care profession

KEY TERMS

Certified pulmonary function technologist
Certified respiratory therapy technician
Clinical practice guidelines
Mechanical ventilation
Perinatal/pediatric specialists
Registered pulmonary function technologist
Registered therapist
Respiration
Respiratory care
Respiratory physiology
Therapist-driven protocols

"Medical history teaches us where we came from, where we stand in medicine at the present time, and what direction we are marching. It's the compass that guides us into the future. If our work is not to be haphazard but to follow a well-laid plan, we need the guidance of history, and it is not by accident that all great medical leaders were fully aware of the value of historical studies."[1]

The quote from medical historian Henry Sigerist sets the theme for this chapter; the outline describes the scope of content. We are all travelers in history. Unlike the Time Traveler in H.G. Wells', *The Time Machine*, we have no vehicle to go into the future. The past can provide the respiratory care practitioner with an explanation for the present and some insight into what lies ahead. This chapter notes remnants of the past and recognizes contributions of those who have gone before. Respiratory care is a relatively young field; many of the pioneers are still with us.

Respiratory care has roots in a diverse history. Biology unraveled "secrets" of the anatomy and function of the cardiopulmonary system. Concurrently, physiologic gases were discovered, and their chemistry, physics, and roles in body function were elucidated. In addition, there is an ongoing evolution of clinical pulmonary medicine, with key technical advances in areas of gas therapy, resuscitation, mechanical ventilation, and cardiopulmonary diagnostics and monitoring. Together with the history of medical science and technology, there is also a legacy of an evolving organized profession. The purpose of this chapter is to review highlights in the history of respiratory care and the structure of the respiratory care profession.

HISTORY OF MEDICINE

Ancient Times

The story of the search for knowledge about respiration goes back to ancient times.

"And he put his mouth upon his mouth . . . and the flesh of the child became warm." (II Kings 4:34)

Twenty-eight centuries ago, the biblical story of the prophet Elisha recounted the restoration to life of the son of a Shunammite woman. He breathed into the mouth of a suffocating child; this set off a series of seven sneezes that relieved the tracheal obstruction. This early concept fit into the practical medicine of the Egyptians and Babylonians. About 3000 B.C., ancient Egyptian science had reached its zenith. The Chinese had a part philosophic and part physiologic concept of breathing in which breath from the air was transmitted into the soul. About 2000 B.C., they had developed acupuncture points, elaborate rituals for taking pulse, and used moxibustion (burning substances on the skin).[2–4]

An important portion of our scientific heritage began with the Greeks, who sought knowledge for its own sake, without need for practical application. Pythagoras (580–489 B.C.) defined life and matter as comprising four basic elements: earth, fire, water, and air. Hippocrates (460–370 B.C.) developed the doctrine of "essential humors." He attributed all diseases to humoral disorders within body fluids and taught that an essential, yet undefined, material derived from the inspired air, entered the heart and was then distributed throughout the body systems. Hippocrates and his contemporaries promoted examination and identification of signs of diseases. Aristotle (384–322 B.C.) recorded the first probable scientific experiment in respiratory physiology when he observed that animals kept in airtight chambers soon died. He ascribed their deaths to the animals' inability to cool themselves by secretion of "phlegm." He also identified the heart as the source of the body's heat and nervous center.[2–4]

Erasistratus worked in Alexandria (about 304 B.C.) and founded the "pneumatic" theory of respiration. He believed that the lungs passed air to the left ventricle, which used air-filled arteries for transport to the body tissues. He apparently understood that heart valves provided one-way flow. After the exodus from Egypt, Moses set up codes for the Jews in matters of public health regarding handling of food, removing contagious cases from homes, and outlawing spitting.

In Asia Minor, Galen *(130–199 A.D.)* dominated the study of respiration longer than any previous scholar. He believed that "pneuma" or "world spirit" from inspired air passed through invisible pores in the heart's intraventricular septum. There, blood became charged with this vital spirit. Against popular thought, Galen believed that blood, not air, was carried by the arterial circulation, and that there were pulmonary and systemic capillaries. By dissection he disproved Aristotle's theories by showing that nerves originate in the brain and spinal cord, not the heart. He worked out the effects of cord transections and hemisection while serving as a physician to gladiators in Rome.

Caesar realized the need for doctors on the battlefield and at remote Roman outposts. Romans applied mechanical inventiveness in building aqueducts, flood control, and other public health measures to control epidemics and make city living possible. However, quacks were prevalent and doctors neglected childbearing women. Sexual freedom resulted in both abortion and increased gynecological problems.[4]

Early Middle Ages

Little new "physiologic" investigation was done in Europe after Galen. Barbarian hordes overran the Roman Empire; frightful pestilences decimated cities. Antisecular and antiscientific feeling during the medieval period resulted from the church taking a firm hold on medicine. There was a gap in progress and the loss of many priceless written documents. Survival of medical ideas from Rome and Greece are credited to Cassiodorus and St. Benedict of Nursia. However, despite Christian strictures, monasteries incorporated infirmaries, leprosaria, and hospices to offer nursing care to both brothers and laymen.[4]

In the 7th century Arabs swept into Persia and accepted the medical wisdom from the Greeks. The bar-

baric Moslems became the purveyors of classic medicine. The golden age of Arab medicine existed from about 850 to 1050 A.D. They are credited with originality in herbal medicines and developing the apothecary. Jewish physician and scholar Moses Maimonides combined the science of Aristotle and Galen with Mosaic Law. Bright lights of this period were naturalists Albertus Magnus (1192–1280) and physicist and mathematician Roger Bacon (1214–1294).[3,4]

Late Middle Ages

With the resurgence of trade in 14th-century Europe, the cities rose in importance. However, city living provided work but also poverty and filth. Garbage and filth were piled high in city streets and pigs roamed at will. Public mixed-gender bathhouses were initially supported to improve personal cleanliness, but resulted as unsanitary centers for public contagion. Physicians formed guilds like other "tradesmen."[4]

One of a series of pandemic plagues occurred in Asia and Europe during the mid and late 1300s. This ushered the end of feudal structure. The bubonic plague or Black Death resulted in disruption of normal life in Asia and Europe. It is estimated that 25 million people perished in Europe alone, about one fourth of the continent's population. The plague's etiology was blamed on comets, or scapegoats such as lepers or Jews, instead of the bacteria *Yersinia pestis*, which inhabited the intestines of fleas. Some lessons were learned in the form of quarantine of ship cargos and controlling water supplies. This helped reduce the impact when the plague returned to Europe in the 15th century. People came to expect more from doctors since they were required to attend formal courses. The plague killed off physicians of the "old school," allowing new ideas to flourish.[4]

The Renaissance

The Renaissance brought a renewed interest in the sciences. In Italy, Leonardo da Vinci (1452–1519) took up human dissection and physiologic experiments on animals. He concluded that subatmospheric (intrapleural) pressure inflated the lungs. Da Vinci observed that fire consumed a component in air, and that animals could not live in an atmosphere that could not support flames.

In 1542, Andreas Vesalius (Fig. 1-1) performed a thoracotomy on a pig and observed the effect of pneumothorax. The pig exhibited "wavelike pulsations of the heart and arteries," which probably was ventricular fibrillation. Vesalius reported that the heart returned to normal after ventilation through a tracheostomy tube made from a reed. He published his great work on anatomy in 1543, contradicting some of Galen's earlier observations. This manuscript and "a cardiac resuscitation" during the autopsy of a "just expired" Spanish nobleman brought on the wrath of the Inquisition. The Spanish anatomist Michael Servetus (1509–1553) was the first to discover that the blood in the pulmonary circulation, after mixing with the air in the lungs, returned to the left side of the heart. Servetus' "heretical" anatomy text resulted in his being burned at the stake.[2–4]

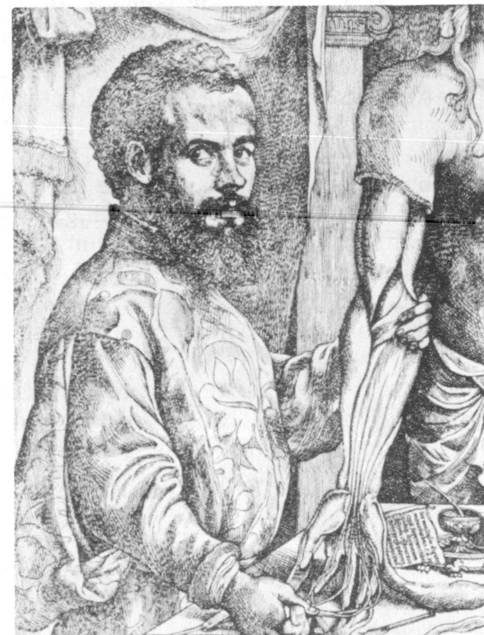

FIGURE 1-1. Andreas Vesalius, founder of modern human anatomy. (Courtesy of History of Medicine Library, Mayo Foundation, Rochester, MN)

75 years passed before the physiology of circulation was correctly clarified. In 1628, William Harvey (1578–1657; Fig. 1-2) described the heart as a muscular pump propelling the blood to the body through the arterial circulation, with return through the venous system. Pharmacists made great strides in keeping up with physicians. Surgeons began techniques of vessel ligature versus cautery, cosmetic surgery, and herniotomy.

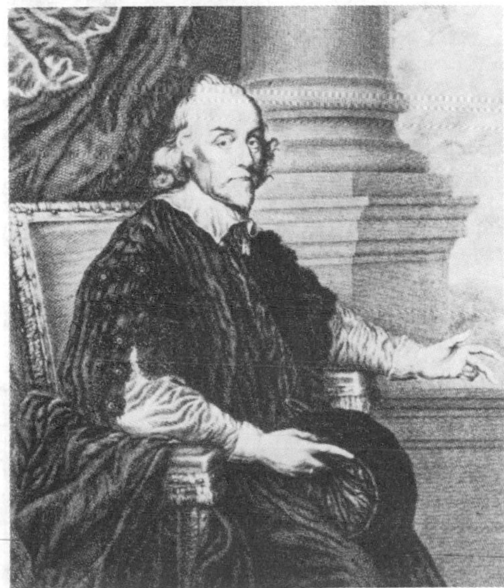

FIGURE 1-2. William Harvey described the circulatory system. (Courtesy of Wellcome Historical Medical Museum, London)

In Italy, Evangelista Torricelli (1608–1647; Fig 1-3) and associates made the first barometer in the 1640s. In France, Blaise Pascal (1623–1662) confirmed the relationship between barometric pressure and altitude. In 1666, England's Robert Boyle (1627–1691; Fig 1-4) speculated that there must be within air:

". . . numberless exhalations of the terraqueous globe . . . The difficulty we find in keeping flame and fire alive . . . without air renders it suspicious that there may be disbursed throughout the rest of the atmosphere some odd substance, either solar, astral, or other foreign nature: on account whereof the air is so necessary to flame."[2–4]

This note from Boyle's *Philosophical Transactions* (1670) surmises that the lack of oxygen, or a similar substance, was also a destructive factor. He recorded the production of aeroembolism by subjecting animals to low pressure. Boyle also developed Torricelli's barometer into the U-shaped form we know today and proposed the relationship between volume and pressure, which we know as Boyle's law. The science of bacteriology began as Anthony van Leeuwenhoek described minute animals he saw through his invention, the microscope, in 1683.[2,3]

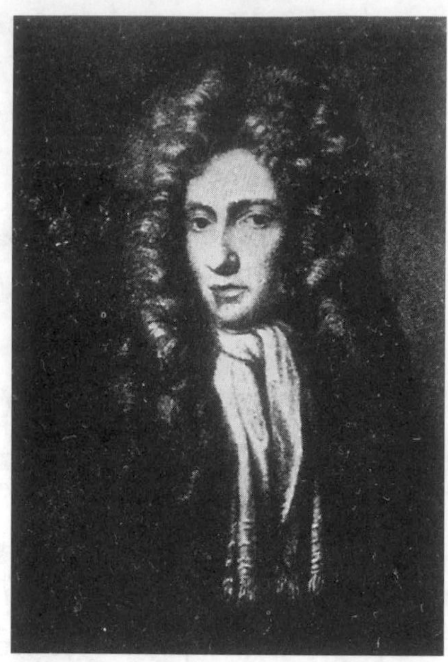

FIGURE 1-4. Robert Boyle. (From Dempster JH: John Locke, physician and philosopher. Ann Med History 4:12, 1932. With permission)

The 18th Century

In 1771, Swedish apothecary Carl Scheele (1742–1786; Fig. 1-5) made oxygen by heating magnesium oxide (MgO_2) with concentrated sulfuric acid (H_2SO_4). He communicated his findings on this "fire air" to others, and a summary of Scheele's findings was published in June 1774. However, Englishman Joseph Priestley (1733–1804; Fig. 1-6) was credited with the discovery of oxygen, although his work was published 3 months later. Priestley described his response to breathing pure oxygen, "phlogisticated air," as follows:

". . . my breath felt peculiarly light and easy for some time afterward. Who can tell but that in time this pure air may become a fashionable luxury. Hitherto, only two mice and myself have had the privilege of breathing it."[3]

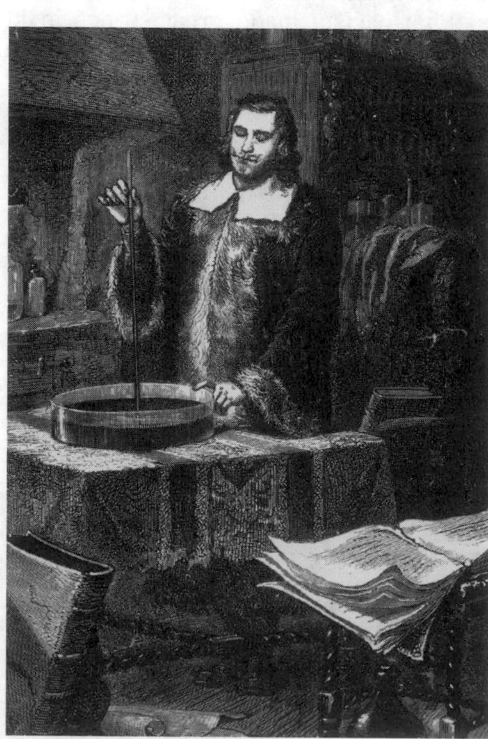

FIGURE 1-3. Evangalista Torricelli with mercury barometer. (From Granger Collection, with permission)

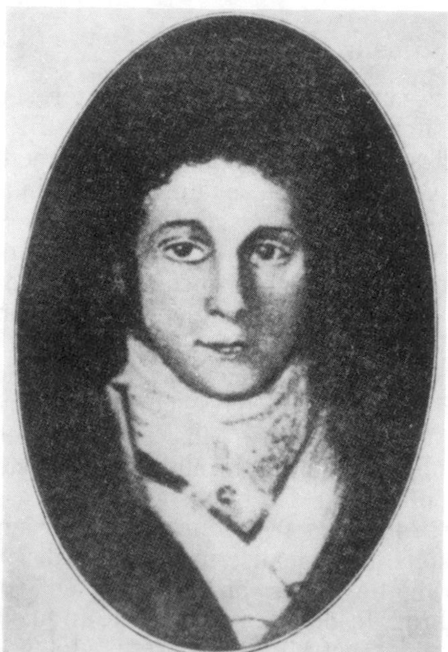

FIGURE 1-5. Carl Wilhelm Scheele, a Swedish apothecary, was the first to synthesize oxygen. (From Am Pharm Soc J 1931; 20:1061, with permission)

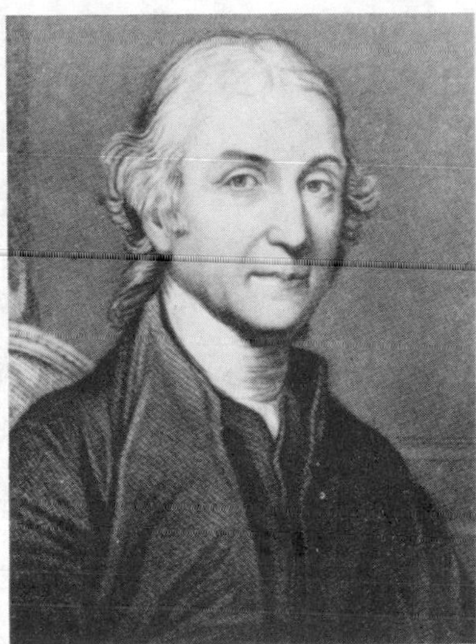

FIGURE 1-6. Joseph Priestley is credited as the discoverer of oxygen. (Courtesy of Wellcome Historical Medical Museum, London)

Both Scheele and Priestley followed the phlogiston theory proposed by the German George Stahl. This theory stated that combustible objects use up phlogiston, which has negative mass when burned. In France, Antoine Lavoisier (1743–1794; Fig. 1-7) published details of his findings on oxygen in 1775. He renamed the gas "oxygen" or "acid maker." Lavoisier appeared to have truly understood the physiologic relationships between oxygen and carbon dioxide. Between 1775 and 1794, his experiments showed that oxygen was absorbed by the lungs and consumed by the body. He further confirmed that carbon dioxide and water vapor were primary components of exhalation and that an inert gas (nitrogen) was essentially unchanged in the process. This work destroyed acceptance of the phlogiston theory. Unfortunately, the knowledge that Lavoisier's laboratory was supported by the French royalty resulted in his death by the guillotine in the prime of his career.[2–4]

Joseph Black (1728–1799; Fig. 1-8) is credited with the discovery of carbon dioxide gas, dephlogisticated "fixed air," which he produced by heating limestone. Actually, Black only rediscovered work done by Jean Baptiste van Helmont 100 years earlier.

During the late 1700s and early 1800s, several scientists provided significant discoveries in essential background physics that applied to pulmonary physiology. Italian physicist Amedeo Avogadro (1776–1856; Fig 1-9) determined the important constant as the basis for expressing the amount of gaseous species. He proposed that equal volumes of gases contain equal numbers of molecules under the same conditions. Jacques-Alexandre-Cesar Charles (1746–1823) and Joseph Louis Gay-Lussac (1778–1850; Fig 1-10) modified Charles' Law to express the relationship of pressure and temperature. English schoolmaster John Dalton (1766–1844; Fig 1-11) laid down his landmark atomic theory between 1803 and 1810, expanding on Avagadro's work. William Henry (1774–1836) and Pierre-Simon de Laplace (1749–1827) provided essential discoveries regarding the circulatory system and surface tension, respectively.[3,4]

Early clinical treatment of lung problems began to take place in the late 1700s in the form of cardiopulmonary resuscitation. Societies for rescuing drowning victims were set up in Denmark, England, and Europe. Several techniques were used: fumigation (blowing smoke into the rectum), chest-belly compression, bloodletting, and administration of stimulants. Reports of successful resuscitation (by now through the air-

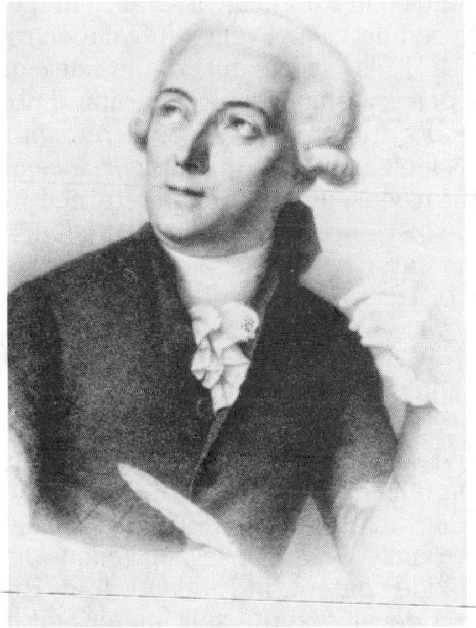

FIGURE 1-7. Antoine Laurent Lavoisier described the relationship of oxygen use with carbon dioxide elimination as respiration. (Courtesy of Wellcome Historical Medical Museum, London)

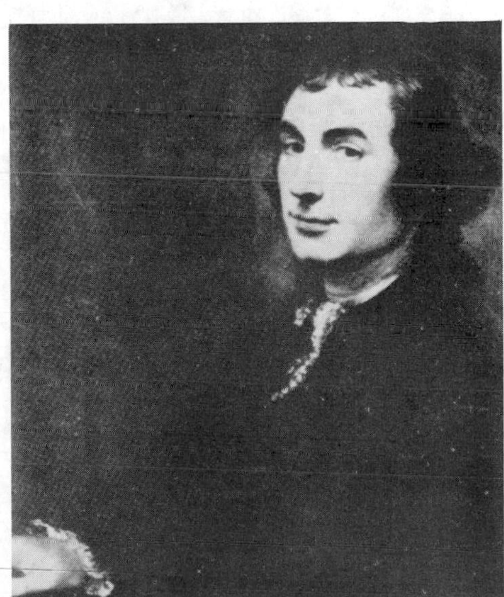

FIGURE 1-8. Joseph Black is credited with the discovery of carbon dioxide. (Courtesy of the University of Edinburgh, Edinburgh)

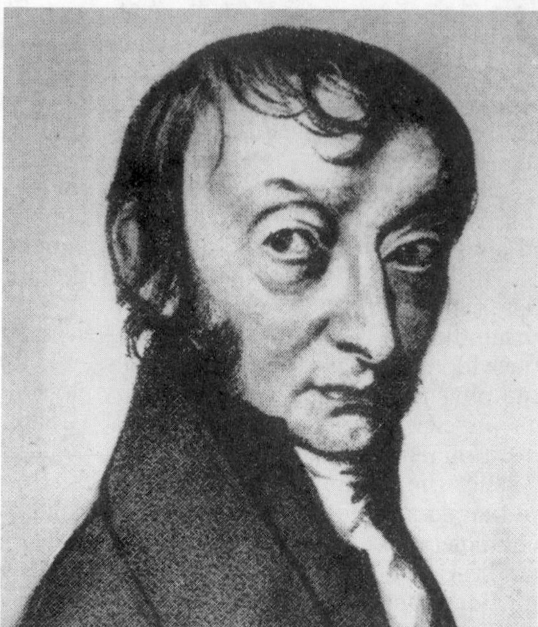

FIGURE 1-9. Amadeo Avagodro. (From Granger Collection, with permission)

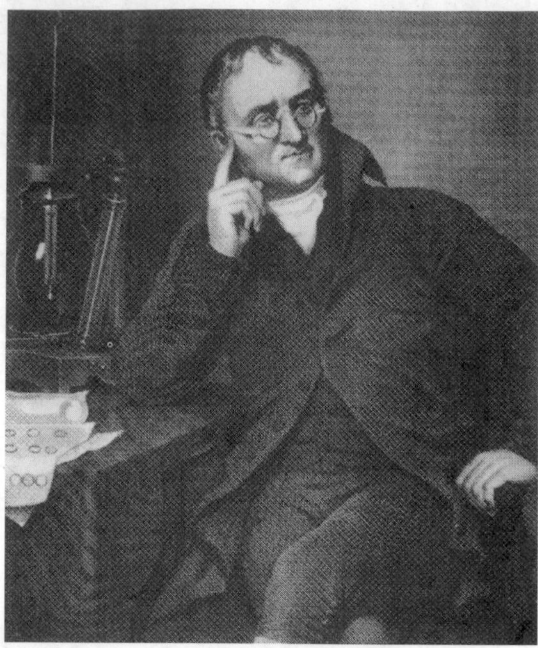

FIGURE 1-11. John Dalton developed atomic theory. (From Granger Collection, with permission)

way!) began in 1744 with John Fothergill of England. In 1776, John Hunter advocated the use of fireplace bellows with oxygen. Later the bellows was abandoned because of cases of complications such as pneumothorax. Tracheal intubation and electrical stimulation of the heart were suggested but were either overlooked or forgotten until years later.[3,4]

In the New World, British- and European-educated William Shippen and John Morgan established the first medical classes in Philadelphia's Independence Hall in 1762. By 1768 King's College (later Columbia University) established a medical school in New York. Basic immunology was known in the East for centuries. In America Reverend Cotton Mather found that one of his negro slaves was protected from smallpox because he was inoculated in Africa. In England, Edward Jenner published his findings on vaccination in 1789.[4]

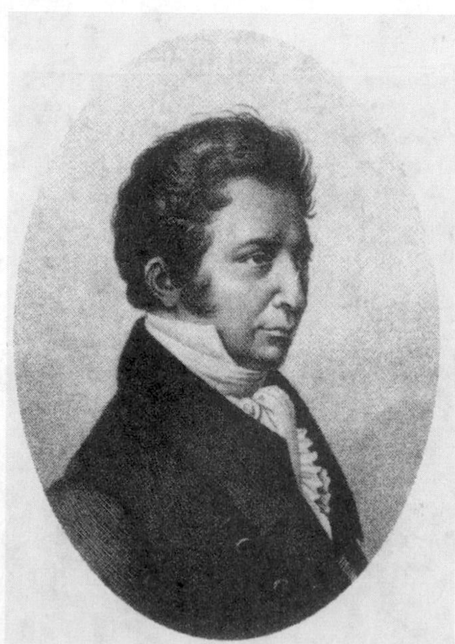

FIGURE 1-10. Joseph Louie Gay-Lussac. (From the Bibliothéque Nationale de France. With permission)

The 19th Century

Paris was the center of medical science in the first half of the 19th century. The French Revolution revised the physician's role as "speculator" of the cause of disease, into more of a pragmatic clinician. Clinical observation of signs and symptoms were compared with autopsy findings. Napoleon realized the importance of medical care for his troops, and surgeons returned home with practical experience from the battlefields of the Napoleonic wars.

Rene T.H. Laennec (1781–1826; Fig 1-12) published *Diseases of the Chest*, based on interrelating clinical findings and disease states. He is also known as the inventor of auscultation and laid the foundations for contemporary chest medicine. Lazzaro Spallazani (1729–1799) was the first scientist to measure oxygen consumption and carbon dioxide production of laboratory animals. By 1837, Heinrich Magnus (1802–1870) made the first quantitative analyses of arterial and venous oxygen and carbon dioxide content. In England, John Hutchinson (1811–1861) developed the spirometer and measured the vital capacity of more than 2000 subjects.

By the 1840s German medicine moved beyond the French approach with emphasis on embryology, mi-

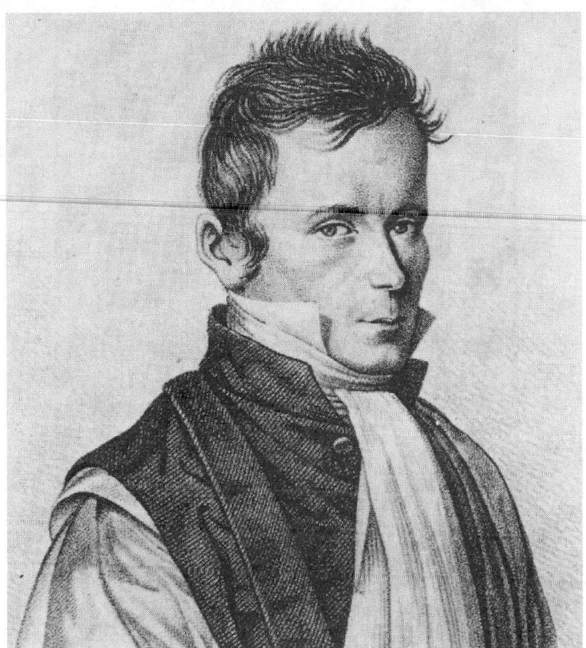

FIGURE 1-12. Rene Laennec developed the science of auscultation. (Courtesy of the Library of the College of Physicians of Philadelphia, Philadelphia)

croscopic anatomy, and physiology. The University system supported laboratory and clinical medicine. German medicine is credited with the development of the laryngoscope, ophthalmoscope, and cystoscope. William Roentgen discovered the "x-ray" in 1895; such devices enabled physicians to see inside the body without surgery. Aspirin was developed in Germany in 1886.

In 1844, American physician Gardner Colton revealed the effects of "laughing gas" in Hartford, Connecticut. Two years later, Dr. William Morton provided the first ether anesthesia in Boston. The Civil War provided a grim lesson to American physicians. Incomplete statistics record a loss of 300,000 Union troops, one third owing to wounds and the balance to sepsis (tetanus), dysentery, and typhoid fever. Elizabeth Blackwell and Civil War-trained Dr. Mary Walker established women's position in medicine in America. The Women's Medical College of Pennsylvania was established in 1850.[4]

Florence Nightingale (1820–1910) demonstrated that nursing skills were critical once the battle surgeons finished. She reduced the death rate of British soldiers from 42% to 2% during the Crimean War. In America, Civil War nurse Clara Barton aroused American interest in the Red Cross which was initiated in Europe in 1864.[4]

With the advent of anesthesia, surgeons were able to be more aggressive. However, wounds rarely healed without infection; 50% resulted in blood poisoning. A germ hunt began. In 1865, Scottish physician Joseph Lister published his theory on antiseptic method. By the mid 1880s, Louis Pasteur had saved the wine industry through his controlled fermentation and developed a vaccine against anthrax and antirabic injections. German physician Dr. Robert Koch determined the cause of tuberculosis in 1876. Paul Ehrlich developed Salvarsan, a synthetic drug against syphilis.[4]

Eduard Pfluger (1829–1910) provided evidence that oxidation occurs in tissues proportional to their needs and devised the term *respiratory quotient*. In 1878, Paul Bert (1833–1886) demonstrated that reduced inspired oxygen tension caused hyperventilation and, in 1885, F. Miescher-Rusch provided evidence that carbon dioxide was the primary stimulus for ventilation. Christian Bohr (1855–1911; Fig. 1-13) constructed the oxyhemoglobin dissociation curve for purified hemoglobin in 1886. Adolph Fick (1829–1901; Fig 1-14) described a means for measuring cardiac output indirectly, but lacked the manometric apparatus to perform the measurement.[3,4]

At the close of the 19th century, the will of Quaker philanthropist Johns Hopkins provided the funds for establishing a medical school and linked university. The theme was to give American doctors a background on a par with European standards. Faculty such as pathologist William H. Welch, surgeon William S. Halsted, gynecologist Howard A. Kelly, and clinician-teacher William Osler established this as a major center for medical education.

The 20th Century

In 1904, Bohr, K. A. Hasselbalch, and August Krogh (1874–1949) linked the processes of oxygen and carbon dioxide transport. In the late 1800s the secretion of materials in the gastrointestinal system were demonstrated; the concept of secretion of oxygen from alveolar gas into the blood was introduced. Christian Bohr and John Scott Haldane (1860–1936; Fig. 1-15)

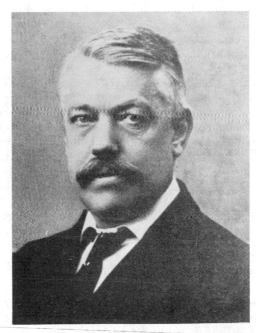

FIGURE 1-13. Christian Bohr established the oxyhemoglobin dissociation curve and oxygen and carbon dioxide's loading—unloading relationship. (Courtesy of Universitets Medicinsk-Historiske Museum, Copenhagen)

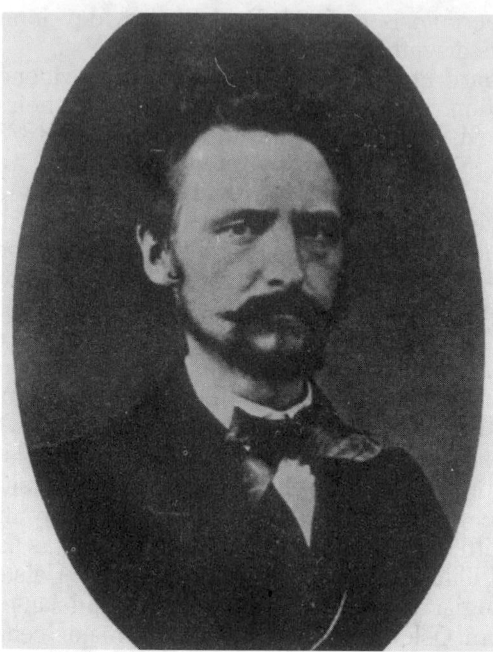

FIGURE 1-14. Adolf Fick. (From Fishman AP: Structure and Function. In Fishman AP: Pulmonary Diseases and Disorders, 2nd ed. New York, McGraw-Hill, 1988, with permission)

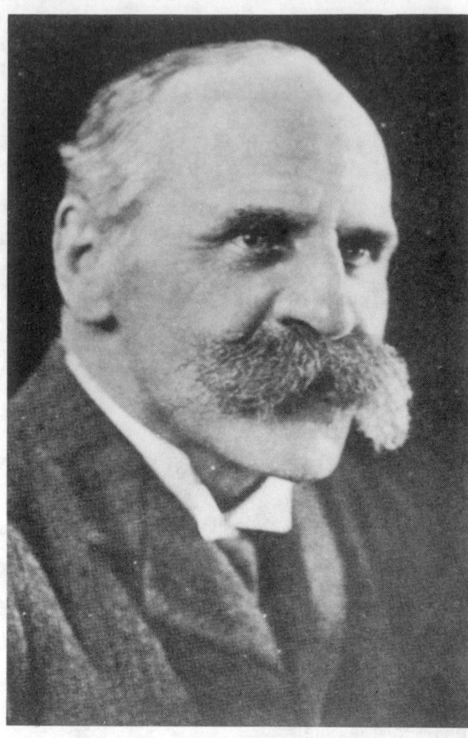

FIGURE 1-15. John Scott Haldane demonstrated that carbon dioxide provides the primary respiratory stimulus and developed oxygen administration devices. (Courtesy of Wellcome Historical Medical Museum, London)

believed oxygen secretion was occurring. August Krogh and Joseph Barcroft (1872–1947) thought oxygen diffusion alone was responsible. Legendary contributions to respiratory physiology were provided by John Gillies Priestly (1880–1941), Yandell Henderson (1873–1944), J. S. Haldane, and Barcroft. The latter two are noted for their high altitude experiments (on themselves) that proved pulmonary alveolocapillary oxygen transfer involves only the simple process of diffusion.

Lawrence J. Henderson (1878–1942; Fig. 1-16) calculated the oxygen dissociation constants for oxygenated and reduced hemoglobin. He also applied the law of mass action to the $CO_2/[HCO_3^-]$ system. In 1917, Hasselbach introduced the logarithmic version, interrelating blood pH, carbon dioxide tension, and bicarbonate ion concentration. The study of acid–base chemistry became intense in the 1920s and 1930s. Wallace O. Fenn (1893–1917) contributed primary research in understanding the mechanics of breathing. He and Herman Rahn developed a diagram for displaying alveolar gas information.[2–5]

Cardiac physiology was also evolving; the electrocardiogram was clinically performed in 1913. In that same year, American endoscopist Chevalier Jackson of Pittsburgh published his instructional work on direct laryngoscopy for the anesthetist and surgeon.

World War I provided yet another horrific lesson for surgeons and internists. Tetanus antitoxin decreased the incidence of that disease in soldiers during the war. From 1918 to 1919 the Spanish Flu infected 5 million Americans and left 500,000 dead. By 1921 the cause of diabetes had been elucidated and insulin therapy begun.

In 1928 Werner Forssmann performed the first central venous catheterization on himself. Mayo Clinic chemist Edward Kendall isolated steroid hormones allowing treatment of Addison's disease and rheumatoid disorders. German chemist Gerhard Domagk discovered antimicrobial properties of an industrial dye that was converted to sulfanilamide in the body.

The synthesis of other sulfa drugs began the antibiotic era. British physician Alexander Fleming rediscovered the antibiotic effect of Penicillium mold on staphylococcal bacteria. American physician Selman Waksman isolated the antituberculosis agent streptomycin in 1944. Antimicrobial science and chemical-warfare work was transferred to antitumor application in 1942 with use of nitrogen mustard at Yale University.

Following World War II, medicine enjoyed exponential growth in basic research, clinical medicine, and technology. Table 1-1 lists major events and contributors. Contemporary issues echo familiar themes. Instead of the Black Plague, the AIDS virus and drug-resistant strains of *Mycobacterium tuberculosis* are infectious concerns as medicine approaches the next millennium. Polio and other curable/preventable infections continue to be concerns for third-world countries. War and defense budgets continue to distract nations from preventing hunger and providing health. Ethical issues are made more difficult with the rising cost of providing health care and involvement by national government.

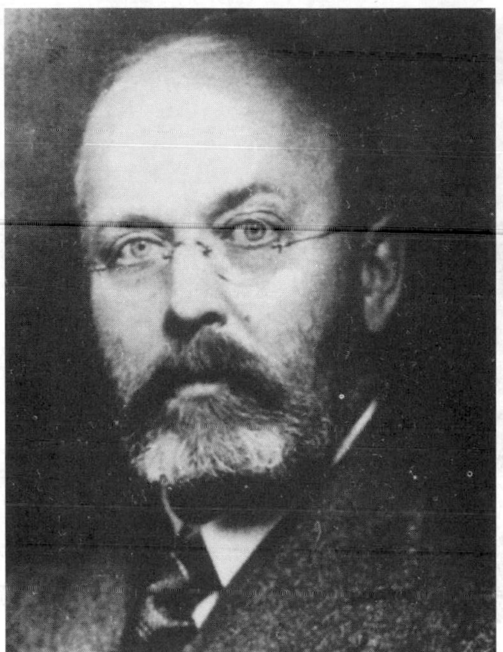

FIGURE 1-16. Lawrence J. Henderson described the interrelationships among carbon dioxide, bicarbonate ion, and pH. (Courtesy of the New York Academy of Medicine, New York)

HISTORICAL EVENTS THAT SIGNALED THE EVOLUTION OF RESPIRATORY CARE

Medical gas therapy (primarily oxygen), and mechanical ventilation including intermittent positive pressure ventilation (IPPV) were the initial specialized services that heralded the development of the multifaceted departments of respiratory care.

Clinical Oxygen Therapy

In 1798, Thomas Beddoes established the Pneumatic Institute in Bristol, England, applying oxygen discovered by Priestly. There he began the use of oxygen to treat heart disease, asthma, and opium poisoning. Beddoes is generally regarded as the father of inhalation therapy. However, he used supplemental oxygen as a panacea for medical problems. Oxygen tents were applied clinically by 1910 (Fig. 1-17). Although it was not until 1920 that a firm physiologic basis for oxygen therapy was established, oxygen orderlies were used to set up equipment and monitor patients.[6–8]

Scientific studies of John Scott Haldane and Joseph Barcroft on oxygen deficiency in humans defined the

TABLE 1-1 **Major Contributions to Modern Medicine Since World War II**

Year	
1945	Inhospital oxygen mask (eg, B-L-B, & Meter) replaces oxygen tent with provision of air condition
	Drs Helen Taussig & Alfred Blalock develop surgical procedure to correct cyanotic congenital heart lesions, eg, Tetralogy of Fallot
1948	Björk develops "disk" extracorporeal oxygenator
1952	58,000 cases of Polio in the United States: Salk and Sabin begin testing vaccines
	Complex cardiac surgery develops need for ICU postoperative care
	Albert Schweitzer wins Nobel Peace Prize
1953	Mayo-Gibbon "vertical screen" cardiopulmonary bypass device
1955	Polio cases are reduced to 5,000
1956	Forsman, Cournand, and Richards receive Nobel Prize for cardiac catheterization
	Linus Pauling receives Nobel Prize for elucidation of sickle cell hemoglobin and other hemoglobinopathies
1958	Raymond Pearl publishes in *Science* that tobacco smoking reduces life span and is associated with a spectrum of diseases
1960	The hospital ship Hope is commissioned
	ECG monitoring available in beds outside operating/recovery room; predecessor of ICU
1963	Hardy performs first lung transplant
	Startle & Moore perform first liver transplant
1967	Favaloro and D. Johnson popularize coronary artery bypass surgery
	Combined pH-Clark-Severinghaus electrodes makes blood gas analysis available
1968	Fiberoptic bronchoscope enters clinical practice
	Bernard performs first successful human heart transplant
	Kantrowitz introduces intra-aortic balloon pumping
1969	ARDS reported by Petty, Ashblaugh, and Bigelow; PEEP therapy recommended; first "test-tube" in vitro fertilization in Great Britain
1970	Pulmonary artery flow-directed catheter developed by Swan & Ganz
	Etiology of "Hyaline Membrane disease" related to inadequate pulmonary surfactant
1971	CPAP described by Gregory
1972	CAT scanner a clinical reality; developed by Houndsfield & Cormack
	High frequency oscillation (HFO) ventilation developed by Lunkenheimer
1973	IMV described by Kirby & Downes
1977	Coronary artery angioplasty developed by Gruentzig
1979	CDC notes first reports of AIDS
	BiPAP® introduced by Respironics
	NIH ECMO trial for ARDS published
1980	Damadian builds first MRI
1982	DeVries implants first Jarvik 7 artificial heart
1983	FDA approves cyclosporin; facilitates organ transplantation surgery
1984	HIV identified by Montagier & Gallo
1989	Identification of the cystic fibrosis conductance regulator gene (CFTR)
1993	FDA approves surfactant replacement

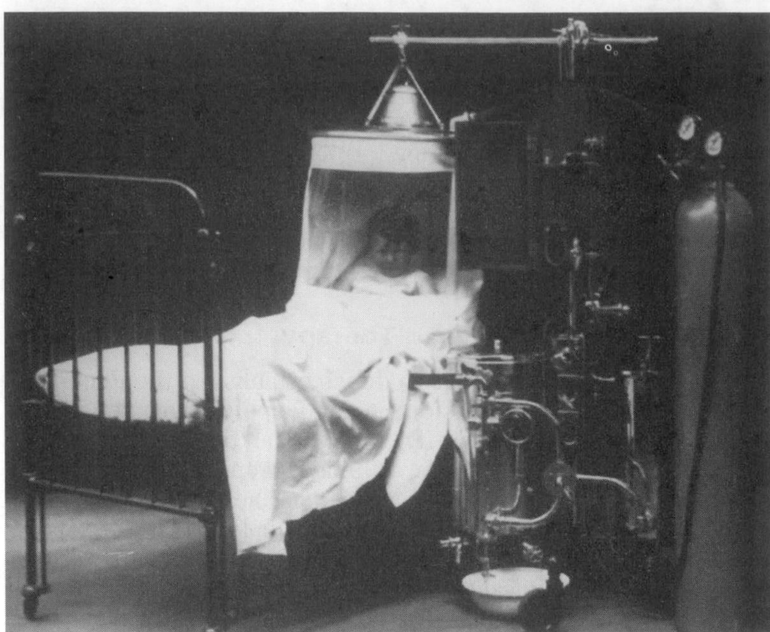

FIGURE 1-17. Oxygen tent, circa 1910; Hospital for Sick Children, Toronto. (From Smolan R, Moffitt P: Medicine's Great Journey: One Hundred Years of Healing. Boston, Little Brown & Co., 1992, with permission)

benefits of oxygen therapy. In a pioneering study conducted in 1920, Barcroft remained for 5 days in a chamber filled with 15% oxygen. In describing the symptoms associated with simulated high-altitude breathing he noted nausea, headache, visual disturbances, rapid pulse, and lassitude. Haldane subjected himself to even lower partial pressures of oxygen and became disoriented. He might have died had his assistants not removed him from the chamber.[6–8]

The development of oxygen devices (face masks, metal/rubber catheters, oxygen chambers) fostered the need for knowledgeable personnel to provide administration. As early as 1907, Sir Arbuthnot Lane advocated the administration of oxygen by a nasal catheter. Haldane perfected an oxygen mask in 1918, which was used to treat patients with poison chlorine gas–induced pulmonary edema in World War I.

Oxygen tents came into clinical use (see Fig. 1-17); in 1920 Sir Leonard Hill developed an oxygen tent used to treat leg ulcers. Although this apparatus had no method for the removal of heat or moisture, it led others to further refine and expand on this mode of therapy. In 1926, New York physician Alvan L. Barach (Fig. 1-18) developed his oxygen tent capable of carbon dioxide removal with soda lime, water vapor extraction using calcium chloride, and thermal control maintained by passing oxygen over a chunk ice refrigeration unit.[8,9]

Large oxygen chambers were also developed by Barcroft in England and W. C. Stadie in the United States. Barach went on to design entire rooms in which patients could be treated with oxygen.[7–9]

During this same period, J. S. Haldane developed a method to dilute gases with room air, used in the therapeutic administration of carbon dioxide. Barach expanded on this concept to develop a meter mask for diluting oxygen with room air. He also began using helium and oxygen mixtures and devised a positive-pressure breathing (CPPB or CPAP) mask capable of developing up to 4 cm H_2O on exhalation.[7–9]

In 1938, Walter Boothby, W. Randolf Lovelace, and Arthur Bulbulian devised the BLB mask at the Mayo Clinic. This mask allowed a high oxygen concentration (80%–100%) with minimal rebreathing. It was developed by Ohio Chemical to provide oxygen to pilots while flying at high altitudes in World War II; commercial units were available for hospital use after the war (Fig. 1-19).[7–9]

Dr. Barach in New York, and Drs. Albert Andrews, Edwin Levine, and Max Sadove in Chicago are credited with providing education to those who were assigned to oxygen therapy. The science and technical needs had exceeded what could be done casually at the bedside. In addition, oxygen orderlies had to be educated in pro-

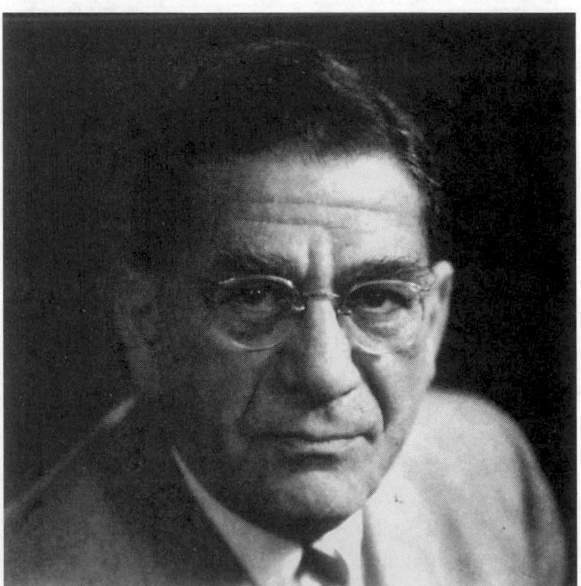

FIGURE 1-18. Alvan Barach. (From Hodgkin JE, Connors GL, Bell CW: Pulmonary Rehabilitation, 2nd ed. Philadelphia: JB Lippincott, 1993, with permission)

fessional patient approach and in recognizing problems associated with oxygen. Physicians and nursing staff needed this 24-hour-per-day support service.

In the late 1940s, the somewhat indiscriminate use of oxygen in premature newborns resulted in a large number of cases of retrolental fibroplasia. There were no clinically efficient ways to quantitate blood oxygen levels in infants or adults.[10] Efforts to provide such technology began with Heinrich Danneel and Walther Nernst, who discovered the electrochemical reduction of oxygen in 1897. Oxygen's polarography was accidentally determined by Jaroslav Heyrovsky in 1922. Leland Clark is credited with constructing a membrane-covered oxygen electrode that was not poisoned by blood in 1954 (Fig 1-20).[7,11]

By the mid-1960s, the Clark and John Severinghaus electrodes allowed clinical blood gas analysis of PaO_2 and $PaCO_2$, respectively. Blood gas analysis was incorporated into departments of inhalation therapy, often an extension of the operating room or pulmonary function laboratory. Blood collection and interpretation skills were added to the respiratory therapists' required abilities. Formal education and credentialing was now in place. The noninvasive ear oximeter using photoximetric principles was initiated by G.A. Millikan in 1942 and clinically available by 1974.

During the late 1970s and early 1980s the Clark and Severinghaus electrodes were adapted for transcutaneous clinical application. Pulse oximetry was discovered by accident by Taku Aoyagi while trying to measure dye indicator cardiac output with an ear probe (Fig 1-21). Since his 1974 abstract, that device has been adopted as a standard for clinical measurement in the operating room, intensive care unit, and hospital floors.[12] The mass spectrometer became a clinical and diagnostic tool for the operating room and pulmonary function laboratory by the 1960s.

To titrate oxygen concentration to physical signs and blood levels, E. J. Moran Campbell developed the Venti-mask in 1960, to provide a high-flow, controlled FIO_2 appliance. This device had the ability to meet tachypneic patients' inspiratory flow demands while reducing the risk of carbon dioxide retention.

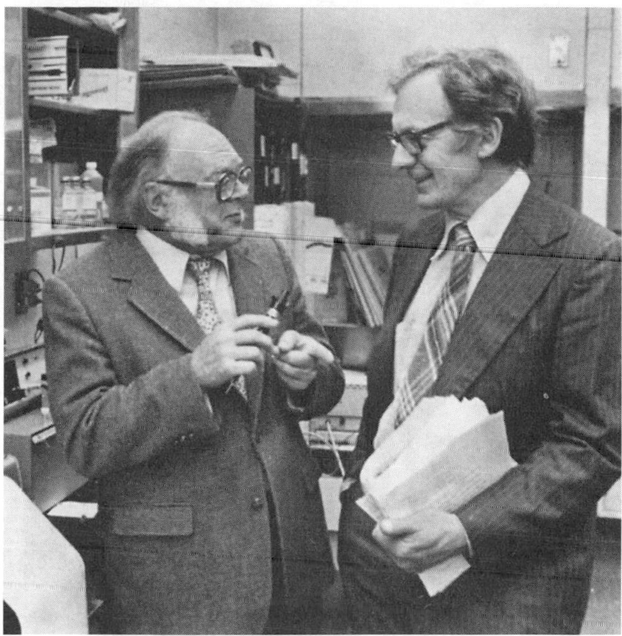

FIGURE 1-20. Leland Clark (*left*) and John Severinghaus (*right*), developers of the oxygen and carbon dioxide blood electrodes. (From Severinghaus JW, Astrup PB: History of Blood Gas Analysis: IV. Leland Clark's Oxygen Electrode. J Clin Monit 1986; 2:125, with permission)

Reliable air–oxygen blenders were developed in the mid 1970s permitting precise FIO_2 for nurseries and intensive care units at a range of flows. Oxygen therapy had evolved from one of merely delivery and set up, to educated practitioners that could evaluate patients needs, recommend care and evaluate its effects. Clinical practice guidelines and therapist-driven protocols define the science and its application.[13,14] Respiratory care practitioners' services included emergency room, delivery and newborn nursery, and intensive care unit. Hyperbaric oxygen is increasingly available and commonly the responsibility of the respiratory care department.

During the 1970s long-term oxygen therapy was shown to reduce mortality in patients requiring supplemental oxygen.[15] Development of oxygen concentrators

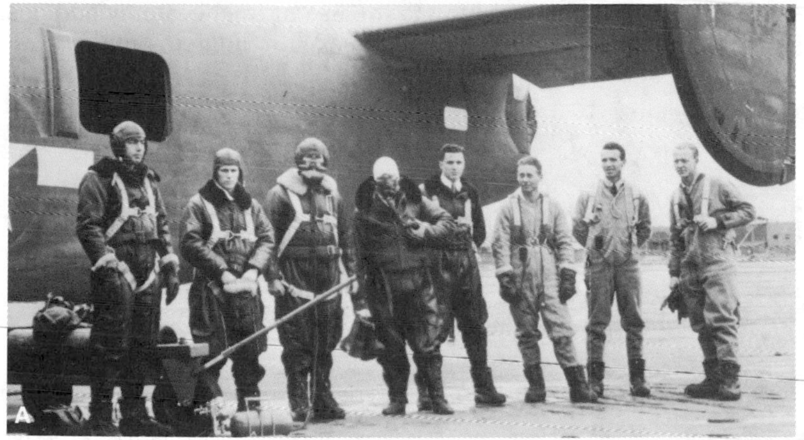

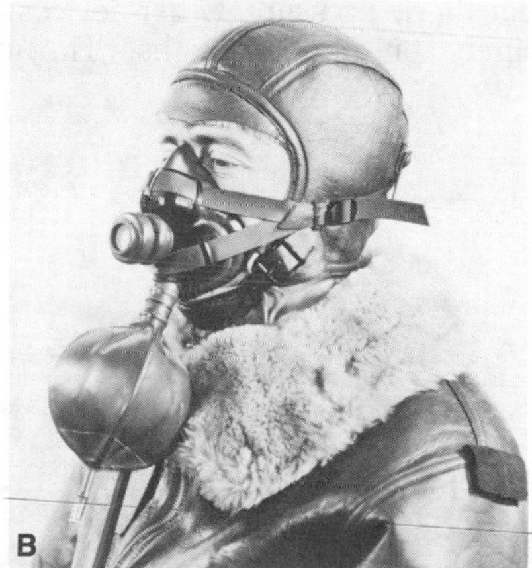

FIGURE 1-19. **(A)** Researchers wearing BLB oxygen masks developed for aviation application during World War II. **(B)** Aviator wearing BLB mask. (Courtesy H. F. Helmholz, Jr., MD)

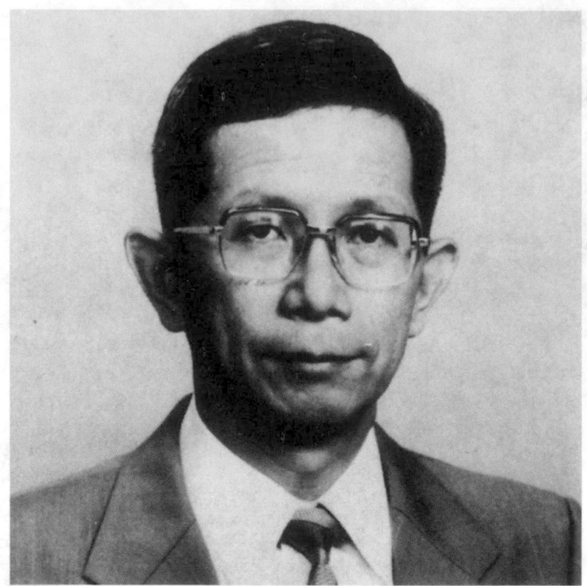

FIGURE 1-21. Taku Aoyagi, inventor of the pulse oximeter. (From Severinghaus JW, Honda, Y: History of Blood Gas Analysis: VII. Pulse Oximetry. J Clin Monit 1987, 3:1410, with permission)

and portable liquid oxygen systems has freed patients and caregivers from awkward cylinders. Conserving devices such as reservoirs, demand pulse units, and tracheal catheters were developed in the 1980s to attempt to save costs in long-term oxygen therapy. Respiratory care practitioners now have expanded their care to extended (subacute) care, nursing homes, and patient homes. In the United States during 1993, approximately 616,000 patients used home oxygen.[16]

Clinical Use of Mechanical Ventilation

A complete historical review of mechanical ventilators is beyond the scope of this introductory chapter. The reader is referred to other sources for a definitive presentation.[17–19] Mechanical-ventilating devices that were more involved than a "fireplace bellows" began appearing in the mid-1800s. Most early devices, such as Woillez's 1876 Spirophore (Fig. 1-22), used a body-enclosing iron lung with a large bellows to create subatmospheric pressure. Other devices resembled steam cabinets or phone booths. The negative-pressure scheme was considered physiologic, and tracheal intubation was not attempted until the 1890s. Surgeons were eager to use their advancing techniques on the chest but were aware of the problems of pneumothorax. To deal with this perioperative problem, some considered positive-pressure ventilation. To accomplish this, an artificial airway was required. By 1900 flexible metallic tubes were available, and Meltzer introduced oral intubation in 1909.

However, in 1904, the German surgeon Ernst Sauerbruch developed a negative-pressure operating chamber (Fig. 1-23). This differential (positive–negative) pressure method caught on and continued to be popular in Europe. In contrast, most American surgeons and anesthetists turned to endotracheal intubation and direct introduction of air into the lungs. By 1913, Chevalier Jackson had developed the laryngoscope and intratracheal catheters in Pittsburgh. However, positive-pressure ventilation by mask continued until the mystique enshrouding intubation technique lessened. This occurred largely because of the work of Ivan Magill and coworkers during World War I.[17–19]

Many positive-pressure devices were developed for surgery or resuscitation. The 1888 Fell-O'Dwyer apparatus combined a laryngeal tube and foot-operated bellows (Fig. 1-24). In 1907 Heinrich Drager developed his Pulmotor in Germany, and in 1910 American Henry Janeway constructed his anesthesia machine.

One of the first poliomyelitis epidemics was in New York, in 1916. By 1928, Philip Drinker, Charles McKhann, and Louis Shaw developed the first iron lung at Harvard, and it was widely used. In 1932 John H. Emerson constructed his iron lung, which improved access to the patient and had a transparent dome to provide positive-pressure ventilation while the tank was opened (Fig. 1-25A). The poliomyelitis epidemic surfaced in England about 1938, and there was an inadequate supply of iron lungs. Epidemics flared in Scandinavia, Europe, and America into the 1950s affecting both adults and children (Fig. 1-25B). This "catastrophic" demand for mechanical ventilation, as well as the increasing need for anesthesia ventilators, prompted a surge of international development. Manufacturers looked to the poliomyelitis centers to guide improved designs.[17–19]

During the catastrophic 1952 poliomyelitis epidemic in Copenhagen, Dr. Bjørn Ibsen effected a change from the iron lung to the use of tracheostomy and positive pressure ventilators. With limited numbers of ma-

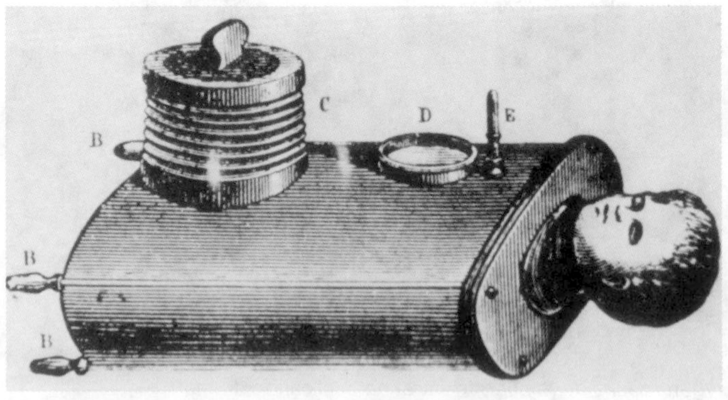

FIGURE 1-22. Woillez's Spirophore negative-pressure ventilator circa 1876. (Mushin WW, Rendell-Baker L, Thompson PW, Mapleson WW: Automatic Ventilation of the Lungs, 3rd ed. London, Blackwell Scientific, 1980, with permission)

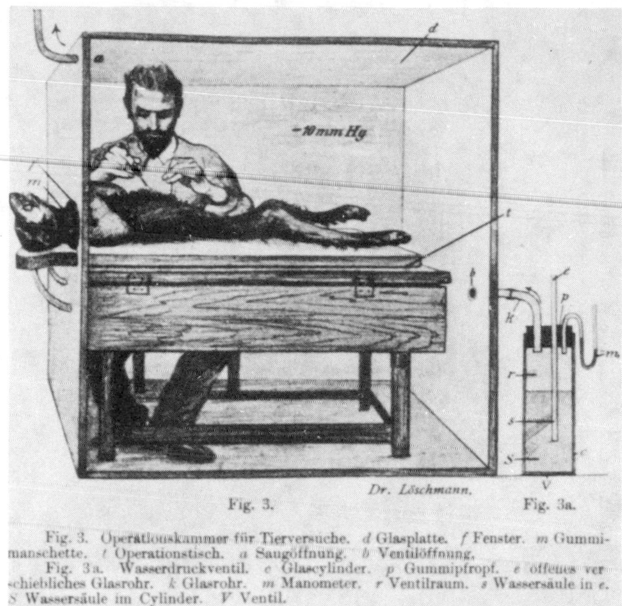

FIGURE 1-23. Ernest Ferdinand Sauerbruch developed a differential-pressure chamber for surgical application, circa 1904. (Mörch ET: History of Mechanical Ventilation In Kirby RR, Banner MJ, Downs JB [eds]: Clinical Application of Ventilatory Support. New York, Churchill Livingstone, 1990, with permission)

chines, vast numbers of medical students (1400) provided manual ventilation. The Ambu-bag (adult manual breathing unit) was developed by Henning Ruben in 1954. The Scandinavians produced positive-pressure devices, such as the Aga Pulmospirator, Engstrom, and Mörch (Fig. 1-26). Mörch's prototype was constructed using a cylinder made from a sewer pipe in German-occupied Copenhagen. British anesthesiologists produced the Beaver, Blease Pulmoflator, and Barnet. In Germany, the Drager Company developed the Poliomat. This international experience with long-term positive-pressure ventilation led to its application during thoracic and cardiac surgery, as well as postoperatively. Swedish surgeons Bjork and Engstrom led the way in addition to British physicians Macintosh and Mushin.

Although Europeans largely abandoned the iron lung, poliomyelitis patients continued to be treated with tank respirators in the United States into the mid-1950s. The National Foundation for Infantile Paralysis was the major force in the effort to eradicate poliomyelitis. As the epidemic of this disease eased in the United States with the introduction of the Salk and, later, Sabin vaccines, the former poliomyelitis facilities' expertise evolved into centers for development of intensive care. The United States then followed the Scandinavians and British in postoperative controlled ventilation. During this time, V. Ray Bennett introduced the TV-2P "assister" in 1948 (Fig. 1-27), and Forrest Bird developed his "clinical magnetic respirator" in 1951 (Fig. 1-28). By the mid-1950s E. Trier Mörch's piston ventilator became clinically available in the United States. First-generation pressure-limited ventilators, such as the Bird Mark 7 and Bennett PR-1, were in large-scale production by 1958 and 1961, respectively. Jack Emerson took the lead with his volume/time-limited Post-Op or 3-PV ventilator in 1964 (Fig. 1-29). Dr. Thomas Petty and colleagues applied Alvan Barach's threshold constant positive pressure breathing (CPPB) for use with ventilators. They termed it positive end-expiratory pressure (PEEP) in 1967 and supported its therapeutic use in the adult respiratory distress syndrome (ARDS).[20]

Over the next 10 years the second-generation volume ventilators followed with the Puritan-Bennett MA-1, Ohio 560, Bourns Bear I, and Siemens 900B. These ventilators became workhorses in growing numbers of intensive care units in the United States. The demand for specialists properly trained in ventilator management paralleled the exponential growth of the respiratory care profession in the 1970s. Table 1-2 lists the chronologic development of modern critical care ventilators.

Breathing modes, adjuncts, and methods of controlling ventilator function have also evolved. Early equipment was operated with pneumatic or basic mechanical switches. Control functions were updated by fluidics, and the transistor was updated with printed circuit boards in the 1970s. Currently, the microprocessor is today's technology for third-generation ventilators. The variety of monitoring and breathing modes has ex-

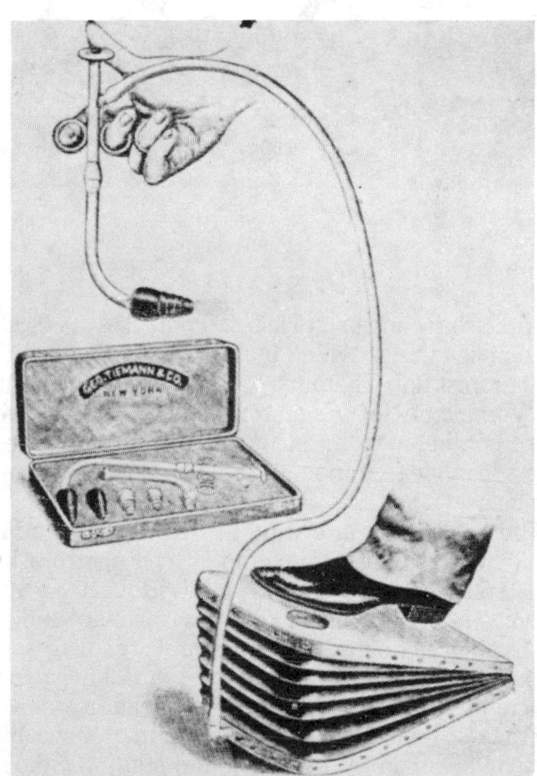

FIGURE 1-24. Fell-O'Dwyer bellows and endotracheal intubating device, circa 1899. (Mörch ET. History of mechanical ventilation. In Kirby RR, Banner MJ, Downs JB [eds]: Clinical Applications of Ventilatory Support. New York, Churchill Livingstone, 1985, with permission)

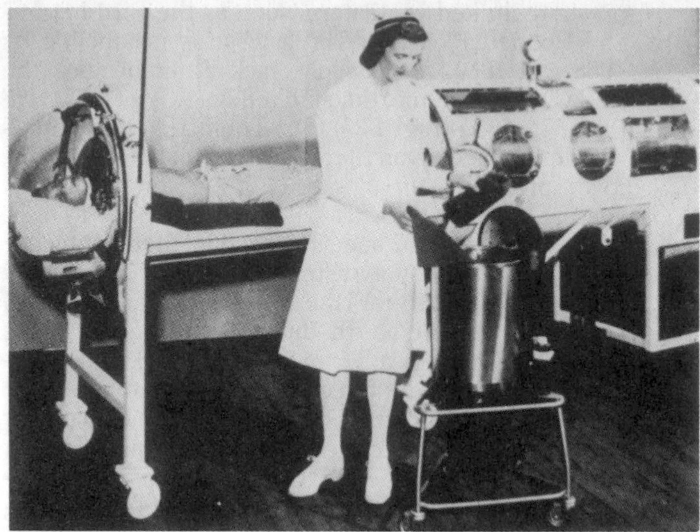

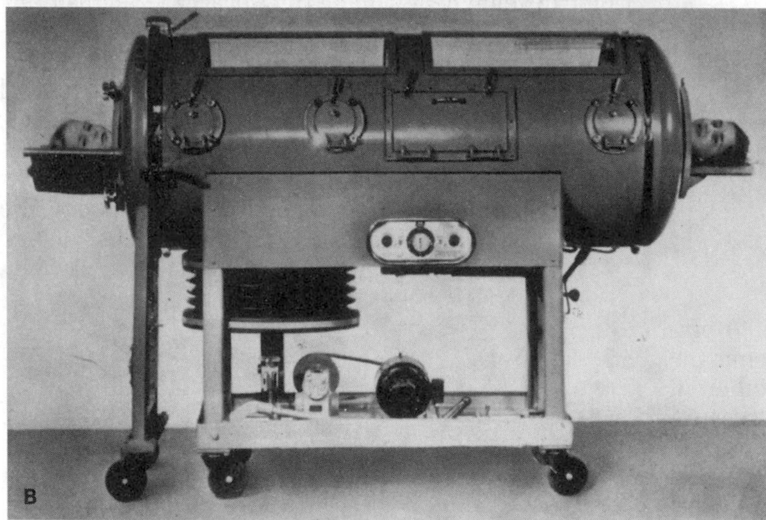

FIGURE 1-25. A, Emerson iron lung with head canopy for ventilation when the body chamber was opened. (Courtesy J. H. Emerson, Cambridge, MA.) **B,** Drinker-Collins tank respirator for treatment of two children. (From Barach AL: Principles and Practices of Inhalational Therapy. Philadelphia, J. B. Lippincott, 1944, with permission)

panded from control and assist/control. A 1960s classification scheme provided by Mushin has been updated by therapist Rob Chatburn to better distinguish the rising complexity of ventilator technology.[21] However, there continues to be inconsistency among manufacturers in mode terminology and their application among clinicians.

The concept of intermittent mandatory ventilation (IMV) was originally developed by Engstrom in the mid-1950s. However, in 1971 Dr. Robert Kirby and coworkers reintroduced this as a primary mode for ventilating neonates with respiratory distress syndrome secondary to prematurity.[22] Dr. John Downs and colleagues followed with the application of IMV in adults as a method to facilitate ventilator weaning.[23] Clinicians began to recognize and study the difficulty patients had signaling IMV demand valve systems and overcoming artificial airway resistance. This fostered the development of pressure support ventilation (PSV) in the mid 1980s. Dr. John Marini and colleagues began objective analysis of patient work of breathing on ventilators.[24]

Other primary modes of adult ventilation have been introduced in the 1980s and 1990s. Pressure controlled ventilation (PCV) has been recommended to limit effects of barotrauma on airways and alveolar tissue, which often occurs in the care of patients with stiff lungs.[25] Other recent interventions to limit pressure damage include airway pressure-release ventilation (APRV), independent lung ventilation (ILV), continuous flow ventilation, and enforced carbon-dioxide retention (permissive hypercapnia). The latter mode has been recommended for use with severe airways obstruction in addition to ARDS.[26]

Inverse (I:E) ratio ventilation (IRV) was originally proposed by E.O.R. Reynolds in 1971 as a method to improve oxygenation in neonates with respiratory distress syndrome. Its application has been extended to adults with ARDS, as a PEEP-like variant to improve oxygenation with limited pressures.[27] Proportional-assist venti-

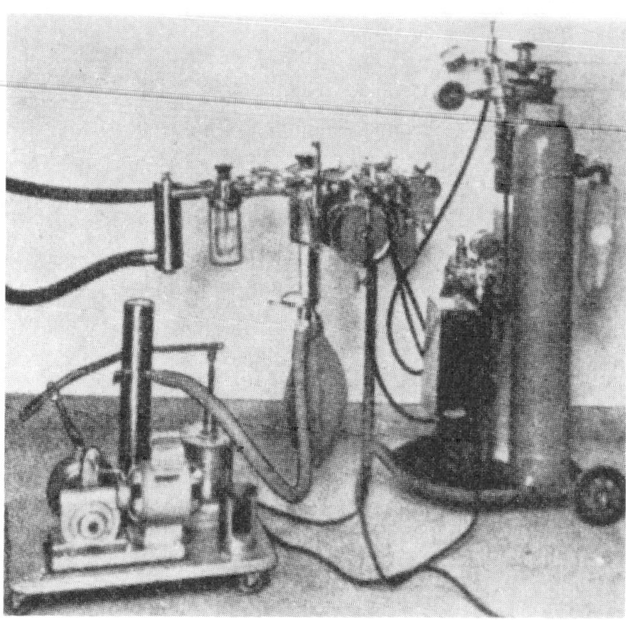

FIGURE 1-26. First piston ventilator designed by Ernst Trier Mörch in 1940. (Mörch ET: History of mechanical ventilation. In Kirby RR, Banner MJ, Downs JB [eds]: Clinical Applications of Ventilatory Support. New York, Churchill Livingstone, 1990, with permission)

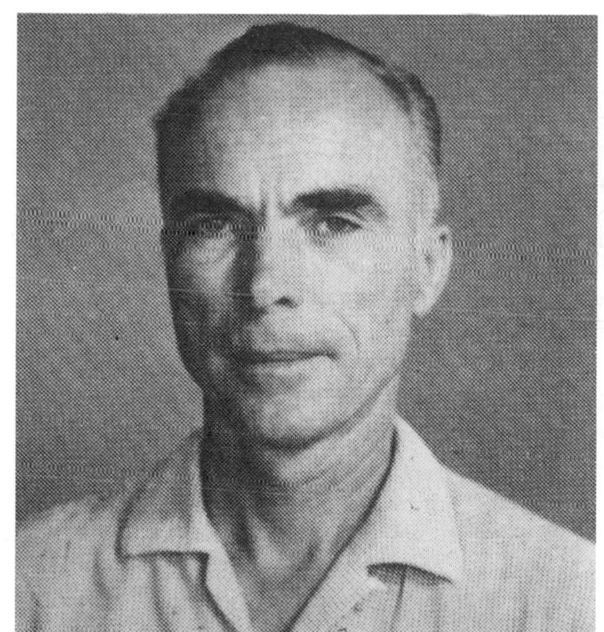

FIGURE 1-27. V. Ray Bennett, developer of the Bennett flow-sensitive valve. (From Mushin WW, Rendell-Baker L, Thompson PW, Mapleson WW: Automatic Ventilation of the Lungs, 3rd ed. London, Blackwell Scientific Publishers, 1980, with permission)

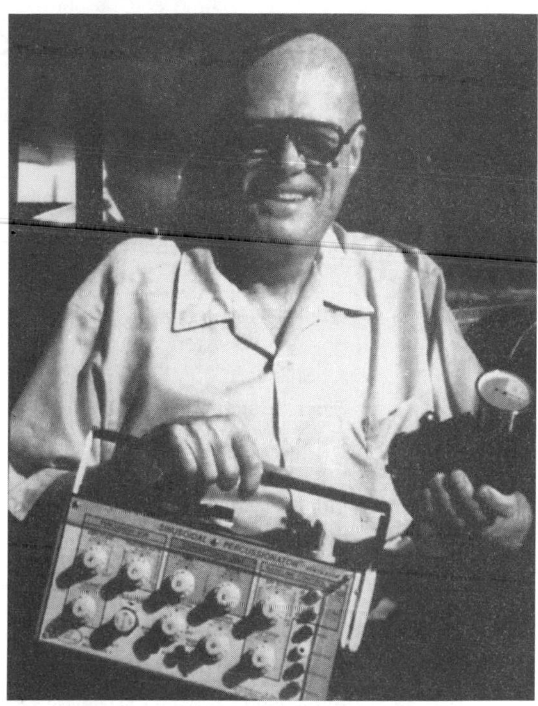

FIGURE 1-28. Forrest Bird, inventor of Bird ventilators. (From Branson RD: Pioneers in Respiratory Care. AARC Times 1990; 14:51, with permission)

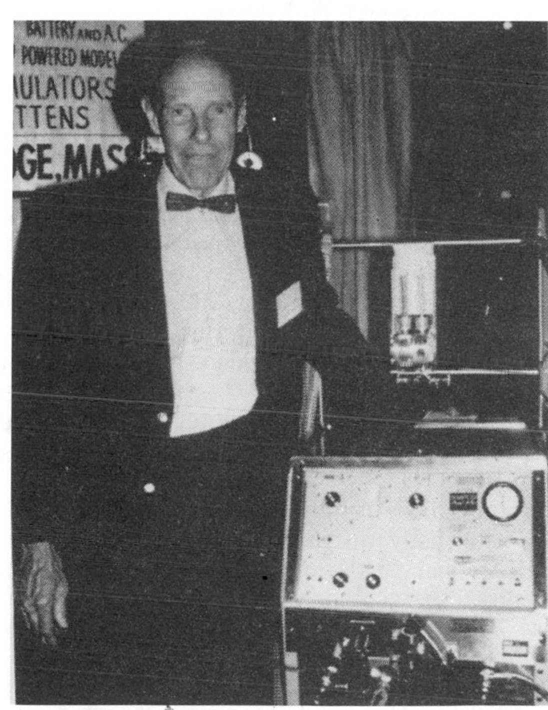

FIGURE 1-29. Jack Emerson, inventor of the Emerson Post-Op and other health-care devices. (From Mushin WW, Rendell-Baker L, Thompson PW, Mapleson WW: Automatic Ventilation of the Lungs, 3rd ed. London, Blackwell Scientific Publishers, 1980, with permission)

TABLE 1-2 **Chronology of Mechanical Ventilator Development**

Year Introduced	Brand/Model	Year Introduced	Brand/Model
1948	Bennett TV-2P	1975	Bourns Bear I
1950	Engstrom 150	1976	Forreger 210
1954	Drager Poliomat	1978	Puritan-Bennett MA-2; MA-2+2
	Thompson Portable Respiratory	1980	Engstrom Erica
1955	Mörch "piston" ventilator		Respironics BiPAP
	Bird Mark 7	1982	Siemens 900C
	Emerson High-Frequency Ventilator		Bear Medical Bear II
1958	Emerson Assistor/Controller	1983	Biomed IC-5
1963	Air-Shields 1000	1984	Puritan-Bennett 7200
	Puritan-Bennett PR-2		Sechrist Adult 2200B
1964	Emerson "Post-Op" 3-PV	1985	Bear Medical Bear 5
	Bourns LS-104-150		Ohmeda CPU
1967	Puritan-Bennett MA-1	1986	Hamilton Veolar
1968	Ohio/Monaghan 560		Bird 6400 ST
	Drager Spiromet		Infrasonics Infant Star
	Engstrom 300	1988	Bear Medical Bear 3
1970	Veriflow CV 2000		Hamilton Amadeus
	Hamilton Standard PAD-1		Bird 8400 ST
1972	Monaghan 225, 225 SIMV		Respironics BiPAP
	Bird-Baby Bird	1989	Bunnell Life Pulse
	Bird-IMV Bird		PPG IRISA/(Drager Evita)
	Siemens 900/900B		Bird VIP
1973	Chemtron Gill 1		Infrasonics Adult Star
1974	Emerson IMV	1991	Siemens Servo 300
	Searle VVA	1993	Bear 1000
	Ohio 550		

lation (PAV) appears to be a promising future mode in which the ventilator generates pressure in proportion to patient effort.[28] A variety of styles of high-frequency ventilation using jets and oscillators have been attempted for both adult and infant disorders in the continuing attempt to ventilate stiff lungs without causing damage. The neonatal applications have proven more successful than adult application.[29] In late 1989, Respironics introduced its bilevel positive airway pressure (BiPAP) device as a noninvasive alternative to standard ventilation, using a nasal mask.

Ventilating patients with dilute concentrations of nitric oxide has shown much promise in assisting gas exchange in severely hypoxemic adults and neonates.[30]

Carbon dioxide removal and oxygenation of blood outside the body (extracorporeal) were first used in the 1930s and 1940s for intraoperative applications. Currently, extracorporeal membrane oxygenation (ECMO), intravascular oxygenation (IVOX), and extracorporeal carbon dioxide removal ($ECCO_2$) have either research or limited roles in respiratory care. Use of fluorocarbon liquid to facilitate respiration has been undergoing research for some time. Limited human trials with premature newborns have shown considerable promise in providing gas exchange without barotrauma.[31]

The use of ventilators for long-term nonhospital (ie, home) use has significant increased since Thompson introduced their portable wheelchair unit in 1954.[32] In recent years, there has been a proliferation of similar devices with DC battery capabilities. Although the negative-pressure ventilators such as the iron lung are rarely used today in the ICU, cuirass-type chest devices and the pneumobelt are still used for long-term ventilation in certain patients to avoid tracheostomy. Perhaps more impressive has been the acceptance of noninvasive ventilatory support using face or nasal mask with portable ventilators or bilevel positive pressure ventilation (BiPAP).[33]

Development of Scientifically Based Respiratory Care Services

The preceding sections reviewed historical advances of only two facets of respiratory care practice. Medical gas therapy and mechanical ventilation are two examples that have proceeded on a relatively clear scientific basis. The job responsibilities have paralleled the advances of technology and its clinical application; training and education were driven by the work-related demands. The historical record shows this has not always been the case.

IPPB therapy is an example of clinical practice that proceeded without adequate documentation of efficacy. During the 1940s, World War II aviation research found that IPPB was less effective than CPPB in increasing pilots altitude tolerance. However, the new technology was applied to treat postoperative hypoventilation, acute asthma, pulmonary edema, and apneic patients by Barach and Motley.[20,34] The Bennett valve IPPB device was also adapted as a positive pressure attachment for the iron lung for polio patient ventilation. During the late 1960s and early 1970s, IPPB turned into a "vast enterprise" as pressure breathing was indiscriminately ordered to deliver bronchodilators, or to treat or provide prophylaxis for postoperative pulmonary complications. A large work effort by respiratory care departments focused on providing IPPB. Patients received therapy without documenting its need or positive benefit. This was despite research literature that identified limitations of this therapy.[35] The practice of IPPB was reviewed at the first Conference on Scientific-Basis for Respiratory Therapy, sponsored by the American Thoracic Society in 1974.[36] Subsequent research has identified appropriate criteria for applying IPPB and methods to assess its benefit.[37–39]

This unfortunate experience confirmed that respiratory care must be founded in science. Furthermore, its practitioners must be diligent in performing only justified care, with appropriate (identified) outcomes and levels of care. Carrying out that approach requires both good information, plus a cooperative, organized, and thoughtful approach. The professional evolution requires that respiratory care practitioners and physicians cooperate in a process of defining care and in its ongoing clinical research. Respiratory care involves care of the critically ill; this mandates a collegial relationship with physicians as medical directors of departments or care of individuals.[40]

During the 1970s the AARC studied and established national roles and delineation of respiratory care. To support evolution of more credible, appropriate, and higher levels of clinical practice in the 1990s, the AARC initiated the formation of **clinical practice guidelines (CPGs).** This was a significant and sustained effort. Effective guidelines, developed with a practical and applicable approach, are reasonable. Continued research should allow additional services to evolve through continued update. Primary goals and likely results of the CPG process are identified in Box 1-1.

The guidelines are outcome oriented; Box 1-2 identifies the standard format for all CPGs.

BOX 1-1

CLINICAL PRACTICE GUIDELINES

- Identify "standards of care"
- Define and justify clinical practice
- Identify appropriateness of care
- Guide education of providers
- Identify future research needs
- Summarize medical literature
- Record current technology details
- Have a source of "clinical indicators" to evaluate/monitor quality of care

BOX 1-2

TYPICAL CLINICAL PRACTICE GUIDELINE ORGANIZATION

- Description/definition
- Setting
- Indications
- Contraindications
- Hazards/complications
- Device limitations/validation of results
- Assessment of need
- Assessment of outcome
- Resources: equipment & personnel
- Monitoring
- Frequency
- Infection control

Approximately 30 guidelines have been prepared to provide up-to-date national consensus on services provided by respiratory practitioners. Box 1-3 identifies currently published CPGs for diagnostic and monitoring techniques and therapies. Additional guidelines continue to be developed and published.

BOX 1-3

PUBLISHED AARC CLINICAL PRACTICE GUIDELINES

Monitoring and Diagnostic

- Pulse oximetry
- Spirometry
- Static lung volumes
- Bronchial provocation testing
- Single-breath carbon monoxide diffusing capacity
- Sampling for arterial blood gas analysis
- In vitro pH and blood gas analysis and hemoximetry
- Exercise testing for evaluation of hypoxemia and/or desaturation

Therapeutic and Life Support

- Oxygen therapy in the acute hospital
- Oxygen therapy in the home or extended care facility
- Resuscitation in the acute care hospital
- Incentive spirometry
- Directed cough
- Nasotracheal suctioning
- Endotracheal suctioning of mechanically ventilated adults and children with artificial airways
- Fiberoptic bronchoscopy assisting
- Postural drainage therapy
- Use of positive airway pressure adjuncts to bronchial hygiene therapy
- Intermittent positive pressure breathing
- Humidification during mechanical ventilation
- Patient-ventilator system check
- Ventilator circuit change
- Tranpsort of mechanically ventilated patients
- Delivery of aerosols to the upper airway
- Selection of aerosol delivery device
- Surfactant replacement therapy
- Application of continuous positive airway pressure to neonates via nasal prongs or nasopharyngeal tube

CONTEMPORARY RESPIRATORY CARE SERVICES

Although the first inhalation therapy departments only assisted with setting up oxygen tents and iron lungs, respiratory care practitioners' acceptance of new opportunities has fostered continued evolution of responsibilities. Diagnostic laboratories (blood gas and pulmonary function) increased in sophistication during the 1970s and 1980s. Therapeutic services became more complete in the areas of airway and ventilator management, bronchial hygiene, and aerosol therapy. During the late 1980s and 1990s, many hospitals increased the scope of services in areas outside the traditional range of inpatient and outpatient respiratory care services.

Appropriate respiratory care delivery is more frequently being guided by **therapist-driven protocols (TDPs).** Therapy and physician staff negotiate algorithm-like decision plans to base therapy on assessment of immediate and continuing needs. Respiratory care departments that provide a wider scope of services in cardiopulmonary care have evolved as a result of increased technology and administrative techniques to conserve both technical and human resources. The direction and pace of diversification varies depending on patient demand, nature of the personnel, and institutional resources. Access to well-educated practitioners, active medical direction, administrative support, and entrepreneurial spirit within the hospital management are all variables in this evolution. Practitioners often possess a mix of educational background and credentialing. The advantage of a multiskilled/credentialed department is most apparent outside the major medical center. At the latter, many of these services are performed by the specific allied health subspecialties. There are several allied health professional organizations who support those providing cardiopulmonary diagnosis, monitoring, and therapeutics in addition to the AARC. Box 1-4 identifies these services and related specialty professional and credentialing organizations.

BOX 1-4

CARDIOPULMONARY CARE SERVICES PROFESSIONAL (◆) & CREDENTIALING ORGANIZATIONS (*)

Monitoring & Diagnostic

- Sleep disorders/polysomnographic monitoring including electroencephalography and electromyography
  - ◆ Association of Polysomnographic Technologists (APT)
  - * Board of Registered Polysomnographic Technologists (BRPT)
  - ◆ American Society of Electroneurodiagnostic Technologists (ASET)
  - ◆ American Association of Electrodiagnostic Technologists
  - * American Board of Registration of Electroencephalographic & Evoked Potential Technologists (ABRET)
- Electrocardiographic services
  - -12-lead ECG
  - -Holter studies
  - -Exercise ECG testing
- Bedside hemodynamic monitoring
  - -Assist insertion of central catheters
  - -Provide ongoing monitoring of central venous, arterial, and pulmonary circulations
  - -Place arterial catheters
- Invasive cardiovascular laboratory services
  - -Cardiac catheterization & electrophysiology
- Noninvasive cardiovascular laboratory
  - -Echocardiography, exercise stress testing
- Noninvasive peripheral vascular studies laboratory
  - -Doppler ultrasonography, thermography, & plethysmography
  - ◆ National Society for Cardiovascular and Pulmonary Technology (NSCPT)
  - ◆ National Alliance of Cardiovascular Technologists (NACT)
  - * Cardiovascular Credentialing International/National Board for Cardiovascular Technology (CCI/NBCVT)
  - ◆ Society of Diagnostic Medical Sonography
  - * American Registry of Diagnostic Medical Sonography (ARDMS)
  - ◆ Society of Noninvasive Vascular Technology (SNIVT)
- Perfusion technology
  - -Intraaortic balloon-pump management
  - -Extracorporeal membrane oxygenation (ECMO)
  - ◆ American Society of Extracorporeal Technology (AmSECT)
  - * American Board of Cardiovascular Perfusion (ABCP)
- Metabolic Assessment

Therapeutic and Life Support

- Cardiopulmonary resuscitation at advanced levels
  - *◆ American Heart Association (ACLS, PALS, & NALS)
  - ◆ National Association of Emergency Medical Technology
  - * National Registry of Emergency Medical Technology
- Hyperbaric oxygenation
  - * National Board of Diving and Hyperbaric Medicine

Education and Other Support Services

- Nicotine dependency clinic/counseling
- Cardiac and pulmonary rehabilitation
  - ◆ American Association for Cardiovascular and Pulmonary Rehabilitation

PROFESSIONAL ORGANIZATIONS

History of the AARC

During the 1940s a group of interested physicians and "oxygen technicians" in the Chicago area began to meet and discuss oxygen therapy, its rationale, and means to improve the care of patients. The physicians, Albert Andrews, Edwin Levine, and Max Sadov, were the prime movers in recognizing the need for a formal organization to promote the education of those involved in the administration of therapeutic gases to patients. Following a meeting at the University of Chicago in 1946, the Inhalational Therapy Association (ITA) was chartered as a nonprofit organization in the State of Illinois on April 15, 1947. There were 59 "charter" members of the new association.

The initial mission of the ITA was based on its members' need for education. From the outset, the theme was to foster a cooperative relationship with physicians and other allied health professions, and to advance the art and science of the work.

In 1948, the name of the association was changed to the Inhalation Therapy Association. Beginning in 1950, the ITA began to publish a quarterly journal titled the *Bulletin*, which was sent without charge to 1500 hospitals in the United States. Throughout that same year the ITA sponsored a series of lectures and educational workshops. In December 1950, 31 certificates were awarded to those who had attended 16 of those workshops and signaled the commitment to education and documenting participation. In 1951, at only 4 years of professional age, the ITA and the American College of Chest Physicians (ACCP) cosponsored a 5-day workshop. This indicated the importance the ACCP placed on the emerging profession and the cooperative relationship between it and other physician groups. The expansion of the membership, now representing 14 states, led to a third name change in 1954, when the ITA officially became the American Association of Inhalation Therapists (AAIT).

During the next 30 years there was an exponential growth in both demand for respiratory therapy services and practitioners. In 1982 the organization again changed its name to the American Association for Respiratory Care (AARC). This name was believed to better reflect the scope of practitioner involvement in diagnostic pulmonary function testing as well as cardiovascular diagnostics.[30] By the mid-1990s the AARC had more than 36,000 members. The AARC is the primary organization; it is both the national and international proponent of the respiratory care profession. The AARC has an approved statement of Code of Ethics for its members.

In 1992 it was estimated that 100,000 practitioners were involved in respiratory care practice. That included 80,000 full-time equivalent positions in hospital respiratory care departments and an additional 20,000 practitioners in educational programs, equipment manufacture, home care, skilled nursing facilities, and other institutions.

Organizational Structure of the AARC

The AARC is governed in corporate-styled structure by an elected group of six officers and a eight-member Board of Directors (BOD). An Election Committee appointed by the President presents a list of officers and BOD candidates for voting by the general membership. A House of Delegates (HOD) is composed of elected representatives from 50 states and Puerto Rico. The House functions in an advisory role making recommendations to the BOD. Another advisory group to the AARC for physician input is the Board of Medical Advisors (BOMA). Physician groups that sponsor members to that board are listed in Box 1-5.

The national office formerly located in Riverside, California, is now in Dallas, Texas. There is an executive director and staff to handle Association business operations. Those include membership, committee support, continuing education and its documentation, a lobbying effort in Washington, DC, and publications. The latter includes the Association's scientific journal *Respiratory Care.*

Much of the AARC work is delegated to a range of committees. Specialty sections identify the specific practitioner interest groups within the AARC. Specific committees and specialty sections are listed in Box 1-6.

The AARC continues with its mission as a source of continuing education for its members. The Continuing Respiratory Care Education (CRCE) system provides standards for approved courses and services for documentation of credits. Many state licensing boards have minimum requirements to maintain licensure. The Association sponsors a national convention in the fall of each year. In addition, each year the AARC sponsors a second major meeting, its Summer Forum which highlights sessions for the management and education section members. The AARC sponsored a series of conferences starting in 1993, as it made an effort to influence formal education standards for the future. Conference proceedings recommended a 2-year/associate's degree as the minimum practice entry level with emphasis towards 4-year training.[41–43]

BOX 1-5

PHYSICIAN GROUPS ON THE AARC BOARD OF MEDICAL ADVISORS

- American Society of Anesthesiologists (ASA)
- American College of Chest Physicians (ACCP)
- American Thoracic Society (ATS)
- Society of Critical Care Medicine (SCCM)
- American Academy of Pediatrics (AAP)
- American College of Allergy and Immunology (ACAI)
- National Association for Medical Directors for Respiratory Care (NAMDRC)

BOX 1-6

AARC COMMITTEES AND SPECIALTY SECTIONS

Standing Committees

- Audit
- Bylaws
- Education
- Health promotion
- Judicial
- Nominating
- RC research council
- Program
- State licensure
- Budget
- Clinical practice guidelines
- Election
- International respiratory care
- Membership & public relations
- Political action
- Position statement review
- RC gerontology
- Task force on professional direction

Specialty Sections

- Diagnostics
- Home care
- Perinatal-pediatrics
- Adult acute respiratory care
- Education
- Management
- Transport

The AARC has increased its political awareness and representation in national matters of health care. The Association continues to monitor legislation that may affect its members, such as antismoking laws, licensure, and medical care reimbursement.

The American Respiratory Care Foundation (ARCF) is a philanthropic organization that provides a wide range of financial support for students, clinicians, and researchers in an effort to enhance growth of the profession through education and research.

The Lambda Beta Society is an independent organization initiated in 1987 as the honor society for the profession of respiratory care. Its role is to recognize excellence in educational accomplishment and to professional contribution and to provide scholarships.

The National Board for Respiratory Care and State Licensure

Credentialing is a generic term that refers to recognition of individuals involved in a specific occupation or profession. The two major forms of credentialing are provided by state licensure and voluntary national certification. Licensing implies permission to practice following some type of demonstration of competency. State legislatures or their medical boards may provide laws that define the right to practice, provide title protection, or require registration/listing of practitioners. At present there are 37 states in the United States with some form of licensure.

In 1960 a separate national voluntary credentialing organization called the American Registry of Inhalation Therapists (ARIT) was incorporated. The purpose was to document practitioners' job knowledge. In 1961, 12 examinees were the first to receive the designation of "registered inhalation therapist."

Because of an unmet demand for registered therapists and large numbers of those not satisfying ARIT admission requirements, many on-the-job trained practitioners continued to work without any credentials. In recognition of the need to examine and certify those with entry-level skills, in 1968 the professional association (AAIT now AARC) established the Technician Certification Board (TCB). The AAIT's decision to established a two-tiered credentialed system (with concomitant educational programs) continues to be controversial to this day. Practitioners who completed that examination were awarded the Certified Inhalation Therapy Technician (CRIT) credential through 1974. Beginning in 1972, the American Association for Respiratory Therapy (ARRT) transferred its credentialing activities to the ARIT to establish a single national credentialing organization for the respiratory care profession. In 1974 the ARIT was reorganized as the National Board for Respiratory Therapy (NBRT), and in 1986 was renamed the National Board for Respiratory Care (NBRC).[44,45] That Board is composed of appointed sponsor members from the respiratory therapy professional organizations, physician groups, and pulmonary function technology. Corporate offices for it and its for profit subsidiary Applied Measurement Professionals are located in Lenexa, KS.

Another finding of the role delineation research of the 1970s, was that there was no real difference in the tasks performed by "technicians" or "therapists" when starting clinical practice. In 1978 it was confirmed by national job analysis that credentialing would best be served by one entry-level examination with a second set of examinations for therapist candidates. Those could be taken 6 months after completing the CRTT examination. The system was put into place in 1983. The soundness of the system is confirmed by the fact that first-time candidates pass rates vary little between CRTT or RRT graduates. The two main credentials are therefore the **registered respiratory therapist (RRT)** and **certified respiratory therapy technician (CRTT)**. Each credential has a determined set of job knowledge/skills that is reviewed on a 5-year basis. The job skills establish a matrix of tasks that determines examination content for each level.[46] The examinations also undergo a validation process as they are evaluated versus clinical practice. This examination is currently being used by most states in their licensure process.

In 1983, the National Board for Cardiopulmonary Technologists (NBCPT) became a sponsor of the NBRC. That Board now provides examinations and credentialing for pulmonary function technologists. Separate job analysis led to test development of **certified pulmonary function technologist (CPFT)** and **registered pulmonary function technologist (RPFT)** examinations. Subsequently another examination has been made available for **perinatal/pediatric specialists**. A credentialing certificate is awarded to those who pass. Currently the NBRC 30-member Board of Trustees is composed of 10 appointees from the AARC, 5 ACCP, 5 ATS, 5 ASA, and 5 NSCPT.

Box 1-7 identifies the numbers of practitioners holding credentials from the NBRC in each category as of

BOX 1-7

NUMBERS OF NBRC CREDENTIALED PRACTIONERS (AS OF JANUARY 1995)

Registered Respiratory Therapists (RRT)	57,100
Certified Respiratory Therapy Technicians (CRTT)	125,152
Certified Pulmonary Function Technologists (CPFT)	8,124
Registered Pulmonary Function Technologists (RPFT)	2,707
Perinatal/Pediatric Specialists	3,375

this writing. The NBRC remains the only nationally recognized voluntary credentialing body in respiratory care. Its Entry-Level Examination is recognized by 37 states in the United States for licensing respiratory care practitioners. Table 1-3 identifies key dates and events in licensing and credentialing.

TABLE 1-3 **Key Events in the Licensure and Credentialing of Respiratory Care Practitioners**

Year	Event
1960	American Registry of Inhalation Therapists (ARIT) incorporated
1961	First group of (12) therapists credentialed
1969	First certification examinations for inhalation therapy technicians given
1974	ARIT and AART's Technician Certification Board merge to form the National Board for Respiratory Therapy (NBRT)
1976	NBRC accredited by National Commission for Certifying Agencies
1977	Last year for OJTs to gain access to NBRT's CRTT examination by the "grandfather clause"
1978	NBRT adopts entry-level concept
	Last year for oral therapist examination
1979	First clinical simulation examinations given
	AART promotes state credentialing
1982	NBRT joins with National Society of Cardiopulmonary Technology for examination/credentialing of pulmonary function
	First state licensure law enacted in California
1983	NBRT becomes NBRC
	Entry level and advanced practitioner examination system put in place
1984	First Certified Pulmonary Function Examination given
1985	California uses NBRC Entry-Level examination for licensure
1986	NBRC & NSCPT agree to transfer registered pulmonary Function Technologist examination
1987	Advanced pulmonary function examination offered
1989	NBRC eliminates 1-year job experience requirement to access RRT examinations
1991	First Perinatal/Pediatrics Specialty Examination
1995	37 states and Puerto Rico have passed licensure laws

History of Respiratory Care Education and School Accreditation

Soon after the formation of the ITA, a formal 16-week course in inhalation therapy was begun in Chicago in 1950. In that same year, Barach and colleagues and the Committee on Public Health Relations of the New York Academy of Medicine formalized minimum standards for training programs.[47] The rapid development and demand for the allied health fields fostered a more organized approach to development of formal training programs and standards for their accreditation. In 1956 an advisory committee of the American Medical Association's Council on Medical Education (AMA's CME) for inhalation therapy was established by the major groups of interested physicians. By 1963, a Board of Schools was established with four physicians and three therapists. That Board was charged with the tasks of reviewing applications and making site-visits to schools desiring formal accreditation. In 1967 the AMA revised guidelines and required a minimum program length of 18 months; schools were largely hospital-based. Because of resistance of the Board of Schools to orient program sponsorship to post-secondary education institutions, it was disbanded in 1969. The Joint Review Committee for Inhalation Therapy Education (JRCITE) took on the Board of Schools accreditation role as it was incorporated in 1970 and later approved by the AMA's CME. The first Committee Chairman was H. Fred Helmholz, MD, a long-term proponent of the profession. He set up a committee to give parity to doctors and therapists; offices were in Rochester, MN.

The JRCRTE became part of the Committee on Allied Health Education (CAHEA), an "umbrella accreditor" which oversaw national programmatic accreditation for 25 other allied health professions, with support from the AMA's CME. In 1976, Dr. Helmholz's retirement established an executive director position and office in Euless, TX; the Committee was renamed the Joint Review Committee for Respiratory Therapy Education (JRCRTE).

Access to educational programs by correspondence was endorsed by the AARC in 1978. This controversial decision required the JRCRTE to adopt Essentials to accommodate "nontraditional" programs. In 1986 the JRCRTE became the first allied health group to base school accreditation criteria on outcome of the educational program, not the training process. Currently there are approximately 190 technician programs that graduate about 4500 students annually. The therapist programs number 300 and have 4400 graduates per year. Table 1-4 identifies key dates and events in education and accreditation. In 1994, the significant AMA sponsorship of CAHEA was withdrawn; 18 professions have regrouped within CAHEA's successor, the Commission of Accreditation of Allied Health Education Program (CAAHEP). Recently conflicts between the JRCRTE and the AARC have been settled. Agreement includes enlarging and reorganizing the committee, plans for future requirement that accredited programs

TABLE 1-4 **Key Dates and Events in Respiratory Care Education**

Year	Event
1950	Barach et al: Minimum standards for Inhalation Therapy. *JAMA* 144:25, 1950.
1956	Emma E, Collins V: Essentials for Inhalation Therapy Schools (reprinted in) *Inhalation Therapy* 1(3), 1956.
1963	Board of Schools formed (4 MDs, 3 RTs) reports to Council on Medical Education (CME) of the AMA as accrediting authority.
1968	Technician Certification Board (TCB) formed by AART
1969	First technician certifying examination given at AAIT annual meeting
1970	JRCITE incorporated: (4 MDs & 4 RTs); later (6 MDs & 6 RTs)
	Study of Accreditation of Selected Health Education Programs (SASHEP)
	62 hours of college coursework required for "registry examination eligibility"
1972	HRA funds "Role Deliniations . . ." done by AART
	JRCITE provides *Essentials* for technician programs
	Conclusion of SASHEP Report recommends formation of Committee for Allied Health Education and Accreditation (CAHEA) to replace CME
1974	AARC suggests discontinuing accredition of technician schools
	ARIT Inc. & TCB combine as NBRT
	AART appoints Director of Education to staff
1975	HRA funds AARC's Second Role Delineations Study; it becomes basis for NBRC Entry Level Examination
1976	"Great Debate" regarding continuance of CRTT programs
1977	Last year of CRTT "Grandfather clause"
	Validity study of JRCRTE revised *Essentials*
1978	AARC endorses nontraditional programs—Biosystems and Ottawa University
1981	AARC Long-range Planning Committee recommends 2-year education minimum entry level
	JRCRTE modifies guidelines to *Essentials* to accomodate nontraditional programs
1986	JRCRTE presents to the profession, *Essentials* providing for development of Product outcome-based programs to meet local and regional needs.
	AARC conducts first Blue Ribbon Panel on new JRCRTE *Essentials*
1987	JRCRTE annual report now requires goals, standards, and outcomes
1992	AARC second Blue-Ribbon Panel on JRCRTE Essentials implementation
	AARC Education Consensus Conference part 1.
	U.S. Department of Education Reauthorization of Higher Education Act specifying "separate & independent" accrediting agencies
	Pew Report reconfirms SASHEP Report; results in formation of Commission on Accreditation of Allied Health Education Programs (CAAHEP) to replace CAHEA.
1993	AARC Education Consensus Conference part 2.
1994	AARC Board of Directors withdraws sponsorship of JRCRTE
	AARC sponsors the Respiratory Care Accrediation Board (RCAB)
	CAHHEP's transition from CAHEA occurs; includes 17 professions
1996	AARC and JRCRTE resolve differences

grant at least the associate degree, and resumption of sponsorship of the committee by the AARC.

The respiratory therapy profession's affairs have been fortunate to operate within a "tripartite" system, the components being the professional association (AARC), credentialing (NBRC), and school accreditation (JRCRTE). By maintaining separateness and independence between groups, there is less occasion to operate at cross purposes and interfere in the roles of the other organizations. History has shown that the evolution of the profession is best served through a pragmatic and scientific approach. Major changes are best made with a collegial approach among concerned respiratory care organizations, physicians, and other allied health specialty groups.

REFERENCES

1. Siegerist HE: In Marti-ImaÑez F (ed): Henry E. Siegerist on the History of Medicine. New York, MD Publications, Inc., 1960
2. Helmholz HF: Early foundations. In Smith GA (ed): Respiratory Care: Evolution of a Profession. Lexena, KS, Applied Measurement Professionals, 15–21, 1989
3. Perkins JF: Historical development of respiratory physiology. In Fenn WO, Rahn H (eds): Handbook of Physiology: Respiration (section 3). Washington, DC, American Physiological Society, 1–58, 1964
4. Bettmann OL: A Pictorial History of Medicine. Charles Thomas Pub. 167, 1956
5. Helmholz HF: Professional champions (1900–1940). In Smith GA (ed): Respiratory Care: Evolution of a Profession. Lexena, KS, Applied Measurement Professionals, 1989
6. Leigh JM: The evolution of oxygen therapy apparatus. Anaesthesia 29:426, 1974
7. Helmholz HF: Oxygen therapy in the 1940's. In Smith GA (ed): Respiratory Care: Evolution of a Profession. Lexena, KS, Applied Measurement Professionals, 1989
8. Barach AL: Inhalation therapy: Historical background. Anesthesiology 23:407, 1962
9. Barach AL: Principles of Inhalation Therapy. Philadelphia, J.B. Lippincott, 1944
10. Silverman WA: The lesson of retrolental fibroplasia. Sci Am 236:100, 1977
11. Severinghaus JW, Astrup PB: History of blood gas analysis IV. Leland Clark's oxygen electrode. J Clin Monit 2:125, 1986
12. Severinghaus JW, Honda Y: History of blood gas analysis. VII. Pulse oximetry. J Clin Monit 3:135, 1987
13. AARC: Clinical practice guideline: Oxygen therapy in the acute care hospital. Respir Care 36:1410, 1991
14. AARC:. Clinical practice guideline: Oxygen therapy in the home or extended care facility. Respir Care 37:918, 1992
15. Nocturnal Oxygen Therapy Trial Group: Continuous or nocturnal oxygen therapy in hypoxemic chronic obstructive lung disease: A clinical trial. Ann Intern Med 93:391, 1980
16. O'Donohue WJ, Plummer AL: Magnitude of usage and cost of home oxygen therapy in the United States. Chest 107:301, 1994
17. Mörch ET: History of mechanical ventilation. In Kirby RR, Banner MJ, Downs JB (eds): Clinical Applications of Ventilatory Support. New York, Churchill Livingstone, 1990

18. Mushin WW, Rendell-Baker L, Thompson PW, Mapleson WW: Automatic Ventilation of the Lungs, 3rd ed. London, Blackwell Scientific, 1980
19. Colice GL: Historical background. In Tobin MJ (ed): Principles and Practice of Mechanical Ventilation. New York, McGraw-Hill, 1994
20. Ashbaugh DG, Bigelow DB, Petty TL: Acute respiratory distress in adults. Lancet 1:319, 1967
21. Chatburn RL: A new system for understanding mechanical ventilators. Respir Care 36:1123, 1991
22. Kirby RR, Robinson EJ, Shulz J, deLemos R: A new pediatric volume ventilator. Anesth Analg 50:533, 1971
23. Downs JB, Klein EF, Desautels D, Model, JH, Kirby, RR: Intermittent mandatory ventilation: A new approach to weaning patients from mechanical ventilation. Chest 64:331, 1973
24. MacIntyre NR: Respiratory function during pressure support breathing. Chest 89:677, 1986
25. Marini JJ: Pressure-controlled ventilation. In Tobin MJ (ed): Principles and Practice of Mechanical Ventilation. New York, McGraw-Hill, 1994
26. Tuxen DV: Permissive hypercapnia. In Tobin MJ (ed): Principles and Practice of Mechanical Ventilation. New York, McGraw-Hill, 1994
27. Marcey TW: Inverse ratio ventilation. In Tobin MJ (ed): Principles and Practice of Mechanical Ventilation. New York, McGraw-Hill, 1994
28. Younes M: Proportional assist ventilation. In Tobin MJ (ed): Principles and Practice of Mechanical Ventilation. New York, McGraw-Hill, 1994
29. Froese AB, Bryan AC: High frequency ventilation: State of the art. Am Rev Respir Dis 135:1363, 1987
30. Abman SH, Griebel JL, Parker DK, Schmidt JM, Swanton D, Kinsella JP: Inhaled nitric oxide in children with severe hypoxemic respiratory failure. J Pediatr 124:881, 1994
31. Wolfson MR, Greenspan JS, Deoras KS, et al: Comparison of gas and liquid ventilation: clinical, physiological and histological correlates. J Appl Physiol 72:1024, 1992
32. Prentice WS: Placement alternatives for long-term ventilator care. Respir Care 31:288, 1986
33. Elliott M, Moxham J: Noninvasive mechanical ventilation by nasal or face mask. In Tobin MJ (ed): Principles and Practice of Mechanical Ventilation. New York, McGraw-Hill, 1994
34. Motley HL: Observations on the use of positive pressure. J Aviat Med 18:417, 1947
35. Fowler WS, Helmholz HF, Miller RD: Treatment of pulmonary emphysema with aerosolized bronchodilator drugs and intermittent positive pressure breathing. Proc Staff Mayo Clin 28:743, 1953
36. Murray JF: Review of the state of the art in intermittent positive pressure breathing therapy. Am Rev Respir Dis 110:193, 1974
37. Intermittent Positive Pressure Breathing Trial Group: Intermittent positive pressure breathing therapy of chronic obstructive pulmonary diseases: A clinical trial. Ann Intern Med 99:612,1983
38. O'Donohue WJ: IPPB past and present. Respir Care 27:588,1982
39. AARC Clinical practice guideline: Intermittent positive pressure breathing. Respir Care 38:1189, 1993
40. Pierson DJ: Respiratory care as a science. Respir Care 33:27, 1988
41. AARC: Year 2001: Delineating the Educational Direction for the Future Respiratory Care Practitioner. Dallas, TX, AARC, 1992
42. AARC. Year 2001: An Action Agenda. Dallas, TX, AARC, 1992
43. Torrington KG: Respiratory care in the 1990s: What will happen in an era of managed care. Clin Pulm Med 2:107, 1995
44. Tomashefski JF: The National Board for Respiratory Therapy. Bull Am Coll Chest Phys 14:9, 1975
45. Smith GA: The 1980's—banner years and trying times. In Smith GA (ed): Respiratory Care: Evolution of a Profession. Lexena, KS, Applied Measurement Professionals, 1989
46. Johnson CB: 1992 Respiratory care job analysis. NBRC Horizons 19:1, 1993
47. Barach AL, Collins, V, Emma E: Minimum standards for inhalation therapy. JAMA 144:25, 1950

2 Respiratory Care in the 1990s

John S. Sabo

SECTION 1 Respiratory Care in the Modern Hospital

PROFESSIONAL SKILLS

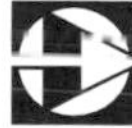

Upon completion of this chapter, the reader will be able to:

- Explain the respiratory care practitioner's role as a leader in the health care environment of the 1900s and beyond
- List and define methods of reimbursement currently being used
- Comment on the results of managed care and how it affects patients and health care personnel
- Define CPR and explain how its use enhances patient care
- List the opportunities identified by the AARC that expand the scope of practice of respiratory therapy
- Name the four foci that make up the "pyramid of focus" and explain how they help increase performance standards
- Understand all aspects of care management: component, outcomes, case, demand, and disease

KEY TERMS

Benchmarking
Case management
Component management
Computerized patient record
Critical pathway
Diagnostic related groups
Disease management
Durable medical equipment
Health maintenance organization
Managed care organization
Mission statement
Outcomes management
Patient-focused care
Preferred-provider organization
Prospective payment
Reimbursement
Ventilator-dependent unit

THE CHANGING ENVIRONMENT

The American health care system, which has evolved with minimal constraints until now, is being scrutinized by employers, consumers, and payers because of its spiraling costs. As we progress into the 1990s, health care consumes 13% of the gross national product (GNP), in comparison with 6% in 1965. It is projected that, by the year 2000, the annual cost of the American health care system will rise to $1.7 trillion.[1] Employers can no longer pass these costs to the consumers. Instead, they are trying to influence health care inflation by pressuring insurance companies to control their costs, forming purchasing coalitions, and negotiating directly with providers.[2]

The health care system has come under the scrutiny of the consumer, as well. No longer are physicians, nurses, therapists, and other health care providers beyond reproach, as evidenced by the fact that malpractice litigation has reached an all-time high. Consumers have been faced with increased personal costs associated with their health care. And the American public has made health care a social issue, ranking with the economy and the environment as a major crisis that must be corrected within our country. Even with the extraordinary expenditure of dollars each year, more than 30 million Americans have no health care coverage. Elections have been lost or won based on the health care issue and the provision of services to the politicians' constituents.

The early 1990s have produced some of the most dramatic changes since the advent of the Medicare system and the move to *diagnostic related groups* (DRGs). California, Tennessee, Hawaii, Pennsylvania, and New Jersey, for example, have become laboratories for national health care reform.[3,4]

Thus, the challenges that face the respiratory care specialty are broad and so diverse that our profession and our provision of service to our patients may be radically different as we approach the year 2000. Change will continue to occur at the present pace if not faster, and the current and future leaders of respiratory care need to understand the health care environment and its trends so they can be responsive. Concepts and strategies discussed in this chapter will assist in shaping the respiratory care service of the future.

The 1990s Leader

Although traditional health care delivery has been unlinked, uncoordinated, and individualized, future delivery will be provided by coordinated and integrated systems.[5] The respiratory care manager and practitioner must be leaders in this new health care environment. These leaders will be customer focused, team oriented, and self-directed. They will identify the customers who will value their successes within their organization, community, and profession. They will possess the capability to understand their organization's vision and management, and they will redesign their systems and processes with full knowledge of the organization's needs. They will recognize that the respiratory care profession's high-priority customers include physicians, nurses, executives, other health providers, external agencies, and—the most vital—patients and their families.

These leaders, while individualistic, must also be proven team players, because teamwork and the team philosophy are already predominant forces for productivity in the 1990s. Attributes of successful leaders will include excellent communication skills, particularly the ability to listen well (see section 2.2). Leaders who demonstrate personal warmth, empathy, and respect build relationships among superiors, peers, and subordinates. They must be able to provide encouragement through celebrations and recognize success within their organizations, both clinical and nonclinical.

These self-directed leaders must be innovative and demonstrate breakthrough thinking outside current practices. They must be able to frame issues in organizational or global terms and understand how best- and worse-case scenarios affect the organization, their areas of responsibility, and themselves. Because a results orientation is taking hold in organizations that are proactively facing the future, leaders will be those who take initiative, accept responsibility, organize well, maintain efficiencies, and focus on goals. Both clinical and managerial decision making must be based on sound judgment, analytical skills, and the ability to deal in facts. Access to information from credible internal and external sources will result in an awareness of the operation, people, and the marketplace. These leaders will be role models who lead by example, live out values, and demonstrate dignity and respect to all they come in contact with. Their overall character must be positive and open minded. Their can-do attitude will be guided by integrity, honesty, and fairness. They will be coaches and enablers, creating an environment for learning and, thus, cultivating knowledge building and sharing. They will motivate, challenge, and empower.[6,7]

Future organizations will stress that leaders should act as if they are CEOs of their own companies and should make the same good, sound judgments they would make for their own companies. Some risk taking will be required of these individuals, although emphasis will be placed on current and future successful outcomes. It is important for these individuals to be actively involved in changes within the organization. And because organizations of today are embracing the attitude that theory is "nice but results are better,"[8] the leaders who deliver on an organization's operational needs **and** fulfill the organization's vision will be successful.

In summary, it is important for each of us to control our own destiny or someone else will. We must face reality and be candid with everyone. We must not compete if we don't have the advantage. We must lead, not manage, and change before we have to. The respiratory care professionals of the 1990s will have to be a force in the conference room as well as at the bedside.

The Science of Change

Survival of both professionals and entire professions in the 1990s is contingent on their ability to adapt to change. Health care continues to change in the 1990s. Although it sounds contradictory, the real source of job security is the ability to adapt to change, while resistance to change ruins careers.[9]

The stress associated with change costs employers $150 billion to $200 billion annually. Surveys show that 44% of office workers indicate job stress has increased in the past 2 years, 52% of workers say work is the main source of stress in their lives, and one in five workers admits taking time off due to work stress.[9,10] Effective leaders are able to balance this stress both within their environment and within themselves. Though change is perpetually happening, there are certain events in which one has no emotional or mental involvement or control, and other situations where one has a level of control and involvement. It is critical to distinguish between the two. We should direct our energy and efforts in areas where we have involvement and control to adapt ourselves and lead others.[11]

A visionary approach to change is proactive and internally driven. Effective leaders adapt to change in a visionary versus a crisis mode. Change driven by crisis is externally motivated, and therefore, we deal with it in a *reactive* fashion to ensure survival. Understanding the health care environment and its current trends helps a person develop a *proactive* vision, transform to be a part of the future, and ensure personal success.

HEALTH CARE TRENDS OF THE 1990S

The unwillingness of public and private payers to continue to financially support the high-cost, inflationary health care system has fueled national health reform and managed care. The constant threat of increasing costs jeopardizes the independence of health care payers and providers. This threat is influencing health care delivery at a magnitude not seen since the advent of the Medicare system in the late 1960s. As a result of the impact of these factors, health care inflation has been lowered, which has in turn resulted in rising numbers of empty hospital beds and declining use of related health care services.[12–15]

Health care has flourished since the late 1960s because of reimbursement policies that allowed consumers the freedom to choose their own providers. The single factor that has had the most profound impact on that thriving health care environment has been the recent transformation from a fee-for-service reimbursement methodology to managed care. Thus, a thorough understanding of reimbursement methodologies is essential to adjusting to the future health care environment.

Reimbursement Methodologies

The most common types of reimbursement have been the following:[16]

1. *Fee-for-service,* in which payment is made by an individual or an insurance carrier at the time services are rendered.
2. *Indemnity without utilization management,* in which a third-party insurance company reimburses for services, often at a discount, with no review of the appropriateness of the services rendered.
3. *Indemnity with utilization management,* in which a third-party insurance company reimburses for services, often at a discount, with review of appropriateness of care before payment. Often prior approval is required before services are delivered.
4. *Cost reimbursement,* which determines the cost of services to be provided and reimbursed at a flat rate or at a slight inflationary margin.
5. *Prospective payment,* the original example of which was the DRG system put in force by Medicare in the early 1980s in an effort to curb the costs of health care. The DRG, based on a specific health condition, was reimbursed at a flat sum regardless of services provided.
6. *Managed care organization* (MCO) *reimbursement,* which provides enrollees with medical and hospital care in exchange for an agreed-upon payment. An MCO may be a *health maintenance organization* (HMO) or a *preferred provider organization* (PPO).

Managed Care

All types of managed care organizations have grown in popularity in the early 1990s. Health maintenance organizations are regulated by federal and state law and are based on one of three physician models:[17]

1. The *staff model,* which employs its care givers.
2. The *group practice model,* in which the HMO contracts with a full-service group practice.
3. The *individual practice affiliates (IPA) model,* which contracts with an alliance of independent providers to perform service.

The PPO was designed to be an alternative to the HMO. In this arrangement, health care services are provided to a defined population at an agreed-upon fee schedule, which may or may not include specialty care. Preferred provider organization physicians are paid on a fee-for-service basis and do not accept risks as the HMO physician does. Current trends in the managed care industry show PPOs and Blue Cross/Blue Shield are converting to HMO models, Medicare and Medicaid are shifting to managed care capitation, HMOs are merging and consolidating, providers are developing new products, and premiums are decreasing.[18–20]

There are four basic stages a health care market experiences during a transformation to managed care:

1. Unstructured
2. Emerging managed care
3. Penetration of managed care
4. Managed competition

The determination of the stage is dependent on the penetration of managed care within the market. The profitability of hospitals is inversely proportional to percent of penetration of managed care in a health care market (Table 2-1).[21,22]

Capitation

The current managed care environment is now evolving to a *capitated* payment system, which pays providers a single fixed sum that covers all or some portions of care delivered by the provider. The enrollee identifies a primary care physician to manage his or her care and has a monthly or annual premium that is paid to the health plan. The provider and health plan negotiate a per-member, per-month (PMPM) payment for specific services to be rendered. "Carve outs," or payment for specialized procedures or conditions, may be negotiated outside the contract.[23]

The integrated delivery system accepts all risks associated with the members of the managed care contract. "Risk pool" funds are set aside for either catastrophic situations or profit sharing at the end of the contract term. These funds are also used as an incentive plan for provider cost-effectiveness. The providers calculate the internal reimbursement rate and police utilization and quality. Thus, profits and losses of a managed care contract are based on the providers' efficiency.[24,25]

Managed Medicare

The government-supported movement toward managed Medicare will be able to reduce Medicare costs. The principle of the program is this: the Medicare recipient assigns his or her Medicare rights to the HMO in exchange for expanded protection. The benefits to the recipient include full coverage, less paperwork, prescription drugs, dental care, no premiums, and the fact that HMOs are paid 95% of the DRG rate and create their own contractual arrangements with providers. Results of the program show a reduction in inpatient and ancillary utilization, decreased acute care length of stay, and increased use of post–acute care settings.[26]

The Managed Care Spiral

Employers and business coalitions are continually demanding decreased HMO premiums. The pressure to decrease premiums is forcing HMOs to hold or cut prices. The choice remaining to the HMO is to lower profits or recoup its losses from providers. The HMO often employs capitation or micromanagement techniques to decrease the patient care costs, resulting in a decrease in provider volumes. The advent of greater managed care penetration gives the provider few opportunities to shift costs to better-paying programs, resulting in weakening of the provider's financial situation. Financial pressures are resulting in the radical rethinking of delivery systems and scrutiny of the people that deliver care, ultimately causing layoffs or restructuring of all professions within many health care organizations.[27]

Hospitals are responding to the managed care trends by reengineering strategies that include integration of systems and services, consolidation, use of automation, and advanced technologies. The goal of these efforts is to respond to the decreased availability of the health care dollar by increasing market share and decreasing costs.

Reengineering

The reengineering of our health care system fosters mergers and partnerships with prudent investors, integration of providers and payers, rethinking of patient care delivery, and the actualization of the computerized patient record (CPR). Hammer and Champy, in their

TABLE 2-1 **Health Care Market Characteristics During Managed Care Stages**

Stages of Managed Care	Unstructured	Emergent	Penetration	Competition	Postreform
HMO	<5%–10%	<10–15%	15%–20%	25%–40%	>40%
Indemnity	>30%	<25%	<15%	<5%	0%
Profits (Hospital)	6%–10%	4%–6%	2%–4%	1%–2%	2%–6%
Ambulatory	<15%	<20%	<15%	>40%	>50%
Hospital Structure	Freestanding	Small system	Multihospital	Regional network	Integrated systems
Physicians' Groups	Solo, small	Few groups	Single specialty	Multispecialty	Megagroups
Quality	TQM, CQI	Benchmarking	Patient focused	Outcomes	Disease management
Employers	Traditional	Data sharing	Direct contracting	Coalitions	Quality purchases

Adapted with permission from Hospital Strategy Report, Vol. 11/No. 6, September, 1994. See Reference 21.

book *Reengineering the Corporation: A Manifesto for Business Revolution,* state, "Forget about what you know about how business should work. Most of it's wrong." The authors state that reengineering involves starting over within a current corporation. It is definitely not modifying the existing systems, keeping current practices in place, and just fine-tuning them. It is actually starting from a blank sheet of paper. Reengineering is formally defined as "fundamental re-thinking and radical redesign of the business process to achieve dramatic improvements and critical contemporary measures of performance such as cost, quality, service, and speed." The engineering process changes business processes, along with jobs associated with those business processes, and the infrastructure of the organization.[28]

The principles of quality management serve as the foundation of reengineering. Management and measurement systems change to support the new business processes, jobs, and structure. Successful reengineering must be customer driven and targeted to radical goals that are company wide. It requires absolute management commitment at all levels. Cross-functional teams composed of staff from all organizational levels assess functional value of processes and structures. Implementation is dramatic, speedy, precisely executed, and measured for long-term results. Major changes in physical layout and job duties can result. The results of reengineering can be more than planned for. It must not be used as an excuse to cut jobs, although entire job classifications and units can be eliminated by the process. The expense for new capital equipment, facilities modification, and enhanced information technology can be massive. An additional, and often unplanned, consequence can be the destruction of a positive organizational culture.[29–31]

Managed care forces health care executives to cut their costs to remain competitive, and reengineering is one option that is being used to accomplish this.[32] No profession is exempt from the effects of this process. Physicians' authority and incomes are declining, nurses are being replaced with nonlicensed personnel, executive positions are being eliminated, and therapists' traditional duties are being modified.[33–40] Mortality and morbidity can be negatively or positively affected by methodologies used to alter patient care delivery.[41,42] The integrated health care delivery system (IHS or IDS), patient care delivery redesign, and automation of processes are types of reengineering efforts. The final impact of these models on the health care system will only be realized in the future.

□ REENGINEERING INTO AN INTEGRATED DELIVERY SYSTEM

Hospital leaders are transforming their organizations into integrated health systems.[43] The health care system is driven by a single corporate vision that positions the system to be the provider of choice. The strategies are the following:[44]

1. A focus on community needs
2. Decreased cost of delivery
3. Superior quality
4. A large network of primary care physicians

The desired result is to build a system with financial strength and integrity that fulfills the community needs for health care.[45,46] The goal of these systems is to provide a comprehensive "vertical integrated continuum of care" to the community. Care delivery is provided by a progression that includes primary care services, ambulatory diagnosis and treatment, mobile services, ambulatory surgery, emergency care, acute care (inpatient hospital), post–acute care (skilled nursing facilities, subacute, and long-term care), home health, rehabilitation, senior care, retirement center, community-based services, and hospice (Fig. 2-1). There is a commitment to enhance human health performance through disease prevention, immunization, health education, health protection and risk reduction, health promotion, and disease management. The final success depends on "horizontal integration" fostering long-term relationships or partnerships that link physicians, payers, and health care providers (Fig. 2-2).[47–53]

□ REENGINEERING THE PATIENT CARE DELIVERY SYSTEM

Hospitals are completely rethinking the organization of inpatient care. This major effort of redesigning the patient care delivery system is often called *patient-focused care* (PFC), or patient-centered care (PCC), because it is modeled after manufacturing processes that bring services closest to the customer. Health care providers often affirm that they are very patient focused, although organizations find the processes that are used to provide the care are often not patient focused. Examination, modification, and improvement of work processes are components of work redesign. The goals of this type of reorganization are to radically

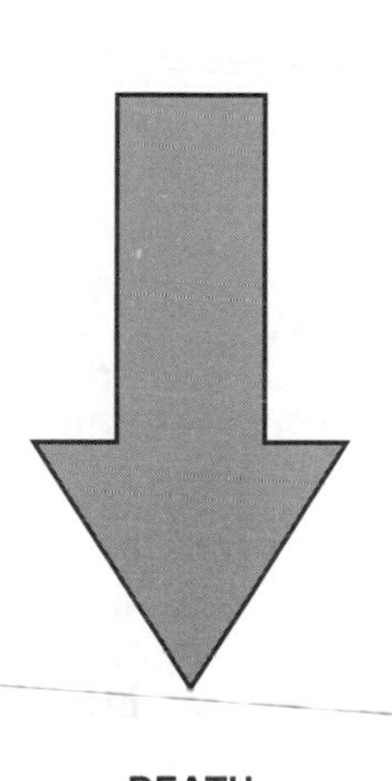
THE CONTINUUM OF CARE
Vertical Integration
BIRTH
DEATH
Prevention/Immunization
Outpatient Centers
Emergency Departments
Immediate (Urgent) Care Facilities
Mobile Services
Ambulatory Care Services
Mental Health Services
Recovery Centers
Acute Care Hospitals
Skilled Nursing Facilities (SNF)
Enhanced Skilled Nursing Facilities
Subacute Care Facilities
Long-term Care Facilities
Rehabilitation Services
Home Care Services
Senior Care Centers
Retirement Centers
Hospices

FIGURE 2-1. The continuum of care, vertical integration.

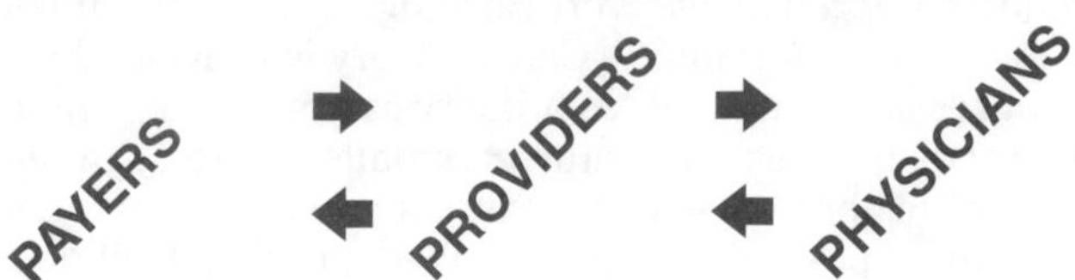

FIGURE 2-2. The continuum of care, horizontal integration.

improve service and quality while reducing costs. Principles associated with patient-focused care are similar to the following:

1. Deliver the highest value of care at the most appropriate cost.
2. Assure appropriate treatment that maximizes desired clinical outcomes.
3. Improve continuity and consistency of patient care.
4. Improve patient and physician satisfaction.
5. Provide a positive environment for employees.
6. Differentiate the health care facility within the marketplace.

Strategies of PFC redesign include the following:[54]

1. Clustering patients with similar medical conditions.
2. Cross training to create multiskilled teams of licensed and nonlicensed care givers, thus converting from an individual to an integrated team approach, which increases actual patient care time.
3. Linking diverse operations with simplified information and documentation, which results in decreased time spent on documentation.
4. Developing new structures, which may include staff redeployment and decentralization of previously centralized services.
5. Redesigning facilities, which includes physical structure changes to accommodate patient-focused care.

Patient-focused care categorizes standard job design in health care as the following:[54]

1. Simplified, where workers perform a small number of narrow tasks and are easily interchanged.
2. Rotational, where workers shift periodically through a set of jobs and can be cross trained to do several tasks.
3. Enlarged, where workers perform a wider variety of similar tasks, making the job more challenging.
4. Enriched, where job tasks are upgraded to increase job depth and scope of decision.

Expanded opportunities for job enlargement and enrichment enhance efficiency, effectiveness, and appropriateness of patient care delivery. The success of redesign efforts can be seen in enhanced staff involvement and commitment, as well as staff use of hard data for decision making.[55]

Although patient-focused initiatives are worthwhile, hospitals should not expect to generate huge, windfall financial savings from this source alone. This effort has decreased costs in some institutions, though patient-focused restructuring can require a major investment, and few hospitals are in a position to spend millions of dollars on it.[56,57] Negatives include decreased hospital use, which causes work-force disruptions including retraining, career alterations, and layoffs.[58]

Reengineering can work if it facilitates professionalism, uses outcomes management and its critical paths, and fosters skill expansion within the educational background and experience of the care giver.[59]

□ REENGINEERING THROUGH AUTOMATION AND TECHNOLOGY

Information systems (IS) are used not only to automate health care but to reengineer it.[60,61] The majority of hospitals in the country are already part of, or plan to be involved in, community health information networks (CHINs). The CHIN expedites the reengineering of the health care system by facilitating the horizontal integration of providers, payers, and physicians to address care delivery across the continuum. The *computerized patient record* (CPR) is the foundation of both the CHIN and its ability to implement the vertical integration of a delivery system.[62,63]

The Computerized Patient Record

The goals of the computerized patient record (CPR) include capturing, accessing, and using data; decision support; optimizing clinical practice; business management; streamlining patient flow; and addressing legal and regulatory requirements.[64,65] The CPR supports patient-focused care by point of care documentation, which increases care givers' time with patients through reduced manual and clerical activities.[66–68] An enhanced continuity of care and concomitant decrease in complications and comorbidities are realized by the CPR's single-source provision, through the CHIN, of information for treatment decisions to a number of providers. Quality and diagnostic data are available to support outcomes research, information control, and audit capabilities.

The information supplied by the CPR improves, concurrently and retrospectively, quality monitoring, management decision making, and reporting capabilities. It improves the use of physicians' time, treatment outcomes, and patient readmission rates. It enhances the opportunity to share information about "best practices" among providers, provides a logical and consistent approach to patient care, and creates the necessary foundation for teaching. Improvement in financial management is realized through the ability to relate clinical status to resource consumption, allowing all parties to negotiate managed care contracts more effectively and to monitor the financial performance of those contracts.[69,70]

Patient satisfaction increases because of scheduling efficiencies that result in decreased patient no-shows and lost customers. Market share can increase through improved communication with referral sources. And patient rights are protected by enhancing patient confidentiality.[68,69]

In conclusion, the CPR facilitates compliance with state and federal regulations for record keeping and reporting, while increasing competitiveness in a managed care environment.

BOX 2-1

PRODUCT LINES AND ASSOCIATED SERVICES

Treatment Modalities
- Small volume nebulizer (SVN) therapy
- Metered dose inhaler (MDI) therapy
- Intermittant positive pressure breathing (IPPB)
- Incentive spirometry (IS)
- Chest physical therapy (CPT)
- Ultrasonic nebulizer (VSN)
- Intrapulmonary percussive ventilation (IPV) therapy

Oxygen Therapy
- Transport
- Routine with and without humidification/aerosol therapy
- Hyperbaric (HBO)

Ventilator Management
- Adult
- Pediatric
- Noninvasive (CPAP, BiPAP)

Physiologic Monitoring and Diagnostics
- ABG sampling and analysis
- Pulmonary function testing
- Venipuncture
- Pulse oximetry
- Capnography
- Exercise and metabolic studies
- $S\bar{v}O_2$
- Cardiac monitoring
- Cardiomuscular monitoring

Specialized Procedures
- Transport
- Cardiopulmonary resuscitation (CPR)
- Airway care
- Selected nursing and physical therapy procedures

RESPIRATORY CARE SERVICES IN THE 1990S

The Respiratory Continuum of Care

Historically, respiratory care services have primarily been provided in an acute care hospital via a centralized department. In the future, respiratory care services will have the opportunity—and the responsibility—to identify various points in a seamless delivery system in which their products can be used.[71] Respiratory care practitioners or teams of practitioners will provide services in work zones that geographically divide the continuum of care. Staffing requirements for the work zone can be formulated by volume of patients, products provided, service requirements, and the acuity of patients located within that zone.[72] Scope of practice of the respiratory practitioner will be defined with the medical leadership of respiratory care.[73]

The integrated delivery system will increase the demand for respiratory care services in diagnostics and treatment, preventive medicine, elder care, and post–acute care (skilled nursing facilities, subacute care, rehabilitation, long-term care, home care), in addition to the acute care facility.

The Respiratory Care Product Lines

Traditionally, service areas of the respiratory care department have been divided into general and critical care. Previously, services such as oxygen therapy, treatment modalities, and pulse oximeter spot checks would have been categorized under general therapy or care. Critical care may have included such interventions as ventilator management, oximetry, and bronchoscopy. Areas of service can be categorized into the five major product lines that are provided by a respiratory care service. These areas of service, or *product lines,* are as follows:

1. Therapy modalities
2. Oxygen therapy
3. Ventilator management
4. Physiological monitoring
5. Specialized procedures and diagnostics

Specific procedures or products rendered by respiratory care professionals can be categorized into these five major product lines (Box 2-1). This type of categorization offers adaptability in the future health care environment. For example, these product lines will be offered in a variety of settings and scopes, all of which will be compatible in an integrated health system. Basic services such as oxygen therapy or particular therapy modalities (eg, incentive spirometry) may be rendered by other professionals with documented competency under the guidance of a respiratory professional. The traditional scope of practice of respiratory care will be examined, and alternatives will be explored for care delivery. This will offer an excellent opportunity for respiratory care practitioners to increase their value to their organizations. Although the respiratory care scope of practice has been focused specifically on the delivery of respiratory care procedures, this scope will be broadened to encompass other patient care duties. The American Association of Respiratory Care (AARC) has already identified opportunities for expansion of the scope of practice of respiratory care practitioners (Box 2-2) into one that is holistic and includes, but is not limited to, cardiopulmonary diagnostics, total airway care, physical therapy procedures, blood sampling, bedside speci-

BOX 2-2

FUTURE SCOPE OF PRACTICE*

1. Mechanical ventilation, management and adjustments of mechanical ventilation, mechanical ventilator support, life-support systems
2. Cardiodiagnostic, hemodynamic monitoring, invasive and noninvasive cardiopulmonary monitoring, critical care monitoring, critical therapeutics, ECG, Holter monitoring, cardiac monitoring, arterial line, indwelling catheter
3. Traditional and current therapies (oxygen therapy, aerosol therapy, humidity therapy, incentive spirometry, etc.)
4. Airway care, airway management, intubation
5. Pulmonary function testing
6. Treatment assessment, outcome assessment
7. Home care
8. CPR, resuscitation
9. Respiratory care of the neonatal and pediatric patient, perinatal pediatrics
10. Acid–base balance, blood gas analysis, arterial puncture, automated lab analysis
11. Rehabilitation, cardiopulmonary, pulmonary rehabilitation
12. Patient education, family counseling, education techniques, teaching the patient
13. Therapist-driven protocols, other protocols
14. Health promotion, disease prevention, health teaching
15. Smoking cessation, nicotine intervention
16. Hyperbaric oxygenation, hyperbaric medicine
17. ECMO, other life-support techniques
18. Management
19. Discharge planning
20. Sleep studies, sleep lab, sleep disorders, sleep apnea, sleep studies therapy
21. Research
22. Medication administration, medication delivery other than aerosol, various routes of administration, IV therapy, cardiac drug delivery
23. Stress testing, exercise testing, exercise physiology assessment
24. Alternate care delivery, long-term care, subacute care, hospice care, physician office and clinic practice
25. Bronchoscopy, bronchoscopy assistance
26. Infection control, cleaning and sterilization
27. Electrolyte analysis, blood lab, stat lab
28. Geriatrics
29. Quality improvement, performance assessment and improvement, quality assessment
30. Case management
31. EEG, neurodiagnostics
32. Computerization, information management
33. Transport, trauma in-flight specialist
34. Metabolic measurements
35. ACLS, NALS, PALS
36. Mechanical cardiac support
37. Ethics, ethical decision making
38. Teach other health care providers, being part of health care team, management of other health professions
39. Patient-focused care
40. Technology assessment
41. Charting and record-keeping

* *Listed in order of importance from group consensus rankings*

men analysis, bedside testing, and arterial and venous line insertion and management.[74]

The Acute Care Work Zone

These services may be rendered by a department that is either centralized or decentralized, or by an *integrated service unit* (ISU).[74a] The centralized service is the traditional hospital department that functions independently from other departments to provide patient care based on physician orders. The decentralized services are of two types:

1. *Unit based,* where practitioners report to a patient care unit. (Some people feel that this can result in loss of professional identity and a decrease in quality of respiratory service rendered.)
2. *Product-line reporting,* which bases respiratory care practitioners and managers in specific product lines (eg, cardiovascular, women's services). In this case, scope of practice will vary depending on the product line.

There can be inefficiencies associated with both centralized and decentralized models. However, an ISU model will maintain a principal structure that coordinates care and ensures quality in the various work zones, as well as validates staff competencies. This will create a customer-focused, outcomes-based, collaborative practice service. Accountability will be to the system's customers (the patient and family, physicians, executives, nurses, and other professionals). The process through which service is delivered will be determined by the desired quality and financial outcomes that determine the value to be received and perceived by its customers. The ISU will complement the continuum of an integrated delivery system (Fig. 2-3).

Thus, the service will conform to the required outcomes of each unique health care organization. In the acute care hospital, it may take the form of cardiopulmonary (respiratory and cardiology) services, therapy (respiratory, physical, occupational, and speech), biotechnology (respiratory, biomedical), diagnostics and therapy (respiratory, hyperbaric oxygen, sleep, imaging, endoscopy, invasive and noninvasive cardiology), or many other configurations.[75,76] Acute care work zones will geographically divide the hospital to promote collaborative patient care delivery among all providers, to maximize the ultimate patient outcome.

The respiratory care service should have a mission that defines where the service and its individual practitioners need to be both today and tomorrow. The mission statement should also state what is important and

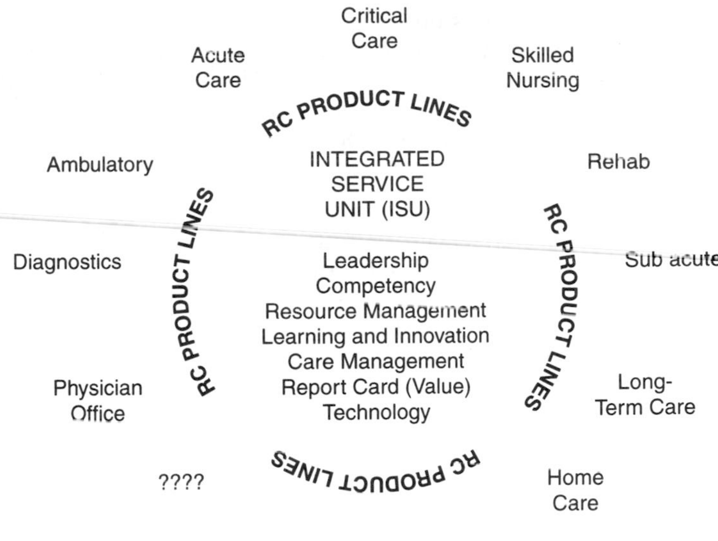

FIGURE 2-3. The integrated service unit.

why for their future success. The department should know where it is, where it is going, and how to communicate organizationally. Input to the mission statement should be obtained from all involved personnel, including both management and staff (Box 2-3).[77] The organization of the new respiratory care service should be process focused, team based, customer driven, flexible, agile, and should be a flat virtual network. The new organization will have multiskilled, complex jobs and direct reporting relationships, and governance will be collaborative and colloquial. The service will be governed by values and beliefs within the system.[78]

The organizational bottom lines, both financial and quality, will equate the value offered to the customer (V = Q/$). (In other words, the Value that is created for the customer is equal to the Quality of the service provided divided by the cost ($) of providing that service.) Institutional values will revolve around goal orientation, integrity, valuing people, and excellence (GIVE). These values are concepts that can be built on to maximize our chance of success within the ever-changing health care environment of the future.

Shared governance, promoted by professional practice councils (PPCs), will create opportunities for staff input in the realm of both customer or patient satisfaction and the operation of the service. The objective of a PPC is to create a structure that will result in enhancement of patient care. The council is empowered with responsibility and authority to optimize cost, quality, and customer service issues and outcomes. This goal is accomplished by using data-driven models that reflect ongoing compliance with JCAHO functional standards and all regulatory and accrediting agencies to improve organizational performance. This council can evolve into a collaborative, self-governed, transprofessional council that includes representation from all professional disciplines. Thus, the professional practice council, the transprofessional council, and functional management will collaborate on improving processes and optimizing outcomes. Continuous quality enhancement (CQE) will be one of the mechanisms that will be used to identify operational quality issues or variances that affect service outcomes.[79,80]

BOX 2-3

MISSION STATEMENT

The mission of the respiratory care service is to provide patient care within the integrated delivery systems continuum documented by patient outcomes. The foundation of this mission is operational expertise, enhanced learning, and innovation, affecting the financial and customer outcomes.

The central focus of the respiratory care service is the patients we serve. The practitioners will act as assistants to the physicians in determining the most appropriate care to be delivered. All staff members will strive to perfect their customer service, team participation, and self-directed leadership.

The goal of this department shall be recognition as a premier respiratory care facility. The value system that will be practiced in our culture will include professionalism, proficiency, productivity, personableness, and pride.

The Post–Acute Care Work Zone

The goal of post–acute care is cost-effective, creative use of health care resources to achieve maximum outcomes. The post–acute care industry is projected to grow because of two factors:

1. The acute care hospital is the most costly component of the health care delivery system; non–acute

care delivery sites offer economically feasible alternatives to acute care.[81–85]
2. The health systems will be faced with increased use by people 65 and older based on an aging population; the majority of inpatient days should fall outside of the acute care hospital environment.[86]

Thus, integrated health care systems will move patients to the appropriate care setting based on acuity to decrease the cost of health care delivery. Post–acute care patients are usually sufficiently stable that they no longer require acute care services, but their care requirements are also usually too complex for the traditional nursing center. So post–acute care programs are focused on outcomes of functional restoration, clinical stabilization, and avoidance of both acute care hospitalization and medical complications.[87]

Post–acute care settings can be divided into five major facilities:[86]

1. The skilled nursing facility (SNF)
2. Enhanced SNF
3. Subacute care
4. Long-term care
5. Home care (see Chap. 24)

The factors that differentiate these five delivery sites include nursing hours per day, rehabilitation requirements, length of stay, and cost within the particular institution (Table 2-2). An increase in total post–acute care use will be realized with a corresponding increase in both long-term care and chronic ventilator care units. In all but the home-care setting, patient requirements include treatment and assessment by a physician; nursing intervention of at least 2.5 hours a day; therapy services such as physical, occupational, respiratory, and psychosocial therapy; ancillary or technology services (which include lab, pharmacy, nutrition, diagnostic, and *durable medical equipment* [DME]); and use of case management and coordination of services.[88]

The post–acute care setting is a major arena in which the respiratory care practitioner's skills will be applied in the future. A major type of post–acute care setting is the long-term care facility that specializes in the ventilator-dependent patient. The National Association of Medical Directors of Respiratory Care (NAMDRC) identifies an effective *ventilator-dependent* unit as a setting where team members have expertise in the relevant areas. In this environment, team members are willing to assist each other in achieving patient goals through the leadership of a strong medical director, as well as lower patient to staff ratios. The environment encourages dedicated unit staff, increased communication frequency, and low staff turnover.[89–93]

Reimbursement varies in a post–acute care center because it uses Medicare ancillary codes in which units of therapy are delivered in 15-minute blocks. Units of therapy are per employee and per shift, based on a Medicare salary equivalency. So reimbursement will vary for a registered respiratory therapist (RRT), certified respiratory care technician (CRTT), and noncredentialed care giver. The facility sends invoices to the bill payers and supplies detailed logs of daily attendance in terms of labor, units, and supplies. Reimbursement is outcomes based for rehabilitation, teaching, and training; chronic therapy is not reimbursed.[93] Accrediting agencies, such as JCAHO and CORF, and trade and industry associations, such as the American Subacute Care Association (ASCA), are promoting use of the post–acute care facility.[94]

Home Care Work Zone

At the turn of the century, most health care was delivered within the home setting. The factors for the reemergence of home care are cost-containment pressures, consumer preferences, and new technologies (see Chap. 24).[95] Home care will grow because of developments in computer linkages between the physician office and patient home, as well. There will be an increased reliance on practitioners such as RNs, respiratory care practitioners, and others to provide care in the home. Advancements in technology will include the following:[96]

1. Home robots for monitoring medication, vital signs, emergencies, ECGs, blood glucose, and other tests.
2. Telephone monitoring of vital signs, blood pressure, and cardiac function.
3. Improved product innovation for room care, incontinence, sleep disorders, pain control, and drug delivery.

Respiratory home care will be used more as an alternative to acute care because it has emerged as a cost-effective way of improving the quality of care of the el-

TABLE 2-2 **Characteristics of Post–Acute Care Settings**

Post–Acute Care Facility Classification	Nursing Hours	Therapy	Length of Stay (LOS)	Cost ($/d)
Home Care	variable	variable	variable	<100
Skilled Nursing Facility (SNF)	2.5	none	240	100
Enhanced Skilled Nursing Facility	3–3.5	1–2 times/wk	45	200–300
Subacute Facility	4–6	2–3 hr/day	20	400–600
Long-Term Facility	7–10	variable	90–120	800–1500

Taken with permission from Madigan, PA: The role of corporate marketing at Mariner Health, New London, CN. Presented at Emerging Issues in Subacute Care. Philadelphia, March 9, 1995

derly and chronically ill. Patients who will benefit from home respiratory care include individuals suffering from AIDS complications, asthma and chronic obstructive disease, pulmonary disease, and sleep disorders.[97]

THE PATIENT-FOCUSED RESPIRATORY CARE PRACTITIONER

The foundation of all professions is their practitioners. Thus, the practitioners of respiratory care will have to be holistic, physician extenders who are customer focused, behave as team players, and act as self-directed leaders with critical-thinking skills. These professionals will have to impact the financial performance of their organizations, be life-long learners, and have impeccable multiskilled clinical expertise that is patient focused.[98]

Health care occupations should reflect the desired outcomes of the organization to be viable. No matter how useful a job might have been in the past, if it does not coincide with future objectives of the organization, it will soon become extinct. A simple example of this is a typewriter repairman living and working in today's computerized environment. Though typewriter repairmen were once very vital to an organization, they no longer have a place because PCs are now the mainstay of word processing within any organization.[99]

The respiratory care practitioner must be committed to quality patient care, use good assessment skills, possess critical-thinking and problem-solving skills, as well as be emotionally adaptable to an ever-changing environment. Such practitioners will be a force at the bedside, thus positively affecting patient care outcomes.[100,101]

Respiratory care practitioners (RCPs) of today are of three basic education origins: RCPs with on-the-job training; CRTTs who are graduates of a technical program or the equivalent; and registered respiratory therapists (RRTs) with a minimum degree from a 2-year technical program, an associate degree, or a bachelor's degree or the equivalent. The organized respiratory care profession is required to promote the highest educational level that is affordable to the health care system.

Personnel Performance Management

Health care professionals must be properly qualified (competent) and satisfy realistic standards of their organizations. Understanding the characteristics of an individual in a given job, role, or culture causes or predicts success. Thus, competency assurance is the responsibility of the principal structure facilitating service. Standards that validate competency will be created and communicated in a balanced, goal-oriented performance plan for all staff members.[102] Whenever possible, objective measurement monitors should be created and used to evaluate individual and team performance.[103,104] Exempt and nonexempt staff should have common denominators of organizational performance.

Increasing Performance Standards: The Pyramid of Focus

The systematic raising of performance standards is a goal of any high-performing organization. Clarity, communication, and measurement of objective standards are the drivers of performance and competency. The "pyramid of focus" (Fig. 2-4) is an instrument that relates competency-performance improvement to quality-cost (value) enhancement. This balanced view of performance for all employees addresses the following four foci:[105,106]

1. Customer focus
2. Financial focus
3. Learning and innovation focus
4. Operational focus

The operational focus is the basis of service delivery and includes the basic skills an individual possesses or the services a unit offers. Learning and innovation form the process from which attitudes and aptitudes are developed and cultivated. The financial (cost) and customer (quality) foci are the results associated with the delivery of operational services or products when enhanced by development through learning and innovation.

□ PERFORMANCE STANDARDS

Performance standards must be strictly based on an individual job description. A role description incorporates the job description and performance standards into a single seamless document. The description should be based on the foci. (Note: The following performance standards are for respiratory care practitioners. However, the standards can be modified for all staff levels.)

The customer focus standards are threefold (Tables 2-3 and 2-4):

1. Patient and customer satisfaction
2. Team member satisfaction (colleagues)
3. Self-directed leadership

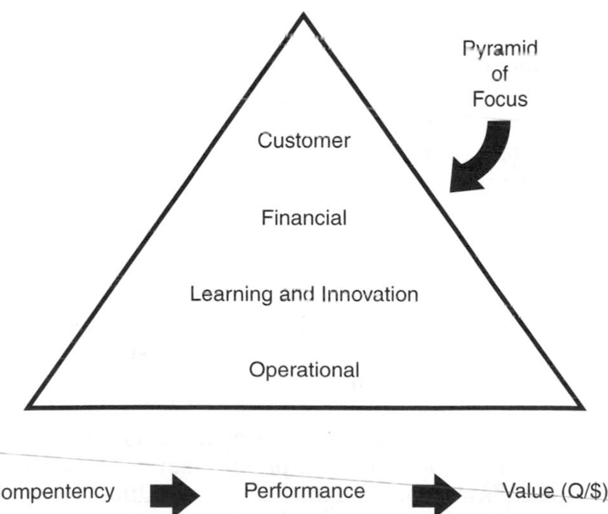

FIGURE 2-4. Pyramid of focus.

TABLE 2-3 **Customer Focus Standards**

Area of Evaluation	Measurement Tool	Component	Scale
Patient and Customer Satisfaction	Press-Ganey Survey (Group) Table 2-4	Analyze results provided by patient care survey for unit. Statistical report used to evaluate performance on the accompanying scale.	> than 3 pts. higher than at last periodic review = 20 2 = 15 1 = 10 0 = 5 <0 = 0
	Customer Principles JCAHO Survey Fire Marshall Department of Health	External review by JCAHO. Responsible for areas that are directly influenced by actions.	Always exceeds = 20 Mostly exceeds = 15 Meets standards = 10 Usually meets = 5 Does not meet = 0
Team Review	Team Principles Council Attendance and Participation Table 2-4	Practices the team behaviors in daily job tasks. Effectiveness is assessed by the manager or designee. Evaluated on stated standards. Evaluation is performed on accompanying scale by statistical reports, identified complications, and observation when indicated. Quality points as per scale.	Always exceeds = 20 Mostly exceeds = 15 Meets standards = 10 Usually meets = 5 Does not meet = 0
Self-Directed Leadership	Leadership Principles Table 2-4	Practices the patient-first behaviors in daily job tasks. Effectiveness is assessed by the manager or designee. Evaluated based on stated standards. Evaluation is performed on accompanying scale by statistical reports, identified complications, and observation when indicated.	Always exceeds = 20 Mostly exceeds = 15 Meets standards = 10 Usually meets = 5 Does not meet = 0

Practicing the principles associated with the customer focus should result in enhanced outcomes and perceptions of quality by the customers. The financial focus standards are applicable to all staff because everyone affects the cost of doing business. The standards not only include performance related to budgets and controlling money, but also to productivity, attendance and punctuality, and performance of duties in a safe and protective manner, because all influence the cost to the institution (Tables 2-5 and 2-6).

The learning and innovation focus standards are the dual responsibility of the employee and the employer. The goals are to enhance operational skills through an ongoing learning process and to encourage innovation in the profession (Table 2-7 and 2-8). Developing a strong set of base skills and cultivating competency in these skills by continual learning will result in positive influences on the financial and customer aspects of service delivery (Table 2-9).

The operational focus includes the traditional skills base of the respiratory care practitioner. These foundational skills are obtained during the educational process and mature during professional practice. The operational focus standards include therapy modalities, oxygen therapy, ventilator management, physiological monitoring, and specialized or diagnostic procedures (Tables 2-10 through 2-15). Selection of the most pertinent areas for evaluation in a given performance year is made based on the operational standards.

A weighted system should be used to ensure a fair evaluation (Table 2-16) where proficiency or competency is specifically outlined and incorporated into all aspects of the performance plan. These standards of performance should be required internally and should be consistent with those competency standards that are externally required by JCAHO.

When possible, the compensation program should truly reflect the performance of an individual within a work unit, although health care has not historically been innovative in compensating its best performers. Compensation programs must center on the high performers or the high-performing teams within the organization to compensate and reward them properly.[107]

□ CODES OF CONDUCT AND PERFORMANCE

A complement to the management of performance is the communication of required performance and conduct standards that explicitly identify actions that may be taken if conduct or performance is not acceptable

TABLE 2-4 **Performance Standards: Principles Expectations**

The Customer Principles Expectation

Motto

"Caring Beyond Expectations"

Creed

"We are caring people who work together to serve our customers."

Points of Service

1. SLEH* exists because of its customers, and **all** positions are created because of those customers.
2. SLEH customers are patients, family, physicians, payers, vendors, agencies, the community, and, most importantly, each other.
3. A colleague is each of the SLEH team members. Each colleague will treat each customer better than he would expect to be treated, emphasizing considerate and respectful communication at all times.
4. Any colleague who receives a customer complaint will own that complaint.
5. Each colleague will help create a healing environment by greeting customers with a smile and a warm attitude, and maintaining the cleanliness of the organization's physical environment.
6. Management will treat nonmanagement staff as their customer.
7. Each colleague will answer telephones and pages in a prompt, professional, courteous manner.
8. Colleagues will practice "On stage–Off stage" behavior.
9. Colleagues will strive to be on the Honor Role, President's Service Award winner, and Employee of the Month.

The Team Principles Expectation

1. Understands, supports, and feels ownership of the team's philosophy.
2. Is willing to put the team's goals ahead of her own goals.
3. Listens to everyone on the team.
4. Maintains "patient" and "team" focus.
5. Will use conflict constructively.
6. Respects all members of the team.
7. Communicates his needs and views openly and honestly.
8. Respects differences and values diversity.
9. Works for defined outcomes.
10. Utilizes the resources of others.
11. Seeks to solve problems on a timely basis.
12. Delegates or accepts delegation with a sense of purpose and a sense of cooperation.
13. Remains flexible about scheduling or staffing based on the patient census and requirements.
14. Accepts suggestions from other team members for improvement with an open mind.
15. Offers help to a team member under stress.
16. Helps cross train other team members, either formally or informally.
17. Applies learned problem-solving skills to keep issues objective and reach resolution.
18. Is patient focused (PFC).
19. Communicates a PFC need when asking for or receiving help from team members.
20. Encourages and praises other team members during difficult times.
21. Motivates team members during difficult times.
22. Meets the needs of doctors, nurses, and other staff, as well as patients, family, and guests.
23. Participates freely in team meetings.
24. Is eager to learn new things to improve the service quality to the patient.
25. Uses his or her time well.
26. Honors holiday commitments.

Leadership Principles Expectations

General

1. Promotes the mission of SLEH.
2. Promotes the mission of SLEH department.
3. Promotes the SLEH two bottom lines, quality and financial.
4. Promotes the four values of GIVE (goal orientation, integrity, valuing people, excellence).
5. Fully commits to the job.
6. Is adaptable to change quickly.
7. Increases speed to provide action.
8. Accepts ambiguity and uncertainty.
9. Behaves as if one is in business for oneself.
10. Continues the learning process.
11. Holds oneself accountable for outcomes.
12. Adds value to the organization.
13. Sees self as a service center.
14. Manages own morale.
15. Practices performance enhancement.
16. Is a fixer not a finger pointer.
17. Is willing to alter expectations.

Specific

1. Is consistently accountable to time scheduling guidelines:
   a. flexibility
   b. coverage of unit during shortage
   c. takes responsibility for shift staffing by making adjustments related to census
   d. assumes responsibility to co-workers in promptly giving and taking report
2. Maintains patient and co-worker confidentiality.
3. Complies with the dress code.
4. Is positive in action and words toward the institution and respectful of fellow employees.
5. Performs special projects.
6. Receives commendations.
7. Provides orientation in services. Educates others regarding his area.
8. Provides advanced skills.
9. Is a leader in unit or zone.
10. Honors holiday commitments.
11. Proactively intervenes with RNs.
12. Participates in rounds and patient conferences.
13. Enhanced outcomes.
14. Exhibits professional conduct.
15. Consults with appropriate persons to develop patient care plans.
16. Volunteers for projects and action teams.
17. Serves as relief supervisor, submits abstracts and papers.

*SLEH: St. Luke's Episcopal Hospital, Houston, TX.

TABLE 2-5 **Evaluation of Performance Standards: Measurement**

Area of Evaluation	Measurement Tool	Component	Scale
Productivity	RCIS Reports Table 2-6	Effectiveness and efficiency are assessed by the manager or designee. Evaluated based on use of resources; takes responsibility for scheduled time; promptly receives report from off-going team members. Evaluation is performed on accompanying scale by statistical reports and observation when indicated.	Always exceeds = 20 Mostly exceeds = 15 Meets standards = 10 Usually meets = 5 Does not meet = 0
Attendance	Personnel T/A Records Table 2-6	Evaluation of attendance records. Based on the performance year.	0–1 occ = 20 2 occ = 15 3 occ = 10 4 occ = 5 >5 = 0
Punctuality	Personnel T/A Records Table 2-6	Evaluation of punctuality records. Based on the performance year.	0–2 occ = 20 3–5 = 15 6–9 = 10 10–19 = 5 >19 = 0
Safety and Infection Control	Reports— Safety Needle sticks Incident Infections Table 2-6	Effectiveness and efficiency are assessed by the manager or designee. Evaluated on performance of duties in a safe and professional manner. Evaluation is performed on the accompanying scale by statistical reports, chart review, and observation when indicated.	Always exceeds = 20 Mostly exceeds = 15 Meets standards = 10 Usually meets = 5 Does not meet = 0

(Tables 2-17 and 2-18). This approach provides a fair, consistent, and equitable system of performance and conduct policies. This requires employees to assume responsibility for their actions and to recognize and correct their deficiencies in knowledge and performance. Corrective action is based on the severity of the violation, the employee's past record, and previous actions taken for the same or similar offenses. Severity of the consequences is based on actual or potential harm to patients, other employees, or others in general. Repeated performance or conduct deficiencies are considered severe in nature. All departmental employees are to be covered by this policy, and it is to be consistent with institutional policy.

RESPIRATORY CARE AUTOMATION: THE RESPIRATORY CARE INFORMATION SYSTEM

New respiratory care information systems (RCISs) offer a variety of managerial, operational, and financial enhancements (Table 2-19). The RCISs are data-manage-

TABLE 2-6 **Evaluation of Performance Standards: Scoring**

Productivity	Attendance	Punctuality	RCIS	Safety and Infection Control
>96% = 20	0–1 occ* = 20	0–2 occ = 20	0 err† = 20	***Infection Control:*** demonstrates consistent compliance in the practice of universal precautions as determined by observation.
90%–95% = 15	2 occ = 15	3–5 occ = 15	1–2 err = 15	Complies with G-Force:
81%–89% = 10	3 occ = 10	6–9 occ = 10	3 err = 10	Gowns ____ Y ____ N ____ N/A
75%–80% = 5	4 occ = 5	10–19 occ = 5	4–5 err = 5	Gloves ____ Y ____ N ____ N/A
<75% = 0	>5 = 0	>19 = 0	>5 = 0	Goggles ____ Y ____ N ____ N/A
				Guards ____ Y ____ N ____ N/A
				Safety: accidents and incidents

*: occurrences
†: errors

TABLE 2-7 **Learning and Innovation Focus Standards: Measurement**

Area of Evaluation	Measurement Tool	Component	Scale	Score
Proficiency review: Areas of operation	Proficiency review Table 2-8	Demonstrates proficiency as outlined by proficiency standards for therapy modalities, oxygen, ventilatory management, physiologic monitoring, specialized procedures, age-specific competency, and general procedures. Fire, Safety, Infection Control, Hazardous Materials. Failure to complete this section results in "0" for entire section.	Always exceeds = 20 Mostly exceeds = 15 Meets standards = 10 Usually meets = 5 Does not meet = 0	
Self Evaluation and Goals	Performance Evaluation and Goals Table 2-8	Uses performance-appraisal program to assess performance, professionalism, and proficiency or competency. States employment and professional goals.	A = 20 B = 15 C = 10 D = 5 E = 0	
Continuous Quality Improvement	CQI Points Table 2-8	CQI reports submitted or action taken to address CQI issues.	Always exceeds = 20 Mostly exceeds = 15 Meets standards = 10 Usually meets = 5 Does not meet = 0	
Education and Council Participation	Education Records Table 2-8	Receive departmental education credits (DECs), contact hours for participation in education programs, HR training by the accompanying scale.	20 = >40 15 = 25–39 10 = 15–24 5 = 5–14 0 = <5	

ment systems that can generate work assignments, reports, bills, and audits, as well as automate clinical data collection, order processing, charge capturing, record keeping, and quality assurance functions. Other capabilities include inventory management, capital equipment tracking, personnel records management, personnel communications, and scheduling. Depending on a particular system's scope and the manipulative ability of its database software, these capabilities may be expanded or reduced. Success of new systems have been demonstrated by increases in charge capture and productivity. Because an RCIS can simplify the operations

TABLE 2-8 **Learning and Innovation Focus Standards: Scoring**

Proficiency and Competency	Self-Evaluation and Goals	CQI	In-Service or Orientation Participation DECs
See Table 2-9	**Evaluation** A = submits objective review with outstanding goals B = submits objective review with goals C = submits review D = submits review with deficiencies E = review not submitted **Goals** A = submits quality goals and achieves 100% completion B = submits quality goals and achieves 75% completion C = submits quality goals and achieves 50% completion D = submits goals and achieves completion E = goals not achieved	2 pt = working on Action Team to solve issue 1.01 pt = submitting CQI issue(s) with suggestion for improvement 1 pt = submitting operational issue(s) or CQI form	8 = ACLS class 8 = CPR instructor (certification) 4 = CPR instructor (recertification) 4 = length of in-service = in-service class instructor 2 = in-service attendance 2 = CPR class (recertification) 2 = teaching CPR class (limit 4 DECs) 1/hour = video tapes (limit 6 DECs) 1/hour = ACLS instructor hour (limit 4 DECs) 1 = council meeting attendance

TABLE 2-9 **Proficiency Review**

Therapy Modalities

HHN, IPPB, CPT, IS
- Demonstrate familiarity with medications, including new meds.
- Demonstrate how to calculate predicted volume and predicted percentage.

Oxygen Therapy

Aerosol
- Demonstrate proficiency by completing equipment proficiency check-off on setting up heated system and charting appropriate set-up dates on equipment.

Nonaerosol
- Demonstrate proficiency by completing equipment proficiency check-off on setting up nonrebreathing mask and charting appropriate set-up dates on equipment.

Ventilator Therapy

Adult
- Puritan-Bennett 7200
- O_2 monitor
- Fisher-Paykel heater
- Interpret ABG, if needed
- Vent change

Nasal CPAP
- Downs Flow Generator
- Fisher-Paykel heater
- Heated wire tubing
- Nasal mask with head straps
- Life Care Pressure Alarm
- Teledyne O_2 analyzer
- 60″ disposable large-bore tubing
- Main-stream bacteria filter
- Set up and explain

BiPAP
- BiPAP system with power cords
- Nasal mask with straps and whisper swivel
- Bore tubing
- Remote control unit and cable
- Set up and explain

Physiological Monitoring

ABG stick
- Complete ABG check-off
- MD approved

ABG line and IABG oximetry
- Demonstrate pulse oximeter set up

Capnography
- Demonstrate capnograph set up

$S\bar{v}O_2$ monitoring
- Demonstrate set up of $S\bar{v}O_2$ monitor and troubleshoot

Specialized Procedures

Transport
- N/A

CPR code blue
- BCLS = 10
- BCLS instructor = 15
- ACLS = 20

Assistance
- N/A

Bronch suctioning
- Demonstrate proper suctioning technique

ECG
- Demonstrate proper ECG technique

Venous puncture
- Demonstrate proper venous puncture technique

Tracheostomy care
- Demonstrate proper tracheostomy care technique

Age-Specific Competency

Infant

Adult
- CPR
- Infant oxyhood

General Procedures

Fire
- Hospital test

Safety
- Hospital test

Infection control
- Hospital test

Hazardous material
- Hospital test

of a respiratory care department, its selection warrants serious consideration. Such a purchase may represent the largest nonclinical capital expenditure of a respiratory care manager's career.

Selection Consideration

A system strategy should consider the following:

1. Replacing existing computer and non–computer systems
2. Selecting proven packages
3. Considering only financially stable vendors
4. Selecting computer solutions for all areas of the department
5. Evaluating leading vendors
6. Selecting and implementing systems
7. Allocating funds
8. Identifying implementation methods
9. Making realization of benefits a central element in the strategy

However, one-stop shopping threatens flexibility and competitive pricing. The department manager should formulate specific business objectives designed to de-

(text continues on page 46)

TABLE 2-10 **Operational Focus Standards**

Area of Evaluation	Measurement Tool	Component	Scale*	Score
Therapy modalities: HHN, IPPB, CPT, IS, USN, IPV	Table 2-11	Observation of administration of modalities by established guidelines. Random review of record(s) to evaluate against documentation standards.	Always exceeds	= 20
			Mostly exceeds	= 15
			Meets standards	= 10
			Usually meets	= 5
			Does not meet	= 0
Oxygen therapy: Nonaerosol and aerosol	Table 2-12	Observation of administration of modalities by established guidelines. Random review of record(s) to evaluate against documentation standards.	Always exceeds	= 20
			Mostly exceeds	= 15
			Meets standards	= 10
			Usually meets	= 5
			Does not meet	= 0
Ventilator management: adult, nasal CPAP, BiPAP	Table 2-13	Observation of administration of modalities by established guidelines. Random review of record(s) to evaluate against documentation standards.	Always exceeds	= 20
			Mostly exceeds	= 15
			Meets standards	= 10
			Usually meets	= 5
			Does not meet	= 0
Physiological monitoring: ABG stick, ABG line, oximetry, capnography, $S\bar{V}O_2$	Table 2-14	Observation of administration of modalities by established guidelines. Random review of record(s) to evaluate against documentation standards.	Always exceeds	= 20
			Mostly exceeds	= 15
			Meets standards	= 10
			Usually meets	= 5
			Does not meet	= 0
Specialized procedures: transport, CPR, assistance, bronchial suction, ECG, venous puncture, tracheostomy care, body mechanics and ambulation See Table 13F	Table 2-15	Observation of administration of modalities by established guidelines. Random review of record(s) to evaluate against documentation standards.	Always exceeds	= 20
			Mostly exceeds	= 15
			Meets standards	= 10
			Usually meets	= 5
			Does not meet	= 0

* See Performance Scoring Table—Performance issues will adjust scale.

TABLE 2-11 **Therapy Modalities**

Administration	Documentation
HHN	
1. Verify physician's orders. Read progress notes, checking patients overall status and physical condition before beginning therapy. 2. Be sure your name badge is readable. 3. Introduce yourself. 4. Check patient arm band. 5. Wash hands. 6. Assemble equipment and medication, and connect to appropriate gas source. 7. Patient education on procedure. 8. Monitor breath sounds and heart rate two times. 9. Cough procedure. 10. Return equipment to proper place and discard disposables. 11. Thank patient. 12. Document in RCIS.	Review of at least one record, to include a. Physician's orders checked b. Medication dosages c. Breath sounds, pretreatment d. Breath sounds, posttreatment e. Tolerated well, adverse reactions f. Cough with secretion production g. Heart rate, respiratory rate (2 each) h. Correct charges generated i. Correct equipment change-out schedule j. Patient education
IPPB	
1. Verify physician's orders. Read progress notes. 2. Be sure your name badge is readable. 3. Introduce yourself. 4. Check patient arm band. 5. Wash your hands. 6. Use IS to determine patient's inspiratory capacity. 7. Connect breathing circuit to IPPB machine and check for proper function before patient use. 8. Prepare equipment and medication. 9. Calculate the patient's predicted tidal volume. 10. Patient education. 11. Position the patient. 12. Monitor heart rate, respiratory rate, tidal volume, machine pressure two times. 13. Thank patient. 14. Document in RCIS.	Review of at least one record, to include a. Physician's orders checked b. Medication dosages c. Breath sounds, pretreatment d. Breath sounds, posttreatment e. Tolerated well, adverse reactions f. Cough with secretion production g. Inspiratory capacity measurements before therapy and % predicted. h. Volumes delivered/pressure given i. Heart rate, respiratory rate (2 each) j. Correct charges generated k. Correct equipment change-out schedule l. Patient education
CPT	
1. Verify physician's orders. Read progress notes, checking patient's overall status and physical condition before beginning therapy. 2. Be sure name badge is readable. 3. Introduce yourself. 4. Check patient arm band. 5. Wash your hands. 6. Continue supplemental oxygen when ordered during CPT. 7. Properly position patient. 8. Instruct the patient to deep breath and cough throughout and following the procedure. 9. Monitor heart rate, respiratory rate, two times. 10. Cough procedure, if applicable. 11. Return patient to proper position. 12. Thank patient. 13. Document in RCIS.	Review of at least one record to include a. Physician's orders checked b. Breath sounds, pretreatment c. Breath sounds, posttreatment d. Areas percussed e. Tolerated well, adverse reactions f. Cough with secretion production g. Heart rate, respiratory rate (2 each) h. Correct charges generated i. Patient education

(Continued)

TABLE 2-11 **Therapy Modalities**

Administration	Documentation
IS 1. Verify physician's order. 2. Be sure name badge is readable. 3. Introduce yourself. 4. Check patient arm band. 5. Wash your hands. 6. Put patients name on device. 7. Determine predicted inspiratory capacity. 8. Mark desired goal with marker on IS device. 9. Position patient. 10. Patient education. 11. Thank patient. 12. Document in RCIS.	Review of at least one record to include a. Physician's orders checked b. Predicted inspiratory capacities c. Observed inspiratory capacities d. Percent predicted capacities e. Cough with secretion production f. Heart rate, respiratory rate (1 only) g. Correct charges generated h. Patient education

TABLE 2-12 **Oxygen Therapy**

Procedure	Documentation
Aerosol 1. Verify physician's orders. Read progress notes, checking patient's overall status and physical condition before beginning therapy. 2. Be sure your name badge is readable. 3. Introduce yourself. 4. Check patient arm band. 5. Wash hands. 6. Assemble equipment and medication, and connect to appropriate gas source. 7. Patient education on procedure. 8. Monitor heart rate one time. 9. Return equipment to proper place and discard disposables. 10. Thank patient. 11. Document in RCIS.	Review of at least one record to include a. Physician's order checked b. Liter flow, FiO_2, and temperature (when applicable) c. Aerosol analyzed d. Oxygen in use or not in use e. SpO_2 chart code scanned with SpO_2 value on new starts f. Appropriate equipment charges g. Equipment change-out schedule followed h. Free text documentation for patients falling out of protocol i. Heart rate, respiratory rate (one time) on new starts
Nonaerosol 1. Verify physician's orders. Read progress notes, checking patient's overall status and physical condition before beginning therapy. 2. Be sure your name badge is readable. 3. Introduce yourself. 4. Check patient arm band. 5. Wash hands. 6. Assemble equipment and medication, and connect to appropriate gas source. 7. Patient education on procedure. 8. Monitor heart rate one time. 9. Return equipment to proper place and discard disposables. 10. Thank patient 11. Document in RCIS.	Review of at least one record to include a. Physician's order checked b. Liter flow and FiO_2 c. Oxygen in use or not in use d. SpO_2 chart code scanned with SpO_2 value on new starts e. Appropriate equipment charges f. Equipment change-out schedule followed g. Free text documentation for patients falling out of protocol h. Heart rate, respiratory rate (one time) on new starts

TABLE 2-13 **Ventilator Management**

Administration	Documentation
Adult Ventilation	
1. Pressure limits. 2. Set alarm limits. 3. Set apnea parameters. 4. Record on flowsheet. 5. Chest x-ray film and ABG.	Chart every 4 hours to include a. Addressograph b. Diagnosis c. Name and professional designation d. ABG and $S\bar{v}O_2$ data e. Noninvasive data f. Equipment changes g. Alarm settings h. Hemodynamic monitoring i. Pulmonary mechanics j. Assessment k. Cuff pressure or minimal occluding volume
Nasal CPAP via Downs Flow	
1. Connect large-bore tubing to Downs Flow Generator. 2. Connect opposite end of large-bore tubing to inlet part of FP humidification chamber. 3. Connect heated wire tubing to outlet of humidification chamber. 4. Connect pressure monitoring line from Life Care pressure alarm to nasal mask. 5. Adjust flow rate control and FIO_2. 6. Occlude mask and observe pressure manometer. 7. Adjust flow rate to achieve desired pressure. 8. Attach disposable bacteria filter to entrainment port. 9. Explain procedure to patient. 10. Place mask squarely over patient's nose and secure with head straps and check for air leaks.	1. Record the following parameters immediately after the initial setup: a. Heart rate b. Respiratory rate c. Blood pressure d. Breathing pattern e. SpO_2 f. Patient compliance g. LOC 2. After 1 hour, record above parameters every 2 hours. 3. Arterial and mixed venous blood samples should be obtained (if possible) after first hour of treatment. 4. Note any adverse reactions.
BiPAP–CPAP	
1. Attach patient circuit to unit. 2. Explain setup to patient and family. 3. Fit patient for mask and adjust head straps. 4. Check for air leaks. 5. Record settings on evaluation sheet.	Include IPAP and EPAP.
BiPAP for Assisted Ventilation	
1. Documented once per shift 2. IPAP and EPAP values 3. Mask sizes 4. O_2 bleed in 5. Reason used 6. Heart rate, respiratory rate, saturation	

termine the capabilities required and the feasibility of the proposed purchase. Once the need for an RCIS has been confirmed, approval should be sought from the administrative and medical staff. Finally, the hospital's information systems department should be consulted to help integrate the respiratory care department's specific requirements with the overall needs and objectives of the institution. These steps allow the respiratory care manager to compare available products and their capabilities and to formulate an initial opinion. No final decision should be made at this point. Such a decision should be made only after a variety of products have been extensively reviewed.

In the end, the purchaser must weigh the product's total benefits against its price. Financial justifications are contingent on a return on investment (ROI) analysis. Associated key factors are net present value (NPV) and internal rate of return (IRR). This information should demonstrate

TABLE 2-14 **Physiologic Monitoring**

Administration	Documentation
ABG Stick 1. Review patient's chart for physician's orders, medications, allergies, FIO_2. 2. Use universal precautions. 3. Introduce yourself. 4. Wash hands and put on gloves. 5. Identify patient by name and number. 6. Patient education. 7. Perform ABG sampling according to department standards. 8. Properly dispose of needle. 9. Properly label specimen. 10. Thank patient. 11. Transport blood to lab. 12. Document in RCIS.	Demonstrate proper documentation as defined by department documentation standards by a review of a minimum of one record, to include the following: a. Physician's order checked b. FIO_2 or liter flow c. Site of stick d. Allen's test performed e. Pressure held f. Pulse check after sample obtained g. Universal precautions followed h. Correct charges i. Lidocaine if used j. Patient education k. Free text if lidocaine not used
ABG Line or IABG 1. Review chart for order. 2. Use universal precautions. 3. Introduce yourself. 4. Wash hands and put on gloves. 5. Identify patient by name and number. 6. Assemble correct equipment. 7. Draw, flush, draw blood, flush line. 8. Check waveform. 9. Properly label specimen. 10. Thank patient. 11. Transport blood to lab. 12. Document in RCIS.	Demonstrate proper documentation as defined by department documentation standards by a review of five records, to include the following: a. Physician's order checked b. Universal precautions followed c. Condition of extremity and arterial cannula after procedure d. Calibration of IABG e. Sensor change out with IABG f. Correct charges
Oximetry 1. Check physician's orders. 2. Introduce yourself. 3. Wash hands. 4. Properly set up oximeter. 5. Vascularize and cleanse site. 6. Allow oximeter to stabilize. 7 Set alarms to no greater than 20% variance.	Demonstrate proper documentation as defined by department documentation standards by review of a minimum of 12 records, to include a. Patient assessment. b. FIO_2, flow rate, and any other oxygen enhancer devices. c. Any patient activity causing variation. d. Document in RCIS. e. Correct charges
Capnography Protocol currently used at this time is per physician's order as measured by QA monitor indicating appropriate alarm settings.	Demonstrate proper documentation as defined by department documentation standards by review of a minimum of 12 records, to include a. Physician's order checked b. Correct equipment charges c. End tidal CO_2 value
$S\bar{v}O_2$ Protocol used at this time includes demonstration of proper technique by measurement of QA monitor for insertion and post–in vivo calibration; 24-hr ± 2-hr daily calibration and correct light intensity; and use of universal precautions as measured by QA monitor.	Demonstrate proper documentation technique by completing the following items in the $S\bar{v}O_2$ notebook in the stat lab: a. Patient's name b. Room number c. Date and time d. Op Mod # e. Stored $S\bar{v}O_2$ f. Measured $S\bar{v}O_2$ g. Charting in RCIS h. Correct charges

TABLE 2-15 **Specialized Procedures**

Administration	Documentation
Transport	
Protocol used at this time is per physician's order.	Demonstrate proper documentation as defined by department documentation standards by review of a minimum of 12 records, to include a. Correct charging for transport b. Free text entry with correct time frames for transport.
CPR Code Blue	
Protocols used follow those standards set up by the American Heart Association or American Red Cross.	Demonstrate proper documentation as defined by department documentation standards by review of a minimum of 12 records, to include a. Correct charging for CPR b. Free text entry with correct time frames for CPR
Assistance	
Protocol used is according to SLEH Respiratory Care policy.	Demonstrate proper documentation as defined by department documentation standards by review of a minimum of 12 records, to include a. Correct charging for assistance b. Free text entry with correct time frames for assistance
Bronchial Suctioning	
Protocols used are those described in SLEH Respiratory Care policy and procedure 30200-03-0011.	Demonstrate documentation by the proper selection of modality as defined in department protocols as measured by review of a minimum of 12 records. a. Department protocols require suctioning within 1–2 hours after initiation of mechanical ventilation and at least every 4 hours afterward. b. Documentation on RCIS charting and ventilator flow sheet at least every 4 hours or explanation why it was not performed.
ECG	
Demonstrate assessment or interaction by ER protocols as measured by completion of ECGs within designated time frames.	Demonstrate proper documentation as defined by department documentation standards by review of 12 records.
Venous Puncture	
Protocols used at this time include demonstration of proper technique and use of universal precautions as measured by QA monitor.	Demonstrate proper documentation as defined by department documentation standards by review of 12 records.
Tracheostomy Care	
Protocols used at this time include demonstration of proper technique and use of universal precautions.	Minimum of one record to include a. Tracheostomy care performed b. RCIS documentation correct c. Charges correct
Body Mechanics	
Demonstrate proper body mechanics when standing, lifting, and transferring patients.	Techniques to be reviewed include transferring a patient from bed to stretcher, chair, or wheel chair and back again.

the potential positive impact of an RCIS. A conservative strategy would include the demonstration of a 12-month system payback. Depending on available funding, the original requirements may be expanded or decreased.

This overview is intended to give the respiratory care manager basic knowledge regarding the purchase of an RCIS and to position the department to receive consideration for this funding. Although the major issues of selecting a system have been touched on, each department considering the purchase of a system should explore the issues in detail to make certain that individual requirements will be met. After selecting and purchasing the RCIS, the respiratory care manager should also expect to deal with issues regarding installation, staff education, and staff acceptance.

Computerizing respiratory care records is no longer a managerial option; it is a necessity. If the institution is not converting to a computerized medical record with a respiratory component in the immediate future, the only decisions left for the respiratory care manager concern the scope of the RCIS's capabilities and the type of system that the department can afford. Though a homegrown system with limited capabilities can cost a great deal in human energy and time, it may be the only choice if funds are limited. If that is the case, the use of a single-station RCIS may be an immediate economical

TABLE 2-16 **Mathematical Model of a Weighted Performance Plan**

			CODE (RRT)	EMPLOYEE (John Doe)	FINANCIAL (0.00)	INNOVATION & LEARNING (0.00)	OPERATIONAL (0.00)	TOTAL (0.00)
Evaluation Division	**Division Wt.**	**Area of Evaluation**	**Area Wt.**	**Section**	**Section Wt.**	**Section Score**	**Section Total**	**Area Total**
Customer Focus	20.00%	Patient Satisfaction		Press Ganey	20%	0.00	0.00	0.00
		Customer Satisfaction		3rd Party Review	20%	0.00	0.00	
		Teamwork		Team Review	20%	0.00	0.00	
		Self-Directed Leadership		Leadership 1	40%	0.00	0.00	
		Self-Directed Leadership		Leadership 2	Bonus	0.00	0.00	
Financial Focus	20.00%	Financial		Productivity	25%	0.00	0.00	0.00
		Financial		Attendance	40%	0.00	0.00	
		Financial		Punctuality	10%	0.00	0.00	
		Financial		RCIS	15%	0.00	0.00	
		Financial		Safety & Infection Control	10%	0.00	0.00	
Innovation & Learning Focus	20.00%	Performance Enhancement		Proficiency	30%	0.00	0.00	0.00
		Self-Development		Self-Evaluation & Goals	30%	0.00	0.00	
		Performance Enhancement		CQI	20%	0.00	0.00	
		Education		Inservice & Councils	20%	0.00	0.00	
Operational Focus	40.00%	Therapeutic Modalities	10%	HNN	20%	0.00	0.00	0.00
				IPPB	20%	0.00	0.00	
				CPT	10%	0.00	0.00	
				IS	20%	0.00	0.00	
				IPV	20%	0.00	0.00	
				USN	10%	0.00	0.00	
		Oxygen Therapy	5%	Aerosol/Non-Aerosol	100%	0.00	0.00	0.00
		Ventilator Management	60%	Flowsheet	20%	0.00	0.00	0.00
				Weaning	40%	0.00	0.00	
				Troubleshooting/Quality	20%	0.00	0.00	
				BiPAP	20%	0.00	0.00	
		Physiologic Monitoring	15%	ABG-Stick	40%	0.00	0.00	0.00
				ABG-Line	0%	0.00	0.00	
				Oximetry	0%	0.00	0.00	
				Capnography	0%	0.00	0.00	
				$S\bar{v}O_2$	60%	0.00	0.00	
		Specialized Procedures	10%	Pacemakers	30%	0.00	0.00	
				CPR	20%	0.00	0.00	0.00
				Patient Education	20%	0.00	0.00	
				Tracheostomy Care	20%	0.00	0.00	
				Bronchial Suction	10%	0.00	0.00	
				Assistance	0%	0.00	0.00	
				EKG	0%	0.00	0.00	
				Transport	0%	0.00	0.00	
				Venous Puncture	0%	0.00	0.00	

Note: The four major areas of focus are weighted in proportion to importance of job function. The relationship of specific subareas to the major focus is also weighted to assure a balanced performance rating. This table is used in conjunction with the written standards and performance criteria.

TABLE 2-17 **Code of Performance**

Purpose

This policy provides a consistent approach to identifying violations of departmental performance standards and initiating appropriate corrective action, up to and including discharge of employees responsible for such violations.

Definitions

Certain performance violations ordinarily result in discharge or possible probation. They are

1. Performing duties outside of the department's scope of practice as identified in job description.
2. Performing assigned duties that seriously compromises a patient's well-being or causes a patient's demise. This includes performing care unsafely.
3. Any orders that do not fall within departmental policy and are considered unsafe practice of respiratory care must not be performed. The supervisor must be notified of the situation. If a practitioner is unsure of an order or unsure of proper equipment setup and chooses to perform therapy, he or she may be held completely responsible.
4. Serious compromise of patient's well-being as reflected in the nurses' notes, physician progress notes in the chart, written incident report, and personal observation.
5. Inappropriate use of equipment without proper supervisory notification that seriously compromises a patient's well-being or causes a patient's demise.

If negligence involves deficiency in equipment usage in ICU areas, then

1. The employee will be removed from ICU setting for either 1 month or the length of probation.
2. The employee must become proficient with the equipment as scheduled by the supervisor.
3. The employee will be checked off on the equipment by clinicians and supervisors before returning to the ICU area.
4. If practitioner cannot function according to the job description, he or she may have a position reassignment.

These steps are followed in addition to the written counseling or probation. If negligence involves deficiency in equipment usage in the acute care areas, then

1. The employee must become proficient with the equipment as scheduled by the supervisor.
2. The employee will be checked off on the equipment by clinicians and supervisors before working with that equipment.
3. If a practitioner cannot function according to the job description, he or she may have a position reassignment.

Certain performance violations ordinarily result in probation or discharge:

1. Continued repeat violations that are in conflict with departmental policy and procedure.

Certain performance violations ordinarily result in written counseling or probation, depending on prior performance record and severity of violation:

1. A repeat violation that an employee had previously made, preceded with a verbal counseling.
2. Performing job duties as identified by the department's scope of practice for which the employee is not qualified.
3. Administering job duties that harm a patient.

Certain performance violations ordinarily result in a verbal counseling depending on severity of violation:

1. Not completing job duties as assigned.
2. Inappropriate use of equipment without proper supervisory notification with no potential harm to a patient.
3. Failure to complete appropriate departmental paperwork as assigned.

solution. On the other hand, if funds are available, a multistation RCIS may be the investment of choice, a choice that will pay future financial and operational dividends.[108]

THE RESPIRATORY CARE REPORT CARD

Appropriateness, Effectiveness, and Efficiency

Reengineering the health care system requires validation of appropriateness, effectiveness (quality), and efficiency (cost) of the changes. The method used to evaluate these outcomes includes the formation of value indicators, benchmarking, and outcomes research.[109,110] The coordination of patient intervention is performed by structured care-management programs. Understanding how reengineering, outcomes measurement, and care-management programs interact with respiratory care is essential for our profession.

□ CARE MANAGEMENT

Component-, outcomes-, case-, demand-, and disease-management are all care-management programs. Respiratory care and other professions historically have flourished in the environment of *component management,* which refers to the uncoordinated treatment of disease episodically with little incentive to treat the entire disease.

Health care reforms of the 1990s have been attempts to minimize costs while maintaining quality by instituting outcomes management. *Outcomes management* is the use of outcomes-assessment information to enhance clinical, financial, and quality outcomes through integration of exemplary practice and services. Outcomes management denotes the commitment to the pursuit of quality in a select population of patients during an acute disease phase.[111] This can be considered an expansion of *case-management* programs that had been developed and implemented in many health care facilities to manage individual patient cases.[112]

In comparison, *demand management* is a triage of services that reduces the need for and use of costly, often unnecessary, medical services, as well as arbitrary managed-care interventions, while enhancing the status of a defined population.[113,114]

Disease management "is a comprehensive, integrated approach to care reimbursement and reimbursement based on the natural course of a disease with treatment designed to address the illness by maximizing the effectiveness and efficiency of care delivered. The emphasis is on preventing the disease and/or managing it aggressively where intervention will have the greatest

TABLE 2-18 **Code of Conduct**

Purpose

This policy provides a consistent approach to identifying violations of departmental conduct standards and initiating appropriate corrective action, up to and including discharge of employees responsible for such violations. Corrective action is to be based on the severity of violation and the employee's past record and previous actions taken for same or similar offense.

Definitions

Certain conduct violations ordinarily result in a verbal counseling, depending on severity of violation.

1. Violation of hospital or departmental dress code or identification badge policy, including failure to wear badge.
2. Parking in an unauthorized area at any hospital location, if so posted.
3. Less than acceptable personal hygiene (conditions or practices not conducive to health) or grooming (neat and attractive).
4. Inappropriate conduct, which results in unprofessional display.
5. Four occasions of absences under the departmental time and attendance policy. (See Points Statement.)
6. Ten occasions of tardiness according to the departmental policy and procedure manual.
7. Five occasions of not badging on time clock.

Certain conduct violations ordinarily result in written counseling or probation.

1. Acceptance of gifts or gratuities from patients or any other person for personal use in excess of nominal amount.
2. Acceptance of cash in any amount from patients or any other person.
3. Unauthorized solicitation of cash, gifts, or gratuities from patients or any other person for any reason.
4. Unauthorized solicitation for any cause or product.
5. Professional misconduct, or inappropriate behavior resulting in negative consequences to an individual, institution, or others.
6. Unauthorized distribution of literature at any hospital location during working hours or in patient care areas at any time.
7. Misuse of hospital bulletin boards or tampering with hospital communication or information systems. All posting requires supervisory approval.
8. Violation of fire, health, sanitation, safety, or security regulations or practices.
9. Taking rest breaks, taking lunch breaks, eating, or drinking in hospital lobbies or other unauthorized areas.
10. Smoking in nondesignated areas on hospital premises.
11. Overstaying rest breaks or performing non-work-related activities on work time.
12. Unauthorized use of hospital property.
13. Six occasions of absences accumulated under the departmental time and attendance policy.
14. Fifteen occasions of tardiness according to the departmental policy and procedure manual.
15. Failure to report absence according to established departmental time limitations.
16. Six occurrences of not badging in.
17. Failure to renew state department of health certificate to practice respiratory care on expiration.

Certain conduct violations ordinarily result in probation or discharge, depending on prior conduct record and severity of offense.

1. Insubordination.
2. Refusal to accept assigned work or perform assigned tasks.
3. Leaving work area without permission or relief, or being in an unauthorized area.
4. Leaving assigned work area without permission or relief, except in emergency situations.
5. Illegal gambling in any form at any hospital location.
6. Sleeping while on duty or if in public view at any time.
7. Any willful violation of professional, technical practices or ethics.
8. Gross professional misconduct, or intentional wrongdoing and improper behavior, including degrading misconduct among peers.
9. Calling in sick and working in another institution while being paid for sick leave.
10. Refusal to accept work assignments or work areas.
11. Seven occasions of absences accumulated under the hospital time and attendance policy (see Points Statement).
12. Twenty occasions of tardiness according to the department policy and procedure manual.
13. Seven occasions of not badging in.

Certain conduct violations ordinarily result in discharge or possibly probation.

1. Willful destruction, abuse, or neglect of hospital property.
2. Indecent, immoral, or violent conduct including threat to do bodily harm to another or horseplay that could result in injury to patients, visitors, or other employees.
3. Sexual harassment complaints must be according to policy and referred to employee relations.
4. Possession, use, or sale of firearms, or dangerous weapons or devices (on hospital property).
5. Illegal possession, use, or unauthorized sale of alcohol, narcotics, hallucinogens, or any medication, or the appearance for work obviously under the influence of any of the foregoing.
6. Patient abandonment and physical or psychological negligence of patients.
7. Failure to report assigned duties that seriously compromise a patient's well-being or causes a patient's demise.
8. Any orders that do not fall within departmental policy are considered unsafe practice of respiratory care.
9. Unauthorized possession of hospital property or the property of patients, guests, or other employees, or an accessory to the unauthorized possession of the aforementioned property.
10. Falsification or misrepresentation of employment application or other work records or documents.
11. Badging another employee's badge on the time clock or allowing one's own badge to be badged on the time clock.
12. Eight occurrences of not badging in.
13. Unauthorized disclosure of any confidential patient information to anyone at any time.
14. Eight occasions of absences accumulated according to hospital time and attendance policy. Non-full-time staff will be governed in accordance with this policy.
15. Twenty-one occasions of tardiness according to the department policy and procedure manual.
16. Violations that include unauthorized access to the respiratory care information system (RCIS), network, or hospital information system(s) as defined by the RCIS and network security policy.

TABLE 2-19 **RCIS Enhancements**

Type of Enhancement	System Capabilities
Managerial	Productivity analysis and reporting
	Employee scheduling
	Patient order and treatment history
	Complete audit trail
	Cost vs revenue analysis
	Cost analysis
	Order list by subject
	Interface to spreadsheets and databases
Operational	Data entry with handheld computers
	Complete order tracking
	Automated computer-assessed charting
	Charge capture and compilation
	Accurate data input
	Work-load forecasting and estimates
Financial	Increased charge and revenue capture
	Decreased missed treatments
	Documentation and charge matching

impact."[115] The basic component of a disease-management program is to understand the disease's natural course and its cost drivers. Disease mapping outlines a realistic model of the disease and interventions based on the disease process, and it is often called critical pathway or clinical pathway development.

Care management is used to manage the pulmonary patient population in the 1990s because of the following:[116]

1. The high resource consumption in acute and chronic pulmonary exacerbations.
2. The chronic nature of many pulmonary problems (eg, asthma, chronic obstructive pulmonary disease, and cystic fibrosis).
3. The opportunity to stress prevention and education in managing pulmonary populations.

Pulmonary Care Management

A goal of care management is to standardize care. The tools of standardization are protocols, algorithms, medical guidelines, standing orders, and pathways. The combination of these tools optimizes care-management goals. A favorite instrument of care, and of outcomes management specifically, is the *critical pathway,* which maps the care of patients with specific DRGs (Fig. 2-5). This critical pathway is based on practice patterns within that organization, and continual analysis of objectives and variances transforms this pathway to an optimal path for that institution. The path may be based on a calculated length of stay (LOS) or phases of intervention based on physiologic status. Typical path components are consultation, diagnostic testing, treatments, interventions, activities, nutrition, teaching, DRG-specific information or outcomes, and discharge planning. The evaluative component of outcomes management is analyzing patient stays for variances that may result in inappropriate use of services and increased length of stays. Use of clinical pathways has increased cost efficiency, improved patient care, and decreased length of stay.[117–120] When appropriate, the integration of therapist-driven protocols (TDPs) formulated from the AARC Clinical Practice Guidelines[121–128] (Box 2-4) are included in clinical pathways for effective and efficient use of respiratory care resources.

The essential elements of the Clinical Practice Guidelines are therapeutic objectives, indications for therapy, and outcome criteria. A TDP based on these guidelines may include patient assessment, ordering procedures, and adjusting and discontinuing treatments on an ongoing basis. In addition, protocols provide physicians and nurses with valuable teaching tools and frequently make the therapist's jobs more interesting. Measurement of outcomes associated with the protocols, such as cost savings without increase in complications, quantifies the effectiveness of the protocol.[129–132] The use of protocols can reduce inappropriate therapy and improve effectiveness of care.[133–135] Successful implementation of TDPs is contingent on strong medical direction, physician support, and administrative and nursing support. The staff must be convinced of the need for protocols. Programs should start small and create respiratory care protocol committees to build staff confidence with continual reinforcement.[136] It is important not to look at TDPs and Clinical Practice Guidelines as independent tools, but as complements to care-management clinical pathways that enhance standardization of patient care.

□ PULMONARY OUTCOMES MANAGEMENT

The initiation of pulmonary outcomes management (POM) programs can result in fiscally manageable hospital stays, early family and patient education, data collection on incidence of complications and use of practice modalities, and improved collaboration with health care professionals who are essential to a positive patient outcome. The goals of POM are an expected patient outcome, appropriate length of stay and use of resources, collaborative practice, continuity of care, consumer satisfaction, staff development, and evidence-based practice. The success of these programs is contingent on medical staff acceptance. Communication and involvement are essential and can be accomplished by a medical staff leader and a physician advisory board. Collaborative practice teams create a seamless system of health care services for the benefit of patients. A collaborative practice team includes medical staff, nursing, physical therapy, nutrition, respiratory therapy, social work, finance, utilization management, and pharmacy. The key to collaboration is clinical competence, credibility, consistency, assertive-

Diagnosis: COPD

DRG:88

Addressograph

DATE	Admit Day	Day 1	Day 2	Day 3
CONSULTS				
DIAGNOSTIC				
TREATMENTS	• Protocol-Driven Respiratory Treatments • O_2 prn • CPT (prn) • Bronchodilators →			
INTERVENTIONS				
ACTIVITY				
NUTRITION				
TEACHING				
D/C PLANNING/ TEACHING				
OUTCOMES				

FIGURE 2-5. A clinical pathway for DAG 88: chronic obstructive pulmonary disease. Note that Therapist-Driven Protocols (TDPs) are imbedded in the clinical pathway. The assumption is made that, from a respiratory care standpoint, TDPs will ensure that appropriate therapy is always given in a timely manner.

BOX 2-4

AARC CLINICAL PRACTICE GUIDELINES

CPG1—Spirometry
CPG2—Oxygen Therapy in the Acute Care Hospital
CPG3—Nasotracheal Suctioning
CPG4—Patient-Ventilator System Checks
CPG5—Directed Cough
CPG6—In Vitro pH and Blood Gas Analysis and Hemoximetry
CPG7—Positive Airway Pressure and Bronchial Hygiene Therapy
CPG8—Sampling of Arterial Blood Gas Analysis
CPG9—Endotracheal Suctioning and Mechanical Ventilation of Adults and Children With Artificial Airways
CPG10—Incentive Spirometry
CPG11—Postural Drainage Therapy
CPG12—Bronchial Provocation
CPG13—Selection of Aerosol Delivery Device
CPG14—Pulse Oximetry
CPG15—Single-Breath CO Diffusing Capacity
CPG16—Oxygen Therapy at Home and in the Extended Care Facility
CPG17—Exercise Testing and Hypoxemia and/or Desaturation
CPG18—Humidification During Mechanical Ventilation
CPG19—Transport of the Mechanically Ventilated Patient
CPG20—Resuscitation in Acute Care Hospitals
CPG21—Bland Aerosol Administration
CPG22—Fiberoptic Bronchoscopy Assisting
CPG23—Intermittent Positive Pressure Breathing (IPPB)
CPG24—Application of CPAP in Neonates With Nasal Prongs
CPG25—Delivery of Aerosols to the Upper Airway
CPG26—Neonatal Time-Triggered, Pressure-Limited, Time-Cycled Mechanical Ventilation
CPG27—Static Lung Volumes
CPG28—Surfactant Replacement Therapy
CPG29—Ventilator Circuit Change
CPG30—Metabolic Measurement and Indirect Calorimetry During Mechanical Ventilation
CPG31—Transcutaneous Blood Gas Monitoring of Neonatal and Pediatric Patients
CPG32—Body Plethysmography
CPG33—Capillary Blood Gas Sampling in Neonatal and Pediatric Patients

ness, and timely decision making. Specific DRGs that impact cost reduction should be analyzed and selected to be included in the POM. There are ideal respiratory-related DRG categories for pulmonary outcomes management (Box 2-5). This list varies between institutions, but DRGs 483, 475, and 88 are good initial candidates.

□ RESPIRATORY DISEASE MANAGEMENT

Disease management is a systems-wide approach of caring for patients throughout the entire course of their disease. Strategies to implement a disease-management program are use of a data-driven approach; focus on a few areas that drive quality and cost from a system-wide perspective; and initiation of physician-care guidelines and customized delivery-system platforms to address issues, giving physicians the opportunity to affect the system design. The objective of disease management is to understand the disease's natural course and its cost drivers. The steps to initiating a disease-management program are as follows:[137]

1. Identification of the appropriate disease areas to improve.
2. Determination of baseline clinical practice patterns.
3. Performing an overall economic analysis of the disease under consideration.
4. Identification of key patients.
5. Identification of critical junctures that have an impact on quality and cost.
6. Creation of a comprehensive disease-management platform.
7. Deployment of the disease-management protocol throughout the organization.

The traditional clinical or care pathway has been used to manage the acute phase of a hospital stay. The disease-management pathways manage the respiratory populations using the entire integrated delivery system. The formation of a multidisciplinary pulmonary-outcomes team is essential to manage the acute disease process associated with pre- and posthospitalization issues and the chronic disease process. The collaborative goal with other health care professionals is to manage wellness of patients who are in a chronic disease state and maximize positive resolution of patients with acute illness. Patient populations that profit from

BOX 2-5

IDEAL DRGS FOR PULMONARY OUTCOMES MANAGEMENT

DRG	Description
079–081	Respiratory infection, inflammation
085	Pleural Effusion with CC
087	Pulmonary edema and respiratory failure
088	Chronic obstructive lung disease
094, 095	Pneumothorax
101, 102	Other respiratory system diagnosis
475	Respiratory system diagnosis with ventilator support
483	Tracheostomy (except for mouth, larynx disorder)

this approach are the asthmatic, chronic obstructive pulmonary disease, cystic fibrosis, and AIDS patient populations.

Understanding the natural course of the disease and the total system cost is essential for respiratory care professionals. Patient education and the need for compliance to improve treatment outcomes is extremely important in the disease management of chronic diseases. Patients are taught about their disease so they can recognize an exacerbation early on. Effectiveness and efficiency of these programs are measured by the quality of life and resource consumption of these patient populations.[137]

THE VALUE EQUATION AND BENCHMARKING

Documentation of valued outcomes is mandated by accrediting agencies (JCAHO), payers (Managed Care Organizations), and providers (integrated delivery systems). Although quality was advocated regardless of cost in the 1970s and 1980s, the changes of the 1990s often brought decreased cost without due regard to quality. Cost and quality must always be considered in tan-dem as value. The value (V) of health care delivery equates to the highest quality (Q) at the most appropriate cost ($):

$$V = Q/\$$$

Value indicators (VIs) measure the performance value of an organization's work unit or a profession's processes, procedures, products, and services.

Benchmarking, the comparison of these VIs with high-performing organizations, is performed by providers, payers, and consumers. The goal of benchmarking is to identify outstanding performance regarding cost-effectiveness, quality of life, and best practices in relation to patient interventions.[138–142] Selection of VIs is an essential part of measuring and evaluating both cost and quality aspects of service, and these value indicators must be pertinent and representative of optimal performance of patient interventions. Relative value indicators for respiratory care are represented in Box 2-6.

The Quality Numerator in the Equation

Adverse events and poor-quality work cause decreased value by increasing costs.[143–146] Health care systems focus on quality to reduce costs associated with poor quality. The improvement of quality is accomplished by identifying an expected outcome, determining the process, measuring the outcome, and acting on the measurement. Quality measures for respiratory care should be related to the areas of service, quality of life, and outcomes of interventions.[147–152]

BOX 2-6

RESPIRATORY CARE REPORT CARD VALUE INDICATORS

Direct Pulmonary Care Outcomes

- Adverse Reaction to Care
  - Ventilation associated pneumonias (VAP)
  - Adverse reactions to medication
- Positive Reaction to Care
  - Improved bronchospasm
  - Decreased atelectasis
  - Decreased length of intubation (LOI)
  - Improved blood gases
  - Decreased mortality & morbidity
- Improvement of Signs and Symptoms
  - Decreased shortness of breath
  - Decreased wheezing
- Improvement of Functional Status and Well-being
  - Impact of a pulmonary rehab program
    - Ability to climb stairs
    - Function with minimal supplemental oxygen

Indirect Pulmonary Care Outcomes

- Patient Satisfaction
  - Increased satisfaction feedback
- Cost of care
  - Cost/admission
  - Length of stay (LOS)
- Revenue Optimization
  - Profitability of pulmonary product line and/or DRG

The Financial Denominator in the Equation

The components that affect this factor of value are those of "cost": productivity, time, and fiscal-performance management.

☐ PRODUCTIVITY MANAGEMENT

Workload measurement is a way to measure performance of an individual or team within a work unit. This type of performance management measures productivity. The *AARC Uniform Reporting Manual*[153] offers a wide range of work standards that are used in productivity measurement. Historically, we have thought of productivity as a measurement of how much work a person did in a time period. Productivity can be categorized into direct, indirect, and non–patient care. Direct, actually administering care (giving a treatment); indirect, performing duties that support patient care (assembling equipment); and non-patient care (breaks, meetings, shift report). Time values were established for direct, indirect, and non-patient care activities. These values are multiplied by the number of activities an individual did in a day, and productivity is calculated. For example, if a treatment took 15 minutes and if an individual did 28 treatments, he or she would have done 7 hours of work; if the same individual spent 1 hour at shift report, breaks, and lunch; he would be 100% productive in an 8-hour shift ((7 + 1)/8 = 100%). This is a relatively simplistic example of how many managers have thought of productivity; it is only one of many aspects that must be taken into account when we think of productivity. Another might be the use of timelines within a department as a useful tool in managing productivity. A timeline for a department is equivalent to a day planner for individuals, which is used to maximize efficiency during the day.

TABLE 2-20 **Relationships Between Unit of Service (Adjusted Admissions) and Revenue, Total Cost, Personnel Cost, and Medical Supply Cost**

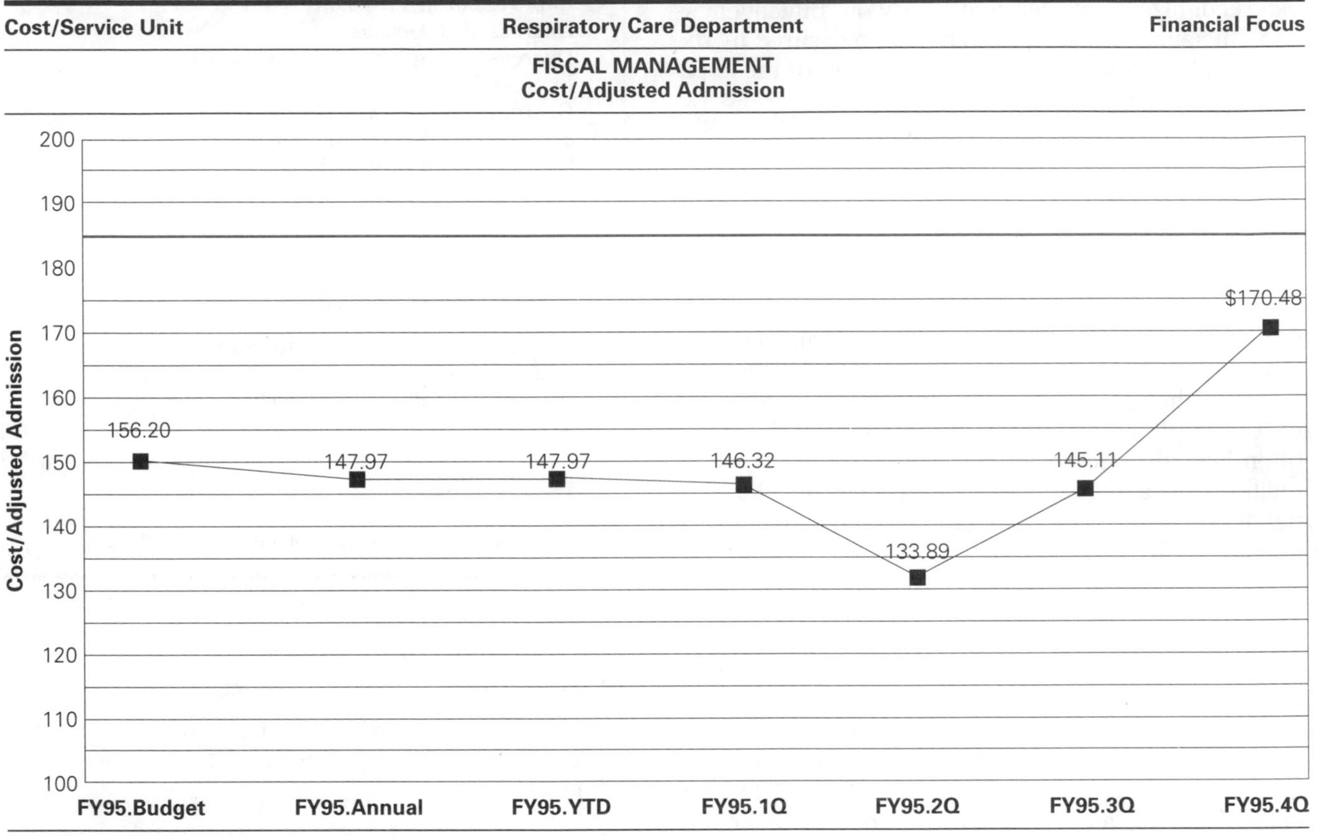

Period: 12

Admissions-Adjusted	FY95 Budget	FY95 Annual	FY95 YTD	FY95 1Q	FY95 2Q	FY95 3Q	FY95 4Q
Total Units	18,000	18,000	18,000	4,000	6,000	5,000	3,000
Gross Revenues	$18,000,000	$18,000,000	$18,000,000	$4,000,000	$6,000,000	$5,000,000	$3,000,000
Revenue/Unit	$1,000.00	$1,000.00	$1,000.00	$1,000.00	$1,000.00	$1,000.00	$1,000.00
Total Expenses	$2,703,615	$2,663,389	$2,663,389	$585,261	$803,343	$725,564	$511,435
% of Gross Revenues	15.02%	14.80%	14.80%	14.63%	13.39%	14.51%	17.05%
Expense/Unit	$150.20	$147.97	$147.97	$146.32	$133.89	$146.11	$170.48
FTEs	50.00	50.50	50.50	48.00	53.00	51.00	50.00
Salaries & Wages & Benefits	$2,022,414	$1,952,655	$1,952,655	$434,680	$583,198	$535,220	$371,701
S&W&B/FTE	$40,448	$38,566	$26,584	$47,811	$47,942	$47,496	$48,310
Wages/FTE	$30,336	$38,888	$38,888	$36,219	$38,510	$115,114	$116,482
Benefits/FTE	$10,112	$9,289	$9,289	$9,592	$9,432	$27,375	$28,449
Wages/Unit	$112.36	$108.48	$108.48	$108.57	$97.20	$107.04	$123.90
Med/Surg. Supplies	$343,856	$341,006	$341,006	$75,433	$111,805	$75,807	$71,121
Supplies/Unit	$19.10	$18.94	$18.94	$18.86	$18.60	$15.16	$28.71

Note: Additional units of service are Patient Days or discharges.

□ TIME MANAGEMENT

Time-management components include attendance, punctuality, scheduling, vacation planning, required overtime (ROT), and required time off (RTO). Absenteeism and tardiness are silent thieves of resources. Hidden costs of absenteeism include downtime, quality issues, missed procedures, overtime, and morale problems.

Attendance must be monitored, and policies must outline corrective action associated with attendance abuse. Although this may vary from institution to institution, there are, unfortunately, attendance abusers in all situations. Most people at a supervisory or managerial level have experienced the negative effects of attendance abuses, or "calling in," within a given work area. A similar situation applies to punctuality problems.

There should be clear-cut policies on scheduling that alert staff members to what the rules are before requesting time off, including both vacation and holiday planning. It is very important for staff members to understand the policies and limits regarding scheduling. In the future, it will also be essential for organizations to flex staff up or down in ensuring appropriate staffing levels at any one time. PRN pools, per diem employees, and part-time employees will become more popular in the future, but guidelines for required overtime, as opposed to required time off, must be stated by the department manager. This will enable the department to flex upward and downward based on workloads. The cry in the 1990s is to do more with less and to optimize resources. Thus, good time-management policies and procedures are essential to the efficiency and success of the respiratory department.

□ FISCAL PERFORMANCE MEASUREMENTS

Historically, respiratory care departments have been revenue centers within their organizations. Prospective payment, managed care, and capitation are transposing all areas of care provision into cost centers. Thus, concurrent monitoring of service costs needs to occur and to be related to an institutional measure such as admissions and discharges. An understandable reporting format that quantifies the efficiency of service provided can enhance communication and understanding of total, personnel, and supply costs (Table 2-20).

CONCLUSION

The changing environment of health care will alter the way respiratory care will be provided. In this chapter, the forces that are the catalyst for this change and strategies that health care will employ to adapt to this changing environment have been outlined. Respiratory care has weathered troubled times in the past because of its adaptability, flexibility, and commitment to the customers it serves.[154–161] The value of RCPs and the service they provide is being displayed in the continuum of care. The profession has demonstrated leadership in acute care, critical care, post–acute care, home health, physician offices, diagnostic and sleep labs, care management, rehabilitation, manufacturing, and management settings.[162–167] The future of RCPs is projected to be excellent if they meet the challenge of change.[168,169]

Breakthrough thinking has been illustrated in the profession's use of automation, with respiratory care information systems and technology advances.[170–173] Departments and practitioners have demonstrated clinical creativity, which has resulted in effective cost and quality outcomes provided by respiratory care.[174–187] The current mission of respiratory leaders (managers, practitioners, educators, medical directors, and the AARC) is to provide and promote customer-focused patient care by practicing respiratory care in the continuum.[188–190] This will champion members of the profession as a viable solution in this changing health care environment.

BIBLIOGRAPHY

1. Congressional Budget Office Report July 26, 1993: Commerce Department as reported in Fortune, May 17, 1993
2. Houston employers form group purchasing co-op. Integrated Health Care Delivery Systems 1(9):1–2, 1994
3. The Governance Committee: The states: Laboratories of federal reform. Washington, DC, Advisory Board Company
4. HHS questions adequacy of TennCare capitation rates, provider networks & start date. Health Care Reform Week 23(42):1–2, 1994
5. Goldstein, DE: The driving forces for change. In: Alliances: Strategies for building integrated delivery systems. Gaithersburg, MD: Aspen Publishers, Inc., 1995, pp 1–16
6. Bebiak, J: Streamline management to reduce costs and strengthen leadership. Strategies for Healthcare Excellence 7(7):8–9, 1994
7. Conger, JA: The brave new world of leadership training. Organizational Dynamics 21(3):46–58, 1993
8. American Productivity & Quality Center: Theory is nice, results are better. Spring 1994 Course Offerings Update
9. Pritchett, P, Pound, R: A Survival Guide–The Stress of Organizational Change. Dallas: Pritchett & Associates, 1995
10. Morrall, K: Employee stress pinches hospitals on the bottom line. UHS Today 10(5):3–4, 1994
11. Covey, SR: The Seven Habits of Highly Effective People: Restoring the Character Ethic. New York: Simon and Schuster, 1989
12. Coile, RC Jr.: Transformation of American healthcare in the post-reform era. Healthcare Executive 9(4):9–12, 1994
13. Coile, RC Jr.: Healthcare 1992: Top 10 trends for the health field. Hospital Strategy Report 4(3):1, 3–8, 1992
14. Coile, RC Jr.: Healthcare 1993: Top 10 trends for the era of health reform. Hospital Strategy Report 5(3):1–8, 1993
15. Coile, RC Jr.: Healthcare 1994: Top ten trends for the era of health reform. Hospital Strategy Report 6(3):1, 3–7, 1994
16. The National Report On Subacute Care: Moving up the reimbursement ladder to the land of risk and capitation. 3(22):3, 1995
17. Bartling, AC: Trends in managed care. Healthcare Executive 10(2):5–11, 1995
18. Coile, RC Jr.: Managed care outlook: "Alternative delivery systems" become dominant health plans. Hospital Strategy Report 4(4):1–8, 1992
19. Managed care glossary. Briefings on Subacute Care 2(4):9–10, 1995

20. Coile, RC Jr.: Managed care outlook 1995–2000: Top 10 trends for the HMO insurance industry. Health Trends 7(5):1, 3–8, 1995
21. Coile, RC Jr.: The five stages of managed care–organizing for capitation and health reform. Hospital Strategy Report 6(11):1–8, 1994
22. Coile, RC Jr.: The sixth stage of managed care: 10 new models for the post-reform era. Hospital Strategy Report 7(1):1–8, 1994
23. Coile, RC Jr.: Eight strategies for capitation. Hospital Strategy Report 6(12):4–8, 1994
24. Miller, MD, Remillard, SL: Preparing for managed care and capitation. In Alliances: Strategies for building integrated delivery systems. Gaithersburg, MD, Aspen Publishers, Inc., 1995, pp 39–71
25. Study: Doctors are making more money in managed care settings. Report on Physician Trends 2(10):304, 1994
26. Implications of managed Medicare. Competitive Insight 2(4):1, 66–68, 1995
27. Coile, RC Jr.: Nursing trends 1995–2000: Advanced practice nurses, case management, and patient-centered care. Health Trends 7(7):1&3, 1995
28. Hammer, M, Champy, J: Reengineering the Corporation–A Manifesto for Business Revolution. New York: Harper Business, 1993
29. Wachel, W: Reengineering . . . beyond incremental change. Healthcare Executive 9(4):17–21, 1994
30. Kennedy, M: Reengineering in healthcare. The Quality Letter for Healthcare Leaders 6(7):2–10, 1994
31. Knight, R: Reengineering: The business buzzword. Sky, January, 22–26, 1995
32. Keegan, AJ: Hospitals become cost centers in managed care scenario. Healthcare Financial Management 48(8):36–39, 1994
33. Traditional hospital medical staff structure may be "doomed." Hospital Peer Review 18(12):185–189, 1993
34. Coile, RC Jr.: Winners and losers under national health reform. Hospital Strategy Report 6(12):2–4, 1993
35. Coile, RC Jr.: Managed medicine: HMOs and managed care put physician incomes under the knife. Health Trends 7(8):1, 1995
36. Johnson, J: Hospital medical staffs: Next managed care casualty? American Medical News 37(39):1, 27–28, 1994
37. Anders, G: Nurses decry cost-cutting plan that uses aides to do more jobs. The Wall Street Journal, B7, Thursday, January 20, 1994
38. Rubbelke, KL: The outsourcing explosion. UHS Today 10(5): 1–2, 1994
39. Bills, SS: Is hospital administration dead? Healthcare Executive 9(6):8–11, 1994
40. Torrington, KG: Respiratory care in the 1990's: What will happen in an era of managed care. Clinical Pulmonary Medicine 2(2):1–6, 1995
41. Murphy, EC: Hospital downsizing has special risks: It may increase mortality. Collins & Company News Release 1–3, October 29, 1993
42. Rightsizing healthcare: What works, what doesn't, and why. Strategies for Healthcare Excellence 7(12):8–10, 1994
43. Deloitte & Touche: U.S. Hospitals and the Future of Health Care, A Continuing Opinion Survey, 5th ed. 1994
44. Kaufman, N: Competing in an integrated healthcare market: Four strategies for success. Healthcare Executive 10(3):18–22, 1995
45. Southwick, K: Culture of visible support for staff and customers underlies TQM gains at 302-bed Butler Memorial. Strategies for Healthcare Excellence 7(7):1–8, 1994
46. Weiss, GD: Implementing total quality management and reshaping delivery systems in a community hospital. Journal for Healthcare Quality 16(2):18–24, 1994
47. Goldstein, DE: A profile of an integrated delivery system. In Alliances: Strategies for building integrated delivery systems. Gaithersburg, MD, Aspen Publishers, Inc., 1995, 73–85
48. Bartling, AC: Integrated delivery systems: Fact or fiction. Healthcare Executive 10(3):7–11, 1995
49. Southwick, K: Putting the pieces in place for regional integration. Strategies for Healthcare Excellence 7(1):1–7, 1994
50. Beckham, JD: The longest wave. Healthcare Forum Journal 36(6):78–82, 1993
52. Griffith, JR: The infrastructure of integrated delivery systems. Healthcare Executive 10(3):12–17, 1995
53. Shortell, SM: Creating organized delivery systems: The barriers and facilitators. Hospital and Health Services Administration 38(4):447–466, 1993
54. Parkman, CA: Understanding the impact of healthcare job redesign. Allied Healthweek 2(13):8–9, 1995
55. Murphy, EC: The quality leader institute work redesign and patient focused restructuring in health care. E.C. Murphy, Ltd., Amherst, 1993.
56. Health Care Advisory Board: Hospital of the future volume I–Toward a twenty-first century hospital-redesigning patient care. Washington DC, The Advisory Board Company, 1992
57. Health Care Advisory Board: Executive report to the CEO–the merits of patient-focused care. Washington DC, The Advisory Board Company, 1992
58. Herrmann, J: Restructuring the healthcare delivery system. Health Systems Review 28(2):18–29, 1995
59. Curtin, LL: Restructuring: What works–and what does not! Nursing Management 25(10):7–8, 1994
60. Hammer, M: Reengineering work: Don't automate, obliterate. Harvard Business Review 68(4):104–112, 1990
61. Bazzoli, F: Designing a place for automation. Health Data Management 3(5):21–28, 1995
62. Clinical information systems enhance continuum of care. Healthcare Management Solutions 10(6):51–52, 1995
63. Dorenfest, S: 1995 & beyond: Stepping around the pitfalls. Healthcare Informatics 12(6):81, 1995
64. Dillon, C: Building an information bridge for integrated delivery systems. Healthcare Informatics 12(7):24, 1995
65. Coddington, DC, Pollard, J: Information systems and integrated healthcare: An essential partnership. Health Management Technology 16(8):38–40, 1995
66. Dick, RS, Andrew, WF: Point of care: An essential technology for the CPR. Healthcare Informatics 12(5):64–78, 1995
67. Hall, J: Midwest hospital selects point-of-care workstations. Healthcare Informatics 12(5):62, 1995
68. Grimm, BC: Wireless communications: Taking healthcare by storm. Healthcare Informatics 12(5):52–54, 1995
69. Understanding and implementing hospital information systems, Part I. ECRI Technology for Respiratory Therapy 15(10):1–7, 1995
70. Understanding and implementing hospital information systems, Part II. ECRI Technology for Respiratory Therapy 15(10):1–8, 1995
71. Tietsort, J, De Marco, FJ: Developing a respiratory care product line. AARC Times 15(5):81–84, 1991
72. Crowley, TP, Rosen, NA, Sabo, JS, Alexander, GD: Audit review and cost containment results of a continuous unit assignment plan in respiratory care. Respiratory Care 24(12):A1199–1200, 1979
73. Scott, F: Doing it right—by getting involved, medical directors can steer departments toward success. Advance for Managers of Respiratory Care 4(8):25–27, 1995
74. The American Association for Respiratory Care: Year 2001: Delineating the educational direction for the future respiratory care practitioner–proceedings of a national education consensus conference on respiratory care education. Dallas, October 2–4, 1992
74a. Giordano SP: The future of respiratory care. Presented at The Future of Respiratory Care Meeting. San Antonio, May 24, 1996
75. Bronson, JG: Hyperbaric therapy: An expanding specialty for RCPs. RT–The Journal for Respiratory Care Practitioners 8(4):39–44, 1995
76. Anderson, C: Hearts and lungs–they work together, but there are big differences in managing a cardiopulmonary and a respiratory care department. Advance for Managers of Respiratory Care 4(5):38–48, 1995

77. Scheffler, S: Mission impossible: Is your mission statement in a state of emergency? Continuous Journey 2(6):30–32, 1994
78. Sharke, G: Playing flat. Holland & Davis Inc. Management Consulting Services—The Management Edge 2, Summer 1995
79. Kerfoot, K: Beyond collaboration: Developing collegial relationships with physicians and other health care professionals. Aspen's Advisor for Nurse Executives 5(10):5–7, 1990
80. Kerfoot, K: From shared governance in nursing to integrated patient care teams. Aspen's Advisor for Nurse Executives 7(1):4–6, 1991
81. Home health care offers patient savings, better quality of life. Managing integration & operation: A guide to quality health care systems 1(5):8, 1995
82. HHS subacute study reports huge savings. Briefings on Subacute Care 2(5):11, 1995
83. Stahl, DA: Subacute care: The future of healthcare. Nursing Management 25(10):34–40, 1994
84. Determining the financial viability of a subacute unit. National Report on Subacute Care 3(9):1–2, 1995
85. Hulet, D, Axene, D: Strategic use of home care services may lower costs system-wide. Managing Integration & Operations: A Guide to Quality Health Care Systems 1(6):1–2, 8, 1995
86. Coile, RC Jr.: Age wave: Organizing integrated care networks for an aging society. Health Trends 7(6):1–8, 1995
87. Cornish, K: Subacute care offers opportunities for RCPs. AARC Times 19(2):22–27, 1995
88. Madigan, PA: The role of corporate marketing at Mariner health care. Presented at Emerging Issues in Subacute Care meeting. Philadelphia, March 9, 1995
89. Thompson, RE: Ventilator management in subacute care. Advance for Managers of Respiratory Care 4(1):20–23, 1995
90. The Gallup Organization and the American Association for Respiratory Care (AARC): A study of chronic ventilator patients in the hospital. Dallas, 1991
91. Criner, GJ, Kreimer, DT: Chronic ventilation. Advance for Managers of Respiratory Care 4(3):21–25, 1994
92. Villa, B: Subacute care centers. Advance for Managers of Respiratory Care 4(2):10–15, 1994
93. Daus, C: RCPs forge new ground in subacute care. RT–The Journal for Respiratory Care Practitioners 8(3):87–88, 1995
94. Anderson, G, Rivera, R: Building top notch subacute teams. Advance for Managers of Respiratory Care 4(3):47–48, 53, 1995
95. Remington, L: 1995 home care predictions and beyond. The Remington Report 3(1):20–23, 1995
96. O'Donnell, KP, Sampson, EM: Home healthcare: The pivotal link in the creation of a new healthcare delivery system. Journal of Health Care Finance 21(2):74–86, 1994
97. Respiratory home health care: A viable option to acute care. Healthcare Management Solutions 10(5):44, 1995
98. Pritchett, P: New work habits for a radically changing world. Dallas, Pritchett & Associates, 1993
99. Murphy, EC: The work image of health care. In The Quality Leader Institute: Work redesign and patient-focused restructuring in health care
100. Thompson, RE: Ventilator management in subacute care. Advance for Managers of Respiratory Care 4(1):20–23, 1995
101. Shrake, K: RCPs and health reform: Demonstrating value, creating opportunity. Respiratory Care 40(2):162–170, 1995
102. Schaffer, S: Demand better results–and get them. Harvard Business Review 69(2):142–149, 1991
103. Milliman, JF, Zawacki, RA, Norman, C, Powell, L, Kirksey, J: Companies evaluate employees from all perspectives. Personnel Journal 99–103, November 1994
104. Zigon, J: Making performance appraisal work for teams. Training Magazine 31(6):58–63, 1994
105. Kaplan, RS, Norton, DP: The balanced scorecard. Harvard Business Review 70(1):71–79, 1992
106. Kaplan, RS, Norton, DP: Putting the balanced scorecard to work. Harvard Business Review 71(5):134–147, 1993
107. Wegmiller, DC: A fresh approach to compensation can lead to a new tool for managing costs. Health Management Quarterly 16(3):21–23, 1994
108. Sabo, JS: The respiratory care information systems guide. AARC Times 16(12):59–64, 1992
109. Burke, G: Healthcare delivery in the 21st century. Health Systems Review 25(2):36–40, 1995
110. Jaklevic, MC: Hospitals tout data with report cards. Modern healthcare 25(19):68, 1995
111. Luquire, R: St. Luke's Episcopal Hospital practices outcomes management. AARC Times 17(7):62–64, 1993
112. Barrett, M: Case management a must to survive managed care. Computers in Healthcare 22–25, June 1993
113. Montrose, G: Demand management may help stem costs. Health Management Technology 16(2):18–21, 1995
114. Croner, G: Can demand management be quantified? Outcomes Measurement & Management 6(8):6, 1995
115. Zitter Group: Disease management, in principle, in practice, in partnership. Parke-Davis Healthcare Systems, 1995.
116. Morrissey, J: Simple asthma-management study produces hard evidence. Modern Healthcare 25(8):40–41, 1995
117. Fields, MA: Clinical pathways: High roads to better patient care. healthcare Informatics 11(8):40–44, 1994
118. Spath, PL: Getting started is the hardest part. Hospital Outcomes Management, 2(2):22–25, February 1995
119. Critical paths can diminish risks, increase accountability. Hospital Risk Management 16(2):17–28, 1994
120. Critical pathways emerge as negotiating tools for hospitals and MCOs. Hospital Case Management 2:12:1–3, 1994
121. Hess, D: The AARC Clinical Practice Guidelines. Respiratory Care 36(12):1398–1401, 1991
122. The American Association for Respiratory Care: AARC clinical practice guidelines. Respiratory Care 36(12):1398–1426, 1991
123. The American Association for Respiratory Care: AARC clinical practice guidelines. Respiratory Care 37(12):855, 856, 882–922, 1992
124. The American Association for Respiratory Care: AARC clinical practice guidelines. Respiratory Care 38(5):495–521, 1993
125. The American Association for Respiratory Care: AARC clinical practice guidelines. Respiratory Care 38(11):1169–1200, 1993
126. The American Association for Respiratory Care: AARC clinical practice guidelines. Respiratory Care 39(8):797–836, 1994
127. The American Association for Respiratory Care: AARC clinical practice guidelines. Respiratory Care 39(12):1170–1190, 1994
128. The American Association for Respiratory Care: AARC clinical practice guidelines. Respiratory Care 40(7):744–768, 1995
129. Tietsort, J: The respiratory care protocol: A management tool for the 90s. AARC Times 15(5):55–57, 1991
130. Therapist-driven protocols special report. Respiratory Manager 8(4):1–20, 1994
131. Phillips, YY: The development of practice guidelines in pulmonary medicine. Clinical Pulmonary Medicine 2(4):224–230, 1995
132. Burton, GG, Tietsort, JA: Therapist-driven respiratory care protocols—a practitioner's guide for criteria-based respiratory care. Los Angeles: Academy Medical Systems, Inc. 1994
133. Stoller, JK: Misallocation of respiratory care services: Time for a change. Respiratory Care 38(3):263–266, 1993
134. Zimcosky, LK, MacDonell, RJ, Sabo, JS, and Larsen, K: Comparison of two bronchial hygiene assessment programs. Respiratory Care 28(10):A1313, 1983
135. Southwick, K: Six steps for adult respiratory distress syndrome. Strategies for Healthcare Excellence 8(8):3–4, 1995
136. Des Jardins, G: Is your staff TDP safe and ready? Here's how to do it. Advance for Managers of Respiratory Care 4(1):33–37, 1995
137. Southwick, K: Disease management broadens focus of care from episodic to long-range. Strategies for Healthcare Excellence 8(6):1–9, 1995
138. Lambertus, T: 26 practical strategies for effective benchmarking. Hospital Benchmarks 2(7):87–90, 1995
139. Sanchez, LA: Pharmacoeconomic principles and methods: An introduction for hospital pharmacists. Hospital Pharmacy 29(8): 774, 777–779, 1994
140. Lambertus, T: How popular is benchmarking? Here's what survey says. Hospital Benchmarks 2(1):7–10, 1995

141. Flower, J: Benchmarking–springboard or buzzword? Healthcare Forum Journal 36(1):14–16, 1993
142. O'Dell, C: Benchmarking–building on received wisdom. Healthcare Forum Journal 36(1):17–18, 1993
143. Greene, J: Software helps hospitals cut back on job, expense of patient-care "rework." Modern Healthcare 25(1):51–52, 1995
144. Brennan, T et al: Incidence of adverse events and negligence in hospitalized patients. New England Journal of Medicine 324(6): 370–376, 1991
145. Bates, D, Cullen, DJ, Laird N, Petersen, LA, Small, SD, Servi, D, Laffel, G, Sweitzer, BJ, Shea, BF, Hallisey, R, Vliet Vander M, Nemeskal, R, Leape, LL: Incidence of adverse drug events and potential adverse drug events. JAMA 274(1):29–43, 1995
146. Neetleman, M, Nelson, A: Adverse occurrences during hospitalization on a general medicine service. Clinical Performance and Quality Health Care 2(2):67–72, 1994
147. Scheckler, WE: Interim report of the quality indicator study group. Infect Control Hosp Epidemiol 15(4):265–268, 1994
148. Davis, A, Doyle, M, Lansky, D, Rutt, W, Stevic, M, Doyle, J: Outcomes assessment in clinical settings: A consensus statement on principles and best practices in project management. The Joint Commission Journal on Quality Improvement 20(1):6–16, 1994
149. Ware, JE Jr., Sherbourne, CD: The MOS 36-item short-form health survey (SF-36). Med Care 30(6):473–483, 1992
150. McHorney, CA, Ware, JE Jr., Raczek, AB: The MOS 36-item short-form health survey (SF-36). Med Care 31(3):247–263, 1993
151. Dean medical center tracks patient outcomes. Inside Ambulatory Care 2(3):6–7, 1995
152. McHorney, CA, Ware, JE Jr., Lu, R, Sherbourne CD: The MOS 36-item short-form health survey (SF-36). Med Care 32(1): 40–66, 1994
153. The American Association for Respiratory Care: Uniform Reporting Manual–Third Edition. Dallas, American Association for Respiratory Care, 1993
154. Sabo, JS, Milligan, S: Reshaping hospitals for the future: Hospital restructuring and respiratory care. AARC Times 17(7):46–59, 1993
155. Revkin, AC: Nurses, doctors decry respiratory staff cut. Los Angeles Times Part 2, 2, July 27, 1986
156. Kedoe, J: Critics hit respiratory therapy cuts at HMNMH. The (Newhall, California) Sunday Signal 68:93, August 3, 1986
157. Revkin, AC: County studying Valencia Hospital's respiratory-staff trims. Los Angeles Times August 8, 1986
158. Thoemmres, L: Hospital gets checkup–County investigating HMNMH respiratory care. The (Newhall, California) Signal November 19, 1986
159. Revkin, AC: Inquiry lifts cloud cast on hospital care in Valencia. Los Angeles Times January 10, 1987
160. Revkin, AC: Valencia hospital death prompts inquiry by county. Los Angeles Times Part 2, November 14, 1987
161. Bunch, D: RCP's and integrated health care systems. AARC Times 19(6):24–28, 1995
162. Bunch, D: Respiratory care career opportunities shift to alternate care sites. AARC Times 19(5):30–42, 1995
163. Bunch, D: Opportunities abound for RCPs in home care. AARC Times 19(4):66–70, 1995
164. Geller, EH: House calls. Advance for Managers of Respiratory Care 5(6):30–33, 1995
165. Bunch, D: Case management holds potential for respiratory care practitioners. AARC Times 19(3):66–70, 1995
166. Gibbons, M: Shape or be shaped. Advance for Managers of Respiratory Care 4(5):25–28, 1995
167. Smith, R: Faces of the future. RT–The Journal for Respiratory Care Practitioners 8(1):53–60, 1995
168. Marable, LM: The fifty hottest jobs in America. Money 24(3):53, 1995
169. Montague, P, Gildersleeve, J, Tomazic, T, McComb, RC: Meeting the challenge of change. Advance for Managers of Respiratory Care 4(5):20–23, 1995
170. Geller, EH: Getting with the program. Advance for Managers of Respiratory Care 4(8):47–49, 1995
171. Ford, RM: Wireless point of care communication. RT–The Journal for Respiratory Care Practitioners 8(4):89–94, 1995
172. Williams, W, Sabo, JS, Hargett, J: Does a respiratory care information system improve charge capture? Respiratory Care 37(11):A1283, 1992
173. Burns, D: Breathing life into respiratory care. Healthcare Informatics 11(5):24–30, 1994
174. Respiratory protocols cut patient charges in NC. Hospital Benchmarks 2(5):64–65, 1995
175. Sabau, DG, Sabo, JS: Weaning protocol evaluation in the cardiovascular recovery room. Respiratory Care 37(11):A1285, 1992
175. Sabo, JS, Sabau, DG: Therapist driven weaning protocol evaluation in the cardiovascular recovery room. Crit Care Med 22(1):A266, 1994
176. Springer, D: Pneumonia pathway gets OK for further LOS reduction. Hospital Case Management 3(9):107–110, 1995
177. Patients breathe easier after open heart surgery. Hospital Benchmarks 2(5):61–62, 1995
178. Gurka, A: Pathway helps ICU staff better manage ventilator patients. Hospital Case Management 1(11):195–198, 1993
179. Ideno, KT, Sabau, D, Randall, C, Kite-Powell, D, Hartgraves, D, Solis, TR, Levy, S: Managing respiratory patients' nutritional outcomes. RT–The Journal for Respiratory Care Practitioners 8(2):111–118, 1995
180. Gibbons, M: Wellness. Advance for Managers of Respiratory Care 4(7):44–46, 1995
181. ED education eliminates repeat admissions. Disease State Management 1(2):16–18, 1995
182. Make, BJ: Patient education. Advance for Managers of Respiratory Care 4(7):55–58, 1995
183. Fink, JB, Covinton, J: Primary patient care task force: A strategy to change utilization patterns, improve quality, and reduce costs outside of the critical care unit. Respiratory Care 37(11):1283, 1992
184. Williams W, Sabo, JS, Kraus, JE: Count the ways–you can save a bundle by keeping close watch on inventory. Advance for Managers of Respiratory Care 4(7):16–19, 1995
185. Ford, RM, Burns, DM: Data-driven cost containment in the patient focused environment. AARC Times 18(5):80–84, 1994
186. Wright, J, Dudley, V: Compiling objective data to prepare for business consultants and the restructuring process. AARC Times 18(12):36–44, 1994
187. Lebouef, L: One respiratory care department's contribution to the bottom line. Respiratory Care 39(7):740–745, 1994
188. Scott, F: A meeting of the minds. Advance for Managers of Respiratory Care 4(7):24–29, 1995
189. Ede, S: How to involve the medical director. AARC Times 19(1): 16–17, 1995
190. Sestito, J: The art of marketing your department: Image–building and business savvy can pay off for respiratory care. Advance for Managers of Respiratory Care 4(8):29–32, 1995

Susan Rickey-Hatfield and Timothy Hatfield

SECTION 2 Effective Interpersonal Communication in Respiratory Care

PROFESSIONAL SKILLS

Upon completion of this chapter, the reader will be able to:

- Note and interpret patients' subjective and attitudinal responses to health problems, the medical environment, and health care provider
- Maintain effective communication with patients and their families, physicians, nursing staff, and other allied health care providers
- Develop interpersonal skills involved in interviewing patients, empathetic listening, and establishing relationships
- Maintain flexibility in communication and a balance in personal and professional life

KEY TERMS

Communication
Empathy
Encoding
Historical context
Information giver
Information seeker
Physical context
Rhetorical sensitivity
Social-psychological context

The relationship between the patient and health care providers is critical to patient satisfaction with the care. It also has a significant impact on whether or not the patient complies with the treatment plan. Because the quality of the provider-patient relationship is a direct result of the quality of communication between the two, an understanding of the dynamics of interpersonal communication is an important part of training for the respiratory care practitioner (RCP). It is important that all medical professionals make a commitment to developing effective and appropriate interpersonal skills during their professional training. As Roter, Hall, and Katz reported, specific communication skills taught to medical students were still evident in their practice 5 years later, and the quality of diagnostic information obtained from their patients was superior to that of other physicians.[1] Because respiratory care practitioners are on the frontline when it comes to treating patients, the development of strong, appropriate, and effective interpersonal skills is essential.

DEFINITIONS AND GOALS OF INTERPERSONAL COMMUNICATION

Interpersonal communication involves two or more people in a transactional process of sending and receiving verbal and nonverbal messages, with the goal of shared meaning. Several aspects of this definition deserve emphasis and explanation.

First, *communication is a transactional process.* The components of the process are interdependent, not independent. A message cannot be understood without some understanding of the message's sender, receiver, and situation. If one were to overhear a statement, but not see the communicators involved or understand their relationship, it would be unlikely that the message could be interpreted correctly.

Next, *communication involves the simultaneous sending and receiving of messages.* Even while we are talking, we are actively interpreting the verbal and nonverbal reactions of the person with whom we are talking and tailoring our message accordingly. An effective communicator is very adept at interpreting his conversational partner's facial expressions, body position, and verbal feedback to determine whether or not the receiver really understands the message.

Finally, *the goal of communication is the creation of meaning or understanding.* Simply sharing information does not always result in effective communication. Even though the person you are talking to may understand the individual words you are using, his understanding of your entire message might be different from the way you had intended your message to be understood. Simply providing information to a patient without checking to make sure he actually understands that information will not promote effective treatment.

BOX 2-7

GUIDELINES FOR EFFECTIVE RESPIRATORY CARE PRACTITIONER–CLIENT INTERACTION

1. Approach each patient and each situation as unique.
2. Create a supportive climate for communication.
3. Seek to understand before being understood.
4. Provide information in a timely, understandable manner.
5. Allow time for patient questions and concerns.
6. Remember: it's not always what you say, but how you say it.
7. Maintain role flexibility.
8. Balance professional and personal lives.

A PRINCIPLES-BASED APPROACH TO THERAPIST-CLIENT INTERACTION

This chapter will use a principles-based approach to help the reader understand the dynamics of the respiratory therapist–patient relationship. It is hoped that this approach will help the student to understand, remember, and apply the concepts discussed. This approach is a significant departure from the more theoretical perspective we used in the previous edition of this text.[2] Although theory is an important base from which to start, unless the concepts are portable (that is, easy to remember and easy to apply), their utility is limited. It is hoped that this principles-based approach will improve the reader's understanding and ability to apply the communication skills and techniques to enhance the quality of respiratory care delivered to patients. Box 2-7 lists important guidelines to achieve effective interaction.

Approach Each Patient and Each Situation as Unique

All communication interactions between an RCP and patient need to be considered as a separate and unique communication situation. As you gain experience as a respiratory therapist, it will be more and more difficult to treat each patient and situation as unique, because you will have treated hundreds of cases similar to each new one. What needs to be remembered is that this kind of thinking is dangerous to the patient's care, as well as disrespectful to the patient. Regardless of how many times you have treated the same symptoms of respiratory distress or answered the same questions, you need to remember that the situation is new—and perhaps frightening—to the patients and their families. Remembering this will increase your ability to provide optimal respiratory care.

The elements of the situation that affect the outcome of the communicative interaction are (1) the physical context, (2) the historical context, and (3) the social-psychological context.[3] These contexts should be considered both separately and collectively, because it is not uncommon for one aspect to affect the others.

□ PHYSICAL CONTEXT

The *physical context* involves the setting in which the interaction takes place. Mark Knapp identified six perceptual frameworks that are characteristic of physical environments. These perceptual frameworks are created by a combination of perceptions of an environment's character, including perceptions of its size, shape, color, temperature, and furnishings.[4] Knapp noted that these physical characteristics of the setting influence the construction and interpretation of messages sent and received within that particular environment. Box 2-8 lists those those characteristics.

For instance, as an RCP, you would probably be more guarded when talking about a critically ill patient with a doctor in a crowded public place (like a cafeteria) than you would in the doctor's office, which affords more privacy. Although the hospital might be familiar to you, it

BOX 2-8

PHYSICAL CHARACTERISTICS OF AN ENVIRONMENT

Formality	Privacy	Distance
Familiarity	Warmth	Constraint

is probably an unfamiliar environment to your patient and the patient's family. This unfamiliarity, coupled with perceptions of hospitals as "cold," lacking privacy, and being highly constraining, are very likely to influence your interactions with the patient, and vice versa.

□ HISTORICAL CONTEXT

The *historical context* refers to the past relationship between the participants in the conversation. Everyone has probably had the uncomfortable experience of having to interact with someone with whom she has recently had an unpleasant experience, such as a disagreement or conflict. These previous encounters shape present and even future interactions. Although historical context certainly affects communication, in professional relationships it is important not to let past interpersonal history get in the way of offering responsible professional respiratory care.

□ SOCIAL–PSYCHOLOGICAL CONTEXT

The *social–psychological context* refers not only to the present emotional states of the persons communicating, but also to the social roles and rules operating in that situation. In terms of psychological context, it is a given that both a respiratory care practitioner and a patient have both good and bad days. It is important to recognize that the way one is feeling influences the way that person formulates and interprets messages.

The social aspect of context concerns the social rules and roles that operate in a specific situation. Status differences are likely to be clearly defined in the hospital or clinical setting, and with those differences come clear sets of communication rules. Communication rules are guidelines for communicative behavior. Whereas some sets of rules are explicit (written down, as, for example, in Robert's Rules of Order), most communication rules are implicit and learned as part of the socialization process. Health care is replete with socially and culturally prescribed rules of interaction. Common communication rules involve forms of address, who initiates conversations, topics permitted to be addressed, and length of conversation. Unfortunately, in health care settings these rules can create a barrier between the client and the health care provider. Patients might be unwilling to discuss the side effects of a particular treatment because discussing the topic would violate rules of etiquette, and yet the health care provider needs to be aware of all pertinent information. Recognizing the barriers created by social rules should prompt a therapist to probe for information in a professional yet caring way that allows patients to express information openly.

Create a Supportive Communication Climate

Communication helps create an understanding or general feeling between people. This general feeling is referred to as a communication climate, and it may range on a continuum from a highly positive climate to an extremely negative climate.

Word choice, sentence structure, and tone of voice taken in combination may help promote a supportive and trusting relationship among the respiratory therapist, colleagues, and patients. Conversely, these same elements also may foster an unproductive relationship marked by distrust and disrespect.

Gibb identified six characteristics of defensive and supportive climates. *Defensive communication climates* are characterized by lack of trust between the individuals and seriously endanger the effectiveness of respiratory care. *Supportive communication climates,* on the other hand, build open, trusting relationships and promote positive therapist-patient relationships, treatment, and care.[5] Box 2-9 lists defensive and supportive environments.

□ EVALUATION VERSUS DESCRIPTION

If the sender of a message seems to be criticizing the other, then the receiver involved in the situation is likely to react by defending herself or her actions. The original issue is lost as both individuals get caught up in the defensive cycle. Communication that focuses on description keeps the conversation specific to the issue and is more likely to lead to productive interaction.

□ CONTROL VERSUS PROBLEM ORIENTATION

Telling a patient what to do (exerting control) isn't helpful unless the patient understands why the particular behavior or therapy is appropriate. When care givers focus on explaining the problem instead of jumping straight ahead into the treatment plan, patients understand more about their health care and are more likely to comply than if they feel like they are simply at the mercy of their provider. As Hall, Roter, and Katz report, the amount of information imparted by the health care provider is a dramatic and significant predictor of patient satisfaction.[6]

□ STRATEGY VERSUS SPONTANEITY

People react negatively when they sense that they are being manipulated or that information is being deliberately withheld. When a patient feels information is not forthcoming (unless he happens to ask a key question), or when information is so jargon laden or technical that it is incomprehensible to anyone without medical train-

BOX 2-9

DEFENSIVE VS SUPPORTIVE CLIMATES

Defensive	Supportive
1. Evaluation	1. Description
2. Control	2. Problem orientation
3. Strategy	3. Spontaneity
4. Neutrality	4. Empathy
5. Superiority	5. Equality
6. Certainty	6. Provisionalism

ing, patients are likely to get the sense that the health care provider knows more than she is willing to share. A spontaneous communication climate, on the other hand, is characterized by openness, honesty, and directness, where appropriate information is communicated willingly and in a way that can be understood.

☐ NEUTRALITY VERSUS EMPATHY

It is easy—and perhaps even tempting—to depersonalize interactions with patients. Referring to patients as sets of symptoms, conditions, or body parts or using nouns (the patient) instead of pronouns (you) removes the patient from the situation and depersonalizes her care. An effective RCP focuses on the patient as a person, not as just a patient with some sort of respiratory distress.

For example, when a patient asks a question about the side effects of a particular treatment, responding with a neutral statement pertaining to the odds of a particular reaction's occurrence is not as helpful as personalizing the response to include the patient ("You may experience these side effects, because a lot of people do.").

☐ SUPERIORITY VERSUS EQUALITY

In a hospital or clinical setting, status differences between health care professionals and patients are clear cut and made obvious through uniforms and name tags. When status differences are made explicit in a communicative interaction, either verbally or nonverbally, patients wind up feeling diminished. Making a conscious effort to reduce the status differential moves the interaction from a therapist-patient level to a more equal, person-person level, allowing for more genuine and productive interaction. The same benefits would accrue if similar efforts were made to reduce status differential among professional staff members.

☐ CERTAINTY VERSUS PROVISIONALISM

A communicative posture of certainty implies that there is only one answer, solution, or way of doing something, and that the person speaking has all the answers. It's a black-and-white, either-or, my-way-or-no-way communicative posture that promotes a defensive climate. However, it has been most people's experience that very few things are really that clear-cut. A climate of provisionalism provides information in a manner that allows for differences among patients and acknowledges that absolute certainly is not the rule in medical practice and health care.

Seek to Understand

One of the most important skills that an RCP can learn is how to get the information necessary to provide appropriate care. Information must be gathered from other health professionals caring for the patient, from the patient's family, and also directly from the patient himself.

In a social setting, the communication roles of sender and receiver are simultaneously occurring. An interview, on the other hand, is a very structured type of interpersonal interaction. In an interview situation, the roles are clearly defined as belonging to the information **seeker** or the information **giver**. In an interview, it is the information seeker (the RCP) who is responsible for the structure and flow of the communicative interaction with the patient. Though respiratory therapists may only do infrequent, targeted interviews with patients, the structure provided for interviews may serve as an informal structure for all interactions with patients.

The actual interview situation contains five parts, the middle three of which directly involve the patient. Box 2-10 lists the interview process steps.

The first step of the process happens before the therapist meets with the patient. *Preparation* includes reading the patient's chart and talking with other providers caring for the patient. Information from these sources should help the RCP identify an information goal for the encounter.

The goal may be to share information related to the patient's treatment or progress, to obtain information from the patient, or a combination of both. It may be as general as finding out how the patient is doing, or as specific as collecting and understanding a list of symptoms that occurred following the last round of treatment. Once the therapist has defined the goal for the interaction, the next three steps occur during the actual interview with the patient.

Although *developing rapport* is important, it should be a relatively brief and focused interaction. At the very least, this stage should be characterized by a greeting, in which the patient is referred to by name, and a self-introduction (if this has not already occurred). If the patient's family is present, all should be acknowledged and greeted. Direct eye contact between the respiratory care professional and those present in the room helps develop rapport. Entering the room reading the chart and greeting the patient while looking down does not establish the interpersonal contact necessary to facilitate information flow between the therapist and patient. Conversation during the rapport stage of the interaction should be kept general and related to the patient's situation. Interestingly, Roter, Hall, and Katz found that interaction that is "off task" may be perceived as reflecting a lack of concentration or a casual attitude of the health care professional.[7] The structure and length of this part of the interaction largely depends on the prior relationship between

BOX 2-10

STEPS INVOLVED IN EFFECTIVE INTERVIEWING

Step 1: Preparation and goal setting
Step 2: Developing rapport
Step 3: Achieving information goals
Step 4: Closing
Step 5: Follow-up

the therapist and client (historical context) and the client's health. During the initial encounter, the rapport stage may last longer than in subsequent interactions.

The third stage of the interview process involves the *achievement of information goal.* Next to information giving, question asking is the most frequent kind of exchange between patients and health care professionals.[8] According to Roter and Hall, health care professions vary greatly in their ability to obtain important facts from patients. The variance is the result of using closed-ended versus open-ended questions as the primary means of obtaining information.[9]

Closed-ended questions are those which have a limited array of possible answers—such as questions that can be answered with a "yes" or "no." In another form of closed-ended question, possible answers are provided from which the patient is to chose the response that most closely approximates her feelings or symptoms. Whereas close-ended questions can reveal important medical information, open-ended questions allow for more in-depth and personal responses. Open-ended questions are questions that allow the patient to answer in her own words. The therapist uses short statements (called probes) to guide the patient's answers to the relevant topic areas.

Open-ended questions allow the respiratory care practitioner a chance to explore psychosocial issues that may be relevant to the patient's illness and treatment. Bertakis, Roter, and Putnam found that between 30% and 85% of patients seen in primary care practice have some relevant psychosocial problem.[10] Identification of these problems—which do not always come to light using closed-ended questions—has the potential to increase treatment compliance and effectiveness. Asking the patient if he has any questions, while pausing to allow for a response, is essential during this stage of the interaction.

But asking the right kind of questions is a futile exercise unless the respiratory care professional also makes a concentrated effort to listen to the patient's answers. Though hearing is a basic physiological function, *listening,* defined as making sense of what is heard, is hard work. In fact, it is estimated that people actually listen to only 25% to 50% of what they hear.[3] Box 2-11 reviews questions that may reveal whether there is a need to improve your own listening skills.[11] Listening is a skill that virtually everyone can improve. In health care situations, learning to be a good listener is key to delivering effective respiratory care.

The fourth stage of the interview sequence is the *closing.* At this point, the RCP should summarize the information presented by both the therapist and the patient, as well as provide necessary information as to what the patient might expect in the future. Roter, Hall, and Katz reported that training health care professionals to implement a 5-minute concluding summary of the visit and a request for patient feedback significantly increased patient satisfaction and recall of information.[1] This stage also allows the patient to ask any additional questions and clarify any information of which she may be uncertain.

For the final stage of the interview, the respiratory care practitioner performs any required or necessary *follow-up* with the health care team, either in consultation or in writing. These follow-up activities should be performed as promptly as feasible.

Provide Information that the Patient and the Patient's Family Can Understand

The RCP's verbal skills can either promote or inhibit effective respiratory care. A therapist who is able to use verbal communication skills effectively can help a patient and the patient's family understand the situation and the steps necessary in the course of treatment. A therapist whose verbal skills are ineffective is likely to create confusion and perhaps resistance. The goal of any communication encounter is the sharing of meaning. Communicating without this goal in mind can leave both parties in the encounter frustrated and feeling misunderstood, render treatment ineffective, or even endanger the patient.

BOX 2-11

COMMON LISTENING MISTAKES

1. Do you tend to avoid discussing difficult material with clients, particularly material that takes time and thought?
2. Do you pretend to listen or show interest when your mind is elsewhere?
3. Do you dismiss the client's discussion as uninteresting?
4. Are you easily distracted? Distractions are always present in health-related settings. Whenever possible, space and time should be designed to eliminate distraction when one-to-one interaction is necessary to develop a good relationship with a client.
5. Do you find fault with the way patients talk, dress, or act? Focusing on ancillary factors can divert your attention from what is being said.
6. Do you listen only for facts and details? If so, you might be failing to take the emotions, behaviors, and intentions of the client into consideration. These would give you the real clues as to what is happening.
7. Do you become angry at what the speaker is saying, particularly if he or she is upset about health care or the way you perform given tasks?
8. If the client uses emotional language, does that antagonize you? If so, you might become defensive and not hear what is being said.
9. Do you become preoccupied with your note taking? Note taking is recognized as important for both the health care practitioner and the client, but it can also be an avoidance technique. Listen and make eye contact before you write.
10. Do you become distracted when it takes the client a long time to speak? Most people speak at approximately 125 words a minute but are capable of listening to 500 spoken words a minute. To really hear what is being said, it is important to learn to concentrate, because it is easy to become distracted.

Encoding is the transforming of ideas and perceptions into symbols that can be transmitted to the other person or persons in the communication situation.[12] The symbol system can be both verbal and nonverbal. For instance, a message may be encoded using a set of verbal symbols that are agreed on by a certain culture (language) or a set of nonverbal gestures that have meaning to a specific audience (eg, sign language for the deaf).

The choice of symbol systems is important, because it is the speaker's responsibility to select symbols that the receivers of the message are likely to understand. Obviously, a speaker would be unwise to encode a message with a symbol system that the receiver might not understand (eg, technical terms or jargon). More subtle encoding errors are made when health care professionals overestimate the patient's level of knowledge or vocabulary, using words that the patient does not understand. Professional jargon is especially problematic. Many professionals are so used to encoding messages in the abbreviated jargon and acronyms of their field that they have difficulty encoding messages for persons outside their field. Respiratory care professionals need to take special care in explaining treatment to patients or nurses and in answering their questions, always remembering that the goal of communication is shared meaning.

The importance of the awareness of the sending of the message was reported by Roter and Frankel, who concluded that physicians who first assessed and then attempted to align themselves with the patient's state of knowledge were more effective in providing information in an acceptable manner. When physicians delivered diagnostic information without respect to the perspective of the recipient, they risked the patient rejecting the critical information and also damaging or destroying trust and compassion in the relationship. Patients who receive undesirable news in such a fashion are likely to seek additional assessments out of a sense of frustration or anger at the style in which the news was delivered.[8]

Sharing meaning is the goal of communication. Box 2-12 lists guidelines to ensure that the message is understood as intended.[13]

BOX 2-12

GUIDELINES TO ENSURE THE INTENDED MESSAGE IS COMMUNICATED

1. Be aware of multiple meanings of words. The same word can have more than one meaning. The word responsibility may mean "take control" to one person, "take blame" to another.
2. Be person minded, not word minded. Frequently ask yourself, "This is what it means to me, what does it mean to the patient?"
3. Paraphrase frequently. Put the other person's statements in your own words. Restate what he or she has said to you in similar but different language.
4. Be approachable. Create a personal atmosphere that invites or encourages the patient or a family member to ask questions if they don't understand your message.
5. Use multiple methods of communication. Try to use a variety of ways to get your message across to another person.
6. Be aware of the contexts (verbal and situational). Verbal context: How was the particular word used in a sentence? Situational context: What was happening in the environment during the interaction with the patient?

Allow Time for Patient Questions and Concerns

A skill at the core of effective interpersonal relationships, as well as any kind of human helping, is the capacity to understand another person's experience from his—not your own—perspective. This involves listening carefully to the total verbal and nonverbal message in all its complexity and communicating your understanding of the message back to the person.

Called *empathy,* or empathic listening, the skill involves a commitment to (1) immersing yourself in the perspective of another to understand the situation from the other's point of view, and (2) communicating your understanding to the other so that he or she knows you understand. Carl Rogers' seminal work on empathy in counseling has had a profound effect on generations of skilled helpers.[14–16] He defined empathic listening as follows:

"Entering the private perceptual world of the other and becoming thoroughly at home in it. It involves being sensitive, moment by moment, to the changing felt meanings which flow in this other person.... It means temporarily living in the other's life, moving about in it delicately without making judgments."[16]

This is the polar opposite of the situation we all have experienced at some time in our life: someone says "I'm listening," yet clearly is not. The basic message conveyed by the person who is not listening is one of disrespect. On the other hand, when a person knows that someone has listened empathically to her, her reaction is apt to be something like, "Yes, that's it exactly! You know what I'm talking about." She feels affirmed, respected, and empowered both to keep exploring her own issues and to allow you to accompany her in that process.

Empathic listening fosters respectful, supportive relationships among colleagues as well as between care giver and patient. It exemplifies the essence of "being there" for someone else, and it is a learnable skill that must be a part of an RCP's repertoire, along with the myriad of technical skills for which he or she is responsible.

Even with the technology in place, it is clear that what a patient often needs most is someone to listen—carefully, sensitively, respectfully—to his own views about his situation. And often the people most available to listen are nurses, respiratory care personnel, or other specialists, rather than the doctor or doctors in charge of the case. Burton has spoken of the important need for physicians to listen and communicate well with respiratory care professionals.[17] Garber, who is, like Burton, a physician, addressed the benefits to physicians and patients alike if physicians were to have better training in basic attending and empathic listening skills.[18] The norm, however, is not in that direction, and vital bedside-manner responsibilities likely will continue to rest with other health care professionals, including the reader of this section.

Roter and Frankel, in fact, reported that patients seldom had the opportunity to have their concerns heard by physicians, who on average interrupted patients only 18 seconds after they began to speak![8] Previously, Roter, Hall, and Katz noted that patients were much more likely to remember what physicians had discussed with them if the interaction was characterized by the kinds of patient-centered empathic interviewing cited above.[7]

Pay Attention to the Nonverbal Message

Although most of the principles discussed to this point have concerned using words to communicate effectively, it is important to know that most research indicates that sometimes only a small percentage of the meaning of a message is conveyed verbally—the rest of the message's meaning is conveyed nonverbally.[19] This is true for messages sent by the therapist, as well as messages sent by the patient. Because of the importance of the nonverbal component of messages, it is important for RCPs to be aware of their own—and their patients'—nonverbal messages.

There are numerous modes of nonverbal messages, and any or all of them can impact the interpretation of the message. For instance, a patient who insists that he is "feeling fine" with a weak voice, slumped posture, and while looking away is not likely to convince anyone that he's ready to be discharged from a hospital. Equally, a therapist probably does not engender much confidence from patients or colleagues if she chooses to stand far away from the patient, look down, nervously fidget, and talk both too fast and too loudly.

Extensive knowledge of appropriate nonverbal communication along with a wealth of scientific and technological expertise does not guarantee that an RCP—or any health care provider—will be either an effective practitioner or a good colleague. The kind of intensive helping implicit in respiratory care demands a real, unambiguous presence on the part of the care giver. At the core of this presence is the capacity and commitment to **attend** to the person.

Egan described the attending process as one that is conveyed, both verbally and nonverbally, and that can help to establish good rapport with a person.[20] The following skills, abbreviated by the acronym SOLER, can help one communicate a positive presence to both patients and colleagues:

1. ***S:** Squarely* face the person, to communicate your involvement nonverbally by orienting yourself to him or her.
2. ***O:** Open* your posture to the person, thus communicating your availability and openness. Although crossing your legs or folding your arms does not close off effective attending per se, the key issue to consider is whether your posture says, "I am open to what you have to say."
3. ***L:** Lean* slightly toward the person at times in appropriate ways, which conveys the nonverbal message, "I'm especially interested in what you're telling me now."
4. ***E:** Eye contact* is essential in telling the person that you are truly present in the conversation. Some happy medium between looking everywhere but at the person and fixing the person in a laserlike stare is the goal of good eye contact in our culture.
5. ***R:** Relaxed* presentation of all the foregoing attending skills in a natural way tells the person, "I am interested in what you have to say, and I am really here for you."

Egan went on to emphasize the importance of using these skills in a nonrigid, nonabsolute way that is sensitive to a person's individual and cultural ways. The goal is to build connections between yourself and the other person because you have paid attention and attended to the person; the goal is **not** to assume that some formula for intimacy is equally effective with everyone.[20]

With practice, these kinds of basic attending skills can provide the foundation for even more effective listening and relationship building—professional and collegial—in your ongoing work in respiratory care. Box 2-13 lists guidelines that summarize a number of helpful and unhelpful nonverbal behaviors for your consideration.[21]

Maintain Role Flexibility

Attending, listening, nonverbal awareness, and empathy skills help one to become a better communicator. These skills, taken collectively, help promote an attitude toward communication known as *rhetorical sensitivity.*

Consider for a moment how you would describe your activities last weekend to (1) your mother or father, (2) your grandmother, (3) your boss, (4) your best friend, and (5) a small child. Chances are that you would change both the structure and the content of the message for each person. Hart and Burks labeled this perspective as an "attitude toward communication."[22] In other words, a person's attitude toward communicating may indeed influence the subsequent communication itself. Hart, Carlson, and Eadie extended this thinking and identified three rhetorical postures.[23] At one end of the continuum is a noble self attitude, narrow in view and very self-oriented. At the other end is a rhetorically reflective attitude, which is strongly oriented to the other person and the situation. The rhetorically sensitive person approaches each situation as unique and weighs all the variables before speaking.

According to Hart and Burks,[22] the rhetorically sensitive person is an ideal communicator, one who does the following:

1. Tries to accept role-taking or role-playing as a normal part of human behavior.

BOX 2-13

GUIDELINES FOR DEVELOPING APPROPRIATE NONVERBAL BEHAVIOR

Eye Behaviors

Positive eye behaviors: Direct eye contact before initiating interaction; sustained eye contact while both talking and listening to patients and colleagues.

Negative eye behaviors: Looking down while talking or listening, exhibiting shifty eyes; looking away from the person with whom you are communicating; keeping eyes downcast, excessive blinking; narrowed eyes, staring.

Gestures

Positive gestures: Gestures that appear spontaneous and relaxed, conversational.

Negative gestures: Gestures that suggest a therapist is nervous, lacks confidence, or is defensive. Hand to face gestures, throat clearing, fidgeting, tugging at clothing, extraneous or continuous head movements.

Facial Expressions

Positive facial expressions: Expressions that are appropriate for the situation, that match the nature of the verbal messages, that appear friendly and spontaneous while at the same time maintain professionalism.

Negative facial expressions: Expressions that are neutral, overintensified, or frozen. Expressions that appear unpleasant or critical.

Postures

Positive postures: Establishing rapport by leaning forward and smiling (when appropriate) as you provide information or listen to another. Speaking to the patient on his or her own level; that is, if the patient is seated, sitting down next to her to avoid speaking down to the patient.

Negative postures: Constricted postures that appear stiff and unnatural. Crossed arms and legs, body tension, and bad posture are apt to impair an RCP's credibility.

Voice

Positive vocal cues: A conversational speaking style with a rate that is appropriate for the message being conveyed (a more technical message requires a much slower rate than less technical information). Appropriate variation in pitch and volume projecting the image of a confident, competent professional. Pausing to allow for questions from the patient or family members.

Negative vocal cues: Dull, monotone delivery. Excessively fast rate that does not facilitate understanding or allow for questions. Interrupting a patient. Using upward intonation at the end of statements, which then sound like questions. Volume that violates the patient's right to privacy. Frequent use of empty words, phrases, or sounds including "ah," "um," "I mean . . . ," and "OK?"

2. Seeks to distinguish between all information available and information acceptable for communication.
3. Tries to understand that an idea can be encoded in several different ways.

Perhaps rhetorical sensitivity can best be understood by examining the ends of the continuum—the noble self and the rhetorical reflector. Darnell and Brockreide[24] describe the noble self as one who

1. Sees any variation from his or her personal norms as hypocritical, as a denial of integrity, and as a cardinal sin.
2. Views the self as the primary basis for making communicative choices. The needs of another person or pressures of a situation are considered to be of secondary importance, if they are taken into account at all.
3. Tends to want control, rather than to share choices. This type of communicator prefers to engage in monologue, rather than dialogue.

The rhetorical reflector, on the other hand, is described by Darnell and Brockreide[24] in the following manner:

1. Rhetorical reflectors have no self to call their own. The self developed for each communication act is inextricably bound up in the situation.
2. Communicative choices from reflectors arise from the perceived needs and wishes of the other person and the situation. They feel their way into the transaction and behave and become what they feel the other needs and wants.
3. Reflectors neither control nor share choices. Rather, from all the frames of reference, the self created plays a passive role and is acted on; it does not assume a proactive role. The only choice a reflector makes is to accommodate the choice of others.

In contrast with the noble self and the rhetorical reflector, the rhetorically sensitive person is one who recognizes that not all messages are suitable for all receivers. With skills such as attending, active listening, and empathy, the rhetorically sensitive person takes into account the receiver's knowledge, background, experiences, emotions, and attitudes when encoding messages.

□ RHETORICAL SENSITIVITY AND RESPIRATORY CARE

Rhetorical sensitivity can help the respiratory therapist balance important professional responsibilities to the patient and to the respiratory care profession. Such a balance leads to professionally responsible respiratory care, as indicated in Figure 2-6. As depicted in the model, the vertical axis is a continuum of knowledge and skills for respiratory care professionals. These would include all the scientific, technical, and general professional issues addressed in respiratory care training programs, along with ongoing learning on the job, through continuing education opportunities. The horizontal axis is a continuum of one's communication and interpersonal skills and sensitivity with patients and colleagues.

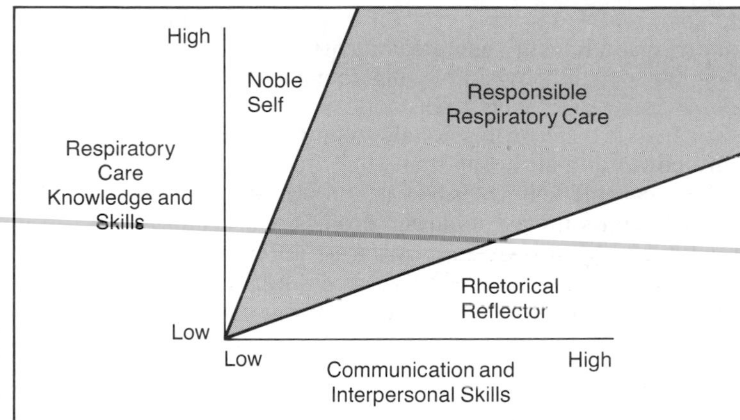

FIGURE 2-6. A model illustrating the balance between technical knowledge and human skills to accomplish "responsible" patient care. When respiratory care practitioners operate outside the stippled area, knowledge and therapeutics are applied without interpersonal skills, or communication occurs without technical substance.

As discussed earlier in this chapter, a high level of knowledge and skills without the communication and interpersonal skills to work well with patients and colleagues does **not** promote professional effectiveness. In rhetorical sensitivity terms, a person with these traits would be more likely to give patients noble self responses, which might be well grounded in science and technology but very insensitive to the patients themselves or to the context of the ongoing work with them. On the other hand, high sensitivity to patients without the requisite professional knowledge and skills certainly would not qualify one to be a respiratory care professional and would be most like a rhetorical reflector posture. However sensitive a communicator this type of person might be, he or she would not belong in the field.

Between these two positions, however, as depicted by the shaded area in Figure 2-6, are those respiratory care professionals who have both the necessary professional skills and the communication and interpersonal skills to deliver them with a view to both the patient **and** the context. In short, they have the skills to provide responsive, responsible respiratory care. This responsible care giver model goes beyond baseline competency levels for entry into the field and accounts for increasing levels of knowledge, expertise, and growth in both areas, through continuing education and commitment to renew and grow in the profession.

Balance Professional and Personal Life: Have a Life to Save a Life

Although this chapter has been intended to stimulate the reader's thinking about the effective delivery of respiratory therapy care, this final section begins with a question that may not at first glance seem to fit with that basic notion.

□ WHERE DOES YOUR WORK LIFE END, AND WHERE DOES THE REST OF YOUR LIFE BEGIN?

As a respiratory care professional, you will be delivering important services to others. You will be giving of yourself constantly. And, paradoxically, your ability to maintain clear personal boundaries between your work life and the rest of your existence will promote more effective professionalism than would be the case if you were on duty constantly. Taking your work home with you—whether in a brief case, in your head, or in your heart—means that you never truly leave work, psychologically speaking. And there is a significant price to pay for this in the long run.

Being well yourself—both inside and outside the workplace—helps sustain you and prevent burnout in this high-intensity care-giving profession. Your own self-care has an important influence on your capacity to keep giving, day after day, in appropriate ways. Maslach, the leading researcher on burnout, titled her book *Burnout: The Cost of Caring.*[25] The very fact that you care about your patients and your profession makes you more vulnerable to burning out, and therefore you need to be actively involved in your own positive self-care.

Although only brief mention of this subject can be made here, managing the inevitable stresses of working in respiratory care enhances the quality of your work, your personal sense of satisfaction in the profession, and your overall enjoyment of life.[26] Listed below are several key concepts, some of which you may wish to pursue in more detail through the sources cited.

□ SELF-CARE AND STRESS MANAGEMENT SKILLS

1. At the most basic level, it is helpful for you to have a clear vision of whether your being in respiratory care truly fits you.

As cited in the model in Figure 2-6, your professional effectiveness depends on both your responsibility to the profession and your responsibility to your patients. Although your very presence in a respiratory care training program may speak to your interest and commitment, it may be that the kinds of training, skills, and professional expectations of a respiratory therapist do not fit nearly as well for you as those of other important roles in health care or other professions.

Can you imagine, for example, having an aversion to highly technical instruments and data, yet still expecting to enjoy work in respiratory care? Or can you imagine having a strong preference for working totally on your own and having absolute control over all decisions affecting a patient, yet knowing that you will be expected to work closely and cooperatively with many other health care professionals, many of whom have more power and authority than you?

Your careful self-assessment and career planning need to be ongoing personal and professional issues for you, both for your own sense of career and life satisfaction as well as for the welfare of the innumerable patients whose lives are often quite literally in your hands. The literature abounds with excellent career-planning and decision-making texts; we refer you to them as a point of departure.[27–30]

2. The **way** in which you think about your work situation strongly affects the amount of stress that you experience in it. For example, to approach the day thinking, "This obviously is going to be a terrible day," has a qualitatively different impact on you than to think, "All my patients and colleagues deserve to have me at my best today."

This is not a new notion—the ancient Greek philosophers wrote about the power of ideas on one's well-being, for example—but it is worth considering as to its impact on your own self-care and your effectiveness in respiratory care. It is a core concept of Frankl's famous book, *Man's Search for Meaning,* about surviving imprisonment in a Nazi concentration camp.[31] It is also a cornerstone of one model of counseling called rational emotive therapy (RET). This model encourages people to look at whether their beliefs are realistic.[32] Woolfolk and Richardson's excellent book, *Stress, Sanity, and Survival,* goes on to say that our perceptions of situations can, all by themselves, trigger stress in our lives.[33]

The work of Kobasa and her colleagues also points out that a person's commitment to a particular line of work and the felt sense of doing something that matters contributes to a hardier, more stress-resistant personality.[34,35] This also speaks to the importance of the way that you think about your work, whether in general or as you approach specific interpersonal situations. Assume, for example, that your respiratory care responsibilities do matter, and that you carry them out in a professional manner to the best of your ability. This work strategy may make it more likely for you to receive negative feedback evenhandedly and respond, "Thanks for the input," rather than to personalize the feedback and respond in a defensive way.

A clear view of the importance of your own respiratory care knowledge and skills also increases the likelihood that you will be able to adopt a positive, respectful perspective on the contributions of all members of the health care team (regardless of whether there is truly a team or the structure of the organization is hierarchical, with physicians on top).

3. Wellness is the process of being actively involved in the integration of one's physical, intellectual, social, emotional, and spiritual well-being. We feel it is important to emphasize the process nature of wellness, because maintaining an ongoing balance among these dimensions of wellness is not achieved in a once-and-for-all way.

Ardell,[36] Travis and Ryan,[37] and the Borysenkos[38] are notable examples of the many authors who have made important contributions to the burgeoning literature on wellness. The key issue is remaining actively involved in one's own self-care as a professional, and, more generally, as a complex human being. The process of balancing may involve placing emphasis, at a given point, on physical fitness, diet, time management, assertiveness skills, difficult relationships, or general stress management skills. Some excellent general resources on this topic include Rice,[39] Greenberg,[40] and Seward.[41]

4. Building and maintaining a support system is an important goal for respiratory care professionals.

From Harlow's early work with laboratory monkeys to Spitz's parallel work with children in foundling homes to more recent applications with a variety of populations, it is becoming increasingly clear that social support can play a crucial role in helping people to cope.[42–47] Coping may involve the expected stresses of everyday life, as well as those of times of higher stress (eg, examination periods or taking national or state board exams). It goes without saying that a sudden illness is extremely stressful for most people, and that is where the work of the RCP is performed.

SUMMARY

This chapter has addressed the need for effective interpersonal communication in respiratory care, presenting eight principles of effective respiratory therapist–patient interaction as a means of promoting the learning and application of the concepts. (1) Considering the physical, historical, and social-psychological contexts of communication helps respiratory therapists to approach each patient and each situation as unique. (2) Taking into account six characteristics of defensive versus supportive climates promotes a better understanding of the importance of creating a supportive communication climate. (3) Interviewing and positive listening skills are at the core of seeking to understand. (4) The sharing of meaning is the goal of all communication, which is central to providing information that the patient and the patient's family can understand. (5) A commitment to empathic listening promotes allowing time for patient questions and concerns.

(6) Besides effective verbal and listening skills, respiratory therapists also need to be aware of the importance of paying attention to nonverbal messages. (7) The research on rhetorical sensitivity speaks to the importance of maintaining role flexibility, depicted in the responsible respiratory care model. (8) Finally, a commitment to balance in one's professional and personal life is discussed by means of four self-care and stress-management modalities.

REFERENCES

1. Roter DL, Hall JA, Katz NR: Patient-physicians communication: A descriptive review of the literature. Patient Education and Counseling 12:99, 1986
2. Hatfield SR, Hatfield T: Effective Interpersonal Communication in Respiratory Care. In G Burton, J Hodgkin, J Ward (eds): Respiratory Care: A Guide to Clinical Practice, 3rd ed. Philadelphia, JB Lippincott, 1991, p 35
3. Verdeber RF: Communicate! Belmont, CA, Wadsworth, 1993
4. Knapp ML: Nonverbal Communication in Human Interaction, 2nd ed. New York, Holt, Rinehart & Winston, 1978
5. Gibb JR: Defensive communication. J Communication 11:143, 1961
6. Hall JA, Roter DL, Katz NR: Meta-analyses of correlates of provider behavior in medical encounters. Med Care 26:657, 1988
7. Roter DL, Hall JA, Katz NR: Relation between physicians' behaviors and analogue patients' satisfaction, recall, and impressions. Med Care 25:437, 1987
8. Roter DL, Frankel R: Quantitative and qualitative approaches to the evaluation of the medical dialogue. Soc Sci Med 34:1097, 1992
9. Roter DL, Hall JA: Physicians' interviewing styles and medical information obtained from patients. J Gen Intern Med 2:325, 1987
10. Bertakis KD, Roter D, Putnam, SM: The relationship of physician medical interview style to patient satisfaction. J Fam Pract 32:175, 1991
11. Kreps GL, Thornton BC: Health Communication Theory and Practice. Prospect Heights, IL, Waveland Press, 1992
12. DeVito JA: The Communication Handbook: A Dictionary. New York, Harper & Row, 1986
13. Northouse PG, Northouse LL: Health Communication: A Handbook for Health Professionals. Englewood Cliffs, NJ, Prentice-Hall, 1985
14. Rogers CR: Client-Centered Therapy. Boston, Houghton Mifflin, 1951
15. Rogers CR: On Becoming a Person. Boston, Houghton Mifflin, 1961
16. Rogers CR: A Way of Being. Boston, Houghton Mifflin, 1980
17. Burton GG: The art of becoming a change agent. Pulmon Med Technol 1:58, 1984
18. Garber JJ: Improved doctor-patient communication: A means of reducing physician stress. Unpublished master's thesis, Winona State University, Minnesota, 1987
19. Mehrabian A: Silent Messages. Belmont, CA, Wadsworth, 1971
20. Egan G: The Skilled Helper, 5th ed. Pacific Grove, CA, Brooks/Cole, 1994
21. Leathers DG: Successful Nonverbal Communication: Principles and Applications. New York, Macmillan, 1992
22. Hart RP, Burks DM: Rhetorical sensitivity and social interaction. Commun Monogr 1972;39:75.
23. Hart RP, Carlson RE, Eadie WF: Attitudes toward communication and the assessment of rhetorical sensitivity. Commun Monogr 17:1, 1980
24. Darnell D, Brockreide W: Persons Communicating. Englewood Cliffs, NJ, Prentice-Hall, 1976
25. Maslach C: Burnout: The Cost of Caring. Englewood Cliffs, NJ, Prentice-Hall, 1982
26. Jaffe DT, Scott CD: Take This Job and Love It. New York, Fireside, 1988
27. Bolles RN: What Color Is Your Parachute? Berkeley, Ten Speed Press, 1994
28. Hagberg J, Leider R: The Inventurers: Excursions in Life and Career Renewal, 3rd ed. Reading, MA, Addison-Wesley, 1988
29. Michelozzi BN: Coming Alive from Nine to Five, 4th ed. Mountain View, CA, Mayfield, 1992
30. Zunker VG: Career Counseling: Applied Concepts of Life Planning, 4th ed. Pacific Grove, CA, Brooks/Cole, 1994
31. Frankl V: Man's Search for Meaning. New York, Washington Square Press, 1963
32. Ellis A, Harper RA: A New Guide to Rational Living. Englewood Cliffs, NJ, Prentice-Hall, 1975
33. Woolfolk RI, Richardson FC: Stress, Sanity, and Survival. New York, Signet, 1979
34. Kobasa S: Stressful life events, personality, and health: An inquiry into hardiness. Person Soc Psychol 37:1, 1979
35. Maddi SR, Kobasa SC: The Hardy Executive: Healthy Under Stress. Chicago, Dorsey, 1984
36. Ardell DB: High Level Wellness, 2nd ed. Berkeley: Ten Speed Press, 1986
37. Travis JW, Ryan RS: Wellness Workbook, 2nd ed. Berkeley, Ten Speed Press, 1988
38. Borysenko J, Borysenko M: The Power of the Mind to Heal. Carson, CA, Hay House, 1994
39. Rice PL: Stress and Health, 2nd ed. Monterey, CA, Brooks/Cole, 1992
40. Greenberg JS: Comprehensive Stress Management, 4th ed. Dubuque, IA, Brown & Benchmark, 1993
41. Seward BL: Managing Stress: Principles and Strategies for Health and Wellbeing. Boston, Jones & Bartlett, 1994
42. Harlow HF: Love in infant monkeys. Sci Am 200:68, 1959
43. Spitz R: Life and dialogue. In HS Gaskill (ed): Counterpoint: Libidinal Object and Subject. New York, International Universities Press, 1963
44. Lynch JJ: The Broken Heart. The Medical Consequences of Loneliness. New York, Basic Books, 1977
45. Albrecht TL, Adelman, MB: Social support and life stress. Hum Commun Res 11:3, 1984
46. Veninga RC: A Gift of Hope. New York, Ballantine, 1985
47. Pearson JE: The definition and measurement of social support. J Counsel Dev 64:390, 1986

Alan L. Plummer and George G. Burton

SECTION 3 The Physician and the Respiratory Care Team

PROFESSIONAL SKILLS

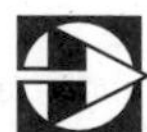

Upon completion of this chapter, the reader will be able to:

- Describe the manner in which a relationship to physicians is implicit in the description of the respiratory care profession
- Understand that all respiratory care services are performed on the basis of specific or generic (protocol) physician orders
- Identify national physician membership organizations involved with the respiratory care profession
- Delineate the roles and responsibilities of RCPs and physicians in the therapist-driven protocol (TDP) and non-TDP setting
- Relate the roles and functions of the medical director in traditional and nontraditional sites
- Relate the roles and functions of the medical director in JRCRTE-approved RCP educational programs

KEY TERMS

Attending physician
BOMA
Institutional certification
JCAHO
JRCRTE
JRCTE Essentials
NAMDRC
NBRC
Physician extender
Physician of record
Physician order
Protocol boundaries
Seamless healthcare delivery
Therapist-driven protocols

THE PHYSICIAN AND THE MODERN RESPIRATORY CARE PRACTITIONER: A CORDIAL RELATIONSHIP

From its earliest beginnings, the respiratory care profession has been identified by its strong relationship with the medical profession. This is reflected in the American Association for Respiratory Care's (AARC's) most recent definition of its members[1] and in no less than 15 current AARC position papers. The relationship of physicians and respiratory care practitioners (RCPs) is reflected in models at the national, state, and local hospital levels; in respiratory care practice in nontraditional sites; with (or without) therapist-driven protocols (TDPs); and most importantly, at the level of individual patient care. The respiratory care profession has historically been careful to recognize the physician as "the captain of the ship" and has distanced itself from any practice patterns that would weaken this relationship. Indeed, in official AARC statements, the various roles and functions of RCPs have consistently been defined in relationship to the medical profession. These relationships have progressively matured and have served both professions well over the last 30 years.

PHYSICIAN–THERAPIST LIAISONS AT THE NATIONAL LEVEL

Official national organizations that formalize interaction between physician organizations and the respiratory care profession include the AARC's Board of Medical Advisors (BOMA), the National Board for Respiratory Care (NBRC), the Joint Review Committee for Respiratory Therapy Education (JRCRTE), and the National Association for Medical Direction of Respiratory Care (NAMDRC). Except for NAMDRC, each of these organizations has membership and representation from the AARC, as well as the American Society for Anesthesia (ASA), the American Thoracic Society (ATS), and the American College of Chest Physicians (ACCP). The Board of Medical Advisors has, in addition, representatives from the American Academy of Pediatrics (AAP) and the Society for Critical Care Medicine (SCCM), American College of Allergy and Immunology (ACAI), and NAMDRC.

AARC Board of Medical Advisors

The Board of Medical Advisors is a consultative body in which the medical profession has formal dialogue with the national AARC membership organization. Though BOMA representatives presently have no voting status in the AARC organization, the advice of this board is usually heeded, and positive dialogue is generally possible. The Board of Medical Advisors advises the AARC on educational program content, on all medical matters and on scientific matters such as position statements and clinical practice guidelines, and on matters such as state licensure and other forms of legal credentialing.

National Board for Respiratory Care

The NBRC is the profession's national credentialing arm. Physicians on the NBRC spend several weeks each year submitting and reviewing items used in the various NBRC credentialing examinations. Thus, the scientific content of the NBRC examinations is medically validated and constantly reflects the changing science of respiratory care. The subject content of NBRC credentialing examinations is periodically validated in the national workplace.

Joint Review Committee for Respiratory Therapy Education

The (as yet unnamed) successor organization to the JRCRTE is the profession's educational accrediting arm, which recommends approval of college-level respiratory care educational programs to the U.S. Department of Education. Currently, such programs are accredited by the American Medical Association through its Commission on Accreditation of Allied Health Education Programs (CAAHEP). The ASA, ATS, and ACCP are physician sponsors of JRCRTE. With educator therapist colleagues from the AARC, physicians from the JRCRTE-sponsoring organizations serve as ombudsmen (referees) for applicant programs and as on-site visitors for the programmatic accreditation visits themselves. Indeed, a physician is part of every JRCRTE site visit team. Among other functions, the task of such physicians is to review medical input into programs' educational process. The JRCRTE was the first allied health educational accrediting body to prepare accreditation standards called *Essentials** for accreditation that were outcome, rather than process, oriented.

National Association for Medical Direction of Respiratory Care

This organization, NAMDRC, was formed in 1977, to educate its members and to address regulatory, legislative, and payment issues that relate to the delivery of health care to patients with respiratory disorders. Based in Washington, DC, the organization has approximately 700 members, almost all of whom are medical directors of respiratory therapy departments or respiratory therapy educational programs. It publishes a quarterly newsletter and sponsors an annual meeting, in which issues of interest to the membership are discussed. The NAMDRC *Handbook* (available only to members) contains a model contract, a job description for medical directors of respiratory care services, various position statements, and an up-to-date analysis of Joint Commission on Accreditation of Health Care Or-

*Copies are available from: JRCRTE, 1701 W. Evless Blvd., Ste. 200, Euless, TX 76040.

ganizations (JCAHO) standards as they affect the role of medical directors of respiratory care services.

Finally, within certain appropriate national medical organizations, there exist sections or officers particularly interested in activities of the respiratory care profession. In the ACCP, there is an active Respiratory Care Steering Committee; in the ATS, the office of the Executive Director fills this role; in the ASA, the Committee on Respiratory Care (part of the section on Clinical Care) is entrusted with this responsibility. As the profession assumes more and more direct patient care responsibility, liaisons with the medical profession become increasingly important, and dialogue assumes greater and greater significance.

THE ATTENDING PHYSICIAN AND THE RESPIRATORY CARE PRACTITIONER

Overall care of patients is the direct responsibility of the physician of record, or *attending physician,* who must assess the patient's condition, perform a physical examination, order appropriate diagnostic tests, integrate this information to reach a correct diagnosis, and outline an appropriate treatment regimen. This basic "assess and treat" paradigm is followed every time that a physician-patient interface occurs, though obviously the physical examination step is overlooked when decisions are reached over the telephone!

In every state, respiratory therapy must be given only on physician order, except in life-threatening emergencies, or when standing orders or hospital medical staff- and board-approved therapist-driven protocols (TDPs) are in place. The respiratory care team member may participate in the patient assessment by performing a physical examination, performing pulmonary function tests including arterial blood gas sampling and analysis, performing exercise tests, monitoring cardiovascular parameters, and so forth. The RCP's major historic function, however, is to provide modalities that **treat** the patient's pulmonary disorder.

The level of expertise of the attending physician in managing patients with pulmonary diseases varies, depending on his or her previous training in caring for such patients. Those with training in internal medicine, with subspecialty training in pulmonary disease and critical care, usually have a more extensive pertinent background than those trained in surgery or the surgical subspecialties, with the exception of thoracic surgery. Extensive, in-depth training in the diagnosis of the vast array of pulmonary diseases and their therapy occurs in pulmonary disease and critical care training programs, but instruction in the actual scope and effectiveness of respiratory care modalities, even there, is often poor. Depending on the residency and fellowship training program, the attending physician's knowledge of the use of respiratory care modalities per se in the treatment of patients with lung diseases may be extensive and detailed or superficial and out of date.

The modern respiratory care practitioner (RCP) can be thought of as a *specialist physician extender.* Because the RCP may see the patient frequently during the day, sudden changes in the patient's condition can be observed by the RCP, and these changes can be communicated quickly to the attending physician. If the patient's condition worsens, intensification of therapy may be indicated; therapeutic needs of the patient frequently diminish as he or she improves. In the latter case, the RCP may well recommend a reduction (down-regulation) in the intensity of therapy. The respiratory care team can monitor the patient's pulmonary function at the bedside by simple measurements of vital capacity, tidal volume, inspiratory and expiratory forces, and arterial blood gas parameters. Not all patients require extensive monitoring, but those who are most ill, particularly those in the ICU, should have extensive monitoring at appropriate intervals. The RCP may suggest to the attending physician that respiratory monitoring be performed if the patient's respiratory condition deteriorates. If monitoring is already being performed, the respiratory therapist should inform the attending physician of any significant deterioration in pulmonary function, as preset boundaries are reached. This is most likely to occur in patients receiving mechanical ventilation. Thus, by effective monitoring and delivery of appropriate therapy, the RCP can be particularly helpful to the attending physician, and cost-effective, timely therapy can be the result.

The Attending Physician in Protocol and Nonprotocol Settings

The Respiratory Care Steering Committee of the ACCP defines TDPs as follows:

"TDPs are defined as patient care plans which are initiated and implemented by credentialed respiratory care workers. These plans are first designed and developed with input from physicians, and are approved for use by the medical staff and the governing body of the hospitals in which they are used. They share in common extreme reliance on respiratory care practitioner assessment and evaluation skills. TDPs are by their nature dynamic and flexible, allowing up- or down-regulation of intensity of respiratory services. They allow the RCP authority to evaluate the patient, initiate care, and to adjust, discontinue, or restart respiratory care procedures on a shift-by-shift, or hour-to-hour basis once the protocol is ordered by the physician. They contain clear strategies for various therapeutic interventions, while avoiding any misconception that they infringe on the practice of medicine."[2]

TDPs were developed in response to the clear perception that respiratory care services were often mislocated,[3] with a net tendency to be overused. A substantial literature, reviewed recently by one of us,[4] has suggested that intelligent use of TDPs goes far toward correcting this pattern of practice. The use of TDPs has been suggested to enrich, rather than disenfranchise, the role of the medical director of respiratory care services.[5]

Therapist-driven protocols empower the medical staff in wise use of respiratory care services. Far from taking the attending physician out of the decision-making loop and reducing the need for pulmonary medicine and critical care consultation, TDPs have done just the opposite. Physicians must order TDPs if they want them started. Fiat management has no place in a mature TDP universe. Physicians may override TDPs, or discontinue them, at any time and for any reason, though the respiratory care staff will take such action seriously and try to ascertain the reason for these actions. Good TDP orders include patient-specific *boundaries,* or situations in which the attending or consultant physician wants to be notified (eg, the decision to intubate or extubate a patient).

Experience has shown that the number of pulmonary medicine and critical care consultations actually increase when many RCP physician extenders are asking the right questions at the right time. The medical staff member who desires and learns interdependence with the health care team, rather than independence from it, thrives in the work ethic of a TDP-mature environment. Use of TDPs has been shown to be helpful in educational settings as well, as therapist students in training, medical residents, and postdoctoral fellows learn best practice approaches to respiratory care use.

Importance of Respect, Trust, and Mutual Confidence

The mutually beneficial association of physicians and RCPs has been present since the first developments of respiratory care (formerly called oxygen or inhalation therapy) departments more than 50 years ago. The common goal of providing optimal care to all patients with cardiopulmonary disease has been the basis for this relationship, which has grown and matured in an atmosphere of mutual trust, respect, and confidence unique in the health care professions. In the TDP paradigm, the importance of professional and personal respect, trust, and mutual confidence has been demonstrated over and over again.

Importance of Communication Skills

Whatever form it takes, and in whichever health care delivery model it must occur, good communication between the RCP, physician, and other members of the health care team is essential. This topic is discussed elsewhere in this chapter.

THE MEDICAL DIRECTOR OF THE RESPIRATORY CARE DEPARTMENT

Though not presently mandated by the JCAHO, a physician is required to be the medical director of respiratory care services by the Medicare Conditions of Participation for Acute Care Hospitals, and thus is still a part of the administrative hierarchy in most health care settings.

Qualifications and Definitions

The medical director of a respiratory care department must have proper qualifications to carry out his or her functions and responsibilities. The National Association of Medical Directors of Respiratory Care (NAMDRC), the American College of Chest Physicians (ACCP), and the Board of Medical Advisors (BOMA) of the American Association of Respiratory Care (AARC) have jointly passed a statement defining a qualified medical director of respiratory care:[6]

"The Medical Director of any inpatient or outpatient respiratory care service, department, or home care agency shall be a licensed physician who has special interest and knowledge in the diagnosis and treatment of respiratory problems. Whenever possible, the medical director should be qualified by special training and/or experience in the management of acute and chronic respiratory disorders. This physician should be responsible for the quality, safety, and appropriateness of the respiratory services provided, and require that respiratory care be ordered by a physician who has medical responsibility for the patient. The medical director should be readily accessible to the respiratory care practitioners and should assure their competency."[2]

A very similar ATS position paper[7] has also been published. The key points of these statements are that medical direction in respiratory care can occur both within and outside the hospital and that the medical director should be a physician who has received specific training in the care and treatment of patients with acute and chronic respiratory diseases. (Medical direction of respiratory care services in home care and at alternative sites will be discussed later in this chapter.)

The vast majority of medical directors of respiratory care are pulmonologists.[8] The next largest group comprises anesthesiologists, who once formed the largest group of medical directors of respiratory care until the large influx of specialists from pulmonary disease training programs in the 1970s and 1980s. Medical direction in respiratory care departments can also be provided by thoracic surgeons, internists, and a few others who have an interest but no specific training in pulmonary diseases. The latter situation tends to occur in small, rural hospitals.

Responsibilities and Functions

Responsibilities and functions of the medical director of respiratory care services are outlined in Boxes 2-14 and 2-15. The hospital, through a contract with the medical director, imparts authority to him or her to carry out its functions. The medical director must be able to make quick decisions in the name of the administration and hospital board of directors, to fulfill these responsibilities, and to satisfy the mission of the respiratory care department.

BOX 2-14

RESPONSIBILITIES OF THE MEDICAL DIRECTOR OF HOSPITAL RESPIRATORY CARE DEPARTMENTS

1. Responsible for the overall function of the respiratory care department and use of its services.
2. Responsible for the quality of care delivered by respiratory care personnel.
3. Responsible for providing support and acting as liaison between the respiratory care department and the medical staff.
4. Responsible for developing mutual respect and being liaison among the respiratory care department, hospital administration, and other hospital departments.
5. Responsible for the in-hospital education of respiratory care personnel.
6. Responsible for the quality of care provided to his or her patients and those patients seen in consultation.
7. Responsible for the respiratory care department's compliance with federal, state, and JCAHO regulations.
8. Shares responsibility with and provides medical expertise to the administrative and technical director(s) of the department in matters regarding the following:
   a. equipment
   b. personnel
   c. supplies
   d. budget
   e. space

Adapted with permission from American Thoracic Society: Position paper: Medical director of respiratory care. Am Rev Respir Dis 138:1082, 1988; NAMDRC Membership Survey, 1994; Miller WF, Plummer AL, et al:[9] Guidelines for organization and function of hospital respiratory care services. Chest 78:79, 1980

The medical director is responsible for the overall function of the respiratory care department. He or she may and should delegate much of the responsibilities for the day-to-day operation of the department to the nonphysician technical director of the department. However, it is the medical director's responsibility to ensure that individual RCP members of the staff perform well, to assure a properly operating respiratory care department that delivers high-quality patient care. If this is seen not to be the case, the medical director should effect the proper changes to ensure a smooth-running, efficient operation.

Quality assurance is one of the principal reasons that a medical director of respiratory care has traditionally been mandated by Medicare. Many of the functions carried out by the medical director (see following section) directly relate to this important responsibility.

Hospital respiratory care services should be provided in accordance with the standards developed by the Joint Commission on Accreditation of Health Care Organizations (JCAHO) and the Medicare Conditions of Participation for Hospitals. The current (1995) JCAHO standards of particular importance when applied to the respiratory care department are those of governance, patient assessment, care of patients, patient rights and organizational ethics, patient education, and continuation of care. The National Association of Medical Directors of Respiratory Care* has recently (1995) prepared a crosswalk of the more department-specific 1994 standards to those currently in force.

The selection of quality personnel is essential; this must be a function of the medical director in concert with the technical director of the department. The medical director should require that only nationally (NBRC) credentialed respiratory care personnel perform respiratory care services, and that other personnel provide only those services for which they have equivalent documented training, experience, and competence. Selection of a new director or assistant directors must be done carefully to assure competence in the management of the day-to-day operations of the department.

The medical director must also have input into the budgetary process to guarantee a cost-effective operation. This is particularly important in determining salaries and the purchase of equipment. The development of an aggressive quality assurance program assists in developing cost-effective budgets.

It is the medical director's responsibility to keep abreast of departmental affairs, and he or she can do this only by spending an adequate amount of time in the department on an almost *daily* basis. This is the best way to effect clear communication and cooperation between the medical director and the technical director of the respiratory care department.

The supervisory functions of the medical director (see Box 2-15) are important to make certain that the quality of care administered to patients is of high caliber. The more complex the care, the more observation is necessary. Those practitioners performing life-critical procedures, such as intubation, arterial puncture and cannulation, mechanical ventilation, and others, should be institutionally certified by the medical director. This certification should be in writing and placed in the employee's file. All therapists who demonstrate competency in TDP assessment and treatment selection skills should be so certified by the medical director as well. Certification should be completed only after the therapist has received proper training and has been directly observed performing the procedure or function by the medical director or his or her designee.

Respiratory care technology continues to expand rapidly. It is an additional responsibility of the medical director to ensure that respiratory care personnel keep abreast of these technological advances, as well as the changes in the therapies offered through the respiratory care department. Departmental in-service education is essential to impart new knowledge to the staff. Education can occur through an ongoing, scheduled program of lectures and conferences, as well as through scheduled rounds with members of the department. The medical director should make sure that department personnel are given time to attend educational

*Copies are available from: NAMDRC, 5454 Wisconsin Ave, Chevy Chase, MD 20815.

BOX 2-15

FUNCTIONS OF THE MEDICAL DIRECTOR OF RESPIRATORY CARE DEPARTMENTS

1. Administrative
   a. Develops and approves all departmental policies.
   b. Develops and approves all department procedures, especially those with high risk.
   c. Reviews and institutes effective new respiratory therapy procedures, including clinical pathways and therapist-driven protocols.
   d. Participates in the selection of new employees and in the dismissal of old employees, as requested by the technical director.
   e. Participates in development of cost-effective departmental budgets and policies.
   f. Participates in the selection and purchase of equipment.
   g. Participates in departmental quality assurance activities.
   h. Participates in the day-to-day activities of the department to the degree necessary to ensure high-quality patient services.
   i. Is available to staff for consultation at all times.
   j. Monitors and prevents misallocation of respiratory care services by appropriate audit techniques.
   k. As indicated, reviews individual medical staff performance in prescribing respiratory therapies, use of indicated therapies, documentation, and outcomes of therapy.
2. Supervisory
   a. Observes the activities of the respiratory care personnel.
   b. Certifies respiratory care personnel for invasive and other procedures.
3. Educational
   a. Reviews all departmental educational programs.
   b. Participates in all educational activities of the department.
   c. Participates in educational activities of medical staff and other hospital departments.
4. Clinical
   a. Provides care for his or her own patients.
   b. Is available for patient consultations as requested by medical staff.
   c. Performs procedures commensurate with training and education.
   d. Interacts directly with RCPs and promotes problem-solving expertise and guidance in the laboratory and at the bedside as needed and requested.
   e. Approves code order policy, definition of brain death determination.
   f. Participates in the development, evolution, and introduction of new respiratory services, equipment, and procedures, and monitors existing respiratory services for their cost-effectiveness and continued medical utility.
   g. May coordinate special respiratory services for other units, which include respiratory intensive care units, pulmonary rehabilitation programs, hyperbaric oxygen therapy units, smoking cessation clinics, transportation of critically ill patients within the hospital and between hospitals, sleep disorders centers, and other programs that appropriately require participation from the respiratory care services department.
5. Research
   a. Approves all clinical research performed in department.
   b. Evaluates and approves all experimental (beta site) testing done in department.

meetings outside the hospital that will upgrade the practitioner's knowledge in respiratory care. A knowledgeable staff is more likely to provide quality patient care.

It is important that the medical director practice medicine and be available for patient consultation by the medical staff. He or she should serve as a model for other physicians to follow in the care of patients with pulmonary diseases. It is very important that the hospital grant the medical director the privilege of practicing medicine within the hospital. Often these functions, if properly structured, allow educational opportunities for respiratory care personnel. The medical director should be available for consultations regarding other physicians' patients, particularly those receiving mechanical ventilation. He or she should have the ability to admit and care for his or her own patients, as well as to perform those procedures (bronchoscopy, thoracentesis, pleural biopsy, chest tube placement, intubation, arterial and venous line placement, and others) for which he or she is qualified by training.

The medical director must be available to the respiratory care department 24 hours a day. In a large department, this function and other responsibilities and duties can be shared with assistant medical directors appointed to the department. In a small department, the medical director should designate a competent physician to handle these responsibilities whenever he or she is away or is otherwise unavailable.

The medical director should be compensated for the time and services he or she provides to the department. The amount of compensation should directly relate to the amount of time spent in the department and should **not** be tied in any way to its productivity (eg, percentage of gross or net revenues, number of patients, and such). Finally, the medical director should have a written contract with the hospital defining his or her authority, responsibilities, functions, and reimbursement.

Hospital Liaisons Important to the Medical Director[10]

Relationships between the medical director and the technical director of the respiratory care department are extremely important. The medical director spends much of his or her time with the technical director, discussing and solving problems concerning the operations of the department. Together they work to set goals and objectives for the department. This interaction can be a mutually rewarding experience. A good working relationship is crucial to the proper functioning of both directors and to their ability to achieve the goals and objectives set.

It is important for the medical director to meet with the technical director on an almost daily basis and with the assistant directors and the supervisory staff on a regular basis. Participation in departmental staff meetings or meetings with the departmental director, assistant director(s), and supervisory staff are a necessity and give the medical director an excellent view of the overall function of the department. Regular discussions with individual members of the department are also very important. This greatly enhances the medical director's familiarity with his or her staff. Often problems with patients are discussed, and these can be solved efficiently and effectively.

The medical director is responsible to the hospital administration for the overall function of the respiratory care department. Often he or she works with a specific hospital administrator. It is very important that the medical director develop a solid working relationship with this administrator. They should meet, along with the technical director of the respiratory care department, on a scheduled basis throughout the year. At times, special projects or events dictate that a meeting be set up with the facility administrator either with or without the technical director present. Communication is crucial to determine solutions for departmental problems and to achieve the goals set.

The medical director interacts with other departments within the hospital, especially nursing. This is particularly important in the TDP setting, where RCPs must work hand-in-hand with the nursing service if good care and excellent outcomes are to be achieved. The medical director is viewed as representing the respiratory care department; hence, it is important that his or her contacts with nursing administration be amiable and constructive. The same can be said about his or her relationship with other hospital departments. In some hospitals, chest physiotherapy (CPT) is under the aegis of the physical therapy department. Timing of respiratory care services (eg, bronchodilator aerosol delivery) with CPT is important and has to be arranged between these two departments if chest physiotherapy is not a function of the respiratory care department. Again, a healthy relationship at the top ensures good cooperation among therapists from both departments.

The medical director should participate in the conferences of the medical staff, to update the medical staff's knowledge in the field of respiratory care. New therapies that are instituted must be communicated to the medical staff so that they may use them. The medical staff may have other services that they wish the respiratory care department to perform, for example, electrocardiograms, exercise testing, or other physiologic studies. Only by effective communication between the medical director and the medical staff can these be accomplished. Medical staff evaluations are periodically necessary to ascertain how well the respiratory care staff is performing the patient care services assigned to it.

The respiratory care department is one department among many in the hospital. Activities of other departments may directly influence activities of the respiratory care department. Similarly, the respiratory care department's functions also impinge on input and output from other hospital departments. It is very important that the medical director ensure that effective communication exists between the respiratory care department and other hospital departments so that activities of one do not compromise or negate the activities of another. If all activities are not coordinated, patient care may be adversely affected. It is the responsibility of the medical director to make certain that this does not happen.

THE MEDICAL DIRECTOR OF THE PULMONARY FUNCTION LABORATORY

The pulmonary function laboratory, sometimes referred to as the pulmonary physiology laboratory, is an essential element in the diagnosis and evaluation of patients with pulmonary diseases. A medical director is required for the proper function of this laboratory, if the physiologic results reported are to be accurate and timely.[11,12] If the pulmonary function laboratory is under the aegis of the respiratory care department, the medical director of the respiratory care department may also function as the medical director of the pulmonary function laboratory. Alternatively, he or she may opt to allow another physician to be the medical director of the pulmonary function laboratory.

The medical director of the pulmonary function laboratory must be a physician, or the equivalent, who has been trained and has expertise in pulmonary physiology. He or she must have in-depth knowledge of the testing instruments, the significance of the data obtained from these devices, and how the data apply to the patient. In addition, he or she should possess the qualifications listed previously for the medical director of the respiratory care department. Responsibilities and specific functions of the medical director of pulmonary function laboratories are outlined in Box 2-16. The medical director of the pulmonary function laboratory is accountable to the hospital administration, the hospital staff, and the medical director of the respiratory care department if the laboratory is under the aegis of that department.

MEDICAL DIRECTION OF RESPIRATORY CARE SERVICES IN THE HOME AND IN ALTERNATE CARE SITES

In recent years, emphasis has been placed on the development of a seamless, vertically integrated health care model (Box 2-17). Although implementation of this model is still not mature, it is clear that patients will not move smoothly along such a continuum. Instead,

BOX 2-16

RESPONSIBILITIES AND FUNCTIONS OF THE MEDICAL DIRECTOR OF PULMONARY FUNCTION LABORATORIES (PFL)

1. Administrative
   a. Is accountable to staff and administration of hospital for PFL activities.
   b. Is responsible for the cost-effective use of the PFL.
   c. Liaises with other hospital units as required, for example, clinical pathology and nursing departments.
   d. Develops and approves all PFL policies, procedures, and testing protocols.
   e. Is responsible for the types of testing performed and PFL equipment used.
   f. Is responsible for assuring that the PFL is in compliance with federal, state, JCAHO, College of American Pathologists (CAP), and American Osteopathic Association regulations and guidelines.
2. Supervisory
   a. Is responsible for the quality of testing performed in the PFL.
   b. Observes the activities of PFL personnel.
   c. Assesses and assures competency of PFL personnel.
   d. Develops, administers, and surveys all quality assurance activities.
   e. Minimizes risks associated with all PFL procedures.
3. Educational
   a. Educates medical and ancillary services staff in appropriate use of PFL.
   b. Ensures optimal knowledge of physiologic testing in students, RCPs, and ancillary and medical staff.
4. Clinical
   a. Assures accurate and timely performance and interpretation of physiologic tests.
   b. Is responsible for the quality of PFL data.
   c. Acts as a consultant to other physicians, advising appropriate test selection and use of PFL facilities.

Adapted with permission from NAMDRC: Position Paper: Responsibilities of the Medical Director of the Pulmonary Physiology Laboratory. Washington, DC, NAMDRC, 1994

BOX 2-17

A SEAMLESS HEALTH CARE DELIVERY MODEL*

Primary care practitioners ("gatekeepers")
Medical specialists
Emergency departments
Acute care hospitals
Subacute care facilities
Specialty-emphasis subacute facilities
Skilled nursing facilities (SNFs)
Hospice, day care, and respite care units
Home care programs

** Patients may pass back and forth between different health care providers.*

patients (and their families) will move in and out and back and forth. As one writer[12] has pointed out, "The key question is not *where* the market will go . . . but how to address this moving target. The answer is the (patient's) physician."

The medical director of respiratory care in the acute care hospital was originally mandated to assure that the respiratory care services provided were appropriate for the patient population and were of high quality. Those who provide respiratory care services in the home and in alternative community sites also have an obligation to provide quality respiratory care services similar to those provided in the acute care hospital. The medical director would seem a logical choice to assure that quality respiratory care services are provided in sites outside the hospital. The American College of Chest Physicians (ACCP), the National Association of Medical Directors of Respiratory Care (NAMDRC), The American Thoracic Society (ATS), and the Board of Medical Advisors (BOMA) of the American Association of Respiratory Care (AARC) all feel strongly that a qualified medical director is needed to supervise respiratory care services outside the hospital.[14–19]

The qualifications, responsibilities, and duties of a medical director of a home care company or an alternative community site have recently been delineated.[16] The medical director should be a licensed physician who has had specialized training and clinical experience in caring for patients with acute and chronic respiratory diseases, particularly those requiring home mechanical ventilation. The roles and functions of the medical director in this setting are outlined in Box 2-18. The roles and functions of the medical director in a subacute unit are very similar to those in the acute care hospital (see Boxes 2-14 and 2-15). He or she should be responsible for the quality and appropriateness of the medical services, which should be delivered in a safe and cost-effective manner. The medical director should be accessible to the respiratory care staff wherever and whenever they practice outside the hospital, as well as to the patients' private physicians. In the absence of TDPs, it is the medical director's responsibility to see that appropriate respiratory care services have been provided as prescribed by the patient's personal physician. The responsibility for the overall care of the patient, however, resides with the attending physician.

The medical director of respiratory care services in home care services and at alternative sites should be involved in activities that lead to the delivery of quality, cost-effective respiratory care. This care must be delivered by qualified practitioners; hence, adequate personnel job descriptions and policies must be in place. All aspects of patient care must be reviewed by the medical director, including patient care policies, treatment protocols, and procedure manuals, to make certain that the care provided by the respiratory care staff is appropriate and of high quality. The equipment used should be safe and reliable. New therapies should be used whenever the staff has the expertise and training to institute their use.

BOX 2-18

THE MEDICAL DIRECTOR OF RESPIRATORY CARE PROGRAMS IN THE HOME AND ALTERNATE SITES

1. Administrative functions
   a. Develops and reviews personnel policies and job descriptions.
   b. Develops and reviews the quality, safety, appropriateness, and cost-effectiveness of patient care, including treatment protocols and procedure manuals.
   c. Reviews and updates all medical services delivered to patients to ensure high quality and cost-effectiveness.
   d. Assesses existing and new equipment and its application for patient use.
   e. Develops and reviews quality assurance measures.
   f. Assists with budgeting and reimbursement from fiscal and regulatory agencies if requested.
   g. Ensures that the respiratory care services provided are in compliance with safety regulations and other regulations dictated by local, state, and federal governments.
   h. Ensures that accreditation standards are met for JCAHO, Medicare, other federal, state, and local agencies as appropriate.
   i. Provides medical expertise to the home health agency or home care disposable medical equipment (DME) vendor in matters relating to program development, compliance with regulations, safety, budgeting, reimbursements, and billing.
2. Educational functions
   a. Develops and reviews all policies, patient programs, and educational materials.
   b. Develops and maintains staff in-service and education programs.
   c. Serves as a medical resource for inquiries from staff, patients, and attending physicians concerning patient care and disease processes.
   d. Educates third-party payers and others regarding the cost effectiveness and importance of providing quality respiratory care outside the hospital.

Used with permission from Plummer AL: Medical direction of home care. Respir Manag 17:9, 1987

A quality assurance program should be designed for these settings to assess the effectiveness of the care provided to patients; this is also necessary because technology continues to advance rapidly in the field of respiratory care. The medical director may be asked to assist in matters of budgeting and reimbursement, depending on his or her interests and expertise. All respiratory care should be in compliance with current safety standards and other regulations dictated by federal, state, and local governments. The JCAHO has developed standards to be met by providers outside the hospital.[17] The purposes of these standards are to protect the patient, assure a high quality of care, and prevent system abuse. This is a voluntary process for any company or facility delivering medical care outside the hospital. If the entity for which the medical director functions decides to seek accreditation, the medical director should be of assistance in any way possible to ensure that the accreditation standards are met.

THE MEDICAL DIRECTOR AS AN EDUCATOR

In Respiratory Care Departments

The medical director should participate in the development and delivery of all the educational functions of the department. Usually, an educational director or a therapist who functions in this capacity develops the department's educational programs. The medical director should deliver some of the conferences, participate in others, and facilitate teaching patient rounds in which respiratory care personnel can participate. The in-service program should be mapped out well in advance. Consideration should be given to videotaping the conferences so that personnel on the evening or night shifts can view them.

In Respiratory Therapy Training Programs

The educational functions of the medical director in the respiratory care department and the medical director in formal school programs of respiratory therapy are outlined in Box 2-19.

BOX 2-19

FUNCTIONS OF THE MEDICAL DIRECTOR AS AN EDUCATOR

1. Directs content of all respiratory care in-service programs.
2. Develops and oversees all therapist competency evaluation programs.
3. Educates medical staff, nursing staff, and others.
4. Develops and approves patient education materials.
5. In an approved school of respiratory therapy
   a. Provides structured, nonconfrontational contacts between students and physicians.
   b. Plans and approves scientific content of curriculum.
   c. Enhances clinical teaching of program faculty.
   d. Provides support for negotiations between program and clinical affiliates.
   e. Encourages and monitors formal and informal medical input at clinical affiliates, including rounds, lectures, and case studies.
   f. Assures timeliness of all medical content taught in program.
   g. Is visible by participation in lectures, case conferences, and direct patient care activities throughout the program.
   h. Is responsible for teaching indications for therapy, awareness of potential harmful effects of therapy, and definitions of boundaries in TDP programs.

The JRCRTE requires medical direction of all the programs that it accredits.[20] One of the most common reasons for failure of educational programs to be approved by the JRCRTE is inadequate input from the medical director of the program and from other physicians involved in the affiliated institutions. The medical director of a school of respiratory care technology should have all the qualifications listed earlier for a qualified medical director of respiratory care, as well as the ability to teach and assist the program director in program development. The medical director must be responsible for the quality and validity of the scientific and clinical content of the program taught by the faculty. It is important that he or she teach at least one course each term and be available for assistance to other faculty in the program.

The medical director of an educational program in respiratory care is responsible for obtaining input from physicians in the hospitals used for the clinical portion of the students' curriculum. Student contact with these physicians is important for the students' growth and development as RCPs. Establishment of good rapport with physicians should be learned as a student and perfected as a graduate RCP.

In Home Care and Alternate Care Sites

The educational functions of the medical director in skilled nursing facilities and other nontraditional sites are very important. The outpatient (home care) programs offered and the educational materials used need to be reviewed and updated for accuracy and applicability to patient care. It is important that the patients and their care givers readily understand the materials. Only those programs that are medically correct and efficacious should be continued. Development of an ongoing, in-service training program for the respiratory care staff is important to keep their knowledge updated and to introduce them to new technology and therapy. The medical director should have a large input in this area. He or she must be available to serve as a resource for inquiries concerning pathophysiology of disease processes, treatment and prognosis, and other aspects of respiratory care from staff, patients, and attending physicians. The medical director may need to discuss the cost-effectiveness and appropriateness of the respiratory care programs offered with third-party payors (including Medicare) and others.

Future Directions for the Medical Director of Respiratory Care Services

Data from our hospitals indicate that there is a shift of medical care from a hospital-centered activity to an outpatient-centered activity. As the number of hospitalized patients decreases, so does the number of procedures performed by RCPs, thus necessitating our hospital respiratory care departments to "right size," to provide cost-effective, high-quality respiratory care. These events are occurring throughout the nation. Because technologic advances will allow it, patients with pulmonary diseases can receive most of their care outside of the hospital. Respiratory care services from subacute care units, skilled nursing facilities, home health agencies, and home care companies are increasing, therefore allowing more RCPs to practice in these venues. As respiratory care outside the hospital becomes more technologically sophisticated and the patients treated are sicker, the need for a qualified medical director of respiratory care in sites outside of the hospital will increase. These events will provide opportunities for RCPs and physicians to work together, to provide the respiratory care necessary for patients with pulmonary diseases. This relationship should be as harmonious in sites outside the hospital as it is within the hospital.

REFERENCES

1. American Association for Respiratory Care: Definition of the Profession. Dallas, 1993
2. American College of Chest Physicians Respiratory Care Steering Committee Working Paper: Therapist-driven respiratory care protocols (Unpublished). Chicago, 1992
3. Stoller JK: Misallocation of respiratory care services: Time of change (Editorial). Respir Care 38:263, 1993
4. Burton GG: A short history of therapist-driven respiratory care protocols. Respir Care Clin North Am 2:15, 1996
5. Burton GG: Therapist-driven respiratory care protocols do not disenfranchise medical direction of respiratory care services. NAMDRC Clin Manag Quart 18(4):2, 1995
6. National Association of Medical Directors of Respiratory Care Position Statement: NAMDRC Definition of a Qualified Medical Director of Respiratory Care. Washington, DC, 1986
7. American Thoracic Society: Position paper: Medical director of respiratory care. Am Rev Respir Dis 138:1082, 1988
8. NAMDRC Membership Survey, 1994
9. Miller WF, Plummer AL, et al: Guidelines for organization and function of hospital respiratory care services. Chest 78.79, 1980
10. Plummer, AL: Hospital liaisons important to the medical director of respiratory care. NAMDRC Newsletter 17(4):5, 1994.
11. ATS Respiratory Care Committee: Position: The director of pulmonary function laboratory. ATS News 4:6, 1978
12. NAMDRC: Position Paper: Responsibilities of the Medical Director of the Pulmonary Physiology Laboratory. Washington, DC, NAMDRC, 1994
13. Tarnove LR: Physicians: The key to the long-term market. Prod Mgt Today July, 1995
14. Plummer AL: Medical direction of home care. Respir Manag 17:9, 1987
15. American Association of Respiratory Care: Medical Direction for Respiratory Care Services Provided Outside of the Hospital. Dallas, AARC, 1989
16. National Association of Medical Directors of Respiratory Care: NAMDRC Position Statement on Medical Direction of Home Health Care. Washington, DC, NAMDRC, 1988
17. Joint Commission on Accreditation of Health Care Organizations: Standards for the Accreditation of Home Care. Chicago, JCAHCO, 1988
18. American Association of Respiratory Care: 1987 Human Resources Survey: Home Health Agencies. Dallas, AARC, 1987
19. American Association of Respiratory Care: 1987 Human Resources Survey: Durable Medical Equipment Companies. Dallas, AARC, 1987
20. American Medical Association: Essentials of an Approved Program for Respiratory Therapy Technician and the Respiratory Therapist. Chicago, Council on Accreditation of Allied Health Education Programs, 1986

Thomas J. DeKornfeld

SECTION 4
Medicolegal Aspects of Respiratory Care

PROFESSIONAL SKILLS

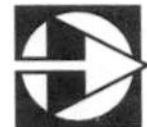

Upon completion of this chapter, the reader will be able to:

- Discuss the health care provider's legal obligations to his or her patient
- List the criteria that a plaintiff must prove in a negligence suit against a health care provider
- Define consent and why it is necessary that it be obtained from a patient
- Explain in what instances a hospital can be held liable
- Understand how the health care provider–technologist relationship may affect respiratory care therapists
- Explain the role of a state licensure board
- Illustrate ways a health care provider can avoid a lawsuit from a patient

KEY TERMS

Abandonment
Breach
Consent
Duty of care
Fraud
Invasion of privacy
Licensure
Malpractice
Negligence
Respondeat superior
Triage

The problems of health care delivery are not limited to the prevention, diagnosis, and treatment of disease. Regretfully, they must also include awareness of the potential legal consequences of all the aspects of current health care provider–health care recipient interaction.

In much of the following discussion, the role of the physician will be emphasized because the physician is still the primary contractor, and most of the other health care personnel function as assistants of the physician and are employees of either the physician or the hospital. There are exceptions to this, and there is an increasing number of nurses and technologists who function as independent contractors and are thus subject to the same legal constraints and liabilities as the physician. Thus, where applicable, one may substitute "health care provider," in its broadest sense, for "physician" in what follows.

THE PHYSICIAN–PATIENT RELATIONSHIP

The physician–patient relationship is the basis of all medical practice. Under the law, this relationship may be considered as either a contractual one or a professional one. Under the former and much less popular one, the physician agrees to render a service for a fee. The professional relationship implies that the physician has accepted the patient and also accepts the responsibility of rendering due and proper care. This relationship is known as the *duty of care.* The relationship, once established, may be terminated by the patient at any time and for whatever reason, but it may be terminated by the physician only under specific circumstances. These include informing the patient in writing of the intent to terminate, giving the patient enough time to find another physician, and getting the patient's concurrence to the termination. Unless these steps are followed, the patient may sue for *abandonment,* if the physician's unilateral withdrawal leads to harm to the patient.

The physician does not have to accept any patient, unless he or she has a contractual or employment obligation to do so. Thus, for instance, an emergency room physician, hired by the hospital to provide care in the emergency room, must attend to all patients who come to the ER for care. Physicians working in any public institution may not refuse care to any patient if in so doing they would violate any of the federal or state antidiscriminatory statutes.

Accepting a patient entails a duty for the physician, namely, to provide services that meet the customary standards of care, and to use reasonable skill and knowledge in providing such services. The law does not require the physician to be perfect, but it does require the physician to perform according to the principles stated by the court in *Blair v Eblen:*[1] "A physician is under a duty to use that degree of skill which is expected of a reasonably competent practitioner in the same class to which he [or she] belongs, acting in the same or similar circumstances."

This definition does not exclude honest differences of opinion, which are so very common in health care. If there are two or more options by which a condition may be diagnosed and treated, any one of these options may be selected, provided that at least a "respectable minority" supports that choice. If, in retrospect, another option may have been preferable, no violation of the standard has occurred, assuming that the option chosen was "reasonable."

Most cases of *malpractice* are tried under the legal concept of *negligence.* For negligence to be proven, four criteria must be satisfied. (1) The plaintiff must show that the health care provider owed a duty, that is, that there was indeed a physician-patient relationship. (2) The plaintiff must show that this duty was violated or, in other words, that the standards of care were breached. This is the most difficult component of a negligence suit, because the standards are rarely defined in writing, and hence, it is difficult to show that they were breached. Consequently, the standards are defined by the "finder of fact," that is, the jury. Because the jury is composed of laypeople with little if any medical knowledge, the court uses experts to explain the intricacies of the situation. In general, national standards apply to almost all health care providers today, and this means that experts may also be recruited from other parts of the country. It also means that local standards cannot be less restrictive than national standards. Conversely, however, local standards may be more restrictive, in which case they are binding on the hospital or community that established the more stringent standards. (3) The plaintiff must show there are damages. If the patient suffers no injury, there is no basis for litigation, regardless of how much the physician may have breached the standards. (4) The plaintiff must show the violation of the standard is the proximate cause of the injury. This means that the injury must ensue directly from the breach of duty, and there can be no intervening steps.

Though negligence is by far the most frequent reason for litigation between patient and physician or hospital, it is by no means the only one. Others include, but are not limited to, assault and battery, breach of confidentiality, invasion of privacy, breach of promise, and fraud.

Assault and battery, in law, does not necessarily mean hitting somebody over the head with a baseball bat but, simply, that one person intentionally tried to touch another person and, in fact, succeeded to do so. In other words, it is the unauthorized touching of another person's body regardless of whatever reason this touching has taken place. It is an absolute right by law that every adult person has the unquestionable privilege to decide what, if anything, is going to be done to them. This very important issue can be put into another context: patients have the right to decide what diagnostic or therapeutic manipulation will be performed on or for them, and hence, no health care provider can do anything to a patient without the patient's specific *consent.* It naturally ensues, therefore, that the patient's consent must be obtained before any diagnostic or therapeutic manipulation may begin.

For the consent to be legally meaningful, it must be (1) valid, (2) free, and (3) informed. For the consent to be valid, it must be given by a person who is legally entitled to do so. This means that it must be given by a competent adult for him- or herself. Adulthood is a matter of age and is determined by statute in all states. Competency is much more difficult to determine, but the assumption is that every adult is competent unless he or she has been declared incompetent by a court. This raises problems, because patients may behave in a bizarre fashion and may even claim to be George Washington or Mother Theresa, but they may still be legally competent. This places the provider in the middle of an awkward dilemma. The usual solution is to seek consent from the family. This may temporarily make the provider feel better, but legally it is totally unacceptable. The family has no standing in this situation, and no adult, regardless of how closely related, may give consent for another, conscious adult who has not been legally declared incompetent.

If the patient is unconscious, physicians may proceed with life-saving measures without any consent whatever. Courts have ruled consistently that this is entirely proper, because it is reasonable to assume that the patient would have consented had he or she been able to do so.

In the case of a minor, only the legal parent or legal guardian may give consent, except in those cases in which the minor is considered legally "emancipated." Minors who are legally married, live away from home, support themselves, serve in the armed forces, or have been declared adults by a court may give consent for themselves, even though they are not technically of legal age. In many states there are also statutory exemptions for minors, but these are usually restricted to reproductive problems or sexually transmitted disease.

Technically, the consent need not be in writing, although from a practical point of view it clearly should be. The consent form should contain information about the proposed procedure and should list the most likely complications. The form should be signed by the consenting person and should be witnessed by a person preferably not directly involved in the patient's care.

The consent must be free; that is, it must be given without any coercion being brought on the patient. Other than in the case of inmates in a penitentiary, this is of little significance, except when the consent is sought for an experimental procedure. In fact the concept of free consent was first formulated in the Nuremberg Declaration,[2] after World War II, when numerous inmates of German concentration camps were forced to participate in so-called medical experiments.

The consent must also be informed, and this is the most complex part of the consent issue. There is clearly no way in which a layperson can truly understand all the possible complications that may ensue from even relatively simple procedures. Fortunately, the law does not expect this, and for the consent to be informed, it is only necessary to acquaint the patient with the nature of the proposed procedure, the purpose for which it is performed, the expected outcome, and the major complications that may occur.

Complications that have a relatively high incidence (> 2% to 5%) should be discussed in some detail, particularly if these complications are disfiguring, sterilizing, or otherwise interfering with the quality of life. The patient must be given an opportunity to ask questions and allowed to make a decision without being unduly influenced by the authoritative presence of a health professional. Under no circumstances should the patient be misled, and lying to a patient is inexcusable. If the patient refuses treatment, this must be respected, and under no circumstances should the patient be talked into undergoing a potentially hazardous procedure (and what procedure is not?). That way lies disaster.

If the patient does refuse, or withdraws a previously given consent, it is incumbent on the health care provider to advise the patient of the risks of such refusal. In a landmark case *(Truman v Thomas)*,[3] the court opined, "If a patient indicates that he or she is going to refuse a risk-free test or treatment, then the doctor has the additional duty of advising of all material risks of which a reasonable person would want to be informed before deciding not to undergo the procedure."

Another cause for litigation may be a breach of confidentiality. Any information obtained from a patient, with very few statutory exceptions (eg, gunshot wounds, some infectious diseases, child abuse), must remain absolutely confidential and may not be revealed without the patient's permission. This applies to all information concerning the patient, including all respiratory care notes and data. Because almost all patients require the services of a number of hospital personnel, information may be shared among these care givers on a "need to know" basis. Obviously, the rule of confidentiality is applicable to this entire group of people.

It is in the nature of the hospital community to discuss interesting cases with each other. Although the ostensible purpose of such discussions is educational, in fact many of these discussions take place in cafeterias, elevators, or other public places, well within the hearing of visitors and other people. This is an almost universal practice, and yet, it is a regrettable one that should be curtailed as much as possible. Even if the patient's name is not mentioned, if the case is really unusual, it would not be difficult for people to find out the identity of the "interesting case." Unless the patient's consent for disclosure is obtained, such breach of confidentiality is actionable.

Invasion of privacy is related to breach of confidentiality, but it deals more specifically with such matters as unauthorized photography or using the patient as a teaching model without the patient's permission.

Breach of promise is rare but not unknown. If the provider is foolish enough to promise a certain outcome, he or she may be held liable under the breach of promise theory if the outcome is not as advertised. All providers should be careful in what they say to the patient. Even an innocuous and frequently heard statement, such as, "Don't worry, everything will be all right," is technically a promise. Fortunately, courts have not held practitioners liable for such vague statements and will consider a breach of promise action only if the promise was made in writing or under circumstances from which the contractual nature of the commitment is obvious.

Fraud is a very distressing type of litigation, because the underlying issue is almost always naked greed. Billing for procedures not performed, double billing, or billing for services not rendered constitutes fraud. Such a case may be handled under the civil law, but if egregious, it may lead to indictment under the criminal law and result in not only a fine but also a prison sentence and the almost-certain loss of one's license.

THE PATIENT–HOSPITAL RELATIONSHIP

Until recently, the relationship of the patient to the hospital was quite similar to that of a guest to a hotel. The hospital was responsible for providing a safe and salubrious environment, room and board, and the personnel and equipment for the physicians to practice their trade. The hospital did not have any responsibility for the quality of medical care practiced within its walls, although traditionally, it participated with the medical staff in administrative decisions pertaining to practice privileges and other similar items. Although the hospital employed the nurses and technologists and was thus responsible for their actions under the legal doctrine of "respondeat superior" (see next section), the employees were frequently held to be under the control of the physician, who thus became responsible for the employees' negligence under the legal doctrine of the "borrowed servant."

This situation has changed dramatically since the precedent-setting case of *Darling v Charleston Community Hospital.*[4] *Darling* established the principle, at least in Illinois, that the hospital as a corporate entity is responsible, through its governing board, for the standards of medical care practiced in the institution. This means that the hospital can be held liable if it permits the physicians having staff privileges to practice below acceptable standards, and if it knows or should have known that a physician is incompetent. Following *Darling,* the hospital boards of trustees (directors, governors, and so forth) must make sure that there is an appropriate staff organization, that there are bylaws governing the activities of the medical staff, that the standards set by the Joint Commission on Accreditation of Health Care Organizations (JCAHO) are rigorously enforced, and that the medical staff properly polices itself according to specific, stated policies and procedures. The *Darling* decision was followed by many others in a number of jurisdictions, so that today the accountability of the hospital is recognized and accepted in all states and territories.

These changing attitudes toward the hospital's legal liabilities make it imperative that the hospital's bylaws, medical staff regulations, and all policies and procedures be carefully reviewed. The steps for admission to the medical staff and the steps necessary for any disciplinary action must be specific and in accordance with the present stringent requirements for due process. Highly desirable disciplinary attempts have been frustrated when the physician or employee could show that due process had not been followed.

The *Darling* decision and others like it have raised awkward problems not only for the hospital, but also for all hospital employees, particularly nurses and technologists. The operative phrase in all decisions like *Darling* was "the hospital knew or should have known." The only way the hospital can know is when somebody tells it. Thus, the hospital must establish quality assurance and other supervisory committees to review records and report staff members who violate the standards set for the institution. Further, any staff person who has information suggesting professional incompetence or impairment has the duty to bring this matter to the attention of the hospital administration in a formal manner. The usual form for such a communication is the incident report that outlines the alleged incident and identifies the person or persons involved.

The employee's duty is clear. Negligent, incompetent, or impaired colleagues or fellow workers must be reported, even though this duty leaves the employee with a difficult dilemma. Nobody likes to blow the whistle, and the traditional hierarchy in the hospital makes it very awkward for a technologist or nurse to "rat" on a physician. In addition, the allegation of professional incompetence or impairment will have to be documented, and failure to do so may make the complainant liable for disciplinary action and even possible dismissal. Legal action for damages can be ruled out in both federal and state action, because it would require that the plaintiff prove malice or the hope for gain on the part of the complainant. This is usually virtually impossible. Yet, the decision to report or not to report deviations from the standard of care remains an individual matter. I believe that reporting is a legal and ethical mandate, and I cite a comment from the opinion of Mr. Justice Goldberg in a California case involving a very bad, impaired physician: "As for the doctors on the Mercy staff, two thoughts keep going through my mind. The one is from Dr. Jones (a physician on the Mercy staff): 'No one told anyone anything.' And the other is from Edmund Burke (an 18th century English politician): 'The only thing necessary for the triumph of evil is for good men to do nothing.' "[5]

Of particular interest in this context is Public Law 99660, the Health Care Improvement Act of 1986. This places heavy responsibility on the hospitals and on the state licensing boards. It grants immunity to those who report on physicians' and nurses' malpractice. It also establishes a federal data bank for all physicians and dentists who have been the target of litigation or of any hospital or state disciplinary action.

THE PHYSICIAN–TECHNOLOGIST RELATIONSHIP

The ethical component of this relationship has undergone significant changes since the last edition of this book and thus requires a more thorough discussion in the next chapter. The legal relationships have not changed to any appreciable degree, and they still depend on the employment conditions of the technologist. If the technologist is employed by the physician, the physician is clearly responsible for the actions of the technologist under the legal doctrine of ***respondeat superior,*** that is, let the "master" be responsible for the actions of the "servant." If the technologist is employed by the hospital, then the hospital is liable under the same doctrine, unless it can be shown that the technologist was under the full control of the physician. In this case, the doctrine of the ***borrowed servant*** applies, and the physician, rather than the hospital, is liable.

There is increasing pressure that certain health care technologists be freed from the burden of working under medical supervision. The JCAHO standards that required this supervision have been modified and no longer make medical direction a requirement for respiratory care services. There has also been considerable pressure from the respiratory care membership organizations to liberate the respiratory care practitioners from physician supervision altogether. Assuming that the requirement that the respiratory care practitioner work under the supervision of a physician were really abolished and the practitioner worked as an independent contractor, there would be no legal relationship between physician and practitioner. The practitioner would be fully responsible for his or her actions and would have to assume both the emotional satisfaction and also the financial risks of such a situation.

As long as the practitioner remained an employee of the hospital, but no longer functioned under medical supervision, the hospital would remain responsible under respondeat superior. I strongly suspect that this would make the hospital administration extremely nervous and that it would lead to a very much tighter job description for the respiratory care practitioner. The therapist-driven protocols would be worded very conservatively, to minimize the potential risks and to immunize the hospital, as far as possible, against litigation.

It remains to be seen whether this arrangement will prove satisfactory to any of the four participants (hospital, physician, respiratory care practitioner, and patient) and how these relationships will be modified under the pressure of legislation on the one hand and litigation on the other. The bottom line in all health-related issues is the welfare and safety of the patient. To what extent this can be reasonably assured by nonphysicians, such as RCPs, making potentially disastrous management decisions on their own also remains to be seen.

It is my opinion (and, as such, not worth more than anybody else's opinion) that independent practice and freedom from medical supervision is likely to be more restrictive to the hospital practice of the respiratory care practitioner than the present system. Outside the hospital, a respiratory care practitioner may do literally anything in the states with no licensing laws, and whatever the laws permit in those states that have them. In both situations, the full fiscal liability rests on the practitioners who would be well advised to protect themselves and their family with substantial malpractice insurance. Currently employed and supervised practitioners require no insurance. It is their employer or supervisor who has to be insured. Once practitioners become fully independent, the awards made against them will be the same as presently made against physicians and hospitals.

THE HOSPITAL–TECHNOLOGIST RELATIONSHIP

I have already referred to the legal relationship between the technologist and the hospital as far as liability is concerned. The employer is responsible for the actions of the employee, provided the employee acted within the general context of his or her responsibilities.

Legal Implications of Employment

Employment is a contract between the employer and the employee that goes into effect as soon as a job offer is made and is accepted by the applicant for the position. Under federal and state law, all job offers must be made in good faith, and the position must be open to all qualified applicants, regardless of age, sex, race, religion, physical handicap, and national origin. There are practically no exceptions to this rule, although the employment of minors is regulated by separate child labor laws.

The Fair Employment Practices Act requires that every job vacancy in a public institution be advertised in suitable media, giving a description of the position, the qualifications for employment, and any other pertinent data that would enable potential candidates to determine their interest in and suitability for the position.

Applicants usually have to complete an application form with personal data and provide letters of recommendation from previous employers. For certain positions, a personal interview is required. Once the employer has made a choice, he or she must prepare a written justification for selecting that particular candidate and, also, for turning down the other candidates who have met the basic requirements for the position. Once the candidate has been selected and a suitable salary is agreed on, the new employee is processed through the various initial stages of employment.

New employees, with few exceptions, are on a probationary status for a period of 3 to 6 months. During this time, orientation and in-service training takes place, and the employer is at liberty to terminate the employment unilaterally, if it becomes evident that the job and the new employee are not well suited to each other. Once the probationary period has elapsed, the new employee becomes a "regular," entitled to all the elaborate mechanisms designed to protect him or her against any capricious or arbitrary actions on the part of the employer.

When the respiratory care practitioner accepts a position, a contract is established. Walking away from the job without proper notice is a reprehensible act and a breach of contract under the law. It places a significant burden on the hospital and on the other members of the department. It may also adversely affect patient care and thereby quite clearly constitutes a violation of the ethical principles that must guide all health professionals.

The contract provides information concerning the salary, fringe benefits, working conditions, grievance mechanism, and numerous other matters. In some hospitals, these matters are negotiated by collective bargaining, and thus, both the employer and the employee have very little room for individual negotiation. There is no question in my mind that collective bargaining does lead to an improvement in salary and working conditions. It serves as a barrier against arbitrary and capricious management decisions and protects jobs in a time of economic constraints. It also may have a negative effect on the institution, because it tends to place an emotional barrier between the institution and the employee and thus may weaken the employee's commitment and loyalty to the job.

LAWS AFFECTING HEALTH CARE DELIVERY

Licensing and Regulation

The right to practice a health profession is considered to be guaranteed under the United States Constitution. It is also clear that the states have the right to protect the public and to enact laws to promote public welfare.

The states may establish properly constituted boards to regulate the practice of medicine and of the other health professions. It is the boards' responsibility to promulgate rules setting the minimum requirements for the entry into the practice of a health profession.

The state boards are also charged with regulating the professionals whom they have licensed. The regulatory power of the boards is an extension of the police powers of the state. Any licensed practitioner who violates a section of the practice act is subject to investigation, hearing, and sanction by the board. The sanctions may range from reprimand, probation, limitation of the license, and fines to a suspension or revocation of the license. The major areas in which practitioners violate the public health code are practice below the accepted standards of care; sexual abuse of patients; criminal behavior; and physical or emotional impairment, that is, the misuse of alcohol or controlled substances.

Unfortunately, in many states, the legislatures have failed to provide the licensing boards with sufficient funds to perform their policing functions thoroughly and effectively. This is a real shame, because it has been shown repeatedly that the professions do not police themselves effectively, and that the half-hearted attempts at voluntary or mandated quality controls, while a step in the right direction, do not accomplish their stated purpose for a variety of reasons. Thus, it is the board and only the board that can make a real contribution in identifying and sanctioning the relatively few, but highly visible, bad apples who give the entire profession a bad name. If the boards are handicapped by lack of personnel and funds, the professionals will continue to ignore them, and it will continue to be business as usual.

The problem of *licensure* in respiratory care is a complex one. Currently, the profession is licensed or otherwise registered and regulated in 44 states, and there are several other states where some form of licensing law is being considered in the legislature. In view of the changing physician-technologist relationships and the strong trend for respiratory care personnel to cast off all forms of medical supervision, at least in some areas of their activities, it becomes essential that states recognize and regulate the profession. Licensure does not seem to improve care, but it is the only way in which the state can maintain some control over the practitioners and sanction substandard providers. In those states where licensure is not yet in place, there is a significant additional burden on the hospital to control the activities of the respiratory care practitioners. If medical supervision is no longer acceptable, hospital administration is left in the unenviable, but inescapable, position of supervising respiratory care personnel. It will be most interesting to see how this will work out.

Federal and State Health Legislation

The entire field of health care delivery in the United States is currently under very severe scrutiny. The enormous increases in the cost of health care, and the persistent problems with providing adequate health care to the uninsured segment of the population, have finally reached a level where most concerned and informed people agree on the need for a major restructuring of the entire system. It is also evident that there are very potent forces that oppose all governmental health legislation for a variety of more or less egotistical and economic reasons. The outcome is impossible to predict with any degree of accuracy. To what extent the federal government can overcome legislative resistance and proceed toward a resolution of the present, untenable conflict depends on the will of the people, as expressed by its behavior at the polls.

Those of us who have followed these matters with increasing concern can only hope that, sooner rather than later, some form of universal health coverage will be available in this country, as it is currently in almost all civilized countries. Some encouraging signs can be seen at the state level. Some state legislatures, tired of waiting for federal action, have started plans of their own. Notable progress has been made in Oregon, Kentucky, Tennessee, and others.

AVOIDANCE OF LITIGATION

Being sued for malpractice is no fun. It is at best a nuisance and at worst an emotional and financial disaster. Whether innocent or not, the defendant's reputation suffers by the mere fact of being sued. Although I feel strongly that patients who have been injured by professional negligence not only have a right to sue, but have an obligation to do so, it is the duty of the health professional to avoid such suits whenever possible and proper.

The most important factors in avoiding malpractice litigation are improved consumer-provider relationships, improved communications, and improved records and risk management. It is axiomatic in malpractice that only an angry patient sues. Patients are usually angry not because of the bad result, but because they feel that they were not treated properly as human beings by the provider. Patients are a great deal smarter than we tend to give them credit for, and they very quickly realize that the provider views them as an "interesting case," a source of revenue, or a damn nuisance. This being the case, a bad result, superimposed on a real or perceived slight, will almost inevitably wind up in litigation.

The answer to this problem is better communication with the patient and the patient's family (see section 2 of this chapter). Making the patient a part of the decision-making process usually pays handsome dividends. With few exceptions, patients want to know and want to participate in the process. Questions should be answered fully and understandably, options should be presented clearly, and risks should be explained in lay terms. Spending 10 minutes with the patient, establishing good relationships and allaying apprehensions, may save very many hours of grief. If the patient likes you, has confidence in you, and believes that you have tried your best, the chances for a suit are minimal, even if the patient is disappointed with the outcome.

Good communications, incidentally, should not be limited to the provider. Patients don't like to be yelled at by secretaries or receptionists either. Because many first contacts are over the telephone, it is critically important that the person answering the phone have impeccable telephone manners. Being kept on hold does little to endear the provider to the consumer.

Good records are also an excellent means of protection against suits. If the record is complete, legible, and reasonable, it may not prevent a suit, but it will be a major factor in having it dismissed or won. Records need not be long, but they must be accurate and must allow a content expert to reconstruct exactly what happened. What was the diagnosis? How was the diagnosis arrived at? What was the indication for the various diagnostic or therapeutic manipulations? What was found? What were the final outcomes? What was the prognosis? Were consultants used? Was their advice followed, and if not, is there justification for not following the consultants' advice? Given this information, even a very bad outcome is unlikely to generate a lawsuit, because many bad results are not the result of ignorance or negligence. A good record should convince the plaintiff's lawyer that he or she does not have a case. If it gets that far, it should also convince a jury to find for the defendant.

There is no excuse for using the record for witticisms; for criticizing another provider; or, worst of all, for making inaccurate or incorrect entries. Faking a record is a very serious offense not only against the ethics of the profession, but it also constitutes fraud and may be actionable not only as a tort, but also as a criminal matter.

The last, but by no means least, protection against malpractice suits is a good risk-management system. Hospitals and other health care facilities routinely establish an office in which specially trained personnel assume the responsibility of dealing with "incidents" that may lead to litigation. The risk managers must be informed promptly of any event that was unforeseen, led to some injury, or was potentially dangerous. The risk manager then contacts all appropriate persons involved, makes sure that the records are in good order, acts as the spokesperson for the institution, and simultaneously acts as ombudsman for the patient and the family. A good risk manager can save the institution huge sums of money and the health care providers infinite grief and aggravation.

MALPRACTICE INSURANCE

All health care providers who function in the system as independent contractors should carry malpractice insurance. In some institutions, it is mandatory for the physicians who have staff privileges to carry insurance.

As indicated above, employees technically need not have individual insurance, because they are fully covered under the policy of the employer. In spite of this, many health professional employees do carry their own insurance. The reason given, usually, is that they do not trust the hospital to provide adequate legal defense. Actually, the insurance for the employed health care provider is nothing more than an expensive security blanket that makes them feel better.

When respiratory care practitioners begin to function as independent contractors, particularly if this is done outside the hospital, they must have insurance, unless they wish to jeopardize their entire financial security. It is important to remember that when independently functioning respiratory care practitioners hire people to work for them, the negligence of these employees becomes their responsibility.

The medical establishment has lobbied very hard, both at the federal and state levels, for some form of tort reform legislation, and indeed some states have passed such legislation. These laws have been helpful in some very limited areas, but they do not resolve the basic conflict. It seems extremely unlikely that legislation will ever be able resolve the "malpractice crisis" or change the fundamental laws governing personal and professional liability.

CONCLUSION

The law has been defined both as an "ass" by Dickens in *Oliver Twist* and also as the "embodiment of everything that's excellent" by Gilbert and Sullivan in *Iulanthe*. Actually it is neither. The law is written by fallible legislatures, is argued by fallible lawyers, and is interpreted by fallible courts, and yet it is the only thing that stands between us and chaos. It is the only recourse of the hurt, injured, and imposed upon. It is the only brake on blind ambition, unbridled greed, dishonesty, and careless disregard for the rights and well-being of others. Even though at times we may disagree with the way a certain case was handled and may be incensed by the seemingly outrageous amount of money a jury awards to a plaintiff, it may be well for all of us to realize that without the law no civilized society can exist. It is our duty as members of both a narrower and broader community to understand the law and, by understanding it, to respect it.

REFERENCES

1. *Blair v Eblen* 461 WE 2d 370, KY, 1970
2. The Nuremberg Code: Trial of the War Criminals Before the Nuremberg Military Tribunals Under Control Council Law No 10, Vol II. Nuremberg, 1946–1949
3. *Truman v Thomas* 611 P 2d 902, CA, 1979
4. *Darling v Charleston Community Hospital* 33 Ill 2d 3213 and 211 NE 2d 252, IL, 1965
5. *Gonzales v Nork* 131 Cal Reptr 717, CA, 1976

Thomas J. DeKornfeld

SECTION 5 Ethical Considerations in Respiratory Care

PROFESSIONAL SKLLS

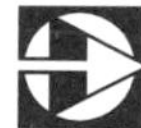

Upon completion of this chapter, the reader will be able to:

- Relate the main reasons for the changes between professionals in the health care delivery system
- Explain the role of ethics committees and institutional review boards
- Discuss the respiratory therapist's role(s) in issues of death and dying
- Elaborate on the ethics of reporting an impaired or dishonest co-worker

KEY TERMS

Abortion
Assisted suicide
Death
Durable power of attorney
Ethics
Euthanasia
Living will
Team concept

Ethics may be defined as that branch of philosophy that deals with the fundamental values of life. Good and bad, right and wrong are the central concerns of the ethicist, and through the ages ethicists have struggled to define these abstract concepts and to apply them to the problems of the everyday world. Every society from the most primitive to the most sophisticated, every religion from the most austere to the most permissive, and, indeed, every learned profession has evolved some set of rules, some moral precepts, or some ethical standards to regulate individual and interpersonal behavior.

Professional ethics have only recently come to be viewed as a subset of general ethics that governs the nontechnical interface between the professional persons and the patient, both individually and societally. The ethics literature of the 19th century accepted as revealed truth that physicians were governed only by "professional ethics" that allowed them to do what others, following "ordinary ethics," could not. The exponential growth of science, the increasingly complex and costly technical and pharmacologic armamentarium of the health professional, and the ghastly revelations of the Nuremberg trials led to the realization that general ethical principles had to apply to all, regardless of profession.

MAJOR TRENDS IN ETHICAL THOUGHT

Formal ethical thinking in the West started in Greece in the 5th and 4th century BC, coming to fruition with Socrates, Plato, and Aristotle. Their writings have influenced ethicists and philosophers to this day.

Roman Catholicism was the dominant force from the 4th to the 16th century of our era and impressed its ethical views on all areas of the known world. The Church equated good and bad, right and wrong with whatever it believed was pleasing or displeasing to a remote Deity, as recorded in writings attributed directly or indirectly to Him. Catholic philosophers tried to harmonize natural law and divine will and put a rational base under the Golden Rule.

The questioning spirit of the 18th century crystallized the two major directions of modern ethical thought, which had been present in more diffuse fashion in the writings of both pagan and early Christian ethicists. These two major strands of ethical thought may be termed utilitarianism and formalism or deontology.

Utilitarianism, most clearly defined in the writings of Jeremy Bentham[1] and John Stuart Mill,[2] holds that an act is good if its results are good, and bad if the results are bad. Thus, an act, in itself neutral or even harmful to an individual, is good if its long-term results benefit a larger group or humanity itself. Although this thinking may be interpreted as endorsing the very dubious principle that the end justifies the means, a modified utilitarianism is one of the basic principles of medical ethics.

Formalism or deontology largely disregards the result of an act and looks at the act itself as being either good or bad. Accordingly, wrongful acts, such as telling lies, are never permissible, even though the results may be beneficial. The foremost proponent of this theory was the German philosopher Immanuel Kant.[3]

Unfortunately, in real life most problems don't lend themselves to simple and pure theoretical solutions. Strict adherence to one or another ethical theory is likely to get the practitioner into trouble with patients or with colleagues.

Instead of worrying about ethical theory, it is best to remember three basic truths: (1) *primum non nocere* (first of all, do no harm); (2) the Golden Rule: "do unto others . . ."; and (3) common sense, good manners, courtesy, and respect for the other person's feelings. These four precepts are the keystones that keep the edifice of society from collapsing.

ETHICAL DYNAMICS OF INTERPERSONAL RELATIONSHIPS: THE TEAM CONCEPT

The traditional interprofessional relationships in the health care delivery system were predicated on a rigid caste system, with the physician at the top, followed in descending order by the nurse, the technologist, the aide, and the orderly. These relationships were paternalistic and authoritarian. Interpersonal relationships were held to a minimum, except between persons on the same level. Personal contentment and professional fulfillment were not major considerations. It is a tribute to human resilience not only that this system was quite efficient, but also that people functioned competently in it and appeared reasonably satisfied with their role. This system was held together by discipline and an unquestioning acceptance of traditional authority.

During the past three decades, these relationships have undergone an accelerating change. The stature of the medical profession has declined, while the education and standing of the other health care providers has increased. It was recognized that nonphysicians could make significant contributions to health care (see Ch. 1). One result of this democratization of the health care system was the development of the team concept.

The basic tenets underlying the *team concept* are that each member has a specific contribution to make, that these contributions are of comparable value, and that all components must collaborate smoothly for the results to be optimal. The traditional roles have undergone changes, and a number of activities, previously considered the exclusive domain of one profession, are now performed by nonphysician and non-nurse technologists.

These changes have had a profound effect on the emotional relationships between the health professions. The caste system required respect from the "lower orders" in return for authoritarian paternalism, quite similar to the Victorian family structure. The father (physician) made all the decisions and bestowed praise or punishment. The mother (nurse) backed the father's authority, but contributed a certain humanizing influence. The children (technologists) were to be seen but not heard and were to "behave" at all times.

Changes came slowly but inexorably. Since the end of World War II, there has been a steadily accelerating trend toward the democratization of all forms of social structures. The health care delivery system was the last bastion of entrenched, feudal authoritarianism to be dragged kicking and screaming into the modern era.

These changes, spurred by both external and internal forces, have led to the gradual evolution of the health care team. The concept is certainly not new. Small teams have functioned in some areas for many years. Psychiatric hospitals have led in this area, and even 40 years ago, teams of physicians, nurses, social workers, occupational therapists, and, more rarely, some non–health professionals met to plan the management of the individual patients in a "case management conference" format. Similar teams became active, much later, in cardiopulmonary resuscitation and in the care of critically ill patients. These teams were still under the nominal leadership of the physician, but individual team members were frequently placed in decision-making roles.

In recent years, the team concept has received a great deal of moral support, but in practice, it has made no appreciable progress. The reasons for this are turf protection and the unwillingness of most people to recognize their own limitations or the abilities of others. The educational institutions are also to blame for this failure of a worthy idea. For a group to function well as a team, the individual members must have a thorough understanding of each others' roles, duties, and competencies. This is not possible unless the members of the team receive at least a part of their training jointly and are exposed to both basic instruction and to clinical experiences as a group. To date, such joint learning opportunities have been few, and where an attempt was made to provide shared learning experiences, these attempts were largely unsuccessful.

Because no change in this unsatisfactory situation can be expected in the foreseeable future, the question remains: what posture should the individual health care provider assume vis-à-vis colleagues in the other health professions? More specifically, what should the attitude of the respiratory care technologist be toward physicians, nurses, physical therapists, and others who may have a direct input into the management of the patients served by respiratory care?

Foremost, the role that each plays in the care of the patient must be understood. The respiratory care practitioner must have a good working knowledge of the medical problems of the pulmonary patient and a thorough understanding of the diagnostic and therapeutic considerations that the physician brings to bear on the problem. The respiratory care practitioner must understand the contributions nurses have to make, both in the narrow sense as providers of bedside care, and in the broader sense as consumer educators and coordinators of the health care team. The same principles apply to working with physical therapists, occupational therapists, social workers, and others.

The recent, and rapidly increasing, trend among respiratory care personnel to assume an independent health care technologist role and to free themselves from medical direction (supervision) raises a new set of legal and ethical issues. The legal aspects of this changing relationship are clear and are discussed in Chapter 2, Section 4.

The ethical implications are much more complex. Respiratory care personnel may be very knowledgeable in a limited and highly focused area of medicine. They may indeed be more knowledgeable than many physicians in setting up and operating sophisticated ventilators. They may be able to follow the patient's respiratory status and recognize changes in either direction, that is, improvement or worsening. Nevertheless, the respiratory care practitioner is not a physician and thus lacks the broad-based knowledge that is required to manage the entire patient. Many, indeed most, patients requiring intensive respiratory care also require numerous other diagnostic and therapeutic manipulations that lie outside the field of respiratory care.

The best interest of a patient demands that all these diagnostic and therapeutic modalities be integrated and controlled by a single source. This source, whether we like it or not, must be the physician, because the physician is the only health care provider trained to provide this service and the only one legally empowered to do so. Technologists, respiratory care personnel, or others can function optimally and in the patient's best interest only if their specialized knowledge and skills are directed by the physician with whom the patient has a professional relationship, and who is ultimately responsible for the patient's total care. Respiratory care is only one facet of total patient care, albeit an extremely important one, and respiratory care personnel wishing to free themselves from all medical direction or supervision are acting irresponsibly and in clear violation of the basic tenet of health care ethics, namely, that the interests of the patient override all petty interpersonal and interprofessional dislikes, jealousies, and frustrations.

Regardless of the final outcome, the physician-therapist relationship will have to continue in some form. It is critical, therefore, that some civilized operational modus vivendi be found. This is critical to the success of new work paradigms, such as the therapist-driven respiratory care protocols. The key to the relationship should be mutual respect; good manners; equanimity; humor; and, most importantly, a single-minded, inflexible devotion to the well-being of the patient.

MAJOR CONTEMPORARY PROBLEMS IN HEALTH ETHICS

Matters of Life and Death

Subsumed under this somewhat pretentious title we find such ethical problems as abortion, care of the defective newborn, death and dying, assisted suicide, and euthanasia.

Death is defined as the total and irreversible loss of brain function, with irreversible loss of both cerebral hemispheric and brain stem functions. Contrary to popular belief, it is not mandatory to perform electroencephalography and brain stem potential studies to confirm brain death. Determination of brain death is a medical issue; family or surrogate approval is not required before this decision is made.[4] With this in mind, let us review these matters of life and death together.

□ ABORTION

Respiratory care personnel have little if any role in decisions on abortion, other than in their personal lives. Thus, a brief discussion of the ethical aspects of abortion should suffice.

Few, if any, of the ethical issues are as replete with emotional content, personal and religious prejudices, and attempts to resolve the insoluble than the problem of abortion. The 1973 U.S. Supreme Court decisions (*Row v Wade*[5] and *Doe v Bolton*[6]) have settled some of the legal aspects of the issue without having touched any of the ethical or moral aspects involved.

The extreme antiabortionists believe that human life begins at conception, and thus any interference with this "human," with the intent to destroy it, is murder and thus forbidden by both divine and human law. The extreme proabortionists believe that the embryo becomes a "person" at some time during intrauterine development and that destroying it before that time is clearly the prerogative of the woman carrying the fetus.

The proabortionist position is clear. The Supreme Court has spoken: abortions are legal. It is an ethical issue only as far as a person's pursuit of happiness and control over her own body is concerned. The only real question is the particular moment when an amorphous number of cells in the uterus becomes a human being, and is thus entitled to all the rights and privileges society has traditionally granted to humans.

The antiabortionists are not a unified group. They include those who condemn abortion under any and all circumstances and those who condemn abortion as means of population control, but who permit it to save the mother's life or sanity or if the pregnancy is the result of rape or incest.

Abortion, like any other societal issue, is influenced greatly by the political leadership of the country and by the composition of the Supreme Court, which in turn is a reflection of the President and Congress responsible for proposing and confirming candidates that ultimately decide these issues. During the 12 years of the Reagan and Bush administrations, the entire weight of the federal government was used to support an antiabortion stand, and this was reflected in certain state court decisions. The Clinton administration is prepared to support the 1973 proabortion decisions of the Supreme Court and has taken steps to protect abortion clinics from the violence of antiabortion extremists. It has always struck me as peculiar that, to prevent the "murder" of the unborn fetus, these people are prepared to murder the personnel working in the clinics, which are legally established to assist the women who lawfully wish to have their pregnancies terminated!

□ THE SEVERELY DEFECTIVE NEONATE

Respiratory care personnel are involved professionally in the next ethical dilemma, the problem of the severely defective neonate. Despite the availability of genetic counseling, intrauterine diagnostics, and legal abortion, many infants are born with severe congenital abnormalities. Some of these abnormalities would be fatal unless corrected surgically, and some would make a decent quality of life impossible, whether corrected or not. The second issue is relatively simple. No newborn who would survive with standard care can be put to death by omission or commission regardless of how grotesque or how severely deformed it may be. Such an act would constitute willful homicide and would properly be prosecuted. The problem becomes much more complicated when sophisticated life support systems or major surgical intervention is necessary to prevent the infant's otherwise inevitable death.

As with most ethical problems, this cannot be discussed intelligently without understanding the legal issues involved. Two cases, admittedly now several years old, illustrate this problem. The "Johns Hopkins case"[7] involved an infant born with intestinal atresia and severe Down syndrome. The atresia was surgically correctable, and the infant would, in all probability, have survived and recovered. The parents, after much discussion with medical and spiritual advisors, refused permission to operate on this mentally deficient infant, and the infant was allowed to die. This process took 2 weeks, during which the infant was given only minimal supportive care and was the center of considerable emotional turmoil among the nurses and other health professionals who were forced to stand by and watch it die. The case was never submitted to a court. Much has been written about it by writers representing a wide spectrum of philosophical and political orientation. The condemnation of the parents and of the Hopkins physicians by these writers was practically unanimous.

The second case concerned a neonate in Maine[8] who suffered from many grossly deforming congenital defects and who also had a tracheoesophageal fistula (TEF). This was the most immediately life-threatening deformity, although the other deformities were such that it was impossible to imagine a satisfactory quality of life for the infant. The parents refused to consent to the TEF repair. The physicians at the Maine Medical Center petitioned the local circuit court to assume guardianship over the infant and to authorize the proposed surgical procedure. The court ruled that the surgery should be performed because "the most basic right enjoyed by every human being is the right to life itself." The court also found that this right began at the moment of birth.

Only the legal parents or guardians can make the decision whether a severely damaged "life" should be saved or whether it should be permitted to die. This decision, made under very great stress, is clearly among the most difficult ethical and moral issues. There are no clear guidelines, and responsible thinkers have expressed their doubt whether such guidelines are even possible. The arguments again range from one extreme, that is, "we always must do everything to maintain life," to the other extreme, that is, "we should save only those who are likely to be fulfilled and fulfilling human beings."

I believe that there is a minimal quality of life, below which existence is at best humanoid. No newborn should be willfully and arbitrarily sentenced to a life of pain, misery, and distress, while at the same time placing an enormous emotional and economic burden on the family and on society as a whole. At the least, the newborn must show some evidence that it is likely to have the cardinal human characteristics of cognition and emotion. Without these, whatever the newborn may be, it is not a human being, and neither law nor morality would be served by maintaining it in a vegetative state.

The parents have the unquestionable right to refuse permission for extraordinary means to salvage what in their opinion would be an unacceptable quality of life. Physicians, by and large, should respect the parents' decision, particularly if the decision is arrived at after thorough discussion with the physicians and with the family's spiritual advisor. If the physician's own set of values is at odds with the family, the only resort is to refer the matter to the local judiciary. The judicial action may have the virtue of appearing dispassionate, but it tends to view the issue entirely from the perspective of the newborn and tends to disregard the burden it may place on the family and on society.

During the 12 years from 1980 to 1992, a new, and to me highly undesirable, development was seen. President Reagan, Attorney General Meese, and Reagan's successor, President Bush, chose to insert their heavy foot into this sensitive ethical web. The federal government decided to regulate what parents and physicians could do in such situations and even invited spying and anonymous reporting of "improper" behavior through a federal hot line, strongly reminiscent of some of the excesses of the Hitler and Stalin eras. Fortunately, American courts, under our wonderful constitution, were able to tell the federal government just exactly how far its authority extended, and in every case that was tried in court, the decision went against the "forces of darkness," as represented by the Reaganites.

A classic example of this type of meddling can be seen in the notorious Baby Jane Doe case.[9] This case involved a newborn with spina bifida and paraplegia. The parents and the physicians at Stonybrook Medical Center agreed not to subject this infant to dangerous and probably unsuccessful surgery. They were dragged into court by an out-of-state lawyer, and indeed, the lower court instructed the physicians to proceed with the surgery. On appeal, the appellate division reversed the lower court in a very strongly worded opinion. At this point, the federal government reopened the issue under the federal antidiscriminatory statute, claiming that Baby Jane Doe had been discriminated against as a handicapped person under the act. The federal judge, in another strongly worded opinion, ruled against the attorney general, finding that the drafters of the antidiscriminatory (civil rights) statute clearly had no such situation in mind when they enacted the law.

Ethics Committees

The only possible benefit of this federal meddling was the mandatory establishment of ethics committees in every hospital where babies were born and cared for. These ethics committees have an advisory role only, but they must be consulted in all cases of an impaired newborn. The committees are usually composed of thoughtful and concerned physicians, other health care providers, the hospital attorney, and one or two laypersons with an interest in ethical issues. Their advice, while not binding, is usually carefully listened to and frequently followed. Similar ethics committees have also been established in adult hospitals, and they are playing an increasingly important role. They are consulted regularly in cases in which the family or the physicians consider the withholding or withdrawing of life support. Members of the committee meet with the family; with the physicians; and, when possible, with the patient. The medical problems are presented and weighed by the committee. After discussion of the salient points, the committee makes a recommendation concerning the ethical and moral justification of instituting or withholding, continuing or withdrawing life support; performing or not performing surgery; and so forth. As indicated above, the committee's recommendations are purely advisory.

□ THE AGED

Another distinct ethical and legal problem exists at the opposite end of human existence. The normal process of aging inevitably leads to physical, mental, and emotional changes, which are usually gradual, but may also be sudden and dramatic. In terminal illnesses, the changes may be primarily physical, but in many patients the changes are also mental when brain damage occurs because of trauma, hypoxia, senility, chronic brain syndrome, Alzheimer's disease, and so on.

The basic problem of how to care for these patients is similar in many ways to the problems of the severely damaged newborn, discussed above. There is, however, one very significant difference. The adult, regardless of age, may be able to make decisions for him- or herself, or may have left instructions about his or her desires for a certain course of action to be taken, should such a catastrophe occur. There are also significant economic and emotional differences between letting a newborn die and letting an old person die. Babies rarely have substantial estates, and inheritance is rarely a consideration. Babies, at least in theory, have the possibility of a long, productive, and happy life before them. Old people can look forward to death as relief from the increasingly intolerable burden of life.

In the conscious, competent adult, the situation is simple. Under constitutional guarantees, a person has the unquestioned right to determine whether diagnostic and therapeutic procedures shall be performed, and every adult has the right to refuse health care, even though such refusal inevitably leads to death. The American Hospital Association has developed a patient code of rights as well, which speaks to the issues of informed consent and the right of the patient to be an active participant in decisions regarding his or her own health. Both court decisions and the overwhelming majority of ethicists clearly distinguish between such refusal of treatment and suicide. Catholic theologians have stated consistently that suicide is a deadly sin, but the refusal to engage in any extraordinary activity to prevent death cannot be considered suicide and, consequently, is not banned by the Church. The key word is "extraordinary."

Theologians and ethicists generally contend, although for different reasons, that a person has the duty to maintain his or her body in good health and to do everything reasonable and proper to avoid illness or to regain health. Where "reasonable and proper" ends and "extraordinary" begins is the question. These terms have never been accurately defined, are subject to individual interpretation, and are certainly changing with the development of new technology. For instance, ventilator care was clearly "extraordinary" 30 years ago, but many would agree that today it is probably "reasonable and proper." Intraaortic balloon pumps or ECMO are probably still "extraordinary," but they may become routine 20 years from now.

□ LIVING WILLS AND DURABLE POWER OF ATTORNEY

If the adult patient is unconscious or otherwise unable to communicate his or her wishes, the situation becomes more complicated, particularly if there are no indications as to the wishes of the person involved. A number of states have enacted "right to die" legislation or at least are willing to recognize a *living will* or a *durable power of attorney*. These documents, while somewhat different in nature and purpose, serve to allow a designated person to make decisions for the incapacitated person. Depending on whether specific limitations have been incorporated into the documents, these decisions may be medical and economic. The person holding the power of attorney may or may not be a family member. He or she may demand that recommended procedures be done or not done or that life support be withheld or withdrawn. These demands carry the same weight as though they were made by the conscious and competent patient. Thus, a person may decide in advance what, if any, means may be used in life support, should he or she become unable to make decisions. To die with dignity is just as much an inalienable right as living in dignity. Yet, otherwise thoughtful and humane physicians, other health practitioners, and allegedly lov-ing family members regularly and commonly deny this right to their patients or nearest and dearest. Again, the choices range widely, from assisted suicide and euthanasia on one end, to the indefinite maintenance of the living dead on the other.

□ ASSISTED SUICIDE

Assisted suicide is a relatively new wrinkle in the fabric of professional relationships that has received a great deal of attention, mainly due to the front-page-news activity of a Michigan pathologist, Dr. Jack Kevorkian. This physician has helped a number of people to commit suicide either by injection or by inhalation. To date, he has done this with patients who had some form of chronic ailment and who wished to end it all. The Michigan legislature has enacted a law that makes assisted suicide illegal, and Kevorkian has been indicted for ignoring this statute. At the time of this writing, the issue is still in legal limbo because the constitutionality of the law has been challenged, and it seems likely that this issue will ultimately be decided by the U.S. Supreme Court. Many physicians are very sympathetic to the concept, and indeed, many patients have their last few hours or days made tolerable by a judicious, but generous use of narcotics. I have no ethical problem with assisted suicide, provided the patients are truly terminal or in such constant severe pain that life becomes an intolerable burden. I strongly object to this being done with patients who are simply neurotic or under circumstances that are at best bizarre.

□ EUTHANASIA

Euthanasia, or mercy killing, is an entirely different matter. To kill another human being knowingly and willfully is homicide. Whether there are circumstances in which a deliberate, positive act, designed solely to produce death, may ever be justified is a question that is very difficult to answer. The proponents of euthanasia feel strongly that the question must be answered in the affirmative. They believe that there are situations in which a conscious, competent adult may reasonably request to be "put to sleep," or in which parents may make the same request for their badly damaged infant or their suffering, terminally ill minor child.

The opponents of euthanasia claim that the answer is categorically and unalterably in the negative. The opponents of euthanasia admit that some people would be much better off dead, and that an unqualified denial of euthanasia condemns some infants and adults to a degrading, quasi-human or subhuman existence for an indefinite period. The arguments against euthanasia usually fall into one of two broad categories. It is claimed that both divine and human law demand that life not be taken except in war, in self-defense, and (perhaps) as the punishment for certain heinous crimes. Or it is claimed that permitting euthanasia is wrong because it would become the thin edge of a wedge that leads inevitably to the elimination of increasing numbers or groups of undesirables. Ultimately, it could lead to political or racial mass murder.

I find this reasoning extremely difficult to accept. Those who truly believe in the divine mandate "Thou shall not kill" should oppose killing absolutely and in all its forms, including self-defense, judicial execution, and war. Once one form of homicide becomes acceptable, it appears totally illogical to deny categorically the potential appropriateness of some other form of equally justifiable homicide. The second argument about the thin edge is even more specious. Making the leap from a carefully circumscribed euthanasia to political or racial genocide is too absurd to deserve serious discussion.

Whatever the arguments may be, it is quite clear that American society is not prepared to accept euthanasia as an option at this time. Let us examine, then, if there is anything short of euthanasia that is acceptable legally and ethically, that will benefit the hopeless sufferer, and that has the support of the health care community.

□ CODE STATUS ORDERS

Comfort Measures Only

The most common suggestion is to change the terminally ill patient's care orders to comfort measures only (CMO) and, for example, to use sufficient narcotics to make the patient comfortable and not to do anything that may prolong the patient's life. Liberal use of morphine and other narcotics is definitely indicated for patients with terminal or preterminal severe pain. How much is given and how often is a medical decision. Given on a regular schedule, morphine is likely to keep such patients quite comfortable and, indeed, may ease and speed the transition from this world into the next one.

Most ethicists agree that this is not euthanasia, although some few maintain that it is just that. Most thoughtful health care providers agree, however, that this method of helping the terminally, desperately, and painfully ill patient is not only ethically permissible, but a mandate of good and compassionate medical care. Legally, it is very unlikely to be questioned unless the narcotic is administered in a single, overwhelming dose.

Withholding Medication

Withholding medication and other therapeutic modalities is a related, but more complicated, issue. Pneumonia was once referred to as the "old person's friend." Now, if an old person gets pneumonia, it can be treated with antibiotics, and the patient can be sentenced to weeks, months, and even years of continued existence that he or she does not want. The question is again the same: is it ethically and legally permissible to withhold antibiotics from these patients, or diuretics from patients with congestive heart failure, thus allowing them to die and by not interfering in a natural process? The reader is referred to the recent suggestions of Raffin[4] regarding the decision-making process in this situation.

Withholding and Withdrawing Life Support

The most recent debate in this area was over the withholding of parenteral nutrition and intravenous (IV) hydration. Recent court decisions and an opinion of the AMA Council on Ethical and Judicial Affairs clearly state that continuation of artificial feeding and hydration, whether through tubes or IVs, was a medical measure that could be terminated, just as artificial ventilation could be terminated.

Do Not Resuscitate

A related issue concerns cardiopulmonary resuscitation. To resuscitate or not to resuscitate is a medical decision. Writing a "no code," do not resuscitate (DNR), or "do not attempt resuscitation" (DNAR) order is legally permissible and ethically desirable. It should be remembered that it is much easier not to start resuscitation than it is to discontinue a ventilator. I believe that resuscitation should be started only if there is a reasonable likelihood that the patient can be reestablished as a functional human being, and that it should be discontinued as soon as evidence of significant central nervous system damage appears. It is very easy to be righteous in this area, but those of us who have resuscitated decerebrate patients and were then involved in their care are inclined to be pragmatic, even to the point of therapeutic nihilism.

The code status of a patient ranges from the full, that is, do everything possible for the patient, to do not attempt resuscitation (DNAR), that is, if the patient stops breathing or cardiac activity becomes imperceptible, make no effort whatever to support either respiration or circulation. Intermediate steps are limited resuscitative efforts, such as endotracheal intubation but no ventilation; vasopressors but no closed chest cardiac compressions; and a wide variety of other combinations and variations on the theme. A relatively recent DNAR concept is the one already alluded to above, namely, comfort measures only.

Behavior Modification and Genetic Engineering

Behavior modification, medically or surgically, was a popular subject of discussion some years ago, and indeed, frontal lobotomies were performed with some regularity. These have been almost entirely abandoned, and now violent and potentially dangerous mental patients are frequently considered "cured" and are let loose on a largely defenseless society. It is not at all uncommon to read in the morning paper about some horrible atrocity committed by a former mental patient, not infrequently on a child. It seems odd that a society that spends so much effort worrying about the poor criminal pays little or no attention to the victim. The civil libertarians are rarely around when the victims of their protégés are brought into the emergency room raped, beaten, stabbed, mutilated, or dead. Constitutional freedoms are important, but I believe that there must be a balance at which individual rights and societal rights are placed in the proper perspective.

The science of human genetics has made enormous strides during the past decade, and now both genetic counseling and genetic engineering have become very real tools in the ongoing battle to protect and improve both individual and societal health. Many diseases have been shown to be hereditary, and these genetically linked illnesses present two major problem areas: the identification and counseling of the carrier and the statutory enforcement of preventive sterilization, amniocentesis, and abortion.

Genetic counseling is a well-recognized discipline. An expert in the field discusses the issues with prospective parents and advises them about the likelihood of producing a child with a genetic defect. The man and woman may then decide whether they will have any children, knowing the risks and the statistical odds. If the woman is already pregnant, amniocentesis should be recommended. If this relatively simple and safe test reveals that the fetus is most probably seriously malformed, the desirability of an abortion must be considered. Not to do so is to deprive the parents of the right to make a decision and may indeed leave them and their medical advisor open to the possibility of "wrongful life" litigation.

Most recently, it has become possible to modify existing genetic patterns and, in essence, create new life forms. Changing the DNA configuration of certain plants or microorganisms could reap immeasurable benefits, both in the production of foods and also in the prevention and treatment of disease. It may, of course, also be possible to create a Frankenstein's monster and let loose, on this already badly managed planet, new life forms of unimaginable ferocity and malignancy. For this reason, thoughtful professional people have argued vigorously against pursuing any studies in this field. Their arguments have been both philosophical and theological.

None of these arguments is convincing. The benefits of creating new life forms may be enormous. The dangers may be real, but they may be minimized and should not be allowed to influence the new technologies. The theological arguments, that the Creator does not wish such research to be done, are unanswerable and, in fact, need no answer. It is safe to assume that if the Creator indeed does not wish such work to go forward, He will make His wishes known in no uncertain terms.

Allocation of Scarce Health Resources: Triage

It has been frequently stated that all residents of the United States are entitled to health care. In fact, roughly 30% of the population has no health insurance and thus has little, if any, access to health care, other than crisis care. Even crisis care is denied to persons with no insurance by some health care providers and health care facilities.

Until very recently, no effort was made to remedy this truly iniquitous situation. Universal coverage was one of President Clinton's principal agenda items to provide health care for all Americans. His attempts to accomplish this have been defeated to date by a coalition of special interest groups and congressional reactionaries. The principal reason for the opposition was political and economic self-interest, but the public justification was the unavailability of funding for such an enormous project.

There is no doubt that health care in the United States is outrageously expensive and that extending it to all residents, at the same cost and same level, would indeed be economically imprudent, if not impossible. There are many reasons why health care is so expensive. The enormous cost of new equipment; the outrageous cost of drugs and supplies; the performance of unnecessary procedures; the inefficiency of many health care facilities; the greed (and dishonesty) of many health care providers; and last, but not least, the expectations of the public are all factors that contribute to the unconscionable cost of even basic medical and surgical care. It is a simple, albeit unpalatable, fact that with present resources it is not possible to provide the very best of everything to everybody. Health resources are limited, and therefore not everybody can possibly be viewed as though he or she was the only recipient of these scarce resources.

To provide at least minimal health care to everybody, it is essential that the allocation of the available resources be managed in a rational manner. The first step would be to eliminate all unnecessary and meddlesome procedures. This would free large amounts of resources that could then be used to provide lower-level care to a larger group. Even indicated procedures would have to be viewed very critically and be made available only if justifiable on the basis of both need and priority.

The problem with allocating scarce resources is that everybody agrees on its necessity, and everybody feels that it is an excellent thing, provided it does not apply to him or her. Assuming for the moment that people are rational and honest, the allocation of resources still presents two major issues that must be resolved. The first issue is the allocation of national resources for specific purposes, and the second issue is the allocation of resources to specific individuals.

The allocation of national resources to specific areas involves such matters, for example, as shunting money from open heart surgery to building hospices for the terminally ill, or stopping the support of renal dialysis and using the money so liberated to set up prenatal walk-in clinics for inner city residents. How these decisions are made concerns us all. They are perhaps not, strictly speaking, ethical or moral issues, but they are fundamental to the second allocation issue. Hence, society in general, and its chosen representatives in particular, cannot delay much longer in making decisions in this area.

The second issue involves people as individuals, and the decisions must be made at the local level. This is known as *triage,* a term well known in military medicine. In that context it means that, when a large number of casualties must be cared for, preference is given to those with minor injuries, who can be treated rapidly and who are likely to recover completely. The severely injured, who would consume a disproportionate amount of the available resources and who would possibly or probably die, are left to the last, even if this means that some of them would die before care can be provided. In civilian practice, triage has not been a necessity to date. Other than in a handful of major disasters, local or regional health facilities have always been sufficient to provide care to all the injured, regardless of the severity of their injury. In most catastrophes, the most severely injured were taken first, and the so-called walking wounded had to wait.

How, then, does triage apply to the future practice of medicine? The issue is rarely one of emergency management of large groups, but usually one of selecting small groups from a large pool for a certain treatment, drug, or other therapy that is not made available by the funding sources in sufficient quantity.

The basic ethical dilemma can be stated very simply: If not all can be saved, who shall be saved? This dilemma was confronted when penicillin was first introduced during World War II, and when renal dialysis first became available in the 1960s. It is very likely that if and when funding sources limit resources for coronary artery bypass surgery, or prevent performance of any of a multitude of diagnostic and therapeutic manipulations, the dilemma of triage will become a very real one. If we assume that all human beings are created equal and have the same intrinsic value, then from a triage point of view, there is no difference between a child with Down syndrome and a Nobel laureate in medicine. It follows, then, that the only reasonable way to choose between them is by chance, either on a first come, first served basis or by some form of lottery.

Because most of us will agree that not all people are equal and that the individual's place in, and value to, society must be a consideration, how then should a choice be made? A thorough discussion of this problem is beyond the scope of this chapter. It will definitely become a major issue in the health care system of the future, and it seems appropriate to start giving it serious consideration now. Precautions will have to be taken so that money does not become a major factor, and the ultimate system of selection will, it is hoped, take into consideration the likelihood of the procedure's success; the continued usefulness of the patient to his or her family and to society; and, to a lesser degree, the past contributions the individual has made. Given a small group of people of approximately equal value by these criteria, chance may well be the final method of selection. Such a system has been recommended by Rescher.[10]

AIDS

The epidemic of AIDS has raised two interesting ethical problems. First, may a health care provider refuse care to a patient if the patient is a known HIV carrier? And second, may testing for HIV be performed without the patient's knowledge or consent?

Both legal and ethical weight is clearly in the negative on both of these issues. Federal legislation has very clearly stated that no discrimination is permissible on the basis of physical handicap. I believe that the ethical considerations are equally binding. Obviously, health care personnel have the duty to protect themselves with gown, gloves, cap, and goggles, but I believe they also have the duty to care for the patient with AIDS or any other infectious disease.

The problem of compulsory testing for HIV is an extremely sensitive area, and there are widely diverging opinions on the propriety and/or legality of such testing. It is my feeling that testing the patient for HIV without the patient's knowing constitutes battery and is actionable. Only a legislature can mandate compulsory testing, and if such a statute were passed, it would have to survive a constitutional challenge.

The Ethics of Experimentation

Because respiratory care personnel are increasingly engaged in research, and because some of this research involves patients, the legal and ethical concerns in human experimentation deserve some discussion.

The findings of the Nuremberg War Crime Tribunal at the end of World War II showed that in the German concentration camps brutal and frequently fatal experiments were conducted on hundreds of prisoners, by trained medical personnel. To prevent the repetition of such barbarity, a code of ethics for human experimentation was issued by the tribunal, known as the Nuremberg code (1946–1949).[11] This code was expanded by the Declaration of Helsinki (1964–1965),[12] a declaration by the World Medical Association, which laid down the principles of ethical medical research and, for the first time, distinguished between clinical research and nontherapeutic biomedical research on human beings.

Following the discovery of some scandalous human experiments in allegedly reputable institutions in the United States, the Surgeon General issued a set of guidelines in 1981. These guidelines, since revised several times, regulate all research done under federal grants, in federal institutions, or in institutions receiving some of their funding from federal sources. In fact, most health facilities today insist that all investigations involving human beings conform to these guidelines, regardless of the funding source of the study. The core of these federal regulations is the establishment of an institutional review board (IRB) that is charged with reviewing all research proposals and with monitoring the progress and results of the approved protocols.

Basically, the rules for clinical research are as follows: no person should be used as an experimental subject, unless he or she consents voluntarily; unless there is no other way in which the same information may be obtained; unless the benefits outweigh the risks; unless the experiments are conducted by experienced and careful scientists, fully aware of their responsibilities; and unless the subject is free to withdraw from the experiment at any time and for whatever reason.

These basic principles are stated in a somewhat different form by Morris et al[13] in connection with computer-controlled ventilation in ICU patients. Morris sets up four ethical principles as criteria for the introduction of an experimental treatment system. The four principles are (1) nonmaleficence (do not harm), (2) beneficence (do good), (3) autonomy (respect for patient self-direction), and (4) distributive justice (be fair). Though Morris limits his considerations to one specific treatment situation, the principles are generally applicable to all new technology, be it diagnostic or therapeutic.

The rules for nontherapeutic, biomedical studies are as follows. (1) The risk of the study to the participants must be minimal and must at no time include the possibility of permanent harm of any kind. (2) The design of the study must be such that the results, positive or negative, have statistical validity. Badly designed, predictably inconclusive studies are never justified. (3) Physiologic studies should not be performed on patients and should be performed only on healthy volunteers. Pathophysiologic studies must be performed on patients, but are legitimate only if there is minimal or no risk, and if the patients understand very clearly that no benefit will accrue to them. (4) Such studies are probably never justified on minors or incompetents. (5) Inducement to participate should never be of a nature to make a rational decision difficult. Studies may produce psychological damage as well as physical damage. Emotional trauma is more difficult to predict and much more difficult to correct. If there is any doubt, the experiment should not be performed.

The review of the protocols and the supervision of all studies is the responsibility of the IRB. It has absolute authority to reject a protocol or demand that it be revised. Having served as the secretary of the IRB at the University of Michigan Medical Center, I can testify to the fact that the establishment of the IRB and the rigorous insistence on scrupulous adherence to the federal guidelines have made a dramatic difference in the human experimentation conducted at one of the nation's major medical centers.

Experimentation in medicine is as old as medicine itself. The entire scope of contemporary health care is based on experiments that were performed by healers, who tried new methods to treat illness. All of us are the beneficiaries of previous human experimentation; indeed, many of us would not be alive if we had not been treated with a drug or a surgical procedure that was experimental at one time. It is therefore absurd to maintain that human experimentation is wrong, that it is the invasion of the sanctity of the human body, or that it should not be permitted under any circumstances. It is not the human experimentation that is wrong, it is that some so-called scientists have been doing human experiments wrong.

Ethics in the Workplace

□ THE IMPAIRED HEALTH PROFESSIONAL

The problem of the impaired health professional is becoming a major issue, and all health care providers must become familiar with it. Most of us have colleagues, co-workers, or associates who are becoming, or have become, incompetent because of senescence, substance abuse (alcohol or controlled substances), mental illness, or other illness affecting the central nervous system. It is our ethical and (perhaps) legal obligation to become familiar with the signs of impairment and to learn what to do when we believe we have noticed such signs.

The signs are sometimes difficult to recognize. They tend to be vague, at least initially, and most of us are insufficiently familiar with or sensitive to them for early recognition. We have to be on the lookout for the telltale signs of changes in the physical and emotional status of our co-workers. Slight, but recurring, changes in behavior or performance; erratic behavior; wide and rapid mood swings; forgetfulness; increasing slovenliness in appearance; increasingly frequent mistakes; and tardiness are all beacons pointing to the inescapable conclusion that the person manifesting them has a serious problem. The surgeon whose tremor becomes less and less controllable, the nurse who forgets to schedule patients, the respiratory care practitioner who suddenly insists on wearing a long-sleeved shirt because he or she is always cold, or the administrator with the odor of alcohol on his or her breath are all people who need help and who constitute a real or potential menace to the patient. That many of these people are our friends, colleagues, or superiors does not make the task any easier. What is our duty as responsible health professionals; what do we do?

If the person is a friend or an employee, the first step may be to schedule a private session to make friendly inquiries, to offer assistance, and to make the person aware that his or her problem has been noted. If we are dealing with what appears to be a problem of substance abuse, such friendly approaches are rarely successful. An occasional substance abuser will readily agree to seek professional help and undergo full therapy to start on the long road to recovery. Most substance abusers will deny any use and may become defensive or angry. In this situation, one must pursue the matter through proper channels, making certain that all allegations are properly documented. All institutions should have a person designated to deal with this problem. This person should be familiar with the therapeutic options; should have ongoing contact with the treatment facilities specializing in the care of the impaired health professional; and should know what local social or health agency to contact, should such assistance become necessary.

If the impaired person is a superior or is outside one's department, the problem must be reported to the appropriate hospital administrator for action. Ignoring a problem is irresponsible toward both the individual and the patients in the hospital.

Substance abuse, if managed properly, is a treatable disease in the health professional. It requires expert and vigorous initial therapy, to be followed by a reentry contract, continued and faithful attendance at AA or NA meetings, and random monitoring of urine or blood. Given this treatment, continuing recovery can be expected in about 80% or more of the patients if the course of therapy is 90 days or more in length. If the initial treatment is less than 90 days, the relapse rate is in the 80% range.

□ THE DISHONEST EMPLOYEE

There are few of us who, on occasion, fail to distinguish between the property of the employer and the perquisites of the employee. The list of minor peccadilloes includes such items as using hospital stationary for personal correspondence, making long-distance calls from the office phone, swiping a few aspirin tablets at the nursing station, taking a bottle of skin-care lotion home, and so forth. More significant thefts include books from the library and scrub suits to be used as pajamas.

Everyone will agree that stealing a patient's pocket book or a hospital television set is reprehensible, and yet most people will see little, if anything, wrong with the minor thefts. From a purely ethical perspective, there is no difference between stealing a sheet of stationery and stealing a television set, even though the law distinguishes on the basis of monetary value, and most employers are willing to look the other way concerning the pettiest of pilfering.

As employees, we have a clear and binding duty to protect our employer's property from others and from ourselves. The excuses that it does not matter, they'll never miss it, or it's only a few penny's worth are at best shabby. Whether we should take any action for the sake of a box of tissue paper is another question. It is ethically clearly wrong, but it may be prudent to look the other way and not antagonize everybody for the sake of trivia. It would almost certainly accomplish nothing, except make a lot of enemies and place us into the invidious position of insufferable righteousness. If we find out about the theft of more costly items, our duty is clear. This must be reported even though apprehension of the thieving co-worker will lead to their loss of employment, and possible legal sanctions.

□ THE WRONG ORDER

In respiratory care, it used to be quite common to find orders that were incomplete, incorrect, or even potentially harmful. Improved medical awareness and, most recently, the therapist-driven protocols have significantly decreased the likelihood of a wrong order. Nevertheless, the possibility exists, and therefore each department must have a written policy outlining the steps that must be taken, should a therapist be confronted with an order he or she considers improper.

The proper way to deal with this problem is to bring the disputed order to the attention of the physician who had given it and to ask for clarification or amendment of the order. If the physician is unavailable, the medical director of the department should be consulted. If the medical director is also unavailable, the therapist has three options: (1) follow the order as written, (2) ignore the order entirely, or (3) modify the order as he or she sees fit. Knowingly following a potentially harmful order is inexcusable and exposes the therapist to justifiable censure. Ignoring an order entirely is also unacceptable and is a dereliction of duty. I believe that in this situation the therapist must use his or her best judgment and do what, by training and experience, appears to be the right action. It is absolutely essential, however, that this action be carefully documented in the record and that written documentation be given for the decision taken.

□ SEXUAL HARASSMENT

An ethical problem as old as humanity itself involves the relationship between the sexes. Women entering the work force in ever-increasing numbers had to overcome prejudice, hostility, and humiliation. They are considered easy prey for the predatory male and are frequently the subject of overt or covert sexual harassment. This may take many forms, from the smutty joke to "accidental" body contact and frank sexual advances, including sexual blackmail. The ethical (and legal) situation is clear and incontrovertible. No woman should ever be made to suffer discrimination or humiliation because she is a woman. Co-workers must be treated with the same courtesy, consideration, and respect regardless whether they are male or female.

Unfortunately, when males and females work together, it is almost inevitable that sooner or later incidents will occur that some consider flattering or amusing, whereas others view them with righteous indignation. There is no ready answer to this problem, and it is the department manager's responsibility to keep interpersonal behavior consistent with professional decorum. Sexual harassment is considered a primarily male problem, but much trouble can be avoided if female behavior is also kept within the same decorous bounds. Unnecessarily provocative behavior or dress is an invitation to trouble, and the woman who flaunts her femininity or who tries to use it for advantage is just as guilty of sexual harassment as the male who is weak enough or stupid enough to fall for it.

More recently, reverse sexual discrimination has become a problem. In respiratory care, as indeed in many other health fields, females are frequently in leadership roles. Female supervisors and female technical directors are not at all uncommon in respiratory care departments. It has been reported that under these circumstances male employees have been subjected to sexual advances and have been punished for failure to comply with the supervisor's explicit or implicit suggestions. This, of course, is sexual harassment as well, and as such it is both unethical and illegal.

Another area of deep ethical concern is the relationship between therapist and patient. Sexual misbehavior between health professionals is regrettable; sexual misbehavior between a health professional and a patient is intolerable. Any health professional guilty of such a serious breach of professional conduct must be reported to the hospital administration and, in the case of licensed personnel, to the licensing agency. He or she must be disciplined with the utmost severity, including dismissal and loss of license.

SUMMARY

Every individual must come to grips with the ethical issues presented all too briefly in this section. Like a discussion of religion or politics, a discussion of ethical issues can clarify the problems, but only very rarely can it change deeply felt convictions or overcome legitimate, conscientious scruples. I hope that this chapter has helped the reader to understand these enormously complex issues a little better. I do not delude myself that I was able to convince anybody of anything, but I do hope that the reader will take one thought with him or her: good manners, good taste, and a profound respect for the other person's point of view accomplish more than rigid rules or the loftiest ethical principles.

REFERENCES

1. Bentham J: In LeFleur K (ed): An Introduction to the Principles of Morals and Legislation. New York, Haffner Press, 1948
2. Mills JS: Utilitarianism and Other Writings. Cleveland, Meridian, 1962
3. Kant I: Groundwork of the Metaphysics and Morals. New York, Harper & Row, 1964
4. Raffin TA: Ethical Issues in Respiratory Care. In DJ Pierson, RM Kacmarek: Foundations in Respiratory Care. Churchill Livingstone, New York, 1992
5. *Roe v Wade* 410 US 113, 1973
6. *Doe v Bolton* 410 US 179, 1973
7. Gustafson JM: Mongolism, Parental Desires and the Right to Life. Perspect Biol Med 16:229, 1973
8. *In re Houle,* 74-145 Supreme Ct, Cumberland County, Maine, Feb. 14, 1974
9. *Weber v Stonybrook Hospital* 469 NYS 2d 63, 1983; and *US v University Hospital* 729 F 2d 144 2nd Circuit, 1984
10. Resher N: The Allocation of Exotic, Medical Lifesaving Therapy. Ethics 79(3):173, 1969
11. The Nuremberg Code: Trial of War Criminals Before the Nuremberg Military Tribunal Under Control Council Law No 10, Vol II. Nuremberg, 1946–1949
12. Declaration of Helsinki, Tokyo, World Medical Association (rev ed), 1965
13. Morris AH et al: Ethical Implications of Standardization of ICU Care with Computerized Protocols. In J Ozbolt (ed): Proceedings of the 18th Annual Symposium on Computer Applications in Medical Care. Philadelphia, Hanley & Belfus, 1994, pp 501–505

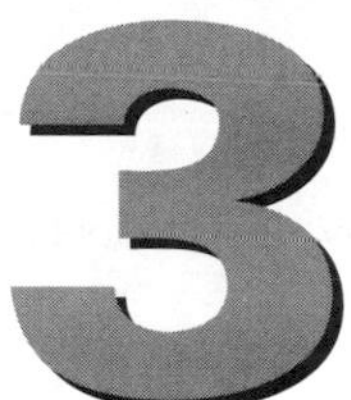

The Future of the Respiratory Care Profession

F. Herbert Douce

PROFESSIONAL SKILLS

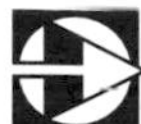

Upon completion of this chapter, the reader will:

- Determine the purpose of managed care contracts
- Identify strategies used for hospital reorganization
- Raise ethical questions regarding the consequences of decreasing health care expenditures
- Predict an expanding role for the respiratory care practitioners in intensive care units, in directing patient care, and in patient education and health promotion services
- Describe the working environment models for respiratory care practitioners that result from hospital reorganization
- Describe alternate care site environments for respiratory care practitioners, such as subacute care and skilled nursing facilities, home care, and physicians' offices
- Explain the role of the respiratory care practitioner who functions as a case manager
- Conclude that the successful respiratory care practitioner of the future must adapt to changing work environments and job roles

KEY TERMS

Capitation	Home respiratory care	Primary care
Consumerism	Intensive respiratory care	Subacute care
Diagnostic-related groups (DRGs)	Managed care contracts	Therapist-driven protocols (TDPs)
Disease state management	Patient-focused care	

There will always be abundant opportunities for well-educated and trained, competent, enthusiastic therapists.

—KEVIN SHRAKE

From its inception, the respiratory care profession has been evolving and changing. During the first 50 years of the respiratory care profession, the respiratory care practitioner (RCP) evolved from an on-the-job-trained worker without formal training or credentialing to a college-educated and licensed allied health professional. The roles and responsibilities of the RCP have changed from equipment maintenance tasks to life-support patient care, sophisticated diagnostic testing, and consultation. The employment settings for RCPs have expanded from hospitals to other patient care settings including outpatient clinics, skilled nursing facilities, and patient's homes. The professional organizations supporting the respiratory care profession have increased in size and scope of services.

In order to adapt to a changing health care environment, each of these aspects of the respiratory care profession will continue to change and evolve. The future of the respiratory care profession will parallel the maturation of other allied health professions and will be greatly influenced by changes in the health care delivery system and the needs of society. The next 50 years will be as dynamic as the first for the respiratory care profession.

DEVELOPMENT OF HEALTH PROFESSIONS

Each health profession has evolved in a predictable pattern, beginning with research and technologic advances that create a new vocation. The evolutionary trend often begins with a technologic advance passed on by unstructured apprenticeships or on-the-job training. Training then becomes more structured and academic, with a more formalized curriculum in an educational institution. Next, education becomes required by employers and consumers; eventually it is required by law, as is credentialing and licensing. Professional organizations begin to set standards for accrediting the educational programs, credentialing and assuring competence of the practitioners, and following professional ethics. Professionalism usually develops from higher standards for education, credentialing, and ethical behavior; research and the creation of a unique body of knowledge; and higher expectations and demands by society. In the nonphysician health professions, the transition to professionalism is often rewarded by medicine and policy makers with delegation of more responsibility, more decision-making authority, and more autonomy. The respiratory care profession has been evolving for half a century and will continue to evolve through the years.

CHANGES IN HEALTH CARE DELIVERY

During recent decades in the United States, health care has changed from a benevolent system to a business. Beginning in 1965 with Medicare, the health care industry has grown to consume almost 13% of the gross domestic product (GDP). Before the 1990s, there were financial incentives in health care to do as much as possible for patients and to provide optimal patient care. More services provided to patients resulted in more fees that providers could charge. This fee-for-service system led to growth in the industry, growth in the respiratory care profession, and to high costs that the government and employers ultimately had to pay for health care services. As the cost of health care and employee benefits increased, the high cost of health care began to have a negative impact on our country's competitiveness in a global economy, and a new approach to providing health care that emphasized *efficiency and cost reduction* began.

Concerns over increasing health care costs will continue to direct the future of our health care delivery system, and the emphasis on reducing health care costs will continue in the future. Third-party payers, such as the government, employers, and insurance companies, will pay less and individual patients will contribute more to payment of their health care bill. Patients will become more interested in their health care services, and there will be a new *consumerism* in health care. Our customers will demand greater accountability and quality for their health care dollar. Managed care and capitation, nonhospital care, and hospital reorganization will be the top trends influencing health care delivery in the 1990s and beyond.[1]

To reduce health care costs in the 1980s, Medicare changed to a reimbursement system based on *diagnostic-related groups* (DRGs) for those citizens over 65 years old. In this system hospitals are paid a set amount based on a patient's diagnosis. Some diagnoses, such as acute respiratory failure with complications, pay more than other diagnoses. If a hospital can provide care and discharge a patient for less than the paid amount, the hospital gets to keep the remainder as a profit. If a hospital spends more treating a patient than it will be paid, the hospital takes a loss on that patient. For Medicare patients, the financial incentives for hospitals changed from providing as much care as possible to reducing costs, providing adequate care, and making profits.

Although the DRG system has not reduced health care costs for the government overall, the system has controlled growth. As a result, other third-party payers, such as private insurance companies, are negotiating similar group contracts with hospitals and other professionals to provide all necessary health care services for their clients at a set fee. Some large employers are negotiating their own health care contracts to provide services directly to their employees. These are called *managed care contracts*, and they provide a set dollar amount per individual whether they require health care services or not. This system is similar to that of health maintenance organizations (HMOs).

Managed care contracts are attractive to insurance companies because they can negotiate lower fees with hospitals in competitive markets and because they can control their costs by setting expenditures in advance. These contracts are also attractive to large employers because they can eliminate the insurance company as a middleman and deal directly with hospitals and primary care physicians. Managed care contracts are attractive to individuals because costs are known and limited in advance. These contracts are attractive to hospitals and other providers because they can count on a set number of patients. To win these contracts, hospitals compete with each other to set the lowest prices, and to remain financially solvent, hospitals must reduce their costs in order to meet the prices negotiated in the contract. Reducing hospital costs usually means reducing staff and eliminating services that are not fully reimbursed or cost-effective.

Managed care contracts are changing the system from a fee-for-service system to a system based on *capitation*. In a capitated system, the provider is paid a flat fee "per covered life." This system is sometimes referred to as a "per member per month" (PMPM) type of reimbursement. Under the capitation system, the financial incentives are to provide the least appropriate services for patients as possible and at the lowest cost. With the new financial incentives, hospitals will continue to cut costs by reorganizing the jobs of health care providers, reducing the number of nonessential hospital admissions and reducing each patient's length of stay in the hospital, scrutinizing medical necessity, reducing the services that a patient receives, and assuring cost-effectiveness of all services. In general, there will be fewer patients in hospitals. They will be sicker because of stricter admission criteria and earlier discharge. In short, hospital patients will be receiving fewer medical services.

Provision of health care services in less expensive settings *outside of hospitals* is increasing. The financiers of health care are emphasizing more primary and preventive care to keep people from needing expensive hospital services. There will be a continuing shift to outpatient care at hospitals and clinics and to home care. New health care institutions that are a hybrid of hospital and nursing home will begin to fill the gap between hospital care and home care. These new institutions are called postacute care or subacute care centers. These facilities are for patients who are well enough to leave a full-service hospital, but who are too sick to go home or to a nursing home. Postacute and subacute care facilities are less costly because they have lower overhead—they do not have operating rooms, emergency rooms, or sophisticated diagnostic laboratories. As a result, these facilities will flourish as the number of full-service acute care hospitals decreases.

Hospital reorganization will occur in multiple forms. In *patient-focused care*, hospitals will reorganize from a structure of departments for every service to a structure of "patient care units." The hospital will reorganize in an effort to provide more friendly and efficient delivery of patient care services. There will be an administrator for each patient care unit instead of a manager for each department. Hospital staff will be assigned to a unit instead of a department, and a variety of medical, nursing, and allied health professionals will work together on a patient care unit. Each caregiver will have multiple skills. Jobs for nurse's aides and orderlies will return to the hospital. Patient-focused care will reduce the number of individuals a patient will encounter in a hospital, and it may provide a more efficient delivery system; however, examples where patient-focused care has reduced overall costs and improved patient satisfaction are currently lacking.

Another model of reorganization is the *multidisciplinary megadepartment* of ancillary services. In this approach, there is one department of ancillary allied health services with one manager. These departments may evolve to include many allied health disciplines; some may include nursing.[2] In this model, multicompetent caregivers who provide care traditionally provided by specialists will prevail. In these and other reorganization models, hospitals are downsizing and reducing the number of administrators, middle managers, and supervisors while maintaining an adequate number of essential staff who provide direct patient care services.

Competition to reduce hospital costs in order to obtain and fulfill managed care group contracts will dominate health care administration. The length of stay will decrease and hospital beds will turn over faster; fewer hospital beds will be needed to meet the future needs of our patients. The number of hospitals, the number of hospital beds, hospital admissions, and occupancy rates will continue to decrease across the country. The number of community hospitals has dropped 9% since 1983. In 1993, 34 community hospitals closed and 18 merged. Rural hospitals have been affected disproportionately: more rural hospitals have closed than urban hospitals, and they have experienced more reductions in the number of staffed beds and fewer admissions. Outpatient services have increased almost 75% since 1983.[3]

This decrease in hospitalizations will decrease the number of health care workers that hospitals employ for inpatient services and will increase opportunities to provide health care services outside the hospital setting. Patient-focused care may make hospitals more attractive to patients, and multiskilling will make hospitals more efficient. In some hospitals, departments for every discipline of caregiver will be eliminated, and only large organizational units will remain.

Reductions of health care services will create new ethical questions, and rationing of health care may evolve. The ethics of setting priorities so that only some patients receive care and providing futile care to the elderly, the premature, and the dying will need to be addressed by policy makers and patient advocacy groups (see Chapter 2). By placing limits on health care expenditures, our society may be indirectly placing limits on medical high technology, on life support, and on medical procedures that may have only marginal success. Limits may create additional risks for patient morbidity and mortality.

IMPACTS ON RESPIRATORY CARE

The impact of managed care on hospitals, on all health care providers, and on patients will be substantial. The managed care system may reduce the hospital census, but the patients' overall acuity level will rise. There may be fewer patients in hospitals, but they will more likely be sick enough to require respiratory care. Some hospitals may initially reduce the number of respiratory care staff in an across-the-board response to a shrinking patient census, but the demand for respiratory care will remain stable. In addition to the continuing problems of cardiopulmonary disease due to smoking, pollution, and obesity, the continuing need for respiratory care services in hospitals will also result from an aging population, an increased prevalence of acquired immunodeficiency syndrome, and a growing population of pediatric patients with chronic lung diseases.

With an increase in patient acuity, hospital intensive care units will flourish. Intensive care units will desire only Registered Respiratory Therapists (RRT), and these RCPs will specialize in *intensive respiratory care* to critically ill patients. Clinical *protocols* (eg, therapist-driven protocols [TDP]) will evolve to the critical care units and cross training will make therapists invaluable to this setting. Fewer RCPs will be needed in hospitals, and those that do work in the intensive care units of the future will be highly trained life-support specialists who are also consultants to the medical and nursing staffs.[4]

RCPs will find a greater role in *directing patient care*. Through clinical protocols and practice guidelines, RCPs will monitor and direct basic care, but may not provide basic care to patients on general hospital floors. RCPs will need to work more independently, without supervisors, and they will need to be more efficient and constantly conscious to cost, medical necessity, and medical effectiveness. They will be expected to determine and assure medical necessity and the appropriateness of medical prescriptions through patient assessment and consultation. They will also be expected to develop and recommend respiratory therapy care plans, evaluate patient response to therapy, assure effectiveness of therapy by evaluating patient outcomes, and recommend and implement changes.[5] These roles will likely be expected of all RCPs working with national clinical practice guidelines and medically endorsed protocols. Routine respiratory care to noncritically ill patients, such as incentive spirometry and medicinal aerosol therapy, will be self-administered or administered by nurses and patient care technicians (aides and orderlies) where allowable by law.

In hospitals that adopt *patient-focused care*, most RCPs will work for a patient care unit such as the medical intensive care unit (MICU) or the emergency department, not a traditional respiratory care department. RCPs will be decentralized, and there will be no specified respiratory care supervisors. The respiratory care department will include fewer RCPs who provide only outpatient services and cardiopulmonary diagnostic testing. In those hospitals that have implemented patient-focused care, many RCPs reported more job satisfaction, at least initially, because they become an important part of an interdisciplinary team and are not as isolated as when they were departmentalized.[6] Patient-focused care presents an opportunity for RCPs to broaden their skills and contribute more to the heath care team.[7] Alternatively, patient-focused care could eliminate traditional respiratory care departments. Depending on the number of hospitals that experiment with patient-focused care, the impact on respiratory care departments, managers, and clinicians could be significant.

Reorganization of hospital departments will decrease the number of managers and supervisors and will create additional opportunities for clinical RCPs. Reorganization may eliminate supervisory and management positions because practitioners will be expected to work more independently. Small respiratory therapy departments, especially in small hospitals, will be changed beyond recognition by coalescing with other health care disciplines, and they will become a component of a *multidisciplinary ancillary department*. The successful respiratory care manager will often become the manager of the multidisciplinary department. The trend of the respiratory therapy department becoming the cardiopulmonary department will continue to expand beyond small hospitals. Clinical RCPs will have the opportunity to learn and perform the multiple services offered by their multidisciplinary departments. Multiskilling and multicredentialing are not new to many RCPs who have earned credentials in advanced cardiac life support (ACLS), pediatric advanced life support (PALS), pulmonary function technology (CPFT or RPFT), cardiac diagnostics (RCVT), or sleep science (RPSGT). In those disciplines in which practitioners qualify for credentialing examinations based on experience, RCPs will earn additional credentials in such areas as electroencephalography (EEG), electromyography (EMG), sonography, and hyperbarics (HBO). The scope of services performed by RCPs may become so broad and diverse that respiratory care could be at risk of losing its identity as an allied health specialty, and the allied health care specialist may supersede respiratory care therapists and technicians.[8]

Some hospital respiratory care departments will provide services under contract to *subacute care* and *skilled nursing facilities* (SNF), and the RCP will be the resident expert with strong assessment skills. With only one or a limited number of staff RCPs on site, RCPs will need to implement protocols more independently because there will be no technical respiratory care supervisors. Subacute care facilities and SNFs will seek RCPs with assessment skills, ventilator management skills, and tracheostomy care skills.

Home care will continue to grow, since patients will be discharged from hospitals and other facilities "sicker and quicker."[9] The new economics of health care will place patients in the least expensive care setting, and this is often the patient's own home (see Chapter 24). Although studies have already demonstrated the cost-effectiveness of *home respiratory care*, additional compelling data will be needed to secure compensation for respiratory home care services.[10,11] RCPs will follow patients to provide respiratory care wherever their care is needed. Respiratory home care encompasses virtually all forms of acute care provided in hospitals including oxygen therapy, bronchopulmonary hygiene therapy, tracheostomy care, and mechanical ventilatory support. In the home environment, invasive and noninvasive, nocturnal and continuous ventilation with appropriate monitoring will become more commonplace for those with chronic lung diseases.[12] Continuous positive airway pressure techniques will support those with obstructive sleep disorders. RCPs will be recognized for more than providing durable medical equipment services in the future. They will coordinate medically prescribed services for pulmonary patients and play a broader role in cardiopulmonary rehabilitation, patient education, and preventing acute exacerbations that might require hospitalization.[13]

RCPs will participate in more *primary care* activities with physician supervision in the offices of primary care physicians and outpatient clinics, and they will serve as physician assistants to pulmonologists. RCPs will perform spirometry, EKG, and other diagnostic tests to assess the ability of individuals with respiratory diseases to be placed in jobs or to retain current jobs under the American Disabilities Act.[14] They will administer medications, provide smoking cessation education and cardiopulmonary fitness activities, and teach patients self-care. RCPs will also find opportunities in independent *diagnostic laboratories* performing cardiopulmonary function testing and sleep testing.

RCPs will become *case managers* for cardiopulmonary patients. Case management is the process of patient care oversight and coordination of care as patients move from acute care hospitals to subacute care facilities and back to their homes. Case managers are patient advocates in matters ranging from filing insurance claims to renting equipment to communicating with the patient's physician. Case managers also monitor costs and reimbursement caps to insure that patient care is cost-effective. As managed care forces shorter patient stays in hospitals, the need for case managers will increase. Although most case managers are nurses who work for insurance companies or HMOs, RCPs may be better prepared to manage cases involving ventilators, artificial airways, and oxygen. For RCPs, case management will most likely be a role within a broader job description instead of a full-time job. The RCP case manager may likely provide the respiratory care as well. Many RCPs who understand the health care delivery system, who have excellent assessment, communications, and team skills will be involved in case management in the future.[15] The concept of "Disease State Management" may become more common, and RCPs with their combination of patient care expertise and management experience will be well-suited to manage the care patients with cardiopulmonary disorders. *Disease State Management* is a holistic approach to patient care, a clinical pathway for life. Because many cardiopulmonary ailments are chronic, in Disease State Management, RCPs will coordinate a plan of prevention and therapeutic care for patients over the course of a lifetime.

FUTURE OF RESPIRATORY CARE PRACTICE

Consistent with the major trends in health care delivery, the future scope of practice of RCPs will continue past trends. The American Association for Respiratory Care (AARC) and the National Board for Respiratory Care (NBRC) have documented an expanding scope of practice, an increased complexity of tasks, and higher job-related expectations for respiratory care clinicians. These trends will continue in the future under managed care and hospital reorganization.

In the future, health promotion and disease prevention will be emphasized more than in the past, and more RCPs will provide patient education and health promotion services. These activities will commonly include nicotine intervention and smoking cessation techniques, asthma education and control,[16] air quality surveillance and management, exercise and fitness, cardiopulmonary resuscitation, normal cardiopulmonary function and the impacts of cardiopulmonary disease, and the proper use of respiratory care equipment for self-care. RCPs will continue to provide noninvasive cardiac diagnostic services, specifically diagnostic electrocardiograms, and in the future may include more sophisticated technology such as performing echocardiograms and Doppler perfusion tests. The trend of an expanding scope of practice which creates a multicompetent RCP will undoubtedly continue in the future. In hospitals, the scope of practice will include a broader range of cardiopulmonary diagnostic testing, invasive and noninvasive cardiology testing, patient assessment and application of clinical protocols.

In 1985 and 1987 the Task Force on Professional Direction of the AARC surveyed hospitals and described an expanding scope of practice of RCPs.[17–20] In addition to providing conventional respiratory care, the task force identified patient education, health promotion services, noninvasive cardiac diagnostic services, and "other nonrespiratory services" as becoming common for RCPs. In their 1986 report, the Task Force predicted that respiratory care was best prepared for the future health care delivery system owing to our adaptability for multiskilling, our educational preparation and recognized clinical competencies, and our presence at the patient's bed side.

In 1987 the AARC surveyed nontraditional employers of respiratory care practitioners; these included skilled nursing facilities, home care agencies, and durable medical equipment suppliers. For oxygen therapy, aerosol therapy, chest physiotherapy, ventilator care, and diagnostic pulmonary tests, the respondents from all three types of alternate care sites reported growth in the number of respiratory care practitioners and services and projected future growth.[21]

In 1989 the Education Committee of the AARC used a panel of 91 experts to identify the knowledge, skills, and attributes that would be needed by future RCPs.[22] In general, the panel's prediction of the future scope of practice for all RCPs would emphasize assessing patients, planning and evaluating respiratory care, providing basic therapeutics, participating more in the therapeutic decisions for patients on mechanical ventilators, and performing pulmonary function testing. Box 3-1 lists the competencies that the experts identified. The experts predicted that advanced level practice would include proficiency in neonatal and pediatric care, pulmonary rehabilitation, respiratory home care, ACLS, quality assurance methods, computer applications, exercise and stress testing, and bedside hemodynamic monitoring skills. In order to adequately prepare future RCPs for their expanded roles, especially in patient assessment and evaluation, the same panel of experts also predicted that 2 years of postsecondary education for entry level would be necessary and that 3 or 4 years would be appropriate in the future to prepare for the advanced level.[23]

BOX 3-1

SKILLS NEEDED BY ALL FUTURE RESPIRATORY CARE PRACTITIONERS

Knowledge
Basic sciences (biology, chemistry, physics, microbiology)
Human anatomy and physiology
Medical terminology
Pathophysiology
Pharmacology
Hemodynamics
Professional roles and functions
Respiratory care theories and procedures
Basic pulmonary function testing
Neonatal and pediatric care
Home care equipment and procedures
Health promotion/disease prevention
Understanding of cost containment
Medical-legal aspects
Ethics
Knowledge of health care regulations
Knowledge of computer science
Knowledge of gerontology

Cognitive Skills
Reading skills
Adequate math skills
Organizational and time management skills
Communication skills (oral, written, and listening)
Critical thinking abilities (analytical skills, problem solving, judgement, decision-making)

Psychomotor and Clinical Skills
Respiratory care implementation, planning and evaluation
Proficiency in basic therapeutics (gases, IPPB, aerosols, etc.)
Proficiency in ventilator management
Proficiency in respiratory mechanics
Proficiency in basic pulmonary function testing
Patient assessment skills (vital signs, breath sounds, etc.)
Blood gas sampling, analysis, and quality control skills
Airway management skills
Patient education skills
Proficiency in infection control
Interview skills, patient oriented
Physical ability to do work
Ability to function in alternate sites

Attributes and Characteristics
Sensitivity to and respect for the needs of others
Dependability/reliability/responsibility (maturity)
Flexibility (ability to adapt to change)
Ability to handle stress
Conscientiousness (hard-working, high standards)
Integrity (honesty, sincerity, ethical behavior)
Compassionate, caring, empathy
Courtesy, tactfulness
Self-motivation (initiative)
Patience and understanding
Desire to help others
Self-direction
People orientation (humanism)
Self-esteem/confidence
Friendliness and being personable
Determination/perseverance
Tolerance
Respect for authority
Health-oriented behaviors
Assertiveness
Interpersonal skills (team work, conflict resolution)
Willingness to learn
Professionalism (image, pride, career versus job attitude)
Commitment/dedication to profession
Motivation for continuing learning
Growth through educational activity
Ability to give and receive criticism
Ability to effect and manage change
Self-directed learning skills
Enjoyment of learning
Credentials
Goal orientation
Loyalty to colleagues and institution
Positive outlook/sense of humor
Willingness to get involved and be proactive
Creative and innovative

In 1992 Arthur Anderson confirmed the observations made by the AARC. They observed again that respiratory care departments in hospitals had expanded beyond traditional respiratory therapy to provide a broader range of services including bronchoscopy, cardiac rehabilitation, sleep studies, and electroencephalograms. Cross-trained and multicompetent RCPs were becoming more customary, especially in small hospitals.[24]

The Coordinating Committee for Educational Advancement of the AARC conducted conferences during 1992 and 1994 to determine if there was a consensus on the future direction of clinical practice and education.[25] The conference participants developed a consensus for the RCP in the year 2001. According to the conference participants, the RCP of the future will be best prepared for the future health care delivery system by having expanded clinical duties, more professional education and attributes, a variety of nonclinical duties, and versatility. The profession will need RCPs "to render care across the entire health care delivery spectrum, from critical care on one extreme to self-care in the home on the other and all points in between, such as transitional care settings, skilled nursing facilities, and all outpatient venues." The essence of the future practitioner is described in Table 3-1.[26]

The NBRC performs job analyses for entry-level and advanced-level RCPs at least every 5 years and makes adjustments in their credentialing examinations to reflect current practice.[27] During more than 10 years of analyzing the jobs of RCPs, the NBRC has demonstrated that job requirements for RCPs have increased significantly (see Figure 3-1: Scope

TABLE 3-1 **Respiratory Care Practitioner 2001**

Clinical Duties

1. Be involved in direct patient care.
2. Furnish monitoring for cardiopulmonary and other systems using sophisticated, high-tech devices.
3. Be positioned on the health care delivery team in such a way as to have the responsibility and authority for refining broad or general physicians' orders within the parameters of predesigned protocols.
4. Administer medications via aerosol, parenteral, intravenous, and intramuscular routes of delivery.
5. Educate other caregivers, patients, and family caregivers on methods of self-administration and other related subjects such as wellness and equipment maintenance.
6. Assess patients and their progress as it relates to the overall care plan.
7. Render clinical interventions over and above the traditional scope of practice, including clinical interventions that rely on qualified patient evaluators; competence with high-tech equipment; and interventions, both therapeutic and diagnostic, that could readily be mastered by qualified respiratory care practitioners.
8. Perform invasive diagnostic and monitoring procedures.

Characteristics

1. Be a product of a multilevel education system, with entry level residing at the associate and advanced identified at the baccalaureate degree levels.
2. Possess training and education in the following areas:
   a. Critical thinking skills
   b. Liberal arts
   c. Basic sciences
   d. Communication skills
   e. Affective skills (dependability)
   f. Computer science
3. Awareness of one's environment and an ability to be flexible and adaptable.
4. Possess human relations skills in order to work as part of a team.
5. Be a licensed professional.

Attributes

1. Possess an ability to practice in all care settings.
2. Have stamina, both physical and mental.
3. Possess a holistic caregiver's perception.
4. Be compassionate.
5. Have an ability to move back and forth between "high tech" and "high touch."
6. Be an innovator and a creator.
7. Be efficient and effective.
8. Be able to respond to change, as well as be a change agent.
9. Possess skills as a negotiator.
10. Act as a mentor.
11. Remain professionally dynamic as manifested by a commitment to being a lifelong student.
12. Be compensated commensurate with skill level, responsibility, and authority
13. Refuse to be a captive of paradigms, and be willing to create new ones as needed.
14. Possess an awareness of cultural sensitivity and diversity.

Nonclinical Duties

1. Discharge planning.
2. Teaching, at both primary and secondary levels, within the context of health care delivery.
3. Be responsible for preventive medicine and wellness interventions.
4. Expand involvement within the infrastructure of the health care delivery system.
5. Possess a leadership role in allied health so as to bring about change in health care practices and health care policy.
6. Expand role in each organization's quality improvement process and data collection in order to improve resource accounting and document efficiency and effectiveness.
7. Expand managerial skill base.
8. Enlarge role in research.
9. Possess a more in-depth familiarity with other allied health procedures and interventions.

Care Settings

1. Possess an ability to render care across the entire health care delivery spectrum, from critical care on one extreme to self-care in the home on the other and all points in between, such as transitional care settings, skilled nursing facilities, and all outpatient venues.

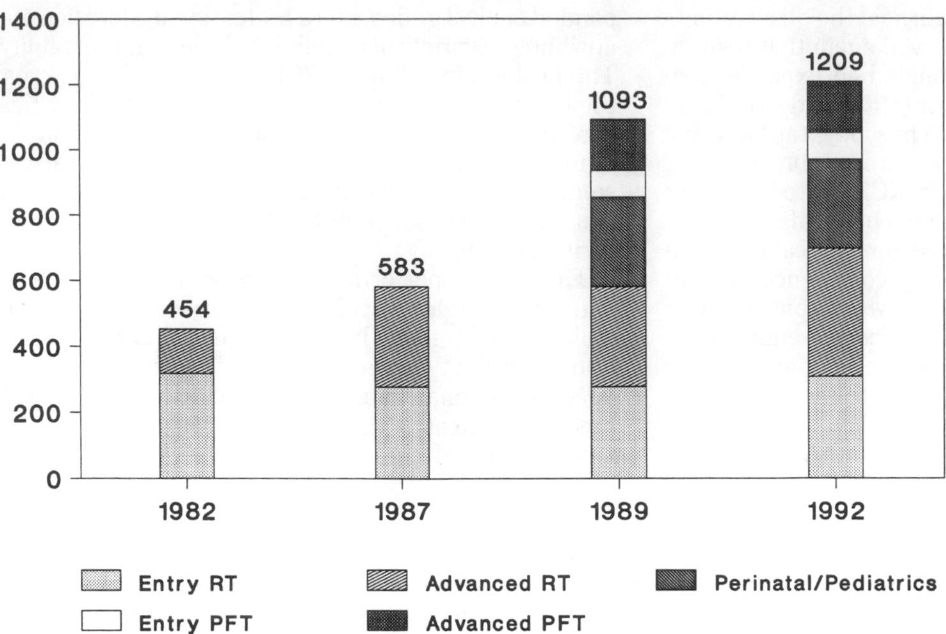

FIGURE 3-1. Scope of RC job tasks.

of RC Job Tasks). Although the number of unique tasks associated with entry-level practice changed little from 1982 to 1992, major change has occurred in advanced-level practice, which expanded from 137 tasks to 391 tasks. The NBRC has also identified pulmonary function technology and perinatal/pediatric care as specialty areas of respiratory care and now administers credentialing examinations in those domains. In 10 years the scope of respiratory care has almost tripled as measured in the increase in the collective number of tasks associated with respiratory care credentialing.

New technology will also present additional opportunities for the respiratory care profession, including liquid ventilation, high-frequency ventilation, noninvasive ventilation and monitoring, new aerosol medications for asthma, cystic fibrosis, and emphysema.

BEING PREPARED FOR FUTURE OPPORTUNITIES

RCPs are well prepared for the future health care delivery system. Table 3-2 provides 10 predictions for the future of respiratory care. RCPs will prosper in the future because they are accustomed to providing direct patient care services 7 days a week and 24 hours a day. RCPs are already used as multiskilled providers in many delivery settings. Certification of RCPs requires some postsecondary education in anatomy, physiology, and other sciences. RCPs have a skills base of more than 100 clinical interventions. RCPs are well trained to use sophisticated high technology medical equipment.[28] The future of the respiratory care profession will reside with (1) educational programs that teach material that coincides with the expanded scope of practice, and (2) the flexibility, expertise, and lifelong learning attributes of RCPs who are currently practicing respiratory care. The respiratory care profession will continue to mature as an allied health profession, will adapt to changes in the health care delivery systems of the future, and will prosper well into the next century.

TABLE 3-2 **Ten Predictions for the Respiratory Care Profession**

1. RCPs will continue to expand their roles and responsibilities in patient care.
2. RCPs will find an increasing number of employment opportunities in nonhospital settings.
3. RCPs will need 2 or more years of postsecondary education to enter the profession.
4. RCPs will be required to have legal credentialing in all 50 states.
5. RCPs will be regulated more closely by state licensing and regulatory boards.
6. RCPs will become known again as respiratory therapists.
7. RCPs will be more recognized and rewarded for their training and expertise.
8. RCPs will be reimbursed directly for their services provided in nonhospital settings.
9. RCPs will become more involved in directing patient care through protocols and case managers.
10. RCPs will be the multiskilled patient care technologist in hospitals of the future.

Abbreviation: RCP, respiratory care practitioner.

REFERENCES

1. Sabo J: Reshaping hospitals for the future: Hospital restructuring for respiratory care. AARC Times 17(7):46–47, 1993
2. Sareen D, Cooney DM: Winds of change force hospitals to batten down hatches. Advances for Respiratory Care Practitioners. Feb 6, 1995, pp 12–13
3. American Hospital Association: AHA hospital statistics, 1994–95 ed. Chicago, American Hospital Association, 1994
4. Miglino B: The survival of respiratory care. Focus Winter:20, 1995
5. White J: Opportunities actually abound for RCPs. Focus Winter:16, 1995
6. Sabo J, Milligan S: Clarkson ventures into "new world" of patient focused care. AARC Times 17(7):48–52, 1993
7. Snyder GM: Patient-focused hospitals: An opportunity for respiratory care practitioners. Respir Care 37(5):448–454, 1992
8. Smith R: Faces of the future. RT—The Journal for Respiratory Care Practitioners 8(2):53–59, 1995
9. Giordano SP: Current and future role of respiratory care practitioners in home care. Respir Care 39(4)321–327, 1994
10. Weimer MP: Home respiratory therapy for patients with chronic obstructive pulmonary disease. Respiratory Care 28(28):1484–1489, 1983
11. Haggerty MC, Stockdale-Wooley R, Nair S: Respi-Care: An innovative home care program for the patient with chronic obstructive pulmonary disease. Chest 100(3):607–612, 1991
12. Elliott MW, Simonds AK, Carroll MP, Wedzicha JA, Branthwaite MA: Domiciliary nocturnal nasal intermittent positive pressure ventilation in hypercapnic respiratory failure due to chronic obstructive lung disease: Effects on sleep and quality of life. Thorax 47(5):342–348, 1992
13. Petty TL: Pulmonary rehabilitation in perspective: Historical roots, present status, and future projections. Thorax 48(8):855–862, 1993
14. Harber P, Fedoruk MJ: Work placement and worker fitness: Implications of the American with Disability Act for pulmonary patients. Chest 105(5):1564–1571, 1994
15. Bunch D: Case management holds potential for respiratory care practitioners. AARC Times 19(3):24–28, 1995
16. Scott F: The business side of asthma. Advances for Respiratory Care Practitioners 8(6):8–9, 1995
17. Walton JR, Sullivan JM: Management Survey Part I Task Force on Professional Direction. AARTimes 9(6):23–25, 1985
18. Walton JR, Sullivan JM: Management Survey Part II Task Force on Professional Direction. AARTimes 9(7):45–47, 1985
19. Walton JR, Sullivan JM: Management Survey Part III Task Force on Professional Direction. AARTimes 9(8):22–24, 1985
20. Bunch D: Task Force Update. AARC Times 11(12):17–19, 1987
21. Giordano S, Walton JR, Gage ML: 1987 Human Resources: A Survey of Respiratory Care Manpower in Alternate Sites. Dallas, TX, American Association for Respiratory Care, 1987
22. O'Daniel C, Cullen D, Douce FH, Ellis GR, Mikles SP, Wiezalis CP, Johnson PL, Lorrance ND, Rinker R: The future educational needs of respiratory care practitioners: A Delphi study. Respir Care 37(2):65–78, 1992
23. Douce FH, Cullen DL: Educational preparation and academic awards for future respiratory care practitioners: A Delphi study. Respir Care 38(9):1014–1019, 1993
24. Arthur Anderson and American Association for Respiratory Care: A study of respiratory care practice. Dallas, TX, AARC, 1992
25. Year 2001: Delineating the educational direction for the future respiratory care practitioner. In Proceedings of a National Consensus Conference on Respiratory Care Education. Dallas, TX, The American Association for Respiratory Care, 1993
26. Dunne PJ: Shaping a vision of the future respiratory care practitioner. AARC Times 16(4):28–30, 1992
27. National Board for Respiratory Care. 1986 Respiratory Therapy Job Analysis/Changes in the NBRC Examination Matrices. Shawnee Mission, KS, National Board for Respiratory Care, 1987
28. O'Daniel C: Health care skill standards and multiskilling. AARC Times 19(3):8–13, 1995

4 The Anatomical Basis for Respiratory Gas Exchange

F. Herbert Douce
J. Robert Kinker

KEY TERMS

Acinus
Alveolus (pl. alveoli)
Alveolar-capillary membrane
Alveolar ducts
Alveolar macrophages
Capacitance
Carina
Carotid and aortic bodies
Chemoreceptors
Choanae
Cilia
Clara cells
Compliance
Dead-space ventilation
Diaphragm
Epiglottis
Eustachian tube
External respiration
Glottis
Glycosaminoglycans
Goblet cells
Internal respiration
Lamina propria
Laryngopharynx
Larynx
Lobar bronchi
Main stem bronchi
Mast cells
Meatus
Medullary respiratory center
Müller's maneuver
Naris (pl. nares)
Nasopharynx
Pleural space
Oropharynx
Respiratory bronchioles
Segmental and subsegmental bronchi
Surfactant
Terminal bronchioles
Trachea
Turbinate(s)
Type I and II alveolar cells
Valsalva maneuver
Vesicular folds
Ventilation to perfusion ratio
Uvula

The primary function of the human lung is to allow for exchange of gases (oxygen and carbon dioxide) between the external environment and internal body cells. Gas transfer occurs by exposing air to the circulating blood at the *alveolar-capillary membrane*. The lung also has secondary functions. These include the following: acting as a reservoir of blood for the left ventricle, serving as a filter in the systemic venous circulation, playing a role in immune function, and synthesis or transformation of biochemical compounds. Abnormalities of gas exchange are the most obvious manifestations of pulmonary disease, but disturbances of the secondary functions of the lung may also occur. The primary purpose of this chapter is to review the anatomy of the structures involved in gas exchange.

In addition to the lungs themselves, other body systems are necessary for gas exchange. The nervous system controls the ventilation process; the musculoskeletal system provides the mechanical work of breathing; the cardiovascular system delivers carbon dioxide to the lungs and oxygen to body tissues; the blood functions as a transport media; the immune system deals with infection of critical tissues; and the renal system complements respiration in maintaining acid-base balance. Each of these body systems plays a role in the gas exchange process demonstrating the complexity and interdependence of many body systems. When the cardiopulmonary system fails, the result is a lack of oxygen and/or an excessive accumulation of carbon dioxide in the blood, which can hinder energy production and utilization, impair mental capability, cause cardiac arrhythmias, and result ultimately in death.

GAS EXCHANGE MODELS

Oxygen and carbon dioxide move between the external air and the metabolizing cells of the body by the processes of bulk flow and simple diffusion from areas of high to low partial pressures. A schematic model shown in Figure 4-1 provides an overview. The delivery of gases from the external atmosphere to the alveolar membrane occurs by passing through the tracheobronchial airways. The bellows pumping action, created by the respiratory musculature, causes bulk gas flow in response to positive and subatmospheric pressure changes (*external respiration*). The heart is a second parallel pump which distributes blood to the pulmonary capillary membrane. The interface of the blood and gas allows intimate contact and diffusion at the *alveolar-capillary membrane*.

Internal respiration occurs as oxygenated blood is distributed to body tissues, and simultaneously carbon dioxide and other cellular metabolic end products are

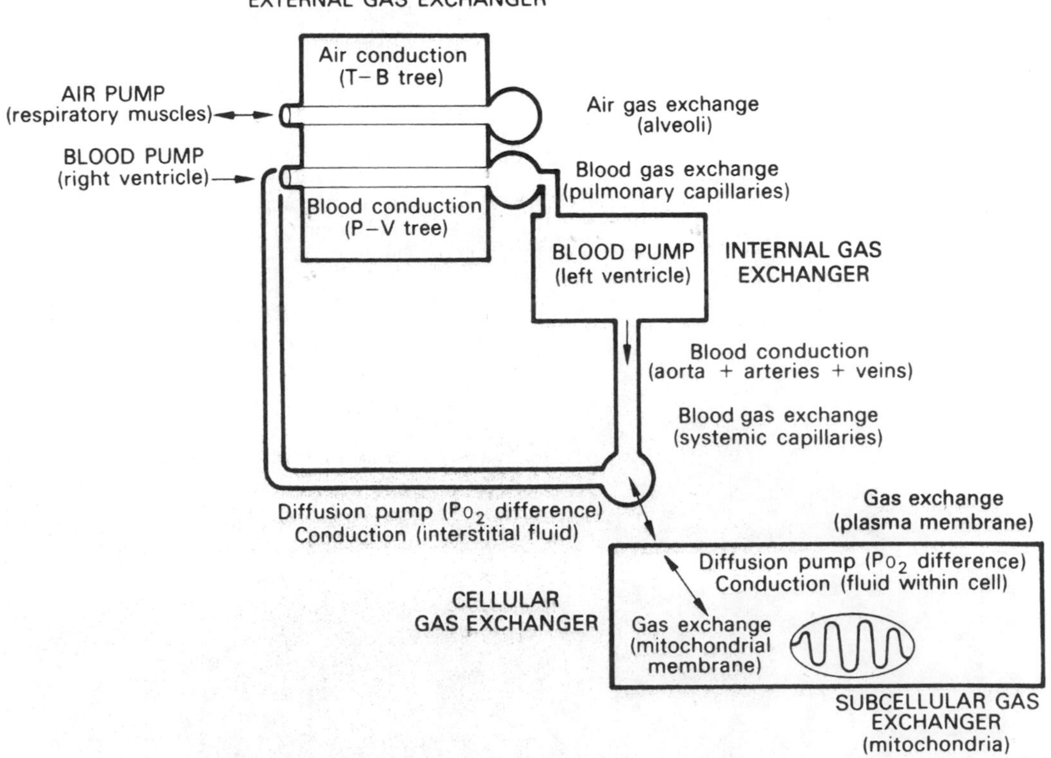

FIGURE 4-1. A model of the respiratory gas exchange mechanism. The respiratory muscles and right ventricle act as two (external gas exchange) parallel pumps to bring air and blood into potential contact within the lung. At the alveolar-capillary membrane (internal gas exchange) begins. The left ventricle and systemic arterial vasculature transport blood to the tissues where gas exchange can be completed at the cellular level. (Modified from Gee JBL, Robin ED: Disorders of respiratory gas transport and metabolism. Scientific Clinician, New York: McGraw-Hill, 1966, with permission)

removed. Gas transport requires the left ventricle and systemic arteries, capillaries, and blood-containing hemoglobin. The internal gas exchanger is in series with the external, cellular, and subcellular gas exchangers. In subcellular gas exchangers, molecular oxygen enters into substrate oxidation by acting as a terminal electron acceptor. For instance, in the metabolism of glucose, the reaction, $C_6H_{12}O_6 + 6O_2 \rightarrow 6CO_2 + 6H_2O +$ ATP (energy), requires an intracellular PO_2 of less than 5 mmHg and is responsible for about 70% of the total oxygen consumption.

A second model illustrated in Figure 4-2 underscores the interdependency of the components of the internal and external exchangers. All pumps, conducting tubes or vessels, and blood must be functioning simultaneously and continuously. If one part of the system begins to fail, even though the others are temporarily functioning adequately, the overall function of the system will be impaired. This model also illustrates the potential compensatory mechanisms that exist. Impairment of gas exchange in the lungs may be partially corrected by increases of the cardiac or hematologic systems.

To understand the gas exchange process, it is first important to understand the normal anatomy of the lung and the gas transport system. The respiratory care practitioner should be familiar with the components of the gas exchange process from the upper airways to the lower airways and from the control of ventilation to the pumping mechanism of air movement. Once normal function is understood, the impact of impairment can be better appreciated. This chapter briefly reviews lung structure. If further details are required, please see the definitive anatomic texts listed in the bibliography at the end of this chapter.

PULMONARY ANATOMY

The components of the pulmonary system consist of the lungs, the upper airways, the central airways, the peripheral airways, the terminal respiratory unit, and

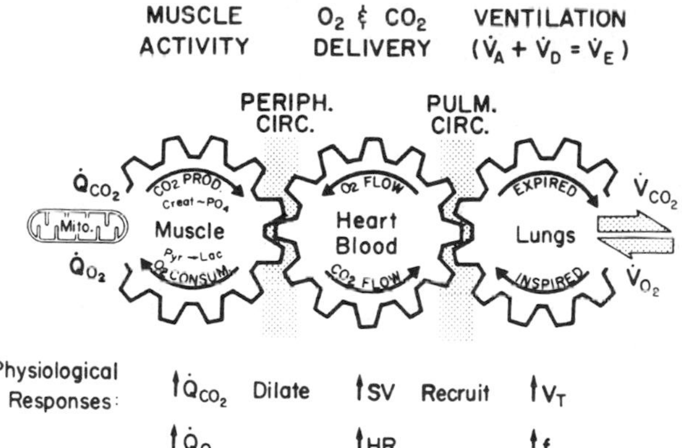

FIGURE 4-2. A model of the key components of gas exchange illustrating the interdependence of the major body system components as well as mechanisms for compensation. (Wasserman K, Hansen JE, Sue DY, Whipp BJ: Principles of Exercise Testing and Interpretation. Philadelphia, Lea & Febiger, 1987, with permission)

the alveolar-capillary units. Effective gas exchange depends on the structure and integrity of each of these components.

The lungs occupy the right and left hemithorax within the chest wall's parietal pleura. In the mature adult they would occupy an average vertical height of 24 cm (at resting exhalation). At that level of inflation, 2.4 L of gas would be contained in the alveolar tissue and airways; at full inflation the lungs might contain 5 to 6 L. The average total weight of the excised lungs would be 900 to 1000 g, of which 40% to 50% is blood. More than 50% of the 300 million gas-exchanging alveoli are located in the peripheral 30% of lung tissue. The general organization of the lung involves gas exchange tissue under loose-binding connective tissue or airways, blood vessels, and pleura. The alveolar wall's interstitium comprises the framework for the lung parenchyma. That tissue is composed of an array of cells, connective tissue composed of fibrils of collagen and elastin. However, the bulk of the lung interstitium is occupied by the ground substance *glycosaminoglycans*.

Upper Airways

The upper respiratory tract begins with the nose, which has an external portion and an internal portion inside the skull (Fig. 4-3). The external nose is made up of skin, bone, cartilage, and fibrous fat tissues, and is lined with mucous membrane. The nasal bones hold the base of the nose in a fixed position and form part of the bridge of the nose with the remainder of the bridge formed from pliable tissues. Paired external nostrils or *nares* (singular: *naris*) are openings of the nose on the under surface, are narrow, and cause significant resistance to air flow. The internal portion of the nose is a cavity composed of a number of bones and soft tissues and is located inferior to the brain and superior to the mouth. Toward the back of the skull, the internal nose connects with the pharynx through two posterior nares (*choanae*), and toward the front of the skull, merging with the external nose. The nasal septum divides both the external and internal nasal cavities into two independent passageways. The anterior portion of the septum is made up of septal cartilage; posteriorly, it is bone (vomer and the perpendicular plate of the ethmoid) and can be deviated at times, potentially leading to a problem of obstruction.

The mucous membranes lining the external and internal chambers of the nose have two different cellular structures. Squamous nonciliated cells line the first third of the passageways, and ciliated columnar epithelial cells line the latter two thirds. The mucous membranes, rich in blood capillaries and goblet cells, line the nasal chambers providing a large surface area to moisten and warm the air. Air passing through the cavity is filtered and warmed to approximately 37°C or 98.6°F at 80% relative humidity. Care must be exercised when inserting catheters into the nasal cavity to prevent tearing the delicate capillaries located within the mucous membranes. The chamber also gives resonance to the voice and is the site for olfactory stimulation (Fig. 4-4).

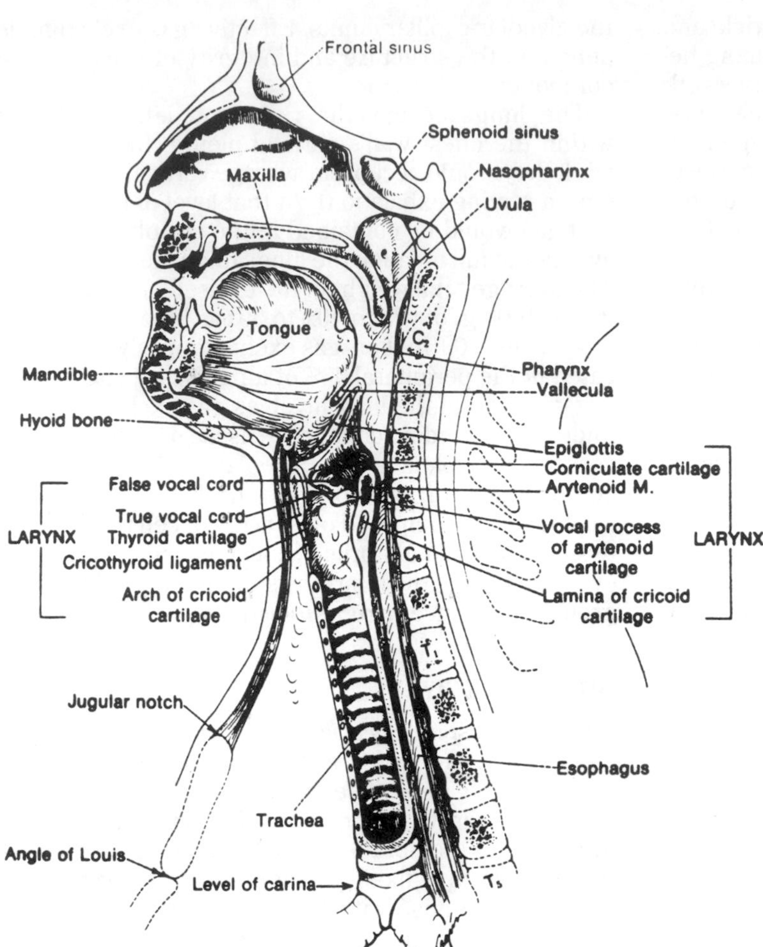

FIGURE 4-3. Saggital section of the normal adult upper airway. (From McCabe BF: Pathologic principles. In Wilkins EW (ed): MGH Textbook of Emergency Medicine (2nd ed.) Baltimore, Williams & Wilkins, 1987, with permission)

Central walls of the interior nose are formed by nasal bones, the frontal processes of the maxilla, and the cribriform plate of the ethmoid bone. The floor of the nasal cavity is the roof of the mouth. The front part of the floor of the interior nose is hard, formed by the palatine process of the maxilla. The posterior surface of the floor of the nasal passages is soft and leads to the nasopharynx. Inside the skull on the lateral walls of the nasal passages, hard bony plates or *turbinates*, project as ridgelike structures into the chambers, creating increased turbulent air motion increasing the potential for filtering particulate matter greater than approximately 10 microns (μm). Cilia transport the particles toward the pharynx for swallowing and elimination from the body. The three sets of turbinates (conchae) are described as superior, middle, and inferior. The depressions between turbinates are referred to as the superior, middle, and inferior *meatuses*. The sensory receptors for olfactory nerves, which also serve to send warning signals regarding airborne irritants, are also found in the area above and near the superior turbinates (see Fig. 4-3).

There are eight paranasal sinuses, which are hollow cavities situated inside the interior bones of the skull. The paired sinuses—frontal, ethmoid, sphenoid, and maxillary sinuses—are named after the bones in which they are located and open into the internal nasal cavities near the turbinates. The sinuses lighten the weight of the bones in the head and may help to control the brain temperature.

The pharynx is a passageway for both food and air. It is a tube approximately 13 cm (5 inches) long, which is composed of skeletal muscle and is lined with mucous membrane. It lies immediately behind the nasal cavities and the oral cavity. There are three sections of the pharynx: the *nasopharynx*, *oropharynx*, and *laryngopharynx* (or hypopharynx). The nasopharynx is a continuation of the nasal cavities and contains openings for the auditory *(eustachian) tubes* responsible for equalizing pressure in the middle ear. The oral pharynx lies behind the mouth and begins with the soft palate and ends at the level of the hyoid bone. The mouth or oral cavity is used primarily for digestion and speech and secondarily for respiration. It is a less effective filter and humidifier than the nasal cavities. Mouth breathing may be essential when either of the two nasal pathways are obstructed or congested, or when the need for ventilation exceeds resting levels.

The oral cavity is defined by the lips and teeth on the anterior side, the teeth and jaws along the bottom and lateral sides, and the uvula and oropharynx on the posterior side. The hard palate is part of the maxilla bone and occupies the anterior two thirds of the roof of the

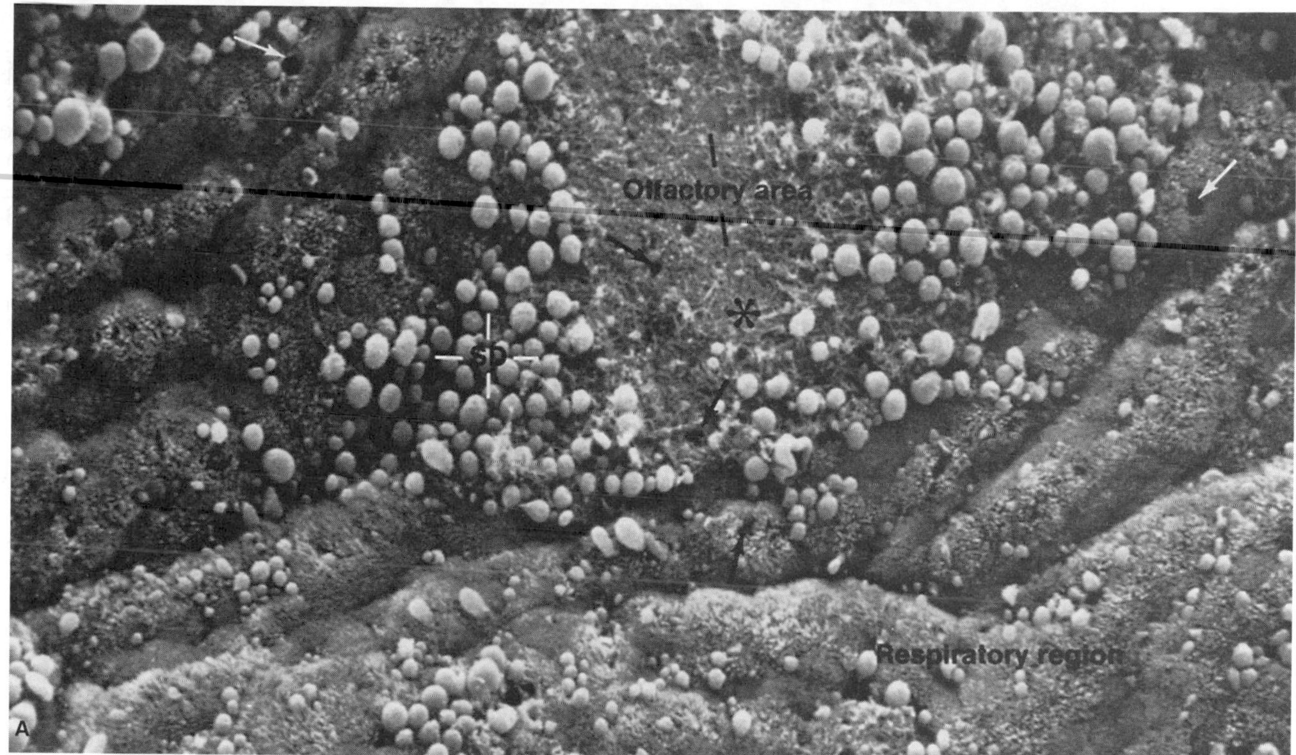

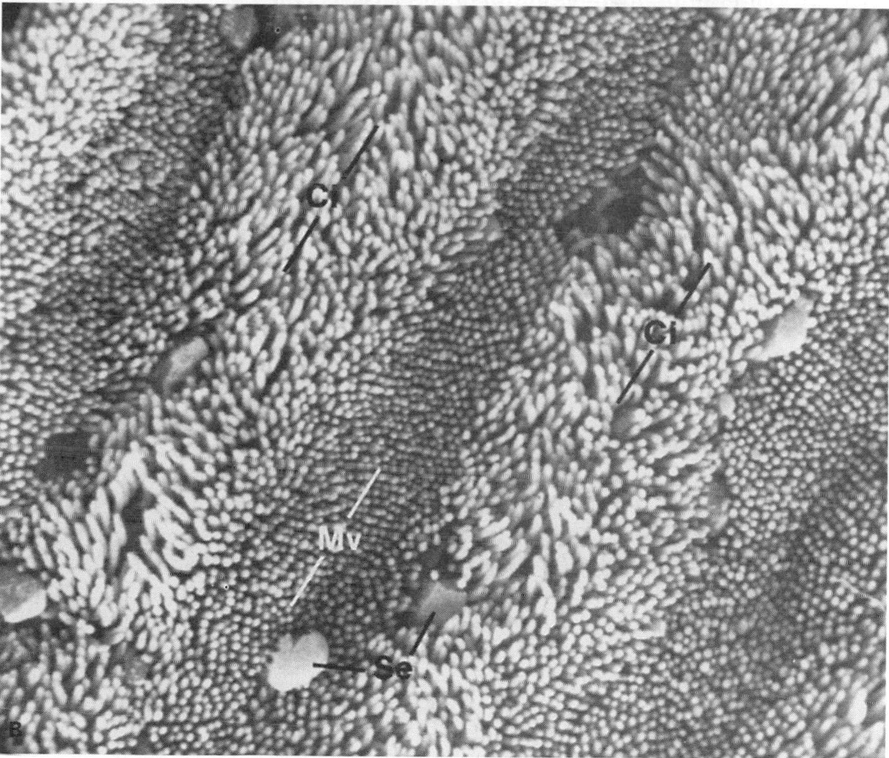

FIGURE 4-4. Scanning electron micrographs of the nasal cavity. The area is lined by a mucous membrane with olfactory and respiratory cells. **(A)** Secretory droplets (SD) from mucous-producing glands are emitted through duct-like orifices *(arrows)*. **(B)** An epithelial cell is illustrated showing apical cilia (Ci) and rows of microvilli (Mv) from nonciliated cells. Secretion from a goblet cell is shown protruding from the surface (Se). (From Kessel RG, Karoon RH: Tissues and organs. In A Text-Atlas of Scanning Electron Microscopy, San Francisco, WH Freeman & Sons, 1979, with permission)

mouth. The soft palate is flexible and fibrous and continues to form the *uvula*, a small piece of fibrous tissue that extends midline from the soft palate. Flexibility of the soft palate allows for a temporary closure between the nasal and oral pharynx. The tongue is a skeletal muscle attached by the hyoid bone and the mandible. It moves food and fluids toward the posterior oral cavity and plays a role in phonation. On the posterior section of the tongue are sensory nerve endings, which activate the protective gag reflex when stimulated.

The laryngopharynx reaches inferiorly from the hyoid bones and connects to the esophagus posteriorly and the larynx anteriorly. The laryngopharynx is both a respiratory and a digestive passage lined by stratified squamous epithelium. This is also the area where contaminants, particulate pollutants, and cellular debris, either drained from the nasopharynx or brought up from the lower airways of the lungs, are expelled or swallowed.

Externally, the *larynx* looks like a pipe with a bulge at its upper portion. Inside it is a complex structure composed of soft tissue and cartilage, with several distinct components, shapes, and functions. It serves as a passageway from the pharynx to the trachea, protects the lower airways from aspirating liquids and solids, and produces vibratory voice sounds. The larynx is composed of nine cartilages. Three of the cartilages are single: the thyroid, the cricoid, and the epiglottic; three are paired: the arytenoid, the corniculate, and the cuneiform. They are held together by membranes, ligaments, and intrinsic and extrinsic muscles. The interior lining of the larynx is a mucous membrane.

The thyroid cartilage is what is commonly referred to as the Adam's apple. It is the largest structure in the larynx. Its fused plates form a double-winged structure that spreads across the anterior portion of the larynx. The upper border has an indentation called the thyroid notch. It attaches to the hyoid bone, a horseshoe-shaped structure at the base of the throat, by the thyrohyoid membrane. Over the thyroid cartilage, at the base of the tongue is the *epiglottis*, a broad, flat leaf-shaped structure lying immediately on top of the larynx. One part, the "stem" of the epiglottis, is connected to the thyroid cartilage, but the "leaf" portion can move fairly freely up and down. The epiglottis diverts food and liquid into the esophagus when swallowing by lifting the larynx in a superior direction.

The paired arytenoid cartilages are shaped like pyramids and lie on the posterior sides of the larynx. On the base of the arytenoid cartilages is a projection called the vocal process. The vocal ligaments, which make up the center of the vocal folds, are attached to the vocal process. The other small cartilages are associated with the arytenoid cartilage. The cricoid cartilage is a "signet ring-shaped" structure that provides a base of support for the larynx. It is attached to the thyroid cartilage via the cricothyroid ligament and to the first cartilaginous ring of the trachea.

Internally, the larynx forms two pairs of folds, each folded inward and covered by mucous membranes. The folds closest to the center are called the true vocal folds, which appear as white bordered veils. The more lateral folds are called false vocal folds or *vesicular folds* and act with the true vocal folds to close off the airway opening or *glottis*. They are involved in the complex coordinated act of coughing or sneezing. The vocal folds attach to the arytenoid cartilage and insert into the posterior surface of the thyroid cartilage. Beside them are the vocal ligaments, which are bands of elastic tissue.

Muscular support is critical in the larynx. The muscles that serve the larynx are intrinsic (or internal) and extrinsic (or external). The extrinsic muscles that move the larynx and the hyoid bone are subdivided into two groups. One group is called the infrahyoid (stemohyoid, stemothyroid, thyrohyoid, and omohyoid) muscles, which pull the larynx and hyoid bone down lower into the neck. The suprahyoid group (stylohyoid, hylohyoid, digasaic, and geniohyoid and stylopharyngeus) pulls the hyoid bone in a complex set of movements anteriorly, superiorly, and posteriorly. Failure of these muscle groups to maintain proper tone when patients are obtunded or during sleep may result in partial or complete airway obstruction.

Distance between the vocal cords changes with adduction (closing) and abduction (opening of the folds). The movement of the folds alters tension on the cords, producing vibratory sound. By varying cord tension, pitch can be altered. By varying the volume of air, the intensity of sound is varied. The cords flatten during normal breathing. During inhalation, the vocal folds move apart, widening the glottis. During exhalation, vocal folds move toward the center, yet still retaining the glottal space. The *Valsalva maneuver* is a means by which both true and false vocal folds close, tightly sealing the airways. It occurs during vomiting, coughing, defecating, childbirth, or when the airways are threatened. The *Müller's maneuver* is the reverse, in that inspiration is attempted with a closed glottis.

The *trachea* is a flexible tube made up of soft muscle tissue and cartilaginous C-shaped rings, and it conducts warmed and humidified air into the lungs. The trachea is found in the middle of the neck, running parallel but anterior to the esophagus and running from the larynx to the fifth thoracic vertebra. Attached to the cricoid cartilage (the base of the larynx), it is about 12 cm long, about 2.5 cm in diameter. It divides into two branches called the *main stem bronchi* at the *carina* (the last cartilage in the trachea) at about the second costal cartilage of the ribs and about the 5th thoracic vertebra on the spinal column. The mucous membrane in the interior trachea is layered with columnar ciliated epithelial tissue, soft muscle tissue, the lamina propria (which is loose fibrous tissue rich in nerves), blood and lymphatic vessels, and an outer cartilaginous layer. *Goblet cells,* serous glands, and mucosal glands produce a mucous blanket that covers the layers. This blanket is part of the filtering system of the airways. The *cilia*, under the mucous blanket, propel bacteria, contaminants, pollutants, and cellular debris upwards toward the pharynx where it can be expelled or swallowed. Figure 4-5 shows the ultrastructure of this epithelial tissue.

The trachea is composed of 16 to 20 horizontal incomplete C-shaped cartilaginous rings piled one on another. Each cartilage is 4- to 5-mm high. On the open side of the "C," the trachealis muscle attaches between the proximal ends of the cartilages. Where the cartilage is incomplete, the trachea and esophagus share a fibroelastic membrane. This structure provides both support and flexibility, allowing for expansion in the lower portion of the trachea and for compression in response to sneezing and coughing. Figure 4-6 illustrates a tracheal wall tissue section.

Central and Lower Airways

As gas exits the trachea, it moves through the descending branches of the airways, which become narrower and more numerous. Most of the airways divide

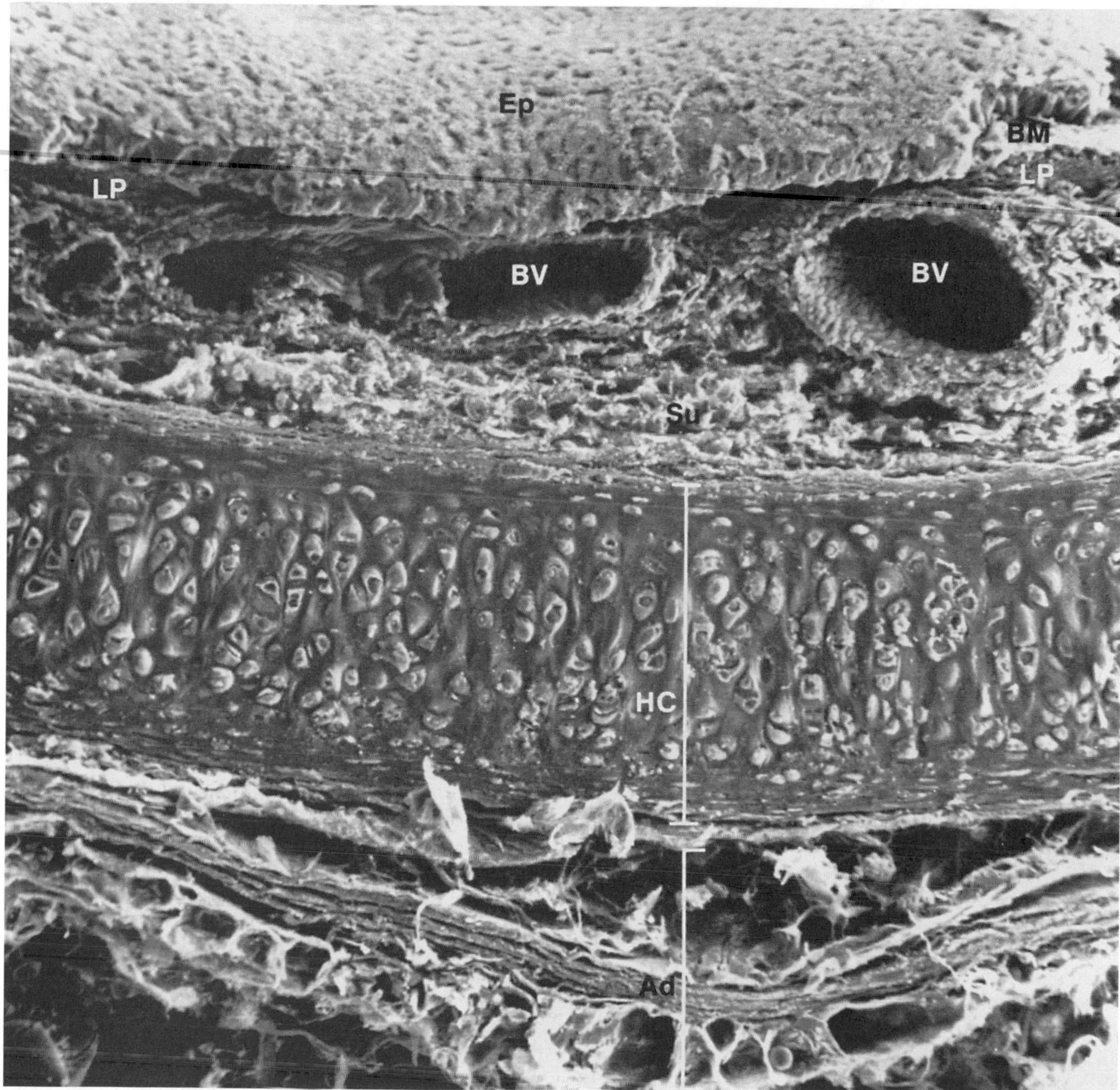

FIGURE 4-5. A section of tracheal wall seen at 300×. The epithelial layer (Ep) and lamina propira (LP) constitute the mucosa. A basement membrane (BM) separates the two. Blood vessels in the connective tissue submucosa are identified as (BV). The outermost layer of connective tissue is the adventitia (Ad). A section of C-shaped cartilage is shown (HC). (From Kessel RG, Karoon RH: Tissues and organs. In A Text-Atlas of Scanning Electron Microscopy, San Francisco, WH Freeman & Sons, 1979, with permission)

into two new branches, a process called bifurcation. The trachea divides into two branches at a site called the *carina,* and the new branches are called main stem bronchi, which open into each lung. The *right main stem bronchus* is about 11 to 19 mm in diameter and branches away from the trachea at a 25-degree angle in the adult. The left main stem bronchus angles at a 40- to 60-degree angle. The trachea and the main stem bronchi have cartilaginous rings that provide structure and substance to reduce deformation or kinking. At each bifurcation of the airways the radius decreases, but the sum of the diameters of all the passageways increases; therefore, resistance to airflow decreases from the trachea to the terminal respiratory bronchioles, the cross-sectional area of which is approximately 1000 cm^2. The pressure required to move air through the large central airways is normally 1.6 $cmH_2O/L/sec$, approximately 80% of the total airways resistance of 2.0 $cmH_2O/L/sec$. Segments of branching are called generations or orders.

The trachea is generation zero; the main stem bronchi are the first generation. The *lobar bronchi* or

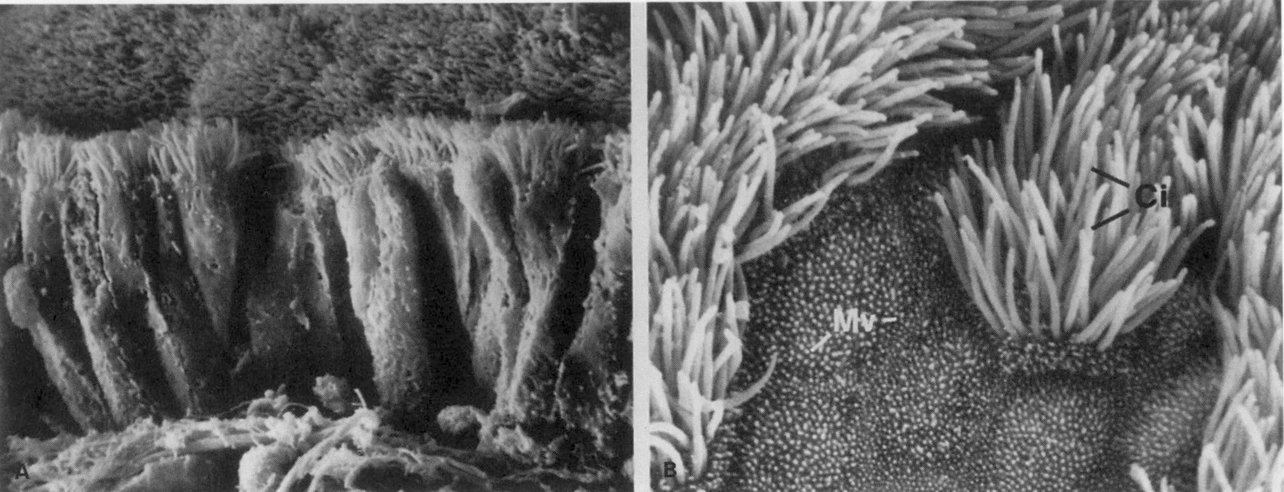

FIGURE 4-6. Scanning electron micrographs of pseudostratified epithelium from the trachea, bronchi or segmental conducting airway. Cells are usually ciliated (Ci) and Goblet cells (GC) are often present. **(A)** Ciliased cells are shown in contact with the basement membrane at their narrow apical ends. **(B)** Goblet cells occupy unciliated areas shown with short microvilli (Mv) on their surfaces. (From Kessel RG, Karoon RH: Tissues and organs. In A Text-Atlas of Scanning Electron Microscopy, San Francisco, WH Freeman & Sons, 1979, with permission)

second-generation bronchi, are 4.5 to 13.5 mm in diameter. The bronchial smooth muscle is innervated by the vagus nerve. When bronchial smooth muscle is stimulated, the muscle contracts and the airway lumen becomes smaller and constricted, causing an increase in airway resistance. The autonomic nervous system is involved in airway caliber. The surface of the cartilaginous central airways is lined with pseudostratified, columnar, ciliated epithelium interspersed with clear goblet cells that secrete thick viscid mucus. Beneath the epithelium, cartilaginous rings, and plates there are nests of mucous glands that connect with the airway lumen by ducts. These glands secrete a mixture of thick and thin mucus, and they secrete their products with vagal stimulation. Both the submucous glands and cartilage gradually disappear distally as the airways become smaller with each bifurcation. Blood supply to the major airways occurs via the bronchial arterial circulation; vessels arise from the aorta. A large portion of the venous drainage from this circulation returns to the left atrium of the heart, thereby contributing to the normal anatomic right-to-left shunt. A shunt is blood that bypasses its normal route through the lungs where gases are normally exchanged.

The surface of the bronchial epithelial cells are coated by a thin, complex layer of mucus secreted by the glands just described. This mucous blanket is propelled toward the pharynx by the hair-like cilia at a rate of about 1000 strokes per minute. Two hundred cilia are found per epithelial cell, and each cilium is about 5 to 7 μm in length. Adverse conditions, such as cigarette smoking, drying of the airways, alcoholism, and hypoxia, interfere with ciliary action and may suppress it altogether. Ciliary function may be overwhelmed by an excessive thickness of the overlying mucous coat in cystic fibrosis or during exacerbations of asthma or chronic bronchitis. The ability of ciliated epithelium to regenerate after damage is not known. At biopsy or autopsy in patients with chronic bronchitis, one often sees replacement of the ciliated epithelium with squamous metaplasia. The only way secretions can pass such damaged areas is by coughing or suctioning, which produces blasts of air shearing off the secretions; postural drainage may also enhance mobilization of secretions in damaged airways.

The *lamina propria* or submucosal layer is a layer of connective tissue that contains blood vessels, branches of the vagus nerve, lymphatic vessels, and two smooth muscle fiber bunches that wrap around each airway in close spirals, one clockwise, the other counter-clockwise. The bronchial smooth muscle tissue forms a thin layer between the epithelial layer and the lamina propria. The bronchial or submucosal glands extend deep into the lamina propria. Also found inside the lamina propria are *mast cells*, which play a significant role in bronchoconstriction of the airways during disease states such as asthma. The cartilaginous layer is the external layer of the tracheobronchial tree. Cartilage becomes progressively thinner as the airways branch into smaller and shorter segments, until it is missing entirely in the bronchioles.

Lobar bronchi feed the primary lobes in each lung, three on the right, two on the left. There is an upper, middle, and lower lobe on the right; an upper and lower lobe on the left, with a central area called the lingula that mirrors the middle lobe in the right lung. The lingula is fed from the left upper lobar bronchus. The lobar bronchi also have cartilage and are part of the conduction airway system. In the bronchi, the cartilaginous rings are replaced by a circumferential structure of cartilaginous plates, which irregularly encircle the airway. These plates are interconnected by a strong fibrous layer intermeshed with circularly arranged smooth muscle. Lung lobes are further divided into bronchopulmonary segments, each with its own airway and arterial and venous circulation. Figure 4-7 illustrates the

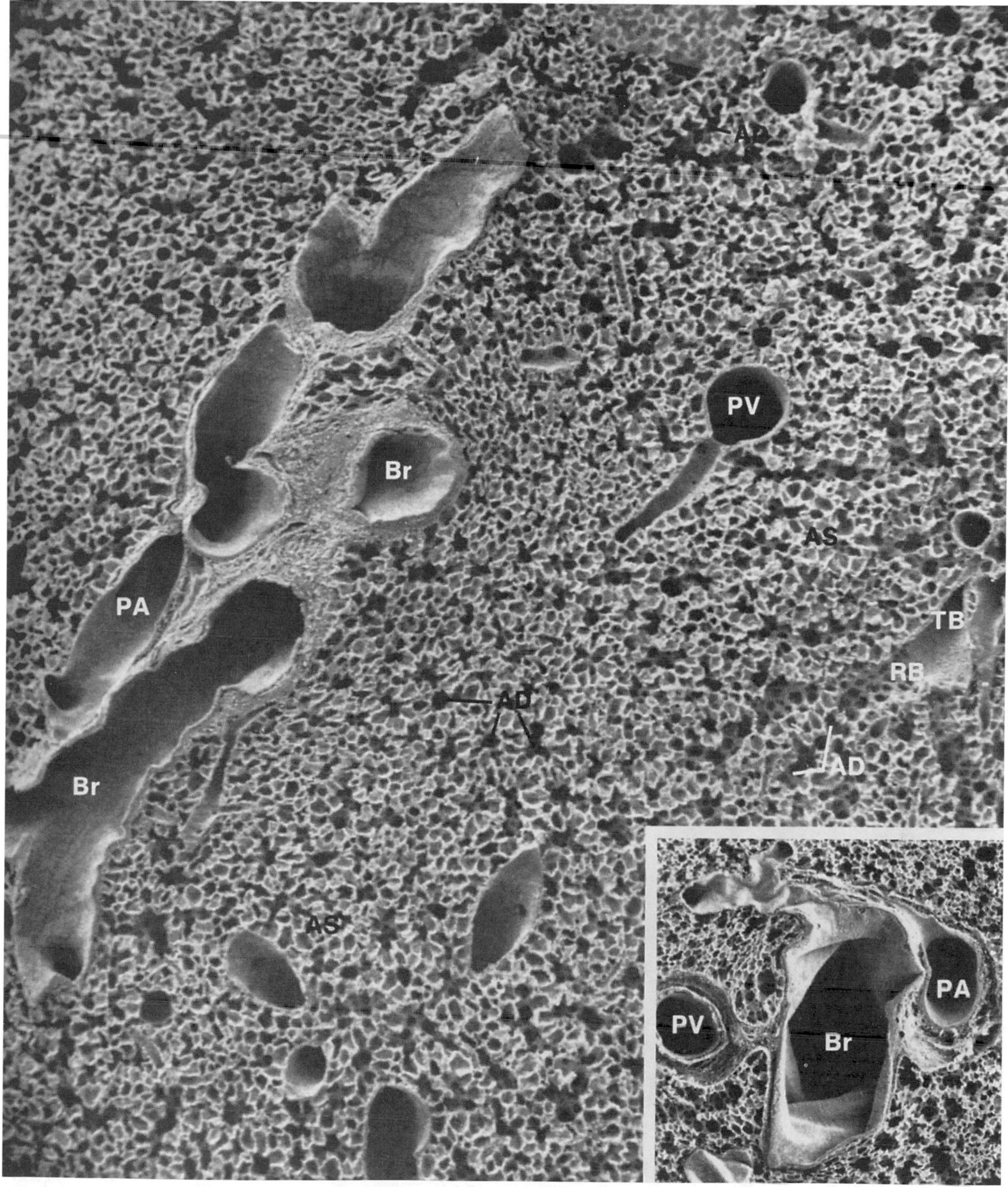

FIGURE 4-7. Micrograph of lung at low (45×) magnification. Alveoli or air sacs (AS) are shown with their shared, thin partitions between adjacent alveoli. Segmental bronchi can be seen (BR), as well as terminal bronchi (TB), respiratory bronchioles (RB) and alveolar ducts (AD). The pulmonary vasculature is shown in structures marked by pulmonary artery (PA), which tend to pass near bronchi and pulmonary veins (PV). (From Kessel RG, Karuon RH: Tissues and organs. In Text-Atlas of Scanning Electron Microscopy, San Francisco, WH Freeman & Sons, 1979, with permission)

organization of airways to adjacent structures. Figure 4-8 shows a transverse section of a bronchus.

Segmental bronchi, each about 4.5 to 6.5 μm in diameter are third-generation airways and divide the lung further into compartments. The right and left lung have 10 segments. Figure 4-9 shows a schematic of the lobar and segmental distribution. The upper right lobe has three: the apical, posterior, and anterior. The upper left lobe also has three: apical, posterior, and anterior. The middle right lobe has two segments: lateral and medial. The lingula has superior and inferior segments, whereas the lower lobes both have only superior segments. The right lower lobe also has medial basal, anterior basal, lateral basal, and posterior basal lobes, and the lower left has anterior, medial, lateral, and posterior basal lobes. The segmental bronchi branch into the subsegmental bronchi; however, both are still part of the cartilaginous airway conduction system.

Subsegmental bronchi compose the 4th through 9th generations, each dividing into two new branches. The number of airways at this level multiples exponentially. These bronchi are about 3 to 6 mm, with their cartilaginous sheath getting thinner. There are approximately 38 subsegmental bronchi.

The bronchioles, the 10th through 15th generations, are the beginning of the noncartilagenous airways, yet they are still considered part of the conduction system. They are primarily smooth muscle and columnar epithelial cells, and the cilia begin to disappear in the terminal bronchioles. Clara cells begin to present in the terminal bronchioles. Because they have thick extensions that intrude into the lumen of the terminal bronchioles, they may contribute to the liquid lining of the bronchioles and alveoli, or they may have enzymes that detoxify inhaled contaminates. Their role in lung function is not completely clear. Bronchioles vary in size, from 0.65 to 1 mm, and they number well over a thousand. The terminal bronchioles compose the 16th through 19th generations. They are at the end of the conduction airways and are a transition stage leading into the airways with gas-exchanging alveoli. There are about 35,000 terminal bronchioles in the adult with a diameter of about 0.65 mm. Although small, the sum of all the diameters, or the cross-sectional area of the terminal bronchioles, is much larger than the central airways. As a result of the relatively large cross-sectional area, the resistance to airflow is relatively low and approximately 20% of the total airway resistance. In com-

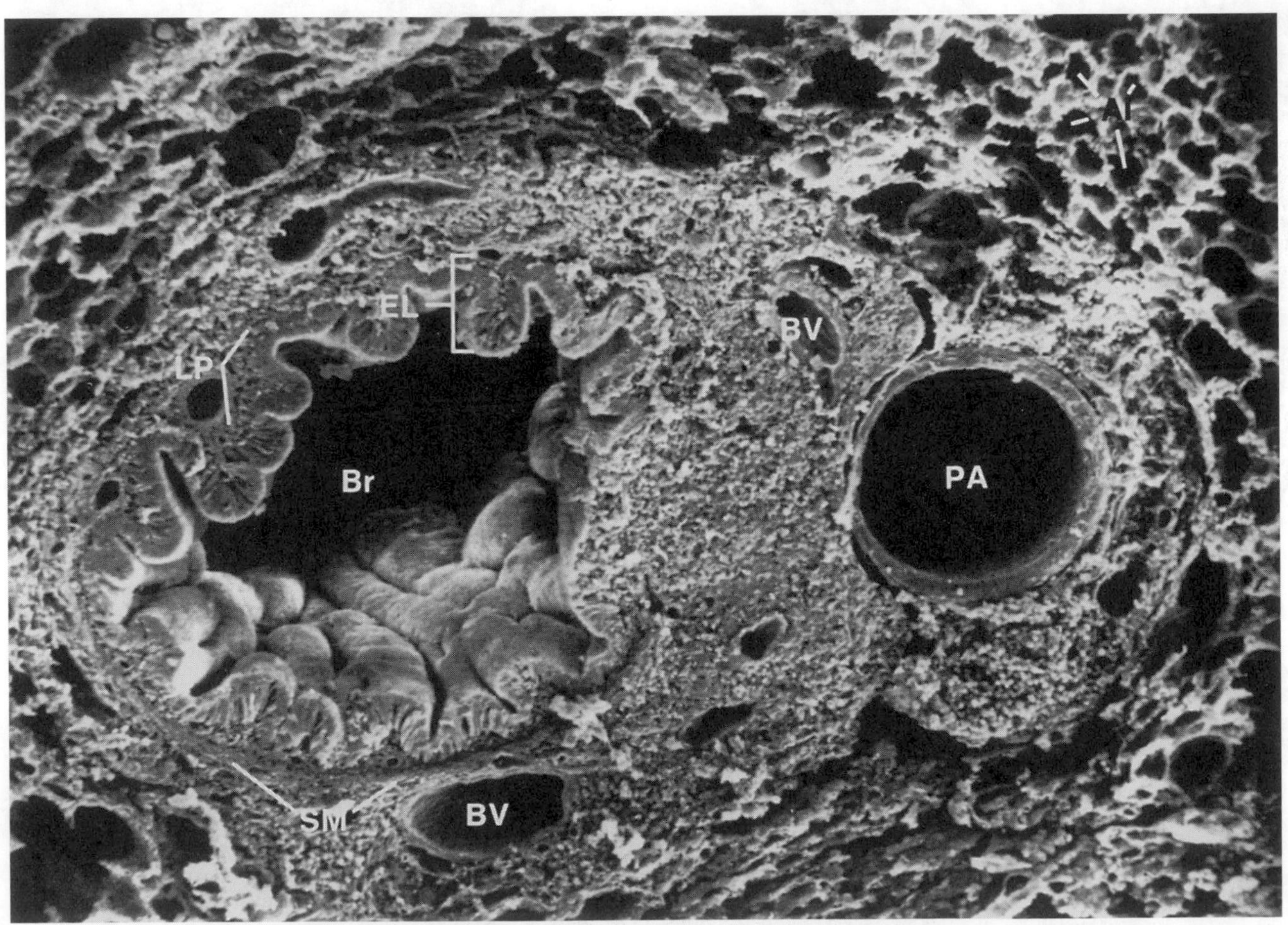

FIGURE 4-8. Transverse section of a bronchus (Br) and adjacent pulmonary artery (PA). The epithelial layer (EL), underlying lamina propira (LP) and smooth muscle are designated, as well as a bronchial vein (BV). (From Kessel RG, Karoon RH: Tissues and organs. In A Text-Atlas of Scanning Electron Microscopy, San Francisco, WH Freeman & Sons, 1979, with permission)

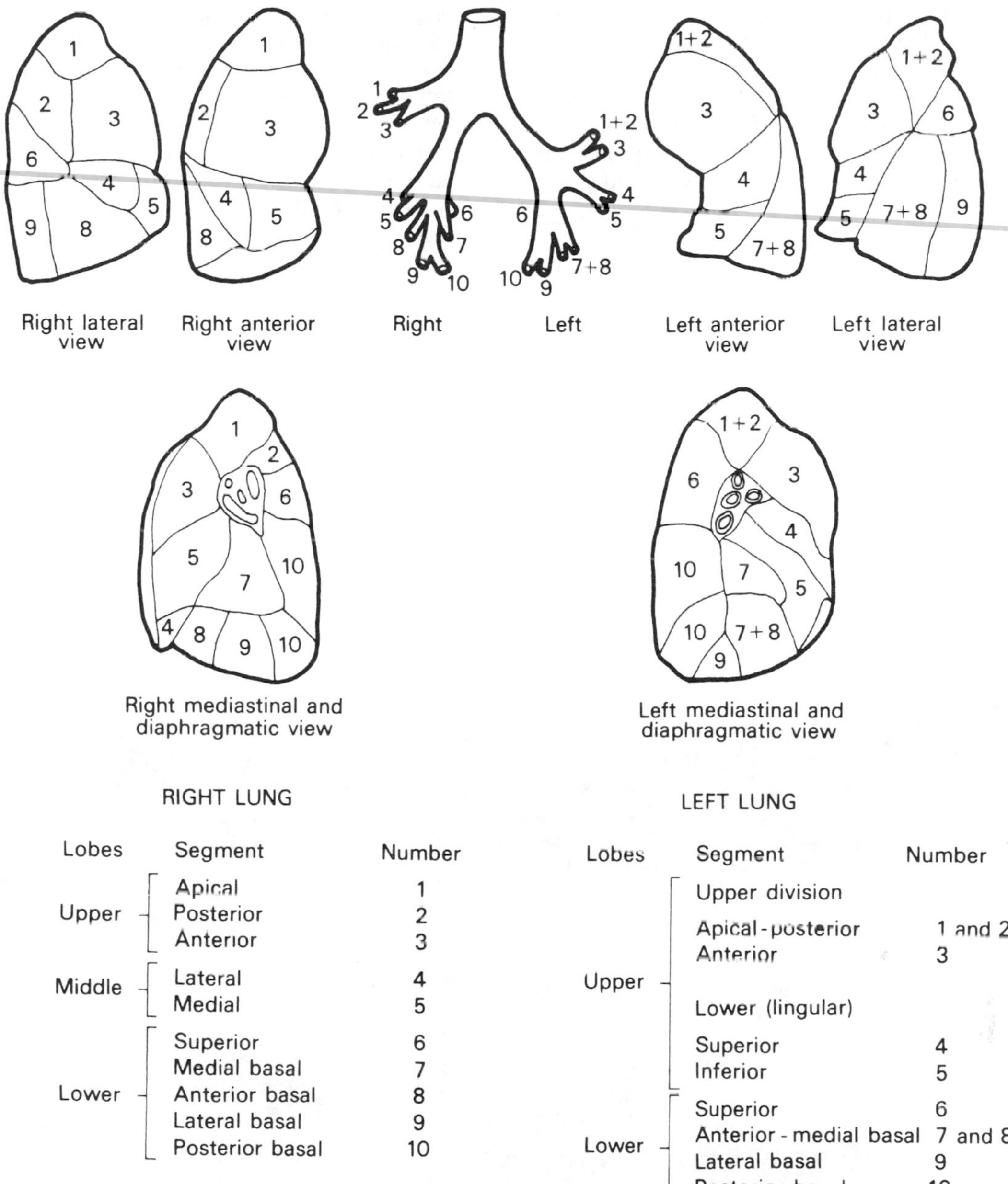

RIGHT LUNG

Lobes	Segment	Number
Upper	Apical	1
	Posterior	2
	Anterior	3
Middle	Lateral	4
	Medial	5
Lower	Superior	6
	Medial basal	7
	Anterior basal	8
	Lateral basal	9
	Posterior basal	10

LEFT LUNG

Lobes	Segment	Number
Upper	Upper division	
	Apical-posterior	1 and 2
	Anterior	3
	Lower (lingular)	
	Superior	4
	Inferior	5
Lower	Superior	6
	Anterior-medial basal	7 and 8
	Lateral basal	9
	Posterior basal	10

FIGURE 4-9. Pulmonary lobes and segments. The diagram views the lungs in the lateral, anterior, mediastinal diaphragmatic projections. The numbered airways correspond to the bronchopulmonary segments.

parison with the central airways, the bronchioles have proportionally more smooth muscle and connective tissue that contains more elastic fibers. With the lack of supporting cartilage, these airways are more susceptible to severe bronchospasm and significant increases in airway resistance.

Gas Exchange Unit

The *respiratory bronchioles*, the 20th through 23rd generations, are the first airways to have alveoli. Alveoli are the structures where gas is exchanged. There are 630,000 respiratory bronchioles with a diameter of approximately 0.45 mm. There are approximately 4×10^6 *alveolar ducts*, and 300×10^6 alveoli. The alveolar ducts are 0.40 mm, and the diameter of the average adult alveolus is 75 to 300 μm. The alveolar surface equates to approximately 70 m^2. Alveoli resemble clusters of grapes on the end of a vine, yet adjacent alveoli share alveolar walls. There are 16 to 20 alveoli sacs at the end of respiratory bronchiole, each fed by an alveolar duct. The respiratory bronchioles, alveolar ducts, and alveolar sacs are also called functional units of the lung parenchyma, or *acinus*. Each gas exchange unit is about 3.5 mm in diameter and there are 130,000 in each lung, with about 2000 alveoli in each functional unit. The blood vessels, lymphatics, and vagal nerves inside lamina propria are in direct contact with the alveoli; all connecting tissue and cartilage have disappeared at this level. Approximately 85% to 95% of alveolar outer walls are covered by pulmonary capillaries. Figure 4-10 illustrates lung tissue at this level. Table 4-1 summarizes anatomic details of the conducting airways down to the alveoli.

The pulmonary capillaries are composed of flattened simple squamous cells. These endothelial cells are thin walled and have an inside diameter only large enough to allow blood cells to flow through in a single file. Intimately adjacent to the outside of the endothelium is a very thin basement membrane. Intercellular junctions where the endothelial cells contact to one another are relatively leaky. This can allow fluid and solutes to move out of the blood into the adjacent interstitial tissue and also into the alveolar cells located next to but beyond the interstitial layer.

The interstitial connective tissue layer lies between the vascular and alveolar tissue, binding the two. Cells of the interstitial layer contain several different types of connective tissue fibers, but the majority is composed of the ground substance or matrix of *glycosaminoglycans.* Entanglements of the large polysaccharide molecules create a gel-like structure to the interstitium. The fibrils composing the connective tissue form a three-dimensional basket-like structure. This allows lungs to expand in all directions without developing excessive tissue recoil. Most of the work to inflate the lungs is caused by alteration of surface tension forces. Evidence of this is shown by liquid-filled lungs inflating at low pressure.

Fibers (connective tissue) within the parenchyma provide elasticity and strength, providing additional structural integrity to the alveolar walls. On inspiration, the airways increase minimally in length and diameter. The alveoli significantly increase in volume. Understanding the role of parenchymal interstitial connective tissue is important because changes in the size of alveoli account for most of the lung's ability to vary the size of a breath. Airways conducting gas to parenchymal areas do change in dimension, but that change accounts for only a small portion of the inhaled volume.

Lungs have two well-defined interstitial connective tissue compartments arranged in series: the parenchymal interstitium (alveolar wall); and the loose-binding connective tissue (peribronchovascular sheaths, interlobular septi, and visceral pleura). Parenchymal inter-

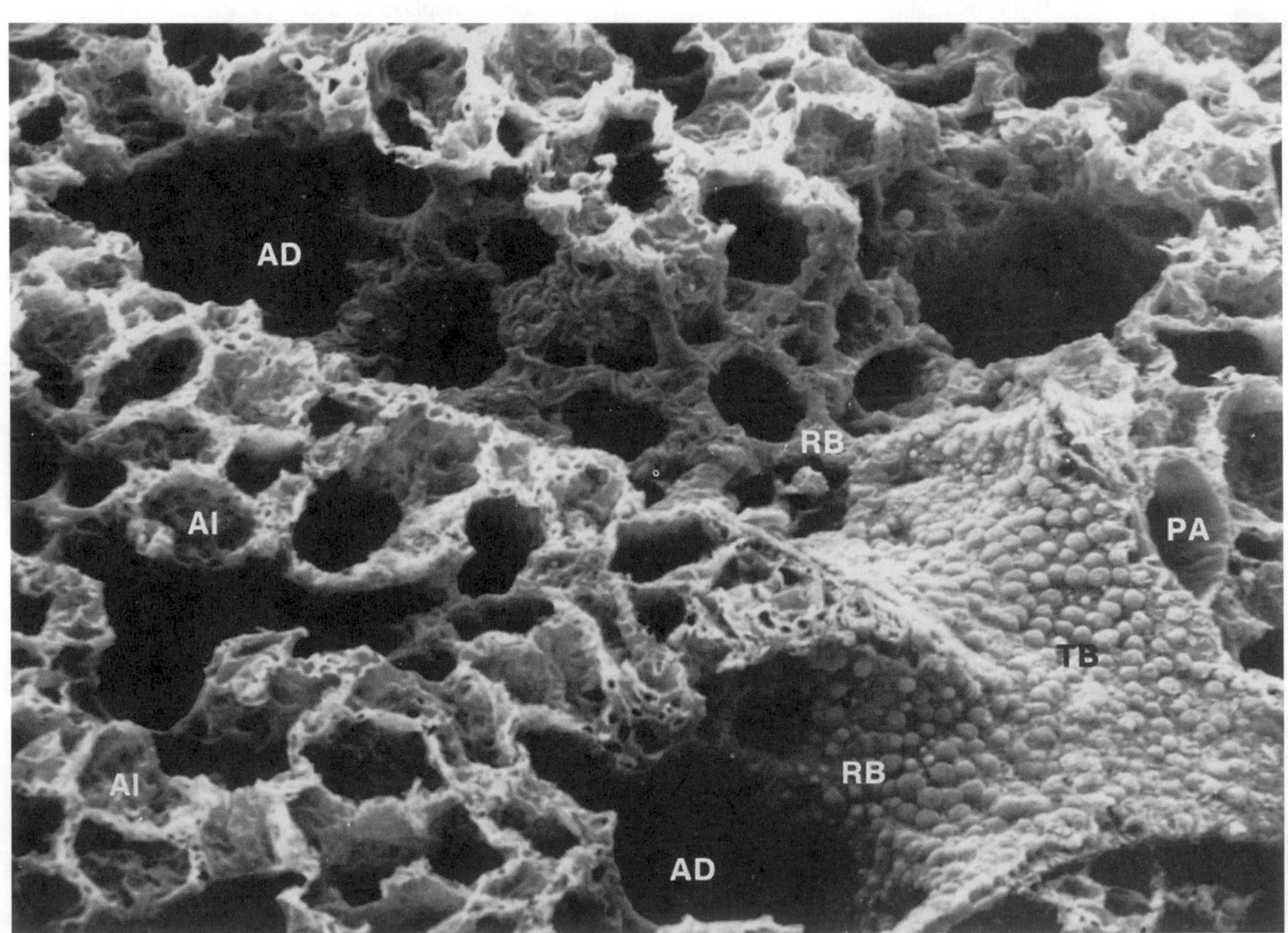

FIGURE 4-10. Scanning electron micrograph of lung showing a primary pulmonary lobule or acinus composed of terminal bronchiole (TB), respiratory bronchioles (RB), and alveolar ducts (AD). A pulmonary arteriole (PA) is also illustrated. (From Kessel RG, Karoon RH: Tissues and organs. In A Text-Atlas of Scanning Electron Microscopy, San Francisco, WH Freeman & Sons, 1979, with permission)

TABLE 4-1 **Airways**

Structure	Units (no.)	Generation	Mean Diameter (mm)	Area Supplied	Cartilage	Smooth Muscle
Conductive Zone						
Mouth Nasopharynx Oropharynx	1	0		Both lungs		
Trachea	1	I	18	Both lungs	U-shaped	Closes open end of cartilage
Bronchus	2	II	13	One lung		
Lobar bronchi	4–5	II–III	7-5	Lobes		
Segmental bronchi	18	III	4	Segments	Irregular helical-shaped	
Smaller bronchi	32 2000	III	3–1	Secondary lobules		Helical bands
Bronchioles						
Terminal bronchioles	4000	IV–XIV				
Respiratory bronchioles	65,000 130,000		1-0.5			
Alveolar ducts	500,000	XV-XX	0.5	Primary lobules	Absent	Muscle bends between alveoli
Alveolar sacs	1,000,000					Thin bands in alveolar septa
	8,000,000	XXIII	0.3			

stitium of the alveolar wall is about one third of the total intestitial volume. Lymphatics are confined to the loose-binding connective tissue. Connective tissue fibrils in the alveolar wall parenchymal connective tissue are extensions of the coarser fibers in the loose-binding connective tissue. Stress forces introduced at the alveolar wall level during inflation are transmitted not only to adjacent alveoli, which abut each other, but also to the surrounding alveolar ducts and bronchioles. Stress forces are also conveyed to the loose-binding connective tissue supporting the whole lobule and ultimately to the outer visceral pleural surface.

Alveolar epithelium is mostly composed of *type I* and *II alveolar cells* (Figs. 4-11 and 4-12). Type I cells form the approximately 95% of the cellular lining of the alveoli. Well suited to provide gas exchange, a type I cell has a large surface area, covering greater than several thousand μm². It also is quite thin, between 0.1 and 0.5 μm. Type II alveolar cells are small and cuboidal in shape. Type II pneumocytes are metabolically active; their primary role is not in gas exchange but in synthesizing and secreting surfactant phospholipids. Type II cells are cuboidal in shape with microvilli.

Alveolar macrophages, or type III cells, phagocytize bacteria and other contaminants that find their way into the alveoli (Fig. 4-13). The macrophages are thought to be produced in the bone marrow and to relocate to the lung via the blood stream. They can move freely about the alveoli or they can be embedded in the extracellular lining of the alveolar epithelial surface. Table 4-2 summarizes alveolar cell types and their function.

Various types of airway intercommunications are important in the pathophysiology of emphysema and in the spread of alveolar disease. The interlobular septa are not clearly defined in the central portions of the lung, and extension of disease through these communications may explain the more rapid spread of alveolar lesions, such as bronchopneumonia. These junctions can pass particles with a molecular weight of up to 60,000 daltons (eg, albumin) in acute pulmonary edema or nearly 500,000 daltons in the adult respiratory distress syndrome (ARDS). The alveolar pores of Kohn and the bronchiolar communication channels of Lambert are largely responsible for the collateral movement of air throughout the lung. When obstruction occurs proximal to these pores and channels, a shunt occurs because of lack of ventilation into this unit, while perfusion to the unit continues.

The alveolar pores of Kohn are smooth, rounded alveolar holes (between 3 and 13 μm diameter) and occasionally reinforced by a ring of elastic tissue. It is believed that they provide a collateral ventilation system to allows gases to move from adjacent alveoli. The number and size of the pores of Kohn increase with age corresponding to the enlargement of the air spaces. With the aging process, the pores of Kohn show a propensity for the lung borders, especially in the apices of the upper and lower lobes. The bronchiolar channels, described by Lambert in 1955, are connections between the bronchioles and adjacent alveoli. They are frequently identified in patches near the hila and also near the larger bronchi, and blood vessels appear to have similar function in preventing atelectasis if local upstream airflow is blocked. These channels are lined with cuboidal epithelium and are one of the prime sites for carbon deposits from smoke or coal dust.

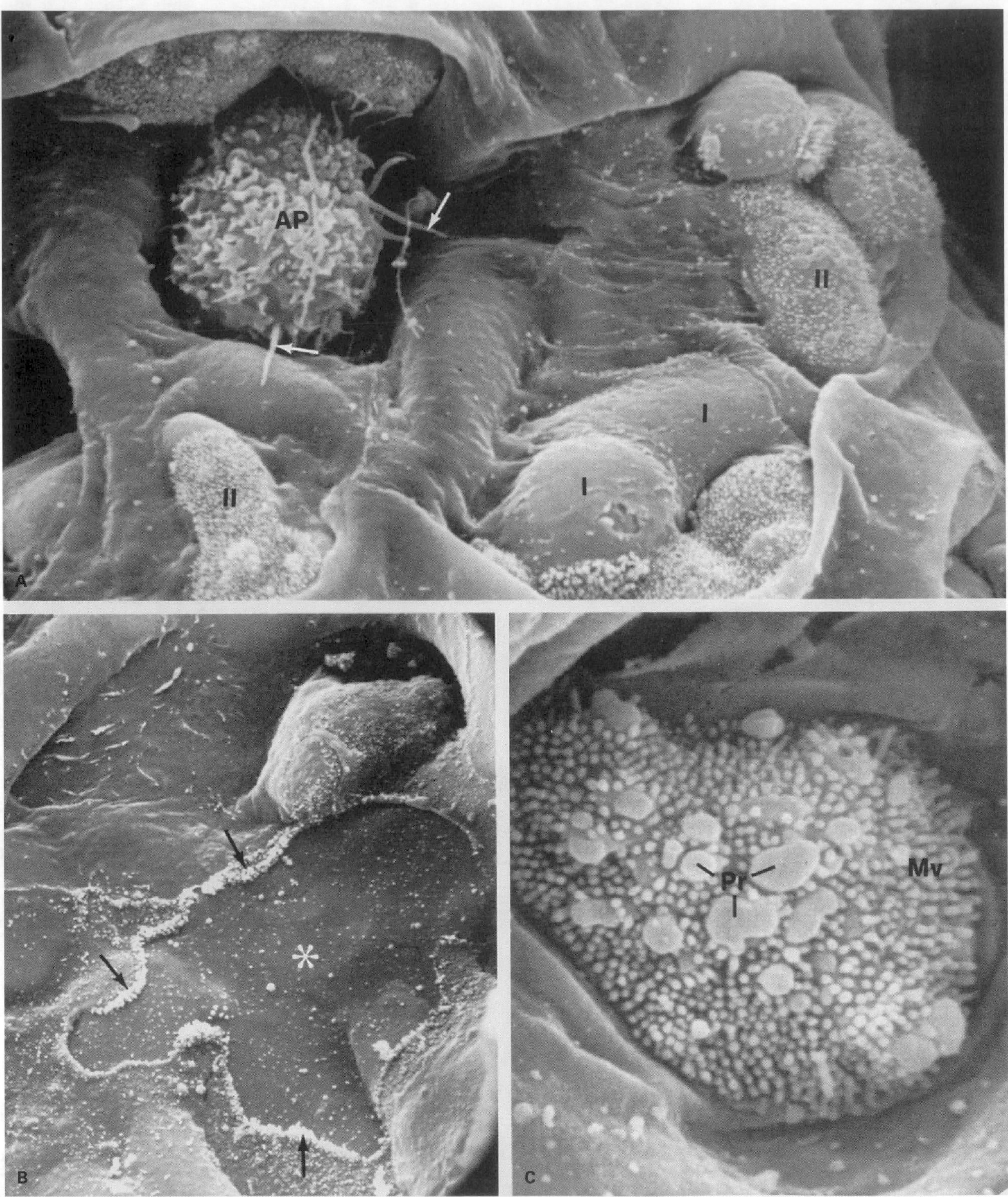

FIGURE 4-11. Scanning electron micrographs of alveoli at high magnification. **(A)** Type I alveolar cells (I) can be easily distinguished from cells (II). **(B)** Intracellular Type I junctions are shown as ridges (arrows) **(C)** A detailed view of a Type II cell showing microvilli (Mv) and projections (Pr) believed to relate to surfactant release. (From Kessel RG, Karoon RH: Tissues and organs. In A Text-Atlas of Scanning Electron Microscopy, San Francisco, WH Freeman & Sons, 1979, with permission)

Oxygen and carbon dioxide molecules pass through the alveolar-capillary membrane with some resistance. It helps that the membrane is very thin, that the cells that make up the membrane are large and flat, and that the total surface area is large. It is estimated that a red blood cell spends 0.75 seconds in transit through the pulmonary capillary.

The barriers to gas diffusion include: the capillary endothelium, the capillary basement, connective tissue, the alveolar epithelium and fluids. In a healthy lung the

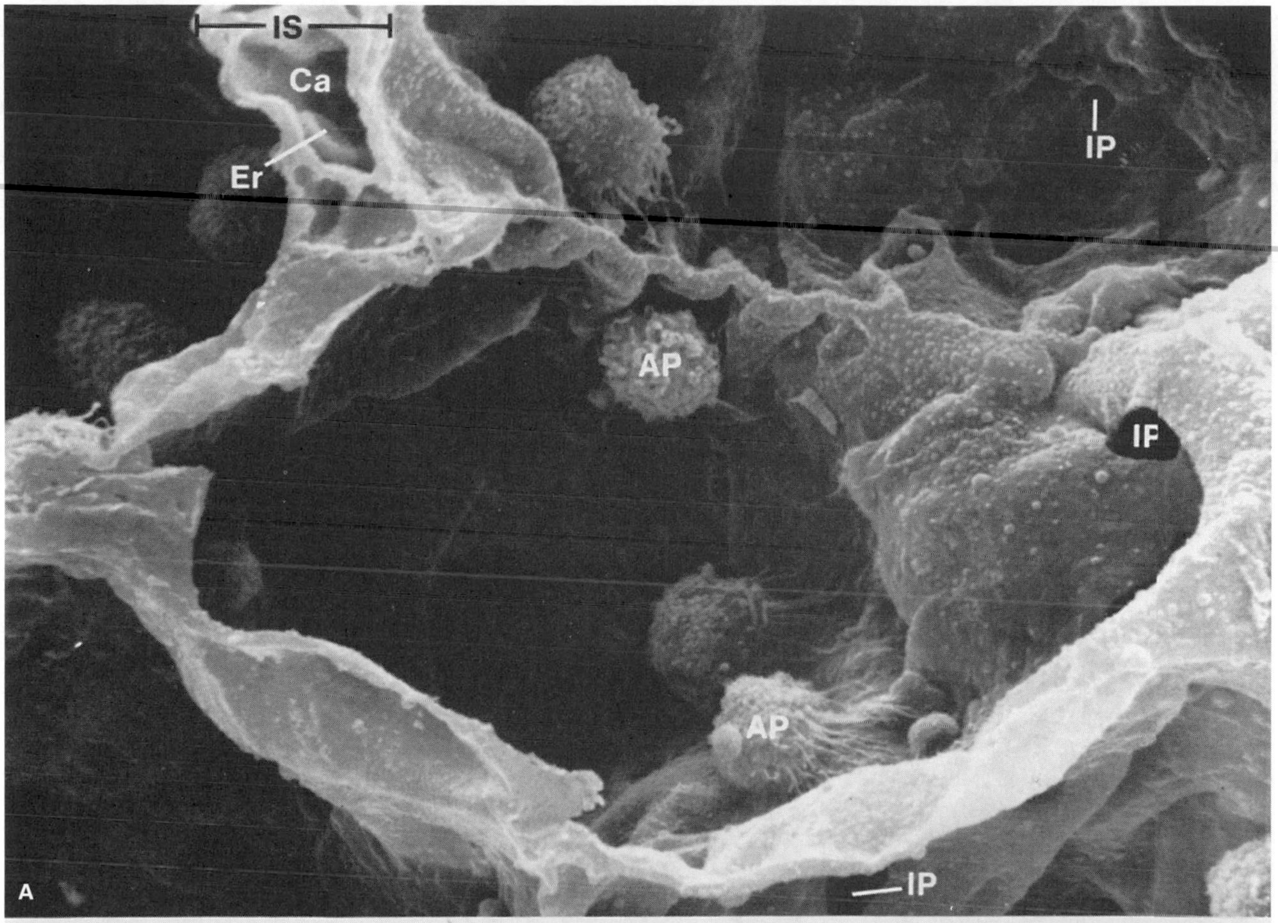

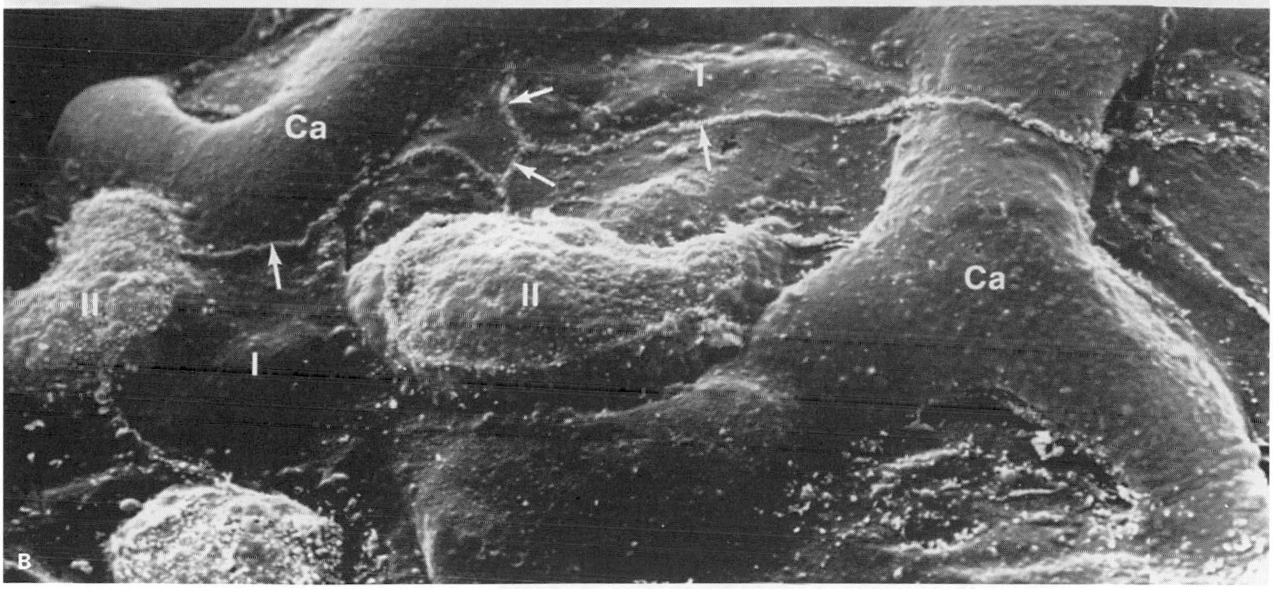

FIGURE 4-12. (A) Scanning electron micrograph of an adjacent alveoli. A pore of Kohn or interalveolar pore (IP) is shown. Such communications allow collateral ventilation and macrophage migration. The intimacy with the capillary endothelium is demonstrated as an erthrocyte (Er) is shown passing through a capillary (Ca) adjacent to 3 alveoli. **(B)** A portion of an alveolar surface is illustrated showing elevated ridges caused by underlying capillaries (Ca). Type II cells are shown as well as intracellular junctions (arrows). **(C)**, **(D)**, Interalveolar septum (Is) is shown oblique sectioned. The area between two alveoli illustrates collagenic and elastic tissue as well as passing erythrocytes (Er). **(E)** Details of the intracellular constituents of the interavolar septum include capillary endothelium (En), basal laminae (Bl) of Type I cells, and a Type II cell (II). (From Kessel RG, Karoon RH: Tissues and organs. In A Text-Atlas of Scanning Electron Microscopy, San Francisco, WH Freeman & Sons, 1979, with permission)

(continued)

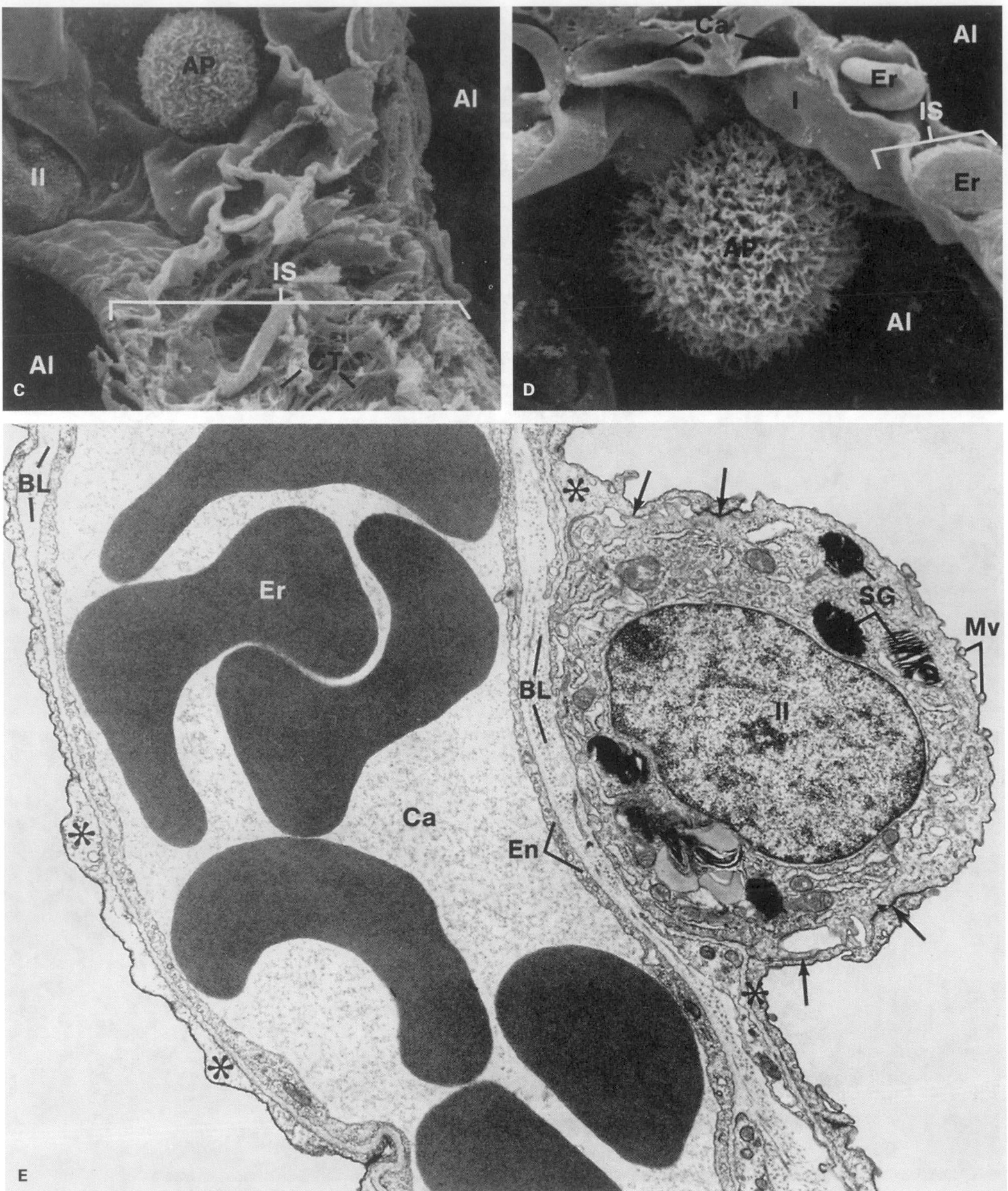

FIGURE 4-12. *(continued)*

distance is about 0.5 μm. The septa has about 25% endothelial tissue, 25% epithelial tissue, 35% connective tissue, and 15% fiber. These barriers are resistant to the exchange of oxygen and carbon dioxide, and each layer provides its own measure of resistance.

Gas and vascular surfaces do not perfectly match. Type I epithelial cells are four times bigger than the endothelial cells, but there are four times more endothelial cells. The alveolar epithelial cells are tightly arranged with little room or spaces, attenuated to one another by cellular leaflets. The alveolar epithelial layer has a selective permeability. The capillary endothelial cells are notoriously leaky, letting particulates, gases, and liquids pass through randomly. Pulmonary arterioles are

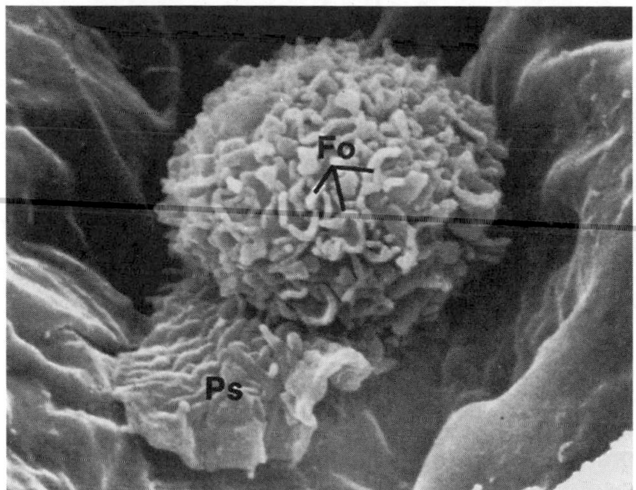

FIGURE 4-13. Micrograph of an alveolar macrophage. (From Kessel RG, Karoon RH: Tissues and organs. In A Text Atlas of Scanning Electron Microscopy, San Francisco, WH Freeman & Sons, 1979, with permission)

muscular and possess the ability to reflexively constrict to limit flow when there are low alveolar oxygen levels.

The fibers of the lung contain collagen and elastic fibers. Both types of fibers are necessary and work together to contract and expand the airways of the lungs. The fiber system works in response to blood, gravity, and gaseous pressure. Collagen fibers are not particularly stretchable, but they are very strong. A collagen fiber 1 mm in diameter can support about 500 g but can only stretch about 2% of its length. Elastic fibers are weaker, but they can extend about 130% of their original lengths before injury occurs. The two fibers together provide both strength and extension to the airways, the capillaries and the interlobular sacs that contain the lung tissue.

In the pulmonary parenchyma, the collagen fibers, in a relaxed state, are longer than the elastic fibers. The collagen fibers bunch up, creating a wavelike appearance. When the elastic fibers unwind, the collagen fibers straighten out. Together they act much like elastic in stockings, in that they only stretch so far.

When the lung is inflated, the fibers expand, creating a bigger airway or alveoli for the passage of air and the exchange of gas. As the tissues deflate, the fibers contract, but recoil forces are reduced by surface tension at the gas-liquid interface. The fiber system provides strength, structure, and support. The collagen and elastic fibers work together providing a flexible, strong superstructure. If one alveoli becomes smaller, the neighboring alveoli stretch to accommodate the air. All of the alveoli are interdependent; when something happens to one alveoli, the adjacent alveoli compensate.

Alveolar collapse at end exhalation is prevented by *surfactant.* Surfactant is an alveolar molecular coating that modifies surface tension inside the alveoli. When the alveoli contract, their surface tension decreases. When they expand, their surface tension increases. This allows the acini to remain stable. Without surfactant the alveoli tend to collapse, as seen in neonatal respiratory distress syndrome secondary to prematurity.

Pulmonary Surfactant and Lung Function

Were it not for the presence of surfactant, alveoli and the bronchioles would collapse during expiration when their size normally becomes smaller. Surfactant is produced by the type II alveolar cell. It is a phospholipid composed mainly of dipalmitoyl lecithin; its production depends on gestational enzyme regulation, an adequate blood supply to the lung parenchyma, and its ability to reduce surface tension may be related to blood pH. The effect of this material is to reduce surface tension, especially as the radii of the alveoli and the small airways decrease at exhalation.

The importance of this material will be appreciated by a consideration of Laplace's law for an alveolar-like structure: $P = 2T/r$, wherein the pressure P inside a spherical bubble with radius r is related to surface tension T. For a given surface tension, the pressure required to keep a sphere from collapsing will be greater as the radius decreases. At end-expiration the alveolar radius decreases, and the alveolar pressure is essentially atmospheric. With the reduction in alveolar radius, surface tension would rise to critical levels causing collapse. Surfactant reduces the amount of surface tension and becomes more concentrated and effective as the alveolus becomes smaller.

Surfactant allows the alveoli and small airways to remain open at low lung volumes and transpulmonary pressures. A reduction in surfactant promotes alveolar instability and atelectasis and may seriously affect gas

TABLE 4-2 **Alveolar Cell Types, Their Function, and Known Metabolic Profile**

Cell Type	Function	Energy Requirement	Substrates
I	Structural support; gas transfer	Low	Glucose
II	Surfactant production	Probably high	Glucose, fatty acids, lipids, amino acids
Macrophages	Scavenger/phagocyte	High	Glucose
Endothelial cells	Gas transfer	High	Biogenic amines Adenine Nucleotides Prostaglandins Polypeptide hormones Lipids

exchange. Depletion of surfactant may occur after repeated bronchial lavage, as in near-drowning victims, after open-heart surgery in which extracorporeal membrane oxygenation is used, after exposure to high concentrations of oxygen, in oxidant air pollution–induced toxicity, and in the neonatal and adult RDS. An excess of surfactant is thought to be present in the relatively rare condition known as pulmonary alveolar proteinosis. The exact nature of the removal and fate of surfactant is unclear at present. Problems of neonatal surfactant deficiency are now treated routinely with artificial or bovine surfactant or surfactant removed from human placentas.

LUNG MECHANICS: THE THORAX AS AN AIR PUMP

The bony thorax and respiratory muscles function as a pump with variable frequency and variable volume displacement to deliver atmospheric air to the alveolar-capillary surface. The components of the bony thorax consist of the thoracic spine, ribs, scapulae, clavicles, and sternum. The respiratory muscles consist of the internal and external intercostals, scaleni, sternocleidomastoids, trapezi, and rhomboids. The primary respiratory muscle of inspiration during tidal breathing is the *diaphragm*.

The diaphragm is a dome-shaped fibromuscular separation between the chest and the abdomen. The central portion of the diaphragm is made up of tendonous tissue and at the periphery consists of skeletal muscle, which attaches to the chest wall. The muscle fiber composition of the diaphragm is 75% high-oxidative fibers, which are highly resistant to endurance fatigue. When high-resistance workloads requiring strength are placed on the diaphragm, these muscle fibers quickly fatigue. In addition, like other skeletal muscles the diaphragm adapts to chronic resistance loads. The diaphragm may function voluntarily when one takes a deep inspiration, or it may function involuntarily during normal breathing at rest or during sleep. The diaphragm is innervated by the phrenic nerve arising from cervical spinal cord roots exiting above vertebral bodies C-3, C-4, and C-5. At the time of diaphragmatic contraction, the transabdominal pressure gradient is increased. During normal breathing, a synchronous interaction occurs between the rib cage, the diaphragm, and to a lesser extent, the abdominal musculature. The diaphragm is the "prime mover" of normal resting ventilation and other muscular movements are secondary.

During inspiration the diaphragm contracts and flattens. It enlarges the thoracic cavity mainly in a longitudinal dimension, but also anteriorly and laterally. The ribs connect to the thoracic spine in such a way as to raise and widen the thorax during inspiration; this movement increases the transverse dimension of the thorax and is called the "bucket-handle" motion. The sternum moves outward from the spine, and this movement increases the anterior to posterior dimension and is called the "pump-handle" motion. Although the ribs are raised during inspiration by contraction of the internal intercostals, contraction of both sets of intercostal muscles provides rigidity to the intercostal spaces. With exercise and in disease states associated with increased work of breathing, the accessory muscles of breathing, including the intercostals, scaleni, sternocleidomastoids, trapezi, and rhomboids, become involved in inspiration.

Exhalation during resting breathing is the result of passive recoil of the lung and chest wall with some modulation by the diaphragm. The abdominal muscles are the major muscle group active during exhalation. When airway resistance is abnormally high, during exercise or forceful expiratory maneuvers (cough or sneezing), the abdominal musculature and internal intercostal muscles contract and depress and lower the thoracic cage, causing positive intra-abdominal and intrapleural pressure. Such events also occur during coughing, sneezing, and the performance of the Valsalva maneuver. The accessory chest and "belly" muscles are innervated by nerves exiting the thoracic and lumbar spine. Thoracic spinal cord injured patients with functioning diaphragms are at risk for pulmonary complications because of reduced ability to cough. By assuming the supine position or using assisted coughing procedures, such patients can use increased abdominal pressure below the diaphragm to aid lung recoil in order to create the greatest exhaled volumes and flows.

The *pleural space* is essentially a closed, potential space delineated by the visceral and parietal pleural. With enlargement of the thorax during inspiration, the intrapleural pressure falls, becoming more subatmospheric, and a pressure gradient develops between the mouth, which is at atmospheric pressure, and the alveoli, which is at subatmospheric pressure. This pressure gradient during tidal breathing is between −3 and −5 cmH_2O and is enough to ensure tidal volumes of between 300 and 750 mL of air per breath, provided that airflow resistance is not abnormally high.

The muscular work of the respiratory air pump is so small that it consumes less than 5% of the total oxygen consumption of the body at rest when the minute ventilation is 6.0 L/min. During severe exercise, when the minute volume is in excess of 100 L/min., 30% of the total oxygen consumption is consumed by the respiratory muscles. The oxygen cost of breathing increases markedly when the airway resistance is high or the compliance of lung is low. In addition, if the ventilation is "wasted" on under-perfused areas of the lung, the normally efficient breathing and gas exchange processes become very inefficient.

When the oxygen cost of breathing or energy demand exceeds the oxygen supply, the gas exchange system must be supported. For example, when the oxygen cost of breathing exceeds approximately 40% of resting oxygen consumption, a mechanical ventilator may be necessary to support the ventilatory muscles.

The mechanical ability of "pumping" air into the lung can be measured as part of an assessment of the lung. Physiologically, the lungs can be divided into four lung volumes and four capacities; a capacity is the sum of two or more lung volumes. The lung volumes and capacities that are most important for gas exchange are the functional residual capacity, tidal volume, and inspiratory reserve volume. The functional residual capacity is the volume of gas in the lungs following a normal exhalation; it serves as a gas reservoir and maintains alveoli in their partially expanded state. With each inspiration the tidal volume delivers new atmospheric gas to the lungs, and with each expiration removes carbon dioxide from the lungs. The inspiratory reserve volume allows us to sigh and reinflate partially collapsed alveoli. The names, abbreviations, normal adult values, and interrelationships of lung volumes and capacities are shown in Figure 4-14.

The balance of elastic forces of the lung and chest wall determine the pulmonary *compliance*, defined as the volume change produced by pressure change across the lung. The normal compliance of lung and chest wall for a spontaneously breathing adult is approximately 0.2 L/cmH_20. That value decreases to about 0.085 L/cmH_20 when respiratory muscles are inactive and positive pressure ventilation is applied.

CONTROL OF RESPIRATION

The arterial pH and PO_2 respond to changing metabolic demands with a fidelity that is relatively unparalleled in nature. From a resting ventilation of 6.0 L/min to maximal exercise of 100 L/min, the normal healthy adult does not demonstrate a significant change in PaO_2. The $PaCO_2$ does not change until the onset of metabolic acidosis, when carbon dioxide is excreted in an attempt to compensate for the lactic acidosis. The complex neural and humoral mechanisms whereby alveolar ventilation is regulated are only now beginning to be understood. The literature on respiratory control is exceedingly complex, and the interested reader should refer to the bibliography and to Chapter 29 for additional information.

Central Neurogenic Control

Attempts to understand respiratory rate and periodicity have caused us to reinterpret studies wherein various portions of the brain or brain stem were transsected or electrically stimulated. When the upper cervical spinal cord is severed, voluntary and rhythmic contraction of the main respiratory muscles is not possible. Breathing is the only automatic function subserved entirely by skeletal muscle. In contrast, the heart continues to pump blood when completely denervated.

The respiratory system is under both voluntary and involuntary control. The behavioral or voluntary centers are located in the motor cortex of the forebrain and the limbic cerebral area. Efferent output fibers descend through the corticospinal and rubrospinal tracts in the dorsal and lateral spinal cord. Certain conscious acts, such as speaking, response to anxiety or fear, voluntary hyperventilation, and breath-holding, interfere with the rhythmic respiratory pattern and are mediated by these pathways. The automatic system has its origins, which are not completely localized, in areas of the lower pons and medulla. The afferents input fibers for this system come from peripheral chemoreceptors, the glossopharyngeal and vagus nerves, and various proprioceptors. The efferent fibers involve the phrenic nerve, which innervates the diaphragm, and cells in the ventral and lateral columns of the upper thoracic spinal cord, which innervate the intercostal muscles. Despite more than a century of study, the exact nature of the cellular organization of those parts of the brain stem (pons and medulla) responsible for respirator rhythmicity still remains one of the mysteries of neurophysiology and respiratory physiology.

To complicate matters further, the way in which the voluntary and involuntary pathways are integrated in the spinal cord is still debatable, although the location of the tracts themselves is well known. The effect of lesions in the cerebral cortex, midbrain, brain stem, and spinal cord on respiratory rate, depth, and periodicity is discussed in Chapter 29.

Humoral Control

Chemoreceptors are located in the *carotid and aortic bodies* and in the medulla. These structures provide the afferent signals for the chemical control of respiration. The respiratory controller responds to these signals by adjusting the level of ventilation to maintain the arterial PCO_2 as constant as possible, combating the effects of increased {H+} or decreased PO_2.

<table>
<tr><td rowspan="4">Total lung capacity (TLC) 6000 mL</td><td rowspan="3">Vital capacity (VC) 4800 mL</td><td>Inspiratory reserve volume (IRV) 3600 mL</td><td rowspan="2">Inspiratory capacity (IC) 3600 mL</td></tr>
<tr><td>Tidal volume (V_t) 500 mL</td></tr>
<tr><td>Expiratory reserve volume (ERV) 1200 mL</td><td rowspan="2">Functional residual capacity (FRC) 2400 mL</td></tr>
<tr><td>Residual volume (RV) 1200 mL</td><td>Residual volume (RV) 1200 mL</td></tr>
</table>

FIGURE 4-14. Terms, abbreviations and normal (adult) values of lung volumes and capacities.

Peripheral Chemoreceptors

Although the peripheral chemoreceptors are stimulated somewhat by an elevation of arterial PCO_2 or elevation of $[H^+]$ (metabolic acidosis), the most important stimulus is a decrease in the oxygen tension of arterial blood. The carotid bodies are found at the bifurcation of the common carotid arteries, and their afferents to the medulla pass through the glossopharyngeal nerve (IX). The aortic bodies are located near the arch of the aorta, with afferents conveyed by the vagus nerve (X). When these structures are denervated in animals, the ventilatory response to hypoxemia is severely blunted. In humans, the aortic bodies respond readily to hypoxemia, with the carotid bodies having less of a role, except in rare instances. The hyperpnea seen with carbon dioxide inhalation is depressed only slightly by denervation of the aortic and carotid bodies. When increased PCO_2 or $[H^+]$ is combined with hypoxemia, however, a considerable increase in ventilation occurs when these centers are intact.

The effects of hyperoxia result in only a mild reduction in ventilation and a clinically insignificant increase in $PaCO_2$ in the normal healthy individual. In the chronically hypoxemic patient, however, hyperoxia may cause a significant increase in $PaCO_2$, resulting in respiratory acidosis and serious side effects (so-called carbon dioxide narcosis.)

Medullary Chemoreceptors

Chemosensitive areas responsive to changes in PCO_2 and $[H^+]$ exist in the medulla. These *medullary respiratory centers* are influenced primarily by the $[H^+]$ of cerebrospinal fluid (CSF), which, unlike blood, has a less effective buffer system, so that changes in PCO_2 produce maximal changes in $[H^+]$. For example, the CSF protein level is low compared with that of blood proteins, which are an important buffer. Furthermore, the concentration of CSF HCO_3 is lower than plasma and does not respond rapidly to changes in arterial PCO_2. The medullary centers respond more slowly to abrupt changes in PCO_2 than do the peripheral chemoreceptors, which respond in seconds.

Miscellaneous Respiratory Control Influences

Nonchemical influences include the voluntary or behavioral system previously discussed, joint proprioceptors, and stretch receptors, which inhibit inspiration, located in the smooth muscle of the airways. In association with this last-mentioned group, deflation receptors exist that stimulate inflation; collectively, these form the Hering-Breuer reflexes.

PULMONARY CIRCULATION

The pulmonary circulation has an intricate role in the exchange of oxygen and carbon dioxide. Several factors determine the effectiveness of the pulmonary circulation in the exchange of respiratory gases. These factors include the total blood volume in the lungs, the regional differences in the capillary blood volume, and the hematocrit of blood in the pulmonary capillaries. In addition, other factors that affect the binding of oxygen to the hemoglobin are important in the exchange and transport of oxygen. A few of the most important factors include the transit time of the erythrocyte in the capillary, the partial pressure of oxygen in the domain of the capillary, and the hemoglobin dissociation curves of oxygen and carbon dioxide. All of these influences of pulmonary circulation form an interweaving network for effective gas exchange.

The lung must also participate in acid-base homeostasis, as well as provide respiratory gas exchange; thus, the respiratory processes are clearly interlocked with circulatory processes, in addition to electrolyte and water balance, temperature control, and metabolism. The lungs, through alveolar ventilation, excrete the major portion of the acid load of the body by eliminating carbon dioxide, which is excreted as a gas through pulmonary ventilation, although it exists transiently as the potent and highly carbonic dissociable acid (H_2CO_3) in the body.

The right ventricle delivers the entire cardiac output to the pulmonary arterial circulation. The right ventricle may be described as a variable-displacement, variable-frequency blood pump that produces a pulsatile flow. By special techniques this pulsatile flow may be theoretically observed in the smallest of pulmonary capillaries, although not all pulmonary capillaries are perfused at resting cardiac output. The output of the right ventricle varies from about 5 L/min at rest to more than 20 L/min during severe exercise.

The lung can be thought of as a network of interlacing capillaries and alveoli separated only by the fine and delicate alveolar-capillary membrane. At any time, the volume of blood in the pulmonary capillaries is between 75 and 150 mL; this increases by about 100 mL during peak exercise, presumably by vascular "recruitment" (opening of normally closed capillaries or distention of underperfused capillaries).

During exercise the normal red blood cells' capillary residence time is shortened considerably. When gas exchange between alveolar and incoming fresh air is incomplete or alveolar-capillary thickening prolongs transmembrane diffusion time, ventilation–perfusion mismatch occurs, and saturation of capillary blood with oxygen is incomplete. These relationships worsen further during exercise and may result in hypoxemia, hypercapnia, or both, limiting exercise performance and increasing dyspnea.

The main pulmonary artery divides at the hilum into a left and right pulmonary artery. These further subdivide, generally paralleling the divisions of the airways, down to about the level of the terminal bronchiole. Unlike the diminishing stiffness of the walls of the branching airway, the pulmonary circulation tends to gain stiffness at its branches, although the pulmonary capillaries are believed to be distensible with increasing blood volumes. The proximal pulmonary arteries make up what is known as the *capacitance* portion of the pulmonary circulation. Here, the vessel walls largely consist of elastic tissue and resemble the aorta and larger systemic blood vessels.

In the normal adult human lung, pulmonary blood vessels 0.1 to 1.0 mm in diameter have media consisting of smooth muscle fibers bounded by internal and external elastic laminae. These vessels and the pulmonary capillary network compose the resistance portion of the pulmonary circulation. The walls of the muscular pulmonary arteries lie close to the bronchioles, respiratory bronchioles, and alveolar ducts. When the blood vessels become smaller than 0.1 mm (at the level of the terminal bronchioles), the walls of the pulmonary arterioles have a large proportion of smooth muscle, which may contract under various stimuli, most notably hypoxemia and acidosis.

Finally, at the level of the pulmonary arterioles (<0.1 mm in diameter), the muscular layer gradually disappears until the vessel wall contains only the endothelium and an elastic lamina. These vessels directly supply the alveolar ducts and alveoli, ending in the pulmonary capillaries. The diameter of the pulmonary capillaries is about 10 μm, just enough for red blood cells to pass through end-to-end. This meshwork of pulmonary capillaries rejoins to form the pulmonary venules, which subsequently drain into the pulmonary veins and the left atrium.

Generally, the pulmonary arterial circulation should be thought of as one with high compliance, for which vascular resistance is less than one fifth that of the systemic circulation. A mean pulmonary arterial pressure of less than 12 mmHg at rest and 15 mmHg during exercise propels the entire cardiac output through the pulmonary circulation. The function of this circulation is to distribute the right ventricular stroke volume over the nearly 100-m^2 surface area of the alveolar-capillary membrane.

A knowledge of normal cardiac chamber and vascular pressures is essential in understanding many of the pathologic conditions that are discussed in later chapters. Figure 4-15 illustrates these relationships. The resting right ventricular pressure is 25/0 mmHg. Cardiac output from this circulation drains into the left atrium, which has a mean pressure of about 5 mmHg. The cause of acute respiratory failure can be separated into pulmonary, cardiac, or combined cardiopulmonary causes by measurement of these chamber and vascular pressures. This can be accomplished in the cardiac catheterization laboratory or at the bedside using the balloon-tipped pulmonary artery (Swan-Ganz) catheter.

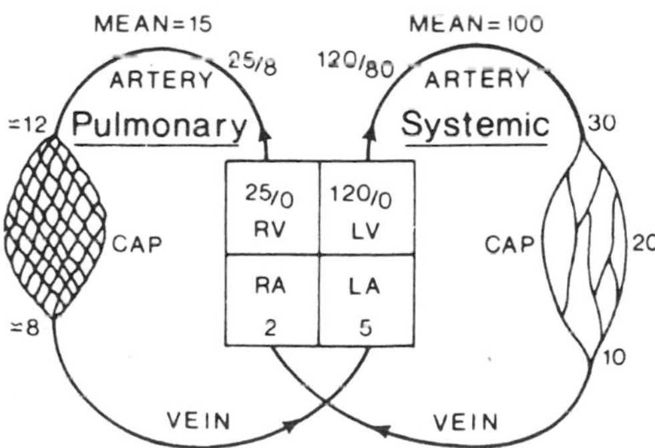

FIGURE 4-15. Normal heart chamber and vascular pressures in the (systemic) and (pulmonary) circulations. To a certain extent, particularly in the lung, these pressures are modified by hydrostatic differences. Note the lung's low resistance as seen by the reduced pressures to provide the same cardiac output. Numbers are mmHg. (From West JB: Respiratory Physiology: The Essentials. Baltimore, Williams & Wilkins, 1974, with permission)

Like the arteries, the pulmonary veins initially are in proximity to the bronchi. At the very periphery of the lung the veins move away from the bronchi and pass between the lobules, whereas the arteries and bronchi travel together down into the center of the lobules. The pulmonary veins possess thinner walls than do the arteries, having a less-developed muscular layer at all stages of life.

GAS EXCHANGE

Matching of Ventilation and Perfusion

Gas exchange occurs optimally if ventilation ($\dot{V}$) and perfusion ($\dot{Q}$) are adequately matched. Blood flow is greatest in the gravity-dependent portions of the lung. Ventilation is also greatest in dependent lung areas, largely because of the geometry of the lung and the greater distending forces (negative intrathoracic pressure) generated in the bases of the lung by the contraction of the diaphragm. The ratio of ventilation to perfusion ($\dot{V}/\dot{Q}$) is highest in the nondependent (upper) parts of the lung, evenly matched in midlung (ie, the level of the third and fourth ribs in the upright position), and lowest in the dependent portions of the lung. The average of these $\dot{V}/\dot{Q}$ ratios is normally 0.8 in the standing adult and varies with body position.

Ventilation-perfusion inequality (or mismatching) is likely the most common cause of hypoxemia. It occurs as a result of a relative or absolute shunt, dead space ventilation, hypoventilation, or a combination of these conditions. When hypoventilation of some alveoli occurs, the carbon dioxide content can be normally maintained by overventilating other alveoli to compensate for the underventilated alveoli. However, it is not possible to compensate for the oxygen deficit caused by underventilated alveoli, because of various considerations including the difference in the solubility and hemoglobin dissociation curves of the two gases.

Pulmonary arterial blood that continues to perfuse non-ventilated alveoli or physically bypasses the lung results in a right-to-left shunt. An example of an anatomical shunt occurs in the congenital heart disease, tetralogy of Fallot. In this disease blood bypasses the lungs, going directly from the right ventricle to the left ventricle through a ventricular septal defect, resulting in venous admixture. No matter how high the PO_2 is in the lungs, there is little improvement in the PaO_2. Some diseases create a relative shunt that is responsive to hyperoxia; an example of such a disease is one involving diffusion impairment across the alveolar-capillary membrane.

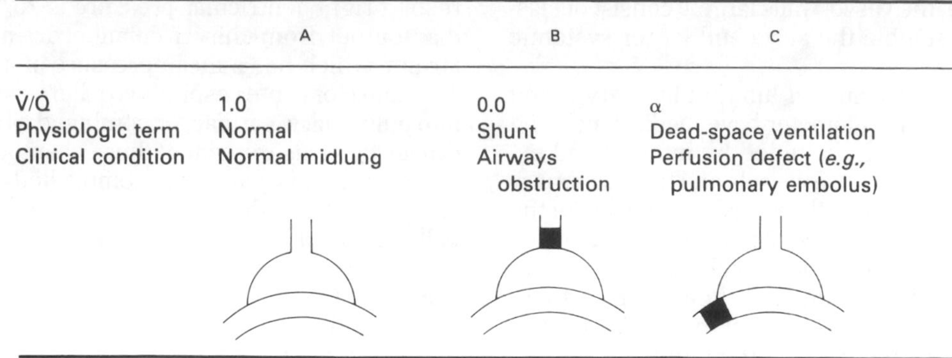

A
B
C
V̇/Q̇
Physiologic term
Clinical condition
1.0
Normal
Normal midlung
0.0
Shunt
Airways obstruction
α
Dead-space ventilation
Perfusion defect (e.g., pulmonary embolus)

FIGURE 4-16. Schematic of ventilation-perfusion relationships in normal **(A)** and diseased lungs. Zones of the lung which are underperfused relative to ventilation **(B)** normally occur in the bases or dependent lung. Some form of airway obstruction causes this pathophysiologic effect. Areas with underperfusion **(C)** occur at the apices (or non-dependent) of normal lung or with interruption of blood flow. Ventilation-perfusion inequality would be a combination of B and C in that there is a relative mismatch of gas and blood.

Dead-space ventilation occurs when alveoli are ventilated but the interfacing capillaries around the alveoli are underperfused or not perfused at all (wasted ventilation or alveolar dead space). Figure 4-16 shows three schematized units in which abnormal $\dot{V}/\dot{Q}$ relationships are compared with normal. Since abnormalities of ventilation/perfusion ratios cause most of the gas exchange abnormalities found in various pulmonary disease states, it is important to consider each clinical problem in terms of the question, "What is the patient's ventilation-perfusion abnormality?" Only when this is understood will the respiratory care practitioner be able to determine the appropriate therapy and the limitations of this therapy for improving the disease state.

LIMITATIONS OF THE GAS EXCHANGE SYSTEM

Several years ago, a young athlete who previously had one entire lung removed for cavitary pulmonary tuberculosis went on to win an international tennis meet in Mexico City, more than 7500 feet above sea level. This is an extreme example of how much respiratory functional reserve normally exists and the extent of loss that must occur before gas exchange impairment and disability become apparent. As mentioned previously, the exchange of oxygen and carbon dioxide is directly or indirectly essential for energy production. The consumption of oxygen is an indicator of the aerobic production of energy. Because energy provides the capacity to perform work, human work performance is highly correlated with the maximal amount of oxygen that can be consumed ($\dot{V}O_2$ max). In the aerobically trained elite athlete, the maximal $\dot{V}O_2$ may be higher than 70 mL/kg/min (5 to 6 L/min). This is an energy expenditure of over 20 times the resting level of 3.5 mL/kg/min.

Maximal work performance is not only limited by the aerobic energy system but also by metabolic acidosis. The less efficient the aerobic system is, the more the reliance on anaerobic energy sources. When the anaerobic system is accelerated to the point that lactic acid is elevated above resting levels (the anaerobic threshold), lactic acidosis ensues, with a blood pH as low as 7.00 and a muscle pH as low as 6.40 at maximal exercise, resulting in fatigue. The quantity of work that can be performed at the anaerobic threshold is closely related to the work rate that can be tolerated for long periods;

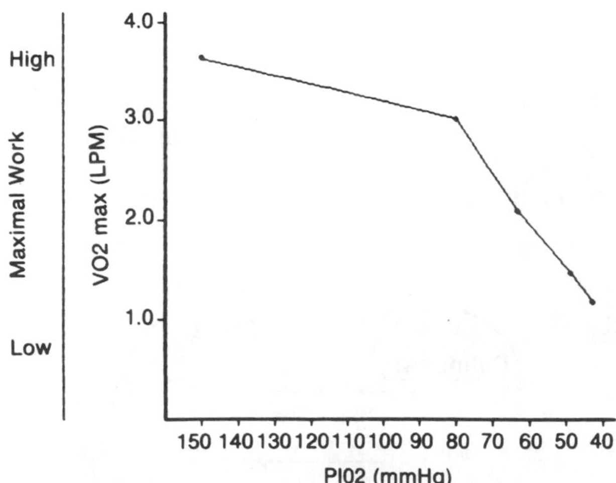

FIGURE 4-17. This figure demonstrates the effect of hypoxia on maximal oxygen consumption ($\dot{V}O_2$ max) and the ability to perform work in young athletes with excellent health. Notice that there is a markedly rapid decline in $\dot{V}O_2$ max below a P_{IO_2} of 80 mmHg. The clinical implications of the effects of hypoxia are important to consider when solving the problems of deficient gas exchange in hypoxemic patients. However, hypoxemia may limit exercise performance because of dyspnea before gas exchange limitations are reached. (Adapted from data in Sutton JR, Reeves JT, Wagner PD et al: Operation Everest II: Oxygen transport during exercise at extreme simulation altitude. J Appl Physiol 64:1309, 1988)

work above the anaerobic threshold rapidly results in fatigue.

Many healthy individuals become dyspneic during stressful work or exercise requirements; their dyspnea is not caused by limited pulmonary gas exchange. The upper limit of gas exchange or maximum oxygen consumption may be limited by the diffusion of oxygen across the alveolar-capillary membrane only in ultra-elite endurance athletes. In these athletes, at maximum exercise, some oxyhemoglobin desaturation is present. The reason for inadequate gas exchange at maximal exercise in these elite athletes is believed to be the tremendous cardiac output, which pushes the blood through the pulmonary capillaries so fast that the oxygen does not have time to completely saturate the hemoglobin. This oxyhemoglobin desaturation may be aggravated by alveolar hypoventilation or $\dot{V}/\dot{Q}$ mismatching. This is similar to the pulmonary-disease patient, who desaturates during exercise or activities of daily living because of hypoventilation, $\dot{V}/\dot{Q}$ mismatching, or alveolar-capillary diffusion defects. The effect of hypoxemia on maximal work performance is illustrated in Figure 4-17.

In normal persons, another extreme stress on gas exchange that is relevant to pulmonary disease occurs at high altitude. As the result of lower inspired and alveolar partial pressures of oxygen, gas exchange at high altitude limits maximal work capacity. At high altitudes the low partial pressure of oxygen results in a lower

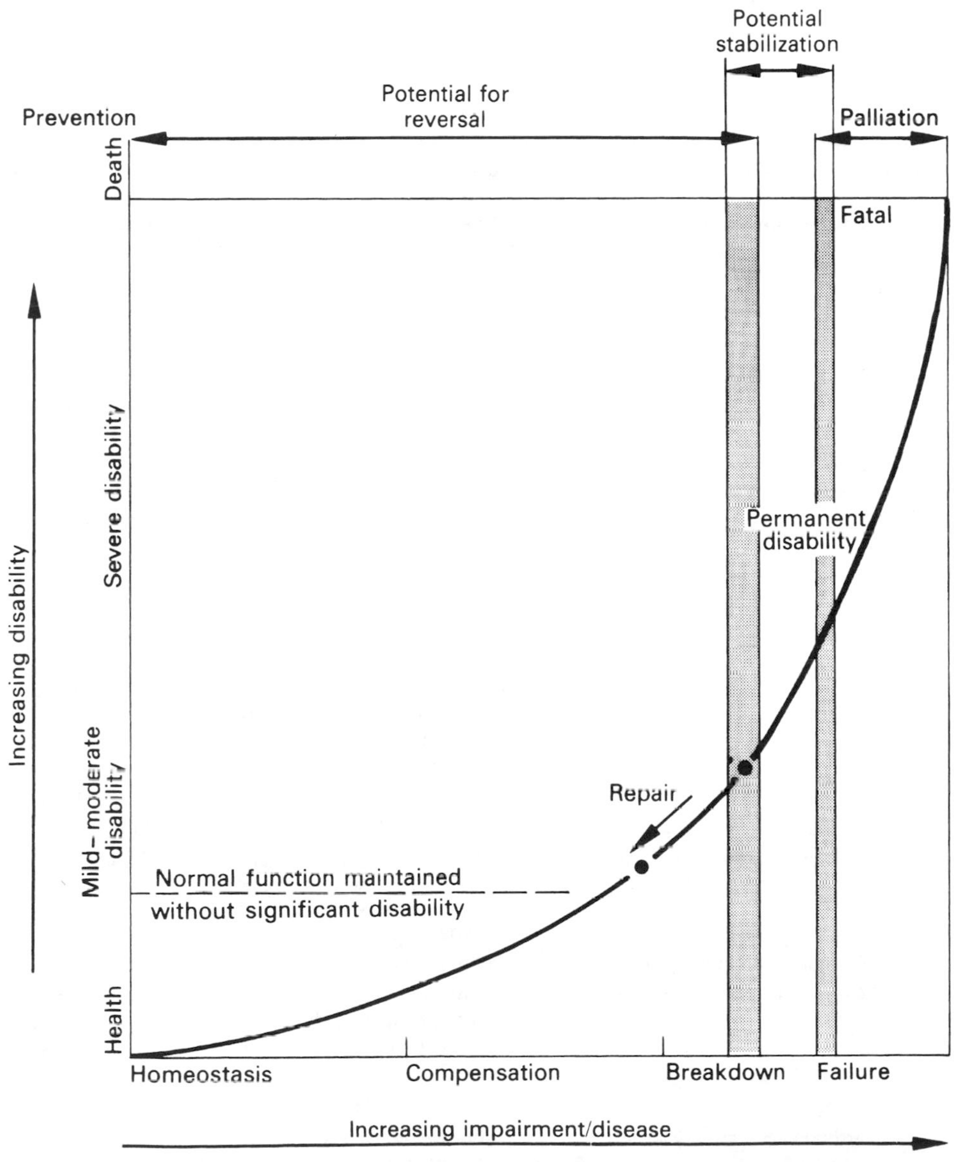

FIGURE 4-18. Early in the course of progressive pulmonary disease, symptoms are scarcely noted by the patient because of the enormous physiologic functional reserve of the lung (see text). With more advanced disease, small exacerbations or complications cause successively more disability (Adapted from Hatch TF: Changing objectives in occupational health. Am Ind Hyg Assoc J 23:1, 1962, with permission)

pressure gradient for oxygen diffusion across the alveolocapillary membrane and, therefore, a lower PaO_2.

SYMPTOM-PATHOLOGY RELATIONSHIPS OF GAS EXCHANGE

All pulmonary pathologic processes can result in impairment of the gas exchange process. Diseased lungs may become a significant impediment to oxygen exchange in all the disease states described in Section V of this text, although the early stages of lung disease may go unnoticed until the disease progresses. In the later stages of lung disease, the delivery of oxygen and removal of carbon dioxide may be impaired to the extent that work production is limited and severe disability may result. In conjunction with impaired gas exchange, the sedentary life-style of lung-disease patients results in a greater than normal demand on the gas exchange process because of atrophied and inefficient muscles.

Figure 4-18 illustrates a hypothetical, yet practical, relationship between increasing pulmonary abnormalities and symptoms. Few symptoms of lung disease are expressed in the early stages of the disease process. When first injured or otherwise affected, the lung remains adequately efficient in performing its task of gas exchange. The effects of cigarette smoking, industrial exposure, or air pollution may continue for years without any significant abnormality in gas exchange or disability on the part of the patient. Furthermore, the most common symptoms of pulmonary disease, shortness of breath and cough, are often considered by the victims of pulmonary disease as the expected effects of air pollution, cigarette smoking, obesity, or age. This is a real tragedy when it occurs in early pulmonary disease that could be diagnosed and stabilized or reversed. The

TABLE 4-3 **Clinical Application of Gas Exchanger Model**

Exchanger Component	Site of Abnormality	Examples of Diseases	Bedside Findings
External			
Air pump	Control of ventilation	Respiratory-depressant drugs, CO_2 narcosis, carotid body excision, sleep apnea	Hypopnea or apnea
	Neuromuscular	Cervical spine injury, poliomyelitis, myasthenia gravis	Hypopnea or apnea; may observe diaphragmatic or chest wall weakness
	Chest wall	Trauma, pleurisy, pleural effusion, kyphoscoliosis, obesity	Restricted chest wall expansion
	Parenchymal	Pulmonary fibrosis, congestive heart failure, respiratory distress syndrome	Shallow rapid breathing, rales
Blood pump	Right ventricle	Infarction (rare)	Elevated CVP
		Failure secondary to pulmonary hypertension	RV gallop, $P_2 > A_2$
Tracheobronchial tree	Airways	Foreign bodies, sputum, bronchospasm, external compression, tumor	Wheezes, rales, sputum production
Terminal respiratory unit	Respiratory bronchioles and alveoli	Emphysema	Decreased breath sounds, expiratory prolongation
		Pulmonary (alveolar) edema	Moist rales, LV gallop
Pulmonary vascular tree	Pulmonary arteries and capillaries	Pulmonary emboli, hypoxia-induced pulmonary vasoconstriction, essential pulmonary hypertension	Signs of cor pulmonale
Air–blood interface	Pulmonary venous system	Pulmonary venous hypertension	Signs of left ventricular failure
	Alveolocapillary membrane	Pulmonary edema, hyaline membrane disease, pulmonary fibrosis, adult respiratory distress syndrome	Signs of left ventricular failure Tachypnea, rales (x-ray and DLCO much more sensitive)
Internal			
Blood conduction	Arteries and capillary lumen	Atherosclerosis (eg, coronary artery disease, emboli, extravascular pressure producing ischemia-plaster casts)	Asymmetrical or absent pulses, arrhythmias, etc.
	Hemoglobin	Anemia hemoglobinopathies, carbon monoxide poisoning	Pallor in anemia, rubor in carbon monoxide poisoning

right side of Figure 4-18 shows the effects of the progression of pulmonary disease to the point that symptoms become apparent.

This brings the chapter back to the theme of a multisystem gas exchange model. Any one of the interdependent gas exchange mechanisms illustrated in Figures 4-1 or 4-2 can be affected by the range of potential disease conditions. Examples of neurologic, vascular, cardiopulmonary, hematologic, and neuromuscular problems listed in Table 4-3 can result in failure of the gas exchange system. For example, with early obstructive lung disease the patient can be medically managed, the disease process can be stabilized, and some symptoms may be reversed. With the insult of secondary complications, such as airways edema, small pneumothoraces, pleural effusions, or segmental pneumonia, the gas exchange impairment may become more severe and may only be reversed if the patient is still within the zone of potential stability. The reversal of this acute secondary disease is limited to the severity of disability caused by the patient's permanent chronic pulmonary disease, which may be further advanced by the secondary disease.

With more advanced disease, severe disability will occur because of the severely impaired pulmonary system limiting the gas exchange process. At this stage in the progression of the disease process, even minor complications will result in exacerbations and failure of the pulmonary system that frequently cannot be reversed, and supportive or palliative care may be all the clinician has to offer the patient. Respiratory care practitioners may be involved in the complete disability–impairment spectrum of pulmonary disease, from smoking cessation education and epidemiologic pulmonary function testing to rehabilitation process. Care of exacerbations that render the patient critically ill can involve multisystem failure as advancing age, artherosclerotic disease, renal failure, anemia, or infections push patients beyond their physiologic limits. The chapters in Section V of this text are in place to review a range of clinical problems that challenge the gas exchange model.

Acknowledgment. The authors would like to thank Conrad Colby for his contribution in the area of pulmonary anatomy.

BIBLIOGRAPHY

The Gas Exchange Process

Johnson RL: The lung as an organ of oxygen transport. Basics RD 2(1), 1973 (published by the American Thoracic Society). An excellent description of the circumstances by which the lungs, whose function at sea level is usually not rate-limiting in exercise, may be so when derangements in alveolar ventilation or pulmonary diffusion occur.

Wasserman K, Whipp BJ: Exercise physiology in health and disease. Am Rev Respir Dis 112:219, 1975. This classic "state-of-the-art" discussion, although tedious reading in spots, will be particularly helpful to the reader who has access to an exercise physiology laboratory, which can be used to advantage in localization of defects in the respiratory–cardiovascular gas transport chain.

West JB: Ventilation/Bloodflow and Gas Exchange, 2nd ed. Oxford, Blackwell Scientific, 1970

Embryology and Growth of the Lung and Surfactant

Avery ME: The Lung and Its Disorders in the Newborn Infant, 3rd ed. Philadelphia, WB Saunders, 1975. Chapters 1 through 4 are pertinent to this section.

England M: Color Atlas of Life Before Birth: Normal Fetal Development. Chicago, Year Book Medical Publishers, 1983. Remarkable color photos of gross fetal cardiopulmonary development.

Hills BA: The Biology of Surfactant. New York, Cambridge University Press, 1988

Scarpelli EM (ed): Pulmonary Physiology of the Fetus, Newborn, and Child. Philadelphia, Lea & Febiger, 1975. A classic.

Thibeault DW, Gregory GA: Neonatal Pulmonary Care, 2nd ed. Norwalk, Conn, Appleton–Century–Crofts, 1986. A literature review with 2213 references, not for the novice.

The Thorax as an Air Pump

Peters RM: The Mechanical Basis of Respiration: An Approach to Respiratory Pathophysiology. Boston, Little, Brown & Co, 1975. Chapters 1, 4, and 9 are concise treatments of complex topics.

Functional Anatomy

Cumming G, Hunt LB: Form and Function in the Human Lung. London, Livingston, 1968

Hayek II: The Human Lung. New York, Hafner, 1960

Murray JF: The Normal Lung: The Basis for Diagnosis and Treatment of Pulmonary Diseases. Philadelphia, WB Saunders, 1976

Negaishi C: Functional Anatomy and Histology of the Lung. Baltimore, University Park Press, 1972. A definitive, beautifully illustrated treatise, well worth including in any departmental library.

Staub NC, Albertine KH: Anatomy of the lungs. In Textbook of Respiratory Medicine, 2nd ed. Murray JF, Nadel JA (eds): Philadelphia, WB Saunders, 1994

5

The Physicochemical Basis for Respiratory Gas Exchange

H.F. Helmholz Jr.

CLINICAL SKILLS

Upon completion of this chapter, the reader will:

- Calculate PaO_2 and explain its components
- Describe an oxyhemoglobin saturation curve and explain how and why it changes when abnormalities are present
- Define oxygen delivery, explain how it is determined, and its significance
- Explain how CO_2 is absorbed, transported, and eliminated
- Explain how the Brønsted-Lowery equation describes acids and bases
- Understand buffers and their function
- Identify how acidosis and alkalosis affect pH
- Understand the relationship of proteins, strong ion differences, pH, and Pco_2 in the body
- Use the Davenport nomogram to locate pH- and Pco_2-determined body conditions

KEY TERMS

Acid
Alveolar oxygen partial pressure
Alveolar ventilation
Anionic shift
Arterial oxygen content
Base
Base deficit
Base excess
Bicarbonate system
Buffer
Buffer base
Carbon dioxide partial pressure
Chloride shift
Haldane effect
Hamburger phenomenon
Metabolic quotient
Mixed venous oxygen content
Oxygen delivery
Oxygen uptake
Oxyhemoglobin dissociation
P_{50}
Standard bicarbonate
Strong ion difference
Ventilation/perfusion matching

Life requires energy that is supplied by oxidation of carbon and hydrogen of food. This supports active transport of ions and substances into, out of, and across cells, as well as synthesis and breakdown of structure and all cellular and tissue activity. The nervous system controls fast actions, and hormones and other modulating substances control slower actions. The source of oxygen for body tissues is the alveolar gas, which is actually a mixture of gases found in the alveoli, the site in the lung where oxygen and carbon dioxide are exchanged.

GAS EXCHANGE IN THE LUNG

The *alveolar oxygen partial pressure* (PaO_2), that is, the portion of the pressure in the lung caused by oxygen delivered via the alveoli, can be estimated by the relationships illustrated in Equations 1 and 2 in Equation Box 5-1. Equation 1 states that the alveolar oxygen pressure is determined by the barometric pressure (PB) reduced by the water vapor pressure of saturated gas at body temperature (47) multiplied by the fraction of oxygen in inspired gas (F_IO_2). (This is the highest oxygen pressure there can be in the lungs.) The oxygen absorbed in the lungs is replaced by carbon dioxide partial pressure ($PaCO_2$), modified by the ratio of carbon dioxide production ($\dot{V}CO_2$), and oxygen utilization ($\dot{V}O_2$) designated by the exchange ratio (R). Note that R has an effect only when inert gas is present ($1 - F_IO_2$). This factor (in final parentheses), used to multiply the partial pressure of CO_2, is 1.2 when air is inhaled gas and the exchange ratio is the average normal of 0.8. R is the combustion quotient (RQ) when the individual is in a "steady state," that is, when carbon dioxide production in and elimination from the body are equal. Note that this correction becomes less as F_IO_2 increases and is 1 when F_IO_2 is 1.

Equation 2 indicates that partial pressure of carbon dioxide in the alveoli ($PaCO_2$) will equal the oxygen consumption ($\dot{V}O_2$) times the exchange ratio (R) divided by the *alveolar ventilation* ($\dot{V}A$), which in turn is equal to the total ventilation ($\dot{V}E$) times 1 minus the ratio of tidal physiological dead space (VD) to volume (VT). The number 0.863 provides correction for the difference in conditions in which values are expressed.

MEASUREMENTS OF O_2

Oxyhemoglobin Saturation

Oxygen passes from the alveoli to capillary blood by diffusion, the capacity for which is dependent on the alveolar area, thus lung size. The membrane of the normal lung allows essential equilibration at end capillary. The oxygen absorbed in the lung is limited by the amount of blood flowing through the lung, the amount of hemoglobin in that blood, and the hemoglobin characteristic affinity for oxygen. In addition, the decrease in oxygen content produced by metabolic utilization affects oxygen absorbed in the lung. Thus oxygen uptake equals pulmonary blood flow ($\dot{Q}$) multiplied by the difference in content between each liter of mixed venous blood from each liter of pulmonary venous blood (Equation 3). The characteristic affinity of hemoglobin for oxygen is illustrated in Figure 5-1. Next to the oxyhemoglobin saturation curve, those factors that change the position of this curve are indicated. Note that increase in temperature and decrease in pH, which take place in active tissues, cause right shift of this curve, which increases the tension of oxygen at any given saturation, thus increasing the gradient from blood to tissue where oxygen is being utilized by the mitochondria. Temperature falls and pH rises in the lung, making hemoglobin affinity for oxygen greater. This tissue decrease in affinity and lung increase in affinity is called the Bohr effect.

When abnormalities such as congenital right to left shunt are present or when individuals climb to high altitude, the low arterial oxygen tension causes red blood cell 2,3-diphosphoglycerate concentration to increase, shifting the affinity to the right favoring oxygen unloading. During fetal development, a hemoglobin is present that has an increased affinity for oxygen. Hemoglobin affinity for oxygen, which is remarkably uniform in humans, is best described by the P_{50}, the oxygen tension at which hemoglobin is 50% saturated at a pH of 7.4 and a temperature of 37°C. The P_{50} is normally 26.5 mm Hg. The amount of oxygen carried by hemoglobin when maximally saturated is 1.34 mL of oxygen per gram of hemoglobin in 100 mL of the containing blood. Inspection of the saturation curve indicates that nearly 90% of the oxygen that will combine with hemoglobin does so at a tension of oxygen of 60 mmHg. At 90

EQUATION BOX 5-1

ALVEOLAR OXYGEN PARTIAL PRESSURE

Equation 1: $$P_AO_2 = (P_B - 47)\,F_IO_2 - P_ACO_2\left(F_IO_2 + \frac{1 - F_IO_2}{R}\right)$$

Equation 2: $$P_ACO_2 = \frac{0.863\,\dot{V}CO_2}{\dot{V}_A} = \frac{0.863\,\dot{V}O_2R}{\dot{V}_E\,(1 - V_D/V_T)}$$

Equation 3: $$\dot{V}O_2 = \dot{Q}\,(CaO_2 - C\bar{v}O_2)\,10$$

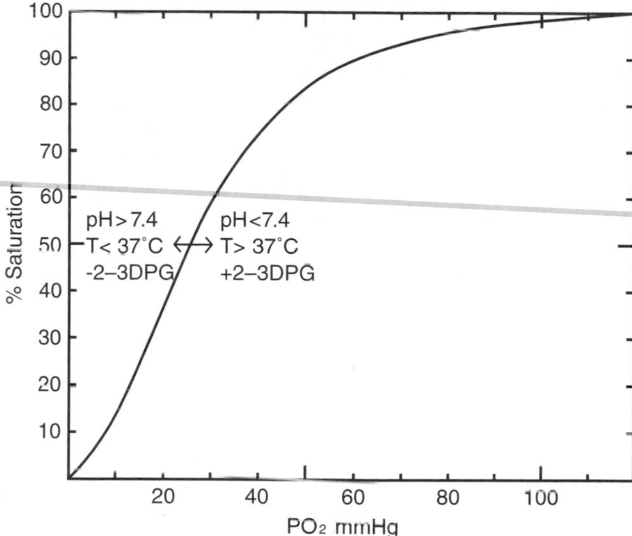

FIGURE 5-1. Hemoglobin saturation curve, with factors that shift the position of the curve indicated.

mmHg the hemoglobin is 95% saturated or better. The content of oxygen in the venous blood entering the pulmonary capillaries determines how much oxygen will be absorbed as long as the ventilation of those alveoli provides it. Oxygen is most soluble in blood at tensions from 0 to above 60 mmHg. Normally, oxygen content of mixed arterial blood is reduced by a small amount of venous blood entering the pulmonary veins from the bronchial circulation and by flow in thebesian veins draining the left ventricular myocardium.

Ventilation/Perfusion Matching and Mismatching

The venous blood requirement for oxygen and the ventilation providing it are nearly equal in the normal lung. With disease, inequalities in the matching of ventilation and perfusion ($\dot{V}/\dot{Q}$) can develop. Figure 5-2 shows the differences in solubilities of oxygen and carbon dioxide. Note that a decrease in ventilation in relation to perfusion can produce a definite deficit in oxygen uptake, whereas an increase in ventilation, though producing an increase in oxygen tension, will produce very little increase in oxygen uptake. On the other hand, the solubility curve of carbon dioxide indicates that any increase in carbon dioxide tension produced by low ventilation relative to perfusion can be completely corrected by the overventilation that must take place in other parts of the lung, washing out extra CO_2. Thus, as long as total alveolar ventilation is normal, ventilation/perfusion mismatching will cause a decrease in arterial oxygen tension but no increase in arterial carbon dioxide tension. For example, in asthma, local decreases in ventilation cause a decrease in arterial oxygen but either no increase or a decrease in carbon dioxide tension produced by increase in total alveolar ventilation because of the stimulus hypoxemia causes through the carotid and aortic bodies.

Oxygen Delivery

Oxygen is delivered to various parts of the body by the output of the left ventricle. The total amount of oxygen available, called *oxygen delivery,* is determined by the cardiac output multiplied by the arterial oxygen content ($\dot{Q} \times CaO_2$). Delivery of oxygen to various parts of the body is determined by the relation of local arterial resistance to total systemic arterial resistance. In critical care, where it would be advantageous to know local as well as total oxygen delivery, methods are not available. During exercise vasoconstriction is blocked in active muscles whereas vasoconstriction in nonactive muscles maintains central arterial pressure. During severe illness, such as adult respiratory distress syndrome (ARDS), whenever flow to a part of the body is reduced, oxygen supply becomes inadequate. Mitochondrial energy production then produces lactic acid, a nonvolatile substance, rather than carbon dioxide, a volatile substance easily eliminated by the lungs. This production of lactic acid causes a metabolic acidosis, which signals lack of oxygen somewhere in the body. Urine flow gives some index of flow to the kidneys, and consciousness gives some index of flow to the brain. Still needed are methods of obtaining indications of lack of blood flow to other parts of the body.

Metabolic Oxidation

Metabolic oxidation produces carbon dioxide and water. The production of carbon dioxide can be measured. Its level in the blood is maintained by the balance of metabolic production and elimination by pulmonary ventilation. Carbon dioxide production divided by oxygen utilization provides indications of fat utilization (exchange ratio of 0.7), carbohydrate utilization (exchange ratio of 1.0), and mixed utilization at levels in between. Thus, so-called *metabolic quotients,* or metabolic ex-

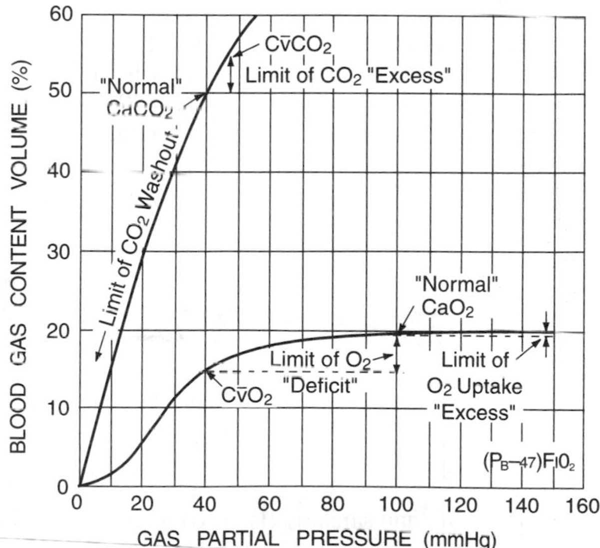

FIGURE 5-2. Oxygen and carbon dioxide solubilities, with limits of maximal and minimal concentrations possible in the lungs with complete right-to-left shunt, or with maximal overventilation.

change ratios, between 0.7 and 1.0 indicate normal metabolism. Ratios outside this range either indicate unsteady state or unusual metabolic activity such as conversion of carbohydrate to fat, which gives exchange ratios above 1.0. In addition to indications of metabolic pathways, levels of arterial carbon dioxide tension indicate adequacy of ventilation and, combined with measurement of pH, provide a readily available index of acid–base balance in the body.

ACID–BASE BALANCE

The major component of living beings is water. The *acids* and *bases* found in water and their various interactions are best understood by the Brønsted–Lowery concept, which describes an acid as a substance that donates a proton to an accepting base.[1] Examples of application of the Brønsted–Lowery concept are illustrated in Equation Box 5-2.

As can be seen in these equations, when dissolved in water, acids stronger than the hydronium ion and bases stronger than the hydroxyl ion will produce hydronium and hydroxyl ions to the same extent, respectively, and thus the acidic and basic properties of all such solutions will be similar. (Heats of neutralization of all strong acids, for example, are the same, as are those of strong bases.) This is called the leveling effect of water.

Buffers

Table 5-1 shows conjugate acid–base pairs arranged to emphasize this with pK[1] values indicated as an index of acidic or basic strength in the range between effective leveling by water. The pK value indicates the pH just above and below which this acid–base pair, when made up by mixing equal concentrations of the acid and the salt of the base, acts as a buffer. *Buffers* are mechanisms that accept or release hydrogen ions; in the human body, these are primarily weak acids. Note that carbonic acid and bicarbonate base will buffer just above and just below a pH of 6.1 (Fig. 5-3). This indicates that at the pH of blood the *bicarbonate system* is not a chemical buffer. Its buffering capacity is caused by the property of carbonic acid to produce carbon dioxide, which is volatile and can be removed by pulmonary ventilation. Thus, it is a system by which the acid product of metabolism is actually removed. Equations 8 and 9 in Equation Box 5-3 indicate the two ways in which carbon dioxide combines chemically in protein-containing solutions, producing bicarbonate and carbamino anions, both of which are treated similarly in theoretically dealing with acid–base balance.

As is indicated in Equation Box 5-3, it is the hydronium ion and not the hydrogen ion that is present in water solutions.[1] The hydrogen atom without its electron (ie, a proton) is very small indeed, some 10,000 times smaller than, for example, a sodium ion. In water, which is a polar substance, such a small unit with a positive charge will be hydrated, thus becoming a much larger complex. This perhaps explains why the hydronium ion does not defuse into and out of the cerebrospinal fluid. Also, the hydronium ion should not be thought of as taking part in exchanges with such ions as sodium or potassium. Figure 5-4 illustrates that to represent hydronium ion concentration at pH 7.0 as 1 cm of the bar of a gamble gram, the total ionic column of positive ions in the blood would have to be 8.75 miles long. At such tiny concentrations, however, the hydronium ion has a remarkable effect on the ionization of compounds such as proteins, which are the major buffers of the body.

Although the body is a complex of cells, extracellular fluid, including the blood, and very slowly modifying components such as bones, for purposes of this discussion the body is treated as tissues in equilibrium with the blood represented by arterial blood samples.

A distinction should be made between a true buffer and a buffering system. A true buffer is a compound or mixture of compounds that minimize the change in pH produced by an added acid that, for example, associates with some of the hydrogen from the hydronium ion that has been added. A buffering system, the bicarbonate system, for example, is one that maintains pH by actually eliminating acid. The properties of proteins as buffers are important in understanding acid–base bal-

EQUATION BOX 5-2

BRØNSTED–LOWRY CONCEPT

The following can be given (*A* and *a* indicate acid, *B* and *b* indicate base). The equation $HCl \leftrightarrow H^+ + Cl^-$ as it applies to aqueous solutions is really only shorthand for:

$$\begin{matrix} A & B & a & b \\ HCl + & H_2O \leftrightarrow & H_3O^+ + & Cl^- \end{matrix}$$

and similarly $H^+ + NH_2^- \leftrightarrow NH_3$ is shorthand for

$$\begin{matrix} B & A & a & b \\ NH_2^- + & H_2O \leftrightarrow & NH_3 + & OH^- \end{matrix}$$

TABLE 5-1 **Conjugate Acid–Base Pairs**

Conjugate Acid		Conjugate Base		pK[1]
Perchloric acid	$HClO_4$	ClO_4^-	Perchlorate ion	
Sulfuric acid	H_2SO_4	HSO_4^-	Hydrogen sulfate ion	
Hydrochloric acid	HCl	Cl^-	Chloride ion	
Nitric acid	HNO_3	NO_3^-	Nitrate ion	
Hydronium ion	H_3O^+	H_2O	Water	1.3
Hydrogen sulfate ion	HSO_4^-	$SO_4^=$	Sulfate ion	1.6
Phosphoric acid	H_3PO_4	$H_2PO_4^-$	Dihydrogen phosphate ion	2.0
Glycine cation	$NH_3CH_2COOH^+$	NH_2CH_2COOH	Glycine	2.3
Succinic acid	COOH CH_2COOH	COOH CH_2COO^-	1 Succinate ion	2.8
Acetoacetic acid	CH_3CO CH_2COOH	$CH_3OCCCH_2COO^-$	Acetacetate ion	3.8
Lactic acid	CH_3CHOH COOH	CH_3CHOH COO^-	Lactate ion	3.9
β-hydroxybutyric acid	CH_3CHOH COOH	CH_3CHOH CH_2COO^-	β-hydroxybutyrate ion	4.4
Acetic acid	CH_3COOH	CH_3COO^-	Acetate ion	4.7
1-Succinate ion	COOH CH_2COO^-	COO CH_2COO^{--}	2-Succinate ion	5.7
Carbonic acid	H_2CO_3	HCO_3^-	Bicarbonate ion	6.1
Dihydrogen phosphate ion	$H_2PO_4^-$	$HPO_4^=$	Hydrogen phosphate ion	6.8
Ammonium ion	NH_4^-	NH_3	Ammonia	9.3
Glycine	NH_2CH_2COOH	$NH_2CH_2COO^-$	Glycine anion	9.7
Bicarbonate acid	HCO_3^-	$CO_3^=$	Carbonate ion	10.4
Methylamine cation	$CH_3NH_3^+$	CH_3NH_2	Methylamine	10.7
Hydrogen phosphate ion	$HPO_4^=$	$PO_4^=$	Phosphate ion	12.0
Water	H_2O	OH^-	Hydroxyl ion	12.7
Ethyl alcohol	CH_3CHOH	CH_3CHO^-	Ethoxide ion	
Ammonia	NH_3	NH_2^-	Amide ion	
Methylamine	CH_3NH_2	CH_3NH^-	Methylamide ion	
Hydrogen	H_2	H^-	Hydride ion	
Methane	CH_4	CH_3^-	Methide ion	

ance and are best understood by referring to Figure 5-5, which shows that the multiple amino groups and organic acid groups of proteins buffer over a wide range of pHs. The properties of protein in buffering can be represented by equations valid for clinical applications[2] (Equation Box 5-3).

ION CONCENTRATION

Equations 4 through 9 in Equation Box 5-3 indicate that the isoelectric point for plasma protein is at pH of 5.08 and for oxygenated hemoglobin is pH 6.81. pH is the point at which the protein is un-ionized. At any

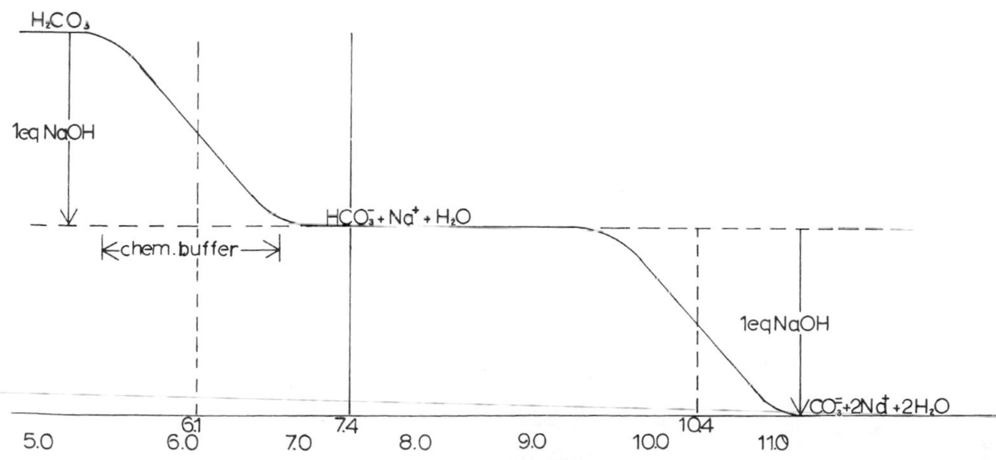

FIGURE 5-3. Carbonic acid carbonate dissociation characteristics.

EQUATION BOX 5-3

BUFFERS AND BUFFERING FORMULAE

Equation 4: $[R_p] = 0.104\ (pH - 5.08)\ (1 - F)10N$

$[R_p]$ = concentration of ions of dissociated plasma proteins (mEq/L); F = fraction of packed red blood cells (hematocrit); N = number of grams of plasma protein in 100 mL plasma

Equation 5: $[R_h] = 2.8\ (pH - 6.81)\ 0.5988N$

$[R_h]$ = concentration of ions of dissociated hemoglobin (mEq/L); N = grams of hemoglobin in 100 mL whole blood

Equation 6: $[R_o] \pm [R_h] = 0.3N$

$[R_o]$ = concentration of anions of dissociated oxygenated hemoglobin in pH range from 7.2 to 7.6. Note: Loss of 1 millimole of oxygen from hemoglobin reduces the anionic concentration in blood at that pH by 0.518 mEq/L; this is the "isohydric change."

Equation 7: $[HCO_3] = \text{antilog}\ (pH - 6.1)\ 0.03\ PCO_2$

Equation 8: $\text{Difference from normal [SID]} = [HCO_3] - \dfrac{N}{1.07}\ (7.4 - pH) - 23.9431$

Equation 9: $\uparrow CO_2 \downarrow + 2H_2O \leftrightarrow H_2CO_3 + H_2O \leftrightarrow H_3O^+ + HCO_3^-$

$\uparrow CO_2 \downarrow + RNH_2 + H_2O \leftrightarrow RNHCOOH + H_2O \leftrightarrow H_3O^+ + RNHOO^-$

pH above this point, a protein ionizes as an anion, thus requiring cations to match. In the blood and tissues the principal matching cations are sodium and potassium

Concentration of ions in human blood can be represented by bar gamble grams, in which the height of the bars represent total cationic and anionic concentrations as illustrated in Figure 5-4 on the left.

A balance of absorption of ions via the gastrointestinal tract and elimination of ions by the kidneys is essential for acid–base balance. This balance controls the difference in *strong ion concentration* (Equation 8). Strong ions are defined as those in which the concentration is unaffected by changes in pH of the containing fluid.[3] Examples are sodium, potassium and calcium cations, and chloride and lactate anions. Living cells are

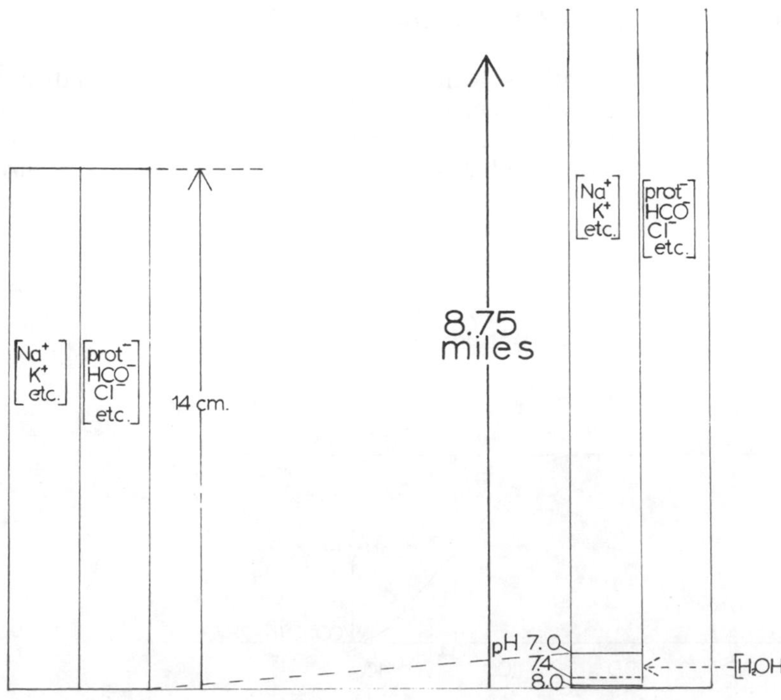

FIGURE 5-4. "Gamble gram" of ionic concentrations enlarged to show hydronium concentration at pH 7.0 as a bar 1cm in height

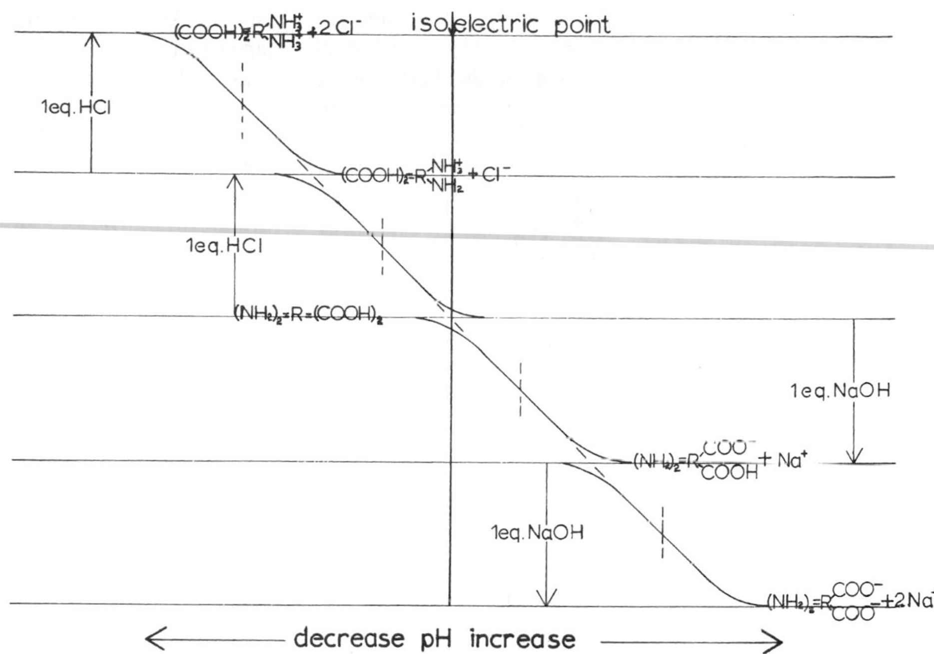

FIGURE 5-5. Protein dissociation characteristics.

capable of actively moving such ions against concentration gradients, as in the maintenance of potential difference between living cells and extracellular fluid, which is responsible for potassium as the primary intracellular cation and sodium as the primary extracellular cation. The anionic strong ion concentration is maintained less than the total strong cation concentration while equality is maintained by bicarbonate and protein anions equal to the strong anion difference. This difference has been called the *buffer base* by several authors.[4,5]

In addition to its importance in relation to metabolism, carbon dioxide, a very soluble gas, diffuses rapidly in the aqueous media and thus is normally present in the entire body at tensions of 40 mmHg in arterial blood, and above that elsewhere. Except during exertion and hypoxemia (reduced blood O_2 tension), the control of pulmonary ventilation is primarily by the pH-sensitive receptors on the ventral surface of the medulla oblongata, which is bathed by cerebrospinal fluid. This fluid contains very little protein and the strong ion relationship is such that changes in carbon dioxide tension produce marked changes in pH because of its poor buffering. Production of cerebrospinal fluid is by the choroid plexuses of the ventricles of the brain, and the composition of the fluid can change as the pH of the blood from which it is produced changes. Respiratory acidosis, in which the base is lower than normal, causes cerebrospinal fluid to change such that its pH at carbon dioxide tension above 40 mmHg causes less drop in pH, whereas respiratory alkalosis, in which the base is higher than normal, causes production of a fluid that approaches normal pH at carbon dioxide tensions below 40 mmHg. This explains why reduction of carbon dioxide tension from chronic hypercapneic levels causes marked decrease in the ventilatory drive, particularly if hypoxic drive is also relieved. Similarly, the removal of the hypoxic drive of high altitude exposure does not decrease ventilation to normal level until the cerebrospinal fluid has been replaced.

Another function of carbon dioxide is to make bicarbonate ions and hydronium ions available wherever acid–base work is required, that is, where acid or alkaline secretions or excretions are taking place. In the parietal cells of the stomach, the cells of the salivary, pancreatic, and intestinal glands, and the tubular cells of the kidney, the presence of carbonic anhydrase speeds the availability of bicarbonate and hydronium ions by rapid hydration of dissolved carbon dioxide. This is, of course, a reversible reaction and provides for the rapid absorption and evolution of carbon dioxide by the blood because of the presence of carbonic anhydrase in the red blood cells. Active transport of chloride ions takes with it the hydronium ion to produce acid in the stomach, whereas active transport of sodium takes with it bicarbonate to produce alkaline secretions and to "regenerate bicarbonate" in the kidney in response to acidosis. This active transport of sodium back to the blood, which allows the hydronium ion to combine with such ions as the hydrogen phosphate in the urine, is one of the mechanisms by which acid urine is produced. The strong ion difference in the blood is changed when the strong ion difference of the blood has been reduced because of some disorder. Thus it is active transport of ions that maintains the *strong ion difference.*

MEASURING VENTILATION AND OXYGENATION WITH ARTERIAL BLOOD SAMPLES

The sampling and analysis of arterial blood can give information concerning ventilation and oxygenation as described above (see Equation Box 5-1), and can properly interpret important information concerning acid–base balance. Various methods of representing relationships of carbon dioxide tension, pH, and bicarbonate are possible. L. J. Henderson in his classic book *The Blood*[5] plotted blood carbon dioxide content on the vertical coordinate and carbon dioxide tension on the horizontal coordinate (Fig. 5-6). Analysis of blood provided the curves indicated. The changes in solubility with changes in strong ion difference are indicated by the *base excess (BE)* ± 5 curves. In 1960 Astrup et al,[6] using a miniature equilibration system, presented a method to determine an acid–base balance of blood by measuring pH of a sample, then pH after equilibration with carbon dioxide tensions above and below that of the sample, then plotted the linear relationship of the log of the carbon dioxide tension on the vertical axis against the pH on the horizontal coordinate. They pointed out that from this method one could derive the *standard bicarbonate*, which was the bicarbonate at a carbon dioxide tension of 40 mmHg. The relationship of carbon dioxide tension and pH describing 45-degree lines of isobicarbonate could be plotted using this method. For normal blood the standard bicarbonate would be at or near 24 milliequivalents per liter, whereas values above 24 indicated alkalosis and below 24 acidosis.

After the Astrup method was introduced, workers in the United States, who were studying human and animal work measuring the effects of equilibration of the whole body with high and low carbon dioxide tension,[7] began the debate[8] over whether the terms BE or standard bicarbonate were the best indication of acid–base status. As a result it became obvious that both methods are valid as long as the standard bicarbonate is near normal, but with marked changes in acid–base balance, the equilibrium represented by the arterial blood sample must be interpreted as that of a less-well-buffered total system. The blood contains more protein than any other part of the body, and the system acts as though roughly three times the blood volume is being buffered by the protein in the blood.

The method of graphing the relationship of carbon dioxide tension, pH, and bicarbonate, introduced by Davenport[9] as a teaching tool, lends itself best to understanding and interpreting blood gas abnormalities, as well as relating blood gas data to the strong ion difference[7,8] to either blood alone or the total body.

As shown in Figure 5-7, using normal values for plasma protein and hemoglobin, the ionic concentration of proteins can be plotted using the reference of the isoelectric point and its pH as zero concentration with anionic concentration plotted downward (Equations 4 and 5). Combining protein concentrations and indicating results of Equation 6, the ionization of blood proteins when hemoglobin is saturated and reduced can be plotted and related to bicarbonate and to the strong ion difference (Fig. 5-8). The relationships of Figure 5-8 can be plotted on the same graph (Fig. 5-9) marked "in vitro." Using a series of curvilinear isopleths of carbon dioxide tension as calculated by the rearranged Henderson-Hasselbalch equation (Equation 7), the relationship of pH carbon dioxide tension and bicarbonate can be graphed (see Fig. 5-9 on page 146).

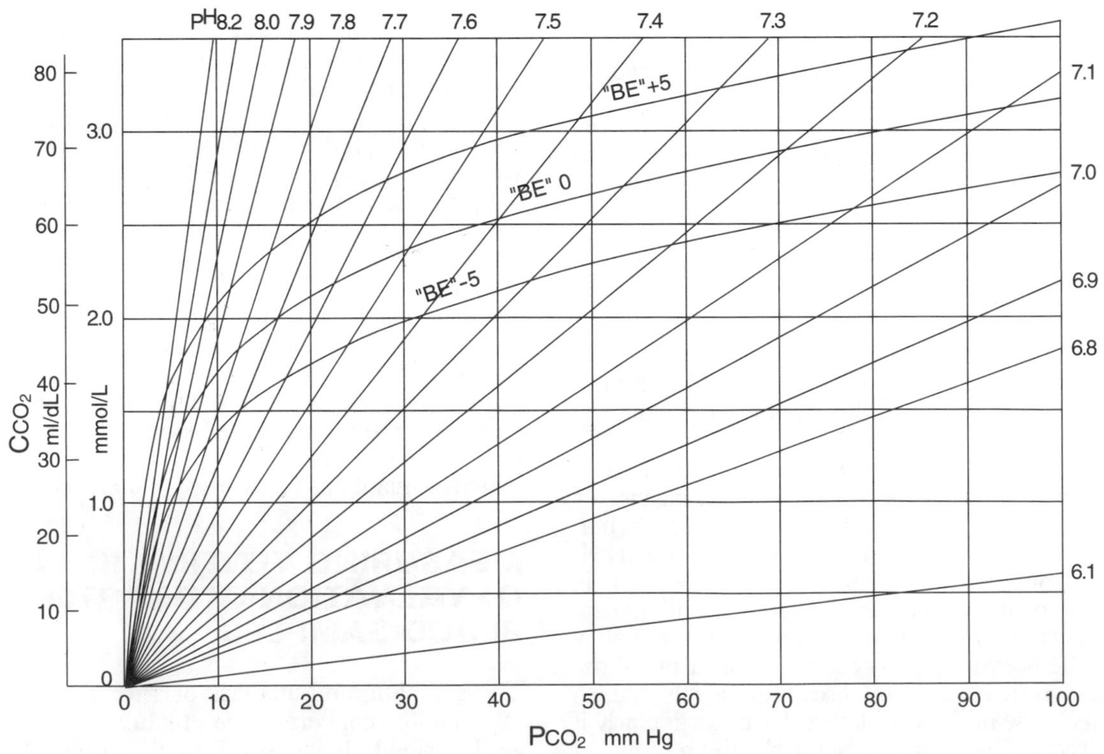

FIGURE 5-6. Carbon dioxide solubilities with changes in "base excess."

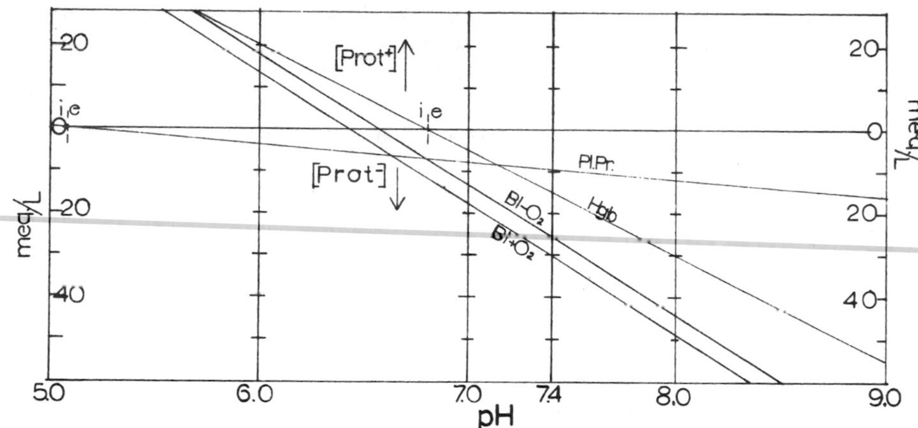

FIGURE 5-7. Protein ionic concentrations at varying pHs.

Note that the slope of the line represents less change in pH with change in carbon dioxide tension than would take place in water. This represents the buffer power of proteins. A best estimate of the buffer power of proteins in the body as a whole as indicated by arterial blood is that the proteins act as though they were only one third of the concentration of that which is found in the blood. Thus one can estimate the normal in vivo effect of changes of equilibrium with changes in the strong ion difference brought about by alkalosis or acidosis, that is, the nonrespiratory effect. Figures 5-10 through 5-12 show the differences in carbon dioxide tensions and pH in the body as a whole normally and with decrease in strong ion difference (*base deficit* [BD]of 6) and increase in strong ion difference (BE of 6).

The advantages of the Davenport method of presentation of relationships are as follows: shift of the zero of bicarbonate concentration shows the effect of increase and decrease of strong ion difference on the position of the PCO_2 to bicarbonate as it shifts in relation to the protein anionic concentration. The relationship of the protein anionic concentration to pH remains constant in relation to total cationic concentration.

Having established the slope of the line representing equilibrium of carbon dioxide tension with the body as a whole (Fig. 5-13), the normal position will be determined by passing through the point indicated by normal values of pH 7.4 and carbon dioxide tension (40 mm Hg). If a subject hypoventilates, the body equilibrium will be represented by pH and PCO_2 along the normal sloped line to the right, whereas hyperventilation will be similarly represented by points along the line to the left. Any points determined by the PCO_2 and pH that lie above the line will indicate BE represented by milliequivalents per liter on the bicarbonate scale, whereas such points falling below the line will indicate base deficit similarly. These points represent the change in strong ion difference in milliequivalents per liter, indicating that the in vivo buffer line has remained fixed relative to total cations, but zero of $[HCO_3^-]$ concentration has shifted.

Finally, since hypoventilation and hyperventilation cause change in pH from normal, the renal mechanism for changing the strong ion difference comes into play. For hyperventilation, the kidney will begin putting out alkaline urine actively excreting cation, which will be

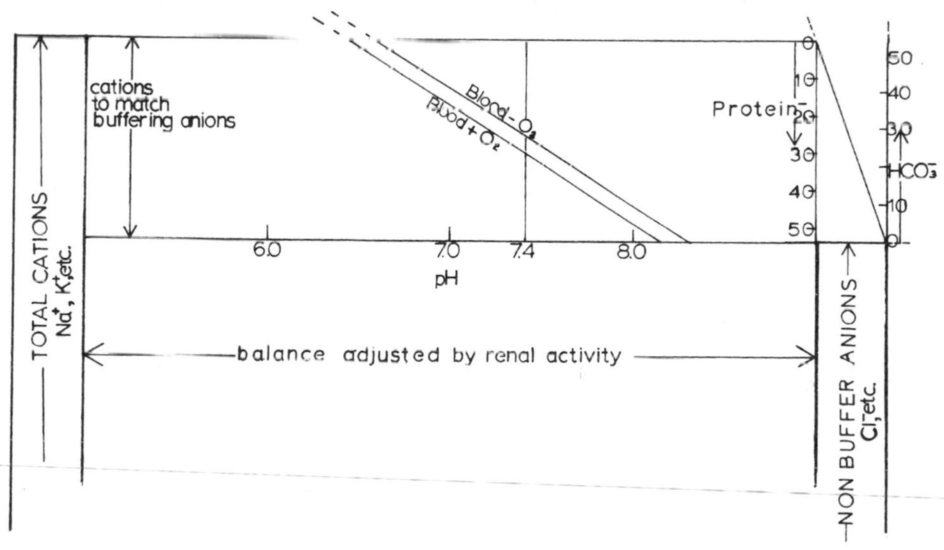

FIGURE 5-8. Blood protein ionization related to strong ion difference, ie, "buffering ions."

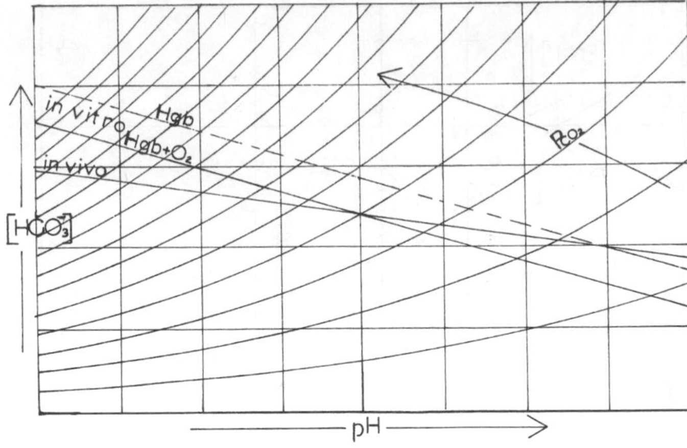

FIGURE 5-9. Characteristics of blood relating $[HCO_3^-]$, Pco_2, and pH.

matched by bicarbonate and a base deficit. In Figure 5-13 and 5-14A and B, the line from the normal point that curves downward is determined from chronic hyperventilation of altitude exposure and indicates the maximal renal compensation that the normal body performs.[10] Similarly from data on chronic exposure to increase carbon dioxide (by research related to submarine personnel) the maximal renal compensation to hypoventilation of which a normal individual is capable is indicated by the curved line upward from the normal point (pH 7.4, PCO_2 40).[11] Thus one can develop a modification of the Davenport diagram with areas of possible interpretation indicated (Fig. 5-14B). These areas indicate the general principle that compensation is never sufficient to remove completely the stimulus producing that compensation. In the upper left-hand corner of this graph are given the slopes of in vitro buffer lines at various concentrations of hemoglobin, major protein buffer of the blood.

It will be noted that points determined by pH and carbon dioxide tension can lie in areas above the buffer slope line to the left in the region of hypoventilation and compensation, or below the line to the right in the region of compensation. Although acidosis will cause shift in pH to the left, the maximal amount of ventilatory compensation cannot be determined because it depends on the ventilatory capacity of the individual, the muscular strength, and the amount of fatigue, that is, the length of time the patient has been maximally hypoventilating. In addition, most individuals do not or only minimally react to metabolic alkalosis by hypoventilation. Thus the important relationship of carbon dioxide tension is illustrated, which decreases the pH as it rises, which in turn reduces protein ionization, providing cationic concentration to match the bicarbonate. Also, with decrease in carbon dioxide tension, pH rises, finally increasing protein anionic concentration to the point where all bicarbonate is converted to carbon dioxide and removed from blood. Thus, whole blood carbon dioxide can be completely removed by bubbling CO_2 free air through it, whereas plasma alone has inadequate protein to provide the anionic concentration nec-

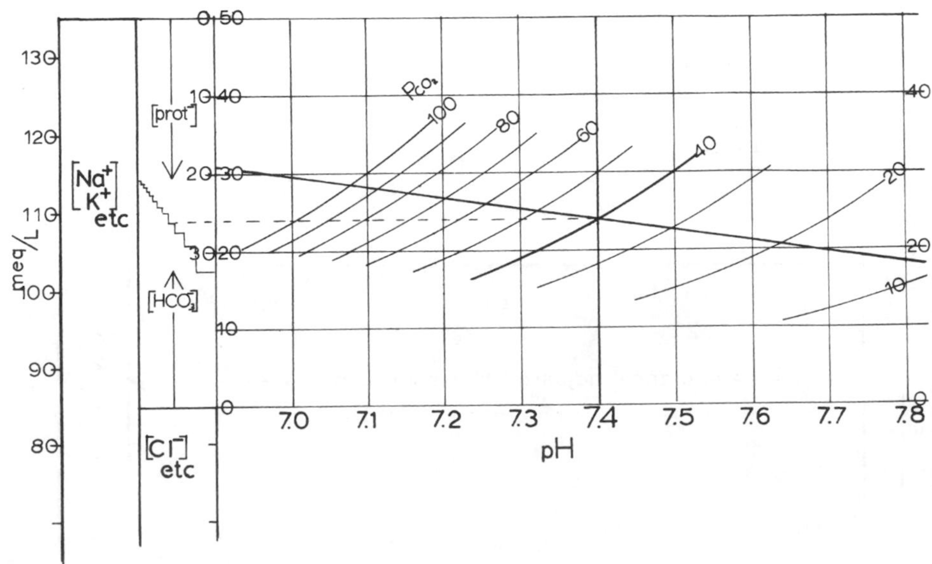

FIGURE 5-10. Relations of Pco_2, $[HCO_3^-]$, and pH with normal strong ion difference.

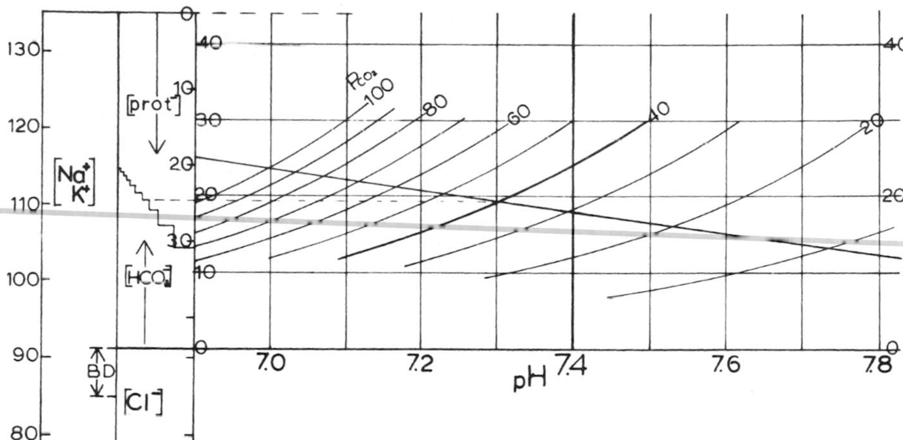

FIGURE 5-11. Relation of P_{CO_2}, $[HCO_3^-]$, and pH with base deficit (BD).

essary as pH rises to the extent that bicarbonate becomes carbonate and will no longer provide volatile carbon dioxide (see Fig. 5-7).

This Davenport method of graphing relationships described above can be used as a nomogram with indications of the effect on arterial blood sample as they indicate the response of the whole body to hypoventilation and hyperventilation alone, the compensation for hyperventilation and hypoventilation, metabolic acidosis and alkalosis with indications of compensation, and those results that cannot be explained without further information (see Figs. 5-14A and B and Box 5-1).

Before presenting examples, details of gas exchange by the blood can now be delineated. During its circulation the blood remains in the vascular system, thus the response to loss and uptake of oxygen and carbon dioxide are as would be expected in the blood alone, that is, in vitro. Therefore, as shown in Figure 5-15, although the body as a whole is equilibrated as indicated by the in vivo line, that equilibrated in lung and tissue is indicated by the in vitro lines for oxygenated and reduced hemoglobin. Thus one can diagram the actual changes that take place as the oxygen delivered reduces saturated hemoglobin to 75%, and carbon dioxide tension rises to 46 mmHg in the tissues. Note that rather than causing a shift in pH to point 1 or even to point 2, the fact that blood remains in the vessels and that oxygen loss from the hemoglobin causes the venous pH to change as indicated at point 3. This explains the lesser drop in pH of venous blood than one might expect.

The effect of changing oxygen saturation of hemoglobin is pertinent to two phenomena, the *Haldane effect* and the *Hamburger phenomenon,* the latter erroneously called the *chloride shift.* Since loss of oxygen from hemoglobin causes association of hydrogen to hemoglobin (reduced hemoglobin is a weaker acid), more cations become available in the red blood cell to match anions. Because water and anions alone diffuse

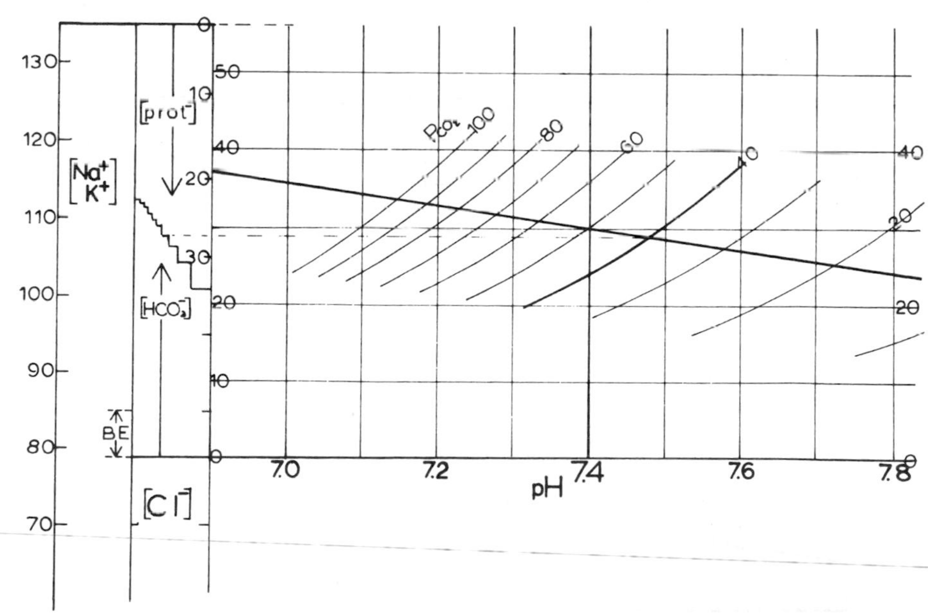

FIGURE 5-12. Relations of P_{CO_2}, $[HCO_3^-]$, and pH with base excess (BE).

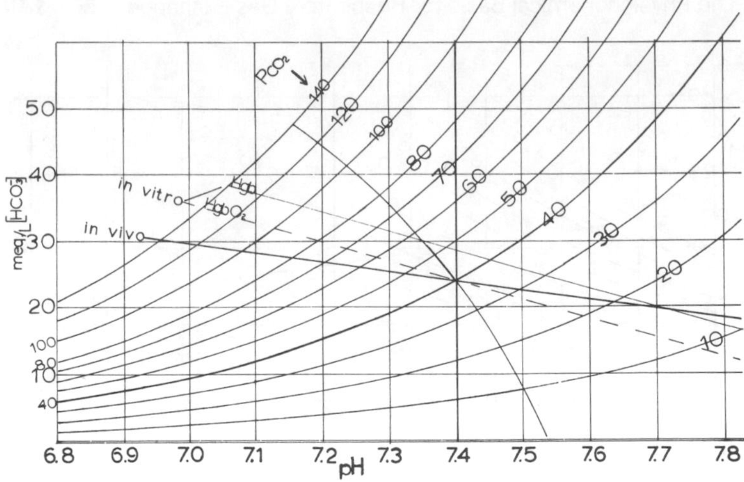

FIGURE 5-13. In vitro and in vivo blood exchange characteristics.

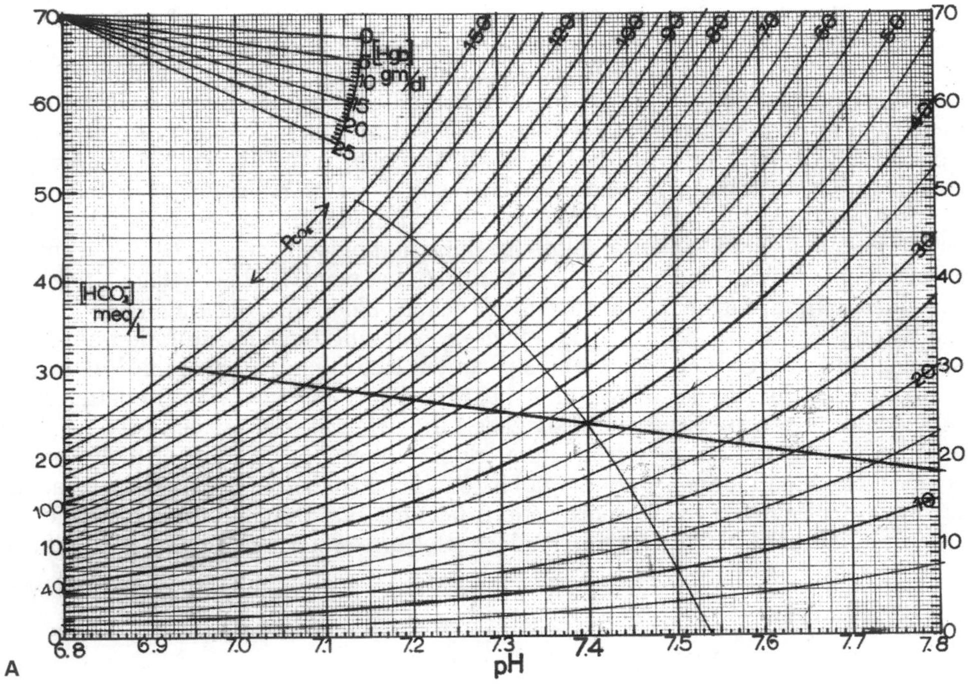

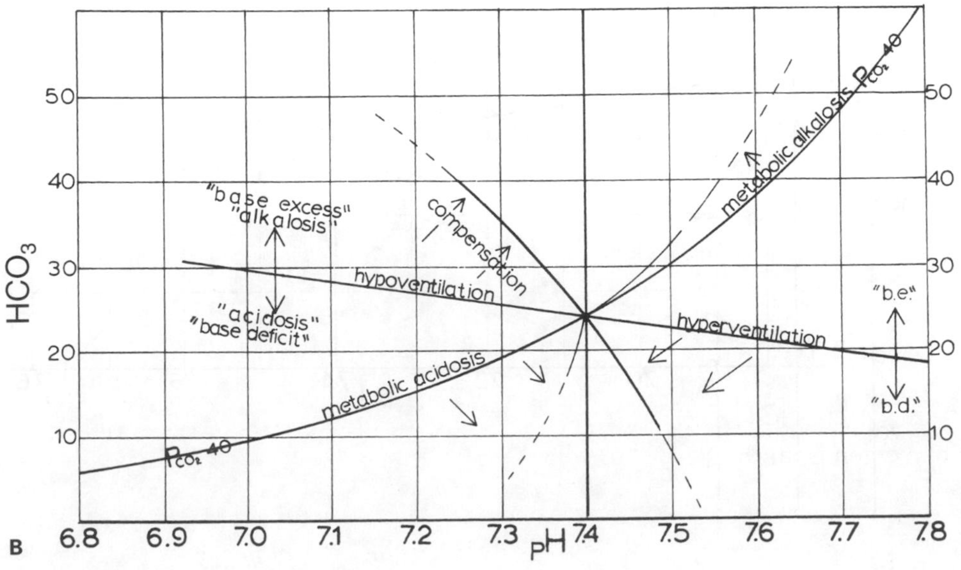

FIGURE 5-14. **(A)** Relationships arranged as a nomogram; identification of "regions." **(B)** Relationships arranged as a nomogram; with units and Hgb effects.

BOX 5-1

INTERPRETATION OF BLOOD DATA (PCO_2 AND pH OF A SAMPLE LOCATED ON NOMOGRAM)

AIR = FIO_2 of 0.2093, others as indicated. PAO_2 calculated by equation No. 1. Tensions are in mmHg (torr), $[HCO_3^-]$ and BE are in mEq/L, saturations are % and Hgbs are in g/dL. All samples except no. 2 are arterial.

1. AIR, PO_2 93, PCO_2 40, pH 7.4, $[HCO_3^-]$ 24, [BE] 0, SO_2 97, Hgb 15. These are the classic normal values. $PAO_2 - PaO_2 = 8$
2. AIR, PO_2 40, PCO_2 46, pH 7.38, $[HCO_3^-]$ 26, [BE] 2, SO_2 73, Hgb 15. These are values typical of a venous sample. PCO_2 is not sufficiently high to explain low PO_2, and $PAO_2 - PaO_2 = 54$ which is not consistent with other findings. PO_2 falls much more than PCO_2 rises in tissue exchanges, because of the differences in solubility.
3. AIR, PO_2 66, PCO_2 65, pH 7.23, $[HCO_3^-]$ 26, [BE] 0, SO_2 87, Hgb 14.8. Low PO_2 can be accounted for by increase in PCO_2. Decreased pH puts point on line of normal acid–base balance. $PAO_2 - PaCO_2 = 5$ indicating normal lungs. This is simple underventilation. More data are needed to explain findings. Drug overdose in a young person would give these findings.
4. AIR, PO_2 55, PCO_2 30, pH 7.48, $[HCO_3^-]$ 22, [BE] −1, SO_2 86, Hgb 15. PCO_2 of 30 indicates overventilation without significant compensation, the explanation for which may be the low PaO_2. $PAO_2 - PaO_2 = 55$. This is typical of severe ventilation–perfusion mismatching. One would ask if the patient is wheezing but had not been given bronchodilator or oxygen. (See example no. 6 for result of failure to treat)
5. AIR, PO_2 62, PCO_2 65, pH 7.33, $[HCO_3^-]$ 33, [BE] 8, SO_2 87, Hgb 15.5. High PCO_2 with only some decrease in pH indicates hypoventilation is chronic leading to compensation. $PAO_2 - PaO_2 = 9$ suggesting normal lungs, ruling out obstructive lung disease such as emphysema. Further data are needed and reveal stridor and history of gradually worsening upper airway obstruction.
6. AIR, PO_2 40, PCO_2 60, pH 7.26, $[HCO_3^-]$ 28, [BE] 1, SO_2 67, Hgb 14.6. High PCO_2 and low PO_2 on nomogram suggesting acute process. $PAO_2 - PaCO_2 = 40$ indicating pulmonary abnormality. Patient is wheezing. This is a medical emergency!
7. AIR, PO_2 115, PCO_2 20, pH 7.33, $[HCO_3^-]$ 10, [BE] −15, SO_2 99, Hgb 14. Low PCO_2 and low pH with base deficit of 16 indicate respiratory response to acidosis in a patient incapable of marked hyperventilation. $PAO_2 - PaCO_2 = 10$. Data are consistent with diabetic ketoacidosis in an otherwise normal individual.
8. AIR, PO_2 105, PCO_2 30, pH 7.44, $[HCO_3^-]$ 20, [BE] −4, SO_2 98, Hgb 6.0. Low PCO_2 and just above normal pH put point in region of compensation for hyperventilation. $PAO_2 - PaO_2 = 8$. Reason for increased ventilation is not hypoxemia but may be decreased oxygen delivery (CO × CaO_2) caused by low hemoglobin.
9. FIO_2 0.6, PO_2 140, PCO_2 75, pH 7.25, $[HCO_3^-]$ 32, [BE] 6, SO_2 99, Hgb 16. High PCO_2 and low pH with BE of 6 indicate compensation for underventilation of a lesser level with further hypoventilation the reason for which may be relief of hypoxemic drive to ventilation by application of too high FIO_2. $PAO_2 - PaO_2 = 205$ consistent with obstructive lung disease.
10. FIO_2 0.6, PO_2 143, PCO_2 40, pH 7.47, $[HCO_3^-]$ 28, [BE] 5, SO_2 99, Hgb 15.8. PCO_2 of 40 and pH of 7.47 indicate point outside area designating predictable causation. BE of 5 indicates PCO_2 may have been high, causing compensation. $PAO_2 - PaO_2 = 240$ indicates pulmonary disease, but explanation for blood gas findings requires further data. Patient has obstructive pulmonary disease, stopped breathing when given oxygen, and was intubated and ventilated. Data suggest better objective of treatment would be normal arterial pH, not PCO_2 of 40 mmHg.
11. AIR, PO_2 93, PCO_2 42, pH 7.5, $[HCO_3^-]$ 30, [BE] 8, SO_2 98, Hgb 14.8. High pH and BE indicates alkalosis. Further data are needed. Suggest asking if excessive antacids are being used or if patient has gastric suction. If not, suggest measuring pH of urine. If acid (with high pH of blood, urine should be alkaline) suggest blood sample for electrolytes, expecting low potassium as cause of alkalosis.[12] $PAO_2 - PaO_2 = 8$.
12. AIR, PO_2 95, PCO_2 15, pH 7.38, $[HCO_3^-]$ 9, [BE] −15, SO_2 97, Hgb 11. Very low PCO_2 with normal pH indicates that marked hyperventilation has brought pH back to normal, which would have removed stimulus to hyperventilate, thus is not reasonable. (Dilution of sample with excessive heparin solution would cause low PCO_2 and Hgb with little effect on PO_2 and pH.)[13]
13. FIO_2 1.0, PO_2 60, PCO_2 30, pH 7.48, $[HCO_3^-]$ 21, [BE] −1, SO_2 90, Hgb 15. PO_2 of only 60 breathing an FIO_2 of 1.0 given $PAO_2 - PaCO_2$ of 623 if barometric pressure is 760 mm Hg. Questions bring out that blood sample was taken from subject exposed in a decompression chamber to PB of 150 mm Hg. In this case $PAO_2 - PaO_2$ is 8, indicating subject has good lungs and is hyperventilating because of hypoxemia.
14. AIR, PO_2 50, PCO_2 25, pH 7.5, $[HCO_3^-]$ 17, [BE] −6, SO_2 85, Hgb 16. Low PCO_2 can be explained by low PO_2. $PAO_2 - PaO_2$ is 69 indicating pulmonary disease. Low PCO_2 indicates pulmonary disease is not obstructive thus some form of restrictive disease such as pulmonary fibrosis is most likely.

readily across the red cell membrane, the total anionic concentration (bicarbonate and chloride) inside the cell increases relative to that in the plasma. Thus the Hamburger shift is an *anionic shift*, not just a chloride shift, and is related only to the loss of oxygen from the hemoglobin. This loss of oxygen makes more cations available to match bicarbonate and thus increases the solubility of carbon dioxide. Therefore, because of decreased saturation of hemoglobin in the tissue, an anionic concentration inside the cells increases the osmotically active particles, and thus water also diffuses into the cell. Because this process is reversed in the lung, the result is that the venous hematocrit is greater than that of the arterial blood and carbon dioxide solubility is increased in the tissues and decreased in the lung. Changes in the acidity of the hemoglobin owing to

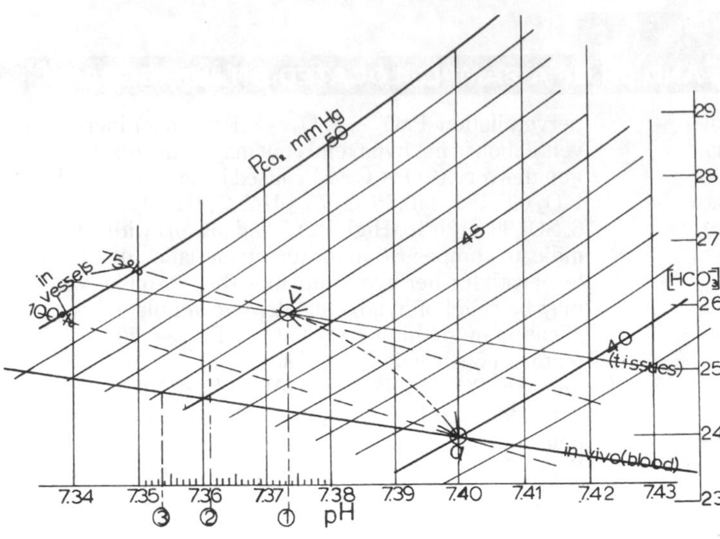

FIGURE 5-15. In vivo CO_2 and O_2 exchange.

oxygen loading and unloading are responsible for the Haldane and Hamburger phenomena.

REFERENCES

1. Vanderwerf CA: Acid Bases and the Chemistry of the Covalent Bond, Chap 2. New York, Reinhold Publishing Corp, 1966
2. Mansfield CW: Topics in Physical Chemistry, Chap 18. Baltimore, Williams and Wilkins, 1948
3. Stewart PA: Modern quantitative acid base chemistry. Can J Physiol Chem 61:1444, 1983
4. Singer RB, Hastings AB: An improved clinical method for the estimation of disturbances of the acid-base balance of human blood. Medicine 27:223, 1948
5. Henderson LJ: The Blood. New Haven, CT, Yale University Press, 1928
6. Astrup P, Jørgensen K, Siggard Anderson O, & Engel K: Acid base metabolism: A new approach. Lancet 278:1035, 1960
7. Schwartz WB, Relman AS: Critique of parameters used in evaluation of acid-base disorders. N Engl J Med 268:1382, 1963
8. Bunker JP: The great transatlantic acid-base debate. Anesthesiology 26:591, 1965
9. Davenport HW: The ABC of acid-base chemistry, 5th ed. Chicago, University of Chicago Press, 1969
10. West JE: Everest—The testing place. Chest 89:625, 1986
11. Schwartz WB, Brackett NC Jr: Response of extracellular hydrogen ion concentration to graded degrees of hypercapnia. Physiologic limits of defense of pH. J Clin Invest 44:291, 1965
12. Schwartz AB, Lyons H: Acid base and electrolyte balance. New York, Grune and Stratton, 1977
13. Bradley JG: Errors in the measurement of blood PCO_2 due to dilution of the sample with heparin solution. Br J Anesthesia 44:231, 1972

SECTION

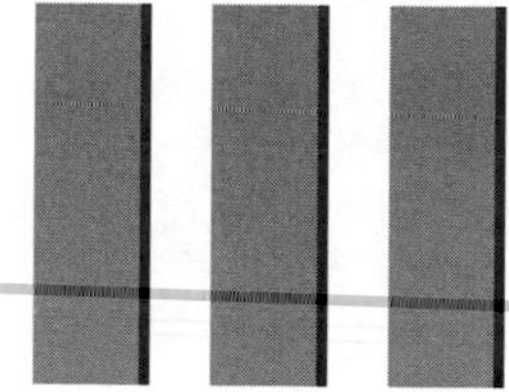

CLINICAL ASSESSMENT OF CARDIOPULMONARY FUNCTION

6 Assessment Skills Core to Practitioner Success

Terry Des Jardins
Judy A. Tietsort

CLINICAL SKILLS

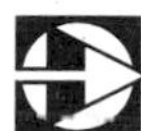

Upon completion of this chapter, the reader will be able to:

- Gather subjective and objective data from the patient history
- Elicit verbal responses from the patient during the interview process and avoid common pitfalls
- Measure and interpret vital signs (body temperature, pulse rate, blood pressure, and respiratory rate)
- Use thoracic cage landmarks and imaginary lines to locate normal chest topography
- Use inspection techniques to assess the patient's breathing pattern, chest configuration, cough, sputum quality, abnormalities of the extremities, and respiratory distress
- Use palpation techniques to assess the patient's tracheal position, chest excursion, tactile and vocal fremitus, and crepitus
- Use percussion techniques to assess the chest and to evaluate diaphragmatic excursion
- Use auscultation techniques to assess normal and adventitious breath sounds
- Describe the use of laboratory tests and other special diagnostic procedures used to obtain assessment data
- Write a problem-oriented medical record progress note

KEY TERMS

Angle of Louis
Assessment
Auscultation
Bronchophony
Clinical Practice Guidelines
Communication
Crackle(s)
Egophony
Percussion
Problem-oriented medical record
Rhonciis (i)
S-O-A-P charting
Therapist-driven protocol
Vital signs
Vocal fremitus or tactile fremitus
Wheezes
Whispered pectoriloqy

Strong assessment skills are vital to good patient care and essential to successful therapist-driven protocol (TDP) programs. The respiratory care practitioner with strong *assessment skills* has the ability to effectively (1) collect pertinent clinical data; (2) assess the data, that is, identify the cause(s) of the data; and (3) select one or more appropriate treatment modalities.

The criterion-referenced bases for TDP programs are the recently published AARC Clinical Practice Guidelines.[1–7] AARC Clinical Practice Guideline: Postural Drainage Therapy is a typical guideline. The boxed portions identified in the clinical practice guideline rely on competent assessment skills. For example, "Difficulty in clearing secretions" is one of the indications for postural drainage therapy. The competent respiratory care practitioner would commonly assess this by visual inspection of the patient's cough effort and sputum production, auscultation of the chest (where rhonchi might be heard), chest x-ray films consistent with atelectasis or mucus plugging, and the deterioration of arterial blood gas values. Protocol 6-1 illustrates a typical assessment flowchart used at a major teaching hospital that uses TDPs. Note how much data is accumulated en route to outlining a treatment plan (the right-hand column).

Before the respiratory care practitioner can have strong assessment skills, however, he or she must first have a basic knowledge and understanding of (1) how each respiratory disease alters the normal anatomy of the lungs; (2) the major pathophysiologic mechanisms resulting from the anatomic alterations; (3) the clinical manifestations caused by the pathophysiologic mechanisms; and (4) the treatment modalities that could be used to offset the clinical manifestations caused by the anatomic alterations and pathophysiologic mechanisms.[8] This chapter assumes that the reader has this basic knowledge and understanding base.

With the above comments in mind, the respiratory care assessment should include (1) patient history; (2) patient interview; (3) a physical examination to identify the cardiopulmonary clinical manifestations demonstrated by the patient; (4) pertinent laboratory data; and (5) a systematic recording method that can be used to effectively gather clinical data, formulate an assessment, and select an appropriate treatment plan.

PATIENT HISTORY

The purpose of the patient history is to gather any pertinent subjective and objective data, which in turn can be used to develop a more complete picture of the patient's past and present health. In most clinical settings, the patient is asked to fill out a printed history form or checklist. The patient should be allowed ample time to recall important dates, health-related landmarks, and family history. The patient interview is then used to validate what the patient has written and collect more data on the patient's health status and life-style. Although history forms vary, most contain the following:

1. Biographical data (age, sex, occupation)
2. The patient's chief complaint or reason for seeking care, including the onset, duration, and characteristics of the signs and symptoms
3. Present health or history of present illness
4. Past health, including childhood illnesses, accidents or injuries, serious or chronic illnesses, hospitalizations, operations, obstetric history, immunizations, last examination date, allergies, current medications, and history of smoking or other habits
5. The patient's family history
6. Review of each body system, including skin, head, eyes, ears, nose, mouth, throat, respiratory system, cardiovascular system, gastrointestinal system, urinary system, genital system, musculoskeletal system, neurologic system, hematologic system, and endocrine system
7. Functional assessment (activities of daily living), including activity and exercise, work performance, sleep and rest, nutrition, interpersonal relationships, and coping and stress management

THE PATIENT INTERVIEW

The interview is a meeting between the respiratory care practitioner and the patient. Its purpose is to collect subjective data about the patient's feelings regarding his or her condition. During a successful interview, the practitioner does the following:

1. Gathers complete and accurate data about the patient's impressions about his or her health, including a description and chronology of any symptoms
2. Establishes rapport and trust so that the patient feels accepted and comfortable enough to share all relevant information
3. Develops and shows an understanding about the patient's health state, which in turn enhances the patient's participation in identifying problems
4. Builds rapport to secure a continuing working relationship, which facilitates future assessments, evaluations, and treatment plans

Interview skills are an art form that takes time—and experience—to develop. The most important components of a successful interview are *communication* and understanding. Understanding the various signals of communication is the most difficult part. When understanding—the conveying of meaning—breaks down between the practitioner and the patient, there is no communication. It cannot be assumed that communication happens just because two people can speak and listen. Communication involves all behaviors, conscious and unconscious, verbal and nonverbal. All these behaviors convey meaning. The following are important factors that enhance the sending and receiving of information during the process of communication.

Internal Factors

Internal factors are those inside the examiner, or what the practitioner brings to the interview in regard to a genuine concern for others, empathy, and the ability to listen. A genuine liking of other people is an essential factor in developing a strong rapport with the patient. This

AARC Clinical Practice Guideline

POSTURAL DRAINAGE THERAPY (PDT)

Indications: Turning is indicated when there is inability or reluctance of patient to change body position (eg, mechanical ventilation, neuromuscular disease, drug-induced paralysis); poor oxygenation associated with position (eg, unilateral lung disease); potential for or presence of atelectasis; and presence of artificial airway. Postural drainage is indicated when there is evidence or suggestion of difficulty with secretion clearance (difficulty clearing secretions with expectorated sputum production greater than 25–30 mL/day [adult] or evidence or suggestion of retained secretions in the presence of an artificial airway); presence of atelectasis caused by or suspected of being caused by mucus plugging; diagnosis of diseases such as cystic fibrosis, bronchiectasis, or cavitating lung disease; and presence of foreign body in airway. External manipulation of the thorax is indicated for sputum volume or consistency suggesting a need for additional manipulation (eg, percussion or vibration) to assist movement of secretions by gravity, in a patient receiving postural drainage.

Contraindications: The decision to use postural drainage therapy requires assessment of potential benefits versus potential risks. Therapy should be provided for no longer than necessary to obtain the desired therapeutic results. (Listed contraindications are relative unless marked as absolute [A].) *Positioning:* All positions are contraindicated for intracranial pressure (ICP) > 20 mmHg; head and neck injury until stabilized (A); active hemorrhage with hemodynamic instability (A); recent spinal surgery (eg, laminectomy) or acute spinal injury; acute spinal injury or active hemoptysis; empyema; bronchopleural fistula; pulmonary edema associated with congestive heart failure; large pleural effusions; pulmonary embolism; aged, confused, or anxious patients who do not tolerate position changes; rib fracture, with or without flail chest; surgical wound or healing tissue. Trendelenburg position is contraindicated for intracranial pressure (ICP) > 20 mmHg, patients in whom increased intracranial pressure is to be avoided (eg, neurosurgery, aneurysms, eye surgery), uncontrolled hypertension, distended abdomen, esophageal surgery, recent gross hemoptysis related to recent lung carcinoma treated surgically or with radiation therapy, uncontrolled airway at risk for aspiration (tube feeding or recent meal). Reverse Trendelenburg is contraindicated in the presence of hypotension or vasoactive medication. *External manipulation of the thorax:* Contraindications in addition to those previously listed include subcutaneous emphysema; recent epidural spinal infusion or spinal anesthesia; recent skin grafts, or flaps, on the thorax; burns, open wounds, and skin infections of the thorax; recently placed transvenous pacemaker or subcutaneous pacemaker (particularly if mechanical devices are to be used); suspected pulmonary tuberculosis; lung contusion; bronchospasm; osteomyelitis of the ribs; osteoporosis; coagulopathy; complaint of chest-wall pain.

Assessment of Need: The following should be assessed **together** to establish a need for postural drainage therapy: excessive sputum production; effectiveness of cough; history of pulmonary problems treated successfully with PDT (eg, bronchiectasis, cystic fibrosis, lung abscess); decreased breath sounds or crackles or rhonchi suggesting secretions in the airway; change in vital signs; abnormal chest x-ray film consistent with atelectasis, mucus plugging, or infiltrates; deterioration in arterial blood gas values or oxygen saturation.

Assessment of Outcome: These represent individual criteria that indicate a positive response to therapy (and support continuation of therapy). Not all criteria are required to justify continuation of therapy (eg, a ventilated patient may not have sputum production > 30 mL/day, but may have improvement in breath sounds, chest x-ray film, or increased compliance or decreased resistance). *Change in sputum production:* If sputum production in an optimally hydrated patient is less than 25 mL/day with PDT, the procedure is not justified. Some patients have productive coughs with sputum production from 15 to 30 mL/day (occasionally as high as 70 or 100 mL/day) without postural drainage. If postural drainage does not increase sputum in a patient who produces > 30 mL/day of sputum without postural drainage, the continuation of the therapy is not indicated. Because sputum production is affected by systemic hydration, apparently ineffective PDT probably should be continued for at least 24 hours after optimal hydration has been judged to be present. *Change in breath sounds of lung fields being drained:* With effective therapy, breath sounds may worsen following the therapy as secretions move into the larger airways and increase rhonchi. An increase in adventitious breath sounds can be a marked improvement over absent or diminished breath sounds. Note any effect that coughing may have on breath sounds. One of the favorable effects of coughing is clearing of adventitious breath sounds. *Patient's subjective response to therapy:* The care giver should ask patient how he or she feels before, during, and after therapy. Feelings of pain, discomfort, shortness of breath, dizziness, and nausea should be considered in decisions to modify or stop therapy. Easier clearance of secretions and increased volume of secretions during and after treatments support continuation. *Change in vital signs:* Moderate changes in respiratory rate and pulse rate are expected. Bradycardia, tachycardia, or an increase in irregularity of pulse, or fall or dramatic increase in blood pressure are indications for stopping therapy. *Change in chest x-ray film:* Resolution or improvement of atelectasis may be slow or dramatic. *Change in arterial blood gas values or oxygen saturation:* Oxygenation should improve as atelectasis resolves. *Change in ventilator variables:* Resolution of atelectasis and plugging reduces resistance and increases compliance.

Monitoring: The following should be chosen as appropriate for monitoring a patient's response to postural drainage therapy, before, during, and after therapy: subjective response—pain, discomfort, dyspnea, response to therapy; pulse rate, dysrhythmia, and ECG if available; breathing pattern and rate, symmetrical chest expansion, synchronous thoracoabdominal movement, flail chest; sputum production (quantity, color, consistency, odor) and cough effectiveness; mental function; skin color; breath sounds; blood pressure; oxygen saturation, by pulse oximetry (if hypoxemia is suspected); intracranial pressure (ICP).

From AARC Clinical Practice Guideline; see Respir Care 36:1418, 1991, for complete text.

requires a generally optimistic view of people, a positive view of their strengths, and an acceptance of their weaknesses. This generates an atmosphere of warmth and caring. The patient must feel accepted unconditionally. Empathy is the art of viewing the world from the patient's point of view while remaining one's self. Empathy entails

RESPIRATORY ASSESSMENT FLOW CHART

Subjective →	Objective →	Assessment →	Plan →
	Vital signs: RR 32 HR 140 BP 155/115		PRESENT PLAN
	Temp. — On antipyretic agent? ☐ Yes ☐ No		
"I've been wheezing for about three days. It appears to be getting worse."	Chest assessment: Insp. Using accessory muscles of inspr. Pursed-lip breathing. Shallow breaths.		
	Palp. —		
	Perc. Hyperresonant bilaterally		
Anterior (R, L)	Ausc. Bilateral wheezing	Bronchospasm	PLAN MODIFICATIONS
			1. Bronchodilator Tx
	Radiography Severely depressed diaphragm	Airtrapping	
Posterior (L, R)	Bedside spir.: PEFR ā 180 p̄ ___ Tx SVC ___ FVC ___ NIF ___		
	Cough: ☐ Strong ☐ Weak Sputum production: ☐ Yes ☒ No Sputum char. ___		
Pt. name Age 46 / Male / Female X Date — / Time —	ABG: pH 7.54 $PaCO_2$ 26 HCO_3^- 20 PaO_2 57 SaO_2 ___ SpO_2 ___ Neg. O_2 transport factors ___	Acute alveolar hyperventilation with moderate hypoxemia. Possible impending ventilatory failure.	2. Oxygen Tx per protocol 3. Ventilator on standby.
Admitting diagnosis Asthma Therapist Hospital	Other:		

PROTOCOL 6-1. Assessment flowchart.

recognition and acceptance of the patient's feelings without criticism. It is sometimes described as feeling *with* the patient rather than feeling *like* the patient.

To have empathy, the practitioner needs to listen. Listening is not a passive process. Listening is active and demanding. Listening requires the practitioner's complete attention. If the examiner is preoccupied with personal needs or concerns, something important will invariably be missed. Active listening is an essential cornerstone to understanding. Nearly everything that the patient says or does is relevant.

During the interview, the examiner should observe the patient's body language and note such things as the patient's facial expressions, eye movement (eg, avoiding eye contact, looking into space, diverting gaze), pain grimaces, restlessness, or sighing. The examiner should listen to the way things are said. For example, is the tone of the patient's voice normal? Does the patient's voice quiver? Are there pitch breaks in the patient's voice? Does the patient say only a few words and then take a breath?

External Factors

A good physical setting enhances the interviewing process. Regardless of where the interview takes place (the patient's bedside, an office in the hospital or clinic, or in the patient's home), efforts should be made to ensure privacy, refuse interruptions, and secure a comfortable physical environment (eg, room temperature, sufficient lighting, absence of noise).

Techniques of Communication

During the interview, the patient should be addressed with his or her surname, and the examiner should introduce himself or herself and the purpose for being there. For example, "Good morning Mr. Jones, I'm Mrs. Smith, and I'm from Respiratory Care. I want to ask you some questions about your breathing so that we can plan your respiratory care here in the hospital."

Verbal skills or techniques used by the examiner to facilitate the interview may include open-ended questions, closed or direct questions, and responses.

☐ OPEN-ENDED QUESTIONS

An open-ended question asks the patient to provide narrative information. The examiner identifies the topic to be discussed but only in general terms. This technique is commonly used to begin the interview, to introduce a new section of questions, or to gather further information whenever the patient introduces a new topic. Here are some examples:

"How are you feeling?"
"Tell me why you have come to the hospital today."
"How has your breathing been getting along?"
"You said that you have been short of breath. Tell me more about that."

The open-ended question is unbiased; it allows the patient freedom to answer in any way. This type of question encourages the patient to respond "in paragraphs" and to give a spontaneous account of his or her condition. As the patient answers, the examiner should stop and listen. Frequently the patient answers in short phrases or sentences, pauses, and then looks at the examiner for some kind of direction as to how to go on. What the examiner does next is often the key to the direction of the interview. If the examiner presents new questions on other topics, much of the initial story may be lost. Ideally, the examiner should first respond by saying such things as "Tell me about it," or "Anything else?" The patient commonly adds important information to the story.

☐ CLOSED OR DIRECT QUESTIONS

A closed or direct question asks the patient for specific information. This type of question elicits a short, one- or two-word answer, a yes or no, or a forced choice. The closed question is commonly used after the patient's narrative, to fill in any details the patient may have left out. Closed questions are also used to obtain specific facts, such as "Have you ever had this chest pain before?" Closed or direct questions also work to speed up the interview. The use of only open-ended questions is unwieldy and takes an unrealistic amount of time, overly stressing the patient. Box 6-1 compares closed and open-ended questions.

☐ RESPONSES—ASSISTING THE NARRATIVE

As the patient answers the open-ended questions, the examiner's role is to encourage free expression, but not let the patient wander off the subject. The examiner's responses work to clarify the story. There are nine types of verbal responses. In the first five responses, the patient leads; in the last four responses, the examiner leads.

BOX 6-1

COMPARISON OF OPEN-ENDED AND CLOSED QUESTIONS

Open-Ended Questions	Direct, Closed Questions
Used for narrative information	Used for specific information
Calls for long-paragraph answers	Calls for short, one- or two-word answers
Elicits feeling, opinions, ideas	Elicits "cold facts"
Builds and enhances rapport	Limits rapport and leaves interaction neutral

The first five responses require the examiner's reactions to the facts or feelings the patient has communicated. The examiner's response focuses on the patient's frame of reference; the examiner's frame of reference does not enter into the response. For the last four responses, the examiner's reactions are not required. The frame of reference shifts from the patient's perspective to the examiner's. These responses include the examiner's own thoughts or feelings. The examiner should only use these responses when merited by the situation. If these responses are used too often, the examiner takes over at the patient's expense. The nine responses are as follows.

1. **Facilitation.** This response encourages the patient to say more, to continue on with the story. For example, "mm-hmm, go on, continue, uh-huh." This type of response shows the patient you are interested in what he or she is saying and will listen further. Maintaining eye contact, or shifting forward in your seat with increased attention, further encourages the patient to continue talking.
2. **Silence.** Silent attentiveness is effective after an open-ended question. It communicates that the patient has time to think, to organize what he or she wishes to say without interruption from the examiner.
3. **Reflection.** This response is used to echo the patient's words. It repeats a part of what the patient has just said to clarify or stimulate further communication. Reflection helps the patient to focus on specific areas and to continue on in his or her own way. Here is an example:

   Patient: "I'm here because of my breathing. It's blocked."

   Examiner: "It's blocked?"

   Patient: "Yes, every time I try to exhale, something blocks my breath and prevents me from getting all my air out."

   Reflection can also be used to express feeling behind the patient's words. The feeling is already present in the patient's statement. The examiner focuses on it and encourages the patient to elaborate. Here is an example:

   Patient: "I have three little ones at home. I'm so worried they're not getting the care they need."

   Examiner: "You feel worried and anxious about your children."

   The examiner acts as a mirror reflecting the patient's words and feelings. This helps the patient to elaborate on the problem.
4. **Empathy.** A physical symptom, condition, or disease frequently has accompanying emotions. Oftentimes, a patient has trouble expressing these feelings. An empathic response recognizes a patient's feelings and allows expression of it. The following is an example:

   Patient: "This is just great! I used to work out every day, and now I don't have enough breath to walk up the stairs!"

   Examiner: "It must be hard—you used to exercise every day, and now you can't do a fraction of what you used to do."

The examiner's response does not cut off further communication, which would occur by giving false reassurance (eg, "Oh, you'll be back on your feet in no time."). Also, it does not deny the patient's feelings, nor does it suggest that the patient's feelings are not justified. An empathic response recognizes the patient's feelings, accepts them, and allows the patient to express them without embarrassment. It strengthens rapport.

5. **Clarification.** This technique is used when the patient's choice of words is ambiguous or confusing. For example, "Tell me what you mean by 'bad air.' " Clarification is also used to summarize the patient's words and to simplify the words to make them clearer. When the examiner simplifies the patient's words, she should then stop and ask if she is on the right track. The examiner is asking for agreement, and this allows the patient to confirm or disagree with the examiner's understanding.
6. **Confrontation.** In this technique, the examiner notes a certain action, feeling, or statement made by the patient and focuses the patient's attention on it. For example, "You said it doesn't hurt when you cough, but when you cough you grimace." Or it may focus on the patient's affect: "You look depressed today," or "You sound angry."
7. **Interpretation.** This technique links events and data, makes associations, or implies causes. It provides the basis for inference or conclusion. "It seems that every time you have a serious asthma attack, you have had some kind of stress in your life." The examiner does run a risk of making the wrong inference. But even if the inference is corrected by the patient, the patient's response often works to prompt further discussion of the topic.
8. **Explanation.** This is used to provide the patient with factual and objective information. For example, "It is very common for your heart rate to increase a bit after a bronchodilator treatment."
9. **Summation.** This is the final overview of what the examiner understands the patient to have said. It condenses the facts and presents an outline of how the examiner perceives the patient's respiratory status. It is a type of validation in that the patient can agree or disagree with the examiner's summary. Both the examiner and the patient should participate in the summary. The summary signals that the interview is about to end.

Nonproductive Verbal Messages

In addition to the nine verbal techniques presented above that are commonly used to enhance the interview, the examiner needs to be aware of, and avoid, nonproductive, verbal messages. These messages restrict the patient's response. They work as barriers to obtaining data and to establishing rapport. During the interview, the examiner should avoid the following common mistakes:

□ PROVIDING ASSURANCE OR REASSURANCE

Patient: "I'm so worried about the mass the doctor found on my chest x-ray. I hope it doesn't turn out to be cancer! What happens to your lung?"

Examiner: "Now don't worry. I'm sure you will be all right. You have a very good doctor."

The above "courage-building" response gives the examiner the false sense of having provided comfort. In fact, this type of response probably does more to relieve the examiner's anxiety than that of the patient. The examiner's response trivializes the patient's concern and effectively closes off any further communication about the topic. Instead, the examiner may have responded in a more empathic way. The following is an example:

Examiner: "You are really worried about that mass on your x-ray, aren't you? It must be very hard to wait for the lab results."

These responses acknowledge the patient's feelings and concerns and, importantly, keep the door open for further communication.

□ GIVING ADVICE

The key here is to know when to give it and when to refrain from it. Often, the patient seeks your professional advice and opinion on a specific topic. Here is an example:

Patient: "What types of things should I avoid to keep my asthma under control?"

This is a straightforward request for information that the examiner has and the patient needs. The examiner should respond directly, and the answer should be based on knowledge and experience.

The examiner should avoid advice based on a hunch or feeling. For example, consider the patient who has just seen the doctor:

Patient: "Dr. Johnson has just told me I may need an operation to remove the mass they found in my lungs. I just don't know. What would you do?"

If the examiner answers with what he or she would do, the accountability for decision making shifts from the patient to the examiner. The examiner is not the patient. The patient has to work this problem out. In fact, it is doubtful that the patient really wants to know what the examiner would do. In this case, it is more likely that the patient is worried about what she might have to do. Instead, a better response could be reflection. An example is the following:

Examiner: "Have an operation?"

Patient: "Yes, and I've never been put to sleep before. What do they do if you don't wake up?"

Now the examiner knows the patient's real concern and can work to help the patient to deal with it. For the patient to accept it, advice must be meaningful and appropriate. For example, in planning pulmonary rehabilitation for a male patient with severe emphysema, the respiratory therapist advises the patient to undertake a moderate walking program. The patient may treat the therapist's advice in one of two ways: either to follow it or not. The patient may choose to ignore it, feeling that it is not appropriate for him (eg, he feels he gets plenty of exercise at work anyway). On the other hand, if the patient does follow the therapist's advice, there are three possible outcomes: the patient's condition stays the same, it improves, or it worsens. If the walking strengthens the patient, the condition improves. However, if the patient was not part of the decision-making process to initiate a walking program, the psychological reward will be limited. This promotes further dependency. If the walking program does not improve his condition, or compromises it, the advice did not work. Because the advice was not the patient's, he can avoid any responsibility for the failure. For example, the patient might say something like this:

"See, I did what you advised me to do, and it didn't help. In fact, I feel worse! Why did you tell me to do this anyway?"

Though it may be quicker just to give advice, the examiner should take the time to involve the patient in the problem-solving process. When the patient is an active player in the decision-making process, the patient is more likely to learn and to modify behavior.

□ USING AUTHORITY

The examiner should avoid responses that promote dependency and inferiority. For example,

Examiner: "Now, your doctor and therapist know best."

Although the examiner and the patient cannot have equality in terms of professional skills and experience, both the examiner and the patient are equally worthy human beings, and each should respect the other.

□ USING AVOIDANCE LANGUAGE

When talking about potentially fearful topics, people often use euphemisms (eg, "passed on" rather than "died") to avoid reality or to hide their true feelings. Though it may appear that the use of euphemisms makes a frightening topic more comfortable, it generally does not. The use of euphemisms does not make the topic or the fear go away. In fact, not talking about a fearful subject suppresses the patient's feelings and, often, makes the subject even more frightening. The use of direct and clear language is the best way to deal with potentially frightening or uncomfortable topics.

□ DISTANCING

Distancing is the use of impersonal conversation that places space between a frightening topic and the speaker. For example, a patient with a lung mass may say, "A friend of mind has a tumor on her lung. She is afraid that she may need an operation," or "There is a tumor in the left lung." By using "the" rather than "my," the patient can deny any association with the tumor. Occasionally, health care workers also use distancing to soften reality. As a general rule, this does not work because it communicates to the patient that the health care practitioner is also afraid of the topic. The use of frank, specific terms usually helps to defuse anxiety, rather than causing it.

□ PROFESSIONAL JARGON

What is called a myocardial infarction by the health care worker is called a heart attack by the patient. The use of professional jargon can sound very exclusionary and paternalistic to the patient. Thus, health care practitioners should always try to adjust their vocabulary to the patient's understanding. Efforts should be made, however, to avoid sounding condescending. Even if the patient uses medical terms, it can not be assumed that he or she fully understands the meaning. For example, patients often think the term "hypertension" means that they are very tense and, therefore, only take their medication when they are feeling stressed, and not when they feel relaxed.

□ ASKING LEADING OR BIASED QUESTIONS

Asking a patient, "You don't smoke anymore, do you?" implies that one answer is better than another. The patient is forced to either answer in a way corresponding to the examiner's values, or feel guilty when admitting the other answer. To respond to this type of question, the patient risks the examiner's disapproval and possible alienation, something the patient does not wish to do.

□ TALKING TOO MUCH

Some examiners feel helpfulness is directly related to verbal productivity. If the air has been full of their sound waves and advice, they leave feeling they have met the patient's needs. In fact, the opposite is true. The patient needs time to talk. As a general rule, the examiner should **listen** more than talk.

□ INTERRUPTING AND ANTICIPATING

While the patient is speaking, the examiner should avoid interrupting or cutting the patient off when she thinks she knows what the patient is about to say. This does not facilitate the interview. Rather, it communicates to the patient that the examiner is impatient or bored with the interview.

Another trap is thinking about the next question while the patient is answering the last one. This is called anticipating the answer. The examiner is not really listening when he is so preoccupied with his role as the interviewer. As a general rule, the examiner should allow for a second or so of silence between the patient's statement and the next question.

□ THE USE OF "WHY" QUESTIONS

The examiner should be careful of the way in which "why" questions are presented. The use of "why" questions often implies blame; it puts the patient on the defensive. For example, "Why did you wait so long before calling your doctor?" or "Why didn't you take your asthma medication with you?" The only possible answer to a "why" question is "Because . . . ," and this places the patient in an uncomfortable position. To avoid this trap, the examiner might say, "I noticed you didn't call your doctor right away when you were having trouble breathing. I'd like to find out what was happening during this time."

Nonverbal Skills

Nonverbal modes of communication include physical appearance, posture, gestures, facial expression, eye contact, voice, and touch. Nonverbal messages are very important in establishing rapport and conveying feelings. Nonverbal messages may either support or contradict verbal messages. Thus, it is important to be aware of the nonverbal messages that may be conveyed by either the patient or the examiner during the interview process.

□ PHYSICAL APPEARANCE

The examiner's general personal appearance, grooming, and choice of clothing send a message to the patient. Professional dress codes vary among hospitals and clinical settings. Depending on the setting, a professional uniform can project a message that ranges from comfortable or casual to formal or distant. Regardless of one's choice in clothing and general appearance, the aim should be to convey a competent and professional image.

□ POSTURE

An open position refers to a posture that demonstrates extension of large muscle groups (ie, arms and legs are not crossed). An open position shows relaxation, physical comfort, and a willingness to share information. A closed position, with arms and legs crossed, sends a defensive and anxious message. The examiner should be aware of any posture changes the patient makes. For example, if the patient suddenly shifts from a relaxed to a tense position, it suggests a discomfort with the topic. In addition, the examiner should try to sit comfortably next to the patient during the interview. Sitting too far away or standing over the patient often sends a negative nonverbal message.

□ GESTURES

Gestures send nonverbal messages. For example, pointing a finger may show anger or blame. Nodding of the head, or an open hand with the palms turned upward, can show acceptance, attention, or agreement. A wringing of the hands suggests worry and anxiety. Patients often describe a crushing chest pain by holding a fist in front of the sternum. When a patient has a sharp, localized pain, one finger is commonly used to point to the exact spot of discomfort.

□ FACIAL EXPRESSION

A person's face can convey a wide range of emotions and conditions. For example, facial expressions can reflect alertness, relaxation, anxiety, anger, suspicion, and pain. The examiner should work to convey an attentive, sincere, and interested expression. Patient rapport will deteriorate if the examiner reflects such facial expressions as boredom, distraction, disgust, criticism, or disbelief.

□ EYE CONTACT

Lack of eye contact suggests that a person may be insecure, intimidated, shy, withdrawn, confused, bored, apathetic, or depressed. The examiner should work to maintain good eye contact, but yet not stare the patient down with a fixed, penetrating look. Generally, an easy gaze toward the patient's eyes with occasional glances away works well. The examiner, however, should be aware that this may not apply when interviewing a patient from a culture that normally avoids direct eye contact. For example, Asian, Native American, Indochinese, Arab, and Appalachian people may consider direct eye contact as impolite or aggressive, and they may divert their own eyes during the interview.

□ VOICE

Nonverbal messages are reflected through the tone of voice, the intensity and rate of speech, the pitch, and long pauses. Often, these messages convey more meaning than the spoken word. For example, a patient's voice may show sarcasm, anxiety, sympathy, or hostility. An anxious patient frequently talks in a loud and fast voice. A soft voice may reflect shyness and fear. A patient with hearing impairment generally speaks in a loud voice. Long pauses may have important meanings. For instance, when a patient pauses for a long time before answering an easy and straightforward question, the honesty of the answer may be an issue. Slow speech with very long and frequent pauses, combined with a weak and monotonous voice, suggests depression.

□ TOUCH

The meaning of touch is often misinterpreted. The meaning of touch is influenced by an individual's age, sex, cultural background, past experiences, and the present setting. As a general rule, the examiner should not touch a patient during an interview unless he or she knows the patient well and is sure how it will be interpreted. When appropriate, touch (such as a touch of the hand or arm) can be very effective in conveying empathy.

To summarize, the nonverbal messages communicated by both the examiner and patient may be extensive during the course of an interview. Thus, the examiner needs to be aware of the various nonverbal messages generated by the patient while, at the same time, working to communicate nonverbal messages that are productive and enhancing to the examiner-patient relationship. Box 6-2 provides an overview of nonverbal messages that can be projected during an interview.

BOX 6-2

NONVERBAL MESSAGES OF THE INTERVIEW

Positive	Negative
Professional appearance	Nonprofessional appearance
Sitting next to patient	Sitting behind a desk
Close proximity to patient	Far away from patient
Turned toward patient	Turned away from patient
Relaxed, open posture	Tense, closed posture
Leaning toward patient	Slouched away from patient
Facilitating gestures—nodding of head	Nonfacilitating gestures—looking at watch
Positive facial expressions	Negative facial expression
Appropriate smiling	Frowning
Interest	Yawning
Good eye contact	Poor eye contact
Moderate tone of voice	Strident, high-pitched voice
Moderate rate of speech	Speech too fast or too slow
Appropriate touch	Too frequent or inappropriate touch

Closing the Interview

The interview should end gracefully. If the session has an abrupt or awkward closing, the patient may be left with a negative impression about the entire interview. This may destroy patient rapport gained during the interview. To ease into the closing, the examiner might ask the patient one of the following questions:

"Is there anything else that you would like to talk about?"

"Do you have any questions that you would like to ask me?"

"Are there any other problems that I should have asked you about?"

The above types of questions give the the patient the opportunity of self-expression. The examiner may choose to give a summary or a recapitulation of what was learned during the interview. This serves as a final statement of what the examiner and patient agree the health state of the patient to be. The examiner should thank the patient for the time and cooperation provided during the interview and outline (if possible) the plan for subsequent interfaces with him. Promising that you, or someone with equal competence, will see the patient again is very comforting.[9–23]

THE PHYSICAL EXAMINATION

Vital Signs

The *vital signs* are used as an initial assessment measurement. The vital signs, which can be obtained quickly in the clinical setting, are an objective evaluation of the patient's immediate condition or response to therapy. Collectively, the vital signs are the body temperature, pulse rate, blood pressure, and respiratory rate (Box 6-3).[24–28]

□ BODY TEMPERATURE

The normal mean body temperature is about 37°C (98.6°F), with a daily variation of 0.5°C (1 to 2°F). At normal body temperature, the metabolic functions of all the body cells are optimal. When the body temperature increases or decreases significantly from the normal range, the metabolic rate and, therefore, the demands on the cardiopulmonary system also change. For example, when the body temperature increases, the metabolic rate increases. This action in turn results in an increased oxygen consumption and carbon dioxide production at the cellular level. It is estimated that for every 1°C increase in body temperature, oxygen consumption increases about 10%. As the metabolic rate increases, the cardiopulmonary system must work harder to meet the additional cellular demands.

An increased body temperature can occur as a result of strenuous exercise or disease. An increased temperature caused by disease is called fever. A patient with a fever is said to be febrile. A fever is commonly seen in patients with viral or bacterial infections. Based on fluctuations over a 24-hour period, a fever may be referred to as continuous, intermittent, or remittent. An intermittent fever has peaks and valleys, with the decreases reaching normal or below normal. A remittent fever is characterized by marked peaks and valleys, but the body temperature does not return to normal between the spikes.

When the patient's temperature falls below the normal range, hypothermia is said to be present. Hypothermia may occur in patients exposed to cold environmental temperatures and in patients with trauma to the hypothalamus. Hypothermia reduces the metabolic rate and cardiopulmonary demand.

BOX 6-3

NORMAL VITAL SIGNS

Vital Sign	Newborn	Adult
Pulse rate	110–160 bpm	60–100 bpm
Respiratory rate	30–60 breaths/min	10–16 breaths/min
Body temperature	36.5–37.5°C	36.5–37.5°C
Blood pressure		
Systolic	50–70 mmHg	95–140 mmHg
Diastolic	30–50 mmHg	60–90 mmHg
Mean	38–52 mmHg	80–100 mmHg
Pulse pressure	15–25 mmHg	35–50 mmHg

The body temperature is most often measured orally. It can also be measured in the axilla, rectum, or ear. Compared to the oral temperature, the rectal temperature is normally about 1°F higher, and the axillary temperature is 1°F lower. Because oxygen therapy via nasal cannula, simple mask, or oxygen entrainment does not significantly affect the oral temperature, it is not necessary to remove the oxygen from the patient receiving such therapies, nor take a rectal or axillary temperature. The oral temperature, however, may be increased in the patient receiving a heated aerosol and decreased in the patient receiving a cool mist aerosol. Measurement of oral temperature should not be attempted in newborns, unconscious patients, or patients with an oral endotracheal tube in place.

□ PULSE RATE

In the normal adult, the pulse rate (or heart rate) is between 60 and 100 beats per minute (bpm). The pulse should be evaluated for rate, strength, and rhythm. A pulse rate greater than 100 bpm is called tachycardia. Tachycardia may occur as a result of hypoxemia, anemia, fever, anxiety, fear, hypotension, and exercise. Tachycardia is also a common side effect in patients receiving certain medications, such as sympathomimetic agents. Bradycardia is a pulse rate below 60 bpm. Bradycardia may be seen in hypothermia and in physically fit athletes.

The strength of the pulse is a reflection of left ventricular contraction. A weak peripheral pulse indicates a decreased cardiac output. Clinically, the strength of the pulse may be recorded on a scale from 0 to 3+ as follows:

0: absent
1+: weak and thready
2+: normal
3+: bounding

□ RESPIRATORY RATE

The normal respiratory rate varies with age. For example, in the newborn, the normal respiratory rate range is between 30 and 60 breaths per minute. In the 1-year-old child, the normal range is between 25 and 35 breaths per minute. The normal range for the preschool child is between 20 and 25 breaths per minute. The normal adolescent and adult range is between 12 and 20 breaths per minute.

Ideally, the respiratory rate should be counted when the patient is not aware. One good method is counting the respiratory rate immediately after taking the pulse, while leaving your fingers on the patient's artery.

An increased breathing rate is called tachypnea. Tachypnea is commonly seen in patients with fever, metabolic acidosis, hypoxemia, pain, or anxiety. A respiratory rate below the normal range is called bradypnea. Bradypnea may occur with hypothermia, head injuries, and drug overdose. In addition to the respiratory rate, the breathing pattern should be assessed. The evaluation of the breathing pattern is discussed later in this chapter.

□ BLOOD PRESSURE

The arterial blood pressure is the force exerted by the circulating volume of blood on the walls of the arteries. Overall, the blood pressure is maintained by the complex interaction of the homeostatic mechanisms of the body, the blood volume, the lumen of the arteries and arterioles, and the force of the cardiac contraction. In the normal adult, the pressure in the aorta and the large arteries is about 120 mmHg during systole and 70 mmHg during diastole. The pulse pressure (the difference between systolic and diastolic pressure) is about 50 mmHg.

Hypertension is defined as a common, often asymptomatic disorder characterized by elevated blood pressure persistently exceeding 140/90 mmHg. Essential hypertension, the most common kind, has no single identifiable cause, but the risk of this disorder is increased with obesity, a high serum sodium level, hypercholesterolemia, and a family history of high blood pressure. Known causes of hypertension include adrenal disorders, such as aldosteronism and Cushing's syndrome, and pheochromocytoma, thyrotoxicosis, toxemia of pregnancy, and chronic glomerulonephritis.

The incidence of hypertension is higher in men than in women, and it is twice as great in blacks as in whites. People with mild or moderate hypertension may be asymptomatic or may experience suboccipital headaches (especially on rising), tinnitus, light-headedness, easy fatigability, and cardiac palpitations. With sustained hypertension, arterial walls become thickened, nonelastic, and resistant to blood flow. This process in turn causes the left ventricle to distend and hypertrophy. Left ventricular hypertrophy may lead to congestive heart failure.

A diastolic pressure higher than 120 mmHg is called malignant hypertension. Malignant hypertension is characterized by severe headaches, blurred vision, and confusion, and it may result in fatal uremia, myocardial infarction, congestive heart failure, or a cerebrovascular accident. A sudden severe increase in blood pressure to a level exceeding 200/120 mmHg is called a hypertensive crisis. A hypertensive crisis is commonly seen in patients who have stopped taking prescribed antihypertensive medication, and it is characterized by numerous signs, which include severe headache, vertigo, diplopia, tinnitus, nosebleed, twitching muscles, tachycardia or other cardiac dysrhythmia, distended neck veins, narrowed pulse pressure, nausea, and vomiting. The patient may be confused, irritable, or stuporous, and the condition may lead to convulsions, coma, myocardial infarction, renal failure, cardiac arrest, congestive heart failure, or stoke.

Hypotension is said to be present when the patient's blood pressure falls below 95/60 mmHg. Hypotension indicates an abnormal condition in which the blood pressure in not adequate for normal perfusion and oxygenation of vital organs. It may be caused by hypovolemia, left ventricular failure, or peripheral vasodilation and is characterized by dizziness, visual blurring, sweating, and occasionally syncope.

The arterial blood pressure commonly fluctuates 2 to 8 mmHg during the normal respiratory cycle, decreasing during inspiration and increasing during expiration. This is because during inspiration the descending diaphragm produces a negative intrapleural pressure, which in turn causes the blood vessels in the lungs to dilate and to pool blood. This action in turn causes the arterial blood pressure to fall. During expiration, the ascending diaphragm causes the intrapleural pressure to rise and the blood vessels in the lungs to narrow. This action enhances left ventricular filling, which in turn increases cardiac output and arterial blood pressure.

Pulsus paradoxus (also called paradoxical pulse) is said to be present when this normal arterial blood pressure fluctuation is greater than 10 mmHg. Pulsus paradoxus may be seen in severe airway obstruction disorders (eg, severe asthma), cardiac tamponade, and constrictive pericarditis. *Pulsus paradoxus* can be detected by using a sphygmomanometer or, in severe cases, by palpating the pulse.

The Systematic Examination of the Chest and Lungs

The physical examination of the chest and lungs should be performed in a systematic and orderly fashion. The most common sequence is as follows:[8,29–35]

- Inspection
- Palpation
- Percussion
- Auscultation

Before the practitioner can adequately inspect, palpate, percuss, and auscultate the chest, however, a good working knowledge of the chest and lung topographical landmarks must first be mastered. Various anatomic landmarks and imaginary vertical lines drawn on the chest are used to identify and document the location of specific abnormalities.

□ LUNG AND CHEST TOPOGRAPHY

Thoracic Cage Landmarks

Anteriorly, the first rib is attached to the manubrium just beneath the clavicle. Once the first rib is identified, the rest of the ribs can easily be located and numbered. The second rib attaches to the sternum at the point where the manubrium and the body of the sternum join. This is the *Angle of Louis*. The sixth rib and its cartilage are attached to the sternum just above the xiphoid process (Fig. 6-1).

Posteriorly, the spinous processes of the vertebrae are useful landmarks. For example, when the patient's head is extended forward and down, two prominent spinous processes can usually be seen at the base of the neck. The top one is the spinous process of the seventh cervical vertebra (C7); the bottom one is the spinous process of the first thoracic vertebra (T1). When only one spinous process can be seen, it is usually C7 (see Fig. 6-1).

Imaginary Lines

Various imaginary vertical lines are used to identify abnormalities on the chest (Fig. 6-2). The midsternal line, which is located in the middle of the sternum, equally divides the anterior chest into left and right hemithoraces. The midclavicular lines, which start at the middle of either the right or left clavicle, run parallel to the sternum.

On the lateral portion of the chest, three vertical lines are used. The anterior axillary line originates at the anterior axillary fold and runs downward along the anterolateral aspects of the chest; the midaxillary line divides the lateral chest into two equal halves; and the posterior axillary line runs parallel to the midaxillary line along the posterolateral wall of the thorax (see Fig. 6-2).

Posteriorly, the vertebral line (also called the midspinal line) runs along the spinous processes of the vertebrae. If only one spinous process can be identified, it is usually C7. The midscapular line runs through the middle of either the right or left scapula and parallels the vertebral line (see Fig. 6-2).

Lung Borders and Fissures

Anteriorly, the apex of the lung extends about 2 to 4 cm above the medial third of the clavicle. Under normal conditions, the lungs extend down to about the level of the sixth rib. Posteriorly, the superior portion of the lung extends to about the level of T1, and the inferior portion extends down to about the level of T10 (Fig. 6-3).

The right lung is separated into the upper, middle, and lower lobes by the horizontal fissure and the oblique fissure. Anteriorly, the horizontal fissure runs from the fourth rib at the sternal border to the fifth rib at the midaxillary line. The horizontal fissure separates the right anterior upper lobe from the middle lobe. The oblique fissure runs laterally from the sixth or seventh rib and the midclavicular line to the fifth rib at the midaxillary line. From this point, the oblique fissure continues to run around the chest posteriorly, and upward, to about the level of T3. Anteriorly, the oblique fissure divides the lower lobe from the lower border of the middle lobe. Posteriorly, the oblique fissure separates the upper lobe from the lower lobe (see Fig. 6-3).

The left lung is separated into the upper and lower lobes by the oblique fissure. Anteriorly, the oblique fissure runs laterally from the sixth or seventh rib and the midclavicular line to the fifth rib at the midaxillary line. The fissure continues to run around the chest posteriorly, and upward, to about the level of T3 (see Fig. 6-3).

□ INSPECTION

The inspection of the patient is an ongoing process that begins with the history taking and the patient interview and should continue throughout the entire physical examination. The inspection of the patient consists of a series of observations that identify general and specific clinical information about the patient's health status. The inspection should include the following:

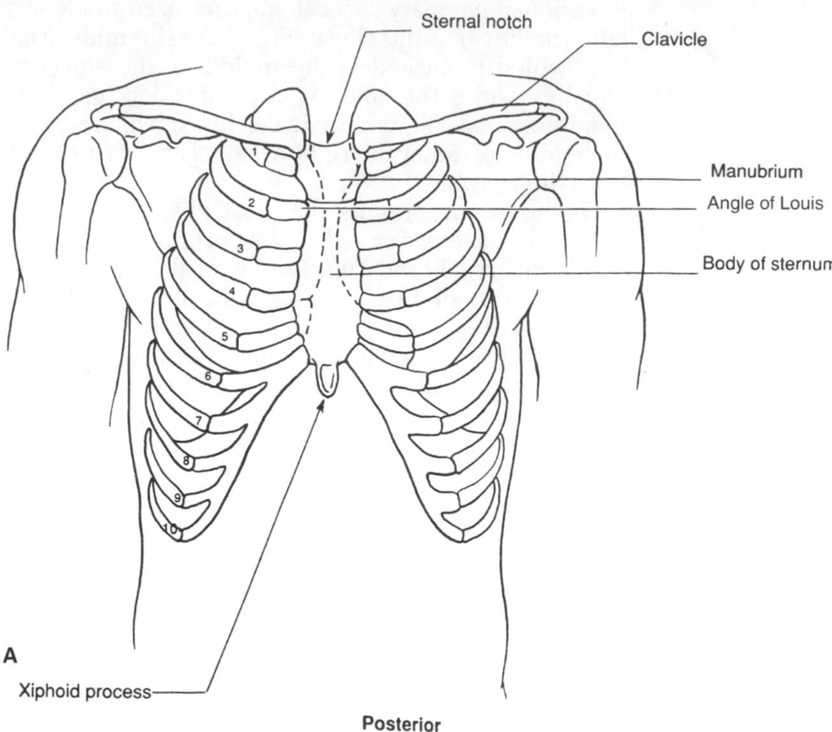

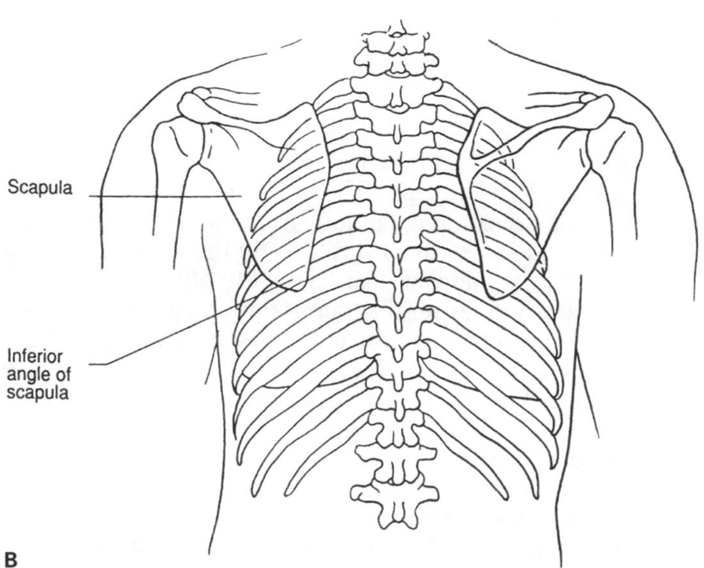

FIGURE 6-1. Anatomic landmarks of the chest. (**A**) Anterior. (**B**) Posterior. (From Matthews: Cardiopulmonary Anatomy and Physiology, Lippincott-Raven Publishers, Philadelphia, 1996.)

Breathing Pattern

The breathing pattern is composed of a tidal volume (V_T), a ventilatory rate, and an inspiratory-expiratory ratio (I:E ratio). In the normal adult, the V_T is about 500 mL (7 to 9 mL/kg), the ventilatory rate is between 12 and 18 breaths per minute, and the I:E ratio is about 1:2. In patients with respiratory disease, however, the breathing pattern is usually abnormal. Box 6-4 lists common abnormal ventilatory patterns associated with respiratory diseases.

Chest Shape and Configuration

The shape and configuration of the chest should be inspected. Does the chest appear normal? Are there any lesions or surgical scars? Is the spine straight? Are the scapulae symmetric? Common chest deformities are the following:

Kyphosis: A "hunchback" appearance caused by curvature of the spine.

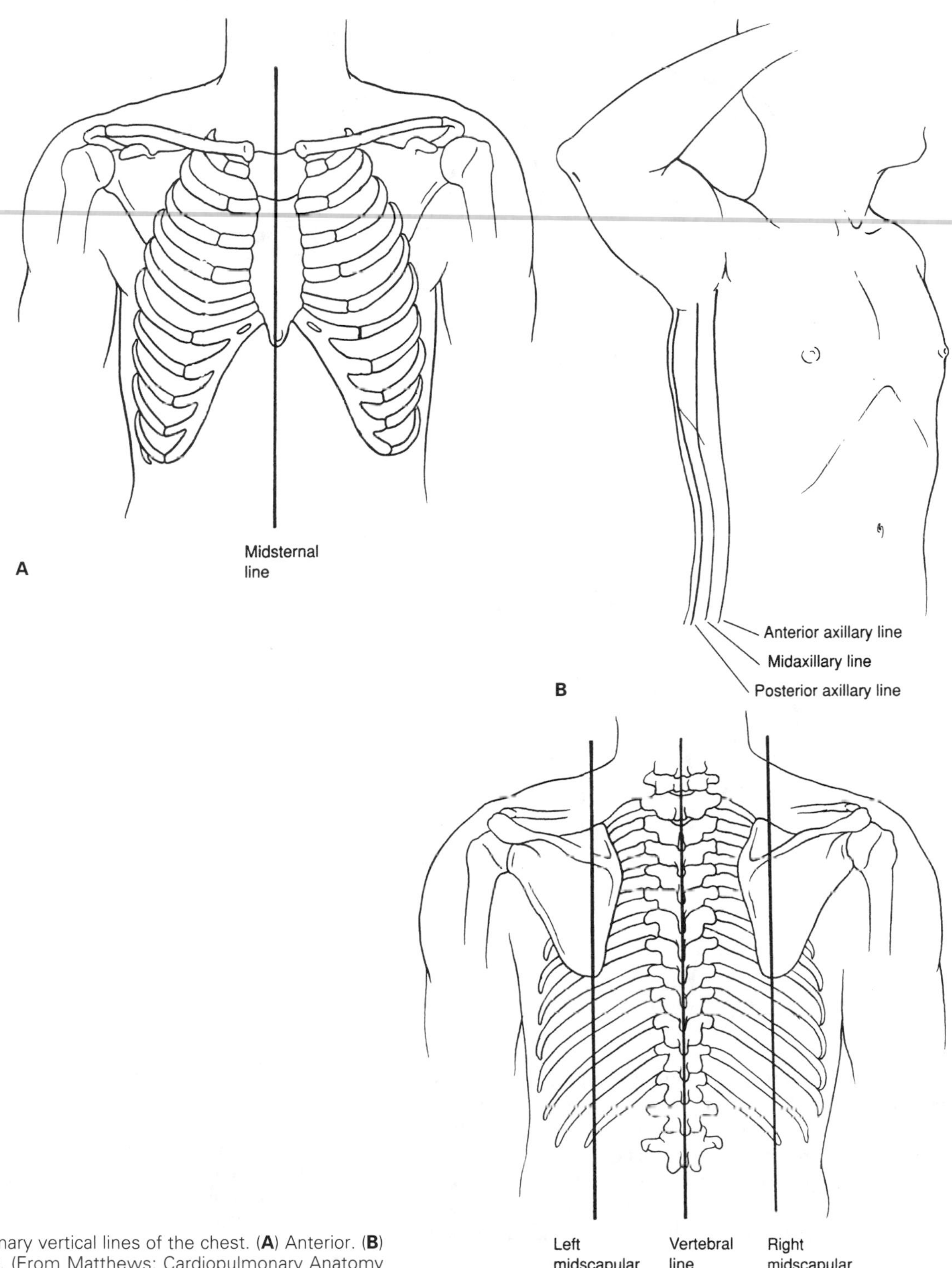

FIGURE 6-2. Imaginary vertical lines of the chest. (**A**) Anterior. (**B**) Lateral. (**C**) Posterior. (From Matthews: Cardiopulmonary Anatomy and Physiology, Lippincott-Raven Publishers, Philadelphia, 1996.)

Scoliosis: A lateral curvature of the spine that results in the chest protruding posteriorly and the anterior ribs flattening out.

Kyphoscoliosis: The combination of kyphosis and scoliosis (Fig. 6-4).

Pectus carinatum: The forward projection of the xiphoid process and lower sternum. Also known as "pigeon breast" deformity.

Pectus excavatum: A funnel-shaped depression over the lower sternum. Also called funnel chest.

Barrel chest: In the normal adult, the anteroposterior diameter of the chest is about half its lateral diameter, that is, a ratio of 1:2. When the patient has a barrel chest, the ratio is nearer to 1:1. It should be noted that the normal infant anteroposterior diameter of the chest has a ratio of about 1:1 (Fig. 6-5).

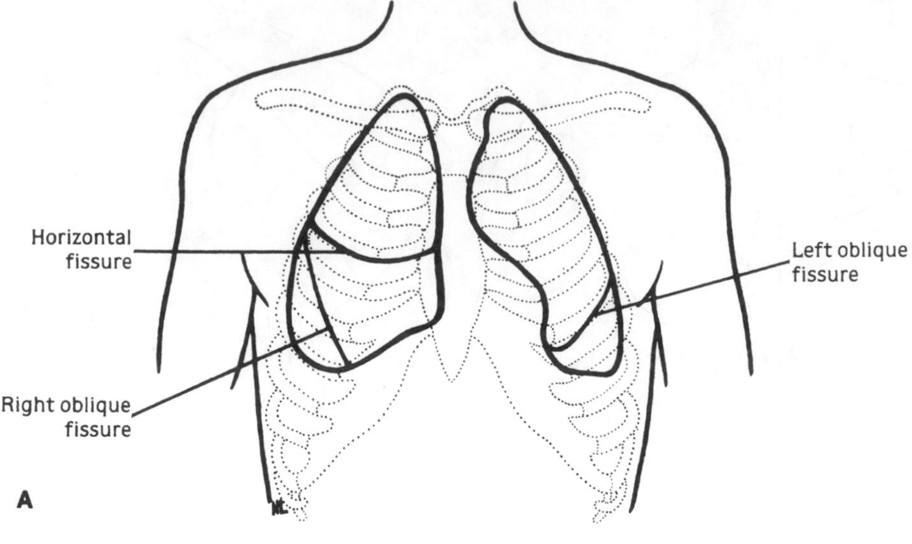

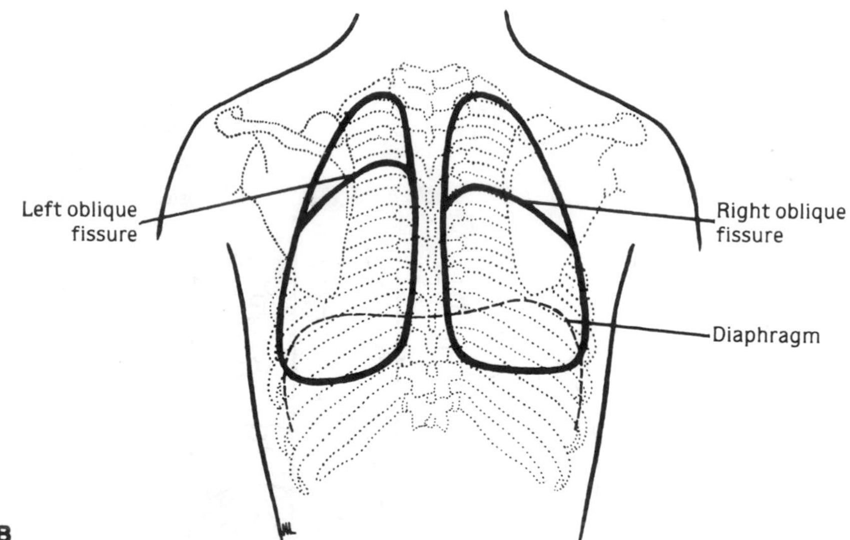

FIGURE 6-3. Topographic location of lung fissures on anterior chest (**A**) and posterior chest (**B**). (Courtesy of Terry Des Jardins.)

Cough

A cough is commonly seen in the patient with respiratory disease. A cough may be voluntary, but it is usually a reflexive response caused by an irritant such as a foreign body (microscopic or larger), infectious agents, or mass of any sort compressing the lungs. A cough is termed productive if sputum is produced, nonproductive when no sputum is produced. The evaluation of the cough should include the following.

Nonproductive Cough

Common causes of a nonproductive cough include (1) irritation of the airway, (2) inflammation of the airways, (3) mucus accumulation, (4) tumors, and (5) irritation of the pleura.

Productive Cough

When the cough is productive, the respiratory practitioner should assess the following:

- Is the cough strong or weak? In other words, does the patient have an adequate or inadequate ability to mobilize bronchial secretions?
- Sputum color
  White and translucent: normal
  Yellow or opaque: indicates acute infection
  Green: old, retained secretions
  Green and foul smelling: *Pseudomonas* or anaerobic infection
  Brown: old blood
  Red: fresh blood

A productive cough should also be evaluated in terms of its frequency of occurrence and pitch and loudness. For example, a "brassy" cough may indicate a tumor, while a "barklike" or "hoarse" cough indicates croup. Finally, the sputum of a productive cough should be monitored and evaluated continuously in terms of amount, consistency, odor, and color.

Inspection of the Extremities

The inspection the patient's extremities should include the following:

Skin color. Is the skin color consistent with the patient's genetic background? Is the skin cyanotic?

BOX 6-4

COMMON ABNORMAL VENTILATORY PATTERNS

Apnea	Complete absence of spontaneous ventilation
Biot's Breathing	Characterized by episodes of rapid, uniformly deep inspirations, followed by long (10 to 30 seconds) periods of apnea. Commonly seen in patients suffering from meningitis or increased intracranial pressure.
Bradypnea	Less than normal rate of breathing
Cheyne-Stokes Breathing	Characterized by a period of apnea lasting 10 to 30 seconds, followed by gradually increasing depth and frequency of respirations. Cheyne-Stokes breathing is associated with cerebral disorders and with congestive heart failure.
Dyspnea	Shortness of breath or a difficulty in breathing, of which the individual is aware
Eupnea	Normal rate and depth of breathing
Hyperpnea	An increased depth (volume) of breathing with or without an increased frequency. A certain degree of hyperpnea is normal immediately after exercise. Hyperpnea is associated with respiratory disease, febrile or cardiac disease, certain drugs, hysteria, or with the hypoxemia experienced at high altitude.
Hyperventilation	An increased alveolar ventilation caused by either an increased ventilatory rate or an increased depth of breathing, or a combination of both, that causes the P_ACO_2 and $PaCO_2$ to decrease
Hypopnea	Decreased depth in rate of breathing
Hypoventilation	A decreased alveolar ventilation caused by either a decreased ventilatory rate or a decreased depth of breathing, or a combination of both, that causes the P_ACO_2 and $PaCO_2$ to increase
Kussmaul Breathing	Both an increased depth (hyperpnea) and rate of breathing (tachypnea). Kussmaul breathing is commonly associated with diabetic acidosis (ketoacidosis).
Orthopnea	A condition in which an individual is able to breathe most comfortably only in the upright position
Tachypnea	A rapid rate of breathing

Used with permission from Des Jardins T, Burton G: Clinical Manifestations and Assessment of Respiratory Disease, *3rd ed. St. Louis, Mosby–Year Book, 1995*

Does the skin appear cold and clammy? Are the nail beds blue?

Digital clubbing. Is there digital clubbing on the patient's fingers or toes (Fig. 6-6)?

Pedal edema. Is there an accumulation of fluid in the subcutaneous tissues of the ankles or face? Bilateral, dependent, pitting edema is frequently seen in the patient with congestive heart failure, cor pulmonale, or hepatic cirrhosis. Pitting edema is graded on a subjective scale of 1+ (mild to slight depression) to 4+ (severe, deep depression).

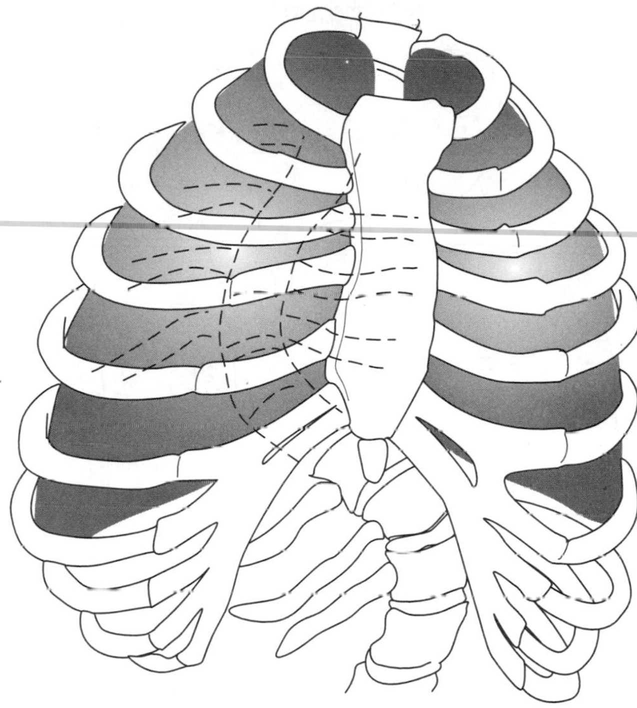

FIGURE 6-4. Posterior and lateral curvature of the spine, causing lung compression and atelectasis.

Signs of Distress

Does the patient appear to be in distress? For example, is the patient using accessory muscles of inspiration (Fig. 6-7)? Is the patient pursed-lip breathing (Fig. 6-8)? Does the patient appear to be in pain or splinting? Are the patient's neck and face veins distended (Fig. 6-9)? Are there substernal or intercostal retractions during inspiration? Is there the presence of audible stridor, wheezing, or rhonchi?

□ PALPATION

Palpation is the process of touching the patient's chest to evaluate the symmetry of chest expansion, the position of the trachea, skin temperature, muscle tone, areas of tenderness, lumps, depressions, and tactile and vocal fremitus. When palpating the chest, the clinician may use the heel of the hand, the ulnar side of the hand, the palms, or the fingertips. As shown in Figure 6-10, both the anterior and posterior chest should be palpated from side to side in an orderly fashion, from the apices of the chest down.

To evaluate the position of the trachea, the examiner places an index finger over the sternal notch and gently moves it from side to side. The trachea should be in the midline directly above the sternal notch. There are a number of abnormal pulmonary conditions that can cause the trachea to deviate from normal. For example,

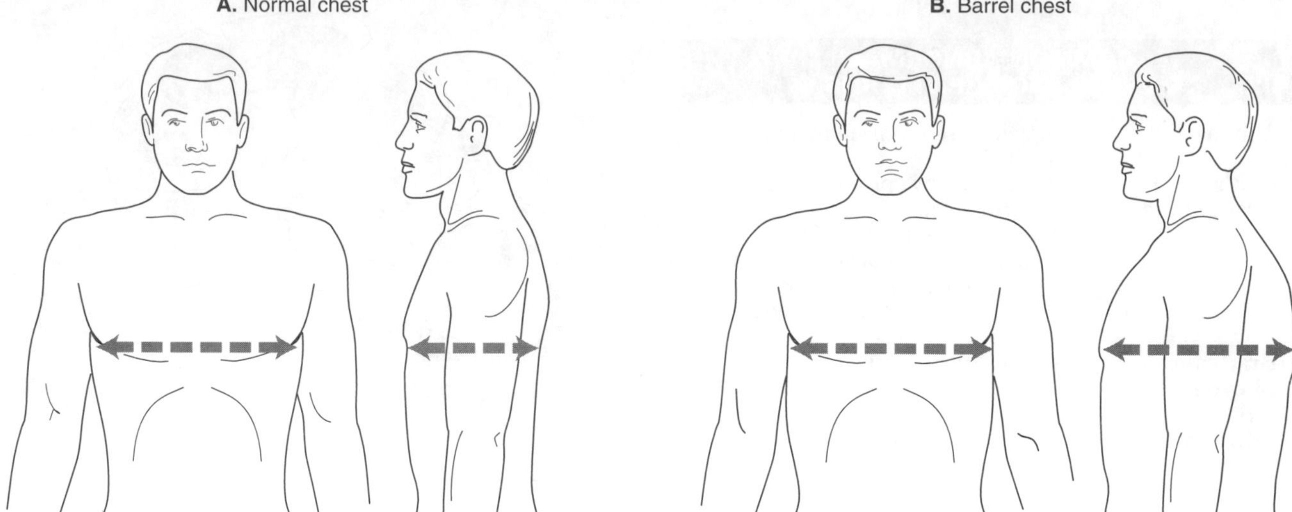

FIGURE 6-5. Normally, the ratio of the anteroposterior chest diameter to the lateral chest diameter is about 1:2 (**A**). In patients who have a barrel chest, however, a ratio nearer to 1:1 is present (**B**).

a tension pneumothorax, pleural effusion, or tumor mass can push the trachea to the unaffected side; atelectasis and pulmonary fibrosis pull the trachea to the affected side.

Chest Excursion

The symmetry of chest expansion is evaluated by lightly placing each hand over the patient's posterolateral chest so that the thumbs meet at the midline at about the T8 to T10 level. The patient is instructed to exhale slowly and completely and then to inhale deeply. As the patient is inhaling, the examiner evaluates the distance that each thumb moves from the midline. Normally, each thumb tip moves equally about 3 to 5 cm from the midline (Fig. 6-11).

Anteriorly, the examiner faces the patient and lightly places each hand on the patient's anterolateral chest so that thumbs meet at the midline along the costal margins near the xiphoid process. The patient is again instructed to exhale slowly and completely and then to inhale deeply. As the patient is inhaling, the examiner observes the distance each thumb moves from the midline (see Fig. 6-11).

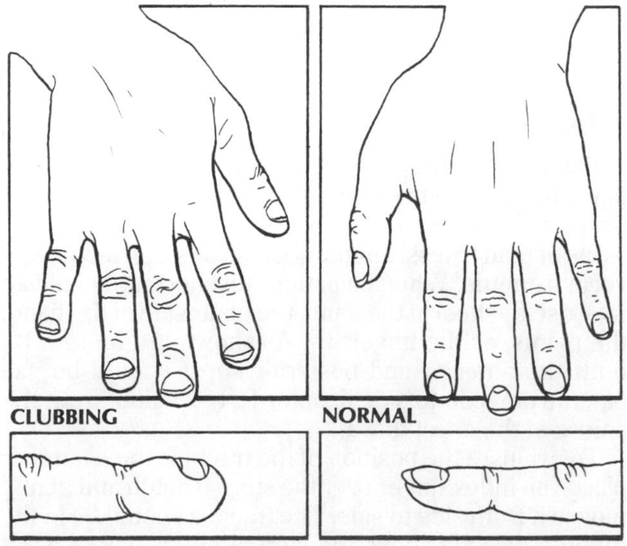

CLUBBING

NORMAL

FIGURE 6-6. Digital clubbing.

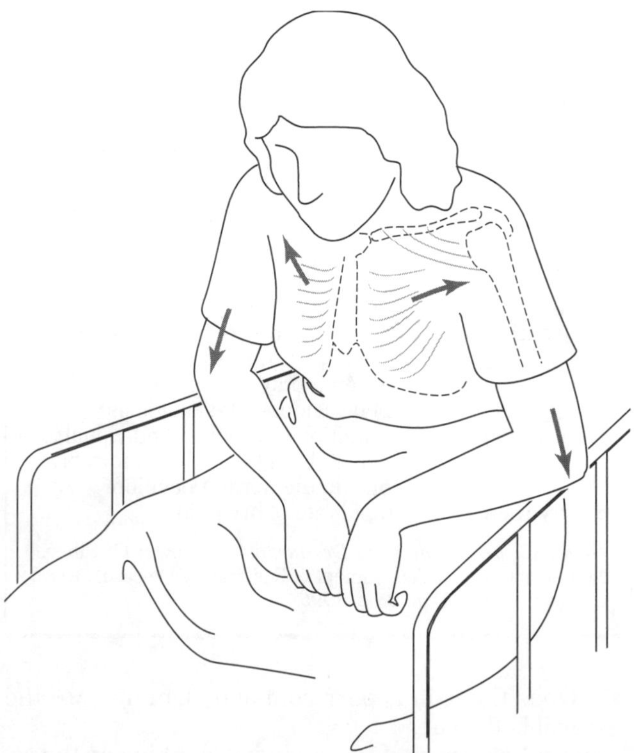

FIGURE 6-7. How a patient may appear when using the pectoralis major muscles.

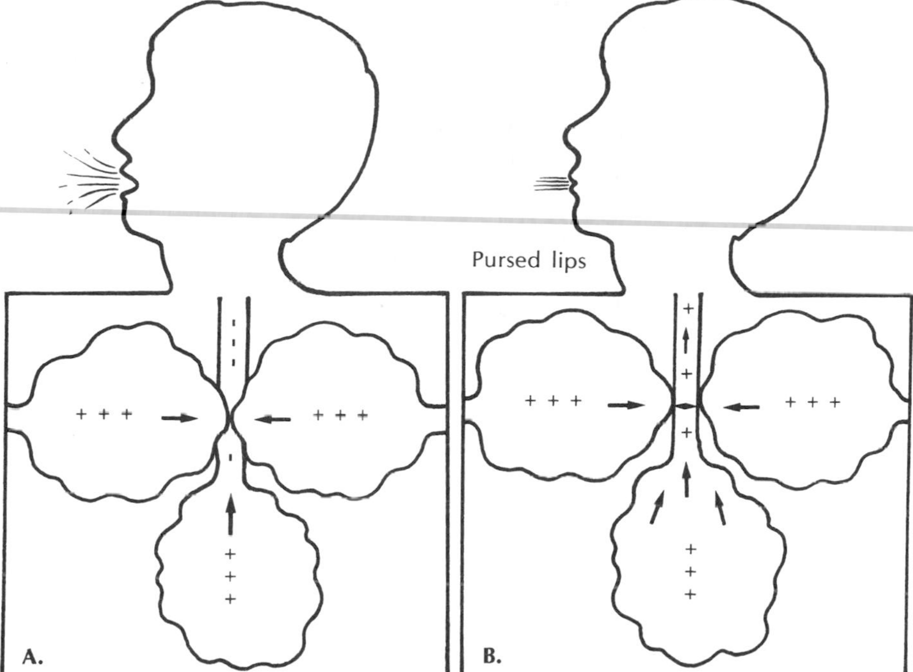

FIGURE 6-8. (**A**) Schematic illustration of alveoli compression of weakened bronchiolar airways during normal expiration in patients with chronic obstructive pulmonary disease (eg, emphysema). (**B**) Effects of pursed-lip breathing. The weakened bronchiolar airways are kept open by the effects of positive pressure created by pursed lips during expiration. (Courtesy of Terry Des Jardins.)

There are a number of pulmonary disorders that can alter the patient's chest excursion. For example, a bilaterally decreased chest expansion may be caused by both obstructive and restrictive lung disorders. An unequal chest expansion may be caused by alveolar consolidation (eg, pneumonia), lobar atelectasis, tension pneumothorax, large pleural effusions, and chest trauma (eg, fractured ribs).

Tactile and Vocal Fremitus

The palpation of vibrations over the chest is called tactile fremitus. *Tactile fremitus* is commonly caused by gas flowing through thick secretions that are partially obstructing the large airways. The palpation of vibrations over the chest during phonation is called vocal fremitus. Sounds produced by the vocal cords are trans-

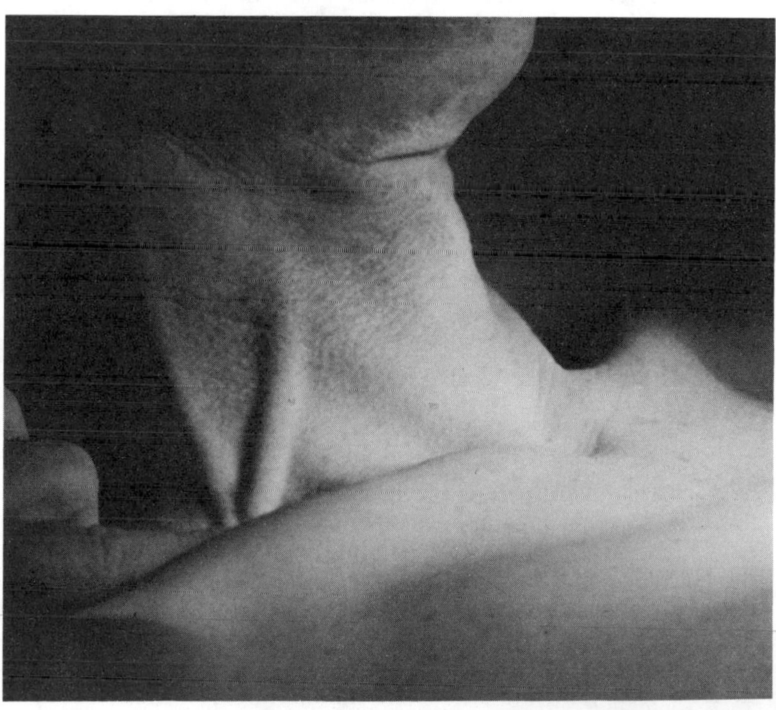

FIGURE 6-9. Photograph of jugular venous distention.

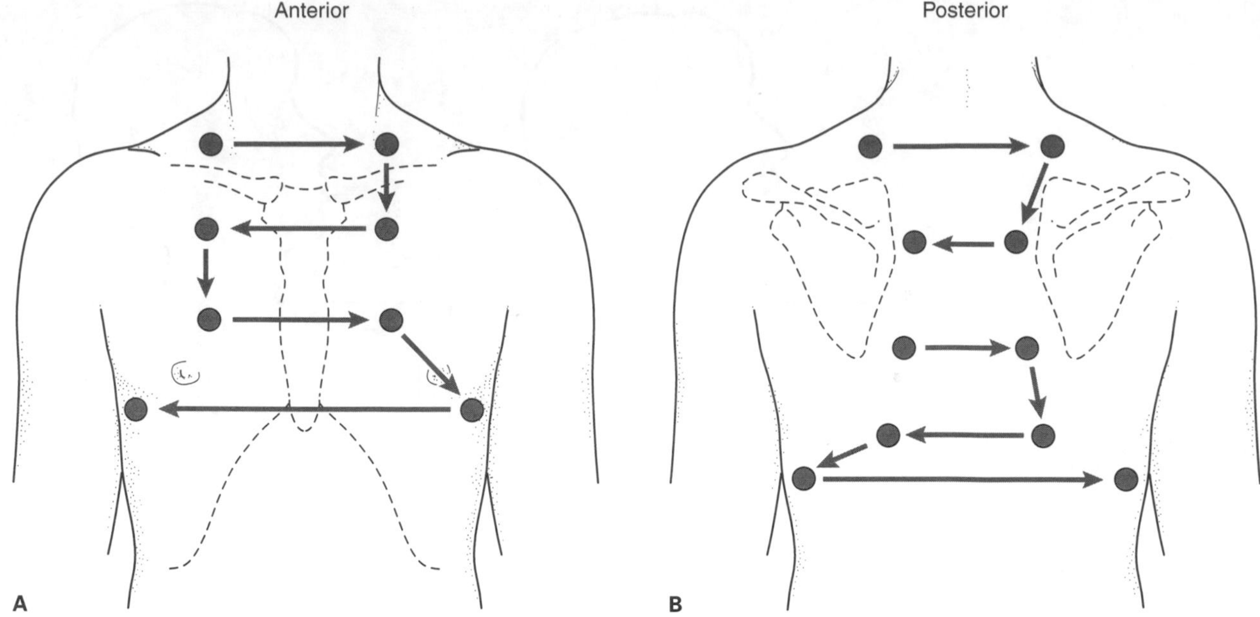

FIGURE 6-10. Path of palpation for vocal or tactile fremitus. (**A**) Anterior. (**B**) Posterior.

mitted down the tracheobronchial tree and through the lung parenchyma to the chest wall where the examiner can feel the vibration. Vocal fremitus can often be elicited by having the patient repeat the phrase "ninety-nine" or "blue moon." These are resonant phrases that produce strong vibrations. Normally, fremitus is most prominent between the scapulae and around the sternum, sites where the large bronchi are closest to the chest wall.

Tactile and vocal fremitus decrease when anything obstructs the transmission of vibration. Such conditions include (1) chronic obstructive pulmonary disease, (2) tumors or thickening of the pleural cavity, (3) pleural effusion, (4) pneumothorax, and (5) a muscular or obese chest wall. Tactile and vocal fremitus increase in patients with (1) alveolar consolidation, (2) alveolar collapse, (3) pulmonary edema, (4) lung tumors, (5) pulmonary fibrosis, and (6) thin chest walls.

Crepitus (also called subcutaneous emphysema) is a coarse, crackling sensation that may be palpable over the skin surface. Crepitus occurs when air escapes from the thorax and enters the subcutaneous tissue. It may also occur following a tracheostomy and mechanical ventilation, or after an open thoracic injury or thoracic surgery.

□ PERCUSSION

Percussion over the chest wall is performed to determine the size, borders, and consistency of air, liquid, or solid material in the underlying lung. When percussing the chest, the examiner firmly places the distal portion of the middle finger of the nondominant hand between the ribs over the surface of the chest area to be examined. No other portion of the hand should touch the patient's chest. With the end of the middle finger of the dominant hand, the examiner quickly strikes the distal joining of the finger positioned on the chest wall and then quickly withdraws the tapping finger (Fig. 6-12). The chest should be percussed in an orderly fashion from the top to the bottom, comparing the sounds generated on both sides of the chest, both anteriorly and posteriorly (Fig. 6-13).

In the normal lung, the sounds produced by percussion are called resonant sounds. The sounds generated by the examiner vibrate freely throughout the large volume of the lungs, producing a sound similar to knocking on a watermelon. Resonant sounds are described as loud, low in pitch, and long in duration. It should be noted that the resonance may be muffled somewhat in the individual with a heavily muscular chest wall and in the obese person.

When percussing the anterior chest, care should be taken to not confuse the normal borders of cardiac dullness with pulmonary pathology. In addition, the upper border of liver dullness is normally located in the fifth intercostal space and midclavicular line. Over the left chest, tympany is produced over the gastric space. When percussing the posterior chest, the examiner should avoid the damping effect of the scapulae.

A dull percussion note is heard when the chest is percussed over areas of pleural thickening, pleural effusion, atelectasis, or consolidation. When these conditions exist, the sounds produced by the examiner do not freely vibrate throughout the lungs. A dull percussion note is described as flat or soft, high in pitch, and short in duration, similar to the sound produced by knocking on a full barrel.

When the chest is percussed over areas of trapped gas, a hyperresonant note is heard. These sounds are described as very loud, low in pitch, and long in duration, similar to the sound produced by knocking on an

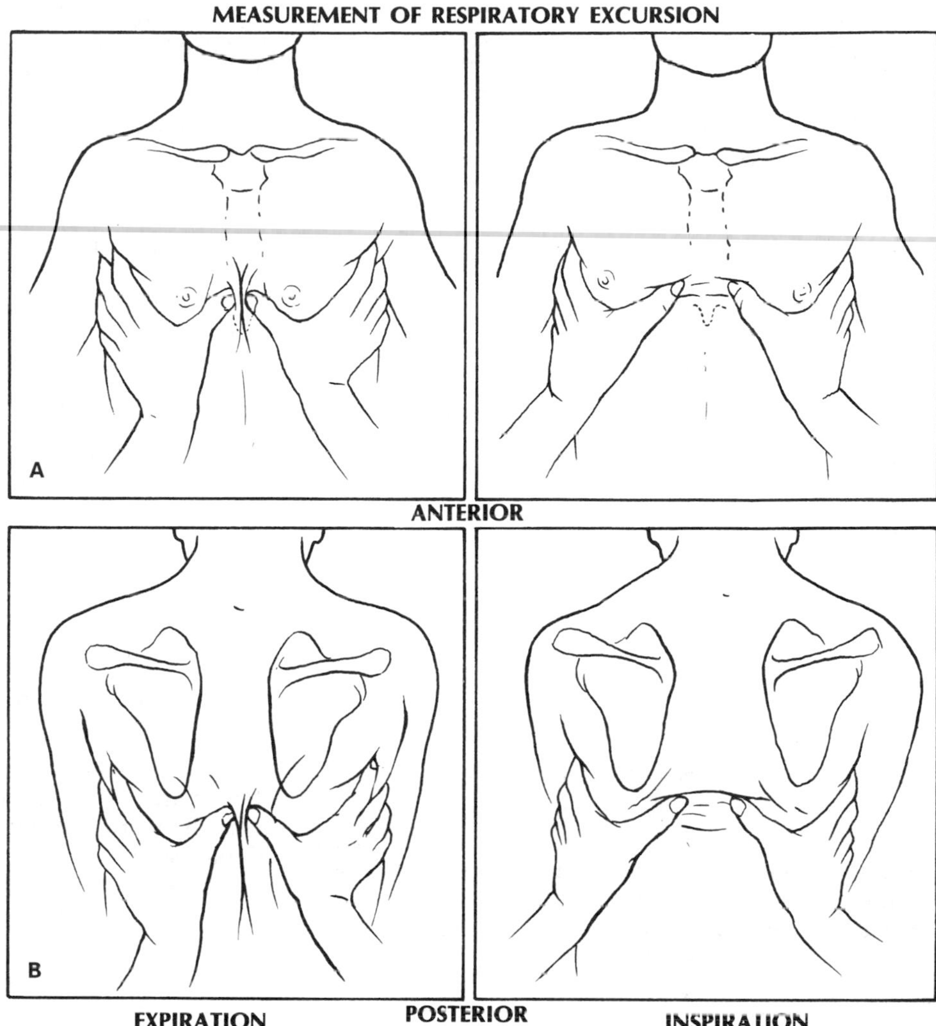

FIGURE 6-11. Assessment of chest excursion. (**A**) Anterior. (**B**) Posterior. (Courtesy of Terry Des Jardins.)

empty barrel. A hyperresonant note is commonly elicited in the patient suffering from a chronic obstructive pulmonary disease or a pneumothorax.

Diaphragmatic Excursion

The relative position and range of motion of the diaphragm can also be determined by percussion. Clinically, this evaluation is called the determination of diaphragmatic excursion. To assess the patient's diaphragmatic excursion, the examiner first maps out the lower lung borders. This is done by percussing the posterior chest from the apex down and identifying the point at which the percussion note definitely changes from a resonant to flat sound. This procedure is then performed at maximal inspiration and again at maximal expiration. Under normal conditions, the diaphragmatic excursion should be equal bilaterally and measure about 4 to 8 cm in the adult.

When severe alveolar hyperinflation is present (eg, severe emphysema or asthma), the diaphragm is low and flat in position and has minimal excursion. Lobar collapse of one lung may pull the diaphragm upward on the affected side and reduce excursion. The diaphragm may be elevated and immobile in neuromuscular diseases that affect the diaphragm.

□ AUSCULTATION

Auscultation of the chest provides information about the heart, blood vessels, and air flowing in and out of the tracheobronchial tree and alveoli. Clinically, a stethoscope is used to evaluate the frequency, intensity, duration, and quality of the sounds. During auscultation, the patient should ideally be in the upright position and instructed to breathe slowly and deeply through the mouth. The anterior and posterior chest should be auscultated in an orderly fashion from the apex to base, comparing the right side of the chest to the left (Fig. 6-14). When examining the posterior chest, the patient should be asked to rotate the shoulder forward so that a greater surface area of the lungs can be auscultated.

Normal Breath Sounds

Three distinctly different breath sounds can be auscultated over the normal chest. They are called bronchial, bronchovesicular, and vesicular breath sounds. Bronchial

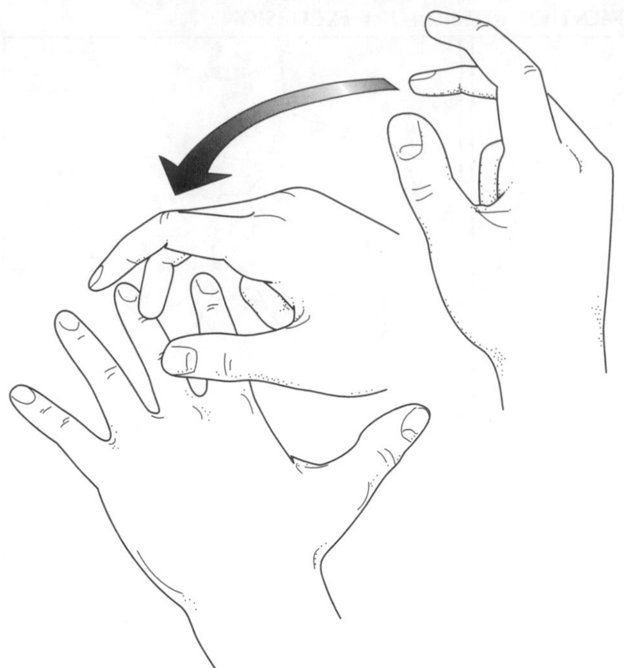

FIGURE 6-12. Chest percussion technique.

breath sounds have a harsh, hollow, or tubular quality. They are loud, high in pitch, and about equal in duration for the length of inspiration and expiration. A slight pause occurs between these two components. Bronchial breath sounds are auscultated directly over the trachea and are caused by the turbulent flow of gas through the upper airway. Clinically, these sounds are also called tracheal, tracheobronchial, or tubular breath sounds.

Bronchovesicular breath sounds are auscultated directly over the main stem bronchi. Bronchovesicular breath sounds are described as softer and lower in pitch than the bronchial breath sounds, and they do not have a pause between the inspiratory and expiratory phase. These sounds are reduced in intensity and pitch as a result of the filtering of the sound that occurs as gas moves between the large airways and alveoli.

Anteriorly, bronchovesicular breath sounds are heard directly over the main stem bronchi between the first and second ribs. Posteriorly, they are heard between the scapulae near the spinal column between the first and sixth ribs, especially on the right side (Fig. 6-15).

The term "vesicular breath sounds" describes the normal sounds of gas rustling or swishing in and out of the small bronchioles and possibly the alveoli. Vesicular breath sounds are described as soft and low in pitch and are primarily heard during inspiration. As the gas molecules enter the alveoli, they are able to spread out over a large surface area and, as a result of this action, create less gas turbulence. As gas turbulence decreases, the breath sounds become softer and lower in pitch, like the sound of the wind in the trees. Vesicular breath sounds are also heard during the initial third of exhalation as gas leaves the alveoli and bronchioles and moves into the large airways (see Fig. 6-15).

Adventitious Breath Sounds

Adventitious (abnormal) breath sounds are added or different sounds that are not normally heard over a particular area of the thorax; for example, bronchial breath sounds heard over an area of the chest that normally demonstrates vesicular breath sounds. There are several different types of adventitious breath sounds, each indicative of a particular pulmonary abnormality. The major adventitious breath sounds are the following.[36–50]

Bronchial Breath Sounds

When alveolar atelectasis or consolidation are present, bronchial breath sounds replace the normal vesicular breath sounds. When atelectasis or consolidation

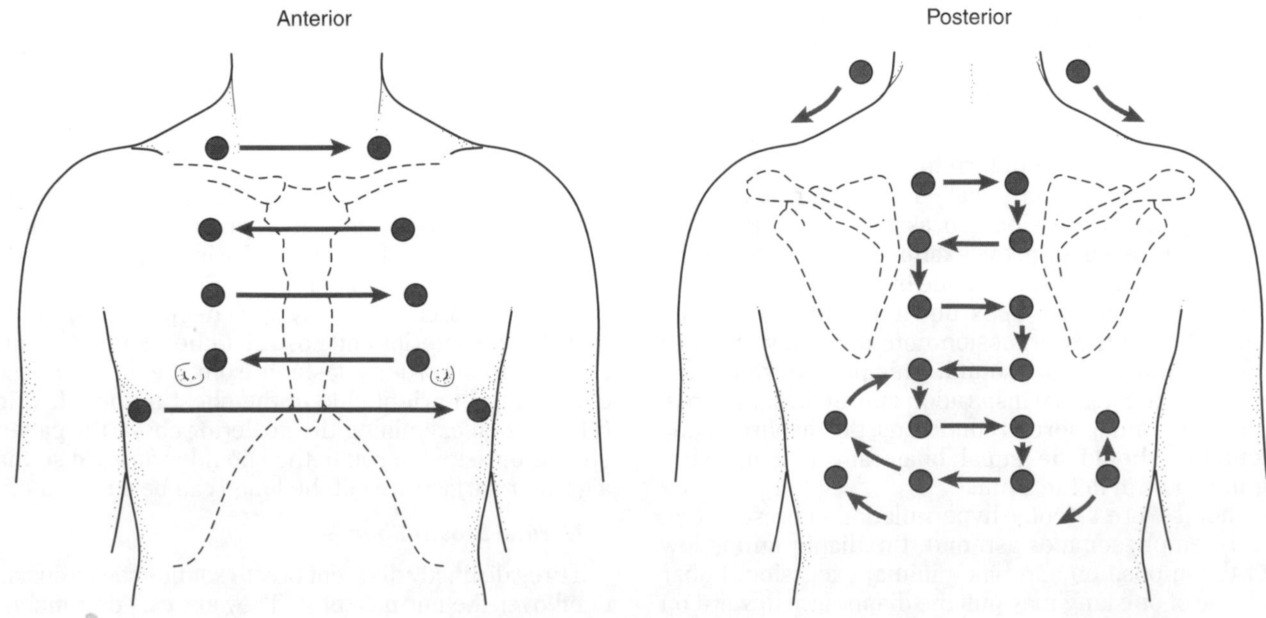

FIGURE 6-13. Path of percussion.

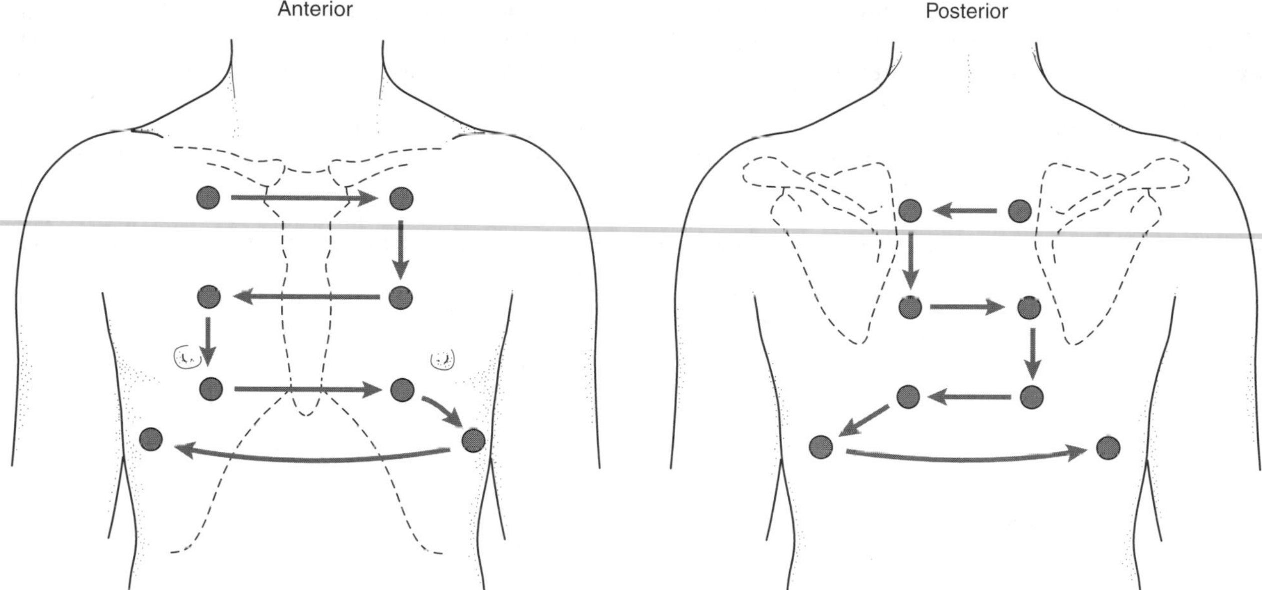

FIGURE 6-14. Path of auscultation.

are present, the gas molecules are only permitted to move (as a turbulent, bronchial gas flow) in and out of the major airways leading to the nonfunctioning alveoli. Under normal conditions, when gas molecules flow into the alveoli, the molecules dissipate throughout the increased alveolar surface area and become less turbulent. Bronchial breath sounds are described as harsh, loud, high-pitched sounds of equal duration during expiration and inspiration—similar to the sound that is normally auscultated directly only over the trachea.

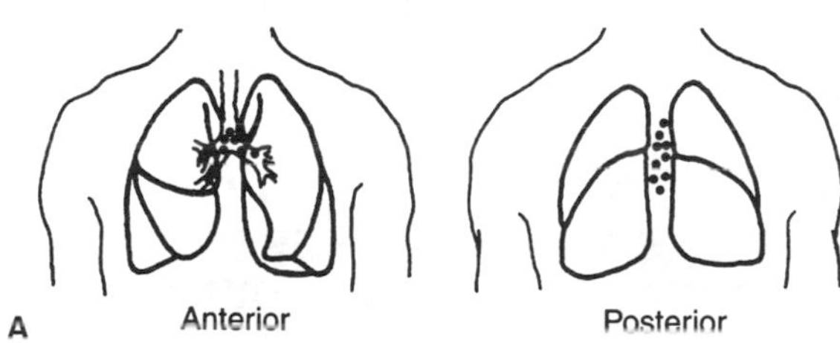

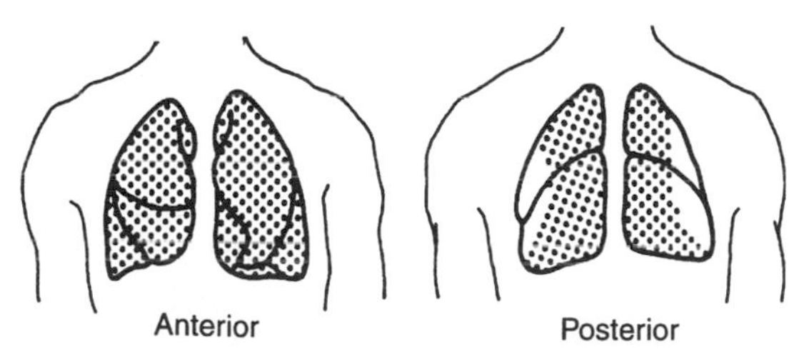

FIGURE 6-15. The locations at which bronchovesicular breath sounds (**A**) and vesicular breath sounds (**B**) are normally auscultated. (Courtesy of Terry Des Jardins.)

Diminished Breath Sounds

When the vesicular breath sound is softer than expected, it is described as diminished, or reduced, or in severe cases absent. Diminished breath sounds may be present in any condition that reduces the sound intensity at the site of production (mainly the large airways) or causes the transmission properties of the lung or chest to decrease. Abnormal conditions that reduce the intensity of a person's sound production include a shallow breathing pattern, a slow breathing pattern, or the complete absence of a breathing pattern (the most ominous of all). Abnormal conditions that reduce the normal transmission of sound through the lungs include obstructed airway disorders (eg, emphysema) and alveolar hyperinflation, pleural effusion, pneumothorax, and obesity.

Wheezes

Wheezes are caused by the vibration of the wall of a narrowed or compressed airway as gas passes through at high velocity. The diameter of the bronchial airway may be narrowed by secretions, bronchospasm, mucosal edema, bronchial tumor, or foreign objects. Wheezes are described as continuous, high-pitched, musical sounds heard primarily on expiration, although in severe cases they can be heard on both inspiration and expiration. The greater the bronchial narrowing, the higher the pitch of the wheeze. Bilaterally auscultated wheezing is commonly caused by bronchospasm (eg, asthma) or mucosal edema (eg, acute or chronic bronchitis). Unilateral or sharply localized wheezing may be caused by an inhaled foreign object or a bronchial tumor.

Rhonchi

Rhonchi (also called sonorous wheezes) are deeper, low-pitched, course, or rumbling sounds that are usually heard on expiration. Although rhonchi, similar to wheezes, can be caused by bronchospasm, bronchial tumors, and external pressure (eg, pneumothorax), they are most commonly associated with conditions that partially obstruct the airways with thick secretions that typically clear after a strong cough.

The more sibilant, higher-pitched rhonchi arise from the smaller bronchi and are commonly heard in patients with asthma. The more sonorous (snoring sound), lower-pitched rhonchi arise from the larger airways and are commonly heard in patients with cystic fibrous, bronchiectasis, or acute or chronic bronchitis. The vibrations set off by rhonchi are often palpable as increased tactile fremitus.

Crackles

Crackles (also known as rales) are described as discontinuous, high-pitched, short, crackling, popping, or bubbling sounds that are usually heard on inspiration and, unlike rhonchi, are not cleared by coughing. Crackles are caused by two major pathophysiologic mechanisms: (1) when inhaled gas enters previously collapsed alveoli, forcing them to pop open, or (2) when inhaled gas flows through distal bronchioles or into alveoli that contain serous secretions, causing the alveoli to expand or open. Crackles are commonly associated with pulmonary edema, pneumonia, early tuberculosis, atelectasis, and pulmonary fibrosis.

Pleural Friction Rub

When the pleural membranes become inflamed, the normal lubricating fluid between the parietal and visceral is lost. As this condition intensifies, sound-generating adhesions develop between the inflamed and roughened pleurae as they rub against each other during the normal breathing process. This action in turn causes a rubbing, grating sound known as a pleural friction rub. The sound is often similar to two pieces of leather being rubbed together. Clinically, this condition is commonly seen in pleurisy. In this condition, pleuritic chest pain may be present.

Voice Sounds

When signs and symptoms of pulmonary disease are present during inspection, palpation, percussion, or auscultation, the respiratory practitioner should evaluate vocal resonance, which is similar to the process of assessing tactile fremitus. The patient is instructed to repeat the words "one, two, three," or "ninety-nine" while the examiner auscultates the chest, comparing one side to the other. The sounds produced by the vocal cords are transmitted down the tracheobronchial tree and through the distal alveolar units to the chest wall.

Under normal conditions, the air-filled alveoli filter the voice sounds, causing them to be diminished, muffled, and unintelligible. When the peripheral lung units are altered by disease, however, vocal resonance is either increased or decreased. For example, alveolar consolidation or atelectasis increases the intensity and clarity of vocal resonance.

Clinically, a loud and more intelligible vocal sound is called *bronchophony*. Even though the increased lung density, caused by alveolar consolidation or atelectasis, may act as a sound barrier and reduce the vocal sounds somewhat, the reduction in sound is not as great as if the sounds were permitted to be filtered throughout the normal lung. Bronchophony is easier to identify when it exists in only one lung. It is commonly associated with increased vocal fremitus, bronchial breath sounds, and dull percussion notes.

Other pulmonary disorders reduce the transmission of vocal vibrations through the distal alveolar units and chest wall, resulting in a decreased vocal resonance. Such conditions include alveolar hyperinflation (eg, emphysema), bronchial obstruction, pneumothorax, and pleural effusion.

Finally, when the vocal resonance increases in intensity and takes on a nasal or bleating quality, it is referred to as *egophony*. Egophony may be identified over areas of the chest that demonstrate bronchophony. It is most easily identified by asking the patient to say "e-e-e" while listening to the suspicious area of the chest with a stethoscope. When egophony is present, the "e-e-e" is heard as "a-a-a." Egophony is commonly heard over an area of consolidated or compressed lung above a pleural effusion.

Whispered pectoriloquy is the transmission of a whisper through the pulmonary structures so that it is clearly heard as normal audible speech on auscultation. Clinically, the assessment for whispered pectoriloquy may be helpful in the identification of patchy areas of alveolar consolidation or atelectasis. For example, having the patient whisper the phrase "one, two, three," normally produces high-frequency vibrations that are filtered by the peripheral lung units and are heard on auscultation as muffled, low-pitched sounds. When alveolar consolidation or atelectasis is present, however, the peripheral lung units lose their filtering ability, and the sounds transmitted to the chest are heard as high-pitched and often clear vocal sounds.

CLINICAL DATA OBTAINED FROM LABORATORY TESTS AND SPECIAL PROCEDURES

In addition to the physical examination of the chest, the clinical data from certain laboratory tests and special procedures are used to more fully evaluate the patient. For the respiratory care practitioner, the most important tests and procedures are discussed below.

Radiology

To fully assess the patient with a respiratory disorder, the information provided by radiologic examination of the chest must be included. Radiography may play an important role in (1) the diagnosis of lung disorders, (2) the assessment of the extent and location of the disease, and (3) the evaluation of the subsequent progress of the disease. The most common radiologic technique is the standard posteroanterior (PA) radiograph of the chest. Other radiologic techniques include fluoroscopy, bronchography, computerized tomography, magnetic resonance imaging, pulmonary angiography, and ventilation-perfusion scanning.[51,52] See Chapter 7 for a more in-depth discussion on these topics.

Sputum Examination

A sputum collection for laboratory analysis must be coughed up from the lungs and expectorated through the mouth. A specimen containing mostly saliva should be discarded. Sputum may contain cellular elements, microorganisms, blood, or pus. The amount, color, and constituents of the sputum are important in the assessment and diagnosis of many respiratory diseases, including tuberculosis, pneumonia, cancer of the lungs, and pneumoconioses.

Yellow or opaque sputum indicates either an infection or inflammatory process. Green sputum is associated with old, retained secretions. Green and foul-smelling secretions are commonly found in patients with anaerobic or *Pseudomonas* bacterial infection. Brown sputum suggests the presence of old blood. Red sputum indicates the presence of fresh blood.

In addition to the general inspection of the sputum, a microscopic examination of the sputum can also identify such characteristics as color, presence of blood, viscosity, and odor. The microscopic examination of a Gram's stained smear of a sputum sample can be used to identify the Gram's stain reaction (gram-positive or gram-negative) and the shape of the organism that is possibly responsible for the infection. Such results are only presumptive. A positive identification of the organism can only be made by isolation of the organism from cultures. Common organisms associated with respiratory disorders that are isolated in the laboratory include the following:[53]

Gram-Positive Organisms

- *Streptococcus* (more than 80% of all bacterial pneumonias)
- *Staphylococcus*

Gram-Negative Organisms

- *Klebsiella*
- *Pseudomonas aeruginosa*
- *Haemophilus influenzae*
- *Legionella pneumophila*

See Chapter 30 for a more thorough consideration of this important topic.

Pulmonary Function Studies

Pulmonary function studies play an important role in the assessment of pulmonary disease. Pulmonary function findings are used to (1) determine the cause of dyspnea, (2) identify obstructive or restrictive pulmonary disorders, (3) evaluate the extent and severity of the pulmonary disorder, (4) monitor the course of a pulmonary disease, (5) assess the effectiveness of bronchodilator therapy, and (6) evaluate the patient's preoperative status.[54–56] For a more in-depth discussion on pulmonary function studies, see Chapter 8.

Arterial Blood Gases

The assessment of the arterial blood gas values is an essential cornerstone in the treatment selection. The pH, $PaCO_2$, and HCO_3 components, also known as the ventilatory acid-base components, of an arterial blood gas (ABG) study are use to identify (1) ventilatory acid-base abnormalities, (2) metabolic abnormalities, or (3) a combination of ventilatory and metabolic acid-base abnormalities. The PaO_2 component of the arterial blood gas value is used to assess the hypoxic state. A short overview follows.[57–59] For a more in-depth discussion of this important topic, see Chapters 5 and 9.

□ VENTILATORY ACID-BASE ABNORMALITIES

The ventilatory acid-base abnormalities and assessments commonly associated with respiratory diseases are listed in Box 6-5.

□ THE NEED FOR MECHANICAL VENTILATION

The pH, $PaCO_2$, and HCO_3 components of an arterial blood gas study are used to assess the patient's need for mechanical ventilation. Mechanical ventilation is indicated when the ventilatory acid-base status shows impending ventilatory failure, acute ventilatory failure, or apnea. For details on initialization of mechanical ventilation, see Ch. 20.

□ METABOLIC ABNORMALITIES

The pH, $PaCO_2$, and HCO_3 components of an arterial blood gas study are used to assess metabolic alkalosis (eg, caused by hypokalemia or hypochloremia), metabolic acidosis (often caused by lactic acidosis, ketoacidosis, or renal failure), or the combination of a respiratory and metabolic problem. Clinical examples of these two metabolic abnormalities are listed in Box 6-6.

BOX 6-5

COMMON CLINICAL ABG ASSESSMENTS

	pH	$PaCO_2$	HCO_3	PaO_2
Acute alveolar hyperventilation with hypoxemia	7.54	29	21	63
Acute ventilatory failure with hypoxemia	7.15	91	28	57
Chronic ventilatory failure with hypoxemia	7.38	88	33	62
Acute alveolar hyperventilation superimposed on chronic ventilatory failure	7.54	57	29	53
Acute ventilatory failure superimposed on chronic ventilatory failure	7.18	103	39	46

BOX 6-6

CLINICAL EXAMPLES OF METABOLIC ABNORMALITIES

Assessment	pH	$PaCO_2$	HCO_3	PaO_2
Metabolic alkalosis	7.57	45	28	95
Metabolic acidosis (lactic)	7.24	36	18	53

☐ ASSESSMENT OF THE HYPOXIC STATE

The PaO_2 and SaO_2 are used in the assessment of the patient's hypoxic state. In the adult on room air, mild hypoxemia is defined as a PaO_2 below 80 mmHg, moderate hypoxemia is a PaO_2 below 60 mmHg, and severe hypoxemia is a PaO_2 less than 40 mmHg.

Oxygen Transport Studies

There are several oxygen transport parameters that can be used to further assess the oxygenation status of the critically ill patient. The major oxygen transport indices are pulmonary shunt ($\dot{Q}s/\dot{Q}T$), total oxygen delivery (DO_2), oxygen consumption ($\dot{V}O_2$), arterial-venous oxygen content difference [$C(a - v)O_2$], oxygen extraction ratio (O_2ER), and mixed venous oxygen saturation ($S\bar{v}O_2$). Table 6-1 lists common oxygen transport study changes seen in common pulmonary diseases.[8]

Skin Testing

Skin testing is useful in the diagnosis of diseases that involve the entire body as well as the lungs. Such diseases include tuberculosis (TB), coccidioidomycosis, histo-

TABLE 6-1. **Oxygen-, Saturation-, and Content-Based Changes Commonly Seen in Respiratory Diseases**

	Oxygenation Indexes					
Pulmonary Disorder	$\dot{Q}_S/\dot{Q}_T$	DO_2†	$\dot{V}O_2$	$C(a - \bar{v})O_2$	O_2ER	$S\bar{v}O_2$
Obstructive airway diseases						
Chronic bronchitis						
Emphysema						
Bronchiectasis	↑	↓	~	~	↑	↓
Asthma						
Cystic fibrosis						
Croup syndrome						
Infectious pulmonary diseases						
Pneumonia						
Lung abscess	↑	↓	~	~	↑	↓
Fungal disorders						
Tuberculosis						
Pulmonary edema	↑	↓	~	↑*	↑	↓
Pulmonary embolism	↑	↓	~	↑*	↑	↓
Lung collapse						
Flail chest						
Pneumothorax	↑	↓	~	↑*	↑	↓
Pleural disease (eg, hemothorax)						
Kyphoscoliosis	↑	↓	~	~	↑	↓
Pneumoconiosis	↑	↓	~	~	↑	↓
Cancer of the lung	↑	↓	~	~	↑	↓
Adult respiratory distress syndrome	↑	↓	~	~	↑	↓
Idiopathic (infant) respiratory distress syndrome	↑	↓	~	~	↑	↓
Chronic interstitial lung disease	↑	↓	~	~	↑	↓
Sleep apnea	↑	↓	~	↑*	↑	↓
Smoke inhalation						
Without surface burns	↑	↓	~	~	↑	↓
With surface burns	↑	↓	↑	↑	↑	↓
Near drowning (wet)	↑	↓	~	~	↑	↓

↑ = increase
↓ = decrease
~ = unchanged
* The increased $C(a - \bar{v})O_2$ is associated with a decreased cardiac output.
† The DO_2 may be normal in the patient with (1) an increased cardiac output, (2) an increased hemoglobin level (polycythemia), or (3) a combination of both. For example, a normal DO_2 is often seen in the patient with chronic obstructive pulmonary disease and polycythemia. When the DO_2 is normal, the patient's O_2ER is usually normal.
Used with permission from Des Jardins T, Burton G: Clinical Manifestations and Assessment of Respiratory Disease, 3rd ed. St. Louis, Mosby–Year Book, 1995

plasmosis, sarcoidosis, blastomycosis, and allergic disorders.[8]

Bronchoscopy

The fiberoptic bronchoscope is used in the further inspection and assessment of abnormal radiographic findings, persistent atelectasis, excessive airway secretions, smoke inhalation trauma, intubation trauma, bronchiectasis, hemoptysis, lung abscess, major chest trauma, stridor or localized wheezing, and an unexplained cough. Specimens can also be obtained for additional laboratory studies with brushings, biopsies, needle aspirations, and washings. A videotape or colored picture can also be obtained through a bronchoscope. See Chapter 10 for additional discussion of this topic.[8]

Pleural Fluid Examination

Under normal conditions, a person's pleural fluid is clear and pale yellow. The total amount of pleural fluid is usually less than 20 mL.

Increased amount of pleural fluid is associated with heart failure, liver disease, infections, and tumors.

Opaque or turbid fluid is associated with infections that produce a large number of white blood cells. Analysis of the cells in the pleural fluid may be helpful in the identification of the type of infection.

Milky fluid is associated with chylous effusion, which is caused by thoracic duct fluid leaking into the pleural space.

Hemorrhage or blood fluid is associated with malignancy, trauma, infection, and pulmonary infarction.

Abnormal protein level. The protein level of the pleural fluid can also provide important information.

- A protein level that is below 3 g/dL is characteristic of a transudate, which is caused by mechanical factors that result in simple effusion of fluid into the pleural space. Transudate is commonly seen in patients with left heart failure or cirrhosis.
- A protein level above 3 g/dL is characteristic of an exudate. An exudate is described as fluid, cells, or other substances that have been slowly exuded, or discharged, into the pleural space.[8]

Electrocardiogram Assessment

The respiratory care practitioner should be able to recognize basic and life-threatening electrocardiogram (ECG) patterns commonly seen in the cardiopulmonary patient. The ECG can be very useful in the identification of the primary cause of the patient's clinical manifestations, the assessment of the impact that lung disease has on the heart, evaluation of the severity of the problem, and the patient's response to therapy.

The respiratory care practitioner should be able to identify and describe the clinical significance of the following abnormal ECG tracings: sinus bradycardia, sinus tachycardia, sinus arrhythmia, paroxysmal atrial tachycardia, atrial flutter, atrial fibrillation, premature ventricular contraction, ventricular tachycardia, ventricular flutter, ventricular fibrillation, and asystole.[60–64] A more complete discussion of these disorders is found in Chapter 12.

TABLE 6-2. **Hemodynamic Values Measured Directly**

Hemodynamic Value	Abbreviation	Normal Range
Central venous pressure	CVP	0–8 mmHg
Right atrial pressure	RAP	0–8 mmHg
Mean pulmonary artery pressure	$\overline{PA}$	10–20 mmHg
Pulmonary capillary wedge pressure (also called pulmonary artery wedge; pulmonary artery occlusion)	PCWP PAW PAO	4–12 mmHg
Cardiac output	CO	4–6 L/min

Used with permission from Des Jardins T, Burton G: Clinical Manifestations and Assessment of Respiratory Disease, 3rd ed. St. Louis, Mosby–Year Book, 1995

Hemodynamic Monitoring

Hemodynamic monitoring (see Chapter 12) is commonly used in the assessment and treatment of the critically ill patient with respiratory disease. Table 6-2 lists the hemodynamic parameters that can be measured directly. Table 6-3 shows the hemodynamic parameters that can be calculated from the direct measurements. Table 6-4 lists common hemodynamic changes seen in pulmonary diseases known to alter the patient's hemodynamic status.[8]

TABLE 6-3. **Hemodynamic Values Calculated From Direct Hemodynamic Measurements**

Hemodynamic Value	Abbreviation	Normal Range
Stroke volume	SV	40–80 mL
Stroke volume index	SVI	40 ± mL/beat/m^2
Cardiac index	CI	3.0 ± 0.5 L/min/m^2
Right ventricular stroke work index	RVSWI	7–12 g · m/m^2
Left ventricular stroke work index	LVSWI	40–60 g · m/m^2
Pulmonary vascular resistance	PVR	50–150 dyne × sec × cm^{-5}
Systemic vascular resistance	SVR	800–1500 dyne × sec × cm^{-5}

Used with permission from Des Jardins T, Burton G: Clinical Manifestations and Assessment of Respiratory Disease, 3rd ed. St. Louis, Mosby–Year Book, 1995

TABLE 6-4. **Hemodynamic Changes Commonly Seen in Respiratory Diseases**

	Hemodynamic Indexes											
Disorder	*CVP*	*RAP*	$\overline{PA}$	*PCWP*	*CO*	*SV*	*SVI*	*CI*	*RVSWI*	*LVSWI*	*PVR*	*SVR*
COPD Chronic bronchitis Emphysema Bronchiectasis Cystic fibrosis	↑	↑	↑	~	~	~	~	~	↑	~	↑	~
Pulmonary edema	↑	↑	↑	↑↑	↓	↓	↓	↓	↑	↓	↑	↑
Pulmonary embolism	↑	↑	↑↑	↓	↓	↓	↓	↓	↑	↓	↑	~
Adult respiratory distress syndrome (ARDS)—severe	~↑	~↑	~↑	~	~	~	~	~	~↑	~	~↑	~
Lung collapse Flail chest Pneumothorax Pleural disease (eg, hemothorax)	↑	↑	↑	↓	↓	↓	↓	↓	↑	↓	↑	↓
Kyphoscoliosis	↑	↑	↑	~	~	~	~	~	↑	~	↑	~
Pneumoconiosis	↑	↑	↑	~	~	~	~	~	↑	~	↑	~
Chronic interstitial lung diseases	↑	↑	↑	~	~	~	~	~	↑	~	↑	~
Cancer of the lung (tumor mass)	↑	↑	↑	↓	↓	↓	↓	↓	↑	↓	↑	~
Hypovolemia (burns)	↓	↓	↓	↓	↓	↓	↓	↓	↓	↓	~	↑

↑ = increase
↓ = decrease
~ = unchanged
Used with permission from Des Jardins T, Burton G: Clinical Manifestations and Assessment of Respiratory Disease, 3rd ed. St. Louis, Mosby–Year Book, 1995

Hematology, Blood Chemistry, and Electrolytes

The assessment of the patient's hematology, blood chemistry, and electrolytes provides the respiratory care practitioner with a greater understanding of the clinical manifestations demonstrated by the patient.[8,65,66]

□ HEMATOLOGY

The most common hematologic laboratory test is the complete blood count (CBC). The CBC includes the counting of red blood cells (RBCs) and white blood cells (WBCs), evaluation of various RBC components that relate to size and hemoglobin content, and counting of the different types of WBCs (called differential count). Box 6-7 shows normal values in the CBC. An increase in the total WBC is called leukocytosis. Box 6-8 lists the common types and causes of leukocytosis.

□ BLOOD CHEMISTRY

The patient's blood chemistry should also be monitored. Table 6-5 lists the blood chemistry tests commonly monitored in respiratory care.

□ ELECTROLYTES

The assessment of the electrolytes should be included in assessment of the patient whose body fluids are being endogenously or exogenously manipulated

BOX 6-7

NORMAL VALUES FOR THE COMPLETE BLOOD COUNT

Test	Normal Values
Red blood cell count (RBC)	
Men	$4.6–6.2 \times 10^6/mm^3$
Women	$4.2–5.4 \times 10^6/mm^3$
Hemoglobin (Hb)	
Men	13.5–16.5 g/dL
Women	12.0–15.0 g/dL
Hematocrit (Hct)	
Men	40%–54%
Women	38%–47%
Erythrocyte index	
Mean cell volume (MCV)	80–96 μm^3
Mean cell hemoglobin (MCH)	27–31 pg
Mean cell hemoglobin concentration (MCHC)	32%–36%
White blood cell count (WBC)	4500–11,500 cells/mm^3
Differential of white blood cells	
Segmented neutrophils	40%–75%
Bands	0%–6%
Eosinophils	0%–6%
Basophils	0%–1%
Lymphocytes	20%–45%
Monocytes	2%–10%
Platelet count	150,000–400,000 platelets/mm^3

BOX 6-8

TYPES OF LEUKOCYTOSIS

Cell Type Increased	Common Causes
Neutrophil	Bacterial infection, inflammation
Eosinophil	Allergic reaction, parasitic infection
Lymphocyte	Viral infection
Monocyte	Chronic infection, malignancies
Basophil	Myeloproliferative disorders

(eg, intravenous therapy, diarrhea, or renal disease). Table 6-6 lists the electrolytes commonly monitored in respiratory care.

Histology and Cytology

When a tissue sample or fluid is obtained during a bronchoscopy (bronchoscopic biopsy), thoracentesis, or during a thoracotomy (open lung biopsy), it is sent to the pathology department for analysis. The tissue is cut into very thin slices, placed on a slide, and stained so that the cells can be viewed under a microscope (study of histologic sections). This process can provide valuable information concerning infectious processes, chronic lung diseases, and benign and malignant tumors. For example, an acid-fast (Ziehl-Neelsen) stain can be used to identify mycobacteria. Fungal organisms can be identified by means of Gomori's methenamine silver (GMS) and periodic acid–Schiff (PAS) stains. Gomori's methenamine silver stain can also be used to identify the *Pneumocystis* organism, which is now commonly seen in patients with acquired immunodeficiency syndrome (AIDS).

When information is needed immediately about a specific specimen during surgery, a frozen section can be obtained. The frozen tissue section can be sliced and examined on a slide under the microscope. The normal processing of tissue is an overnight procedure. The frozen section allows the pathologist to examine the tissue and relay the appropriate diagnostic information to the surgeon while the operation is in progress.[65]

Cytology is the study of the cellular components of fluids, secretions, and other substances that contain cellular material but that do not have actual pieces of intact tissue (as in biopsies). The cells are smeared on a slide (Papanicolaou [Pap] smear) and examined under a microscope. This process can identify a malignancy and even the type of malignancy. Cytological examination is used to examine sputum, bronchial washings, bronchial brushings, and pleural fluid. Another procedure used in cytology is fine needle aspiration (FNA). In FNA, a relatively small needle (typically 22 gauge) is inserted into a mass, and some of the cells are aspirated and examined under a microscope. Radiologic guidance is used when FNA of a lung mass is performed. The information provided by the FNA procedure may avoid the need to perform surgery.

TABLE 6-5. **Blood Chemistry Tests Commonly Monitored in Respiratory Care**

Chemical	Normal Value	Common Abnormal Findings
Glucose	70 to 110 mg/dL	Hyperglycemia (excess glucose level) Diabetes mellitus Acute infection Myocardial infarction Thiazide and "loop" diuretics Hypoglycemia (low glucose level) Pancreatic tumors or liver disease Pituitary or adrenocortical hypofunction
Lactic dehydrogenase (LDH)	80 to 120 Wacker Units	Increases are associated with Myocardial infarction Chronic hepatitis Pneumonia Pulmonary infarction
Serum glutamic oxaloacetic transaminase (SGOT)	8 to 33 U/mL	Increases are associated with Myocardial infarction Congestive heart failure Pulmonary infarction
Bilirubin	Adult: 0.1 to 1.2 mg/dL Newborn: 1 to 12 mg/dL	Increases are associated with Massive hemolysis Hepatitis
Blood urea nitrogen (BUN)	8 to 18 mg/dL	Increases are associated with Acute or chronic renal failure
Serum creatinine	0.6 to 1.2 mg/dL	Increases are associated with Renal failure

Used with permission from Des Jardins T, Burton G: Clinical Manifestations and Assessment of Respiratory Disease, 3rd ed. St. Louis,. Mosby–Year Book, 1995

TABLE 6-6. **Electrolytes Commonly Monitored in Respiratory Care**

Electrolyte	Normal Value	Common Abnormal Findings	Clinical Manifestations
Sodium (Na^+)	136 to 142 mEq/L	Hypernatremia (excess Na^+)	
		Dehydration	Desiccated mucous membranes Flushed skin Great thirst Dry tongue
		Hyponatremia (low Na^+)	
		Sweating Burns Loss of gastrointestinal secretions Use of some diuretics Excessive water intake	Abdominal cramps Muscle twitching Poor perfusion Vasomotor collapse Confusion Seizures
Potassium (K^+)	3.8 to 5.0 mEq/L	Hyperkalemia (excess K^+)	
		Renal failure Muscle tissue damage	Irritability Nausea Diarrhea Weakness Ventricular fibrillation
		Hypokalemia (low K^+)	
		Diuretic therapy Endocrine disorder Diarrhea Reduced intake or loss of K^+ Chronic stress	Metabolic alkalosis Muscular weakness Malaise Cardiac arrhythmias Hypotension
Chloride (CL^-)	95 to 103 mEq/L	Hyperchloremia (excess Cl^-)	
		Renal tubular acidosis	Deep, rapid breathing Weakness Disorientation
		Hypochloremia (low Cl^-)	
		Alkalosis	Metabolic alkalosis Muscle hypertonicity Tetany Depressed ventilation (respiratory compensation)
Calcium (Ca^{++})	4.5 to 5.4 mEq/L	Hypercalcemia (excess Ca^{++})	
		Malignant tumors Bone fractures Diuretic therapy Excessive use of antacids or milk consumption Vitamin D intoxication Hyperparathyroidism	Increased skeletal density Mental deterioration
		Hypocalcemia (low Ca^{++})	
		Respiratory alkalosis Pregnancy Vitamin D deficiency Diuretic therapy Hypoparathyroidism	Decreased skeletal density

Used with permission from Des Jardins T, Burton G: Clinical Manifestations and Assessment of Respiratory Disease, 3rd ed. St. Louis, Mosby-Year Book, 1995

THE SYSTEMATIC COLLECTION OF CLINICAL DATA, ASSESSMENT, TREATMENT SELECTION, AND DOCUMENTATION

To effectively and efficiently assess and treat the patient with a respiratory disorder, the practitioner must be able to collect and document pertinent clinical data in a systematic and orderly fashion. Clinically, this is commonly accomplished with the use of the *problem-orientated medical record* (POMR). The POMR is used to (1) systematically gather clinical data, (2) formulate an assessment, and (3) select an appropriate treatment plan.[8,67–71]

There are a number of good POMR methods used in the hospital setting. Regardless of which method is used, it is critical that one method is selected and used on a continuous basis. One of the most popular POMR

TABLE 6-7. **Assessments Commonly Made by the Respiratory Care Practitioner**

Objective Clinical Data *(Examples)*	**Assessments** *(Cause of Objective Clinical Data)*	**Plan** *(Common Treatment Selections)*
Vital Signs		
↑ breathing, ↑ blood pressure, ↑ pulse	Respiratory distress	Treat underlying cause
Airway		
Wheezing	Bronchospasm	Bronchodilator Tx
Inspiratory stridor	Laryngeal edema	Cool mist
Rhonchi	Secretions in large airways	Bronchial hygiene Tx
Crackles	Secretions in distal airways	Treat underlying cause—eg, CHF
Cough		
Strong cough	Good ability to mobilize secretions	None
Weak cough	Poor ability to mobilize secretions	Bronchial hygiene Tx
Secretions		
Amount: >30 mL/24 hr	Excessive bronchial secretions	Bronchial hygiene Tx
White and translucent sputum	Normal sputum	None
Yellow/opaque sputum	Acute airway infection	Treat underlying cause
Green sputum	Old, retained secretions and infections	Bronchial hygiene Tx
Brown sputum	Old blood	Bronchial hygiene Tx
Red sputum	Fresh blood	Bronchial hygiene Tx
Frothy secretions	Pulmonary edema	Treat underlying cause—eg, CHF
Alveoli		
Bronchial breath sounds, Dull percussion note, Opacity on chest x-ray, Restrictive PFT values	Atelectasis, Infiltrates, Fibrosis	Hyperinflation Tx, oxygen Tx
	Consolidation	No specific, effective respiratory care Tx
Depressed diaphragm on x-ray	Air trapping and hyperinflation	Treat underlying cause
Pleural space		
Hyperresonant percussion note	Pneumothorax	Evacuate air†
Dull percussion note	Pleural effusion	Evacuate fluid†
Thorax		
Paradoxical movement of the chest wall	Flail chest	Mechanical ventilation†
Barrel chest	Air trapping (hyperinflation)	Treat underlying cause—eg, asthma
Posterior and lateral curvature of spine	Kyphoscoliosis	Bronchial hygiene Tx
Arterial Blood Gases—Ventilatory		
pH ↑, $PaCO_2$ ↓, HCO_3 ↓	Acute alveolar hyperventilation	Treat underlying cause
pH N, $PaCO_2$ ↓, HCO_3 ↓↓	Chronic alveolar hyperventilation	Generally none
pH ↓, $PaCO_2$ ↑, HCO_3 ↑	Acute ventilatory failure	Mechanical ventilation†
pH N, $PaCO_2$ ↑, HCO_3 ↑↑	Chronic ventilatory failure	Low-flow oxygen, bronchial hygiene
Sudden Ventilatory Changes on Chronic Ventilatory Failure (CVF)		
pH ↑, $PaCO_2$ ↑, HCO_3 ↑↑, PaO_2 ↓	Acute alveolar hyperventilation on CVF	Treat underlying cause
pH ↓, $PaCO_2$ ↑↑, HCO_3 ↑, PaO_2 ↓	Acute ventilatory failure on CVF	Mechanical ventilation†
Metabolic		
pH ↑, $PaCO_2$N or ↑, HCO_3 ↑, PaO_2N	Metabolic alkalosis	Give potassium†—Hypokalemia Give chloride†—Hypochloremia
pH ↓, $PaCO_2$N or ↓, HCO_3 ↓, PaO_2 ↓	Metabolic acidosis	Give oxygen—Lactic acidosis
pH ↓, $PaCO_2$N or ↓, HCO_3 ↓, PaO_2N	Metabolic acidosis	Give insulin†—Ketoacidosis
pH ↓, $PaCO_2$N or ↓, HCO_3 ↓, PaO_2N	Metabolic acidosis	Renal therapy†
Indication for Mechanical Ventilation		
pH ↑, $PaCO_2$ ↓, HCO_3 ↓, PaO_2 ↓	Impending ventilatory failure	Mechanical ventilation†
pH ↓, $PaCO_2$ ↑, HCO_3 ↑, PaO_2 ↓	Ventilatory failure	
pH ↓, $PaCO_2$ ↑, HCO_3 ↑, PaO_2 ↓	Apnea	
Oxygenation Status		
PaO_2 <80 mmHg	Mild hypoxemia	Oxygen Tx and treat underlying cause
PaO_2 <60 mmHg	Moderate hypoxemia	
PaO_2 <40 mmHg	Severe hypoxemia	
Oxygen Transport Status		
↓ PaO_2, anemia, ↓ cardiac output	Inadequate oxygen transport	Oxygen Tx and treat underlying cause

† Physician ordered

Used with permission from Des Jardins T, Burton G: Clinical Manifestations and Assessment of Respiratory Disease Workbook. St. Louis, Mosby, to be published 1996

methods is the *SOAP* progress note. The acronym SOAP stands for the following:

S: Subjective data provided by the patient regarding his or her feelings or concerns.

O: Objective data that can be measured, factually described, or collected from other professional reports or test results.

A: Assessment is the determination of the cause of the subjective and objective data. For example, wheezing would be the objective datum for the assessment of bronchospasm (the cause of the wheezing). See Table 6-7 for assessments commonly documented by the respiratory care practitioner.

P: Plan is the treatment selection used to remedy the cause identified in the assessment. For example, the assessment of bronchospasm would justify the selection of a bronchodilator.

After the treatment plan has been implemented, another SOAP should be performed to collect measurable data and evaluate the patient's response to the treatment plan. Based on this evaluation, the patient's treatment plan may be regulated up or down. For example, if the wheezing does not decrease appropriately after the administration of a bronchodilator, the respiratory care practitioner might select to increase the frequency or dose of the bronchodilator until the desired effect is reached.

For the student, a predesigned SOAP form may be used to enhance the rapid collection and organization of clinical data, the assessment (ie, the cause of the clinical data), and the development of a treatment selection or selections. For example, note how the subjective and objective data in the following case example is collected and used in the predesigned SOAP document shown in Protocol 6-1.

Case Example

(Subjective and objective data are presented in bold type.)

A **46-year-old female** with a long history of **asthma** presented in the emergency room in respiratory distress. On observation, her arms were braced on the arms of a chair, she was using her **accessory muscles of inspiration,** and she was **pursed-lip breathing.** The patient stated, **"I've been wheezing for about 3 days. It appears to be getting worse."** Her **heart rate** was **140 beats per minute,** and her **blood pressure** was **155/115.** Her **respiratory rate** was **32 breaths per minute and shallow. Hyperresonant percussion notes** were elicited **bilaterally. Auscultation** revealed **wheezing bilaterally.** Her **chest x-ray film** showed a severely **depressed diaphragm.** Her **PEFR** was **180.** Her **arterial blood gas** values showed a **pH of 7.54,** a **$PaCO_2$ of 53,** an **HCO_3 of 31,** and a **PaO_2 of 46** (on room air).

The experienced respiratory care practitioner can typically condense and abbreviate a SOAP note in just a few minutes at the patient's bedside. For example, the information shown in Figure 6-16 may be written in the patient's chart in the following abbreviated form:

S: "I've been wheezing for about 3 days. It appears to be getting worse."

O: RR 32, HR 140, BP 155/115. Using accessory muscles of inspiration. Hyperresonant and wheezing bilaterally. Severely depressed diaphragm. PEFR 180. ABGs (rm air): pH 7.54, $PaCO_2$ 26, HCO_3 20, PaO_2 57.

A: Bronchospasm
Air trapping
Acute alveolar hyperventilation with moderate hypoxemia
Possible impending ventilatory failure

P: Bronchodilator Tx per protocol. Oxygen Tx per protocol. Place ventilator on standby.

Finally, it should be noted that after the treatment plan has been administered, another abbreviated SOAP note should be made to determine if the therapy should remain the same, be regulated up, be regulated down, be revised, or be discontinued.

In summary, the core to a successful TDP program is the **quality** of the respiratory practitioner's assessment skills and her or his ability to recognize and appropriately communicate when physician-determined patient-specific severity indicators have been reached or exceeded. The respiratory care practitioner with competent assessment skills will have mastered the techniques to (1) develop a complete patient history; (2) conduct a patient interview; (3) perform a complete and systematic physical examination of the chest and lungs; (3) obtain important information from various laboratory tests and special procedures; and (4) systematically collect all the clinical data, formulate an assessment, develop a treatment plan, and appropriately document the entire assessment process.

REFERENCES

1. Hess D: The AARC clinical practice guidelines. Resp Care 36: 1398, 1991
2. American Association for Respiratory Care: Clinical practice guidelines. Resp Care 36:1402, 1991
3. Hess D: More clinical practice guidelines: Now what? Resp Care 37:855, 1992
4. American Association for Respiratory Care: Clinical practice guidelines. Resp Care 37:882, 1992
5. American Association for Respiratory Care: Clinical practice guidelines. Resp Care 38:495, 1993
6. American Association for Respiratory Care: Clinical practice guidelines, Resp Care 38:1173, 1993
7. American Association for Respiratory Care: Clinical practice guidelines. Resp Care 39:797, 1994
8. Des Jardins T, Burton GG: Clinical Manifestations and Assessment of Respiratory Disease, 3rd ed. St. Louis, Mosby, 1995
9. Jarvis C: Physical Examination and Health Assessment. Philadelphia, WB Saunders, 1992
10. Bates B: A Guide to Physical Examination and History Taking, 5th ed. Philadelphia, JB Lippincott, 1991
11. Christensen BL, Kockrow EO: Foundations of Nursing. St. Louis, Mosby–Year Book, 1991
12. Craven RR, Hirnle CJ: Fundamentals of Nursing: Human Health and Function. Philadelphia, JB Lippincott, 1992
13. Harkness-Hood G, Dincher JR: Total Patient Care: Foundations and Practice of Adult Health Nursing. St. Louis, Mosby–Year Book, 1992

14. Lewis L, Timby B: Fundamental Skills and Concepts in Patient Care, 4th ed. Philadelphia, JB Lippincott, 1988
15. Benjamin A: The Helping Interview, 3rd ed. Boston, Houghton Mifflin, 1980
16. Bernstein L, Bernstein RS: Interviewing: A guide for Health Professionals, 4th ed. Norwalk, CT, Appleton-Century Crofts, 1985
17. Dirckx JH: Talking with patients, the art of history-taking. Clin Nurse Practitioner 3:13, 1985
18. Grimes J, Iannopollo E: Health Assessment in Nursing Practice, 3rd ed. Monterey, CA, Wadsworth Health Sciences Division, 1992
19. Malasanos L, Barkauskas V, Stoltenberg-Allen, K: Health Assessment, 4th ed. St Louis, Mosby–Year Book, 1990
20. Lane W: Patient Interview and History Taking. In JA Spittel (ed): Practice of Medicine, vol 1. New York, Harper & Row, 1972
21. Morton PG: Nurse's Clinical Guide to Health Assessment. Springhouse, Pa, Springhouse, 1990
22. Mengel A: Getting the most from patient interviews. Nursing 12:46, 1982
23. Okun BF: Effective Helping: Interviewing and Counseling Techniques, 3rd ed. Monterey, CA, Brooks/Cole, 1986
24. Daily Ek, Schroeder JP: Techniques in Bedside Hemodynamic Monitoring, 4th ed. St. Louis, Mosby–Year Book, 1989
25. Milewski A, Ferguson KL, Terndrup TE: Comparison of pulmonary artery, rectal, and tympanic membrane temperatures in adult intensive care unit patients. Clin Pediatr (Phila) (Suppl):13, 1991
26. Chamberlain JM, et al: Comparison of a tympanic thermometer to rectal and oral thermometers in a pediatric emergency department. Clin Pediatr (Phila) (Suppl):24, 1991
27. Talo H, Macknin ML, Medendorp SV: Tympanic membrane temperatures comparted to rectal and oral temperatures. Clin Pediatr (Phila) (Suppl):30, 1991
28. Gravelyn TR, Weg JG: Respiratory rate as an indicator of acute respiratory dysfunction, JAMA 244:1123, 1980
29. Op't Holt TB: Assessment Based Respiratory Care. New York, John Wiley & Sons, 1986
30. Wilkins RL, et al: Clinical Assessment in Respiratory Care, 3rd ed. St. Louis, Mosby–Year Book, 1995
31. Stevens SA, Becker KL: How to perform picture-perfect respiratory assessment. Nursing 18:57, 1988
32. Cherniack RM, Cherniack L: Respiration in Health and Disease, 3rd ed. Philadelphia, WB Saunders, 1983
33. Judge RD, Zuidema GD: Clinical Diagnosis: A Physiological Approach, 5th ed. Boston, Little, Brown, 1988
34. Malasanos L, Barkauskas B, Stoltenberg-Allen K: Health Assessment, 4th ed. St. Louis, Mosby–Year Book, 1990
35. Seidel HM, et al: Mosby's Guide to Physical Examination, 2nd ed. St. Louis, Mosby–Year Book, 1991
36. Andrews JL, Badger TL: Lung sounds through the ages. JAMA 241:2625, 1979
37. Report of the ACCP-ATS joint committee on pulmonary nomenclature. Chest 67:583, 1975
38. Report of the ATS-ACCP ad hoc subcommittee on pulmonary nomenclature. ATS News 3:5, 1977
39. Report of the ATS-ACCP ad hoc subcommittee on pulmonary nomenclature. ATS News 2:8, 1981
40. Wilkins RL, et al: Lung sound nomenclature survey. Chest 98:886, 1990
41. Murphy RLH, Holford Sk: Lung sounds. Basics of RD (March) 8:3, 1980
42. Forgacs P: The functional basis of pulmonary sounds. Chest 73:399, 1978
43. Forgacs P: Lung sounds. Br J Dis Chest 63:1, 1969
44. Forgacs P: Lung Sounds. London, Balliere Tindall, 1978
45. Wilkins RL, Hodgkin JE, Lopez B: Lung Sounds: A Practical Guide. St. Louis, Mosby–Year Book, 1988
46. Lehrer S: Understanding Lung Sounds. Philadelphia, WB Saunders, 1984
47. Loudon RG: The lung exam. Clin Chest Med 8:265, 1987
48. Wilkins RL, Dexter JR, Smith JR: Survey of adventitious sound terminology in case reports. Chest 85:523, 1984
49. Wilkins RL, Dexter JR: Comparing RCPs to physicians for the description of lung sounds: Are we accurate and can we communicate? Respir Care 35:969, 1990
50. Forgacs P: Crackles and wheezes. Lancet 2:203, 1967
51. Armstrong P, et al: Imaging of Diseases of the Chest. St. Louis, Mosby–Year Book, 1990
52. Gurley LT: Introduction to Radiologic Technology, 3rd ed. St. Louis, Mosby–Year Book, 1992
53. Finegold M, Martin J: Diagnostic Microbiology, 7th ed. St. Louis, Mosby–Year Book, 1986
54. Madama VC: Pulmonary Function Testing and Cardiopulmonary Stress Testing. Albany, NY, Delmar Publishers, 1993
55. Ruppel G: Manual of Pulmonary Function Testing, 6th ed. St. Louis, Mosby–Year Book, 1991
56. Miller WF, Scacci R, Gast LR: Laboratory Evaluation of Pulmonary Function. Philadelphia, JB Lippincott, 1987
57. Malley WJ: Clinical Blood Gases: Application and Noninvasive Alternatives. Philadelphia, WB Saunders, 1990
58. Shapiro BA, et al: Clinical Application of Blood Gases, 5th ed. St. Louis, Mosby–Year Book, 1994
59. Jones NL: Blood Gases and Acid-Base Physiology, 2nd ed. New York, Thieme-Stratton, 1987
60. Conover MH, Zalis EG: Understanding Electrocardiography: Physiological and Interpretive Concepts, 6th ed. St. Louis, Mosby–Year Book, 1992
61. Brown KR, Jacobson S: Mastering Dysrhythmias: A Problem Solving Guide. Philadelphia, FJ Davis, 1988
62. Davis D: How to Quickly and Accurately Master ECG Interpretation. Philadelphia, JB Lippincott, 1985
63. Huszar RH: Basic Dysrhythmias: Interpretation and Management. St. Louis, Mosby–Year Book, 1988
64. Thaler MS: The Only ECG Book You'll Ever Need. Philadelphia, JB Lippincott, 1988
65. Tilkian SM, Conover MG, Tilkian AG: Clinical Implications of Laboratory Tests, 4th ed. St. Louis, Mosby–Year Book, 1987
66. Wintrobe MM: Clinical Hematology, 9th ed. Philadelphia, Lea & Febiger, 1993
67. Bergerson S: More about charting with a jury in mind. Nursing 18:51, 1988
68. McPhee A: Teaching students how to chart. Nurse Educator 12:33, 1987
69. Philpott M: 20 Rules for good charting. Nursing 16:63, 1986
70. Weed LL: Medical Record, Medical Education, and Patient Care: The Problem-Oriented Record as a Basic Tool. Cleveland, OH, Case Western Reserve University Press, 1971
71. Weed LL: Medical Record, Medical Education and Patient Care. St. Louis, Mosby–Year Book, 1969

7 Imaging Assessment

Glen A. Lillington
A. Janelle Burton
Elizabeth Moore

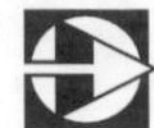

CLINICAL SKILLS

Upon completion of this chapter, the reader will:

- Understand basic concepts pertaining to chest imaging
- Become familiar with common radiologic/roentgenographic terminology
- Understand the various imaging techniques and the indications for their use
- Acquire some familiarity with the normal radiologic anatomy of the lungs
- Appreciate the concept and implications of unavoidable observer error
- Understand the problems in obtaining suitable images in seriously ill patients
- Define or briefly describe the major chest roentgenologic patterns
- Identify some important underlying etiologies for these patterns
- Recognize basic roentgen patterns on examination of chest radiographs, including the following: diffuse alveolar filling, interstitial and miliary patterns, uncomplicated pleural effusion, lobar consolidation, lobar atelectasis, large pneumothorax, hydropneumothorax, lung abscess, bullous emphysema, congestive heart failure, tubes and lines in the thorax, ventilator barotrauma, and pneumomediastinum.

KEY TERMS

Atelectasis
Barotrauma
Central venous catheters
Chest tubes
Chronic pulmonary hypertension
Diffuse alveolar disease
Diffuse interstitial disease
Endotracheal
Fat embolism
Fiberoptic bronchoscopy
Flail chest
Goodpasture's syndrome
High-resolution CT
Hyperinflation
Interlobar effusion
Lung abscess
Lung fields
Positron emission tomographic (PET) scans
Pseudomonas
Radiation
Radiation fibrosis
Radiation pneumonitis
Radiolabeled gallium
Radiolucent
Radiopaque
Swan-Ganz catheters

BASIC PRINCIPLES OF CHEST ROENTGENOGRAPHY

Roentgenographic visualization of body structures depends on the perception of contrast between tissues of different radiodensities. As the roentgen beam passes through the tissues to register on the radiographic film, differential attenuation (absorption) of the beam by different tissues occurs. The greater the radiodensity of the tissue, the greater the absorption of the beam; as a result, the film image of the tissue or organ will be relatively white or *radiopaque*. Less dense tissues appear blacker on the film and are less radiopaque and more *radiolucent*.

The detection of diagnostically useful images by chest roentgenography is made possible by the widespread distribution in the lung of the relatively radiolucent intra-alveolar air. This provides contrast to the denser opacities of the normal intrapulmonary and extrapulmonary tissues, and the abnormal tissues resulting from disease.

As calcium has the greatest radio-opacity of any endogenous material, calcified structures are usually easily detected on the roentgenogram. Certain exogenous substances (tin, iodine, barium), which may occasionally appear in the thorax, have a "metallic density" similar to or greater than that of calcium. Body fluids and most tissues have a lesser degree of radio-opacity, usually referred to as "water density" or "tissue density." Tissue fat has a somewhat lesser attenuation than other tissues. The "air density" of the air-filled lung is partially attenuated by the normal intrapulmonary tissues and the overlying chest wall.

The degree of radio-opacity also depends on the *thickness* of tissue through which the beam has penetrated. For example, the heart, which is large, will appear more opaque than the much smaller right or left pulmonary artery.

In the majority of lung diseases, the air density of the affected area of lung is replaced (or displaced) by the tissue or water density of the disease process, resulting in the appearance of increased radio-opacity. Such abnormalities are commonly referred to as "shadows" or "infiltrates." The size, shape, distribution, location, and homogeneity of such opacities form patterns that provide clues to the radiologist in predicting the possible nature of the abnormality.

Certain thoracic diseases produce increased radiolucency, owing to an increase in the air-tissue ratio in the affected area. This is most commonly caused by a focal loss of lung tissue (emphysema, bullae, cavities), diffuse obstructive hyperinflation (asthma or a check-valve bronchial obstruction), or a collection of air in an abnormal location (pneumothorax or pneumomediastinum).

VALUE AND LIMITATIONS OF CHEST ROENTGENOGRAPHY

The chest roentgenogram is very sensitive, that is, it is highly effective in the detection of abnormalities in the lungs. Routine chest roentgenography often reveals evidence of disease in asymptomatic patients with no abnormal signs on physical examination.

In addition to the detection of disease, the chest roentgenogram displays the pattern of the abnormality. Pattern analysis provides valuable clues in determining the cause of the disorder. Only occasionally is the roentgenographic pattern specifically diagnostic. More commonly, the abnormal pattern suggests a limited number of diagnostic possibilities, which must be clinically correlated and which often will require further investigation by other imaging techniques or nonimaging tests.

Serial chest roentgenograms obtained at appropriate intervals provide a dynamic portrait of the disease process. Information of this type has diagnostic value and prognostic implications and permits monitoring of the effectiveness of therapy.

In assessing the diagnostic implications of a normal chest roentgenogram, one must be constantly aware of the limitations of the technique. In patients with bronchial asthma or chronic bronchitis, for example, the chest roentgenogram may appear entirely normal even when the disease is severe. Emphysema may cause little change in the chest roentgenogram until an advanced stage has been reached. Bronchogenic carcinomas usually cannot be detected by standard roentgenography until the tumor mass has reached a diameter of 1 cm or greater, at which time the tumor may have already been present for 10 years or longer. Relatively large lesions may be virtually undetectable on the chest roentgenogram if they are located in the "blind" areas where the lung tissue is obscured by overlapping opaque structures such as the heart, great vessels, or subdiaphragmatic solid organs.

Disorders of the ventilatory pump of neurological or musculoskeletal origin may cause respiratory failure, yet the chest roentgenogram may appear completely normal unless pulmonary complications secondary to sputum retention occur. Causes include chest wall trauma, overdosage of sedative drugs leading to respiratory center depression, trauma to the brain or spinal cord, and neuromuscular disorders such as poliomyelitis, amyotrophic lateral sclerosis, and myasthenia gravis.

Conversely, variations in the roentgenographic appearances of normal structures may be mistakenly interpreted as evidence of disease. Thus, both false-negative and false-positive results are encountered.

Moderate or even extensive abnormalities on the chest roentgenogram are not always accompanied by severe symptoms or marked abnormalities in pulmonary function. This dichotomy between radiologic appearance and pathophysiologic reality tends to occur most commonly in sarcoidosis and in some forms of pneumoconiosis.

STANDARD CHEST ROENTGENOGRAMS

The standard chest roentgenographic study includes two views, each obtained with the subject in the upright position: a film obtained in the posteroanterior projection (the PA film), and a lateral projection, either right or left (the lateral film). The exposures should be made with respiration suspended in the full inspiratory position, with the subject properly positioned so that there is no rotation in either frontal or lateral projection, and with appropriate exposure techniques to enhance contrast without underpenetration or overpenetration.

When the patient is seriously ill, many of these ideal circumstances may be unattainable. The physician will often be required to examine and interpret a supine anteroposterior (AP) film that is badly overpenetrated or underpenetrated, obtained on a subject who was rotated and was in a state of submaximal inspiration and breathing at the time of exposure. A lateral film is rarely obtainable under such circumstances.

Normal Radiologic Anatomy

A full description of the normal radiologic anatomy of the thorax is beyond the scope of this chapter, and the reader is referred to the classic descriptions in the standard texts.[1–3] Some pertinent data are included in the following description of the techniques of inspecting the radiographic film.

Inspection of the Posteroanterior Chest Radiograph

A roentgenographic abnormality cannot be interpreted unless it has been detected. Many factors are operative in the unavoidable observer error that occurs in radiology,[4] but failures in perception can be reduced by following a standard search pattern in which the different areas and anatomic components of the chest roentgenogram are systematically inspected during the interpretative process (Fig. 7-1). The precise order in which one studies the various structures is less important than the consistency with which one applies the method.

The proper positioning of the patient is verified by comparing the relationship of the medial ends of the clavicles to the midline. Relatively minor degrees of rotation may create a spurious appearance of tracheal deviation, cardiac displacement, cardiomegaly, or widening of the vascular pedicle.

The extrathoracic soft tissues should be inspected briefly. If the patient is female, the breast shadows should be identified. Absence of one breast will result

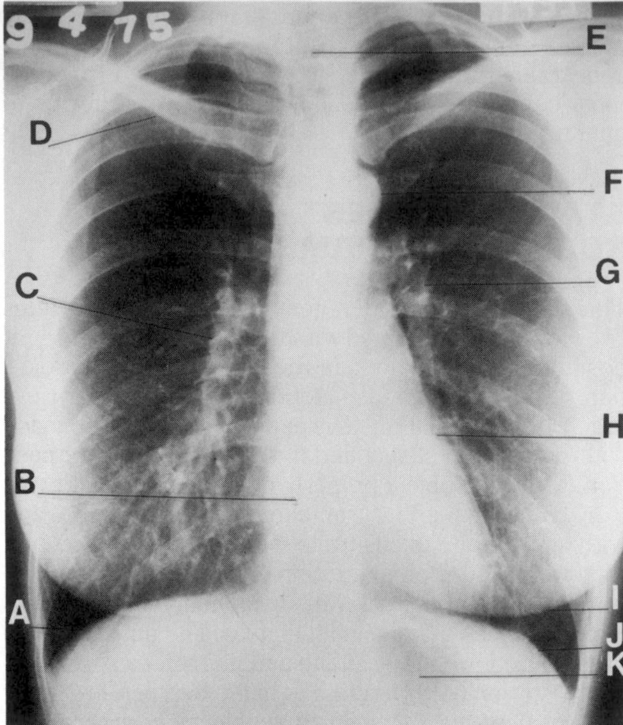

FIGURE 7-1. Posteroanterior (PA) chest roentgenogram of a young woman. **(A)** Right hemidiaphragm, convex upwards with a clear costophrenic angle; **(B)** Thoracic spine; **(C)** Right hilum (the hilar opacity is due to the central pulmonary vessels); **(D)** Right clavicle; **(E)** Midline lucency due to intratracheal air; **(F)** Aortic knob (this becomes more prominent in older persons); **(G)** Left hilum, usually higher than the right hilum; **(H)** Left heart border (interface between left ventricle and left lung); **(I)** Interface representing the inferior margin of left breast; **(J)** Left hemidiaphragm, usually a little lower than the right; **(K)** Gas bubble within stomach.

in relative hyperlucency over the lower lung on the affected side. Large breasts cause considerable haziness over the lower lung fields that may simulate pneumonia or pulmonary congestion. Nipple shadows may be mistaken for solitary nodules. The presence of subcutaneous emphysema may be apparent in the neck or lateral chest wall.

The bony thorax is inspected, including ribs, spine, manubrium, scapulae, and shoulders. A cervical rib is present in 1% to 2% of normal persons. One should search for rib fractures, arthritic changes, and lytic lesions of bone. Scapulae that overlie the lung may be confused with pleural or extrapleural lesions. The presence of kyphosis or scoliosis makes interpretation of the chest roentgenogram more difficult.

The diaphragms should have a fairly smooth rounded contour that is convex upwards. The costophrenic angles should be clear. The right diaphragm is usually 2 cm higher than the left, and normally the dome is at the level of the anterior end of the sixth rib. Unilateral or bilateral elevation of the hemidiaphragms may have diagnostic significance. Flattening of the diaphragms suggests hyperinflation seen in the obstructive pulmonary diseases.

The mediastinal contour should be inspected for shifting of the mediastinum from the midline position, cardiomegaly, abnormalities in position or size of the large vessel shadows, focal areas of mediastinal widening, and the presence of air or calcium within the mediastinum.

The hilar areas are inspected with particular attention to changes in size or position. The left hilum is usually about 2 cm higher than the right. Vertical displacement of the hilum, either cephalad or caudad, strongly suggests volume loss of a lobe of the lung on that side.

The vascular pattern in the lungs is assessed, tracing the vessels from the hilum to the periphery. The vascular shadows should progressively branch and diminish in size as one follows the vessels outward from the hilum to the periphery. Changes in the vascular pattern may be localized or generalized. Minor increases or decreases in vascularity are difficult to identify with certainty.

The *lung fields* are then searched for localized areas of increased or decreased translucency. The lung fields should be inspected in a systematic fashion from top to bottom, comparing one side with the other. The pattern of the abnormality should be identified, where possible.

The Lateral Chest Roentgenograph

The lateral chest roentgenograph (Fig. 7-2) is customarily obtained in conjunction with the standard PA film, although there is some evidence to suggest that the incremental diagnostic value of the lateral film is relatively low if the patient is asymptomatic. Nevertheless, this view may yield important information about the mediastinum and hilar areas,[5] and may detect pulmonary lesions not visible on the PA film.

By convention, the view obtained is a left lateral, with the film cassette against the left axilla. A right lateral roentgenogram is preferred if there is clinical reason to suspect that the right lung harbors the dominant abnormality.

Anteroposterior Supine Chest Roentgenograph

This is considered here, as it often, by necessity, replaces the standard PA and lateral films. As previously noted, the AP supine (or semi-erect) chest roentgenograph has inherent disadvantages that must be recognized if erroneous interpretations are to be minimized. The most common clue that the film was exposed with this technique is the absence of a companion film affording a lateral view. Other radiologic clues that the projection was AP include high clavicles and transverse course of ribs (because the path of the roentgen beam often has a cephalad angulation) and the tendency of the scapulae to overlie the lung fields.

Assessment of heart size is difficult because there is a 15% to 20% magnification effect of the heart and a concomitant apparent widening of the superior mediastinum.[6] The position-induced apparent diaphragmatic elevation and the frequent failure of critically ill patients

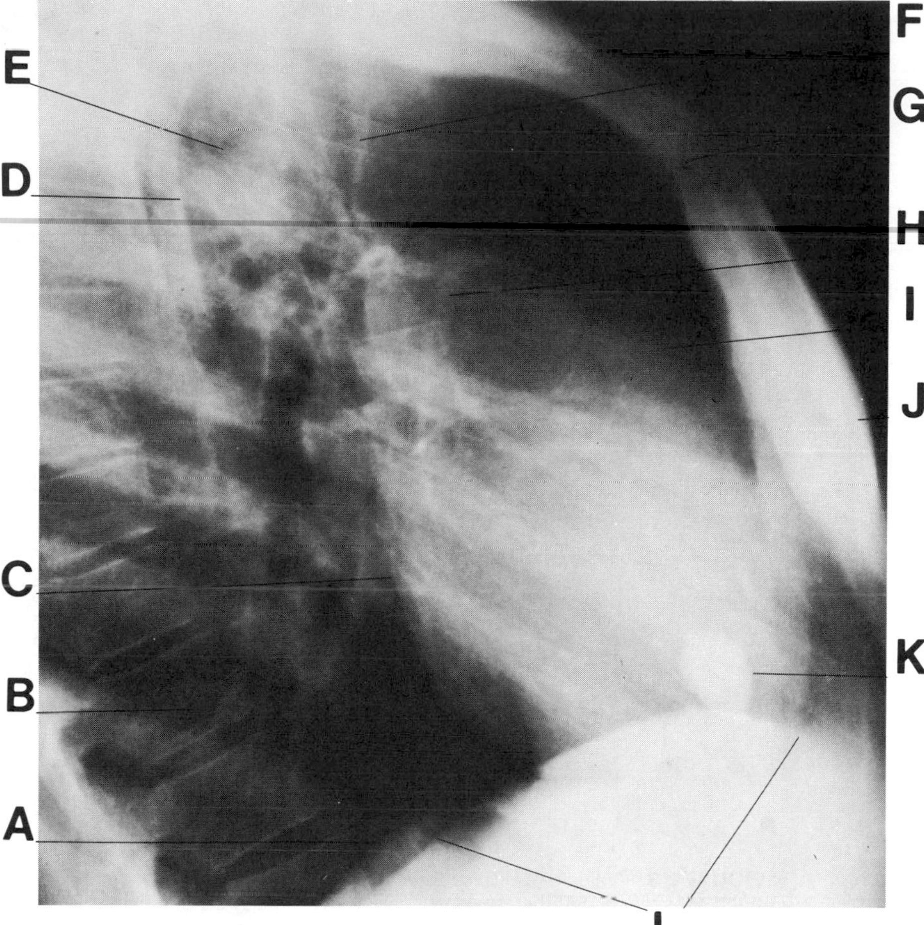

FIGURE 7-2. Chest roentgenogram in the right lateral projection. **(A)** Left hemidiaphragm, the laterality of which is suggested in this particular case because the gastric air bubble can be seen; **(B)** Thoracic spine (the intervertebral disc spaces are shown clearly); **(C)** Posterior wall of the heart; **(D)** Scapulae; **(E)** Upper margin of the aortic arch; **(F)** Anterior wall of the trachea (posterior to this is the vertical tracheal air lucency); **(G)** Sternum. The manubriosternal joint is visible; **(H)** Right hilum, which is anterior to the left hilum in the lateral projection; **(I)** Anterior border of the heart; **(J)** Breast opacities; **(K)** Rounded opacity due to the presence of a small benign (fibrous) mesothelioma within the oblique fissure on the right (this is, of course, not a normal structure); **(L)** Right hemidiaphragm.

to perform a maximal inspiration often result in basilar haziness, which may be confused with pulmonary congestion or pleural effusion. Obscuration of the left hemidiaphragm is commonly noted.[7]

SPECIAL RADIOLOGIC TECHNIQUES

Special techniques may enhance the radiologic examination.[8] The most important are included here and discussed briefly.

Digital Radiography

Digital radiography is particularly useful in improving the image quality and diagnostic value of portable chest radiography, particularly in its applications in the critical care unit.[9] Film digitization is a two-step procedure: a conventional film image is obtained and then digitized and is subsequently manipulable by computer techniques. Conversely, with the use of photostimulable phosphor plates instead of the standard film cassette, a direct digital image can be obtained. Digital images can be transmitted to bedside video monitors, although "hard copy" films provide more optimal images.[6]

Changes in Position of the Patient

In addition to the standard PA and lateral projections, other views are sometimes helpful. Oblique projections aid in localizing lesions and at times detect evidence of disease that was not apparent on the standard films. The apical lordotic projection allows an improved view of the apical and subapical areas of the lungs (Fig. 7-3) and is particularly helpful in detection of chronic tuberculous disease. The lateral decubitus view is usually obtained with the affected side dependent and is particularly valuable in detecting the presence of small pleural effusions and in demonstrating that some large opacities seen on standard roentgenograms are caused by free pleural fluid and not by parenchymal consolidation. The shift in position will also shift fluid levels within pulmonary cavities, which at times is diagnostically helpful. The dependent lung appears smaller and more opaque; if larger and hyperlucent, partial airway obstruction, ie, an aspirated foreign body, may be present. This finding is of great importance in children.

The end-expiratory PA chest roentgenogram is mentioned here for convenience. The end-expiratory film is compared with the standard end-inspiratory film. The comparison provides an objective measurement of diaphgramatic excursions and is valuable in detecting air trapping within a lobe or an entire lung. If a mediastinal

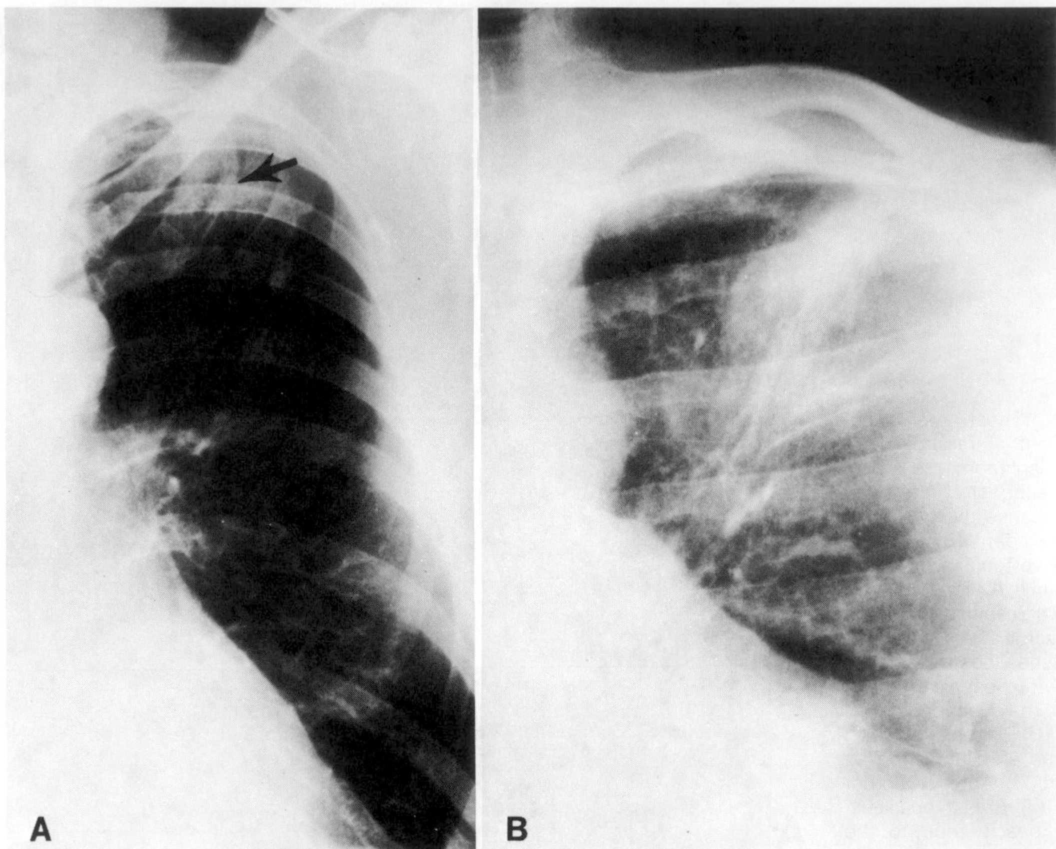

FIGURE 7-3. Value of the apical lordotic projection. **(A)** Posteroanterior chest film showing poorly defined consolidation in the upper left lung below the clavicle and overlying the first rib, the second rib, and the first anterior interspace. **(B)** Apical lordotic view more clearly shows large ovoid mass in left upper lung field. Final diagnosis, established by biopsy, was bronchogenic carcinoma.

shift is present, as in atelectasis or in obstructive hyperinflation, a change in the degree of shift may occur between inspiration and expiration, which is useful in determining which hemithorax is the abnormal one: the mediastinum appears to move toward the normal side on expiration. The end-expiratory film is also useful in the detection of a small pneumothorax.

Changes in Radiologic Contrast

On occasion it is useful to alter the technical factors affecting exposure and radiation density to produce an "overpenetrated" film that delineates certain abnormalities more clearly. This complements the standard chest roentgenogram and is rarely a substitute for it. Digitized images may be easily manipulated to provide a variety of contrasts.

Standard Tomography

Body-section roentgenography (standard tomography, planigraphy, laminography, stratigraphy) was used extensively in the past to facilitate the study of intrathoracic lesions obscured in standard chest roentgenograms by the superimposed opacities of overlying structures. The images obtained were axial rather than cross-sectional. Standard tomography has been replaced almost completely by computed tomography (CT).

Bronchography

Bronchography requires the instillation of a radiopaque substance into the tracheobronchial tree. This adheres to the bronchial mucosa and allows radiologic visualization of the bronchi (Fig. 7-4). The standard bronchographic media contain iodine, although barium has been used occasionally, and inhalation of tantalum dust has been used in research studies. Bronchograms in bronchiectasis clearly show narrowing, dilatation, or closure of the bronchi. Bronchography causes some discomfort to the patient and increases hypoxemia and airway resistance, which involves an element of risk to the patient with diminished pulmonary function. The main contraindication to bronchography is allergy to the local anesthetic or to the bronchographic medium. The CT scan has largely replaced bronchography.

Bronchography of localized areas of lung can be accomplished by instillation of contrast through a fiberoptic bronchoscope that has been positioned in the bronchus serving the region of interest.

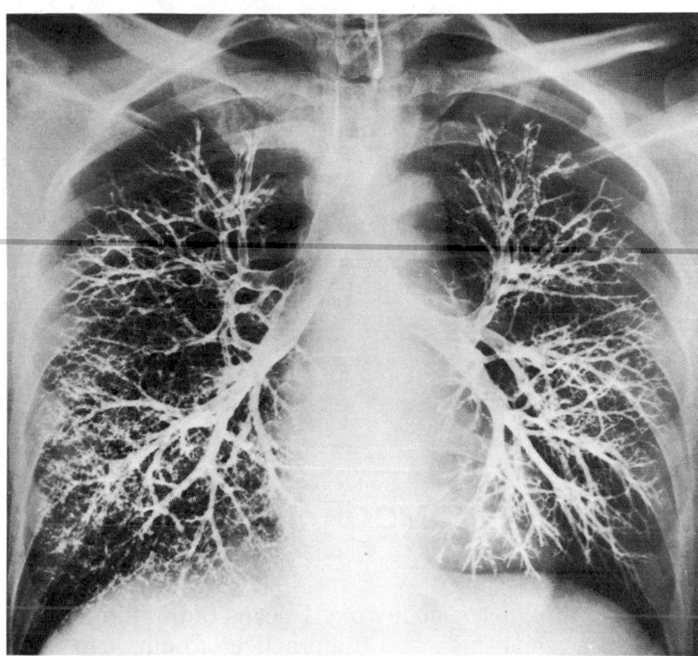

FIGURE 7-4. Normal bilateral bronchogram (posteroanterior view). Note the progressive diminution of airway caliber moving from the carina peripherally. The opaque medium coats the inner walls of the trachea and the bronchial trees.

Angiography

Angiography is a contrast enhancement obtained by injection of a radiopaque medium into the vascular tree to determine the size, patency, and pattern of the blood vessels that are "downstream" from the point of injection. In the investigation of pulmonary diseases, injections of angiographic medium into appropriate areas may be used to opacify one or more of the following: the lower extremity veins, the inferior vena cava, the superior vena cava and its tributaries, the cardiac chambers, the pulmonary trunk and pulmonary arteries, the pulmonary veins, and the aorta and its branches in the thorax or abdomen (including the bronchial arteries).

Pulmonary arteriography is probably the most commonly used of these procedures. It is employed primarily in diagnosing pulmonary embolism but has other uses as well. Bronchial arteriography is sometimes used in the investigation and treatment of hemoptysis of unknown type; arteriography often localizes the site of bleeding and provides guidance for therapeutic embolization of the bleeding vessel.[10]

Contrast venography is the "gold standard" technique for detection of deep vein thrombosis in leg, thigh, and iliac veins and the inferior vena cava. Less commonly, the arm veins are examined by contrast injections. Superior vena cavalgrams are useful to confirm the presence and location of the obstruction in patients with clinical evidence of superior vena cava obstruction.

Fluoroscopy

Fluoroscopy presents a continuous moving image of the area being examined. It provides a dynamic picture of the thorax and its contents during inspiration and expiration and throughout the cardiac cycle. Cinefluoroscopy will provide a permanent recording of the abnormalities visualized. Fluoroscopy is less sensitive than standard roentgenograms in detecting certain pulmonary lesions; it is therefore an adjunct to standard chest roentgenograms, not a substitute for them. In addition, fluoroscopic examination entails a much greater radiation exposure than standard chest roentgenograms.

Fluoroscopy provides valuable information about the motion of the diaphragms and mediastinum and detects the presence of air trapping. The relative expansion of the two lungs during inspiration is well shown. Mediastinal lesions can be better defined in terms of movement during breathing and swallowing. It is difficult, however, to differentiate the pulsatile expansion of a vascular mediastinal mass from the transmitted movement of a nonvascular mass adjacent to a large arterial vessel.

Fluoroscopic monitoring is used during a barium swallow to detect abnormalities and displacements of the esophagus, and during needle aspiration biopsy of lung or mediastinum to guide needle emplacement. Fluoroscopy is sometimes used as a guide during bronchoscopic procedures, particularly during biopsy of lesions beyond the visual field of the instrument, and for emplacement of bronchial stents. Fluoroscopy helps monitor the passage of *central venous* and *Swan-Ganz catheters*.

Radiologic Assessments of Pulmonary Function

Numerous attempts have been made to use roentgenographic techniques for estimating some of the various functions measured by standard pulmonary function tests. The standard fluoroscopic methods obviously provide some information about the total expansibility of the lungs and the relative volume contributions of the two sides, but quantitation is extremely difficult. The specialized techniques of roentgen kymography and roentgen densitometry have shown a fairly good correlation with spirometric measurements of vital capacity and flow rates and have an advantage in that regional variations in these parameters are detectable. Similar information is obtainable with quantitative CT scans. These methods have not found widespread application.

Total lung capacity can be measured fairly accurately from the standard end-inspiratory PA and lateral chest roentgenograms.[11] The method is tedious, however, and is not commonly used.

COMPUTED TOMOGRAPHIC SCANS

The widespread availability of CT scans of the thorax has had a major impact on the practice of pulmonary medicine. The method provides a series of cross-sectional (transverse) "tomographs" of the body structures at multiple levels. Each image is generated by the computer and represents what a thin "slice" through the thorax at that particular level would look like (Fig. 7-5). It is also possible to reconstruct composite images in other planes, particularly with the helical technique.

The CT scan is a supplement to, and not a replacement for, conventional chest radiography. It is particularly helpful in detecting or confirming the presence of a mediastinal mass and in determining its size, shape, location, and radiodensity. In the lungs, CT helps differentiate pleural from parenchymal masses, detects pulmonary nodules and subpleural lesions not visible on standard films or tomograms, and provides excellent demonstrations of the patterns of the abnormalities. Lesions in the bones and thoracic wall are seen very clearly. *High-resolution CT* is particularly valuable in the assessment of diffuse lung parenchymal diseases.[13]

Thoracic CT has been used widely for staging of bronchogenic carcinoma, although recent studies have shown that it is less sensitive and specific than previously thought.[14,15] Procedures such as needle biopsy of pulmonary or mediastinal lesions can be carried out with CT guidance of needle emplacement.[16]

With modern scanning devices, it is possible to perform the examination on critically ill patients maintained on controlled ventilation (Fig. 7-6).

RADIOISOTOPIC IMAGING

Ventilation and Perfusion Scintiscans

Pulmonary scintiscanning is not, strictly speaking, a roentgenologic technique; the image is generated by the radiation emitted from radioisotopes introduced into the lungs.

Pulmonary scintiscans measure the volume and spatial distribution of ventilation and perfusion in the lungs.[17] The standard lung perfusion scintiscan utilizes albumin particles that are tagged or labeled with a radioactive marker, such as iodine or technetium. This material is injected intravenously, and during its pas-

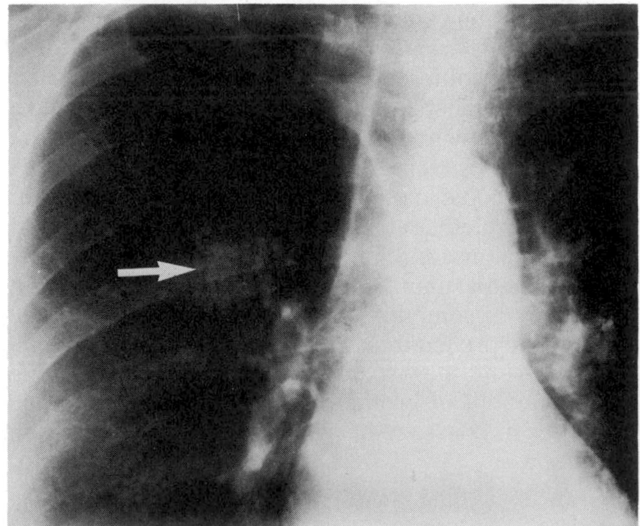

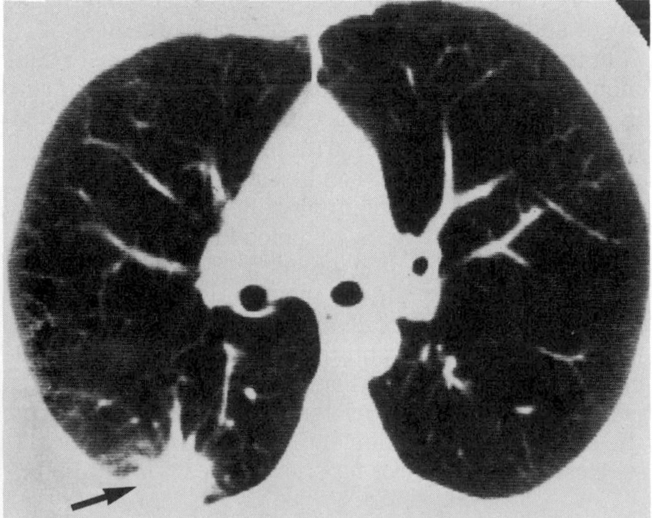

FIGURE 7-5. Advantages of the thoracic CT scan. The standard PA chest film *(left)* shows a poorly demarcated mass *(arrow)* in the right lung. It was not clearly identified in the lateral projection film. The CT scan *(right)* shows the mass *(arrow)* in the right lung adjacent to the right posterior chest wall. The "sunburst" effect is due to tendrils of malignant tissue radiating outward from the main tumor mass—also called the *corona radiata.* This view is a transverse section made at the level just below the carina. The patient is lying supine and the observer is looking cephalad. The right lung is therefore on the left side of the picture.

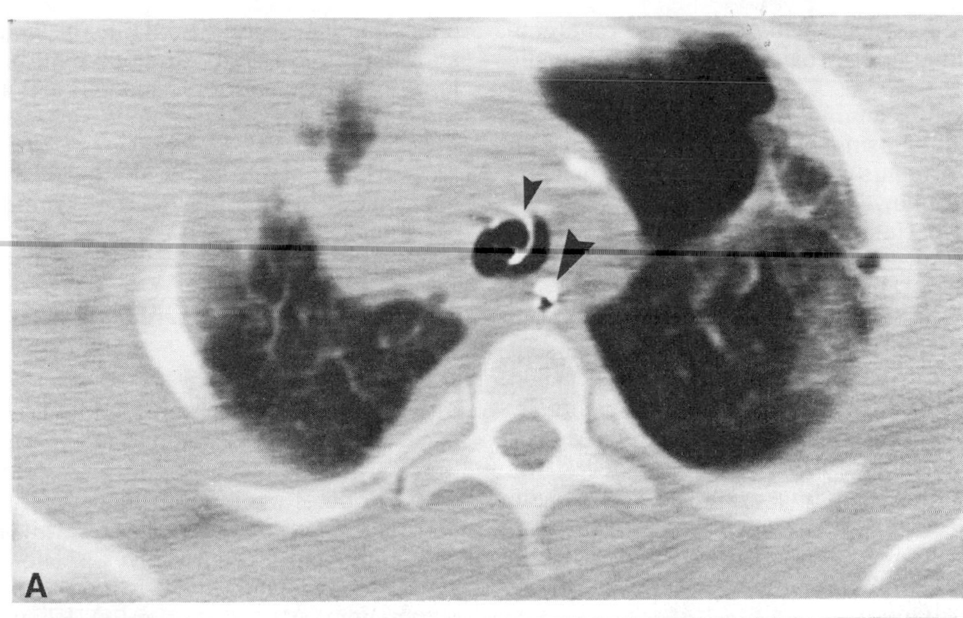

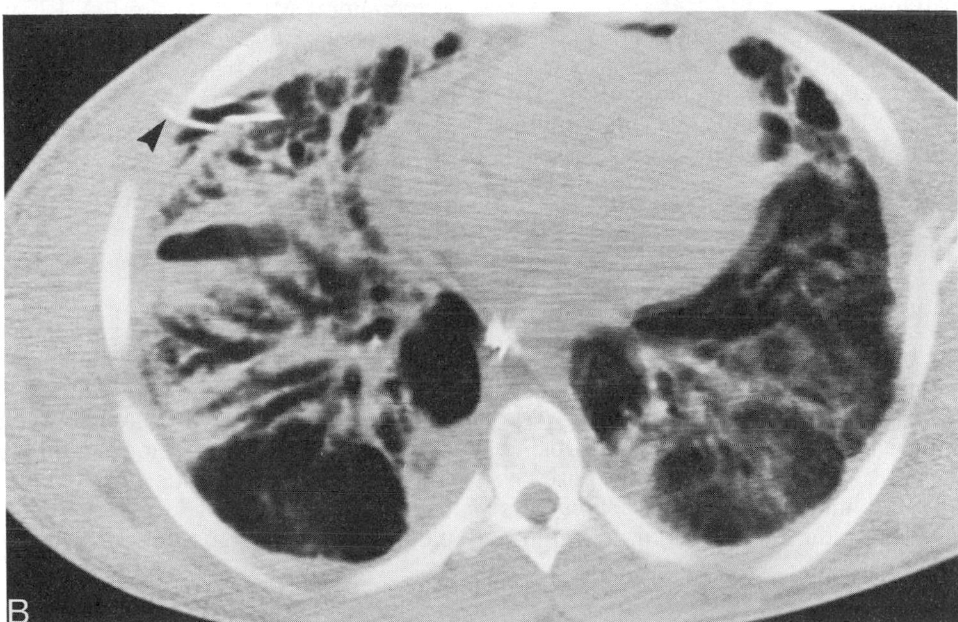

FIGURE 7-6. Thoracic CT scans of a young man with chest and head trauma from a motorcycle accident. **(A)** This upper level section ("cut") shows an endotracheal tube *(upper arrowhead)* within the lumen of the trachea, and a small opaque gastric tube *(lower arrowhead)* within the esophagus. The patchy opacities in the anterior half of the right lung are due to pneumonia. An air-filled bulla occupies the anterior portion of the left lung. **(B)** The lower section, a few centimeters above the dome of the diaphragm, shows a pleural drainage tube *(arrowhead)* entering the right pleural cavity anteriorly. There is extensive opacification throughout the right lung, with prominent air bronchograms. This indicates an alveolar-filling process called consolidation, which in this case was due to pneumonia. The gastric tube is still visible within the lower esophagus.

sage through the lungs some of the albumin particles impact in the small pulmonary capillaries. A scanning device is then passed over the thorax, and the pattern of gamma radiation provides a recorded image of the distribution and volume of perfusion in the lungs.

Similarly, the ventilation scintiscan assesses both the distribution pattern and the volume of ventilation within the lungs, measured by scanning the thorax while the patient takes one or several breaths of radioactive gas, usually xenon. Radioaerosols labeled with technetium can also be used and have some technical advantages over the xenon inhalations.

The diagnostic usefulness of ventilation and perfusion scintiscans lies in the fact that a number of pulmonary diseases will give rise to abnormalities in either ventilation or perfusion, or both. Although the pattern that emerges is not entirely specific for any single process, it does delineate the abnormality in physiology that can then be correlated with clinical and roentgenographic information to provide improved diagnostic precision.

Pulmonary scintiscanning is used most commonly in detecting and diagnosing pulmonary embolism. The lodgment of an embolus within a lobar or segmental pulmonary artery is followed by a marked decrease or complete absence of perfusion in the involved area. Ventilation to the area, however, is often fairly well maintained, at least for the first 24 to 48 hours. Ventilation/perfusion scans taken within the first 48 hours will often show a highly characteristic pattern of diminished or absent perfusion with normal ventilation. These are called "nonmatching" defects. If the embolized area eventually undergoes infarction, ventilation will also decrease or disappear in the region of the perfusion defect. This type of combined or "matching" ventilation/perfusion defect is not specific for pulmonary infarction; however, it may also be seen with many other conditions, including pneumonia, asthma, emphysema, atelectasis, and bronchogenic carcinoma.

Ventilation/perfusion scintiscans have some application in cases of bullous emphysema, particularly in selecting those patients who might benefit by surgical resection of the bullae. The technique has some limited usefulness in other pulmonary parenchymal and vascular conditions.

Other Radioisotopic Techniques

Radiolabeled gallium localizes in tissues that are inflamed or have been invaded by malignant tumors. The gallium scan has been used to detect metastatic lung tumor in mediastinal lymph nodes, but CT is more sensitive and specific. Gallium is most commonly used to determine if diffuse lung diseases such as fibrosing alveolitis or sarcoidosis are "active" and therefore potentially treatable. In individuals with *Pneumocystis carinii* pneumonia secondary to the acquired immunodeficiency syndrome (AIDS), the gallium scan may show a diffuse increase in uptake of the isotope in the lungs before radiographic changes are clearly visible on the standard chest radiographs.

Positron emission tomographic (PET) scans appear to have great value in differentiating benign from malignant pulmonary nodules and in staging bronchogenic carcinomas.[18]

MAGNETIC RESONANCE IMAGING

Although the images generated by the magnetic resonance imaging (MRI) technique superficially resemble those produced by CT, the processes are quite different. MRI detects the radiosignals emitted when hydrogen nuclei in the body are placed within a magnetic field and stimulated by radio waves.[19] The images may be viewed in any plane (Fig. 7-7).

In general, MRI is inferior to CT in imaging most intrapulmonary disorders, but the two processes are about equally effective in the study of lesions in the hilar areas or mediastinum.[20] MRI is particularly valuable in the study of mediastinal vascular disorders, such as aneurysms, and in detecting the presence and degree of invasion of apical (Pancoast) tumors of the lung.

DIAGNOSTIC ULTRASOUND

Ultrasonography is an important diagnostic tool in the investigation of certain cardiac abnormalities, but the applications of the technique in other forms of intrathoracic diseases are more limited, for technical reasons.[21]

Sonography is often helpful in the assessment of intrapleural fluid collections, both to detect free fluid and to localize pockets of loculated fluid within massive pleural densities. This may provide guidance for the

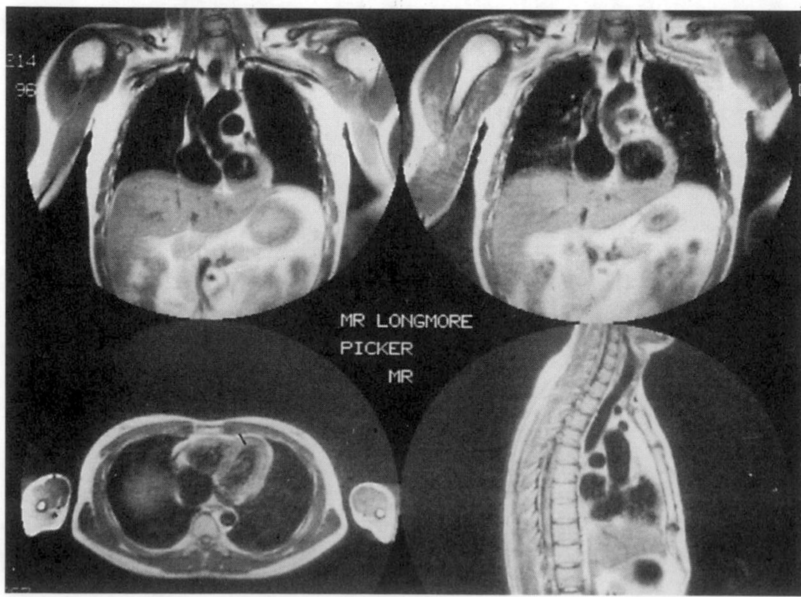

FIGURE 7-7. MRI scans of the thorax. The two upper images are coronal sections, with the one on the right being slightly more posterior. Note that the subcutaneous and intra-abdominal fat deposits are white, and the trachea, blood vessels, and heart chambers appear black. Intrapulmonary structures are poorly defined. The two lower images are a supradiaphragmatic transverse section *(left)*, and a midline sagittal section *(right)*.

placement of thoracentesis needles or intercostal drainage tubes. Subpulmonic and subphrenic collections of fluid may also be detected in this fashion. The position and degree of movement of the right hemidiaphragm can usually be determined. In some cases, sonography may provide guidance for needle aspiration biopsy of certain pulmonary and mediastinal lesions.

Doppler (duplex) ultrasonography is now the noninvasive technique of choice for the detection of deep vein thrombosis in the lower extremities in patients believed to have suffered a pulmonary embolic episode.[22]

INTERVENTIONAL (INVASIVE) RADIOLOGY

Imaging techniques, such as fluoroscopy, CT, and sonography, can be used to guide or monitor the performance and effectiveness of a number of diagnostic or therapeutic invasive procedures in and around the thorax, and the performance of these techniques has given rise to the newest radiologic subspecialty.[23] Most of these that pertain to the thorax have already been mentioned.

LOCALIZED OPACIFICATIONS

Localized (focal) opacifications in the lungs may be single or multiple. The distribution of the opacities may be lobar, segmental, or nonsegmental.[24] There are four major underlying causes of localized opacities.

Consolidation

This is an opacification owing to displacement of alveolar air by fluid, tissue, or exudate, resulting in solidification of the involved area of lung.[1] The distribution is lobar or segmental in some instances. There is usually little or no loss or gain of volume in the consolidated area. The lung tissue itself is relatively preserved.

Consolidation typically manifests a radiologic appearance called alveolar filling. An early radiologic sign is blurring of the normal vascular patterns in the consolidating area, with increasing loss of vessel outlines as the opacification increases. The opacification is caused by the presence of multiple areas of alveolar filling, which are poorly circumscribed and often confluent. Consolidation is usually nonhomogeneous even when extensive, giving a patchy radiologic appearance (Fig. 7-8). Air bronchograms are often detectable in nonobstructive alveolar-filling processes (see Fig. 7-6).

Ground glass opacification (Fig. 7-9) is a lesser degree of consolidation, manifested by a diffuse haziness on standard radiographs, and by increased opacity without air bronchograms or marked blurring of bronchovascular bundles on high-resolution CT.[20]

Areas of consolidation may be single or multiple, unilateral or bilateral. Common causes include pneumonia (infectious or noninfectious), pulmonary edema, posttraumatic pulmonary contusion, intra-alveolar hemorrhages, certain chronic granulomatous diseases, localized alveolar cell carcinoma, and the early stages of pulmonary infarction.[24]

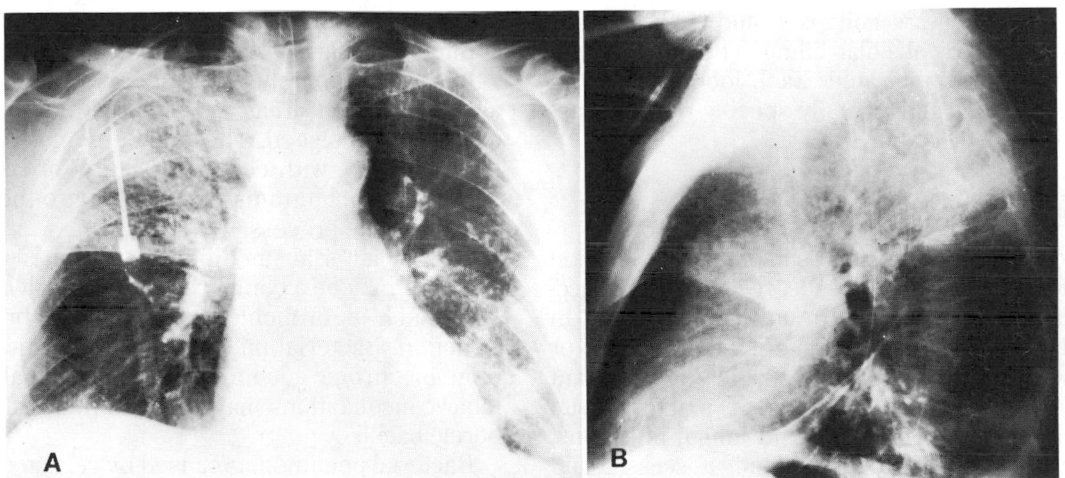

FIGURE 7-8. Bacterial pneumonia, causing consolidation of the right upper lobe. This localized alveolar-filling process occupies most of the right upper lobe. Lucent "air bronchograms" can be seen within the consolidation, indicating that the opacity is alveolar-filling in type, and that the upper lobe bronchus is patent. **(A)** PA projection with the consolidation sharply limited inferiorly by the horizontal fissure. Overlying the right hemithorax is a catheter taped to the anterior chest wall which then passes down the right subclavian vein and into the superior vena cava. The tip is obscured within the mediastinal opacity. Patchy, confluent, poorly circumscribed opacities can be seen in the lower left hemithorax. These are areas of bronchopneumonia. **(B)** Left lateral projection. The sternum is to the left, and the spine to the right. The pneumonic consolidation is sharply demarcated inferiorly by the horizontal fissure (anteriorly) and by the oblique fissure (posteriorly). Foci of bronchopneumonia can be seen above the left hemidiaphragm posteriorly. The left diaphragm can be identified by its proximity to the gastric air bubble.

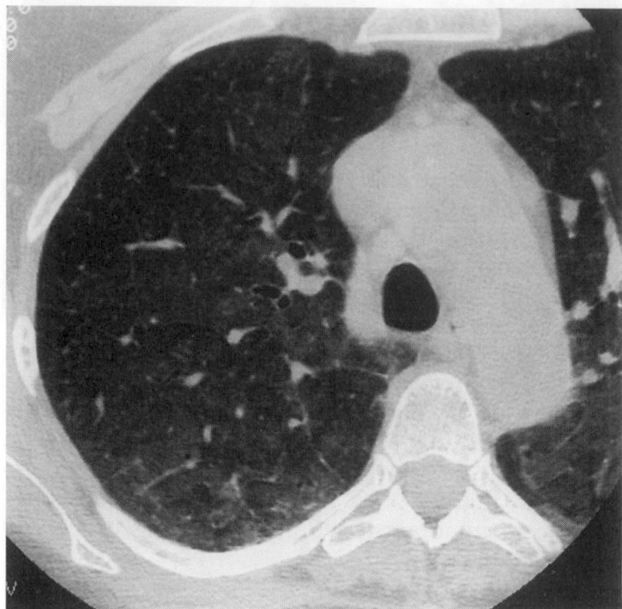

FIGURE 7-9. CT scan showing "ground glass" type of alveolar opacity. Note the diffuse haziness without obliteration of the bronchovascular markings. No air bronchograms are seen.

Atelectasis

Atelectasis signifies an opacification with loss of volume (collapse) in a segment or lobe.[1,2,25] With complete obstruction of a bronchus, the collapse results from progressive resorption of air in the lung distal to the obstruction; the opacification will be homogeneous in appearance without air bronchograms (see Fig. 7-9), and the entire lobe or segment will be involved. Pathologically, the alveoli are collapsed and airless rather than consolidated by alveolar filling. The vascular pattern is completely obliterated. Each lobe or segment has a characteristic and virtually specific roentgen appearance when atelectatic.[25]

Replacement Opacity

A localized opacity may be the result of focal destruction or distortion of normal lung tissue, resulting in replacement by inflammatory tissue, tumor, or scar tissue. In some instances, the normal tissue is pushed aside or compressed by a growing mass, usually a malignant tumor. In other instances, there has been actual tissue necrosis, owing to tuberculous and fungal infections, necrotizing pneumonias, undrained lung abscesses, and complete infarcts. Such lesions, single or multiple, tend to be rather homogeneous in density and often sharply circumscribed, although the outline may be irregular.

Pleural Effusion

A collection of pleural fluid presents as a homogeneous opacity, which is generally gravity dependent. A moderate sized, uncomplicated effusion in an individual who is in the upright position occupies the lower hemithorax, blurs out the diaphragm-lung interface, and has a poorly demarcated upper border, which is generally concave upwards.[1,2]

PNEUMONIA

Pneumonia is an inflammatory consolidation of the lung, most commonly caused by an infection with microorganisms. Other causes include auto-immune processes and inhalation or aspiration of toxic substances. Most pneumonias are acute in onset, bacterial in origin, and alveolar-filling in radiologic presentation. The opacification is usually nonhomogeneous, provided that the bronchus to the area is not completely obstructed.[1,2] Pneumonia sometimes shows lobar/segmental distributions (Figs. 7-8 and 7-10), but the involvement is incomplete in many instances and multilobar in some. Small and multiple poorly circumscribed pneumonic opacities are called bronchopneumonia.

The radiologic appearances do not permit identification of the origin, although certain features provide clues, particularly when considered in conjunction with clinical criteria.

Bacterial Pneumonias

Bacterial pneumonias may be caused by a variety of pathogenic microorganisms that reach the lung through inhalation or aspiration of infected secretions (commonly) or by hematogenous spread from an infection elsewhere (less commonly). Primary bacterial pneumonias caused by the pneumococcus *(Streptococcus pneumoniae)*, Friedlander's bacillus *(Klebsiella pneumoniae)*, or the staphylococcus *(S. aureus)* are commonly lobar or segmental in distribution (see Fig. 7-8). Most commonly, one lobe or segment is involved, although several areas of disease within different lobes are sometimes seen. These pneumonias are alveolar-filling in type, with confluent "fluffy" areas of opacity and "air bronchograms" contributing to the nonhomogeneity of the process.[26]

Lobar bacterial pneumonias are often primary in type, but may be a complication of underlying lung disease, such as bronchiectasis or partial bronchial obstruction. Bacterial pneumonias are particularly common in chronic alcoholics. In occasional instances, lobar consolidations may result from infection with tubercle bacilli or fungi.

Bacterial pneumonias caused by certain other microorganisms usually present as "bronchopneumonia," characterized by multiple nonsegmental opacities. Organisms that commonly present in this fashion include *Streptococcus pyogenes, Hemophilus influenzae, Mycoplasma,* the coliform bacilli, *Pseudomonas, Proteus, Serratia,* anaerobic bacteria, and *Staphylococcus.*

Necrosis may occur with bacterial pneumonias, particularly those caused by *Staphylococcus aureus,* aerobic gram-negative bacilli, and anaerobic organisms. Drain-

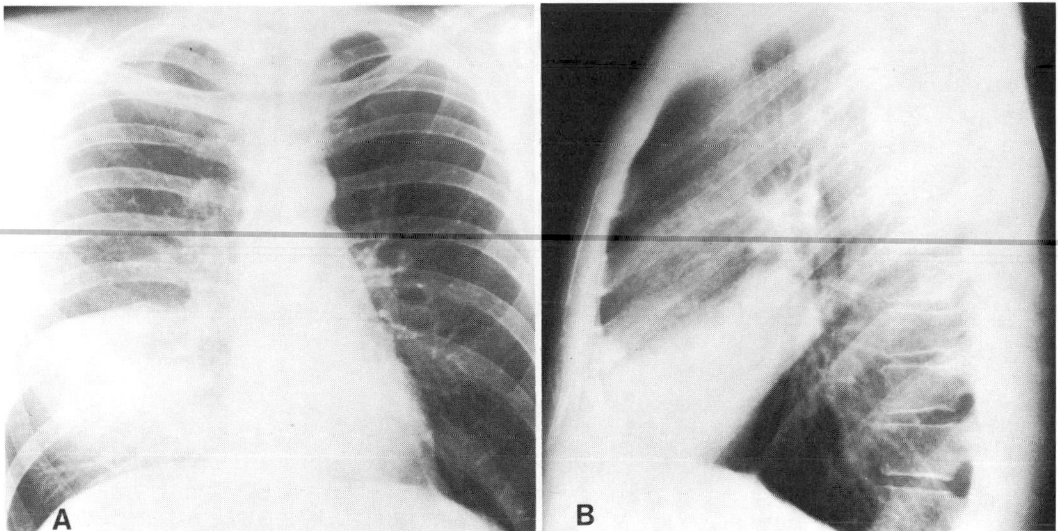

FIGURE 7-10. Right middle lobe pneumonia. **(A)** PA projection showing the consolidation with its characteristic triangular configuration. The sharp interface of the upper border is limited by the horizontal (minor) fissure. The lateral border is limited by the oblique fissure, but there is no sharp interface, as the x-ray beam in the PA projection is not parallel to the fissure. Note that the costophrenic angle is clear and the right heart border is blurred (the silhouette sign). **(B)** Lateral view showing the roughly triangular opacity (with the apex at the hilum) overlying the cardiac opacity. The upper margin is often more sharply outlined than this.

age of the necrotic material results in the appearance of air-filled hyperlucent areas called cavities (see Fig. 7-11). A cavity secondary to necrotizing pneumonia is termed a *lung abscess.* A cavity that changes rapidly in size (a pneumatocele) is a common complication in staphylococcal infections.

Bacterial aspiration pneumonia presents with single or multiple consolidation of dependent portions of the lungs caused by aspiration of infected pharyngeal secretions; it is most common in alcoholics and in patients with poor oral hygiene, particularly if obtunded. The infecting organisms are usually anaerobes or gram-negative aerobic bacilli; necrosis and abscess formation are common. Bacterial pneumonias are commonly accompanied by parapneumonic pleural effusions. Occasionally frank empyema develops.

Certain bacterial pneumonias may initially appear to be nonbacterial because the organisms are rarely seen in sputum smears and are difficult to culture. These include mycoplasma pneumonia, a common form of community-acquired pneumonia. Other examples are psittacosis (parrot fever), legionellosis (Legionnaire's disease), and the pneumonia caused by *Chlamydia pneumoniae.* Diagnosis is serologic or by lung biopsy. The radiologic pattern is usually bronchopneumonic.[26–28] The clinical term "atypical pneumonia" is often applied in such cases.

Viral Pneumonias

Viral pneumonias may present with a diffuse interstitial or alveolar-filling pattern.[27] This is particularly common with influenzal (Fig. 7-12) and cytomegalovirus infections, which may be accompanied by severe hypoxemia and increased lung stiffness sufficient to qualify these diseases as examples of adult respiratory distress syndrome (ARDS).

Many or most viral pneumonias, however, present roentgenographically as a patchy bronchopneumonia, which may be complicated by secondary bacterial infection. These illnesses may be only a temporary inconvenience to a previously healthy person, but can produce a life-threatening respiratory insufficiency in the patient with chronic obstructive lung disease. Adenovirus pneumonia is often epidemic in young adults.

Viral pneumonias caused by measles or varicella may appear on the roentgenogram as miliary lesions or multiple nodules rather than as an obvious alveolar-filling process. Mortality is high.

Noninfectious Pneumonias

Pneumonic consolidation may be caused by physical or chemical irritation of the lung rather than by infection. Such pneumonias may be diffuse or localized in distribution.

The inhalation of noxious fumes, such as nitrogen dioxide (silo-fillers' disease), chlorine, sulfur dioxide, or phosgene, may cause a diffuse pneumonic process that is acute, extensive, and often fatal. The aspiration of low-pH gastric juice may cause a widespread pneumonic process called peptic (acid) pneumonitis. This syndrome is discussed in the section on diffuse alveolar diseases.

Lipoid pneumonia (oil granuloma, paraffinoma) results from aspiration of mineral oil or oily nose drops and presents radiologically as a localized chronic consolidation stimulating carcinoma. Localized noninfec-

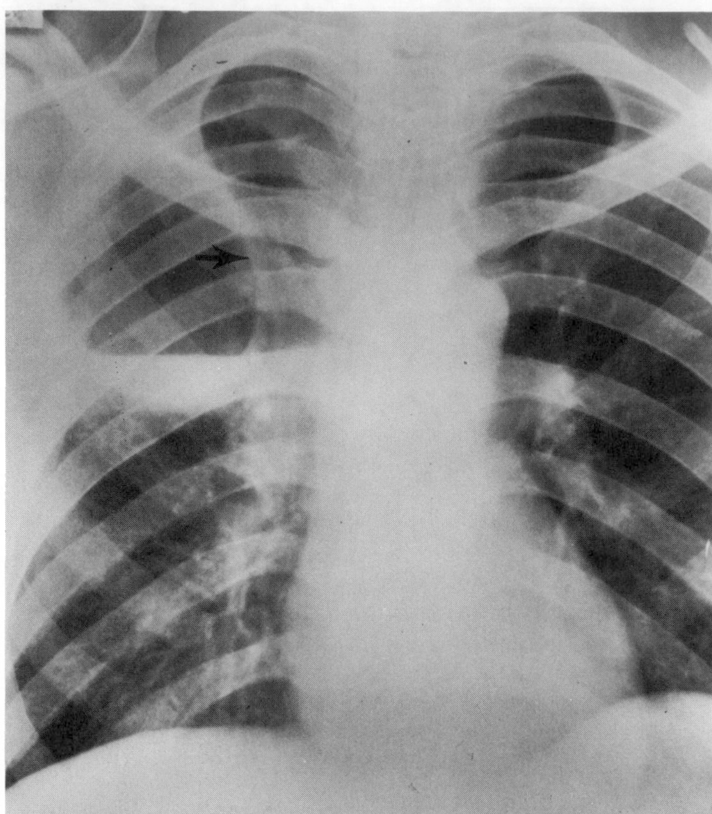

FIGURE 7-11. Lung abscess. A large thin-walled cavity containing a small amount of fluid is seen in the upper right lung. Note the horizontal air-fluid interface, indicating that the x-ray beam is tangential to the interface, as the subject was in the upright position. The medial wall of the cavity is marked *(arrow)*. The superior wall is hidden by the clavicle and the lateral wall is obscured by the ribs of the lateral chest wall. The antecedent necrotizing pneumonia which caused the cavity has largely cleared.

tious pneumonias, with solitary or multiple lesions, may occur in collagen-vascular diseases.

The term hypersensitivity pneumonitis (allergic alveolitis) encompasses a group of diseases caused by inhalation of organic antigens. Examples include farmers' lung and bird-fancier's lung. The early stage of the reaction of the lung to *radiation* is pneumonic in type, although a rather dense interstitial fibrosis may eventually develop in the involved area.

Atypical Pneumonias

This term dates back to a time when microbiologic sciences had developed sufficiently to permit the recognition that some cases of pneumonia were both clinically and microbiologically different from the "typical" bacterial pneumonias, and were then classified as examples of "primary atypical pneumonia."

In current usage, the term denotes pneumonias that tend to have a gradual onset. Clinically, upper respiratory symptoms and systemic symptoms such as fever and malaise are prominent. The pneumonia, which is sometimes an unexpected chest radiographic finding, is usually nonsegmental. Sputum is scanty and nonpurulent, and examination of sputum by smears and standard bacterial cultures commonly fails to identify an obvious bacterial cause.

Common forms of atypical pneumonia include mycoplasma pneumonia, psittacosis, rickettsial pneumonia, legionellosis, and viral pneumonias.[27,28] In some cases, primary tuberculous and fungal infections may present with this syndrome of atypical pneumonia.

Aspiration Pneumonias

This term is applied to three different types of pneumonia, which have already been mentioned: the acute chemical pneumonitis caused by massive aspiration of gastric fluids, the chronic lipoid pneumonia caused by chronic or recurrent aspiration of lipids, and anaerobic bacterial pneumonia with lung abscess, caused by aspiration of infected pharyngeal secretions in obtunded patients.

TUBERCULOSIS, FUNGAL, AND PARASITIC DISEASES

Tuberculosis

In the early (primary) stage of tuberculous infection, before the body develops resistance, single or multiple areas of pneumonia may occur, usually accompanied by regional lymphadenopathy. These usually heal, but a positive tuberculin skin test and sometimes one or two small calcific areas persist as evidence of infection. However, small infected foci, not roentgenographically apparent, may remain and may give rise to progressive tuberculous disease months or years later.[29] This process is called endogenous reactivation and may be triggered

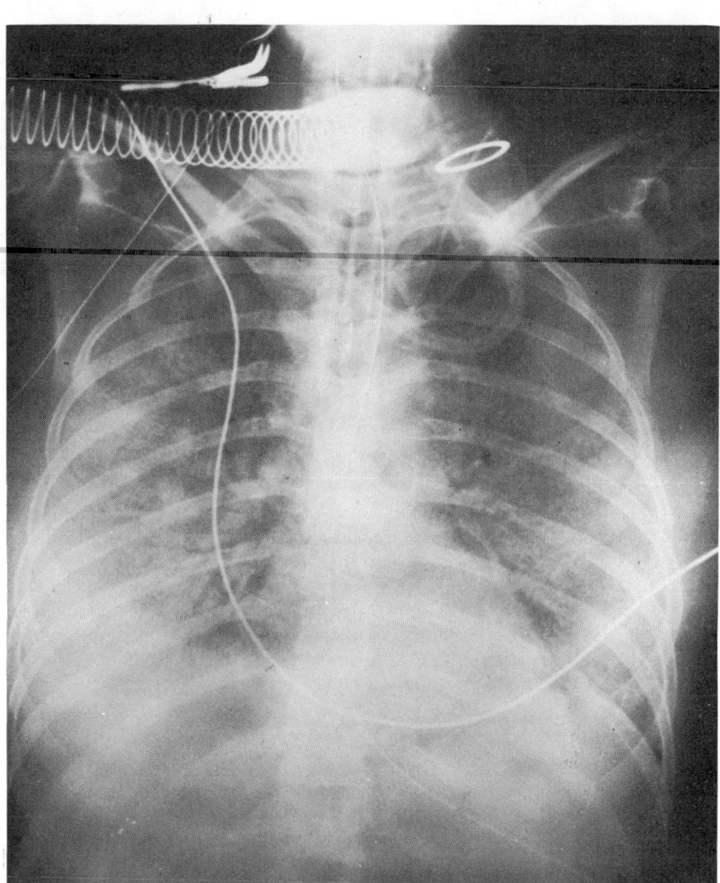

FIGURE 7-12. Extensive bilateral alveolar consolidation due to influenzal pneumonia. The diagnosis was proven by open lung biopsy and cultures. The lesions are variable in size, confluent, and poorly demarcated. The main involvement is in the lower lungs.

by a number of factors, including silicosis, use of immunosuppressive drugs, or the development of AIDS.[30]

Reactivation tuberculosis may be rapidly progressive but more commonly presents as a somewhat indolent destructive granulomatous process in which consolidation, cavitation, fibrosis, and calcification are often present simultaneously. The irregular lesions usually involve apical and subapical areas of the lungs (Fig. 7-13), and the disease is often bilateral. Tuberculosis in AIDS patients often has atypical clinical and roentgenologic features.[29]

Fungal Diseases

Lung disease caused by certain fungi, particularly *Coccidioides immitus* and *Histoplasma capsulatum,* may resemble tuberculosis radiologically.[31] Nodules and thin-walled cavities are common in coccidioidomycosis (Fig. 7-14).

Other fungi may cause pneumonic consolidations, sometimes rapidly spreading, if the host defenses have been compromised. Fungi that often behave in this fashion include *Cryptococcus neoformans,* the Phycomycetes, *Candida albicans* and *Aspergillus fumigatus.* Infection with phycomycetes (mucormycosis) is most commonly seen in diabetic patients. Candidiasis and aspergillosis may follow long-term antibiotic therapy and often occur in granulocytopenic patients and after the use of immunosuppressive drugs.

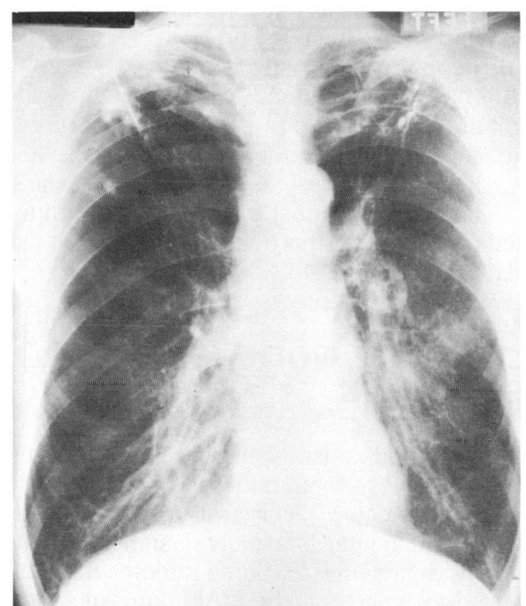

FIGURE 7-13. Bilateral apical and subapical tuberculosis. The lesions are opaque, clearly calcified in some areas and probably fibrotic in others. However, active infection may be present in lesions such as this that appear healed. This patient also has emphysema, proven by pulmonary function tests, and suggested by the loss of lung markings in many areas of the lungs. Note the upward retraction of the left hilum, due to fibrotic scarring and volume loss in the left upper lobe.

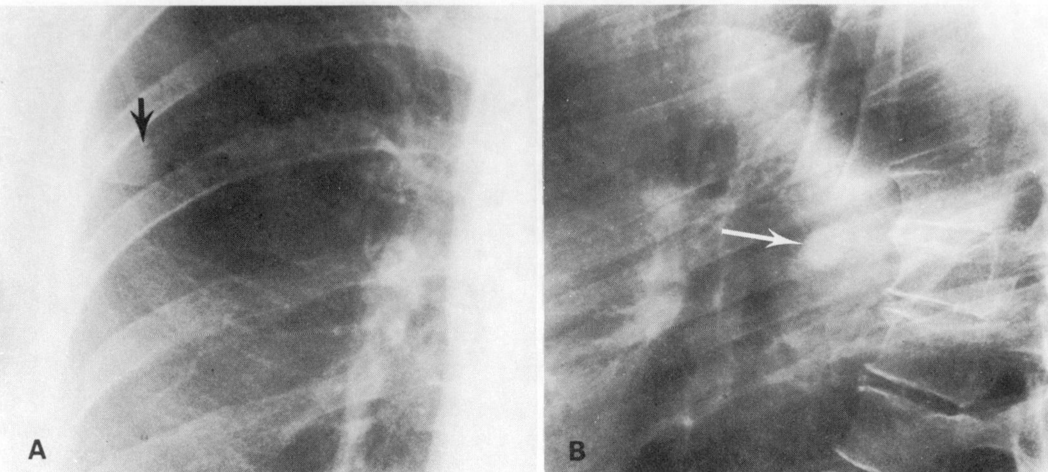

FIGURE 7-14. Solitary pulmonary nodule due to coccidioidomycosis. **(A)** PA view of right hemithorax showing the 1.5-cm nodule situated far laterally *(arrow)* in the upper lung. **(B)** In the lateral view, the nodule is clearly seen overlying the shadow of the aortic arch, halfway between the hilar opacity and the thoracic spine. The nodule is calcified *(arrow)*. This lesion was a 4-cm area of pneumonia when first detected, and gradually evolved into the nodule over a 3-month period. (Lillington GA: A Diagnostic Approach to Chest Diseases, 3rd ed. Baltimore, Williams & Wilkins, 1987.)

Nocardiosis and actinomycosis may also behave similarly and are commonly included among the fungal diseases, even though the causative organisms are now classified as bacteria rather than fungi.

Parasitic Infestations

Pulmonary consolidations caused by parasitic infestations are rarely seen in nontropical climates, with two exceptions. Amebic infection in the liver may spread upward through the diaphragm to involve the right lower hemithorax; the roentgenographic changes include pneumonic consolidation, pleural effusion, or pulmonary cavitation. Pneumonia caused by infection with *Pneumocystis carinii* presents as a diffuse alveolar-filling process and occurs almost exclusively in immunosuppressed patients.[32] It is particularly common in patients with AIDS.

PULMONARY NODULES AND MASSES

A pulmonary nodule is a well-circumscribed, roughly spherical, opaque intrapulmonary lesion usually greater than 1 cm in diameter.[33] A circumscribed lesion greater than 4 cm in diameter is usually designated a mass lesion rather than a nodule. Some nodules develop cavitation, and many are calcified. Although most nodules are solid, the appearance may be mimicked by a small loculated effusion.

Solitary Pulmonary Nodule

The solitary nodule is most commonly a healed or healing infectious granuloma that may result from tuberculosis, coccidioidomycosis, histoplasmosis, or other infections. Less commonly the solitary nodule is a lung tumor, either benign or malignant. Primary malignant tumors are usually bronchogenic carcinomas, but occasionally the malignant lung nodule is a solitary metastasis from an extrapulmonary primary tumor. Other disease processes may occasionally present as a solitary nodule.[33]

If serial chest roentgenograms show that the nodule has not increased in size over 2 years or if it exhibits extensive calcification, it is very likely that the lesion is benign (see Fig. 7-14). A nodule that fails to meet these criteria is potentially malignant and is usually subjected to needle biopsy or exploratory thoracotomy. Malignant nodules usually have lobulated or spiculated margins; these features are best analyzed by CT.

Multiple Pulmonary Nodules

These are usually intrapulmonary metastases from an extrapulmonary primary malignant lesion. Other causes include tuberculosis, fungal diseases, sarcoidosis, silicosis, and necrotizing granulomatous conditions such as Wegener's syndrome or lymphomatoid granulomatosis.[33] The appearance of multiple pulmonary nodules in an immunosuppressed host strongly suggests opportunistic infection with fungi. The smaller miliary nodules are discussed in the section on diffuse lung diseases.

BRONCHOGENIC CARCINOMA

Bronchogenic carcinoma, the commonest cause of cancer death in both males and females, may present radiologically in many fashions.[34] Occult lung cancer refers to a tumor not visible on standard chest roentgenograms but detected by positive sputum cytology. Most cases of bronchogenic carcinoma present as a solitary nodule or lung mass. Other roentgen presentations include atelectasis, persistent or recurrent pneumonic consolidation, an enlarging apical opacity, hilar enlargement, pleural effusion, and mediastinal enlargement.

Radiologic imaging plays a major role in determining the stage of lung cancers,[35] although CT is now known to be less sensitive and specific than previously considered.[14,15]

ATELECTASIS AND LOSS OF VOLUME

Atelectasis is a loss of volume of part (or all) of a lung. The airless atelectatic area is usually opaque and is lobar/segmental in location. Although atelectasis may result from several different mechanisms, the term is used most commonly in reference to those losses of volume caused by bronchial obstruction or cicatrization (scar formation).

Obstructive Atelectasis

Obstructive atelectasis may result from (1) extrabronchial compression from tumors or enlarged lymph nodes, (2) endobronchial diseases such as bronchial tumors (Fig. 7-15) or inflammatory strictures (Fig. 7-16), or (3) an intrabronchial mass such as an exogenous foreign body or a large mucus plug (Fig. 7-17). A movable intrabronchial mass may act as a "ball valve" that allows the air to be pumped out from the affected segment within minutes. More commonly, atelectasis results from the slow resorption of air in the bronchioles and alveoli distal to the completely obstructed bronchus.

Cicatrization Atelectasis

Cicatrization (scar) atelectasis may occur in the absence of significant bronchial obstruction. It is sometimes a complication of lobar or segmental pneumonia, which fails to resorb and becomes "organized" and fibrotic. Contraction of the parenchymal fibrosis decreases the lung volume. It may also develop as a complication of chronic fibrocaseous tuberculosis, usually involving an upper lobe.

Signs of Atelectasis

The *indirect* signs of atelectasis are secondary to the collapse of a lobe or an entire lung.[25] They are usually detectable on the chest roentgenogram and will suggest that volume loss has occurred, even if the opacification of the atelectatic segment or lobe is not clearly seen. These signs include elevation of the hemidiaphragm on the affected side, shift of the mediastinum towards the affected side, a decrease in size of the rib interspaces over the affected hemithorax, and in many

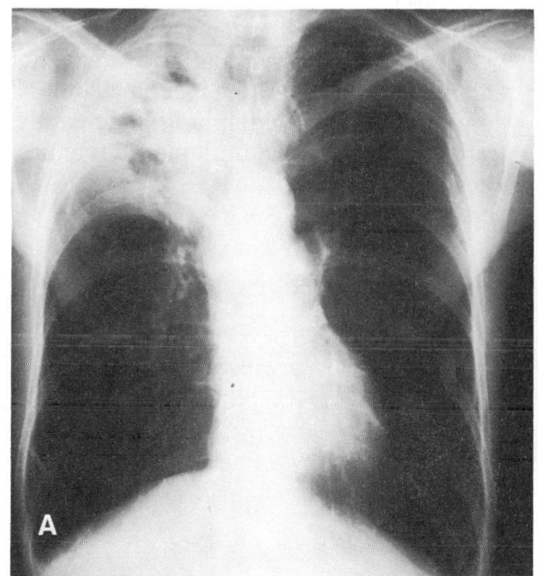

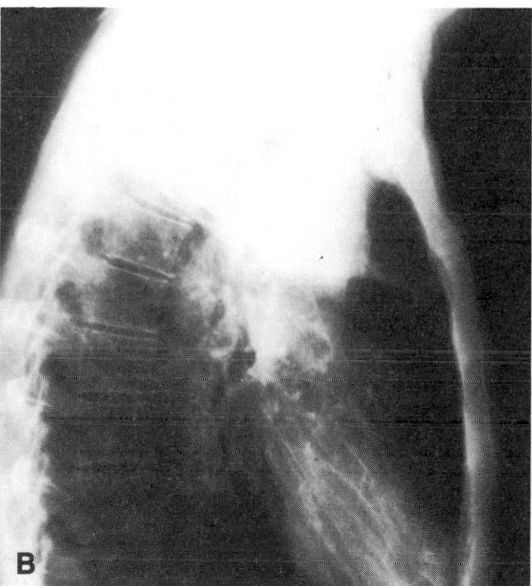

FIGURE 7-15. Obstructive pneumonitis of the right upper lobe secondary to bronchial occlusion by bronchogenic carcinoma. **(A)** In the PA view, the lobe has lost some volume, as shown by the elevation of the horizontal fissure, which demarcates the consolidation inferiorly, but the fissure has not completely rotated to the diagonal position that would be expected if the more marked loss of volume due to complete atelectasis was present. Intralobar cavitation is secondary to necrotizing pneumonitis. **(B)** Lateral view shows fissures elevated but retaining their normal angulation.

This man also has advanced pulmonary emphysema. In the PA view, the lungs are hyperlucent from hyperinflation and from widespread destruction of the pulmonary parenchyma and vessels. The diaphragms are low and flat and the small heart appears to be "hanging" in the mediastinum above the left hemidiaphragm. In the lateral view, the diaphragms are flat and scalloped, and the sternodiaphragmatic angle is considerably greater than 90°. The retrosternal air space is large and markedly hyperlucent.

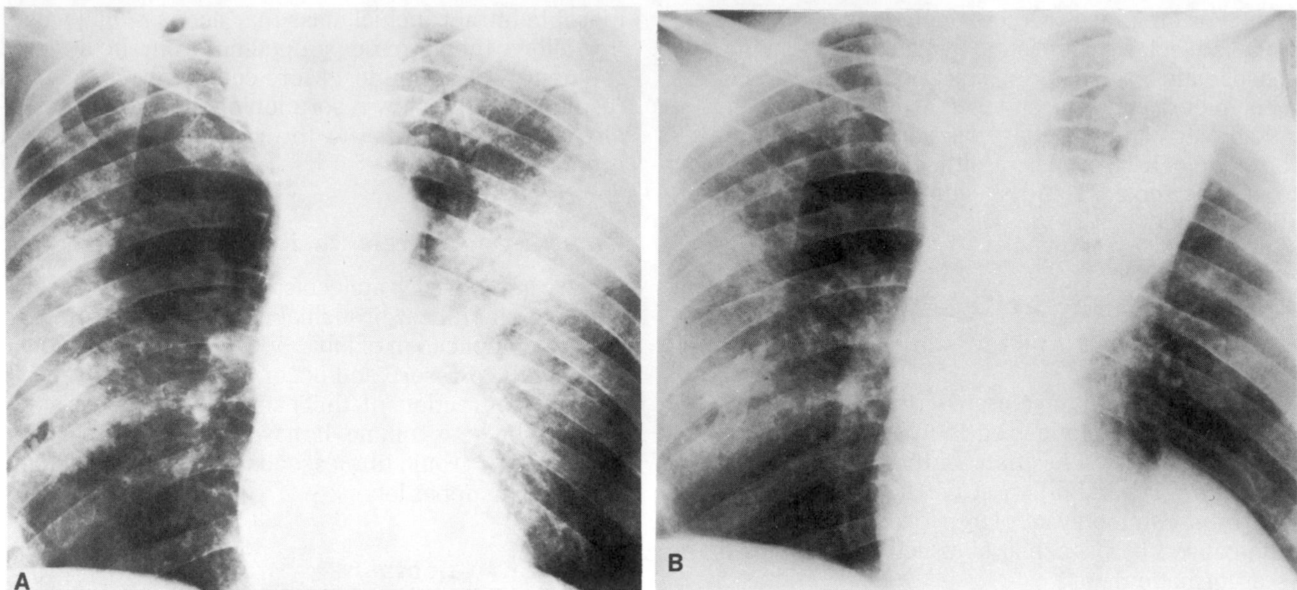

FIGURE 7-16. Consolidation of the left upper lobe, followed by atelectasis, in a case of active pulmonary tuberculosis. **(A)** PA view showing a fairly dense alveolar consolidation in the left upper lobe, with sparing of the apical segment but involvement of the lingula. There is little loss of volume. In the right lung are several areas of tuberculous bronchopneumonia. **(B)** Two weeks later. The left upper lobe bronchus has become occluded by tuberculous endobronchitis, and the left upper lobe is now atelectatic, being smaller and denser. There is still some aeration within the apical segment. The left hemidiaphragm is now markedly elevated due to loss of volume in the left lung.

instances a compensatory hyperinflation of the adjacent lobes or of the opposite lung. A shift of the hilum, either upward or downward, is sometimes present.

The *direct* signs of atelectasis are the characteristic appearances[1,2,25] on the standard chest roentgenograms of the collapsed opaque segment, lobe, or lung (Figs. 7-15 through 7-17). The margins of the collapsed lobes are usually sharp and smooth, as the interfaces are delineated by interlobar fissures.

Other Types of Decreased Lung Volumes

Decreased volume of the entire lung occurs when the stability of the chest wall is impaired, allowing the elastic recoil of the lung to pull the affected area inwards and thus effect a decrease in lung volume. Common examples include hemidiaphragmatic paralysis or eventration (Fig. 7-18) and multiple rib fractures with a flail chest.[36]

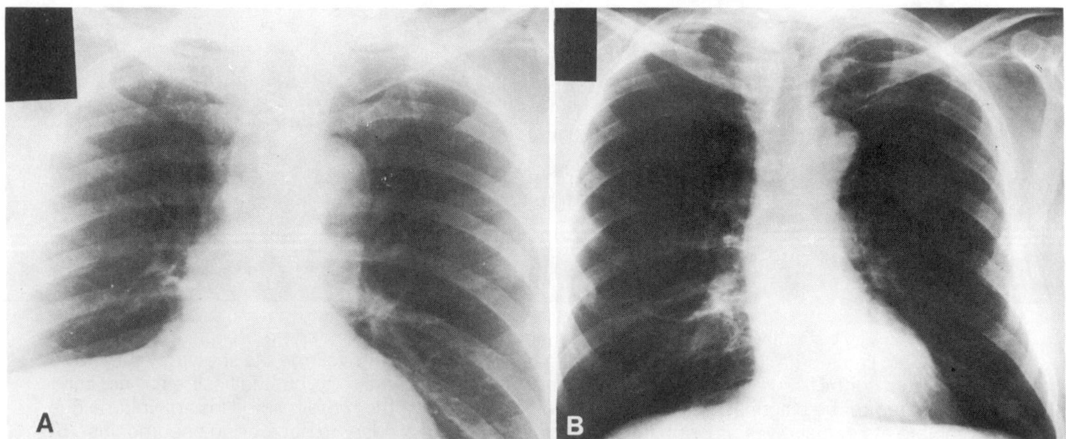

FIGURE 7-17. Atelectasis of the right lower lobe due to sputum plug retention after intracranial sugery in an 18-year-old boy. **(A)** The PA view shows a collapsed and airless right lower lobe that mimics an elevated right hemidiaphragm. The interface is at the level of the oblique (major) fissure which is pulled downwards by the collapse. **(B)** The same patient, 1 hour after bronchoscopic aspiration of the plug. The right lower lobe has reexpanded, and the diaphragm is now visible at its normal level.

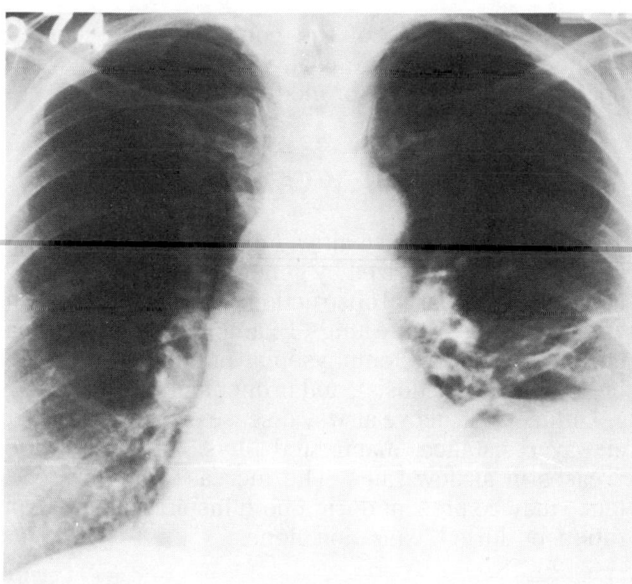

FIGURE 7-18. Eventration of the left hemidiaphragm. The elevated hemidiaphragm showed paradoxical movement on sniffing. Usually the upper margin of the eventrated hemidiaphragm maintains a sharp convex contour. In this case, a previous pulmonary infection has resulted in pleural adhesions between the diaphragm and the lung. Horizontal streaks of "discoid" atelectasis can be seen. (Lillington GA: A Diagnostic Approach to Chest Diseases, 3rd ed. Baltimore, Williams & Wilkins, 1987.)

The development of extensive pleural scarring (fibrothorax) renders the affected hemithorax smaller and less expansile. Finally, an expanding lesion within the lung, such as a rapidly growing tumor, a lung abscess, or an expanding tension cyst, may cause some compression of the adjacent normal lung. Although loss of the volume of the lung is a feature of all these conditions, the term atelectasis is not usually used in these circumstances.

The appearance in the pleural space of air (pneumothorax) or fluid (hydrothorax, pleural effusion) allows the lung to retract towards the hilum into a partially collapsed position.[1,2] In these cases the loss of volume is generalized, not localized, is partial and not complete, and the radiologic picture is dominated by the primary intrapleural disturbance.

Other Manifestations of Bronchial Obstruction

Bronchial obstruction will have differing effects on the distal lung depending on the degree of obstruction and the rapidity with which it develops. Minor degrees of obstruction that have no major effect on airway dynamics will not result in roentgenologic changes. However, the presence of the localized obstruction may be clinically apparent on auscultation over the affected area. A persistent localized wheeze or reduced breath sounds may be noted.

An obstruction large enough to impair the clearance of mucoid secretions from the distal lung predisposes towards pneumonia in the affected segment or lobe. This pneumonic consolidation will have the usual roentgenologic characteristics of a segmental or lobar alveolar-filling process caused by nonobstructive pneumonia and will often demonstrate air bronchograms.

If, however, the obstruction increases and becomes complete while the pneumonia is still present, the affected segment or lobe becomes completely airless. However, it cannot shrink in volume because the alveoli are filled with inflammatory exudate. In such cases of obstructive pneumonitis ("drowned lung"), air bronchograms will be absent, allowing one to infer the presence of bronchial obstruction as the cause of the homogeneous opacification of the lobe without loss of volume (see Fig. 7-15). A complete bronchial obstruction that develops without secondary infection intervening will show the signs of *atelectasis* described previously (see Fig. 7-17).

Another important manifestation of a partial bronchial obstruction is obstructive *hyperinflation,* which occurs when the location and magnitude of the obstruction is such that it allows air to enter the lobe as the bronchus increases in size during inspiration but prevents egress of air as the bronchus decreases in size during expiration. The hyperinflated lobe or segment is hyperlucent and virtually functionless. It may cause some compressive loss of volume in adjoining or contralateral nonobstructed lung segments or lobes. Although bronchography can be used to confirm the presence and site of obstruction, bronchoscopic visualization with biopsy of the obstructing lesion is the most effective diagnostic tool.

CAVITIES AND CYSTS

A cavity is a hole within the lung parenchyma.[1,2] It usually results from destruction of lung tissue, although sometimes it follows the bronchial evacuation of the contents of a congenital fluid-filled cyst. The terminology of cavitary lesions of the lung is confusing and somewhat inconsistent.

A *lung abscess* is a localized area of lung destruction caused by liquefaction necrosis, usually within an area of necrotizing pneumonitis caused by pyogenic bacteria. A lung abscess may present initially with the roentgenographic appearance of a solid mass; if the liquefied material then drains into a bronchus and is expectorated, the lung abscess will appear as a thick-walled, round cavity containing air and often an air-fluid level (see Fig. 7-11). Hematogenous spread of infection to the lungs may result in multiple abscesses. Hemorrhage, often life-threatening, may occur within cavitary lesions. A lung abscess may be a source of dissemination of infection throughout the body, resulting in septicemia or sometimes brain abscesses.

Obstruction of a bronchus, usually from foreign body or tumor, may cause a necrotizing process in the distal lung that eventually forms an abscess. Conversely, a large neoplastic mass may undergo central necrosis resulting in a thick-walled malignant abscess. Both primary and secondary tumors may undergo cavitation.

Cavitation may occur within noninfectious granulomas, and occasionally within an infarcted area secondary to pulmonary embolism.

Cavitation occurs commonly in pulmonary tuberculosis and in fungal infections of the lungs. These cavities may have thick or thin walls. There are usually other lesions in neighboring portions of the lungs as well.

Bullae are thin-walled, focal areas of emphysema. They vary in size but may be several centimeters in diameter in some cases. The wall of the bulla may not be roentgenographically visible or may present as one or more "hairline" shadows that form part of the wall that are not always continuous around the entire air-containing structure (Fig. 7-19). Bullae may occasionally occur in otherwise normal lungs, but are usually a manifestation of diffuse obstructive emphysema. Secondary infection may result in the development of air-fluid levels.

A pneumatocele is a bulla that results from a check-valve obstruction of a bronchus, which causes the bulla to increase or decrease rapidly in size. It occurs most commonly as a complication of staphylococcal pneumonia.

A cyst is a thin-walled cavity, usually congenital in origin. Many cysts are originally fluid-filled and contain air only if drainage of the contents has occurred. Bronchogenic cysts are oval, well-circumscribed and opaque, and often hilar or mediastinal in location.

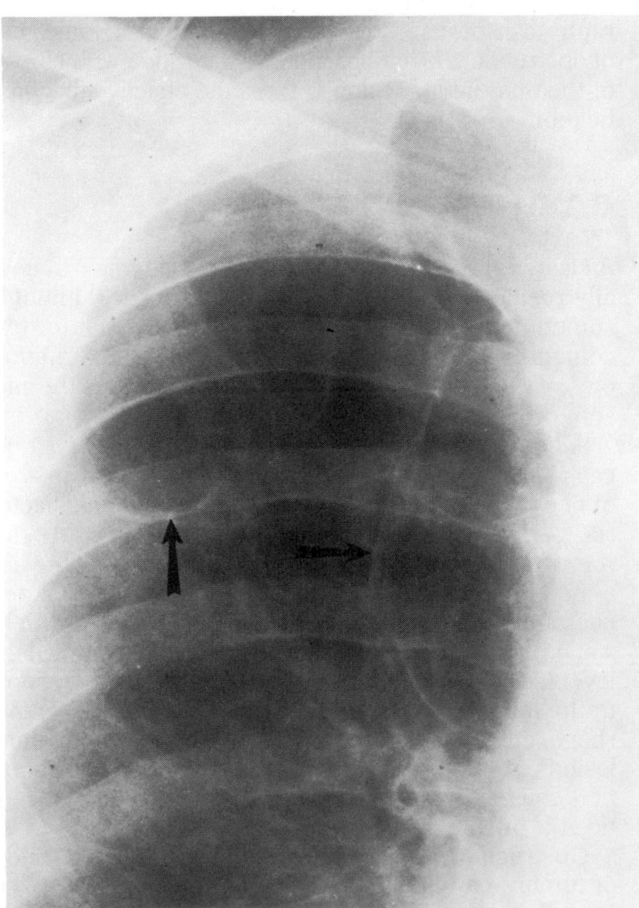

FIGURE 7-19. Bullae in the upper right lung. Thin hairline shadows bordering the bullae are shown *(arrow)*. Within the bullae, there is little or no lung substance. This is a chest roentgenogram of a 76-year-old male with panacinar emphysema with bullous transformation.

DIFFUSE AIRWAY OBSTRUCTION

The diffuse obstructive airway diseases are a group of conditions characterized by generalized airway narrowing resulting in partial obstruction of most of the bronchi and bronchioles in the lungs. Examples include asthma, chronic bronchitis, emphysema, pulmonary cystic fibrosis (mucoviscidosis), and bronchiolitis obliterans.

Diffuse obstructive airway disease leads to increased airway resistance, manifested physiologically by decreases in airflow rates. The increased airway resistance may be present during both inspiration and expiration, or during expiration alone.

Roentgenologic Changes

These may be very obvious or fairly subtle. These changes, manifested in varying degrees by the different disease processes, include the following:

1. *Hyperinflation.* An increase in the total lung capacity as shown on standard end-inspiratory chest roentgenograms. The roentgenographic signs are depression and flattening of the diaphragms, a generalized increased translucency of the lung fields, and an increased size of the retrosternal air space as seen on the lateral projection. The flattening of the diaphragms is the most reliable sign.
2. *Air trapping.* A decreased ability to evacuate alveolar air during expiration. Detection of air trapping requires an end-expiratory roentgenogram to compare with the standard end-inspiratory roentgenogram. Fluoroscopic examination will supply similar information.
3. *Loss of interstitial tissue and pulmonary vessels.* The loss of interstitial tissue is most apparent if bullae are present; demonstration of diminution in vasculature may require "full chest" tomograms or pulmonary angiography. It is now known that so-called "high-resolution" CT is the most sensitive and accurate modality for the identification and quantitation of lung destruction.[37]
4. *Increased lung markings.* This occurs in some cases and is presumed to be caused by bronchial wall inflammation with thickening, and by peribronchial fibrosis secondary to previous bronchopneumonic infections. This appearance is often referred to as the "dirty lung" and is commonly seen in chronic bronchitis, cystic fibrosis, and widespread bronchiectasis.

Asthma

Asthma is an intermittent or reversible form of diffuse airway obstruction characterized by bronchospasm, eosinophilic inflammation of the bronchial mucosa, and plugging of the airways with tenacious mucus. In about

40% of cases, the disease is associated with atopic allergy and is called extrinsic asthma; in the remainder of cases (intrinsic asthma), no definite allergic features can be identified, and the onset is often in middle age or later.

During symptom-free periods, the chest roentgenogram appears entirely normal in most instances. During an acute asthmatic attack, in which the airway obstruction is manifested clinically by severe dyspnea and wheezing, the chest roentgenogram is usually normal, particularly in patients with adult onset asthma. In asthmatic children, the reversible hyperinflation may cause some depression of the diaphragm and increased hypertranslucency.[38] Destructive changes in the interstitial tissue do not occur, and the pulmonary vasculature is essentially normal. In short, an asthmatic attack may cause acute deterioration of pulmonary function with relatively little radiographic change. In such cases the physical signs are diagnostic and more helpful than the roentgen features.

Complications of asthma may give rise to roentgenographic abnormalities.[10] Recurrent infections result in thickened bronchial walls and a "tram-line" appearance. Atelectasis may occur because of mucus plugs. Pneumomediastinum and pneumothorax may occasionally complicate asthma. Radiologic abnormalities in allergic bronchopulmonary aspergillosis (ABPA) include perihilar masses, consolidations, tram line shadows, nodules, and ring shadows.[38]

Chronic Bronchitis

Chronic bronchitis is a chronic low-grade inflammation of the bronchi manifested by persistent cough and sputum production. Diffuse airway obstruction may be absent, mild, or severe. The chest roentgenogram is often normal but may show the pattern of "increased lung markings."[37] In some instances there is a superimposed reversible or asthmatic component (chronic asthmatic bronchitis), and in these cases hyperinflation and air trapping are sometimes noticeable. Unless complicated by emphysema, chronic bronchitis is not associated with destruction of interstitial tissue or loss of pulmonary vasculature.

Emphysema

Emphysema is a destructive process in the pulmonary parenchyma, and the roentgenologic signs listed above, including loss of interstitial tissue and pulmonary vessels, hyperinflation, and bullae, are most marked in emphysema (Figs. 7-13, 7-15, 7-19). The detection of bullous disease is the most reliable sign of emphysema on the standard chest roentgenogram. In advanced cases, hyperinflation is usually quite apparent on roentgenographic studies. In many cases of emphysema, the chest roentgenogram appears normal.

CT is considerably more sensitive and accurate than standard roentgenography in the imaging of emphysema.[36] Chronic bronchitis and emphysema have the same cause (tobacco smoking) and often coexist in a given patient. The term "chronic obstructive pulmonary disease" (COPD) is commonly applied to denote this association.

PNEUMOTHORAX

Pneumothorax denotes the presence of air within the pleural cavity. Air may gain access to the pleural cavity through the chest wall, diaphragm, mediastinum, or from the lung through the visceral pleura. Pneumothorax may be traumatic, iatrogenic, or spontaneous.

The roentgenographic sign of pneumothorax is the patternless hypertranslucency of intrapleural air separating the partially collapsed lung from the chest wall.[2] A "hairline" linear shadow representing the visceral pleura forms the interface between pleural air and lung (Fig. 7-20). The partially collapsed lung contains less air and appears a little more opaque.

A small pneumothorax may be difficult to detect on the standard end-inspiratory roentgenogram. The pneumothorax is always more obvious if films are taken in the end-expiratory position, and this is a very useful diagnostic maneuver in questionable cases. The presence of underlying lung disease may be detected by the chest roentgenogram. The concomitant presence of blood, pus, chyle, or serous effusion will result in an air-fluid level.

With a small pneumothorax the air may be visible only in the apical and subapical areas. Pleural adhesions may prevent the retraction of portions of the lung, and this may result in a loculated pneumothorax in which the intrapleural air is localized to one or more discrete areas instead of involving the entire pleural space (Fig. 7-21).

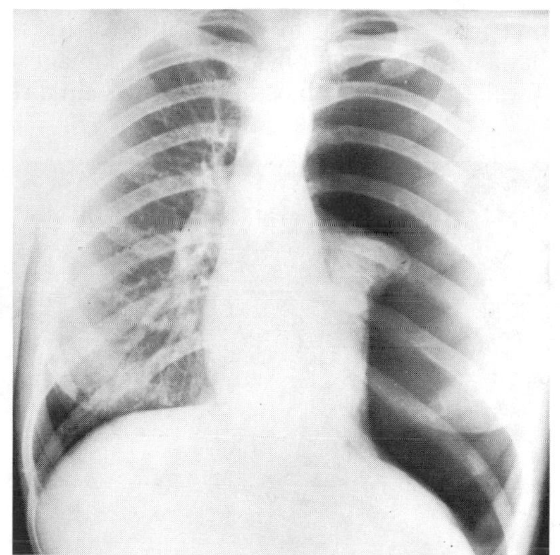

FIGURE 7-20. Massive left spontaneous pneumothorax in a young woman. The collapsed left lung forms a small opaque ball in the hilar area, whereas the rest of the hemithorax is filled with the patternless hypertranslucency of pleural air. Usually the lung does not collapse to this degree in cases of spontaneous pneumothorax unless the air communication remains widely open, or there is a "tension" pneumothorax. The marked depression of the left hemidiaphragm suggests the latter, although one might expect greater contralateral mediastinal shift.

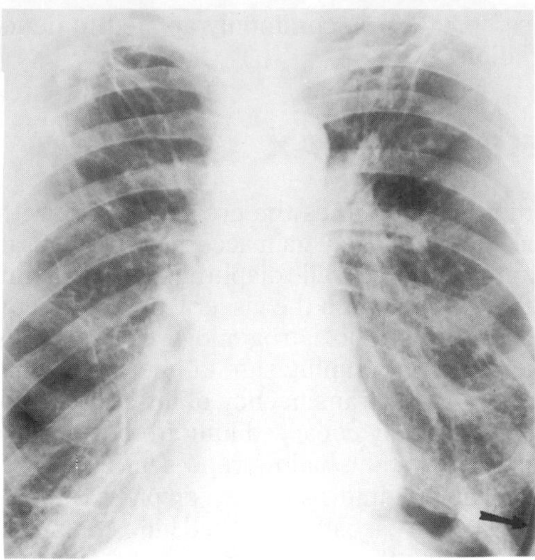

FIGURE 7-21. Small loculated pneumothorax at the left base. Compare with Fig. 7-13, which is a previous x-ray of the same patient. Apparently an emphysematous bleb has ruptured, allowing leakage of air into the pleural space which is bound down by adhesions in most areas except laterally and inferiorly at the left base.

If a patient already has impaired pulmonary function, the development of a pneumothorax, even one that is small in degree, may cause serious respiratory difficulty, which can, however, be quickly relieved once the correct diagnosis has been established by roentgenography and the air evacuated by closed intercostal drainage. Pneumothorax should be considered whenever there is an acute increase in dyspnea, particularly if unilateral chest pain is present.

Traumatic Pneumothorax

Trauma may give rise to pneumothorax by several mechanisms, the most obvious being damage to the chest wall that allows atmospheric air to gain direct access to the pleural space. More commonly the underlying lung is lacerated, either from a penetrating foreign body or from injury to the lung by rib fracture.[36] Another mechanism is traumatic fracture of a bronchus with resulting air leakage. An air-fluid level caused by pleural blood is often visible in traumatic cases.

Iatrogenic Pneumothorax

This is now the most common cause of intrapleural air. Such pneumothoraces may be intentional (as in the induction of pneumothorax for diagnostic purposes), unavoidable (as in needle biopsy of the lung), or unintentional.

Iatrogenic pneumothorax may result from inadvertent perforation of the lung during various diagnostic or therapeutic procedures, including thoracentesis, liver biopsy, pericardiocentesis, intercostal nerve block, stellate ganglion block, transbronchial or percutaneous lung biopsy, attempted cannulation of a subclavian vein, and surgical procedures (such as tracheostomy) at the base of the neck. Procedures such as transtracheal needle aspiration and endoscopic injury of the thoracic esophagus may result in mediastinal emphysema, which may subsequently rupture into the pleural space. Pneumothorax is, unfortunately, a rather common complication of barotrauma (Fig. 7-22) owing to mechanical ventilation.[39]

Spontaneous Pneumothorax

Spontaneous pneumothorax may occur as a complication of intrapulmonary or mediastinal disease processes. Most commonly it is seen in young smokers and is caused by rupture of a bleb at the apex of a lung (see Fig. 7-20). It is essentially a benign disorder that may, however, be recurrent and eventually require surgical correction. Tuberculosis must be ruled out if the condition is recurrent. Pneumothorax resulting from in-

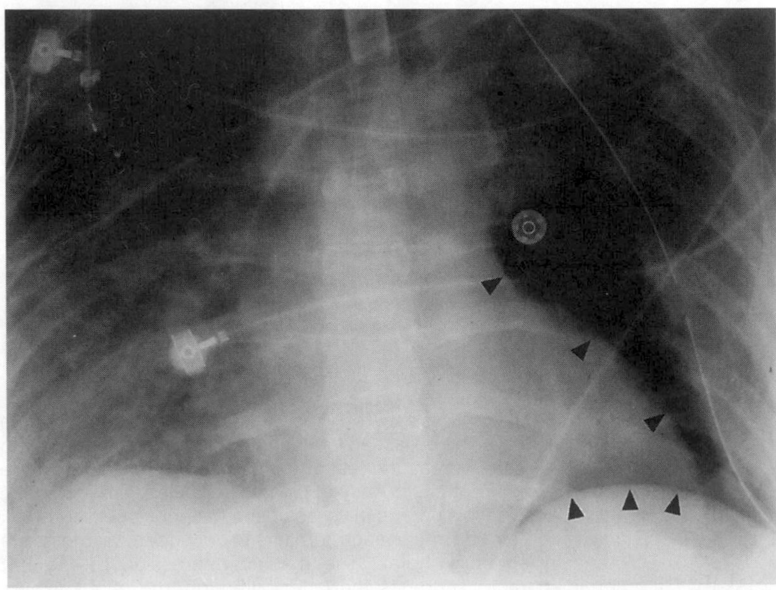

FIGURE 7-22. Anterior, medial and subpulmonic pneumothorax in an ARDS patient with barotrauma. Note overly sharp definition of left heart border and diaphragm, which indicates that the interface is being formed by pneumothorax air rather than by the lung.

trapulmonary infectious diseases may be complicated by empyema (pyopneumothorax).

MEDIASTINAL EMPHYSEMA

Free air within the mediastinum is termed mediastinal emphysema (pneumomediastinum). It may result from rupture of a major bronchus or the esophagus, or from the passage of air upward through the diaphragm or downward from the neck. Most commonly it is secondary to an intrapulmonary rupture of alveoli with subsequent dissection of air centrally along the bronchovascular sheaths into the mediastinum.[40] This may occur as the result of trauma or from spontaneous rupture of alveoli (seen most often in asthmatic and diabetic patients, and pregnant women). It is a commonly encountered complication of mechanical ventilation (ventilator barotrauma), particularly with the use of positive end-expiratory pressure (PEEP).[39]

Mediastinal emphysema is manifested by the presence within the mediastinum of one or more vertical linear hyperlucent streaks, most easily identified as a separation of the mediastinal pleura from the underlying structures (Fig. 7-23). The roentgenographic changes are often subtle and frequently escape recognition. The air may pass upward into the soft tissues of the neck and thoracic wall (subcutaneous emphysema), where it is easily visible on roentgenographic examination and equally easily detectable by palpation. Mediastinal emphysema often causes chest pain but usually has little deleterious effect on pulmonary function.

DIFFUSE LUNG DISEASES

A large number of lung diseases (more than 100) may present with diffuse pulmonary opacifications. Differential diagnosis is somewhat simplified by the recognition that there are three basic radiologic patterns of diffuse lung disease: the alveolar-filling pattern, the interstitial pattern, and the miliary (small nodular) pattern.[1,2,41] Less commonly recognized are the bronchial pattern and the vascular pattern, which often resemble the interstitial pattern.

The Alveolar-Filling Pattern

The diffuse alveolar-filling pattern is characteristically comprised of "soft," fluffy, poorly demarcated and confluent opacities, which are multifocal but widely distributed throughout the lungs. In the early stages, there are individual opacities (acinar nodules), which are 0.5 cm to 1 cm in diameter; but they become sufficiently profuse to overlap on the radiograph and also to coalesce, resulting in the appearance of larger, irregular, poorly demarcated opacities that may be several centimeters in diameter. The normal vascular pattern becomes blurred and eventually obliterated, as the alveolar opacification reduces the contrast between the air density of the lung and the water density of the vessels. At the same time, the alveolar opacifications provide contrast to the hyperlucent air within the bronchial tree, revealing a characteristic arborizing pattern called an "air bronchogram." These appearances are called consolidation.[13]

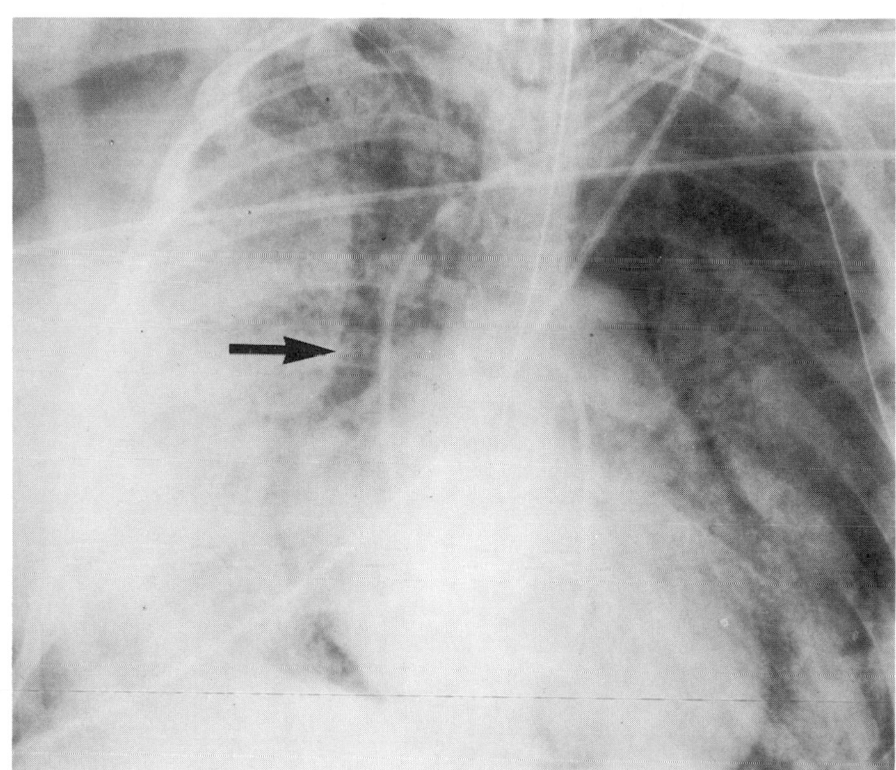

FIGURE 7-23. Mediastinal emphysema. PA view of a 16-year-old woman with ARDS and barotrauma. Note the tracheostomy tube, the Swan-Ganz catheter and the chest tube draining air from the left pleural space. The mediastinal pleura *(arrow)* is lifted off by the air. Subcutaneous air can be seen in the lateral chest wall, and streaks of air are visible within the pectoralis muscles.

A bilateral perihilar (butterfly wing, bat wing) distribution is sometimes seen when an alveolar-filling process diffusely involves the lungs (Fig. 7-24). Diffuse alveolar filling may also show a ground-glass appearance of diffuse fine granularity in some cases.[13] On CT, ground-glass opacities do not show air bronchograms or obliteration of the bronchovascular markings (see Fig. 7-9).

The nature of the substance that is filling the alveoli can rarely be determined from the radiologic characteristics of the abnormality. Blood, pus, water, or cells can produce a diffuse, alveolar-filling pattern. Differential diagnosis, on which successful treatment is based, depends on the associated clinical features and, at times, the results of bronchoalveolar lavage or lung biopsy.

□ FUNCTIONAL ABNORMALITIES

Pulmonary function is usually markedly impaired with diffuse lung disease. Clinically such patients are usually very dyspneic. Pulmonary function studies show the typical restrictive pattern: significant reductions in vital capacity (VC), residual volume (RV), and total lung capacity (TLC) without evidence of diffuse airway obstruction. The FEV_1/FVC ratio is normal or high. The lung is stiff and has a low compliance. The diffusing capacity is usually markedly reduced, and the arterial blood gases typically show severe hypoxemia associated with hypocapnia owing to secondary hyperventilation. In advanced cases, widespread involvement of alveoli may also be associated with carbon dioxide retention. The arterial hypoxemia may be very profound, and even high-flow oxygen supplementation may fail to raise the arterial oxygen tensions to levels that will alleviate the tissue hypoxia. The hypoxemia is primarily caused by shunting of blood within the lungs.

The acute development of a diffuse alveolar-filling process frequently necessitates intubation and controlled mechanical ventilation, often with PEEP. Generally the severity of the physiologic abnormality mirrors the extensiveness of the radiologic findings; progressive changes in the radiologic picture are useful indices to the success or failure of prevention or treatment.

□ ETIOLOGY

The most common forms are cardiogenic pulmonary edema and ARDS. In AIDS patients, diffuse alveolar filling is very likely to be caused by *Pneumocystis carinii* pneumonia.

The important causes of diffuse alveolar filling are shown in Tables 7-1 and 7-2. Some of these are discussed below.

□ PULMONARY EDEMA

Acute pulmonary edema is the most common cause of acute alveolar filling (see Fig. 7-24). Hydrostatic pulmonary edema is caused by elevated pressures in the pulmonary capillaries or marked decreases in osmotic pressure. Cardiogenic pulmonary edema, the most common form of hydrostatic edema, usually results from left ventricular failure (which may have various causes) or from pulmonary venous hypertension, usually owing to mitral valve disease (see Chapter 35).

Roentgen characteristics of cardiogenic edema include cardiac enlargement, predominance of the pulmonary opacities in the lung bases bilaterally, Kerley B lines (thickened interlobular septa at the lung periph-

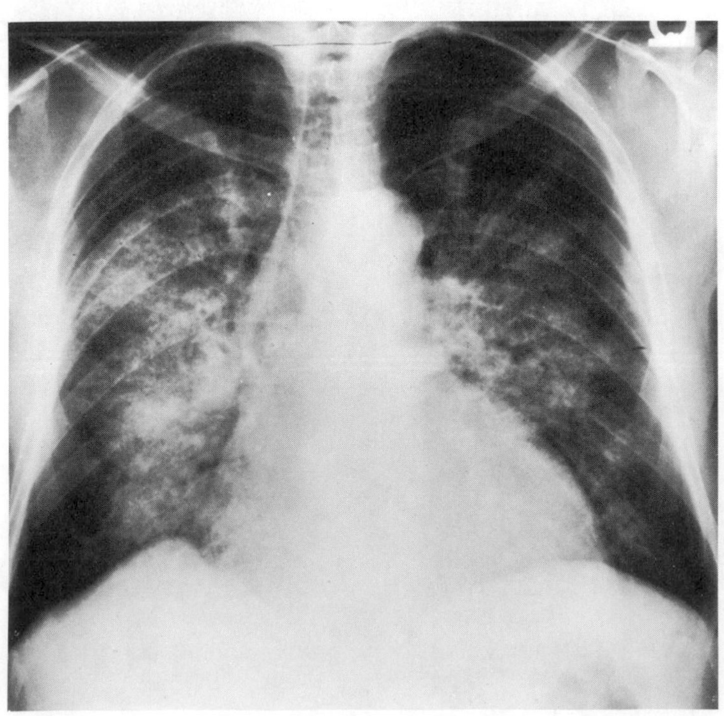

FIGURE 7-24. Bilateral perihilar distribution of pulmonary edema (the "batwing" or "butterfly" distribution). The soft, fluffy, poorly circumscribed and confluent alveolar-filling lesions are seen clearly. This appearance may occur with cardiogenic edema, but is even more characteristic of edemas due to fluid overload or renal failure. In this case, the patient had renal failure.

TABLE 7-1 **Diffuse Alveolar-Filling Processes**

Pulmonary Edema
Hydrostatic edema
  Cardiogenic
  Renal, fluid overload
Capillary leak edema
  ARDS
  Others

Diffuse Inflammatory Processes
Infectious pneumonias
  Viral pneumonias
  Pneumocystis carinii pneumonia (PCP)
  Other pneumonias
Noninfectious pneumonias
  ARDS
  Aspiration (peptic) pneumonitis
  Toxic gas inhalation
  Fat embolism syndrome
  Drug-induced
  Amniotic fluid embolism
  Acute interstitial pneumonitis (Hamman-Rich syndrome)

Intra-Alveolar Hemorrhage
Hemorrhagic disorders
Idiopathic pulmonary hemosiderosis (IPH)
Goodpasture's syndrome
Wegener's granulomatosis

Chronic Alveolar-Filling Diseases
Pulmonary alveolar proteinosis
Bronchoalveolar carcinoma
Sarcoidosis (rarely)

ery), redistribution of pulmonary blood flow towards the upper lung fields, and pleural effusions in many cases.[42] Examination of the heart will usually reveal tachycardia and a gallop rhythm, and heart murmurs are often present. Occasionally, when the diagnosis is in doubt, the demonstration of an elevated pulmonary wedge pressure on right heart catheterization will strongly suggest the cardiogenic origin of the disorder.[43]

Other types of hydrostatic pulmonary edema include fluid overloads caused by renal failure or excessive administration of intravenous fluids. In such cases, the roentgen pattern is a little different in that the distribution of the intrapulmonary fluid is often more central (paramediastinal), and significant widening of the "vascular pedicle" of the upper mediastinum is almost invariably apparent.[42]

Capillary leak pulmonary edema may result from acute cerebral disorders (neurogenic edema), high altitudes, uremia, intravenous overdosage of narcotic drugs such as heroin, aspirin overdose, transfusion reactions, near-drowning, and allergic reactions to drugs. The most common form is ARDS, which is discussed later.

Pulmonary edema may result from prolonged exposure to elevated inspiratory tensions of oxygen. Because diffuse alveolar-filling diseases are among the most common indications for the use of high-inspired oxygen concentration, it is usually difficult to determine how much of the pulmonary abnormality is caused by oxygen toxicity and how much by the underlying disease process.

In these syndromes of capillary-leak edema, the heart is often normal sized and the alveolar opacities are scattered throughout all areas of the lung. The vascular pedicle is usually normal sized and pleural effusions are rare.[42] The diagnosis can usually be established from a careful analysis of the history and surrounding clinical circumstances.

Unilateral pulmonary edema may occur if the patient has been lying for a prolonged time in one lateral decubitus position during the period when the edematous state developed. In rare instances unilateral pulmonary edema may occur after a rapid re-expansion of the lung by aspiration of a pneumothorax or pleural effusion.

□ ADULT RESPIRATORY DISTRESS SYNDROME

A diffuse hemorrhagic inflammatory intra-alveolar exudation may occur after such stresses as shock, extrathoracic trauma, septicemia, and intra-abdominal catastrophes (see Table 24-2). The pulmonary abnormality usually begins 24 to 48 hours after the traumatic episode and is associated with severe dyspnea and profound hypoxemia. The roentgen characteristics are those of capillary leak edema.[42,43] This syndrome is discussed in detail in Chapter 34.

The common name for this condition, ARDS, emphasizes the profound physiologic disturbances in these patients. The term "shock lung" emphasizes a common mechanism, and the term "diffuse alveolar damage" pertains to the pathologic changes. Although ARDS is usually classified in the category of noncardiogenic pulmonary edema, the alveolar inflammation is a major factor.

TABLE 7-2 **Causes of Acute Respiratory Distress Syndrome**

Traumatic shock
Septic shock
Aspiration
  Peptic pneumonitis
  Near-drowning
Inhaled irritants and fumes
Drugs (paraquat, narcotic overdose, salicylate overdose)
Others
  Fat embolism
  Neurogenic pulmonary edema
  Uremia
  Intravascular coagulation syndrome
  Diffuse pneumonias

□ DIFFUSE INFECTIOUS PNEUMONIAS

Diffuse viral pneumonitides may result in a widespread alveolar-filling process and severe hypoxemia. Influenza virus (see Fig. 7-12), cytomegalovirus, and herpesvirus are the most common causes of diffuse viral pneumonias.[26]

Pneumocystis carinii pneumonia is typically diffuse and has both interstitial and alveolar-filling characteristics. The most common underlying mechanism is the presence of AIDS.[32]

□ DIFFUSE NONINFECTIOUS PNEUMONIAS

Diffuse alveolar damage may result from massive aspiration of gastric juice with a low pH. The consequent peptic (acid) pneumonitis usually causes enough damage to be classified as a form of ARDS. The opacification is usually widespread and bilateral (Fig. 7-25).

Diffuse alveolar damage may result from inhalation of toxic gases such as chlorine, SO_2, and NO_2 (silo-fillers' disease). Ingestion of paraquat may result in diffuse pneumonia, which is usually rapidly fatal.

Fat embolism is a post-traumatic syndrome that is considered to be secondary to embolization of fat globules into the pulmonary capillaries, followed by enzymatic breakdown of the fats with the release of fatty acids that irritate the lung. Presumably the fat globules originate from traumatized tissues. The condition occurs almost exclusively in association with bone fractures. Although the radiologic abnormalities are similar to those in shock lung, fat embolism has some special clinical characteristics that usually allow its identification, and it usually responds more readily to therapy.

□ INTRA-ALVEOLAR HEMORRHAGE

Widespread intra-alveolar bleeding may result from spontaneous hemorrhagic states or from anticoagulant drug overdosage. In many instances, diffuse alveolar hemorrhages are manifestations of idiopathic pulmonary hemosiderosis, which occurs primarily in children and adolescents, and is not associated with involvement of other organs, or *Goodpasture's syndrome,* which typically occurs in young male adults and is caused by an autoimmune disorder that damages the kidneys as well as the lungs. Clinical findings include the rapid development of a diffuse alveolar-filling process associated with a sudden fall in hemoglobin and, usually, hemoptysis. Recurrent attacks eventually may lead to diffuse interstitial fibrosis.

Diffuse alveolar hemorrhages may occur in cases of uremia and in patients with mitral stenosis. Diffuse bleeding can also be a manifestation of Wegener's granulomatosis or of systemic lupus erythematosus.

□ CHRONIC ALVEOLAR FILLING DISEASES

A number of diseases may occasionally present as a persistent diffuse alveolar opacification, including sarcoidosis, infectious granulomas, alveolar cell carcinoma, and "alveolar" lymphoma. An unusual cause of chronic alveolar disease is pulmonary alveolar proteinosis. Most of these conditions require lung biopsy for diagnosis.

Diffuse Interstitial Pattern

The interstitial tissue of the lung includes the alveolar walls, the intralobular vessels, the interlobular septa, and the connective tissue framework that surrounds the pulmonary arteries, veins, and bronchial tree. Opacifications resulting from diseases, which primarily involve interstitial tissues, have certain characteristics that often allow fairly confident recognition of the roentgenographic pattern.[1,13,41]

Diffuse interstitial diseases often show a pattern of linear streaks throughout the lungs. This phenomenon is primarily caused by thickening of the interlobular septa and may be caused by fibrosis, granuloma, lymphangitic carcinoma, or interstitial edema. These linear streaks are called Kerley lines, which may be further differentiated into "A" lines (long linear streaks), "B"

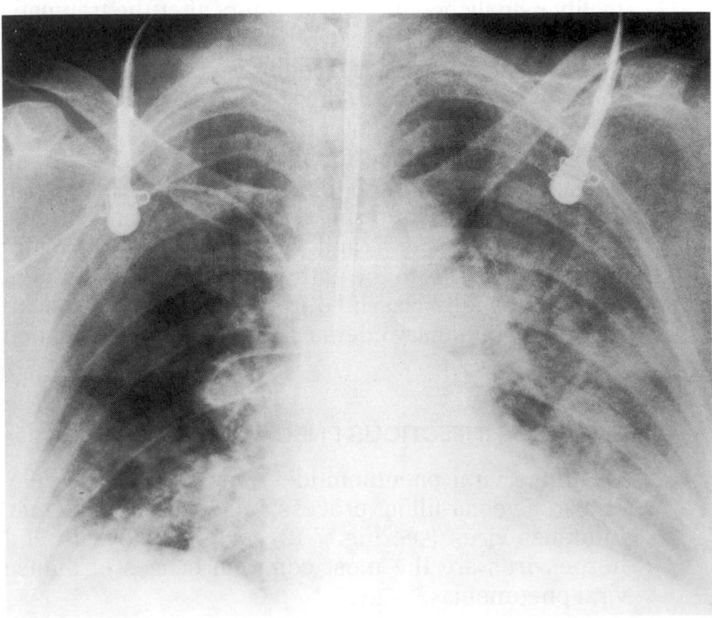

FIGURE 7-25. Peptic (acid) pneumonitis. A diffuse patchy alveolar opacification secondary to massive aspiration of gastric acid. Diagnosis depends on the history, as radiologic differentiation from other causes of diffuse alveolar filling is usually difficult. This roentgenogram also shows artifacts peculiar to the intensive care unit: a midline tube passed down the esophagus for gastric decompression, two ECG leads, and a Swan-Ganz catheter inserted in the right arm, which passes through the subclavian vein, superior vena cava, right atrium, right ventricle, the pulmonary trunk, and the right pulmonary artery.

lines (short horizontal transverse streaks) best seen at the periphery of the lower lung fields (Fig. 7-26), and "C" lines (a diffuse reticular network) caused by the overlapping of linear streaks running in different directions (Fig. 7-27).

Perhaps the most characteristic feature of interstitial disease is honeycombing, which consists of multiple rounded lucent areas, usually 5 to 10 mm in diameter, outlined by the surrounding dense interstitial opacifications (Fig. 7-28). The presence of honeycomb cysts, and their typical subpleural location, are best seen on CT scans.

The air bronchogram effect is usually absent or not prominent in interstitial disease. Other interstitial processes in which cystic changes may be prominent include histiocytosis X and lymphangiomyomatosis.

Many types of diffuse lung disease have both alveolar and interstitial components, with manifestations of both patterns radiologically. This is usually described as a "mixed" pattern. For example, cardiogenic pulmonary edema begins as septal thickening caused by edema (manifested by Kerley "B" lines) and then evolves into diffuse alveolar filling. In other cases, such as fibrosing alveolitis, ARDS, or desquamative interstitial pneumonitis, the initial manifestation is alveolar filling, which evolves into an interstitial pattern caused by fibrosis.

Many diseases may give rise to a diffuse interstitial pattern (Table 7-3).

□ DIFFUSE INTERSTITIAL PNEUMONITIDES

The most common condition in this category is usual interstitial pneumonitis (UIP), which is also known as fibrosing alveolitis or diffuse pulmonary fibrosis. Many cases are idiopathic, but some are secondary to (or associated with) underlying conditions, such as rheumatoid arthritis, scleroderma, inhalation of high oxygen concentrations (oxygen pneumonopathy), and the administration of drugs such as methotrexate, cyclophosphamide, busulfan, and others. In most cases, UIP is a slowly progressive disorder that results in a fibrotic "end-stage" lung (see Fig. 7-28). In UIP, the distribution of the scarring and honeycomb cysts is typically peripheral (subpleural).[13]

Less common are desquamative interstitial pneumonitis (DIP) and lymphocytic interstitial pneumonitis (LIP). These may also progress to diffuse "end-stage" honeycomb lung in some instances. Diagnosis requires biopsy.

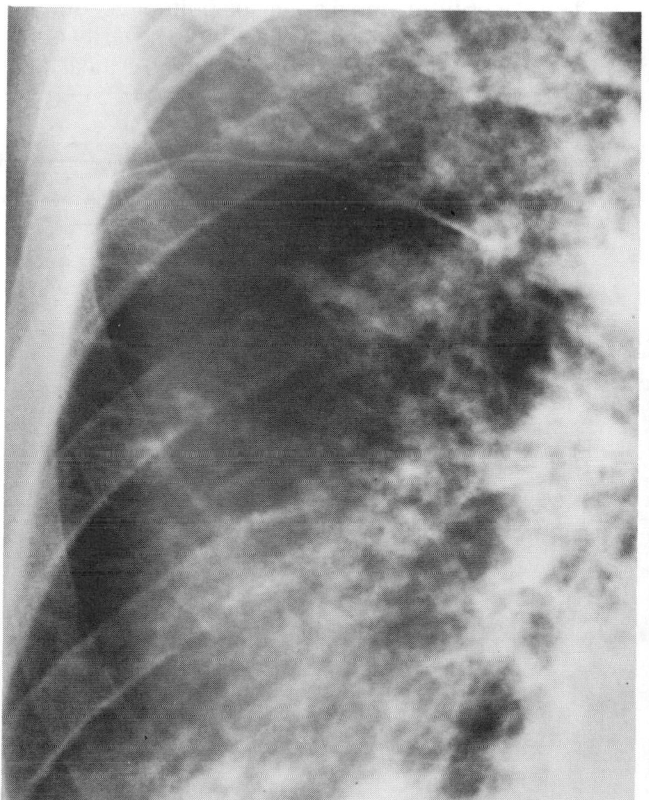

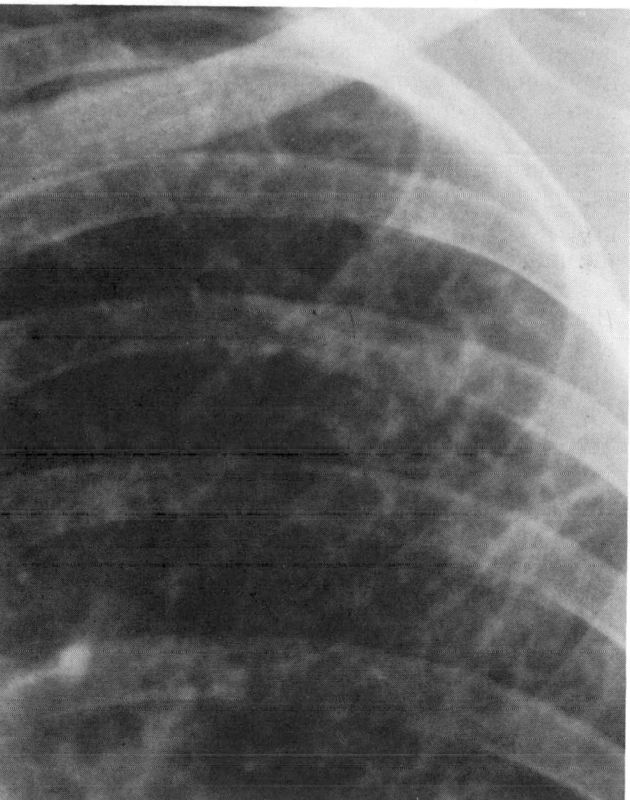

FIGURE 7-26. *(left)* Kerley B lines. These thin lines extend horizontally for 1–2 cm inwards from the pleural surface and represent thickened interlobular septa. They result in this case from interstitial edema due to pulmonary venous hypertension. Note scattered areas of alveolar filling medially, which represent pulmonary edema of cardiogenic origin. *(right)* PA view showing upper left lung in a 32-year-old woman with biopsy-proven eosinophilic granuloma (Histiocytosis X). A reticular pattern is present, intermixed with blebs. A somewhat similar pattern may occur with cystic fibrosis.

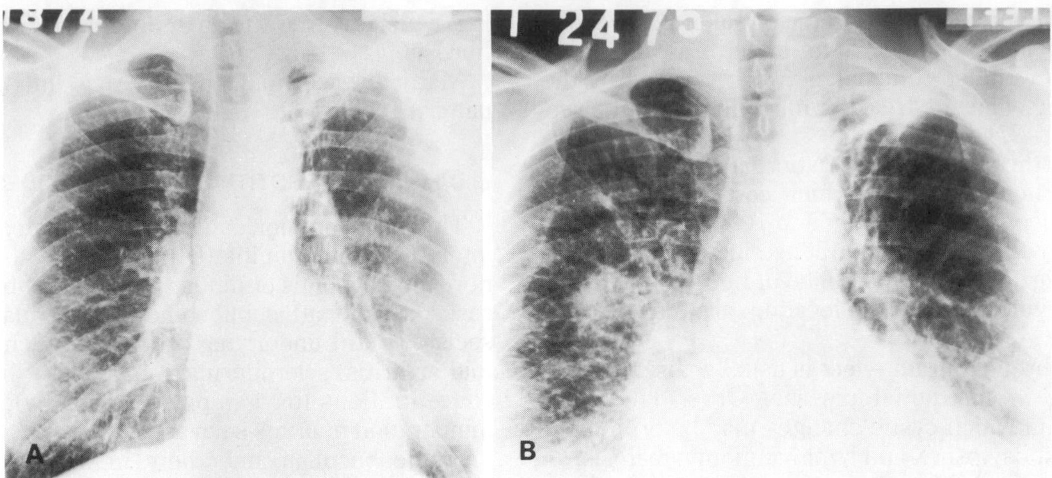

FIGURE 7-27. Congestive heart failure. **(A)** PA chest film at a time when cardiac function was normal. In the left hemithorax, apical scarring and elevation of the left hilum have resulted from previous active tuberculosis, with loss of volume in the left upper lobe during the healing process. **(B)** Two months later, this man has suffered an acute myocardial infarction, and has developed left heart failure. The heart is enlarged. The hilar shadows are larger and have hazy margins. Pulmonary edema is present, manifested by a reticular pattern (Kerley B and C lines) and frank alveolar filling at the bases. The vascular shadows in the upper lung are accentuated due to cephalad redistribution of blood flow.

☐ OTHER FORMS OF DIFFUSE INTERSTITIAL DISEASE

Sarcoidosis is perhaps the most common diffuse interstitial process.[2,13] Other conditions that commonly present with an interstitial pattern include asbestosis, hypersensitivity pneumonitis, lymphangitic carcinomatosis, and eosinophilic granuloma (histiocytosis X) (see Fig. 7-26).

In most of these conditions, lung biopsy is needed to establish the diagnosis. In some instances the CT appearances and the related clinical features will suggest the underlying origin with considerable assurance.

Physiologically, the diffuse interstitial diseases are characterized by small, stiff lungs with a reduced diffusing capacity and hypoxemia, usually without carbon dioxide retention. In fact, hypocapnia is common, caused by secondary hyperventilation. The hypoxemia can usually be relieved by a moderate enrichment of inspired air with oxygen. Generally, the severity of the physiologic abnormality is proportional to the extensiveness of the radiologic changes. There may, however, be gross disparity between clinical status and radiologic abnormalities in sarcoidosis, with the patient being much less ill than his or her chest radiograph would suggest.

Miliary Pattern

This is a variant form of the interstitial pattern, in which the chest roentgenogram shows profusion of small nodules about 2 mm to 4 mm in diameter (Fig. 7-29).[1,2,13] The prototype is miliary tuberculosis, but a diffuse fine nodularity of this type may also occur with fungal infections, sarcoidosis, certain pneumoconioses, metastatic tumors to lung, and varicella pneumonia (Table 7-4). The distinction between the interstitial and miliary patterns is often elusive, in which case the term "reticulonodular" disease may be used to denote that the roentgenogram shows features of both patterns.

The severity of impairment of pulmonary function does not always correlate well with the severity of radiologic impairment in miliary disease. The critical task is

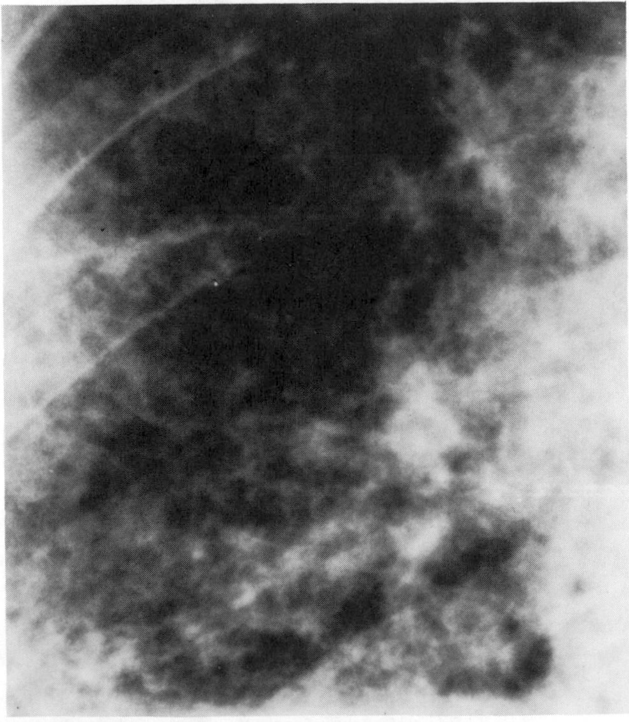

FIGURE 7-28. Honeycomb lung in a patient with fibrosing alveolitis. The honeycomb cysts form dozens of rounded lucent areas, 5 mm to 10 mm in diameter, separated from each other by opaque fibrous tissue. These cysts are particularly well seen with CT.

TABLE 7-3 **Diseases With a Diffuse Interstitial Pattern**

Diffuse Interstitial Pneumonitis/Fibrosis
Fibrosing alveolitis (usual interstitial pneumonitis)
Cryptogenic (idiopathic pulmonary fibrosis)
Secondary
Collagen vascular diseases
Drug-induced pneumonopathy
Desquamative interstitial pneumonitis (DIP)
Lymphocytic interstitial pneumonitis
End-stage ARDS (in some cases)
Conditions Involving Lymphatics
Sarcoidosis
Lymphoma
Lymphangitic carcinomatosis
Inhalational Disorders
Asbestosis
Hypersensitivity pneumonitis (allergic alveolitis)
Miscellaneous
Histiocytosis X (eosinophilic granuloma)
Lymphangioleiomyomatosis

to determine the cause, particularly in infectious cases. Lung biopsy is often indicated.

Vascular Pattern

The pulmonary arteries and veins, as previously noted, form a somewhat indistinct branching pattern radiating peripherally from the hilum on the normal chest roentgenogram. Increases in the size of the pulmonary vessels cause an accentuation of this pattern. This accentuation superficially resembles interstitial disease, and may be confused with it.

A generalized increase in vascularity may result from polycythemia, fluid overloads, left heart failure, or congenital heart disease with left-to-right shunts. A striking feature of left heart failure is increased prominence of the vessels in the upper lung fields owing to cephalization of blood flow (see Fig. 7-27). A spurious pattern of increased vascularity, particularly at the bases, may appear in normal lungs if the roentgenogram was obtained with the chest in the end-expiratory position.

Localized increases in vascularity in cases of pulmonary emphysema are caused by redistribution of blood flow from avascular areas to the vascular beds in the more normal areas of lung.

Decreased vascularity may be focal, as in emphysema or pulmonary embolism, or diffuse, as in right-to-left shunts, pulmonic stenosis, and obstructive pulmonary hypertension. The central hilar vessels are often enlarged in obstructive pulmonary hypertension.

Bronchial Pattern

Diffuse involvement of the bronchial tree by inflammatory disease may result in roentgen abnormalities, which somewhat resemble the diffuse interstitial pattern. This can result from thickened bronchial walls (as in chronic bronchitis, asthma, bronchiectasis), from peribronchial scarring (as in mucoviscidosis or allergic bronchopulmonary aspergillosis), or from mucoid impactions within the bronchial tree. In patients with COPD, this appearance is often referred to as the "dirty lung"[37] and usually indicates that chronic bronchitis is a

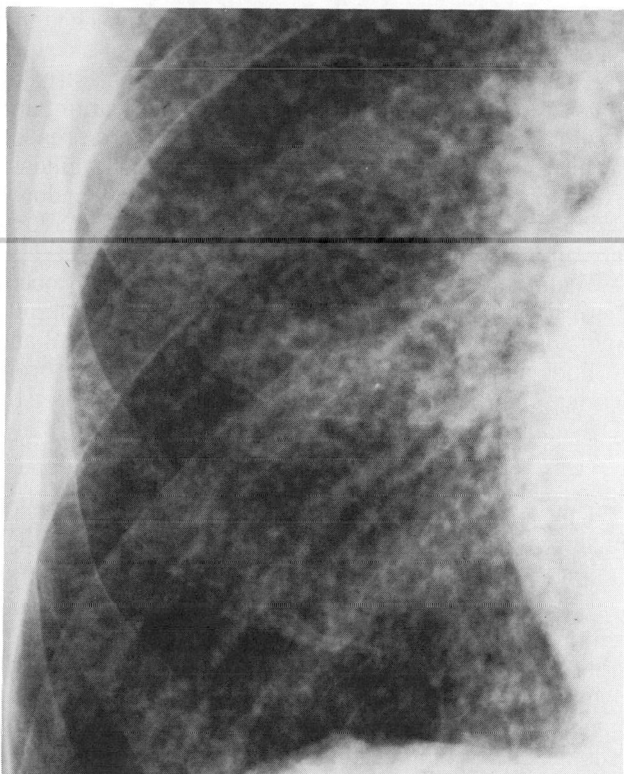

FIGURE 7-29. Diffuse miliary nodules in a patient with disseminated coccidioidomycosis. The innumerable tiny nodules are well circumscribed and are 2 mm to 4 mm in diameter. A similar appearance occurs in miliary tuberculosis and is sometimes seen in certain fungal diseases, sarcoidosis, coal-worker's pneumoconiosis, and metastatic tumors.

TABLE 7-4 **Diffuse Miliary Processes**

Inhalational
Silicosis
Coal workers' pneumoconiosis
Berylliosis
Hair-spray thesaurosis
Hematogenous/Lymphogenous
Metastatic tumors
Miliary infections
Tuberculosis
Fungal diseases
Lymphangitic carcinomatosis (some cases)
Talc granulomatosis
Sarcoidosis

major component of the obstructive complex. The term "increased markings pattern" is also used.

The roentgen changes include focal linear streaks, fine ring shadows, irregular foci of opacification, and "tramline" shadows. If mucoid impactions are present, as in cases of allergic bronchopulmonary aspergillosis, such picturesque terms as "toothpaste" shadows, "gloved hand" shadows, and "frond of grapes" shadows are often used.

Widening of the bronchovascular bundles may occur with lymphomas, sarcoidosis, and lymphatic carcinomatosis. This is usually accompanied by Kerley B and C lines as well as the nodular thickening of the bronchovascular markings. These features are best seen on CT scans.[13]

PLEURAL EFFUSIONS

Fluid within the pleural space may be blood (hemothorax), pus (empyema), chyle (chylothorax), or, most commonly, a relatively clear serous fluid, which is either a transudate or an exudate. The nature of the fluid cannot be determined from the roentgenographic appearance; its identification is dependent on microscopic, bacteriologic, and chemical analysis of aspirated fluid.

Pleural effusions of any type will reduce pulmonary function to the extent that the intrapleural fluid volume reduces lung volume. In addition, pleuritic pain, when present, impairs the patient's ability to take a deep breath and cough effectively, and the latter may lead to sputum retention, which may eventually result in pneumonia or atelectasis.

Roentgen Appearances

The roentgen appearance of a pleural effusion depends on the amount of fluid and whether loculations are present.[1,2] A small effusion may show only haziness or obliteration of a costophrenic angle, sometimes seen better on the lateral view than on the PA projection. A moderate-sized effusion presents as a homogeneous opacity in the dependent portion of the thorax, with an irregular and poorly defined upper border that is generally concave and higher laterally along the chest wall (Fig. 7-30). The contour of the diaphragm is obliterated both in the upright PA and lateral projections. A very large pleural effusion causes relatively complete opacification of the hemithorax, with relatively less opacity at the top than at the bottom and usually with evidence of mediastinal shift towards the normal hemithorax.

The appearances just described above are those with the subject in the upright position and with a pleural space not bound down to any major degree by adhesions. If the exposure is made with the subject in the supine position, the pleural fluid layers out posteriorly, causing a diffuse haziness throughout the hemithorax. A subpulmonic effusion forms between the lung and diaphragm with the patient in the upright position. It simulates elevation of the hemidiaphragm. An *interlobar effusion* collects within an interlobar fissure and resembles a mass lesion in the PA projection, but in the lateral view usually has a characteristic fusiform appearance. In all these cases a film taken in the lateral decubitus position will usually show movement of fluid to the most dependent portions of the hemithorax, establishing the true nature of the opacity (Fig. 7-31).

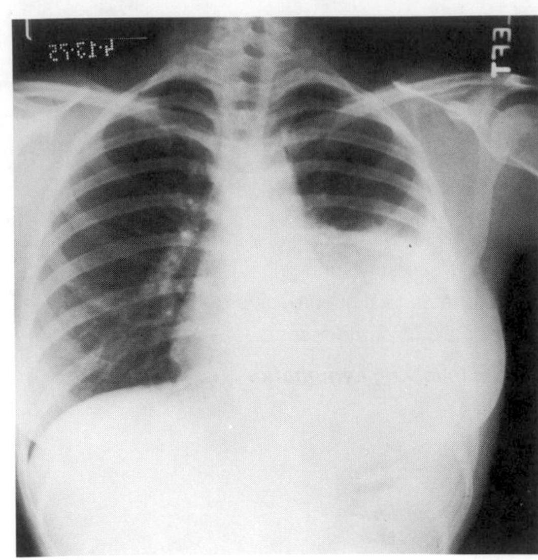

FIGURE 7-30. Moderately large pleural effusion due to tuberculosis. There is a large homogeneous opacification in the lower half of the left hemithorax, with the upper border of the opacity being concave upwards. There is some shift of the heart to the right.

Types of Pleural Effusions

Transudative effusions result from changes in the hydrodynamic forces in the circulation and may be regarded as localized manifestations of a general tendency to form edema fluid. It is most commonly caused by left heart failure. Other causes include cirrhosis and the nephrotic syndrome. Exudative effusions result from irritation of the pleural membranes, secondary to inflammatory or malignant processes. Most inflammatory effusions are caused by an infection within the adjacent lung, including pneumonias, mycobacterial infections, and fungal diseases.

Malignant pleural effusions are most commonly caused by metastatic involvement of the pleura from bronchogenic carcinoma, an extrapulmonary primary malignancy such as breast cancer, or a lymphoma. The most common primary malignant tumor of the pleural space is the diffuse pleural mesothelioma, usually secondary to asbestos exposure.

Empyema is a purulent pleural effusion, usually secondary to pneumonia or lung abscess. Other causes of empyema include tuberculosis, fungal diseases, mediastinal abscess, and subphrenic abscess. Hemothorax denotes the presence of blood in the pleural space, usually resulting from chest trauma, either penetrating wounds or laceration of the lung by fractured ribs (Fig. 7-32).

Chylothorax results from leakage of chyle from the thoracic duct and is usually caused by chest trauma or

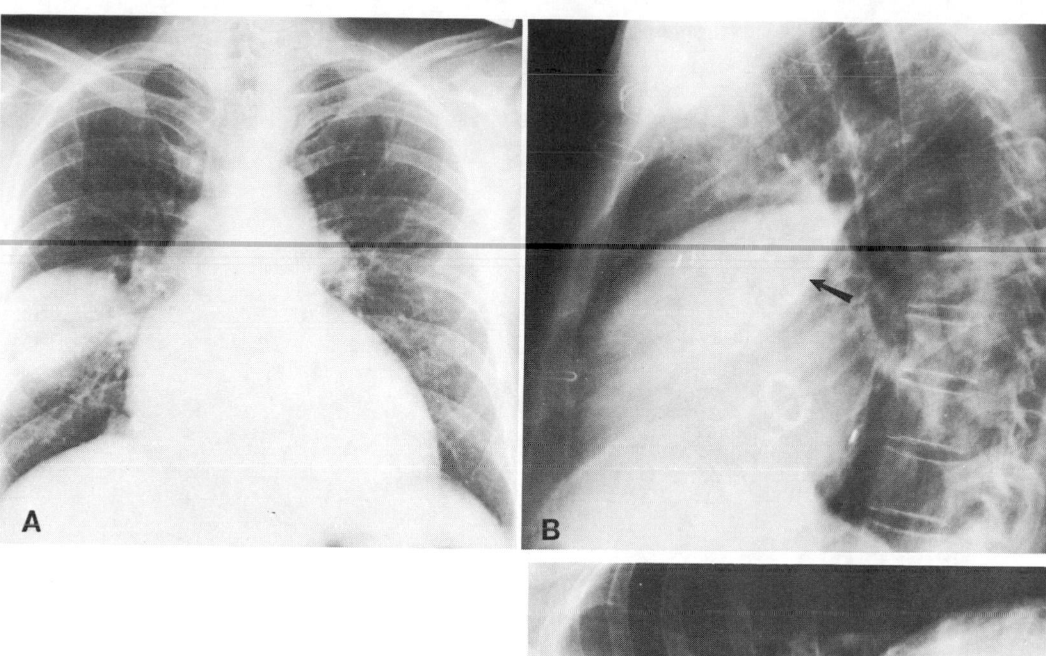

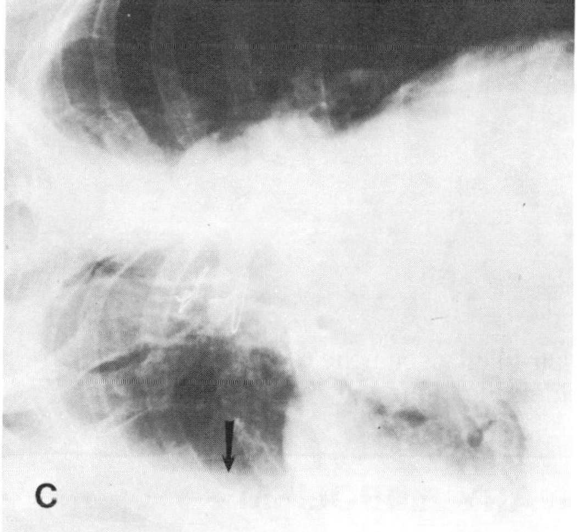

FIGURE 7-31. Loculated interlobar effusion. **(A)** PA chest film shows the fluid as a rounded opacity in the right hemithorax, resembling a tumor mass (pseudotumor). **(B)** Lateral film shows the characteristic fusiform appearance of an interlobar effusion *(arrow)*, continuing upwards as a thin diagonal line representing the upper portion of the oblique fissure. An artificial heart valve can be seen within the heart shadow, and surgical wires are seen encircling the sternum. **(C)** Right lateral decubitus film showing some passage of the pleural fluid out into the "lateral gutter," which is now the most dependent portion of the hemithorax.

by malignant obstruction of the thoracic duct. The fluid usually has a characteristic milky appearance, but in questionable cases, the determination of the true nature of the fluid may require chemical studies. Chyliform and pseudochylous effusions resemble true chyle on gross inspection but result from the endogenous formation of lipids within a chronic and highly cellular exudative effusion or empyema.

DIAPHRAGMATIC ABNORMALITIES

The diaphragm is subject to relatively few primary disorders but is often affected by disease processes above or below it. Bilateral depression of the diaphragm is an important sign of hyperinflation and usually indicates emphysema or severe asthma. Bilateral elevation of the diaphragm may result from obesity, ascites, painful breathing, or inability of the patient to take a deep breath. It is a common finding in cases of bilateral pulmonary embolism (Fig. 7-33) and in roentgenograms obtained on obtunded patients lying in the supine position.

Unilateral elevation of the diaphragm may be an important sign of disease in or near the diaphragm and should never be ignored. Supradiaphragmatic disorders causing unilateral elevation include inflammatory or irritative processes in the adjacent lung and visceral pleura, for example, pulmonary embolism (with or without infarction), pneumonia, atelectasis, or pleurisy of any cause. Diaphragmatic disorders that cause unilateral elevation include paralysis owing to phrenic nerve dysfunction, and eventration, which is a loss of diaphragmatic muscle with thinning of the organ, probably congenital in origin (see Fig. 7-18). Infradiaphragmatic processes causing diaphragmatic elevation include subphrenic abscess (usually secondary to abdominal surgery or perforation of an abdominal viscus) and a large cyst or hematoma in the upper abdomen. On occasion, gross enlargement of the liver may cause diaphragmatic elevation. In most cases of an elevated hemidiaphragm the respiratory excursions are reduced and will actually show paradoxical movement with phrenic nerve palsy.

A diaphragmatic hernia may simulate unilateral elevation of the diaphragm. In many instances, the hernia

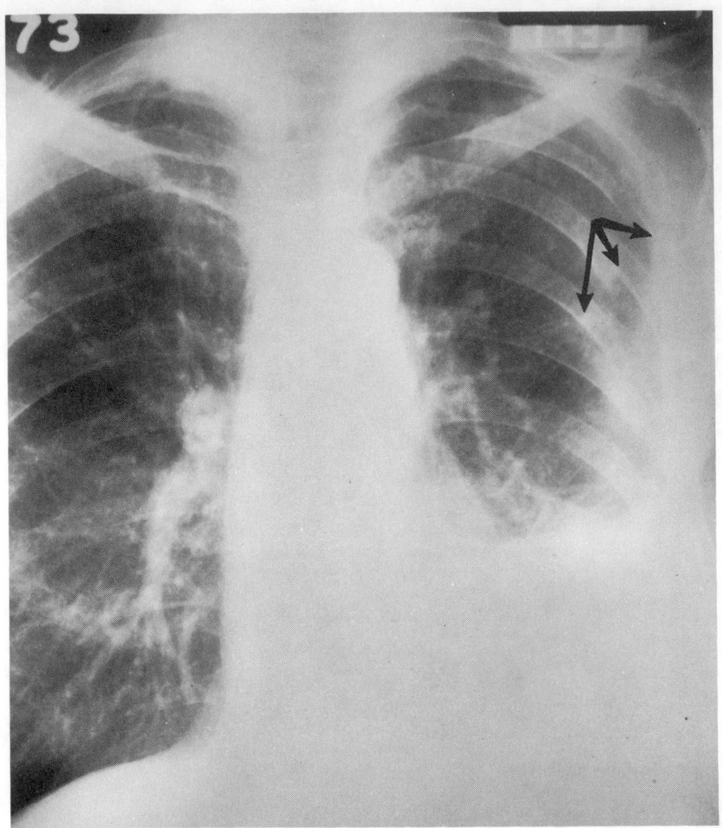

FIGURE 7-32. Left hemothorax secondary to rib fractures *(arrows)*. The intrapleural opacity of the hemothorax cannot be distinguished from other types of fluid effusion.

contains an air-filled viscus, the roentgen appearance of which aids identification.

PULMONARY EMBOLISM

The radiologic changes that accompany pulmonary embolism are never distinctive, but they will often suggest the diagnosis and thus indicate the need for more specific studies to identify positively the presence of the pulmonary embolus.[2] In many instances pulmonary scintiscans will establish the diagnosis with a high degree of assurance, and in other cases pulmonary angiography is needed. It is critically important to recognize the clinical and roentgenographic findings that will suggest the possibility of pulmonary embolism.

Massive pulmonary embolism is caused by the impaction of one or more large thrombi in the pulmonary outflow tract or main pulmonary arteries. If the patient survives long enough for appropriate diagnostic studies to be performed, the standard frontal projection chest roentgenogram will usually show relatively clear or even oligemic lung fields, usually with unilateral or bilateral increased hilar size, secondary to enlargement of the capacitance portion of the pulmonary arterial circulation. Pulmonary angiography in such circumstances is almost invariably diagnostic, but echocardiography is also helpful and has the advantage of being noninvasive. The differential diagnosis includes acute myocardial infarction and leaking thoracic aortic aneurysms.

Pulmonary infarction is ischemic necrosis of an area of lung, which occurs in 10% to 20% of cases of embolism. Infarcts are often multiple and appear on the chest roentgenogram as one or more areas of consolidation, large or small, always abutting on a visceral pleural surface (peripheral or interlobar) and often pre-

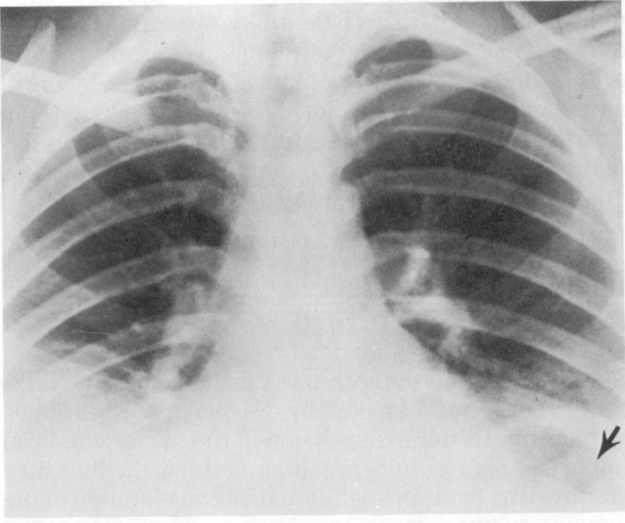

FIGURE 7-33. Bilateral pulmonary emboli in a young woman. The degree of elevation of the left hemidiaphragm is indicated by the position of the gastric bubble. *(arrow)*. On the right, the hemidiaphragm is probably elevated as well, but it cannot be seen clearly due to overlying pleural fluid. The thick horizontal curved linear opacity in the right third anterior interspace is discoid atelectasis.

senting a rounded contour on the margin facing the hilum (Fig. 7-34).[44] Pleural effusion is often present, and ipsilateral hilar enlargement with hemidiaphragmatic elevation is usually apparent. Infarcts occasionally undergo cavitation. Pulmonary scintiscanning is of limited value in such cases, because an infarct will show a matching ventilation-perfusion defect similar to that occurring with any type of pulmonary consolidation. However, because emboli are commonly multiple, the scans may show one or more nonmatching defects in other nonconsolidated areas of lung that have been embolized but have not undergone infarction. Segmental pulmonary angiography is usually diagnostic. The differential diagnosis of pulmonary infarction includes pneumonia, atelectasis, and pleural effusion of other types.

Unexplained dyspnea is the presenting syndrome in patients who have single or multiple embolic occlusions in medium-sized branches of the pulmonary arteries without the development of infarction. Pleuritic chest pain is unusual in these cases. The chest roentgenogram occasionally shows one or more oligemic, hyperlucent areas, but commonly is interpreted as being normal. Careful review of such cases may show unilateral enlargement of the hilum or the lobar vessels, often associated with elevation of ipsilateral hemidiaphragm and the presence of discoid atelectasis, also called Fleischner's lines (see Fig. 7-33). Discoid atelectasis appears as one or more transverse linear shadows, 1 mm to 3 mm in diameter and extending 2 cm to 4 cm in length, usually horizontal in position and mainly in the lower lung fields. The appearance of discoid atelectasis is not pathognomonic of pulmonary embolism but should always suggest the diagnosis. It may also result from any condition causing painful chest movement, including rib fractures, pleurisy, and upper abdominal surgery. The differential diagnosis of the "unexplained dyspnea" syndrome includes asthma, exacerbation of COPD, metabolic dyspnea, and psychogenic dyspnea.

Chronic pulmonary hypertension, with right ventricular enlargement, bilateral hilar enlargement, and clear or oligemic lung fields may be caused by pulmonary embolism. Exertional dyspnea and exertional chest pain are often present. Although the syndrome may result from recurrent showers of small emboli, many cases result from persistence of large-vessel embolic occlusions—a syndrome known as chronic thrombo-embolic pulmonary hypertension (CTEPH).[45] Clinical differentiation from primary pulmonary hypertension (plexogenic pulmonary hypertension, PPH) is often difficult. However, pulmonary scintiscans are virtually normal in PPH but show moderate to high probability patterns in embolic cases, and pulmonary angiography is diagnostic. Pulmonary endarterectomy is life-saving in patients with CTEPH.[45]

HILAR ENLARGEMENT

The hila contain bronchi, lymph nodes, and blood vessels, but only the blood vessels are sufficently large and radiopaque to contribute to the normal hilar opacity. Increased size of the hilum may be caused by vascular dilatation, enlargement of the hilar lymph nodes, or development of a mass lesion, such as a bronchogenic carcinoma, within the hilum. The differentiation between lymphadenopathy and vessel enlargement as the

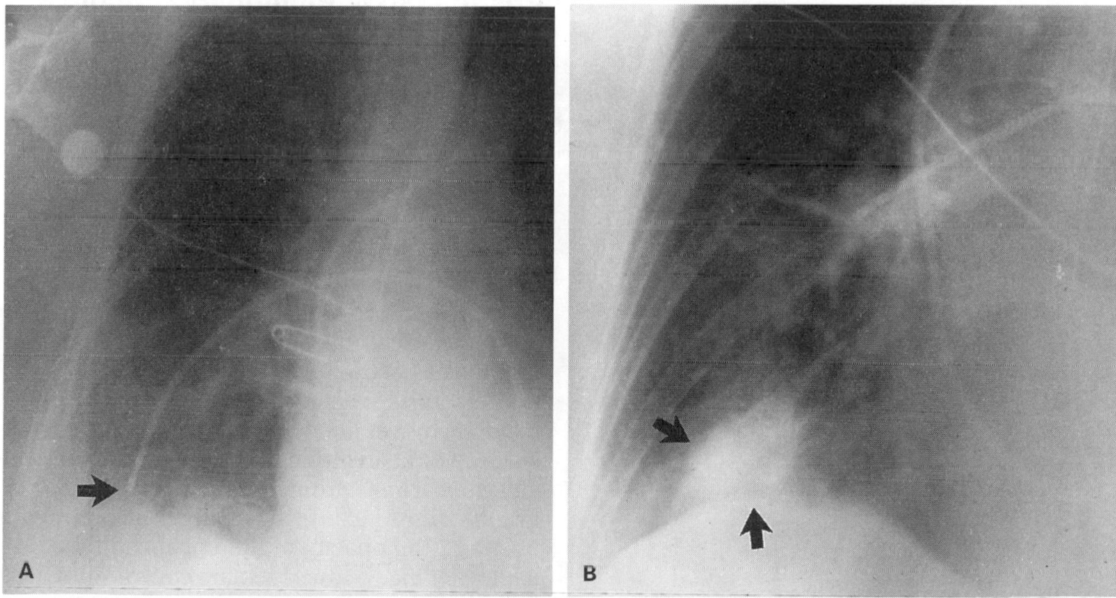

FIGURE 7-34. **(A)** Swan-Ganz catheter tip *(arrow)* is lying approximately 5 cm from right hilum, a position that is excessively peripheral. **(B)** Resulting pulmonary infarct presents as a wedge-shaped pleural based density *(arrows)* seen adjacent to the right hemidiaphragm. Film B was obtained 2½ hours after film A.

cause of hilar enlargement may require pulmonary angiography, CT or MRI.

Unilateral nonvascular hilar enlargement may result from the development of an intrahilar mass lesion (tumor, bronchogenic cyst) or from the lymphadenopathy of tuberculosis, bronchogenic carcinoma, certain fungal diseases, and lymphoma.[2] Unilateral enlargement is rare in sarcoidosis.

Unilateral vascular hilar enlargement is most commonly caused by pulmonary embolism, but there are several rare causes, including pulmonary artery aneurysms and poststenotic dilatation related to pulmonic stenosis.

Bilateral nonvascular hilar enlargement is most commonly caused by the lymphadenopathy of sarcoidosis (Fig. 7-35). Other causes of bilateral hilar adenopathy include lymphoma, leukemia, some fungus infections, and certain pneumoconioses.

Bilateral vascular hilar enlargement from dilated central pulmonary vascular shadows suggests pulmonary embolism, congestive heart failure (see Fig. 7-27), mitral stenosis, plexogenic pulmonary hypertension, cor pulmonale (pulmonary arterial hypertension owing to chronic lung disease), and congenital heart diseases associated with a left-to-right shunt. In most instances the peripheral intrapulmonary arteries are also distended and prominent, although in pulmonary embolism and in PPH, the lungs are more commonly oligemic.

IATROGENIC LUNG DISEASE

An iatrogenic disease is one caused by some action (or occasionally a lack of action) of the physician. The increasing incidence of iatrogenic disease has now become a major medical problem. These "diseases" are related to relentless increase in the number of invasive and potentially hazardous diagnostic procedures now available, and to the many toxic side-effects of the powerful drugs and complicated therapeutic procedures in current use. Many iatrogenic diseases are unavoidable but predictable, and their prompt recognition depends on the physician's realization of their possible occurrence in certain clinical situations. The lungs are particularly susceptible to various iatrogenic diseases.

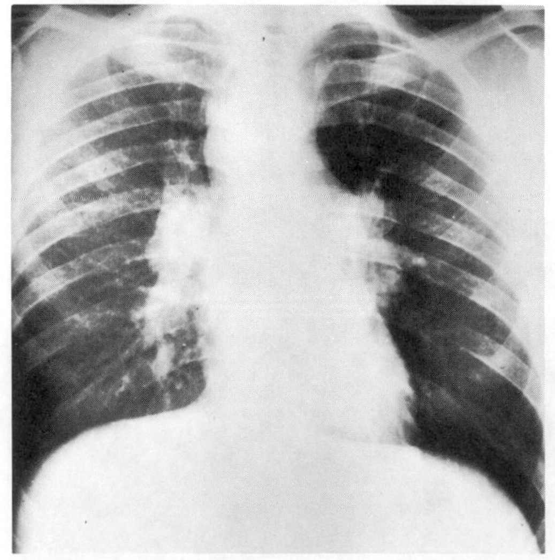

FIGURE 7-35. Bilateral hilar adenopathy in sarcoidosis. Such well-circumscribed, lobulated masses have been aptly described as having a "potato node" appearance. Compare with the poorly demarcated vascular hilar enlargements seen in Fig. 7-27.

Nosocomial Infections

Pulmonary infections developing in hospitalized patients may result from invasion by the indigenous pathogenic microbiologic flora of the hospital or may be a manifestation of infection by "saprophytic" organisms normally present in the body but which develop invasive potential because of reduced resistance in patients exposed to various diagnostic or therapeutic maneuvers.[46] Predisposing factors include recent surgery, the use of broad-spectrum antibiotics or immunosuppressive drugs, invasive diagnostic or therapeutic procedures, swallowing difficulties allowing aspiration of food or infective pharyngeal secretions, tracheal intubation, and contaminated respiratory therapy equipment. The site of the infection may be tracheobronchial, alveolar, or both.

Common infecting organisms include *Staphylococcus, Pseudomonas*, and other aerobic gram-negative bacilli, anaerobic organisms, and bacteria and fungi normally of low pathogenicity, including *Aspergillus* and *Candida.* The roentgenographic features of nosocomial pneumonia are not characteristic except that the lesions are less likely to be lobar or segmental in distribution and commonly are multiple, bilateral, and poorly circumscribed (bronchopneumonia). Common complications include cavitation and pleural effusion or empyema.

Postoperative Pulmonary Complications

Pulmonary complications are a major cause of morbidity and mortality after surgical procedures, and their incidence is greatly increased if pre-existing pulmonary disease is present (see Chapter 36). Chronic obstructive airway diseases present the greatest hazard, since pulmonary function may already be borderline and the inability of the patient to generate an effective cough predisposes to postoperative sputum retention. Surgical procedures on the thorax itself or on the upper abdomen are more likely to be followed by postoperative pulmonary complications than procedures involving other areas of the body.

Atelectasis caused by obstruction of one or more bronchi by retained mucus plugs may occur during surgery or at any time in the postoperative period, usually appearing within the first few days. Roentgenographic signs include the changes indicating loss of volume and the opacity of the collapsed lobe or segment itself (see Fig. 7-17). The main contributing factor is the inability or unwillingness of the patient to cough effectively because of postoperative pain. In most instances postoperative atelectasis can be prevented by a vigorous program of pulmonary toilet both before and after surgery. Treatment for atelectasis is simple and effective provided the condition is recognized.

Postoperative pulmonary embolism may occur at any time in the postoperative period but most commonly appears several days after the surgical procedure. The clinical and radiologic signs of pulmonary embolism have already been reviewed. Predisposing factors include obesity, polycythemia, heart disease, malignancy, and orthopedic procedures to the limbs, particularly the treatment of hip fractures. In most instances clear-cut evidence of underlying thrombophlebitis will not be detectable on physical examination.

Postoperative respiratory insufficiency has become increasingly common with the use of complicated surgical procedures on elderly or seriously ill patients. Chronic obstructive lung disease is the main predisposing factor. In many patients who develop respiratory insufficiency in the postoperative state, the chest roentgenogram shows no particular change from the preoperative film. The diagnosis primarily depends on arterial blood gas measurements. Prolonged, complicated surgical procedures associated with hypovolemic shock or sepsis may lead to the development of ARDS, in which case the chest roentgenogram reveals a diffuse patchy alveolar-filling process that develops 24 to 48 hours after the procedure.

Drug-Induced Lung Disease

A wide variety of drugs may cause acute or chronic lung diseases.[47] The diagnosis is critically dependent on the history of exposure, supplemented in some cases by toxicologic tests.

Certain drugs may have a direct toxic effect on the lungs. The prolonged use of high concentrations of oxygen in the inspired gas leads to diffuse alveolar damage, which is often not recognized because of the extensive radiographic abnormalities resulting from the underlying pulmonary disease that necessitated the oxygen therapy. Allergic reactions to drugs may cause pulmonary edema, asthmatic attacks, pulmonary vasculitis, or eosinophilic pneumonia.

Certain drugs (bleomycin, busulfan, methotrexate, and several others) may cause a diffuse interstitial pneumonitis/fibrosis. Methysergide may cause mediastinal fibrosis with compression of the superior vena, the main bronchi, or the pulmonary veins. The prolonged use of adrenal corticosteroids often results in mediastinal lipomatosis; the fat deposits cause generalized mediastinal widening. The anti-arrythmic drug amiodarone may cause a progressive pneumonitis, possibly due to hypersensitivity and detectable on standard radiographs or CT.

Noncardiogenic pulmonary edema may result from salicylate overdoses or the intravenous use of narcotic drugs such as heroin. Beta-adrenergic drugs used in the therapy of premature labor may cause pulmonary edema, particularly in cases in which adrenal steroids are also used.[48] However, eclampsia is the most common cause of acute pulmonary edema in pregnancy.

Fluid Overload

Hospitalized patients, particularly those in intensive care units, sometimes develop generalized fluid retention and pulmonary edema from vascular overloading with intravenous fluids. This possibility must be considered in any patient receiving intravenous fluids who develops a diffuse alveolar-filling process. Congestive heart failure or renal failure are predisposing causes in some cases (see Figs. 7-26 and 7-27). The chest radiograph will usually show widening of the "vascular pedicle."[42] The diagnosis can be confirmed in most instances by a careful study of intake/output data and serial body weights. In most cases, the central venous pressure and the pulmonary capillary wedge pressure are elevated.

Complications of Mechanical Ventilation

Mechanical ventilation, commonly used for maintaining life during episodes of respiratory insufficiency or respiratory failure, carries certain inherent hazards.[49] Oxygen toxicity has already been mentioned. The inspired oxygen concentration must be maintained at the lowest level that will yield an arterial oxygen tension of 60 to 80 mmHg.

Endobronchial infections are common in intubated patients. Bacterial colonization of the upper tracheobronchial tree is unavoidable when an endotracheal tube is in place, but the incidence and severity of secondary infections can be minimized by strict adherence to appropriate technique. Endobronchial infections are manifested by purulent bronchial secretions, often without any radiologic abnormality indicative of parenchymal pneumonia. Inadequate sterilization of respiratory therapy equipment may result in a serious or even fatal pulmonary infection that is often bilateral and sometimes necrotizing (associated with cavity information).

Displacement of the endotracheal tube into the right main bronchus usually results in the rapid development of atelectasis of the left lung. Atelectasis is easily recognized by stethoscopic examination, and a chest roentgenogram is confirmatory. This disorder can be avoided by radiographic monitoring of the tube placement and by routine stethoscopic examination of the lungs of the intubated patient at appropriate intervals.

Pneumomediastinum and subcutaneous emphysemas are infallible indices that air leakage is occurring (see Fig. 7-23).[40] If a tracheostomy has been performed, the leakage of air may be occurring from the tracheal incision or from the surgical site. Air leakage may occur from transtracheal needle aspiration, even without barotrauma (Fig. 7-36).

In patients with *barotrauma,* alveolar rupture probably occurs first, with subsequent dissection of the air in a centripetal fashion along the bronchovascular bundles into the mediastinum and up into the subcutaneous tissues of the neck. This is commonly followed by development of a pneumothorax, and the appearance of subcutaneous air should indicate the need for immediate chest radiographic examination. Other clinical signs that indi-

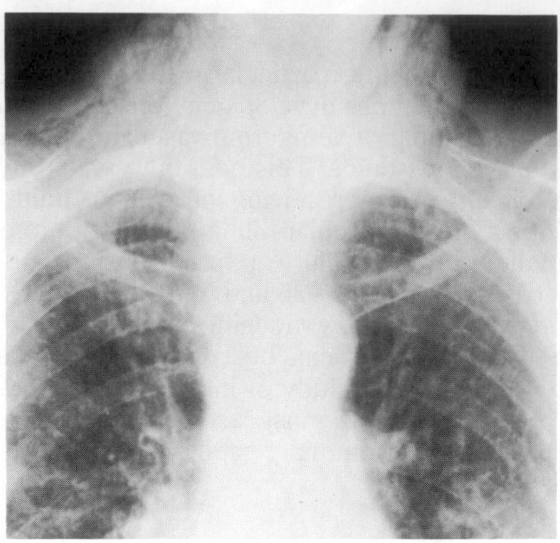

FIGURE 7-36. Subcutaneous emphysema in the neck secondary to diagnostic transtracheal aspiration. Multiple linear lucencies represent air within subcutaneous fat and cervical muscle bundles. The patient also has diffuse interstitial lung disease.

cate a pneumothorax include tachycardia, shock, and decline of arterial blood gas values. The intubated and sedated patient cannot always complain of chest pain or dyspnea. Roentgenographic recognition of a pneumothorax is simple if the collapse is massive, but the demonstration of a small amount of intrapleural air may require that the patient assume a somewhat upright position for the exposure of the film. The occurrence of interstitial emphysema and pneumothorax is not uncommon with volume-limited ventilation, particularly if high pressures and PEEP are used.

Radiation Lung Disease

Radiation therapy in or near the lungs may result in acute radiation pneumonitis or chronic radiation fibrosis. *Radiation pneumonitis* appears within 1 or 2 months from the start of therapy and is manifested roentgenographically as a soft, fluffy alveolar process usually localized to the areas exposed to the radiation, although on occasion it may become generalized. *Radiation fibrosis* may be a sequela of radiation pneumonitis or may develop independently some months after radiation therapy has been completed. It is interstitial in its roentgenographic appearance and is characterized by its strict localization to the field of radiation exposure and its lack of segmental distribution. Secondary bronchiectasis within the involved area gives the infiltrate a nonhomogeneous character.

Endoscopic Trauma

Fiberoptic bronchoscopy is relatively atraumatic to the lung. Bronchoscopic biopsy of bronchial lesions may result in hemorrhage, more commonly with the larger-sized biopsies that are possible with the rigid bronchoscope. Bronchial bleeding may produce evidence of alveolar-filling consolidation in the affected lung area. Transbronchoscopic biopsies of peripheral lung may result in traumatic pneumothorax caused by disruption of the visceral pleura by the biopsy forceps (Fig. 7-37).

Esophageal endoscopic examination or bougienage may cause esophageal rupture, leading to acute mediastinitis. Roentgenographic findings include mediastinal widening, mediastinal emphysema, and often pneumothorax or hydropneumothorax. The esophageal perforation resulting from violent vomiting ("spontaneous" perforation of the esophagus) has identical radiologic characteristics.

Misplaced Tubes and Lines

Misplaced endotracheal tubes can cause several problems. In adults, the tip of the tube should be at least 2.5 cm above the carina and 3 cm below the vocal cords. In-

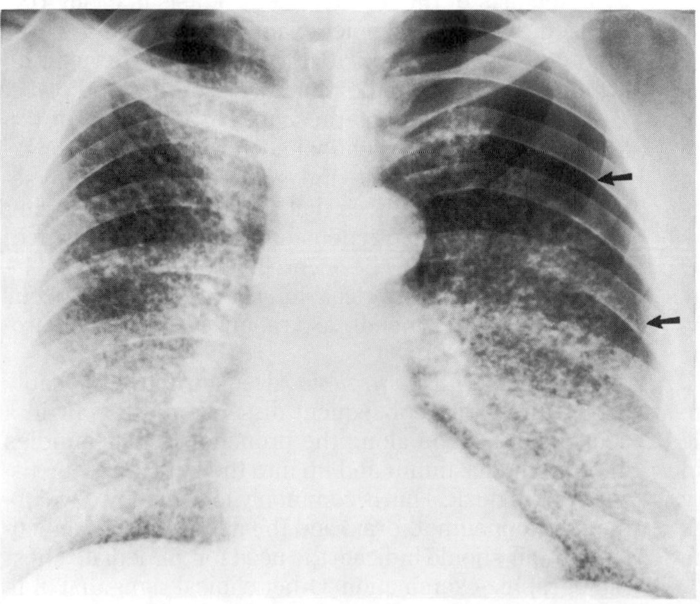

FIGURE 7-37. Left pneumothorax secondary to perforation of the visceral pleura during transbronchial lung biopsy with the fiberoptic bronchoscope. This complication occurs in 5% of such biopsies. The diagnosis of miliary tuberculosis was established by the lung biopsy and the patient was treated successfully. Lung edge is marked *(arrows)*. Note the absence of miliary lesions in the area of pneumothorax gas.

advertent intrusion of the tube into the right main bronchus occurs in 10% of cases and may cause left lung hypoventilation or even atelectasis. Proximal intubation may damage the larynx and predisposes to accidental extubation. Inadvertent esophageal intubation can be confirmed by the aberrant position of the balloon and severe gastric distension with air (Fig. 7-38).

Central venous catheters are malpositioned on insertion in one third of cases.[6] The tip should be proximal to the right atrium and beyond the venous valves. Intracardiac positioning may result in cardiac perforation or arrhythmias. Extravascular extrusion usually is first suspected by the roentgen detection of unexplained mediastinal or pleural fluid collections.

Esophageal feeding tubes may be placed inadvertently in the tracheobronchial tree, resulting in such complications as pneumothorax, atelectasis, pneumonia, lung abscess, or empyema. The malposition of the tube is readily apparent on chest roentgenograms.

Swan-Ganz catheters are subject to shearing during insertion and excessive looping or coiling. Pulmonary ischemic complications, which occur in up to 7% of patients, usually result from persistent wedging of the catheter tip within a small pulmonary artery or persistent balloon inflation after wedging. The consequent infarct has a subpleural location (see Fig. 7-34). The catheter tip should be no more than 2 cm lateral to the hilum.

Chest tubes for pleural space drainage may function poorly if improperly placed. Detection of tube misplacement usually requires both PA and lateral fims, and CT is often necessary.

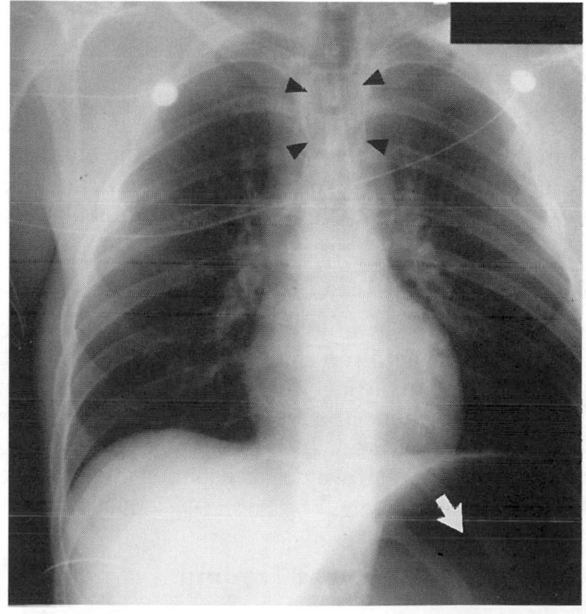

FIGURE 7-38. Esophageal intubation with endotracheal tube. Note that the ET tube does not follow the contours of the trachea, the gastric air bubble is dramatically distended *(white arrow)*, and the ET tube balloon is well visualized around its entire oval contour *(black arrows)*.

OPPORTUNISTIC INFECTIONS

Opportunistic infections occur in patients with impaired host defenses. The "compromised host" may owe his or her vulnerability to his or her underlying disease (diabetes, impaired cellular or humoral immunity, granulocytopenia, splenectomy), to mechanical conduits (endotracheal tubes, intravenous catheters) that provide access for microorganisms, or to the effects of drugs (adrenal steroids, cytotoxic drugs).

The lungs are commonly the site of opportunistic infections. The organisms may have low pathogenicity under ordinary circumstances and are often normal body flora. The development of immune compromise gives the organisms the opportunity to give rise to infection. A given opportunistic infection may be caused by several organisms present simultaneously.

In the clinical and radiologic assessment of such patients, it must be remembered that the roentgenographic abnormality is not invariably caused by an infectious process.[32,50] It may also be a manifestation of the primary underlying disease, an untoward reaction to treatment, or a nonspecific abnormality such as lymphocytic interstitial pneumonitis (Table 7-5).

The radiologic appearance of the lungs does provide some etiologic clues. Lobar/segmental consolidation suggests bacterial, fungal, or mycobacterial infections. Multiple nodules are often caused by fungal infections, and sometimes by metastatic tumors. *Diffuse alveolar disease* suggests pneumocystis or cytomegalovirus infection, alveolar hemorrhage, oxygen toxicity, or drug reaction. *Diffuse interstitial disease* in a compromised host may result from viral infection, lymphoma, or the chronic stage of drug reactions, radiation fibrosis, and oxygen-damaged lung. Miliary lesions suggest mycobacterial and fungal infection, or talc granulomas due to intravenous drug abuse.

PULMONARY MANIFESTATIONS OF AIDS

AIDS caused by infection with human immunodeficiency virus (HIV) eventually manifests pulmonary manifestations in almost all cases.[32] The most common abnormality is *Pneumocystis carinii* pneumonia, but other infectious processes may be present, and noninfectious disorders may also develop in the lungs (see Table 7-5). More than one disease process may be present in the lungs simultaneously.

RADIOLOGY IN THE INTENSIVE CARE UNIT

Bedside radiography comprises about 50% of all chest radiographic examinations,[9] and in such cases, the examination is clinically useful about 50% of the time.

Because patients in intensive care units tend to have life-threatening and rapidly changing pulmonary ab-

TABLE 7-5 **Pulmonary Diseases in Compromised Hosts**

Opportunistic Infections
Drug-Induced Pulmonary Disease
Infections from drug-induced immunosuppression
Drug reactions
Radiation pneumonitis/fibrosis
Transfusion reactions
Oxygen toxicity
Underlying Disease in Lungs
Metastatic tumor growth
Lymphomas and leukemias
Fibrosing alveolitis in collagen–vascular diseases
Complications of the Underlying Disease
Hematogenous infections
Diffuse alveolar hemorrhages
Graft versus host disease
Pulmonary edema
Kaposi's sarcoma in AIDS
Nonspecific Interstitial Pneumonitis
Lymphocytic interstitial pneumonia in AIDS
Heart–lung transplants
Marrow transplants

normalities, accurate interpretation is critically important, but the technical quality of the AP supine chest roentgenograms is often unavoidably suboptimal.[51] New technical advances, which improve the quality of the images obtained by bedside radiography, have already been mentioned.[7,9] Errors can arise from overinterpretation of "abnormalities" that may be spurious and caused by positional factors or differences in exposure on serial films. It has been wisely suggested that interpreters of such roentgenograms attempt primarily to provide answers to the following questions:[52]

1. Is the film technically adequate?
2. Are there any rib fractures?
3. Are the endotracheal tube and intravenous lines correctly positioned?
4. Is there pulmonary consolidation? Has it changed from prior roentgenograms? Attempts to predict causes may be seriously misleading.
5. Is pleural fluid present?
6. Is atelectasis present?
7. Is a pneumothorax present?

The interpreter must constantly remember that pneumothoraces and pleural effusions often have atypical appearances on AP supine films (see Fig. 7-22) and that the variations in penetration and contrast from film to film may be misinterpreted as changes in the course of the disease.

Roentgenographic examinations in seriously ill patients should be interpreted rapidly, with written reports easily available. The roentgenograms should be easily accessible for review by the attending physicians.

THORACIC TRAUMA

Thoracic trauma may result in various physiologic and roentgenographic abnormalities in the thorax, the prompt recognition of which is imperative for successfully managing the patient. In most instances the fact that trauma to the thoracic cage has occurred is apparent from the history or from superficial inspection of the thorax; however, if an unconscious patient is brought to the hospital emergency room and inspection of the thorax reveals no obvious evidence of injury, traumatic lung damage may go unrecognized. Thoracic trauma must be suspected in all such cases and appropriate roentgenographic studies carried out.[36] The mechanisms of production of thoracic trauma and the nature of the resulting lesions are extremely varied. Some of the more common abnormalities are mentioned.

Rib Fractures

Rib fractures may have a variety of possible consequences. One or two undisplaced rib fractures may have no deleterious effect other than pain and may be difficult to detect on standard roentgenograms. Special rib films may be needed to detect their presence. If the patient has COPD, the cough suppression induced by the pain of the fractures may result in atelectasis, pneumonia, or acute respiratory failure.

Multiple rib fractures will create an instability of the chest wall, known as *flail chest,* which may cause severe respiratory embarrassment. The modern treatment of flail chest with intubation and mechanical ventilation (internal pneumatic stabilization) represents one of the more important advances in managing thoracic trauma. Flail chest is easily recognized on physical examination by the paradoxical movement of the traumatized unstable chest wall and can be confirmed radiographically by inspiration and expiration films.

Rib fractures may lacerate vessels and cause hemothorax (see Fig. 7-32) or may lacerate the lung and cause pneumothorax. The presence of air and fluid within the pleural space is manifested by the characteristic air-fluid interface, which cannot be seen, however, unless the roentgen beam is in the horizontal plane.

Penetrating Wounds

Penetrating chest wounds cause pneumothorax by virtue of entry of air through the chest wall wound or by leakage of air from the lacerated lung. Intrapleural hemorrhage is common, and chylothorax appears if the thoracic duct is injured. Intrapulmonary hemorrhage occurs along the pathway of the penetrating foreign body within the lung.

Nonpenetrating Chest Trauma

Nonpenetrating trauma may result in the formation of an intrapulmonary hematoma (pulmonary contusion), which appears roentgenographically as a poorly circumscribed opaque consolidation without localization to segmental boundaries. The opacity appears within hours after the injury and clears spontaneously within 1 or 2 weeks. Occasionally closed-chest trauma may tear the lung internally to produce a pulmonary laceration—a cystlike hyperlucent space that may contain an air-fluid level because of intracavitary hemorrhage. Tracheobronchial rupture caused by nonpenetrating trauma results in pneumothorax, often accompanied by mediastinal and subcutaneous emphysema and frequently associated with fractures of the upper three ribs. Nonpenetrating trauma may cause hemothorax or chylothorax in some instances.

Mediastinal structures may be affected by nonpenetrating trauma. Traumatic pericarditis is often secondary to steering wheel injuries of the anterior chest. Traumatic rupture of the descending portion of the aortic arch may lead to formation of a false aneurysm, which presents on the chest roentgenogram as a left-sided mediastinal mass. Mediastinal hematoma resulting from traumatic injury of one or more small vessels causes generalized or diffuse mediastinal widening.

LUNG TRANSPLANTATION

The radiologic changes appearing in the transplanted lung may result from several causes, which can be differentiated with reasonable confidence from the clinical features and radiologic characteristics.[53] The reimplantation response develops in the first 3 to 4 days after surgery and is characterized by reticular interstitial changes plus alveolar filling. It gradually subsides over periods of weeks or months. Acute rejection has a similar appearance but develops later; fever and dyspnea are usually present and small pleural effusions are common. There is usually a dramatic response to intravenous steroids.

Bronchiolitis obliterans will develop in 50% of long-term survivors of heart-lung transplantation. Radiologic changes are minor and nonspecific; peripheral bronchiectasis on CT seems to be the most typical. Airway problems include dehiscence (resulting in mediastinal emphysema) and bronchial strictures; both are best seen with CT. Lung infections, which are very common, may be bacterial, viral, or fungal. The radiographic features are nonspecific.

REFERENCES

1. Fraser RG, Paré JAP, Paré PD, Fraser RS, Genereux GP: Roentgenologic signs in the diagnosis of chest disease. In Diagnosis of Diseases of the Chest Vol I, 3rd ed, Chap 4. Philadelphia, WB Saunders, 1988, pp 458–687
2. Blank N: Chest Radiographic Analysis. Churchill Livingstone, New York, 1989
3. Greenspan RH, Sostman HD: Radiographic techniques. In Murray JF, Nadel JA (eds): Textbook of Respiratory Medicine, 2nd ed, Chap 24. Philadelphia, WB Saunders, 1994, pp 610–681.
4. Fraser RG, Paré JAP, Paré PD, Fraser RS, Genereux GP: Perception in chest roentgenology. In Diagnosis of Diseases of the Chest, Vol I, 3rd ed. Philadelphia, WB Saunders, 1988, pp 291–296
5. Proto AV, Speckman JM: The left lateral radiograph of the chest. Med Radiogr Photogr Part I, 55:30, 1979, Part II 56:38, 1980
6. Weiner MP, Garay SM, Leitwen BS, Wiener DN, Ravin CE: Imaging of the intensive care unit patient. Clin Chest Med 12:169–198, 1991
7. Zylak CJ, Littleton JT, Durizch ML: Illusory consolidation of the left lower lobe: A pitfall of portable radiography. Radiology 167:653–55, 1988
8. Glazer HS, Muka E, Sagel SS, Jost RG: New techniques in chest radiography. Radiol Clin North Am 32:711–717, 1994
9. Wandtke JC: Bedside chest radiography. Radiology 190:1–10, 1994
10. Pinet F, Clermont A, Michel C, Celard P, Lagrange C: Embolization of the systemic arteries of the lung. J Thorac Imag 2(2):11–14 1987
11. Miller RD, Offord KP: Roentgenologic determination of total lung capacity. Mayo Clin Proc 55:694, 1980
12. Zerhouni EA (ed): CT and MRI of the Thorax. Churchill Livingstone, New York, 1990
13. Webb WR, Müller NL, Naidich DP: High Resolution CT of the Lung. Raven Press, New York, 1992
14. Friedman PJ: Lung cancer staging: efficacy of CT. Radiology 182:307–309, 1992
15. Colice GJ: Chest CT for known and suspected lung cancer. Chest 106:1539–1550, 1994
16. Westcott JL: Transthoracic needle biopsy of the hilum and mediastinum. J Thorac Imag 2(2):41, 1987
17. Gottschalk A, Alderson PO, Sostman HD: Nuclear medicine techniques and applications. In Murray JF, Nadel JA (eds): Textbook of Respiratory Medicine, 2nd ed, Chap 25. Philadelphia, WB Saunders, 1994, pp 682–710
18. Dewan NA, Gupta NC, et al: Diagnostic efficacy of PET-FDG imaging in solitary pulmonary nodules—potential role in evaluation and management. Chest 104:997–1002, 1993
19. Weinreb JC, Naidich DP: Thoracic magnetic resonance imaging. Clin Chest Med 12:33–54, 1991
20. Webb WR: Mediastinum and Hila. In Partain CL, et al (eds): Magnetic Resonance Imaging, 2nd ed. Philadelphia, WB Saunders, 1988
21. Sistrom CL, Reiheld CT, Wallace KK: Ultrasound for diagnosis and intervention in thoracic diseases. Postgrad Radiol 14:21–49, 1994
22. White RH, McGahan JP, Daschback MM, Hartling RP: Diagnosis of deep vein thrombosis using duplex ultrasound. Arch Intern Med 111:297–304, 1989
23. Tarver RD, Conces DJ: Interventional chest radiology. Radiol Clin North Am 32:689–709, 1994
24. Naidich DP, Garay SM: Radiographic evaluation of focal lung disease. Clin Chest Med 12:77–95, 1991
25. Proto AV, Toscino I: Radiographic manifestations of lobar collapse. Semin Roentgenol 15:117, 1980
26. Genereux GP, Stilwell GA: The acute bacterial pneumonias. Semin Roentgenol 15:9, 1980
27. Janower ML, Weiss EB: Mycoplasmal, viral and rickettsial pneumonias. Semin Roentgenol 15:25, 1980
28. Lynch DA, Armstrong DA: A pattern-oriented approach to chest radiographs in atypical pneumonia syndromes. Clin Chest Med 12:203–222, 1991
29. Miller WT, Miller WT Jr.: Tuberculosis in the normal host: Radiological findings. Semin Roentgenol 28:109–119, 1993
30. Davis SD, Yankelewitz DF, Henschke CI: Pulmonary tuberculosis in immunocompromised hosts: Epidemiological, clinical and radiological assessment. Semin Roentgenol 28:119–130, 1993
31. Sarosi GA: Community-acquired fungal diseases. Clin Chest Med 12:337–347, 1991
32. Kuhlman JE: Pulmonary manifestations of acquired immunodeficiency syndrome. Semin Roentgenol 29:242–274, 1994
33. Lillington GA, Caskey CI: Evaluation and management of solitary and multiple pulmonary nodules. Clin Chest Med 14:111–119, 1993
34. White CS, Templeton PA: Radiologic manifestations of bronchogenic cancer. Clin Chest Med 14:5567, 1993
35. Moore EH, Templeton PA: Imaging the advancing frontier of lung cancer operability. Semin Resp Med 13:293–308, 1992
36. Dee PM: Radiology of chest trauma. Radiol Clin North Am 30:291–306, 1992
37. Thurlbeck WM, Müller NL: Emphysema: Definition, imaging, and quantification. Am J Roentgenol 163:1017–1025, 1994

38. Palmer PES: Radiologic considerations in asthma. In: Gershwin ME, GM Halpern (eds): Bronchial Asthma, 3rd ed. Totowa, NJ, Humana Press, 1994, pp 237–271
39. Jantz MA, Pierson DJ: Pneumothorax and barotrauma. Clin Chest Med 15:75–91, 1994
40. Pierson DJ: Pneumomediastinum. In Murray JF, Nadel JA (eds): Textbook of Respiratory Medicine, 2nd ed, Chap 80. WB Saunders, Philadelphia, 1994, pp 2250–2265
41. Groskin SA: Pattern recognition in pulmonary radiology. In Heitzman's The Lung—Radiologic-Pathologic Correlations, 3rd ed, Chap 5. St. Louis, Mosby, 1993 pp 76–105
42. Milne ENC, Pistolesi M, et al: The radiologic distinction of cardiogenic and noncardiogenic edema. Am J Roentgenol 144:879, 1985
43. Aberle DA, Brown K: Radiologic considerations in the adult respiratory distress syndrome. Clin Chest Med 11:737–754, 1990
44. Fleischner FG: Roentgenology of the pulmonary infarct. Semin Roentgenol 2:61, 1967
45. Fedullo PF, Auger WR, Channick RN, Moser KM, Jamieson SW: Chronic thromboembolic pulmonary hypertension. Clin Chest Med 16:353—374, 1995
46. Rubin SA, Winer-Muram, Ellis JV: Diagnostic imaging of pneumonia and its complications in the critically ill patient. Clin Chest Med 16:45–59, 1995
47. Ahmad M, Demeter SL: Drug-induced pulmonary disease. In Baum GL, Wolinsky E (eds): Textbook of Pulmonary Disease, 5th ed. Boston, Little, Brown & Co, 1994 pp 775–787
48. Pisani RJ, Rosenow EC III: Pulmonary edema associated with tocolytic therapy. Ann Intern Med 110:714, 1989
49. Zwillich CW, et al: Complications of assisted ventilation: A prospective study of 354 consecutive episodes. Am J Med 57:161, 1974
50. Moore EH: Diffuse lung disease in the current spectrum of immunocompromised hosts (non-AIDS). Radiol Clin North Am 30:525–554, 1991
51. Lefcoe MS: Basic principles of chest x-ray interpretation in a critical care unit. In WJ Sibbald (ed): Synopsis of Critical Care 3rd ed, Chap 9. Baltimore, Williams & Wilkins, 1988
52. Adams FG: A simplified approach to the reporting of intensive therapy unit chest radiographs. Clin Radiol 30:214, 1979
53. Herman SJ: Radiologic assessment after lung transplantation. Radiol Clin North Am 32:663–678, 1994

8 Pulmonary Function Tests

Paul L. Enright
John E. Hodgkin

CLINICAL SKILLS

Upon completion of this chapter, the reader will:

- Know indications for testing lung function
- Understand equipment needed, procedure, quality assurance, and calculations for the various lung tests
- Interpret pulmonary function tests

KEY TERMS

Forced vital capacity (FVC) maneuver
Forced expiratory flow (FEF)
Forced expiratory volume
Forced inspiratory vital capacity (FIVC) test
Functional residual capacity (FRC)
Lung compliance testing
Maximal voluntary ventilation (MVV)
Maximal expiratory pressure (MEP)
Maximal inspiratory pressure (MIP)
Peak expiratory flow (PEF)
Residual volume (RV)
Slow vital capacity (SVC)
Static lung compliance
Total lung capacity (TLC)

Respiratory therapists are often asked to perform pulmonary function (PF) testing at the bedside or in the emergency room, and they are frequently responsible for operating the hospital's pulmonary function laboratory. Pulmonary function testing offers many opportunities for a respiratory therapist because the indications for testing are many and the tests are currently underused by most physicians.

Evaluation of pulmonary function benefits many types of patients.[1] Pulmonary disease may frequently be detected by PF tests years before the onset of signs or symptoms. Early detection of pulmonary disease helps the physician convince patients to stop smoking, reducing the risk of both cardiovascular and pulmonary disease. Test comparison helps the physician to determine whether a specific therapeutic regimen is beneficial. Shortness of breath is a common complaint for which PF tests can help differentiate between a cardiac and a pulmonary cause. The PF tests performed before planned surgery help to reduce the incidence of postoperative pulmonary complications by identifying patients at increased risk. Finally, patients who feel that their ability to work is limited by shortness of breath can be objectively evaluated by PF tests. The results often carry considerable legal and economic consequences.

This chapter first introduces the reader to the most important and most frequently performed PF tests. The tests described at the end of this chapter are not usually available in smaller laboratories. For each test, you will learn why physicians order the test (indications), what equipment is necessary to perform the test (because you will often be asked to specify and purchase instruments), how to perform the test, how to calibrate the instruments and obtain accurate results (quality assurance), how to calculate the results and normal values, and, finally, what the results mean clinically (interpretation).

AARC Clinical Practice Guideline

SPIROMETRY

Indications: The indications for spirometry include the need for detecting the presence or absence of lung dysfunction suggested by history or physical indicators (eg, age, smoking history, family history of lung disease, cough) or the presence of other abnormal diagnostic tests (eg, chest x-ray films, arterial blood gases); quantifying the severity of known lung disease; assessing the change in lung function over time or following administration of or change of therapy; assessing the potential effects or response to environmental or occupational exposure; assessing the risk for surgical procedures known to affect lung function; assess impairment and/or disability.

Contraindications: Relative contraindications to performing spirometry are hemoptysis of unknown origin; untreated pneumothorax; unstable cardiovascular status; thoracic, abdominal, or cerebral aneurysms; recent eye surgery (eg, cataract); presence of an acute disease process that might interfere with test performance; recent surgery of the thorax or abdomen.

Assessment of Need: Determination that valid indications are present.

Assessment of Test Quality: Spirometry performed for the listed indications is valid only if the spirometer functions acceptably and the subject is able to perform the maneuvers in an acceptable and reproducible fashion. All reports should contain a statement about the technician's assessment of test quality and specify which ATS standards were not met.

Monitoring: The following should be evaluated during the performance of spirometric measurements to ascertain the validity of the results: test data of repeated efforts (ie, reproducibility of FVC, FEV_1), level of effort and cooperation by the subject, equipment function or malfunction (eg, calibration). The final report should contain a statement about test quality.

From AARC Clinical Practice Guideline; see Respir Care 41:629, 1996, for complete text.

SPIROMETRY

Several types of tests can be performed with a spirometer. We first consider the most frequently performed test—the *forced vital capacity (FVC) maneuver.*

Indications

Spirometry is the most commonly performed PF test because it is quick, safe, and inexpensive (see AARC Clinical Practice Guideline: Spirometry). It is a screening test for pulmonary disease, just as blood pressure measurement is a screening test for hypertension. All current and former cigarette smokers over the age of 40 should be tested; 15% to 33% of them have abnormal spirometry results, and their abnormal lung function will probably improve if they stop smoking.[2,3] Box 8-1 lists the indications for spirometry, which is usually performed before any of the other PF tests.

Equipment

Several types of spirometers are available—from $300 hand-held spirometers to $5000 computerized spirometers (Table 8-1). Manual spirometers should be avoided for frequent testing because manual calculations are time consuming and error prone. Independent evaluations of commercial spirometers[4] show that only half of the volume-sensing spirometers and half of the flow-sensing spirometers meet the American Thoracic Society's (ATS) spirometry standards (Table 8-2).[5]

Procedure

The FVC maneuver requires considerable cooperation from the patient. You must first explain the test and then demonstrate the maneuver. The patient must then perform at least three acceptable and two reproducible maneuvers while you provide enthusiastic coaching.

BOX 8-1

INDICATIONS FOR PULMONARY FUNCTION TESTS

Diagnostic

To evaluate symptoms, signs, and abnormal results of laboratory tests
- Symptoms: cough, dyspnea, wheezing, orthopnea, or chest pain
- Signs: overinflation, expiratory slowing, cyanosis, chest deformity, wheezing, or unexplained crackles
- Abnormal results of laboratory tests: hypoxemia, hypercapnia, polycythemia, or abnormal chest radiographs

To measure the effect of disease on pulmonary function

To screen persons at risk for pulmonary disease
- Smokers
- Persons with occupational exposure to injurious substances
- Some persons at the time of a routine physical examination

To assess preoperative risk

To assess prognosis

Monitoring

To assess effectiveness of therapeutic interventions
- Bronchodilator therapy
- Steroid treatment for asthma, interstitial lung disease, and the like
- Management of congestive heart failure
- Other

To provide information on the course of diseases affecting lung function
- Pulmonary disease, such as obstructive airways disease and interstitial lung disease
- Cardiac disease, such as congestive heart failure
- Neuromuscular disease, such as Guillain-Barré syndrome

To assess current status of persons with occupational exposure to injurious substances

To detect adverse reactions to drugs with known pulmonary toxicity

Evaluation of disability or impairment

To assess patients as part of a rehabilitation program
- Medical
- Industrial
- Vocational

To assess risks for an insurance evaluation

To assess the condition of persons for legal reasons
- Social security or other program involving government compensation
- Personal-injury lawsuits
- Other

Public health

Epidemiologic surveys

Used by permission from Crapo RO: Current concepts: Pulmonary function testing. N Engl J Med 331: 25, 1994.

A traditional volume-time tracing is depicted in Figure 8-1. Submaximal initial effort is best detected by viewing the flow-volume curves produced by an automated spirometer (Fig. 8-2), and volume-time tracings are best for detecting premature termination at the end of a test. If three acceptable maneuvers are not produced after eight attempts, testing should be rescheduled.

TABLE 8-1 **Types of Spirometers and Examples**

Type	Examples
Volume Sensing	
Water sealed	Collins Survey
Bellows	Med Science Wedge
Dry rolling seal	Spirotech, Sensor Medics
Flow Sensing	
Fleisch pneumotachometer	Welch Allyn Pneumocheck
Metal screen	Vitalograph Alpha
Disposable screen	Puritan Bennett Renaissance
Vortex shedding	Riko Spiromate

The primary advantage of volume-sensing spirometers is better long-term accuracy if calibration is not done regularly. Flow-sensing spirometers are smaller, less expensive, and easier to clean, but must be calibrated every day to maintain accuracy. Both types may be automated with a microprocessor or a personal computer. Hand-held spirometers are flow sensing. Nonautomated, manually operated spirometers are volume sensing.

Quality Assurance

Submaximal FVC efforts mimic disease patterns, potentially resulting in false-positive interpretations. Vigorous coaching and close observation of the patient's body language during his or her efforts is essential. You must

TABLE 8-2 **ATS 1994 Spirometry Standards**

1. Minimum graph

	RANGE	SIZE
Volume	7 L	7 cm
Flow	12 L/sec	6 cm
Time	15 sec	40 cm

2. Daily calibration check with a 3-L syringe for >3% accuracy
3. Daily leak check for volume spirometers with no volume change after 1 minute
4. Quarterly speed check for volume spirometers with 1% accuracy using a stopwatch
5. Less than 1.5 $cmH_2O/L/sec$ back pressure
6. Temperature measured in the spirometer within 1°C for each subject (test only between 17–40°C)

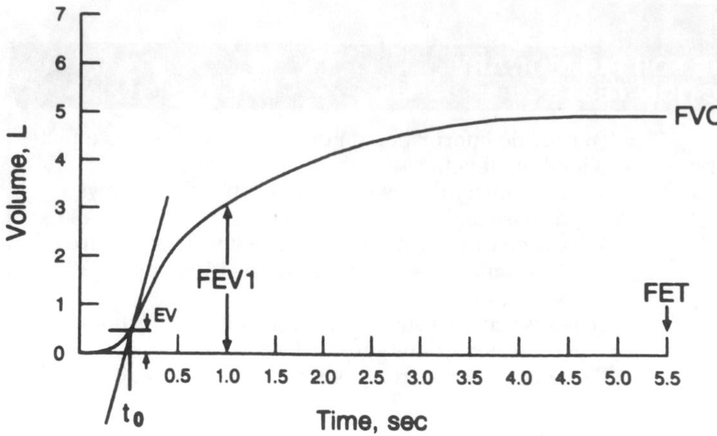

FIGURE 8-1. Traditional volume–time spirogram. The FVC maneuver starts at the lower left corner at full inhalation. The FVC is the total exhaled volume at the end of the maneuver's plateau (FVC = 5.0 L in this example). The start of the maneuver is determined by "back extrapolation:" a tangent is drawn through the steepest portion of the maneuver, intersecting the baseline at the time zero (t_0). The FEV_1 occurs 1 second after time zero (FEV_1 = 3.0 L here). The extrapolated volume (EV = 0.5 L here) and the forced expiratory time (FET = 5.5 sec here) are measured as quality control checks. (© Mayo Foundation)

also learn to recognize the patterns of unacceptable maneuvers (Fig. 8-3).[6] After three acceptable maneuvers are obtained, you must then check them for reproducibility. The two highest FEV_1s should match within 0.2 L, and the two highest FVCs should match within 0.2 L. If a flow-volume display is available, the peak expiratory flows (PEFs) give an excellent index of effort and should match within 10%.

The accuracy of all types of spirometers should be checked using a 3.00-L syringe at least daily. The resulting volumes should be within 3% of 3.00 L. Volume spirometers should also be checked daily for leaks by placing a weight on the bell or piston and watching for at least 1 minute to be sure that it does not change position. At least quarterly, further quality assurance checks should include a linearity check over the entire range of flows (0 to 12 L/sec) and volumes (0 to 7 L or more); a stopwatch should be used to ensure that the chart speed is accurate to within 1%.

To reduce the risk of cross contamination from spirometers, always use a new mouthpiece and a clean breathing tube for each patient, avoid inhalation from the spirometer, and dry the inside of the spirometer at the end of each day. Consider the use of disposable flow sensors or a separate spirometer for infectious patients, such as those with tuberculosis, hepatitis, or acquired immunodeficiency syndrome (AIDS). After testing such patients, wipe all surfaces exposed to exhaled air with a detergent solution while wearing rubber gloves, soak all hoses and the spirometer interior in an activated glutaraldehyde solution for at least 20 minutes, then dry all surfaces before using the spirometer to test another patient.

Calculations

The FVC maneuver measures both flow and volume. Flow is best represented by the FEV_1, which is the average flow during the first second. Its name, *forced expiratory volume in 1 second,* comes from the old method of measuring it directly from a spirogram (see Fig. 8-1). A method called back extrapolation is used to determine the onset (zero time) of the maneuver. The many other indexes of flow that can be measured from FVC maneuvers are generally unnecessary or misleading.

The *forced vital capacity* (FVC) is the volume of air exhaled during the FVC maneuver. It is measured from

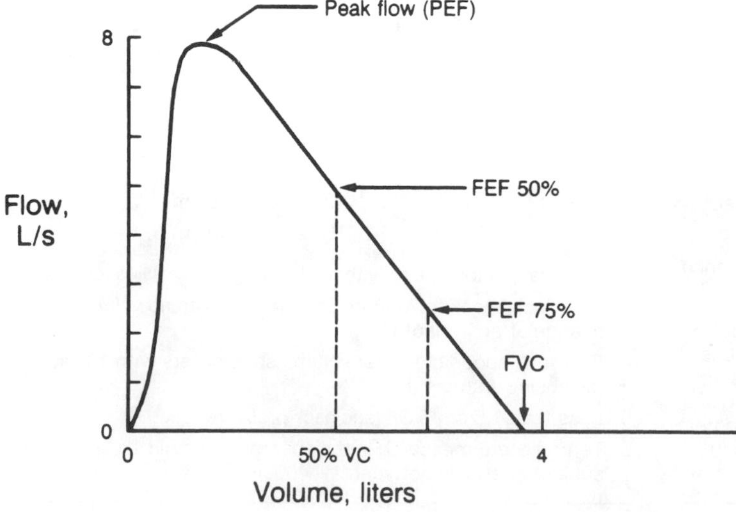

FIGURE 8-2. Flow–volume curve from a healthy person. The maneuver starts at the lower left corner. Flow increases rapidly to a peak expiratory flow (PEF) and then decreases evenly until all of the forced vital capacity (FVC) is exhaled. Instantaneous flows at 50% and 75% of the FVC are sometimes measured. The FEV_1 and the forced expiratory time (FET) cannot be measured directly from a flow–volume curve. (© Mayo Foundation)

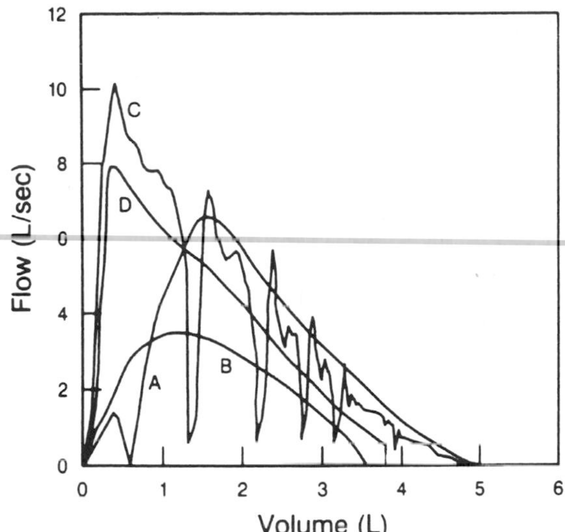

FIGURE 8-3. Unacceptable FVC maneuvers. Maneuver A shows a hesitating start. Maneuver B shows poor peak flow effort; the patient did not blast out the air quickly. The jagged lines of maneuver C are due to coughing throughout the maneuver. The vertical drop at the end of maneuver D occurred when the patient quit too soon (premature termination of effort). (© Mayo Foundation)

the point of maximal inhalation to the point at which the patient cannot exhale any more air. This may take only 3 seconds in normal children, but more than 20 seconds in adults with emphysema.

The FEV_1 is often divided by the FVC to obtain the FEV_1/FVC ratio. This ratio is a sensitive index of borderline-to-mild airways obstruction and is also helpful in differentiating obstructive from restrictive pulmonary disease. It is decreased in obstruction and is normal or increased in restriction. Normal adults are able to exhale more than 70% of the FVC in the first second (this ratio decreases with age). The maximal midexpiratory flow rate or forced expiratory flow between 25% and 75% of the FVC ($FEF_{25\%-75\%}$) is also used by some physicians as a sensitive (but highly variable) index of borderline-to-mild obstruction.

The maximum flow that can be achieved during the FVC is known as the *peak expiratory flow* (PEF). The PEF is a good index of the amount of effort (blast) during the first part of the FVC maneuver, but is not a good measure of obstruction because of this effort dependence. The PEF is not easily measured by volume spirometers and must be determined either by flow-volume curves or by using a peak flowmeter.

Normal values for spirometry results are determined from large studies of supposedly normal subjects. Older studies were flawed by including smokers, using obsolete equipment or techniques, or not including enough subjects from wide ranges of age or height. The studies of Miller,[7] Crapo,[8] and Knudson,[9] done since 1980, provide accurate predicted-values equations and normal ranges for white adults, ages 20 to 65. The recent Six Cities Study provides accurate predicted values for black and white children ages 6 to 18,[10] and the Cardiovascular Health Study provides predicted values for the elderly, ages 65 to 85.[11] The lower limit of the normal range for FEV_1 and FVC is about 80% of the mean predicted value. It is more accurate, however, to define the normal range as excluding the bottom 5% of the healthy population. Use of this 95% confidence interval is necessary to define the normal range of the FEV_1/FVC ratio, the $FEF_{25\%-75\%}$, and most other pulmonary function variables.

The predicted values for nonwhites are not well established, but they are estimated by multiplying the white-adult predicted values by 0.88 for blacks, Asians, and East Indians. Predicted values depend largely on height, which must be measured accurately in stocking feet.

Interpretation

Submaximal efforts must always be excluded by inspection of the spirometry tracings before attempting to interpret the results. When selecting tests for interpretation, select the largest values for FVC and FEV_1 from an acceptable maneuver. For indexes of average or instantaneous flow, use values from the maneuver with the largest value for FVC and FEV_1 combined.[3] The most common spirometry abnormality is airways obstruction, demonstrated by reduced flow rates, a reduced FEV_1/FVC ratio, and a reduced FEV_1 (Fig. 8-4).[12] The degree of impairment (abnormality) is determined by the percentage achieved of the predicted FEV_1 value, because the FEV_1 decreases linearly with worsening obstructive lung disease (Fig. 8-5). Most adults with an FEV_1 below 1 L are short of breath with only mild exertion and meet the American Thoracic Society (ATS)[13]

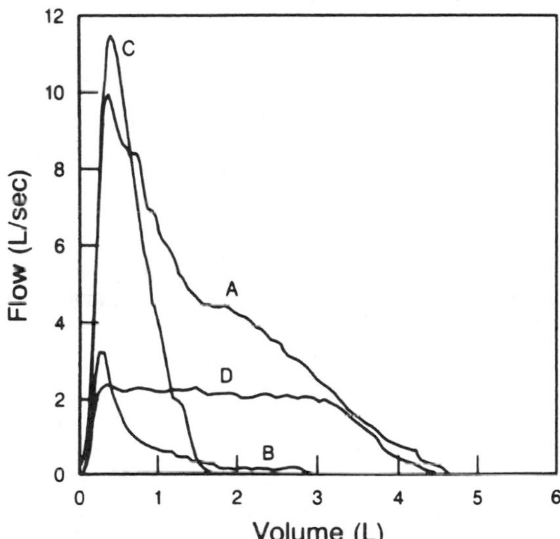

FIGURE 8-4. Flow–volume patterns of spirometric abnormality. Patient A is normal. Patient B has severe obstruction (COPD) resulting in small flows. Patient C demonstrates moderate restriction caused by interstitial fibrosis, resulting in high flows but a low volume. Patient D has a fixed upper airways obstruction (UAO) from tracheal stenosis; his expiratory flow is limited to a maximum of about 2 L/sec, causing a plateau pattern. (© Mayo Foundation)

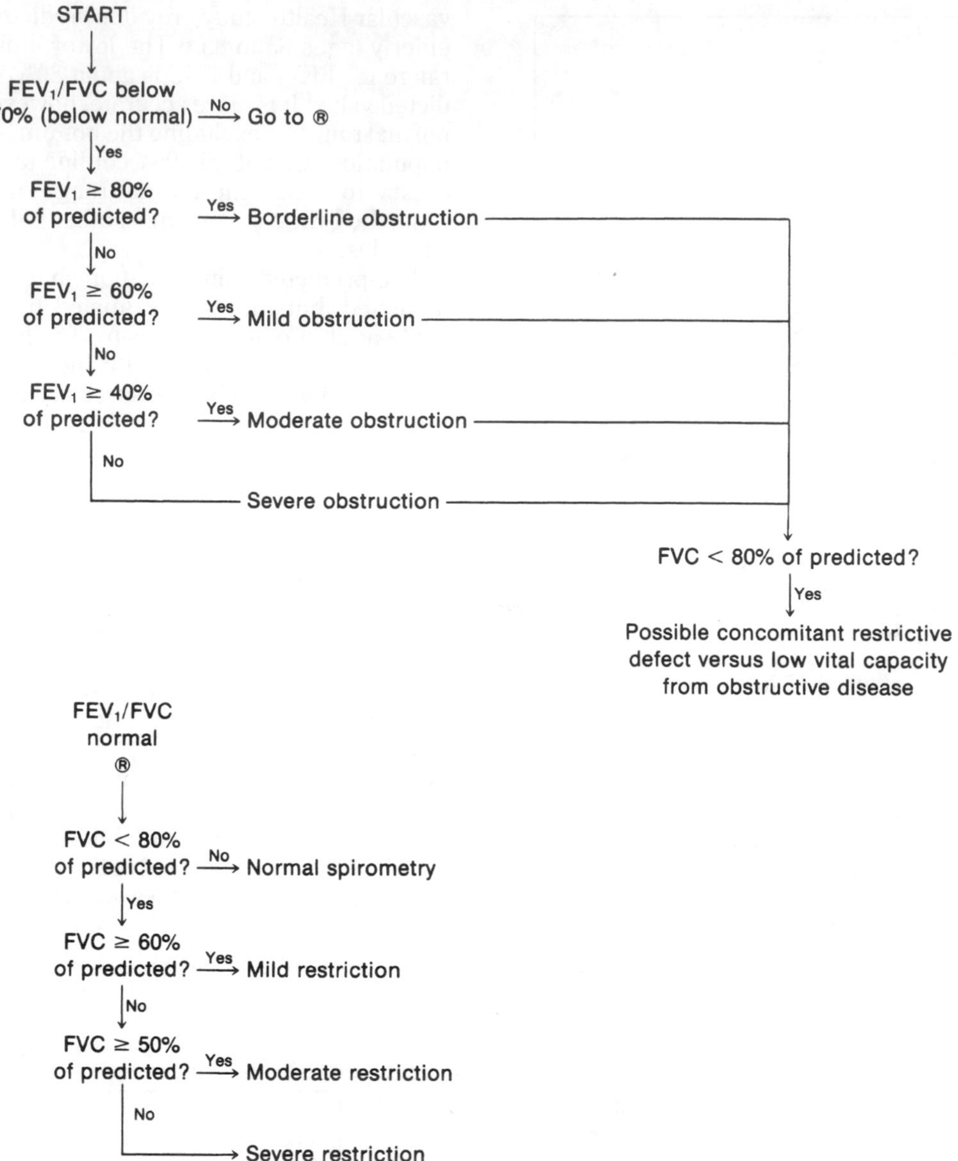

FIGURE 8-5. Spirometry interpretation. Always start by using the FEV_1/FVC ratio to determine if obstruction exists. Grade the degree of obstruction using the percent of predicted FEV_1. If the FEV_1/FVC ratio and the FVC are above the lower limit of normal range (LLN), spirometry is normal. (© Mayo Foundation)

and Social Security Administration's criteria for total disability from chronic obstructive pulmonary disease (COPD).[14]

A reduction of the FVC below 80% of the predicted value with a normal FEV_1/FVC ratio is probably caused by one of many kinds of restrictive lung disorders (Table 8-3). When obstruction is present (a reduced FEV_1/FVC ratio) *and* the FVC is also reduced, the tendency to interpret a mixed pattern of obstruction and restriction should be avoided without measurement of absolute lung volumes, because the low FVC is frequently caused by air trapping secondary to the obstructive disease rather than to a concomitant restrictive disorder. (See Fig. 8-5 for a flow diagram for interpretation of spirometry results.)

COMPARISON STUDIES

Indications

Because the normal range for spirometry values is so wide (80% to 120% of predicted values), it is often useful to compare a patient's current results with his or her own previous results (Table 8-4). Pertinent information regarding comparison tests can be found in AARC Clinical Practice Guideline: Bronchial Provocation.

Isoproterenol given by metered-dose inhaler (MDI) is a bronchodilator (BD) commonly used for testing because its onset of action is rapid and its effects short-lived. If a patient is known to have heart disease, it is prudent to substitute a β_2-adrenergic bronchodilator such as albuterol.

TABLE 8-3 **Types of Pulmonary Disease**

I. Obstructive Pulmonary Disease
   1. Emphysema
   2. Chronic bronchitis
   3. Bronchial asthma
   4. Bronchiectasis
   5. Cystic fibrosis
   6. Tracheobronchomalacia

II. Restrictuve Pulmonary Disease
   A. Intrapulmonic
      1. Interstitial fibrosis
      2. Pulmonary edema
      3. Pneumonia
      4. Vascular congestion
      5. Adult respiratory distress syndrome
      6. Pneumoconioses
      7. Sarcoidosis
   B. Extrapulmonic
      1. Thoracic
         a. Kyphoscoliosis
         b. Multiple rib fractures
         c. Rheumatoid spondylitis
         d. Thoracic surgery
         e. Pleural effusion
         f. Pneumothorax or hemothorax
      2. Abdominal
         a. Abdominal surgery
         b. Ascites
         c. Peritonitis
         d. Obesity
      3. Neuromuscular defects
         a. Poliomyelitis
         b. Guillain-Barré syndrome
         c. Myasthenia gravis
         d. Tetanus
         e. Drugs (eg, pancuronium, kanamycin)
      4. Respiratory center depression
         a. Narcotics
         b. Barbiturates
         c. Anesthesia

Methacholine is a bronchoconstricting agent that should normally be given only to patients with normal baseline spirometry (or borderline obstruction) in whom asthma is suspected but not confirmed.[15] These patients often have chronic cough, chest tightness, or wheezing only during upper respiratory infections or after exercise in cold weather. Exercise testing for exercise-induced bronchospasm (EIB) is probably unnecessary if a methacholine challenge test is negative.

Equipment

Several nebulizers and a compressor and dosimeter are useful for methacholine challenges. Drugs and oxygen for treating an acute asthma attack should be readily available. A treadmill or bicycle ergometer and electrocardiogram (ECG) monitor are used for exercise testing. Simple metered-dose inhalers are used for post-BD testing.

Procedure

The FEV_1 is the most reproducible PF parameter; hence, when the patient has airways obstruction, the FEV_1 should be followed. When following up on patients with restrictive disorders, serial FVC's are compared. The $FEF_{25\%-75\%}$ and FEV_1/FVC should not be used for comparisons.

The technique for administering drugs from a metered-dose inhaler is important. You should first explain and demonstrate the correct maneuver. It is better for you (not the patient) to actuate the MDI. Consider using a spacer if the patient cannot inhale slowly. Be sure to wait for maximal bronchodilation before repeating the FVC maneuvers: 5 minutes after isoproterenol, 15 minutes after albuterol, and 45 minutes after ipratropium.

Methacholine is mixed from a commercially available powder, and serial dilutions are added to nebulizers.[15] Starting with the smallest concentration, five deep inhalations are administered, followed by two reproducible FVC maneuvers. Exhalation need continue only 3 to 4 seconds because only the FEV_1 is measured. If the FEV_1 decreases less than 20%, the next higher concentration is administered, and so on, up to a maximum concentration of 25 mg/mL.

Isoproterenol or albuterol is given if FEV_1 decreases more than 20% following methacholine. You should also make a note of any symptoms of coughing, wheezing, dyspnea, or chest tightness provoked by the methacholine; however, disturbing asthma attacks almost never occur.

The goal of exercise testing for EIB is to raise the patient's heart rate to greater than 85% of the predicted value for at least 6 minutes using a treadmill, bicycle, or free running. Noseclips are recommended to bypass the "air-conditioning" of the nose.

TABLE 8-4 **Spirometry Comparison Studies**

Study	Indication	Agent	Time Interval
Pre- and post-BD	Baseline obstruction, bronchodilator response	Isoproterenol	5 min
		Albuterol	15 min
		Ipratropium	45 min
Methacholine challenge	Suspect asthma but normal baseline spirometry	0.1–25 mg/mL methacholine	1 min after each dose
Exercise	Suspect exercise-induced bronchospasm	6–10 min of exercise	6 and 20 min after exercise
Therapeutic intervention	Evaluate effectiveness of chronic therapy	Steroids and bronchodilators	6–8 wk
Work shift	Suspect occupationally induced asthma	Dusts, chemicals	8-hr work shift
Trend analysis	Evaluate effects of chronic exposures	Time	Annually × 5 yr

AARC Clinical Practice Guideline

BRONCHIAL PROVOCATION

Indications: The need to diagnose or to confirm a diagnosis of airway hyperreactivity (asthma), the need to follow changes in hyperresponsiveness, the need to document the severity of hyperresponsiveness, the need to determine who is at risk in the military or workplace, the need to establish a control or baseline before a series of environmental or occupational exposures.

Contraindications: Relative contraindications are existence of ventilatory impairment at the time of the proposed challenge, $FEV_1 \leq 80\%$ of previously recorded best value, $FEV_1/FVC\% \leq 70\%$, $SGaw < 0.09\ s^{-1} \cdot cmH_2O^{-1}$, $FEV_1 \leq 1.0$ L in adults, significant response to the diluent (>10% fall in FEV_1 from baseline), upper- or lower-respiratory-tract infection within previous 6 weeks, specific antigen exposure within previous 1 week, exposure to high atmospheric pollution levels within previous 1 week, pregnancy (the effect on the fetus is unknown), subject's inability to perform acceptable spirometry at baseline or during postdiluent measurements (eg, variability in $FEV_1 > \pm 5\%$), failure to withhold medications that may affect the bronchial reactivity test. Recommended periods for withholding medications are β_2-adrenergic aerosols—12 hours, anticholinergic aerosols—12 hours, disodium cromoglycate—8 hours, oral β_2-adrenergic agonists—12 hours, theophyllines—48 hours, H_1-receptor antagonists—48 hours, antihistamines—72 to 96 hours. Corticosteroids, inhaled or oral, have been shown to decrease hyperresponsiveness, duration of effect is unknown but may be prolonged. Beta blockers may increase response, but duration of effect is unknown. Other factors that may confound results include ingestion of cola drinks, chocolate, and other agents containing caffeine or theobromines; smoking; occupational exposure to antigens.

Assessment of Need: Need is established by documenting in a subject the presence of one or more of the listed indications.

Assessment of Test Quality: Factors that affect the size of the dose received and thus the response and its interpretation include nebulizer output, particle size, inspiratory flow rate, lung volume at beginning of inspiration, and breath-hold time. These factors must be held constant across the testing procedure and from one test to another. Excessive variability in measured values including a nonreproducible baseline (FEV_1 variation of more than 5% after repeated efforts) makes test results unacceptable.

Monitoring: The FEV_1 is the primary variable to be monitored, and the results of spirometry should meet all recommendations proposed by the American Thoracic Society, with reproducibility of FEV_1 and FVC within ±5% for each set of maneuvers associated with a given dose. The test should be administered according to the specific protocol, with the number of breaths and the breathing pattern documented. Periodic auscultation, pulse rate, or blood pressure may be monitored to assist in patient evaluation and test interpretation. In the case of a positive response to provocation (ie, >20% fall in FEV_1), bronchodilator may be administered to speed recovery. Spirometry should be repeated after bronchodilator administration to ensure that ventilatory function has returned to near baseline.

From AARC Clinical Practice Guideline; see Respir Care 37:902, 1992, for complete text.

Quality Assurance

Optimal accuracy is needed for comparison studies because 10% or 0.2-L changes in the FEV_1 are often considered significant. Repeat tests should be performed by the same technician with the same spirometer, and calibration must be done daily. Maximal efforts should be confirmed by watching for maximal inhalations and by obtaining reproducibly high PEFs; otherwise, apparent changes in the FEV_1 could be caused by only a difference in effort.

Calculations

The percentage change in FEV_1 should be calculated compared with the baseline value. Because measurement errors of up to 0.2 L are common, the absolute change in liters should be calculated when severe obstruction was present at baseline. For instance, an increase from 1.00 L to 1.15 L is a +15% change, but the 0.15-L improvement could have been caused by measurement errors. Normal subjects improve their FEV_1 by up to 9% following a bronchodilator. Normal subjects can be given five breaths of 25 mg/mL methacholine with less than a 20% decrease in their FEV_1.

The normal annual change in FEV_1 caused by aging alone is about −30 mL/yr after age 30, whereas cigarette smokers developing COPD have an accelerated decline of −60 to −120 mL/yr.[2] At least five annual measurements of the FEV_1 are usually necessary before an individual's rate of decline can be accurately estimated. Trend analysis involves calculating the slope of the regression line of these annual FEV_1 measurements over time (Fig. 8-6).

Interpretation

When baseline spirometry shows airways obstruction, both an acute increase in FEV_1 or FVC of 12% and an absolute increase of 0.2 L after a bronchodilator inhalation is considered a significant response, indicating "reversible" airways obstruction.[1,12,16] This suggests the presence of asthma, although a response may sometimes also be seen in patients with COPD. Lack of an acute response, however, does not rule out benefit from long-term therapy with bronchodilators or steroids.

For methacholine challenge tests, a positive response is a 20% or greater reduction in the FEV_1 following inhalation of 8 mg/mL or less of methacholine (Fig. 8-7).[17] A 20% or greater reduction in the FEV_1 at concentrations between 8 and 10 mg/mL is considered borderline, and above 16 mg/mL is considered negative. A positive response is evidence of "airways hyperreactivity." Almost all asthmatics have a positive response if their bronchodilator and antihistamine medications are withheld; however, a few persons without any asthma-like symptoms also have a positive response.

A 15% or greater fall in the FEV_1 at 6 and 20 minutes after exercise is considered positive for EIB and is seen in most patients with asthma.[18] However, a negative response does not rule out asthma.

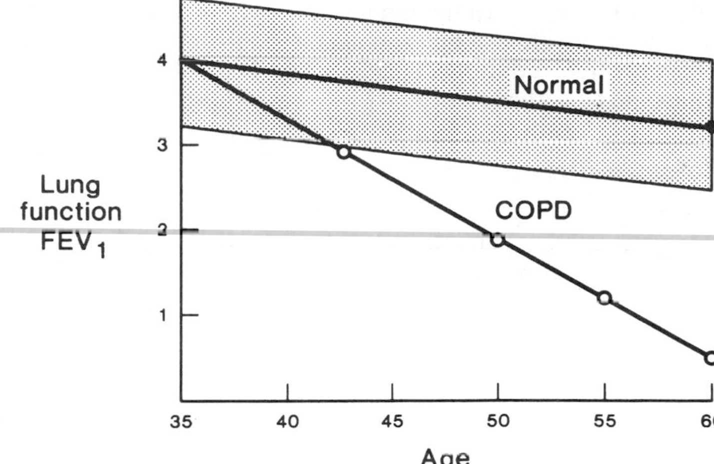

FIGURE 8-6. Trend analysis of annual changes in pulmonary function. The normal rate of FEV_1 decline for adults is 30 mL/y. Smokers developing COPD have declines greater than 60 mL/y. Smoking cessation can alleviate this abnormal rate of decline. (© Mayo Foundation)

A reproducible 15% reduction in the FEV_1 after an 8-hour work shift indicates work-induced bronchospasm, according to cotton dust standards. For long-term trend analysis in adults, a greater than 60 mL/yr decrease in the FEV_1 is considered an abnormal rate of decline (significantly greater than the 30 mL/yr expected from aging alone).

FORCED INSPIRATORY FLOWS

Indications

The *forced inspiratory vital capacity* (FIVC) test is indicated whenever an upper airway obstruction is suspected, especially in patients with inspiratory stridor (Table 8-5). The FIVC test is not useful for routine outpatient screening.

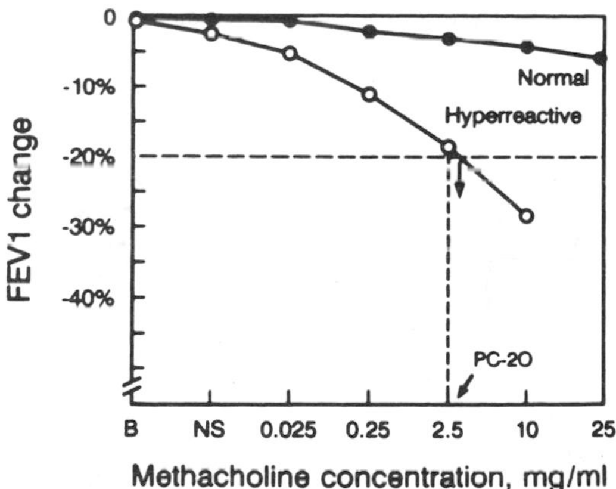

FIGURE 8-7. Methacholine challenge results. The patient inhales increasing concentrations of nebulized methacholine with the FEV_1 measured after each dose. The FEV_1 of normal subjects will not drop 20% even after the highest concentration. The FEV_1 of patients with airways hyperreactivity (and of all patients with asthma) will drop by 20% or more, indicating a positive response at concentrations of 8 mg/ml or less. The test may be summarized by the PC-20, the concentration that causes a 20% fall in the FEV_1 (about 2.5 mg/mL in this example from a patient with moderate asthma). (© Mayo Foundation)

Equipment

The FIVC can be performed on spirometers that allow forced inhalation maneuvers to be graphed on a flow-volume curve. Volume spirometers that return to zero volume automatically (using gravity or a spring) cannot be used. A volume-time spirogram is not adequate for judging the degree of effort or for interpreting the results.

Procedure

Forced inspiratory maneuvers are started by a slow complete exhalation followed by a maximally rapid deep inhalation. The common practice of performing FIVC maneuvers immediately after FVC maneuvers should be avoided, as the subject may not exhale completely because of air trapping, and the best FIVC maneuver often does not follow the best FVC maneuver. The FIVC results are very dependent on effort, much more so than FVC results. It is useful to almost scare the patient into inhaling quickly by coaching loudly. At least three reproducible maximal maneuvers should be obtained.

Quality Accurance

The FIVC maneuver graphs should be displayed superimposed at the onset of inhalation and checked for reproducibility. The inspiratory volumes should match within 5%, and the peak inspiratory flows should match

TABLE 8-5 **Indications for FIVC Test**

Suspected upper airways obstruction
Stridor (noise on forced inspiration)
Hoarseness
Recent general anesthesia, then dyspnea
Neck surgery
Neck masses
Normal spirometry but low MVV

within 10%. The spirometer's inspiratory flow calibration should be checked by simulating inhalation with a 3.00-L syringe at different speeds. The FIVCs obtained should all be within 3% of 3.00 L.

Calculations

The shape of the FIVC curves is most important. Although some instruments measure parameters from the FIVC, there are no good predicted values available. The inhaled volume and peak inspiratory flows should be used primarily for quality assurance to check for maximal and reproducible efforts.

Interpretation

A reproducible plateau of forced inspiratory flow may indicate an upper airway obstruction (UAO) (Fig. 8-8)[19] If a similar plateau exists during exhalation, the obstruction is *fixed* (as in tracheal stenosis), but if there is a sharp peak flow during exhalation, the obstruction is *variable* and extrathoracic (as in vocal cord paralysis). False-positive results occur frequently because of submaximal efforts. A plateau during forced exhalation with maintenance of peak flow during forced inhalation is indicative of a *variable* intrathoracic obstruction. Confirmation of a UAO is necessary, with tracheal radiographs, computed tomography scans, or direct visualization.

MAXIMAL RESPIRATORY PRESSURES

Indications

Measurement of *maximal inspiratory pressure* (MIP) and *maximal expiratory pressure* (MEP) is indicated when respiratory muscle weakness is suspected clinically or to follow-up on patients with neuromuscular diseases that may involve the diaphragm. These pressures may be markedly decreased in the presence of normal lung volumes and blood gas levels. Maximal respiratory pressures are also useful as an index of a patient's ability to be weaned from mechanical ventilation.

Equipment

Maximal respiratory pressures are measured using simple mechanical or electronic pressure gauges (0 to 100 cmH_2O for MIP and 0 to 300 cmH_20 for MEP). A large rubber mouthpiece must be pressed *against* the lips for MEP maneuvers. A 1-mm diameter leak is introduced intentionally to reduce the effect of the patient generating pressure with his or her cheeks. A tracheostomy tube fitting with the breathing hole plugged during measurements is used for intubated patients.

Procedure

The maximal inspiratory pressure maneuver starts by complete exhalation, then a maximal attempt to inhale from the pressure gauge, sustained for 2 seconds (like trying to suck up a thick milkshake through a narrow straw). At least two reproducible maneuvers should be obtained and the best reported. Maximal expiratory pressure starts with complete inhalation, followed by a maximal attempt at exhalation (like trying to blow up a small balloon). Always make a note of the patient's apparent degree of effort.

Quality Assurance

Maximal respiratory pressures are very effort dependent. False-positive results often occur because of poor coaching or malingering. The pressure gauges should

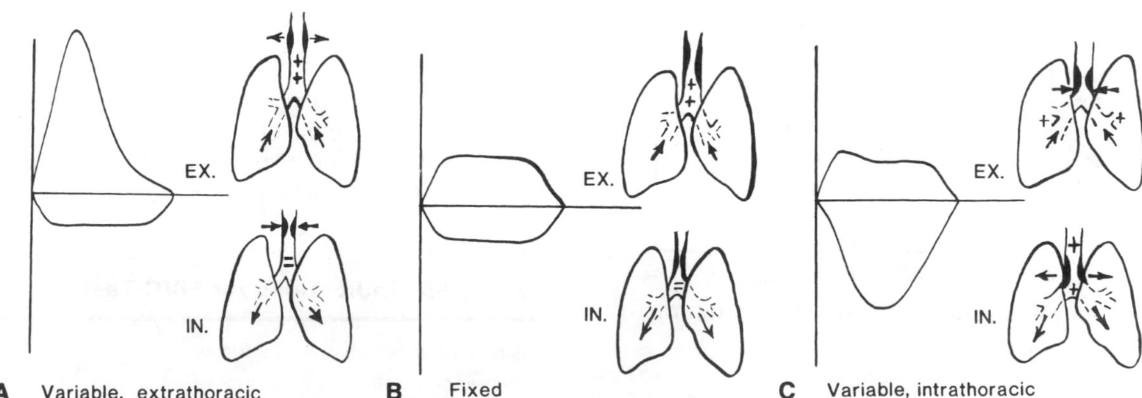

FIGURE 8-8. Flow–volume loop patterns caused by three types of upper airways obstruction (UAO). **(A)** A variable, extrathoracic UAO is commonly due to vocal cord paralysis. The vocal cords are forced wider during forced exhalation but narrow during forced inhalation (because of negative pressure in the airway), creating an inspiratory plateau. **(B)** A fixed UAO, such as tracheal stenosis, is unaffected by pressure differences across the airway, resulting in limited flow (a plateau) during both forced exhalation and inhalation. **(C)** Less commonly, a variable, intrathoracic UAO, such as a tumor near the carina, opens during forced inhalation, but narrows during forced exhalation, limiting expiratory flow. (© Mayo Foundation)

be calibrated regularly with a mercury manometer (blood pressure type) before use. Five percent accuracy at 100 cmH_2O is acceptable. A large, firm rubber mouthpiece is necessary for MEP measurements to allow a firm seal against the lips; otherwise, MEP is underestimated. The pressures should be sustained for 1 second because short peaks may be caused by only cheek muscles being used.

Calculations

The average normal MIP for adults is about 100 cmH_2O for men and 70 cmH_2O for women. The average normal MEP for adults is about 200 cmH_2O for men and 140 cmH_2O for women. The lower limit of the normal range is about 65% of the predicted value.[20]

Interpretation

Reduction of MIP indicates diaphragm (inspiratory muscle) weakness, whereas a reduced MEP indicates expiratory muscle weakness. Respiratory pressures may be reduced by generalized weakness, malnutrition, unilateral diaphragm paralysis, myasthenia gravis, amyotrophic lateral sclerosis (ALS), muscular dystrophy, hypothyroidism, and steroid myopathy.

MAXIMAL VOLUNTARY VENTILATION

Indications

The *maximal voluntary ventilation* (MVV) maneuver has traditionally been used for preoperative testing and disability determinations, but it is losing favor because of its lack of specificity. Patients who are debilitated or who have heart disease should probably not have MVV tested. The MVV is not a screening test, because it is insensitive to both obstructive and restrictive pulmonary diseases; however, the MVV is useful when performed before exercise testing so that it may be compared with the exercise ventilation. Avoid performing MVV maneuvers on patients known to have asthma because it may provoke bronchoconstriction.

Equipment

The MVV tests can be performed on many but not all spirometers. A 15-second volume-time graph is necessary. Volume spirometers are preferred because their large dead-space volume tends to prevent hypocarbia during the rebreathing maneuver.

Procedure

The MVV maneuver simulates breathing during strenuous exercise, but it only lasts for 15 seconds. Rapid, deep breaths usually give the best results (Fig. 8-9). Vigorous coaching is necessary throughout the maneuver. Several minutes of rest are necessary to avoid fatigue and hyperventilation before the maneuver is repeated.

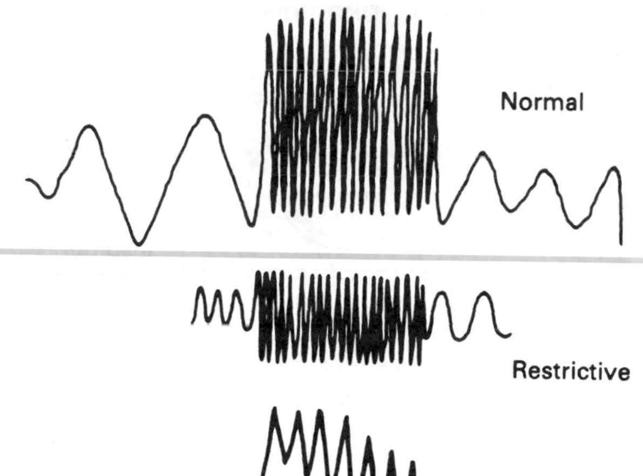

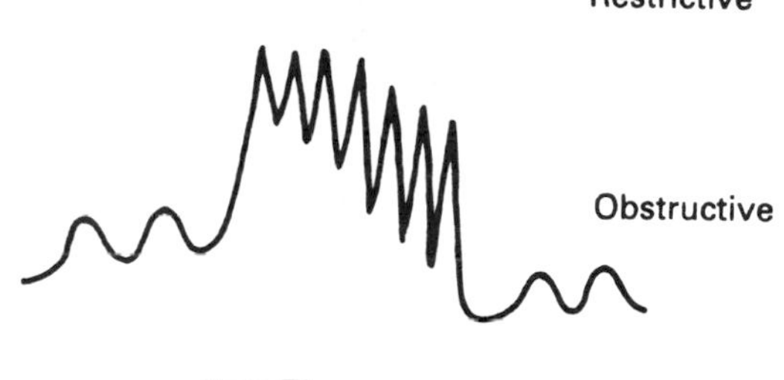

FIGURE 8-9. Maximal voluntary ventilation (MVV) maneuver tracings. The patient breathes rapidly in and out of a spirometer for 15 seconds. Note the lower tidal volumes produced by the patient with a restrictive disorder and the slower breathing rate, with increasing lung volume, produced by the patient with airways obstruction. The MVV is an estimate of the maximal ventilation that could be achieved in 1 minute. The normal MVV for an adult male is about 150 L/min.

Quality Assurance

The MVV is very effort dependent. The MVV maneuvers must last for at least 10 seconds to avoid overestimation of the MVV. The breathing pattern should be relatively regular.

Calculations

The MVV is calculated by multiplying the accumulated exhalation volume during 12 seconds by 5. The respiratory rate should also be reported. The predicted MVV can be quickly estimated by multiplying the predicted FEV_1 value by 40. Because of its wide variability, the lower limit of the normal range is about 65% of the predicted value.

Interpretation

A reduction of the MVV is nonspecific—it may be caused by upper or lower airways obstruction, restriction, muscle weakness, or poor effort.

LUNG VOLUMES

Indications

Traditionally, four lung volumes have been recognized. Combining these volumes results in four *capacities* (Fig. 8-10). Those that cannot be measured with only a spirometer are the *total lung capacity* (TLC), *residual vol-*

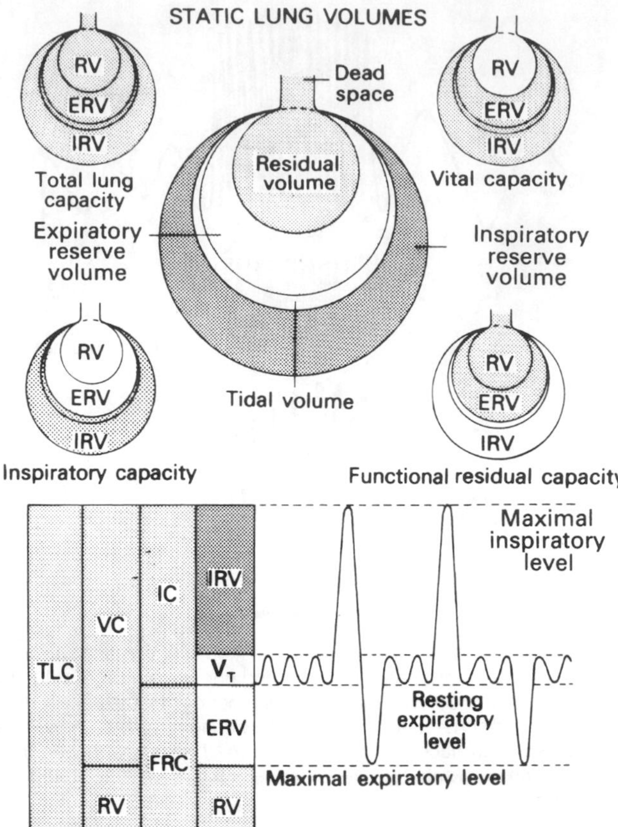

FIGURE 8-10. Division of total lung capacity into lung volumes and lung capacities. In the small diagrams surrounding the large central one, the shaded areas outline the volumes that constitute the various lung capacities. (Adapted from Comroe JH Jr et al: The Lung: Clinical Physiology and Pulmonary Function Tests, 2nd ed. Chicago, Year Book Medical Publishers, 1962)

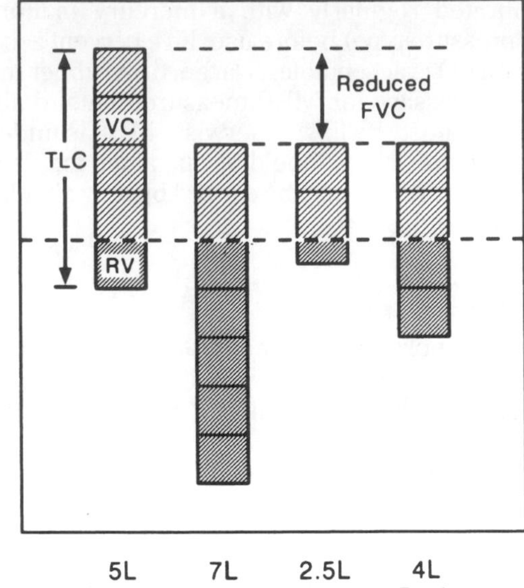

FIGURE 8-11. Spirometry measures only the vital capacity (VC, above the dashed line). The residual volume (RV) and, therefore, the total lung capacity (TLC) are absolute lung volumes, usually measured with a body box or inert gas technique. For comparison, the first patient in this example has normal lung volumes, but the latter three patients all have a VC of only half normal. Knowledge of their absolute lung volumes allows a diagnosis of COPD when the TLC is increased (hyperinflation), restriction when the TLC and RV are reduced, and a mixed pattern when the TLC is reduced but the RV is enlarged. (© Mayo Foundation)

ume (RV), and *functional residual capacity* (FRC). Measurement of these absolute lung volumes may be useful when the vital capacity is reduced. Because the FVC maneuver often causes airways to collapse in patients with obstruction, when reduction of the FVC is noted, the *slow vital capacity* (SVC) should also be measured. If the SVC is normal, a coexisting restrictive pattern is ruled out; if the SVC is also reduced, absolute lung volumes may be measured to evaluate for a coexisting restriction of lung volumes (Fig. 8-11). (See also AARC Clinical Practice Guideline: Static Lung Volumes.)

Equipment

Four methods are available for determining absolute lung volumes (Table 8-6). Equipment costs range from $300 for a simple planimeter to $40,000 for an automated body plethysmograph (body box) system. (See Ref. 21 for a good description of methods of measuring lung volumes.)

Body boxes are of three types: variable pressure, variable volume, and flow. Variable-pressure boxes are used more commonly because they are easier to keep accurately calibrated. The body box method is faster than the other methods, and gives accurate measurements in the presence of obstructive airway disease. A minor drawback is that some patients are claustrophobic in a box.

Procedures and Calculations

□ BODY BOX PROCEDURE

See AARC Clinical Practice Guideline: Body Plethysmography for details regarding the body box procedure.

The patient sits quietly breathing through a pneumotachometer inside the box (Fig. 8-12). At the end-tidal position (FRC), a shutter is occluded in the breathing tube. The patient continues momentarily to try to breathe against this obstruction, and the changes in mouth pressure and box pressure are measured. The shutter is then opened and the patient is asked to inhale completely (to TLC) through the pneumotach, as inspiratory capacity (IC) is measured by integrating the pneumotach flow.

□ BODY BOX CALCULATIONS

The principle of measurement of thoracic gas volume in the body plethysmograph is based on Boyle's law:

$$P_1V_1 = P_2V_2$$

The starting alveolar pressure, P_1, new alveolar pressure, P_2, and change in alveolar volume, V_2, are measured when the shutter is closed. From these data, the starting volume, V_1, is calculated. The volume measured when the shutter is closed is the FRC (also called the

AARC Clinical Practice Guideline

STATIC LUNG VOLUMES

Indications: Indications include but are not limited to the need to differentiate between obstructive and restrictive disease patterns; to assess response to therapeutic interventions (eg, drugs, transplantation, radiation, chemotherapy, lobectomy); to aid in the interpretation of other lung function tests; to make preoperative assessments in patients with compromised lung function when a surgical procedure is known to affect lung function; to evaluate pulmonary disability; to quantify the amount of nonventilated lung.

Contraindications: No apparent absolute contraindications exist. The relative contraindications for spirometry include the following: hemoptysis of unknown origin, untreated pneumothorax, unstable cardiovascular status, thoracic and abdominal or cerebral aneurysms. With respect to whole-body plethysmography, such factors as claustrophobia, upper body paralysis, obtrusive body casts, or other conditions that immobilize or prevent the patient from fitting into or gaining access to the body box are a concern. In addition, the procedure may necessitate stopping intravenous therapy or supplemental oxygen.

Assessment of Need: Determination that valid indications are present.

Assessment of Outcome and Test Quality: Outcome and test quality are determined by ascertaining that the desired information has been generated for the specific indication and that validity and reproducibility have been assured. Results are valid if the equipment functions acceptably and the subject is able to perform the maneuvers in an acceptable and reproducible fashion. Report of test results should contain a statement by the technician performing the test about test quality (including patient understanding of directions and effort expended) and, if appropriate, which recommendations were not met.

Monitoring: The following should be monitored during lung-volume determinations: test data of repeated efforts (ie, reproducibility of results) to ascertain the validity of results. The patient should be monitored for any adverse effects of testing; patients on supplemental oxygen may require periods of time to rest on oxygen between trials.

From AARC Clinical Practice Guideline; see Respir Care 39:830, 1994, for complete text.

TABLE 8-6 **Methods of Measuring Absolute Lung Volumes**

Method	Accuracy	Cost ($)	Time (min)	Sensors
Body box	++++	40,000	5	Pressure transducers
Helium dilution	++	20,000	20	Helium analyzer
Nitrogen washout	++	20,000	20	Nitrogen analyzer
CXR planimetry	+++	300	10	Planimeter

AARC Clinical Practice Guideline

BODY PLETHYSMOGRAPHY

Indications: Body plethysmographic determination of thoracic gas volume (Vtg), airways resistance (Raw), and airways conductance (SGaw) may be indicated for measurement of lung volumes to distinguish between restrictive and obstructive processes; for evaluation of obstructive lung diseases, such as bullous emphysema and cystic fibrosis, which may produce artifactually low results if measured by helium dilution or N_2 washout (an index of trapped gas [ie, $FRC_{plethysmograph}/FRC_{He\ dilution}$] can be established); for measurement of lung volumes when multiple repeated trials are required, or when the subject is unable to perform multibreath tests; for evaluation of resistance to airflow; for determination of the response to bronchodilators (Raw, SGaw, and Vtg); for determination of bronchial hyperreactivity in response to methacholine, histamine, or isocapnic hyperventilation (Vtg, Raw, and SGaw); for following the course of disease and response to treatment.

Contraindications: Relative contraindications to body plethysmography are mental confusion, muscular incoordination, body casts, or other conditions that prevent the patient from entering the plethysmograph cabinet or adequately performing the required maneuvers (ie, panting against a closed shutter); claustrophobia that may be aggravated by entering the plethysmograph cabinet; presence of devices or other conditions, such as continuous IV infusions with pumps or other equipment that do not fit into the plethysmograph, that should not be discontinued, or that might interfere with pressure changes (eg, chest tube, transtracheal O_2 catheter, or ruptured eardrum); continuous oxygen therapy that should not be temporarily discontinued.

Assessment of Test Quality: Each laboratory should standardize procedures and demonstrate intertechnician reliability. Test results can only be considered valid if they are derived according to and conform to established laboratory control and quality assurance protocols. These protocols should address test standardization and reproducibility criteria that include the methodology used to derive and report Vtg and airways mechanics. Results are valid if the equipment functions acceptably and the subject is able to perform the maneuvers in an acceptable and reproducible fashion. Vtg maneuvers may be considered acceptable when the displayed or recorded tracing indicates proper panting technique; the P_{mouth}/P_{box} loop (closed shutter) should be closed or nearly so. The patient should support his or her cheeks with the hands to prevent pressure changes induced by the mouth. This should be done without supporting the elbows or elevating the shoulders. Recorded pressure changes should be within the calibrated pressure range of each transducer. The entire tracing should be visible. Pressure changes that are too large or too small may yield erroneous results. There should be evidence of thermal equilibrium; tracings should not drift on the display or recording. The panting frequency should be approximately 1 Hz. Nonpanting maneuvers may be acceptable if the plethysmograph system is specifically designed to perform such a maneuver. The reported Vtg should be averaged from a minimum of three to five separate, acceptable panting maneuvers; should be calculated using tangents or angles that agree within 10% of the mean; should be averaged when tangents or angles vary widely and reported as variable; should indicate whether the thoracic volume was at FRC or at another level; should be compared with other lung volume determinations (He dilution, N_2 washout) if performed; should be corrected for patient weight for some systems. A slow vital capacity (VC) maneuver and its subdivisions, inspiratory capacity (IC) and expiratory reserve volume (ERV), should be performed during the same testing session. The ERV, IC, and inspiratory vital capacity (IVC) can be measured before disconnecting the patient from the measuring system. Alternatively, the patient can be disconnected and the ERV, IC, and IVC performed immediately afterward. The largest VC obtained should be used for calculation of derived lung volumes (ie, total lung capacity (TLC); residual volume, or RV; and RV/TLC%). The IC and ERV from the largest acceptable VC should be used to calculate derived volumes. TLC may be calculated from the FRC determined plethysmographically: TLC = FRC + IC or TLC = RV + VC. RV may be calculated from the FRC determined plethysmographically: RV = FRC − ERV, or RV = TLC − VC. Raw and SGaw maneuvers may be considered acceptable if they meet the criteria above. The open shutter panting maneuver should show a relatively closed loop, particularly in the range of +0.5 to −0.5 L/sec. The panting frequency during serial measurements in a given patient should be kept the same to aid interpretation (1.5–3.0 Hz). The reported Raw and SGaw should be calculated from the ratio of closed and open shutter tangents for each maneuver. Airway resistance and lung volume are interdependent in a nonlinear fashion; should be averaged from three to five separate, acceptable maneuvers; should be calculated from maneuvers with a reproducibility within 10%; should have the open shutter tangent (V/P_{box}) measured between flows of +0.5 and −0.5 L/sec. For loops that display hysteresis, the inspiratory limbs may be used; the SGaw should be calculated using the Vtg at which the shutter was closed for each individual maneuver. Report of test results should contain a statement, by the technician performing the test, about test quality and, if appropriate, which recommendations were not met.

Monitoring: The final report should contain a statement regarding test quality. The final report should contain the Vtg, Raw, and SGaw, if performed. If the Vtg is measured at a lung volume other than FRC, both values should be reported. If the FRC is measured by more than one method, the report should indicate how lung volumes are reported.

From AARC Clinical Practice Guideline; see Respir Care 39:1184, 1994, for complete text.

thoracic gas volume, VTG) and is added to the IC measured when the shutter opens to obtain the TLC.

□ HELIUM DILUTION PROCEDURE

The study starts with about 10% helium in a bag-spirometer system (Fig. 8-13). Helium is used because it is relatively inert and does not leave the alveoli to dissolve in lung tissue or blood. The starting concentration of helium in the lungs is zero. The patient is switched from breathing room air to breathing into the bag-

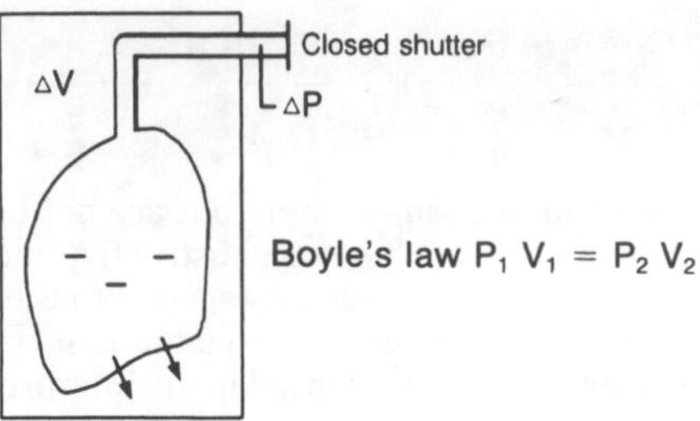

FIGURE 8-12. Body plethysmography. The patient sits in a box and attempts to inhale when the shutter closes. The change in pressure at the mouth (ΔP) and change in the box volume (ΔV) are measured with electronic transducers. The air in the thorax when the shutter was closed is calculated from Boyle's law. (© Mayo Foundation)

spirometer system at the end-tidal position (FRC). He or she then rebreathes the helium mixture from the bag-spirometer system until equilibration between the lungs and bag-spirometer system is reached.

□ HELIUM DILUTION CALCULATION

By knowing the new concentration of helium in the system, F_E, along with the starting volume of gas, V_S, and helium fraction in the equilibrated bag-spirometer system, F_S, the starting lung volume, FRC, can be readily calculated:

$$VFRC = V_S(F_S - F_E)/F_E$$

□ NITROGEN WASHOUT PROCEDURE

The patient begins to breathe 100% oxygen at the end-tidal position (FRC). The concentration of nitrogen is measured at the mouth (Fig. 8-14). The gas in the lungs at the start of the test contains about 80% nitrogen. As the patient breathes 100% oxygen, the nitrogen is washed out of the lungs.

□ NITROGEN WASHOUT CALCULATION

By measuring the volume of gas exhaled during the study and the fraction of nitrogen in this gas, the volume

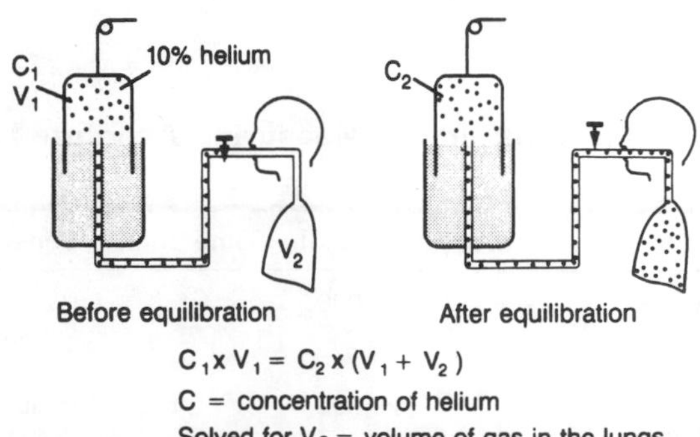

FIGURE 8-13. Helium dilution method. The patient begins to breathe air from a spirometer containing 10% helium. The helium is diluted by the air in the patient's lungs but is not absorbed by the body. The helium concentration of the system is monitored until it stops changing (equilibration). (© Mayo Foundation)

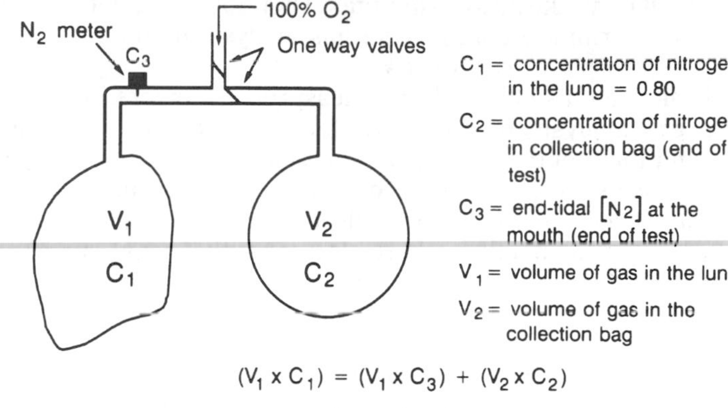

FIGURE 8-14. Nitrogen washout. The patient begins to inhale 100% oxygen with each breath, thereby washing out all of the nitrogen in the lungs. All of the exhaled nitrogen is collected and measured. (© Mayo Foundation)

of nitrogen in the lungs at the start of the test can easily be calculated. Because this represents approximately 80% of the gas, FRC can be calculated. A minor correction is made for the small amount of nitrogen present in the "100%" oxygen that passes from the blood and lung tissue into the alveoli during the washout study.

☐ CHEST X-RAY PLANIMETRY

A good estimate of the TLC can be easily obtained from a standard posteroanterior and lateral chest x-ray (CXR) film taken at full inhalation. One technique involves making 28 measurements with a ruler, and the other uses a drafting instrument called a planimeter. The separate outlines of the right and left lungs are traced on the posteroanterior view, and then the area of both lungs is traced on the lateral view with the planimeter, which measures the enclosed areas (Fig. 8-15). The three areas are then used in a simple, empirically determined equation to estimate the TLC. The results are usually within 5% of the body box technique in both children and adults.

Quality Assurance

The major disadvantage of the gas analysis methods for determining lung volumes is that some alveolar gas is usually trapped in the lungs of patients with moderate-to-severe obstructive airway diseases; therefore, all of the nitrogen does not wash out during the short time that the test is performed, or the alveolar gas does not reach true equilibration for helium. The standard length of time for the nitrogen washout test is 7 minutes; however, in patients with COPD, complete

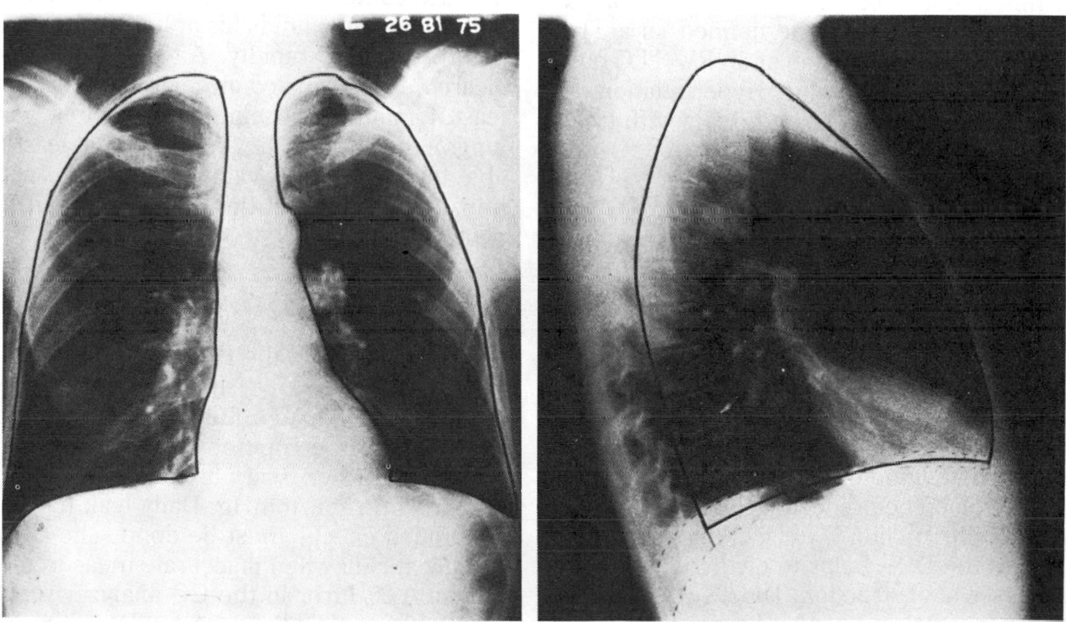

FIGURE 8-15. Determination of total lung capacity (TLC) by chest radiograph planimetry. The areas outlined in the PA and lateral chest films are measured with an inexpensive planimeter, and simple calculations are made to determine the TLC. (Harris TR, Pratt PC, Kilburn KH: Total Lung Capacity Measured by Roentgenograms. Am J Med 1971; 50:756)

washout may take 20 to 30 minutes. Therefore, lung volumes determined using these gas analysis methods may be gross underestimates.

Leaks can also cause large measurement errors in the gas analysis methods. Leaks commonly occur around the mouthpiece, through cracks in the tubing, and because of punctured eardrums. The vacuum pumps used by nitrogen analyzers can lose their efficiency, the needle valves clog, and the sensors get dirty. These problems can be detected by daily calibrations using at least two known concentrations of test gas.

The body box pressure transducers are very sensitive to temperature changes and overpressure. A small, 30-mL sine wave pump should be used at least daily to calibrate the box pressure, and a water manometer should be used to calibrate the mouth pressure to within 5% accuracy. A 1.00- or 3.00-L syringe emptied at several rates should calibrate the pneumotachometer to within 3% accuracy.

Interpretation

Normal adults' TLC should not decline as they grow older, but their RV slowly increases, resulting in a gradual decline in their vital capacity. The lower limit of the normal range for the TLC is about 80% of the mean predicted value—a decrease in TLC below this indicates a restrictive process. A restrictive process usually reduces all lung volumes proportionately. (Refer back to Table 8-3 for a list of causes of restriction.) Prediction equations for lung volumes are available.[12]

Even mild degrees of airways obstruction often cause the RV to increase. As obstruction worsens, the TLC increases, eventually seen as hyperinflation on the chest x-ray film and as a barrel chest on physical examination. Hyperinflation may be defined as a TLC above 140% of the predicted value, or an RV/TLC ratio above 140% of the predicted value. Hyperinflation occurs both with asthma (decreasing rapidly with treatment) and emphysema.

DIFFUSING CAPACITY

Indications

Diffusing capacity measured with carbon monoxide (DL_{CO}), also called *transfer factor* in Europe, determines the ability of gases to cross the alveolar-capillary membrane. Carbon monoxide (CO) is used because of its great affinity for hemoglobin and its normally low concentration in the blood before testing.

When airways obstruction is present on spirometry, measurement of the DL_{CO} helps to distinguish among the various causes of obstruction. The DL_{CO} is reduced in emphysema, normal in simple chronic bronchitis, and normal or increased in asthma.

When spirometry and lung volumes show restriction, DL_{CO} measurement helps to distinguish between chest wall and interstitial disease. The diffusing capacity test is probably the most sensitive indicator of early interstitial lung disease (such as the *Pneumocystis* pneumonia seen in patients with AIDS) and vasculitis, and it is also used to determine response to specific therapy. In patients with cancer, the DL_{CO} is sensitive for detecting lymphangitic spread of cancer to the lungs and lung fibrosis caused by radiation therapy and chemotherapy.

Equipment

The DL_{CO} measurement requires one of three types of carbon monoxide analyzers: infrared, fuel cell, or gas chromatograph. All three require that water vapor and carbon dioxide be removed first (Fig. 8-16). A thermal conductivity helium analyzer is usually used to simultaneously measure alveolar volume. Most laboratories have finally replaced "homemade," Rube Goldberg–like apparatus with an automated system that costs between $15,000 and $30,000 and also measures spirometry and lung volumes.

Procedure

The technique most widely used is the single-breath method (DL_{CO}-SB) (see AARC Clinical Practice Guideline: Single-Breath Carbon Monoxide Diffusing Capacity). The exact procedure has recently been standardized by the American Thoracic Society.[22] The patient should be asked to refrain from smoking for 24 hours before the test and should not eat or exercise for 1 hour before the test.

Explain the test and demonstrate the breathing maneuver. The patient must be seated wearing noseclips. Starting at RV, the patient rapidly inhales to TLC a gas mixture containing 0.3% carbon monoxide (CO) and 10% helium, then holds his or her breath for 10 seconds before exhaling rapidly. After 1 L of dead space is cleared, 1 L of exhaled alveolar gas is sampled. Wait at least 4 minutes (to eliminate the test gas from the lungs), then repeat the test. Obtain at least two acceptable tests with DL_{CO} values that match within 3 mL/min/mm Hg. Report the mean DL_{CO} and V_A of all acceptable tests.

Quality Assurance

Many factors affect the DL_{CO}, often causing differences in the reported DL_{CO} between laboratories testing the same individual. A fully automated system with recently updated computer software, as well as careful tech-nique, is necessary to obtain results reproducible within 3 mL/min/mmHg. Daily leak tests and volume calibration checks must be done. The CO analyzer is usually at fault when inaccurate measurements are obtained. A 2% error in the CO analyzer results in more than a 10% error in the reported DL_{CO}; therefore, the accuracy and linearity of the CO analyzer must be checked at least quarterly and found to be within 1%. The chemical absorbers frequently used to prevent carbon dioxide

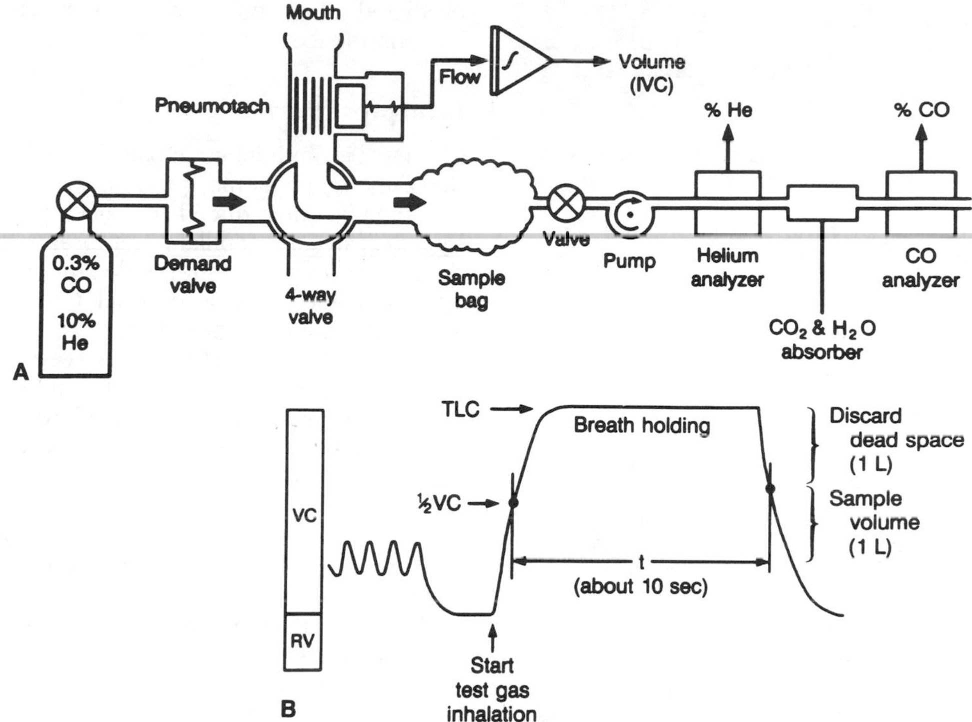

FIGURE 8-16. (A, B) Measurement of diffusing capacity. The patient inhales a full breath of a test gas containing 0.3% carbon monoxide (CO) and 10% helium. He holds the test gas in his lungs for 10 seconds. Some of the CO is taken up by his red blood cells and the helium is diluted. As he exhales, dead-space gas is discarded and the next liter of air (exhaled into the sample bag) is analyzed for CO and helium.

and water from entering the CO analyzer must also be checked daily.

A "biologic control" is also necessary to check D_{LCO} instruments. Test yourself or another nonsmoker without lung disease every week. After at least five measurements, determine the mean and standard deviation (SD) of the results. Thereafter, plot the results; if the current D_{LCO} is greater than 2 SD from the mean of the previous results, recheck the D_{LCO} system thoroughly, fix the problem, and repeat the test to validate the repair.

Individual D_{LCO} maneuvers are unacceptable (and should be discarded) if any of the following occurs:

- The volume of test gas inhaled is less than 90% of a previously measured slow vital capacity.
- Inspiratory time is more than 2.5 seconds.
- Breath-hold time is less than 9 seconds or more than 11 seconds.
- Washout volume is less than 500 mL.
- Sample size is less than 500 mL.
- Sample collection time is more than 3 seconds.

Calculations

Think of D_{LCO} as the uptake of carbon monoxide. It is reported in milliliters of CO that diffuse per minute across the alveolar-capillary membrane per millimeter of mercury pressure (mL/min/mmHg). The pressure is the difference in the partial pressure of CO between alveoli (the driving pressure) and the blood in pulmonary capillaries (the back pressure).

Some laboratories also report the ratio of D_{LCO}/V_A, where V_A is the alveolar volume at which D_{LCO} was measured. (This ratio is called Krogh's constant in Europe.) The V_A is equivalent to the TLC; because it is measured by the single-breath helium dilution method, however, the V_A measured in severely obstructed patients is somewhat lower than the TLC measured by other methods. The D_{LCO}/V_A tends to remain normal in restriction caused by chest wall disorders, in patients following the surgical removal of a significant amount of lung tissue, and in individuals with small lungs. A reduced D_{LCO}/V_A implies abnormality in function; however, a normal D_{LCO}/V_A should not be assumed to indicate that the lung tissue present is normal. For example, the D_{LCO}/V_A may be normal or reduced in people with a decreased TLC caused by significant interstitial lung disease.[23]

Because the uptake of CO also depends on the number of red cells in the blood, D_{LCO} decreases in people with anemia with no lung disease. For example, an anemic patient with a hemoglobin value of 7 g/dL and a measured D_{LCO} value of 20 mL/min/mmHg would have a D_{LCO} value of 30 mL/min/mmHg if he or she were transfused to reach a normal hemoglobin (Hb) of 15 g/dL. Consequently, if the patient's hemoglobin value is available, both the uncorrected D_{LCO} and Hb-

AARC Clinical Practice Guideline

SINGLE-BREATH CARBON MONOXIDE DIFFUSING CAPACITY

Indications: Tests of diffusing capacity may be indicated in evaluation and follow-up of parenchymal lung diseases associated with dusts (eg, asbestos) or drug reactions (eg, amiodarone) or related to sarcoidosis; evaluation and follow-up of emphysema and cystic fibrosis; differentiating among chronic bronchitis, emphysema, and asthma in patients with obstructive patterns; evaluation of pulmonary involvement in systemic diseases (eg, rheumatoid arthritis, systemic lupus erythematosus); evaluation of cardiovascular diseases (eg, primary pulmonary hypertension, pulmonary edema, acute or recurrent thromboembolism); prediction of arterial desaturation during exercise in chronic obstructive pulmonary disease; evaluation and quantification of disability associated with interstitial lung disease; evaluation of the effects of chemotherapy agents, or other drugs known to induce pulmonary dysfunction; evaluation of hemorrhagic disorders.

Contraindications: Relative contraindications to performing a diffusing capacity test are mental confusion or muscular incoordination preventing the subject from adequately performing the maneuver; a large meal or vigorous exercise immediately before the test; smoking within 24 hours of test administration. Smoking may have a direct effect on DL_{CO} independent of the effect of carboxyhemoglobin.

Assessment of Test Quality: Individual test maneuvers and results should be evaluated according to the ATS recommendations. In particular, the inspiratory volume should exceed 90% of the largest previously measured vital capacity. Breath-hold time should be between 9 and 11 seconds, with a rapid inspiration. The washout volume (dead space) should be 0.75 to 1.00 L, or 0.50 L if the subject's vital capacity is less than 2.0 L. If a washout volume other than 0.75 to 1.00 L is used, it should be noted. Two or more acceptable tests should be averaged; the maneuvers should be reproducible to within 10% or 3 mL $CO \cdot min^{-1} \cdot torr^{-1}$, whichever is greater. The subject should have refrained from smoking for 24 hours prior to the test. Correlation for Hb and COHb should be included. Correction for tests performed at altitude is recommended. If Hb correction is made, both the corrected and uncorrected DL_{CO} values should be reported.

Monitoring: The final report should contain a statement about test quality. The final report should contain the DL_{CO}, the corrected DL_{CO} (Hb, COHb, altitude), and the Hb value used for correction. The alveolar volume (VA) and DL/VA (ie, the ratio of diffusing capacity to the lung volume at which the measurement was made) may be included in the report.

From AARC Clinical Practice Guideline; see Respir Care 38:511, 1993, for complete text.

corrected DL_{CO} values are reported. The formula for adjusting the DL_{CO} for anemia is the following:[22]

$$DL_{CO}\text{ (Hb-corrected)} = (10.22 + Hb)\ DL_{CO}\text{ measured}/1.7\ Hb$$

The DL_{CO} normally declines with aging in adults. The lower limit of the normal range is about 80% of the mean predicted value, but it is more accurately defined by the 95% confidence interval.[12,24]

Interpretation

The DL_{CO} is diminished in patients with interstitial lung diseases, emphysema, pulmonary vascular diseases, and anemia. The reduced DL_{CO} of emphysema is caused by loss of alveolar-capillary membrane area (permanent destruction of lung tissue). A declining DL_{CO} in a patient with sarcoidosis or interstitial pneumonitis–fibrosis suggests a poor response to the therapy initiated (usually corticosteroids). The DL_{CO} is a very sensitive test for early interstitial lung disease. It is often reduced in pulmonary sarcoidosis, vasculitis, scleroderma, and *Pneumocystis* pneumonia, when the chest x-ray films, lung volumes, and resting arterial blood gas values are still within normal limits.

An increase in the DL_{CO} above 120% of the predicted value may occur in asthma (for unknown reasons), polycythemia (because of the increased number of red cells in the lungs), during or immediately following exercise, and in patients with left-to-right cardiovascular shunts.

EXERCISE TESTING

Indications

Cardiopulmonary exercise testing was previously confined to research laboratories, but it is now clinically useful for the following (see AARC Clinical Practice Guideline: Exercise Testing for Evaluation of Hypoxemia and Desaturation).

- To measure a person's ability to perform work (disability evaluation)
- To measure cardiovascular fitness for vigorous sports (maximal oxygen uptake)
- To help differentiate between cardiac and pulmonary causes of dyspnea
- To determine the need for and dose of ambulatory oxygen
- To assist in developing a safe exercise prescription for patients with cardiovascular or pulmonary disease
- For predicting the morbidity of lung resection

Contraindications include recent heart attack, severe hypertension, aortic stenosis, or worsening angina.

Equipment

The minimum equipment necessary includes a treadmill with 0 to 5 mph and 0% to 20% grade adjustments (or a calibrated bicycle ergometer), ECG monitor, and pulse oximeter. For noninvasive oxygen uptake measurement, add a low-resistance breathing valve, mixing chamber, pneumotachometer, and oxygen analyzer (Fig. 8-17). Complete breath-by-breath computerized systems add fast-responding O_2 and CO_2 gas analyzers and cost up to $60,000. Cardiac output may be estimated using a CO_2 rebreathing or acetylene method. Invasive studies may add radial artery cannulation for blood gas and lactate mea-

AARC Clinical Practice Guideline

EXERCISE TESTING FOR EVALUATION OF HYPOXEMIA OR DESATURATION

Indications: Exercise testing may be indicated to assess and quantify the adequacy of arterial oxyhemoglobin saturation during exercise in patients who are clinically suspected of desaturation (eg, dyspnea on exertion, decreased DL_{CO}, decreased PaO_2 at rest); to quantitate the response to therapeutic intervention (eg, oxygen prescription, medications, smoking cessation); to titrate the optimal amount of supplemental oxygen to treat hypoxemia or desaturation during activity; for preoperative assessment for lung resection or transplant; to assess the degree of impairment for disability evaluation (eg, pneumoconiosis, asbestosis).

Contraindications: Absolute contraindications include acute electrocardiographic changes of myocardial ischemia or serious cardiac dysrhythmias; unstable angina; recent myocardial infarction (within the previous 4 weeks) or myocarditis; aneurysm of the heart or aorta; uncontrolled systemic hypertension; acute thrombophlebitis or deep venous thrombosis; second- or third-degree heart block; recent systemic or pulmonary embolus; acute pericarditis. Relative contraindications include situations in which pulse oximetry may provide invalid data (eg, elevated HbCO); situations in which arterial puncture or arterial cannulation may be contraindicated; a noncompliant patient or one who is not capable of performing the test because of weakness, pain, fever, dyspnea, incoordination, or psychosis; severe pulmonary hypertension (cor pulmonale); known electrolyte disturbances (hypokalemia, hypomagnesemia); resting diastolic blood pressure $\geq$110 torr or resting systolic blood pressure $\geq$200 torr; neuromuscular, musculoskeletal, or rheumatoid disorders that are exacerbated by exercise; uncontrolled metabolic disease (eg, diabetes, thyrotoxicosis, or myxedema); SaO_2 or SpO_2 $\leq$85% with the subject breathing room air; untreated or unstable asthma.

Assessment of Need: Exercise testing for evaluation of hypoxemia or desaturation may be indicated for the following reasons: the presence of a history and physical indicators suggesting hypoxemia or desaturation, or both; the presence of abnormal diagnostic test results; the need to titrate or adjust a therapy (eg, supplemental oxygen).

Assessment of Test Quality: Arterial blood gases or SpO_2, or both, should confirm or rule out oxygen desaturation during exercise to validate the patient's clinical condition. Documentation of results, therapeutic intervention (or lack of), and clinical decisions based on the exercise testing should be placed in the patient's medical record. The exercise should have a symptom-limited or physiologic end point documented (eg, heart rate or onset of dyspnea).

Monitoring: Recommended monitoring equipment includes electrocardiograph with strip recorder, preferably with multiple leads; pulse oximeter (heart rate correlated with electrocardiograph if available); oxygen delivery devices with documented F_DO_2; treadmill or cycle ergometer calibrated according to the manufacturer's recommendations, with periodic reverification; blood gas sampling and analysis equipment. Recommended patient monitors during testing include physical assessment (chest pain, leg cramps, color, perceived exertion, dyspnea); respiratory rate; cooperation and effort level; Borg or modified Borg dyspnea scale; blood gas sampling; heart rate, rhythm, and ST-T wave changes; blood pressue.

From AARC Clinical Practice Guideline; see Respir Care 37:907, 1992, for complete text.

surements, or right heart catheterization with monitoring of PA and wedge pressures.

The technician should have CPR certification and a resuscitation cart with a defibrillator; oxygen must be in the room. A physician should be present for any individual with symptoms or signs of cardiac disease to monitor the ECG for signs of ischemia (ST segment depression) or malignant arrhythmias (which are more likely to occur during the recovery period). A 12-lead ECG system is best for detecting ischemia.

Procedure

Attach the ECG electrodes securely, calculate the predicted maximal heart rate (HR) for the patient (220 minus age), adjust the cycle seat height (for a cycle ergometer), then instruct the patient that maximum effort is required for a valid test. Monitor the HR, blood pressure (BP), oxygen saturation (SpO_2), and ventilation ($\dot{V}e$) during an initial 3- to 5-minute resting period. Start the workload at a level judged to be easy for the patient (1.7 mph at 0 grade or 50 watts), and then increase it at 1- to 3-minute intervals, measuring HR, BP, SpO_2, and $\dot{V}_E$ at the end of each interval. Automated systems are available that gradually increase the workload, referred to as a *ramp protocol*, so that there are no sudden jumps in work intensity. Return the workload back to the lightest level for a cool-down period only when the patient is exhausted, has chest pain suggesting angina, or develops serious arrhythmias. Record the symptoms that limited further exercise and continue monitoring for 5 minutes.

Quality Assurance

Before each test, check the pneumotachometer for 3% accuracy at high- and low-flow rates using a 3.00-L syringe. Gas analyzers must also be calibrated to within 0.1% accuracy before each test, using at least two calibrated reference gases. The delay times of gas analyzer outputs in breath-by-breath computerized systems can be a major source of error and should be remeasured periodically and whenever tubing changes are made.

Perform a biologic control by testing a laboratory technician each week or month, depending on test volume. Collect exhaled gas in large Douglas bags during 1-minute intervals at high and low work loads. The volume and gas concentrations in the bags must then be checked with a large-volume spirometer (Tissot) and mass spectrometer or gas chromatograph, respectively, and compared with results from the pneumotachometer and gas analyzers. Keep a log of the results at each work load—the variability in one subject of $\dot{V}_E$ and $\dot{V}O_2$ max measurements should be less than 10%.

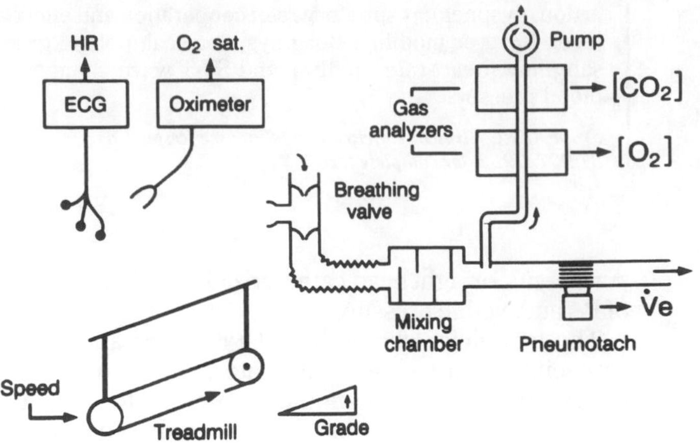

FIGURE 8-17. Exercise-testing equipment. The speed and grade of the treadmill control the workload. The ECG is monitored for arrhythmias and heart rate (HR). Oxygen saturation may be monitored noninvasively with a pulse oximeter. The patient inhales room air through a low-resistance breathing valve. Exhaled air is mixed and then sampled for oxygen and carbon dioxide concentrations. A pneumotach measures exhaled airflow and the signal is integrated to give minute ventilation ($\dot{V}e$). Alternately, a bicycle ergometer may replace the treadmill, a radial artery cannula may be placed to measure arterial blood gas and lactate levels, and a mass spectrometer may replace the individual gas analyzers.

Every 2 months, check the indicated treadmill speed for 1% accuracy by measuring the length of the belt and counting the number of cycles per minute, using a stopwatch at two different speeds. Also check the indicated grade for 1% accuracy. Ask hospital safety engineers to check the electrical current leakage of the instruments at least yearly.

Calculations

The best overall indicator of cardiopulmonary health and physical fitness is the maximum oxygen uptake ($\dot{V}O_2$ max), which is usually normalized for body weight in kilograms (mL/kg/min). Predicted $\dot{V}O_2$ max and other exercise variables should be calculated from data from a large study.[25] The $\dot{V}O_2$ max is about 30 to 45 mL/kg/min in sedentary persons, whereas athletes may achieve an oxygen consumption of more than 80 mL/kg/min. The $\dot{V}O_2$ max from a bicycle ergometer is about 90% of that achieved by the same person on a treadmill. In some patients with cardiac disease, it may be risky to perform "maximal" exercise; thus, various submaximal exercise test regimens have been developed.

The O_2 pulse ($\dot{V}O_2$/HR) at maximum exercise should be greater than 8 mL O_2/beat in women and 12 mL O_2/beat in men. Maximum ventilation ($\dot{V}_E$) achieved should be about 60% of the previously measured MVV. (If the MVV is less than 40 times the FEV_1, poor MVV effort should be suspected.) The ratio of dead space to tidal volume (V_D/V_T) should be less than 0.25 during exercise (this calculation requires arterial blood gas measurements). The anaerobic threshold, the $\dot{V}O_2$ at which blood lactate increases, should normally be reached at or above a $\dot{V}O_2$ of 40% of the predicted $\dot{V}O_2$ max.

Interpretation

Maximal effort probably has been obtained if any of the following occurs at the end of exercise:

HR > 90% predicted max
$\dot{V}_E$ max ≥ 80% of MVV
$\dot{V}O_2$ max ≥ 85% predicted value
Blood lactate > 8 mM/L

The test result is considered normal if the patient achieves an oxygen consumption ($\dot{V}O_2$ max) of 85% or more of the predicted value (Table 8-7).[26] The most common cause of low oxygen consumption is deconditioning, indicated by normal ventilation, normal oxygen saturation, and a normal-to-low O_2 pulse response to exercise. Cardiovascular diseases generally cause a high heart rate for a given workload, a low O_2 pulse, and sometimes angina or abnormal ECG findings. A cardiovascular limitation to exercise should also be suspected if the anaerobic threshold is reached at a lower oxygen consumption than expected.

Exercise limitation caused by moderate COPD or restriction is accompanied by a high minute ventilation relative to workload, which quickly approaches the resting MVV, and oxygen desaturation, while the ECG and HR respond normally. Pulmonary vascular diseases (such as primary pulmonary hypertension) are noted

TABLE 8-7 **Exercise Response Interpretation**

	Deconditioning	Cardiac	COPD	Fibrosis	Pulmonary Vascular
$\dot{V}O_{2max}$	Low	Low	Low	Low	Low
HR/work load	High	High			High
MVV − $\dot{V}E_{max}$	High	High	Low	Low	
O_2 sat			Low	Low	++Low
O_2 pulse		Low			Low
V_D/V_T			High	High	++High

for an increased V_D/V_T at rest that does not fall with exercise and considerable oxygen desaturation.

LUNG COMPLIANCE

Indications

Lung compliance testing measures the elastic recoil or stiffness of the lungs. It is more invasive than other PF tests because the patient must swallow an esophageal balloon. Lung compliance is usually measured to distinguish lung abnormalities from those of the chest wall.

Equipment

Lung compliance studies are often performed in a body box because the necessary mouth shutter, pneumotachometer, and 60-cmH_2O range pressure transducer are already available; only an esophageal balloon needs to be added. However, lung compliance can be measured without a body box.

Procedure

Lung compliance is normally measured under static conditions (no airflow) as the change in volume produced by a unit change in pressure: $C = \Delta V/\Delta P$. Prepare the esophageal balloon, mark the position 50 cm from the tip, and fill it with 0.5 mL of air. Give the patient a glass of water. Dip the balloon in 4% lidocaine jelly and gently guide it straight backward through the more patent nostril. When it reaches the back of the throat, tell the patient to quickly drink the water as you advance the catheter. The balloon is usually swallowed down the esophagus. Advance it to the 50-cm mark and have the patient breathe to and from the spirometer or pneumotachometer as you watch the volume and pressure changes. Withdraw the balloon 10 cm if the pressure is positive during inspiration, indicating that it is in the stomach. Tape the catheter to the nose when it is correctly positioned.

Ask the patient to inhale to TLC and then close the shutter for 3 seconds several times as he or she slowly exhales. The patient should relax each time you close the shutter. Repeat this procedure two or three more times.

To measure *static lung compliance* in mechanically ventilated patients, apply an inspiratory hold after the tidal volume has been delivered, either by using a prolonged inspiratory plateau or by occluding the exhalation port. Note the mouth pressure obtained and the tidal volume. Repeat the procedure twice and report the average values.

Quality Assurance

Before each test, calibrate the spirometer with a 3.00-L syringe for 3% accuracy, and calibrate the pressure transducer with a U-tube manometer at 50 cmH_2O for 5% accuracy. Check the balloon for patency and leaks. Check the mouthpiece and shutter assembly to be sure it does not leak when the shutter is closed. Ignore any occlusions when the volume changes or the pressure does not remain constant.

Calculations

Two components contribute to overall compliance of the respiratory system (C_{RS}): the lung itself (C_L) and the chest wall (C_W). Pressure-volume (PV) curves can be made by measuring the pressure developed at many lung volumes. The driving pressure (Prs) equals alveolar pressure (Palv) minus atmospheric pressure or pressure at the body surface (Pbs): Prs = Palv − Pbs. The pressure used to develop the PV curve of the lung itself is the transpulmonary pressure (ie, alveolar pressure minus pleural pressure): P_L = Palv − Ppl. Alveolar pressure is equivalent to pressure at the mouth when there is no airflow (Palv = Pm).

Compliance is often reported as a single value from that portion of the PV curve 1 L above end-tidal volume, but you should plot all of the pressure and volume pairs from each valid occlusion and draw a line between them. The normal static compliance for the lung and the chest wall systems is the same (ie, 0.2 L/cmH_2O). The compliances of the total respiratory system, lung, and chest wall are related in a reciprocal fashion: $1/C_{RS} = 1/C_L + 1/C_W$. Normal C_{RS} = 0.1 L/cmH_20.

Compliance is related directly to lung volume and, thus, is meaningless unless related to the patient's lung volume. For example, the compliance of a newborn lung is almost the same as the compliance of an adult lung when expressed as liters per cmH_2O per liter of lung volume. When the difference in lung volume is not taken into account, the neonate's lung compliance is about 0.006 L/cmH_2O, whereas the adult's lung compliance is about 0.2 L/cmH_2O. Therefore, it is helpful to divide lung compliance (C_L) by the lung volume at which the measurement is made (V_L), to give a parameter known as *specific compliance.*

Compliances of the chest wall and total respiratory system are not routinely measured because they are affected by skeletal muscle contraction. Therefore, unless the muscles are totally relaxed, the measurements are invalid. Lung compliance, on the other hand, can be determined readily, even if the subject is not relaxed.

Interpretation

An abnormally high lung compliance in a patient with obstructive pulmonary disease indicates the presence of anatomic emphysema, which destroys lung tissue, making the lungs easy to distend. Lung compliance is normal in chronic bronchitis and bronchial asthma. Reduced lung compliance suggests the presence of interstitial or alveolar filling lung disease, which makes the lungs stiffer (Fig. 8-18).

Chest wall compliance (C_W) may be decreased in patients who have kyphoscoliosis, ankylosing spondylitis, prominent obesity, severe pectus excavatum, and neu-

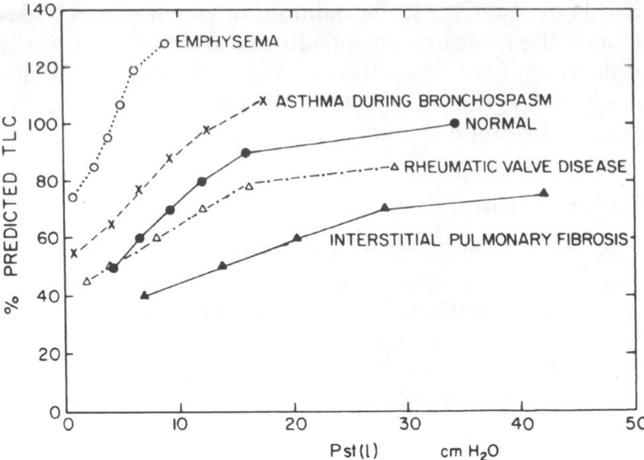

FIGURE 8-18. Pressure–volume curves for the lungs. The pressure is measured by an esophageal balloon when a shutter is closed at different lung volumes. The change in lung volume on the vertical axis is measured by a spirometer. Examples include a normal curve, a curve demonstrating the increased compliance of emphysema, and curves showing reduced compliance as seen with interstitial and alveolar lung disease. (Bates DV, Macklem PT, Christie RV: Respiratory Function in Disease, 2nd ed. Philadelphia, WB Saunders Co., 1971).

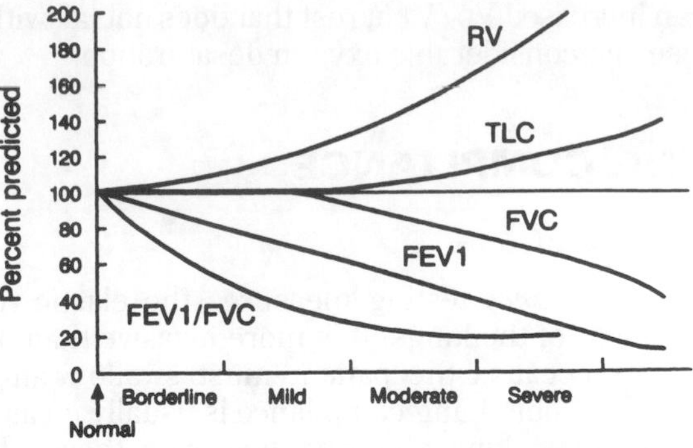

FIGURE 8-19. Changes in pulmonary function parameters as the degree of airways obstruction worsens from borderline to very severe. The FEV_1/FVC ratio becomes abnormal first (is most sensitive). Note the linear decline in FEV_1. As the patient becomes short of breath with moderate obstruction, the FVC decreases and the TLC increases (with emphysema) as progressive air trapping occurs. (© Mayo Foundation)

romuscular disorders associated with spasticity of the muscles. A reduced compliance of the lung or chest wall results in increased work of breathing because the pressure required to produce a volume change is increased.

In mechanically ventilated patients, changes in respiratory system stiffness are usually the result of pulmonary edema or pneumonitis, but may also be caused by factors other than lung compliance, such as changes in chest wall compliance secondary to muscle spasm or abdominal distension.

CONTROL OF BREATHING

Factors that stimulate the ventilatory drive and, thereby, control breathing include hypoxemia, hypercapnia, and acidosis. Some patients partially or completely lose the ability to respond to these ventilatory stimuli. The response to these factors can be measured in a few laboratories.[7,21]

PATTERNS OF IMPAIRMENT

Obstructive Pattern

Refer to Figure 8-19 for a diagram of how pulmonary function parameters change as an obstructive airways disease progresses over time, from mild to severe. During the asymptomatic early stages, the FEV_1/FVC ratio becomes abnormal first, followed by a linear decline in the FEV_1. As the patient becomes symptomatic with moderate obstruction, air trapping causes an increase in the RV and a decrease in the FVC. In the late stages of emphysema, the TLC increases (hyperinflation) because of further air trapping. If the obstruction is caused by emphysema, the DL_{CO} decreases. Refer to Table 8-8 for patterns of pulmonary function abnormality.

Restrictive Pattern

All lung volumes are reduced in restrictive disorders. Expiratory flow rates that are more reduced than the reduction in vital capacity (VC) suggest the presence of concomitant obstructive airways disease. Although the FEV_1 and FVC are reduced, the FEV_1/FVC ratio is normal or increased in pure restrictive disease. This helps to differentiate the reduced FEV_1 of obstructive disease from that of restrictive disease. The RV/TLC ratio is usually normal in pure restrictive disease.

TABLE 8-8 **Patterns of Pulmonary Function Abnormality**

	Normal	Obstruction	Restriction	Mixed
FEV_1/FVC	≥90% predicted	Low	Normal to high	Low
FEV_1	≥80% predicted	Low	Low	Low
FVC	≥80% predicted	Normal to low	Low	Low
TLC	80%–120% predicted	Normal to high	Low	Normal to low
RV/TLC	25%–40%	High	Normal	High

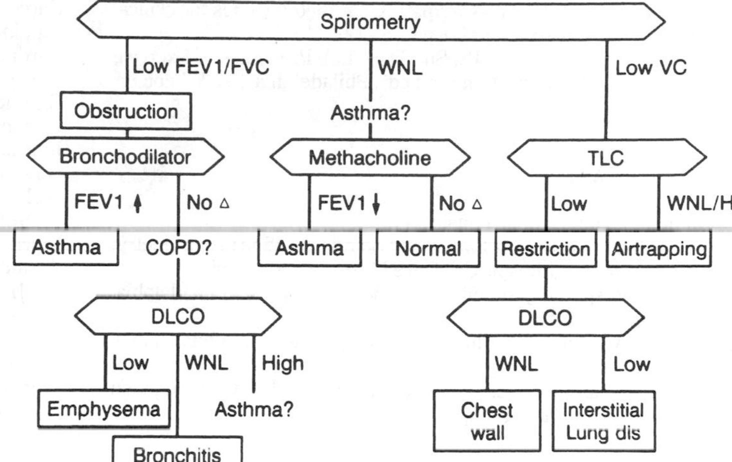

PROTOCOL 8-1. Flow chart for efficient evaluation of pulmonary function. Start with spirometry. Obstruction is probably due to asthma if the FEV_1 increases to near normal (following bronchodilator inhalation), and is probably due to emphysema if the diffusing capacity (DL_{co}) is low. If spirometry is normal in a patient with symptoms suggesting asthma, a positive methacholine challenge supports a diagnosis of asthma. Restriction is probably due to an interstitial lung disease if the DL_{co} is low. (© Mayo Foundation)

Combined Obstructive and Restrictive Pattern

Patients occasionally have more than one disorder, which may result in a combined obstructive and restrictive pulmonary function abnormality. Examples include emphysema (obstructive) with mild congestive heart failure (restrictive), or tracheal stenosis (obstructive) with obesity (restrictive). The VC is reduced in combined obstructive and restrictive disease. The flow rates are reduced disproportionately to the reduction in VC, reducing the FEV_1/FVC ratio.

A common error is to assume that a reduced FVC indicates the presence of restrictive pulmonary disease. The FVC (and slow VC) may be reduced solely because of air trapping from obstructive airways disease. To be certain that restrictive disease is present, in association with a reduced VC and reduced FEV_1/FVC ratio, one should demonstrate that a reduced TLC is present. Serial changes in the TLC might be helpful. For instance, the TLC in a patient with emphysema may change from above normal to normal as a concomitant restrictive process is developing. The RV/TLC ratio increases in the presence of combined obstructive and restrictive disease.

Refer to Protocol 8-1 for an efficient method of evaluating pulmonary function. This method starts with simple screening spirometry; other, more expensive tests are added depending on the spirometry results.

REFERENCES

1. Crapo RO: Pulmonary-function testing. N Engl J Med 331:25, 1994
2. Camilli AE, Burrows B, Knudson RJ, et al: Longitudinal changes in FEV_1 in adults: Effects of smoking and smoking cessation. Am Rev Respir Dis 135:794, 1987
3. The Lung Health Study Research Group: Effects of smoking intervention and the use of an inhaled anticholinergic bronchodilator on the rate of decline of FEV_1. JAMA 272:1497, 1994
4. Nelson SB, Gardner RM, Crapo RO, Jensen RL: Performance evaluation of contemporary spirometers. Chest 97:288, 1990
5. American Thoracic Society Statement: Standardization of spirometry—1987 update. Am Rev Respir Dis 136:1285, 1987
6. Enright PL, Hyatt RE: Office Spirometry: A Practical Guide to the Selection and Use of Spirometers. Philadelphia, Lea & Febiger, 1987
7. Miller A: Pulmonary Function Tests in Clinical and Occupational Lung Disease. Orlando, Grune & Stratton, 1986
8. Crapo RO, Morris AH, Gardner RM: Reference spirometric values using techniques and equipment that meet ATS recommendations. Am Rev Respir Dis 123:659, 1981
9. Knudson RJ, Lebowitz MD, Holberg CJ, Burrows B: Changes in the normal expiratory flow–volume curve with growth and aging. Am Rev Respir Dis 127:725, 1983
10. Wang X, Dockery DW, Wypij D, et al: Pulmonary function between 6 and 18 years of age. Pediatr Pulmonol 15:75, 1993
11. Enright PL, Kronmal RA, Higgins M, et al: Spirometry reference values for women and men 65–85 years of age: Cardiovascular Health Study. Am Rev Respir Dis 147:125, 1993
12. American Thoracic Society: Lung function testing: Selection of reference values and interpretative strategies. Am Rev Respir Dis 144:1202, 1991
13. American Thoracic Society Statement: Evaluation of impairment/disability secondary to respiratory disorders. Am Rev Respir Dis 133:1205, 1986
14. Disability Evaluation under Social Security: A Handbook for Physicians. Washington, DC, HEW Publication No 05-10089, 1986
15. Chatham M, Bleecker ER, Norman P, et al: A screening test for airways reactivity. Chest 82:15, 1982
16. American Thoracic Society: Guidelines for the evaluation of impairment/disability in patients with asthma. Am Rev Respir Dis 147:1056, 1993
17. Juniper EF, Cockcroft DW, Hargreave FE: Histamine and methacholine inhalation test: Tidal breathing method, laboratory procedure and standardization. Lund, Sweden, AB Draco, 1991
18. Spector SL: Update on exercise-induced asthma. Ann Allergy 71:571, 1993
19. Acres JC, Kryger MH: Clinical significance of pulmonary function tests: Upper airway obstruction. Chest 80:207, 1981
20. Enright PL, Kronmal RA, Schenker M, et al: Correlates of respiratory muscle strength, and maximal respiratory pressure reference values in the elderly. Am Rev Respir Dis 149:430, 1994
21. Clausen JL: Pulmonary Function Testing Guidelines and Controversies. New York, Academic Press, 1982
22. American Thoracic Society Statement: Single breath carbon monoxide diffusing capacity (transfer factor): Recommendations for a standard technique. Am Rev Respir Dis 136:1299, 1987
23. Kanengiser LC, Rapoport DM, Epstein H, Goldring RM: Volume adjustment of mechanics and diffusion in interstitial lung disease: Lack of clinical relevance. Chest 96:1036, 1989
24. Knudson RJ, Kaltenborn WT, Knudson DE, Burrows B: The single-breath carbon monoxide diffusing capacity: Reference equations derived from a healthy nonsmoking population and effects of hematocrit. Am Rev Respir Dis 135:805, 1987

25. Hansen JE, Sue DY, Wasserman K: Predicted values for clinical exercise testing. Am Rev Respir Dis 129:S49, 1984
26. Wasserman K, Hansen JE, Sue DY, et al: Principles of Exercise Testing and Interpretation (2nd ed). Philadelphia, Lea & Febiger, 1994

BIBLIOGRAPHY

Additional resources to be considered:

American Thoracic Society Statement: Standardization of spirometry: 1994 update. Am J Respir Crit Care Med 152:1107, 1995

Bates DV: Respiratory function in disease (3rd ed). Philadelphia, WB Saunders, 1989

Cherniak RM: Pulmonary function testing (2nd ed). Philadelphia, WB Saunders, 1992

European Respiratory Society Statement: Standardized lung function testing. Eur Respir J 6(Suppl 16):1, 1993

Gardner RM, Clausen JL, Cotton DJ, et al: Computer guidelines for pulmonary laboratories. Am Rev Respir Dis 134:628, 1986

Gardner RM, Clausen JL, Epler G, et al: Pulmonary function laboratory personnel qualifications. Am Rev Respir Dis 134:623, 1986

Gardner RM, Clausen JL, Crapo RO, et al: Quality assurance in pulmonary function laboratories. Am Rev Respir Dis 1134:625, 1986

Journal Conference, St Petersburg, Florida: Pulmonary function testing. Respir Care 34:647, 1989

Mahler DA (ed): Pulmonary function testing. Clin Chest Med 10(2):129, 1989

Morris AH, Kanner RE, Crapo RO, Gardner RM: Clinical pulmonary function testing: A manual of uniform laboratory procedures (2nd ed). Salt Lake City, Intermountain Thoracic Society, 1984

Quanjer PH, Helms P, Bjure J, Ganltier C (eds): Standardization of lung function tests in paediatrics. Eur Respir J 2(Suppl 4):121S, 1989

Wanger J: Pulmonary function testing: A practical approach. Baltimore, Williams & Wilkins, 1991

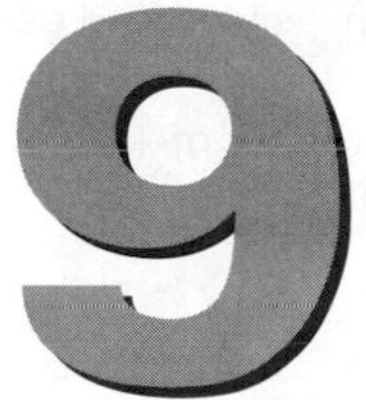

9 Arterial Blood Gas Analysis

John J. Mahoney
John E. Hodgkin
Antonius L. Van Kessel

CLINICAL SKILLS

Upon completion of this chapter, the reader will:

- Describe the chemical and physical basis of oxygen and carbon dioxide transport
- Define hypoxemia and its five primary causes
- Interpret blood gas reports and be proficient in their validation
- State the normal arterial blood gas values
- Interpret arterial blood gases for acid–base disturbances and postulate possible causes
- Explain the correct procedure for the safe collection of arterial blood-gas samples
- Identify potential pre-analytical errors associated with blood gas collection and their probable impact on results

- Describe the uses and limitations of data from noninvasive blood gas monitors
- Apply the Clinical Laboratory Improvement Ammendment of 1988 (CLIA-88) criteria to blood gas instrument calibration and quality control

KEY TERMS

Anion gap	Carbon dioxide	Noninvasive estimations of blood gases
Arterial puncture	Hemoglobin	Oxygen content
Bicarbonate ion	Hemoglobin derivatives	Oxygenation
Blood gas measurement	Hypoxemia	P_{50}
Blood gas sensors	Mixed venous PO_2	pH

Arterial blood gas analyses are used to assess (1) oxygenation, (2) ventilation, and (3) acid–base status; therefore, they are crucial for the proper treatment of respiratory or metabolic disorders.[1] Blood gas values provide information that is used to determine oxygen (O_2) therapy, ventilatory support, and pharmacologic interventions and are especially crucial for patients on life-support. Therefore, blood gas measurements should be closely monitored so that they meet clinical needs.[2]

This chapter discusses the chemical and physiological basis of blood gas analysis. It also reviews the various methods of blood gas analysis and describes how to interpret blood gas data as they relate to possible patient conditions.

GAS LAWS

The amount of pressure a pure gas exerts is caused by the constant motion of its constituent molecules and is dependent on temperature and volume. Not all gases behave the same because of differences in their molecular size and bond enthalpy. The ideal gas law combines Boyle's Law, Charles' Law, and Gay-Lussac's Law and states that pressure (P), volume (V), and absolute temperature (T) of a gas are related to the number of moles (n) of gas by the universal gas constant (R):

$$PV = nRT \qquad (1)$$

If pressure is measured in millimeters of mercury (mmHg), volume is measured in liters (L), and temperature is measured in degrees Kelvin (°K, where 0°C = 273.16°K), then R has the value 62.36 mmHg · L/°K/mole.[3] It can be deduced that 1 mole of an ideal gas at standard temperature and pressure dry (STPD) occupies 22.4 L, when standard temperature and pressure are 273.16°K and 760 mmHg, respectively.

Dalton's Law of Partial Pressure

Dalton's Law states that for a mixture of different gases, each gas exerts the same pressure that it would exert if it alone occupied the whole volume, and the pressure each gas exerts is called its partial pressure. From this, it follows that (1) the total pressure of a gas mixture is the sum of the partial pressures of its constituent gases; and (2) each constituent gas in the mixture exerts the same proportion of the total pressure as its volume is of the total volume.

The partial pressure of ambient gas is a direct function of its atmospheric concentration. For O_2 in dry air, the inspired pressure of O_2 (P_{IO_2}) can be calculated by:

$$P_{IO_2} = P_B \times F_{IO_2} \qquad (2)$$

where P_B is the barometric pressure in mmHg and F_{IO_2} is the fraction of inspired O_2. At sea level, P_B is 760 mmHg and the F_{IO_2} of ambient air is 0.21 (rounded off from 0.2093), so the dry air P_{IO_2} would be equal to 159.6 mmHg.

Dissolved gas in the solution exerts a pressure that is called the tension of that gas in solution. For O_2 and carbon dioxide (CO_2), the tensions are denoted PO_2 and PCO_2, respectively. When the solution is arterial blood, PaO_2 and $PaCO_2$ denote the partial pressure of O_2 and CO_2 dissolved in the plasma of arterial blood. Partial pressures are commonly expressed in mmHg or torr. One mmHg is equal to one torr (in honor of Torricelli, the inventor of the barometer). However, under the SI (Systéme International d'Unités) listings of physicochemical quantities and units in clinical chemistry, partial pressure is expressed in pascals (newtons per square meter). The kilopascal (kPa) unit has been recommended as a replacement for mmHg and torr. Table 9-1 shows how pressure in mmHg is converted to kPa.

The molecules in a liquid, like those of a gas, are in constant motion and those at the liquid-gas interface tend to escape into the gas above the liquid. The kinetic energy of water molecules increases as temperature rises, thus increasing the tendency of the water molecules to escape from the liquid. The pressure of the water vapor above the liquid surface therefore directly depends on temperature and is independent of P_B. At body temperature, the partial pressure of water vapor (P_{H_2O}) is referred to as the saturated vapor pressure (SVP). At its boiling point, the SVP of water is equal to P_B.

The SVP plays a special role in blood gas physiology. Inspired air, when fully saturated with water vapor, has a P_{H_2O} of 47 mmHg. Because the total gas pressure

TABLE 9-1 **Blood Gas Symbols, Definitions, Units, and Conversions**

Symbol	Definition	Normal Values*
pH	Negative log of hydrogen ion activity	7.40 ± 0.05 pH units
$PaCO_2$	Partial pressure of CO_2 in arterial blood	40 ± 5 mmHg[§]
HCO_3^-	Bicarbonate ion	24.0 ± 2.0 mEq/L[†]
PaO_2	Partial pressure of O_2 in arterial blood	70 to 100 mmHg[‡]
O_2Hb	Oxyhemoglobin	≥94.5%[‖,¶]
COHb	Carboxyhemoglobin	<1.5%[‖,#]
MetHb	Methemoglobin	<1.5%[‖]
HHb	Deoxyhemoglobin	<2.0%[‖]
ctHb	Concentration of total hemoglobin	males: 15.8 ± 2.3 g/dL females: 14.0 ± 2.0 g/dL
SO_2	Hemoglobin O_2 saturation	>94.5%[¶]
$ctO_2(Hb)$	O_2 content of hemoglobin	15 to 23 vol%
P_{50}	Partial pressure of O_2 at 50% saturation	27.0 ± 2.0 mmHg

Conversions: 1 mEq/L = 1 mmol/L; 1 kPa (kilopascal) = 7.5 mmHg; 1 mmHg = 0.133 kPa.
* NOTE. Normal values are for arterial blood.
† Calculated from pH and plasma PCO_2 from Reference 5.
‡ Normal values for PaO_2 are age-dependent [see References 6–8 and Equations 21 through 23 in text].
§ Reference 9 uses a normal range of 40 ± 4 mmHg for $PaCO_2$.
‖ Hemoglobin derivatives are fractions of the concentration of total hemoglobin and are expressed as percentages.
¶ From Reference 10.
\# For nonsmoking adults; smoking adults have COHb as high as 10% (from Reference 4).

cannot exceed atmospheric pressure (eg, 760 mmHg), only 760 − 47 = 713 mmHg is available for the sum of the partial pressures of O_2, CO_2, and nitrogen (N_2). As a result, Equation 2 can be modified as follows:

$$P_IO_2 = (P_B - P_{H_2O}) \times F_IO_2 \quad (3)$$

Therefore, at sea level, the P_IO_2 in humidified air (ie, in the trachea) is (760 − 47) × 0.21 = 149.7 mmHg. At high altitude, where P_B is less, P_IO_2 will decrease. Table 9-2 lists (1) the P_IO_2 and P_B at various altitudes, (2) the theoretical maximum for the sum of the PaO_2 and $PaCO_2$, and (3) the normal values for P_AO_2 (assuming normal ventilation). It can be deduced from Dalton's Law that, for a patient breathing room air at sea level, the sum of the PaO_2 plus $PaCO_2$ can never exceed the theoretical maximal limit (149.7 mmHg). Because the PaO_2 is always determined by both P_IO_2 and P_B, a patient placed in a hyperbaric chamber set to 2 atmospheres of pressure may have a theoretical PaO_2 of 309 mmHg while breathing room air and 1473 mmHg while breathing 100% O_2!

Solubility of Gases in Liquids

Solubility coefficients quantify the amount of gas that can be dissolved at a given temperature in a given quantity of liquid (commonly 1 mL or 100 mL of liquid) when a given pressure of that gas (often 760 mmHg) exists above the liquid surface. Solubility is dependent on the type of gas, the fluid in which it is dissolved, and the

TABLE 9-2 **Relationship Between Altitude, Barometric Pressure (P_B), Ambient (21%) P_IO_2, Maximum Calculated Sum of PaO_2 + $PaCO_2$, and Normal Alveolar P_AO_2**

Altitude (feet)	P_B (mmHg)	Ambient P_IO_2 (mmHg)	Maximum PaO_2 + $PaCO_2$* (mmHg)	Normal P_AO_2† (mmHg)
0	760	159	149	102
5,000	630	132	122	75
8,000	564	118	108	63
10,000	523	110	100	57
12,000	483	101	91	54
15,000	412	90	80	52
20,000	349	73	63	35
30,000	226	47	37	9

* During hyperventilation, the P_AO_2 and PaO_2 can increase but neither can ever exceed the calculated maximum sum for PaO_2 + $PaCO_2$ when the F_IO_2 is 21% at the given P_B. This information is sometimes useful for internal (within-patient sample) quality control.
† This normal P_AO_2 estimate is based on normal ventilation.

temperature of the fluid. The solubility coefficient of O_2 in plasma is quite low (0.00314 mL [STPD]/dL × mmHg),[11] whereas the coefficient for CO_2 is about 24 times higher.[5]

VENTILATION

Air moves in and out of the lungs as pressure gradients are created between the external atmosphere and the alveoli by the action of the respiratory muscles. The volume of the chest is increased by the movements of the diaphragm and chest wall. According to Boyle's Law, increasing volume (V) reduces pressure (P). The negative alveolar pressure produced during inspiration allows air to flow into the lungs.

The main function of ventilation is to exchange O_2 and CO_2 between blood and alveolar gas and thus maintain an optimal level of PaO_2 and $PaCO_2$. Alveolar gas can be thought of as a compartment of gas lying between atmospheric inspired air and alveolar capillary blood. Oxygen is continuously removed from the alveolar gas and CO_2 is added to it by diffusion. Inspired air normally contains only 0.03% CO_2. Therefore, almost all the alveolar CO_2 (P_ACO_2) comes from diffusion as capillary blood equilibrates rapidly with the alveolar air. For normal subjects, $PaCO_2$ can be assumed to be the same as P_ACO_2 of 40 ± 5 mmHg (see Table 9-1).

Respiration is maintained by the activity of the respiratory center in the medulla oblongata. This center is constantly stimulated by the peripheral chemoreceptors (the carotid bodies, located in the bifurcation of the common carotid arteries, and the aortic bodies, located above and below the aortic arch) and also by the central chemoreceptors (located on the ventral surface of the medulla). The peripheral chemoreceptors respond to decreases in PaO_2, increases in hydrogen ions (H^+), and increases in $PaCO_2$. They are responsible for the increase in ventilatory rate that occurs in response to low O_2 concentration in the blood (hypoxemia). The central chemoreceptors respond to changes in H^+ concentration. An increase in H^+ stimulates the respiratory center and a decrease inhibits it. The most important factor in the control of ventilation under normal conditions is the $PaCO_2$, and the role of the hypoxic (below normal tissue oxygenation) stimulus in day-to-day control of ventilation is small. However, for patients with chronic obstructive pulmonary disease (COPD) with chronic hypercapnia ($PaCO_2$ > 45 mmHg) or for normal subjects at high altitudes, arterial hypoxemia becomes the main stimulus for ventilation.

OXYGENATION

Oxygen is transported around the body by the pumping action of the heart. The cardiac output (Q) is defined as the quantity of blood ejected from the heart during each beat, multiplied by the heart rate. The normal value for Q in humans is about 5.0 L/min. The quantity of O_2 transported by the blood per minute can be calculated by multiplying $\dot{Q}$ by the quantity of O_2 carried by each mL of blood. This is termed the available O_2, that is, the quantity of O_2 transported to the body tissues. The relationship can be written as follows:

$$\text{Available } O_2 = \dot{Q} \times O_2/\text{mL blood} \quad (4)$$

A conscious resting adult human consumes about 250 mL O_2/min. The circulating blood therefore loses 25% (250 mL O_2/min/1000 mL O_2/min) of its O_2, leaving mixed venous blood approximately 75% saturated. This 75% of remaining O_2 forms an "O_2 reserve," which can be used in cases of stress. The reason why humans do not need a very large blood volume, or massive $\dot{Q}$, is because the hemoglobin in blood can chemically combine with large quantities of O_2. In fact, most of the O_2 is carried by blood in this way. The actual amount of O_2 dissolved or carried in the plasma is very small and is not sufficient to support human life without the presence of hemoglobin.

Hemoglobin

Hemoglobin, a large tetramer molecule (molecular weight = 64,458) found in erythrocytes, consists of four polypeptide iron porphyrin heme groups (identified α_1, α_2, β_1, β_2) attached to a single globin protein. Each of the four heme groups, located at the corners of an irregular tetrahedron-shaped molecular structure, can combine reversibly with one O_2 molecule.[12] In the fully oxygenated state, hemoglobin exists in the smaller 'R' (relaxed) high-affinity quaternary structure. In the completely deoxygenated state, hemoglobin exists in the larger quaternary 'T' (taut or tense) low O_2 affinity structure.[13] The 'T' structure is stabilized by salt bridges at the carboxy terminals of the peptide chains and by 2,3-diphosphoglycerate (2,3-DPG).

In the presence of appropriate pressures of O_2, the salt bridges are broken, 2,3-DPG is displaced, O_2 attaches to the binding sites, and H^+ is released. This reversible reaction is expressed by:

$$HHb \cdot H^+ + O_2 \leftrightarrow O_2Hb + H^+ \quad (5)$$

where $HHb \cdot H^+$ represents hydrogen ions bound to deoxyhemoglobin (HHb) and O_2Hb is oxyhemoglobin. Equation 5 also shows how hemoglobin can act as an important buffer for H^+ in the blood.

Because hemoglobin is a carrier protein, it can be characterized by the attached ligand or by the chemical state of the binding site. The concentration of total hemoglobin (ctHb) in the blood is the sum of these hemoglobin species and is expressed as:

$$ctHb = O_2Hb + COHb + MetHb + HHb \quad (6)$$

where carboxyhemoglobin (COHb) and methemoglobin (MetHb) are common hemoglobin derivatives that are unable to bind O_2 (ie, dyshemoglobins). Table 9-1 lists the normal ranges for ctHb and these hemoglobin derivatives.

When carbon monoxide (CO) binds with hemoglobin to form COHb there is an immediate decrease in the number of hemoglobin binding sites. Carbon monoxide has a high affinity (217 times O_2) for hemoglobin binding sites.[14] CO also alters the geometric configuration of the hemoglobin molecule,[15] which increases the affinity of hemoglobin for O_2 and decreases the release of O_2 to the metabolizing tissues.[16,17]

The erythrocyte uses several metabolic pathways to ensure that the iron in hemoglobin is maintained in the reduced (ferrous [Fe^{2+}]) state so that it can readily combine with O_2. When these pathways either fail or become defective, MetHb is formed as the iron is oxidized to the ferric state (Fe^{3+}).[13] MetHb is produced in normal cells at a rate of about 0.5% to 3.0% per day. Increased production of MetHb can seriously hinder O_2 transport because MetHb cannot bind O_2. Table 9-3 lists the genetic abnormalities, oxidant drugs, or chemical toxins that can cause abnormal increases in MetHb formation.

Erythrocytes contain a number of different types of hemoglobin (A, A_2, F, Gower I, Gower II, and Portland) depending on the age of the individual.[13] The predominant hemoglobin in neonates is fetal hemoglobin (HbF), whereas in adults the predominant hemoglobin is HbA.

Oxyhemoglobin and Oxygen Saturation

O_2Hb is defined as a percentage of ctHb as follows:

$$(\%)\ O_2Hb = (O_2Hb/ctHb) \times 100 \quad (7)$$

It should not be confused with O_2 saturation (SO_2), which is defined as the amount of hemoglobin that is bound to O_2 divided by the amount of total hemoglobin that is *available* to bind with O_2 as follows:

$$(\%)\ SO_2 = (O_2Hb/O_2Hb + HHb) \times 100 \quad (8)$$

Table 9-1 gives the normal range for SO_2. There are instances when, in the presence of large quantities of dyshemoglobins (eg, as seen in carboxyhemoglobinemia, methemoglobinemia, or sulfhemoglobinemia), a person can be hypoxic and still have an SO_2 within normal limits.

Oxyhemoglobin Dissociation Curve

The outstanding characteristic of hemoglobin is its unique ability to reversibly bind ligands to their respective binding sites: O_2 to the iron atoms in the heme groups, CO_2 to the four N-terminal valines, H^+ to the imidazolyl groups, and 2,3-DPG to the space between the phosphate groups and the positively charged amino acid residues located at the entrance of the central cavity.[18] The binding of O_2 (or any ligand) to its respective binding site increases the affinity and binding rates for remaining sites. This has been termed ***subunit cooperativity***.[13]

The sigmoidal shape of the oxyhemoglobin dissociation curve (Fig. 9-1) illustrates this subunit cooperation. The lower (or steep) portion of the curve (between 10 and 40 mmHg) depicts what occurs at the tissue level where, at a low PO_2, small changes in PO_2 produce large changes in SO_2. The upper portion of the curve (between 80 and 100 mmHg) depicts what occurs at the alveolar level where increases in PO_2 rapidly saturate the hemoglobin. At the flat portion of the curve, large increases in PO_2 do not materially increase SO_2. Because the upper portion of the curve is relatively flat, SO_2 will change only slightly at first as PO_2 decreases, thus PaO_2 is a more sensitive indicator of mild hypoxemia than is SO_2.

TABLE 9-3 **Genetic or Congenital Factors, Chemicals, and Drugs That Can Cause Increased Levels of Methemoglobin**

Genetic or Congenital Factors	Chemicals	Drugs
Hemoglobin M	Nitrates	Nitroglycerin
Enzyme deficiency ($NADH_2$ reductase)	Nitrites	Nitric oxide
	Chlorates	Phenacetin
	Quinones	Sulfonamides
	Aminobenzenes	
	Nitrobenzene	
	Ferrous sulfate	

P_{50}

The standard P_{50} identifies the PO_2 (in mmHg) where hemoglobin is 50% saturated with O_2 ($SO_2 = 50\%$) at pH = 7.40, PCO_2 = 40 mmHg, and a temperature of 37.0°C. The P_{50} is a convenient way to numerically describe the relative affinity of a specific hemoglobin type for O_2. Figure 9-2 depicts the normal P_{50} for HbA.

Changes in hemoglobin affinity can be demonstrated by deviations in that portion of the curve below the normal P_{50} intersection point.[19] Figure 9-3 shows that the amount of O_2 available to the metabolizing tissues is changed when the position of this curve is shifted to the left (ie, when hemoglobin has an increased affinity for O_2) or to the right (ie, when hemoglobin has a decreased affinity for O_2) by various factors (Table 9-4).

Both the pH (proton Bohr effect) and PCO_2 (carbamate Bohr effect)[20] can affect hemoglobin affinity and cause a shift in the position of the oxyhemoglobin dissociation curve. For example, an exercising muscle metabolizes O_2 and produces CO_2 and H^+, which in turn, causes a decrease in hemoglobin affinity for O_2 and a release of additional O_2. This is depicted by a rightward shift in the curve. In contrast, in the lungs where O_2 is taken up and CO_2 is excreted, the decreased blood acidity causes an increased hemoglobin affinity for O_2 and, as a result, O_2 uptake is maximized.

The amount of 2,3-DPG can also affect hemoglobin affinity. During hypoxemia, acute exposures to high altitude, anoxia resulting from cardiopulmonary disease, or anemia, HHb binds 2,3-DPG in a molar ratio of 1:1, a reaction that causes a shift to the right and improves O_2 delivery to tissues.

The predominant hemoglobin present in the blood is a major determinant of the affinity of hemoglobin for O_2. For example, in the fetus, the high affinity of HbF for O_2 permits maximal O_2 extraction from the small amounts that cross the placental barrier. Of 154 genetic hemo-

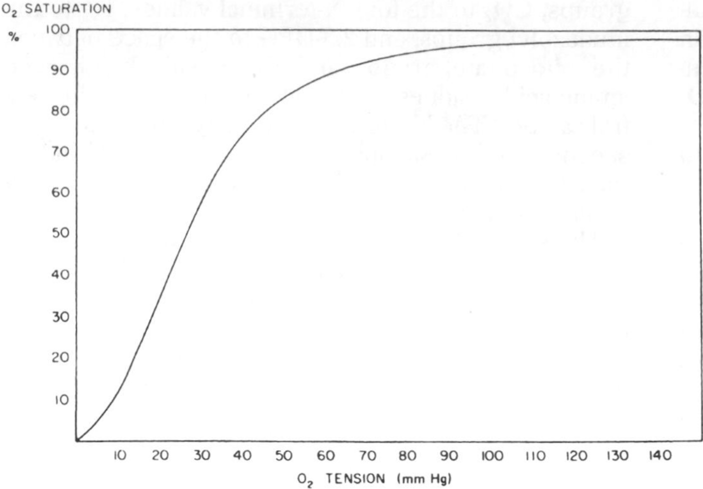

FIGURE 9-1. Oxyhemoglobin dissociation curve, showing relationships between PO_2 and O_2 saturation. (Bates DV, Macklem PT, Christie RV: Respiratory Function in Disease, 2nd ed. Philadelphia, WB Saunders, 1971)

globin abnormalities, 118 have been characterized by their increased affinity for O_2 and 36 by their decreased affinity.[21]

P_{50} Measurement

The P_{50} of blood can be determined in vitro. The measurement is not accurate in patients who have received intravenous transfusions of whole blood or packed cells within 2 months before testing. Also, patients who smoke must refrain for 8 to 12 hours before the test so that their COHb will be at near-normal levels. Heparinized, venous blood is usually drawn from the patient, and the blood sample should be tested shortly after collection in order to minimize MetHb formation.

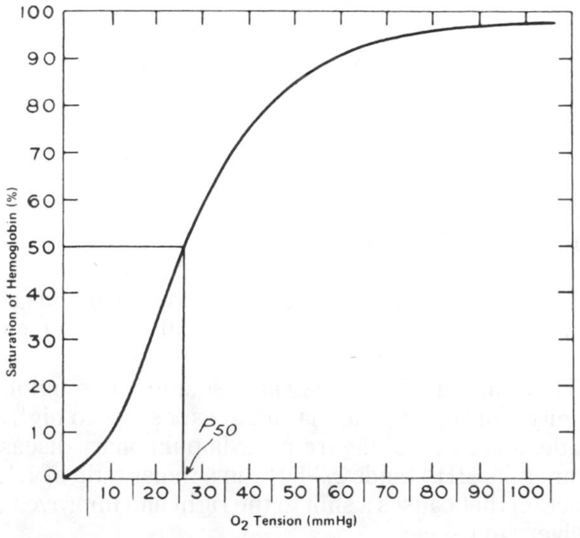

FIGURE 9-2. Oxyhemoglobin dissociation curve depicting the P_{50} at 50% O_2 saturation). The P_{50} is normally 27.0 ± 2.0 mmHg. (Comroe JH Jr: Physiology of Respiration. Chicago, Year Book Medical Publishers, 1974. Data of Mohler, et al: in Clausen [ed]: Pulmonary Function Testing Guidelines and Controversies, New York, Academic Press, 1982:223.

The blood is equilibrated to various O_2 concentrations at 37.0 ± 0.1 °C with a tonometer connected to a gas mixer or to certified gas mixtures. The PCO_2 is maintained at a constant value of 40 mmHg to minimize the carbamate Bohr effect. On completion of the equilibration procedure, the blood is analyzed for pH, PCO_2, PO_2, and SO_2, and appropriate correction factors are applied.[22] The final value for P_{50} can be measured directly or interpolated from a Standard Oxyhemoglobin Dissociation Curve.

Oxygen Capacity of Hemoglobin (Hüfner's Factor)

The O_2 binding capacity of hemoglobin (βO_2) is defined as the maximal amount of O_2 that can bind to 1 g of hemoglobin when it is fully saturated. The molecular mass of hemoglobin (64,458 g/mol), the volume of an ideal gas (22.4 L/mol), and the number of O_2 binding sites per molecule (4) are used to calculate the upper theoretical limit for this value as follows:

$$\begin{aligned} \beta O_2 &= 4 \times 22.4 \text{ L/mol} \div 64{,}458 \text{ g/mol} \\ &= 0.00139 \text{ L/g} = 1.39 \text{ mL/g} \end{aligned} \tag{9}$$

This value (1.39 mL/g) for βO_2 has been adopted for use by the National Committee of Clinical Laboratory Standards (NCCLS) for the calculation of oxygen content.[11] Other numerical values for βO_2 seen in the literature (including Hüfner's original result of 1.34 mL/g, which is still found in many medical textbooks) are less than 1.39 mL/g because dyshemoglobins were present in the blood when the βO_2 was calculated from the ctHb.[23]

Oxygen Content

The oxygen content (ctO_2) quantifies the amount of O_2 present in the blood. It can be a more important indicator of oxygenation than either the PaO_2 or SO_2 whenever a patient is anemic or when high concentrations of dyshemoglobins are present in the blood. The ctO_2 is reported as "mL of O_2 per 100 mL of whole blood" or as

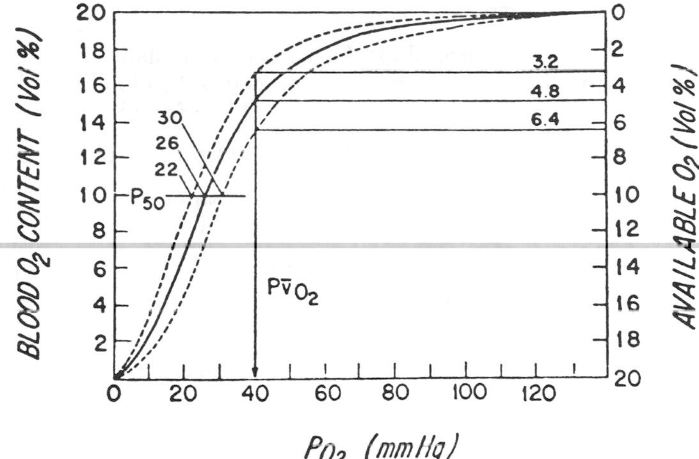

FIGURE 9-3. Effect of shifts of the O_2 dissociation curve on O_2 content and the amount of oxygen available to the tissues (assuming a $P\overline{V}O_2$ of 40 mmHg). The isopleths represent different P_{50} values, ranging from 22 to 30 mmHg. A reduced P_{50} is associated with an increased O_2 content in the venous blood, indicating that less oxygen has been released to the tissue (low A–V O_2 difference). (Snider GL: Clinical Interpretations of Blood Gases. Audiographic series, Vol 1. American College of Chest Physicians)

"volumes percent." There are two components that comprise ctO_2:

1. The amount of O_2 dissolved in plasma:

$$PO_2 \times 0.003 = \text{mL } O_2 \text{ dissolved per 100 mL whole blood} \quad (10)$$

2. The amount of O_2 bound to hemoglobin:

$$\text{Hemoglobin g/dL} \times 1.39 \text{ mL/g} \times SO_2 = \text{mL } O_2 \text{ bound to hemoglobin} \quad (11)$$

Therefore, calculation of the normal ctO_2 for arterial blood with a PO_2 of 100 mmHg, a hemoglobin of 15 g/dL, and a SO_2 of 98% would be as follows:

1. The amount of O_2 dissolved in the plasma:

$$100 \text{ mmHg } PaO_2 \times 0.003 \text{ mL} = 0.3 \text{ mL } O_2 \text{ per 100 mL blood}$$

2. The amount of O_2 bound to hemoglobin:

$$15 \text{ g/dL} \times 1.39 \text{ mL/g} \times 0.98 = 20.4 \text{ mL } O_2 \text{ bound to hemoglobin per 100 mL blood}$$

Therefore, the total ctO_2 is the sum of the O_2 dissolved in the plasma and the hemoglobin bound O_2:

$$0.3 + 20.4 = 20.7 \text{ mL } O_2 \text{ per 100 mL whole blood}$$

Mixed Venous PO_2

The mixed venous PO_2 ($P\overline{V}O_2$) is the measurement of the PO_2 in blood withdrawn from a central venous or pulmonary artery catheter. If the sampling is done correctly,[24] this measurement can be used to determine the adequacy of tissue oxygenation, $\dot{Q}$, or shunt measurements. At rest, the normal $P\overline{V}O_2$ is 35 to 45 mmHg. A value less than 35 mmHg in a critically ill patient suggests that O_2 extraction is increased and/or tissue O_2 delivery may be inadequate. One must then look at the multiple factors involved in oxygenation to determine the cause for the tissue hypoxia. Unfortunately, the $P\overline{V}O_2$ may occasionally be normal despite serious tissue hypoxia (eg, with septicemia). In septic patients, arteriovenous shunting occurs so that blood bypasses tissues and less O_2 is extracted from the blood. If tissue metabolism is markedly reduced, as occurs in cyanide poisoning (which inhibits cytochrome oxidase of the respiratory transport chain), the difference between arterial and venous O_2 content and PO_2 narrows, even though severe hypoxia is present. Because $P\overline{V}O_2$ mostly represents blood returning from tissue with higher perfusion, it does not adequately represent the O_2 extraction in tissues with low perfusion.

The implementation of positive end-expiratory pressure (PEEP) can occasionally reduce $\dot{Q}$ and worsen tissue O_2 delivery. If the PaO_2 improves with the introduction of PEEP but the $P\overline{V}O_2$ decreases, worsening of tissue oxygenation has occurred, most likely as a result of reduced $\dot{Q}$. One of the techniques for determining the optimal level of PEEP is to select the amount of PEEP that results in the highest $P\overline{V}O_2$.[25] The $P\overline{V}O_2$ can also be very helpful in determining the amount of supplemental O_2 needed (ie, the FIO_2 needed to provide satisfactory oxygenation to the tissues).

TABLE 9-4 **Factors That Can Cause the Affinity of Oxygen for Hemoglobin to Change and, Therefore, Cause a Shift in the Position in the Oxyhemoglobin Dissociation Curve**

Shifts to the Left (Increased Affinity)	Shifts to the Right (Decreased Affinity)
Alkalosis	Acidosis
Hypothermia	Hyperthermia
Hypocapnia	Hypercapnia
Decreased 2,3-DPG	Increased 2,3-DPG
Hexokinase deficiency	Pyruvic kinase deficiency
Myxedema	Thyrotoxicosis
Hemoglobinopathy (eg, HB Zürich)	Hemoglobinopathy (eg, Hb Kansas)
Fetal hemoglobin	Hypoxia
Carboxyhemoglobin	Anemia

The Fick Equation

When the O_2 content of blood (ctO_2) can be measured in both arterial (CaO_2) and mixed venous ($C\bar{v}O_2$) blood, perfusion ($\dot{Q}$) can be determined by the Fick Equation:

$$\dot{Q}\ (\text{L/min}) = \dot{V}O_2/(CaO_2 - C\bar{v}O_2) \qquad (12)$$

where $\dot{V}O_2$ is O_2 consumption and can be assumed to be 250 mL/min in normal (70 kg) individuals or it can be calculated by:

$$\dot{V}O_2 = (V_I\ \text{STPD} \times 0.21) - (V_E\ \text{STPD} \times FeO_2) \qquad (13)$$

where V_I STPD is the volume of inspired O_2 and V_E STPD $\times$ FeO_2 is the volume of expired O_2 over 1 minute.

The O_2 content difference between arterial and mixed venous blood ($CaO_2 - C\bar{v}O_2$) represents the amount of O_2 extracted (in mL) per 100 mL of blood and is reported in units of vol%. A difference of greater than 5 vol% would suggest that delivery of O_2 to the tissues may be inadequate. The ($CaO_2 - C\bar{v}O_2$) difference can assist in the early detection of cardiovascular problems and changes in $\dot{Q}$. Assuming that a patient has adequate O_2-carrying capacity, effective perfusion, adequate alveolar ventilation, and normal acid–base status, the ($CaO_2 - C\bar{v}O_2$) difference can reflect the adequacy of $\dot{Q}$ in relation to metabolic O_2 demand. In addition, in nonseptic patients who have a stable temperature and do not exhibit excessive movement (eg, seizures, shivering), a constant O_2 consumption ($\dot{V}O_2$) can be assumed, and therefore serial determinations of ($CaO_2 - C\bar{v}O_2$) difference can reliably reflect changes in $\dot{Q}$ (as [$CaO_2 - C\bar{v}O_2$] difference increases, $\dot{Q}$ decreases) by the Fick equation where:

$$(CaO_2 - C\bar{v}O_2) = \dot{V}O_2/\dot{Q} \qquad (14)$$

Alveolar-Air Equation

If there is no CO_2 in the inspired gas, the P_AO_2 may be calculated from the alveolar-air equation as follows:

$$P_AO_2 = P_IO_2 - P_ACO_2/R + [P_ACO_2 \times F_IO_2 \times (1-R)/R] \qquad (15)$$

where R is the respiratory exchange ratio that represents the ratio of CO_2 production to O_2 consumption uptake. Because the term in the brackets is a small correction factor and P_ACO_2 is assumed to be equivalent to $PaCO_2$, the formula can be reduced to the following:

$$P_AO_2 = P_IO_2 - (P_ACO_2/R) \qquad (16)$$

If R is assumed to be 0.8, then this becomes:

$$P_AO_2 = P_IO_2 - (PaCO_2 \times 1.25) \qquad (17)$$

The factor 1.25 (1/0.8) changes slightly with changes in F_IO_2. Again, assuming P_ACO_2 is equal to $PaCO_2$, the alveolar air equation can also be represented as follows:

$$P_AO_2 = P_IO_2 - PaCO_2 \times [(1/R) - F_IO_2 + (1-R)/R] \qquad (18)$$

This can be rewritten as:

$$P_AO_2 = P_IO_2 - PaCO_2 \times [F_IO_2 + (1-F_IO_2)/R] \qquad (19)$$

Assuming an R of 0.8, while the patient breathes room air, this equation simplifies to:

$$P_AO_2 = P_IO_2 - (PaCO_2 \times 1.20) \qquad (20)$$

If R is not measured, it is assumed to be 0.8 (from the estimation that CO_2 production [$\dot{V}CO_2$] is 200 mL/min and O_2 consumption uptake [$\dot{V}O_2$] is 250 mL/min at rest, so $\dot{V}CO_2/\dot{V}O_2 = 200/250 = 0.8$). The R value can range from about 0.7 with fat metabolism to 1.0 with carbohydrate metabolism and even higher when total body endogenous production of CO_2 ($\dot{V}CO_2$) is elevated. However, inserting different values into the alveolar air equation changes the actual P_AO_2 very little. Therefore, under most clinical situations the simplified equation, which assumes an R of 0.8, will suffice. In our laboratory (Stanford University Hospital), we tend to use Equation 20 rather than Equation 17 because of the simpler mathematics. However, because $1 \div 0.8 = 1.25$, Equation 17 and the use of the multiplier 1.25 is theoretically more correct. Remember to calculate P_IO_2 from Equation 3 and to directly measure the $PaCO_2$.

Alveolar-Arterial Oxygen Tension Gradient

The alveolar-arterial oxygen tension gradient [$P(A-a)O_2$] is the difference between the P_AO_2 and the PaO_2. As a person ages, normal PaO_2 *decreases* owing to worsening ventilation-perfusion ($\dot{V}/\dot{Q}$) mismatch and the [$P(A-a)O_2$] difference increases. Therefore, normal values for PaO_2 should always take the age of the patient into account. Table 9-5 gives examples of age-predicted PaO_2 and [$P(A-a)O_2$] values.

Investigators have confirmed this age-related PaO_2 phenomenon in groups of normal subjects and have developed regression equations for the estimation of PaO_2 based on age. All of these equations have relatively large standard errors for the estimate because of (1) biological variation and (2) the measuring methods used. Also important is the positioning of the subject during the collection of the arterial blood sample. In general, supine PaO_2 is normally lower than upright or seated PaO_2.

TABLE 9-5 **Normal, Supine PaO_2 and the Alveolar-Arterial Oxygen Tension Gradient [$P(A - a)O_2$] at Sea Level for Various Ages**

Age (years)	PaO_2 (mmHg)	$P(A - a)O_2$ (mmHg)
20	96–104	<5
30	92–100	<9
40	88–96	<13
50	84–92	<17
60	79–87	<22
70	76–83	<26
80	71–79	<30
90	66–74	<35

For the *supine* position at 760 mmHg, the PaO_2 can be predicted by the following equation[6]:

$$PaO_2 = 109 - (0.43 \times \text{age}) \pm 4 \quad (21)$$

For the *seated* position, the PaO_2 can be predicted by the following equation[7]:

$$PaO_2 = 104.2 - (0.27 \times \text{age}) \pm 6 \quad (22)$$

When combining data from patients in both *seated and supine* positions, the PaO_2 can be predicted by the following equation[8]:

$$PaO_2 = 103.7 - (0.24 \times \text{age}) \pm 7.9 \quad (23)$$

Arterial/Alveolar O_2 Tension Ratio

The arterial/alveolar O_2 tension ratio is the ratio of the PaO_2 to the estimated P_AO_2.[26] Whereas the $[P(A-a)O_2]$ varies as the F_IO_2 is changed, the arterial/alveolar O_2 ratio remains relatively stable. One can use the arterial/alveolar O_2 ratio as an index to lung function status when the F_IO_2 being delivered to the patient is altered. The arterial/alveolar O_2 ratio can also be used to predict what a new PaO_2 should be when the F_IO_2 is changed or to help choose the F_IO_2 needed to obtain a desired PaO_2. To determine a new F_IO_2:

$$\text{New } F_IO_2 = \frac{[\text{Desired } PaO_2/(PaO_2/P_AO_2)] + (P_ACO_2/R)}{(P_B - 47)} \quad (24)$$

Hypoxemia

Hypoxemia refers to a low O_2 concentration in the blood and should not be confused with tissue hypoxia, which is an inadequate availability of O_2 for tissues and may be present despite a normal ctO_2. The measurement of PaO_2 is commonly used to determine whether hypoxia is present; however, the ctO_2 may be significantly reduced owing to anemia despite a normal PaO_2. In contrast, ctO_2 may be normal, despite a reduced PaO_2, when hemoglobin is increased. There are basically five causes of hypoxemia: (1) altitude, (2) overall hypoventilation, (3) $\dot{V}/\dot{Q}$ mismatch, (4) diffusion defect, and (5) shunt.

□ ALTITUDE

An obvious cause for reduced PaO_2 is a decrease in P_IO_2. This most commonly results from high altitude. When patients with pulmonary disease are discharged from a hospital located at low altitude (eg, at sea level) and return to their homes at a higher altitude (eg, at 5000 feet elevation), their PaO_2 may drop significantly. This must be kept in mind when determining whether supplemental O_2 will be needed for the patient at discharge. Furthermore, the P_IO_2 in a pressurized aircraft is equivalent to that found at approximately 5000 to 8000 feet elevation, and this must be taken into account should the patient plan to travel in airplanes. Table 9-2 shows the relationship between altitude, P_B, P_IO_2, and P_AO_2.

□ OVERALL HYPOVENTILATION

The minute ventilation ($\dot{V}_E$) may be decreased as a result of a reduction in tidal volume, a slowing of respiratory rate, or both. Decreased alveolar ventilation ($\dot{V}_A$) owing to decreased minute ventilation ($\dot{V}_E$) results in hypoxemia and hypercapnia. The differential diagnosis of hypoventilation includes respiratory center depression owing to drug overdose (eg, morphine, barbiturates), effects of anesthesia during the early postoperative period, excessive postoperative analgesia, the pickwickian syndrome, thoracic deformities (eg, kyphoscoliosis and rheumatoid spondylitis), and neuromuscular disturbances.

□ $\dot{V}/\dot{Q}$ MISMATCH

$\dot{V}/\dot{Q}$ mismatch is the most common cause of hypoxemia. When units of lung are underventilated relative to their perfusion (low $\dot{V}/\dot{Q}$), the pulmonary capillary blood that leaves these units is underoxygenated, and hypoxemia results. Examples include bronchospasm, mucoid obstruction of the airway with resultant atelectasis, obstruction of airways associated with chronic bronchitis and emphysema, pneumonia, and pulmonary edema. High $\dot{V}/\dot{Q}$ units do not directly cause hypoxemia because the blood perfusing these units becomes well-oxygenated.

□ DIFFUSION DEFECT

The alveolar-capillary membrane may occasionally be thickened to the extent that diffusion is reduced enough to result in hypoxemia. However, this is unusual because, normally at rest, the hemoglobin in the pulmonary capillary is fully saturated by the time the blood is one third of the way past the alveolus. The alveolar-capillary membrane can be widened substantially before resting hypoxemia occurs.

□ SHUNT

Anatomic (or congenital) right-to-left shunts (eg, the tetralogy of Fallot and the transposition of the great vessels) result in hypoxemia. Physiologic shunts also cause hypoxemia; for example, in lobar atelectasis resulting from a mucous plug obstruction, if the collapsed area of the lung continues to be perfused, this functions as a shunt (ie, the blood does not come in contact with ventilated alveoli).

□ DETERMINING THE CAUSE OF HYPOXEMIA

With proper evaluation, the cause of a patient's hypoxemia may be determined. A "rule of thumb" that works reasonably well for determining the cause of hypoxemia in adult patients is to calculate the sum of the PaO_2 and the $PaCO_2$. If, when inhaling room air, the sum is between 110 and 130 mmHg, the cause of the hypoxemia is overall hypoventilation. If the sum is less than 110 mmHg with room air or when receiving supplemental O_2, the cause is $\dot{V}/\dot{Q}$ mismatch, diffusion defect, or shunt. If the sum is more than 130 mmHg in adults when the patient was supposedly inhaling room air, one should suspect an error; either the patient was receiving supplemental O_2 or an error was made in the PaO_2 or $PaCO_2$ measurements. In children or teenagers, the sum of the PaO_2 and $PaCO_2$ may normally be above 130 mmHg.

Measurements such as the N_2 washout and helium dilution tests give evidence for the presence of $\dot{V}/\dot{Q}$ mismatch and nonuniform ventilation. Comparison of ventilation and perfusion in lung scans can give a semiquantitative analysis of $\dot{V}/\dot{Q}$ matching over the lung fields. The CO diffusing capacity test can evaluate the patient for the presence of a diffusion defect. The diffusing capacity is a fairly sensitive indicator of the presence of interstitial lung disease. In the presence of obstructive airway disease, a reduced diffusing capacity is usually indicative of emphysema.

The presence of a shunt can be detected by giving the patient 100% O_2 for about 20 minutes and then obtaining an arterial blood gas sample. For a patient at sea level, there is about a 5% shunt for every 100 mmHg the PaO_2 is below 550 to 600 mmHg. This rule of thumb works reasonably well down to a PaO_2 of 100 mmHg. One should remember that everyone normally has about a 2% to 4% shunt. Unfortunately, the administration of 100% O_2 to detect a shunt in patients with diseased lungs has a major drawback: when alveoli that are supplied by partially obstructed airways are filled with a high percentage of O_2, they are prone to collapse. Alveoli that normally contain a large amount of N_2 resist collapse because N_2 is not significantly absorbed by the blood perfusing the alveolus; however, when this N_2 is replaced by O_2, which is readily absorbed by the blood that comes in contact with the alveolus, the alveolus can rapidly collapse (absorption atelectasis), resulting in a shunt. Therefore, administration of 100% O_2 in diseased patients may, ironically, produce a significant shunt. In patients with hypoxemia resulting from overall hypoventilation, $\dot{V}/\dot{Q}$ mismatch, or diffusion defect, inhalation of 100% O_2 can correct the hypoxemia—that is, the PaO_2 should reach the level expected for normal subjects inhaling 100% O_2.

CARBON DIOXIDE TRANSPORT

The majority of CO_2 excretion is accomplished by normal pulmonary gas exchange. CO_2 rapidly diffuses out through the alveolar membrane during the brief (0.75 seconds) time period when blood is in contact with alveolar air.[5] As we have seen previously (Equations 16 through 20), near equilibrium develops between the CO_2 in the blood and normal alveoli such that $PaCO_2 = P_ACO_2$.

CO_2 is transported in blood as dissolved gas, as bicarbonate ion (HCO_3^-), and in combination with carrier proteins as carbamino compounds. The equilibrium between CO_2 and acid (H^+) can be visualized by the equation:

$$CO_2 + H_2O \leftrightarrow H_2CO_3 \leftrightarrow HCO_3^- + H^+ \leftrightarrow CO_3^{-2} + 2H^+ \quad (25)$$

Figure 9-4 summarizes the major reactions in the transport of CO_2 in the body. Carbon dioxide can be transported to the lungs from the tissues in six forms. When CO_2 enters the plasma, it may: (1) remain dissolved in plasma; (2) become bound to plasma proteins to form carbamino compounds; or (3) join with water to form carbonic acid and then H^+ and HCO_3^-. However, most CO_2 enters the erythrocyte where it again may be: (1) present as dissolved CO_2; (2) become bound to the globin portion of hemoglobin; or (3) join with water to form carbonic acid and then H^+ and HCO_3^-. When CO_2 binds with the N-terminal amino group of HHb, carbaminohemoglobin is formed:

$$Hb \cdot NH_2 + CO_2 \leftrightarrow Hb \cdot NH \cdot COOH \text{ (carbaminohemoglobin)} \quad (26)$$

The formation of H_2CO_3 (Equation 25) occurs slowly in the plasma. The bulk of the CO_2 readily moves into the erythrocyte (CO_2 is freely permeable to all body compartments) because there is a pressure gradient favoring its diffusion in that direction. Inside the erythrocyte, carbonic anhydrase rapidly helps convert CO_2 to H^+ and HCO_3^-. This enzyme allows the reaction to occur 13,000 times faster than it would otherwise. The HCO_3^- then rapidly diffuses out of the erythrocyte into the plasma because there is now a greater concentration of HCO_3^- inside the erythrocyte than outside in the plasma, and the erythrocyte membrane is fairly permeable to this ion. To maintain electroneutrality, chloride ions (Cl^-) diffuse into the cell from the plasma (the so-called *chloride shift*). About 60% to 90% of the CO_2 is transported from the tissues to the lung in the form of HCO_3^-, with most of this having been formed within the erythrocyte, but then transferred out into the plasma for transport. Some 10% to 20% of the CO_2 is transported as carbamino compounds, with less than 10% being transported as dissolved CO_2.

HCO_3^- concentration is regulated by the kidneys and by nonbicarbonate buffers. However, it takes hours or days for the kidney to substantially change the HCO_3^- level in the plasma. In hypercapnia, the kidney will attempt to compensate for the increased acidosis by generating additional HCO_3^-. Therefore, increases in CO_2 (eg, owing to hypoventilation) will present as acidosis until the kidney can eventually compensate for the hypercapnia. A person is considered hypocapnic when the level of $PaCO_2$ is lower than normal limits (Table 9-1).

pH AND HYDROGEN IONS

The strength of an acid may be expressed in terms of its chemical potential (μH^+), the concentration of hydrogen ions (cH^+), or its relative molal activity (aH^+).[5] Hydrogen ion activity is commonly converted to pH (puissance hydrogen) by:

$$pH = -\log_{10} aH^+ \quad (27)$$

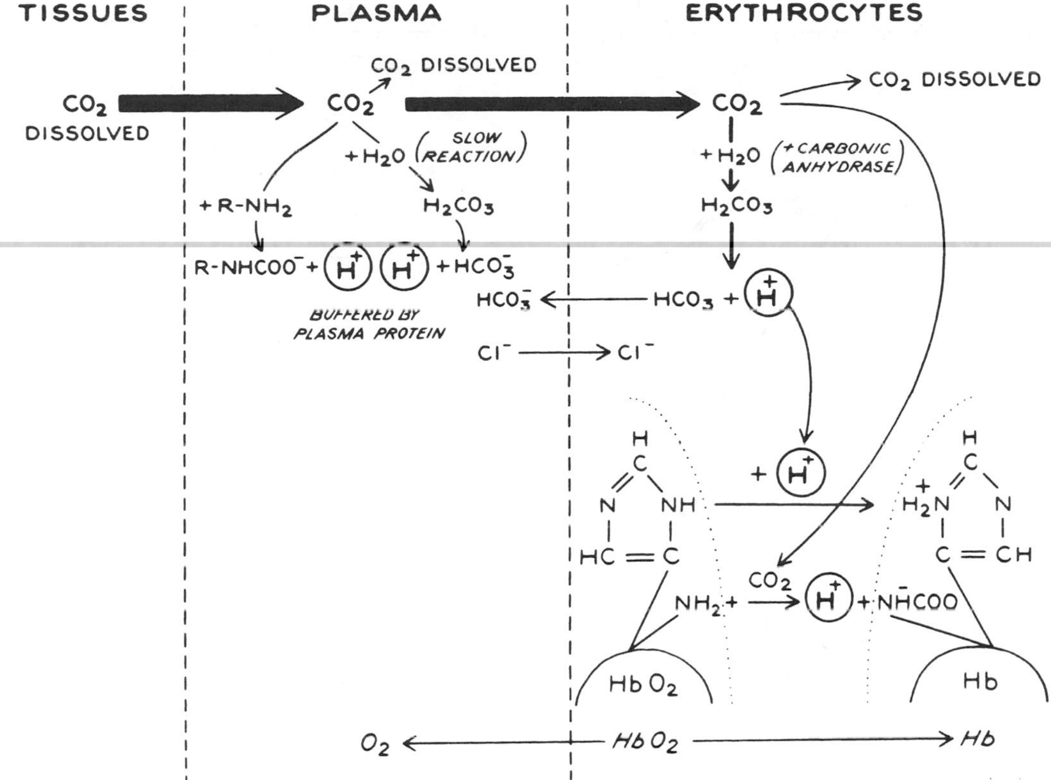

FIGURE 9-4. Carbon dioxide transport in blood. About 70% to 80% of CO_2 is transported as HCO_3^- in the plasma; 10% is carried as carbamino compounds both inside and outside the cell; and about 7% as dissolved CO_2. The reverse of these reactions occurs when the blood reaches the lungs, allowing rapid elimination of CO_2 (Comroe JH Jr: Physiology of Respiration. Chicago, Year Book Medical Publishers, 1974. Redrawn from Davenport H: The ABC of Acid-Base Chemistry, 5th ed. Chicago, University of Chicago Press, 1969)

Some investigators prefer to use concentration rather than activity and routinely convert pH to cH^+ by:

$$cH^+ = [\text{antilog } (9 - pH)] \text{ nmol/L} \quad (28)$$

Because enzymes require a narrow pH range to catalyze biochemical reactions, the body strives to maintain extracellular pH between 7.35 and 7.45. Any deviations from this range can have dire biological consequences. The buffering system of the body incorporates HCO_3^-, hemoglobin, proteins, and phosphate (PO_4^-). Because all of these buffers are in equilibrium, changes in one concentration will affect all the others.

The exact relationship between pH, PCO_2, and HCO_3^- is represented by the Henderson-Hasselbalch equation:

$$pH = pK + \log [HCO_3^-]/[H_2CO_3] \quad (29)$$

where pK is the negative logarithm of the HCO_3^- dissociation constant. For HCO_3^-, $pK = -\log [7.85 \times 10^{-7}] = 6.1$. The concentration of H_2CO_3 can be expressed by multiplying the $PaCO_2$ by the CO_2 solubility constant: $[0.03 \times PaCO_2]$. The Henderson-Hasselbalch equation can thus be reduced to:

$$pH = 6.1 + \log [HCO_3^-]/[0.03 \times PaCO_2] \quad (30)$$

Assuming a normal $PaCO_2$ of 40 mmHg ($0.03 \times 40 = 1.2$ mEq/L) and a normal HCO_3^- of 24 mEq/L, the pH of a sample will be:

$$pH = 6.1 + \log (24/1.2) = 7.40 \text{ pH units} \quad (31)$$

HCO_3^- should always be calculated from the measured pH and $PaCO_2$, which can be performed by the blood gas instrument, by using a nomogram (see Figure 9-5), or by the following equations:

$$[HCO_3^-] = \text{antilog } (pH - 6.1)\ 0.03\ CO_2 \quad (32)$$

or

$$[HCO_3^-]_p = 10^y \quad (33)$$

where y = pH + log10 $PaCO_2$ − 7.604; where 7.604 is the apparent pK, which includes the pH electrode correction factor of 0.01 pH units. The plasma HCO_3^- (also known as actual HCO_3^-) is the preferred index of metabolic acid–base status.[5]

The plasma HCO_3^-, to a small degree, is quickly affected by respiratory changes. Many experienced physicians simply make a quantitative mental correction of the HCO_3^- for the respiratory effect. The effect is never greater than about 4 mEq/L of HCO_3^-.

In general, the kidneys regulate HCO_3^- and the lungs regulate $PaCO_2$. If any two of the three principal acid–base parameters (pH, $PaCO_2$, or HCO_3^-) are known or can be estimated, the third can be accurately determined by equations or by nomogram. Therefore, the

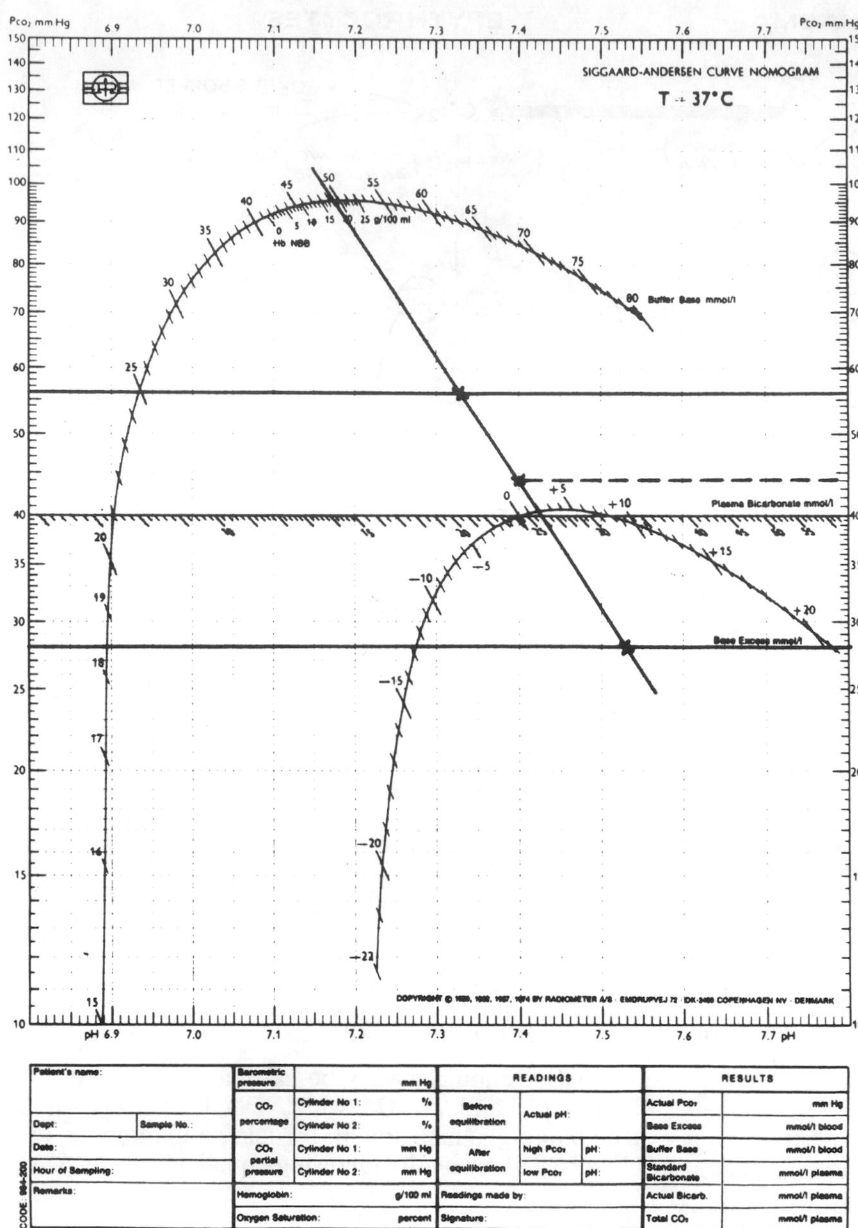

FIGURE 9-5. Siggaard–Andersen curve nomogram: **(1)** pH values are measured after equilibration, and the two points are plotted versus known PCO_2; **(2)** a line is drawn between the two points and extended to intersect the buffer base and base excess curves (these values are read directly); **(3)** an approximate hemoglobin for purposes of quality control can be interpolated by subtracting the value of the BE curve from the BB curve reading directly below BB on the hemoglobin scale; **(4)** actual pH is plotted along this line, and the PCO_2 is read off the vertical axis; **(5)** the line itself intersects HCO_3^- at a PCO_2 of 40 mmHg, thus indicating the standard HCO_3^-; **(6)** to determine actual plasma HCO_3^-, a 45° angle must be constructed through the actual pH until it intersects the HCO_3^- scale. Calculation of buffer base, base excess, and standard bicarbonate uses another modification of the Siggaard–Andersen nomogram. (Reproduced, with modifications, by permission of Siggaard–Andersen O and Radiometer A/S, Copenhagen, 1962)

Henderson-Hasselbalch equation can be conceptualized as:

$$pH \sim HCO_3^-/PaCO_3 \sim \text{kidney/lung} \sim \text{metabolic component/respiratory component} \quad (34)$$

CLINICAL APPLICATIONS

Normal Values

Blood gas measurements are affected by numerous factors such as: gender, the position of the body during the collection procedure, altitude, level of anxiety (ie, changes in $\dot{V}$), and diet.[27] Other important factors are the temperature within the blood vessel, the FIO_2, the site from which the blood sample is drawn, and the method of analysis. Ranges for normal values for arterial blood gases are shown in Table 9-1. These normal values for blood gases and hemoglobin derivatives are based on a group of normal adult subjects at sea level where the source of blood is from a peripheral artery.

Panic Values

Panic values, shown in Table 9-6, are those values that represent imminent life-threatening conditions. The Clinical Laboratory Improvement Amendment of 1988 (CLIA-88) mandates that laboratories have a procedure in place to communicate panic values to the medical team. It should always be remembered that blood gas values should be interpreted collectively and with regard to the patient's underlying condition because an accurate diagnosis is seldom dependent on a single measured parameter. A pH value that represents an extreme acidotic or alkalotic condition, whether caused by metabolic or res-

TABLE 9-6. **Suggested "Panic Values" Ranges (Values That May Require Immediate Therapeutic Intervention) for Arterial Blood Gas Results**

pH	<	7.20 pH U
pH	>	7.60 pH U
PCO_2	>	65 mmHg*
PO_2	<	50 mmHg†
COHb	>	20%
MetHb	>	10%

NOTE. Clinicians should remember to interpret all blood gas values collectively and with regard to the patient's underlying condition because an accurate diagnosis is seldom dependent on a single measured parameter.

* Only in cases with a marked decrease in pH; check HCO_3^- to see if renal compensation has occurred.

† Except for patients who have been diagnosed with some congenital cardiac malformations.

piratory failure, is potentially life-threatening. Therefore extreme pH values (pH < 7.20 or pH > 7.60) are considered to be panic values. A PaO_2 that denotes extreme hypoxemia represents a critical situation except for patients who have been diagnosed with congenital cardiac abnormalities. An elevated $PaCO_2$ is life-threatening above 65 mmHg when it is associated with a marked decrease in pH as in acute respiratory failure. However, an elevated $PaCO_2$ measurement taken alone does not necessarily indicate an imminent life-threatening condition. For example, this same $PaCO_2$ is not life-threatening if the kidneys have compensated to bring the pH to near-normal levels (as is commonly seen in patients with COPD). A COHb concentration >20% represents a serious condition, especially in persons diagnosed with cardiac disease as does an elevated MetHb concentration (>10%); both will reduce the number of potential hemoglobin binding sites. Elevated concentrations of PaO_2 (hyperoxemia) are potentially toxic but they do not represent imminent life-threatening patient conditions.

Acid–Base Disturbances

Respiratory acidosis is caused by H^+ accumulation as a result of hypercapnia. Respiratory acidosis may be caused by overall hypoventilation associated with respiratory center depression and neuromuscular disturbances in the presence of normal lungs, or it may indicate respiratory failure associated with COPD or other lung diseases. Respiratory acidosis may be acute or chronic depending on duration. An acute *respiratory alkalosis* is a sudden primary loss of CO_2 (eg, hyperventilation). Chronic respiratory alkalosis is the primary loss of H_2CO_3 or CO_2 of sufficient duration to allow for renal adjustment. Respiratory alkalosis is commonly associated with hyperventilation, interstitial lung diseases, pulmonary embolism, asthma, and severe hypoxemia. *Metabolic acidosis* is the primary accumulation of noncarbonic acid (eg, in diabetic ketoacidosis and lactic acidosis), the reduction in excretion of acids (eg, in renal failure), or the exogenous addition of acids in the blood. In chronic metabolic acidosis, an equilibrium of slowly permeable electrolytes (eg, HCO_3^-) occurs along with respiratory compensation. Metabolic acidosis is likely when the pH is less than normal, the HCO_3^- is either low or less than normal, and the $PaCO_2$ is at near-normal levels. Metabolic acidosis may also result from a loss of HCO_3^- and a resultant loss of HCO_3^- buffering (eg, diarrhea, excess renal loss, ileostomy loss). If a primary metabolic acidosis occurs, within minutes the lungs will begin to compensate by altering alveolar $\dot{V}$ to change the $PaCO_2$. It may take up to 12 hours for the lungs to compensate maximally. *Metabolic alkalosis* is primarily caused by a loss of H^+. This is associated with hypokalemia (decreased serum potassium) or increased HCO_3^- (eg, exogenous IV or oral $NaHCO_3$ administration).

Table 9-7 summarizes the causes for the conventional acid–base disturbances. There are also combined or mixed acid–base disturbances that include elements of both metabolic and respiratory disorders. For example, a patient can have a chronic respiratory acidosis that is superimposed on a metabolic alkalosis.

In Vitro and In Vivo Buffer Systems

The effectiveness of a buffer system is proportional to its concentration. Most of the nonbicarbonate buffers of the extracellular fluid (ECF) are concentrated in the blood, but PCO_2 and HCO_3^- are rather evenly distributed in the interstitial fluid as well as in the blood plasma. Because the ECF volume is about three times the blood volume in an adult, the effective concentration and, hence, the buffering power of nonbicarbonate buffers in the entire ECF are only about a third of that

TABLE 9-7 **Causes of Conventional Acid-Base Disturbances**

Respiratory Acidosis

- Hypoventilation (drug overdose, head injury, neuromuscular disturbance, kyphoscoliosis)
- Chronic obstructive pulmonary disease (COPD)
- Pulmonary edema

Respiratory Alkalosis

- Neurogenic hyperventilation
- Interstitial lung disease
- Pulmonary embolism
- Acute asthma
- Hyperventilation syndrome

Metabolic Acidosis

- Increased metabolic acid formation (eg, diabetic ketoacidosis, uremic, and lactic acidosis)
- Exogenous acid (ammonium chloride, hydrochloric acid)
- Loss of bicarbonate (diarrhea, ileostomy loss, renal tubular acidosis)
- Exogenous administration of acetazolamide (Diamox)

Metabolic Alkalosis

- Loss of H^+ (nasogastric suction, vomiting, diuretic therapy, steroid therapy)
- Exogenous bicarbonate administration

in the blood. It is these considerations that cause the arterial blood in a living subject to react differently than the same blood in a test tube when subjected to changes in PCO_2. In vitro corrections are calculations based on the buffering power of whole blood in the test tube.

Blood Gas Parameters

Through the years, opinions have changed regarding what are the most clinically relevant parameters in acid–base physiology. They have partly depended on the particular acid–base disorder and partly on the availability of analytical methods. Today, for a nearly complete description of the oxygenation, ventilation, and acid–base status, blood gases (eg, pH, $PaCO_2$, and PaO_2) and the calculated plasma (actual) HCO_3^- are generally sufficient. If information regarding O_2 transport and content is required, the levels of ctHb and percentages of hemoglobin derivatives (ie, CO-oximetry) are also important.

The literature contains literally hundreds of calculated parameters that incorporate these basic quantities, and the actual clinical benefit for most of them has not been adequately demonstrated. However, some of these are discussed in this chapter.

□ STANDARD BICARBONATE

The standard HCO_3^- has been defined as the plasma HCO_3^- concentration when the blood has been equilibrated at a PCO_2 of 40 mmHg, a temperature of 37 °C, and the hemoglobin is 100% saturated with O_2. This measurement theoretically allows one to look at the "metabolic component" of a plasma HCO_3^-, eliminating the "respiratory component." For example, in acute respiratory failure, with a $PaCO_2$ of 85 mmHg, the plasma HCO_3^- may be slightly increased; however, the standard HCO_3^- would, in theory, still be normal. The acute elevation in plasma HCO_3^- as a result of the hypercapnia is caused by an increased respiratory component rather than by a metabolic increase in HCO_3^-. The normal standard HCO_3^- is 22 to 26 mEq/L. The standard HCO_3^- works fairly satisfactorily to correct for the respiratory component of HCO_3^- when hypocapnia ($PaCO_2 < 35$ mmHg) is present. However, in the presence of hypercapnia it is unreliable, as explained in the discussion of "In Vivo Corrections" below.

□ BLOOD BUFFER BASE

The blood buffer base (BB_b) includes the total concentration of anions in the blood available to buffer the H^+ chemically or by elimination of CO_2. The buffer base thus includes HCO_3^-, hemoglobin, plasma proteins, and phosphates. The normal buffer base with a hemoglobin value of 15 g/dL is 48 mEq/L.

In pure respiratory acid–base disturbances, the buffer base theoretically should remain normal. For example, in acute hypercapnia:

$$\uparrow CO_2 + H_2O \rightarrow H_2CO_2 \rightarrow \underset{\substack{+ \\ BUF^- \\ \downarrow \\ HBUF}}{H^+} + HCO_3^- \qquad (35)$$

The BUF^- includes hemoglobin, plasma proteins, and phosphate buffers. An increased $PaCO_2$ results not only in an increased H^+ level, but also in an increased plasma HCO_3^- level as well. However, the interaction with the other buffer systems results in an equal reduction in the nonbicarbonate buffers (BUF^-). Because the buffer base comprises HCO_3^- and the other buffers (BUF^-), the total buffer base should remain normal in the presence of a pure respiratory acid-base disorder. However, in vitro and in vivo changes in buffer base in response to changes in $PaCO_2$ are different, as described later in this chapter. In vitro determinations are fairly satisfactory in the presence of hypocapnia, as is explained in "In Vivo Corrections" below. Changes in buffer base are commonly described in terms of base excess.

□ BASE EXCESS OF BLOOD

Base excess of the blood (BE_b) is another way of reflecting an increase or decrease in the buffer base. Normally, the BE_b is -2 to $+2$ mEq/L. A BE_b greater than $+2$ means that acid has been removed or that base has been added; and a BE_b less than -2 means that acid has been added or that base has been removed. The BE_b represents the amount of fixed acid needed to titrate the blood pH to 7.40 after the blood has been equilibrated to a PCO_2 of 40 mmHg. The negative BE_b would require titration with a base, which can be calculated accurately from Figure 9-6.

This is an elegant way to quantify the metabolic component of the blood, but unfortunately it is an in vitro measurement. The BE_b will not change if CO_2 is added to the blood in vitro, but if it is added to the blood in vivo, the BE_b will decrease, as shown in Figure 9-7. Therefore, this test is of limited usefulness in the presence of hypercapnia. When hypocapnia is present, BE_b is a fairly reliable indicator of plasma HCO_3^-.

□ IN VIVO CORRECTIONS

In vivo corrections have the theoretical advantage of representing the state of the entire ECF compartment, not just blood. The T_{40} bicarbonate (discussed below) and the base excess of the ECF (BE_{ECF}) are available in vivo measurements and are calculated essentially the same way as the standard HCO_3^- and BE_b, but the buffer value of the ECF is used instead of that of blood. An acute elevation of $PaCO_2$ owing to alveolar hypoventilation does result in an increase in plasma HCO_3^- and a decrease in the other buffers; however, because the capillary wall is permeable to HCO_3^- but not to the principal nonbicarbonate buffers (ie, proteins), some of the HCO_3^- formed in response to acute hypercapnia diffuses through the capillary wall and into the interstitial fluid. The HCO_3^- formed as a direct result of the buffer response to acute hypercapnia is distributed throughout the ECF space; thus, the increase in blood HCO_3^- is only about one third of what would be seen in an in vitro system with a single volume of distribution. Therefore, the in vivo increase in plasma HCO_3^- in response to acute CO_2 retention is less than would occur in vitro, making

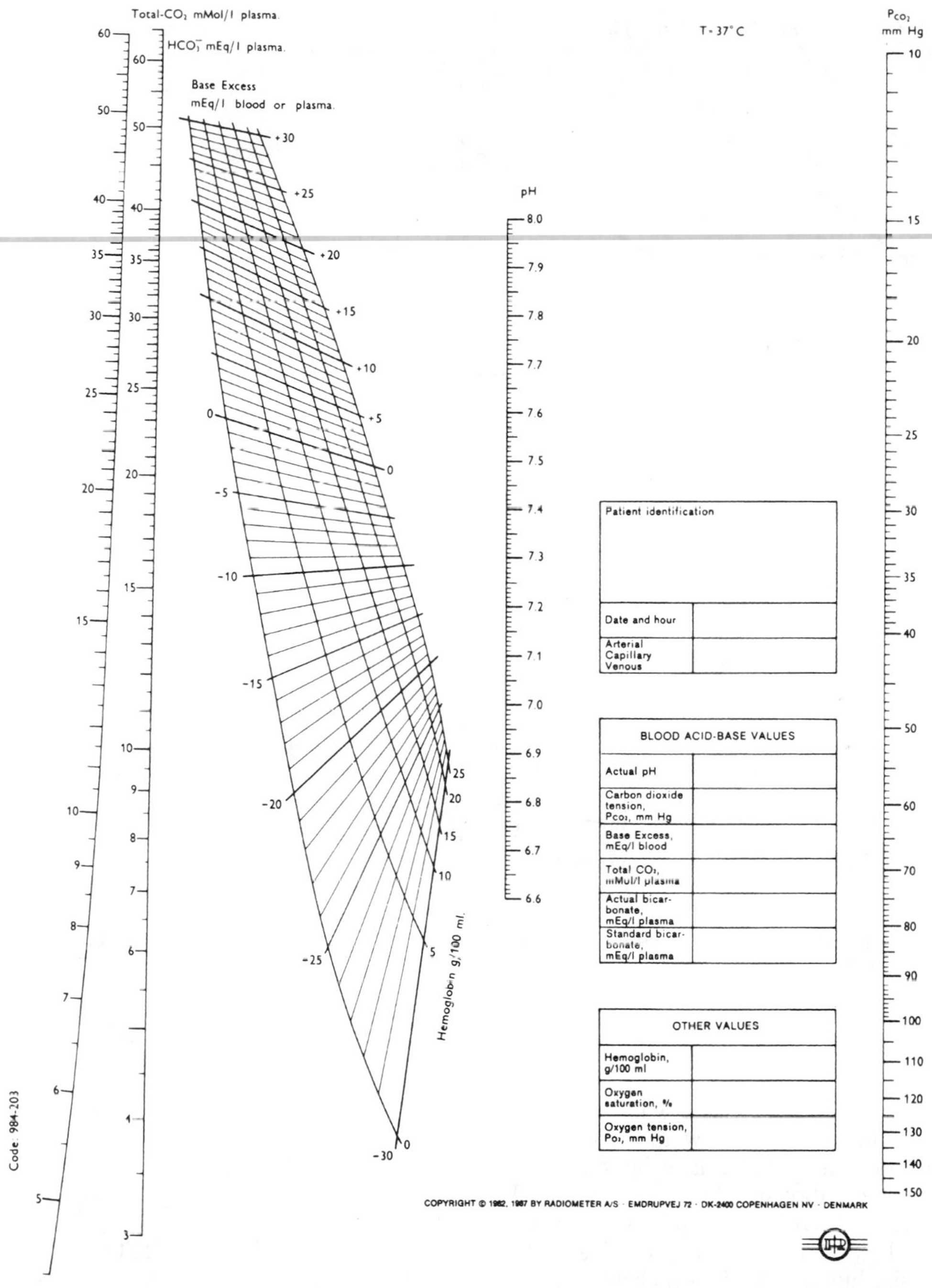

FIGURE 9-6. Siggaard–Andersen alignment nomogram: (1) a line is constructed between pH and PCO_2; (2) actual plasma HCO_3^- is read directly at the intersection of the line; (3) BE_b is hemoglobin-dependent and can be read at the intersection of the constructed line and the patient's Hb value; (4) standard HCO_3^- can be determined by constructing another line through the BE_b–Hb point, and a PCO_2 of 40 mmHg, and by reading the HCO_3^- scale; (5) buffer base can be computed from the equation $BB = 41.7 + (0.42 \times Hb) + BE$; (6) BE_{ECF} is calculated similarly to the BE_b, but the BE_{ECF} is read off at the intersection of the constructed line and one-third of the patient's Hb value; (7) T_{40} HCO_3^- can be determined by constructing another line through the BE_{ECF}, Hb/3 point, and a PCO_2 of 40 mmHg, and by reading the HCO_3^- scale. (Reproduced with modifications, by permission of Siggaard–Andersen O and Radiometer A/S, Copenhagen, 1963)

the standard HCO_3^-, BB_b, and BE_b unreliable indicators of the metabolic component of the plasma HCO_3^- during acute hypercapnia. Because the reduction in nonbicarbonate buffers is the same but the increase in plasma HCO_3^- is less than would occur in vitro, the total BB_b or BE_b may, in fact, decrease in association with acute hypercapnia. In this situation, the decrease in BB_b or BE_b would not then represent a superimposed metabolic disturbance (eg, metabolic acidosis), but would be related only to the in vivo response to acute CO_2 retention.

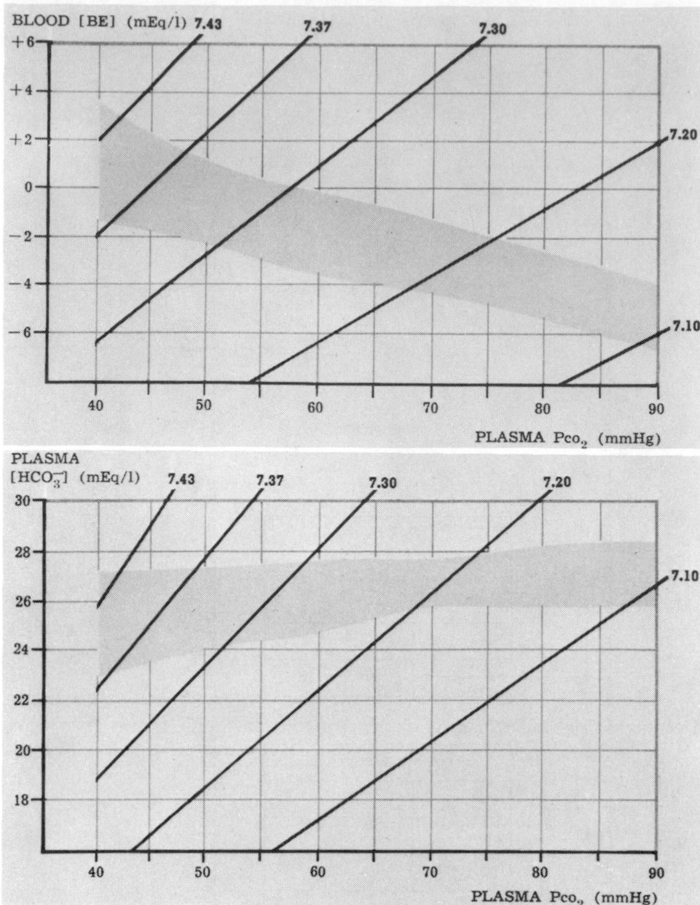

FIGURE 9-7. Ninety-five percent confidence-limit bands for acute CO_2 retention. Note that the blood base excess does drop below −2 with acute CO_2 retention even though there has been no change in "metabolic component." (Winters RW et al: Acid–Base Physiology in Medicine. 2nd ed. Cleveland, London Co, 1969)

Superficially, it appears that the pathway of acute hypocapnia is the same for in vitro blood as for a living subject. The effect of acute hypocapnia on in vitro blood is exactly what would be predicted by extrapolation from hypercapnia experiments. Frequently, in the living subject, a true superimposed metabolic acidosis is caused by lactic acidosis. The lactic acidosis may be produced by a reduced blood flow to some tissues caused by hypocapnia and alkalemia or by reduced excretion or reduced metabolism of lactate owing to the same causes. The T_{40} bicarbonate and base excess of ECF (discussed below) reveal the presence of this metabolic acidosis, but the in vitro measures do not show it. With hypocapnia, in vitro and in vivo changes in standard HCO_3^-, buffer base, and base excess are similar.

□ T_{40} BICARBONATE

Because it was recognized that, with acute hypercapnia, the increase in plasma HCO_3^- that occurs in vivo is less than that which occurs in vitro, and therefore, that in vitro nomograms used to calculate standard HCO_3^- might be invalid, a new calculation, known as the T_{40} bicarbonate was developed.[28] A method of calculating it graphically is shown in Figure 9-6. A bedside estimation can be done by assuming that an acute increase in $PaCO_2$ of about 15 mmHg will increase the plasma HCO_3^- by about 1 mEq/L. The change in plasma HCO_3^- expected to occur with acute CO_2 retention would be:

$$\Delta HCO_3^- = (\text{observed } PaCO_2 - 40)/15 \qquad (36)$$

The T_{40} bicarbonate is equal to the observed plasma HCO_3^- minus the HCO_3^- expected to occur secondary to the acute CO_2 elevation. For example, if the $PaCO_2$ equals 85 mmHg, then:

$$\Delta HCO_3^- = (85 - 40)/15 = 3 \text{ mEq/L} \qquad (37)$$

If the observed plasma HCO_3^- = 28 mEq/L, then in this example, it follows that:

$$T_{40} \text{ bicarbonate} = 28 - 3 = 25 \text{ mEq/L} \qquad (38)$$

Therefore, in this example, the slightly elevated HCO_3^- was caused by acute CO_2 retention and did not indicate increased metabolic HCO_3^-.

Because changes in plasma HCO_3^- with acute CO_2 retention are different in vivo than in vitro, T_{40} bicarbonate is a more reliable measure than is the standard HCO_3^- in patients with acute hypercapnia. In acute hypocapnia, T_{40} bicarbonate may also be more reliable than standard HCO_3^- because it can detect the concomitant lactic acidosis better than the standard HCO_3^- does.

For estimating the decrease in T_{40} bicarbonate in the presence of acute CO_2 reduction ($PaCO_2$ less than 35 mmHg),[29] a ratio of 5:1 ($PaCO_2$/plasma HCO_3^-) should be used. The T_{40} bicarbonate becomes more inaccurate when a large metabolic component is also present.

□ BASE EXCESS OF EXTRACELLULAR FLUID

The BE_{ECF} is easy to calculate accurately, even at the bedside, and is a measure of the metabolic component of the entire ECF, provided the patient has been in a quasi-steady state for about 10 minutes. It can be defined as the titratable basicity of the ECF. In other words, it represents the amount of fixed base or acid that would have to be added to the ECF to bring the pH to 7.40 after the $PaCO_2$ has been brought to 40 mmHg.[30]

The calculation is shown graphically in Figure 9-6. The BE_{ECF} is the deviation from the ECF buffer line. The BE_{ECF} can also be calculated using a quite accurate bedside calculation:

$$BE_{ECF} = \Delta HCO_3 + 10\ \Delta pH, \tag{39}$$

where

$$\Delta HCO_3^- = \text{actual } HCO_3^- - 24 \tag{40}$$

and

$$\Delta pH = \text{actual pH} - 7.40 \tag{41}$$

The approximate slope of the ECF buffer line is 10 mEq/L HCO_3^- per pH unit. (The slope depends on the hemoglobin concentration of the blood and on the ratio of blood volume to ECF volume). A slope of 11.6 was obtained in a group of normal subjects. The value of 10 makes the calculation easier.

□ COMPARISON OF IN VITRO AND IN VIVO MEASURES

By using the following set of numbers from an arterial blood analysis, the in vitro and in vivo measures are compared:

	MEASURED	NORMAL
pH	7.14	7.35–7.45
$PaCO_2$	85 mmHg	35–45 mmHg
Plasma HCO_3^-	28 mEq/L	22–26 mEq/L
Standard HCO_3^-	21 mEq/L	22–26 mEq/L
$T_{40}HCO_3^-$	25 mEq/L	22–26 mEq/L
BB_b	44 mEq/L	46–50 mEq/L
BE_b	−4 mEq/L	−2 to +2 mEq/L
BE_{ECF}	1.4 mEq/L	−2 to +2 mEq/L

The BE_{ECF} in this example, is derived as follows:

$$\begin{aligned} BE_{ECF} &= (\Delta HCO_3^-) + 10\ (\Delta pH) \\ &= (28 - 24) + 10(7.14 - 7.40) \\ &= (4) + 10(-0.26) \\ &= 4 - 2.6 \\ &= 1.4 \text{ mEq/L} \end{aligned}$$

The plasma HCO_3^- is slightly elevated; however, the T_{40} HCO_3^- and the BE_{ECF} are normal, which indicates that the increased plasma HCO_3^- is of respiratory origin, from the hypercapnia, rather than of metabolic origin. The reduced standard HCO_3^-, BB_b, and BE_b are inaccurate because they are derived from in vitro observations that are different from in vivo observations in acute hypercapnia. The reduced BB_b and BE_b result from the leakage of HCO_3^- from the blood into perivascular tissues, which occurs in vivo with acute hypercapnia. The normal BE_{ECF} accurately indicates that this is a pure respiratory acidosis, with a normal metabolic component.

□ INTERPRETATION OF ACID–BASE DISORDERS

In attempting to properly interpret acid–base disorders, one must remember the basic relationship implied in the Henderson-Hasselbalch equation (Equation 34). Two of the three factors (pH, $PaCO_2$, and/or HCO_3^-) in this relationship must be known to properly evaluate the acid–base disturbance.

When interpreting acid–base data, one should look at the pH to determine whether acidemia or alkalemia is present, remembering that a normal pH does not rule out an acid–base disorder. If the pH is in the normal range (7.35 to 7.45) and the $PaCO_2$ and HCO_3^- are in their normal ranges, then the acid–base status is normal. If the pH is below 7.35, then an acidemia exists. If the pH is above 7.45, an alkalemia exists.

When the pH is outside the normal range, the cause must be determined. One must then look at the $PaCO_2$ value to see if it is above or below its normal range (35 to 45 mmHg). The same must then be done with the HCO_3^- value to see if it is above or below its normal range (22 to 26 mEq/L). Whichever parameter is out of the normal range will reveal the system responsible. For example, if the pH is on the acid side (below 7.35) and the $PaCO_2$ is greater than 45 mmHg, a respiratory acidemia exists. If the kidneys are functioning normally, they will start retaining HCO_3^- to offset the respiratory acid (CO_2). If the HCO_3^- is still in the normal range when the arterial blood gas was obtained, the respiratory condition would be identified as an acute respiratory acidemia. However, if the pH was in the normal range with the $PaCO_2$ above 45 mmHg, most likely the body has compensated for the hypercapnia. Because the kidney takes a while to respond to changes in CO_2, this second condition would be termed chronic or compensated respiratory acidemia. When the pH is in the normal range, but the $PaCO_2$ and HCO_3^- are not, the primary problem can usually be determined by noting the direction the pH has moved from 7.40. Any value above 7.40 is toward the alkaline side. Any value below a pH of 7.40 is toward the acid side. Because the body will not overcompensate, finding the pH on the acid side (below 7.40) suggests that the primary problem is too much "acid." Since, in our chronic respiratory acidosis example, the CO_2 is also on the "acid side" (ie, $>$ 45 mmHg), the respiratory system is likely responsible for the primary problem. Remember that large changes in pH (from normal) suggest an acute process. Small changes in pH, with large deviations in $PaCO_2$ or HCO_3^- suggest a chronic process.

Not all acid–base disturbances are as straightforward as the preceding example. The use of acid–base nomograms or acid–base rules of thumb (Table 9-8) can help

TABLE 9-8 **Rules of Thumb to Determine If Simple or Mixed Acid–Base Disorder Exists***

Condition	$PaCO_2$ (mmHg)	HCO_3^- (mEq/L)
Acute hypercapnia	↑10	↑1
Chronic hypercapnia	↑10	↑3.5
Acute hypocapnia	↓10	↓2
Chronic hypocapnia	↓10	↓4.5
Metabolic acidosis†	↓12	↓10
Metabolic alkalosis	↑ 6	↑10

* The changes (increase or decrease as indicated by the arrows) are from normal values, $PaCO_2$ of 40 mmHg and HCO_3^- of 24 mEq/L. For a "simple" disorder to exist, a given change in $PaCO_2$ will result in the predicted change in HCO_3^-. If the suggested change is not present, then a mixed acid–base disorder is very likely.

† The formula: $PaCO_2 = (1.54 \times HCO_3^-) + 8.36$ can be used for determining the expected $PaCO_2$ for a "simple" metabolic acidosis.

one decide whether a given change in CO_2 or HCO_3^- alone will account for the change in pH.

When evaluating the metabolic component, the plasma HCO_3^- is what one should consider first. However, because there is a small respiratory component to the plasma HCO_3^-, the T_{40} bicarbonate and the BE_{ECF} more accurately reflect the metabolic component of the plasma HCO_3^- in the presence of hypercapnia.

One should decide whether "compensation" is present. If a primary respiratory acidosis has occurred, for example, within hours the intracellular buffers will contribute to an increase in plasma HCO_3^- and BE_{ECF}. Also within hours, the kidney will begin to alter the plasma HCO_3^- in an attempt to compensate for the respiratory disturbance. The kidney response is slow, requiring 72 hours or more for maximal effect. If a primary metabolic disorder occurs, within minutes the lungs will begin to compensate for the metabolic disorder by altering the alveolar ventilation to change the $PaCO_2$. It may take up to 12 hours for the lungs to compensate maximally. In the past, the presence or absence of compensation has been categorized as follows:

1. Uncompensated. The presence of an abnormal pH owing to deviation of one component ($PaCO_2$ or HCO_3^-), with the other component still within normal limits (eg, presence of metabolic acidosis with a $PaCO_2$ still within the normal range).
2. Partially compensated. Deviation of one component with the other component changing appropriately to compensate for the acid–base disorder. However, the pH is still abnormal.
3. Completely compensated. Deviation of one component with an appropriate change of the other component so that the pH has been restored to normal (ie, between 7.35 and 7.45).

It is now well recognized that with a major deviation from normal of one component, it is not possible for the other component to restore the pH to normal; for example, with severe diabetic ketoacidosis, it is impossible for the lungs to increase alveolar ventilation sufficiently to reduce the $PaCO_2$ to the extent by which the pH would be restored to normal. Also, in the presence of severe chronic respiratory failure, the normal kidney will not regenerate enough HCO_3^- to return the pH to the normal range.

Because physiologic compensatory mechanisms are unable to fully return the pH to normal for major deviations in acid–base status, it has become apparent that determining the extent to which one could maximally return the pH toward normal would be more appropriate. Studies in animals and humans have helped determine the degree of compensation that can be expected for any given disturbance.

One way of evaluating the compensation is to consider the acid–base data from such studies. In a group of 100 subjects, the results are distributed in a bell-shaped curve. It has become acceptable to compare a patient's acid–base data with the middle 95% of the curve, recognizing that 2.5% of patients will fall below and 2.5% will fall above the middle 95%. These data have been developed into 95% confidence-limit bands that aid in the proper interpretation of various acid–base disturbances. These bands have been developed for both acute and chronic acid–base disturbances. For example, in the presence of acute hypercapnia, one can determine the appropriate pH, plasma HCO_3^-, BE_b (see Figure 9-7), or BE_{ECF} (Figure 9-8) for any given $PaCO_2$. In the presence of chronic hypercapnia, one can determine the expected pH to be achieved for a given level of $PaCO_2$ (see Figure 9-8); for example, a $PaCO_2$ of 85 mmHg and a pH of 7.38, under the old acid–base terminology, would be interpreted as a completely compensated respiratory acidosis. However, examination of this point on Figure 9-8 reveals that it lies considerably to the right of the 95% confidence band for chronic hypercapnia, indicating that the level of plasma HCO_3^- and BE_{ECF} is inappropriately high for this $PaCO_2$ and that the patient has a chronic respiratory acidosis with a superimposed metabolic alkalosis.

The proper terminology for compensation using 95% confidence-limit bands would express the compensation as "maximal" or "less than maximal" (see Figure 9-8 for further examples of 95% confidence-limit bands). It is impossible to interpret acid–base disorders accurately and completely without a knowledge of: (1) the duration of the acid–base disturbance (observation of serial arterial blood gas values are often helpful for this); (2) patient's clinical condition (ie, whether disorders are present that could lead to respiratory or metabolic acid–base disturbances); and (3) the electrolytes (ie, the anion gap). Occasionally, one will have a "combined" or "mixed" acid–base disturbance; for example, if changes in both the $PaCO_2$ and plasma HCO_3^- would result in acidosis, the patient would have a combined respiratory and metabolic acidosis. Mixed respiratory and metabolic alkalosis may also occur (see Table 9-7 for some causes of acid–base disturbances). Familiarity with the various causes of altered acid–base balance will facilitate proper treatment. To facilitate rapid bedside interpretation of acid–base disturbances when an acid–base nomogram is not available, Table 9-8 lists

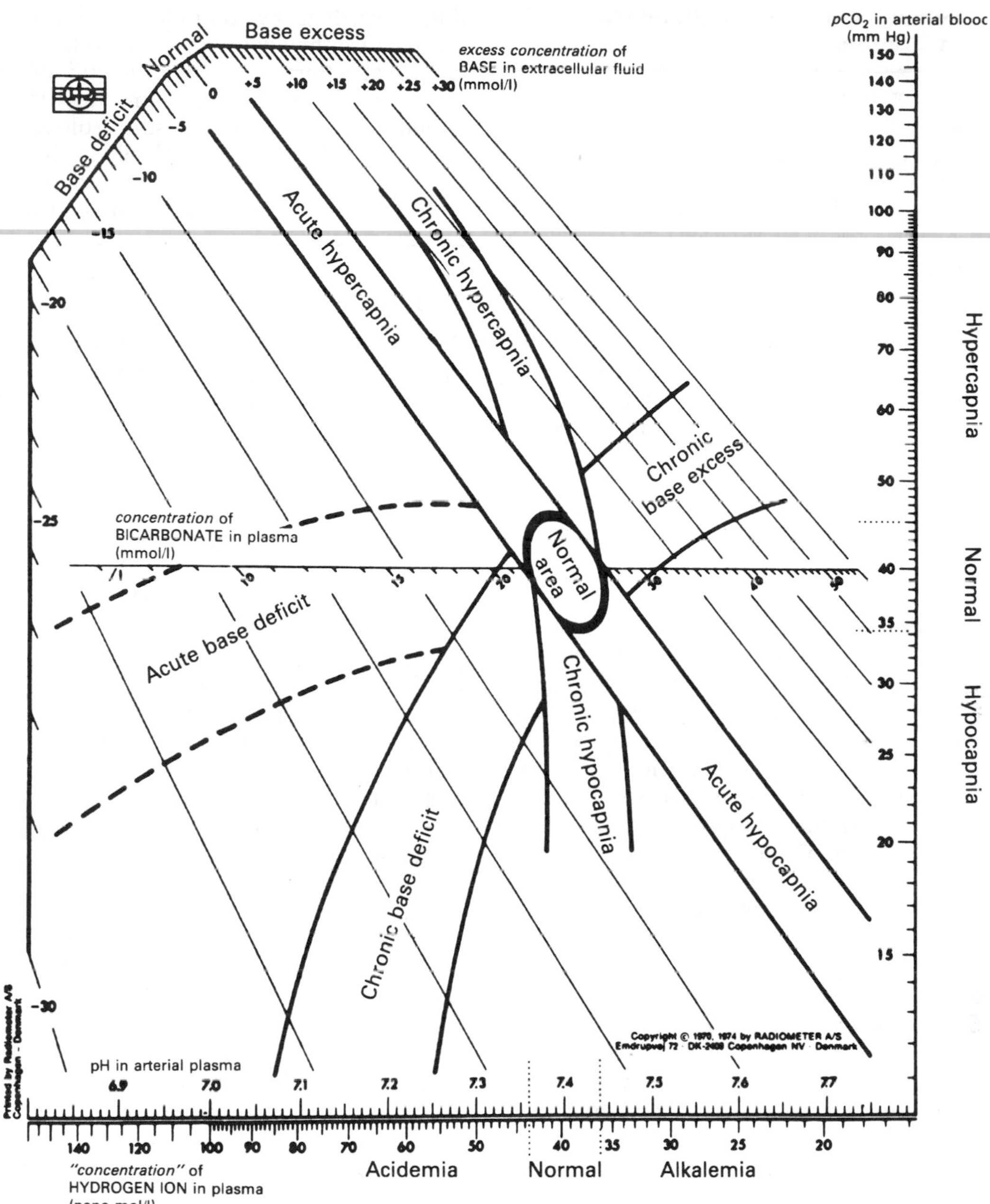

FIGURE 9-8. Depiction of 95% confidence-limit bands by Siggaard–Andersen. (Reproduced by permission of O. Siggaard–Andersen and Radiometer A/S, Copenhagen, 1971.) Note that extracellular fluid base excess (BE_{ECF}) is depicted on this in vivo nomogram.[17]

rules of thumb for determining if a simple acid–base disorder or mixed disorder exists. If the CO_2 or HCO_3^- values do not follow the rules, then there is a mixed acid–base disturbance present.

Table 9-9 summarizes the steps necessary for most blood gas interpretations. It is important to develop the habit of interpreting each blood gas report in a systematic way so as to not overlook important diagnostic information.

For useful guidelines relating to oxygenation and acid–base disorders, see Appendix A.

□ ANION GAP

According to the law of electroneutrality, the sum of the concentrations of positively charged ions (cations: Na^+, Ca^+, K^+, and Mg^+) must equal the concentrations of the negatively charged ions (anions: Cl^-, Pr^-, HCO_3^-, HPO_4^{-2}, SO_4^{-2}, and organic anions) so that a constant ionic balance in the ECF is maintained. However, only three of these ions (Na^+, Cl^-, and HCO_3^-) are generally used in the calculation of anion gap. As seen in Figure 9-9, the value for Na^+ (140 mEq/L) is used exclusively to represent the cations because it accounts for 95% of all the

TABLE 9-9. **Summary of Arterial Blood Gas Interpretation Guidelines**

1. Evaluate oxygenation status.
2. Check pH, then $PaCO_2$ and HCO_3^-.
3. Check if blood gas data is consistent with a simple disorder (use rules of thumb or nomogram).
4. Check anion gap, if a metabolic acidemia is present.
5. Compare interpretation with clinical history.

cations present. In this same figure, values for Cl^- (100 mEq/L) and HCO_3^- (25 mEq/L) are used to represent the anion concentration because they account for 85% of all anions present. As a result, there is a normal constant difference between the cations (+140) and measured anions (−125), which is termed the "anion gap."

The normal anion gap can vary between 8 and 16 mmol/L. Plasma albumin normally is responsible for about 11 mmol/L of the anion gap. Unlike cations, excess amounts of anions can occur frequently. If the sum of Cl^- and HCO_3^- decreases while the Na^+ concentration remains constant (see Fig. 9-9), the calculated difference or "gap" between the two types of charges will widen. Because no actual change in charge occurs (electroneutrality is always maintained), this means that an increase in negative charge must have been produced from some unknown source. By knowing that an increase in the anion gap exists, the source of the increased anions can be investigated. The "anion gap" concept may be helpful in identifying the cause of the metabolic acidosis. Table 9-10 lists some common causes that can affect the anion gap.

PRE-ANALYTICAL GUIDELINES FOR BLOOD GAS SAMPLES

According to CLIA-88, laboratories must monitor and evaluate their criteria for sample handling and collection. More than any other clinical laboratory test, blood gas data can be adversely affected by a variety of pre-analytical factors. Consequently, guidelines for proper specimen collection and handling have been published.[31,32] For optimal results, blood gas samples should be collected anaerobically in gas-tight syringes, anticoagulated with a minimum amount of heparin, and analyzed before cellular metabolism can adversely affect the results.

Heparin

Excessive amounts of heparin salts can adversely affect blood gas results. Sodium heparin is an acid (6.39 pH units) and, in liquid form, its PCO_2 (7.6 mmHg) and PO_2 (134.6 mmHg) values approach those of ambient air.[33] One study showed a 25% decrease in $PaCO_2$ values when 0.25 mL of heparin was mixed with 1.0 mL of blood.[34] In another study, when 0.5 mL of 1000 U/mL heparin was mixed with 2 mL from different patient blood samples, the $PaCO_2$ subsequently decreased by an average of 12.9 mmHg, the PaO_2 decreased by an average of 9.3 mmHg, while the pH remained unaffected.[35] The reason the pH did not change may be because of the buffering characteristics of hemoglobin.[36] In general, a marked decrease in $PaCO_2$ measurements is the major pre-analytical error associated with excessive amounts of heparin. The PaO_2 value may be affected depending on the O_2 gradient that exists between the blood sample and the heparin.

Adequate anticoagulation of the blood, however, is also important because even microscopic blood clots can adversely affect the performance of blood gas instruments.[31] Therefore, when liquid heparin is used, 0.05 mL (of heparin concentration 1000 U/mL) should be used to anticoagulate 2.5 mL of blood.[37] The minimum amount of heparin to anticoagulate blood is much less than these amounts, but because it is difficult to adequately disperse the heparin in the syringe, it is advisable to use these stated amounts.

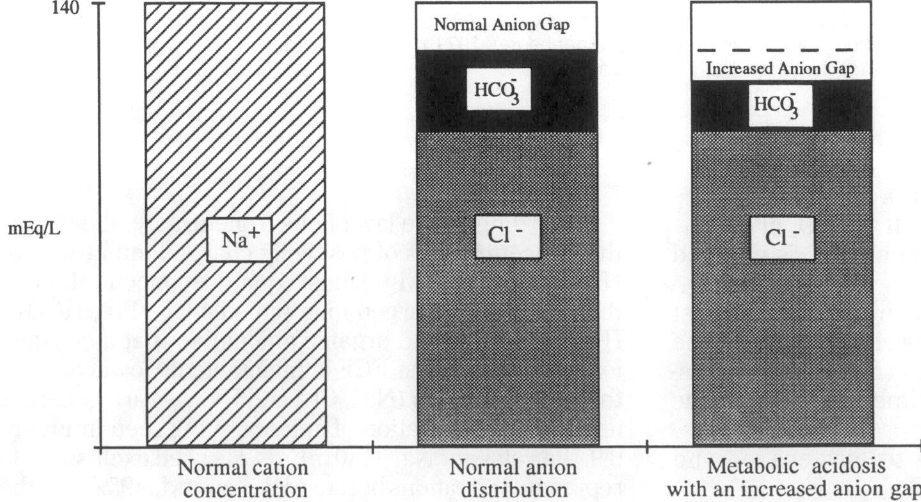

FIGURE 9-9. The graph shows the normal cation concentration (Na^+ ions), the normal distribution of anions with a normal anion gap, and a decreased HCO_3^- concentration caused by a concomitant increase in unmeasured anions and resulting in an abnormal anion gap. (Reprinted by permission of the Western Journal of Medicine: Haber RJ: A Practical Approach to Acid-Base Disorders, 1991, 155:149.)

TABLE 9-10 **Possible Causes for Increases or Decreases in the Anion Gap**

Causes of Increased anion Gap

- Increased unmeasured anion
  - Organic anions
    - Lactate
      - Shock
      - Severe hypoxemia
      - Carbon monoxide poisoning
      - Severe anemia
      - Adult respiratory distress syndrome
      - Severe exertion
      - Renal failure
      - Malignancies
    - Ketones
      - Diabetes mellitus
      - Starvation
      - Inherited metabolic defects
      - Alcohol
    - Urea
      - Uremic acidosis
  - Inorganic anions: phosphate, sulfate
  - Proteins: Increased albumin
  - Exogenous anions: salicylate, formate, nitrate, penicillin
  - Other: Ingestion of methanol, paraldehyde, ethylene glycol
- Decreased concentrations of cations (eg, K^+, Mg^{2+}, Ca^{2+})

Causes of Decreased Anion Gap

- Increased concentrations of cations (eg, K^+, Mg^{2+}, Ca^{2+})
- Retention of other abnormal cations
- Decreased albumin

Air Bubbles

Blood gas samples should be collected anaerobically because air bubbles left in the blood sample can cause changes in PaO_2 and $PaCO_2$.[38] When a small (55 µL or 2.75% of the volume of the blood sample) air bubble was injected into 2-mL blood samples, no increase in PaO_2 was found as long as the bubble was expelled within 30 seconds. When this same size air bubble was left in the syringe for 30 minutes, mean PaO_2 increased by 13.5 mmHg whereas mean $PaCO_2$ decreased by 1.2 mmHg.[39]

Time Delay

If the blood gas sample is anaerobically stored in an air-tight syringe before analysis, the degree of increased $PaCO_2$, decreased PaO_2, and increased acidity will correlate with storage temperature, time,[40] and the number of leukocytes in the blood.[41] Therefore, even anaerobically collected samples must be analyzed as quickly as possible. A pneumatic tube system is ideal for the transport of blood gas samples. In our institution (Stanford University Hospital), we found that most samples can be transported to the laboratory by pneumatic tube within 5 minutes. The effect of pre-analytical time delay is often dependent on the storage device used (type of syringe) as well as the storage temperature.

Blood Gas Syringes

Until the last decade, blood gas samples were typically drawn via in-dwelling catheters or a one-time needle puncture into a sterile, heparinized all-glass syringe. Because leukocytes continue to consume O_2 and excrete CO_2, blood gas samples drawn in glass syringes were placed in ice (0° C) during the pre-analytical storage period to slow the metabolism of these cells. Glass provides a very good barrier against leakage or intrusion of gases for up to 2 hours.[42,43] Glass syringes also provide for easy sample inspection and removal of air bubbles, permit minimal contamination, fill freely under arterial pressure, and provide for anaerobiosis during and after the collection process. In terms of biosafety, however, glass syringes are a considerable threat to staff because of the risk of breakage and possible skin puncture. In addition, the liquid sodium heparin anticoagulant, which is used as a lubricant for the glass, may make the sample susceptible to excessive heparin contamination if care is not taken.[34]

Plastic syringes, mostly made of polypropylene, have been widely accepted as a substitute for glass for clinical use. The O_2 permeability value for polypropylene (150 $cm^3/mL \cdot day \cdot 100\ in^2 \cdot atm$) is relatively high when compared with other barrier polymers,[44] and there was some concern regarding the clinical efficacy of plastic syringes for blood gas testing. Early studies were confusing as some investigators found clinical errors with the use of plastic,[39,43,45] whereas other studies found no clinically significant differences between plastic and glass.[46,47] In 1991, our laboratory (Stanford University Hospital) found that polypropylene syringes did indeed cause blood gas errors—but only under certain conditions.[48] The explanation was based on: (1) the relative strength of the chemical relationship between O_2 and hemoglobin (dependent on initial PO_2); (2) the amount of storage time in the syringe; and (3) the storage temperature. When iced, the PO_2 of blood temporarily decreased owing to a leftward shift in the oxyhemoglobin dissociation curve and an increased O_2 solubility in the plasma. These two factors act like an O_2 sink that attracts O_2 from the walls of the plastic.[43] Therefore, we advised laboratories not to ice blood gas samples in plastic syringes because they would be risking O_2 permeation, which might lead to sample contamination and errant blood gas reporting. In 1992, a European group reported comparable results and reached similar conclusions.[49] Based on this new evidence, the NCCLS warns laboratories of possible blood gas errors when polypropylene syringes are iced.[31]

To minimize the effects of cellular metabolism, blood gas samples collected in plastic syringes should be kept at room temperature and should be analyzed within 30 minutes of collection.[31] When blood samples are drawn for special studies that require accurate determinations of PaO_2 values above the normal physiologic range (eg, shunt studies), they should be kept at room temperature and analyzed within 10 minutes of collection to minimize changes in gas tensions.[31] If a prolonged pre-analytical storage period is anticipated

(>30 min), sterile glass syringes with close-fitting plungers should be used and the syringes should be placed in ice to minimize changes in the blood gas sample results.

OBTAINING BLOOD GAS SAMPLES

Safety

It is strongly recommended that all personnel comply with appropriate infection prevention policies and procedures in order to minimize the risk of transmission of nosocomial (hospital-associated) infections. Personnel should handle all blood specimens as if they are biohazardous and wear latex gloves (and other barrier protections if necessary) to minimize the risk of biohazard exposure. For further information, readers are referred to Centers for Disease Control (CDC) publications.[50]

Arterial Catheter

When multiple blood gas samples are needed, indwelling catheters provide rapid sampling and reduced physiologic stresses (hyperventilation or hypoventilation from pain is usually absent) and are usually well-tolerated. However, complications can occur, so strict placement and infection control protocols should be followed to avoid necrosis, infection,[51] and thrombosis.[52]

When aspirating blood gas samples, it is important that the catheter line be void of any anticoagulants, lipids, or saline solutions before collection. This is usually accomplished by the use of a secondary "waste" syringe that is used to clear approximately five times the dead space volume of the catheter line. The arterial blood sample (we currently draw 2 mL for adults [0.5 mL for neonates]) can then be aspirated into a heparinized blood gas syringe. All air bubbles should be immediately removed from the sample, the syringe should be capped with a neoprene cap, gently mixed to ensure thorough anticoagulation, and analyzed within 30 minutes.

Arterial Puncture

The appropriate artery should be selected after the patient is resting comfortably and the area is well-lighted. It is desirable to have the patient supine in order to minimize the risk of a vasovagal syncopal episode. Outpatients can be accommodated through the use of a six-position recliner that has fold-out tables on each side. Radial or brachial arteries are the preferred sites for arterial punctures.[53] (Femoral artery punctures should be used only as a last resort because of the risk of undetected postpuncture bleeding).

For a radial artery, a modified Allen's Test should always be performed to ascertain if there is adequate ulnar artery perfusion to the palmar atrial arch of the hand.[54] After the patient has made a fist to force blood from the hand, pressure is applied to compress both the ulnar and radial arteries. When the hand is relaxed, the palm and fingers are blanched. Obstructing pressure is then removed from the ulnar artery while the radial artery remains compressed. If the ulnar artery is patent, the hand should quickly become flushed within 10 to 15 seconds. If the modified Allen's Test reveals poor ulnar perfusion to the hand, the radial artery in that wrist should not be used for arterial puncture and the contralateral wrist or a brachial artery should be considered.

Once adequate collateral circulation has been demonstrated, the patient is prepared for the puncture of the radial artery. A rolled towel placed under the wrist with the hand hyperextended should bring the radial artery closer to the subdermal skin layer to facilitate the puncture. For the brachial artery, the arm should be extended and the hand pronated. The brachial artery should be palpated on the medial side of the biceps tendon 1 to 2 cm distal to the antecubital fossa. Punctures should not be made through infected skin or other lesions.

Unless contraindicated, a local anesthetic (eg, lidocaine HCl 1% 10 mg/mL, without epinephrine) should be used in the noncomatose patient. Arterial punctures can be painful and a properly infiltrated anesthetic often minimizes anxiety-induced changes in the patient's respiratory status as well as arterial spasm during the puncture. (Arterial punctures are painful primarily owing to the needle entering the richly innervated arterial vessel walls). One milliliter of anesthetic is aspirated into a 1-mL tuberculin syringe fitted with either a 25- or 27-gauge needle. The artery is located by palpating the site for maxmial arterial pulse. The puncture site is cleaned with an alcohol swab, iodophor solution, or other appropriate disinfectants. The needle is passed into the skin and the syringe is aspirated slightly before injection so that an intra-arterial injection of lidocaine can be identified and avoided. A small amount of anesthetic is first injected subcutaneously before more is injected deeper on the side of the artery. If performed correctly, the drug will not only anesthetize the nerve endings but will also help to immobilize the artery.

The arterial puncture is performed using either: (1) an all-glass syringe lubricated with a minimum amount of liquid heparin or (2) a special, vented, heparinized (100 to 200 IU) plastic syringe. The blood gas syringe should be fitted with a 1-inch 21- to 23-gauge ultra-thin wall needle. The point of maximal arterial pulse is located in the anesthetized area and used as a reference point. The syringe is held at a 45° angle pointing in the opposite direction of arterial flow with the needle bevel up. The skin is punctured and the artery is entered. If the needle must be repositioned, it should be pulled back only to the subdermal layer before it is redirected. After the artery is entered, a flash of arterial blood will be seen in the needle hub. Approximately 2 to 3 mL of arterial blood is collected as the arterial pressure fills the syringe. Aspiration should not be necessary. (If there is a flash of blood in the hub but the syringe fails to passively fill, or fills very slowly, a vein may have been punctured or the needle may not be centered within the artery). After the proper volume has been obtained, the needle is withdrawn from the artery and the site is compressed for a minimum of 5 minutes. This will decrease the possibility of hematoma formation, compartment syndromes, and ecchymosis, which may interfere with future arterial punctures. Longer compression times may be necessary for patients receiving therapeutic doses of heparin (or other anticlotting therapy) or who are significantly thrombocytopenic (platelets < 50,000).[4] After the bleeding has been stopped, an elastic bandage is applied with moderate pressure. If possible, the patient should apply 5 additional minutes of pressure for complete hemostasis.

The exposed needle should be disposed of safely (in a puncture-resistant container), air bubbles, if any, should be removed, and the syringe should be sealed with a neoprene rubber tip cap. The syringe should be gently mixed for a few seconds and the blood analyzed within 30 minutes.

Most individuals can tolerate an arterial puncture without any ill effects. Rare complications from the arterial puncture can include hematoma, arteriospasm, thrombosis, and anaphylaxis.[32] Others experience reactions ranging in severity from a feeling of "uneasiness" to vasovagal syncopal reactions, shocklike symptoms, fainting, or convulsions. Early recognition of these symptoms by the puncturist can help lessen the severity of these reactions.

Peripheral Venous Blood Gases

Peripheral venous blood provides an estimation of tissue acidity and oxygenation, but the information is specific to the exact site where the blood is collected. Therefore, blood gas values from peripheral veins are rarely clinically useful and are not recommended.[36]

Capillary Blood Gases

The ear lobe (for adults) or the sides of the heel (for neonates) are typical collection sites for capillary blood gases. These sites are generally warmed to increase arterial blood perfusion before the blood is collected in a glass capillary tube. This "arterialized" capillary blood is a mixture of both arterial and venous blood.

Capillary blood is used for blood gas determinations only when arterial punctures are not feasible. Capillary blood gas values are inaccurate and meaningless when collected from poorly perfused patients.[27] Even for well-perfused patients, the PO_2 of capillary blood correlates poorly with PaO_2.[55] Capillary pH and PCO_2, however, may be helpful for estimations of acid–base status.

ANALYTICAL CONSIDERATIONS

Blood Gas Analyzers

Under CLIA-88, most blood gas analyzers have been classified as "moderately complex" whereas others, mainly older manual models, are "highly complex." The sensors (either electrochemical or potentiometric) used in these analyzers are inherently unstable and require frequent calibration and quality control checks for optimal performance. The complexity of the newer automated systems has been applied to such things as autocalibration, membrane integrity checks, drift and stability checks, and calculation of secondary results. The new sensors have longer lifetimes and are smaller (requiring smaller sample volumes), disposable, and need little maintenance (ie, no membranes), but the basic science of the original pH, PCO_2, and PO_2 electrodes has remained relatively unchanged.[56] In recent models, manufacturers have incorporated algorithms into the instrument software that automatically extrapolate to the end of the sensor output curve (before the actual sensor response is achieved) in order to speed up analyzer throughput. In addition, most manufacturers offer analyzers that incorporate ion-selective sensors that can simultaneously analyze (Na^+, K^+, Cl^-, ionized Ca^{2+}, glucose, lactate) as well as pH, PCO_2, and PO_2. Regulations and the demands of the laboratory may determine which system is most appropriate. This present level of sophistication in equipment, however, should never be expected to compensate for unqualified or inexperienced personnel.

The major manufacturers of laboratory-based blood gas analyzers are: AVL Scientific Corp. (Roswell, GA), Ciba Corning Diagnostics Corp. (Medfield, MA), Instrumentation Laboratory (Lexington, MA), Nova Biomedical (Waltham, MA), and Radiometer A/S (Copenhagen, Denmark). In addition, several other manufacturers have produced portable blood gas analyzers, with miniaturized components and automated features, designed for point-of-care blood gas testing.[57,58]

Oxygen Electrode (Clark Electrode)

The first polarographic electrodes for the measurement of O_2 were developed in the late 1930s. However, the development in the 1950s of an electrode for measuring O_2 in blood and other solutions is attributed to Clark. Thus the PO_2 electrode is commonly referred to as a Clark electrode.

Measurements are made on whole blood, which is brought into contact with a thin plastic membrane (usually polypropylene), about 1 mm thick, which covers the tip of the electrode. This membrane has two functions: it serves as a barrier between the blood and the electrode, keeping the electrode and its electrolyte free of contamination; and it is a semipermeable barrier that permits diffusion of O_2 molecules. Accordingly, equilibration between blood and electrolyte occurs while variables such as temperature, contamination, and calibration can be closely controlled.

The O_2 electrode consists of a platinum cathode and a Ag-AgCl anode, with a polarizing voltage of 0.5 to 0.6 volts and completion of the circuit by a KCl electrolyte bridge. O_2 molecules present in the plasma diffuse through the semipermeable membrane until equilibrium between plasma and the electrolyte solution occurs. As the O_2 diffuses through the electrolyte solution to the platinum electrode surface, it is reduced, altering the conductivity of the electrolyte solution. This causes a change in the current between the cathode and the anode, which is proportional to the PO_2 in the sample.

The output can be significantly altered by exposure to low concentrations of halothane, an anesthetic agent.[59]

pH Electrode

A reference method for the determination of pH in blood has been published.[60] Measuring the chemical potential of H^+ with an electrode is only possible by using a glass electrode comprised of two half cells. One half cell is a silver-silver chloride-measuring electrode in contact with a liquid of known pH (usually pH 6.840). Its function is to convey the potential difference across the pH-sensitive glass to the electronic circuitry. The other half cell is a mercury-mercurous chloride (calomel) reference anode that supplies a constant reference voltage. The reference half cell is connected to the measuring half cell by the liquid junction or potassium chloride salt bridge that completes the circuit. Two measurements are required at the same temperature to determine the pH of any solution. The first measurement is made to determine the pH of a known solution for standardization of the instrument and the second to determine the pH of the unknown solution or, for our application, the pH of blood. Therefore, each pH determination is actually the difference between two separate measurements.

PCO_2 Electrode (Severinghaus Electrode)

The modern-type PCO_2 electrode was first developed by Stowe in the mid-1950s. It was further modified by Severinghaus in 1958.

Although physically resembling a PO_2 electrode, the PCO_2 electrode is, in principle, a modified pH electrode. The tip is covered by a membrane that acts as a diffusion barrier between blood and the sodium bicarbonate buffer solution. When blood is brought into contact with the membrane, CO_2 molecules diffuse across the membrane into the electrolyte solution and react with a small amount of buffer. Diffusion of CO_2 from the blood into the buffer solution produces an equilibrium of PCO_2; the result is a proportional change in the H^+ concentration of the buffer solution (Equation 25), which is then easily measured by the pH electrode.

Diffusion proceeds until equilibrium has been reached. The resultant change in H^+ concentration in the buffer solution is measured by the pH-type electrode and is proportional to the amount of CO_2 that has diffused into the buffer.

Quality Control

For blood gas testing, CLIA-88 requires that one sample of control material must be analyzed every 8 hours of testing and that the controls be rotated to check normal, alkalosis, and acidosis levels. The laboratory must also test one sample of calibration or control material each time patient samples are tested unless automatic calibrations occur every 30 minutes. The laboratory must use a combination of calibrators and control materials that include both low and high values on each day of testing (C-161 Interpretive Guidelines; 493.1245, Federal Register). The Joint Commission on Accreditation of Healthcare Organizations (JCAHO) also requires that the laboratory assay at least three levels of control on each day of individual testing and at least one level of control for each 8 hours of individual testing.[61]

The operator of blood gas analyzers should strictly adhere to the maintenance, calibration, and troubleshooting protocols that are recommended by each instrument manufacturer. It is extremely important that the temperature of the sensor block be accurately thermostatted. Users should perform all maintenance procedures at the frequency recommended by the manufacturer. Regular cleaning of the sample path, use of calibration reagents with the same quality as recommended by the manufacturer, and the monitoring of electrode drifts and error messages are all important.

Tonometry

Because of the unique O_2-binding characteristics of hemoglobin and the complex viscosity characteristics of normal fresh blood, whole blood must be carefully tonometered so that exact gas tensions can be prepared for analysis by a blood gas instrument. A tonometry reference method has been developed and recognized as the internationally accepted standard method for the determination of PCO_2 and PO_2 measurements.[62] Gas mixtures or gas mixers can be used to equilibrate the blood to theoretical gas values by the following equation:

$$\text{mmHg} = (\%\text{Gas}\ [P_B - 47])/100 \qquad (42)$$

Guidelines for tonometry methods have been extensively described elsewhere.[31,62] Blood should be fresh (less than 24 hours old), from asymptomatic donors, nonhemolyzed, and without leukocytosis or high lipid levels. Rapid gas flow rates may cool the sample and the temperature should be strictly maintained at 37 °C. Gas mixture compositions should be verified with a mass spectrometer or with CO_2 and O_2 gas analyzers (eg, Ametek, Pittsburgh, PA).

Tonometry can be used for routine quality control,[63] but the use of human blood is problematic because it is not always safe or in sufficient supply. Bovine hemoglobin solutions have been successfully used as substitutes for human blood in the tonometry reference method and have yielded excellent data when compared with human blood.[64,65] These bovine preparations (both the reduced and oxygenated forms) closely match the O_2-binding characteristics of fresh human whole blood and are sensitive to temperature malfunctions in blood gas analyzers.[64] In addition to assessing the inaccuracy of PaO_2 and $PaCO_2$, these solutions can also be formulated to provide precision data for the pH, ctHb, and electrolytes.

Commercial Blood Gas Controls

The use of commercial controls in sealed ampules eliminates the time and technical demands required for tonometry. Aqueous buffers and perfluorocarbon emulsions, factory equilibrated with CO_2 and O_2, are widely used as blood gas controls because of their convenience and biosafety. However, these tertiary controls only provide information on data imprecision and are not checks for inaccuracy.[62] Aqueous buffers are susceptible to variations in room storage temperature[66] and, unlike human or bovine blood, cannot detect temperature or protein errors in blood gas analyzers.[67,68] Perfluorocarbon materials have the same O_2-buffering capacity as blood at 98 mmHg[69] and are more precise than aqueous controls,[70] but overall, they are relatively poor O_2 buffers in comparison with human blood.[67] Perfluorocarbons are also temperature insensitive and cannot detect analyzer temperature malfunctions.[64] Also, intermodel differences for both aqueous and perfluorocarbon materials, especially for PO_2, have been regularly observed and can be quite large.[71] These intermodel differences are not seen with whole blood tonometry.[72]

Blood Comparisons

CLIA-88 mandates that laboratories perform periodic split-sample testing between instruments that are not currently enrolled in interlaboratory proficiency testing. However, for laboratories that have two or more analyzers, split-sample testing is also an excellent way to routinely confirm the validity of independently calibrated and controlled analyzers.[73] Unlike controls that are used to generate performance data for a single instrument, split-sample blood comparisons can be used to quantify overall laboratory imprecision. This procedure can better monitor the imprecision of laboratory measurements, especially in laboratories where nonblood matrices are used as control materials. If the results from all the analyzers with split-sample blood are in relative agreement (we use maximal differences for PO_2 and $PCO_2 \leq 3.0$ mmHg; pH ≤ 0.03 pH units; ctHb ≤ 0.3 g/dL), the operator can be assured that interinstrument biases do not exist and that all instruments are capable of comparable measurements. However, this method does not yield information regarding absolute accuracy nor does it identify which instrument is in error if the results differ significantly. The performance of a reference method or the testing of controls or calibrations is necessary to obtain this information.

Calibration

CLIA-88 requires that all categories of blood gas equipment perform calibration and calibration verification in accordance and at the frequency recommended by the manufacturer. If a blood gas is performed with an instrument that does not automatically verify a calibration at least every 30 minutes, then a calibrator or control must be tested each time a patient specimen is tested (Federal Register 493.1245). According to JCAHO, blood gas calibrations are required to be performed in accordance with manufacturers' instructions with the frequency predicated on use (eg, check calibration each time a specimen is tested unless automated calibrations verifies internally at least every 30 minutes).

All electrodes (or sensors) require periodic checks of their electronic output as a function of known analyte concentration, but blood gas sensors are highly susceptible to drift and require frequent electronic checks. Most manufacturers recommend calibrations every 30 minutes of operation, but one manufacturer has installed a mechanism for continuous calibration checks for its models (KD Fallon, personal communication, Instrumentation Laboratory Co., Lexington, MA). The isopotential (zero) points of the pH and PCO_2 sensors and the nonzero calibration point of the PO_2 sensor require the most frequent calibrations. The nonzero calibration points, for the pH and PCO_2, and the isopotential point for the PO_2 electrode are more stable and require less-frequent (usually every 2 hours) calibrations.[74]

Calibration reagents are usually standard CO_2 and O_2 gases for PO_2 and PCO_2 sensors and phosphate buffers for pH. These reagents are referenced to the National Institute of Standards and Technology (NIST). Laboratories should be cautioned not to unconsciously modify their blood gas systems. Changing the manufacturer's calibration set points, changing the calibration or control value, or using a different calibration material may be interpreted as method modification under CLIA-88 and, therefore, the blood gas instrument may be reclassified as "highly complex". Use of products from a different manufacturer is not considered method modification as long as the Food and Drug Administration (FDA) has cleared a manufacturer's reagents and calibration materials (Interpretive Guidelines C-105).

Temperature Corrections

Blood gas values change with variations in body temperature by the gas law equations (Equation 1). For blood gases in the normal range, the PaO_2 of the blood rises or falls about 7% per degree Celsius, for $PaCO_2$ the change is 4% per degree, and for pH the change is 0.0146 units per degree.[4] For blood gases outside of the normal range, complex temperature algorithms can be applied.[75] During analysis, blood gas instruments heat and maintain the blood sample at a constant 37 °C. The operator has the option to apply correction factors to the results so that they can reflect the actual body temperature of the patient. However, there is considerable debate concerning the efficacy of this practice.

The most compelling reason to adjust the results to the patients' body temperature is that corrected results more accurately reflect the true oxygenation and acid–base status of the body. In addition, when pulmonary gas values are considered, these temperature corrections are especially crucial because pulmonary gases are in a "dynamic equilibrium" with the gases dissolved in the blood. Therefore, using pulmonary gases in the same expression as blood gas values requires that the blood gas values be corrected to body temperature.[75–77]

However, several good arguments can be made against the practice of routinely correcting blood gas values to body temperature. These are: (1) the pH and $PaCO_2$ values at 37°C reliably reflect the in vivo acid–base status of the patient; (2) the pH and $PaCO_2$, when adjusted for temperature, do not affect the HCO_3^-; (3) most acid–base nomograms are valid only at 37°C and very large errors will occur if thermally adjusted blood gas data are used;[76] and (4) data reliably quantifying the balance between O_2 delivery and uptake at temperatures other than 37°C are unavailable. In addition, most physicians do not remember "normal" values other than those at 37°C[36] and that temperature corrected values do not improve the ability to make clinical decisions.[27] For these reasons, we recommend that, for values that are not to be used in pulmonary gas equations, routine blood gas measurements be consistently reported at 37°C.

CO-OXIMETRY

CO-oximeters are specialized spectrophotometers that are relatively easy to operate, require no sample preparation (except, in most cases, for adequate sample mixing), and display rapid and simultaneous readouts of all of the clinically important hemoglobin derivatives (COHb, HHb, MetHb, and O_2Hb), ctHb, and the calculation of SO_2 and ctO_2. (The ctHb is a regulated analyte under CLIA-88 and, therefore, all CO-oximeters that are used to test patient samples must be operated according to federal regulations.) The absorbance of a "zeroing" or blank solution at multiple wavelengths (shown in Fig. 9-10) is subtracted from the resulting absorbance values of the blood sample. Then, four or more equations are used to calculate the concentration of each species of hemoglobin to the characteristic absorption of light at each frequency.

The COHb and ctHb measurements by CO-oximeter have been compared with the more selective gas chromatograph and cyanmethemoglobin methods.[78] For ctHb, spectrophotometric measurements were found to be reliable. However, for COHb, CO-oximeters were found to be inaccurate when small concentrations were measured. Their inaccuracy (about ±1.0% COHb [full scale 0%–100%]) is acceptable for measurements of COHb levels above 5% but problematic for COHb levels below 5% COHb in certain applications. Relative to gas chromatographic values (a recognized reference method for COHb measurement), CO-oximeters overestimate COHb measurements below 2.5% and underestimate results above 5.0%.[78]

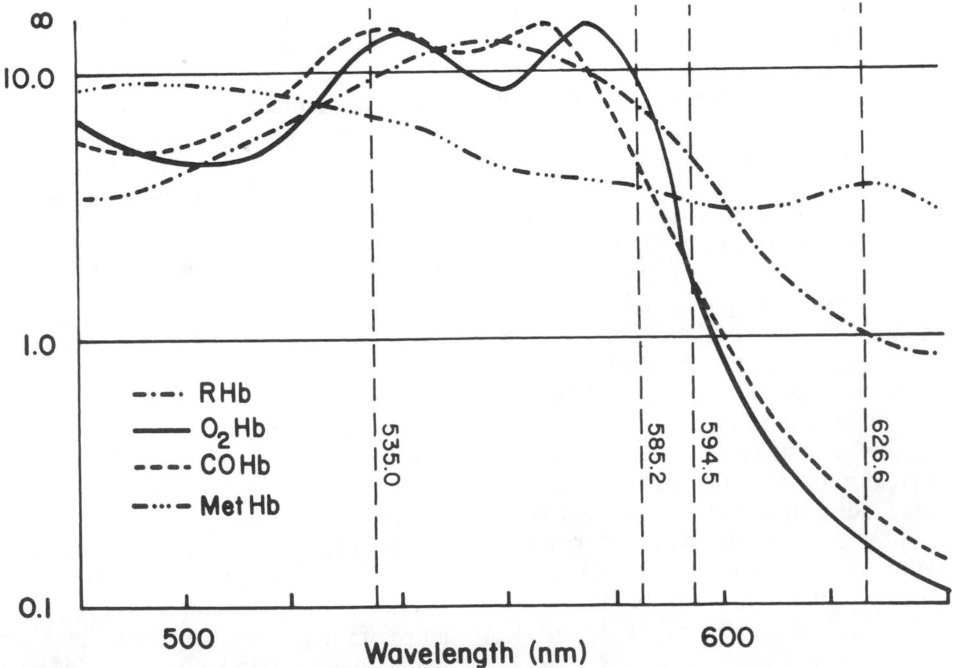

FIGURE 9-10. Many two-wavelength methods have been published for determining either carbon monoxide- or oxygen-bound hemoglobin. The wavelengths that are used vary. Typically, the wavelengths are either at an inflection or at an isosbestic point of two or more of the species. It is common to select one wavelength at which the absorbance difference between species is at a maximum and the other at which this difference approaches zero. Because the absorbance of these species generally changes differently and abruptly as a function of wavelength, the spectrophotometer must have the smallest possible bandwidth, and the center wavelength must be positioned accurately and reproducibly. This figure shows hemoglobin spectra for four species of hemoglobin. Furthermore, in two-wavelength methods, unmeasured species must be absent, or the wavelengths must be chosen to minimize spectral interference from unmeasured species. This has frequently been overlooked in determining oxyhemoglobin in the presence of small but varying levels of endogenous and environmentally generated carbon monoxide. (Courtesy of Instrumentation Laboratory, Inc. from the IL-282 Operators Manual)

A possible explanation for the COHb measurement errors with CO-oximeters may be that these instruments are highly susceptible to a wide variety of interfering substances. Fetal oxyhemoglobin can cause errors in COHb measurements in direct proportion with its concentration[79] unless the CO-oximeter is specially designed so that fetal oxyhemoglobin does not adversely affect the results.[80] Bilirubin,[81] methylene blue cardiac dye, and sulfhemoglobin are also capable of adversely affecting spectrophotometric measurements (Operators Manual, Corning 270 CO-oximeter, Ciba Corning Diagnostics Corp, Medfield, MA). Even components of the same analysis, O_2Hb[82] and MetHb,[83] can contribute to the inaccuracy of the COHb results if they are present in certain quantities. Levels of MetHb above 10% may cause errors in O_2Hb and COHb determinations.

The only user adjustable calibration is the ctHb value, which is often tested using a dye-based propylene glycol solution. For accurate results on patient blood, it is essential that hemolysis is complete, that there are no air bubbles in the cuvette, and that the temperature of the cuvette is properly thermostatted. It is also crucial that samples be adequately mixed for homogeneous dispersion of cells in the plasma if accurate ctHb measurements are desired.[11] Recently, a two-wavelength oximeter has been developed that does not require hemolysis and generates results in just 9 seconds.[84]

NONINVASIVE BLOOD GAS MONITORS

Pulse Oximeters

In vivo measurements of O_2 saturation by pulse oximeter (SpO_2), have been widely accepted as a standard of care in many hospitals because they are noninvasive, easy-to-use, and provide continuous readouts.[85] Pulse oximeters use a probe that measures the absorption of two wavelengths; one for O_2Hb and one for HHb. As a light is shined through the pulsating vascular bed, the absorbances are measured and any light scattering (from skin and muscle tissues) is corrected after the establishment of baseline absorbance.

The pulse oximeter has questionable accuracy, especially at high and low physiologic extremes, but it is considered useful as a trending device and in the detection of marked desaturation.[86,87] For many patients being weaned from supplemental O_2, the use of SpO_2 can shorten the days of O_2 use and decrease the number of arterial blood gas determinations.[88] However, the manufacturer's inaccuracy claim ($SpO_2 \pm 3\%$) is excessive and problematic for use with neonatal patients.[89]

Although their clinical utility has been demonstrated, pulse oximeters are still subject to numerous errors and their limitations should be recognized. Pulse oximeters are subject to motion artifact, hypothermia, vasopressor drugs, stray ambient lighting,[56] low pulse pressure (hypotension, peripheral vascular disease), low light transmission owing to opaque tissues (edema, dark skin pigment,[90] and abnormal concentrations of hemoglobin. The presence of dyshemoglobins (eg, carboxyhemoglobinemia, methemoglobinemia) can lead to erroneous and artifactually high SpO_2 measurements.[91] This is because the pulse oximeter measures the dyshemoglobin fractions as if they were oxyhemoglobin. If the patient blood has a high concentration of dyshemoglobins, the displayed SpO_2 will be artifactually high and true patient SO_2 will be lower.[92] Therefore, in order to prevent clinical errors, data from pulse oximeters or other two-wavelength devices should be used only after their limitations have been considered and after baseline SO_2 and dyshemoglobin fractions have been measured.[93]

Transcutaneous Monitors

Transcutaneous sensors are miniaturized versions of conventional blood gas analyzer sensors (eg, Clark PO_2 electrode, Severinghaus PCO_2 electrode). Transcutaneous $PO_2[P_{TC}O_2]$ values at 44 °C are approximately equal to PaO_2 values at 37 °C in newborn infants. Large biases in $P_{TC}O_2$, however, are common in adults. Transcutaneous $PCO_2[P_{TC}CO_2]$ values at 42 °C to 45 °C are higher than $PaCO_2$ at 37 °C, but the relative difference between the two measurements is more stable than for $P_{TC}O_2$ and, therefore, more clinically useful.

The variables affecting transcutaneous measurements are the actual PaO_2 and $PaCO_2$ of the blood, capillary blood flow in the skin under the sensors, O_2 consumption and CO_2 production by the skin, O_2 consumption by the electrode, temperature gradients in the skin, structure and diffusive properties of the skin, and interference from anesthetic gases. The $P_{TC}O_2$ and $P_{TC}CO_2$ measurements can be used as a trending device but, because of the large imprecision of the $P_{TC}O_2$ data, should not be used to replace PaO_2 measurements.[88]

Capnometers and Capnographs

Capnometers are noninvasive devices used to measure end-tidal $CO_2(EtCO_2)$ in breath for the purpose of estimating $PaCO_2$. A capnometer projects an infrared beam through the gas sample to continuously measure the CO_2 absorbance in either sidestream or mainstream breath. The results are graphically displayed on a capnograph.

The relationship between $EtCO_2$ and $PaCO_2$ is good when there is stability and normality in the capnographic wave form, cardiovascular function, and the body temperature.[27] If any one of these parameters is unstable, capnography provides an unreliable estimate of $PaCO_2$. The routine use of capnography as a substitute for actual $PaCO_2$ measurements has been discouraged.[87]

Near-Infrared Spectrophotometry

Near-infrared spectrophotometry is an experimental method designed to estimate the adequacy of the O_2 delivery to the cytochromes. It measures the color change of cytochrome a_3 at two or more wavelengths of light as it becomes oxidized or reduced. This method may prove useful in the diagnosis of general hypoxic episodes or for ascertaining the adequacy of cerebral oxygenation.[94,95]

Magnetic Resonance Spectroscopy

Magnetic resonance spectroscopy is an experimental method designed to estimate O_2 delivery to cells by measuring the energy reserves and pH within the cell. This technique may also be useful for estimating the effects of tissue hypoxia[91] and blood clots.[96]

Magnetic Resonance Saturation Imaging

Magnetic resonance saturation imaging generates images of the resonant differences between O_2Hb and HHb to estimate blood saturation and takes advantage of the different responses of HHb and O_2Hb within magnetic fields. This method may also be useful for the detection and imaging of blood clots for the diagnosis of deep venous thrombosis and coronary artery occlusion.[97]

Time-of-Flight and Absorbance Spectrophotometry

Time-of-flight absorbance (TOFA) spectrophotometry is an experimental method designed to estimate deep-tissue saturation and construct saturation images from light scattering through tissues.[98] It measures the distribution of the paths traveled by photons (ie, the intensity of the light as it returns from the tissue) by emitting a short pulse of light. Current work suggests that a two-dimensional saturation image can be produced,[99] although complexities, such as changing path length, need to be overcome.

INVASIVE BLOOD GAS MONITORS

Fiberoptic Blood Gas Sensors

Fiberoptic intravascular sensors for PO_2 contain an O_2-sensitive fluorescent dye immobilized in a gas permeable polymer matrix. For PCO_2, the sensors contain a pH sensitive fluorescent dye in a HCO_3^- buffer. Excitation light is transported via optical fibers and causes the compounds inside the internal sensors to fluoresce. The consequent light emission is collected by co-linear filters and the subsequent measurements by the monitor's photodetectors are proportional to the respective analyte concentration. Algorithms are used to convert the amount of emitted fluorescent light intensity to blood gas values.[100] A 20-gauge cannula containing the sensors is inserted into an artery and electrically connected to a multichannel detection system that measures the resultant electrical voltage signals and provides a continuous display of pH, PCO_2, and PO_2 readouts.[101] Another model of similar design incorporates a bent-fiber light path.[102] The major problems with this technology have been inconsistent sensor fabrication, measurement interference owing to thrombus formation, and sensor failure during clinical trials.[103,104] When compared with blood gas instruments, measurements from these devices compare well for pH, but the agreement is less favorable for $PaCO_2$ and PaO_2.[105] However, good correlations have been reported in a study with hypercapnic patients.[106]

Some of these sensors have been used during extracorporeal circulation with some success.[104,107] The measurements from another fluorescent fiberoptic sensor is used as an intermittent monitor that is placed ex vivo in the patient's arterial line tubing. The measurements of this monitor have been successfully compared with tonometry targets for bovine blood in vitro and with conventional blood gas analyzers for normal human subjects.[100]

Other Invasive Sensors

Miniaturized electrochemical sensors have also been designed to fit into a 20-gauge radial artery cannula.[108] In general, however, sensors based on electrochemical principles perform poorly in the harsh environment of intravascular monitoring.[109]

Ion-selective field-effect transistors for intravascular monitoring have shown some success[110] but are susceptible to thrombosis formation and moisture.

FUTURE OF BLOOD GASES

Under CLIA-88, most types of diagnostic measurements are strictly regulated regardless of where they are performed. For blood gas testing, the trend is toward "point-of-care" (ie, at the bedside of the patient) testing.[111] Yet, little progress has been achieved in the attempt to transfer laboratory sensor technology to bedside instrumentation despite much effort and large investments. Invasive in vivo technologies, although potentially accurate, require improvements in measurement stability and in the protection of the sensor's chemistry from the arterial environment.[112] Noninvasive blood gas technologies hold great promise; however, improvement in the reliability of the data from these devices is still needed. The goal of future blood gas systems is to provide continuous, noninvasive, and accurate readouts of both the acid–base and oxygenation status of the patient.

SUMMARY

Blood gas determinations, whether in vitro or in vivo, remain an essential part of modern patient care.[36] To be useful, blood gas results should accurately reflect the true status of the patient. To accomplish this, three main areas need to be addressed. First, a strict blood collection protocol should be followed to minimize changes in the ongoing physiologic status of the patient. Second, a blood gas sample handling protocol should eliminate or, at least, minimize all potentially adverse pre-analytical errors (time-delay, metabolism, air bubbles, type of syringe, and heparin contamination). If care is not taken during and after sample collection, the blood gas results, even from a perfect laboratory, will not accurately reflect the condition of the patient. Third, the inaccuracy and imprecision of blood gas instruments should be monitored so that these data will meet medical needs. Unfortunately, because reference methods are seldom used, the inaccuracy of blood gas systems is rarely known. Many hospital laboratories test commercially prepared, nonblood control materials for quality control without realizing that these tertiary controls are only limited to the assessment of instrument imprecision. Tonometry of bovine solutions (both the reduced and oxygenated forms) may be an alternative that can be used to accurately assess analyzer performance without the drawbacks associated with human blood tonometry.

Data from any technology need to be properly understood, interpreted, and acted on before any patient benefit can be realized. With an understanding of acid–base chemistry, gas laws, and the physiology of gas exchange, the validity of blood gas results can be properly evaluated and patient conditions can be appropriately treated.

Acknowledgment

The authors thank Ronald J. Wong for his contributions and critical review of this manuscript.

REFERENCES

1. Raffin TA: Indications for arterial blood gas analysis. Ann Intern Med 105:390, 1986
2. Clausen JL, Murray KM: Clinical applications of arterial blood gases: How much accuracy do we need? J Med Tech 2(1):19, 1985
3. Adams AP, Hahn CEW: Principles and practice of blood gas analysis. ISBN 0906534054 Franklin Scientific Projects, London, England, 1979
4. Mohler JG, Collier CR, Brandt W, Abramson J, Verkaik G, Yates S: Blood gases. In Clausen JL (ed): Pulmonary Function Testing Guidelines and Controversies, Chap 21. New York, Academic Press, 1982, p 223
5. Siggaard-Anderson O: The acid-base status of the blood, 4th ed, Baltimore, Williams & Wilkins, 1974
6. Sorbini CA, Grassi V, Solinas E: Arterial oxygen tension in relation to age in healthy subjects. Respiration 25:3,1968
7. Mellemgaard K: The alveolar-arterial oxygen difference: Its size and components in normal man. Acta Physiol Scand 67:10,1966
8. Raine JM, Bishop JM: A-a difference in O_2 tension and physiological dead space in normal man. J Appl Physiol 18(2):284,1963
9. Turino GM, Cugell DW, Goldring RM, et al: Workshop on assessment of respiratory control in humans: VII. Measurements of the responsiveness of the respiratory apparatus in disease. Am Rev Respir Dis 115:883,1977
10. Nunn JF: Applied Respiratory Physiology, 2nd ed, Woburn, MA, Butterworths Inc., 1977, p 405
11. National Committee of Clinical Laboratory Standards: Fractional oxyhemoglobin, oxygen content and saturation, and related quantities in blood: Terminology, measurement, and reporting; tentative guideline. NCCLS document C25-T (ISBN 1-56238-160-1). NCCLS, 771 East Lancaster Avenue, Villanova, PA 19085, 1992
12. Antonini E, Brunori M: Hemoglobin and myoglobin in their reactions with ligands. Amsterdam, Holland, North-Holland Publishing Company, 1971
13. Wintrobe MM: The diagnostic and therapeutic approach to hematologic problems. In Wintrobe's Clinical Hematology, 9th ed, Chap 1. Malvern, PA, Lea & Febiger, 1993, p 3
14. Engel RR, Rodkey FL, O'Neal JD, Collison HA: Relative affinity of human fetal hemoglobin for carbon monoxide and oxygen. Blood 33(1):37, 1969
15. Collman JP, Brauman JI, Doxsee KM: Carbon monoxide binding to iron porphyrins. Proc Natl Acad Sci 76(12):6035, 1979
16. Roughton FJW, Darling RC: The effect of carbon monoxide on the oxyhemoglobin dissociation curve. Am J Physiol 141:17, 1944
17. Zwart A, Kwant B, Oeseburg B, Zijlstra WG: Human whole-blood oxygen affinity: Effect of carbon monoxide. J Appl Physiol 57(1):14, 1984
18. Garby L, Meldon J: The respiratory functions of blood. New York, Plenum, 1977
19. Haab P: The effect of carbon monoxide on respiration. Experientia 46:1202, 1990
20. Zijlstra WG, Kwant G, Oeseburg B, Zwart A: The Bohr effect in human blood: Terminology and numerical values. Proceedings from International Federation of Clinical Chemistry, Methodology and Clinical Applications of Blood Gases, pH, Electrolytes and Sensor Technology. IFCC/WGSE-AACC/EBGD Symposium, Monterey. IFCC, Copenhagen, Denmark, 1990, p 29
21. Lukens JN, Lee GR: The abnormal hemoglobins: General principles. In Wintrobe's Clinical Hematology, 9th ed, Chap 36. Malvern, PA, Lea & Febiger, 1993, p 1023
22. Severinghaus JW: Blood gas calculator. J Appl Physiol 21:1108, 1966
23. Zwart A: Spectrophotometry of hemoglobin: Various perspectives. Clin Chem 39(8):1570, 1993
24. Suter PM, Lindauer JM, Fairley HB, Schlobohm RM: Errors in data derived from pulmonary artery blood gas values. Crit Care Med 3(5):175, 1975
25. Suter PM, Fairley HB, Isenberg MD: Optimum end-expiratory airway pressure in patients in acute pulmonary failure. N Engl J Med 292:284, 1975
26. Gilbert F, Keighley JF: The arterial/alveolar oxygen tension ratio: An index of gas exchange applicable to varying inspired oxygen concentrations. Am Rev Respir Dis 109:142, 1974
27. Shapiro BA, Peruzzi WT, Kozelowski-Templin R: Clinical application of blood gases, 5th ed. St. Louis, Mosby–Year Book, 1994
28. Armstrong BW, Mohler JG, Jung RC, et al: The in vivo carbon dioxide titration curve. Lancet 1:759, 1966
29. Armstrong BW: Rapid changes in $PaCO_2$ and HCO_3^-. Respir Care 21:808, 1976
30. Siggaard Anderson O: An acid-base chart for arterial blood with normal and pathophysiological reference areas. Scand J Clin Lab Invest 27:239, 1971
31. National Committee of Clinical Laboratory Standards: Blood gas pre-analytical considerations: specimen collection, calibration, and controls; approved guideline. NCCLS document C-27A (ISBN 1-56238-190-3). NCCLS, 771 East Lancaster Avenue, Villanova, PA 19085, 1993
32. National Committee of Clinical Laboratory Standards: Percutaneous collection of arterial blood for laboratory analysis; approved guideline. NCCLS document H11-A, Vol 5, No. 3 (ISBN 0273-3099). NCCLS, 771 East Lancaster Avenue, Villanova, PA 19085, 1993
33. Dake MD, Peters J, Teague R: The effect of heparin dilution on arterial blood gas analysis [letter]. West J Med 1984;140(5):792.
34. Hansen JE, Simmons DH: A systematic error in the determination of blood PCO_2. Am Rev Respir Dis 115:1061, 1977
35. Ordog GJ, Wasserberger J, Balasubramanian S: Effect of heparin on arterial blood gases. Ann Emerg Med 14:233, 1985
36. Hansen JE: Arterial blood gases. Clin Chest Med 10(2):227, 1989
37. Christiansen TF: Heparin and blood sampling for pH, blood gases and direct potentiometric electrolyte analysis. AS96, ISBN 87-88138-08-9, Radiometer A/S Copenhagen, Denmark, 1986
38. Biswas CK, Ramos JM, Agroyannis B, Kerr DNS: Blood gas analysis: Effect of air bubbles in syringe and delay in estimation. BMJ 284:923, 1982
39. Harsten A, Berg B, Inerot S, Muth L: Importance of correct handling of samples for the results of blood gas analysis. Acta Anaesthesiol Scand 32:365, 1988
40. Eldridge F, Fretwell LK: Change in oxygen tension of shed blood at various temperatures. J Appl Physiol 20(4):790, 1965
41. Hess CE, Nichols AB, Hunt WB, Suratt PM: Pseudohypoxemia secondary to leukemia and thrombocytosis. N Engl J Med 301:361, 1979

42. Fletcher G, Barber JL: Effect of sampling technique on the determination of PaO_2 during oxygen breathing. J Appl Physiol 21(2):463, 1966
43. Scott PV, Horton JN, Mapleson WW: Leakage of oxygen from blood and water samples stored in plastic and glass syringes. BMJ 3:512, 1971
44. Aminabhavi TM, Aithal US: Molecular transport of oxygen and nitrogen through polymer films; JMS—Rev Macromol Chem Phys C31(2&3):117, 1991
45. Janis KM, Fletcher G: Oxygen tension measurements in small samples. Am Rev Respir Dis 106:914, 1972
46. Evers W, Racz GB, Levy AA: A comparative study of plastic (polypropylene) and glass syringes in blood gas analysis. Anesth Analg 51:92, 1972
47. Winkler JB, Huntington CG, Wells DE, Befeler B: Influence of syringe material on arterial blood gas determinations. Chest 66:518, 1974
48. Mahoney JJ, Harvey JA, Wong RJ, Van Kessel AL: Changes in oxygen measurements when whole blood is stored in iced plastic or glass syringes. Clin Chem 37:1244, 1991
49. Müller-Plathe O, Heyduck S: Stability of blood gases, electrolytes and haemoglobin in heparinized whole blood samples: Influence of the type of syringe. Eur J Clin Chem Clin Biochem 30:349, 1992
50. Centers for Disease Control: Guidelines for preventing the transmission of tuberculosis in health-care settings, with special focus on HIV-related issues. CDC August 1991, Vol 39, No. RR-17
51. Stamm WE, Colella JJ, Anderson RL, Dixon RE: Indwelling arterial catheters as a source of nosocomial bacteremia. N Engl J Med 292:1099, 1975
52. Downs JB, Rackstein AD, Klein EF, Hawkins IF: Hazards of radial artery catheterization. Anesthesiology 38:283, 1973
53. Hallett W, Jung RC: Arterial puncture—techniques for collection of arterial blood gas analysis (pH, PCO_2, PO_2)—LAC/USC Medical Center. In Training Manual of the Respiratory Care Committee of the California Thoracic Society (Tustin, CA).
54. Greenhow DE: Incorrect performance of Allen's test—ulnar artery flow erroneously presumed inadequate. Anesthesiology 37:356, 1972
55. Van Kessel AL: The blood gas laboratory. An update: 1979. Lab Med 10(7):419, 1979
56. Burritt MF: Current analytical approaches to measuring blood analytes. Clin Chem 36(8B):1562, 1990
57. Wong RJ, Mahoney JJ, Harvey JA, Van Kessel AL: StatPal® II pH and blood gas analysis system evaluated. Clin Chem 40(1):124, 1994
58. Jacobs E, Nowakowski M, Colman N: Performance of Gem Premier blood gas/electrolyte analyzer evaluated. Clin Chem 39(9):1890, 1993
59. Severinghaus JW, Weiskopf RB, Nishimura M, Bradley AF: Oxygen electrode errors due to polarographic reductions of halothane. J Appl Physiol 31:640, 1971
60. Maas AHJ, Weisberg HF, Burnett RW, et al: Approved IFCC methods. Reference method (1986) for pH measurement in blood. Clin Chim Acta 165:97, 1987
61. Accreditation Manual for Pathology and Clinical Laboratory Services—Standards and Scoring Guidelines. Joint Commission on Accreditation of Healthcare Organizations. ISBN: 0-86688-346-0, 1993, JCAHO, Oakbrook Terrace, IL 60181, PA. 6.3.4.1:98
62. Burnett RW, Convington AK, Maas AHJ, et al: International Federation of Clinical Chemistry, IFCC Method (1988) for theory of blood: Reference materials for PCO_2 and PO_2. IFCC document Stage 3, Draft 1, 1989. Ann Biol Clin 47:373, 1989
63. Elser RC, Sitler J, Garver C: A flexible and versatile program for blood-gas quality control. Am J Clin Pathol 78:471,1982
64. Mahoney JJ, Wong RJ, Van Kessel AL: Reduced bovine hemoglobin solution evaluated for use as a blood gas quality-control material. Clin Chem 39(5):874, 1993
65. Sprokholt R, van Ooik S, van den Camp RAM, Bourma BN, Zijlstra WG, Maas AHJ: Evaluation of a quality control material containing hemoglobin for blood gas and pH measurement. Scand J Clin Lab Invest 47(Suppl 188):101, 1987
66. Ong ST, David D, Snow M, Hansen JE: Effect of variations in room temperature on measured values of blood gas quality-control materials. Clin Chem 29(3):502, 1983
67. Leary ET, Graham G, Kenny MA: Commercially available blood-gas quality controls compared with tonometered blood. Clin Chem 26:1309, 1980
68. Abramson J, Verkaik G, Poltl K, Mohler JG: Evaluation and comparison of commercial blood gas quality controls and tonometry. Respir Care 25:441, 1980
69. Feil MC, Cormier AD, Legg KD: Perfluorocarbon emulsions as pH/blood-gas controls. Clin Chem 28(10):2187, 1982
70. Itano M: CAP blood gas survey—1981 and 1982. Am J Clin Pathol 80(Suppl):554, 1983
71. Hansen JE, Clausen JL, Levy SE, Mohler JG, Van Kessel AL: Proficiency testing materials for pH and blood gases, the California Thoracic Society experience. Chest 89(2):214, 1986
72. Van Kessel AL, Eichhorn JH, Clausen JL, Stone ME, Rotman HH, Crapo RO: Inter-instrument comparison of blood gas analyzers and assessment of tonometry using fresh heparinized whole human blood. Chest 92:418, 1987
73. Elser RC, Hess DR, Moran RF: Is multi-level, multi-shift QC necessary for blood gas analyzers? Proceedings from International Federation of Clinical Chemistry, Methodology and Clinical Applications of Blood Gases, pH, Electrolytes and Sensor Technology. IFCC/WGSE-AACC/EBGD Symposium, Monterey. IFCC, Copenhagen, Denmark, 1990, p 19
74. Moran RF, Bradley F: Blood gas systems—major determinants of performance. Lab Med 12(6):353, 1981
75. Ashwood ER, Kost G, Kenny M: Temperature correction of blood-gas and pH measurements. Clin Chem 29(11):1877, 1983
76. Severinghaus JW: Respiration and hypothermia. Ann NY Acad Sci 80(2):384, 1959
77. National Committee of Clinical Laboratory Standards: Definitions of quantities and conventions related to blood pH and gas analysis; approved standard. NCCLS document C-12A (ISBN 1-56238-242-X). NCCLS, 771 East Lancaster Avenue, Villanova, PA 19085, 1994
78. Mahoney JJ, Vreman HJ, Stevenson DK, Van Kessel AL: Measurement of carboxyhemoglobin and total hemoglobin by five specialized spectrophotometers (CO-oximeters) in comparison with reference methods. Clin Chem 39(8):1693, 1993
79. Vreman HJ, Ronquillo RB, Ariagno RL, Schwartz HC, Stevenson DK: Interference of fetal hemoglobin with the spectrophotometric measurement of carboxyhemoglobin. Clin Chem 34:975, 1988
80. Vreman HJ, Stevenson DK: Carboxyhemoglobin determined in neonatal blood with a CO-oximeter unaffected by fetal hemoglobin. Clin Chem 40(8):1522, 1994
81. Koch MJ, Casucci GM, Koch DD: Evaluation of the Corning 2500 CO-oximeter [Abstract]. Clin Chem 31:921, 1985
82. Allred EN, Bleecker ER, Chaitman BR, et al: Acute effects of carbon monoxide on individuals with coronary artery disease. HEI Res Rep 25. Cambridge, MA, Health Effects Institute, 1989
83. Rem J, Siggaard-Anderson O, Norgaard-Pedersen B, Sorenson S: Hemoglobin pigments: Photometer for oxygen saturation, carboxyhemoglobin, and methemoglobin in capillary blood. Clin Chim Acta 42:101, 1972
84. Freeman GL, Steinke JM: Evaluation of two oximeters for use in cardiac catheterization laboratories. Cathet Cardiovasc Diagn 30(1):51, 1993
85. Fairley HB: Changing perspectives in monitoring oxygenation. Anesthesiology 70:2, 1989
86. Severinghaus JW: History and recent developments in pulse oximetry. Scand J Clin Lab Invest 53(Suppl 214):105, 1993
87. Technology Subcommittee of the Working Group on Critical Care: Noninvasive blood gas monitoring: A review for use in the adult critical care unit. Can Med Assoc J 146(5):703, 1992
88. King T, Simon RH: Pulse oximetry for tapering supplemental oxygen in hospitalized patients. Evaluation of a protocol. Chest 92:713, 1987
89. Wimberley PD, Helledie NR, Friis-Hansen B, Siggaard-Anderson O, Fogh-Anderson N: Some problems involved using hemoglobin oxygen saturation in arterial blood to detect hypoxemia and hyperoxemia in newborn infants. Scand J Clin Lab Invest 48(Suppl 189):45, 1988
90. Zeballos RJ, Weisman IM: Reliability of noninvasive oximetry in black subjects during exercise and hypoxia. Am Rev Respir Dis 144(6):1240, 1991

91. Benaron DA, Benitz WE, Ariagno RL, Stevenson DK: Noninvasive methods for estimating in vivo oxygenation. Clin Pediatr 31(5):258, 1992
92. Seidler D, Hirschl MM, Roeggla G: Limitations of pulse oximetry. Lancet 341:1600, 1993
93. Craft JA, Alessandrini E, Kenney LB, et al: Comparison of oxygenation measurements in pediatric patients during sickle cell crises. J Pediatr 124:93, 1994
94. Wyatt JS, Cope M, Delpy DT, et al: Quantitation of cerebral blood volume in human infants by near-infrared spectroscopy. J Appl Physiol 68(3):1086, 1990
95. Brazy JE, Lewis DV, Mitnick MH, van der Vliet FFJ: Noninvasive monitoring of cerebral oxygenation in preterm infants: Preliminary observations. Pediatrics 75(2):217, 1985
96. Reynolds EOR, Wyatt JS, Azzopard D, et al: New non-invasive methods for assessing brain oxygenation and haemodynamics. Br Med Bull 44:1052, 1988
97. Bryant RG, Marill K, Blackmore C, Francis C: Magnetic relaxation in blood and blood clots. Magn Res Med 13:133, 1990
98. Benaron DA, Lenox MA, Stevenson DK: 2-D and 3-D images of thick tissue using time constrained times-of-flight and absorbance (tc-TOFA) spectrophotometry. Proceedings of Physiological Monitoring and Early Detection Diagnostic Methods. SPIE Vol 1641. Society of Photo-optical Instrumentation Engineers, Bellingham, WA, 1992, p 35
99. Singer JR, Grunbaum FA, Kohn P, Zubelli JP: Image reconstruction of the interior of bodies that diffuse radiation. Science 248:990, 1990
100. Mahutte CK, Holody M, Maxwell TP, Chen PA, Sasse SA: Development of a patient-dedicated, on-demand, blood gas monitor. Am J Respir Crit Care Med 149:852, 1994
101. Divers S, Larson CP, Riccitelli S, et al: A continuous intravascular oxygen and carbon dioxide monitor. Proceedings from International Federation of Clinical Chemistry, Methodology and Clinical Applications of Blood Gases, pH, Electrolytes and Sensor Technology. IFCC/WGSE-AACC/EBGD Symposium, Monterey. IFCC, Copenhagen, Denmark, 1990, p 51
102. Costello DJ, Salter JR, Schlain LA, Kosa N: Design of an optical biosensor using a bent-fiber light path for continuous in vivo monitoring. Proceedings from International Federation of Clinical Chemistry, Methodology and Clinical Applications of Blood Gases, pH, Electrolytes and Sensor Technology. IFCC/WGSE-AACC/EBGD Symposium, Monterey. IFCC, Copenhagen, Denmark, 1990, p 41
103. Venkatesh B, Brock THC, Hendry SP: A multiparameter sensor for continuous intra-arterial blood gas monitoring: A prospective evaluation. Crit Care Med 22(4):588, 1994
104. Gøthgen IH, Siggaard-Anderson O, Rasmussen JP, Wimberley PD, Fogh-Anderson N: Fiber-optic chemical sensors (Gas-Stat) for blood gas monitoring during hypothermic extracorporeal circulation. Scand J Clin Lab Invest 47(Suppl 188):27, 1987
105. Haller M, Kilger E, Briegel J, Forst H, Peter K: Continuous intra-arterial blood gas and pH monitoring in critically ill patients with severe respiratory failure: A prospective, criterion standard study. Crit Care Med 22(4):580, 1994
106. Pappert D, Rossaint R, Gerlach H, Falke K: Continuous monitoring of blood gases during hypercapnia in a patient with severe lung failure. Intensive Care Med 20:210, 1994
107. Siggaard-Anderson O, Gøthgen IH, Wimberly PD, Rasmussen JP, Fogh-Anderson N: Evaluation of the Gas-STAT® fluorescence sensors for continuous measurement of pH, PCO_2, and PO_2 during cardiopulmonary bypass and hypothermia. Scand J Clin Lab Invest 48(Suppl 189):77, 1988
108. Nikolchev JN, Thapliyal H: Micromachined electrochemical sensor for in-vivo monitoring of arterial blood gases. Proceedings from International Federation of Clinical Chemistry, Methodology and clinical applications of blood gases, pH, electrolytes and sensor technology. IFCC/WGSE-AACC/EBGD Symposium, Monterey. IFCC, Copenhagen, Denmark, 1990, p 63
109. Halbert SA: Intravascular monitoring: Problems and promise. Clin Chem 36(8B):1581, 1990
110. Oeseburg B, Ligtenberg HCG, Schepel SJ, Zijlstra WG: Intravascular pH-ISFET, a method of the future. Scand J Clin Lab Invest 47(Suppl 188):31, 1987
111. Chernow B (Ed): Bedside diagnostic testing. Chest 97(5) [Suppl]:183S, 1990
112. Fogt EJ: Continuous ex vivo and in vivo monitoring with chemical sensors. Clin Chem 36(8B):1573, 1990

10 Fiberoptic Bronchoscopy

W. Mark Brutinel
Denis A. Cortese

CLINICAL SKILLS

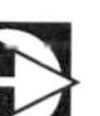

Upon completion of this chapter, the reader will:

- Recognize indications for diagnostic and therapeutic bronchoscopy
- Understand complications of bronchoscopy
- Recognize absolute and relative contraindications for bronchoscopy
- Follow personnel safety considerations in bronchoscopy
- Prepare patients for bronchoscopic procedures
- Monitor patients during bronchoscopic procedures
- Understand conscious sedation policy
- Prepare, handle, and transport specimens obtained during bronchoscopy
- Assist in performance of transbronchial biopsy procedures
- Assist in performance of bronchoalveolar lavage
- Decontaminate/sterilize equipment used in bronchoscopic procedure

KEY TERMS

Acute hypercapnia
Acute inhalation injury
Asthma
Brachytherapy
Bronchiectasis
Bronchoalveolar lavage
Bronchopleural fistulas
Broncholithiasis
Conscious sedation
Cough
Diaphragmatic paralysis
Endotracheal intubation
Hemoptysis
Laryngeal edema
Laser resection
Lung abscess
Photodynamic therapy
Transbronchial biopsy

Bronchoscopy is an established and useful tool in patient care and medical research. The ability to visualize the tracheobronchial tree has been available since the development of rigid bronchoscopy. However, until the introduction into clinical practice of the flexible fiberoptic bronchoscope in 1968, this procedure was limited to specialists, most often surgeons, and was performed in operating suites or dedicated bronchoscopy suites. The flexible fiberoptic bronchoscope has proved to be easy to use and highly portable. Once its efficacy was established, a wide range of medical specialists found it useful in their practice and have taken bronchoscopy out of the operating room and into the intensive care units, procedural rooms, and even outpatient settings away from the hospital.

In this chapter, we give an overview of the clinical indications and contraindications to the use of the flexible fiberoptic instrument. Also presented is a more detailed discussion of necessary equipment; the procedure itself; how to set up for a bronchoscopy, assist the bronchoscopist, and collect specimens; and how to clean the bronchoscope after the procedure. Unless otherwise stated, the discussion deals with the flexible fiberoptic bronchoscope.

PROCEDURE

The procedure begins with a thorough inspection of the upper and lower respiratory tract through the bronchoscope. This should include the nasal passages, pharynx, hypopharynx, larynx, vocal cords, and the subglottic area. Next a complete inspection of the tracheobronchial tree is performed, including the trachea, bronchi, lobar bronchi, and segmental bronchi down to the third or fourth divisions. If abnormalities are seen, diagnostic maneuvers are done, which may include any or all of the following: brushings, biopsies, needle aspirations, and washings. If no abnormalities of the visible airways are seen, then fluoroscopy may be used to direct the brush, needle, and biopsy forceps to the area of interest.[1] With these maneuvers the diagnosis and extent of disease frequently can be determined for various disorders. These include cancer, sarcoidosis, infection, foreign bodies, and other more unusual disorders of the lung parenchyma and bronchial tree.

INDICATIONS

The diagnostic and therapeutic indications for bronchoscopy are shown in Box 10-1 and 10-2[1–5]; details can be found in American Association for Respiratory Care (AARC) Clinical Practice Guideline: Fiberoptic Bronchoscopy Assisting. The decision to perform a bronchoscopy must be undertaken with a full knowledge of the patient's history, physical findings, and laboratory data. The appropriate timing and selection of the most effective diagnostic maneuvers cannot be done without detailed information about the patient. Care and attention must always be directed to the overall medical condition

BOX 10-1

DIAGNOSTIC INDICATIONS FOR BRONCHOSCOPY

- Abnormal radiographic findings
  - Localized lesion
    - Mass lesion
    - Recurring pulmonary infiltrates
    - Unresolved pulmonary infiltrates
    - Persistent atelectasis/collapse
      - Segmental
      - Lobar
      - Lung
    - Mediastinal and hilar abnormalities
    - Malignant pleural effusions
    - Abnormalities of the tracheobronchial air shadow
  - Diffuse parenchymal lung disease
    - Immunocompetent host
    - Nonimmunocompetent host
- Acute inhalation injury
- Aspiration
- Assessment of endotracheal and tracheostomy tubes
  - Tracheal damage
  - Airway obstruction
  - Tube placement
- Assessment of rejection of transplanted lung
- Bronchiectasis
- Bronchopleural fistulas
- Broncholithiasis
- Diaphragmatic paralysis
- Foreign body
- Hemoptysis
- Lung abscess
- Major thoracic trauma
- Positive sputum cytology for malignancy
- Recurrent laryngeal nerve (vocal cord) paralysis
- Stridor or localized wheezing
- Unexplained cough
- Upper esophageal lesions

BOX 10-2

THERAPEUTIC INDICATIONS FOR BRONCHOSCOPY

- Endotracheal intubation
- Retained secretions or mucus plugs
- Foreign body aspiration
- Management of life-threatening hemoptysis
- Bronchopleural fistulas
- Drainage of lung abscess
- Bronchial strictures
  - Dilatation (rigid bronchoscopy)
  - Placement of stents (rigid bronchoscopy)
  - Laser therapy (rigid and flexible bronchoscopy)
- Endobronchial malignant obstruction
  - Dilatation (rigid bronchoscopy)
  - Placement of stents (rigid bronchoscopy)
  - Laser therapy (rigid and flexible bronchoscopy)
    - Photodynamic therapy
    - Carbon dioxide laser
    - Neodymium: YAG laser
- Brachytherapy

AARC Clinical Practice Guideline

FIBEROPTIC BRONCHOSCOPY ASSISTING

Indications: Indications include but are not limited to the presence of lesions of unknown cause on chest radiograph or the need to evaluate recurrent or persistent atelectasis or pulmonary infiltrates; the need to assess patency or mechanical properties of the upper airway; the need to investigate hemoptysis, persistent unexplained cough, localized wheeze, or stridor; suspicious or positive sputum cytology results; the need to obtain lower respiratory tract secretions, cell washings, and biopsies for cytologic, histologic, and microbiologic evaluation; the need to determine the location and extent of injury from toxic inhalation or aspiration; the need to evaluate problems associated with endotracheal or tracheostomy tubes (tracheal damage, airway obstruction, or tube placement); the need for aid in performing difficult intubations; the suspicion that secretions or mucus plugs are responsible for lobar or segmental atelectasis; the need to remove abnormal endobronchial tissue or foreign material by forceps, basket, or laser; and the need to retreive a foreign body.

Contraindications: Flexible bronchoscopy should be performed only when the relative benefits outweigh the risks. Absolute contraindications include absence of consent from the patient or his or her representative unless a medical emergency exists and the patient is not competent to give permission; absence of an experienced bronchoscopist to perform or closely and directly supervise the procedure; lack of adequate facilities and personnel to care for such emergencies as cardiopulmonary arrest, pneumothorax, or bleeding; and inability to adequately oxygenate the patient during the procedure. The danger of serious complications from bronchoscopy is especially high in patients with the following disorders and these conditions are usually considered absolute contraindications unless the risk:benefit assessment warrants the procedure: coagulopathy or bleeding diathesis that cannot be corrected, severe obstructive airways disease, severe refractory hypoxemia, and unstable hemodynamic status including dysrhythmias. Relative contraindications (or conditions involving increased risk), according to the American Thoracic Society Guidelines for Fiberoptic Bronchoscopy in adults, include lack of patient cooperation; recent myocardial infarction or unstable angina; partial tracheal obstruction; moderate to severe hypoxemia or any degree of hypercarbia; uremia and pulmonary hypertension (possible serious hemorrhage after biopsy); lung abscess (danger of flooding the airway with purulent material); obstruction of the superior vena cava (possibility of bleeding and laryngeal edema); debility, advanced age, and malnutrition; respiratory failure requiring mechanical ventilation; disorders requiring laser therapy, biopsy of lesions obstructing large airways, or multiple transbronchial lung biopsies; and known or suspected pregnancy because of radiation exposure. The safety of bronchoscopic procedures in asthmatic patients is a concern, but the presence of asthma does not preclude the use of these procedures.

Assessment of Need: Need is determined by the presence of clinical indicators and contraindications as previously described.

Assessment of Outcome: Patient outcome is determined by clinical, physiologic, and pathologic assessment. Procedural outcome is determined by the accomplishment of the procedural goals as previously indicated.

Monitoring: The following should be monitored before, during, and after bronchoscopy, continuously, until the patient returns to his pre-sedation level of consciousness. *Patient:* level of consciousness; medications administered, dosage, route, and time of delivery (termed *conscious sedation* by the JCAHO); subjective response to procedure (eg, pain, discomfort, dyspnea); blood pressure, heart rate, rhythm, and changes in cardiac status; SpO_2 and FIO_2; tidal volume, peak inspiratory pressure, adequacy of inspiratory flow, and other ventilation parameters if subject is being mechanically ventilated; lavage volumes (delivered and retrieved); documentation of site of biopsies and washings and tests requested on each sample; periodic postprocedure follow-up monitoring of patient condition is advisable for 24 to 48 hours for inpatients. Outpatients should be instructed to contact the bronchoscopist regarding fever, chest pain or discomfort, dyspnea, wheezing, hemoptysis, or any new findings presenting after the procedure has been completed. Oral instructions should be reinforced by written instructions that include names and phone numbers of persons to be contacted in emergency. *Technical Devices:* bronchoscope integrity (fiberoptic or channel damage, passage of leak test); strict adherence to the recommended procedures for cleaning, disinfection, and sterilization of the devices, and the integrity of disinfection or sterilization packaging; and smooth, unhampered operation of biospy devices (forceps, needles). *Recordkeeping:* quality assessment indicators as determined appropriate by the institution's quality assessment committee; identification of bronchoscope used for each patient; annual assessment of the institutional or departmental bronchoscopy procedure, including an evaluation of adequacy of bronchoscopic specimens (size or volume for accurate analysis, sample integrity), review of infection control procedures and compliance with the current guidelines for semicritical patient-care objects, synopsis of complications, control washings to assure that infection control and disinfection/sterilization procedures are adequate and that cross-contamination of specimens does not occur, annual review of the bronchoscopy service and all of the above listed records with the physician bronchoscopists.

From AARC Clinical Practice Guideline, see Respir Care 38:1173–1178, 1993, for complete text.

of the patient and, particularly, to the patient's respiratory reserve. The relative contraindications to bronchoscopy must be kept in mind and suitable decisions made for the patients to whom they apply (see Box 10-3).[3]

Diagnostic

The most common indication for a bronchoscopic procedure is an abnormal roentgenographic study. Chest roentgenograms, tomograms, computed tomograms (CT scan), and magnetic resonance imaging (MRI) scans can all show abnormalities. The approach to these lesions depends on their location and the clinical situation.[2]

BOX 10-3

CONTRAINDICATIONS TO BRONCHOSCOPY

Absence of informed consent (Unless a medical emergency exists)
Absence of an experienced bronchoscopist
Lack of emergency facilities for:
- Cardiopulmonary arrest
- Pneumothorax
- Bleeding

Inability to adequately oxygenate the patient
Relative contraindications
- Hypoxemia
- Hypercapnia
- Cardiovascular instability
  - Hypotension
  - Uncontrolled angina
  - Myocardial infarction
  - Malignant arrhythmias
- Uncontrolled asthma
- Coagulopathy
- Partial tracheal obstruction
- Uremia
- Pulmonary hypertension
- Superior vena cava obstruction
- Patient unable to cooperate with the procedure
- Known or suspected pregnancy

The bronchoscopist is commonly called upon to diagnose diffuse lung disease. In the *immunocompetent host*, the procedure is most effective in diagnosing neoplastic and infectious causes of diffuse disease.

In the immunocompromised host, the bronchoscope is highly efficacious in diagnosing infectious causes of new pulmonary infiltrates.[6–15]

Bronchoalveolar lavage (BAL) is now routinely used in an attempt to diagnose bacterial, fungal, mycobacterial, *Pneumocystis*, *Legionella*, and viral infections that can occur in these patients. If a diagnosis is not made in both immunocompetent and immunocompromised patients, after physical examination, initial laboratory testing, and analysis of the patient's sputum,[9,16] bronchoscopy is performed and a segment of the lung containing the infiltrate is lavaged. Appropriate microbiologic tests are then performed on the aspirated fluid. If appropriate, brushing and biopsies can be performed. The yield on these procedures is excellent and helps avoid an open-lung biopsy. Because of the efficacy of bronchoscopy with BAL, the bronchoscopist is often asked to perform the procedure on patients who are very ill and with little respiratory reserve. This requires care on the part of the medical team to ensure the patient's comfort and safety.

Acute inhalation injury from toxic or heated gases can be a life-threatening situation. Initially, judgments need to be made about the degree of respiratory support that will be needed. A bronchoscopic examination of the upper and lower airways can be helpful in judging the extent of the damage and planning therapy. One of the most immediate dangers is *laryngeal edema* causing upper airway obstruction, usually at the level of the vocal cords. An experienced observer can judge the degree of laryngeal damage and proceed to elective intubation with the help of the bronchoscope before the edema can make intubation difficult or impossible to accomplish. Knowledge of the degree and extent of mucosal damage can help determine whether careful observation or early therapy with steroids and possibly antibiotics is indicated.[17–21]

Endotracheal intubation carries with it the risk of damage to the larynx, vocal cords, and trachea. The bronchoscope is an excellent tool to assess the possibility of damage to these areas. Hemoptysis from an endotracheal tube or postintubation shortness of breath, stridor, or wheezing are reasons to perform a bronchoscopy. The bronchoscope is also an excellent tool to assess the patency of the airway in a patient who is intubated or has a tracheostomy. A quick examination can aid in the discovery of whether the endotracheal tube is placed correctly and whether any mucus, blood, or foreign body is obstructing the endotracheal tube. Difficulty ventilating the patient without obvious cause and difficulty passing a suction catheter are reasons to examine the airway.[22–24]

Bronchiectasis is fortunately less common in this age of antibiotic therapy, but it still occurs. It is important to assess the bronchial anatomy in individuals with bronchiectasis to rule out an endobronchial cause and look for the extent of involvement. *Bronchopleural fistulas* with persistent leakage of air into the pleural space can be troublesome. The bronchoscope can be used to attempt to locate the fistula. Particularly after a lung resection, inspection of the bronchial suture line for dehiscence is important. *Broncholithiasis* presenting as hemoptysis, lithoptysis, or bronchial obstruction can be diagnosed with the bronchoscope in conjunction with appropriate roentgenographic studies.[25] Unfortunately, it is not as useful for removal of the broncholiths because of the dangers of massive hemorrhage.[26]

Diaphragmatic paralysis can be idiopathic or iatrogenic from surgical manipulation. However, it can also be caused by neoplasms of the airway, and some clinicians have recommended a bronchoscopic examination to look for endobronchial lesions. The advent of CT scanning has made this less necessary in our view. The likelihood of there being a visible endobronchial lesion causing a phrenic nerve paralysis in the face of a negative CT scan of the chest is quite small.

Foreign bodies in the airway almost always can be removed with bronchoscopy. The flexible fiberoptic bronchoscope is excellent for diagnosing the presence of a foreign body, and some authors feel that they can be removed with the flexible instrument.[25] However, when the foreign body cannot be easily withdrawn through an endotracheal tube, the rigid bronchoscope is the instrument of choice for removal of the foreign body.[27,28] In children, the rigid bronchoscope allows ventilation of the patient under general anesthesia; in both children and adults, the rigid bronchoscope facilitates safe delivery of large foreign bodies through the subglottic area and the larynx.[29–32]

Most patients with *hemoptysis* have benign bronchitis. Unfortunately, hemoptysis is also a sign of bronchiectasis, broncholithiasis, foreign body aspiration, endobronchial tumor, and bronchogenic carcinoma. In patients who are older, have a smoking history, have had hemoptysis longer than 1 week, or have an abnormal chest radiograph, the risk of a significant pathologic cause of the hemoptysis is increased. Bronchoscopy is indicated in selected patients with increased risk factors for cancer or in whom the clinical situation suggests a diagnosis that can be investigated by a visual inspection of the airway.[33–37]

A *lung abscess* is a strong indication for a bronchoscopic examination. The abscess may be a result of endobronchial obstruction, which may be due to a foreign body, tumor, extrinsic compression, or mucosal lesions. The bronchoscopist can also help therapeutically by attempting to establish drainage from the abscessed area of the lung. Clinical judgment must be exercised in attempting drainage of a lung abscess. The potential exists to flood the airway with purulent material, and the bronchoscopist must weigh the benefit:risk ratio to decide if attempting to drain the abscess cavity is clinically indicated.[38,39]

Major blunt thoracic trauma can result in a pulmonary contusion as well as a laceration or disruption of the tracheobronchial tree. The disruptions can range from small tears to complete transection and can occur in the trachea and major bronchi. They may present as pneumothorax, pneumomediastinum, and subcutaneous emphysema. Airway obstruction and asphyxia can occur with transection of the trachea. The bronchoscope is invaluable in determining the integrity of the tracheobronchial tree.[40]

A patient who has *cancer cells* on cytologic examination of the sputum and a negative result on chest roentgenogram or CT scan presents a diagnostic dilemma. An ear, nose, and throat examination will rule out an upper airway cause; bronchoscopy will then be needed to search for a cancer of the tracheobronchial tree. If this is negative, a repeat examination is performed under general anesthesia with selective brushing of all 20 lobar segments. If malignancy is confirmed by biopsy, positive brush cytology on two separate occasions, or both, the cancer is considered localized and treatment begins. If the malignancy cannot be localized, careful observation with repeat roentgenographic and bronchoscopic studies is advised. Localization with hematoporphyrin fluorescence is another technique that can be used, but it is performed in only a few medical centers.[41]

Recurrent laryngeal nerve (vocal cord) paralysis suggests the possibility of a lesion along the distribution of the recurrent laryngeal nerve. Imaging of the chest with a CT scan is appropriate. If the CT scan is abnormal, bronchoscopy can be performed to look for an endobronchial lesion (most commonly malignant) to make the diagnosis for the cause of the nerve dysfunction. A transbronchial needle aspiration could be performed if the diagnosis cannot be made with inspection of the tracheobronchial tree and if a mediastinal mass is present on the CT scan.[42] Bronchoscopy performed when the result of the CT scan is negative has less chance of finding the cause of the nerve paralysis, but it can be performed to be sure there is no occult extra-bronchial lesion.

Stridor or localized wheezing suggests a functional or structural narrowing of the airway from various causes. Pulmonary function tests can be helpful, along with roentgenographic studies, in attempting to localize the point of narrowing. Asthma should be considered, but care must be taken not to confuse a localized obstruction with the more diffuse bronchial narrowing of asthma. Bronchoscopy is an excellent technique to look for vocal cord paralysis, laryngeal pathology, tumors (benign and malignant), and extrinsic compression of the tracheobronchial tree.[43–45]

Unexplained *cough* can be a diagnostic dilemma. Once common causes such as respiratory infections, chronic obstructive pulmonary disease, and asthma have been ruled out, bronchoscopy should be considered. Occult endobronchial lesions can cause chronic persistent coughing and are often small and treatable. A careful evaluation for treatable causes of cough should be undertaken and appropriate therapy should be instituted. If no cause for the cough is found and no significant improvement occurs in 2 to 3 months, bronchoscopy should be considered.[46,47]

Cancer of the upper esophagus can invade the tracheobronchial tree. It is important for the thoracic surgeon attempting to resect this type of cancer to know the extent of the spread of the tumor. A bronchoscopic examination of the trachea and main bronchi can accomplish this.[48–52]

Therapeutic

The bronchoscope is also an excellent therapeutic tool. It is extremely useful in *placing endotracheal tubes* by the oral or nasal route. It is the instrument of choice to assist with difficult intubations. It can help with assessment of the position of tracheostomy tubes. Patients who cannot move their necks or who have unusual upper airway anatomy can be intubated safely while awake with this technique.[22–24]

Probably the most frequent therapeutic use of the bronchoscope is to *remove retained secretions.* In a hospitalized patient in whom new atelectasis or collapse of a lung or its segments develops and who has not responded to aggressive chest physiotherapy and suctioning, bronchoscopy is indicated to assess the airway for retained secretions and to remove them. If the patient is stable and has an adequate blood oxygen tension, increasing those measures that improve pulmonary toilet is as likely to resolve the atelectasis and collapse as bronchoscopy. These include instituting or increasing chest physical therapy, cough, deep inspiratory maneuvers, pain relief, and ambulation. If these measures are already in place, or if after 12 to 24 hours of intensive treatment there is no improvement, bronchoscopy is indicated. If the patient is hypoxemic despite oxygen supplementation and it is judged that relief of the presumed obstruction caused by secretion retention will improve the hypoxemia, then bronchoscopy should be done promptly while the oxygen saturation is monitored.[53,54]

Management of life-threatening hemoptysis is a difficult clinical problem.[26,55–60] The degree of danger to the patient depends on the amount of hemorrhage and the patient's pulmonary reserve. Therapy should be directed toward protecting what pulmonary function remains. The flexible instrument can be used to attempt to localize the site of bleeding, remove blood and clot from the airway, place single- and double-lumen endotracheal tubes,[61] and place balloon catheters to tamponade that portion of the lung that is bleeding.

However, in massive hemoptysis, the flexible instrument is often not adequate. Its small fiberoptic bundle is quickly obscured, making vision difficult if not impossible, and the relatively small suction channel is easily clogged with fibrin clot. *Rigid bronchoscopy* has the advantage of being able to simultaneously ventilate the patient through the instrument and maintain a clear airway. Larger instruments can be passed through the scope. This permits the use of large suction catheters, and more than one suction catheter can be used at once.

In addition, the bronchus leading to the bleeding area of the lung can be packed with umbilical tape soaked in epinephrine.[59] The rigid bronchoscope cannot examine the upper lobes well, but if required the flexible bronchoscope can be passed through the rigid scope to examine these areas. The optimum management of massive hemoptysis is with a combination of flexible and rigid instruments.

Bronchial strictures, other than thin webs, are treated definitively with surgical resection. In patients in whom this is not possible, dilatation with a rigid bronchoscope can be a temporizing measure. Placement of *Silastic bronchial stents* can be tried,[62,63] and *laser resection* with the neodymium:YAG or carbon dioxide laser has been used.[64]

Endobronchial malignant obstruction is best treated with surgical resection, but when that is not possible, bronchoscopic techniques can help in palliation of respiratory symptoms and prolongation of life. Dilatation can be performed with the rigid bronchoscope. Laser therapy with either the neodymium:YAG or carbon dioxide laser has been helpful.[65] Endobronchial Silastic stents can be placed to maintain airway patency.[62,63] Photodynamic therapy with hematoporphyrin has been used by some clinicians to treat malignant airway obstruction.[66–69]

Photodynamic therapy is also used to treat small-airway carcinomas for cure in patients who are not candidates for surgical resection.[70] *Brachytherapy* performed with small plastic tubes temporarily placed in the airways with bronchoscopic guidance can help decrease malignant obstruction in patients who have received maximal external beam radiation therapy. The catheters are subsequently loaded with iridium-192 beads on a wire, and local radiation therapy is delivered to the airway obstruction.[71]

COMPLICATIONS

Fortunately, complications from a fiberoptic bronchoscopy examination are rare. These complications include adverse effects of medications administered before and during the procedure, hypoxemia, hypercarbia, wheezing, hypotension, laryngospasm, bradycardia, and increased airway resistance.[72] Overall mortality should be less then 0.1%. All complications should be fewer than 8.1%. Other complications not leading to death have been reported, including fever (1.2%), pneumonia (0.6%), vasovagal reaction (2.4%), obstruction of the airways (0.9%), respiratory arrest (0.1%), cardiac arrhythmias (0.9%), pneumothorax (0.7%), nausea and vomiting (0.2%), psychotic reaction (0.1%), and aphonia (0.1%).[73] Bacteremias can occur after bronchoscopic examination. Infective endocarditis prophylaxis with antibiotics is recommended for rigid bronchoscopy.[74] Laser bronchoscopy increases the risk of death to 2%.[65]

Complications can be minimized if thought is given to the clinical status of the patient. For example, before the procedure the asthmatic should be treated for bronchospasm, the unstable cardiac patient stabilized medically, and the hypoxic chronic lung disease patient adequately oxygenated. With careful preparation and monitoring, bronchoscopy can be made safe.

CONTRAINDICATIONS

The contraindications to bronchoscopy are shown in Box 10-3.[1–3,72,75] They are all relative. If after careful evaluation it is thought that the possible benefit of bronchoscopy outweighs the risks, then the procedure should be performed by an experienced bronchoscopist. Bronchoscopy frequently can cause a decrease in the arterial oxygen tension, both during and after the procedure. Oxygen supplementation should be provided, and a finger pulse oximeter to monitor the need for oxygen before, during, and after the procedure should be used.[76–81] If the patient is already significantly hypoxemic despite medical management, oxygen supplementation, and mechanical ventilation, bronchoscopy *may worsen the hypoxemia* and could be a serious risk to the patient. Patients who have borderline or low arterial oxygen tensions should continue to receive supplemental oxygen after the procedure until their oxygen saturation is at an acceptable level.

Acute hypercapnia with acidosis is a significant contraindication. Bronchoscopy will increase airway resistance and the work of breathing and can quickly worsen the situation. If it is thought that the procedure is necessary, mechanical ventilation will be required. If the patient is hypercapnic and acidotic on a ventilator, the procedure should be performed if the potential benefit is judged to be high. In a patient with stable compensated respiratory acidosis, bronchoscopy can be performed, depending on the degree of hypercapnia, with careful attention to the use of premedication, sedation during the procedure, and the amount of oxygen supplementation.

Cardiac instability should be treated before the bronchoscopy. Elective bronchoscopy should not be performed until the situation is stabilized. However, if the cause of cardiac instability can be corrected by the bronchoscopy, then the risks of the procedure must be weighed against the benefits.

Asthma is a relative contraindication because bronchoscopy can stimulate or worsen bronchospasm. If the asthma is adequately treated and controlled, asthmatics can be examined safely.[82]

Coagulopathies are contraindications only to brushings, needle aspirations, and biopsies. Patients can safely undergo a bronchoscopy while receiving full anticoagulation therapy as long as care is taken not to irritate the mucosa. Bronchoalveolar lavage can be performed with low platelet counts, and it is useful in the immunocompromised hematologic patient, who often has a coagulopathy. Uremia increases the risk of bleeding owing to platelet dysfunction, and the serum creatinine level should be routinely measured; if the creatinine level is increased, a blood urea nitrogen measurement is indicated before a bronchoscopy in which brushings, needle aspirations, or biopsies are planned.

If the patient is unable to cooperate with the procedure, then consideration can be given to performing the bronchoscopy under heavy sedation or general anesthesia. This is best done in an operating room, outpatient surgical area, or intensive care unit, with assistance from an anesthesiologist or nurse anesthetist.

PERSONNEL SAFETY

All members of the bronchoscopy team should use universal precautions at all times and wear approved masks, eye protection, and gloves. Personnel safety is increased with identification of patients with pathogens that can be potentially transmitted to health care workers. These pathogens include hepatitis A, B, and C, *Mycobacterium tuberculosis* and HIV. With the increase in the incidence of active *M. tuberculosis* infections and the appearance of multiple drug-resistant *M. tuberculosis* associated with the HIV epidemic, much more attention must be paid to the potential for transmission of this pathogen by the airborne route. All bronchoscopy procedures that are performed on patients who may have infectious tuberculosis should be performed in rooms that meet the ventilation requirements for tuberculosis isolation. Approved high-efficiency particulate air (HEPA) filter mask should be worn by health care workers on all cases suspected of having *M. tuberculosis* infection. After the procedure, patients suspected of having infectious tuberculosis should be kept in isolation rooms that meet the ventilation requirements for tuberculosis isolation. The patient should also be given an approved mask when traveling outside the isolation room. Transmission can also be reduced by giving the patient tissues and asking them to cover their mouth and nose when coughing.[83,84] Hepatitis B vaccine is recommended.[72] It is good practice to use nonsterile protective gowns to keep secretions and blood off clothes and bodies. The entire procedure should be done carefully to prevent contamination of the bronchoscopy team with secretions. With the advent of the acquired immunodeficiency syndrome (AIDS), there has been concern that the virus could be transmitted by the patient's respiratory secretions. Fortunately, there is no documented case of human immunodeficiency virus (HIV) transmission to bronchoscopy personnel. Of more concern is contact with the patient's blood. Care with handling of blood products should be exercised at all times, but particularly when handling the needle catheters used for cytologic aspiration. They should be handled in the same manner as any contaminated sharp instrument. Because the needle is passed from the bronchoscopist to the assistant, special care must be taken not to puncture the person receiving the needle catheter.[85]

EQUIPMENT

The proper selection of equipment is important to ensure a safe and effective procedure. Box 10-4 lists suggested equipment that can be placed on a portable cart and moved to wherever the bronchoscopy is to be performed (Figs. 10-1, 10-2). If possible, a system should be devised to store the bronchoscopes on the side of the cart such that they hang straight and are protected from injury (Fig. 10-3). Particular attention should be paid to avoid catching the scope in the hinges of a door, drawer, or case. Oxygen, suction, and a cardiac monitor should be available where the procedure is to be performed. A regular program of inspection and stocking of the bronchoscopy cart should be instituted, especially in the situation in which more than one physician uses the equipment.

ASSISTING IN THE PROCEDURE

Before a bronchoscopy is performed, a certain amount of preparation is required to ensure a safe and smooth procedure. The patient's history should be carefully reviewed for possible contraindications to the procedure. Special attention should be directed to the patient's mental status, cardiovascular status, history of asthma, respiratory reserve, and arterial blood gas values. A recent hemoglobin value, platelet count, electrolyte values, and creatinine level should be available. If there is any concern about the patient's respiratory reserve, an arterial blood gas measurement and possibly pulmonary function testing should be done. If the history or laboratory results suggest a coagulopathy, then a prothrombin time, activated partial thromboplastin time, and if indicated, a bleeding time should be measured. These need to be performed only if brushings, aspirations, or biopsies are contemplated.

The bronchoscopist selects the appropriate instruments for the procedure planned. The bronchoscopy cart should be set up close to the patient so that the

BOX 10-4

BRONCHOSCOPY EQUIPMENT

- Portable cart
- Light source
- Bronchoscopes
  - Adult scope (5.0-mm OD)
  - Adult lavage scope (6.0-mm OD)
  - Pediatric scope (3.5-mm OD)
  - Suction adapters, valves, and caps
- Bite block
- Oxygen source
  - Tubing, nasal cannulas, close-fitting mask
- Assortment of endotracheal tubes
- Swivel adapters with rubber diaphragms
- Cardiac monitor
- Pulse oximeter
- Isotonic saline
- Syringes (non–Luer-lock)
  - 10–12 mL
  - 30–50 mL
- Sterile needles
- Lidocaine
  - Viscous 2%
  - Injectable 2%
  - Injectable 4%
- Benzocaine 20% oral spray
- Direct laryngoscopes
- Laryngeal mirror
- Laryngeal cannula
- Head lamp
- Wall suction
- Suction tubing and connectors
- Specimens
  - Secretion traps
  - Glass slides
  - Cytology jars
  - Formalin jars
  - Sterile containers
- Cytology brushes
- Transbronchial aspiration needles
- Double-sheathed protected catheter brush
  - Sterile capped plastic tubes with 1 mL of isotonic saline
  - Sterile scissors
  - Sterile wire cutters
- Biopsy forceps
  - Cup forceps
  - Alligator forceps
- Foreign body forceps
  - Basket
  - Grasping
- Bronchoalveolar lavage kit
  - Tubing
  - Stopcock
  - Connectors
  - Specimen containers

bronchoscope's light guide is not under tension. The patient should have a cardiac monitor and finger-pulse oximeter attached and supplemental oxygen given by nasal cannula or close-fitting mask. If a close-fitting mask is used, a small hole can be cut in the disposable mask to allow insertion of the bronchoscope. If the patient is intubated or is going to be intubated, a swivel adapter with a rubber diaphragm should be available. Also, if the patient is to be intubated, an appropriate-sized endotracheal tube, 7.5 or larger, should have its balloon tested, lubricated, and placed over the bronchoscope before intubation. A means to hand-ventilate the patient during the procedure should be ready, and a mechanical ventilator should be available.

On the top of the bronchoscopy cart a sterile towel is spread and the basic items required for the procedure are placed (Fig. 10-4). These may vary somewhat with the individual requirements of each physician. A clear, water-soluble lubricant is needed to lubricate the insertion tube of the scope. Four-by-four sponges are helpful to apply the lubricant and wipe off excess lubricant and secretions. Isotonic saline is used to clear the suction channel and to fill the lavage syringes. Two 50-mL non–Luer-lock syringes filled with 30 mL of isotonic saline and 10 mL of air are needed for lavage. For instilling local anesthetic, two 10-mL non–Luer-lock syringes filled with 1 mL of 2% lidocaine and 9 mL of air should be prepared. Wall suction should be available and, if secretions are to be collected, a secretion trap should be inserted in the suction line. The trap must be held upright or taped to an object to prevent tipping and losing secretions.

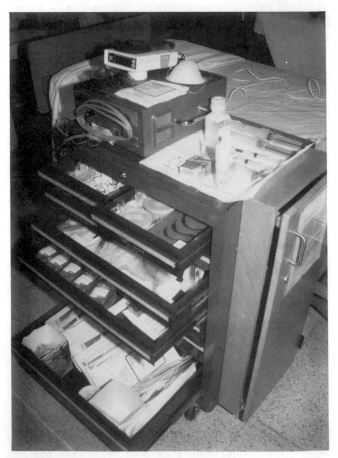

FIGURE 10-1. Portable bronchoscopy equipment cart at bedside.

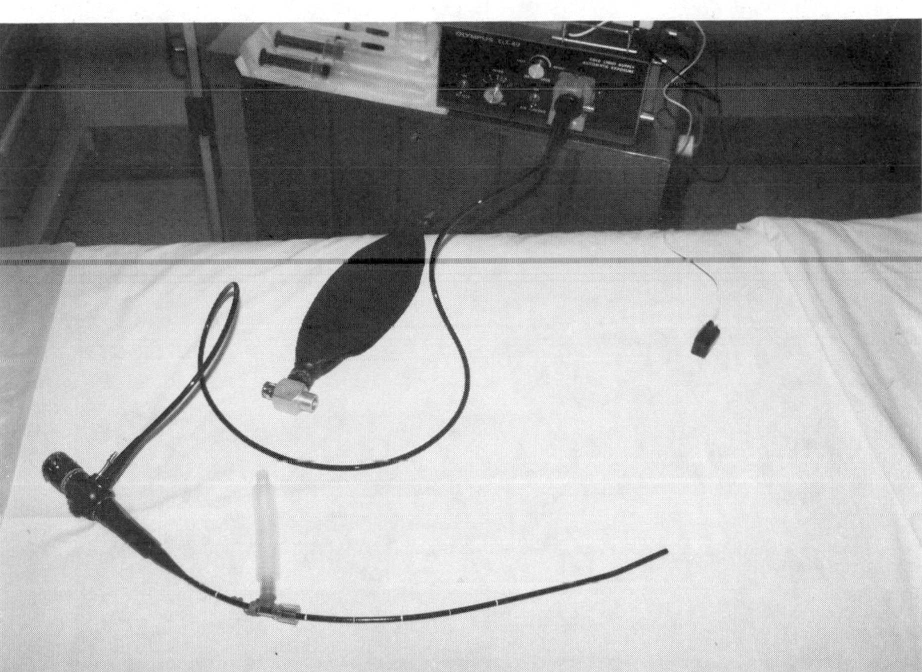

FIGURE 10-2. Flexible fiberoptic bronchoscope with swivel adaptor and anesthesia bag.

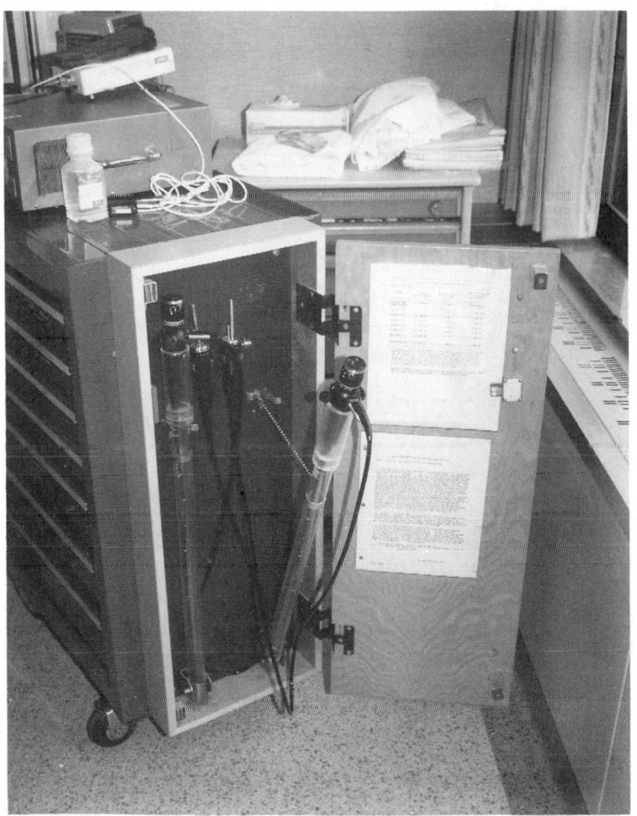

FIGURE 10-3. Storage cabinet for flexible fiberoptic bronchoscopes attached to a portable bronchoscopy equipment cart. This allows the scopes to be stored in a straight position and reduces the chance of damage to them.

Depending on the diagnostic procedures planned (Table 10-1), the appropriate instruments should be readily available (see Box 10-4). Wire brushes are needed for cytologic specimens. Transbronchial needle catheters vary according to the type of aspiration planned. Flexible biopsy forceps should be tested to ensure that the jaws work smoothly. If BAL is planned, it is best to have a kit available (see Box 10-4).

Preoperative medications to be given before the bronchoscopy should be selected by the bronchoscopist and can include benzodiazepines, anticholinergic agents, and narcotics. Most bronchoscopists in this country will perform the procedure while facing a sitting patient who is receiving supplemental oxygen. The bronchoscope is inserted through an anesthetized naris, without an endotracheal tube, and 2% lidocaine is given through the suction channel of the scope to anesthetize the hypopharynx, larynx, vocal cords, and tracheobronchial tree, as needed. Other alternatives used are an endotracheal tube placed through the naris or through the mouth. When performing the bronchoscopic examination through the mouth, the use of an endotracheal tube is also optional. Endotracheal tubes may be used when the patient will need ventilatory support during the procedure, when thick tenacious secretions are expected, or when there is a risk of hemorrhage. A swivel adapter is used to allow assisted ventilation while bronchoscopy is performed (Fig. 10-5). If one elects to examine the patient through the mouth, local anesthetic can be in stilled in the back of the throat and tongue with a spray, such as 20% benzocaine, and the hypopharynx, larynx,

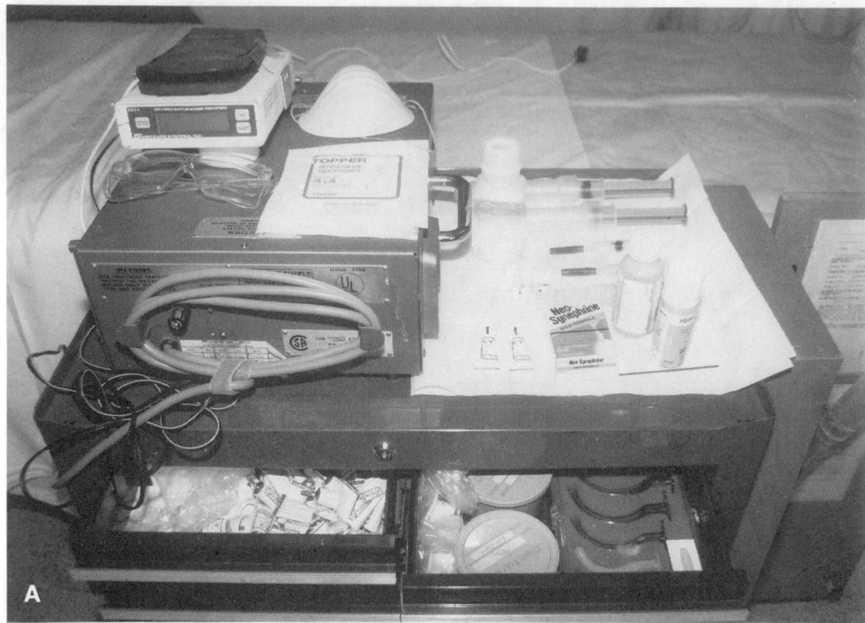

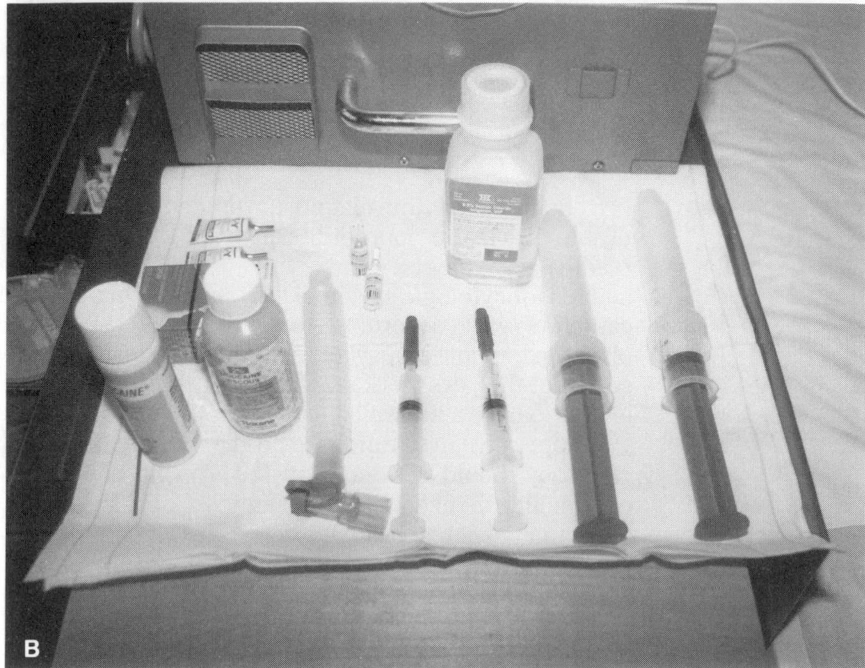

FIGURE 10-4. Portable bronchoscopy equipment cart setup with equipment needed for a basic bronchoscopic examination.

and vocal cords can be anesthetized with 2% lidocaine by using a laryngeal mirror and cannula. Other techniques include the use of 5 mL of 4% lidocaine delivered by nebulizer, superior laryngeal nerve block, and direct instillation of 2 mL of 2% lidocaine through the cricothyroid membrane into the trachea with a syringe and a small-gauge needle.

If secretions are being collected for culture, suction should not be attached to the bronchoscope until it is inside the trachea. This prevents aspiration of saliva and pharyngeal contents. The bronchoscopist asks for lidocaine and isotonic saline when needed, and the syringes should be handed to his or her free hand. In older bronchoscopes the suction should be interrupted during injection of small volumes of liquid into the suction channel to prevent the liquid from being drawn into the suction tubing. The current generation of bronchoscopes have been designed so that this is not necessary as long as the suction trigger is not being depressed during injection.

Specimen Handling and Collection

The handling of specimens depends on the requirements of the microbiologist, pathologist, and cytopathologist who will interpret the results. What follows is a description of how specimens are handled in our institution.

TABLE 10-1 **Diagnostic Procedures Performed in Fiberoptic Bronchoscopy**

Inspection
Collection of secretions
Fungal cultures
Mycobacterial cultures
Cytology
Brushings
Bacterial culture
Double-sheathed protected catheter brush
Cytology
Needle aspirations
Cytology
Biopsy
Culture
Bacterial cultures
Fungal cultures
Mycobacterial cultures
Aspiration of cystic structures
Biopsy
Bronchoalveolar lavage
Research
Cultures
Bacterial
Fungal
Mycobacterial
Legionella
Pneumocystis carinii
Viral

If brushings are performed for cytologic examination, the brush is handed to the bronchoscopist such that it can be grasped just behind the bristles. The brush is inserted through the suction channel, and the area of interest is brushed. After this the brush will either be pulled back through the suction channel and handed to the assistant, or the scope will be removed from the patient and the brush removed by grasping the wire behind the bristles and pulling it out of the distal tip of the bronchoscope's suction channel. The brushings should be smeared on a series of slides and placed in the fixative. At some institutions the end of the brush is clipped off and also placed in the fixative.

A *double-sheathed protected catheter brush* is used to obtain specimens for sterile bacterial cultures. There are several available; instructions on how to use them are included in their packaging. In general, the procedure is performed before applying any suction to the suction channel. Consequently, this catheter brush is often used first, even before inspecting the airways. The tip of the catheter should be treated in a sterile manner. The catheter brush is advanced, as is, into the area of interest. Then the inner catheter is advanced out of the outer catheter sheath, pushing the glycerol plug into the airway where it melts and is absorbed. The brush is advanced out of the inner catheter sheath. The brush is pulled back into the inner catheter sheath, and the whole catheter brush is removed from the bronchoscope channel. The inner catheter sheath is cleaned with alcohol and its tip is cut off with sterile scissors. The brush is advanced out of the inner catheter sheath and, with a sterile wire cutters, is clipped into a small container with 1 mL of isotonic saline. This is tightly sealed and transported to the microbiology laboratory, where it can be quantitatively cultured for aerobic and anaerobic bacteria.

Transbronchial Biopsy

Transbronchial needle aspirations are performed with needle catheters, which come in various sizes and styles. The bronchoscopy assistant should be familiar with, and have practiced with, the needle catheters that are used. All needle catheters are inserted through the suction channel of the scope. The needle is prepared by either withdrawing the stylet or extending and locking the needle. The bronchoscopist punctures the bronchial wall and asks for suction, which is created by using a syringe attached to the end of the needle catheter. A stylet will need to be withdrawn slightly from the proximal end of the catheter to allow the suction to reach the needle tip. The syringe should contain a small amount of isotonic saline. The needle is agitated in the bronchial wall and then withdrawn through the suction channel of the scope. The assistant flushes the needle catheter and needle with the saline in the syringe. If a small needle is used, the aspirations are placed on a cytologic slide and submitted in fixative. Excess fluid is separately submitted in a jar for cytologic examination. If a large biopsy needle was used, the core of tissue is flushed into a fixative jar to be submitted for histologic analysis. The catheter is then prepared for the next aspiration. Usually several aspiration/biopsies will be done in the area of interest.

The assistant also should be familiar with the control and function of the biopsy forceps. The forceps jaws should work smoothly. The forceps is handed to the bronchoscopist in the closed position. It will be inserted in the suction channel and directed to the area of interest; then the assistant is asked to open and close the jaws as needed. Once the sample is acquired, either the forceps is removed from the suction channel or the entire bronchoscope, with the forceps still in place, is removed from the patient. The forceps jaws are then opened and the sample is removed. The sample is placed either on a glass slide with isotonic saline, if frozen sections are desired, or in formalin for histologic examination. If the forceps is shaken in formalin to remove the specimen, then that part of the forceps should be washed with isotonic saline before being inserted again into the suction channel.

If BAL is to be done, it should be performed before aspirating secretions through the suction channel. If we are also using a double-sheathed protected catheter brush, we perform the BAL after the brushings are done. The wall suction should be set at 80 mmHg for BAL. The bronchoscopist inserts the bronchoscope in

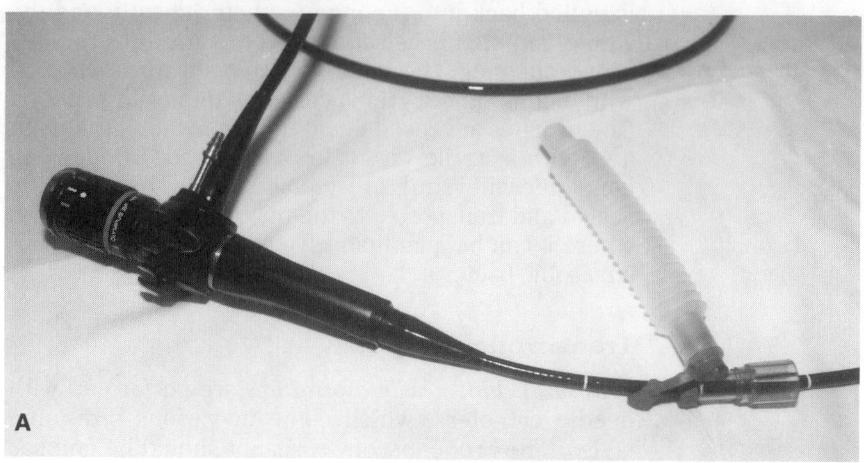

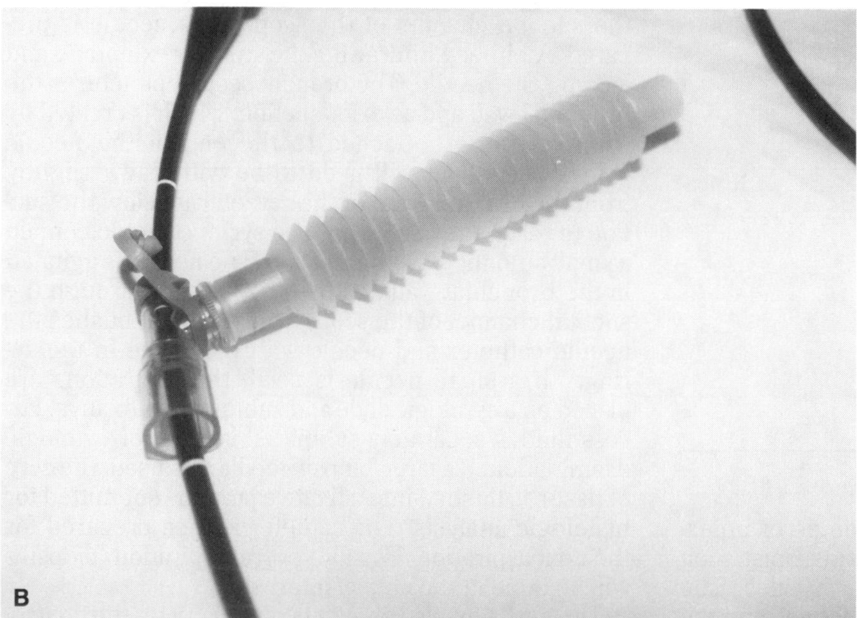

FIGURE 10-5. (**A** and **B**) Flexible fiberoptic bronchoscope with swivel adaptor. The swivel adaptor is used to ventilate an intubated patient during a bronchoscopic examination.

the airway and, without suction, advances it until it is wedged into a segmental bronchus that has been selected. The suction tubing is attached with a three-way stopcock between the scope and the collection jar. The stopcock is initially turned off to suction. We use five 30-mL syringes filled with 20 mL of isotonic saline and 10 mL of air. The contents of one syringe are then injected slowly. The syringe points down so that at the end of the injection the line is flushed with air. The stopcock is then turned off to the syringe and opened to suction. A new syringe is inserted into the stopcock after the return of isotonic saline has stopped. The maneuver is repeated with each of the subsequent four syringes until 100 mL of saline is instilled. The actual amount of isotonic saline used may vary and will depend on the bronchoscopist's preference. The volume of lavage fluid aspirated by the end of the procedure should be 40 mL or more if a total of 100 mL of lavage fluid was injected. The BAL fluid is sent to laboratories where standard protocols are followed to be sure that all appropriate tests are performed on the specimen. The actual laboratory tests done will depend on the clinical situation and should be specified by the bronchoscopist.

CLEANING UP

At the end of the procedure the suction channel should be cleansed immediately by suctioning clean water or saline through it. The bronchoscope should be cleaned carefully following the manufacturer's instructions. Transmission of infectious agents to patients by bronchoscopes is possible. Also, outbreaks of pseudoinfections due to contaminated bronchoscopes are frequently reported.[86] A protocol should be established for each institution and followed routinely to protect both the patients and the bronchoscopes. Currently, we use a soaking time of 45 minutes in glutaraldehyde, and the scope can be ready for use in approximately 1 hour.[83,87,88] It is helpful to have a designated area for cleaning, with all necessary equipment and solutions available. In contaminated cases, if exposure to tuberculosis, hepatitis virus, or HIV is known or suspected, the bronchoscope should be gas sterilized. This requires 24 hours to complete; manufacturer's instructions should be followed to prevent damage to the bronchoscope. When planning more than one bronchoscopy in 24 hours, depending on the number of bronchoscopes available, consideration needs to be given to examining contaminated cases last. Biopsy forceps also need to be cleaned carefully to keep their mechanisms working smoothly. Gas sterilization of biopsy forceps will also be needed in contaminated cases.

CONCLUSION

Bronchoscopy is a safe and efficacious procedure that has become a routine part of respiratory care. Understanding the indications and contraindications for the procedure, how to set up and assist the bronchoscopist, and how to care for the equipment will increase the respiratory care practitioner's usefulness, patient's comfort, and physician's satisfaction with the procedure.

REFERENCES

1. Shure D: Fiberoptic bronchoscopy—diagnostic applications. Clin Chest Med 8:1–13, 1987 [published erratum appears in Clin Chest Med 8(2):following xii, 1987]
2. Fulkerson WJ: Current concepts. Fiberoptic bronchoscopy. N Engl J Med 311:511–515, 1984
3. Van Gundy K, Boylen CT: Fiberoptic bronchoscopy. Indications, complications, contraindications [Review]. Postgrad Med 83:289–294, 1988
4. Green CG, Eisenberg J, Leong A, Nathanson I, Schnapf BM, Wood RE: Flexible endoscopy of the pediatric airway. Am Rev Respir Dis 145:233–235, 1992
5. Prakash UB, Offord KP, Stubbs ES: Bronchoscopy in North America: The ACCP survey. Chest 100:1668–1675, 1991
6. de Blic J, Blanche S, Danel C, et al: Bronchoalveolar lavage in HIV infected patients with interstitial pneumonitis. Arch Dis Child 64:1246–1250, 1989
7. Frankel LR, Smith DW, Lewiston NJ: Bronchoalveolar lavage for diagnosis of pneumonia in the immunocompromised child. Pediatrics 81:785–788, 1988
8. Heurlin N, Lonnqvist B, Tollemar J, Ehrnst A: Fiberoptic bronchoscopy for diagnosis of opportunistic pulmonary infections after bone marrow transplantation [Review]. Scand J Infect Dis 21:359–366, 1989
9. Luce JM, Clement MJ: Pulmonary diagnostic evaluation in patients suspected of having an HIV-related disease. Semin Respir Infect 4:93–101, 1989
10. Martin WJ II, Smith TF, Sanderson DR, et al: Role of bronchoalveolar lavage in the assessment of opportunistic pulmonary infections: Utility and complications. Mayo Clin Proc 62:549–557, 1987
11. Pattishall EN, Noyes BE, Orenstein DM: Use of bronchoalveolar lavage in immunocompromised children with pneumonia. Pediatr Pulmonol 5:1–5, 1988
12. Pedersen U, Hansen IM, Bottzauw J: The diagnostic role of fiberoptic bronchoscopy in AIDS patients with suspected *Pneumocystis carinii* pneumonia. Arch Otorhinolaryngol 246:362–364, 1989
13. Xaubet A, Torres A, Marco F, et al: Pulmonary infiltrates in immunocompromised patients. Diagnostic value of telescoping plugged catheter and bronchoalveolar lavage. Chest 95:130–135, 1989
14. Salzman SH, Schindel ML, Aranda CP, Smith RL, Lewis ML: The role of bronchoscopy in the diagnosis of pulmonary tuberculosis in patients at risk for HIV infection. Chest 102:143–146, 1992
15. Abadco DL, Amaro-Galvez R, Rao M, Steiner P: Experience with flexible fiberoptic bronchoscopy with bronchoalveolar lavage as a diagnostic tool in children with AIDS. Am J Dis Child 146:1056–1059, 1992
16. Obrien RF, Quinn JL, Miyahara BT, et al: Diagnosis of *Pneumocystis carinii* pneumonia by induced sputum in a city with moderate incidence of AIDS. Chest 95:136–138, 1989
17. Bingham HG, Gallagher TJ, Powell MD: Early bronchoscopy as a predictor of ventilatory support for burned patients. J Trauma 27:1286–1288, 1987
18. Desai MH, Rutan RL, Herndon DN: Managing smoke inhalation injuries. Postgrad Med 86(8):69–76, 1989
19. Robinson L, Miller RH: Smoke inhalation injuries. Am J Otolaryngol 7:375–380, 1986
20. Schneider W, Berger A, Mailander P, Tempka A: Diagnostic and therapeutic possibilities for fibreoptic bronchoscopy in inhalation injury. Burns Incl Therm Inj 14:53–57, 1988
21. Masanes MJ, Legendre C, Lioret N, Maillard D, Saizy R, Lebeau B: Fiberoptic bronchoscopy for the early diagnosis of subglottal inhalation injury: Comparative value in the assessment of prognosis. J Trauma 36:59–67, 1994
22. Edens ET, Sia RL: Flexible fiberoptic endoscopy in difficult intubations. Ann Otol Rhinol Laryngol 90(4 part 1):307–309, 1981
23. Messeter KH, Pettersson KI: Endotracheal intubation with the fiber-optic bronchoscope. Anaesthesia 35:294–298, 1980
24. Rogers SN, Benumof JL: New and easy techniques for fiberoptic endoscopy-aided tracheal intubation. Anesthesiology 59:569–572, 1983
25. Lan RS, Lee CH, Chiang YC, Wang WJ: Use of fiberoptic bronchoscopy to retrieve bronchial foreign bodies in adults. Am Rev Respir Dis 140:1734–1737, 1989
26. Rees JR: Massive hemoptysis associated with foreign body removal. Chest 88:475–476, 1985
27. Mantor PC, Tuggle DW, Tunell WP: An appropriate negative bronchoscopy rate in suspected foreign body aspiration. Am J Surg 158:622–624, 1989
28. Wood RE, Gauderer MW: Flexible fiberoptic bronchoscopy in the management of tracheobronchial foreign bodies in children: The value of a combined approach with open tube bronchoscopy. J Pediatr Surg 19:693–698, 1984
29. McGuirt WF, Holmes KD, Feehs R, Browne JD: Tracheobronchial foreign bodies. Laryngoscope 98(6 part 1):615–618, 1988
30. Pasaoglu I, Dogan R, Demircin M, Hatipoglu A, Bozer AY: Bronchoscopic removal of foreign bodies in children: retrospective analysis of 822 cases. Thor Cardvasc Surg 39:95–98, 1991
31. Wolach B, Raz A, Weinberg J, Mikulski Y, Ben Ari J, Sadan N: Aspirated foreign bodies in the respiratory tract of children: Eleven years experience with 127 patients. Int J Pediatr Otorhinolaryngol 30:1–10, 1994
32. Black RE, Johnson DG, Matlak ME: Bronchoscopic removal of aspirated foreign bodies in children. J Pediatr Surg 29:682–684, 1994
33. Johnston H, Reisz G: Changing spectrum of hemoptysis. Underlying causes in 148 patients undergoing diagnostic flexible fiberoptic bronchoscopy. Arch Intern Med 149:1666–1668, 1989
34. Lederle FA, Nichol KL, Parenti CM: Bronchoscopy to evaluate hemoptysis in older men with nonsuspicious chest roentgenograms. Chest 95:1043–1047, 1989
35. Poe RH, Israel RH, Marin MG, et al: Utility of fiberoptic bronchoscopy in patients with hemoptysis and a nonlocalizing chest roentgenogram. Chest 93:70–75, 1988
36. Set PA, Flower CD, Smith IE, Chan AP, Twentyman, OP, Shneerson JM: Hemoptysis: comparative study of the role of CT and fiberoptic bronchoscopy. Radiology 189:677–680, 1993
37. O'Neil KM, Lazarus AA: Hemoptysis: Indications for bronchoscopy. Arch Intern Med 151:171–174, 1991

38. Schmitt GS, Ohar JM, Kanter KR, Naunheim KS: Indwelling transbronchial catheter drainage of pulmonary abscess. Ann Thorac Surg 45:43–47, 1988
39. Sosenko A, Glassroth J: Fiberoptic bronchoscopy in the evaluation of lung abscesses. Chest 87:489–494, 1985
40. Hara KS, Prakash UB: Fiberoptic bronchoscopy in the evaluation of acute chest and upper airway trauma. Chest 96:627–630, 1989
41. Edell ES, Cortese DA: Bronchoscopic localization and treatment of occult lung cancer [Review]. Chest 96:919–921, 1989
42. Shure D: Transbronchial biopsy and needle aspiration [Review]. Chest 95:1130–1138, 1989
43. Filston HC, Ferguson TB Jr, Oldham HN: Airway obstruction by vascular anomalies. Importance of telescopic bronchoscopy. Ann Surg 205:541–549, 1987
44. Hirschler-Schulte CJ, Postmus PE, van Overbeek JJ: Endoscopic treatment of a whistling middle-lobe bronchus. Chest 88:635–636, 1985
45. Zalzal GH: Stridor and airway compromise. Pediatr Clin North Am 36:1389–1402, 1989
46. Poe RH, Israel RH, Utell MJ, Hall WJ: Chronic cough: Bronchoscopy or pulmonary function testing? Am Rev Respir Dis 126:160–162, 1982
47. Sen RP, Walsh TE: Fiberoptic bronchoscopy for refractory cough. Chest 99:33–35, 1991
48. Choi TK, Siu KF, Lam KH, Wong J: Bronchoscopy and carcinoma of the esophagus II: Carcinoma of the esophagus with tracheobronchial involvement. Am J Surg 147:760–762, 1984
49. Choi TK, Siu KF, Lam KH, Wong J: Bronchoscopy and carcinoma of the esophagus I: Findings of bronchoscopy in carcinoma of the esophagus. Am J Surg 147:757–759, 1984
50. Inculet RI, Keller SM, Dwyer A, Roth JA: Evaluation of noninvasive tests for the preoperative staging of carcinoma of the esophagus: A prospective study. Ann Thorac Surg 40:561–565, 1985
51. Leipzig B, Zellmer JE, Klug D: The role of endoscopy in evaluating patients with head and neck cancer: A multi-institutional prospective study. Arch Otorhinolaryngol 111:589–594, 1985
52. Weaver A, Fleming SM, Knechtges TC, Smith D: Triple endoscopy: A neglected essential in head and neck cancer. Surgery 86:493–496, 1979
53. Jaworski A, Goldberg SK, Walkenstein MD, et al: Utility of immediate postlobectomy fiberoptic bronchoscopy in preventing atelectasis. Chest 94:38–43, 1988
54. Marini JJ, Pierson DJ, Hudson LD: Acute lobar atelectasis: A prospective comparison of fiberoptic bronchoscopy and respiratory therapy. Am Rev Respir Dis 119:971–978, 1979
55. Conlan AA: Massive hemoptysis—diagnostic and therapeutic implications [Review]. Surg Annu 17:337–354, 1985
56. Garzon AA, Gourin A: Surgical management of massive hemoptysis: A ten-year experience. Ann Surg 187:267–271, 1978
57. Imgrund SP, Goldberg SK, Walkenstein MD, et al: Clinical diagnosis of massive hemoptysis using the fiberoptic bronchoscope. Crit Care Med 13:438–443, 1985
58. McCollun WB, Mattox KL, Guinn GA, Beall AC Jr: Immediate operative treatment for massive hemoptysis. Chest 67:152–155, 1975
59. Noseworthy TW, Anderson BJ: Massive hemoptysis [Review]. Can Med Assoc J 135:1097–1099, 1986
60. Porter DK, Van Every MJ, Anthracite RF, Mack JW Jr: Massive hemoptysis in cystic fibrosis. Arch Intern Med 143:287–290, 1983
61. Shivaram U, Finch P, Nowak P: Plastic endobronchial tubes in the management of life-threatening hemoptysis. Chest 92:1108–1110, 1987
62. Cooper JD, Pearson FG, Patterson GA, et al: Use of silicone stents in the management of airway problems. Ann Thorac Surg 47:371–378, 1989
63. Tsang V, Goldstraw P: Endobronchial stenting for anastomotic stenosis after sleeve resection. Ann Thorac Surg 48:568–571, 1989
64. Shapshay SM, Beamis JF Jr, Hybels RL, Bohigian RK: Endoscopic treatment of subglottic and tracheal stenosis by radial laser incision and dilation. Ann Otol Rhinol Laryngol 96:661–664, 1987
65. Brutinel WM, Cortese DA, McDougall JC, et al: A two-year experience with the neodymium-YAG laser in endobronchial obstruction. Chest 91:159–165, 1987
66. Balchum OJ, Doiron DR, Huth GC: HpD photodynamic therapy for obstructive lung cancer. Prog Clin Biol Res 170:727–745, 1984
67. Balchum OJ, Doiron DR: Photoradiation therapy of endobronchial lung cancer: Large obstructing tumors, nonobstructing tumors and early-stage bronchial cancer lesions. Clin Chest Med 6:255–275, 1985
68. Lam S, Muller NL, Miller RR, et al: Predicting the response of obstructive endobronchial tumors to photodynamic therapy. Cancer 58:2298–2306, 1986
69. McCaughan JS Jr, Hawley PC, Bethel BH, Walker J: Photodynamic therapy of endobronchial malignancies. Cancer 62:691–701, 1988
70. Edell ES, Cortese DA: Bronchoscopic phototherapy with hematoporphyrin derivative for treatment of localized bronchogenic carcinoma: A 5-year experience. Mayo Clin Proc 62:8–14, 1987
71. Schray MF, McDougall JC, Martinez A, et al: Management of malignant airway compromise with laser and low dose rate brachytherapy: The Mayo Clinic experience. Chest 93:264–269, 1988
72. Shrake K, Blonshine S, Brown B, Kochansky M, Ruppel G, Wanger J: AARC Clinical Practice Guideline: Fiberoptic bronchoscopy assisting. Respir Care 38:1173–1178, 1993
73. Pereira W Jr, Kovnat DM, Snider GL: A prospective cooperative study of complications following flexible fiberoptic bronchoscopy. Chest 73:813, 1978
74. Dajani AS, Bisno AL, Chung KJ, Durack DT, Freed M, Gerber MA, Karchmer AW, Millard HD, Rahimtoola S, Shulman ST, et al: Prevention of bacterial endocarditis: Recommendations by the American Heart Association. JAMA 264:2919–2922, 1990
75. American Thoracic Society Medical Section of the American Lung Association: Guidelines for fiberoptic bronchoscopy. Am Rev Respir Dis 136:1066, 1987
76. Breuer HW, Charchut S, Worth H: Effects of diagnostic procedures during fiberoptic bronchoscopy on heart rate, blood pressure, and blood gases. Klin Wochenschr 67:524–529, 1989
77. Brutinel WM, McDougall JC, Cortese DA: Bronchoscopic therapy with neodymium–yttrium–aluminum–garnet laser during intravenous anesthesia. Effect on arterial blood gas levels, pH, hemoglobin saturation, and production of abnormal hemoglobin. Chest 84:518–521, 1983
78. Hendy MS, Bateman JR, Stableforth DE: The influence of transbronchial lung biopsy and bronchoalveolar lavage on arterial blood gas changes occurring in patients with diffuse interstitial lung disease. Br J Dis Chest 78:363–368, 1984
79. Lennon RL, Hosking MP, Warner MA, et al: Monitoring and analysis of oxygenation and ventilation during rigid bronchoscopic neodymium-YAG laser resection of airway tumors. Mayo Clin Proc 62:584–588, 1987
80. Macgillivray RG, Zulu S: Oxygen saturation after bronchography under general anaesthesia. S Afr Med J 76:151–152, 1989
81. Matsushima Y, Jones RL, King EG, et al: Alterations in pulmonary mechanics and gas exchange during routine fiberoptic bronchoscopy. Chest 86:184–188, 1984
82. Van Vyue T, Chanez P, Bousquet J, Lacoste JV, Michel FB, Godard P: Safety of bronchoalveolar lavage and bronchial biopsies in patients with asthma or variable severity. Am Rev Respir Dis 146:116–121, 1992
83. Dooley SW, Castro KG, Hutton MD, Mullan RJ, Polder JA, Snider DE: Guidelines for preventing the transmission of tuberculosis in health-care settings, with special focus on HIV-related issues. MMWR Morb Mortal Wkly Rep 39:1–29, 1990
84. CDC: Draft guidelines for preventing the transmission of tuberculosis in health care facilities, second edition: Notice of comment period. Fed Reg 58(195):52810–52854, 1993
85. Hanson PJ, Collins JV: AIDS and the lung. 1: AIDS, aprons, and elbow grease: Preventing the nosocomial spread of human immunodeficiency virus and associated organisms [Review]. Thorax 44:778–783, 1989
86. Maloney S, Welbel S, Daves B, Adams K, Becker S, Bland L, Arduino M, Wallace R Jr, Zhang Y, Buck G, et al: Mycobacterium abscessus pseudoinfection traced to an automated endoscope washer: Utility of epidemiologic and laboratory investigation. J Infect Dis 169:1166–1169, 1994
87. Elford B: Care and cleansing of the fiberoptic bronchoscope. Chest 73(suppl 5):761–763, 1978
88. Tablan OC, Anderson LJ, Arden NH, Breiman RF, Butler JC, McNeil MM: Guideline for prevention of nosocomial pneumonia. Respir Care 39(12):1191–1236, 1994

11 Sleep-Disordered Breathing

Donna L. Arand
Michael H. Bonnet

CLINICAL SKILLS

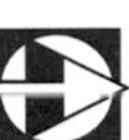

Upon completion of this chapter, the reader will:

- Understand the importance of sleep staging
- Recognize symptoms of obstructive sleep apnea
- Understand types and causes of sleep-related breathing disorders
- Understand treatment options for sleep-related breathing disorders as well as their limitations and possible side effects
- Understand the physiologic effects of nasal continuous positive airway pressure (CPAP) therapy
- Become familiar with major nonrespiratory sleep disorders
- Become familiar with types of sleep tests available, including their purpose and usual results

KEY TERMS

Apnea
Cataplexy
Central hypopnea
Central sleep apnea
Circadian
Continuous positive airway pressure (CPAP)
Electroencephalogram (EEG)
EEG arousals
Electrocardiogram (ECG)
Electromyogram (EMG)
Electro-oculogram (EOG)
Fatigue
Hypersomnia
Hypnagogic hallucinations
Hypopnea
Insomnia
k-complexes
Mixed apnea
Narcolepsy
Obstructive hypopnea
Obstructive sleep apnea
Periodic limb movements
Polysomnogram
Positional sleep apnea
Rapid eye movement
Restless legs syndrome
Sleep apnea syndrome
Sleep latency
Sleep paralysis
Sleep spindles
Slow-wave sleep
Snoring
Stroke
Upper airway resistance syndrome

Even thus last night, and two nights more, I lay,
And could not win thee, Sleep, by any stealth:
So do not let me wear tonight away:
Without thee, what is all the morning's wealth?

—WORDSWORTH

In the past, sleep was generally regarded as a state of quiescence and absence. People who fell asleep during the day were considered to be lazy. With the discovery of rapid eye movements (REMs), which were associated with dreaming during sleep in 1953,[1] people began to realize that sleep was not a unitary state and that significant physiologic changes occurred during the night. In the next 20 years, examination of the physiologic processes of sleep led directly to the discovery of sleep apnea and other disorders of sleep. In 1971, the first Sleep Disorders Center was established to perform objective evaluations of sleep disorders. In the last 20 years, the number of Sleep Centers has grown, and they can now be found in most large hospitals. More importantly, the public now realizes that sleep disorders not only cause a poor night of sleep but also result in poor ability to function during the next day. Disturbed or shortened nocturnal sleep has inevitable consequences the next day.

HISTORICAL NOTES

The importance of the relationship between reduced sleep and decreased ability to function is evident in such catastrophic events as the disaster at Chernobyl, the near disaster at Three Mile Island, the Space Shuttle Challenger accident, and the grounding of the Exxon Valdez, all of which have been attributed in part to the effects of sleepiness.[2] Such spectacular events are rare, but there are more common sleep-related accidents that occur each day. For example, it has been estimated that *fatigue* was a factor in 57% of accidents leading to the death of truck drivers.[3] Such truck accidents typically result in the death of three or four other people and large monetary expense. An average of more than 13 fatal truck accidents occur in the United States every 24 hours. Because truck driving accidents are carefully examined by the National Transportation Safety Board, data are readily available and causes are well delineated. However, there is every reason to believe that a similar degree of fatigue-related accidents or mistakes would be found in all other jobs involving shift work, sleep deprivation, or in individuals with untreated sleep disorders.

SLEEP PHYSIOLOGY

Sleep can be measured by either behavioral or electrophysiologic means (see AARC Clinical Practice Guideline: Polysomnography). Over the past 30 years, it has become increasingly common to define sleep based on changes in brain electrical activity. Stages of sleep were initially defined based on the correlation between depth of sleep, as measured by the intensity of an auditory

AARC Clinical Practice Guideline

POLYSOMNOGRAPHY

Indications: Polysomnography may be indicated in patients with COPD whose awake PaO_2 is >55 mmHg, but whose illness is complicated by pulmonary hypertension, right heart failure, polycythemia, or excessive daytime sleepiness; with restrictive ventilatory impairment secondary to chest-wall and neuromuscular disturbances whose illness is complicated by chronic hypoventilation, polycythemia, pulmonary hypertension, disturbed sleep, morning headaches, or daytime somnolence and fatigue; with disturbances in respiratory control whose awake $PaCO_2$ is >45 mmHg or whose illness is complicated by pulmonary hypertension, polycythemia, disturbed sleep, morning headaches, or daytime somnolence and fatigue; with nocturnal cyclic bradyarrhythmias or tachyarrhythmias, nocturnal abnormalities of atrioventricular conduction, or ventricular ectopy that appear to increase in frequency during sleep; with excessive daytime sleepiness or insomnia; with snoring associated with observed apneas or excessive daytime sleepiness; with other symptoms of sleep-disordered breathing as described in *International Classification of Sleep Disorders;* with symptoms of sleep disorders described in *International Classification of Sleep Disorders.*

Contraindications: There are no absolute contraindications to polysomnography when indications are clearly established. However, risk:benefit ratios should be assessed if medically unstable inpatients are to be transferred from the clinical setting to a sleep laboratory for overnight polysomnography.

Assessment of Need: Those patients who are believed to have sleep-related respiratory disturbances, periodic-limb-movement disorder, or other sleep disorders described in *The International Classification of Sleep Disorders, Diagnostic and Coding Manual.* Polysomnography is used to assess and quantify the presence and severity of such disturbances and their effect on oxygenation, cardiac status, and sleep continuity.

Assessment of Test Quality: With respect to sleep-related respiratory disturbances, polysomnography should either confirm or eliminate a diagnosis. Documentation of findings, suggested therapeutic intervention, or other clinical decisions resulting from polysomnography should be noted. Each laboratory should devise and implement indicators of quality assurance with respect to equipment calibration and maintenance, patient preparation and monitoring, scoring method, and intertechnician scoring variances.

Monitoring: Intervention is required if the physiologic signals are lost owing to problems with instrumentation or become obscured by artifact. Infrared or low-light video cameras and recording equipment should permit visualization of the patient throughout the procedure. Patients undergoing polysomnography are being evaluated for the presence of a chronic disease; therefore, their clinical status is unlikely to deteriorate acutely. However, the center-based polysomnographic studies described in this guideline require the presence of a technician throughout the study. Therefore, the technician should intervene if an acute change in physiologic status occurs and should communicate these changes to appropriate medical personnel.

(From AARC Clinical Practice Guideline: For complete text see Respir Care 40:1336–1343, 1995.)

stimulus required to awaken a sleeper, and increased amplitude and decreased frequency of the electroencephalogram (EEG) (Fig. 11-1).

An awake individual has a low-voltage, fast frequency, irregular EEG pattern. As people relax and close their eyes, they typically produce a more regular rhythm of 8 to 12 cycles per second called *alpha*. Sleep onset is defined as the disappearance of the alpha pattern and its replacement by slower frequency *theta* waves in conjunction with a decrease in muscle activity. This pattern, called stage 1, serves as a transition to the appearance of higher frequency bursts called *sleep spindles* and low-frequency, high-amplitude *k-complexes*, which define stage 2 sleep. The stage 2 pattern accounts for about 50% of a normal adult's night of sleep. Early in the night, high-amplitude, 0.5 to 3 cycles per second frequency waves begin to appear in stage 2. When 20% to 50% of an epoch is made up of these slow *delta* waves, it is called stage 3. When the delta waves predominate the sleep epoch, it is stage 4. In humans, stages 3 and 4 are called deep sleep, delta sleep, or *slow-wave sleep* (SWS).

After about 90 minutes of sleep, the low-voltage EEG pattern of Stage 1 reappears, but it is accompanied by REMs and very low EMG levels; this pattern is therefore named stage 1 REM (or just REM) sleep.

The sleep stage distribution of a typical normal night of sleep in a young adult is shown in the histogram in Figure 11-2. Normal young adults have 90-minute cycles, in which they progress from stage 1 to stage 2 to stage 3 to stage 4 (collectively called non-REM or NREM sleep) followed by REM. Delta sleep occurs almost exclusively in the first half of the night, whereas most of the REM sleep occurs in the second half of the night. REM periods get progressively longer across the night. In older individuals, delta sleep is greatly reduced, there are more awakenings, and the pattern of sleep is generally more irregular than in young adults. A typical histogram for a 65-year-old man is seen in Figure 11-3A.

During SWS, people are difficult to awaken and may be groggy after awakening. Respiration is usually slow and regular at a rate of 16 to 17 breaths per minute, and there is a 15% decrease in minute ventilation and tidal volume.[4] Alveolar and arterial P_{CO_2} increase 3 to 7 mm Hg.[5] Upper airway resistance doubles.[6] Heart rate and blood pressure are decreased and growth hormone is

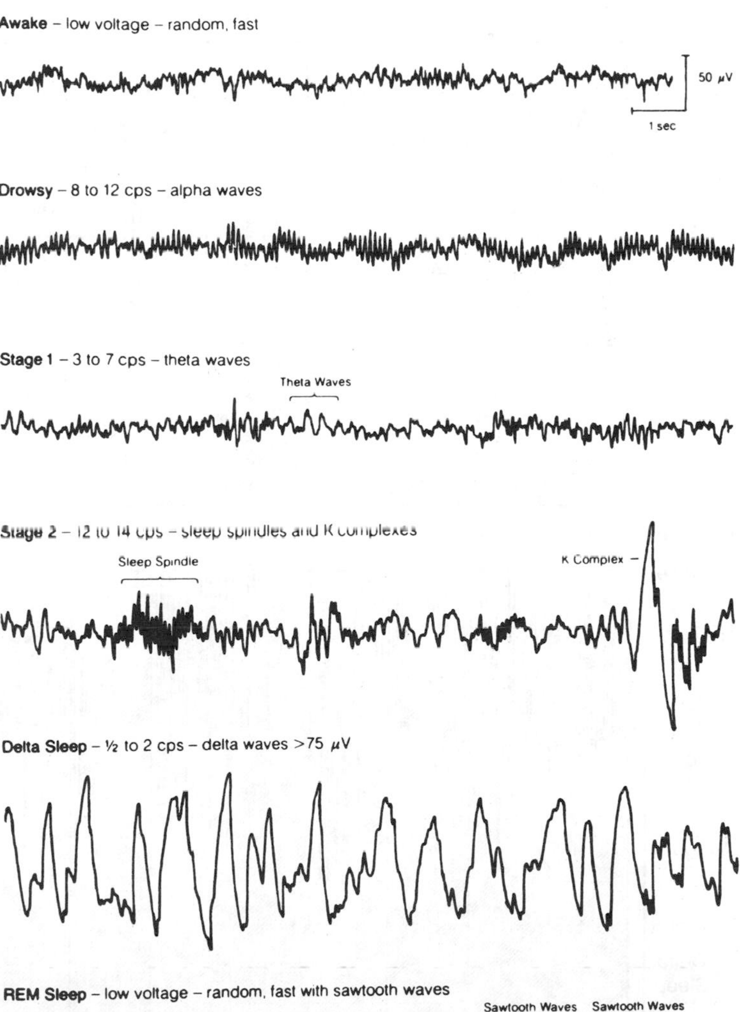

FIGURE 11-1. Human sleep stages (Hauri, P.: The Sleep Disorders [Current Concepts 8800-18], 2nd ed, pp. 1–20. Kalamazoo, Michigan, The Upjohn Company, October, 1982. By permission of the publisher.)

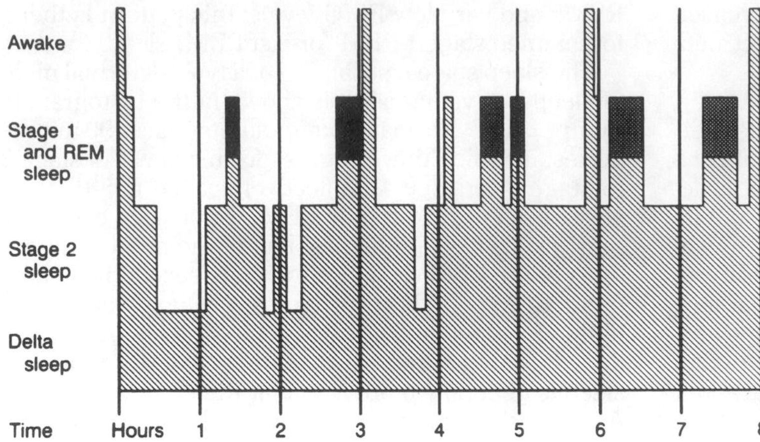

FIGURE 11-2. Typical sleep pattern of a young adult: Solid black area, REM sleep. (Hauri, P: The Sleep Disorders [Current Concepts 8800-18], 2nd ed, pp. 1–20. Kalamazzo, Michigan, The Upjohn Company, October, 1982. By permission of the publisher.)

secreted. During REM sleep, which may also be called "active" sleep, there is a flaccid paralysis of all skeletal muscle activity. In addition, activity of the upper airway and genioglossus muscles[7] is greatly decreased. All physiologic activity becomes extremely variable. Bursts of eye movements are often accompanied by sudden changes in blood pressure, heart rate, and respiratory rate and amplitude.[8] Irregular breathing or brief hypopnea may be seen. Average minute ventilation, tidal volume, and respiratory rate probably do not differ from

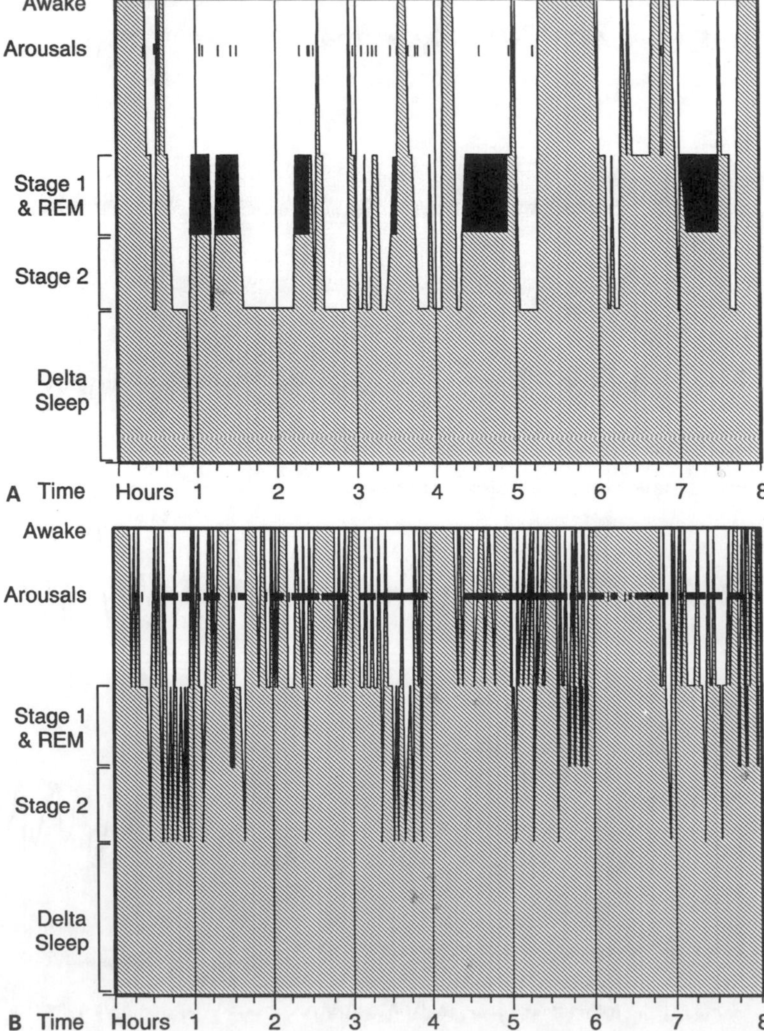

FIGURE 11-3. **(A)** Typical sleep pattern in a normal elderly individual. Solid black area, REM sleep; lines at the top indicate brief arousals during sleep. **(B)** Typical sleep pattern in a normal elderly individual with sleep apnea. Solid black area, REM sleep; lines at the top indicate brief arousals during sleep (bar appearance indicates very frequent, repetitive arousals).

NREM sleep despite the shift in variability.[4] Penile erections occur in males during REM sleep. If awakened during REM, reports of dream activity are common.

The daily sleep requirement varies substantially as a function of age. In general, total sleep time varies from 16 or more hours per day in newborns to 6 to 7 hours in the elderly.[9] However, at all ages, each individual has a unique sleep requirement. As a result, sufficient sleep is usually defined as the amount of sleep that allows the individual to maintain required alertness during the day. Because the definition of sufficient sleep has evolved to include reference to daytime alertness, an objective test, the Multiple Sleep Latency Test (MSLT) has been developed to measure sleepiness.[10] An MSLT is always preceded by a nighttime sleep study in the sleep center to ensure an adequate amount of normal sleep is attained. During the day, the patient is given naps at 10 AM, 12 PM, 2 PM, 4 PM, and 6 PM, and the length of time taken to fall asleep (*sleep latency*) is measured. The shorter the sleep latency, the sleepier the patient. If the average sleep latency is 10 minutes or more on the MSLT, alertness is considered in the normal range. If the average sleep latency is less than or equal to 5 minutes, a diagnosis of Excessive Daytime Sleepiness is considered.[10] It has been found that the length of time taken to fall asleep varies systematically with many factors including time of day, amount of prior sleep deprivation,[11] amount of sleep disturbance,[12] and clinical sleep pathology. For example, after one night of sleep loss, normal young adults fall asleep in about half the time it takes them under baseline conditions.[13]

Alertness and virtually all physiologic parameters vary not only as a function of sleep but also as a function of time of day. Each of us has an internal *biologic clock*, and most physiologic systems follow a general 24-hour (*circadian*) pattern of increasing throughout the day to a peak in the afternoon (about 2 PM) followed by a decrease through the period of sleep onset to a low point in the middle of the night (about 4 AM). Most functions, like becoming sleepy in the evening, follow this underlying pattern. The internal clock is normally a good mechanism for keeping people in synchrony with the rest of the world, but it can become a serious problem if one chooses to work at night, has irregular sleep patterns, or loses synchrony with the rest of the world.

In summary, the sleep and wakefulness cycle is one of several biologic rhythms. In normal individuals each night of sleep is characterized by an orderly progression of electrophysiologic changes in brain activity accompanied by changes in each major physiologic control system. The interaction of the circadian rhythm with sleep and altered physiologic function cause several unique sleep states, each prone to possible irregularity or pathology.

SLEEP PATHOLOGY

Pathologies of sleep are clinically identified through a *polysomnogram*, which is an all-night recording of several physiologic variables usually including *electroencephalogram (EEG)*, *electro-oculogram (EOG)*, *electromyogram (EMG)*, *electrocardiogram (EKG)*, blood oxygen saturation, air flow, and chest movements. Examination of EEG parameters provides information about the stages and continuity of sleep. Examination of the air flow, chest movement, and oxygen saturation channels allows detection of respiratory pathology during sleep. Examination of the EMG channels helps in the diagnosis of abnormal muscle activity during sleep (eg, periodic limb movements). Because sleep, respiration, and muscle activity interact, simultaneous information from within all of these parameters is essential in diagnosing sleep pathologies.

The American Sleep Disorders Association has published the *International Classification of Sleep Disorders*,[14] which contains almost 100 unique sleep-related pathologies. Differential diagnosis of these many disorders is beyond the scope of this chapter, but the methods described here have been developed, in part, to diagnose the many pathologies.

RESPIRATORY PATHOLOGY

Several types of respiratory disorders may be seen during sleep. They may be divided into upper airway disorders such as *snoring*, *upper airway resistance syndrome*, *obstructive sleep apnea*; central disorders such as *central sleep apnea*; and exacerbation of existing pulmonary disease.

Snoring

Snoring is a primarily inspiratory noise produced by vibration of the oropharyngeal walls.[15] About 20% of the adult population snores, and snoring occurs in as many as 60% of males over 50 years of age.[15] There is a normal increase in intrathoracic airway resistance and upper airway resistance during sleep.[16] In addition, snorers display an increased negative endothoracic pressure, which creates a suction mechanism that narrows the oropharyngeal isthmus. It is unclear at exactly what point snoring becomes pathologic in a physiologic sense. However, it has been shown that snoring is associated with various diseases including hypertension, stroke, and heart disease.[17] [10]

Snoring is more prevalent in males than females at all ages.[15] This difference might be mediated either by progesterone or testosterone effects. Snoring is increased in the supine sleep position, possibly as a function of gravity causing the tongue to fall back across the airway. Sleep deprivation and the use of alcohol increase the severity of snoring. Snoring may appear or increase in severity with weight gain. Many individuals with a recent onset of snoring may respond favorably to weight loss, a side sleep position, and avoidance of alcohol in the evening.

The mechanics that induce a narrowed airway in snorers also predispose them to developing complete airway closure during sleep. Historic evidence indicates that over a period of years, some snorers will develop airway narrowing sufficient to significantly limit airflow (obstructive hypopnea) or completely block airflow (obstructive sleep apnea).

Upper Airway Resistance Syndrome

Snoring is associated with increased supraglottic pressure and airway resistance.[20] This means that some snorers struggle to maintain airflow at the cost of increased work of breathing. As long as airflow is not reduced, such patients will not be diagnosed as having apnea or hypopnea even though they report loud snoring. Guilleminault and associates[21] have reported such a group of snoring, nonapneic patients who had frequent *EEG arousals* secondary to increased airway resistance and resulting daytime sleepiness.[21] When treated with CPAP, the EEG arousals disappeared and the daytime sleepiness was reversed. This syndrome, called upper airway resistance syndrome, has been recently identified, and very little data concerning its prevalence or possible progression exist. The patients may be overlooked in sleep centers because their airflow and chest tracings appear "normal" in the polysomnogram. However, a more thorough analysis of arousals and snoring in conjunction with their daytime sleepiness aids in diagnosis.

Sleep Apnea

In adults, an apnea is commonly defined as a cessation of airflow for 10 seconds or longer. Reduction in airflow by 50% or more for 10 seconds with some residual airflow maintained is classified as *hypopnea*. In a polysomnogram, respiration during the night is examined and each apnea and hypopnea is counted and classified. When the reduction or elimination of airflow is secondary to the development of airway obstruction, the event is called an *obstructive hypopnea* or apnea. When the reduction or elimination of airflow is secondary to decreased or absent chest movement, the event is called a *central hypopnea* or apnea. In some patients, an airway obstruction will apparently develop during a period of central apnea so that obstructed respiratory movements will directly follow a central pause in respiration. Such an event has been called a *mixed apnea*. These three types of apneic events are illustrated in Figure 11-4. Hypopneas, which may also be obstructive, are illustrated in Figure 11-5. To compare apnea frequency among patients with different amounts of sleep, the number of apneas observed is typically divided by the total hours of sleep to produce an *apnea index (AI)* or an *apnea/hypopnea index (AHI)* if hypopneas are also included. Initial normative studies with healthy asymptomatic middle-aged adult subjects revealed that the male subjects averaged about seven apneas and the females about two apneas per 8-hour recording.[22] As a result of this and another study of 213 sleep disorder patients without clinical indication of sleep apnea,[22] a rate of apneas in excess of 5 per hour of sleep was defined as a clinical entity called *sleep apnea syndrome*.

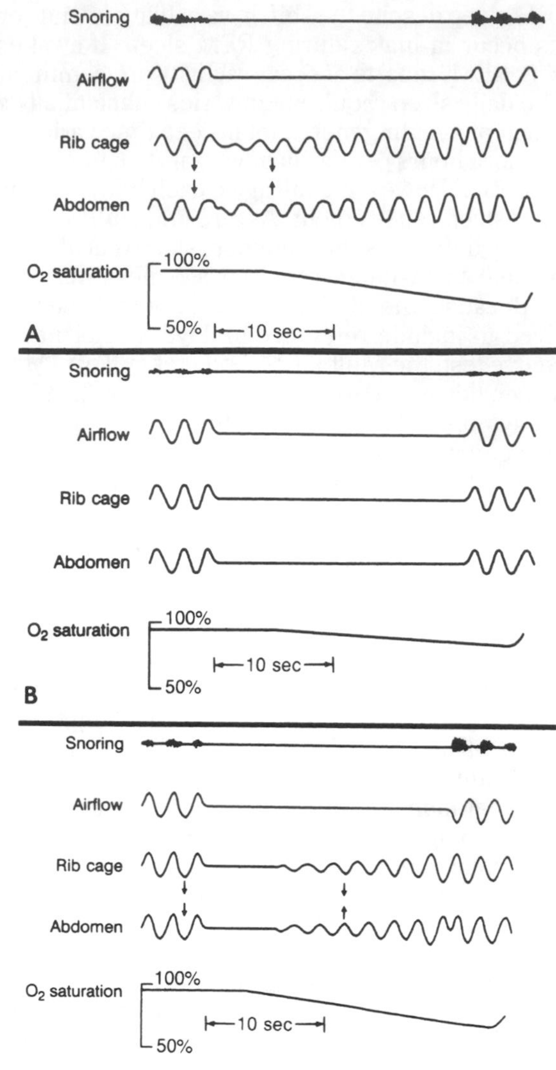

FIGURE 11-4. Types of sleep apnea. **(A)** Obstructive apnea: This is characterized by loud intermittent snoring, complete cessation of airflow, paradoxic movement of the chest and abdomen, and moderate to severe oxygen desaturation. **(B)** Central apnea: The features are simultaneous cessation of airflow and respiratory effort and mild to moderate oxygen desaturation. **(C)** Mixed apnea: An initial central apnea is followed by an obstructive apnea that usually produces moderate to severe oxygen desaturation.

☐ OBSTRUCTIVE SLEEP APNEA SYNDROME

Obstructive apneas are characterized by increasing chest movement associated with a closed airway. A typical event (see Fig. 11-4A) is 20 to 30 seconds in length and is accompanied by oxygen desaturation, which may range from a 5% drop in SaO_2 during short apneas in healthy patients to a 50% drop during long apneas in patients with compromised heart or lung function. During the course of the apnea (again dependent on the factors mentioned above), there is an approximate 25% increase in blood pressure, which peaks shortly after the termination of the apnea.[23] During apneas, there is also a decrease in left ventricular stroke volume and heart rate resulting in decreased cardiac output.[24] Immediately on termination of the apnea, there is a rapid increase in heart rate and cardiac output.

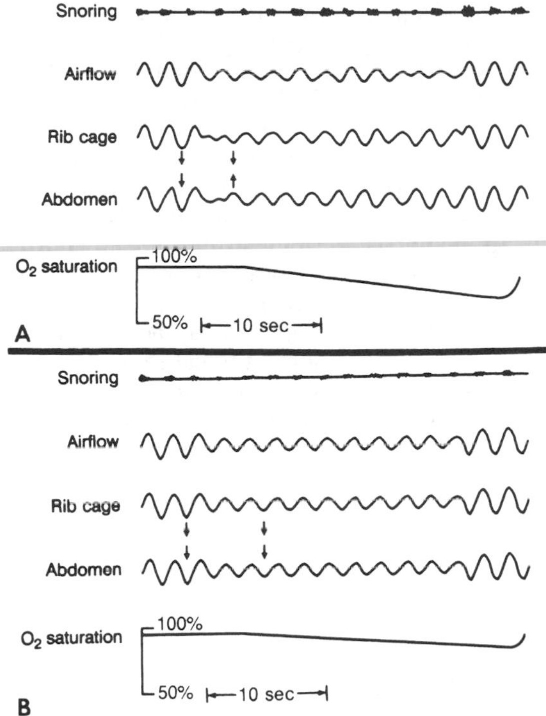

FIGURE 11-5. Hypopnea. **(A)** Obstructive type characterized by persistent snoring, decreased airflow, paradoxic movement of the rib cage and abdomen, and mild to moderate oxygen desaturation. **(B)** Nonobstructive type characterized by diminished snoring, persistent but decreased airflow, and rib cage and abdominal movements in phase; this usually is associated with mild oxygen desaturation.

The termination of an apnea generally includes an EEG arousal, an increase in muscle activity, and a snort or other sound indicating resumed airflow. The frequent EEG arousals result in significant changes in the sleep distribution (see Figure 11-3B for a histogram of a night of sleep in a patient with sleep apnea), including large decreases in SWS and REM. Frequent arousals have been linked to daytime sleepiness and performance deficits[25] and probably account for these symptoms in obstructive apnea patients. In general, apneas that occur during REM sleep are 25% to 50% longer than those in NREM sleep[23] and are accompanied by greater physiologic change in all parameters.

Following the arousal or awakening that terminates an apnea, the patient quickly returns to sleep, but the muscles maintaining the airway may collapse again causing another apnea. As such, it is not unusual for patients to develop cycles of obstructed breathing followed by arousals that may continue for much of the night. In some patients, obstruction only occurs in the supine position (*positional sleep apnea*) or during REM sleep. In such patients, the cycle of apneas will continue until the patient changes position or sleep stage.

About 2% of adults have obstructive apnea.[26] However, the incidence is higher in males and increases with age and weight so that 24% of a random sample of 65 year olds were found to have sleep apnea.[27] Typical symptoms associated with obstructive sleep apnea can be found in Table 11-1. Loud snoring with intermittent silent periods followed by snorts is the hallmark identifier. However, some patients may not describe this pattern because no one has reported it to them. Such patients may deny a specific sleep disorder and may maintain that, if anything, they are "too good" at sleeping. Patients with moderate to severe sleep apnea will report some loss of daytime function, usually becoming sleepy in sedentary situations such as watching television or driving.

Other common symptoms consistent with sleepiness include memory loss, irritability, or loss of motivation. Several studies have shown that the brief arousals associated with resumption of respiration in these patients decrease the restorative power of sleep so that patients with moderate to severe apnea become increasingly sleepy. In many patients, the severity of symptoms increases with weight gain and may be reversed to some extent with weight loss. Obstructive apneas, like snoring, are increased by alcohol and fatigue and may be more frequent in some patients when sleeping in the supine position. Periods of apnea and desaturation are associated with wide swings in blood pressure and may be related to the presence or development of hypertension.

About 33% of patients with essential hypertension have been found to also have obstructive sleep apnea.[28] These patients tend to have higher blood pressure early in the morning rather than late in the afternoon as normally would be expected, and they often have a significant reduction in daytime blood pressure after their apnea is effectively treated. Periods of apnea and desaturation may also be associated with cardiac arrhythmias in some patients. In one large study, 48% of patients with obstructive sleep apnea were found to have cardiac arrhythmias during the night. The most common arrhythmias were sinus arrest (greater than 2.5

TABLE 11-1. **Symptoms of Obstructive Sleep Apnea**

Symptom	%
Loud snoring	100
Abnormal motor activity in sleep	100
Excessive daytime sleepiness	78
Intellectual deterioration	78
Automatic behavior	58
Hypertension	52
Personality change	48
Impotence	42
Obesity	40
Morning headache	36
Enuresis	30

Guilleminault C, van den Hoed J, Mitler M: Clinical overview of the sleep apnea syndromes. In: Guilleminault C, Dement WC (eds): Sleep Apnea Syndromes. New York, Alan R. Liss, 1978, pp 1–12. Reproduced with permission.

seconds), which was found in 11% of patients and sinus bradycardia (below 30 beats per minute), which was found in 7% of patients.[29] Other arrhythmias, including atrial or ventricular tachycardia, atrial flutter, and atrial fibrillation were seen in 1% to 7% of the patients. Such arrhythmias were more frequent toward the end of apneas and when oxygen saturation dropped below 70% SaO_2.[29] An apnea index of more than 20 has been associated with increased mortality.[30,31] Survival rate at 8 years was 96% for a group with more normal respiration during sleep compared with 63% for patients with severe apnea.

Conditions associated with a higher than usual preponderance of obstructive sleep apnea include (1) any malformation of the upper airway (tonsillar hypertrophy (Fig. 11-6), deviated septum, macroglossia, micrognathia or retrognathia, large neck; (2) obesity; (3) hypertension; (4) hypothyroidism; (5) acromegaly; or (6) spondylolysis.

Treatments for obstructive sleep apnea are related to the cause and severity of the breathing disorder. A high number of patients with sleep apnea are overweight. In fact, 40% of a random sample of obese men were found to have significant obstructive sleep apnea.[32] Several studies have shown that weight loss will reduce the severity of sleep apnea,[33,34] and weight loss is therefore a frequent treatment recommendation. Elimination of alcohol use in the evening can also provide immediate benefit. Some apneic patients only display events when sleeping in the supine position. For these patients with positional sleep apnea, methods to avoid the supine sleep position may be effective and the only treatment needed.[35] Unfortunately, many patients will not respond sufficiently to these behavioral interventions.

Currently, the recommended treatment for a majority of patients with obstructive sleep apnea is *continuous positive airway pressure* (*CPAP*). In CPAP treatment (Fig. 11-7), a sealed mask (Fig. 11-8A) or nasal pillow (Fig. 11-8B) is placed over the nose, and pressurized room air is inspired through the nose to provide a "pressure splint" to prevent collapse of the upper airway (see Fig. 11-9). Patients typically are scheduled for an all-night CPAP titration study to determine the appropriate CPAP pressure and to note any adjustment difficulties to the CPAP apparatus or air pressure. On the titration night, CPAP pressure is slowly increased as the patient sleeps until apneas, periodic arousals, and snoring no longer occur in any sleep position or stage of sleep. In some cases, if the maximally effective pressure is exceeded, the number of apneas can actually increase. Therefore it is very important to carefully monitor respiration as CPAP pressures are increased. When the "correct" pressure is reached, there is often a long period of REM sleep as patients recover from previous deprivation. CPAP has been shown to be extremely effective in eliminating obstruction during sleep and in reversing the symptoms associated with sleep apnea.[36] However, CPAP therapy is not tolerated by a small percentage of patients, usually because the patient has difficulty breathing through his or her nose. Others are unable to tolerate CPAP because of claustrophobia, which may be aggravated by the face mask, or sensitivity to the air pressure. Common side effects of CPAP include dry mouth or throat (52%), sore eyes, headache, and nasal problems and rhinorrhea (14%).[37] Significant long-term negative consequences of CPAP use have not been reported. However, 19% of patients will cease to use their CPAP machines, and another 16% will seek an alternative treatment rather than continuing CPAP.[37] Patients who stop using CPAP will typically have a return of symptoms and need to be considered for another treatment modality.

The "gold standard" treatment for sleep apnea has historically been tracheotomy. Clearly, the insertion of an artificial airway below the site of airway obstruction should eliminate the problem of obstructive sleep

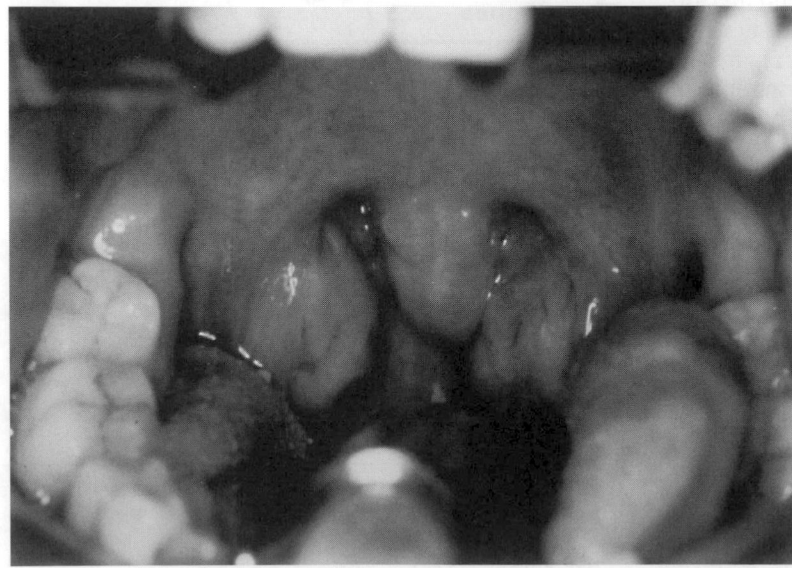

FIGURE 11-6. An example of significant tonsillar hypertrophy with airway compromise.

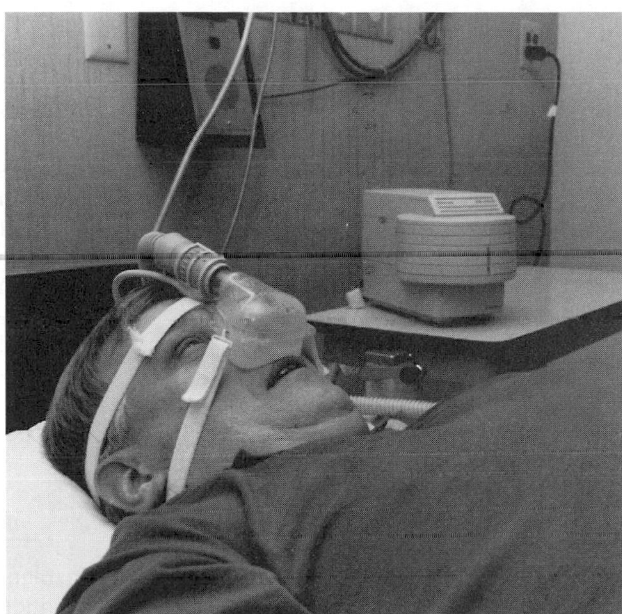

FIGURE 11-7. Continuous positive airway pressure (CPAP) including a standard CPAP machine (background) and attached mask on an adult model.

apnea. This is usually the case, although selected patients can block the tracheotomy tube with secretions or excess fatty neck tissue. Currently, tracheotomy is rarely used as a treatment for sleep apnea because of the required surgery and discomfort as well as the care required to maintain the tracheotomy opening.

A surgical procedure called *uvulopalatopharyngoplasty* (*UPPP*) was developed to remove redundant tissue at the site of obstruction. UPPP surgery promised improved respiration without the drawbacks of tracheotomy or nightly discomfort of CPAP. Unfortunately UPPP and other airway corrective procedures have not been very effective. They have resulted in a 20% to 50% reduction in respiratory events, but this may still leave a significant number of apneic events in many patients.[38] In addition, long-term follow-up studies in many patients with initially successful postoperative outcomes have shown a return of symptoms several months to years later. Because of the uncertain success rate, questionable long-term effectiveness, required hospital stay, and occasional nasal regurgitation problems, UPPP is not the first choice of treatments and is recommended less frequently than CPAP.

Recently, the development of laser-assisted uvulopalatoplasty (LAUP) has eliminated the hospital stay and bleeding problems sometimes associated with UPPP. This procedure is frequently performed to eliminate snoring. However, an early study has suggested that 90% of patients referred for the LAUP based on a history of snoring also had sleep apnea. Unfortunately, data on the effectiveness of the procedure to reduce apnea is still not available, so the procedure should not be considered a snoring therapy[39] unless sleep apnea has already been ruled out.

Another treatment, the use of a dental appliance to advance the tongue or mandible to increase airway space, has been shown to produce limited benefits in selected patients with obstructive sleep apnea. In examining data from 29 different experiments, Lowe[40] reported that the apnea index from the studies as a whole was reduced from 43 to 19. As with UPPP, these results indicate that although some patients will benefit substantially, others will improve but still have significant residual sleep apnea, and some patients will not improve at all.

□ CENTRAL SLEEP APNEA SYNDROME

A central apnea episode in adults is defined as a pause in breathing lasting 10 seconds or longer in which there is no respiratory effort (see Fig. 11-4B). Generally, patients with central apnea tend to be older, have a normal body habitus, snore mildly, and complain of insomnia more than typical obstructive sleep apnea patients.[41] Central sleep apnea is much less common than obstructive apnea and accounts for less than 10% of apnea patients seen in most sleep centers.[41] The majority of central sleep apneas occur during stage 1 sleep at transitions from wake to sleep or sleep to wake.[42] Patients

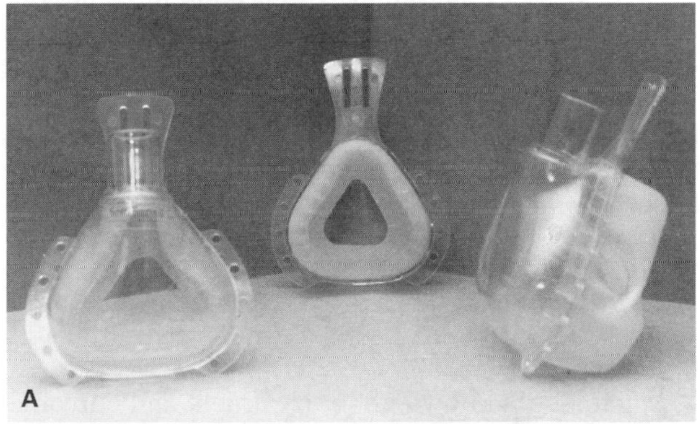

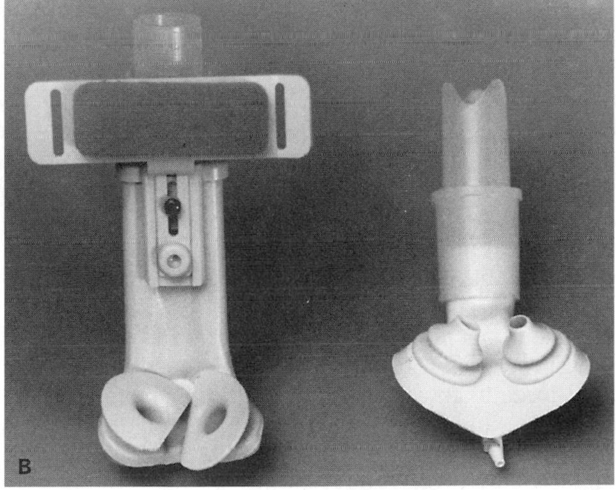

FIGURE 11-8. **(A)** Standard adult nasal CPAP masks. **(B)** Nasal pillow CPAP masks.

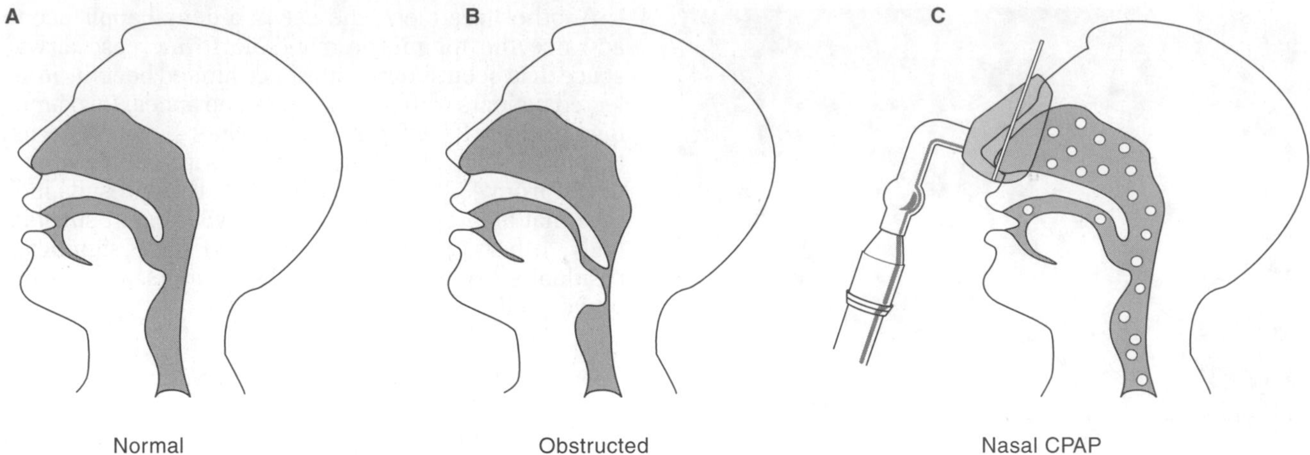

FIGURE 11-9. Schematic of airway with nasal CPAP applied.

with central apnea tend to have normal respiration during deep sleep and REM.

Central apnea is often found secondary to other medical disorders. Neurologic disorders that tend to be associated with central apnea include polio, muscular dystrophy, and myasthenia gravis. Some patients with tumor, hemorrhage, or infarction causing damage in the medullary area of the brain may display central apnea. *Congestive heart failure* can be associated with Cheyne-Stokes respiration. The waning of respiratory effort during Cheyne-Stokes respiration in sleep produces a period that meets the definition of central apnea (ie, no chest movements). It is similar to a central apnea in that changes in PaO_2 and $PaCO_2$ along with frequent arousals from sleep are seen. However, the cause appears to be different. In congestive heart failure, it is hypothesized that the periodic changes in respiration are secondary to increased circulation time. In central apnea, the periodic apneas are more likely due to decreased neural control than to increased circulation time.

Much less is known about treatment and outcomes for patients with central sleep apnea compared with obstructive sleep apnea because the patient population is smaller, older, and generally less symptomatic. Central apneas, like obstructive apneas, are more frequent in the supine sleep position, and therefore some patients can benefit from positioning therapy.[43] Many patients have both obstructive and central apneas, and in these patients, treatment is based on the predominant type of events. Patients with nocturnal oxygen desaturation and central apnea can benefit from low flow oxygen, which results in fewer central events and better oxygenation.[44] Some success has also been reported with the use of nasal CPAP. However, because high CPAP pressures are frequently required in these patients who may already have some difficulty sleeping, effective treatment and long-term use is less likely than for obstructive apnea patients. Medications including theophylline, medroxyprogesterone acetate, or acetazolamide have not shown significant effectiveness in the treatment of central apnea. Several recent studies[45,46] have indicated that benzodiazepines such as triazolam or temazepam improve sleep and may actually reduce central apneas in patients with central apnea or Cheyne-Stokes respiration. This is probably secondary to reduction in light sleep and sleep transitions where the apneas predominate. However, because these medications can be depressants and have not been shown to be helpful in obstructive apnea, they should be used cautiously. Patients with central apnea can also be treated by mechanical ventilation or diaphragmatic pacing, but these therapies are typically reserved for severe disease.

Pulmonary Disease and Sleep

As mentioned earlier, airway resistance is increased during sleep, and the ventilatory response to such resistance is diminished. In REM sleep, there is a decrease in muscle tension, including that of the intercostal muscles. Minute ventilation is decreased during sleep in control and in chronic obstructive pulmonary disease (COPD) patients, and the reduction is greatest during REM sleep.[8] In normal patients, alveolar ventilation is about 40% lower during eye movements in REM.[8] When patients with COPD begin rapid, shallow breathing during REM, hypoxemia without apnea often results. COPD patients have more ventricular ectopic beats during sleep,[47] and pulmonary arterial pressure increases as oxygen saturation decreases.[48] In addition, patients with COPD frequently report *insomnia* and shortness of breath during the night. Nocturnal death is more common in hypoxic COPD patients breathing room air than in those receiving nocturnal oxygen.[49]

There is no evidence to suggest that the incidence of sleep apnea is greater in patients with COPD than in other groups, but the prevalence of both disorders in older men assures that apnea does exist in many patients with COPD and may exacerbate the disease. In a study of a large series of patients with obstructive sleep apnea,[50] 11% were found to have COPD (defined as FEV_1/VC ratio \lt 60%). These patients with overlapping COPD and obstructive sleep apnea were more than twice as likely to develop respiratory insufficiency and pulmonary hypertension than COPD patients without obstructive sleep apnea.[50]

Correlation of daytime and nighttime oxygen saturation levels with survival rates in patients with COPD has not shown increased survival rates due to prescribing oxygen based on nocturnal oxygen saturation parameters when not also indicated from daytime blood gas values. The general use of polysomnograms in COPD patients without signs of apnea is not recommended unless the patients have polycythemia or cor pulmonale while maintaining a daytime PO_2 greater than 60 mmHg.[51] However, polysomnograms should by done promptly in COPD patients who snore and have symptoms of obstructive apnea because even short periods of apnea may cause tremendous oxygen desaturation in a compromised pulmonary system, and supplemental oxygen is of little use in an obstructed airway.

It is common for patients with *asthma* to complain of increased cough or wheeze secondary to bronchoconstriction at night. FEV_1 and peak flow rates may fall over 50% in some asthma patients.[52] In asthma patients recovering from recent exacerbation, about two thirds have their lowest flow rate at night,[53] and there is increased likelihood of death in asthmatics at night.[52] Several studies have shown that asthma patients who wheeze at night have decreased ability to sleep, and it is hypothesized that the resulting fatigue may exacerbate ventilatory impairment on the nights that follow. Snoring or apnea may worsen asthma. However, CPAP therapy can greatly improve peak expiratory flow rate[54] while treating apnea in these patients. Also, nocturnal treatment with long-acting bronchodilators is generally effective. However, oral β_2 agonists such as sustained release terbutaline are less likely to cause insomnia than oral theophylline.[55]

In summary, sleep is a time of increased risk for patients with significantly compromised respiratory systems and for patients with unfavorable anatomy owing to the recumbent position, gravity, and the loss of muscle tone. Increased work of breathing or an obstructed airway can lead to significant medical problems or death in some patients. In addition, patients unable to maintain respiration during sleep are prone to fragmented sleep and subsequent daytime sleepiness, which can also be a significant threat. Respiratory disorders during sleep are common, but effective treatments are available.

Nonrespiratory Sleep Disorders

Sleep disorders historically have been divided into those that disturb or reduce sleep at night (*insomnia*) and those that cause increased sleepiness during the day (*hypersomnia*).

Insomnia is an extremely frequent complaint in the general population. It is secondary to other underlying disorders including depression, anxiety, sleep apnea, chronic pain, use of or withdrawal from drugs or alcohol or caffeine, or other medical illness. Medications, such as theophylline and some beta antagonists (eg, propranolol, metoprolol, and pindolol) may cause poor sleep.[56] Insomnia may also be caused by irregular sleep patterns or habits. Aging is accompanied by a decrease in sleep requirement and an inability to maintain sleep across the entire night. As such, normal changes in sleep as a function of age may be interpreted as insomnia.

Everyone has occasional nights of poor sleep usually due to transient stress. Therefore, to be considered pathologic, poor sleep should be chronic and should be related to decreased ability to function during the day. It is important that treatments for insomnia be related to the underlying cause. In cases where multiple underlying causes may exist, referral to a sleep disorders center may be necessary. However, most patients with insomnia can benefit from improved sleep hygiene including regularity of wake time and bedtime, avoidance of caffeine and alcohol, avoidance of naps and bed rest during the day, and increased activity during the day. Medical disorders that may precipitate or exacerbate insomnia include any condition causing pain, any disorder causing chronic movement, peptic ulcer disease, osteoarthritis or rheumatoid arthritis, cystic fibrosis, chronic renal failure, hyperthyroidism, menopause, allergies, and chronic fatigue syndrome. In most of these disorders, treatment of the underlying medical problem can help to alleviate the associated sleep problem.

One movement disorder frequently associated with difficulty in initiating or maintaining sleep is *restless legs syndrome* and the associated periodic limb movements. Restless legs syndrome consists of an irresistible urge to move the legs. It may be described as creepy, crawling, or tingling sensations in the legs. It is briefly reversed by leg movement but returns again in increasing intensity until the legs are moved again. Because it occurs primarily in the evening and upon lying down, it is frequently associated with difficulty in falling asleep or remaining asleep. Restless legs is reported by 5% or more of the population.[57] Almost all patients with restless legs also have frequent twitching or jerking in their legs or arms while they sleep.

These sleep-related movements, called *periodic limb movements in sleep (PLMS)* also occur independently of restless legs. The incidence of PLMS has been estimated at 5% of the population between 30 and 50 years of age, 29% of the population over 50 years of age, and 44% of the population over 65 years of age.[58,59] Patients with PLMS are usually restless sleepers who may have been told that they jerk their arms or legs while they sleep. Both restless legs and PLMS occur more frequently in patients with diabetes mellitus, anemia, uremia, pulmonary disease, rheumatoid arthritis, and fibromyositis.[58] Restless legs and PLMS are frequently treated with benzodiazepines or dopaminergic agents, which reduce the limb jerks somewhat and improve sleep.

Hypersomnia is a less frequent complaint than insomnia, but it is a much more disabling problem. As a result, a majority of patients seen in sleep disorder centers complain primarily of daytime sleepiness. Sleepiness is defined as the propensity to actually fall asleep when sedentary (eg, in waiting rooms, church, meetings) and needs to be differentiated from fatigue or tiredness, which frequently are not related to actually falling asleep. Seven common signs of sleepiness are summarized in Table 11-2. Studies suggest that 4% to 5% of the population complain of excessive sleepiness.[26,60] The people who frequently claim to be sleepy include: 25% of shift workers,[61] as a result of the juxtaposition of their circadian rhythm and their actual sleep/wake schedule; undiagnosed patients with sleep apnea and severe PLMS; a minority of patients with major depression (10%–15%) and some patients with bipolar and seasonal affective disorder (1%–2% of the population[62,63]); and otherwise normal people who get insufficient sleep as a result of sacrificing sleep for other endeavors. Sleepiness may be secondary to infectious disease or metabolic, neoplastic, or endocrine conditions. Sleepiness may also be related to the use of medications including antidepressants, antihistamines or antihypertensives such as clonidine.[56]

A small group of sleepy patients, about 5 in 10,000,[64] suffers from narcolepsy. *Narcolepsy* is a condition in which symptoms usually appear between the ages of 15 and 30 years. The first symptom to appear is usually sleepiness, described as irresistible, short sleep episodes. Other symptoms including emotion-triggered muscle weakness (*cataplexy*), vivid dreams at sleep onset (*hypnagogic hallucinations*), and inability to move at awakening (*sleep paralysis*) may appear later and are useful in differentiating narcolepsy from other hypersomnias. The symptoms—cataplexy, hypnagogic hallucinations and sleep paralysis—are all related to the muscle inhibition and mental activity of REM sleep. Patients with narcolepsy often begin REM sleep within 15 minutes after falling asleep, rather than 90 minutes as normal sleepers do. The MSLT is considered an objective test for narcolepsy because it can document the REM sleep onsets shortly after sleep onset as well as determine the degree of pathologic sleepiness. Recently, it has been shown that narcolepsy is actually a genetic disease and that close to 100% of patients with the disorder show a common tissue type, HLA DR2.[65] HLA DR2 positivity by itself is not considered specific to narcolepsy (it is a common tissue type), but the absence of this tissue type can serve as a "narcolepsy rule out." The irresistible sleepiness associated with narcolepsy can be treated with stimulants such as methylphenidate or pemoline. The other symptoms, which seem to be associated with REM sleep, can be treated with medications such as tricyclic antidepressants, which are strong REM suppressors.

TABLE 11-2. **Seven Signs of Sleepiness**

1. Yawning or head nodding
2. Drooping eyelids, frequent eye closure, dull expression in the eyes, inability to keep eyes focused
3. Irritability or emotional outbursts
4. Poor memory, lapses in attention
5. Lack of motivation, unwillingness to become involved in activities, poor performance at work or school, poor personal hygiene, careless dress
6. Inordinate use of caffeinated beverages such as coffee, tea, or soft drinks
7. Hyperactivity

Not all disorders of sleep can be classified as causes of insomnia or excessive sleepiness. There are many transitory disorders that occur during sleep that do not have an obvious impact on daytime function. Many of these conditions, such as enuresis, somnambulism, nightmares, and sleep talking, are grouped together as parasomnias. Other disorders, such as the combined insomnia and sleepiness caused by shift work or travel across time zones ("jet lag"), are secondary to disturbance of underlying circadian rhythms. These and other disorders are covered more completely in other sources.[14,66]

In summary, the ability to function well during the day and sleep well at night is influenced by behavior, pharmacology, medical status, age, and circadian rhythms. Identifying the cause of a sleep disorder from these many factors can be difficult. Sleep disorder centers evolved to deal with the wide range of sleep-related pathology and many underlying causes.

SLEEP IN OTHER MEDICAL DISORDERS

Any disease that causes pain, limits movement, or requires frequent treatment or attention will have a negative impact on sleep. A review of these many conditions is beyond the scope of this chapter. However, comments on common medical problems that are found in respiratory care and involve sleep components are examined.

Patients with *congestive heart failure* (CHF) have been found to have reduced total sleep time with increased arousals. These patients frequently demonstrate Cheyne-Stokes respiration during light sleep. However, although such respiration was not associated with significant oxygen desaturation during wakefulness, desaturation to about 80% SaO_2 was seen during sleep.[67] Arousals occurred frequently at the end of periods of shallow breathing. Treatment with low-flow oxygen at 2 to 3 L/min decreased the duration of Cheyne-Stokes respiration, improved oxygen saturation, and increased total sleep.[68] Arousals were decreased and daytime alertness improved without significant changes in respiration when patients with CHF were treated with benzodiazepines in two studies.[46,69] In a study of patients with CHF and sleep apnea, CPAP therapy resulted in an improved ejection fraction in addition to improved SaO_2 and sleep.[70]

Myocardial infarction and stroke have a similar circadian pattern with a peak incidence between 6 AM and noon.[71] It has been suggested that increased sympathetic tone and platelet aggregability, which occur on awakening and when standing, contribute to the incidence peak. The use of β-blocking agents and aspirin seems to reduce the number of events primarily by reducing the morning peak. Nocturnal use of these medications provides maximum early morning effect. Some studies report an increased incidence of *angina* between 4 and 6 AM when REM sleep predominates. This may reflect increased heart rate and sympathetic activity during REM sleep. However, because obstructive sleep apnea is associated with large changes in blood pressure, heart rate, oxygen, and carbon dioxide levels, the potential for sudden death may be greatly increased during sleep in patients with sleep apnea and potential for myocardial infarction or stroke.[72] In a group of post–myocardial infarction patients,[73] 38% were found to have sleep apnea (versus 8% in a control group). Patients with an apnea index of greater than 5.3 had 23 times the risk of having a myocardial infarction compared with a group of patients with an apnea index of less than 1.0.[74]

In summary, in addition to several primary disorders that occur during sleep, many primary medical conditions influence or are influenced by sleep. Sleep apnea clearly can interact in a detrimental fashion with major disorders of both the pulmonary and cardiac systems. Respiratory therapists can provide key input into the identification of sleep apnea in a broad range of patients. Respiratory therapy can also be a valuable background for the specialized training required to become certified as a registered polysomnographic technician.[75]

REFERENCES

1. Aserinsky E, Kleitman N: Regularly occurring periods of eye motility, and concomitant phenomena, during sleep. Science 118:273–274, 1953
2. Mitler MM, Dinges DF, Dement WC: Sleep medicine, public policy, and public health. In Kryger MH, Roth T, Dement WC (eds): Principles and Practice of Sleep Medicine, 2nd ed, Philadelphia, WB Saunders, 1994, pp 453–462
3. US Congress Office of Technology Assessment: Gearing up for safety: Motor carrier safety in a competitive environment. Washington, DC, OTA-SET-382, U.S. Government Printing Office, 1988
4. Krieger J: Breathing during sleep in normal subjects. In Kryger MH, Roth T, Dement WC (eds): Principles and Practice of Sleep Medicine, 2nd ed, Philadelphia, WB Saunders, 1994, pp 212–223
5. Rist KE, Daubenspeck JA, McGovern JF: Effects of non-REM sleep upon respiratory drive and the respiratory pump in humans. Respir Physiol 63:241–256, 1986
6. Lopes JM, Tabachnik E, Muller NL, Levison H, Bryan AC: Total airway resistance and respiratory muscle activity during sleep. J Appl Physiol 54:773–777, 1983
7. Orem J: Control of the upper airways during sleep and the hypersomnia-sleep apnea syndrome. In Orem J, Barnes CD (ed): Physiology in Sleep. New York, Academic Press, 1980, pp 273–314
8. Gould GA, Gugger M, Molloy J, Tsara V, Shapiro CM, Douglas NJ: Breathing pattern and eye movement density during REM sleep in humans. Am Rev Respir Dis 1988;138:874–877, 1988
9. Williams L, Karacan I, Hursch C: Electroencephalography of Human Sleep: Clinical Applications. New York, John Wiley & Sons, 1974, pp 1–169
10. Carskadon MA: Guidelines for the Multiple Sleep Latency Test (MSLT): A standard measure of sleepiness. Sleep 9:519–524, 1986
11. Carskadon MA, Dement WC: Effects of total sleep loss on sleep tendency. Perceptual and Motor Skills 48:495–506, 1979
12. Podszus T, German Society of Pneumology, Study Group of Disorders of Nocturnal Respiration and Circulation: Recommendations for nocturnal nasal respiratory therapy in respiratory disorders. Pneumologie 47:333–335, 1993
13. Bonnet MH: Sleep deprivation. In Kryger M, Roth T, Dement WC (eds): Principles and Practice of Sleep Medicine, 2nd ed. Philadelphia, WB Saunders, 1994, pp 50–68
14. American Sleep Disorders Association: The International Classification of Sleep Disorders. Lawrence, KS, Allen Press, 1990
15. Lugaresi E, Cirignotta F, Montagna P, Sforza E: Snoring: Pathogenic, clinical, and therapeutic aspects. In Kryger M, Roth T, Dement W (eds): Principles and Practice of Sleep Medicine, 2nd ed. Philadelphia, WB Saunders, 1994, pp 621–629
16. Vincent NJ, Knudson R, Leith DE, Macklem PT, Mead J: Factors influencing pulmonary resistance. J Appl Physiol 29:236–243, 1970
17. Koskenvuo M: Cardiovascular stress and sleep. Ann Clin Res 19:110–113, 1987
18. Koskenvuo M, Partinen M, Kaprio J: Snoring and disease. Ann Clin Res 17:247–251, 1985
19. Telakivi T, Partinen M, Koskenvuo M, Kaprio J: Snoring and cardiovascular disease. Compr Ther 13:53–57, 1987
20. Skatrud JB, Dempsey JA: Airway resistance and respiratory muscle function in snorers during NREM sleep. J Appl Physiol 59:328–335, 1985
21. Guilleminault C, Stoohs R, Clerk A, Cetel M, Maistros P: A cause of excessive daytime sleepiness: The upper airway resistance syndrome [see comments]. Chest 104:781–787, 1993
22. Guilleminault C, Dement WC: Sleep apnea syndromes and related sleep disorders. In Williams RL, Karacan I (eds): Sleep Disorders: Diagnosis and Treatment. New York, John Wiley & Sons, 1978
23. Shepard JW: Cardiorespiratory changes in obstructive sleep apnea. In Kreiger M, Roth T, Dement WC (eds): Principles and Practice of Sleep Medicine, 2nd ed. Philadelphia, WB Saunders, 1994, pp 657–668
24. Tolle FA, Judy WV, Yu PL, Markand ON: Reduced stroke volume related to pleural pressure in obstructive sleep apnea. J Appl Physiol 55:1718–1724, 1983
25. Bonnet MH: Effect of sleep disruption on sleep, performance, and mood. Sleep 8:11–19, 1985
26. Lavie P: Sleep habits and sleep disturbances in industrial workers in Israel: Main findings and some characteristics of workers complaining of excessive daytime sleepiness. Sleep 4:147–58, 1981
27. Ancoli-Israel S, Kripke DF, Klauber MR, Mason WJ, Fell R, Kaplan O: Sleep-disordered breathing in community-dwelling elderly. Sleep 14:486–495, 1991
28. Partinen M: Epidemiology of sleep disorders. In Kryger M, Roth T, Dement WC (eds): Principles and Practice of Sleep Medicine, 2nd ed. Philadelphia, WB Saunders, 1994, pp 437–452
29. Guilleminault C, Connolly S, Winkle R: Cardiac arrhythmia during sleep in 400 patients with obstructive sleep apnea. Am J Cardiol 52:490–494, 1983
30. He J, Kryger MH, Zorick FJ, Conway W, Roth T: Mortality and apnea index in obstructive sleep apnea: Experience in 385 male patients. Chest 94:9–14, 1988
31. Partinen M, Jamieson A, Guilleminault C: Long-term outcome for obstructive sleep apnea syndrome patients: Mortality. Chest 94:1200–1204, 1988
32. Vgontzas AN, Tan TL, Bixler EO, Martin LF, Shubert D, Kales A: Sleep apnea and sleep disruption in obese patients. Arch Intern Med 154:1705–1711, 1994
33. Browman CP, Sampson MG, Yolles SF, Gujavarty KS, Weiler SJ, Walsleben JA, Hahn PM, Mitler MM: Obstructive sleep apnea and body weight. Chest 85:435–438,1984
34. Harman EM, Wynne JW, Block AJ: The effect of weight loss on sleep disordered breathing and oxygen desaturation in morbidly obese men. Chest 82:291–294, 1982
35. Cartwright RD, Lloyd S, Lilie J, Kravitz H: Sleep position training as treatment for sleep apnea syndrome: A preliminary study. Sleep 8:87–94, 1985
36. Sullivan CE, Grunstein RR: Continuous positive airway pressure in sleep-disordered breathing. In Kryger MH, Roth T, Dement WC (eds): Principles and Practice of Sleep Medicine, 2nd ed. Philadelphia, WB Saunders, 1994, pp 694–705
37. Crowe-McCann C, Nino-Murcia G, Guilleminault C: Nasal CPAP: The Stanford experience. In Guilleminault C, Partinen M (eds):

Obstructive Sleep Apnea Syndrome: Clinical Research and Treatment. New York, Raven Press, 1990, pp 119–128
38. Fujita S: Pharyngeal surgery for obstructive sleep apnea and snoring. In Fairbanks D, Fujita S, Ikematsu T, Simmons FB (eds) Snoring and Obstructive Sleep Apnea. New York, Raven Press, 1987, pp 101–128
39. Keidar A, Zammit GK, Krespi YP: The relationship between polysomnographic findings and self-reported symptoms in laser assisted uvulopalatoplasty (LAUP) candidates. Sleep Research 23:271, 1994
40. Lowe AA: Dental appliances for the treatment of snoring and obstructive sleep apnea. In Kreiger M, Roth T, Dement WC (eds): Principles and Practice of Sleep Medicine, 2nd ed. Philadelphia, WB Saunders, 1994, pp 722–735
41. White DP: Central sleep apnea. In Kreiger M, Roth T, Dement WC (eds): Principles and Practice of Sleep Medicine, 2nd ed. Philadelphia, WB Saunders, 1994, pp 630–641
42. Bradley TD, McNicholas WT, Rutherford R, Popkin J, Zamel N, Phillipson EA: Clinical and physiologic heterogeneity of the central sleep apnea syndrome. Am Rev Respir Dis 133:1163–1170, 1986
43. Orr WC, Stahl ML, Duke J, McCaffree MA, Toubas P, Mattice C, Kroush HF: Effect of sleep stage and position on the incidence of obstructive and central apnea in infants. Pediatrics 75:832–835, 1985
44. McNicholas W, Carter J, Rutherford R, Zamel N, Phillipson EA: Beneficial effect of oxygen in primary alveolar hypoventilation with central sleep apnea. Am Rev Respir Dis 125:773–775, 1982
45. Bonnet MH, Dexter JR, Arand DL: The effect of triazolam on arousal and respiration in central sleep apnea patients. Sleep 13:31–41, 1990
46. Biberdorf DJ, Steens R, Millar TW, Kryger MH: Benzodiazepines in congestive heart failure: Effects of temazepam on arousability and Cheyne-Stokes respiration. Sleep 16:529–538, 1993
47. Flick JW, Block AJ: Nocturnal versus diurnal cardiac arrhythmias in patients with chronic obstructive pulmonary disease. Chest 75:8–11, 1979
48. Boysen PG, Block AJ, Wynne JW, Hunt LA, Flick MR: Nocturnal pulmonary hypertension in patients with chronic obstructive pulmonary disease. Chest 76:536–542, 1979
49. Douglas NJ, Flenley DC: Breathing during sleep in patients with obstructive lung disease. Am Rev Respir Dis 141:1055–1070, 1990
50. Chaouat A, Weitzenbaum E, Krieger J, Ifoundza T, Oswald M, Kessler R: Association of chronic obstructive pulmonary disease and sleep apnea syndrome. Am J Respir Crit Care Med 151:82–86, 1995
51. Douglas NJ: Breathing during sleep in patients with chronic obstructive pulmonary disease. In Kreiger M, Roth T, Dement WC (eds): Principles and Practice of Sleep Medicine, 2nd ed. Philadelphia, WB Saunders, 1994, pp 758–768
52. Douglas NJ: Asthma. In Kreiger M, Roth T, Dement WC (eds): Principles and Practice of Sleep Medicine, 2nd ed. Philadelphia, WB Saunders, 1994, pp 748–757
53. Connolly CK: Diurnal rhythms in airway obstruction. Br J Dis Chest 73:357–366, 1979
54. Chan CS, Woolcock AJ, Sullivan CE: Nocturnal asthma: Role of snoring and obstructive sleep apnea. Am Rev Respir Dis 137: 1502–1504, 1988
55. Stewart IC, Rhind GB, Power JT, Flenley DC, Douglas NJ: Effects of sustained release terbutaline on symptoms and sleep quality in patients with nocturnal asthma. Thorax 42:797–800, 1987
56. Nicholson A, Bradley C, Pascoe P: Medications: Effect on sleep and wakefulness. In Kryger M, Roth T, Dement WC (eds): Principles and Practice of Sleep Medicine, 2nd ed. Philadelphia, WB Saunders, 1994, pp 364–372
57. Ekbom KA: Restless legs syndrome. Neurology 10:868–873, 1960
58. Montplaisir J, Godbout R, Pelletier G, Warnes H: Restless legs syndrome and periodic limb movements during sleep. In Kreiger M, Roth T, Dement WC (eds): Principles and Practice of Sleep Medicine, 2nd ed. Philadelphia, WB Saunders, 1994, pp 589–597
59. Ancoli-Israel S, Kripke DF, Klauber MR, Mason WJ, Fell R, Kaplan O: Periodic limb movements in community-dwelling elderly. Sleep 14:496–500, 1991
60. Bixler EO, Kales A, Soldatos CR, Kales JD, Healey S: Prevalence of sleep disorders in the Los Angeles metropolitan area. American Journal of Psychiatry 136:1257–1262, 1979
61. Akerstedt T, Torsvall L, Gillberg M: Sleepiness in shiftwork. A review with emphasis on continuous monitoring of EEG and EOG. Chronobiology International 4:129–140, 1987
62. Reynolds CF: Sleep in affective disorders. In Kryger MH, Roth T, Dement WC (eds): Principles and Practice of Sleep Medicine. Philadelphia, WB Saunders, 1989, pp 413–415
63. Benca RM: Mood Disorders. In Kryger MH, Roth T, Dement WC (eds): Principles and Practice of Sleep Medicine, 2nd ed. Philadelphia, WB Saunders, 1994, pp 899–913
64. Dement WC, Zarcone V, Varner V, Hoddes E, Nassau S, Jacobs B, Brown J, McDonald A, Horan K, Glass R, Gonzales P, Friedman E, Phillips R: The prevalence of narcolepsy. Sleep Res 1:148, 1972
65. Guilleminault C: Narcolepsy syndrome. In Kryger M, Roth T, Dement WC (eds): Principles and Practice of Sleep Medicine, 2nd ed. Philadelphia, WB Saunders, 1994, pp 549–561
66. Kryger MH, Roth T, Dement WC: Principles and Practice of Sleep Medicine. Philadelphia, WB Saunders, 1994, pp 1–1067
67. Hanly PJ, Millar TW, Steljes DG, Baert R, Frais MA, Kryger MH: Respiration and abnormal sleep in patients with congestive heart failure. Chest 96:480–488, 1989
68. Hanly PJ, Millar TW, Steljes DG, Baert R, Frais MA, Kryger MH: The effect of oxygen on respiration and sleep in patients with congestive heart failure. Ann Intern Med 111:777–782, 1989
69. Guilleminault C, Clerk A, Labanowski M, Simmons J, Stoohs R: Cardiac failure and benzodiazepines. Sleep 16:524–528, 1993
70. Takasaki Y, Orr D, Popkin J, Rutherford R, Liu P, Bradley TD: Effect of nasal continuous positive airway pressure on sleep apnea in congestive heart failure. Am Rev Respir Dis 140:1578–1584, 1989
71. George CFP: Cardiovascular disease and sleep. In Kryger M, Roth T, Dement WC (eds): Principles and Practice of Sleep Medicine. 2nd ed. Philadelphia, WB Saunders, 1994, pp 835–846
72. Guilleminault C: Natural history, cardiac impact, and long-term follow-up of sleep apnea syndrome. In Guilleminault C, Lugaresi E (eds): Sleep/Wake Disorders: Natural History, Epidemiology, and Long-term Evolution. New York, Raven Press, 1983, pp 107–125
73. Partinen M, Alihanka J, Lang H, Kalliomaki L: Myocardial infarction in relation to sleep apneas. Sleep Res 12:272, 1983
74. Hung J, Whitford EG, Parsons RW, Hillman DR: Association of sleep apnoea with myocardial infarction in men. Lancet 336: 261–264, 1990
75. Decker MJ, Smith BL, Strohl KP: Center-based vs patient based diagnosis and therapy of sleep-related respiratory disorders and the role of the respiratory care practitioner. Respir Care 39: 390–395, 1994

SUGGESTED READING

Guilleminault C, van den Hoed J, Mitler M: Clinical overview of the sleep apnea syndromes. In Guilleminault C, Dement WC (eds): Sleep Apnea Syndromes. New York, Alan R. Liss, 1978, pp 1–12

12 Respiratory Care Monitoring

Dean Hess

CLINICAL SKILLS

Upon completion of this chapter, the reader will know how to:

- Conduct a proper patient examination, including obtaining all pertinent respiratory tests (blood gas analysis, indices of oxygenation and ventilation, respiratory monitoring, pulse oximetry, transcutaneous oxygen and carbon dioxide monitoring, capnography, hemodynamic monitoring, mechanical ventilator wavetorms and mechanics, indirect calorimetry and/or resting energy expenditure, and gastric intramural pH.
- Review existing data in patient record, including medical history, and recommend diagnostic procedures or monitoring.
- Select, assemble, and check monitoring equipment (pulse oximeters, capnometers, mechanical ventilator airway pressure and exhaled volume measuring systems, mechanical ventilator graphics, transcutaneous oxygen and carbon dioxide monitors, indirect calorimetry systems, and arterial, central venous, and pulmonary artery pressure catheters) for proper function, operation, and cleanliness.
- Explain goals of monitoring to patients.
- Maintain records of patient monitoring.
- Protect patients from nosocomial infection.
- Make modifications in therapeutic procedures and recommend care plan modifications based on patient response.

KEY TERMS

Afterload
Airway resistance
Alveolar PO_2
Capnography
Carbon dioxide production
Cardiac output
Central venous pressure
Contractility
Dead space
End-tidal PCO_2
Esophageal pressure
Flow-volume loop
Gastric intramural pH
Intra-arterial blood gas monitoring
Indirect calorimetry
Lung compliance
Mixed venous blood gas monitoring
Oxygen consumption
Preload
Pressure-volume loop
Pulmonary artery pressure
Pulmonary capillary wedge pressure
Pulse oximetry
Shunt
Transcutaneous monitoring
Work of breathing

Respiratory monitoring may be invasive or noninvasive, continuous or intermittent. It can be used to evaluate arterial or venous oxygenation, transcutaneous O_2 and CO_2, exhaled CO_2, O_2 consumption and CO_2 production, and hemodynamics. One of the characteristics of all monitoring devices is real-time assessment, which allows rapid detection of abnormalities and evaluation of therapeutic interventions. Arterial blood gases vary in critically ill patients and serial measurements may reflect this variability rather than a physiologic change.[1–3] Monitors, on the other hand, should allow detection of trends in physiologic parameters before they would be detected by intermittent measurements. Another feature of monitors is that they cause little or no blood loss from the patient, reducing the risk of blood exposure for the clinician.

A concern related to monitors is their proliferation in critical care units. The result of this is many false-positive alarms.[4,5] The result of false-positive alarms is that they are ignored, which decreases the impact of the monitor. The role of some monitors is not firmly established, particularly in areas other than critical care and anesthesia.

NONINVASIVE MONITORING OF OXYGENATION, VENTILATION, AND METABOLIC RATE

Pulse Oximetry

Pulse oximeters are available as small hand-held units, as semiportable units with alarms and waveform display, in combination with other monitors such as capnography and transcutaneous PCO_2, and as part of the bedside critical care monitoring system. Pulse oximeters are used for continuous monitoring and intermittent spot checks in prehospital care, in the emergency department, in outpatient clinics, in neonatal and pediatric critical care, in adult critical care, and in general patient care wards. Pulse oximetry is generally considered safe, but burns (owing to defective probes) and pressure necrosis may occur.

The pulse oximeter passes two wavelengths of light (660 nm and 940 nm) through a pulsating vascular bed (Fig. 12-1). This is accomplished using two light-emitting diodes (LEDs) and a photodetector. Although reasonably specific, there is some error in the wavelength of light emitted by the LEDs (±30 nm) that can affect accuracy. Also, the photodetector is not specific (ie, it will respond to any wavelength of light, which can result in interference). Although some of the light emitted from the LEDs is absorbed by each constituent of the tissue, the only variable absorption is caused by arterial pulsations. This is translated into a plethysmographic waveform, and the ratio of the amplitudes of these two waveforms is translated into a display of O_2 saturation (SpO_2).

A probe is used to pass light from the LEDs through a pulsating vascular bed. A variety of probes are available and include finger probes, ear probes, and nasal probes. Probes are available in disposable and reusable designs.

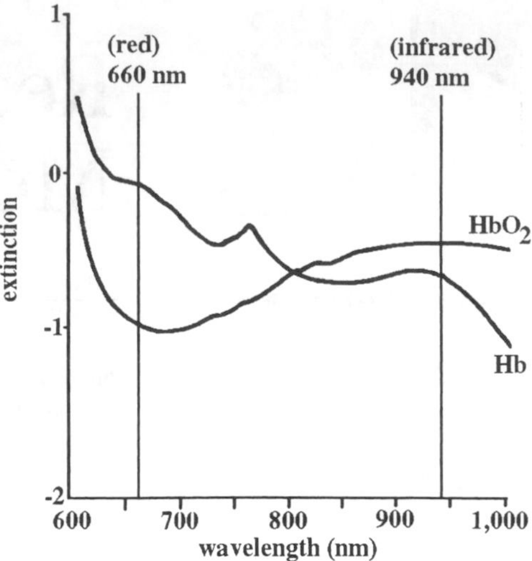

FIGURE 12-1. Light absorption spectra for oxyhemoglobin and deoxyhemoglobin. Pulse oximeters use wavelengths of 660 nm and 940 nm.

Although most pulse oximeters use transmission oximetry (ie, the light from the LEDs is transmitted through the tissue and the photodetector is opposite the LEDs), other designs use reflectance oximetry (ie, the light from the LEDs is reflected from the tissue and the photodetector is on the same side of the tissue as the LEDs).

The limitations of pulse oximetry should be recognized, appreciated, and understood by everyone who uses pulse oximetry data.[6–11] Most pulse oximeter errors can be explained as too little signal (eg, low perfusion, improper probe placement) or too much noise (eg, motion, ambient light).

- *Accuracy:* Pulse oximeters use empiric calibration curves developed from studies of healthy volunteers. At saturations greater than 80%, the accuracy of pulse oximetry is about ±4% to 5%. The accuracy is not as good at saturations less than 80%, but the clinical importance of this is questionable. The accuracy of pulse oximetry relates to the oxyhemoglobin dissociation curve (Fig. 12-2). If the pulse oximeter displays a SpO_2 of 95%, the true saturation could be as low as 90% or as high as 100%. If the true saturation is 90%, the PO_2 will be about 60 mmHg. If the true saturation is 100%, however, the PO_2 could be very high (>150 mmHg).
- *Saturation versus PO_2:* At a SpO_2 greater than 90%, PaO_2 is a more sensitive indicator of lung function than SpO_2. Owing to the shape of the oxyhemoglobin dissociation curve, pulse oximetry does not detect hyperoxemia very well. However, pulse oximetry may be a useful indicator of desaturation and has been considered by some clinicians to be a desaturation monitor. Owing to the limits of inaccuracy of pulse oximetry and the shape of the oxyhemoglobin dissociation curve, PaO_2 cannot be precisely predicted from SpO_2.
- *Differences between devices and probes:* The pulse oximeter is unique in that it requires no user cali-

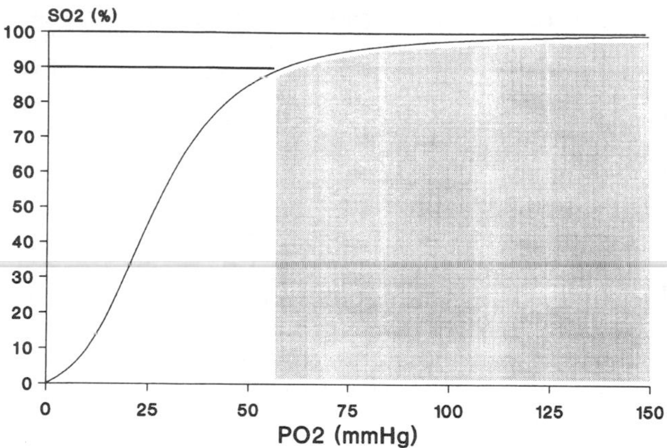

FIGURE 12-2. Oxyhemoglobin dissociation curve. When the SpO_2 is 95%, the SaO_2 could be in the range of 90%–100%; this could result in a very large range of PaO_2.

bration. However, manufacturer-derived calibration curves programmed into the software vary from manufacturer to manufacturer and can vary among pulse oximeters of a given manufacturer. The output of LEDs can vary from probe to probe. The result of these factors is that the accuracy of pulse oximetry varies among devices. To decrease costs, some hospitals have adopted the practice of reusing disposable pulse oximeter probes, which could affect the accuracy of the probe over time. For these reasons, the same pulse oximeter and probe should ideally be used for each SpO_2 determination on a given patient. When SpO_2 is not consistent with the patient's clinical condition, an arterial blood gas sample should be obtained.

- *Penumbra effect:* If the pulse oximeter probe does not fit correctly, light can be shunted from the LEDs directly to the photodetector. Theoretically, this will cause a falsely low SpO_2 if SaO_2 is greater than 85% and a falsely elevated SpO_2 if SaO_2 is less than 85%.
- *Dyshemoglobinemias:* Because commercially available pulse oximeters use only two wavelengths of light, they only evaluate O_2Hb and deoxyhemoglobin. Pulse oximeters assume that COHb and metHb concentrations are low. Abnormal elevations of COHb and metHb each result in significant inaccuracy in pulse oximetry, which should not be used when elevated levels of either are present. COHb always produces a SpO_2 greater than the O_2Hb and metHb causes the SpO_2 to move towards 85%. Fetal hemoglobin may affect the accuracy of CO oximetry, but it does not affect the accuracy of pulse oximetry.
- *Endogenous and exogenous dyes and pigments:* Vascular dyes can affect the accuracy of pulse oximetry, with methylene blue having the greatest effect. Nail polish can also affect the accuracy of pulse oximetry and should be removed when pulse oximetry is used. Hyperbilirubinemia does not affect the accuracy of pulse oximetry. Vascular infusions of intralipids do not affect pulse oximetry, although they affect in vitro measurements of O_2 saturation (by CO-oximetry) and in vivo monitoring of mixed venous O_2 saturation.
- *Skin pigmentation:* The accuracy and performance of pulse oximeters are affected by deeply pigmented skin.
- *Perfusion:* Under conditions of low flow (eg, cardiac arrest or severe peripheral vasoconstriction), pulse oximetry becomes unreliable. Under these conditions, an ear probe may be more reliable than a finger probe. The plethysmographic waveform displayed by the pulse oximeter may be a useful indicator for the arterial blood flow to the site of the oximeter probe—a dampened plethysmographic waveform suggests poor signal quality.
- *Anemia:* Although pulse oximeters are generally reliable over a wide range of hemoglobin levels, they become less accurate and reliable with conditions of severe anemia (Hb <8 g/dL at low saturations and hematocrit <10% at all saturations).
- *Motion:* Motion of the probe can produce considerable artifact with unreliable and inaccurate pulse oximetry readings. This may be corrected by using an alternate probe site (such as the ear or toe rather than the finger) and a longer sample averaging time.
- *High-intensity ambient light:* Because the photodetector of the pulse oximeter is nonspecific, high-intensity ambient light can produce interference. This can be corrected by wrapping the probe with a light barrier.
- *Abnormal pulses:* Venous pulses and a large dicrotic notch have been shown to affect the accuracy of pulse oximetry.

Pulse oximetry is indicated in unstable patients likely to desaturate, in patients receiving a therapeutic intervention that is likely to produce hypoxemia (such as bronchoscopy), and in patients having interventions likely to produce changes in arterial oxygenation (such as changes in F_{IO_2} or PEEP; see AARC Clinical Practice Guideline: Pulse Oximetry). The pulse oximeter is probably no better at detection of a disconnect than the alarms already available on the ventilator. The pulse oximeter may actually be more likely to produce annoying false-positive alarms and there may be a relatively long time between disconnect and desaturation (particularly if the Pa_{O_2} is high before the disconnect). Despite its limitations, pulse oximetry has become a standard of care for mechanically ventilated patients.

Although pulse oximetry may improve the detection of desaturation, there are few data to support that it makes a difference in morbidity and mortality. A large study (>20,000 patients)[12,13] of pulse oximetry use during anesthesia and postanesthesia care found no difference in outcome. Interestingly, hypoxemia and related respiratory events were more likely to be detected with the use of pulse oximetry, but the detection and treatment of these events did not affect outcome. Similar studies have not been reported for other patient popu-

AARC Clinical Practice Guideline

PULSE OXIMETRY

Indications: The need to monitor the adequacy of arterial oxyhemoglobin saturation, the need to quantitate the response of arterial oxyhemoglobin saturation to therapeutic intervention or to a diagnostic procedure (eg, bronchoscopy), the need to comply with mandated regulations or recommendations by authoritative groups.

Contraindications: The presence of an ongoing need for measurement of pH, $PaCO_2$, total hemoglobin, and abnormal hemoglobins may be a relative contraindication to pulse oximetry.

Device Limitations/Validation of Results: Factors, agents, or situations that may affect readings, limit precision, or limit the performance or application of a pulse oximeter include motion artifact, abnormal hemoglobins (primarily carboxyhemoglobin [COHb] and methemoglobin [metHb]), intravascular dyes, exposure of measuring probe to ambient light during measurement, low perfusion states, skin pigmentation, nail polish or nail coverings with finger probe, inability to detect saturations below 80% with the same degree of accuracy and precision seen at higher saturations, and inability to quantitate the degree of hyperoxemia. Hyperbilirubinemia has been shown not to affect the accuracy of SpO_2 readings. To validate pulse oximeter readings, incorporate or assess agreement between SpO_2 and arterial oxyhemoglobin saturation (SaO_2) obtained by direct measurement—these measurements should be initially performed simultaneously and then periodically re-evaluated in relation to the patient's clinical state. To assure consistency of care (between institutions and within the same institution) based on SpO_2 readings, assess selection of proper probe and appropriate placement (the probe is attached to its intended site); for continuous, prolonged monitoring, the hi/low alarms must be appropriately set, specific manufacturer's recommendations complied with; the device is applied and adjusted correctly to monitor response time and electrocardiographic coupling; confirm strength of plethysmograph waveform or pulse amplitude strength; and assure that device is detecting an adequate pulse. SpO_2 results should be documented in the patient's medical record and should detail the conditions under which the readings were obtained: date, time of measurement, and pulse oximeter reading; patient's position, activity level, and location; during monitoring, assure that patient's activity is according to physician's order; inspired oxygen concentration or supplemental oxygen flow, specifying the type of oxygen delivery device; probe placement site and probe type; model of device (if more than one device is available for use); results of simultaneously obtained arterial pH, PaO_2, and $PaCO_2$, and directly measured saturations of COHb, MetHb, and O_2Hb (if direct measurement was not simultaneously performed, an additional, one-time statement must be made explaining that the SpO_2 reading has not been validated by comparison to directly measured values); stability of readings (length of observation time and range of fluctuation, for continuous or prolonged studies, review of recording may be necessary); clinical appearance of patient—subjective assessment of perfusion at measuring site (eg, cyanosis, skin temperature); agreement between patient's heart rate as determined by pulse oximeter and by palpation and oscilloscope. When disparity exists between SpO_2, SaO_2 readings, and the clinical presentation of the patient, possible causes should be explored before results are reported. Discrepancies may be reduced by monitoring at alternate sites or appropriate substitution of instruments or probes. If such steps do not remedy the disparity, results of pulse oximetry should not be reported; instead, a statement describing the corrective action should be included in the patient's medical record, and direct measurement of arterial blood gas values should be requested. The absolute limits that constitute unacceptable disparity vary with patient condition and specific device. Clinical judgment must be exercised.

Assessment of Need: When direct measurement of SaO_2 is not available or accessible in a timely fashion, an SpO_2 measurement may temporarily suffice if the limitations of the data are appreciated. SpO_2 is appropriate for continuous and prolonged monitoring (eg, during sleep, exercise, bronchoscopy). SpO_2 may be adequate when assessment of acid-base status or PaO_2 is not required.

Assessment of Outcome: SpO_2 results should reflect the patient's clinical condition (ie, validate the basis for ordering the test). Documentation of results, therapeutic intervention (or lack of), or clinical decisions based on the SpO_2 measurement should be noted in the medical record.

Monitoring: The monitoring schedule of patient and equipment during continuous oximetry should be tied to bedside assessment and vital signs determinations.

(From AARC Clinical Practice Guideline: For complete text see Respir Care 36:1406–1409, 1991.)

lations (eg, critical care). Whether pulse oximetry reduces the number of blood gas analyses and the cost of care is unclear, and conflicting results have been published.[14–16]

Pulse oximetry is useful in titrating supplemental O_2 in critically ill ventilator-dependent patients.[17] A SpO_2 of 92% has been shown to be reliable in predicting a PaO_2 $\geq$ 60 mmHg in white patients ($\geq$ SpO_2 of 95% in black patients).[17] Although pulse oximetry is useful to titrate a level of arterial oxygenation that does not produce hypoxemia, it does not eliminate the need for periodic arterial blood gases. When pulse oximetry is used to titrate FIO_2, the final FIO_2 setting should *always* be confirmed by arterial blood gases. Because of the accuracy limits of pulse oximetry, it should be used cautiously to determine the need for long-term O_2 because it may exclude patients from O_2 who would qualify based on PaO_2 criteria.[18]

Although pulse oximetry is now commonly used, many clinicians do not understand the basic principles of pulse oximetry and make serious errors in the interpretation of pulse oximetry readings.[19,20] Further, pulse oximetry is often used with inadequate attention to the presence of significant events[21]—the use of a monitor without attention to the information provided is worthless!

Capnography

Capnometry is the measurement of CO_2 at the airway during the ventilatory cycle, and capnography is the measurement of CO_2 with display of a waveform called the capnogram. Capnography (ie, display of PCO_2 and a waveform) is superior to capnometry (ie, display of PCO_2 without a waveform), not only because it provides additional clinical information but also because it allows the quality of the signal to be assessed (see AARC Clinical Practice Guideline: Capnography/Capnometry).

CO_2 can be measured at the airway using either mass spectrometry or infrared capnography.[11,22,23] Most bedside capnographs measure CO_2 by infrared absorption, which takes advantage of the principle that CO_2 has an absorption peak at 4.26 μm (Fig. 12-3). With the mainstream capnograph, the measurement chamber is placed at the airway and with the sidestream capnograph, gas is aspirated through fine-bore tubing to the measurement chamber inside the capnograph (Fig. 12-4). There are advantages and disadvantages of each design (Table 12-1), and neither is clearly superior.

There are numerous technical problems related to the use of capnography. These include the need for periodic calibration and interference from gases such as N_2O. Water is particularly a problem, because it occludes sample lines in the sidestream capnograph and condenses in the cell of mainstream devices. Manufacturers use a number of features to overcome these problems, including H_2O traps, purging of the sample line, construction of the sample line with H_2O-vapor permeable Nafion, and heating of the mainstream cell.

The normal capnogram is illustrated in Figure 12-5. During inspiration, PCO_2 is zero. At the beginning of exhalation, PCO_2 remains zero as gas from anatomic dead space leaves the airway (Phase I). The PCO_2 then sharply rises as alveolar gas mixes with dead space gas (Phase II). During most of exhalation, the curve levels and forms a plateau (Phase III). This represents gas from alveoli and is called the "alveolar plateau." The PCO_2 at the end of the alveolar plateau is called end-tidal PCO_2 ($P_{ET}CO_2$). In patients with abnormal lung function, the shape of the capnogram may be abnormal, which can be diagnostic in some cases (Figs. 12-6 and 12-7).

The $P_{ET}CO_2$ presumably represents alveolar PCO_2 (P_ACO_2). P_ACO_2 is determined by the rate at which CO_2 is added to the alveolus and the rate at which CO_2 is cleared from the alveolus. Thus, P_ACO_2 is the result of the $\dot{V}/\dot{Q}$ (Fig. 12-8). With a normal $\dot{V}/\dot{Q}$, the P_ACO_2 will approximate the P_aCO_2. If the $\dot{V}/\dot{Q}$ decreases, P_ACO_2 increases toward $P\bar{v}CO_2$. With a high $\dot{V}/\dot{Q}$ (ie, dead space), P_ACO_2 will approach the P_ICO_2, which is usually zero. Theoretically, $P_{ET}CO_2$ could be as low as the P_ICO_2 (zero) or as high as the $P\bar{v}CO_2$.

An increase or decrease in $P_{ET}CO_2$ can be the result of changes in $\dot{V}CO_2$ (ie, metabolism), changes in CO_2 delivery to the lungs (ie, circulation), or changes in $\dot{V}_A$). However, because of homeostasis, compensatory changes may occur so that $P_{ET}CO_2$ does not change. In

AARC Clinical Practice Guideline

CAPNOGRAPHY/CAPNOMETRY

Indications: On the basis of available evidence, capnography should not be mandated for all patients receiving mechanical ventilatory support, but it may be indicated for evaluation of exhaled CO_2, especially end-tidal CO_2, which is the maximum partial pressure of CO_2 exhaled during a tidal breath (just before the beginning of inspiration) and is designated $P_{ET}CO_2$. Monitoring severity of pulmonary disease and evaluating response to therapy, especially therapy intended to improve the ratio of dead space to tidal volume (V_D/V_T) and the matching ventilation to perfusion ($\dot{V}/\dot{Q}$), and possibly to therapy intended to increase coronary blood flow; determining that tracheal rather than esophageal intubation has taken place (low or absent cardiac output may negate its use for this indication); continued monitoring of the integrity of the ventilatory circuit, including the artificial airway; evaluation of the efficiency of mechanical ventilatory support by determination of the difference between the P_aCO_2 and the $P_{ET}CO_2$ reflecting CO_2 elimination; monitoring adequacy of pulmonary and coronary blood flow; monitoring inspired CO_2 when CO_2 gas is being therapeutically administered; graphic evaluation of the ventilator-patient interface. Evaluation of the capnogram may be useful in detecting rebreathing of CO_2, obstructive pulmonary disease, waning neuromuscular blockade (curare cleft), cardiogenic oscillations, esophageal intubation, cardiac arrest, and contamination of the monitor or sampling line with secretions or mucus.

Contraindications: There are no absolute contraindications to capnography in mechanically ventilated adults provided that the data obtained are evaluated with consideration given to the patient's clinical condition.

Assessment of Need: Capnography is considered a standard of care during anesthesia. The Society of Critical Care Medicine has suggested that capnography be available in every ICU. Assessment of the need to use capnography with a specific patient should be guided by the clinical situation. The patient's primary cause of respiratory failure and the acuteness of the condition should be considered. Patients with severe dynamic disease, such as adult respiratory distress syndrome, should be considered candidates for capnography.

Assessment of Outcome: Results should reflect the patient's condition and should validate the basis for ordering the monitoring. Documentation of results (along with all ventilatory and hemodynamic variables available), therapeutic interventions, or clinical decisions made based on the capnogram should be included in the patient's chart.

Monitoring: Ventilatory variables: tidal volume, respiratory rate, positive end-expiratory pressure, inspiratory-to-expiratory ratio, peak airway pressure, and concentrations of respiratory gas mixture. Hemodynamic variables: systemic and pulmonary blood pressures, cardiac output, shunt, and ventilation-perfusion imbalances.

(From AARC Clinical Practice Guidelines: For complete text see Respir Care 40:1321–1324, 1995.)

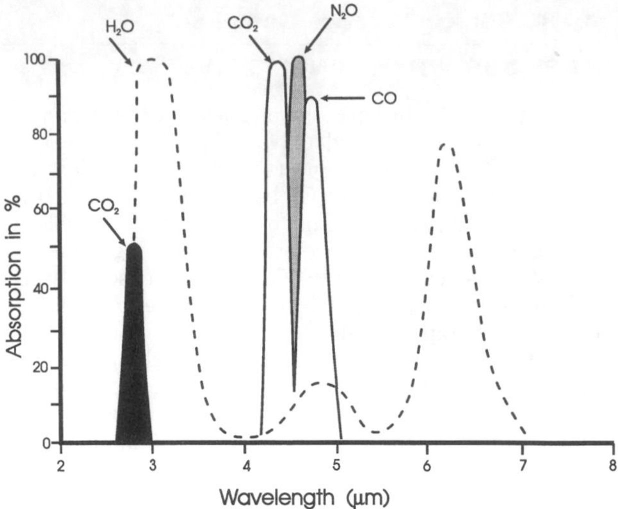

FIGURE 12-3. Light absorption spectra for CO_2, H_2O, CO, and N_2O.

practice, $P_{ET}CO_2$ is a nonspecific indicator of cardiopulmonary homeostasis and usually does not indicate a specific problem or abnormality.

The gradient between P_ACO_2 and $P_{ET}CO_2$ [$P(a-ET)CO_2$] is often calculated. This gradient is usually small (<5 mmHg). However, in patients with dead space-producing disease (eg, pulmonary embolism with high $\dot{V}/\dot{Q}$), the $P_{ET}CO_2$ may be considerably less than P_ACO_2. Although not commonly appreciated, the $P_{ET}CO_2$ may occasionally be greater than the P_ACO_2.

There is considerable intra- and inter-patient variability in the relationship between P_ACO_2 and $P_{ET}CO_2$. The $P(a-ET)CO_2$ is often too variable to allow precise prediction of P_ACO_2 from $P_{ET}CO_2$ (Figs. 12-9 and 12-10).[24,25] $P_{ET}CO_2$ is useful for monitoring iatrogenic hypocapnia in head-injured patients, probably because these patients often have relatively normal lung function.

A useful application of capnography is the detection of esophageal intubation. Because there is normally very little CO_2 in the stomach, intubation of the esophagus and ventilation of the stomach result in a very low $P_{ET}CO_2$ (Fig. 12-11).[26,27] Of the methods available to detect esophageal intubation, measurement of $P_{ET}CO_2$ is regarded as the most reliable. A potential problem with the use of capnography to confirm endotracheal intubation occurs during cardiac arrest, with false results because of very low $P_{ET}CO_2$ values related to decreased blood flow. A relatively low-cost disposable device for detecting esophageal intubation is commercially available (Fig. 12-12), which produces a color change in the presence of exhaled CO_2.[28–30]

Capnography may be potentially useful to evaluate pulmonary blood flow during resuscitation.[31,32] During resuscitation, changes in blood flow are reflected by changes in $P_{ET}CO_2$; low pulmonary blood flow results in low $P_{ET}CO_2$ and vice versa. It has also been found that patients likely to be resuscitated have a higher $P_{ET}CO_2$ (<15 mmHg) than patients who cannot be resuscitated ($P_{ET}CO_2$ >15 mmHg).[32] The use of $P_{ET}CO_2$ as a real-time objective indicator of resuscitation effectiveness is promising, but it is premature to recommend its routine use during resuscitation.

Use of capnography in the operating room has become a standard of care. However, the use of capnography in the critical care unit has not been as enthusiastically supported. Part of this relates to the fact that capnometers are technically more difficult to use than other monitors such as pulse oximeters. More importantly, $P_{ET}CO_2$ has often been found to be an imprecise predictor of P_ACO_2, particularly in patients with lung disease—precisely those in whom its use might be most desirable. Although the use of capnography has been advocated as a backup disconnect alarm, there is no evidence that it is any better than the alarms currently available on ventilators. Although its use in anesthesia of infants and children has been described,[33] the role of capnography in neonatal and pediatric critical care is unclear.

Transcutaneous Monitoring

Transcutaneous PO_2 ($P_{TC}O_2$) and transcutaneous PCO_2 ($P_{TC}CO_2$) has been commonly monitored in the neonatal intensive care unit (ICU) (see AARC Clinical Practice Guideline: Transcutaneous Blood Gas Monitoring for Neonatal and Pediatric Patients), but it has had limited acceptance in the care of adult patients.[6,26,11,34–36] Since the introduction of pulse oximetry, $P_{TC}O_2$ monitoring has also decreased in the neonatal ICU. Most commercially available transcutaneous monitors use a combination $P_{TC}O_2/P_{TC}CO_2$ electrode.

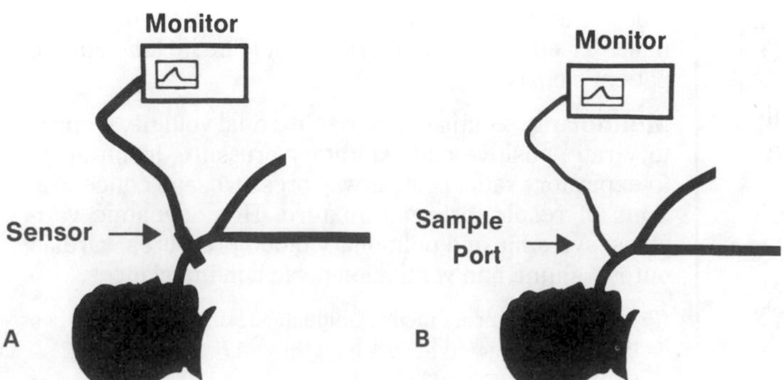

FIGURE 12-4. **(A)** Mainstream capnometer; **(B)** Sidestream capnometer.

TABLE 12-1. **Mainstream Versus Sidestream Capnography**

Advantages	Disadvantages
Mainstream	
Sensor at patient airway	Secretion/condensation blocks sensor
Fast response (real-time readings)	Window
No volume loss from system	Bulky sensor at patient airway
	Difficult to use with nonintubated patients
Sidestream Capnograph	
No bulky sensors at airway	Secretions/condensation blocks sample tubing
Use with nonintubated patients	Trap required to remove H_2O from sample
	Slow response; lag time
	Volume loss owing to sample flow

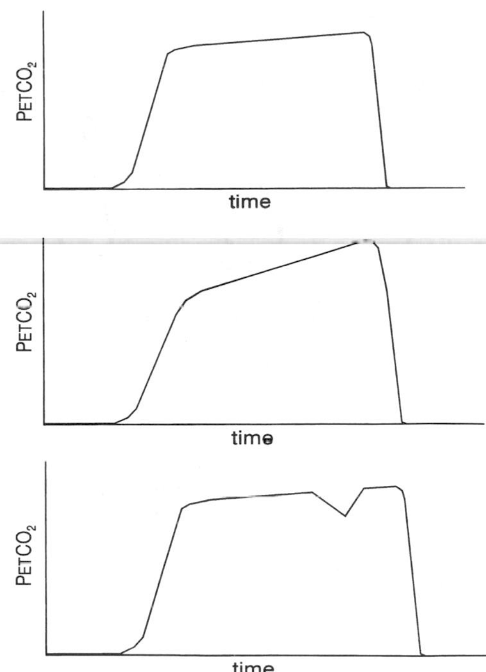

FIGURE 12-6. *Top*—normal capnogram; *middle*—capnogram with airflow obstruction (eg, COPD or asthma); *bottom*—capnogram with curare cleft (eg, patient recovering from paralysis or not breathing in synchrony with the ventilator).

The $P_{TC}O_2$ electrode (Fig. 12-13) uses a polarographic principle similar to that used in blood gas analyzers and O_2 analyzers. To produce a $P_{TC}O_2$ approximating PaO_2, the electrode must be heated to approximately 44° C. The close relationship between PaO_2 and $P_{TC}O_2$ in neonates is the result of a complex set of physiologic events. The increase in PO_2 caused by heating roughly balances the decrease in PO_2 caused by skin O_2 consumption and the diffusion of O_2 across the skin. The close relationship between PaO_2 and $P_{TC}O_2$ that occurs in neonates is probably more coincidental than physiologic. This creates the illusion that $P_{TC}O_2$ is the same as PaO_2. Particularly in adults, the $P_{TC}O_2$ is frequently less than PaO_2 (Fig. 12-14). $P_{TC}O_2$ is also affected by perfusion and may reflect O_2 delivery (the product of cardiac output and arterial O_2 content) to the skin under the electrode. $P_{TC}O_2$ has been used in adults to monitor the results of vascular surgery and hyperbaric O_2 therapy, the intent being to evaluate perfusion rather than PO_2 per se.

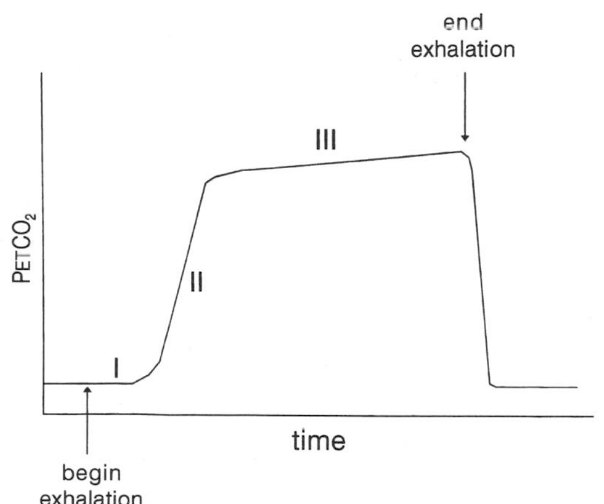

FIGURE 12-5. Normal capnogram.

$P_{TC}CO_2$ uses a Severinghaus electrode similar to that used in the blood gas analyzer. Unlike the $P_{TC}O_2$ electrode, reasonably good correlation can be obtained at a temperature of 37°C. The $P_{TC}CO_2$ is consistently greater than P_ACO_2, and for this reason manufacturers incorporate a correction factor so that the $P_{TC}CO_2$ displayed approximates the P_ACO_2. Like $P_{TC}O_2$, the closeness with which $P_{TC}CO_2$ approximates P_ACO_2 is the result of a complex set of physiologic events, and thus it is incorrect to think of $P_{TC}CO_2$ as P_ACO_2. Decreased perfusion causes the $P_{TC}CO_2$ to increase. $P_{TC}CO_2$ monitoring may be more useful than $P_{TC}O_2$ in adults (Fig. 12-15), but it has not had widespread acceptance owing to the limitations listed in Table 12-2.

Indirect Calorimetry

The relationship between metabolism, $\dot{V}O_2$, and $\dot{V}CO_2$ depends on the specific substrate that is metabolized.[37] Respiratory quotient ($RQ = \dot{V}CO_2/\dot{V}O_2$) is 1.0 for car-

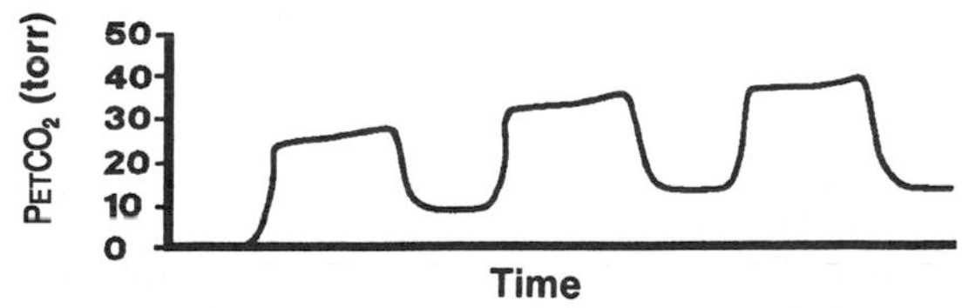

FIGURE 12-7. Capnogram with rebreathing. Note the inspired $P_{ET}CO_2$ greater than zero.

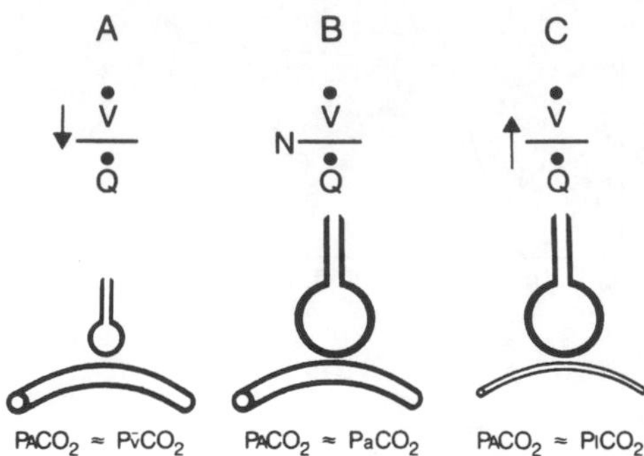

FIGURE 12-8. The P_ACO_2 is determined by the $\dot{V}/\dot{Q}$.

bohydrate metabolism, 0.71 for fat metabolism, 0.81 for protein metabolism, 8.7 for lipogenesis, and 0.25 for ketogenesis. RQ is normally between 0.7 and 1.0, and will be about 0.8 with a balance of metabolism. Carbohydrate metabolism will raise the RQ toward 1.0 and fat metabolism will lower it toward 0.7. With lipogenesis, the whole-body RQ may be greater than 1.0 (but seldom exceeds 1.2), and the whole-body RQ may be less than 0.7 (but seldom less than 0.65) with ketogenesis. An increase in metabolic rate (ie, energy expenditure) results in an increased $\dot{V}O_2$ and $\dot{V}CO_2$, which requires an increase in ventilation.

Indirect calorimetry is the calculation of energy expenditure by the measurement of $\dot{V}O_2$ and $\dot{V}CO_2$, which are converted to energy expenditure (kcal/day) by the Weir Method (Equation Box 12-1). Indirect calorimetry also allows calculation of the RQ. Indirect calorimeters use either an open-circuit method or a closed-circuit method.[11,37–40]

The open-circuit method measures the concentrations and volumes of inspired and expired gases to determine $\dot{V}O_2$ and $\dot{V}CO_2$ (Equation Box 12-1). $\dot{V}O_2$ and

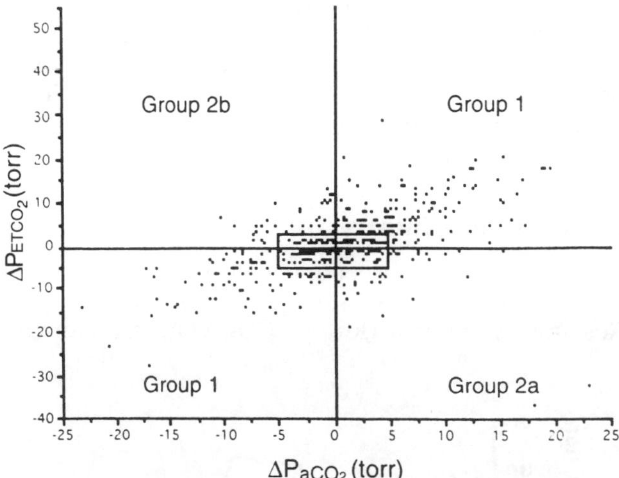

FIGURE 12-9. Relationship between changes in $P_{ET}CO_2$ and $PaCO_2$ in 80 ICU patients. Note that there are a number of cases in which the $P_{ET}CO_2$ increases and the $PaCO_2$ decreases and vice versa. (From Graybeal JM, Russell GB: Capnometry in the surgical ICU: An analysis of the arterial-to-end-tidal carbon dioxide difference. Respir Care 1993;38:923–928.)

$\dot{V}CO_2$ can be measured by collecting expired gas into a large collection bag, and then measuring F_IO_2, $F_{\bar{E}}O_2$, $F_{\bar{E}}CO_2$, and $\dot{V}_E$. With this method, gas collection time is limited by the volume of the bag. This can result in short collection times and incorrect estimates of caloric requirements. Also, O_2 analyzers and volume monitors commonly used in bedside respiratory care are not accurate enough for this application.

The principal components of an open-circuit calorimeter are the analyzers (O_2 and CO_2), a volume measuring device, and a mixing chamber. The analyzers must be capable of measuring small changes in gas concentrations, and the volume monitor must be capable of accurately measuring volumes from 0.05 to 1.0 L. The open-circuit method can be used with spontaneously breathing subjects (canopy, mouthpiece, or mask) and those requiring mechanical ventilation (Fig. 12-16). Exhaled gas from the patient is directed into the mixing chamber. At the end of the mixing chamber, a vacuum pump aspirates a small sample of gas for measurement of O_2 and CO_2. After analysis, this sample is returned to the mixing chamber. The entire volume of gas then exits through a volume monitor. Periodically, the analyzer also measures the F_IO_2. A microprocessor performs the necessary calculations.

Several points must be observed in order for the open-circuit technique to work properly:

- The F_IO_2 must be stable (± 0.005%). An external air-O_2 blender may be used to prevent fluctuations caused by the instability of gas-mixing systems in some mechanical ventilators.
- The F_IO_2 must be less than 0.60. Open circuit calorimeters measure $\dot{V}O_2$ inaccurately at high F_IO_2 (see AARC Clinical Practice Guideline: Metabolic Measurement Using Indirect Calorimetry During Mechanical Ventilation).
- The entire system must be leak free. Loss of gas from the system results in incomplete gas collection as may occur with uncuffed airways, bronchopleural fistulae, sidestream capnography, or dialysis.
- Inspired and expired gases must be completely separated. This can be a problem with continuous flow systems (eg, flow triggering).

A variation on the open-circuit technique is the breath-by-breath technique (Fig. 12-17). With this method, $\dot{V}O_2$ and $\dot{V}CO_2$ are measured on a breath-by-breath basis. Gases are sampled directly at the airway using a sidestream technique, and the volume of exhaled gas is measured using a pneumotachometer. This method can be used with mechanically ventilated patients and with spontaneously breathing patients.

The key components of the closed-circuit calorimeter are a volumetric spirometer, a mixing chamber, a CO_2 analyzer, and a CO_2 absorber (Fig. 12-18). The spirometer is filled with a known volume of O_2 and is connected to the patient. As the patient rebreathes from the spirometer, O_2 is consumed and CO_2 is produced. The CO_2 is removed from the system by the CO_2 absorber before the gas is returned to the spirometer. The decrease in

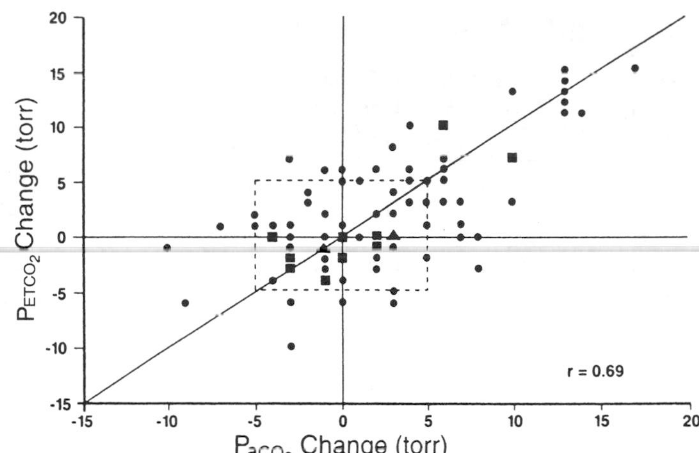

FIGURE 12-10. Relationship between changes in P_{ETCO_2} and $PaCO_2$ in patients weaning from mechanical ventilation following cardiothoracic surgery. Note that there are a number of cases in which the P_{ETCO_2} increases and the $PaCO_2$ decreases and vice versa. (From Hess D, Schlottag A, Levin B, Mathai J, Rexrode WO: Evaluation of the usefulness of end-tidal PCO_2 to aid weaning from mechanical ventilation following cardiac surgery. Respir Care 1991;36:837–843.)

the volume of the system equals $\dot{V}O_2$. Gas from the patient flows into the mixing chamber and a sample is aspirated for analysis of $F\bar{E}CO_2$. From the mixing chamber, gas flows through a CO_2 absorbent (such as barium hydroxide) and then to the spirometer. Changes in the volume of the spirometer are used to measure tidal volume. The difference between end-expiratory volumes is calculated to determine $\dot{V}O_2$. If the patient is mechanically ventilated, a bag-in-the-box system is used as a part of the inspiratory limb of the calorimeter. The bellows is pressurized by the ventilator, resulting in ventilation of the patient. Measurement time is limited by FIO_2 and the volume of the spirometer. When the volume of the spirometer decreases to a critical level, the measurement is interrupted to refill the spirometer.

Leaks from the closed-circuit calorimeter will result in erroneously high $\dot{V}O_2$ (uncuffed airway, bronchopleural fistula, sidestream capnograph). Another problem with this technique is related to ventilatory support, where compressible volume is increased and trigger sensitivity is affected. The major advantage of the closed-circuit method over the open-circuit method is its ability to make measurements at a high FIO_2 (up to 1.0).

During indirect calorimetry, the patient should be undisturbed, motionless and at rest, supine, and aware of his or her surroundings (unless comatose). The patient should either be on continuous nutritional support or fasting for several hours before the measurement. Before indirect calorimetry is performed, there should have been no changes in ventilation for at least 90 minutes, no factors that affect $\dot{V}O_2$ for at least 60 minutes (eg, fever, activity), and stable hemodynamics for at least 2 hours. The validity of the measurements should be assessed by direct observation rather than relying on a "steady state" indicator from the calorimeter.

Resting energy expenditure (REE) is similar, but not equivalent to, basal energy expenditure (BEE). BEE is measured in a neutral thermal environment after 12 hours of fasting. Because REE is measured with the patient at rest, calories must be added owing to patient activity. There may be considerable fluctuation in REE throughout the day and from day to day.

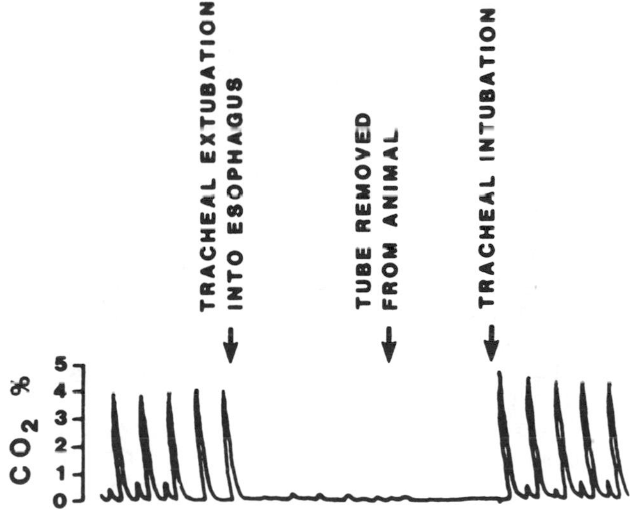

FIGURE 12-11. Differences in P_{ETCO_2} with endotracheal tube in the trachea and in the esophagus. (Murray IP, Modell JH. Early detection of endotracheal tube accidents by monitoring carbon dioxide concentration in respiratory gas. Anesthesiology 1983; 59:344–346.)

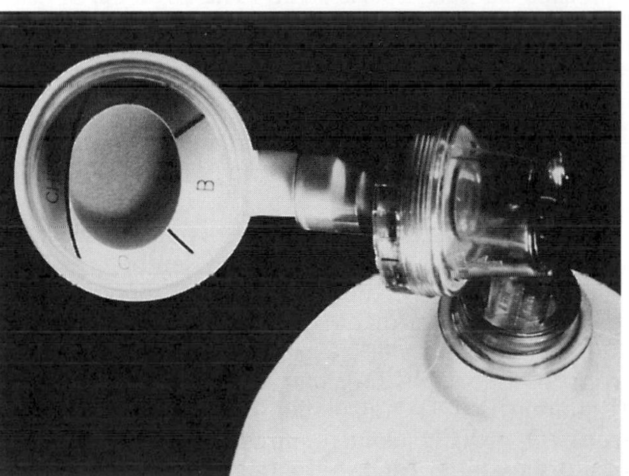

FIGURE 12-12. Small disposable CO_2 detector used to confirm endotracheal tube position in the trachea.

AARC Clinical Practice Guideline

TRANSCUTANEOUS BLOOD GAS MONITORING FOR NEONATAL AND PEDIATRIC PATIENTS

Indications: The need to monitor the adequacy of arterial oxygenation or ventilation. The need to quantitate the response to diagnostic and therapeutic interventions as evidenced by $P_{TC}O_2$ or $P_{TC}CO_2$ values.

Contraindications: In patients with poor skin integrity or adhesive allergy, transcutaneous monitoring may be relatively contraindicated.

Assessment of Need: When direct measurement of arterial blood is not available or accessible in a timely fashion, $P_{TC}O_2$ or $P_{TC}CO_2$ measurements may temporarily suffice if the limitations of the data are appreciated. Transcutaneous blood gas monitoring is appropriate for continuous and prolonged monitoring during mechanical ventilation, continuous positive airway pressure (CPAP), and supplemental oxygen administration. $P_{TC}O_2$ values can be used for diagnostic purposes as in the assessment of functional shunts (eg, persistent pulmonary hypertension of the newborn, PPHN, or persistent fetal circulation) or to determine the response to oxygen challenge in the assessment of congenital heart disease.

Assessment of Outcome: Results should reflect the patient's clinical condition (ie, validate the basis for ordering the monitoring). Documentation of results, therapeutic intervention (or lack of), and clinical decisions based on the transcutaneous measurements should be noted in the medical record.

Monitoring: The monitoring schedule of patient and equipment during transcutaneous monitoring should be integrated into patient assessment and vital signs determinations. Results should be documented in the patient's medical record and should detail the conditions under which the readings were obtained: the date and time of measurement, transcutaneous reading, patient's position, respiratory rate, and activity level; inspired oxygen concentration or supplemental oxygen flow, specifying the type of oxygen delivery device; mode of ventilatory support, ventilator, or CPAP settings; electrode placement site, electrode temperature, and time of placement; results of simultaneously obtained PaO_2, P_ACO_2, and pH when available; and clinical appearance of patient, subjective assessment of perfusion, pallor, and skin temperature.

(From AARC Clinical Practice Guideline: For complete text see Respir Care 39:1176–1179, 1994.)

In critically ill patients who have a pulmonary artery (Swan-Ganz) catheter in place, $\dot{V}O_2$ can be calculated from arterial O_2 content (CaO_2), mixed venous O_2 content ($C\bar{v}O_2$), and cardiac output: $\dot{V}O_2$ = cardiac output × ($CaO_2 - C\bar{v}O_2$). Caloric expenditure can be calculated from $\dot{V}O_2$ alone, $\dot{V}CO_2$ alone, or both $\dot{V}O_2$ and $\dot{V}CO_2$ (Equation Box 1). Calculation of energy expenditure from $\dot{V}O_2$ or $\dot{V}CO_2$ alone requires an estimation of respiratory quotient (RQ). Although this is acceptable for clinical estimates of REE, it may be desirable to know RQ to evaluate substrate metabolism.

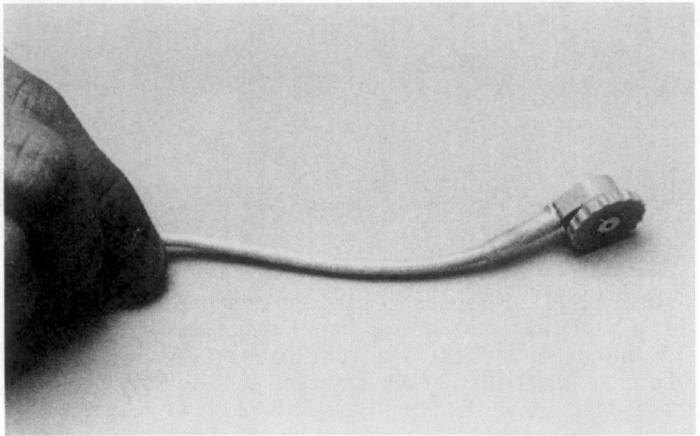

FIGURE 12-13. $P_{TC}O_2$ electrode.

WAVEFORMS AND MECHANICS DURING MECHANICAL VENTILATION

Respiratory mechanics (eg, resistance, compliance, and work of breathing) can easily be estimated in mechanically ventilated patients using only the aneroid pressure gauge and spirometer available on all ventilators.[41] Additional information can be gained by observing a graphic waveform display of pressure, volume, and flow (Fig. 12-19). Commercially available systems (eg, Bicore, Ven-Trak) can be used to assess waveforms and mechanics on mechanically ventilated patients, and this capability is incorporated into the design of many current generation ventilators. The airway pressure waveform can be displayed using the bedside critical care monitoring system and a pressure transducer (such as that used for hemodynamic measurements) attached at the proximal airway.

An illustrative pressure waveform (measured at the proximal endotracheal tube) for a ventilator-delivered breath is shown in Figure 12-20. The peak inspiratory pressure (PIP) is the result of the force necessary to overcome resistive work (endotracheal tube and airways) and elastic work (lung and chest wall compliance). An end-inspiratory pause of 0.5 to 1.5 seconds produces a plateau pressure (Pplat) which is a reflection of mean peak alveolar pressure. An end-expiratory pause demonstrates the presence of end-expiratory alveolar pressure (auto-PEEP). Some ventilators have a built-in feature that allows an end-expiratory pause and auto-PEEP measurements. A Braschi valve (Fig. 12-21) can be used to measure auto-PEEP using any ventilator system.

Much qualitative information can be obtained by observing the airway pressure waveform. Active patient effort often continues after the initiation of an assisted breath, which produces scalloping of the airway tracing during an assisted breath. This suggests that the inspiratory flow of the ventilator should be increased. The depth and duration of the negative pressure deflection before a patient-assisted breath indicates the sensitivity of the ventilator, and the depth and duration of the negative pressure deflection during a spontaneous breath (ie, during synchronized intermittent mandatory venti-

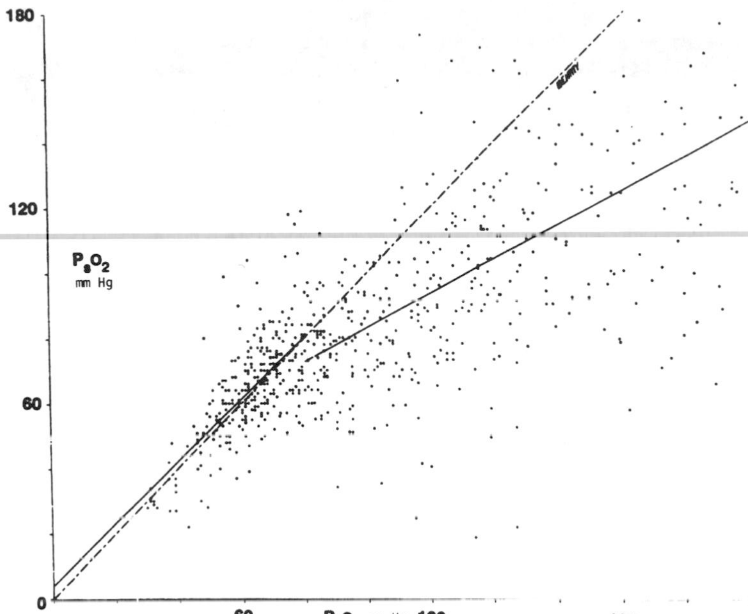

FIGURE 12-14. Relationship between transcutaneous PO_2 (PsO_2) and PaO_2. (From Palmisano BW, Severinghaus JW: Transcutaneous PCO_2 and PO_2: A multicenter study of accuracy. J Clin Monit 1990; 6:189–195.)

lation [SIMV]) indicates the effort required to obtain flow from the ventilator demand valve. Airway pressure monitoring may also be useful to calculate mean airway pressure (Equation Box 12-2).[42–44] Many of the beneficial and adverse effects of positive pressure ventilation may be the result of mean airway pressure (see Chapter 20).

A typical flow waveform during mechanical ventilation is shown in Figure 12-22. Inspiratory flow is above baseline (positive) and represents the flow setting on the ventilator for mandatory breaths. Flow below baseline (negative) is expiratory flow. Expiratory flow that does not return to baseline suggests that auto-PEEP is present. During pressure support ventilation, a flow that does not return to baseline during inhalation represents a leak. A positive dip in the expiratory flow waveform suggests a patient effort that is insufficient to overcome auto-PEEP and fails to trigger the ventilator (Fig. 12-23).

A typical volume waveform during mechanical ventilation is shown in Figure 12-24. If the expiratory volume does not return to baseline, this suggests that there is a leak in the system. The difference between inspiratory volume and expiratory volume can be used to quantify the amount of leak (eg, bronchopleural fistula).

With a passive inflation during mechanical ventilation, total compliance (lung and chest wall) can be calculated (Equation Box 12-2). This is often referred to as static compliance. When static compliance is calculated,

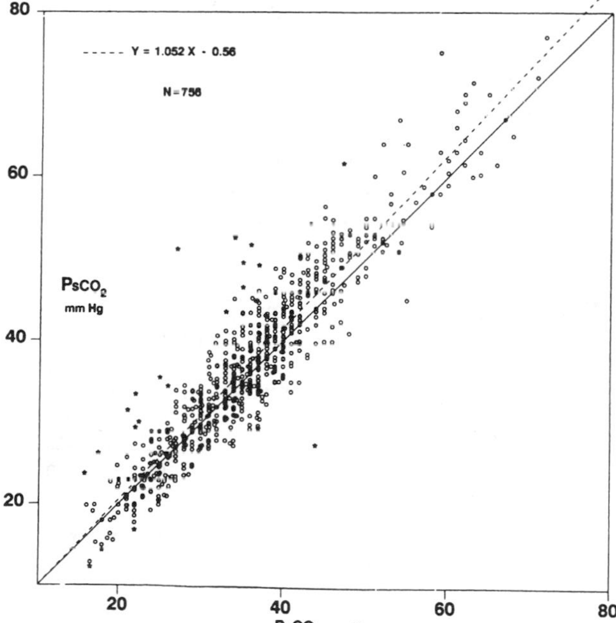

FIGURE 12-15. Relationship between transcutaneous PCO_2 ($PsCO_2$) and $PaCO_2$. (From Palmisano BW, Severinghaus JW: Transcutaneous PCO_2 and PO_2: A multicenter study of accuracy. J Clin Monit 1990; 6:189–195.)

TABLE 12-2. Limitations of Transcutaneous Monitoring

Frequent calibration required
Frequent position changes of electrode required
Long equilibration time following electrode placement
Insufficient electrode temperature may adversely affect performance
Performance may be suboptimal over poorly perfused areas
$P_{TC}O_2$ underestimates PaO_2 and $P_{TC}CO_2$ overestimates $PaCO_2$ (particularly in adults)
Compromised hemodynamics causes underestimation of PaO_2 and overestimation of $PaCO_2$
Heated electrode may cause skin burns
Frequent membrane/electrolyte changes and electrode maintenance required
Performance more reliable in neonates than adults (at least for $P_{TC}O_2$)

EQUATION BOX 12–1

INDIRECT CALORIMETRY

The Weir Equation is used to calculate REE from oxygen consumption ($\dot{V}O_2$) and carbon dioxide production ($\dot{V}CO_2$).

$$REE = (\dot{V}O_2 \cdot 3.94) + (\dot{V}CO_2 \cdot 1.11)) \cdot 1440 \text{ (min/day)}$$

The following equations are used to calculate $\dot{V}CO_2$ and $\dot{V}O_2$:

$$\dot{V}CO_2 = (\dot{V}_E \cdot F\bar{E}CO_2) - (\dot{V}_I \cdot F_ICO_2)$$

$$\dot{V}O_2 = [(((1 - F\bar{E}O_2 - F\bar{E}CO_2) \cdot F_IO_2) \div (1 - F_IO_2)) - F\bar{E}O_2] \cdot \dot{V}_E$$

When REE is estimated from $\dot{V}O_2$ or $\dot{V}CO_2$ alone, the following equations can be used:

$$REE = \dot{V}O_2 \cdot 4.83 \cdot 1440 \text{ (min/day)}$$

$$REE = \dot{V}CO_2 \cdot 5.52 \cdot 1440 \text{ (min/day)}$$

REE = resting energy expenditure.

it is important that the tidal volume be corrected for the effect of gas compression in the ventilator circuit. PEEP should be the total PEEP (set PEEP + auto-PEEP). In mechanically ventilated adult patients, normal static compliance is 50 – 100 mL/cmH_2O. Causes of decreased static compliance include the following: tension pneumothorax, main stem intubation, congestive heart failure, acute respiratory distress syndrome, pleural effusion, atelectasis, consolidation, hyperinflation, pulmonary fibrosis, and abdominal distention.

Inspiratory and expiratory resistance can also be calculated (Equation Box 12-2). Airways resistance is increased with secretions and bronchospasm. In intubated patients, a major site of resistance is the endotracheal tube. For this reason, significant changes can occur in airways resistance, with little change in the calculated resistance because of the relatively high fixed resistance of the endotracheal tube. In mechanically ventilated patients, expiratory resistance may be significantly greater than inspiratory resistance.[45]

If volume and pressure are measured at the proximal airway, then inspiratory work of breathing can be calculated by integrating the area under the pressure-volume

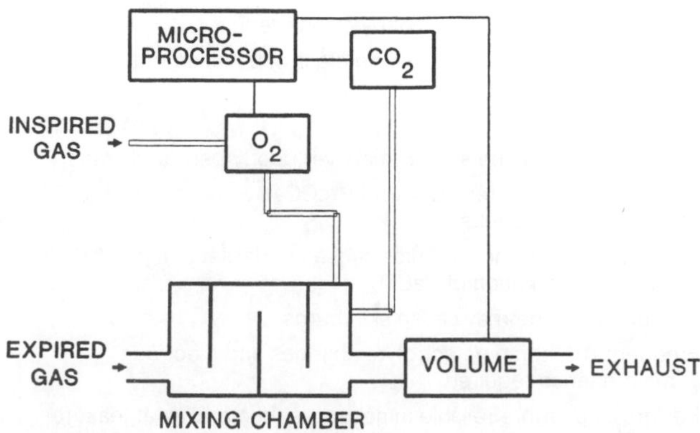

FIGURE 12-16. Open circuit indirect calorimeter.

AARC Clinical Practice Guideline

METABOLIC MEASUREMENT USING INDIRECT CALORIMETRY DURING MECHANICAL VENTILATION

Indications: Metabolic measurements may be indicated in patients with known nutritional deficits or derangements; multiple nutritional risk and stress factors that may considerably skew prediction by Harris-Benedict equation include neurologic trauma, paralysis, COPD, acute pancreatitis, cancer with residual tumor burden, multiple trauma, amputations, patients in whom height and weight cannot be accurately obtained, patients who fail to respond adequately to estimated nutritional needs, new patients on home total parenteral nutrition, patients who are unable to eat and who require mechanical ventilation for ≥5 days, transplant patients, morbidly obese patients, severely hypermetabolic or hypometabolic patients; when the desire or perceived need is present to measure the O_2 cost of breathing in mechanically ventilated patients; when the need exists to assess the VO_2 in order to evaluate the hemodynamic support of mechanically ventilated patients.

Contraindications: When a specific indication is present, there are no contraindications to performing a metabolic measurement using indirect calorimetry unless short-term disconnection of ventilatory support for connection of measurement lines results in hypoxemia, bradycardia, or other adverse effects.

Assessment of Need: Metabolic measurements should be performed only on the order of a physician after review of indications and objectives.

Assessment of Test Quality and Outcome: Test quality can be evaluated by determining whether RQ is consistent with the patient's nutritional intake; RQ rests in the normal physiologic range (0.67 to 1.3); measured VO_2 is within ±10% of the mean value and measured VCO_2 within ±6% of the mean value; REE has been defined as the value obtained with the patient lying in bed, awake and aware of his or her surroundings, and observed for 10 to 15 minutes. Outcome may be assessed by the interpretation and confirmation/manipulation of patient nutritional support regimen by a physician or nutritionist based on the measurement results. Outcome may be assessed by the successful manipulation of the mechanical ventilator settings or hemodynamic management based on the measurement of the VO_2.

Monitoring: The following should be evaluated during the performance of a metabolic measurement to ascertain the validity of the results: clinical observation of the resting state; patient comfort and movement during testing; values in concert with the clinical situation; equipment function. Measurement data should include a statement of test quality and list the current nutritional support, ventilator settings, and vital signs.

(From AARC Clinical Practice Guideline: For complete text see Respir Care 39:1170–1175, 1994.)

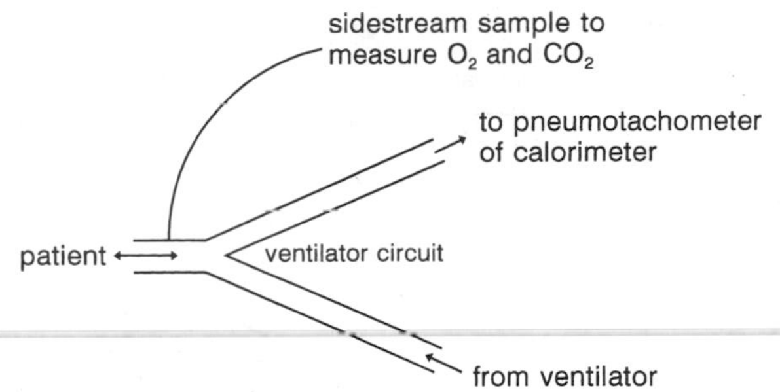

FIGURE 12-17. Breath-by-breath indirect calorimeter.

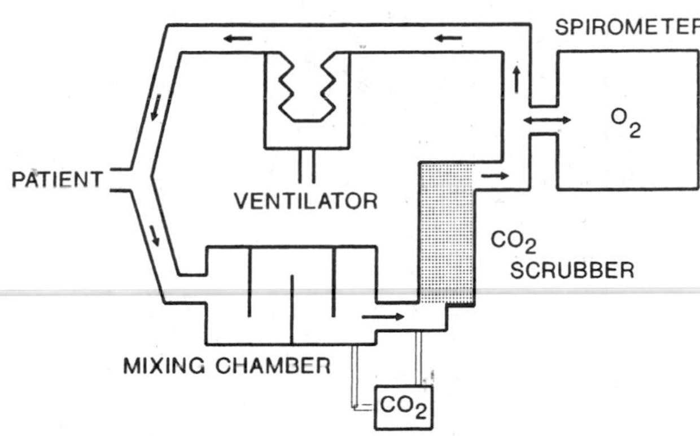

FIGURE 12-18. Closed-circuit indirect calorimeter.

curve (Fig. 12-25). This requires accurate and simultaneous measurement of flow (integrated to volume) and pressure at the proximal airway, and the patient must be relaxed and breathing in synchrony with the ventilator. Inspiratory work of breathing can be calculated during constant flow passive inflation of the lungs using measurements commonly available on the ventilator (Equation Box 12-2).[46] Note that the units for work of breathing are kilogram-meter or joules (0.1 kilogram-meter = 1.0 joule). Work of breathing will be increased with an increase in resistance, a decrease in compliance, or an increase in tidal volume. Work of breathing is often normalized to the tidal volume (work/L).

Esophageal pressure measurements can be used to estimate changes in pleural pressure during the respiratory cycle. Esophageal pressure measurements are made from a balloon containing 0.5 to 1.0 mL of air that has been placed into the lower esophagus. During controlled ventilation, esophageal pressure can be used to calculate chest wall compliance (Table 12-3 and Fig. 12-26).[47,48] During spontaneous breathing, esophageal pressure monitoring allows calculation of resistance, compliance, work of breathing, and auto-PEEP. Esophageal pressure monitoring also allows patient effort during spontaneous breathing modes to be evaluated (Fig. 12-27).[49] Esophageal pressure is not commonly performed and is probably only of value in a few select patients who are difficult to manage using conventional monitoring techniques.[50] In the absence of an esophageal balloon, respiratory variation in the central venous pressure (CVP) can be used to estimate changes in pleural pressure during the respiratory cycle.

During controlled mechanical ventilation, pressure-volume loops can be displayed (Fig. 12-28). The slope of the pressure-volume loop represents dynamic compliance and the area within the pressure-volume loop represents resistive work. During constant flow ventilation, the shape of the pressure-volume loop can be used to identify the need for a higher PEEP level or the presence of over-distention.

The flow-volume loop during mechanical ventilation can be used to evaluate expiratory airflow obstruction. The flow-volume loop can also be used to assess the response to a bronchodilator (Fig. 12-29).

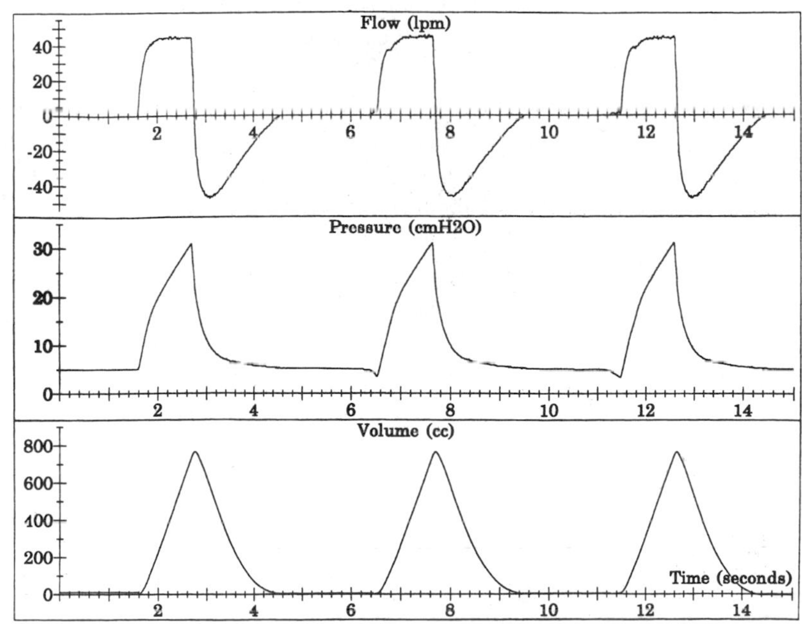

FIGURE 12-19. Waveforms of flow, pressure, and volume during mechanical ventilation.

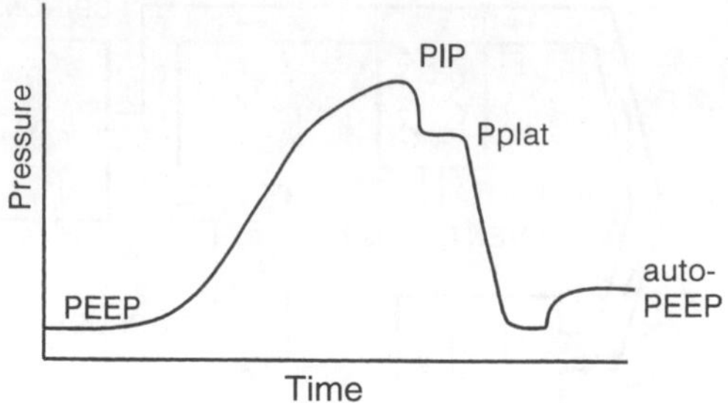

FIGURE 12-20. Airway pressure waveform illustrating end-inspiratory pause (Pplat) and end-expiratory pause (auto-PEEP).

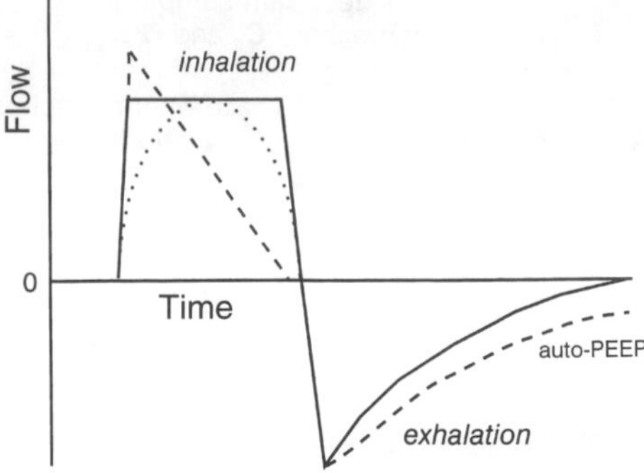

FIGURE 12-22. Airway flow waveform with volume ventilation. The flow during inhalation represents the flow setting on the ventilator, and the flow during exhalation is determined by the characteristics of the patient's lungs.

HEMODYNAMIC MONITORING

Direct Measurements

Arterial pressure should be monitored continuously in unstable patients (Table 12-4). A pressure transducer attached to an indwelling arterial catheter can provide continuous pressure monitoring. Indications for an arterial catheter include hypotension, low cardiac output, administration of potent vasoactive drugs, and the need for frequent arterial blood gas determinations. Common sites for indwelling arterial catheters are the radial, brachial, axillary, and femoral arteries. The radial artery is usually the vessel of choice. Potential complications of an indwelling arterial catheter include infection, air embolism, thromboembolism, inadvertent catheter dislodgement, electrical microshock, hemorrhage, and impaired peripheral circulation.

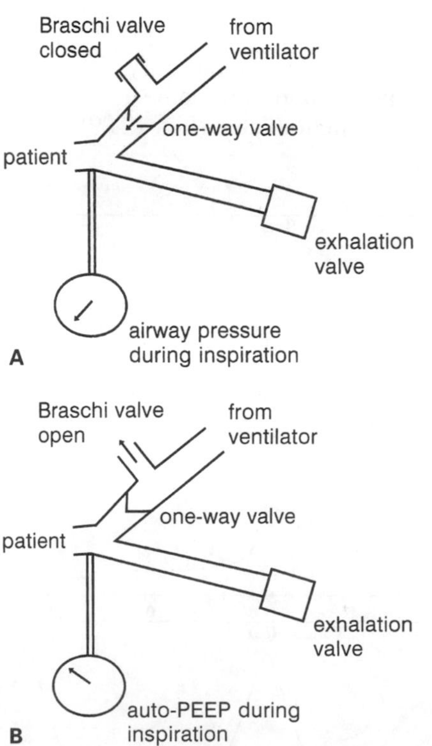

FIGURE 12-21. Braschi valve. (**A**) With valve capped, ventilator operates in its usual fashion. (**B**) When the cap is removed during exhalation, and end-expiratory pause is created that is equal in duration to the inspiratory time set on the ventilator.

Following insertion of the arterial catheter, a pressure transducer is attached and connected to the oscilloscope to produce a visual display. The arterial waveform that is displayed consists of the anacrotic limb, the systolic peak, the dicrotic notch, and the diastolic pressure. The system consists of the catheter, a flush solution, a series of stopcocks, and a pressure transducer. By changing the stopcock position, blood can be drawn from the catheter, the pressure tracing can be displayed on the oscilloscope, or the transducer-catheter system can be flushed with solution.

Automated systems to noninvasively measure arterial blood pressure use the oscillometric method or the Penaz method.[51] As its name implies, the oscillometric method depends on the detection of oscillations and their quantification during stepwise decrements of pressure in a standard blood pressure cuff. The systolic blood pressure is the cuff pressure at which the amplitude of oscillations increases rapidly and the diastolic blood pressure is where the amplitude decreases rapidly. The Penaz method uses a finger cuff to provide continuous blood pressure and an arterial waveform display. Although convenient, these devices have not gained widespread acceptance because their accuracy and reliability is questionable, particularly when circulatory instability exists.

CVP monitoring is used to assess the hemodynamic status and the need for fluid replacement. The CVP catheter can also be used to administer medications,

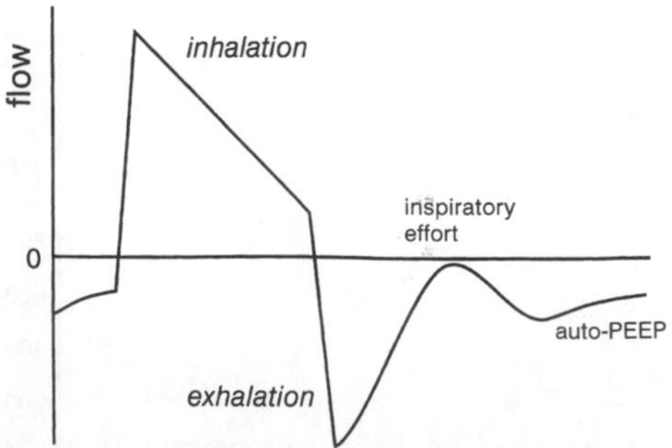

FIGURE 12-23. Flow waveform during pressure support ventilation in a patient with auto-PEEP.

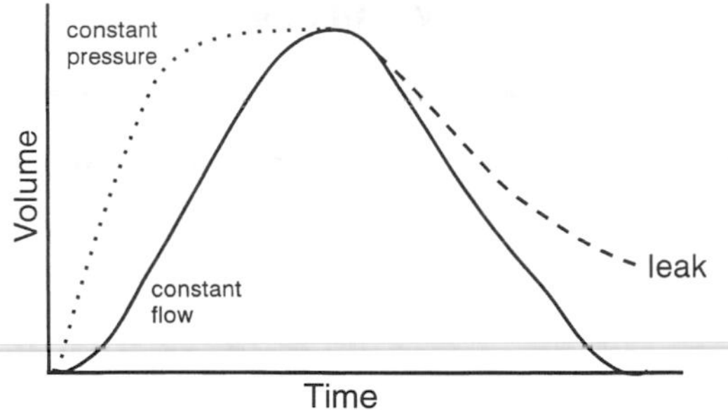

FIGURE 12-24. Volume waveform during mechanical ventilation.

to administer hyperalimentation solutions, and to obtain blood samples. Fluid replacement can be managed using CVP monitoring as a guide. In patients with normal cardiac reserve and pulmonary vascular resistance, CVP reflects the ability of the heart to pump blood.

The CVP catheter is located in the superior vena cava or right atrium. When properly positioned, CVP reflects the pressure of the right atrium. Right atrial pressure, in turn, reflects right ventricular end-diastolic pressure and the performance of the right ventricle. The CVP catheter may be inserted through the jugular (internal or external), subclavian, femoral, or antecubital vein. Insertion using the subclavian vein has the potential complication of pneumothorax during the insertion procedure. Additional complications of a central line include pulmonary emboli, phlebitis, pneumothorax, malposition of the catheter, arrhythmias, fluid overload, air emboli, and electrical microshock. CVP may be monitored continuously with a pressure transducer or intermittently with an H_2O manometer. Because positive pressure ventilation alters CVP, pressure should be measured at end-exhalation. If PEEP is used, it should be considered in the interpretation of CVP.

Pulmonary artery pressure (PAP) monitoring[52–54] is used to evaluate intravascular volume, cardiac output, pulmonary artery occlusion pressure (PAOP), and pulmonary vascular resistance. The pulmonary artery (Swan Ganz) catheter is a balloon-tipped, flow-directed catheter used for PAP and PAOP monitoring. The standard pulmonary artery catheter consists of a proximal port (at the level of the right atrium to infuse fluids, measure CVP, and inject cold solution for cardiac output), distal port (in the pulmonary artery), a balloon (which is inflated for PAOP measurements), and a thermistor (to measure temperature and calculate cardiac output).

Some pulmonary artery catheters can also be used to continuously measure $S\bar{v}O_2$, to provide temporary cardiac pacing, and to measure right-ventricular ejection fraction. The catheter is floated through the superior vena cava, right atrium, right ventricle, and into the pulmonary artery. The position of the catheter determines the pressure being measured. With the catheter tip in the pulmonary artery, measurement of the pulmonary artery pressure can be obtained. When the balloon of the pulmonary artery catheter is inflated, the catheter floats forward to a small branch of the pulmonary artery. Blood flow past the balloon is thus obstructed, and PAOP is measured (Figure 12-30). PAOP (also called pulmonary artery wedge pressure or pulmonary capillary wedge pressure) is a reflection of left atrial pressure. Monitoring PAOP is preferred to CVP because the

EQUATION BOX 12-2

MECHANICS DURING MECHANICAL VENTILATION

Mean airway pressure ($\bar{P}aw$) is calculated from the following equations:

$$\bar{P}aw = [(PIP - PEEP) \cdot Ti/Ttot] + PEEP$$
(constant pressure ventilation)

$$\bar{P}aw = [0.5 \cdot (PIP - PEEP) \cdot Ti/Ttot] + PEEP$$
(constant flow ventilation)

For example, if PIP = 30 cmH_2O, PEEP = 10 cmH_2O, Ti/Ttot = 0.5 (I:E = 1:1), then $\bar{P}aw$ is 20 cmH_2O for constant pressure ventilation and 15 cmH_2O for constant flow ventilation.

Compliance is calculated as:

$$C = V_T \div (Pplat - PEEP)$$

For example, a tidal volume of 800 mL, a Pplat of 50 cmH_2O, and a PEEP of 10 cmH_2O results in a compliance calculation of 20 mL/cmH_2O.

Inspiratory airways resistance is calculated as:

$$R_I = (PIP - Pplat) \div \text{end-inspiratory flow}$$

For example, if PIP is 30 cmH_2O, Pplat is 20 cmH_2O, and end-inspiratory flow is 60 L/min (1 L/sec), then the calculated resistance is 10 cmH_2O/L/sec.

Expiratory airways resistance can also be calculated:

$$R_E = (Pplat - PEEP) \div \text{peak expiratory flow}$$

For example, if Pplat is 25 cmH_2O, PEEP is 10 cmH_2O, and peak expiratory flow is 30 L/min (0.5 L/sec), then R_E is 30 cmH_2O/L/sec.

Work of breathing can be calculated using the following equation during constant flow volume ventilation:

$$W = [(PIP - (0.5 \cdot Pplat)) \div 100] \cdot V_T$$

For example, if PIP = 40 cmH_2O, Pplat = 30 cmH_2O, and tidal volume = 0.8 L, then W = 0.2 kg-m.

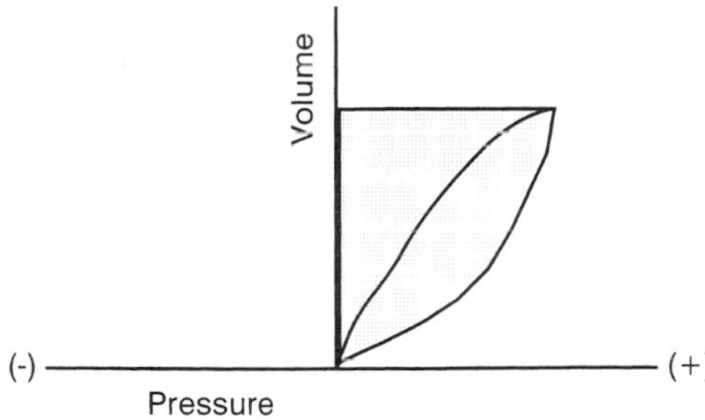

FIGURE 12-25. Pressure-volume curve during mechanical ventilation. The shaded area represents the work of breathing performed by the ventilator.

TABLE 12-3. **Influence of the Site of Pressure Measurement and Mode of Ventilation on Measurements of Work of Breathing and Compliance**

Site of Pressure Measurement and Mode of Ventilation	Area of the Pressure-Volume Loop = Work Done to Overcome	Slope of the Pressure-Volume Loop
Esophageal pressure during spontaneous ventilation	Pulmonary inspiratory and expiratory resistance	Lung compliance
Esophageal pressure during mechanical ventilation	Chest-wall inspiratory and expiratory resistance	Chest-wall compliance
Pressure at tracheal (carinal) end of endotracheal tube during spontaneous ventilation	Imposed inspiratory and expiratory resistance of the total breathing apparatus (i.e., endotracheal tube, breathing circuit, and the ventilator)	Compliance of the total breathing apparatus
Pressure at the tracheal (carinal) end of endotracheal tube during mechanical ventilation	Pulmonary and chest-wall inspiratory and expiratory resistance	Compliance of the respiratory system (lungs plus chest wall)
Pressure at airway opening (between "Y" piece of breathing circuit and endotracheal tube) during spontaneous ventilation	Imposed inspiratory and expiratory resistance of the breathing circuit and ventilator	Compliance of the breathing circuitry
Pressure at airway opening during mechanical ventilation	Pulmonary and chest-wall inspiratory and expiratory resistance, plus resistance of the endotracheal tube	Compliance of the respiratory system (lungs plus chest wall)

(From Banner MJ, Jaeger MJ, Kirby RR: Components of the work of breathing and implications for monitoring ventilator-dependent patients. Crit Care Med 22:515–523, 1994; Reproduced with permission.)

CVP is not always a reliable guide to left ventricular filling pressure or left atrial pressure, whereas PAOP reflects left atrial pressure and the adequacy of left ventricular function.

An elevated PAP may indicate left-to-right shunt, left ventricular failure, mitral stenosis, or pulmonary hypertension. An elevated PAOP may indicate left ventricular failure, mitral stenosis, or cardiac insufficiency. During mechanical ventilation, the effects of positive pressure ventilation on PAP and PAOP should be considered. Vascular pressures are typically measured at end-exhalation to avoid the confounding effects of respiratory changes in intrathoracic pressure on PAP and PAOP.

With a thermodilution pulmonary artery catheter positioned in the pulmonary artery, it is possible to determine cardiac output. Cardiac output is measured by injecting a cold solution into the central circulation (right atrium). The downstream change in temperature in the pulmonary artery allows cardiac output to be calculated. Cold solution (room temperature or iced) is introduced into the right atrium via the catheter. A thermistor located near the tip of the catheter measures the blood temperature in the pulmonary artery. The temperature of the patient, the injection solution, and the change in blood temperature are the variables used to compute cardiac output. The infusate temperature change is inversely proportional to cardiac output.

Derived Indices

From the measured hemodynamics, a number of derived (ie, calculated) parameters can be determined (Table 12-4). Cardiac output is often normalized to patient size [ie, body surface area (BSA)] by calculating cardiac index (CI). The volume of blood ejected from the ventricle with each contraction is stroke volume (SV), which can be normalized to patient size to produce stroke volume index.

Hemodynamic monitoring allows preload, afterload, and contractility to be assessed. This provides information to assess cardiac output (Fig. 12-31). Preload is determined by the amount of myocardial stretch at end-diastole (end-diastolic tension). An increase in blood volume and an increase in vascular tone increase preload. A decrease in blood volume, such as with diuretic administration, decreases preload. CVP is an indicator of right ventricular preload, and PAOP is an indicator of left ventricular preload.

Afterload is the resistance against which the ventricle must eject blood. The afterload of the right ventricle is pulmonary vascular resistance. The afterload of the left ventricle is systemic vascular resistance. Afterload is determined primarily by arterial tone; an increase in arterial tone increases afterload and a decrease in arterial tone decreases afterload. Thus, vasodilating agents (eg, nitroprusside, nitroglycerine, hydralazine) decrease afterload, whereas vasoconstricting agents (eg, dopamine, norepinephrine, phenylephrine) increase afterload.

Contractility is the intrinsic ability of the heart to contract independent of preload and afterload. The contractility of the right ventricle is determined by the right ventricular stroke work indexed. The contractility of the left ventricle is determined by the left ventricular stroke work indexed. Contractility is manipulated by use of inotropic and beta-blocking agents. Inotropic agents (eg, dopamine, dobutamine) increase contractility and beta-blocking agents (eg, propanolol, metoprolol) decrease contractility.

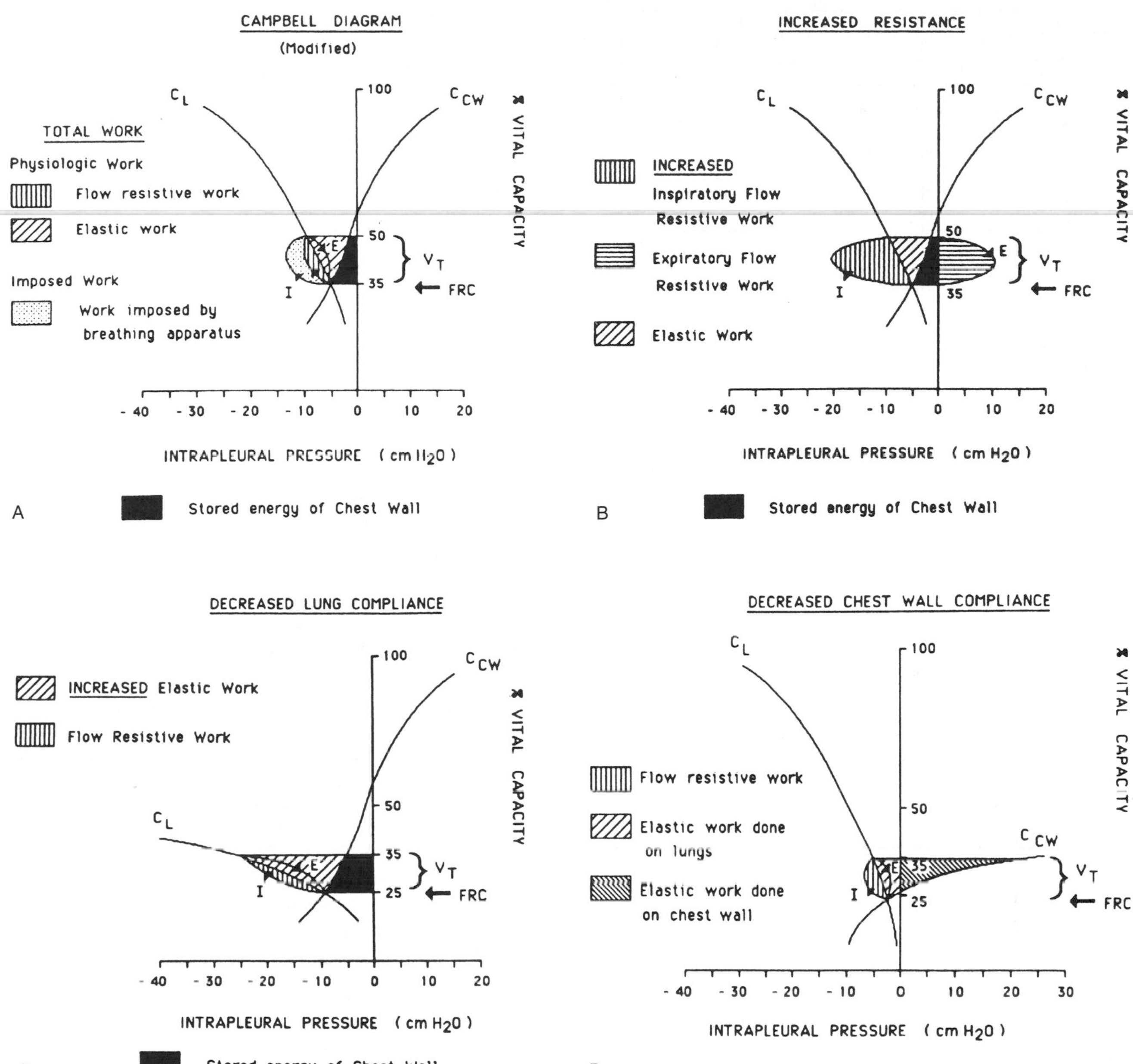

FIGURE 12-26. (**A**) Campbell diagram showing chest wall compliance curve (C_{cw}), lung compliance curve (C_L), and work of breathing. (**B**) Campbell diagram with increased airway resistance. (**C**) Campbell diagram with decreased lung compliance. (**D**) Campbell diagram with decreased chest wall compliance. (From Banner MJ, Jaeger MJ, Kirby RR: Components of the work of breathing and implications for monitoring ventilator-dependent patients. Crit Care Med 1994;22:515–523.)

INVASIVE MONITORING OF OXYGENATION AND VENTILATION

Intra-arterial Blood Gas Monitoring

In vivo blood gas systems use optical biosensors called fluorescent optodes.[55–62] The optode consists of a miniaturized probe containing a fluorescent dye in conjunction with an optic fiber (Fig. 12-32). The fluorescent dye will augment fluorescence as the hydrogen ion concentration or CO_2 increases within the dye and quench fluorescence as the O_2 concentration increases within the dye. Photosensors are used to quantify the amount of quenching, and a microprocessor is used to translate the signal into a display of PO_2. Optode systems are presently available to measure PO_2, PCO_2, and pH. The accuracy of these systems has not been completely characterized, but it may be acceptable for monitoring and clinical decision making.

Several approaches can be taken to blood gas monitoring in conjunction with an arterial catheter. The first uses a probe that passes through the arterial catheter and resides directly within the arterial lumen. This sys-

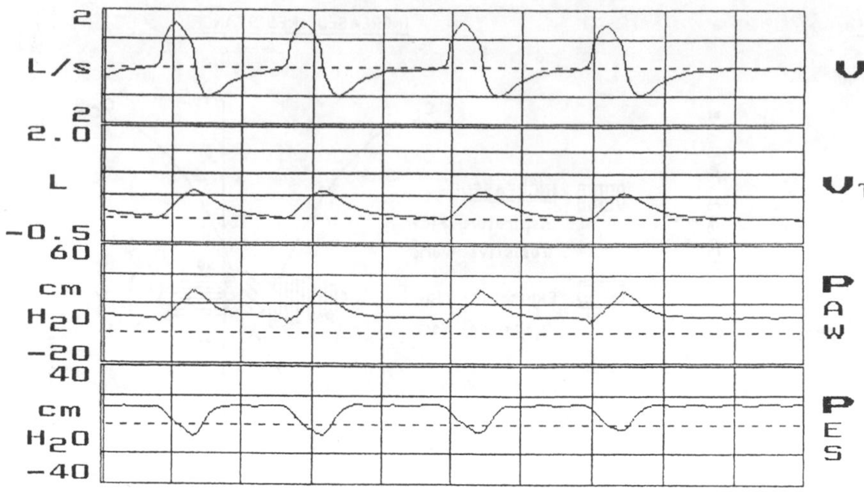

FIGURE 12-27. Flow, volume, airway pressure, and esophageal pressure waveforms for a patient breathing spontaneously with CPAP mode.

tem is miniaturized to fit through a 20-gauge arterial catheter without affecting blood pressure measurements. With the second approach, the optode is connected to the proximal arterial line, but does not pass through the catheter. With this method, when blood gas and pH levels are desired, blood is drawn into a chamber containing the optodes. After analysis, the blood is flushed back into the artery. Thus frequent (but *not* continuous) blood gas measurements are possible without blood loss.

Despite considerable clinical interest, the future of in vivo measurement of arterial blood gases is unclear. One problem with these systems is their cost. Although blood gas analyzers are equally expensive, they are not dedicated to a single patient. Manufacturers are striving to design user-friendly systems that are easy to use, but the amount of technical attention that these systems are likely to require in a busy ICU may be high. The life of the optode and its effect on the function of the arterial catheter system (eg, blood pressure measurements) in a busy ICU also remains to be seen. The quality control and quality assurance requirements for clinical and regulatory purposes are currently unclear. Whether or not the benefits of continuous (or on-demand) blood gas and pH measurements will outweigh the costs and technical support required has yet to be determined.

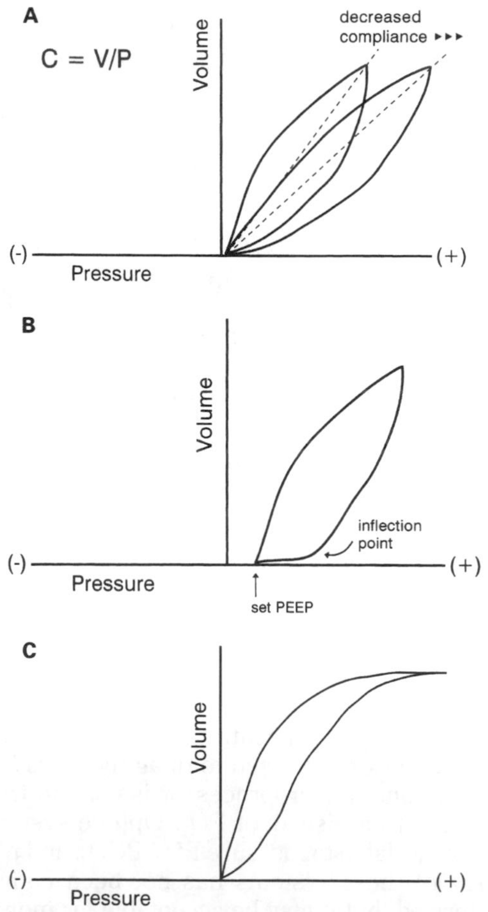

FIGURE 12-28. (A) Effect of compliance on the pressure-volume curve during mechanical ventilation. **(B)** Pressure-volume curve illustrating an inflection point. PEEP should be set above the inflection point on the pressure-volume curve. **(C)** Pressure-volume curve with overdistension. The tidal volume (or pressure control setting) should be decreased to avoid this overdistension.

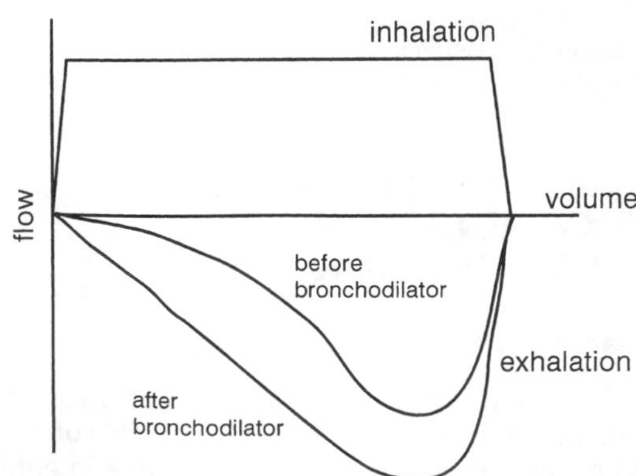

FIGURE 12-29. Flow-volume curve during mechanical ventilation before and after administration of a bronchodilator to an asthmatic patient.

TABLE 12-4. **Normal Values for Hemodynamic Parameters**

Parameter	Abbreviation	Normal Value	Equation
Heart rate	HR	60–100/min	Measured directly
Systolic arterial blood pressure	SBP	90–140 mmHg	Measured directly
Diastolic arterial blood pressure	DBP	60–90 mmHg	Measured directly
Mean arterial blood pressure	MAP	80–100 mmHg	(SBP + 2 · DBP) ÷ 3
Central venous pressure	CVP	1–6 mmHg (3–1 cmH$_2$O)	Measured directly
Systolic pulmonary artery pressure	SPAP	4–10 mmHg	Measured directly
Diastolic pulmonary artery pressure	DPAP	20–30 mmHg	Measured directly
Mean pulmonary artery pressure	MPAP	10–20 mmHg	(SPAP + 2 · DPAP) ÷ 3
Pulmonary artery occlusion pressure (wedge)	PAOP (PCWP)	4–12 mmHg	Measured directly
Cardiac output	CO	4–8 L/min	Measured directly
Cardiac index	CI	2.5–4 L/min/m^2	CI = CO ÷ BSA
Stroke volume	SV	60–80 mL	SV = CO ÷ HR
Stroke volume index	SVI	35–45 mL/min^2	SVI = CI ÷ HR
Pulmonary vascular resistance	PVR	<250 dynes-sec/cm^5	PVR = ((PAP − CVP) ÷ CO) · 80
Pulmonary vascular resistance index	PVRI	200–450 dynes-sec/cm^5	PVRI = PVR · BSA
Systemic vascular resistance	SVR	1200–1400 dynes-sec/cm^5	SVR = (MAP − PCWP) ÷ CO) · 80
Systemic vascular resistance index	SVRI	1700–2600 dynes-sec/cm^5	SVRI = SVR · BSA
Right ventricular stroke work index	RVSWI	5–10 g · m/m^2	RVSWI = SVI · (PAP − CVP) · 0.0136
Left ventricular stroke work index	LVSWI	35–55 g · m/m^2	LVSWI = SVI · (MAP − PCWP) · 0.0136

Mixed Venous Blood Gas Monitoring

Mixed venous O_2 can be used to evaluate tissue oxygenation.[6] $P\bar{v}O_2 < 30$ mmHg (or $S\bar{v}O_2 < 60\%$) has been associated with a high likelihood of tissue hypoxia (ie, hyperlactemia). Mixed venous blood gases can be assessed by obtaining a sample from the distal part of the pulmonary artery catheter (with the balloon deflated). If the pulmonary catheter is positioned in a distal branch of the pulmonary artery, rapid aspiration can contaminate the mixed venous blood with pulmonary capillary blood (Fig. 12-33). Therefore, a slow aspiration rate (<1 mL/30 sec) should be used when blood is sampled from a pulmonary artery catheter.

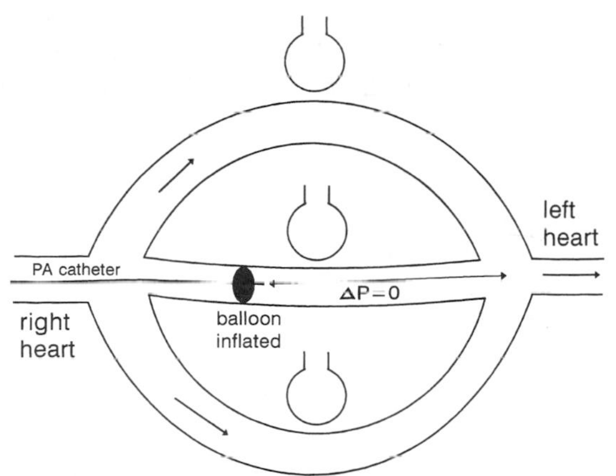

FIGURE 12-30. Measurement of PAOP. With the balloon inflated, flow past the catheter tip stops so that pressure measured at this point is the same as the downstream pressure in the left atrium.

$P\bar{v}O_2$ (or $S\bar{v}O_2$) is an average from many vascular beds and does not necessarily reflect the $P\bar{v}O_2$ ($S\bar{v}O_2$) of any individual tissue. With septic shock, peripheral arteriovenous shunts open, resulting in a $P\bar{v}O_2$ ($S\bar{v}O_2$) higher than expected. In some patients, tissue $\dot{V}O_2$ may decrease in proportion to O_2 delivery. In such cases, $P\bar{v}O_2$ ($S\bar{v}O_2$) may not be an adequate indicator of tissue oxygenation. $P\bar{v}O_2$ ($S\bar{v}O_2$) will also be falsely elevated (ie, *not* reflect tissue oxygenation) in patients with ventricular septal defect or cyanide poisoning.

$S\bar{v}O_2$ can be mathematically derived from the Fick Equation (Equation Box 12-3),[63] which illustrates that $S\bar{v}O_2$ is determined by the balance between oxygen consumption ($\dot{V}O_2$) and oxygen delivery ($\dot{D}O_2$). The relationship $\dot{V}O_2/\dot{D}O_2$ is known as the O_2 utilization coefficient or the O_2 extraction ratio. Continuous measurement of $S\bar{v}O_2$ via oximetric methodology uses a microprocessor, an optical module with light sources and photodetectors, and a flow-directed pulmonary

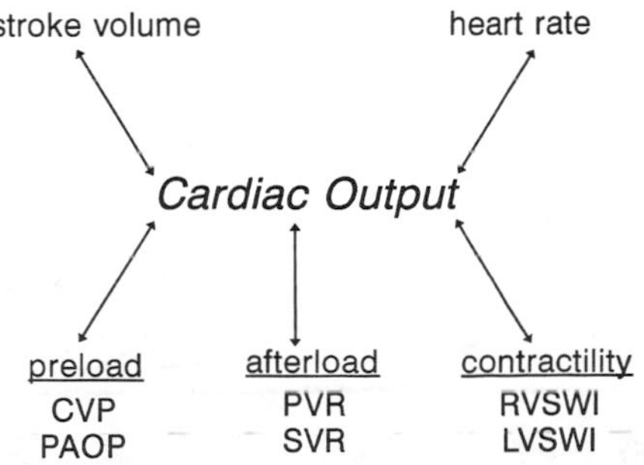

FIGURE 12-31. Relationship between cardiac output and preload, afterload, and contractility.

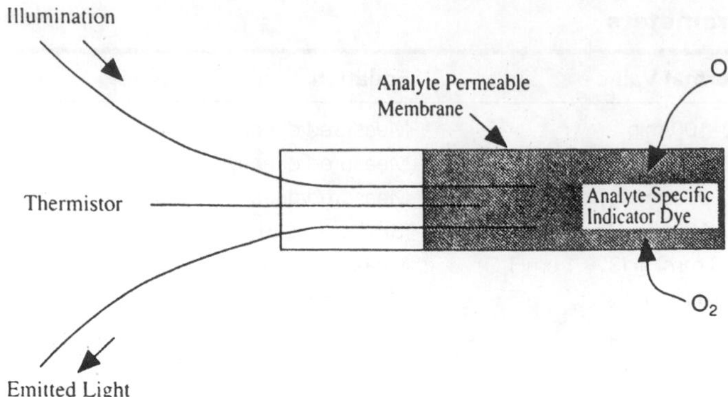

FIGURE 12-32. Optode to measure PO_2. Similar optodes can be used to measure PCO_2 and pH.

artery catheter.[6] Using fiberoptics, wavelengths of light between 650 nm and 1000 nm are pulsed into the pulmonary artery (Fig. 12-34). This light is reflected off red blood cells in the pulmonary artery and returned to the optical module via another fiberoptic bundle. $S\bar{v}O_2$ is determined by the ratio of transmitted and reflected light. Before insertion, the system is calibrated using an in vitro calibration standard and calibration can be updated periodically by in vivo calibration using a CO-oximetry determined $S\bar{v}O_2$. Factors that affect the measurement of $S\bar{v}O_2$ using this method include temperature, pH, blood flow velocity, hematocrit, occlusion of the catheter tip (eg, clot or vessel wall), and intralipid infusions.

Several systems are commercially available to measure $S\bar{v}O_2$ by oximetry.[64,65] The Edwards Sat-One Catheter (American Edwards) uses two reference wavelengths and one detecting fiberoptic filament and allows the user to manually update the hematocrit to control its effects on $S\bar{v}O_2$ measurements. The Oximetrix Opticath Catheter (Abbott Critical Care) uses three reference wavelengths and one detecting filament, with the third wavelength supposedly improving the accuracy of the system in the face of physiologic effects such as changes in hematocrit. The Spectramed Spectracath Catheter (Spectramed) uses two reference wavelengths and two detecting filaments, with the second detecting filament supposedly improving the accuracy of the system when hematocrit changes. Regardless of their technical performance, the overall clinical usefulness of $S\bar{v}O_2$ monitoring remains unclear. Although the accuracy and performance of these systems has been reported, there has been relatively little reported regarding their effect on patient outcome.

$P\bar{v}CO_2$ can also be measured on mixed venous blood. During cardiac arrest, $P\bar{v}CO_2$ (and thus tissue PCO_2) may be very high despite a normal (or decreased) PCO_2. P_ACO_2 is affected primarily by alveolar ventilation, whereas $P\bar{v}CO_2$ is affected primarily by perfusion (Fig. 12-35).

Gastric Intramural pH

Gastric tonometry has been suggested as a minimally invasive method to assess tissue oxygenation in critically ill patients.[66–68] Perfusion of the gut is affected early in the course of systemic hypoxia. Theoretically, tissue hypoxia should result in a decrease in gastric intramucosal pH (pHi). Normal pHi is 7.38 ± 0.03. A low pHi (<7.32) has been associated with increased mortality. A decrease in pHi has been suggested to be an early indicator of sepsis. However, others have suggested that pHi is no more useful than other clinical data that are readily available.[69] Gastric intramural pH has also been used to assess weaning from mechanical ventilation.[70]

The gastric tonometer consists of a nasogastric tube with a distal CO_2-permeable balloon (Fig. 12-36).[6] The balloon is filled with 2.5 to 3 mL of saline. An equilibration time of 1 to 2 hours is allowed for CO_2 in the gastric lumen to equilibrate with the saline inside the balloon. After discarding 1 to 1.5 mL of aspirate from the gastric tube (dead volume), the remaining 1 to 1.5 mL is ana-

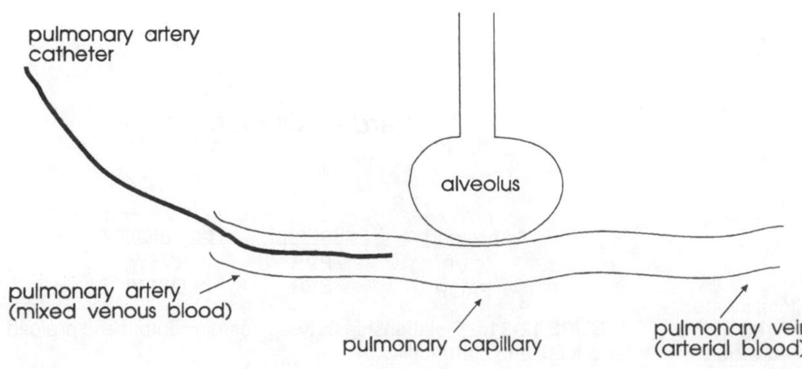

FIGURE 12-33. Tip of pulmonary artery catheter in the pulmonary circulation. Rapid aspiration of blood can aspirate oxygenated blood from the pulmonary venous circulation.

EQUATION BOX 12-3

FICK EQUATION TO DETERMINE $S\bar{v}O_2$

$S\bar{v}O_2$ can be mathematically derived from the Fick Equation:

$$S\bar{v}O_2 = 1 - \dot{V}O_2/\dot{D}O_2$$

where $\dot{V}O_2$ is O_2 consumption and $\dot{D}O_2$ is O_2 delivery. The relationship $\dot{V}O_2/\dot{D}O_2$ is known as the O_2 utilization coefficient or the O_2 extraction ratio.

lyzed for PCO_2 using a blood gas analyzer. A simultaneous arterial blood sample is analyzed to determine HCO_3^-. Gastric pHi is then calculated from the Henderson-Hasselbach equation, using the PCO_2 of the saline from the gastric balloon and the HCO_3^- of arterial blood.

INDICES OF OXYGENATION AND VENTILATION

Indices of Oxygenation

P_AO_2 is derived using the alveolar gas equation (Equation Box 12-4). An increase in the difference (gradient) between P_AO_2 and PaO_2 [$P(A-a)O_2$] can result from $\dot{V}/\dot{Q}$ disturbances, shunt, or diffusion limitation. Changes in P_ACO_2 will not affect the $P(A-a)O_2$ because P_ACO_2 is taken into account in the calculation of P_AO_2. A problem with the use of the $P(A-a)O_2$ is its tendency to change as the F_IO_2 changes. The normal $P(A-a)O_2$ is 5 to 10 mmHg breathing room air and 30 to 60 mmHg when breathing 100% O_2. This variability when the F_IO_2 is changed limits its usefulness as an indicator of pulmonary function when the F_IO_2 is changed, and invalidates it as a predictor of the change in PaO_2 if the F_IO_2 is changed.

The PaO_2/P_AO_2 is calculated by dividing the PaO_2 by P_AO_2. Unlike the $P(A-a)O_2$, the PaO_2/P_AO_2 remains relatively stable when F_IO_2 changes. A $PaO_2/P_AO_2 < 0.75$ indicates pulmonary dysfunction owing to $\dot{V}/\dot{Q}$ abnormality, shunt, or diffusion abnormality. The PaO_2/P_AO_2 is more useful than the $P(A-a)O_2$ for comparing the pulmonary function of patients on different F_IO_2 and following pulmonary function as F_IO_2 is changed.

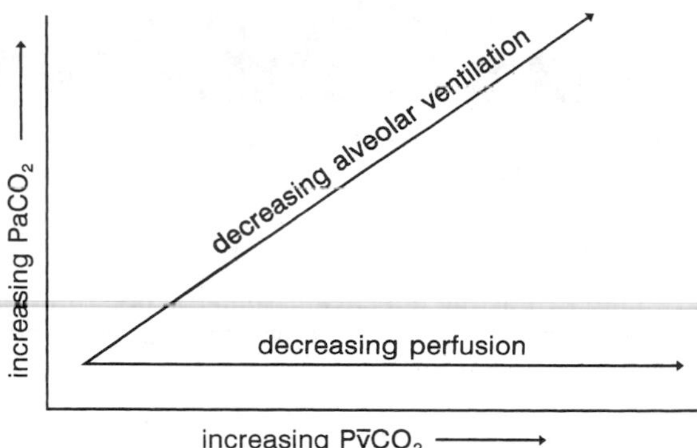

FIGURE 12-35. $PaCO_2$ is affected by alveolar ventilation and $P\bar{v}CO_2$ is affected by cardiac output.

The PaO_2/F_IO_2 is easier to calculate than $P(A-a)O_2$ and PaO_2/P_AO_2 because it does not require calculation of P_AO_2. A PaO_2/F_IO_2 of less than 200 is associated with significant shunt in patients with acute respiratory failure. The PaO_2/F_IO_2 is affected by changes in P_ACO_2. Compared with the $P(A-a)O_2$ and PaO_2/P_AO_2, the PaO_2/F_IO_2 is a cruder index of pulmonary dysfunction.

Shunt is calculated from the O_2 content of pulmonary end-capillary ($Cc'O_2$), arterial (CaO_2) and mixed venous ($C\bar{v}O_2$) blood (Equation Box 12-5).

Indices of Ventilation

Dead space ventilation is that portion of the minute ventilation that does not participate in gas exchange, and consists of anatomic dead space and alveolar dead space. Dead space is calculated using the Bohr equation (Equation Box 12-6). Normal V_D/V_T is 0.2 to 0.4. Causes

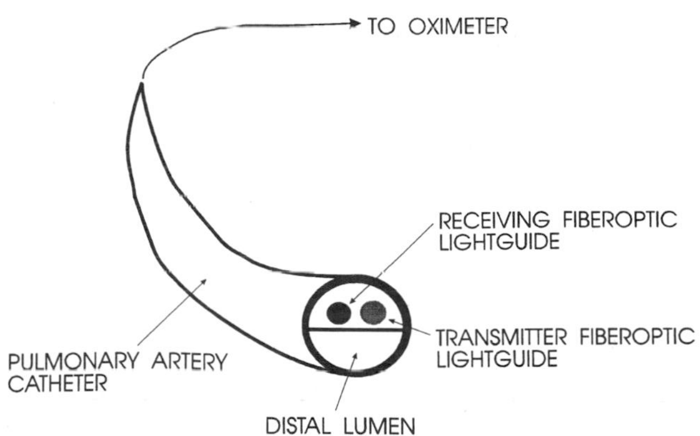

FIGURE 12-34. Venous oximetry catheter.

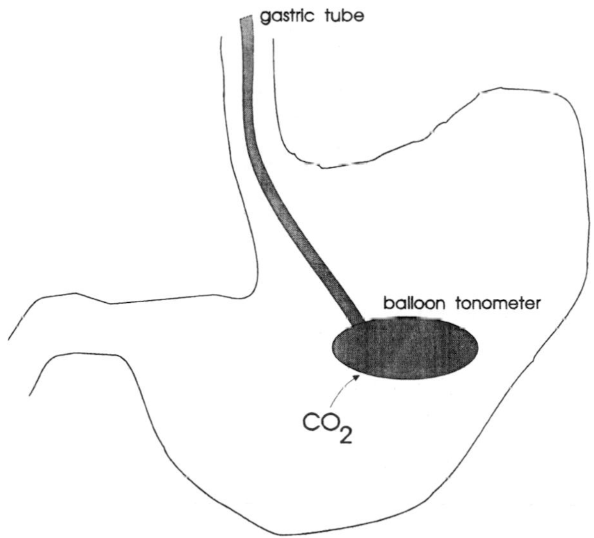

FIGURE 12-36. Gastric tonometer.

EQUATION BOX 12-4

ALVEOLAR GAS EQUATION

The alveolar PO_2 (PAO_2) is calculated from the alveolar gas equation:

$$PAO_2 = (FIO_2 \cdot EBP) - [(PaCO_2 \cdot FIO_2 + ((1 - FIO_2) \div RQ))]$$

where EBP is the effective barometric pressure (barometric pressure minus H_2O vapor pressure), and RQ is the respiratory quotient ($\dot{V}CO_2/\dot{V}O_2$). For calculation of PAO_2, an RQ = 0.8 is commonly used. For $FIO_2 \geq 0.6$, the effect of RQ on PAO_2 becomes negligible, and the alveolar gas equation becomes

$$PAO_2 = (EBP \cdot FIO_2) - PaCO_2$$

For $FIO_2 < 0.6$, the alveolar gas equation becomes

$$PAO_2 = (EBP \cdot FIO_2) - (1.2 \cdot PaCO_2)$$

For example, if barometric pressure is 760 mmHg (EBP = 713 mmHg), FIO_2 = 0.80, and $PaCO_2$ = 40 mmHg, then PAO_2 = 520 mmHg. If barometric pressure is 700 mmHg (EBP = 653 mmHg), FIO_2 = 0.40, and $PaCO_2$ = 60 mmHg, then PAO_2 = 189 mmHg.

EQUATION BOX 12-5

PULMONARY SHUNT EQUATION

Pulmonary shunt ($\dot{Q}_S/\dot{Q}_T$) is calculated using the shunt equation:

$$\dot{Q}_S/\dot{Q}_T = (Cc'O_2 - CaO_2) \div (Cc'O_2 - C\bar{v}O_2)$$

where $\dot{Q}_S$ is shunted cardiac output, $\dot{Q}_T$ is total cardiac output, $Cc'O_2$ is pulmonary end-capillary O_2 content, CaO_2 is arterial O_2 content, and $C\bar{v}O_2$ is mixed venous O_2 content. Oxygen content in pulmonary end-capillary, arterial, or mixed venous samples is calculated by the following equation:

$$O_2 \text{ content (vol\%)} = (Hb \cdot HbO_2 \cdot 1.34) + (0.003 \cdot PO_2)$$

where Hb is hemoglobin content, HbO_2 is hemoglobin O_2 saturation, and PO_2 is the partial pressure of O_2. The O_2 content is expressed in milliliters of O_2 per 100 mL of blood (vol%).

CaO_2 is calculated from arterial blood gas values and $C\bar{v}O_2$ is calculated from pulmonary artery blood gas values. $Cc'O_2$ is calculated based on the assumption that pulmonary end-capillary PO_2 is equal to the alveolar PO_2. When $PAO_2 > 150$ mmHg, it is assumed that the end-capillary blood is maximally saturated with O_2. Because small fractions of carboxyhemoglobin (COHb) and methemoglobin (metHb) are present in the blood, the end-capillary saturation becomes:

$$Sc'O_2 = 1 - COHb - metHb$$

Thus:

$$Cc'O_2 = (Hb \cdot Sc'O_2 \cdot 1.34) + (0.003 \cdot PAO_2)$$

When a pulmonary artery catheter is not in place to sample mixed venous blood, shunt can be estimated from the equation:

$$\dot{Q}_S/\dot{Q}_T = (Cc'O_2 - CaO_2) \div (3.5 + (Cc'O_2 - CaO_2))$$

When the patient has a high PaO_2 (>100 mmHg), the modified shunt equation can be used:

$$\dot{Q}_S/\dot{Q}_T = [(PAO_2 - PaO_2) \cdot 0.003] \div [3.5 + (PAO_2 - PaO_2) \cdot (0.003)]$$

EQUATION BOX 12-6

DEAD SPACE EQUATION

Dead space (V_D/V_T) is calculated from the Bohr Equation:

$$V_D/V_T = (PaCO_2 - P\bar{E}CO_2) \div PaCO_2$$

where V_D/V_T is the fraction of total ventilation that is dead space, and $P\bar{E}CO_2$ is partial pressure of CO_2 in mixed expired gas. For example, if $PaCO_2$ = 50 mmHg and $P\bar{E}CO_2$ = 20 mmHg, then V_D/V_T = 0.60.

$\dot{V}_D$ can be calculated:

$$\dot{V}_D = (\dot{V}_E \cdot V_D/V_T)$$

$\dot{V}_A$ can also be calculated:

$$\dot{V}_A = \dot{V}_E - (\dot{V}_E \cdot V_D/V_T)$$

or

$$\dot{V}_A = \dot{V}_E \cdot (P\bar{E}CO_2 \div PaCO_2)$$

of increased V_D/V_T include pulmonary embolism, positive pressure ventilation, pulmonary hypoperfusion, and high rate–low tidal volume ventilation.

Calculation of V_D/V_T requires the measurement of mixed expired PCO_2 ($P\bar{E}CO_2$). To determine $P\bar{E}CO_2$, mixed exhaled gas is collected for 5 to 15 minutes. During this gas collection period, the patient should be undisturbed and have a stable $\dot{V}_E$. $PACO_2$ via an arterial blood gas measurement is determined during this time. $P\bar{E}CO_2$ can be estimated by measuring the PCO_2 of H_2O that accumulates in the expiratory H_2O trap of the ventilator circuit. Water is sampled anaerobically from the H_2O trap and its PCO_2 is measured using a blood gas analyzer to estimate $P\bar{E}CO_2$.[71] However, further clinical evidence of effectiveness is necessary before the water trap method can be endorsed.

REFERENCES

1. Hess D, Agarwal NN: Variability of blood gases, pulse oximeter saturation, and end-tidal carbon dioxide pressure in stable, mechanically ventilated trauma patients. J Clin Monit 8:111–115, 1992.
2. Thorson SH, Marini JJ, Pierson DJ, Hudson LD: Variability of arterial blood gas values in stable patients in the ICU. Chest 84:14–18, 1983
3. Sasse SA, Chen PA, Mahutte CK: Variability of arterial blood gas values over time in stable medical ICU patients. Chest 106:187–193, 1994
4. Hess D: Noninvasive monitoring in respiratory care—present, past, and future: An overview. Respir Care 35:482–498, 1990
5. Hess D, Kacmarek RM, Stoller JK: Perspectives on monitoring in respiratory care. In Kacmarek RM, Hess D, Stoller JK (eds): Monitoring in Respiratory Care (pp. 1–11). St. Louis, Mosby-Year Book, 1993
6. Hess D, Kacmarek RM: Techniques and devices for monitoring oxygenation. Respir Care 38:646–671, 1993
7. Welch JP, DeCesare R, Hess D: Pulse oximetry: Instrumentation and clinical applications. Respir Care 35:584–601, 1990
8. Kelleher JF: Pulse oximetry. J Clin Monit 5:37–62, 1989
9. Severinghaus JW, Kelleher JF: Recent developments in pulse oximetry. Anesthesiology 76:1018–1038, 1992
10. McCarthy K, Decker MJ, Strohl KP, Stoller JK: Pulse oximetry. In Kacmarek RM, Hess D, Stoller JK (eds): Monitoring in Respiratory Care (pp. 309–347). St. Louis, Mosby-Year Book, 1993
11. Hess DR, Branson RD: Noninvasive respiratory monitoring equipment. In: Hess DR, Branson RD, Chatburn RL (eds): Respiratory Care Equipment (184–216). Philadelphia, JB Lippincott, 1995
12. Moller JT, Pedersen T, Rasmussen LS, Jensen PF, Pedersen BD, Ravlo O, Rasmussen NH, Espersen K, Johannessen NW, Cooper JB: Randomized evaluation of pulse oximetry in 20,802 patients. I. Design, demography, pulse oximetry failure rate, and overall complication rate. Anesthesiology 78:436–444, 1993
13. Moller JT, Johannessen NW, Espersen K, Ravlo O, Pedersen BD, Jensen PF, Rasmussen NH, Rasmussen LS, Pedersen T, Cooper JB: Randomized evaluation of pulse oximetry in 20,802 patients. II. Perioperative events and postoperative complications. Anesthesiology 78:445–453, 1993
14. Bierman MI, Stein KL, Snyder JV: Pulse oximetry in the postoperative care of cardiac surgical patients: A randomized controlled trial. Chest 102:1367–1370, 1992
15. Inman KJ, Sibbald WJ, Rutledge FS, Speechley M, Martin CM, Clark BJ: Does implementing pulse oximetry in a critical care unit result in substantial arterial blood gas savings? Chest 104:542–546, 1993
16. King T, Simon RH: Pulse oximetry for tapering supplemental oxygen in hospitalized patients: Evaluation of a protocol. Chest 92:713–716, 1987
17. Jubran A, Tobin MJ: Reliability of pulse oximetry in titrating supplemental oxygen therapy in ventilator-dependent patients. Chest 97:1420–1425, 1990
18. Carlin BW, Clausen JL, Ries AL: The use of cutaneous oximetry in the prescription of long-term oxygen therapy. Chest 94:239–241, 1988
19. Rodriquez LR, Kotin N, Lowenthal D, Kattan M: A study of pediatric house staff's knowledge of pulse oximetry. Pediatrics 93:810–813, 1994
20. Stoneham MD, Saville GM, Wilson IH: Knowledge about pulse oximetry among medical and nursing staff. Lancet 344:1339–1342, 1994
21. Bowton DL, Scuderi PE, Harris L, Haponik EF: Pulse oximetry monitoring outside the intensive care unit: Progress or problem? Ann Intern Med 115:450–454, 1991
22. Hess D: Capnography: Technical aspects and clinical applications. In Kacmarek RM, Hess D, Stoller JK (eds): Monitoring in Respiratory Care (375–405). St. Louis, Mosby-Year Book, 1993
23. Hess D: Capnometry and capnography: Technical aspects, physiologic aspects, and clinical applications. Respir Care 35:557–576, 1990
24. Graybeal JM, Russell GB: Capnometry in the surgical ICU: An analysis of the arterial-to-end-tidal carbon dioxide difference. Respir Care 38:923–928, 1993
25. Hess D, Schlottag A, Levin B, Mathai J, Rexrode WO: Evaluation of the usefulness of end-tidal PCO_2 to aid weaning from mechanical ventilation following cardiac surgery. Respir Care 36:837–843, 1991
26. Hess D, Eitel D: Monitoring during resuscitation. Respir Care 37:739–768. 1992
27. Murray IP, Modell JH: Early detection of endotracheal tube accidents by monitoring carbon dioxide concentration in respiratory gas. Anesthesiology 59:344–346, 1983
28. Anton WR, Gordon RW, Jordan TM, Posner KL, Cheney FW: A disposable end-tidal CO_2 detector to verify endotracheal intubation. Ann Emerg Med 20:271–275, 1991
29. MacLeod BA, Haller MB, Gerard J, Yealey DM, Menegazzi JJ: Verification of endotracheal tube placement with colorimetric end-tidal CO_2 detection. Ann Emerg Med 20:267–270, 1991
30. Kelly JS, Wilhoit RD, Brown RE, James R: Efficacy of the FEF colorimetric end-tidal carbon dioxide detector in children. Anesth Analg 75:45–50, 1992
31. Falke JL, Rackow EC, Weil MH: End-tidal carbon dioxide concentration during cardiopulmonary resuscitation. N Engl J Med 318:607–611, 1988
32. Sanders AB, Kern KB, Otto CW, et al: End-tidal carbon dioxide monitoring during cardiopulmonary resuscitation: A prognostic indicator for survival. JAMA 262:1347–1351, 1989
33. Cote CJ, Rolf N, Liu LM, Goudsouzian NG, Ryan JF, Zaslavsky A, Gore R, Todres TD, Vassallo S, Polaner D: A single-blind study of combined pulse oximetry and capnography in children. Anesthesiology 74:980–987, 1991
34. Koff PB, Hess D: Transcutaneous oxygen and carbon dioxide measurements. In Kacmarek RM, Hess D, Stoller JK (eds): Monitoring in Respiratory Care (349–374). St. Louis, Mosby-Year Book, 1993
35. Palmisano BW, Severinghaus JW: Transcutaneous PCO_2 and PO_2: A multicenter study of accuracy. J Clin Monit 6:189–195, 1990
36. Martin RJ: Transcutaneous monitoring: Instrumentation and clinical applications. Respir Care 35:577–583, 1990
37. Hess D, Mundorff J: Assessment of metabolic and nutritional status. In Pierson DJ, Kacmarek RM (eds): Foundations of Respiratory Care. New York, Churchill Livingstone, 1992, pp 541–554
38. Ritz R, Cunningham J: Indirect calorimetry. In Kacmarek RM, Hess D, Stoller JK (eds): Monitoring in Respiratory Care. St. Louis, Mosby–Year Book, 1993.
39. Branson RD: The measurement of energy expenditure: Instrumentation, Practical Considerations, and Clinical Application. Respir Care 35:640–659, 1990
40. Kemper MS: Indirect calorimetry equipment and practical considerations of measurement. Prob Respir Care 2:479–490, 1989
41. Marini JJ: Lung mechanics determinations at the bedside: Instrumentation and clinical application. Respir Care 35:669–696, 1990

42. Marini JJ, Ravenscraft SA: Mean airway pressure: Physiologic determinants and clinical importance—Part 1. Physiologic determinants and measurements. Crit Care Med 20:1461–1472, 1992
43. Marini JJ, Ravenscraft SA: Mean airway pressure: Physiologic determinants and clinical importance—Part 1. Clinical implications. Crit Care Med 20:1604–1616, 1992
44. Primiano FP, Chatburn RL, Lough MD: Mean airway pressure: Theoretical considerations. Crit Care Med 10:378–383, 1982
45. Hess D, Tabor T: Comparison of six methods to calculate airway resistance during mechanical ventilation. J Clin Monit 9:275–282, 1993
46. Marini JJ, Rodriquiez M, Lamb V: Bedside estimation of the inspiratory work of breathing during mechanical ventilation. Chest 89:56–63, 1986
47. Banner MJ, Jaeger MJ, Kirby RR: Components of the work of breathing and implications for monitoring ventilator-dependent patients. Crit Care Med 22:515–523, 1994
48. Blanch PB, Banner MJ: A new respiratory monitor that enables accurate measurement of work of breathing: A validation study. Respir Care 39:897–905, 1994
49. Banner MJ, Jaeger MJ, Kirby RR: Components of the work of breathing and implications for monitoring ventilator-dependent patients. Crit Care Med 22:515–523, 1994
50. Kacmarek RM, Hess D: Routine measurement of work of breathing: Is it necessary? Respir Care 39:881–882, 1994
51. Meeker DP, Wiedemann HP: Cardiovascular function. In Kacmarek RM, Hess D, Stoller JK (eds): Monitoring in Respiratory Care (443–477). St. Louis, Mosby-Year Book, 1993
52. Connors AF: Hemodynamic monitoring. In Kacmarek RM, Hess D, Stoller JK (eds): Monitoring in Respiratory Care (227–265). St. Louis, Mosby-Year Book, 1993
53. Marini JJ: Obtaining meaningful data from the Swan-Ganz catheter. Respir Care 30:572–585, 1985
54. O'Quin R, Marini JJ: Pulmonary artery occlusion pressure: Clinical physiology, measurement, and interpretation. Am Rev Respir Dis 128:319–326, 1983
55. Shapiro BA: In-vivo monitoring of arterial blood gases and pH. Respir Care 37:165–169, 1992
56. Shapiro BA, Mahutte CK, Cane RD, Gilmour LJ: Clinical performance of a blood gas monitor: A prospective, multicenter trial. Crit Care Med 21:487–494, 1993
57. Zimmerman JL, Dellinger RP: Initial evaluation of a new intra-arterial blood gas system in humans. Crit Care Med 21:495–500, 1993
58. Haller M, Kilger E, Briegel J, Forst H, Peter K: Continuous intra-arterial blood gas and pH monitoring in critically ill patients with severe respiratory failure: A prospective, criterion standard study. Crit Care Med 22:580–587, 1994
59. Venkatesh B, Brock THC, Hendry SP: A multiparameter sensor for continuous intra-arterial blood gas monitoring: A prospective evaluation. Crit Care Med 22:588–594, 1994
60. Mahutte CK, Holody M, Maxwell TP, Chen PA, Sasse SA: Development of a patient-dedicated, on-demand, blood gas monitor. Am J Respir Crit Care Med 149:852–859, 1994
61. Larson CP, Vender J, Seiver A: Multisite evaluation of a continuous intraarterial blood gas monitoring system. Anesthesiology 81:543–552, 1994
62. Lumsdent T, Marshall WR, Divers GA, Riccitelli SD: The PB3300 intraarterial blood gas monitoring system. J Clin Monit 10:59–66, 1994
63. Nelson LD: Continuous venous oximetry in surgical patients. Ann Surg 203:329–333, 1986
64. Rouby JJ, Poete R, Bodin L, Bourgeois J, Arthaud M, Viars P: Three mixed venous saturation catheters in patients with circulatory shock and respiratory failure. Chest 98:954–958, 1990
65. Scuderi PE, Bowton DL, Meredith JW, Harris LC, Evans JB, Anderson RL: A comparison of three pulmonary artery oximetry catheters in intensive care unit patients. Chest 102:896–905, 1992
66. Gutierrez G, Bismar H, Danzker DR, Silva N: Comparison of gastric intramucosal pH with measures of oxygen transport and consumption in critically ill patients. Crit Care Med 20:451–457, 1992
67. Gutierrez G, Palizas F, Doglio G, Wainsztein N, Gallesio A, Pacin J, Dubin A, Schiavi E, Jorge M, Pusajo J, Shottlender J, San Roman E, Dorfman B, Shottlender J, Giniger R: Gastric intramucosal pH as a therapeutic index of tissue oxygenation in critically ill patients. Lancet 339:195–199, 1992
68. Chang MC, Cheatham ML, Nelson LD, Rutherford EJ, Morris JA: Gastric tonometry supplements information provided by systemic indicators of oxygen transport. J Trauma 37:488–494, 1994
69. Boyd O, Mackay CJ, Lamb G, Bland JM, Grounds RM, Bennett ED: Comparison of clinical information gained from routine blood-gas analysis and from gastric tonometry for intramural pH. Lancet 341:142–146, 1993
70. Mohsenifar Z, Hay A, Hay J, Lewis MI, Koerner SK: Gastric intramural pH as a predictor of success or failure in weaning patients from mechanical ventilation. Ann Intern Med 119:794–798, 1993
71. von Pohle WR, Anholm JD, McMillan J: Carbon dioxide and oxygen partial pressure in expiratory water condensate are equivalent to mixed expired carbon dioxide and oxygen. Chest 101: 1601–1604, 1992

SECTION

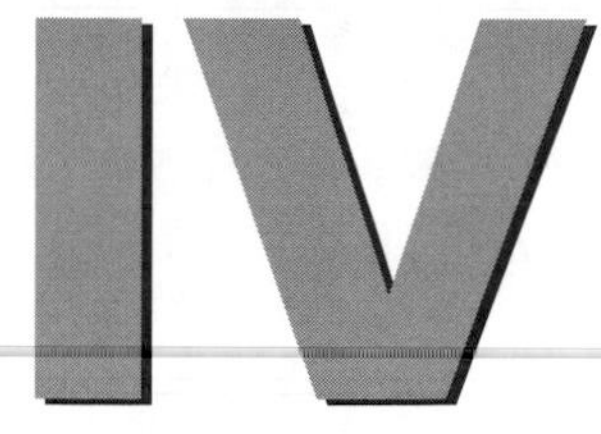

RESPIRATORY CARE MODALITIES AND EQUIPMENT

13 Medical Gas Therapy

Jeffrey J. Ward

CLINICAL SKILLS

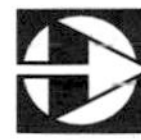

Upon completion of this chapter, the reader will be able to:

- Review existing data in the patient record to determine whether any childhood or adult diseases are likely to manifest in hypoxemia/hypoxia
- Conduct a physical examination, including a CNS examination, checking for pulmonary or cardiovascular signs of hypoxia and hypoxemia
- Perform pulmonary function testing, including arterial blood gas and pulse oximetry
- Recommend and perform other procedures to obtain additional oxygen transport data
- Interview the patient to determine the level of dyspnea, the need for medical gas therapy, and any other circumstances that would suggest specific systems or delivery devices
- Select, assemble, and check equipment for proper function, operation, and cleanliness; identify problems and take action to correct malfunctions of all

equipment, including regulators, reducing valves, flowmeters, oxygen/air blenders, gas cylinders, portable liquid and bulk systems, oxygen administration appliances or systems, and gas-analyzing and patient-monitoring devices

- Explain therapeutic goals, maintain records and communication
- Protect patients from nosocomial infection
- Conduct a therapeutic plan to achieve adequate arterial and/or tissue oxygenation
- Evaluate and monitor patient's response to gas therapy
- Modify oxygen, helium oxygen, carbon dioxide/oxygen therapy based on observed or measured patient response
- Initiate medical gas therapy in an emergency situation

KEY TERMS

Absorption atelectasis
Adult respiratory distress syndrome (ARDS)
Boiling point
Carboxyhemoglobinemia (HbCO)
Chronic obstructive pulmonary disease (COPD)
Circulatory (stagnant) hypoxia
Critical pressure
Critical temperature
Dalton's law
Demand hypoxia
Diameter Index Safety System (DISS)
Electrolysis
Fick principle
Fractional distillation
Hemic hypoxia
Histotoxic hypoxia
Hypercarbia
Oxygen concentration
Pascal principle
Pin Index Safety System
Retinopathy of prematurity (ROP)
Triple point

The purpose of this chapter is to review the therapeutic use of inhaled medical gases, including supplemental oxygen, mixtures of helium–oxygen and carbon dioxide–oxygen and nitric oxide. The chapter outline shows the broad scope of content. Gases that are considered anesthetic, or used for diagnostic purposes, or invasive oxygenation using intravascular (IVOX) and extracorporeal membrane (ECMO) techniques are not discussed.

Clinical skills needed in initiating those services are summarized as follows:

- Select, review, obtain and interpret data relative to medical gas therapy:
  - Review existing data in patient record:
    History—childhood and/or adult diseases likely to manifest in hypoxemia/hypoxia
    Physical examination—CNS, pulmonary, or cardiovascular signs of hypoxia and hypoxemia
    Laboratory—pulmonary-function testing including arterial blood gas and pulse oximetry
  - Recommend and perform procedures to obtain additional data
  - Interview patient to determine:
    Level of dyspnea and need for medical gas therapy
    Circumstances that would suggest specific systems or delivery devices

This list of job-oriented tasks or matrices is determined by the National Board for Respiratory Care Inc., via national survey for the certified (CRTT) and registered respiratory therapist (RRT).[1] The roles and responsibilities of a respiratory care practitioner in medical gas therapy are also listed in Box 13-1.

Scientifically based medical gas therapy requires both knowledge and skills. There is the gas-specific data related to its manufacture, storage, and means of making it available for use. Therapy begins with the initial assessment of the patient and the understanding of the pathologic manifestations requiring gas therapy. As therapeutic goals are determined, practitioners can enlist established clinical practice guidelines (CPGs) and protocols to assure that goals are attained. Respiratory care practitioners should also be aware of the hazards and limitations of medical gas therapy and/or its equipment. This rational approach to oxygen therapy is well documented because of consensus data.[2–4] Guidelines for clinical practice offer a framework for current and future practice. Those presented in this chapter were developed by the American Association for Respiratory Care (AARC)—Clinical Practice Guidelines: Oxygen Therapy in the Acute Care Hospital and Oxygen Therapy in the Home or Extended Care Facility.[3,4] A systematic approach to therapy is suggested using examples of critical pathways or therapist-driven protocols (TDPs). A review of equipment used for gas delivery and monitoring concludes this chapter.

HISTORICAL NOTES

The historical record allows us to look back and recognize the important contributors and events that have shaped current medical gas therapy. Box 13-2 summarizes key events and contributions.

BOX 13-1

ROLES AND RESPONSIBILITIES OF RESPIRATORY CARE PRACTITIONERS IN OXYGEN AND MIXED GAS THERAPY

- Recognize how supplemental oxygen can effect oxygen transport
- Identify signs and symptoms of hypoxemia, hypoxia, or upper airway narrowing/obstruction provided by history, interview, or patient examination
- Recognize pathologic disorders that commonly present with indications for oxygen, CO_2/O_2, He/O_2, or nitric oxide (NO) medical gas therapy
- Solve equations to determine: estimate of PaO_2 over age, $P(A\text{-}a)O_2$, duration of cylinder contents, peak flow estimate, and air/O_2 ratio to create an FIO_2 mixture
- Select equipment appropriate for therapy
- Assemble gas therapy equipment, check for proper function, and take action to correct malfunctions
- Initiate oxygen and other medical gas therapy (Heliox [He/O_2] and carbogen [CO_2/O_2]) to achieve adequate arterial tissue oxygenation, reduced work of breathing, or other desired physiologic response
- Evaluate, monitor, and record patient's response to medical gas therapy
- Modify therapy based on patient response (alternative device, flow, or FIO_2 adjustment)
- Initiate/conduct, monitor, and modify medical gas therapy for use in home or for transport
- Explain and instruct patient and patient's family in home medical gas therapy

AARC Clinical Practice Guideline

OXYGEN THERAPY IN THE ACUTE CARE HOSPITAL

Indications: Documented hypoxemia in adults, children, and infants older than 28 days, PaO_2 <60 mmHg or SaO_2 <90% in subjects breathing room air or with PaO_2 and/or SaO_2 below desirable range for specific clinical situation; in neonates, PaO_2 <50 mmHg and/or SaO_2 <88% or $PtcO_2$ <40 mmHg. An acute care situation in which hypoxemia is suspected (substantiation of hypoxemia is required within an appropriate period of time following initiation of therapy)—severe trauma, acute myocardial infarction, short-term therapy (eg, post-anesthesia recovery).

Contraindications: No specific contraindications to oxygen therapy exist when indications are judged to be present.

Assessment of Need: Need is determined by measurement of inadequate oxygen tensions and/or saturations, by invasive or noninvasive methods, and/or the presence of clinical indicators as previously described.

Assessment of Outcome: Outcome is determined by clinical and physiologic assessment to establish adequacy of patient response to therapy.

Monitoring: Clinical assessment including but not limited to cardiac, pulmonary, and neurologic status; assessment of physiologic parameters—measurement of oxygen tensions or saturation in any patient treated with oxygen in conjunction with the initiation of therapy or within 12 hours of initiation with FIO_2 >0.40, within 8 hours with $FIO_2 \geq 0.40$ (including postanesthesia recovery), within 72 hours in acute myocardial infarction, within 2 hours for any patient with the principal diagnosis of COPD, within 1 hour for the neonate. All oxygen delivery systems should be checked at least once per day. More frequent checks by calibrated analyzer are necessary in systems susceptible to variation in oxygen concentration (eg, hoods, high-flow blending systems) applied to patients with artificial airways, delivering a heated gas mixture, applied to patients who are clinically unstable or who require an FIO_2 of 0.50 or higher. The standard of practice for newborns appears to be continuous analysis of FDO_2 with a system check at least every 4 hours, but data to support this practice may not be available.

(From AARC Clinical Practice Guideline; For complete text see Respir Care 36:1410–1413, 1991; with permission.)

The ancient records note that the Chinese and Greeks believed that the air contained a substance required for life. Little was written until 1500 A.D. when Leonardo da Vinci found that animals required something in the atmosphere to sustain life. In 1660 Robert Boyle suggested that combustion of a flame and respiration both required a common substance found in air. About that same time, Evangelista Torricelli and Blaise Pascal worked on physical relationships of atmospheric pressure, and they developed the barometer. In 1670 Robert Hook, working with Boyle, surmised that the primary purpose of respiratory movements was to provide a fresh supply of air to the lungs.

Instead of building on the work by Boyle and others of that time, George Stahl proposed a chemical theory he called the "phlogiston theory." According to Stahl, air supported combustion by "taking up" the phlogiston given off by the burning object.

During the late 1700s, many investigators almost simultaneously discovered oxygen and carbon dioxide. In 1771 Swedish apothecary Carl Scheele heated magnesium oxide (MnO_2) with concentrated sulfuric acid (H_2SO_4), generating oxygen, which he called "fire air." Apparently understanding the significance of his finding, he communicated by letter in 1773 to others working in this area. England's Joseph Priestly made his discovery of oxygen in August 1774. Being a true phlogiston man, he named oxygen "dephlogisticated air." Until 1962 it was believed that Priestly preceded Scheele's published findings. However, though a summary of Scheele's work was published by Torbern Bergman in 1775, it was originally printed in June of 1774, 3 months before Priestly.[5] In France, Antoine Lavoisier published details of his findings on oxygen in 1775. Of interest is the fact that these three researchers nearly simultaneously and independently came to similar conclusions about oxygen. Lavoisier, however, appeared to have a better understanding of the gases' (CO_2 and O_2) physiological roles. He reported that "respiration is a combustion . . . similar to the combustion of charcoal," with knowledge of oxygen as a participant

AARC Clinical Practice Guideline

OXYGEN THERAPY IN THE HOME OR EXTENDED CARE FACILITY

Indications: In adults, children, and infants older than 28 days: $PaO_2 \leq 55$ mmHg (or $SaO_2 \leq 88\%$ in subjects breathing room air) or PaO_2 of 56 to 59 mmHg (or SaO_2 or $SpO_2 \leq 89\%$) in association with specific clinical conditions (eg, cor pulmonale, congestive heart failure, or erythrocythemia with hematocrit >56). Some patients may not qualify for oxygen therapy at rest but will qualify for oxygen during ambulation, sleep, or exercise. Oxygen therapy is indicated during these specific activities when SaO_2 is demonstrated to fall to ≤88%.

Contraindications: No absolute contraindications to oxygen therapy exist when indications are present.

Assessment of Need: *Initial assessment:* Need is determined by the presence of clinical indicators as previously described and the presence of inadequate oxygen tension and/or saturation as demonstrated by the analysis of arterial blood. Concurrent pulse oximetry values must be documented and reconciled with the results of the baseline blood gas analysis if future assessment is to involve pulse oximetry. *Ongoing evaluation or reassessment:* Additional arterial blood gas analysis is indicated whenever there is a major change in clinical status that may be cardiopulmonary related. Arterial blood gas measurements should be repeated in 1 to 3 months when oxygen therapy is begun in the hospital in a clinically unstable patient to determine the need for long-term oxygen therapy. Once the need for long-term oxygen therapy has been documented, repeat arterial blood gas analysis or oxygen saturation measurements are unnecessary other than to follow the course of the disease, to assess changes in clinical status, or to facilitate changes in the oxygen prescription.

Assessment of Outcome: Outcome is determined by clinical and physiologic assessment to establish adequacy of patient response to therapy.

Monitoring: Clinical assessment should routinely be performed by the patient and/or the caregiver to determine changes in clinical status. Patients should be visited/monitored at least once a month by credentialed personnel unless conditions warrant more frequent visits. Measurement of baseline oxygen tension and saturation is essential before oxygen therapy is begun. These measurements should be repeated when clinically indicated or to follow the course of the disease. Measurements of SO_2 also may be made to determine appropriate oxygen flow for ambulation, exercise, or sleep. *Equipment Maintenance and Supervision:* All oxygen delivery equipment should be checked at least once daily by the patient or caregiver. Facets to be assessed include proper function of the equipment, prescribed flowrates, F_DO_2, remaining liquid or compressed gas content, and backup supply. A respiratory care practitioner or equivalent should during monthly visits reinforce appropriate practices and performance by the patient and caregivers and assure that the oxygen equipment is being maintained in accordance with manufacturers' recommendations. Liquid systems need to be checked to assure adequate delivery. Oxygen concentrators should be checked regularly to assure that they are delivering 85% oxygen or greater at 4 L/min.

(From AARC Clinical Practice Guideline; For complete text see Respir Care 37:918–922, 1992; with permission.)

BOX 13-2

MEDICAL GAS THERAPY HISTORICAL EVENTS

- 1774—Discovery of oxygen (Scheele, Priestly)
- 1775—Understanding roles of O_2 and CO_2 in respiration (Lavoisier)
- 1798—"Pneumatic Institute" (Beddoes)
- 1800–1920s—Early administration devices
- 1900—Toxic effects of high oxygen %s reported
- 1900–1940s—Fundamental physiological studies including WWII high altitude research (Henderson, Bohr, Haldane, Krogh, et al)
- 1930s—Devices for specific needs and F_IO_2s, oxygen tent, "meter-mask," heliox, and CPAP (Barach)
- 1940–1950s—"Epidemic" of retrolental fibroplasia
- 1960–1970s—Methods to measure "oxygenation and ventilation" (Clark, Severignhaus, Millikan & Aoyagi)
- 1960–1990s—Methods to match F_IO_2 and flows: Venti-mask, O_2/air blenders, high-flow systems
- 1980—Benefits of long-term oxygen therapy and access to home O_2
- 1970–1990s—Consensus Conferences, Clinical Practice Guidelines and Regulations: ATS, ACCP, AARC, HCFA, et al

in the two processes. Lavoisier also renamed the gas "oxygen," or "acid generator." Joseph Black is credited with the discovery of carbon dioxide. Black heated limestone and found that it lost weight due to loss of "fixed air." He discovered that burning charcoal and fermenting beer produced this substance. Actually, Black's work was a rediscovery of Jean Baptiste van Helmont's work performed 100 years earlier.[6]

Thomas Beddoes and J. Watt are credited with the early clinical use of oxygen. In the late 1790s they established the Pneumatic Institute in Bristol, England and began treating patients with oxygen for heart disease, asthma, opium poisoning, and "anything else." The Institute failed to flourish because of the less-than-scientific approach. Lacking a clear understanding of oxygen transport physiology, Beddoes prescribed it indiscriminately. Early oxygen appliances used by Beddoes and Watt resembled the mouth piece with silk valves and reservoir shown in Figure 13-1A. Fresh oxygen was "manufactured" on location using electrolysis, available from local apothecaries. By 1868 Barth was able to compress the gas in 15-gallon copper cylinders at 450 psig so that a supply could be transported for later use.[7,8]

The first medical gas administration devices appeared during the 1800s and early 1900s. Some were original, whereas others were modifications of anesthetic devices. Besides mouth-pieces (Fig. 13-1B), cheek-pieces (Fig. 13-1C), and masks of oiled canvas (Fig. 13-1D), leather, glass funnels, and velveteen (Fig. 13-1E) were also used. Early versions of the contemporary face tent were initially developed for anesthetic gases (Fig. 13-1F). Sir Arbutnot Lane introduced the nasal catheter using a simple rubber tubing in 1907, which was used for sick children and adult victims of World War I gas poisoning. During the early 1900s,

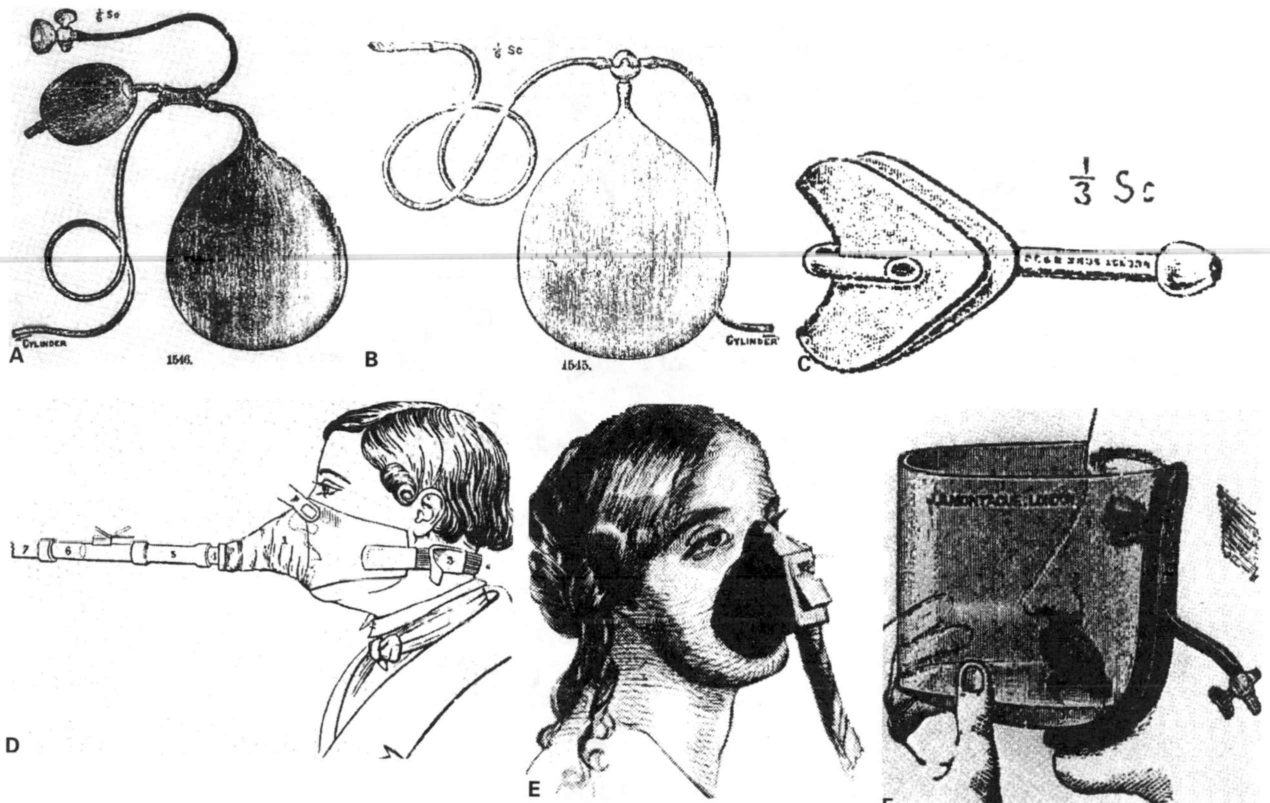

FIGURE 13-1. **(A)** Reservoir oxygen inhaler, circa 1914. (From Leigh JM. The evolution of the oxygen therapy apparatus.); **(B)** Vintage oxygen inhaler with glass mouthpiece. (From Leigh JM. The evolution of the oxygen therapy apparatus.); **(C)** Cheekpiece oxygen inhaler (From Leigh JM. The evolution of the oxygen therapy apparatus.); **(D)** Mask of oiled canvas (From Leigh JM. The evolution of the oxygen therapy apparatus.); **(E)** Nonreservoir oxygen mask with flap for exhaled gas, circa 1847. (From Leigh JM. The evolution of the oxygen therapy apparatus. Anaesthesia 1974;29:462. Reproduced by permission.); **(F)** Anesthesia open face tent originally used for nitrous oxide, circa 1899. (From Leigh JM. The evolution of the oxygen therapy apparatus. Anaesthesia 1970;25:210. Reproduced by permission of the publisher, Academic Press, LTD., London.)

Christian Bohr, August Krogh, Karl A. Hasselbalch, Lawrence Henderson, and others made significant strides in understanding pulmonary physiology, including oxygen transport.[6] In addition, the first reports on the toxic effects of oxygen in high concentration first appeared around 1900.[9]

During World War I, John Scott Haldane, Sir Joseph Barcroft, and others performed fundamental studies on anoxia and pathophysiology of respiration. Haldane developed an oxygen mask with 2-L rubber reservoir bag in 1918 for treating pulmonary edema caused by gas poisoning (Fig. 13-2A). In 1920, Haldane and Barcroft researched the effects of hypoxia by placing themselves in chambers filled with 15% oxygen. In 1926, American physician Alvan Barach developed a "closed system" oxygen tent with CO_2-absorbing calcium chloride canisters and chunk ice for cooling (Fig. 13-2B).[10] During the 1920s and 1930s Barach developed a variety of delivery appliances and promoted oxygen's scientific application. Both Haldane and Barach constructed masks that would provide consistent F_{IO_2}s by diluting oxygen with specific flows of room air (Fig. 13-2C).[7,11,12] Barach also experimented with helium–oxygen mixtures (heliox) with constant positive pressure breathing (CPPB a.k.a. CPAP) in 1934 (Fig. 13-2D)[13,14] In 1938, William Boothby, W. Randolf Lovelace, and Arthur Bulbulian developed the BLB mask at the Mayo Clinic. This reservoir-style mask permitted oxygen concentrations of 80% to 100% for high altitude flying World War II pilots (Fig. 13-2E).[7,15] Metal nasal cannulas were improvements on rubber masks and tents (Fig. 13-2F).

There was continued clinical research in identifying patient pathologies that would benefit from this "drug," such as myocardial infarction, pulmonary edema, pneumonia, atelectasis of the newborn, and asthma. A similar process occurred in realizing oxygen's toxic effects and how to measure physiologic levels. The first reports of pulmonary oxygen toxicity occurred in the late 1890s; by the mid-1940s more than 350 references had been collected in the literature.[16]

In the early 1940s, treatment of premature infants with excessive oxygen concentrations in incubators resulted in an "epidemic" of retrolental fibroplasia. Quantitating oxygen levels in gas or blood by chemical analysis was slow and tedious. The development of the membrane-covered oxygen electrode is credited to Leland Clark in the mid-1960s. Analysis of both gaseous and blood oxygen levels had a profound effect on oxygen therapy. Clinicians could easily and objectively evaluate both the levels of hypoxemia and titrate the appro-

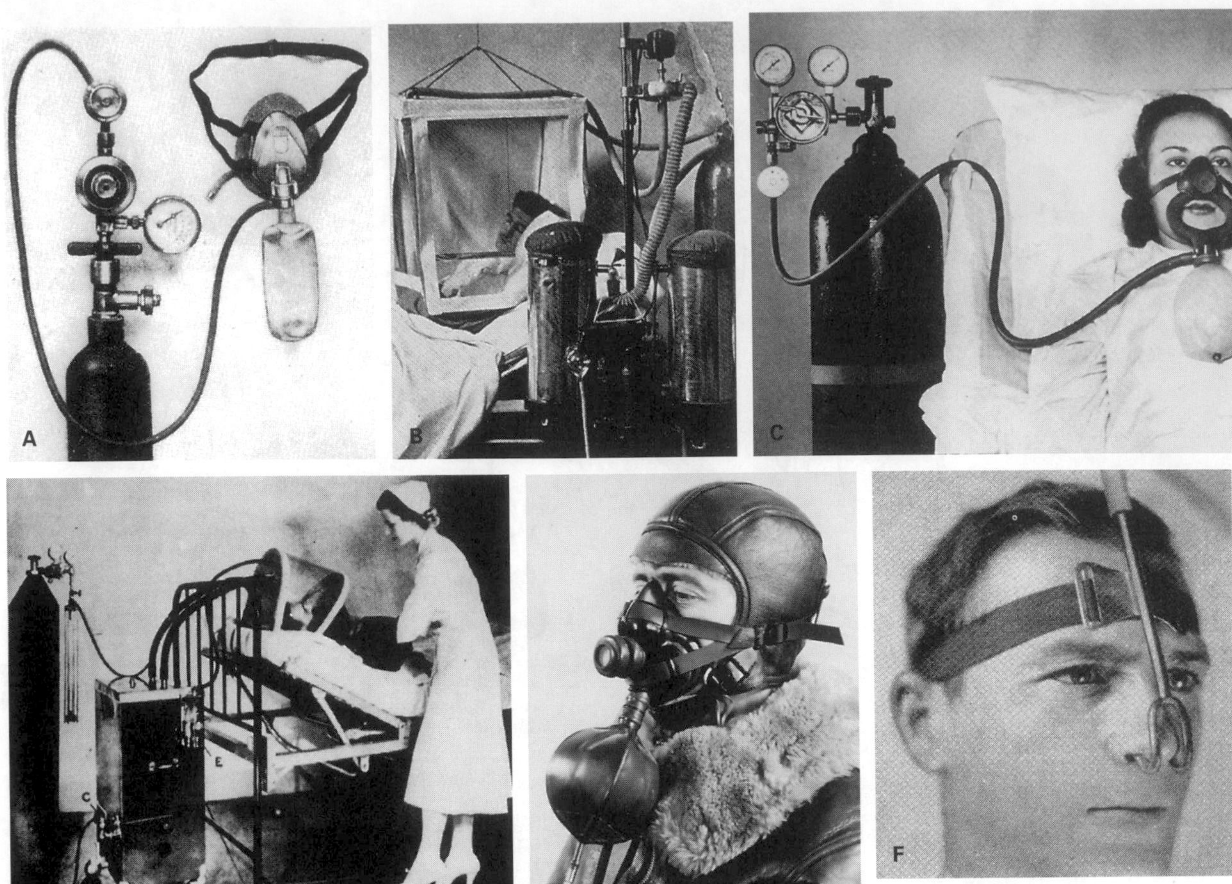

FIGURE 13-2. **(A)** Haldane's oxygen mask and reservoir, circa 1919. (From Leigh JM. The evolution of the oxygen therapy apparatus. Anaesthesia 29:462–485, 1974. Reproduced by permission.); **(B)** Barach's oxygen tent, circa 1926. Metal cannisters contained soda lime and ice. (From Barach AL. Symposium—inhalation therapy historical background. Anesthesiology 1962;23:407. Reproduced by permission.); **(C)** Barach's "mix-o-mask". (From Barach AL, Eckman M. A mask apparatus which provides high concentration with accurate control of oxygen in the inspired air and without accumulation of carbon dioxide. Aviat Med 1941;12:39. With permission); **(D)** Barach's heliox constant positive airway pressure device. (From Barach AL. Principles and Practices of Inhalation Therapy. Philadelphia, PA: J.B. Lippincott, 1944. With permission); **(E)** World War II aviator with BLB mask. (From personal collection H.F. Helmholz, Jr. MD); **(F)** Metallic nasal cannula. (From Barach AL. Principles of Inhalation therapy. Philadelphia, PA: J.B. Lippincott. 1944. With permission)

priate dosage of oxygen via a blood sample.[17] Another medical milestone was introduction of the "noninvasive" oximeter by G. A. Millikan in 1942.[18] Early ear oximeters were expensive and not easy to use continuously; they became common in pulmonary function laboratories by the early 1970s. The pulse oximeter followed in the late 1970s after its development by Takuo Aoyagi.[19] The clinical use of pulse oximeters proliferated beyond the pulmonary function testing (PFT) laboratory since they facilitated the noninvasive continuous monitoring of oxyhemoglobin saturation because of the ease, portability, and reduced cost. Although not a complete substitute for arterial blood gas analysis, this noninvasive monitoring of the "fifth vital sign" has had a major impact on oxygen administration.

In 1960, E.J. Moran Campbell developed the "Venti-mask," which was a nonreservoir bag version of Barach's "meter-mask." Campbell realized that dyspneic patients with COPD hypoventilated with excessive oxygen levels and patients required controlled and consistent F_{IO_2} by meeting their inspiratory flow needs.[20] The first mechanical ventilators with air/oxygen blending proportioner valves appeared in the late 1960s. Free-standing blenders became available in the early 1970s.

In the 1980s, long-term oxygen therapy was shown to have a positive effect on hypoxemic patients with COPD.[21] This prompted development and use of specially adapted appliances such as the reservoir cannulas and transtracheal catheter. The need for effective home oxygen therapy promoted the use of oxygen concentrators and portable liquid systems. Governmental regulations directing reimbursement for long-term oxygen prescription soon followed.[22] There is continued interest to make long-term therapy devices more efficient and cost effective.[23]

Carbon dioxide–oxygen and helium–oxygen mixtures have enjoyed only minor historical highlights compared with pure oxygen. Mixtures of carbon dioxide (5% to 15% in oxygen) were used to promote hyperventilation to aid in the postoperative removal of inhalation agents, such as ether, from the body; to treat hiccoughs and syncopal attacks; to improve regional blood flow (particularly to the brain); and to induce convulsions in psychoneurosis therapy. Because of the frequent complications from carbon dioxide–oxygen, its therapeutic application is largely historical except for its use in cardiopulmonary bypass in preventing total carbon dioxide washout.

The low-density properties of helium have intrigued clinicians since Alvan Barach's work in the mid-1930s.[13,14] He developed the approach and devices for treating asthma and obstructions of the larger airways. Heliox continues to have a small role in current practice but only as palliative care until more definitive therapy can correct the primary problem.

During the 1970s to 1990s, interest in optimizing oxygen therapy continued. Instead of developing new oxygen masks and the like, the focus has been on improving application and assessment of therapy. Scientific summaries, clinical practice guidelines, and rules for health care reimbursement have been developed by a number of groups including the following: National Heart, Lung and Blood Institute (NHLB), American College of Chest Physicians (ACCP), American Thoracic Society (ATS), American Association for Respiratory Care (ARRC), and Health Care Financing Association (HCFA).[2–4] The theme for the future is based on improved patient care using established guidelines, protocols with frequent patient assessment, and appropriate use of resources.

In 1987 Palmer and associates determined that nitric oxide (NO) was synthesized in the vascular endothelial cells.[24] Biologic research has since demonstrated that this gas acts as a biologic messenger in many cells, mediating neurotransmission, vasodilation, bronchodilation, and immune response. At present, nitric oxide inhalation therapy remains experimental but promising therapy for adults with pulmonary hypertension or the adult respiratory distress syndrome (ARDS) and newborns with persistent pulmonary hypertension of the neonate (PPHN) or congenital heart lesions.[25,26]

PHYSICAL AND CHEMICAL CHARACTERISTICS AND SOURCES OF MEDICAL GASES

Oxygen

PHYSICAL CHARACTERISTICS

Table 13-1 lists the specific physical data for oxygen, carbon dioxide, helium, and atmospheric air. Oxygen's concentration or fraction (F_{IO_2}) in air normally remains constant at 0.2095 to an altitude of 60 miles (96.5 km) above sea level. The partial pressure of oxygen gas available for respiration varies with changes in barometric pressure, which decreases at higher or lower altitudes compared to sea level. Equation Box 13-1 identifies Dalton's law, which determines oxygen's portion of the total atmospheric gas pressure, that is, its partial pressure (PO_2).

Although the fraction of atmospheric oxygen does not normally change, the partial pressure will vary considerably. On Mount Everest the total pressure is about 220 mmHg (29.26 kPa), the PO_2 is only 47 mmHg (6.25 kPa), and the equivalent F_{IO_2} is 0.062. Below sea level, 1 atm is added for each 33 ft (10 m) of sea water. Therefore, for a diver 66 ft below sea level (or patient in a hyperbaric chamber at 3 atmospheres) the total gas pressure is 2280 mmHg (303.24 kPa). The PO_2 is 478 mmHg (64 kPa) and the equivalent F_{IO_2} is 0.63. For an example of how to calculate equivalent F_{IO_2}, see Equation Box 13-2.

The atomic weight of oxygen is 16 g/mole and the gram molecular weight is 32 g/mole. There is some difference in proportion of atomic and molecular oxygen with altitude. At about 20 km, photodissociation produces atomic oxygen. Also there is an increase in ozone. Each reaches its maximum concentration at 30 km (0.003%) and 90 km (7%), respectively. Radiation

TABLE 13-1. **Physical Characteristics of Medical Gases**

	Oxygen	Air	Carbon Dioxide	Helium
Symbol	O_2	—	CO_2	He
Molecular weight	31.99	28.97	44.01	4.00
Percent by mole	20.946	—	0.0335	—
Partial pressure (ATPD)	158 mmHg	—	0.25 mmHg	—
Density*	1.32 kg/m^3	1.2 kg/m^3	1.833 kg/m^3	0.165 kg/m^3
Viscosity*	201.8×10^{-6}	182.7×10^{-6}	148×10^{-6}	194.1×10^{-6}
Specific gravity	1.1049	1	1.524	0.138
Boiling point	−183°C	−194.3°C	−29°C	−268.9°C
Critical temperature	−118.6°C	−140.7°C	31.1°C	−267.9°C
Critical pressure	731.4 psia	547 psia	1070.6 psia	731.4 psia
Triple point	218.8°C at .220 psia	—	−56°C at 75.1 psia	—

* Values referenced to 21.1°C and 1 atmosphere.

EQUATION BOX 13-1

CALCULATION OF PARTIAL PRESSURE

$$P_{O_2} = (P_B)F_{IO_2}$$

where
PB = barometric pressure (mmHg or torr)
P = partial pressure (mmHg or torr)
F = fractional concentration
I = inspired

At average sea level barometric pressure, the partial pressure of oxygen is:

$$P_{O_2} = (760)0.21$$
$$= 159 \text{ mmHg or torr*}$$

* *Units of pressure in the MKSs metric system are mmHg or torr; the kilopascal, kPa, is used in the system internationale (SI). The text will attempt to present both; practitioners should be able to compute conversion as follows:*

1 mmHg = 0.133 kPa

1 kPa = 7.5 mmHg

strips off an electron from atomic oxygen, producing ionized species O^+ and O^{++}. However, the atomic form is quite reactive, occurring only at high altitudes, and oxygen most commonly exists in molecular form. Oxygen is interesting in its molecular bonding characteristics. The atom's outer 2p orbit of the L shell has "room" for six electrons, but only four are filled. In its molecular form, the 2p orbit achieves stability by "filling" the orbit, by each atom sharing one of its electrons. In addition, the outermost orbit is occupied by two electrons, one from each atom. This outer orbit configuration provides the basis for the "paramagnetic" or magnetic-like quality in which higher concentration intensifies the force of a magnetic field. It is the only naturally occurring gas with this characteristic that is used as the basis for the design of one type of gas analyzer.[27]

Oxygen's normal physical state is as a gas. However, most hospitals and many patients have liquid supplies. To convert a gas to a liquid, it must be compressed and/or cooled. The *critical pressure* is defined as the pressure required for liquefaction (at the critical temperature). For oxygen it is 716 psig (4937 kPa). The *critical temperature* is the temperature required to cause a gas to change to a liquid at the critical pressure. That temperature for oxygen is −118°C; above that level, no amount of pressure can cause liquefaction. Oxygen will stay in liquid form only if its temperature is kept below −183°C at atmospheric pressure, which is its boiling point. The *boiling point* is the temperature above which gas could not be converted back to a liquid, regardless of pressure applied. The *triple point* is defined as the pressure and temperature conditions that allow solid, liquid, and vapor to exist in equilibrium. For oxygen it is −362°F (−218°C), at 0.022 psia (0.152 kPa).

EQUATION BOX 13-2

EQUIVALENT F_{IO_2}

$$\text{Equivalent } F_{IO_2} = \frac{\text{Barometric pressure at ambient altitude}}{\text{Barometric pressure at sea level}}$$

Example: Determine the equivalent oxygen concentration at altitude using the following formula. For Ledville, Colorado (10,000 ft or 3048 m) the Equation Box 13-5 follows with the calculation of Equivalent F_{IO_2}:

$$\text{Equivalent } F_{IO_2} = \frac{P_B \text{ at altitude}}{P_B \text{ at sea level}} \times F_{IO_2}$$
$$= \frac{522.9 \text{ mmHg}}{760 \text{ mmHg}} \times 0.21$$
$$= 0.14 \text{ or } 14\% \text{ oxygen}$$

□ SOURCES OF SUPPLEMENTAL OXYGEN

The process of biologic photosynthesis is the main source and regulator of oxygen levels in the atmosphere. Photosynthesis is the process whereby light energy from the sun converts carbon dioxide and water into glucose and oxygen. Chlorophyll is the chemical agent necessary for this transformation. A normal human consumes 2 to 5 lb of oxygen/day (4.5 to 11.2 kg) as required to convert carbohydrates, fats, and proteins into heat and energy.

Laboratory or commercial manufacture of oxygen uses four methods: (1) heating metallic oxides, (2) electrolysis, (3) fractional distillation, and (4) filtration by membrane or molecular sieve.

Scheele and Priestly generated oxygen by heating metallic oxides of mercury, silver, or barium. The following formula demonstrates the chemical reaction:

$$2HgO \xrightarrow{\text{Heat}} 2Hg + O_2$$

Since water is 33% oxygen by volume and 88% by weight, it is a source of oxygen. The process, called *electrolysis*, occurs by passing an electric current through water (with a trace of acid to improve conduction). Oxygen can be collected in a glass chamber above the anode. For every 1 mL of oxygen, 2 mL of hydrogen is obtained at the cathode. This process is only used for laboratory applications.

The most common commercial source uses a complex technique termed *fractional distillation* of air, or the Joule-Kelvin method. According to this principle, gases under pressure lose kinetic energy when released into a vacuum. This loss results in a loss of temperature. It then removes the constituents of air by using their different boiling points. Karl von Linde first used this process commercially in 1907. The following is a simplified explanation of three basic steps of fractional distillation. A schematic diagram is presented in Figure 13-3.

Fractional Distillation

Atmospheric air is first filtered and compressed to 1500 psig (10,341 kPa), then further to 2000 psig (13,789 kPa) (see Fig. 13-3). During each pressurization, the heat built up by molecular compaction is reversed by

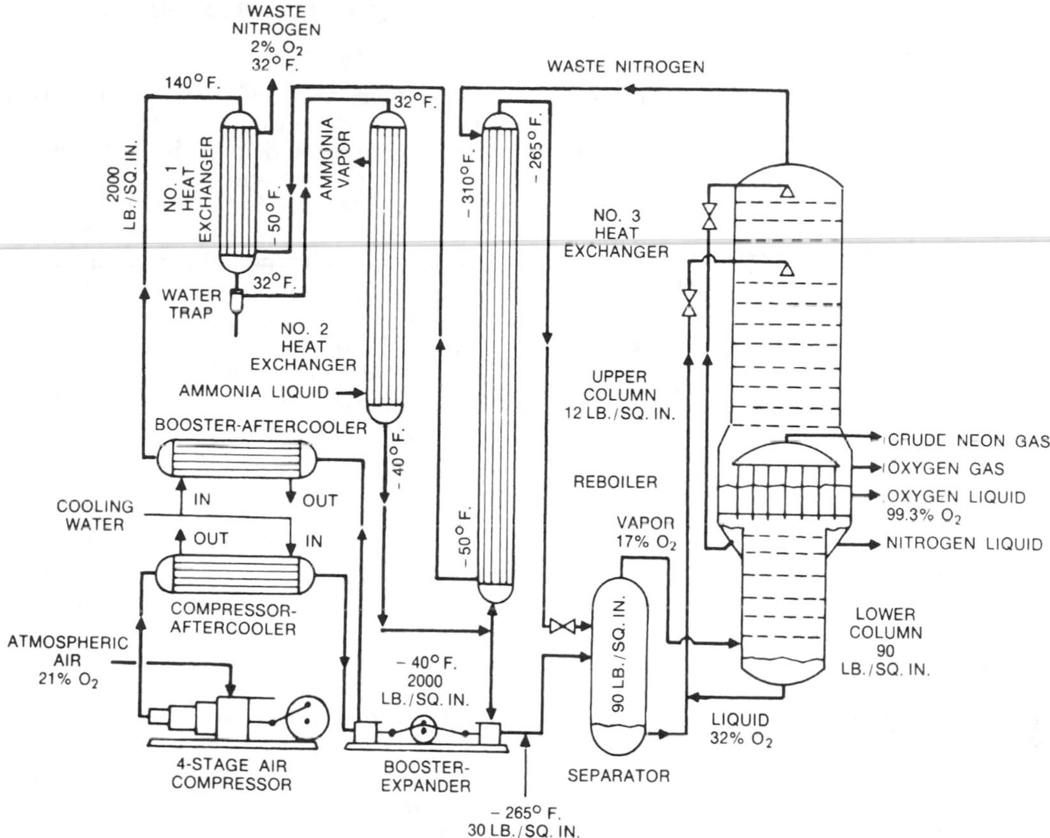

FIGURE 13-3. Schematic of fractional distillation plant for the production of liquid oxygen from air. (Courtesy of Union Carbide Corporation, Linde Division, Indianapolis.)

water-cooled aftercoolers. Next, three countercurrent heat exchangers purify and liquefy the compressed air, partially through a refrigeration process. Waste nitrogen is used as a coolant in #1 exchanger, dropping the temperature to −50°F (−45.5°C), which removes water vapor through condensation. Gas enters exchanger #2 at 32°F (0°C). It uses evaporating liquid ammonia to cool the purified air to approximately −40°F (−40°C), which removes any remaining water vapor. Exchanger chamber #3 extends cooling to −265°F (−160°C) and compression to 200 psig (1379 kPa). At this pressure (below the 530 psig critical pressure) air cannot liquefy. The compressed gas–liquid mixture is next expanded into a "relative vacuum" of 90 psig causing separation of liquid and gas. The air and gas are pumped in separate streams into the distillation column.

Filtration

Liquid air is expanded further by a pressure drop of 12 psig as it enters the vertically stacked distillation columns. Nitrogen and rare gases in the liquid have lower boiling points than oxygen. Nitrogen boils off the top at −320°F (−196°C) as it descends down the column, and the liquid increases its pure oxygen content as it reaches the bottom. Near the base the oxygen-rich liquid is boiled again, releasing rare gases, such as argon and krypton.

The most recent devices used to make oxygen for medical purposes using a process termed *oxygen concentration*. This term is somewhat generic in that the devices filter out gas molecules *other* than oxygen. The most common is the molecular sieve or pressure swing absorbent method (Fig. 13-4). A vacuum draws room air into cylinders packed with crystallized zeolite, a silicate with ion exchange properties. The air is compressed (100 to 300 psig [690 to 2069 kPa]) and environmental nitrogen is filtered out, that is, temporarily absorbed by the zeolite. The process is reversed by switching to a depressurization phase, which causes the crystals to release the nitrogen as exhaust. The final concentration of oxygen as well as the flow setting exiting the sieve varies among manufacturers. Most concentrators deliver oxygen in the 1 to 5 L/min range at between 0.95 and 0.98 but fall to 0.92 to 0.95 when run at higher flows. The increasing concentration of argon gas causes this decrease in oxygen concentration.[28]

The other type of commercial device is the membrane oxygen concentrator that uses a set of plastic polymer membranes through which air is filtered. A pump provides the pressure gradient across the membrane cells. Oxygen and water vapor are more permeable than nitrogen and move through the membranes to be collected. These concentrators are less popular commercially because they produce only 30% to 40% oxygen and are not currently being manufactured. Concentrators require routine mechanical maintenance and should be periodically checked in either the home or

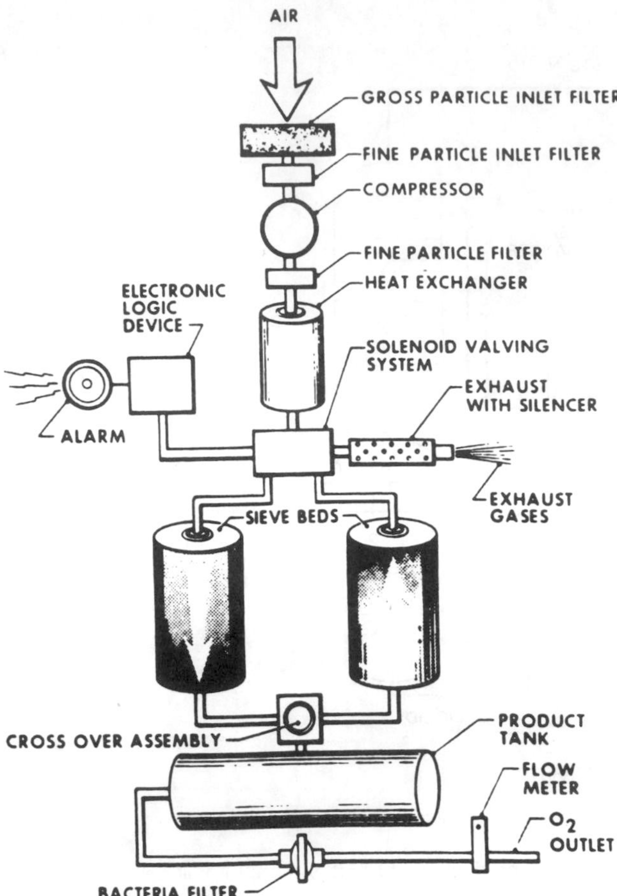

FIGURE 13-4. Molecular sieve oxygen concentrator. (From Lucas J, Golish J, Sleeper G, O'Rayne J. Home Respiratory Care. Norwalk, CT: Appleton & Lange, 1987. With permission.)

hospital setting to confirm proper flow setting and oxygen concentration. Testing of home units of both designs of concentrators shows a reduction of the F_{IO_2} expected from membrane units.[29] Because the limited driving pressure from some units is 5 to 10 psig (34 to 69 kPa), manufacturers suggest limiting the maximum total distance of small bore tubing from the concentrator to about 50 feet (15.2 m).

Compressed Air

□ PHYSICAL CHARACTERISTICS

At normal atmospheric conditions air exists as a colorless, orderless, and tasteless gas mixture. Trace elements are not significant physiologically. The largest component, nitrogen, serves no metabolic function yet aids in maintaining the inflation of gas-filled body cavities such as alveoli, sinus cavities, and the middle ear. The Compressed Gas Association specifies the oxygen concentration in air to be from 0.195 to 0.235 and limits the concentration of trace constituents for medical grade air (Grade J). Aside from its medical applications, compressed air is used for underwater breathing, aerospace technology, industry, and fire fighting self-contained breathing devices.[30]

□ SOURCES OF COMPRESSED AIR

Piped Air Systems

Piped compressed air is commonly provided in hospital medical gas systems for use in areas such as the operating room and intensive care units. Many mechanical ventilators and O_2/air blenders require separate sources of both medical air and oxygen. Various designs of large compressors are available, but the piston type appears to be the industrial standard. A pressure-sensitive switch senses pressure levels and turns the compressor on and off to maintain line pressures of 50 psig (345 kPa). Normally a holding reservoir is added into the system to provide a ready supply and prevent the compressor from running all the time. In large institutions, it is common to have two compressors that alternate, prolonging compressor life.[31]

Portable Compressors

Smaller versions are also available for hospital or home use that require a portable air compressor. Since the source of these systems is the hospital ambient air, high humidity causes considerable condensation. It is important that a compressed air system incorporate condensers to scavenge water during cooling after the gas is warmed during the compression phase. Water trap drains must be religiously maintained to prevent wet air from fouling flowmeters and ventilators. The federal specifications BB-A-1034 for source II grade C breathing air permits a maximum of 0.3 mg/L for total water content. Inline desiccant dryers or filters may also be needed, especially in humid months.[30,32]

Carbon Dioxide

□ PHYSICAL CHARACTERISTICS

Under normal atmospheric conditions, carbon dioxide gas has a concentration of 0.03% by volume (F_{ICO_2} of 0.003 in atmospheric air). Since it is a by-product of human and animal metabolism and the burning of carbonaceous fuels, the concentration may increase in certain environments. The current Occupational Safety and Health Act (OSHA) standard for maximal allowable concentration is 0.5% for 8 hours of continuous exposure or 3% carbon dioxide over a 10-minute period.[33] Carbon dioxide and oxygen therapy gas mixtures, commonly 5% CO_2, 95% O_2, are used for short treatment intervals (about 10 minutes), during which the patient must be carefully monitored.

In gaseous form, carbon dioxide is relatively nonreactive, nontoxic, and "blocks" combustion. Carbonic acid (H_2CO_3), which forms when carbon dioxide dissolves in water, is corrosive to metals. Nonmedical uses include carbonated beverage bottling, food preservation, refrigeration, and fire extinguishing. Solid carbon dioxide (dry ice) exists at temperatures below its triple point of 69°F (21°C) and at a pressure above 60 psig (416 kPa). At temperatures below its triple point, −70°F (−56°C) and 1 atm pressure, dry ice will sublime or "smoke" into a gas without passing through a liquid phase. Carbon dioxide also has a low thermal conductivity, which allows dry ice to remain relatively stable.[33]

Cylinders of CO_2 commonly contain both liquid and gas if the temperature is below 31°C with pressures above 60 psig (414 kPa). This possibility requires that cylinders be weighed to determine the quantity of remaining gas. This phenomenon does not occur with medical mixtures of 95%/5% and 90%/10% oxygen–carbon dioxide. There is significant difference in the density and viscosity of carbon dioxide when compared with oxygen or air (see Table 13-1). Accurate metering of gas through tubes and orifices must accommodate this factor.

☐ SOURCES OF CARBON DIOXIDE

Carbon dioxide in an unrefined form is obtained from combustion of coal, coke, natural gas, oil, steam hydrocarbon reformers, lime kilns, the fermentation process, and natural springs. Refining removes carbon monoxide, hydrogen sulfide, nitric acid, water, and other impurities. For medical purposes the purity is 99.5% or better. Three types of carbon dioxide are available: type 1 (cylinders at ambient temperatures), type 2 (liquid at subambient temperatures), and type 3 (solid carbon dioxide).[30]

Helium

☐ PHYSICAL CHARACTERISTICS

Helium is the second lightest element in the atmosphere (see Table 13-1). It is a rare gas, having a concentration of only 5 ppm. Helium is chemically inert, nontoxic, tasteless, and nonflammable. Low concentrations (<5%) of helium are used in pulmonary function laboratories as a test gas in lung volume and diffusing testing. In higher concentration (>50%) it is used medically for its low density properties in palliative treatment of large airway obstruction. Commercially, helium is used as a nuclear reactor coolant, in cryogenic research, as a shield in arc welding, in silicon and germanium crystal-growing atmosphere, in lighter-than-air craft, and for breathing mixtures in deep-water diving.[30] Helium/oxygen, or heliox, is more expensive and far less frequently used than oxygen.

☐ SOURCES OF HELIUM

Natural gas containing up to 2% helium is found in wells in the southern United States. Other wells are located in Canada and the Black Sea.

Nitric Oxide

☐ PHYSICAL CHARACTERISTICS

Nitric oxide or nitrogen monoxide (NO) is an unstable free radical (N=O or NO^1) that was originally regarded as an environmental pollutant (eg, found in smog and cigarette smoke) and an impurity of nitrous oxide manufacture. In 1987 it was found to normally biosynthesize in vascular endothelial cells. It is an important mediator of physiologic functions, including vasodilation, neurotransmission, long-term memory, and immunologic defense.[25]

The molecule is highly diffusable and lipid soluble. Its half life ranges from 3 to 50 seconds as its conversion to nitrates, nitrites, and higher oxides of nitrogen increases with higher oxygen tensions. The superoxide anion rapidly inactivates NO. Its biologic reactivity and properties depend on its interrelated redox forms:

- neutral nitric oxide (NO^1)
- nitrosonium cation (NO^+)
- nitrosyl anion (NO^-)

In solution NO is oxidized to nitrites (NO_2^-) and nitrates (NO_3^-). Neutral nitric oxide (NO^1) can react to produce tissue-damaging oxidants or bind with hemoglobin to cause cytotoxic effects. The cation form (NO^+) reacts to produce metallo-nitrosyl compounds, which mediate physiological responses such as vasodilation. This effect on the pulmonary vascular bed is seen when small concentrations are inhaled 18 to 36 parts per million (ppm). The greatest clinical interest to date is in treatment of PPHN and hypertension-associated congenital heart disease in infants. There is also interest in treatment of ARDS or primary pulmonary hypertension. The role of nitrosyl anion (NO^-) is unknown; it is rapidly converted to nitrous oxide (N_2O) in water. A detailed review of the biologic and physiologic aspects can be found in other sources; a summary of its properties is found in Box 13-3.[24,25] A discussion of clinical administration and complications follows later in this chapter.

☐ SOURCES OF NITRIC OXIDE

The manufacture of nitric oxide for research/clinical purposes occurs during the commercial production of the anesthetic gas nitrous oxide. For in-hospital application, NO is supplied in high-pressure cylinders. Nitric oxide at 800 to 2200 ppm is balanced with nitrogen (N_2) for a 99.0% purity. It is available in 1800 cuft volume aluminum cylinders containing 4000 L of gas at 2000 psig. In a cylinder, NO will remain in stable form and not convert to nitrogen dioxide for over 18 months.[25]

BOX 13-3

PROPERTIES OF NITRIC OXIDE

Atomic weight—40 g
Physiochemistry
  Half life 3–50 sec
  Highly lipid soluble
  Highly diffusible
Fate:
  Gaseous—Oxidized to NO_2 and higher oxide
  Solution—Oxidized to nitrites (NO_{2-}) and nitrates (NO_{3-})
NO activity inhibited by:
  Hemoglobin, myoglobin, methyl blue, superoxide anion
NO activity potentiated by:
  Superoxide dismutase
  Cytochrome C
  H^+ ions

SYSTEMS FOR GAS STORAGE AND DISTRIBUTION

Main and Reserve Storage Systems

Today medical gases are available to medical consumers in portable high-pressure gas cylinders, bulk (liquid) cylinders, and fixed liquid systems that feed pipelines for gas supply. Because of the potential hazards to the general public during transportation and to handlers and patients, a fairly complex array of regulatory and recommending agencies have become involved. Each group provides extremely detailed information, specifications, regulations, and safety procedures. A detailed presentation of guidelines and regulations is beyond the scope of this text. Readers are referred to the summary in Box 13-4 and references for details.[30]

☐ LIQUID BULK SYSTEMS

The American Society for Mechanical Engineers (ASME) establishes the standards for liquid oxygen storage vessel construction and safety. The liquid reservoirs are similar to a cold/hot beverage Thermos bottle. A vacuum between inner and outer walls provides the insulation. Standards are quite complex because they are composed of two systems. System A is the primary supply, and system B is the reserve, or backup, supply. Liquid oxygen is transported to the facility by truck or rail and filled at location No. 1 as shown in Figure 13-5. To provide positive pressure within the system, liquid oxygen is drawn off at locations #6 and #7, where a pressure regulator and vaporizer reintroduce gaseous oxygen to the tank. As the atmosphere warms the liquid passing through the vaporizer, the internal pressure is increased. Liquid oxygen continuously vaporizes and is fed into the liquid pipeline in an economizer circuit at location #4. The main liquid supply leaves the tank and is led to the main vaporizers and location #9. Following the vaporizers, gas flows to the main supply regulators, a primary and backup, location #11, #11a, and #11b. A pressure relief valve will vent off pressure if the pressure exceeds the normal level, 55 psig, by 50%, or 80 psig (552 kPa).

A reserve supply of a second liquid bulk reservoir may be used (see Fig. 13-5). In the diagram, it is shown as a parallel design to the main unit. Besides acting as a backup, it also continuously adds a small amount of gas as normal vaporization occurs. Check valves, one-way valves, prevent any leaks in either system from inadvertently draining the other. Facilities with less volume demand may only need a reserve bank of large gas cylinders. The NFPA requires that the reserve supply be equal to 1 day's average supply.[34–36]

Incidents involving bulk oxygen systems are not rare. Often maintenance is not done in a preventive manner, or poor communication between the maintenance and the respiratory care departments leads to problems. An oxygen system that abruptly stops is a major emergency. Oxygen loss in the operating room or critical care unit must be quickly corrected with backup cylinder gas that is easily available. Unless there are predetermined protocols, the response will usually be slow and disorganized. An anesthesia-based algorithm (Fig. 13-6) demonstrates a coping strategy for oxygen system supply failure.[37] Alarms to alert personnel to problems in a bulk system traditionally consist of the following:

- Low liquid level in either primary or reserve systems
- Reserve in use following a switchover when the main supply falls to approximately 85 psig (586 kPa)
- Main supply line pressure variations exceed ±20%

A report of incidents in a 500-bed hospital noted fairly numerous problems when the hospital's bulk system was followed for 1 year. The following were most significant:[38]

BOX 13-4

GOVERNMENTAL AND NONGOVERNMENTAL AGENCIES THAT REGULATE STANDARDS

Governmental Agencies	Responsibility/Authority
Department of Transportation (DOT)	Compressed gas cylinders, inspection, and transport
Department of Health and Human Services (DHHS) Food and Drug Administration (FDA)	Purity of medical gases
Bureau of Medical Devices	Classification, provision of standards, and regulation of medical devices
Federal Department of Labor, Occupational Safety and Health Administration (OSHA)	Safety in workplace related to gases
Nongovernmental	**Responsibility/Authority**
Compressed Gas Association (CGA)	Specification, recommendations in gas manufacture, containers, regulation, and safety systems
National Fire Protection Association (NFPA)	Codes and safety regulations for storage
International Standards Organization (ISO)	Manufacturing standards
American National Standards Institute and its Z-79 Committee (ANSI)	Coordination of standards for health devices
American Society for Testing and Materials (ASTM)	Coordination of standards for health devices (airways, adaptors, ventilatory equipment, etc.)
Association for the Advancement of Medical Instrumentation (AAMI)	Biomedical standards related to medical equipment
American Society of Mechanical Engineers (ASME)	Standards and safety regulations for bulk liquid reservoirs

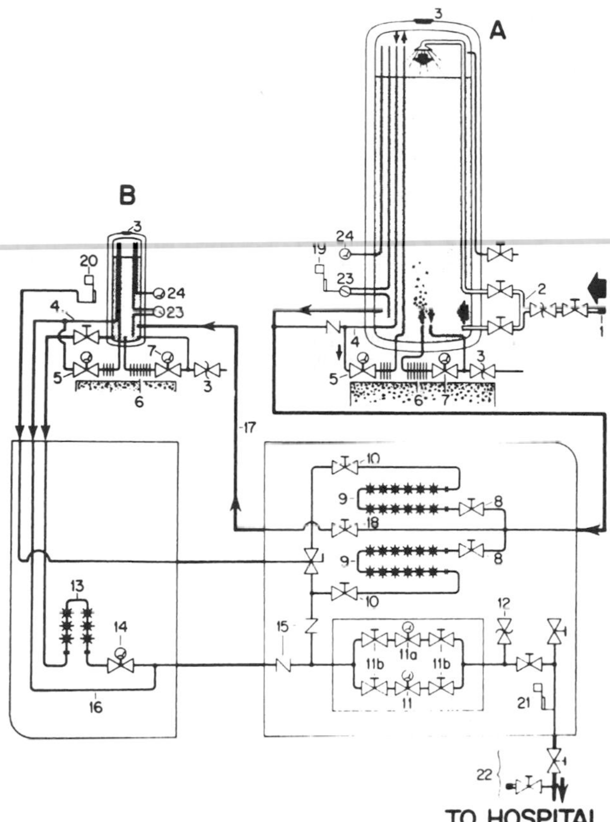

FIGURE 13-5. Schematic of main and reserve liquid oxygen reservoirs. (From Bancroft ML, du Moulin GC, Hedley-Whyte J. Hazards of hospital bulk oxygen delivery systems. Anesthesiology 1980;52: 504. Reproduced by permission.)

- False alarms caused by calibration drift of pressure sensors
- Excessive depletion of the reserve supply because of pressure imbalance between the main and reserve supply
- Failure of the vacuum seal on the reserve supply
- Inappropriate manipulation of supply valves
- Leakage around valves and ruptured piping
- Failure of monitoring personnel to notify appropriate service personnel.
- Occlusion of pressure sensors with foreign substance

Other potentially serious problems include the following:

- Filling bulk tanks with the wrong gas
- Misconnection of pipelines following remodeling
- Damage from high winds, tornadoes, earthquakes, and fires.

☐ HOME LIQUID/PORTABLE SYSTEMS

Miniature versions of hospital bulk liquid systems are used in homes or where a large-volume supply is needed. Instead of the fin-type external vaporizer coils found on large reservoirs, these reservoirs use coils of tubing inside a protective housing. Commercial examples are the Linde PCU-500/Walker (Union Carbide) and the Liberator/Stroller (Cryogenics Associates) (Fig. 13-7A). The basic designs for both involve a two-part system. A cross-sectional diagram of a portable container is shown in Figure 13-7B. The fixed reservoir is identical in design to larger hospital units except that the pressure within the vessel is commonly about 20 psig (137 kPa). However, the Linde unit operates at 90 psig (621 kPa). A major advantage of all systems is that small, portable reservoirs can be transfilled from the larger home-based unit. The portable liquid containers provide 8 to 12 hours of oxygen (depending on the flow). Patients who can only ambulate with continuous supplemental oxygen are freed from having to use small cylinders of compressed gas. Liquid systems are also convenient for air transport vehicles where space and weight are at a premium. However, even when not being used, these reservoirs lose oxygen owing to warming and subsequent pressure venting.

Technical problems for portable liquid containers are similar to those of large volume liquid devices.[39]

- Need for well-educated users
- Hazard of freezing exposed tissue (need gloves & goggles)
- Fire hazard (no petroleum lubricants/products)
- Tipped-over containers spill/spurt contents
- Increased level of contaminants as oxygen vaporizes.

Duration of Contents

To estimate duration of portable liquid reservoirs, contents must be weighed to determine their remaining capacity. Some manufacturers have built-in scales to allow a spot determination. Equation Box 13-3 follows the two-step calculation with an example of a liquid supply duration problem (if the user has access to a scale).

Pipeline Supply Systems

☐ DESIGN CONSIDERATIONS

Bulk medical gas liquid reservoirs or banks of compressed gas cylinders provide a source for multiple supply outlets in medical facilities. Pipeline supply outlets for one or several different medical gases offer convenience and prevent safety problems and significant human resource needs related to cylinders. The National Fire Protection Association (NFPA) regulates the gas "plumbing" of a hospital or clinic. They provide numerous guidelines and specifics for construction, materials, and maintenance.[33–36] Most hospitals use a primary bulk liquid source and a reserve system of either a compressed gas cylinder bank or portable liquid cylinders or a second fixed liquid supply. The reserve is used only if the main unit fails or is depleted (Fig. 13-8A). An alternating system can use a pair of compressed gas cylinder banks or portable liquid reservoirs. They are filled on an alternating use schedule (Fig. 13-8B). Check valves prevent gas from draining any side of the system if a leak occurs in another area.

Once a supply system enters the facility, it divides into a labyrinth of pipes that are sent to all locations requir-

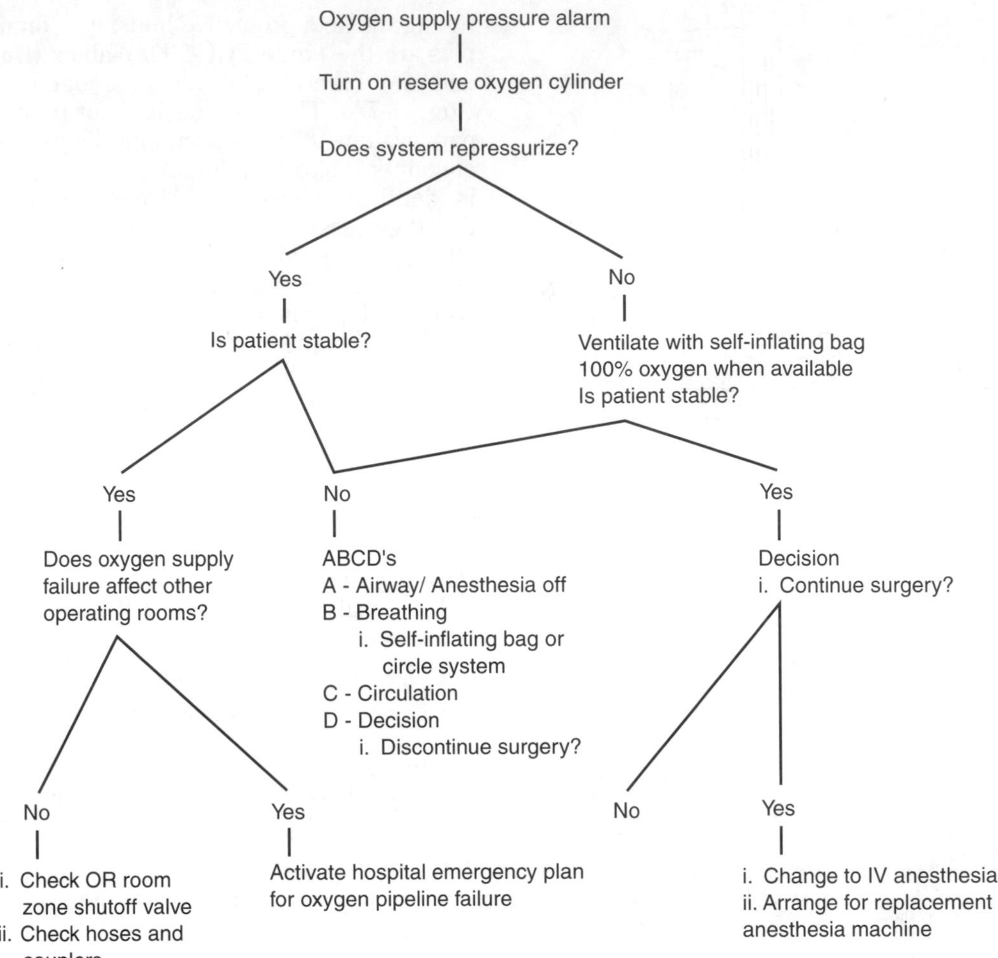

FIGURE 13-6. Strategy algorithm to deal with gas supply problems. (From Anderson WR, Brock-Utne JG: Oxygen pipeline supply failure: A coping strategy. J Clin Monit 7:39, 1991, reproduced with permission.)

ing compressed gas (Fig. 13-9). Main line piping carries gas to secondary piping that directs gas vertically up "risers" or across branch "lateral" lines. Engineers use smaller diameter pipe as outlets are placed further from the main inlet to maintain a constant pressure of 50 psig.

□ ZONE VALVES

A system of partitioning off branches of the system is required. Zone valves are strategically installed to allow isolation of outlets in a certain area or zone (Fig. 13-10). Valves are required immediately adjacent to anesthetizing areas, life-support rooms, or intensive care units, to shut down in case of leak, for repair, or in case of a fire. Practitioners must secure alternative gas sources for patients before closing a zone valve.

□ POTENTIAL PROBLEMS

Following regulations prevents most problems that occur in pipeline systems; for example, the use of seamless type K or L copper or brass pipe, secured by independent supports. Soldered or brazed connections must first be inspected and tested to insure that they are leak free. New or modified systems require a special cleaning procedure to remove bits of flux, corrosion, or rust. Each gas system is individually tested to confirm its capability by charging it to 1.5 times its working pressure and confirming that it can hold pressure for 24 hours. Adding a new section to an existing system requires making multiple measurements to confirm the proper gas flows from the specific labeled outlet. Errors have occurred and are the source of litigation and unsatisfactory publicity if one gives critically ill patients air or nitrous oxide instead of oxygen.

□ STATION OUTLETS

Station outlets provide individual access to pipeline gas. Numerous types of connectors provide access to the gas; most common are the quick connect style. The NFPA and CGA regulations have caused the development of noninterchangeable gas connectors incorporating automatic shutoff valves. Most manufacturers have some sort of plunger that is inserted into a spring-loaded station outlet. Normally the male connector is

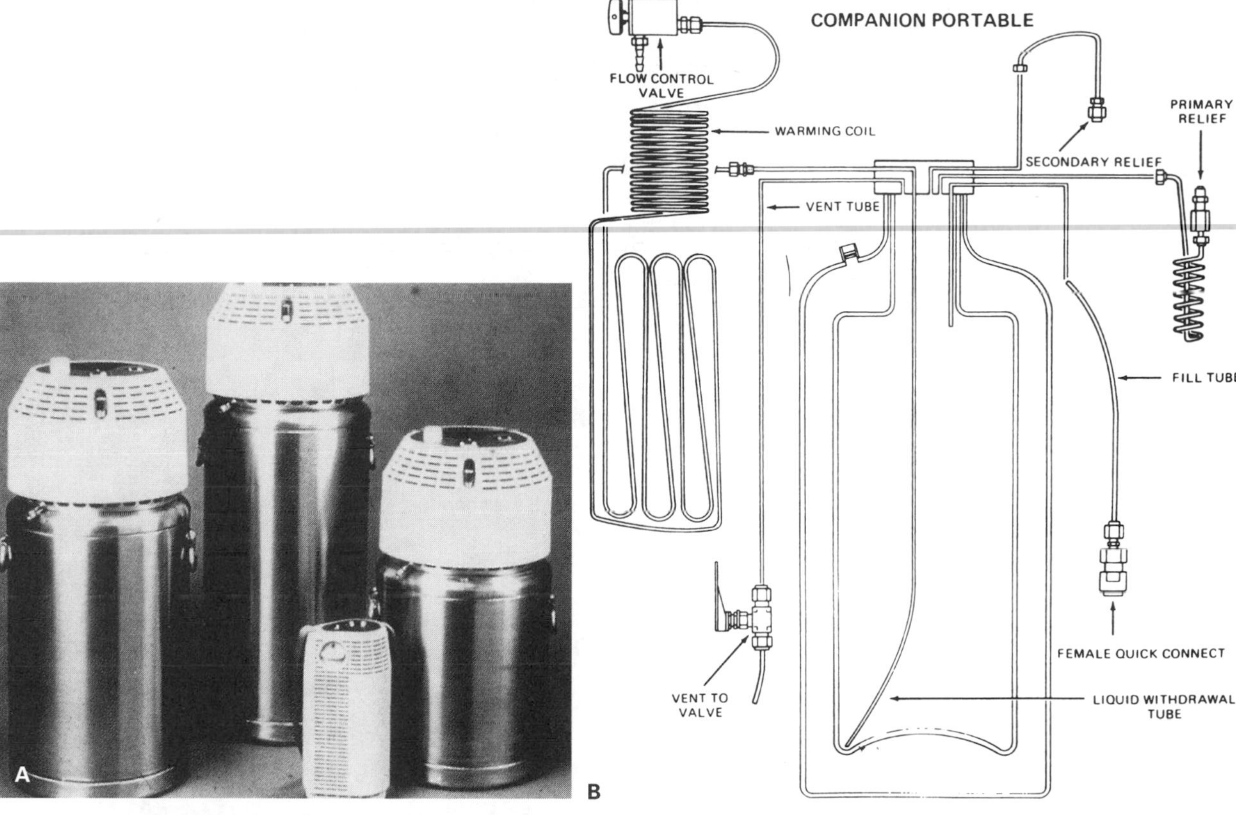

FIGURE 13-7. **(A)** Home liquid oxygen reservoir and portable reservoir. **(B)** Schematic of portable reservoir (From Langenderfer R, Branson R. Compressed Gases: Manufacture, storage and piping systems. In: Branson RD, Hess DR, Chatburn RL. (eds) Respiratory Care Equipment. Philadelphia: JB Lippincott, 1995. With permission.)

held in place until a button or collar is activated to allow release. Adapters that allow different types of outlet connectors to be used are available. Also, many of the connectors are color coded similar to cylinders, and all have the specific gas type printed on them.

Medical Gas Cylinders

As early as the 1890s, cylinders were used to store compressed oxygen and other gases. They continue to be used substantially in medical care today despite piped gas supply systems. Properly handled, they are quite safe, and small cylinders offer portability for patient transport or ambulation. Today the cost of cylinder gas is quite reasonable; however, the cylinders themselves are expensive. The containers, their storage, handling, and fittings are carefully regulated because of potential hazards. Danger is present if gas under considerable pressure is suddenly released, or if flammable gases or gases that augment combustion are released in a fire.

□ CONSTRUCTION

Oxygen cylinders are constructed of high-quality alloy steel and usually spun into shape while the steel is still hot. A 3A designation indicates non–heat-treated and 3AA

EQUATION BOX 13-3

CALCULATING DURATION OF LIQUID RESERVOIR

Constants:
One volume of liquid expands to 860 volumes of gaseous oxygen.
One liter of liquid oxygen weighs 2.5 lb (1.1 kg).

$$\text{Step 1. Gas remaining (L)} = \frac{\text{liquid weight (lbs)} \times 860}{2.5 \text{ lbs/L}}$$

$$\text{Step 2. Duration of contents (min)} = \frac{\text{gas remaining (L)}}{\text{flow (L/min)}}$$

Example: A patient adds 2 lb of liquid oxygen to his or her portable reservoir. How long will this last if the oxygen appliance is set at 1.5 L/min?

$$\text{Step 1. Gas remaining} = \frac{2 \text{ lbs} \times 860}{2.5 \text{ lb/L}} = 688 \text{ L}$$

$$\text{Step 2. Duration of contents} = \frac{688 \text{ L}}{2 \text{ L/min}} = 344 \text{ min}$$

$$\text{Duration of contents (h)} = \frac{344 \text{ min}}{60 \text{ min/h}} = 5 \text{ h } 44 \text{ min}$$

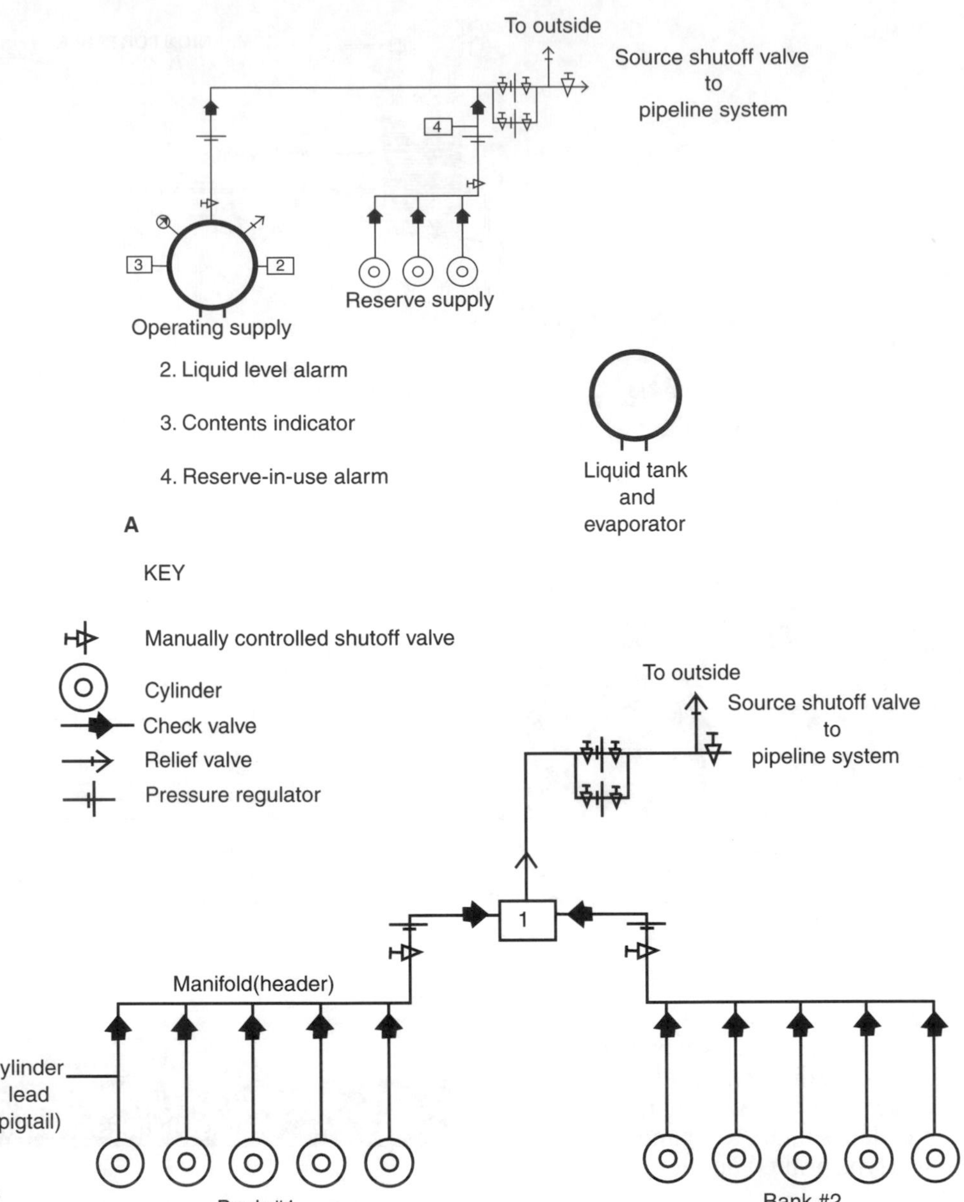

FIGURE 13-8. **(A)** Schematic of bulk oxygen supply with cylinder reserve. A fixed liquid oxygen reservoir serves as the main supply. A reserve supply is composed of either liquid or compressed gas cylinders or a fixed second bulk system. (From Dorsch JA, Dorsch SE: Understanding Anesthesia Equipment. 3rd ed. Baltimore, MD: Williams & Wilkins, 1994. With permission.) **(B)** Diagram of a double cylinder bank pipeline supply with alternating supply. The operator selects either bank by control #1. The alternate bank will automatically function as a reserve supply.

heat-treated steel. Aluminum cylinders have become popular recently because their weight is one half that of steel cylinders. They are also labeled 3A yet they too have a working pressure of 2015 psig (13,893 kPa). However, if aluminum cylinders are exposed to high temperatures (more than 400°F [204°C]), the metal loses its elastic properties and is more subject to rupture than steel. Aluminum cylinders must be retested every 5 years.

The Federal Department of Transportation (DOT) requires that all cylinder gas contents be identified by label, and unlabeled cylinders should be returned to the vendor. In addition, the cylinder itself is identified by stampings on the front and back shoulders below the cylinder valve (Fig. 13-11).[30]

☐ SAFE HANDLING

The DOT and the CGA offer the following general rules for safe handling of high-pressure gas cylinders:[30]

- No petroleum-based lubricants should come in contact with cylinder valves, regulators, high-pressure gas hoses, or fittings.
- Never use open flames to detect leaks, but use solutions of a leak detector or soapy water.

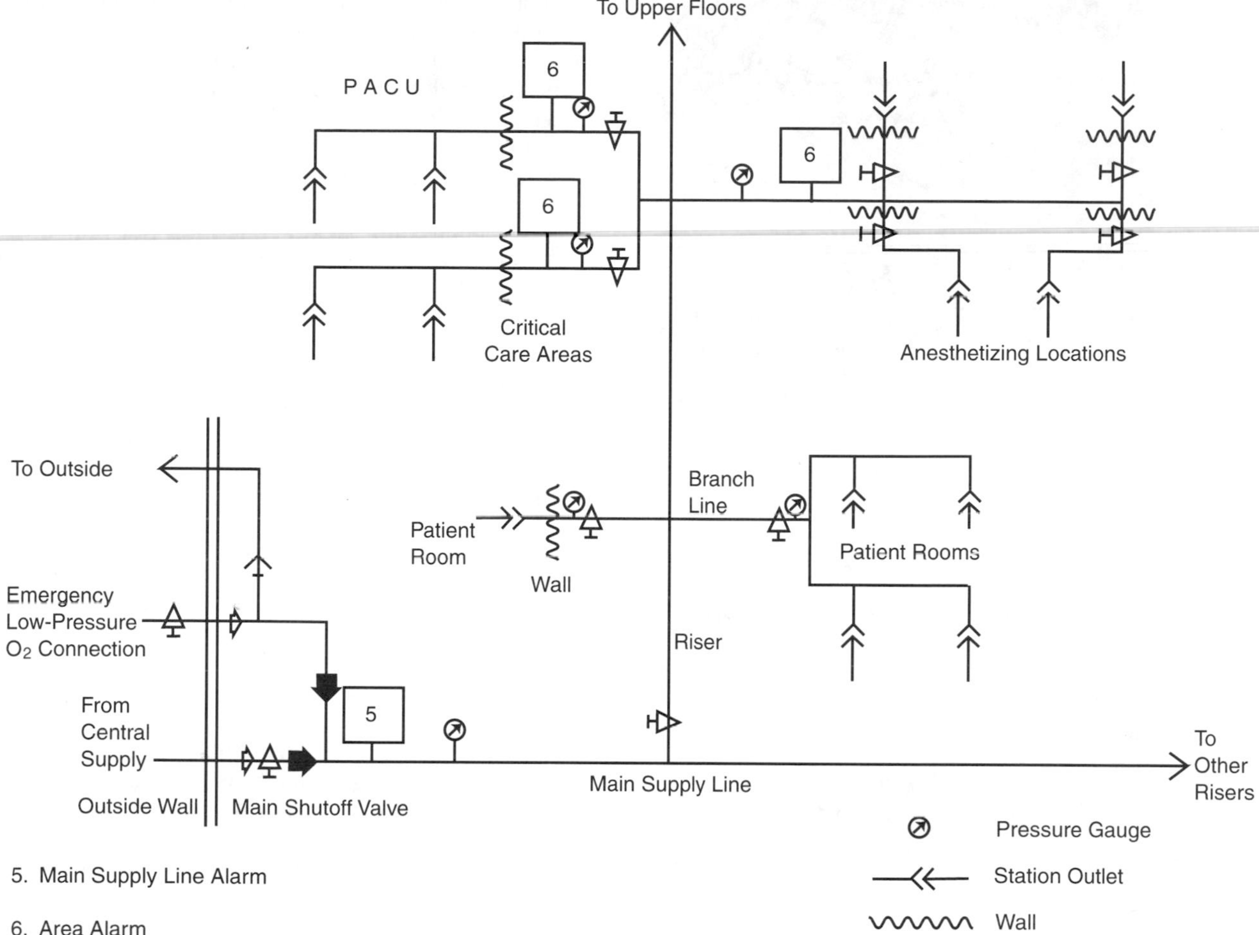

FIGURE 13-9. Schematic diagram of a typical hospital pipeline system showing check and zone valving. (From Dorsch JA, Dorsch SE: Understanding Anesthesia Equipment. 3rd ed. Baltimore, MD: Williams & Wilkins, 1994. With permission.)

- Never interchange regulators that are not intended for use with that specific gas or gas blend.
- Open valves on cylinders or regulators slowly to allow dissipation of heat. Valves should be opened fully for use.
- Unlabeled cylinders should be returned to the vendor.
- Cylinders should not be subjected to temperatures exceeding 54.4°C or put in areas with flames or sparks.
- Do not attempt to modify or repair cylinders.
- Cylinder valves should remain in the closed position when not in actual operation.
- Cylinder valve caps (found on larger cylinders) should remain on when in storage or when being transported.
- Do not drop cylinders, and move them only with suitable carts with capability of securing the cylinder via chain.

☐ STORAGE

The following are guidelines from the NFPA regarding proper storage of high-pressure medical gas cylinders:[34]

- Cylinders should be stored in locations that meet NFPA standards with regard to physical construction and materials. The area should be cool, dry, and well ventilated.
- Full and empty cylinders should be stored in separate areas to prevent confusion as to their status.
- Flame-resistant wall partitions should be used.
- Large cylinders should be restrained from being knocked over by chain or other style of physical restraint.
- Cylinder areas should be locked to prevent unauthorized use or tampering.

☐ SIZE DESIGNATIONS, SPECIFICATIONS, AND CAPACITIES

Cylinder manufacturers designate letter codes to indicate the size and potential gas capacity (Table 13-2). The most common sizes are the H or K and the E cylinders (Fig. 13-12). Those sizes with letter designation AA through E are used a great deal because they are relatively portable sources of medical gas. The operating room uses AA through E for anesthetic gases and the

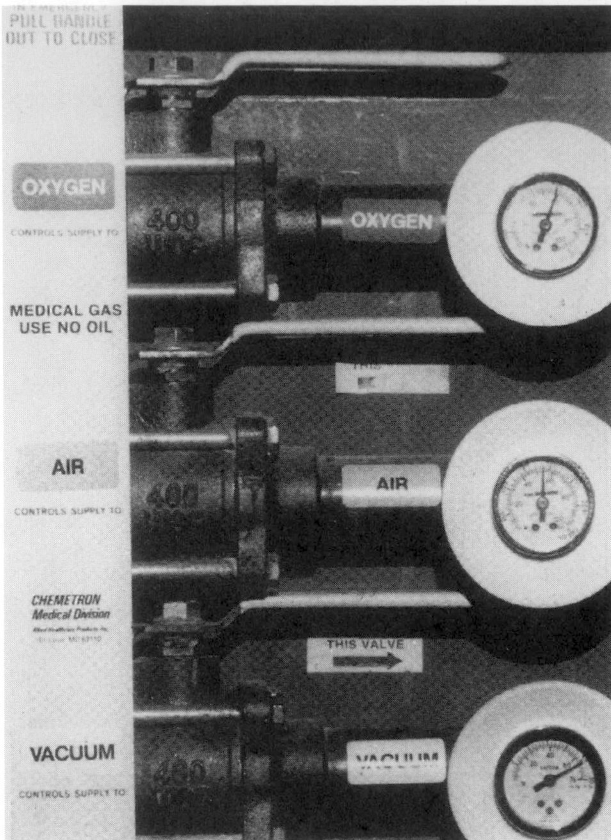

FIGURE 13-10. Zone valves for air, oxygen, and vacuum. (From Langenderfer R, Branson R. Compressed Gases: Manufacture, storage and piping systems. In: Branson RD, Hess DR, Chatburn RL. eds. Respiratory Care Equipment. Philadelphia: JB Lippincott, 1995. With permission.)

laboratory uses them for calibration gases. This group employs a yoke-style connection to mount regulators on the cylinder valve (Fig. 13-13A). Manufacturers have agreed on a system of varying the position of yoke alignment pins for various types of gases (Fig. 13-14). Only regulators for that gas can be mounted. A hand-tightening screw forces the yoke inlet into the cylinder valve outlet, with a plastic ring gasket helping to provide a seal (Fig. 13-14). Large cylinders use a threaded connection (see Fig. 13-14), different threads, sizes of connecting nipples, and thread direction on the valve outlets to guard against misconnection (Fig. 13-15).

Using different colored paint is another method of identifying cylinder gases used in the United States and Canada (Table 13-3), although the cylinder label is a more reliable guide.[38] Cylinders are tested and checked for their integrity every 5 years (3A and 3AA high-pressure containers) unless the markings are followed by a star, in which case they are tested every 10 years. All aluminum cylinders are inspected every 5 years.

The owner of the cylinder is required to follow DOT standards for cylinder inspection, several of which are presented below:[31]

- Visual inspection of external and internal surfaces is used to detect arc burns, dents, bulging, gouges, rust, or corrosion. Loose scale should be removed from the cylinder interior.
- Hammer or dead ring testing (upon each refilling) is used to detect any dampening of the normal 2- to 3-second ring when struck with a hammer. If dampening occurs, fire damage, corrosion, or oil or water contamination should be suspected.
- Hydrostatic testing involves immersing a cylinder in a special water jacket container, both filled with water. An initial water level is noted when the water-filled cylinder is under no pressure. Water pressure inside the cylinder is increased to an excess of 3000 psig (20,685 kPa), and the amount of water displaced by the cylinder expansion is measured. Loss of the compliance of the steel or aluminum is a sign of aging. The elastic expansion information is stamped following the test along with the date and inspector's mark.

Filling a gas cylinder from another gas cylinder, usually portable cylinders from larger ones, is called transfilling. This procedure differs from the practice of most medical gas vendors who use large stores, usually liquid, to fill a group of cylinders at one time. Transfilling has met with some resistance, and some older publications (eg, the CGA) forbade the practice by hospital or nonprofessional workers. Problems occur because of the tremendous energy release as gas passes from the full to empty cylinder, causing heat due to recompression. In addition, there is risk of contamination of gas. Labels and inspection of the cylinder being transfilled must be in accordance with DOT standards. They suggest using a gas control unit to (1) isolate the supply cylinder, (2) limit the filling rate to 200 psig/min, and (3) offer calibrated pressure gauges on the cylinder being filled. They also suggest that the system be mounted on a wall or installed on a portable cart.[40]

□ DURATION OF CYLINDER GAS FLOW

Providers of gas therapy cannot always expect a pipeline outlet to be readily available, and cylinders must be used in transport, during pipeline failure or inaccessibility of wall outlets. To calculate the remaining volumes of cylinder gas, or duration at a specific flow, requires data in both English and metric units. Cylinders are commonly sized by cubic foot, (ft^3); gas is administered in liters per minute (L/min). Cylinders of pure carbon dioxide and nitrous oxide contain a mixture of liquid and gas and must be weighed to determine remaining contents. Their cylinder pressures will remain constant until the last bit of liquid evaporates. Equation Box 13-4 describes the two-step calculation for gaseous (only) cylinders. Table 13-4 lists factors for cylinder duration calculation.

□ GAS CYLINDER SAFETY

To decrease the possibility for inadvertent administration of the wrong therapeutic gases, a system using color coding, labels, and connection devices is used. However, despite such measures, problems have oc-

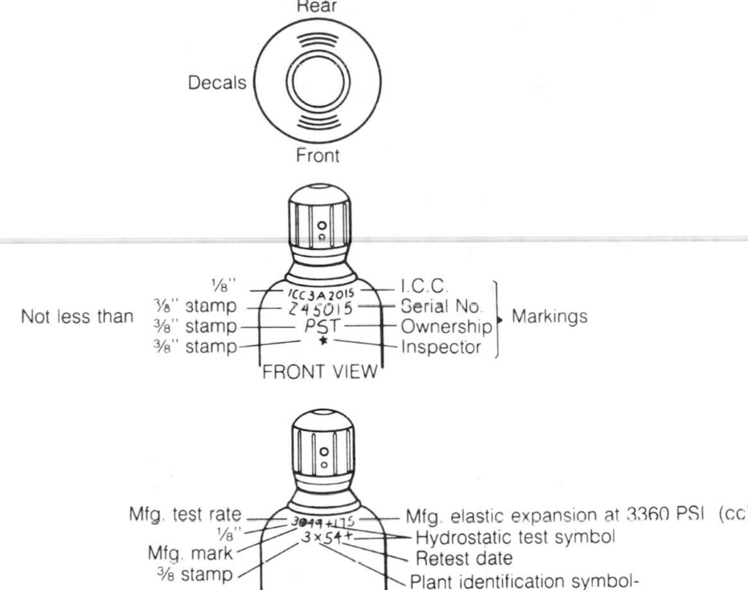

FIGURE 13-11. High-pressure medical gas cylinder stampings and their significance. (From Ward JJ. Equipment for mixed gas and oxygen therapy. In: Barnes TA. (ed) Core Textbook of Respiratory Care Practice, 2nd ed. St. Louis: CV Mosby, 1994. With permission.)

curred because of difficulties with the manufacturer, gas distributor, or user. Box 13-5 identifies such incidents.

Much of the safety system involves the manufacturer's use of the cylinder valve. The most common high-pressure type of valve is the direct-acting style. As the operator turns the outer stem or valve wheel, the screw-like movement is reflected in the opening or closing of the area above the valve seat. A threaded needle-type valve plunger moves away from or toward the valve seat as the valve wheel turns.

For cylinder safety in hazardous environmental conditions, the body of the valve contains a built-in pressure-release device. If a cylinder is exposed to fire or heat that raises its internal pressure to 1.5 times its working pressure (normal working pressure 2025 psig), a safety valve opens and vents the gas. This response prevents the cylinder wall from exploding. Some valves use a frangible (breakable) or fusible (meltable) metal plug or a combination of the disk and the plug. Wood's metal is commonly used for the fusible plug material. It is an alloy of bismuth, lead, cadmium, and tin. It will yield when the temperature reaches 208°F (97.8°C) to 220°F (104°C). Copper is used as frangible disk material.

TABLE 13-2. **Medical Gas Cylinder Code Designations, Specifications, and Capacities**

Letter Designation	Dimensions (in)	Weight (lb)	Volume (ft³/L)
A	3 × 10.5	2.5	2.5/75.7
B	3.75 × 16.5	5.75	5/151
D	4.2 × 20	7	12.6/356
E	4.2 × 30	9	22/622
M	7 × 47	27	106/3000
G	8.5 × 55	100	186/3000
H or K	9 × 55	132	244/6900

Data from Reference 30. Cylinder capacities and dimensions may vary slightly among manufacturers.

Standard Valve Outlet Connections

The outlets of cylinder valves are manufactured so that only the regulator or connector specific for that gas or mixture can be attached (see Fig. 13-15). The American Standards Association specifies indexing for the cylinder connections (larger than E), and the CGA publishes these industry standards. For example, an oxygen cylinder with 0.903-14-RH Ext. indicates:

- Diameter of the threaded outlet in inches
- Number of threads per inch
- Whether it's right- or left-handed threaded
- Whether the regulator's mating nut is internal or external to the cylinder's outlet.

Left-handed threads are reserved for gases such as carbon monoxide, hydrogen, pure helium, and mixtures with less than 20% oxygen (toxic gases or those not capable of supporting life). Recently the CGA and DOT have implemented new connection standards for laboratory gases. In the past, cylinder valve to regulator connectors were available. "Cheaters" allowed the use of one regulator on almost any mixture. Because of the danger involved in this practice, the CGA 504 or 500 series connections were developed.

Pin Index Safety System

Small cylinders (AA through E) that use the yoke and post-type of valve use the Pin Index Safety System (PISS) (see Fig. 13-14).

Diameter Index Safety System

Practitioners who work with medical gas systems must be familiar with the *Diameter Index Safety System (DISS)*. The CGA system is based on the diameter of

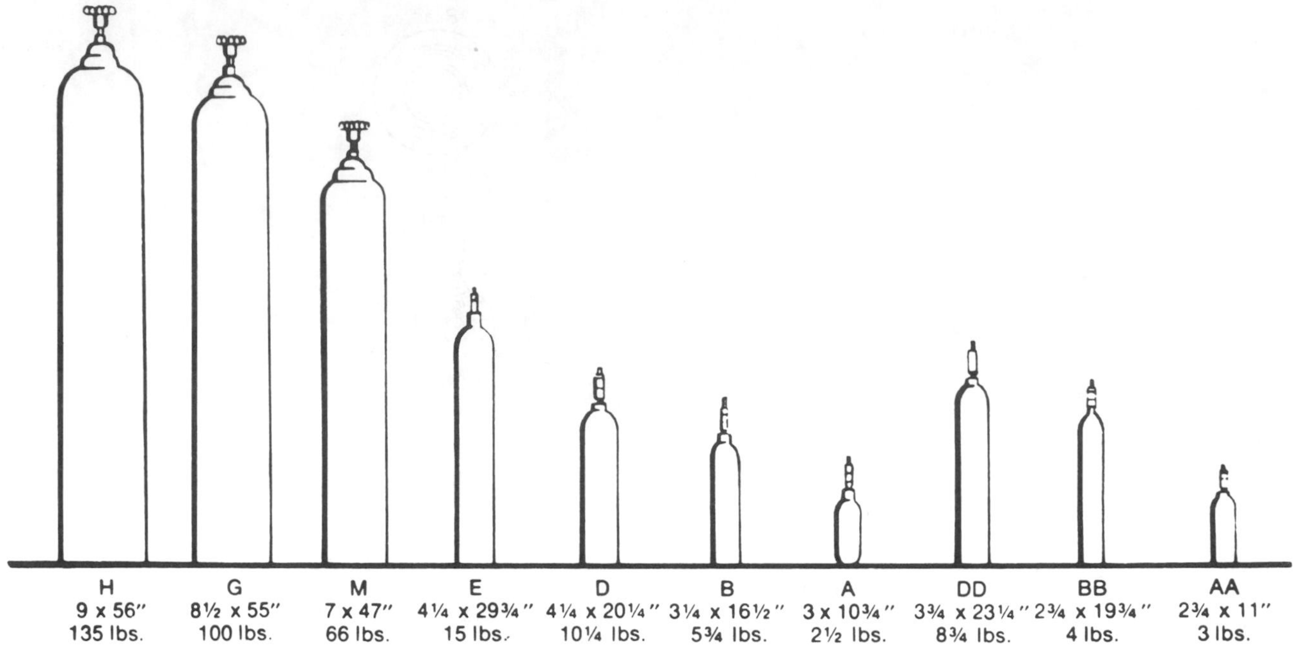

FIGURE 13-12. Letter designation and approximate dimensions of high-pressure medical gas cylinders. (From Ward JJ. Equipment for mixed gas and oxygen therapy. In: Barnes TA. (ed) Core Textbook of Respiratory Care Practice, 2nd ed. St. Louis: CV Mosby, 1994. With permission.).

threaded gas connections subjected to 200 psig or less. Hence, the fittings from medical gas regulators, flowmeters, oxygen concentrators, and high-pressure hoses have specific-diameter threaded connections. The CGA No. 022 DISS 9/16"-diameter threaded swivel fitting allows connection of either air or oxygen flowmeters to nipple adaptors, humidifiers, and/or mainstream nebulizers. Clinicians must be aware that potential misconnection is possible. When two gases are used on a single piece of equipment, such as an oxygen-air blender or mechanical ventilator, the DISS connections have noninterchangeable fittings unique to that gas or gas mixture.

Regulators (Pressure-Reducing Valves)

Gas pressure regulators or reducing valves are used throughout medical gas pipeline systems and with high-pressure gas cylinders. They step down inlet pressures to specific pressure requirements such as 50 psig for U.S. medical facilities. Regulators also modulate the effect of pressure decay as a cylinder is depleted of its gas.

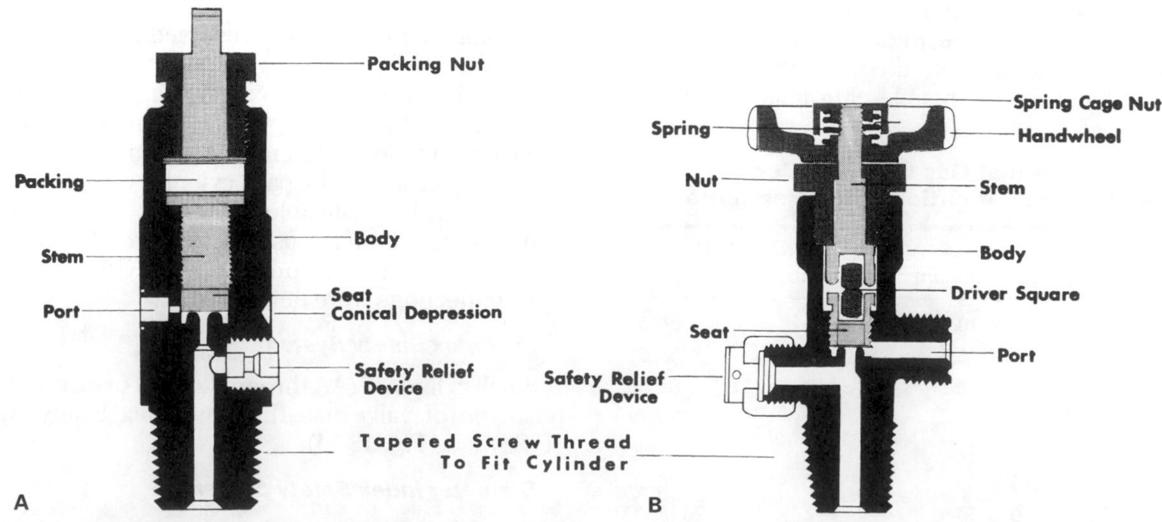

FIGURE 13-13. **(A)** Diagram of small yoke-style valve (sizes AA-E) and **(B)** Large American Standard Cylinder valve (sizes M-H). (From Dorsch JA, Dorsch SE. Understanding Anesthesia Equipment. 3rd ed. Baltimore, MD: Williams & Wilkins, 1994. With permission.)

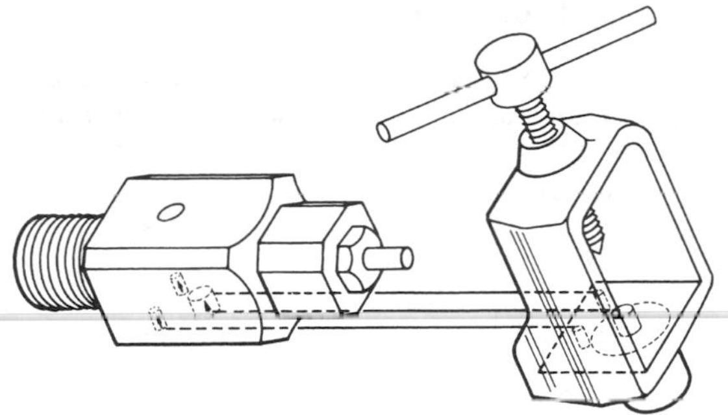

FIGURE 13-14. Diagram of Pin Index Safety System pin alignment. (From Ward JJ: Equipment for mixed gas and oxygen therapy. In: Barnes T (ed) Core Textbook of Respiratory Care Practice. 2nd ed. St. Louis: Mosby, 1994:382. With permission.)

TABLE 13-3. **Color Markings**

Intended Gas	Color
Oxygen (O_2)	Green
Carbon dioxide (CO_2)	Gray
Nitrous oxide (N_2O)	Blue
Cyclopropane ($(CH_2)_3$)	Orange or chrome
Helium (He)	Brown
Ethylene (C_2H_4)	Red
Carbon dioxide and oxygen (CO_2/O_2)	Gray and green
Helium and oxygen (He/O_2)	Brown and green
Nitrogen (N_2)	Black
Air	Yellow
Mixtures of nitrogen and oxygen	Black and green

□ THEORY OF OPERATION

The principle of regulator design is known as the *Pascal principle*, and operation can be explained simply by a playground teeter-totter. By varying the distance of the lever arms on either side of a balance point, a lighter child can balance a heavy one. In regulators, instead of different lengths of lever arms, the size of two different surface areas are varied, each being exposed to different gas pressures.

A cylinder's high gas pressure (P_c), is balanced by a lower regulated pressure (P_r) because the area subjected to the high pressure (A_1) is very small compared with the area (A_2) of a flexible diaphragm (Fig. 13-16). As the orifice at A_1 opens, gas fills a chamber, and it can exert force on only one side, the diaphragm A_2. P_r indicates the level of reduced pressure. V represents a needle valve or on/off valve, allowing gas to flow from the regulator. Equation Box 13-5 describes the calculation of the reduced pressure.

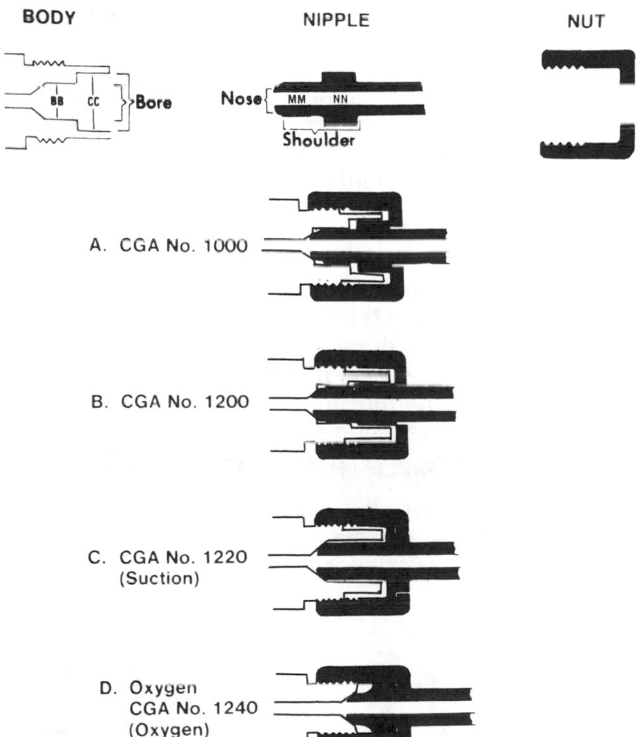

FIGURE 13-15. Valve outlet connections for large cylinders showing use of nut, thread, and nipple to set specifications for different gases. (From Dorsch JA, Dorsch SE. Understanding Anesthesia Equipment. 3rd ed. Baltimore, MD: Williams & Wilkins, 1994. With permission.)

There are limits to the areas used because of the flexibility of metal diaphragms. Various improvements are used in commercially manufactured regulators. By adding springs to counteract the diaphragm distortion and to seal nozzle jets, the regulator maintains a more constant pressure as it empties.

Regulators are categorized as either direct- or indirect-acting as well as single and multiple stage. A direct-acting regulator is shown in Figure 13-17A in the closed and open positions. As the pressure-adjusting screw is tightened, the diaphragm is displaced and gas is allowed to flow. As the cylinder pressure lessens with use, the operator must reduce spring tension or the gas flow will also decrease. The indirect style is shown in Figure 13-17B. Its operation is similar, but because of the inverted placement of the thrust pin connected to the diaphragm, gas flow will slightly increase as gas pressure decays. Single stage regulators are sufficient for simple medical gas applications. Multiple stages in regulators of either type modulate the changes and offer smoother operation.

□ REGULATOR RELIEF SYSTEMS

Because of the high pressures to which the contents of a regulator are subjected, manufacturers build in pressure relief valves or similar devices. Usually there is one for each stage of the regulator. Normally, increased pressure in the regulator chamber tends to close the nozzle that holds pressure constant. However, if debris or a mechanical failure prevents this normal valve closure, the device connected to that regulator could be exposed to higher pressure than normal. Also, rupture of metallic parts may discharge shrapnel toward the operator or patient.

EQUATION BOX 13-4

CALCULATING DURATION OF CYLINDER GAS

A key piece of information is the factor to convert from cubic feet to liters (patient administration units):

$$1 \text{ ft}^3 = 28.3 \text{ L}$$

Step 1. Find the factor that converts cylinder pressure drop to liters of gas released. The factor varies with cylinder volume. (Table 13-4)

$$\text{Conversion factor (any cylinder)} = \frac{\text{ft}^3 \text{ in full cylinder} \times 28.3 \text{ L/ft}^3}{\text{pressure in full cylinder (psig)}}$$

for an "E-size" cylinder

$$\text{Conversion factor (E size)} = \frac{22 \text{ ft}^3 \times 28.3 \text{ L/ft}^3}{2200 \text{ psig}} = 0.28 \text{ L/psig}$$

$$\text{Conversion factor (Using SI units)} = \frac{22 \text{ ft}^3 \times 28.3 \text{ L/ft}^3}{15{,}168 \text{ kPa}} = 0.041 \text{ L/kPa}$$

Step 2. Multiplying the cylinder factor by the remaining gas pressure determines total liters available. Dividing that product by the flow (L/min) results in the remaining time (min).

$$\text{Time remaining (minutes)} = \frac{\text{actual cylinder pressure} \times \text{conversion factor}}{\text{oxygen flow}} = \frac{\text{psig} \times \text{L/psig}}{\text{L/min}} \text{ or } \frac{\text{kPa} \times \text{L/kPa}}{\text{L/min}} = \text{min}$$

Example: How long will a full E cylinder (2200 psig) last at a CPR event, if flow to the resuscitation bag is 10 L/min?

$$\text{Time remaining (minutes)} = \frac{2200 \text{ psig} \times 0.28 \text{ L/psig}}{10 \text{ L/min}}$$

$$\text{or } \frac{15{,}168 \text{ kPa} \times 0.41 \text{ L/kPa}}{10 \text{ L/min}}$$

$$= 308 \text{ min} = \frac{308 \text{ min}}{60 \text{ min/hr}} = 5.13 \text{ h or 8 h and 8 min}$$

There are two basic types of regulator relief systems. The most obvious is the external spring-loaded valve with an adjustable stud. It allows venting the reduction chamber to the atmosphere. Adjustment is made with an Allen wrench. Leak detector solution is placed over the safety valve, and the wrench loosens the spring until it begins to leak gas. The wrench is advanced just until bubbles cease.

An internal pressure relief system uses a second spring located near the main spring. When pressures exceed safe levels, the diaphragm is allowed to lift away from the regulator chamber body, thus releasing the gas. It is not easily adjustable. Leakage may indicate a damaged or dirty diaphragm sealing gasket or warn spring. Relief pressures for either type of relief valve are commonly set in the 140 to 200 psig range.

TABLE 13-4. **Factors to Compute Cylinder Duration**

Letter Size Designation	Factor (L/psig drop)
D	0.16
E	0.28
M	1.36
G	2.41
H or K	3.14

$$\text{Duration} = \frac{\text{actual gauge pressure (psig)} \times \text{factor (L/psig)}}{\text{flow (1/min)}}$$

Another necessary component of a pressure regulator are the gauges that indicate the remaining pressure in the cylinder and/or in its reduction chamber. Only adjustable regulators require a second gauge. The typical gauge registers pressure by converting the movement of a "crooked," dead-ended, compliant metal tube. The straightening, reflecting higher pressure is referred by a connecting rod to a set of gears. They turn an indicator needle on a calibrated background scale. Different ranges of pressure reading can be designed by varying the stiffness of the metal.

A range of different applications of cylinder gases require several different options for regulators and outlets. For a regulator to provide high-pressure gas to operate a mechanical ventilator, only a quick-connect connection is needed. However, if oxygen appliances require gas flows to be measured, a flowmeter can be temporarily or permanently attached to the regulator.

Flowmeters

Flowmeters are devices that permit controlled release of gas and metering of the flow (volume per time). The indication of flow is done indirectly by various techniques. The major types of flowmeter vary by the physical principles of their design.

☐ PHYSICAL PRINCIPLES RELATED TO ORIFICES

Flowmeters are designed based on physics of gas flow through holes (orifices) and tubes. An orifice can be thought of as tube with hardly any length. The type

BOX 13-5

REPORTED HAZARDOUS INCIDENTS INVOLVING CYLINDERS

- Incorrect cylinder color coding[41]
- Incorrect cylinder label[42]
- Incorrect gas filling/contents[43]
- Incorrect valve/yoke[44]

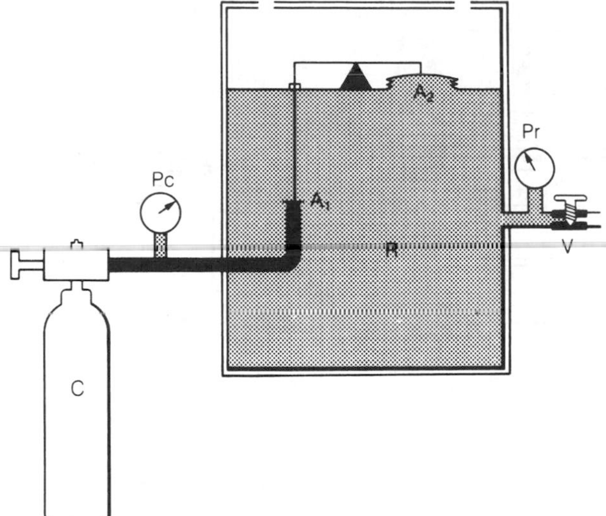

FIGURE 13-16. Schematic drawing of basic regulator. (From Ward JJ. Equipment for mixed gas and oxygen therapy. In: Barnes TA (ed.) Core Textbook of Respiratory Care Practice, 2nd ed. St. Louis: CV Mosby, 1994. With permission.)

of flow seen through a fixed-orifice device may be turbulent or laminar depending on a number of variables. Six factors determine or effect the behavior of gases flowing through an orifice.

1. Reynold's number (N_R) predicts the type of flow pattern that results for any given flow and tube or orifice. It is the ratio of the force of momentum within the fluid (gas) to the force of viscous friction.

$$N_R = \frac{4 \times \text{density} \times \text{flow}}{\pi \times \text{viscosity} \times \text{diameter}}$$

   Reynold's number is dimensionless yet indicates whether the flow is laminar (<2300) or turbulent (>2500). Intermediate values show a mixed pattern. Density plays a greater role in orifices, and viscosity determines flow patterns in tubes.[45]

2. The flow of gas through an orifice is proportional to the square root of the pressure difference across the orifice, that is, the head of pressure.

$$\text{Flow} \propto \sqrt{P_1 - P_2}$$

   Flow increases or decreases, respectively, if upstream source pressure applied to the proximal side of the orifice (P_2) is changed. The pressure distal (downstream) to the orifice in most medical applications will approximate atmospheric pressure. However, if an additional device is attached to the orifice, which increases P_2 by impeding flow, the $P_1 - P_2$ relationship will be distorted. The outlet flow decreases proportionally to this decrease in the pressure gradient. This concept identifies limitations of the Bourdon gauge and non-pressure compensated Thorpe tube flowmeters, which are described later.

3. Flow through an orifice is proportional to the square of the diameter of the opening. If pressures at P_1 and P_2 are constants, the flow varies exponentially as the opening is increased or decreased. This principle forms the basis of flowmeters using a constant source pressure with either fixed or variable orifices.

$$\text{Flow} \propto (\text{Diameter})2$$

4. Flow through an orifice is proportional to the inverse of the square root of the density of the gas. If pressure and the diameter are constant, flow increases with lower-density gases and vice versa.

$$\text{Flow} \propto \frac{1}{\sqrt{\text{Density}}}$$

   This relationship involving density is important to consider if clinicians administer gases of different densities when using oxygen flow devices. Helium/oxygen mixtures (Heliox) are the most significant, although carbon dioxide/O_2 blends and

EQUATION BOX 13-5

CALCULATION REGULATOR PRESSURE

The following expression explains the balance of forces (note: pressure = force/unit area, and force = pressure × unit area).

$$P_c \times A_1 = P_r \times A_2$$

Solving for P_r, the reduction pressure is equal to the ratio of valve seat/diaphragm areas and the level of the pressure in the cylinder.

$$P_r = \frac{A_1}{A_2} \times P_c$$

Therefore, if the valve seat is very small and the diaphragm is made quite large (producing a small number), a substantial reduction in cylinder pressure occurs.

Example 1: What is the reduction in cylinder pressure (P_r)?

Given:

P_c = 2,200 psig

$A_1 = 2\ mm^2$

$A_2 = 4\ mm^2$

$$P_r = \frac{2\ mm^2}{4\ mm^2} \times 2200\ \text{psig}$$

P_r = 1000 psig

Example 2: What is the reduction in cylinder pressure (P_r) when the ratio of valve seat to diaphragm is greater?

Given:

P_c = 2200 psig

$A_1 = 1\ mm^2$

$A_2 = 44\ mm^2$

$$P_r = \frac{1\ mm^2}{44\ mm^2} \times 2200\ \text{psig}$$

P_r = 50 psig

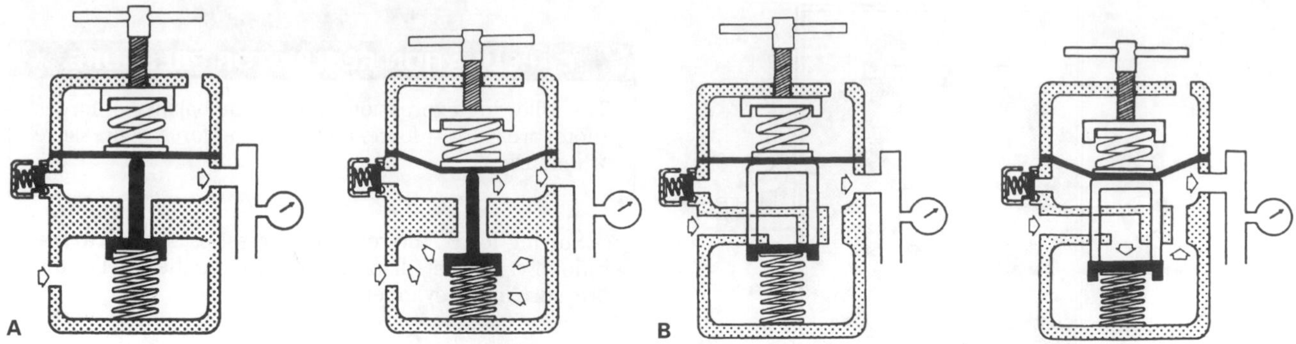

FIGURE 13-17. **(A)** Contemporary direct regulator. **(B)** Indirect regulator. (From Branson RD. Gas delivery systems: Regulators, flowmeters, and therapy devices. In: Hess DR, Chatburn RL. (eds) Respiratory Care Equipment, Philadelphia, PA: J. B. Lippincott, 1995. With permission.)

air will also vary. Equation Box 13-6 describes the calculations needed if a specific helium/oxygen flowmeter is not available and accurate flows are needed.

5. Temperature changes affect the viscosity and density of a gas. Although the effect is slight, density of a gas varies proportionally with the absolute pressures.
6. Flowmeters used at significantly different altitudes may require correction. A rough approximation of the error involved has been calculated to be about 1% for each 1000 feet (304 m) of variance from sea level. Equation Box 13-7 describes the calculation as follows:

EQUATION BOX 13-6

CALCULATING HELIUM/OXYGEN FLOW THROUGH AN OXYGEN FLOWMETER

The following illustrates the basic relationships:

Density of 80%/20% He/O_2

$$= \frac{0.80\ (\text{GMW He}) + 0.20\ (\text{GMW O}_2)}{22.4\ \text{L}}$$

$$= \frac{0.80\ (4\ \text{g}) + 0.20\ (32\ \text{g})}{22.4\ \text{L}} = 0.43\ \text{g/L}$$

$$\text{Density of 100\% oxygen} = \frac{1.0\ (\text{GMW O}_2)}{22.4\ \text{L}}$$

$$= \frac{1.0\ (32\ \text{g})}{22.4\ \text{L}} = 1.43\ \text{g/L}$$

Example: A mixture of 80%/20% helium-oxygen is being substituted in a flowmeter calibrated for oxygen. The flow of pure oxygen was 10 L/min. What will be the actual flow of heliox if no changes are made to the needle valve (orifice diameter) or gas inlet pressures (ie, 50 psig)?

$$\text{Actual flow} = \text{indicated flow} \times \frac{\sqrt{\text{density for which calibrated}}}{\sqrt{\text{density of alternate gas mixture}}}$$

$$= 10\ \text{L/min} \times \frac{\sqrt{1.43}}{\sqrt{0.43}}$$

$$= 10\ \text{L/min} \times \frac{1.20}{0.66}$$

$$= 18\ \text{L/min}$$

Therefore, for each liter of oxygen flowing through the orifice, 1.8 L of heliox exits. The actual flow of the 80%/20% He/O_2 mixture is 18 L even though the oxygen flowmeter indicates a lower value.

Fixed Orifice and Constant Pressure

The most basic flowmeter is commercially known as a flow restrictor. It is a carefully machined orifice attached to a 50-psig gas source. There are no adjustments and no gauges (Fig. 13-18A). They are of value when a fixed flow is required, a specific gas is always used, and the pressure source is stable. The most common use is in home oxygen concentrators. Other applications would be in emergency resuscitation packs where a compact, lightweight device is needed to provide relatively high flows to a bag-valve-mask device. Because there is no way to indicate to the operator what the actual flow is, flow restrictors must be periodically checked by calibration flowmeter or volume versus time spirometer. However, they are quite stable and have no moving parts. Multiple fixed-orifice flowmeters are an extension of the basic unit, with several restric-

EQUATION BOX 13-7

EQUATION TO CORRECT FLOW AT ALTITUDE

$$\text{Actual flow} = \frac{\text{Indicated flow} \times \text{Barometric pressure at sea level}}{\text{Actual barometric pressure}}$$

Example: An oxygen flowmeter calibrated at sea level is used in Denver where the barometric pressure measures 600 mmHg (80 kPa). When the indicator ball registers 5 L/min, what is the actual flow?

$$\text{Actual flow} = 5\ \text{L/min} \times \frac{760\ \text{mmHg}}{600\ \text{mmHg}}$$

$$= 5\ \text{L/min} \times 1.267$$

$$= 6.3\ \text{L/min}$$

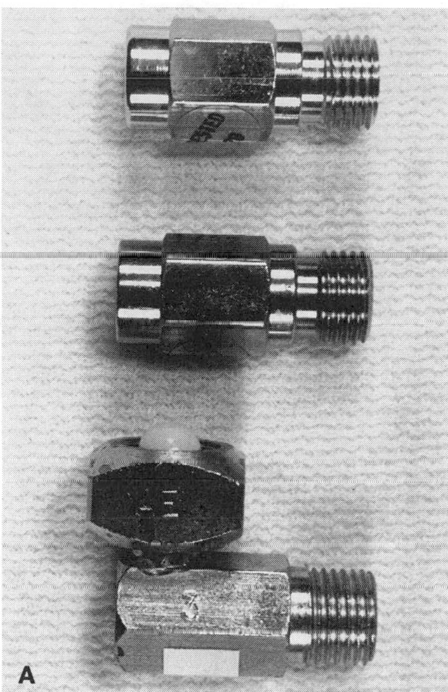

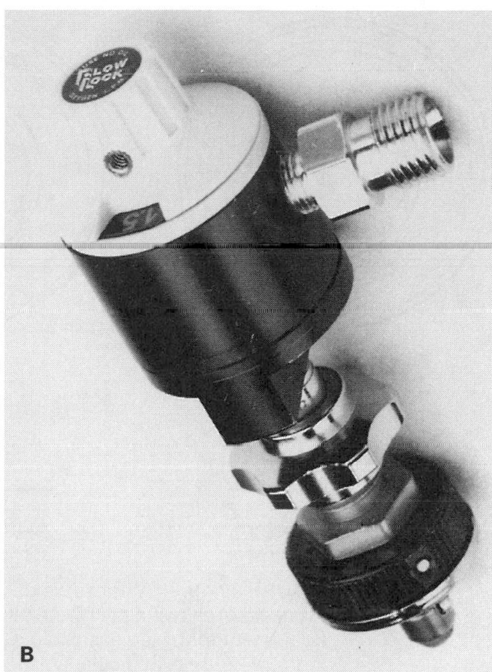

FIGURE 13-18. (A) Single-flow flow restrictors. (From Branson RD. Gas delivery systems: regulators, flowmeters, and therapy devices. In: Branson RD, Hess DR, Chatburn RL. (eds) Respiratory Care Equipment. Philadelphia: JB Lippincott, 1995. With permission.) **(B)** Adjustable flow restrictor.

tors in combination. The operator can make a selection by rotating a knob that directs gas to that orifice. Although more expensive, it offers a variety of therapeutic flows (Fig. 13-18B).

Fixed Orifice and Variable Pressure

The term Bourdon gauge flowmeter is clinically used to describe a fixed orifice placed downstream from an adjustable pressure regulator (Fig. 13-19A and B). In this design, the operator manually increases or decreases the pressure upstream to the orifice by increasing spring pressure on a variable pressure regulator. Therefore, flow varies as the square root of the pressure difference. The term "gauge" refers to the use of a recalibrated pressure gauge (identical to those recording cylinder pressure), to reflect flow as pressure changes upstream to the orifice. Clinical devices frequently have two gauges; one indicates cylinder pressure, the other flow (Fig 13-19C). Accurate flow indication is performed unless (1) the density of the gas is different from designed, or (2) impedance to gas flow out of the orifice causes an increase in distal pressure (P_1). In clinical practice, attaching a device that has an orifice smaller than that in the flowmeter itself upsets the pressure relationship used at calibration, and the crooked tube distends out of proportion to the actual flow. Thus, the indicated flow could be higher than actual. Pneumatic nebulizers are an example of such a device that should not be used with a Bourdon gauge, if accurate indication of flow rate is necessary.

Bourdon gauges are commonly used on medical gas cylinders for transport and when masks or nasal cannulas are used. These compact flowmeters are handy because flow can be changed (in contrast to flow restrictors), and they can be read correctly without being held in a vertical (gravity-dependent position).

Variable Orifice and Constant Pressure

The most common type of medical gas flowmeter has a needle valve for adjustment of flow and a hollow tube with an indicator float device. They are called a Thorpe tube or rotameter. The name rotameter implies use of a rotating bobbin or float instead of a spherical-type indicator. Rotameters are often used to administer anesthetic gases, which require greater accuracy in flow indication. Ball floats are read at their center, rotameter floats are read at the top.

The location of the needle valve in the system is the critical component of this type of device, and the flow indicator merely reflects the level of gas flow. The physics involved in confirming accurate flow indication is quite complex. It relates to Reynold's number, density and viscosity of gas, and Stokes' law of gravitational sedimentation.[45–48] The most common type of Thorpe tube positions the flow indicator tube/ball between the inlet pressure source and the needle valve (Fig. 13-20B). This position defines a design called pressure-compensated. Internal pressure changes within the float tube are not affected if the operator attaches an appliance (eg, nebulizer) with an orifice smaller than that set by the needle valve. Adding a smaller orifice, which increases impedance to flow, is similar to reducing the diameter of the flowmeter's needle valve. The actual flow decreases, and the indicator drops to a lower level reflecting new equilibrium of forces. The operator is correctly informed of the actual output flow. The pressures above and below the float were altered from the previous conditions, but the forces acting on the indicator were not distorted.

Pressure-compensated Thorpe flowmeters indicate actual flow unless:

- The source gas pressure varies from 50 psig (345 kPa).
- The flowmeter is set to deliver a higher flow than is available from its gas supply source.

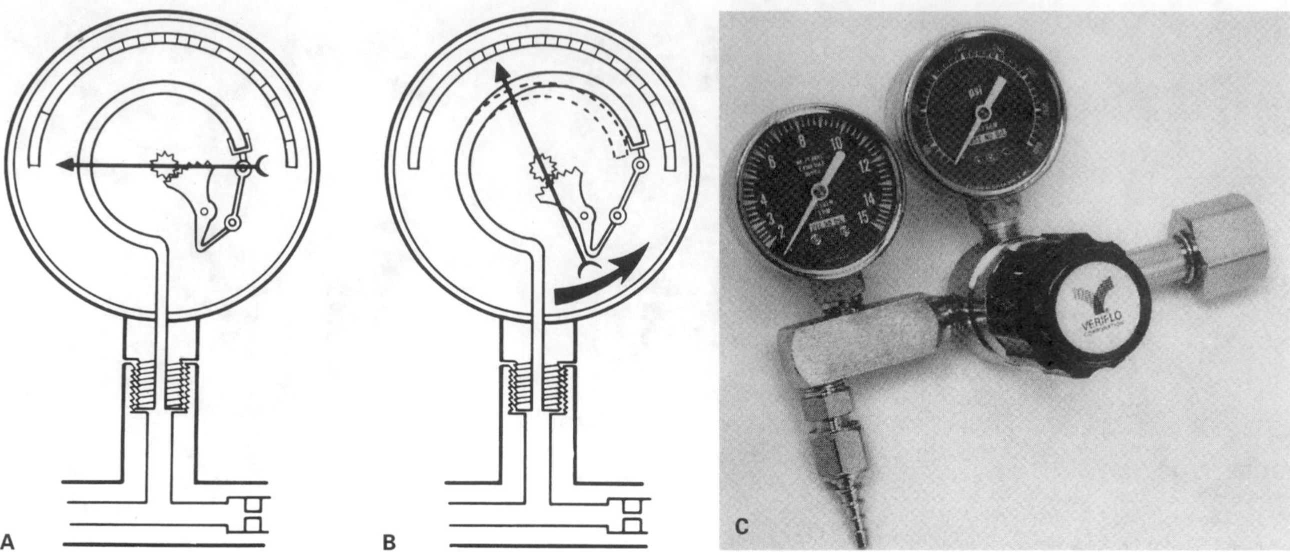

FIGURE 13-19. **(A)** Pressure gauge (back view) showing crooked tube and gearing. **(B)** Same gauge (front view) showing how tube "straightening" is translated to alter the needle position (From Ward JJ. Equipment for mixed gas and oxygen therapy. In: Barnes TA. (ed.) Core Textbook of Respiratory Care Practice, 2nd ed. St. Louis: CV Mosby, 1994. with permission). **(C)** Clinical example of a contemporary Bourdon gauge flowmeter. The gauge on the left registers flow; the one on the right provides pressure in the cylinder.

- The float tube is not set in the vertical position allowing the influence of added frictional forces.

A simple test determines if a flowmeter is pressure compensated. With the needle valve closed, connect it to the pressure source and activate the gas. If the ball jumps, it is pressure compensated, because the gas has to pass through the indicator tube before it reaches the needle valve (see Fig. 13-20).

In the past, non–pressure-compensated flowmeters were commonly used for medical applications. They are still used for laboratory or industrial applications. The difference in design is the placement of the indicator tube downstream from the needle valve (see Fig. 13-20A). Although a subtle change, the pressure and other physical factors related to flow can cause the unit to incorrectly read flow if a high resistance device is attached. This change elevates the pressure above the float and alters the physical relationships from those the manufacturer used when calibrating the flow scale. This may result in a depression of the float and an underestimation of the actual flow. There are no problems in accurate indication of flow if only low resistance devices are used, for example, nasal cannulas.

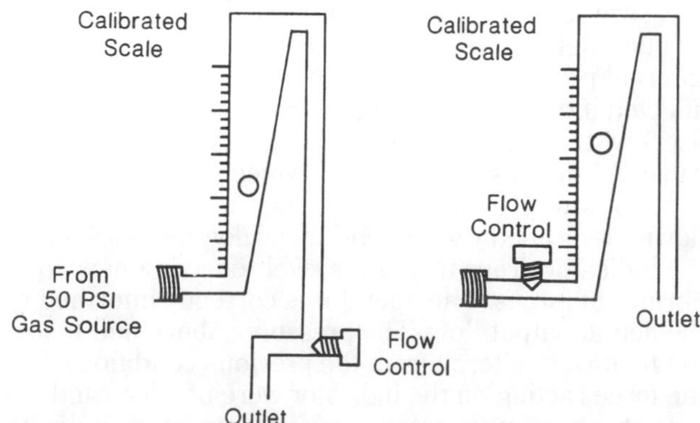

FIGURE 13-20. Pressure compensated *(left)* and non-compensated Thorpe tube flowmeter *(right)*. (From Branson RD. Gas delivery systems: Regulators, flowmeters, and therapy devices. In: Branson RD, Hess DR, Chatburn RL. (eds) Respiratory Care Equipment. Philadelphia: JB Lippincott, 1995. With permission.)

Ball-type float flowmeters should be interpreted by sighting the center of the ball against the background scale. The scale should be read at eye level to eliminate error caused by parallax. Thorpe tube flowmeters are usually quite accurate, but should be checked against another flowmeter initially and periodically when in service. The handiest method is to connect the clinical flowmeter to a calibration flowmeter designed for this purpose. They are available as electronic devices or very accurate float tube flowmeters. The flow over several different settings on the clinical unit should be identical to that on the calibration unit. Another approach is to let a flowmeter fill a volume displacement type of spirometer, commonly found in pulmonary function laboratories. Since flow is volume per time, read the flow directly or calculate it as the slope of the tracing on a volume/time kymographic recording.

If a flowmeter reads differently than its actual output, it should be repaired. Fouled sintered metal inlet filters, leaky O-rings, and cracked float tubes are components that result in inaccuracy. Needle valve seats are the most common area for wear. Needle valves should be closed before the units are connected to gas sources to avoid additional wear.

The majority of clinical flowmeters are scaled from 0 to 16 L/min. Setting such flowmeters at 1 to 2 L/min to

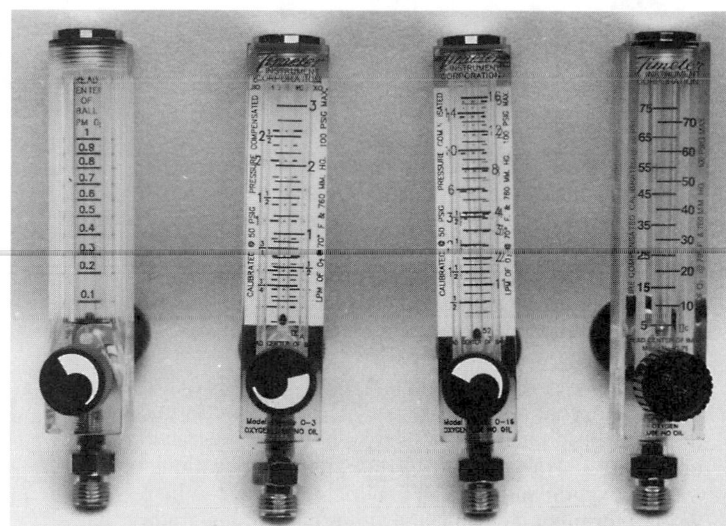

FIGURE 13-21. Examples of pressure-compensated Thorpe tubes. (from left to right: 0-1 L/min, 0-3 L/min, 0-16 L/min and 0-75 L/min.)

administer low concentrations via nasal cannula requires a delicate touch. Need for more accurate reading of low flows for infants and oxygen-sensitive adult patients fostered development of 0 to 1 L/min or 0 to 5 L/min units. Manufacturers also provide units with dual or expanded scales for more accurate reading at low-flows. Most Thorpe type flowmeters also have a flush position beyond the calibrated range. There is no industry standard; most provide greater than 60 L/min. High-flow oxygen delivery systems (requiring calibrated flow measurements) have prompted manufacturers to develop 0 to 75 L/min Thorpe tubes. They are popular in continuous positive airway pressure (CPAP) systems or with oxygen-air blenders. Dual high-flow air and oxygen flowmeters can set the FIO_2 as well as guarantee adequate total flows to meet or exceed patient's inspiratory flow needs. Figure 13-21 shows examples of Thorpe tube flowmeters with differing calibrated ranges.

☐ OXYGEN-AIR BLENDING AND PROPORTIONERS

Precise delivery of oxygen fractions is required to supply therapeutic levels of oxygen and hopefully avoid complications. Several methods exist for control of FIO_2 and delivery of adequate flow to meet inspiratory demands. One method is use of a jet nebulizer or Venturi system with internal mixing of room air with a stream of oxygen. Dilution devices cannot be reliably used with mechanical ventilators and often do not deliver the variety of concentrations and flows that are possible with true oxygen–air blenders (proportioner valves) or dual air-oxygen flowmeters.

☐ DUAL AIR-OXYGEN FLOWMETERS

Dual flowmeters are the simplest and most economical method to deliver a specific FIO_2 and total flow. Applications include continuous flow systems for intermittent mandatory ventilation (IMV) or CPAP. Basic algebra can be used to aid respiratory care practitioners in set-up; actual oxygen analysis should confirm calculated settings. Equation Box 13-8 describes the mathematics for clinical applications.

The previous equations will allow you to adjust dual flowmeter applications with oxygen and air flows to arrive at desired total flow and FIO_2 (see Table 13-5). Nomograms have also been developed to allow clinicians to quickly determine appropriate settings.[49]

Practitioners can use "mainstream" nebulizers (that mix gases in predetermined ratios) with additional oxygen or air flowmeters to create a wider range of FIO_2 values at higher flows than normally available. On some commercial nebulizers it is not possible to deliver FIO_2 less than 0.35 to 0.40 when driving the nebulizer by oxygen flowmeter. However, the nebulizer can be run off an

TABLE 13-5. **Air/Oxygen Mixing Ratios**

FIO_2	Air/Oxygen Ratio
0.24	25.1/1
0.25	18.75/1
0.30	7.78/1
0.35	4.64/1
0.40	3.17/1
0.45	2.29/1
0.50	1.72/1
0.55	1.32/1
0.60	1.03/1
0.65	0.79/1
0.70	0.61/1
0.75	0.46/1
0.80	0.34/1
0.85	0.23/1
0.90	0.145/1
0.95	0.065/1

EQUATION BOX 13-8

EQUATIONS FOR MIXING OXYGEN AND AIR

The first premise:

$$\text{Fraction of gas } x \text{ in a system} = \frac{\text{Volume of gas } x \text{ in a system}}{\text{Total volume of all gas in the system}}$$

This relationship can be expanded into a generic mixing equation that can be used to mix oxygen and air or any other substance:

$$F_x(\dot{V}_a + \dot{V}_b) = F_x(\dot{V}_a) + F_x(\dot{V}_b)$$

The total volume of gas equals $(\dot{V}_a + \dot{V}_b)$; it is assumed that x can be found in both $\dot{V}_a$ and $\dot{V}_b$; F_x equals the fraction of gas x in a volume. A common application is mixing oxygen and air. The generic equation can be rewritten for mixing oxygen and air for clinical respiratory care:

$$F\text{IO}_2(\dot{V}O_2 + \dot{V}_{air}) = F\text{IO}_2(\dot{V}O_2) + F\text{IO}_2(\dot{V}_{air})$$

$$\dot{V}_{Total} = \text{total gas flow}$$

$$\dot{V}O_2 = \text{flow of pure oxygen}$$

$$\dot{V}_{air} = \text{flow of room or medical compressed gas}$$

Because the $F\text{IO}_2$ of pure oxygen and air are 1.0 and 0.21, respectively, the equation can be further simplified:

$$F\text{IO}_2(\dot{V}_{Total}) = (\dot{V}O_2) + 0.21(\dot{V}_{air}) \quad [1]$$

A second equation can be written that relates volumes of gases.

$$\dot{V}_{Total} = \dot{V}O_2 + \dot{V}_{air} \quad [2]$$

By rearranging equation 2, any gas volume can be algebraically isolated, and substituted in place of unknown volumes into equation 1. All clinical gas mixing problems can be solved using the combination of equations 1 and 2. Several clinical examples will demonstrate the application.

Example 1: Determine the (ratio) of air to oxygen so the mixture produces a desired $F\text{IO}_2$. What is the air/O_2 ratio for an $F\text{IO}_2$ of 0.40?

$$F\text{IO}_2(\dot{V}_{Total}) = (\dot{V}O_2) + 0.21(\dot{V}_{air}) \quad [1]$$

$$0.4(\dot{V}_{Total}) = (\dot{V}O_2) + 0.21(\dot{V}_{air})$$

By convention, the expression for air/O_2 ratio is x:1, therefore substitute 1 for $\dot{V}O_2$.

$$0.4(\dot{V}_{Total}) = 1 + 0.21(\dot{V}_{air})$$

To eliminate one of the unknown total flow, use equation 2 to substitute, since $1 + \dot{V}_{air} = \dot{V}_{Total}$.

$$0.4(1 + \dot{V}_{air}) = 1 + 0.21(\dot{V}_{air})$$

$$0.4 + 0.4(\dot{V}_{air}) = 1 + 0.21(\dot{V}_{air})$$

Combining terms

$$0.19(\dot{V}_{air}) = 0.6$$

$$\dot{V}_{air} = 3.16$$

Therefore, the air/O_2 ratio for $F\text{IO}_2$ of 0.4 equals 3.16:1. (See Table 13-5 for common air/O_2 ratios listed by $F\text{IO}_2$)

(continued)

EQUATION BOX 13-8 *(CONTINUED)*

Example 2: Determine the $F\text{IO}_2$ knowing the flows of air and oxygen. What is the $F\text{IO}_2$ if $\dot{V}O_2$ equals 10 L/min and $\dot{V}_{air}$ equals 10 L/min?

$$F\text{IO}_2(\dot{V}_{Total}) = (\dot{V}O_2) + 0.21(\dot{V}_{air})$$

$$F\text{IO}_2(10 + 10) = 10 + .21(10)$$

$$F\text{IO}_2 = \frac{12.1}{20}$$

$$F\text{IO}_2 = 0.6$$

Example 3: Solve for the $\dot{V}O_2$ and $\dot{V}_{air}$ flows to provide a specific $F\text{IO}_2$ as well as required total flow to match the patient's inspiratory needs. To what level should the O_2 and air flowmeters be set if the clinician estimates the patient requires a maximum of 40 L/min and the $F\text{IO}_2$ needed is 0.70?

$$F\text{IO}_2(\dot{V}_{Total}) = (\dot{V}O_2) + 0.21(\dot{V}_{air})$$

$$0.7(40 \text{ L/min}) = (\dot{V}O_2) + 0.21(\dot{V}_{air})$$

Substitute for $\dot{V}_{air}$:

$$\dot{V}_{Total} = \dot{V}O_2 + \dot{V}_{air} \quad [2]$$

$$\dot{V}_{air} = \dot{V}_{Total} - \dot{V}O_2$$

$$F\text{IO}_2(\dot{V}_{Total}) = (\dot{V}O_2) + 0.21(\dot{V}_{Total} - \dot{V}O_2)$$

$$0.7(40 \text{ L/min}) = (\dot{V}O_2) + 0.21(40 \text{ L/min} - \dot{V}O_2)$$

$$28 \text{ L/min} = \dot{V}O_2 - 0.21(\dot{V}O_2) + 8.4 \text{ L/min}$$

$$19.6 \text{ L/min} = 0.79(\dot{V}O_2)$$

$$25 \text{ L/min} = \dot{V}O_2$$

Since

$$\dot{V}_{air} = \dot{V}_{Total} - \dot{V}O_2$$

$$\dot{V}_{air} = 40 \text{ L/min} - 25 \text{ L/min}$$

$$\dot{V}_{air} = 15 \text{ L/min}$$

The general mixing equation can be solved for each of its four component factors. Practitioners can quickly solve problems by "plugging" known data into the following equations:

$$F\text{IO}_2 = \frac{\dot{V}O_2 + 0.21(\dot{V}_{air})}{\dot{V}_{Total}} \quad [3]$$

$$\text{or } F\text{IO}_2 = 0.79\left(\frac{\dot{V}O_2}{\dot{V}_{Total}}\right) + 0.21 \quad [3']$$

$$\dot{V}O_2 = \frac{\dot{V}_{Total}(F\text{IO}_2 - 0.21)}{0.79} \quad [4]$$

$$\dot{V}_{air} = \frac{\dot{V}O_2(1 - 0.21)}{F\text{IO}_2 - 0.21} \quad [5]$$

$$\dot{V}_{Total} = \frac{\dot{V}O_2(0.79)}{F\text{IO}_2 - 0.21} \quad [6]$$

air flowmeter to generate the aerosol, and a separate oxygen flow is injected into the system (in the top of the nebulizer) or with a "Tee" in the delivery tubing. Recently the Medical Moulding Corporation of America made a commercial version of this concept termed a "gas-injection nebulizer" (Fig. 13-22).

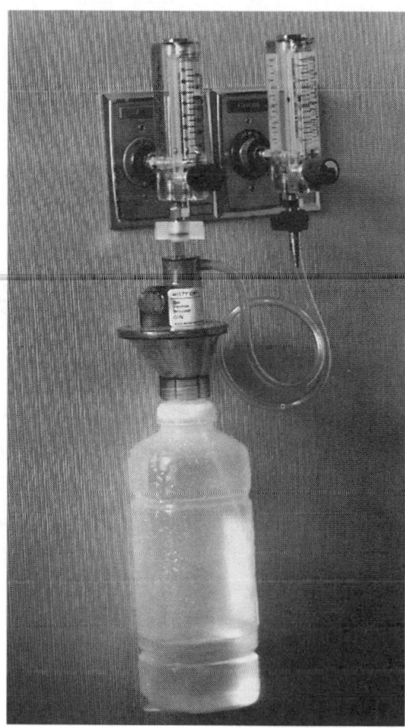

FIGURE 13-22. Mainstream nebulizer with high-flow capabilities.

Equation Box 13-9 describes further development of the general mixing equation for this specific application.

During clinical practice, all air-oxygen systems should have the F_{IO_2} confirmed by direct oxygen analysis. Although the previously listed equations are valid, errors in calculations and inaccurately calibrated equipment may effect the delivered oxygen fraction, sometimes abbreviated as F_{DO_2}.

EQUATION BOX 13-9

FURTHER CALCULATIONS OF OXYGEN/AIR MIXING FOR USE WITH MAINSTREAM NEBULIZERS

$$\dot{V}O_2 = \frac{\dot{V}^{s}_{air}[0.79(F_{DO_2} - 0.21)}{(F^{s}{IO_2} - 0.21)(1 - F_{DO_2})]}$$

$\dot{V}^{s}_{air}$ = Flow of air from flowmeter driving nebulizer

F_{DO_2} = Oxygen concentration delivered to the patient

$F^{s}{IO_2}$ = Dilution setting on the nebulizer

$\dot{V}O_2$ = Supplemental oxygen that should be added to produce the F_{DO_2} needed.

Example: If an air driven nebulizer is set on 0.40 dilution ($F^{s}{IO_2}$) and the air flowmeter running it is set at 14 L/min ($\dot{V}^{s}_{air}$), how much supplemental oxygen ($\dot{V}O_2$) should be added to produce a F_{DO_2} of 0.28?

$$\dot{V}O_2 = 14\left[\frac{0.79(0.28 - 0.21)}{(0.40 - 0.21)(1 - 0.28)}\right]$$

$$= 14\frac{(0.0553}{0.1368)}$$

$$= 14(0.404)$$

$$= 5.7 \text{ L/min}$$

Oxygen–Air Blenders (Proportioners)

Oxygen–air blenders, or proportioners, provide a convenient compact device to premix gases by dialing in a specific oxygen concentration (Fig. 13-23). They are commonly used to mix gas for mechanical ventilators (eg, Siemens-Elema Servo 900 series and the Sechrist infant ventilators), continuous-flow CPAP systems, add-on IMV systems, heart–lung bypass machines, and controlled oxygen therapy.

It is difficult for manufacturers to build blenders with desired accuracy over the complete range of flows needed clinically. Low-flow blenders are most accurate at low-flow applications requiring less than about 20 L/min. High-flow blenders must be accurate in providing controlled F_{IO_2} levels at flows in the 80 to 100 L/min range.

Oxygen–air proportioners receive each gas separately from a pipeline or compressed gas cylinder. Ideally the supply pressures of both gases are nearly equal, usually 50 psig (344.75 kPa). In clinical practice this does not always occur, so blenders have internal pressure-regulating systems. Air and oxygen enter the blender and pass through check valves (Fig. 13-24A). Then gas flows through spool-shaped valves separated by a flexible diaphragm (Fig. 13-24B). They lower and balance the inlet pressures. This process should produce similar pressures for air and oxygen. If that is the case, a dual orifice needle valve controls the proportion of each gas flowing out of the orifices. For higher concentrations, the valve would simultaneously open for more oxygen flow as it decreased air flows. Blender manufacturers have built-in alarm systems and, in some, pressure gauges to allow clinicians to confirm proper inlet pressures.

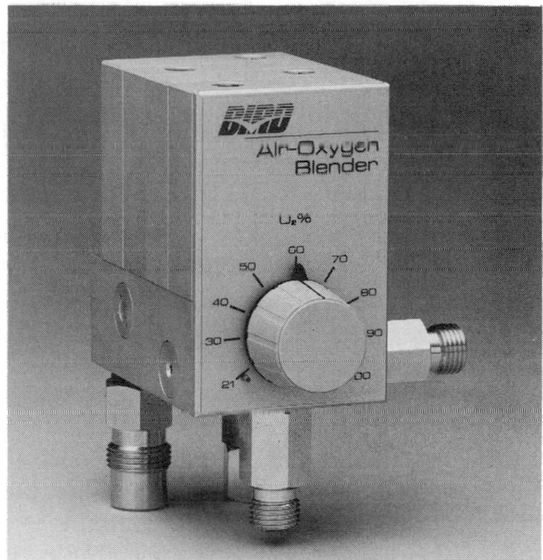

FIGURE 13-23. Air–oxygen blender (From Branson RD. Gas delivery systems: Regulators, flowmeters, and therapy devices. In: Branson RD, Hess DR, Chatburn RL. (eds) Respiratory Care Equipment. Philadelphia: JB Lippincott, 1995. With permission.)

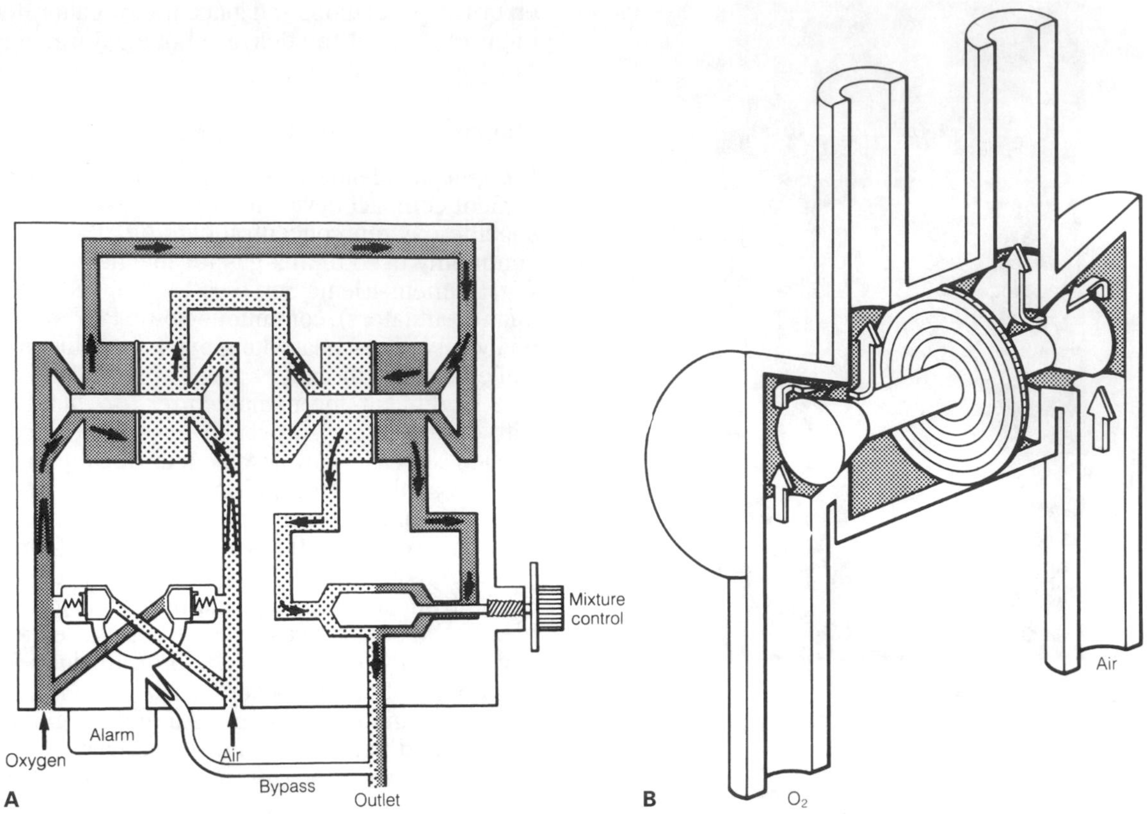

FIGURE 13-24. **(A)** Schematic of typical air–oxygen blender showing proportioner valve system, **(B)** Close-up of parallel diaphragms. (From Ward JJ. Equipment for mixed gas and oxygen therapy. In: Barnes TA. (ed) Core Textbook of Respiratory Care Practice, 2nd ed. St. Louis: CV Mosby, 1994. With permission.)

□ CLINICAL USE AND TROUBLESHOOTING

Evaluations of commercially available medical oxygen–air blenders have found that all blenders were quite accurate when both inlet pressures were 50 psig (345 kPa). Units should be able to mix with an accuracy of ±3% over an FIO_2 range of 0.21 to 1.00. High-flow blenders tend to have greatest inaccuracy at low flow rates and low-flow blenders at high flows. Some high-flow commercial units are not able to meet the 80 L/min criteria established by the Emergency Care Research Institute (ECRI).[50]

All blenders should be calibrated initially and periodically by oxygen analyzers. With an in-line analyzer, operators should be able to adjust the FIO_2 within 0.01 increments over the 0.21 to 0.35 range and 0.05 in the 0.4 to 1.0 range.

Besides imbalance of inlet gas pressure supply lines, one of the most common problems involves contamination of one gas supply by another because of retrograde flow. This problem has been reported when blenders are connected to gas inlets but not running to patient systems. The higher pressure gas (usually oxygen) can flow into the medical air gas lines if inlet check-valves are defective. When blenders are not in use, the path of least resistance for the higher pressure oxygen is the piped air system. Contaminates from gas lines can prevent these pressure valves from sealing properly. Corrosion due to moisture and particulate matter can build up and restrict flow or prevent sealing of check valves. Routine inspection and cleaning are recommended twice a year. Replacement of inlet sintered metal filters and use of water trap filters should reduce this problem. In more serious cases, more complex filter systems may be required.[50,51]

□ HIGH-FLOW GENERATOR

A modern version of the classic "Venturi tube" provides gas mixing by oxygen-driven air-entrainment (Fig. 13-25A). Commercially known as a Down's Flow Generator, it was initially designed to be incorporated in mask CPAP systems.[52] In contrast to other Venturi mixing systems (eg, all-purpose nebulizers), this device was designed to provide gas at high flows. CPAP systems must meet or exceed patient's inspiratory flow demand to maintain the therapeutic threshold pressure in the system. It would appear that the flow generator's application is not limited to only mask-applied CPAP systems. When passed through a humidifier, it can be used to produce a variable FIO_2 at high flows as an alternative to all-purpose nebulizers or air/oxygen blenders. Asthmatics with high-flow demands may not tolerate the bronchospastic particulate water.

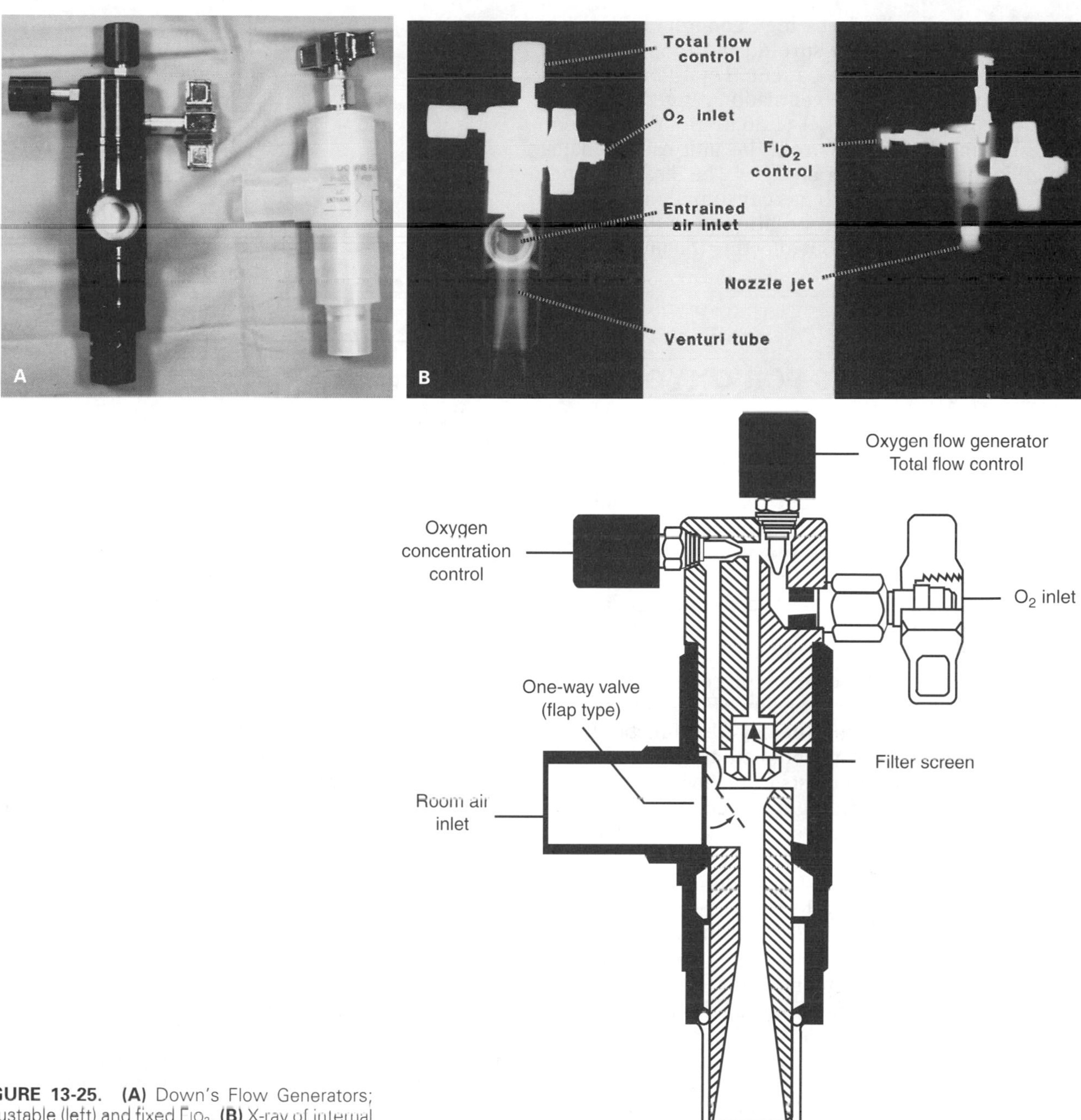

FIGURE 13-25. **(A)** Down's Flow Generators; adjustable (left) and fixed F_IO_2. **(B)** X-ray of internal components, **(C)** Schematic diagram. (Courtesy of Vital Signs Corp, Towanda N.J.)

Two styles are currently available: a fixed F_IO_2 (see Fig. 13-25A, right side) and a model that can independently adjust flow and F_IO_2 (see Fig. 13-25 A, left side). The fixed F_IO_2 unit delivers oxygen concentrations of approximately 0.33 and greater at flows up to 100 L/min when the output is unrestricted. However, with downstream pressure of 15 cmH_2O (1.36 kPa), the total output falls and the F_IO_2 increases to 0.37. Both units can be connected to any oxygen flowmeter or directly to a 50-psig DISS outlet.

The adjustable flow generator provides an F_IO_2 of 0.3 to 1.0 and maintains output flows of 100 L/min. This is in contrast to many mainstream nebulizers, which decrease output flow as F_IO_2 is increased. In that unit the flow of incoming oxygen stays constant, and the amount of the entrained air is manipulated by changing orifices. The flow generator's F_IO_2 adjustment directs the oxygen inlet flow (see 13-25B and C). When it is opened, more oxygen bypasses the Venturi jet and passes through a channel. By shifting greater proportions of source oxygen away from the jet, the F_IO_2 can increase. Higher flows of pure oxygen compensate for lesser amounts of entrained room air. The needle valve at the top of the tube controls the total amount of source oxygen into the system. It is adjusted to supply the appropriate total flow of mixed gas into a CPAP system. Flow ideally should be high enough to minimize drops in the system pressure during the most rapid inspiratory efforts of the patient. Total flows are adjustable to accommodate ventilation ranges of infants to adults. With a 15 cmH_2O (1.36 kPa) CPAP system pressure, maximum flow from the unit can be maintained in the 100 L/min. range.[52–54] The disadvantages of these units include high gas consumption and noise level. Bacterial filters can be fitted over the air inlet port to reduce noise without affecting the unit's performance significantly.

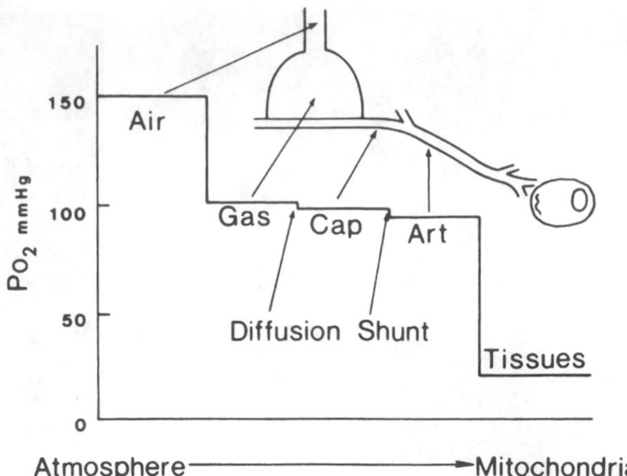

FIGURE 13-26. Oxygen pressure "cascade" from atmosphere to tissues. (From West JB. Respiratory Physiology, 4th ed. Baltimore, MD: Williams & Wilkins, 1990. Reproduced with permission.)

SCIENTIFIC BASIS FOR OXYGEN THERAPY

Oxygen Transport Physiology

Normal gas transport to (and from) body tissues requires proper function of key physiologic events and systems. Box 13-6 identifies the factors that determine successful transport of oxygen.

Oxygen that diffuses into blood at the alveolar-capillary membrane is transported to body tissues by the cardiovascular system and the blood. The tissues have the opportunity to take up the oxygen. Alveolar oxygen pressure (P_AO_2) and arterial tension (PaO_2) establish a "head of pressure." Blood (hemoglobin function), cardiac, and tissue perfusion complete the gas transport. The pressure "cascade" exists from environmental gas to tissues as is shown in Figure 13-26. The removal of carbon dioxide from tissues by the cardiopulmonary system occurs simultaneously.

Oxygen consumption ($\dot{V}O_2$) is defined as the total amount of oxygen used by the body. Resting normal levels are 250 to 300 mL/min (STPD) but can exceed 16 L/min in athletic extremes. Carbon dioxide production ($\dot{V}CO_2$) describes the amount of CO_2 the body "exhausts" through the lungs; normal resting levels are 200 to 250 mL/min. The respiratory exchange ratio ($\dot{V}CO_2/\dot{V}O_2$ or R) relates the overall metabolic relationship of the two gases. The ratio, or molecule-for-molecule exchange, depends on diet and activity level. For example, when a balance of fat and carbohydrate is eaten, the R will be approximately 0.8 (eg, normal at rest: $\dot{V}CO_2/\dot{V}O_2 = 250/300$ mL/min). When fat is the primary fuel, the ratio approaches 0.7; with high carbohydrate intake, the exchange ratio will move towards 1.0.

Acute and serious problems at any stage of the oxygen transport cycle may require medical intervention. Normal intracellular oxygen tensions are estimated to range from 5 to 40 mmHg depending on tissue and activity level. Under normal rates of cellular oxygen consumption there is a safety margin. Cellular oxygen levels below 1 to 3 mmHg limits normal hydrolysis of adenosine triphosphate (ATP).

The body's normal immediate physiologic response to dangerously low blood/tissue oxygen is to increase cardiac output, improve perfusion to the tissue, and improve the blood's oxygen transporting characteristics (oxyhemoglobin dissociation curve changes). Oxygen delivery ($D\dot{V}O_2$) is the product of the cardiac output (or cardiac index) and the available amount of oxygen being transported. Equation Box 13-10 expresses the relationship mathematically.

Under normal conditions previously described, a total body oxygen need of 250 to 300 mL/min would be met by a significant margin of safety. Oxygen content (CaO_2) determines the quantity of oxygen that can be made available to cells. O_2 content and pressure are inseparably related aspects of the same system. Cardiac output relates to the movement of the oxygen from lung to tissues and back to lung. The arterial oxygen content

BOX 13-6

KEY FACTORS IN OXYGEN TRANSPORT

- Ventilation and perfusion of the lungs (airways, vascular, and neuromuscular)
- Diffusion of gases into blood (PaO_2, lung parenchyma)
- Transport of gas in arterial blood (blood volume, hemoglobin level and function, and cardiac output)
- Arterial vasculature and blood pressure (vessels and cardiac output)
- Diffusion and utilization by cells (cellular biochemical)

EQUATION BOX 13-10

OXYGEN DELIVERY CALCULATION

Oxygen delivery = cardiac output × arterial oxygen content

$$DV_{O_2} = \dot{Q} \times CaO_2$$

Example: cardiac output 4000 mL/min

- arterial oxygen content = 19 mL/100 mL
  DV_{O_2} = 760 mL/min

(CaO_2) is normally composed of oxygen that is physically dissolved in the water of the plasma and in the erythrocyte plus that combined with hemoglobin. The measuring units of convention are mL/100 mL of blood or mL/dL. The dissolved oxygen quantitatively depends on the solubility of oxygen, temperature, and atmospheric pressure. The Bunsen solubility coefficient for oxygen at body temperature and a barometric pressure of 760 mmHg is 0.023 mL O_2/mL blood. The value would be 2.3 mL O_2/dL of blood. A clinically more useful relationship is the quantity of dissolved oxygen (only), for each mmHg or torr of oxygen gas tension in blood as shown in Equation Box 13-11.

The dissolved oxygen level follows the linear relationship described above and plays a small part in oxygen transport. Under normobaric conditions breathing 100% oxygen, the maximal contribution would be approximately 2 mL/dL. However, this level can provide about one third of the body's resting tissue requirements. The following example in Equation Box 13-12 illustrates this point and identifies supplemental oxygen's role in anemic patients.

The vast majority of oxygen is transported to tissues via its loose chemical bond with hemoglobin. One molecule of hemoglobin has four heme groups, each has the capacity to bind one oxygen molecule. One gram of hemoglobin can potentially bind 1.34 mL of oxygen in each 100 mL of blood. To quantify the hemoglobin oxygen binding, the percentage of oxygen filled sites is determined by spectrophotometer. The following Equation Box 13-13 calculates content, combining both dissolved and hemoglobin-bound oxygen.

Factors That Modify the Oxygen-Carrying Capability of Blood

The oxyhemoglobin dissociation curve describes the nonlinear bonding relationship between hemoglobin and oxygen. The S-shaped curve shown in Figure 13-27 describes hemoglobin's chemical binding characteristics as oxygen partial pressure/tension varies. The curve provides a physiologic adaption for loading and unloading oxygen. At oxygen tensions found in the lung (eg, >90 mmHg), the association is high. This results in levels of bonding producing high percentages of saturation on the flat portion of the curve. At lower tensions (eg, <40 mmHg) reflecting the oxygen's unloading from hemoglobin, there is much less chemical attraction demonstrated by the steep-sloped portion of the curve. If the hemoglobin level is given, the arterial and venous content levels can be determined. Box 13-7 summarizes the factors involved in the dynamic binding relationship, demonstrated by the curve's shape and relative position.

EQUATION BOX 13-11

CALCULATING DISSOLVED OXYGEN CONTENT

Dissolved oxygen = $PO_2 \times 0.003$ mL O_2/dL

Example: For a patient with a PaO_2 of 90 mmHg at sea level

$$= 90 \text{ mmHg} \times .003$$

$$\text{Dissolved oxygen} = 0.27 \text{ mL/dL}$$

EQUATION BOX 13-12

EFFECT OF 100% OXYGEN BREATHING ON THE DISSOLVED OXYGEN CONTENT

Example: For a patient with a hemoglobin of 7 g/dL (normal, 15 g/dL) breathing 100% oxygen at 1 atmosphere. PaO_2 of 55 mmHg at 1 atmosphere.

$$\text{Dissolved oxygen content} = 550 \times .003$$

$$= 1.65 \text{ mL/dL}$$

Interrelationships in Oxygen Transport: The Fick Principle

As arterial blood completes a full cardiovascular cycle, oxygen is consumed ($\dot{V}O_2$) by body tissues. The change in oxygen content between arterial and venous levels is variable depending on tissue need and level of blood flow (cardiac output). The arteriovenous content difference ($C(a-\bar{v})O_2$) is normally approximately 4.5 ml/dL (CAO_2= 19 mL/dL, $C\bar{v}O_2$ = 14.5 mL/dL). Oxyhemoglobin shows a total body desaturation from 97% to 75% as oxygen is delivered to tissues. Mixed venous blood is obtained from the pulmonary artery and is a net reflection of all body tissue oxygen "extraction" from a dL of blood in one cardiac cycle. The *Fick principle* provides a relationship that "bridges" body oxygen consumption ($\dot{V}O_2$), cardiac output ($\dot{Q}$), and the arterio-

EQUATION BOX 13-13

OXYGEN CONTENT CALCULATION

$$\text{Arterial oxygen content } CaO_2 = [\text{Hb} \times 1.34 \times SO_2] + [0.003 \times PO_2]$$

Example: The arterial content for a patient with the following data:

PaO_2 = 90 mmHg, Hb = 14 g/dL, and SaO_2 = 95%

$$CaO_2 = [14 \times 1.34 \times 0.95] + [0.003 \times 90]$$
$$= [17.8] + [0.27]$$
$$= 18.07 \text{ mL/dL}$$

Example: The venous content for a patient with the following data:

PvO_2 = 40 mmHg, Hb = 14 g/dL, and SvO_2 = 75%

$$CvO_2 = [14 \times 1.34 \times 0.75] + [0.003 \times 40]$$
$$= [14.7] + [0.12]$$
$$= 14.8 \text{ mL/dL}$$

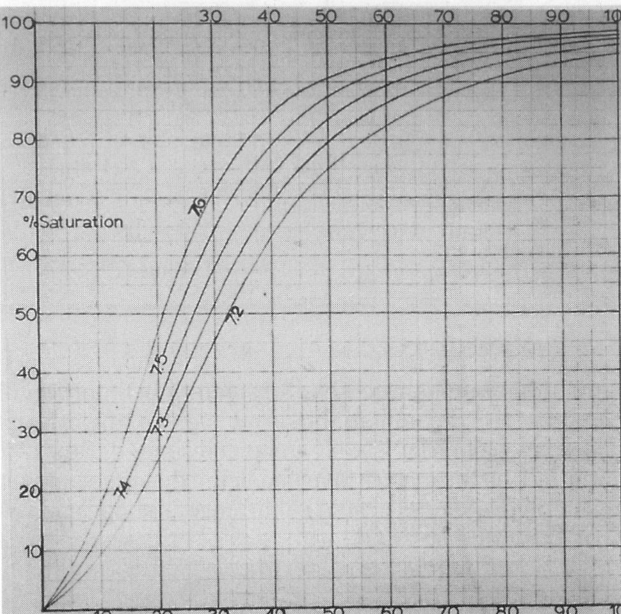

FIGURE 13-27. Oxyhemoglobin dissociation curve (Courtesy H.F. Helmholz, Jr. MD.)

venous oxygen content difference ($C(a-\bar{v})O_2$). The formula is presented in Equation Box 13-14. In clinical practice an "indirect" oxygen consumption estimate can be made if systemic arterial and pulmonary artery catheter data provide cardiac output and $C(a-\bar{v})O_2$. (Note: 0.1 is used to correct units so cardiac output will be in L/min)

The indirect Fick method of oxygen consumption calculation is less accurate when applied to the critically ill. Unfortunately those patients may have abnormal oxygen consumption that must be directly measured by more deliberate methods. In addition to increased oxygen consumption, the critically ill often have difficulty in oxygen transport and impaired ability to extract oxygen at tissue sites.[56] Also, tissues vary in their oxygen consumption (eg, CNS and cardiac muscle have high levels). Others may not have adequate perfusion (eg, coronary artery occlusion or shock-like cardiovascular collapse). Increased tissue demand for oxygen will require an increase in cardiac output, if the arteriovenous content difference is to remain normal. A widening of the normal arteriovenous content difference can reflect either a decrease in cardiac output or increase in tissue oxygen consumption. Box 13-8 summarizes these interrelationships.

Pathology of Hypoxemia and Rationale for Supplemental Oxygen

Following an overview of oxygen transport physiology, the focus will switch to the pathologic problems in oxygenation that result in hypoxemia, hypoxia, or both. Hypoxemia is defined as abnormally low arterial oxygen tension, PaO_2. The rationale for ambient (nonhyperbaric) oxygen therapy devices, applied to the face or artificial airway, is to elevate the oxygen partial pressure in the lung. This occurs by elevating the inspired (P_IO_2) and therefore alveolar gas (P_AO_2).

In the acute care setting, supplemental oxygen is indicated when hypoxemia is suspected by history, physical examination, or documented by laboratory data. Classic signs and symptoms relate to dyspnea, tachypnea, use of accessory muscles, or other signs of increased effort in breathing. In adults, children, and in-

BOX 13-7

FACTORS THAT MODIFY HEMOGLOBIN-OXYGEN BINDING AND RELEASE

Blood pH or PCO_2	Lower from normal pH (or increasing H^+ concentration) decreases the affinity of hemoglobin for oxygen. Elevations of carbon dioxide produce a similar effect. This is seen as a rightward shift. More oxygen is released at the same level of oxygen tension. This is a physiologic advantage for tissue regions with high metabolic activity. The reverse occurs with alkaline pH or hypocarbia.
Blood temperature	Increase in temperature reduces the affinity of hemoglobin for oxygen. This improves oxygen unloading in areas of active metabolism. Cold produces the opposite effect.
2,3-Diphosphoglycerate (2,3-DPG)	Polyphosphate compounds such as ATP and 2,3-DPG effect the affinity of hemoglobin by stabilizing the unoxygenated configuration of the hemoglobin molecule. This reduces its affinity for oxygen. Physiologic levels increase in chronic hypoxic states such as residence at high altitude, chronic cyanotic heart diseases, chronic anemias, and hypoxemia from lung disease. Decreased 2,3-DPG is associated with hyperoxia ($PaO_2 > 260$ mmHg), septic shock, and stored blood bank blood.
Carbon monoxide	Hemoglobin avidly combines with carbon monoxide at 200 to 300 times its affinity for oxygen. By decreasing access to binding sites, it induces a functional anemia. This can be illustrated by the compression of the content versus oxygen tension relationship (see Fig. 13-28). Note, however, that the tension of dissolved oxygen is not affected. In addition, CO induces a leftward curve shift, further interfering with the oxygen loading from functioning binding sites.
Hemoglobin concentration	Anemias (Hb <12 mL/dL) or polycythemias (Hb >16 mL/dL) directly affect the potential oxygen-carrying capability as was demonstrated previously in the calculation of arterial oxygen content (see Box 13-17).

EQUATION BOX 13-14

CALCULATING OXYGEN CONSUMPTION AND CARDIAC OUTPUT USING THE FICK EQUATION

The "Fick equation" $\dot{Q} = \frac{\dot{V}O_2(0.1)}{Ca - \bar{v}O_2}$

Example: Calculate the oxygen consumption using the "indirect" Fick method, for a patient with the following data:

$$(PaO_2 = 90 \text{ mmHg}, SaO_2 = 97\%$$
$$P\bar{v}O_2 = 40 \text{ mmHg}, SvO_2 = 75\%$$
$$Hb = 14 \text{ g/dL}, \dot{Q} = 5 \text{ L/min})$$

Step 1. Calculate both CaO_2 and $C\bar{v}O_2$ and the $Ca - \bar{v}O_2$.

$$CaO_2 = [1.34 \text{ m/g} \times 14 \text{ g/dL} \times 0.97\%] + [0.003 \times 90 \text{ mmHg}]$$
$$= [18.2] + [0.27]$$
$$= 18.5 \text{ mL/dL}$$
$$C\bar{v}O_2 = [1.34 \times 14 \times 0.75] + [0.003 \times 40]$$
$$= [14.1] + [0.12]$$
$$= 14.3 \text{ mL/dL}$$
$$Ca - \bar{v}O_2 = 18.5 - 14.3 = 4.2 \text{ mL/dL}$$

Step 2. Calculate $\dot{V}O_2$

$$\dot{Q} \text{ L/min} = \frac{\dot{V}O_2 \text{ mL/min} \times 0.1}{C(a - \bar{v})O_2 \text{ mL/dL}}$$
$$5 = \frac{\dot{V}O_2 \times 0.1}{4.2}$$
$$5 \times 4.2 = \dot{V}O_2 \times 0.1$$
$$\frac{21}{0.1} = \dot{V}O_2$$
$$\dot{V}O_2 = 210 \text{ mL/min}$$

(Note: the normal resting oxygen consumption is 200–300 mL/min (STPD).)

Example: Calculate the cardiac output for a patient with the following data.

$$(PaO_2 = 90 \text{ mmHg}, SaO_2 = 97\%$$
$$P\bar{v}O_2 = 28 \text{ mmHg}, S\bar{v}O_2 = 48\%$$
$$pH = 7.3 \; Hb = 14 \text{ g/dL}$$
$$\dot{V}O_2 = 210 \text{ mL/min})$$

Step 1. Calculate both CaO_2 and $C\bar{v}O_2$ and the $C(a - \bar{v})O_2$.

$$CaO_2 = [1.34 \text{ m/g} \times 14 \text{ g/dL} \times 0.97\%] + [0.003 \times 90 \text{ mmHg}]$$
$$= [18.2] + [0.27]$$
$$= 18.5 \text{ mL/dL}$$
$$C\bar{v}O_2 = [1.34 \times 14 \times 0.48] + [0.003 \times 28]$$
$$= 9 + [0.08]$$
$$= 9.8 \text{ mL/dL}$$
$$C(a - \bar{v})O_2 = 18.5 - 9.8 = 8.7 \text{ mL/dL}$$

(continued)

EQUATION BOX 13-14 *(CONTINUED)*

Step 2. Calculate $\dot{Q}$ L/min

$$\dot{Q} \text{ L/min} = \frac{\dot{V}O_2 \text{ mL/min} \times 0.1}{C(a - \bar{v})O_2 \text{ mL/dL}}$$
$$\dot{Q} = \frac{210 \times 0.1}{8.7}$$
$$\dot{Q} = 2.41 \text{ L/min}$$

fants (older than 1 month) at rest, breathing room air, documentation is less than 60 mmHg (7.98 kPa) or SaO_2 or SpO_2 less than 90%. In neonates PaO_2 less than 50 mmHg (6.7 kPa) or SaO_2 less than 88% or capillary oxygen PCO_2 tension of less than 40 mmHg (5.33 kPa).[3] In the non–critically-ill patient, the history and previous laboratory record are key data.

Categories of Hypoxemia

The following are the classic categories of hypoxemia. Table 13-6 provides a summary of clinical data relating $P(A-a)_2$ and likely responses to 100% oxygen breathing.

1. Rarefied atmosphere due to altitude, accidental suffocation, or iatrogenic omission of oxygen from closed breathing circuits
2. Hypoventilation causing alveolar carbon dioxide to displace oxygen
3. Increased mismatching of pulmonary blood to pulmonary ventilation $\dot{V}/\dot{Q}$, decreasing the efficiency of gas exchange
4. Increased shunting of blood through pulmonary, vascular, or cardiac areas, bypassing functioning ventilated alveoli. This may be termed arteriovenous or right-to-left shunting and is an extreme of $\dot{V}/\dot{Q}$
5. Increased defect in gaseous diffusion across the alveolar capillary membrane

It should be noted that *only* with hypoxemia due to rarified atmosphere or hypoventilation is there a normal gradient of alveolar oxygen pressure in lung to arterial blood tension $P(A-a)_2$. In the last three categories, the pathology of the hypoxemia is reflected in a widened alveolar to arterial oxygen gradient. Further differenti-

BOX 13-8

SUMMARY OF OXYGEN TRANSPORT

Availability of the cardiopulmonary system to load, transport, and deliver oxygen requires the following factors:

- Adequate amount of hemoglobin
- Functioning hemoglobin-binding sites
- Adequate pressure/tensions of oxygen gas in lung and blood
- Appropriate conditions for hemoglobin dissociation (eg, pH, temperature, and 2,3-DPG)
- Adequate cardiac output and vascular perfusion of tissues

TABLE 13-6. **Characteristics of the Categories of Hypoxemias**

Category	Clinical Example	$P(A\text{-}a)O_2$ (FIO_2 = 0.21)	$P(A\text{-}a)O_2$ (FIO_2 = 1.0)	PaO_2 Response to FIO_2 = 1.0
Hypoventilation	Narcotic drug overdose	5–30 torr (normal)	100–150 torr (normal)	Variable: up to or >400 torr
Ventilation/perfusion mismatch	Asthma (low V/Q)	Increased	Increased	Slow: up to or >400 torr
	pulmonary embolism (high V/Q)	Increased	Increased	Rapid: less than 400 torr
Shunt (pulmonary or anatomic)	Atelectasis, pneumonia, or R → L (eg, atrial septal defect)	Increased	Increased	Rapid: to <400 (<200 torr if room air PaO_2 <50 torr)
Diffusion defect	Pulmonary interstitial fibrosis (eg, sarcoidosis)	Increased	Increased	Delayed: to ≈ 400 torr

Adapted from Ziment I: Respiratory Pharmacology and Therapeutics. Philadelphia, PA, WB Saunders, 1978, 452; reprinted with permission.

ation requires either testing after 100% oxygen breathing or carbon monoxide diffusion lung testing.

The net improvement in PaO_2 when supplemental oxygen is given to a patient with one or more of the above hypoxemias is quite variable.[57,58] The response depends on the category and severity of the problem. Patients with predominant $\dot{V}/\dot{Q}$ mismatching or diffusion defect normally achieve 400 mmHg or more, although the response may be slow. Normal subjects given 100% oxygen can achieve a PaO_2 of more than 500 mmHg (66.65 kPa).[58] Those patients with significant shunt may not show substantial improvement to increasing FIO_2. When given high concentrations (ie, 0.6 to 1.0), those with sizable shunts (20% to 50%), usually do not increase PaO_2 beyond about 400 mmHg (53.32 kPa). By increasing the fraction of inspired oxygen, the partial pressure of inspired oxygen (PIO_2) is elevated beyond normal atmospheric levels.

$$PIO_2 = (P_B - PH_2O)FIO_2$$

The effect of elevating the PIO_2 directly influences the partial pressure of oxygen in the alveolar gas (PAO_2). By increasing the head of oxygen pressure across the alveolar capillary membranes, the arterial oxygen tension (PaO_2) should increase. This can hopefully compensate for defects in oxygen transport that are expressed as an increased gradient between alveolar and arterial oxygen levels ($P(A-O_2)$). The normal $P(A-a)_2$ on room air ranges from 10 to 16 mmHg (1.33 kPa).[59] Equation Box 13-15 identifies a calculated estimate of PAO_2 and provides calculation of the normal level.

An abbreviated version of the alveolar oxygen equation also appears in the literature.

$$PAO_2 = (PB - PH_2O)FIO_2 - \left(\frac{PaCO_2}{R}\right)$$

This may present a simpler calculation but consistently underestimates PAO_2 at any concentration of inspired oxygen above room air.[60,61]

☐ HYPOXEMIA SECONDARY TO HYPOVENTILATION

When patients hypoventilate, increased alveolar carbon dioxide level causes displacement of oxygen in alveolar gas. A larger gas pressure, $PACO_2$, must be subtracted from the potential oxygen pressure, PIO_2. Supplemental oxygen can raise the FIO_2, increasing PAO_2 sufficiently to potentially compensate for elevations of $PaCO_2$ if the primary hypoventilation cannot be corrected. Equation Box 13-16 provides examples to illustrate this concept.

The effect of increasing levels of supplemental oxygen on the alveolar oxygen partial pressures can be estimated for variable levels of arterial carbon dioxide tension (Table 13-7). Of clinical importance is the knowledge that under average barometric conditions, patients cannot tolerate the arterial hypoxemia resulting from carbon dioxide levels over 90 mmHg (11.9 kPa) without oxygen-enriched atmospheres.

Quantitative indices to describe the severity of hypoxemias and separate them into categories are useful to those evaluating oxygen therapy. For example, hypoventilation causing hypoxemia can be separated from shunt and other lung disorders by calculating the $P(A-a)O_2$. Of the calculated indices commonly used in clinical practice are PaO_2/FIO_2 and PaO_2/PAO_2 ratio, the latter has the greatest clinical value.[62] The reader is referred to Equation Box 13-17 for an example of using

EQUATION BOX 13-15
ALVEOLAR AIR EQUATION

$$PAO_2 = (PB - PH_2O)FIO_2 - PaCO_2\left(FIO_2 + \frac{1 - FIO_2}{R}\right)$$

(R = respiratory quotient = $\dot{V}CO_2/\dot{V}O_2$) and can be estimated to be 0.8 for most clinical calculations if not actually determined by metabolic measurement)

Example: The estimate for average alveolar oxygen partial pressure under normal atmospheric and physiologic conditions, ie, P_B = 760 mmHg, PH_2O = 47 mmHg, $PaCO_2$ = 40 mmHg, respiratory quotient = 0.8, and FIO_2 = 0.21.

$$PAO_2 = (760 - 47)0.21 - 40\left(0.21 + \frac{1 - 0.21}{0.8}\right)$$
$$= (713)0.21 - 40(0.21 + 0.99)$$
$$= 149.73 - 48$$
$$= 101.73 \text{ mmHg or } [13.56 \text{ kPa}]$$

EQUATION BOX 13-16

CORRECTING HYPERCAPNIC HYPOXEMIA WITH SUPPLEMENTAL OXYGEN

Example: What is the estimated PAO_2 of a drug overdose patient with hypoventilation? He has a $PaCO_2$ of 80 mmHg [10.6 kPa], a PaO_2 of 44 mmHg [5.86 kPa] and the barometric pressure is 760 mmHg [101.3 kPa].

$$PAO_2 = (PB - PH_2O)FIO_2 - PaCO_2\left(FIO_2 + \frac{1 - FIO_2}{R}\right)$$

$$PAO_2 = (760 - 47)0.21 - 80\left(\frac{0.21 + 1 - 0.21}{0.8}\right)$$

$$= (760 - 47)0.21 - 80(0.21 + 0.8)$$

$$= 149.73 - 95$$

$$= 54 \text{ mmHg or } [7.19 \text{ kPa}]$$

Assuming a normal oxygen tension loss or gradient from alveolar gas to arterial blood ($PA - aO_2$) of 10 mmHg, one would estimate the arterial oxygen to be approximately 44 mmHg [5.86 kPa]:

$$\text{Estimated } PaO_2 = PAO_2 - PA - aO_2$$

$$= 54 - 10$$

$$= 44 \text{ mmHg or } [5.9 \text{ kPa}]$$

Example: If supplemental oxygen with a FIO_2 of 0.3 oxygen is given to the patient with a $PaCO_2$ of 80 mmHg [10.66 kPa], what is the estimated PAO_2? What is the estimated PaO_2?

$$PAO_2 = (760 - 47)0.3 - 40\left(0.3 + \frac{1 - 0.3}{0.8}\right)$$

$$= 213.9 - 94$$

$$= 120 \text{ mmHg or } [15.99 \text{ kPa}]$$

Assuming the same $P(A - a)O_2$ of 10 mmHg, the estimated PaO_2 after oxygen administration would be 110 mmHg [14.66 kPa].

the PaO_2/PAO_2 ratio to mathematically predict supplemental oxygen levels to correct hypoxemia.

Categories of Hypoxia

Hypoxia refers to subnormal tissue oxygen content; anoxia has become a synonymous term. Hypoxia expands the definition of oxygen transport beyond in addition to problems that are pulmonary based; hypoxia includes other factors that can influence blood transport and delivery to tissues. The term normoxemic hypoxia covers conditions that result in tissue hypoxia despite a normal PaO_2. Those conditions involve either abnormalities in amount or function of hemoglobin, inadequate delivery, or utilization of oxygen by tissues. Box 13-9 lists classic categories of hypoxias and associated conditions and/or circumstances. Figure 13-28 illustrates the corresponding causes schematically.

In humans, tissue hypoxia is estimated to occur when mitochondrial PO_2 is less than 7 mmHg (0.93 kPa).[62] The direct clinical analysis of oxygen at the tissue sites is not possible clinically. Clinicians must use physical

TABLE 13-7. **Effect of $PaCO_2$ and Oxygen Concentration on Calculated PAO_2**

FIO_2	0.21	0.28	0.35	0.50	0.80	1.0
			PAO_2			
$PaCO_2$						
20	126	176	226	333	549	693
40	102	152	203	311	528	673
60	78	129	180	289	507	653
80	54	105	157	266	486	633
100	30	82	133	243	465	613
120	6	58	110	221	444	593

EQUATION BOX 13-17

PREDICTING NEEDED FIO_2 TO ACHIEVE A DESIRED PaO_2

Example: What is the estimated FIO_2 needed to treat a COPD patient who has a $PaCO_2$ of 80 mmHg [10.6 kPa], a PaO_2 of 30 mmHg [5.86 kPa] at a barometric pressure of 760 mmHg [101.3 kPa]? A desired PaO_2 is 60 mmHg; the $PaCO_2$ level is to remain constant.

Step 1. Calculate the initial PAO_2

$$PAO_2 = (PB - PH_2O)FIO_2 - PaCO_2\left(FIO_2 + \frac{1 - FIO_2}{R}\right)$$

$$PAO_2 = (760 - 47)0.21 - 80\left(0.21 + \frac{1 - 0.21}{0.8}\right)$$

$$= (760 - 47)0.21 - 80(0.21 + 0.98)$$

$$= 149.73 - 96$$

$$= 54 \text{ mmHg or } [7.19 \text{ kPa}]$$

Step 2. Calculate the PaO_2/PAO_2 ratio

$$= 30/54$$

$$= 0.55$$

Step 3. Calculate the new PAO_2 to achieve the desired PaO_2 of 60 mmHg.

$$\frac{\text{desired } PaO_2}{\text{new } PAO_2} = 0.81$$

$$\frac{60}{\text{new } PAO_2} = 0.55$$

$$\text{new } PAO_2 = 109 \text{ mmHg}$$

Step 3. Calculate the new FIO_2 that would create a PAO_2 = 109 mmHg assuming no change in $PaCO_2$.

$$PAO_2 = (760 - 47)\text{new } FIO_2 - 80(1.2)$$

$$\text{new } FIO_2 = \frac{109 + 96}{713}$$

$$= 0.28$$

BOX 13-9

CATEGORIES AND EXAMPLES OF HYPOXIAS

Categories	Clinical Example
Hypoxic hypoxia	
1. Low P_{IO_2} due to F_{IO_2} <0.21 or reduced barometric pressure	Anesthetic circuit without oxygen flow Altitude
2. Impaired ventilation	Narcotic drug overdose Neuromuscular weakness
3. Impaired oxygenation	Pulmonary fibrosis
4. Venous → arterial shunts	ARDS
Circulatory hypoxia	
5. Impaired circulation	Myocardial infarction
Hemic hypoxia	
6. Decreased O_2-carrying capacity	Anemia Carbon monoxide poisoning
Demand hypoxia	
7. Increased $\dot{V}O_2$	Fever
Histotoxic hypoxia	
8. Abnormal utilization	Cyanide toxicity

signs, symptoms, and other data with blood gases to "infer" that patients are hypoxic.

Anoxic (hypoxic) hypoxia refers to pulmonary conditions that would cause low tissue levels caused by inadequate arterial oxygen tensions (PaO_2). Disorders would include all four categories of hypoxemic causes. Figure 13-29A identifies an oxyhemoglobin curve showing a depressed oxygen content caused by low oxygen tension in arterial blood. The arteriovenous content difference is normal but the venous level $P\bar{v}O_2$ and $S\bar{v}O_2$ may be depressed because of a low arterial starting point. The short-term compensation would involve increasing cardiac output and supplemental oxygen. Long-term adaption would involve increasing levels of hemoglobin and 2,3-DPG.

Circulatory (stagnant) hypoxia involves inadequate pumping of blood from lungs to tissues. This can occur in cardiovascular disorders including decreased cardiac output from myocardial infarction (MI), reduced fluid volume, systemic hypotension, and poor arterial vascular supply. With reduced circulation yet normal tissue oxygen consumption, tissues extract more oxygen per blood volume. This is displayed as a widened arteriovenous content difference, $C(a-\bar{v}))_2$. A below-normal oxygen content, $P\bar{v}O_2$ and $S\bar{v}O_2$ will be a typical finding if pulmonary blood is analyzed. Figure 13-29B identifies the typical oxyhemoglobin curve and pattern of physiologic data. PaO_2 levels may be in the normal range until severe failure. Primary therapy is restoration of fluid volume or cardiac function. If myocardial dysfunction is caused by hypoxia, supplemental oxygen would be indicated. However, in patients with myocardial ischemia that is critically limited by coronary stenosis, supplemental oxygen is of less benefit.[63]

Demand hypoxia refers to an above-normal tissue consumption of oxygen in hypermetabolic states. The net result is a similar presentation to circulatory hypoxia, in that there is a disparity between oxygen supply and need. Such conditions occur in significant fever, sepsis, malignant hyperthermia, hyperthyroidism, and pheochromocytoma. The oxygen transport system may be normal, but it is unable to meet the abnormally high metabolic demands. The oxyhemoglobin dissociation curve for this category will resemble that of circulatory hypoxia (Figure 13-29B).

Hemic hypoxia describes conditions in which the hemoglobin content is decreased (anemia, hemorrhage, hemolysis, or sickling), or in the presence of hemoglobin-

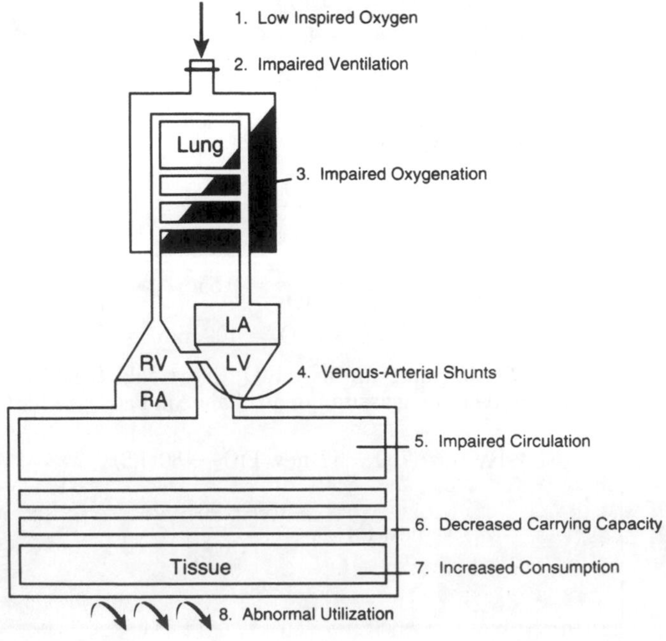

FIGURE 13-28. Schematic diagram illustrating the potential areas for defects leading to problems in oxygen transport (From Higgins TL, Yared JP. Clinical effects of hypoxemia and tissue hypoxia. Respir Care 1993;38:603. Reproduced with permission.)

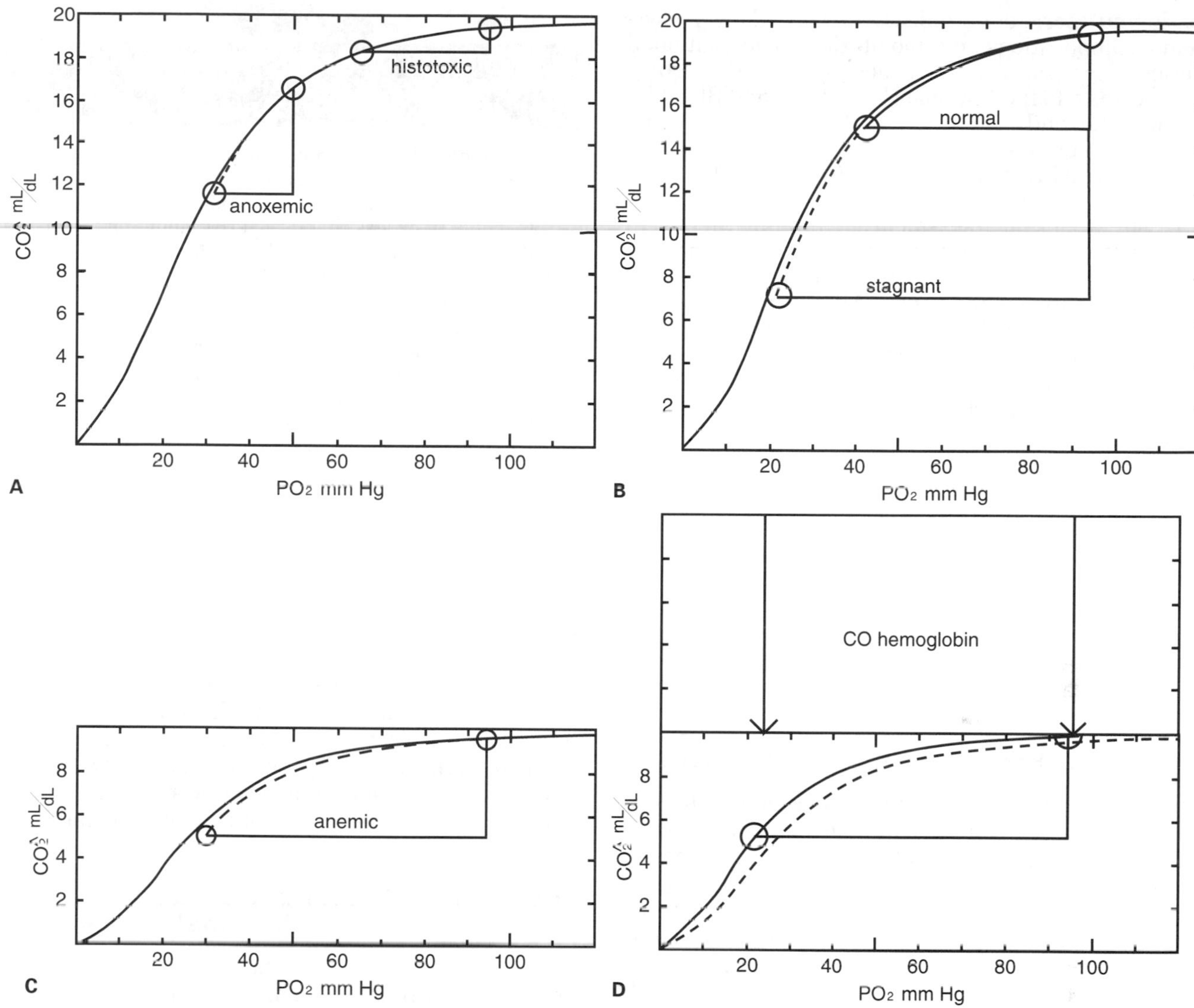

FIGURE 13-29. Oxygen dissociation curves illustrating abnormal patterns of hypoxias. Oxygen content is compared to oxygen tension. **(A)** Hypoxic (anoxic) **(B)** Circulatory "stagnant" hypoxia, **(C)** Anemic hypoxia, and **(D)** Hypoxia produced by hemoglobinopathy, eg, carbon monoxide toxicity and histotoxic hypoxia. (Courtesy HF Helmholz, Jr. MD.)

opathies (carboxyhemogobinemia, methemoglobinemia, and sulfhemoglobinemia). The oxyhemoglobin dissociation curve for anemia shows a vertically compressed "content" curve as seen in Figure 13-29C. In either anemia or hemoglobinopathy, there is no interference with alveolar oxygen pressures; therefore arterial tensions (PaO_2) or pulse oximetry (SpO_2) will be normal despite a decreased oxygen content (CaO_2). (Pulse oximetry spectrophotometric analysis will not discriminate the abnormal hemoglobin absorption.) The key information in anemic-hemic hypoxia is the laboratory value of hemoglobin (g/dL). In hemic hypoxia caused by hemoglobinopathies, a multiband spectrophotometric blood analysis will reveal a decreased SaO_2 owing to increased carboxyhemoglobin (COHb) or methemoglobin (MetHb) (Fig. 29-D).

Histotoxic hypoxia is the tissue's inability to use oxygen. Cyanide toxicity is included in this category. Cyanide poisons the cytochrome electron exchange of the final pathway to generate ATP. Consequently, the venous tissue levels ($P\bar{v}O_2$ and $S\bar{v}O_2$) and $C(a-\bar{v})_2$ will all be higher than normal (Fig. 13-29A). In addition, carbon monoxide toxicity also causes a malfunction in tissue oxygen utilization in addition to oxygen-binding sites on hemoglobin molecules.[64]

GUIDELINES AND PROTOCOLS TO DIRECT RATIONAL MEDICAL GAS THERAPY

Respiratory therapy practitioners are frequently asked to integrate patient information and recommend an approach to medical gas therapy. It is possible to devise a plan to approach most patient problems. Alvan Barach was an early proponent for rational oxygen prescription in the United States. In the mid-1970s, an effort was made to reach consensus and provide scientifically based approaches to supplemental oxygen therapy.[65] Since then, physician-sponsored national groups have held conferences to review the scientific basis and therapeutic efficacy, oxygen delivery systems, complications, and monitoring.[2] The continued series is sponsored by the American College of Chest Physicians and the National Heart, Lung and Blood Institute.[66] Recently the American Association for Respiratory Care targeted respiratory care practitioners with their Clinical Practice Guidelines (CPGs).[3,4] The CPGs were designed to provide a national consensus for therapy. They focus on assessment and titrating therapy to patient response (laboratory and physical examination) and relate to either the acute hospital-based care or long-term care setting. See AARC Clinical Practice Guideline: Oxygen Therapy in the Acute Care Setting (Box 13-10) and AARC Clinical Practice Guideline: Oxygen Therapy in the Home or Extended Care Facility (Box 13-11) for details.

Indications for Oxygen Therapy

Common signs and symptoms of hypoxia and hypoxemia are presented in Table 13-8. The short-term application even of high concentrations of oxygen is relatively free of complications; withholding oxygen can have grave consequences. Hypoxemia often progresses to tissue hypoxia, acidosis, cardiac dysrhythmia, and vital organ failure.

Conditions Requiring Nitrogen Washout

High concentrations of oxygen have been used to treat patients who have collection of air in body cavities or tissues. Such conditions would include pneumothorax, pneumomediastinum, subcutaneous emphysema, postpneumoencephalography, and distended bowel. Oxygen in gas pockets is usually absorbed, leaving mainly nitrogen. When pure oxygen is breathed, nitrogen is displaced from the lung and blood. The elimination of nitrogen results in the total gas tension of end-systemic capillary being reduced from approximately 706 mmHg (101 kPa) (breathing air at sea level) to about 150 mmHg (19.95 kPa).[158] The lowered gas tension in the venous side of the capillary will favor absorption of gas molecules from closed spaces. This phenomenon can be undesirable in the case of the middle ear with a blocked eustachian tube or paranasal sinuses with blocked ostia. Pulmonary atelectasis is also more likely to occur during high-concentration oxygen breathing.

BOX 13-10

SUMMARY OF AARC CPGS INDICATIONS FOR OXYGEN THERAPY IN THE ACUTE CARE SETTING

Documented hypoxemia: In adults, children, and infants (older than 1 month) at rest, breathing room air, documentation is: PaO_2 less than 60 mmHg (7.98 kPa) or SaO_2 or SpO_2 less than 90%. In neonates: PaO_2 less than 50 mmHg (6.7 kPa) or SaO_2 less than 88% or capillary oxygen PcO_2 tension of less than 40 mmHg (5.33 kPa). The goal of therapy would be to restore blood gas tension and saturations to the baseline values and above critical levels, eg $\geq PaO_2$ 60 mmHg (7.98 kPa) or SaO_2 or $SpO_2 \geq 90\%$.[3]

Suspected acute hypoxemia or hypoxia: Clinical information based on physical examination, patient symptoms, or other laboratory data should guide respiratory care practitioners to initiate and/or modify oxygen therapy. There may be limited history. Oxygen can be provided before procedures such as tracheal suctioning or bronchoscopy that commonly cause arterial desaturation. Pre- and post-procedure oxygen therapy can prevent or limit iatrogenic hypoxemia.[3]

BOX 13-11

SUMMARY OF AARC CPG INDICATIONS FOR OXYGEN THERAPY IN THE HOME OR EXTENDED CARE FACILITY

Documented hypoxemia: Home oxygen therapy is indicated when there is evidence that the resting PaO_2 is equal to or less than 55 mmHg (6.67 kPa) or SaO_2 or SpO_2 equal to or less than 88%. Prescribing physicians in the United States must deal with the Health Care Financing Administration (HCFA) to certify the necessity for home therapy. Medicare regulations and reimbursement grants greater flexibility in allowing PaO_2s of 56 to 59 mmHg (7.44–7.84 kPa) or SaO_2 of 89% if patients have evidence of cor pulmonale by electrocardiogram and erythrocytosis (hematocrit >56%). Oxygen is indicated during sleep, ambulation, or exercise if there is demonstration that the SaO_2 drops to 88% or less.[4, 22]

Limitations in Treating Hypoxic Conditions With Supplemental Oxygen

Oxygen therapy may be of limited value for a number of nonpulmonary problems. Patients with hypoxic conditions produced by acute anemia, that is, lack of hemo-

TABLE 13-8. **Signs and Symptoms of Hypoxemia/Hypoxia**

Organ System	Clinical Signs/Symptoms
Pulmonary	Tachypnea
	Dyspnea
	Hyperpnea
Cardiovascular	Tachycardia
	Changes in pulse
	Dysrhythmias
	Palpitations
	Hypertension
Hematology	Anemia
	Polycythemia (sign of compensation)
CNS	Restlessness, disorientation, lethargy, and coma
	Paresthesias
	Apnea
Other	Digital clubbing
	Cyanosis

globin (Hb <10 g/dL) can be temporarily supported by high-concentration supplemental oxygen. Primary immediate therapy involves increasing hemoglobin levels by transfusion. Their hemoglobin should be fully saturated, and supplemental oxygen used to increased the dissolved oxygen content. However, only a portion of resting oxygen needs can be met. An increase in cardiac output has a more impressive role in increased oxygen transport in anemia. Chronic anemia is often better tolerated.

Hypoxia produced by low cardiac output or tissue perfusion primarily depend on the degree of tissue demand versus delivery inadequacy. The goal of oxygen therapy during periods of low cardiac output is to maximize the blood's oxygen content. If lack of oxygen to the myocardium is the cause of low cardiac output, oxygen therapy has a more direct role in therapy. However, in coronary ischemia in critical coronary artery stenosis, oxygen therapy may not yield significant benefit.[63]

Patients with large cardiac or pulmonary right-to-left shunts will have a disappointing response to oxygen therapy. In pulmonary shunts, increasing the P_{AO_2} in the areas of good $\dot{V}/\dot{Q}$ matching cannot "supersaturate" hemoglobin to overcompensate for poorly saturated blood from areas with shunting.

Supplemental oxygen should not be used as substitute for those patients needing mechanical ventilation as primary therapy.

Patient Conditions Commonly Warranting Oxygen Therapy

Acute MI with cardiac arrest requires resuscitative efforts with 100% oxygen. The efficacy of oxygen therapy post MI to reduce myocardial ischemia has been shown in laboratory animals.[2] However, there is lack of data to suggest it alters mortality in uncomplicated post-MI care. It is rational to use supplemental oxygen to avoid hypoxemia and decrease incidence of dysrhythmias. Tissue hypoxia (circulatory) and lactic acidemia is often the result of reduced cardiac output.[2,56]

Cardiogenic pulmonary edema commonly require high concentration oxygen therapy while cardiotonic drugs, diuretics, and vasoactive drugs treat manifestations of the left ventricular failure. If present, tissue hypoxia is commonly the result of reduced cardiac output, as well as hypoxemia from $\dot{V}/\dot{Q}$ mismatching, shunting, and diffusion defect in the lung. Oxygen therapy is indicated. It can be administered in conjunction with intermittent positive pressure breathing (IPPB) or constant positive airway pressure breathing (CPAP) to reduce venous return. Cor pulmonale is a common manifestation of chronic hypoxemia. Low alveolar oxygen pressures induce hypoxic pulmonary vasoconstriction. Oxygen administration can reverse the arteriolar constriction unless the vascular changes have become fixed or there is destructive vascular disease. One of the goals of long-term oxygen therapy is to reverse or prevent cor pulmonale.

The use of 100% oxygen is essential therapy in *carboxyhemoglobinemia (HbCO)* in addition to support of vital signs. Red cell degradation produces a small amount of HbCO normally. The majority of cases involve accidental inhalation of gas from incomplete combustion. Hemoglobin has a 200-fold greater attraction for carbon monoxide than oxygen. This can greatly reduce blood's oxygen transport function. There is also a direct neurophysiologic effect of CO. In addition, the oxyhemoglobin dissociation curve is shifted left, hindering oxygen unloading to tissues. Symptoms including weakness, headache, nausea, vomiting, chest or abdominal pain, and dizziness or confused behavior can occur with 20% HbCO. With levels of 40% to 60% there is stupor, coma, and death caused by widespread organ hypoxia.[67] Supplemental oxygen can fully saturate functional hemoglobin and speed removal of the CO from binding sites. High-level oxygen can reduce the HbCO half-life from 320 minutes without treatment to 137 minutes.[68] The neurologic sequelae from toxic exposures can be severe and persistent. The efficacy of hyperbaric versus normobaric oxygen therapy treatment requires careful patient selection and further research.[69] High oxygen concentrations are a valuable temporizing measure in severe acquired methemoglobinemia (HbMET). Specific therapy involves oral or intravenous methylene blue.

The perioperative state often predisposes to the need for supplemental oxygen. General anesthesia commonly causes a decrease in PaO_2, secondary to increased $\dot{V}/\dot{Q}$ mismatching and decreased functional residual capacity.[70] The effects are greatest with thoracic and abdominal surgery, the elderly, obese, and in preexisting pulmonary disease. Hypoxemia usually responds to intraoperative or postoperative supplemental oxygen. General anesthetics can also reduce the normal respiratory center's responsiveness to hypoxemia.[2,70]

Chronic obstructive pulmonary diseases (COPD) such as asthma, chronic bronchitis, emphysema, bronchiectasis, and cystic fibrosis often require supplemental oxygen during acute exacerbations or during end-stage disease. In this pathologic grouping hypoxemia is caused by mismatching with or without hypercapnia. The use of high, moderate, or low oxygen concentrations is dictated by individual patient presentation. Efficacy for continuous long-term use of oxygen therapy in emphysema has been well documented.[22,66,71,72] (see Box 13-11) Use during exercise or during sleep for sleep-related hypoxemia has not been as well established.

Patients with *interstitial pulmonary fibrosis* may require supplemental oxygen if a diffusion defect becomes significant.

Adult respiratory distress syndrome is a nonspecific pulmonary response to a range of pulmonary and nonpulmonary insults. The exact mechanisms are not completely understood. ARDS is characterized by interstitial infiltrates, alveolar hemorrhage, diffuse atelectasis, and reduced functional residual capacity. Intrapulmonary shunting results in hypoxemia that is difficult to correct with supplemental oxygen. Patients often require high F_{IO_2}s, CPAP, and mechanical ventilation with positive end-expiratory pressure (PEEP). Although it is based on different etiology, the respiratory distress syndrome of the newborn (RDS) also results in pulmonary atelectasis causing increased work of breathing and hypoxemia.

Supplemental oxygen is used to correct the pulmonary (and/or intracardiac) R→L shunting and mismatching; adjuncts of CPAP or PEEP with mechanical ventilation are added as indicated.

Complications and Hazards of Oxygen Therapy

Supplemental oxygen is a relatively benign drug. Far more adult patients die of hypoxia than suffer complications from acute oxygen therapy. However, clinicians must be aware of precautions and complications and make efforts to minimize untoward effects. Precautions and possible complications caused by supplemental oxygen are summarized in Box 13-12.[3]

Pulmonary oxygen toxicity refers to cellular injury of lung parenchyma and airway epithelium. When intracellular PO_2 is elevated, cytotoxic free radicals are generated in excessive amounts. The free radicals include superoxide anion (O_2^-), singlet oxygen $^1O_2$, hydroxyl radical ($OH^\cdot$), and partially reduced oxygen metabolites like hydrogen peroxide (H_2O_2). Some free radical production occurs as a normal aspect of cellular metabolism; intracellular enzymes like superoxide dismutases and catalase eliminate most toxic products. Nonenzymatic antioxidants include vitamin A, ascorbate, cysteine β-carotene, α-tocopeherol, and hemoglobin.

Cellular elements most sensitive to oxygen pressures are proteins containing free sulfhydryl groups that act as intracellular enzymes. This results in a decrease in ATP production. In addition, both protein and DNA synthesis is inhibited. Pulmonary types I and II epithelial and endothelial cells are affected structurally and ultimately may result in death. Toxic effects result in thickening of the intracellular space, replacement of type I by type II cells, and inhibition of surfactant production. There is histologic resemblance of oxygen toxicity and diffuse alveolar injury from other causes that result in ARDS.[73,74]

Clinical manifestations of high-concentration oxygen breathing include symptoms of mild to severe substernal pain, dyspnea, fatigue, and paresthesias. There is tracheobronchitis, and ciliated airway cells have depressed activity within 6 hours of 100% oxygen exposure. Clinical signs of gas exchange abnormalities can occur within 24 to 48 hours at an F_{IO_2} of 1.0. They include hypoxemia caused by R→L shunting from atelectasis, decreased lung compliance, and infiltrates on chest radiograph reflect the cellular pathology. Inflammatory changes, edema, and fibrosis occur with exposure longer than 72 to 96 hours.[75]

Toxic effects depend on the concentration, length of exposure to oxygen, and underlying lung condition. Since cellular levels cannot be directly measured, dosage relationships can only be presumed. To date, no exact threshold concentration has been established at which toxicity occurs. Multiple factors affect tolerance, including hormones, catecholamine levels vitamin E levels, and drugs such as paraquat poisoning. Exacerbation of bleomycin therapy remains controversial because of the difficulty in human research.[76,77]

In clinical practice, high-concentration oxygen should not be withheld from critically ill patients or for transport. Breathing concentrations up 0.5 for 2 to 7 days does not result in clinically significant lung impairment.[2] Extended exposure to F_{IO_2}s ≥ 0.6 should be avoided when possible. A goal of respiratory care practitioners is to use the minimum concentration required to achieve adequate tissue oxygenation. CPAP and mechanical ventilation with PEEP should be considered to increase the alveolar volume for improving oxygenation.[2,74]

Absorption atelectasis can occur with high-concentration oxygen breathing, secondary to "washout" of nitrogen from the lungs. During room air breathing, the partial pressure of nitrogen in the lung is approximately 570 mmHg. Nitrogen molecules are replaced with oxygen in the alveoli. Any airway obstruction or reduction in ventilation may result in oxygen being removed by pulmonary blood. Alveolar collapse is likely without the resident nitrogen, and hypoxemia from increased physiologic shunting will result.

Oxygen-induced hypercarbia or apnea may occur in spontaneously breathing patients with elevated baseline $PaCO_2$. Traditionally, the mechanism has been postulated to reflect medullary centers of patients with COPD who are no longer responsive to carbon dioxide levels. These patients breathe in response to hypoxic stimulation of aortic and carotid receptors. Sufficient supplemental oxygen has been thought to suppress the hypoxic ventilatory drive. More recently, oxygen-induced hypercarbia has been attributed to changes in ventilation-perfusion relationships, resulting in an increased dead space to tidal volume ratio (V_D/Vt)[78] and/or the Haldane effect. Regardless of the mechanisms, clinicians must be alert to this complication. If patients do underventilate or become apneic, ventilation with reduced F_{IO_2}s should be initiated. Oxygen should be titrated to produce a PaO_2 in the 50 to 60 mmHg range with SaO_2 **or** SpO_2 in the 84% to 90% level. Oxygen must never be withdrawn in the face of high or rising $PaCO_2$.

Fire hazard is a concern when dealing with normobaric oxygen and a major hazard in hyperbaric applications. There is risk with oxygen-enriched atmospheres in patient enclosures, during laser bronchoscopy, and

BOX 13-12

COMPLICATIONS AND HAZARDS OF OXYGEN THERAPY

- Pulmonary oxygen toxicity including alteration of ciliary and/or leukocyte function ($F_{IO_2} \geq 0.5$)
- Absorption atelectasis ($F_{IO_2} > 0.5$)
- Oxygen-induced hypercarbia in chronically hypercapnic patients ($PaO_2 > 60$ mmHg)
- Increased fire hazard and during laser bronchoscopy
- Microbial contamination from humidifier or nebulizer gas administration systems.

Newborns would require additional precautions for the following:

- Retinopathy of prematurity (retrolental fibroplasia) ($PaO_2 > 80$ mmHg)
- Unwanted closure of the ductus arteriosus in ductus-dependent congenital heart lesions.

during head and neck surgery. Ignition can result in a flash flame via fine surface fibers of fabric or body hair. Combustible materials (eg, cigarettes), sparking friction toys, and electric razors should be avoided in enclosures or close to open sources of oxygen.

Retinopathy of prematurity (ROP) is an insult to the developing retinal vasculature from elevated PaO_2s. It was first described in 1942 and termed retrolental fibroplasia (RLF) by Terry.[79] Oxygen radicals attack the incompletely developed retinal tissue and result in vasoconstriction, which can progress to complete obliteration and retinal detachment (see Fig. 13-30). In RLF it was initially thought that supplemental oxygen was the "iatrogenic culprit." However, elevated PaO_2 in retinal vessel walls is only one of several predisposing factors that can result in visual defects, which can progress to total blindness. Low birth weight, sepsis, gestational age, apnea, acidemia/hypercarbia, level of oxygen, and length of exposure all interact as multiple causes. ROP is seen in low-birth-weight babies who never received supplemental oxygen. Occurrence of blindness vary from 1% to 3% in all live births and 40% to 70% in infants weighing less than 1000 kg.[80] The incidence is inversely proportional to birth weight and highest in neonates weighing less than 1 kg.[81] In the 1940s and 1950s, the incidence of ROP reached "epidemic" proportions since oxygen was used without monitoring. Arbitrary guidelines of limiting to oxygen concentration of 0.4 resulted in increased mortality and cerebral palsy births.[82] The development of blood gases and pulse oximetry has helped reduce this complication. Dietary supplementation with vitamin E can ameliorate the effect and reduce the incidents of ROP through its antioxidant action.[83] Critically ill infants' FIO_2 should be analyzed; PaO_2 and SaO_2/SpO_2 are monitored both by periodic blood gases and continuous pulse oximetry. Supplemental oxygen should be given to keep the PaO_2 higher than 50 mmHg. However, the safe upper level is unknown and not likely to be studied. Guidelines stipulate no greater than 80 to 90 mmHg. Not only is the PaO_2 important, but the duration is also critical in developing ROP.[3,84]

Neonates with congenital heart lesions depend on patency of the ductus arteriosus for either pulmonary or systemic blood flow. Those with pulmonary atresia form the majority of cases but also include coarctation of the aorta, tricuspid atresia, and aortic arch interruption. Many newborns will have profound hypoxia or circulatory collapse as the ductus closes spontaneously. Use of prostaglandin E_1 has been an important management drug. Increasing oxygen tension is the chief trigger of ductal smooth muscle contraction. Therefore, "modest" PaO_2s are also indicated as a palliative measure or until corrective surgery can be carried out.[85]

Humidification and nebulization equipment, as adjuncts to oxygen delivery systems, have been associated with nosocomial contamination. Water reservoirs, resuscitation bags, and oxygen analyzer probes can be come contaminated by the hands of personnel, unsterile humidification fluids, or inadequate sterilization/disinfection between uses.[86]

Initial Oxygen Therapy Recommendations and Dosage Guidelines

The simple algorithm in Figure 13-31 diagrams the initial decision-making process.

The process begins after determining the patient has a problem that oxygen or other medical gas may assist in treating (see Fig. 13-31A). Either there is a suspicion based on clinical circumstances or specific signs or symptoms suggest hypoxemia or hypoxia. Sometimes

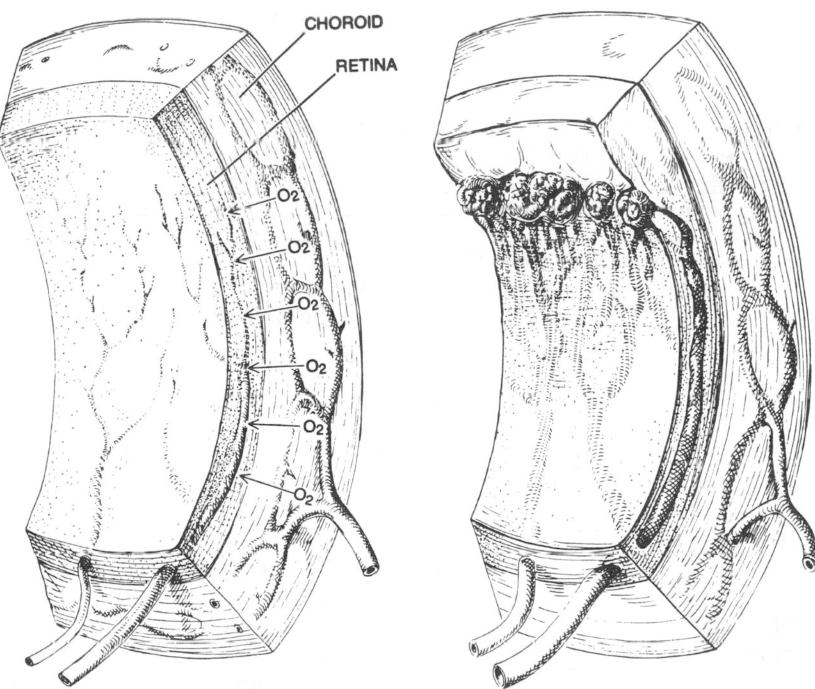

FIGURE 13-30. Diagram of pathologic changes of the developing retina seen in retinopathy of prematurity (aka retrolental fibroplasia). (From Silverman WA. The lesson of retrolental fibroplasia. Scientific American 1977;236:100. Reproduced with permission.)

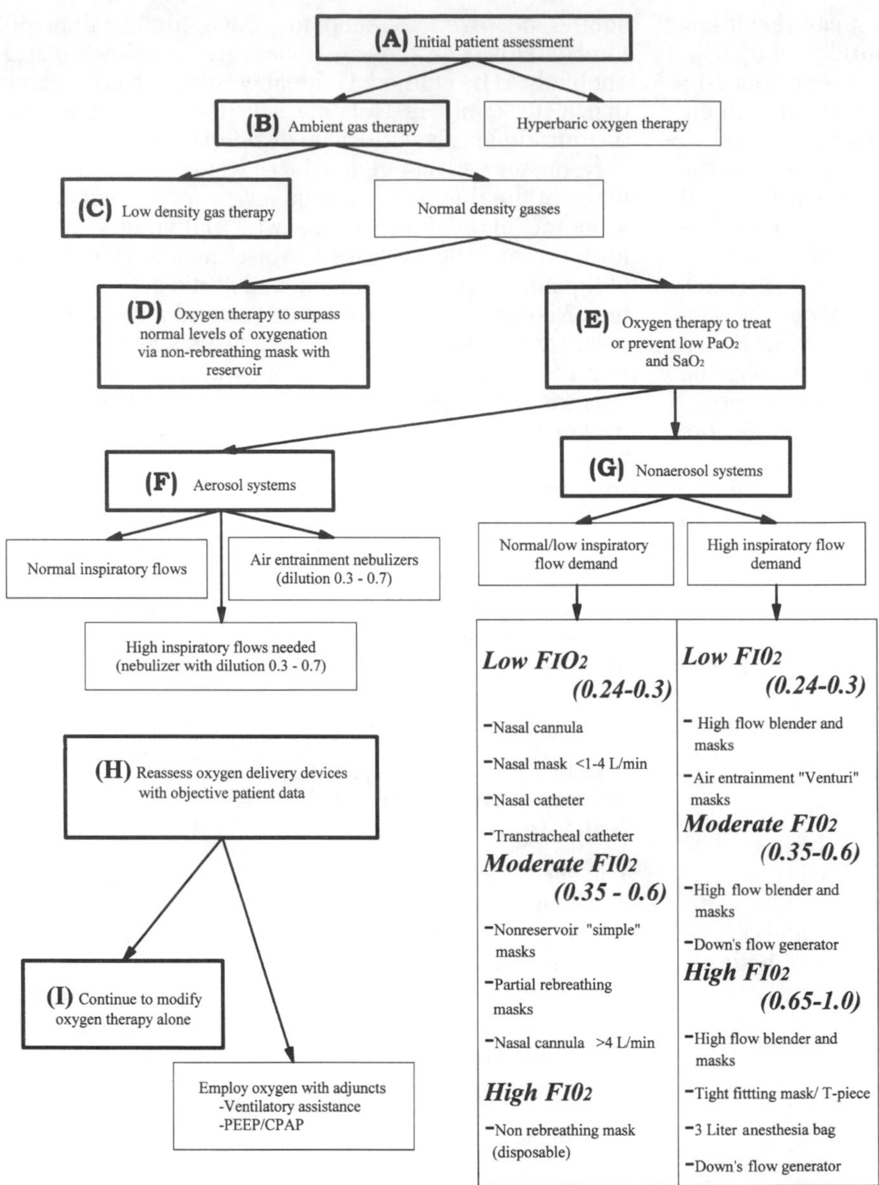

FIGURE 13-31. Guide to assist medical gas therapy.

laboratory data (eg, blood gases) reveal a surprise problem. The many factors related to oxygen transport tend to make the decision-making process more complex. In summary, there may be problems in:

- Ventilation (removal of CO_2)
- Oxygen content of arterial blood (eg, hemoglobin, gas tensions, saturation levels, oxyhemoglobin dissociation curve position)
- Central or local perfusion

A complete history and laboratory profile are commonly absent when patients have acute problems indicating medical gas therapy. Clinical signs and symptoms may be the only guides. As a general guideline, it is usually safer to provide liberal flows and concentrations than to restrict oxygen. There are always exceptions, but side effects are usually less significant than profound brain damage secondary to hypoxia. In the past there was undue emphasis on withholding oxygen because of a relatively small number of COPD patients with chronic hypercarbia. They may hypoventilate when given enough oxygen to produce a PaO_2 above 60 to 65 mmHg (7.9 − 8.64 kPa). Having to ventilate a patient is a problem, but you can manage if the patient is carefully monitored.

Following the initial assessment, you should separate patients into those requiring hyperbaric therapy and those needing only ambient medical gas therapy (see Fig. 13-31B). Usually the situations demanding hyperbaric therapy are obvious, or the hyperbaric therapy is a planned event. You can treat severe carbon monoxide poisoning with hyperbaric therapy if there is immediate access to a chamber.[69]

The initial assessment may provide information about the cause of the dyspnea or hypoxemia. It may be caused by acute asthma, worsening chronic bronchitis or emphysema, or obstructed upper airway. If this diagnosis is confirmed, helium–oxygen therapy (see Fig. 13-31C) is an option for their care. Heliox breathing may allow time to further evaluate the pathology and/or prepare definitive therapy, or await effects of pharmacologic therapy.

The next decision for those receiving ambient oxygen therapy is related to the concentration of oxygen needed to surpass normal levels, or to the treatment or prevention of abnormally low oxygen tensions or saturations (see Fig. 13-31D). Examples are victims of carbon monoxide poisoning, absorption of air pockets (pneumothorax), and recent post-MI victims.

History and laboratory data may not be immediately available for many patients, especially those arriving in the emergency room. Clinicians should immediately apply oxygen, based on empiric judgment. A room air blood gas analysis is quite valuable if it can be obtained without significant delay. Besides assisting with the diagnosis, arterial blood data can guide selection of the level of oxygen concentration needed. The room air blood gas can be compared with an estimate of normal values based on the patient's age. The following equations will allow an estimate for clinicians:[57]

$$\text{Normal (supine)} = 103.5 - 0.42\ (\text{age}) \pm 4\ \text{mmHg}$$

$$\text{Normal (sitting)} = 104.2 - 0.27\ (\text{age}) \pm 4\ \text{mmHg}$$

Guidelines suggest minimum PaO_2 levels be kept above 60 mmHg (7.9 kPa) with a saturation near 90%.[3]

An oxygen therapy system should be selected based on the apparent need and the patient's inspiratory flow requirement. High-flow or fixed-performance devices allow more consistent levels with patients who have rapid respiratory rates or gasping respiratory patterns (Fig. 13-31E). Those with normal breathing can usually receive low-flow or variable-performance systems.

Further discrimination should allow you to rule out or involve aerosol delivery devices to provide oxygen (Fig. 13-31F). Aerosol therapy may be part of gas therapy for treatment of secretion retention. If there is concern that asthmatic patients may develop or have worsening bronchospasm, you should consider an oxygen/air blender or Venturi humidifier systems. In addition, patients who have high inspiratory flows requirements and need FIO_2s greater than 0.60 will probably exceed the output from usual nebulizer systems. Practitioners should perform oxygen analysis to correlate blood gases with the FIO_2 and titrate the FIO_2 to achieve desired blood or pulse oximetric levels.

The options for patients with normal inspiratory flow requirements are those commonly used (see position G, Fig. 13-31). Respiratory care practitioners might select specific low-flow devices with several factors in mind, for example, patient comfort, perceived duration of therapy, and blood levels. Because analysis of inspired oxygen concentrations may be clinically difficult, arterial blood analysis or noninvasive methods may be used to assess effect of therapy. Pulse oximetry and transcutaneous oxygen monitoring can provide valuable information, especially in documenting trends. However, they do have limitations that should be recognized.[87]

As patients begin to respond to oxygen therapy, inspiratory flow and breathing rates may decrease, and blood oxygen levels should increase. The converse may also occur. Those administering initial therapy should carefully observe patients and modify therapy, as new information (physical signs and blood data) dictates (Fig. 13-31H). Clinicians should remove from aerosol systems those patients who show signs of bronchospasm. Also uncomfortable facial masks can be replaced with more comfortable nasal cannulas. Toxic levels are a concern, and you should reduce FIO_2 below 0.60 when possible. Certain COPD patients may develop increased arterial CO_2 tensions if given excessive oxygen fractions. The PaO_2 or SpO_2 should be used to carefully reduce flow settings or oxygen concentrations.

As was previously mentioned, various mathematical relationships may be used to help estimate new FIO_2 values to produce desired blood levels in patients such as the PaO_2/PAO_2 ratio.[88,89]

Each application makes certain assumptions and has limitations. Their value is in lending a quasi-scientific approach, which may reduce frequent blood gas analysis and hit-or-miss guesswork.

Oxygen therapy alone may not correct hypoxemia, hypoxia, or both in all patients (see Fig. 13-31I). Patients with profound hypercapnia with hypoxemia must frequently receive mechanical ventilatory assistance. PEEP or CPAP may be needed to augment high-concentration oxygen inhalation. The type of primary cardiopulmonary or hematologic disorder will determine the potential response to oxygen. Those with large right-to-left shunts, for example, will not show dramatic improvement in PaO_2 regardless of level of FIO_2 applied.

Clinicians should note that the schematic presentation in Figure 13-31 guides initial therapy. Other authors have provided algorithms to support decisions based on patient response.[90] More recently, the use of TDPs as illustrated in Protocol 13-1, allows clinicians to apply oxygen therapy within a predetermined decision making algorithm.[91] However, each patient must be considered as a special case, and clinicians should only use these guidelines as reasonable approaches.

AMBIENT OXYGEN THERAPY EQUIPMENT

Classifying Oxygen Therapy Equipment

Oxygen therapy devices are commonly grouped by their ability to provide both total gas flow levels and range of FIO_2. The purpose is to assist practitioners in understanding capabilities and limitations of their equipment, so they may better match patient's needs. Box 13-13 describes the most useful classification system:

Variable-Performance Equipment

☐ NASAL CATHETER

The catheter is a remnant from the early history of oxygen therapy and rarely used in adult care. It consists of a soft plastic tube with small outlet holes at the distal tip. It is sized using outside diameter (OD) French (F); an adult would use F 12 to 14 and pediatric patients F 8 to 10. The catheter is lubricated with water-soluble material before insertion to reduce or prevent adherence

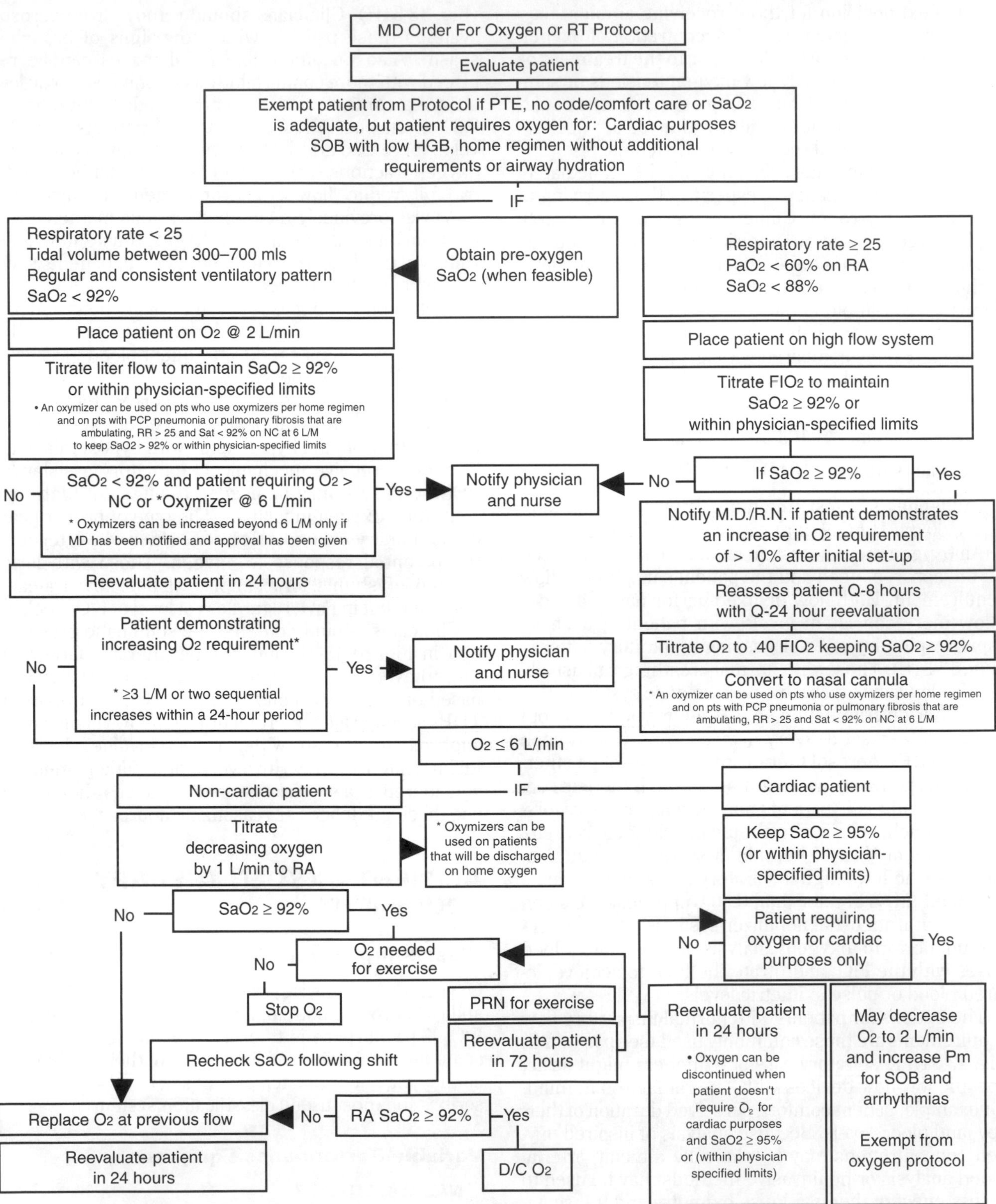

PROTOCOL 13-1. Therapist-driven protocol for oxygen therapy. (From Phillips JE: Oxygen protocol. AARC Times 19:56, 1995, with permission.)

BOX 13-13

CLASSIFICATION OF OXYGEN EQUIPMENT

Low-flow or variable-performance equipment: Supply oxygen at a fixed flow that is only a portion of all inspired gas. As ventilatory demands change, variable amounts of room air will dilute the oxygen flow. Low flow systems are adequate for patients with:

- Minute ventilations less than approximately 8 to 10 L/min
- Breathing frequencies less than 20 breaths/min
- Tidal volumes less than 0.8 L
- Normal inspiratory flow (10 to 30 L/min)

High-flow, or fixed-performance equipment: Supply all inspired gas at a preset FIO_2. Generally, the patient's FIO_2 is not affected by variations in their ventilatory demands or breathing patterns. Exceptions will be reviewed. High-flow systems are indicated for patients who require:

- Consistent FIO_2 and/or
- Large inspiratory flows of gas (≥40 L/min)

Reservoirs, demand valves, or high continuous flow are clinical options. With the latter system, the minimum gas flow to the patient is about 40 L/min but must be adjustable to accommodate greater flow needs. Profoundly dyspneic and hypoxemic patients may need flows of 100% oxygen in excess of 100 L/min.

to mucosal surfaces. Patency of the tubes distal outlets should be confirmed before insertion.

Placement

The catheter is inserted into either external naris and along the floor of the nasal cavity. It is designed to be inserted to just behind the uvula in the oropharynx. This procedure produces some discomfort in all patients. It can be complicated if there is nasal pathologic condition or the catheter is inserted upward, injuring the nasal turbinates. A defect in the blood clotting mechanism would be a contraindication since catheter insertion/removal may cause nasal bleeding. Deviated septum, severe mucosal congestion, and nasal polyps may prevent passage of the catheter. The alternative naris or (more likely) a different appliance should be selected. The catheter is held in place by taping it to the external nose.

The clinician can determine the appropriate distance to pass the catheter into the nose by two techniques, that is, use direct vision to locate the catheter. After the catheter is advanced into the nose, the conscious patient should be asked to open his or her mouth, and then with the tongue depressed, visualize the catheter with a light as it emerges from behind the uvula. The catheter is located to a position where it just disappears behind that structure.

The nasal catheter is usually inserted blindly and the appropriate distance for insertion is estimated by measuring the length from the nose to the external ear. Inserting the catheter for that distance should place it in the approximate location. The catheter is usually changed periodically (eg, every 8 hours) to prevent secretions from encasing the catheter, which causes problems on withdrawal.

Performance

Nasal catheters are best suited to provide a modest FIO_2. They appear to be most useful with patients breathing with stable, low rates and normal or small tidal volumes. Actual delivered FIO_2 will be substantially influenced if there is profound hypoventilation or hyperventilation. Also, the amount of open-mouth breathing will potentially vary the balance of room air and oxygen. The literature varies greatly regarding the actual performance of catheters. Adult tracheal FIO_2s of 0.22 to 0.24 with therapeutic flows of 2 to 5 L/min are reasonable expectations. Because of the ability of the nasal catheter to be firmly secured in position, and because infants require lower flows than adults, catheters have been favorably used in pediatric practice. Nasal catheters have largely negative factors that should be considered before being used to administer oxygen therapy.

Complications and Troubleshooting

The two major problems deal with insertion and removal, and with catheter positioning. It is an uncomfortable procedure. Trauma to the nasal area can occur if the catheter is forced into a blocked nasal passage. Nosebleeds may occur at this point or on later removal. The other major concern is oxygen passing into the esophagus if the catheter is placed or moves in the lower pharynx. To guard against this complication, patients should be observed initially and later for gulping movements or epigastric distention. The stomach filling with oxygen can lead to gastric rupture or at least mechanical resistance to diaphragm descent. The nasal cannula and other less "invasive" oxygen appliances have replaced the catheter because of the frequency of complications with its use.

□ NASAL CANNULAS

In 1929 Barach developed a dual nasal catheter and later a bifurcated metal cannula (see Fig. 13-2F).[92] Today the nasal cannula is a blind-ended soft plastic tube with either an over-the-ear elastic or lariat with under-the-chin adjustment (Fig. 13-32). Sizing is available for adults, children, and infants (Fig. 13-33A and B). Cannulas are connected to the flowmeter with small-bore tubing and may be used with bubble humidifier.

Placement

The nasal cannula can be rapidly and comfortably placed on most patients. An elastic headband or ear lariat holds the prongs in the nares and prevents twisting or kinking. The tension should be firm yet comfortable enough to avoid pressure sores on the ears, cheeks, and nose.

Performance

Actual FIO_2 levels that nasal cannulas can achieve at specific oxygen flows have been debated in the literature for many years. The fact that investigators using human subjects and bench tests have found a wide

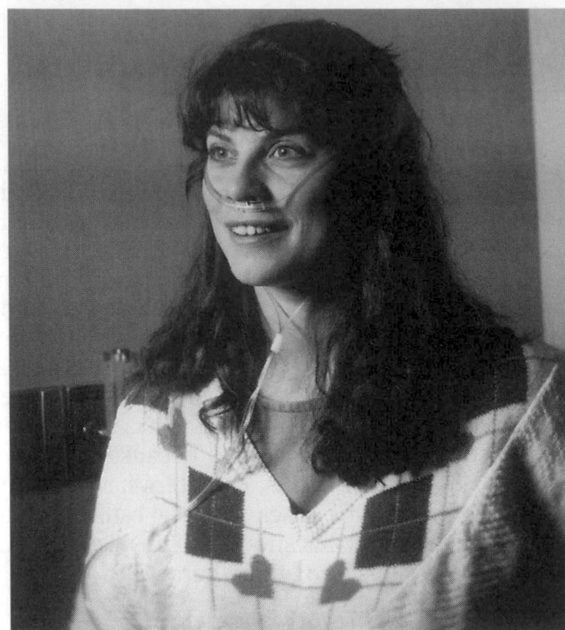

FIGURE 13-32. Adult nasal cannula

range of FIO_2s delivered to the trachea points to the variability of this device. Discrepancies in research findings also appear owing to the difficulty in obtaining accurate measurements of the inspired gas, breathing pattern, level of inspiratory flow, and level of minute ventilation. Such data influenced early practitioners and textbooks to overestimate the capabilities of the cannula.[93] Some authors suggest an estimated FIO_2 can be made based on a calculation of cannula flow and patient data or breathing-simulated mannequins.[94,95] Investigators who have analyzed gas using human subjects with rapid response sampling from trachea or hypopharynx found lower FIO_2s compared with either historical or calculated figures.[96,97] These in vivo studies have documented FIO_2s to range from 0.22 to 0.26, with normal breathing rates and patterns using flows of 2 to 5 L/min, respectively (Table 13-9). Flows of 10 and 15 L/min can achieve tracheal concentrations of 0.35 to 0.44; however, that level of flow is uncomfortable and should only be considered for short term. Data from "normal breathing subjects" may not be accurately transferred to acutely ill patients. Increasing volumes and short inspiratory times will dilute the small flow of oxygen during tachypnea and hyperventilation. Different levels of mouth-only versus nasal-only breathing patterns and varied inspiratory flow can vary FIO_2s up to 40%.[98]

In clinical practice, research estimates are valuable only as rough guides. The flow should be titrated using the following: clinical (vital) signs, pulse oximetric, and arterial blood gas measurements. Aggressiveness in monitoring levels of supplemental oxygen is determined by the patient's condition and importance of knowing the estimated level. At a minimum, respiratory care practitioners should monitor the patient by recording the oxygen flow and respiratory rate. Some patients with COPD tend to hypoventilate with even modest oxygen flows, yet are hypoxemic on room air. They may do well with the cannula at flows of <1 to 2 L/min. Patients on long-term oxygen therapy most commonly use the nasal cannula.[23]

Troubleshooting

Clinicians should confirm actual flow from the distal prongs by feeling for gas flow. Absent or low flows should prompt the operator to check (1) flowmeter accuracy, (2) twisted cannula or connecting tubing, or (3) leaky humidifier bottle seal (if humidifier is used). Most humidifiers are equipped with audible pop-off valves, which alert to obstructions causing pressure of about 40 mmHg.

Foam or gauze padding can be added to protect pressure points on the ears or over the cheekbones. Critically ill patients who become tachypneic or change their

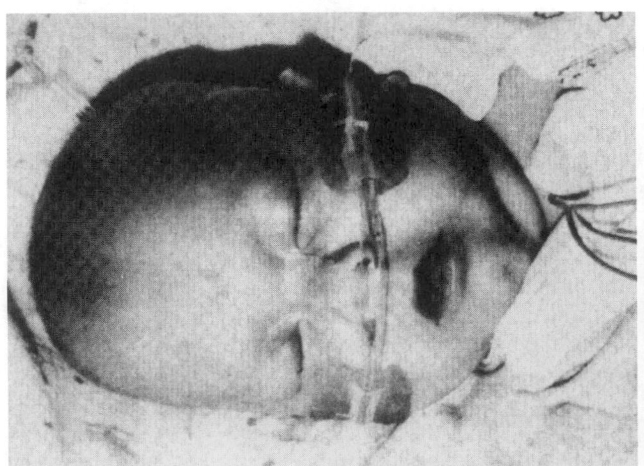

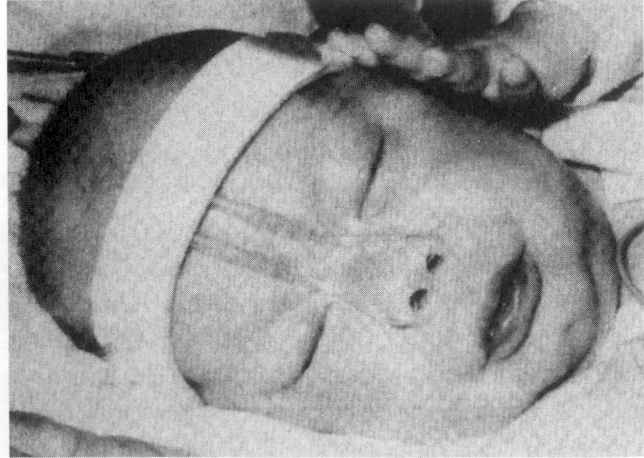

FIGURE 13-33. Infant nasal cannulas. (From Rotschild A, Schapira D, Kuyek N, Solimano A. Evaluation of nasal prongs of new design for low-flow oxygen delivery to infants. Respir Care 34:801, 1989. Reproduced with permission.)

TABLE 13-9. **Oxygen Concentrations for Delivery Systems***

System	O_2 Flow Rate (L/min)	FIO_2 Range
Nasal cannula	1	0.21–0.24
	2	0.23–0.28
	3	0.27–0.34
	4	0.31–0.38
	5–6	0.32–0.44
Venturi masks	4–6 (total flow = 105)†	0.24
	4–6 (total flow = 45)	0.28
	8–10 (total flow = 45)	0.35
	8–10 (total flow = 33)	0.40
	8–12 (total flow = 33)	0.50
Simple masks	5–6	0.30–0.45
	7–8	0.40–0.60
Masks with reservoirs	5	0.35–0.50
Partial rebreathing	7	0.35–0.75
	10	0.65–1.00
Nonrebreathing	4–10	0.40–1.00

* Values listed in this table are approximate.
† Values for total gas delivered are for the Accurox Venturi Mask.

tidal volume should be reevaluated by blood gas analyses or oximetry. Flow to the cannula may need to be readjusted to achieve desired blood levels. Alternative devices should be substituted if blood levels are critical and the patient appears to require higher oxygen concentrations. Fixed-performance or high-flow systems may be more appropriate for a COPD patient who is in distress but who hypoventilates at FIO_2s greater than 0.3. Blenders, dual-oxygen air flowmeters, or Venturi masks with high-flow systems are high flow/low FIO_2 options. Some clinicians combine a cannula with an oxygen mask (eg, aerosol face mask) in an attempt to provide high flows with greater FIO_2 reliability.

Infant Application

Pediatric-sized nasal cannulas are available for infants, and their clinical use has become increasingly common for patients with prolonged oxygen requirements. This practice has simplified nursing care, and facilitated ambulation and use at home. Because of the inherently reduced minute ventilation of infants, flow requirements to the cannula must be proportionately reduced. This generally requires a pressure-compensated Thorpe tube flowmeter with pure oxygen flows of 0 to 1 or 0 to 3 L/min range. Clinicians should limit oxygen flows to a maximum of 2 L/min.[3] Hypopharyngeal oxygen sampling from infants breathing with cannulas reveals mean FIO_2s of 0.35, 0.45, 0.6, and 0.68 with flows of 0.25, 0.5, 0.75, and 1 L/min, respectively.[99] Some clinicians use such flowmeters coupled with oxygen blenders for in-hospital care. Independent reduction of flow (at fixed blender FIO_2s) may facilitate smoother weaning versus reduction of flows of 100% oxygen. Cannulas for infants are available in various designs (see Fig. 13-33A and B). Some allow patients to nurse normally and subject the babies to less trauma of the face and nose.[100]

Clinical aspects of the nasal cannula are summarized in Box 13-14.

☐ OXYGEN-CONSERVING MODIFICATIONS OF NASAL CANNULAS

Cannulas can be combined with spectacle frames for convenience or to improve acceptance by improving cosmesis. Oxygen-conserving cannulas equipped with inlet reservoirs are available for patients receiving long-term oxygen. Since oxygen flows continuously, approximately 80% of the gas is wasted during expiration. This concept has resulted in the use of valved reservoir devices to allow storage of incoming oxygen until inspiration occurs.[101–103]

The "mustache cannula" (Oximizer) and pendant storage device (Oximizer Pendant) are contemporary storage cannulas (Figs. 13-34A and B; 13-35). The Oximizer can store 20 mL of oxygen in a space between a membrane and the back wall of the flexible reservoir body. Any deadspace gas exhaled into the reservoir is displaced by entering oxygen. The pendant holds 40 mL plus 20 mL in a conduit leading to a standard-appearing cannula. The oxygen savings with either device varies from 2:1 to 4:1 compared with continuous oxygen flow cannulas in the 1 to 2 L/min flow range. Both conserving devices can achieve similar supplemental oxygen performance compared with a standard nonstorage cannula but at a reduced oxygen flow. Patients must be taught to exhale through their nose to reset the membrane, which may interfere with pursed-lip breathing. Oxygen savings during rest and exercise is in the 50% to 75% range depending on flow levels. Pulse oximetry is commonly used to titrate flows.[104–107] Box 13-15 summarizes the conserving cannulas.

☐ OXYGEN PULSE-DEMAND DELIVERY SYSTEMS

Oxygen pulse-demand delivery systems can be used with standard cannulas, reservoir cannulas, or tracheal catheters to reduce oxygen costs; oxygen is delivered

BOX 13-14

SUMMARY OF THE NASAL CANNULA CLINICAL CONSIDERATIONS

FIO_2 range ≈ 0.22 to 0.3

Advantages	Disadvantages
Technically simple	Performance varies with patient's V_T and f
Usually well tolerated	Difficult to determine delivered FIO_2
"Unobtrusive"	Flows >4 to 5 L/min tend to irritate nasal mucosa
Nonclaustrophobic	Tubing can kink or become obstructed
Modifications for infant and oxygen conservation	Limited FIO_2 range

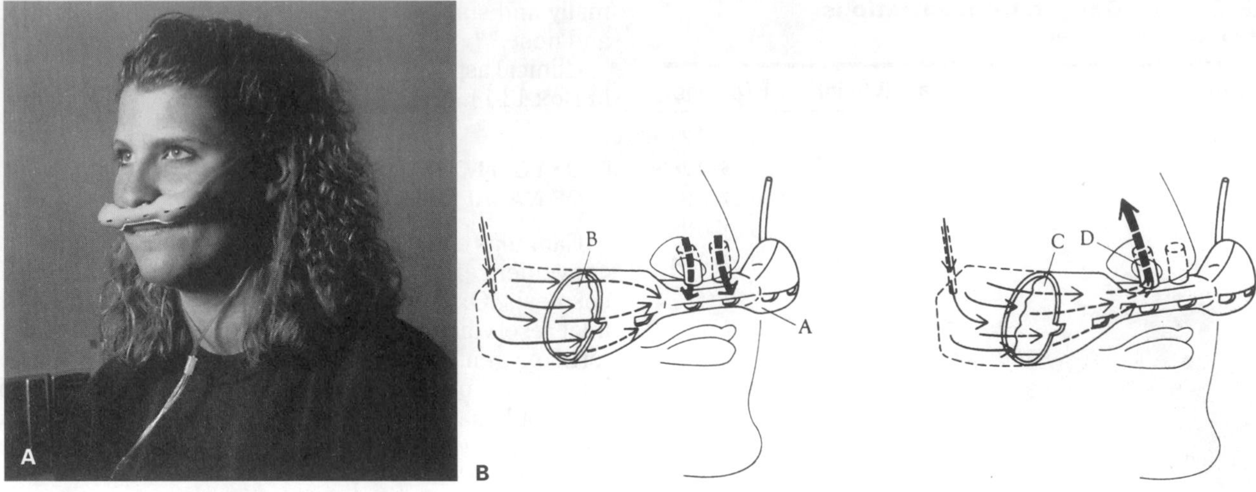

FIGURE 13-34. **(A)** Storage cannula. **(B)** Cross-sectional detail *(left)* showing internal membrane during expiratory phase and *(right)* during inspiration. (From Tiep BL, Belman MJ, Mittman C, Phillips RE, Ostap B. A new oxygen-conserving delivery device. Woodland Hills, CA: Chad Therapeutics, Inc. 1983. Reproduced with permission.)

only during inspiration (Fig. 13-36). Most designs use a battery-powered fluidic valve attached to a gaseous or liquid portable supply. The cannula tip senses flow at inspiration and rapidly initiates a bolus of oxygen via a solenoid valve. The size of the pulsed dose or flow can be adjusted. Commercially available oxygen pulsing devices report oxygen savings from 50% to 86% compared with continuous flow cannulas.[107–109] Reduced oxygen flows also favor ambulation and exercise because patient's oxygen supplies last longer or smaller vessels need be carried. However, costs for demand systems may offset some of the oxygen savings and potential technical problems are disadvantages that should be considered. There is little data on the long-term efficacy of the device.[107,109–112] Box 13-16 summarizes clinical aspects of demand pulse devices.

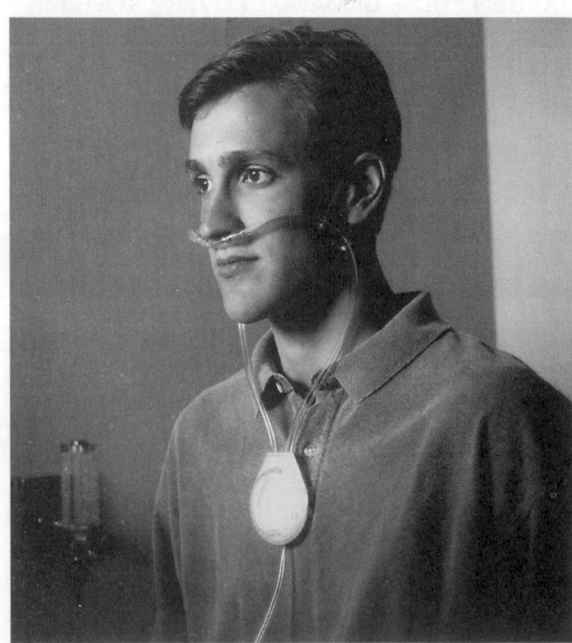

FIGURE 13-35. Pendant reservoir cannula.

□ TRANSTRACHEAL OXYGEN CATHETERS

Instillation of oxygen directly into the trachea by percutaneous catheter was first performed by Heimlich in the early 1980s.[113] The Scoop (Transtracheal Systems) and MicroTrachr (Inmedco) are commercially available catheters (Fig. 13-37). Transtracheal oxygen (TTO) catheters are thought to reduce the oxygen flow requirement by reducing waste through dilution of inspired oxygen and using the large airways as a reservoir during the expiratory phase. These catheters are not to be confused with those used to provide an emergency airway via cricothyrotomy. Those devices provide oxygen under pressure (with or without ventilation) for acute upper airway obstruction.[114]

Transtracheal oxygen catheters have been advocated for the following reasons: improved compliance because of cosmetic appearance, decreased nasal irritation, reduced cost of oxygen because of longer duration of portable oxygen supply, or improved patient function. Some patients experience relief of refractory hypoxemia (versus standard cannula) and improved exercise tolerance because of the increased efficiency of TTO. Oxy-

BOX 13-15

SUMMARY OF OXYGEN CONSERVING CANNULA CLINICAL CONSIDERATIONS

FIO_2 range ≈ 0.22 to 0.3

Advantages	Disadvantages
Technically simple 50% to 75% reduction in oxygen flow or higher PaO_2 or SaO_2 at same flow of standard cannula Modest FIO_2 increase over standard cannula	Performance varies with patient's V_T and f Some may be obtrusive Difficult to determine FIO_2 May interfere with pursed-lip breathing

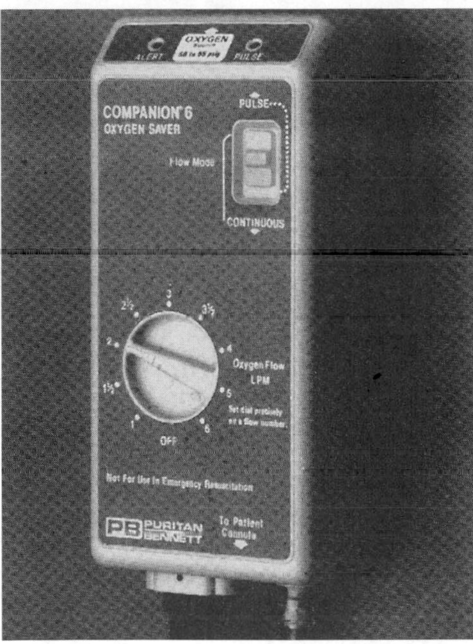

FIGURE 13-36. An electronic pulsed-demand oxygen delivery system (Courtesy of Puritan-Bennett Corp. Kansas City, MO.)

gen flows to the catheter may be reduced approximately 40% to 50% of cannula levels yet maintaining the same oxygen performance. Transtracheal oxygen catheters have also been used with electronic pulsed demand devices for further efficiency.[107,109,115–117,119]

Complications of TTO therapy include hemoptysis, subcutaneous emphysema, cough, site infection (cellulitis), catheter dislodgment, cephalad displacement, portions of the catheter breaking off, and mucous obstruction.[107,113,120] Most complications occur when the tract is immature. Although minor complications can occur in 10% to 60% of patients, they seldom require hospitalization. A serious complication is formation of mucous balls on the distal tip due to inspissated secretions. Proper patient selection and education are extremely important with this device. Severe respiratory tract infections have occurred secondary to the catheter.[121] There are reports of excessive stomal granulation tissue that required Nd:YAG laser bronchoscopy to reestablish tracheal patency.[122] A backup nasal cannula should be available to use if the tracheal catheter fails. In addition, if oxygen was supplied by fixed-flow restrictor, a device to give higher flow (approximately double) should be available. Patients requiring tracheal intubation should have the endotracheal tube placed with the catheter left in place and the TTO capped. Medical insurers support part of the cost of the surgical insertion and of the catheter replacement (approximately $100).

BOX 13-16

SUMMARY OF OXYGEN DEMAND FLOW DEVICES

Advantages	Disadvantages
Technically simple	Expensive
50% to 85% reduction in oxygen flow or higher PaO_2 or SaO_2 at same flow of standard cannula	Technical problems
Portable supplies last longer, allowing greater mobility	May not accommodate to increased needs during exercise

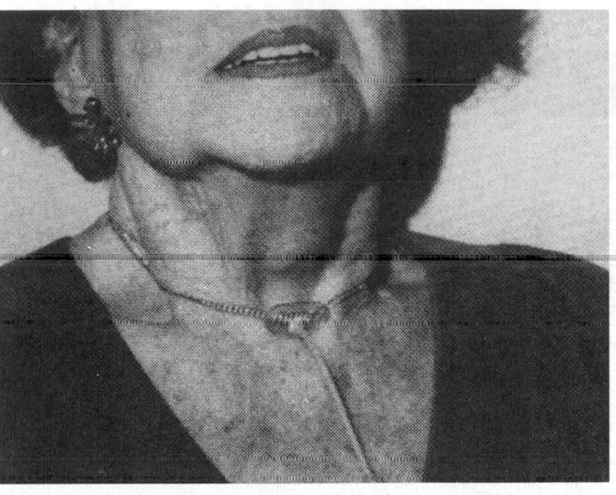

FIGURE 13-37. Patient with TTO catheter. (From Johnson JT, Ferson PF, Hoffman LA, Weismiller SW et al. Transtracheal delivery of oxygen: Efficacy and safety for long-term continuous therapy. Ann Otol Rhinol Laryngol 100:108, 1991. Reproduced with permission.)

Equipment Placement and Performance

Initially metallic and standard vascular catheters were used; however, specialized TTO catheters are now available. The Transtracheal Systems' SCOOP catheter is an example of a commercial system that provides patient and caregiver education plus maintenance recommendations. Initial placement is done as an in-hospital surgical procedure with strict attention to sterile technique. A nonfunctioning stent tube is initially placed through the tracheal cartilage to facilitate tract formation. After 1 week, the stent is removed over a wire guide and a functioning (9F) catheter is inserted. The catheter is held in place by a neck-chain. After 8 weeks from the initial surgery, patients return to receive instruction for daily care of the mature tract and catheter. Catheter replacement is recommended at 90 days, or earlier if the catheter cracks, breaks, kinks, or appears grossly fouled with pus. Patients may have problems replacing the catheter even after a well formed "tract" has formed. Routine care includes site cleaning, lavage, and use of a cleaning rod to remove mucus from the lumen and distal tip. Box 13-17 summarizes the transtracheal oxygen catheter.

□ NASAL MASK

The first "nasal-only" masks appeared in the 1930s to 1940s with a hat-like reservoir and headband or under-the-chin reservoir version of the BLB oronasal mask.[123,124] Currently, a nasal mask is available in the United States (Fig. 13-38) and Great Britain.

BOX 13-17

SUMMARY OF TRANSTRACHEAL OXYGEN CATHETER

Advantages	Disadvantages
Reduced nasal drying and irritation	Expense (surgery and catheter)
Cosmetic concealment of oxygen device	Requirement for routine care and patient education
Oxygenation in refractory hypoxemia	Increased risk of complications
Reduced oxygen flow and/or longer duration of gas supplies	Increased need for medical follow-up

Placement and Performance

The current nasal masks are applied to the face either by over-the-ear lariat or headband strap. The lower edge of the mask's flanges rest on the upper lip, surrounding the external nose. The nasal masks have been shown to provide supplemental oxygen equivalent to the nasal cannula under low-flow conditions for patients at rest.[123,124]

The primary advantage of the nasal mask appears to be patient comfort. Sores can develop around the external nares of long-term cannula wearers. Oxygen is not "jetted" into the nasal cavity like the cannula. Consider the nasal mask under these circumstances, especially if comfort improves patient compliance in wearing the oxygen device.

Troubleshooting

The nasal mask is subject to technical problems similar to those for the cannula: malpositioning, kinked tubing, and limited F_{IO_2} range. Blocked nasal passages and unstable breathing patterns may require an alternative device. Box 13-18 summarizes the nasal mask.

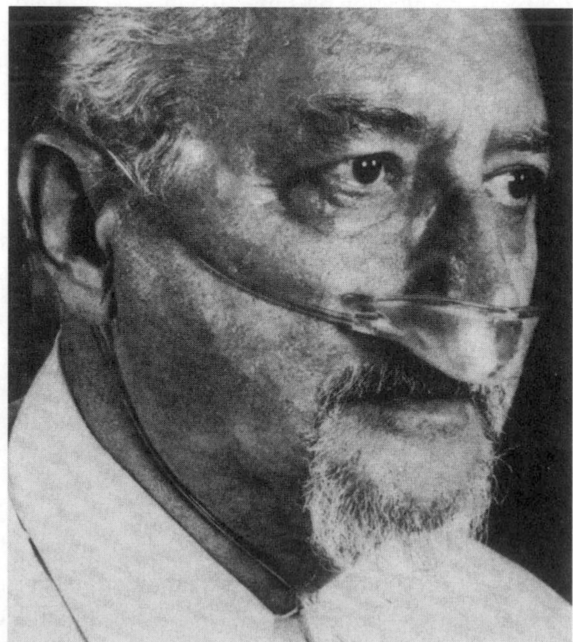

FIGURE 13-38. Nasal mask.

□ NONRESERVOIR OXYGEN MASK

This oxygen mask is a disposable lightweight plastic device that covers both nose and mouth (Fig. 13-39). The face seal is not easily fitted to ensure a leak-free system. The patient receives a mixture of pure oxygen and entrained room air, depending on mask fit, oxygen flow, and breathing pattern. Exhaled air exits through holes in the side of the mask but largely between the face and mask. Oxygen enters the mask from the flowmeter and bubble humidifier (if used) via small-bore tubing. Some brands of the simple mask connect tubing to a standard tapered fitting; others have a small room air-entrainment hole at the connection.

The body of the mask functions as a reservoir for both oxygen and expired carbon dioxide. A minimum oxygen flow of 5 L/min is sent to the mask in order to avoid rebreathing and excessive respiratory work.[125]

Placement

Masks are fastened to the patient's face by adjustment of an elastic headband; some manufacturers provide a malleable metal nose bridge adjustment device. Those applying masks must secure a tight seal but not cause facial pressure sores at the mask edges, especially where they pass over cheek bones. Wearing a mask for long periods is uncomfortable and hot. Speech is muffled and drinking and eating difficult.

Performance

The amount of oxygen enrichment of the inspired air depends on mask volume, pattern of ventilation, and the oxygen flow to the mask. It is difficult to predict delivered F_{IO_2}s at specific flows. During normal breathing, it is reasonable to expect a range from 0.3 to 0.6 with flows of 5 to 10 L/min, respectively. Oxygen levels can be higher with small tidal volumes or slow breathing rates.[125,126] With higher flows and ideal conditions, F_{IO_2}s may approach 0.7 or 0.8.

The nonreservoir mask may be best suited to patients who require higher level of oxygen than cannulas yet need oxygen therapy for fairly short periods. Examples

BOX 13-18

SUMMARY OF CLINICAL CONSIDERATIONS FOR THE NASAL MASK

F_{IO_2} range ≈ 0.22 to 0.3

Advantages	Disadvantages
More comfortable than nasal cannula	Performance varies with patient's V_T and f
	Difficult to determine delivered F_{IO_2}
	Tubing can kink or become obstructed
	Limited F_{IO_2} range

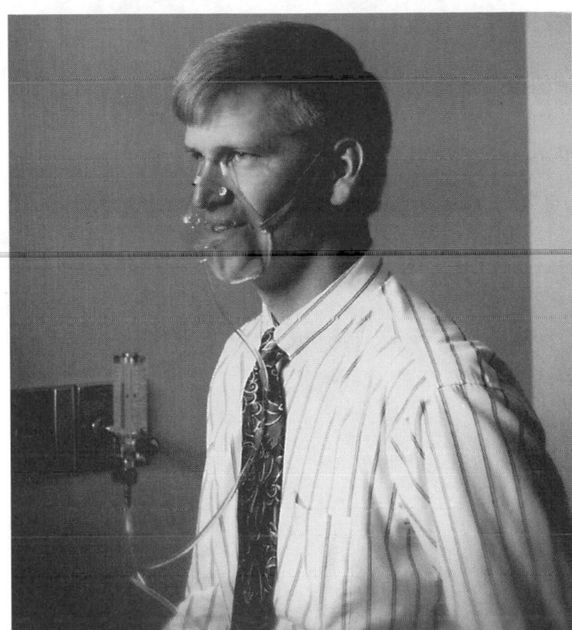

FIGURE 13-39. Nonreservoir mask.

would include medical transport or interim therapy in the emergency room. Successful use of the simple mask has been described in the post-anesthesia recovery area.[127]

Troubleshooting

The problems of mask dead space have been mentioned as well as those associated with pressure on facial skin. There also is potential for worsening the extent of aspiration if a patient vomits while a mask is in position. Those applying the mask to unconscious victims or to profoundly hypoxic obtunded patients should not strap the mask to the face. The mask should be held in place by hand or just set on the face.

The simple mask is suited to patients with mild to moderate hypoxemia, needing higher concentration than the nasal cannula. It is not the device of choice for patients with severe respiratory disease who are profoundly hypoxemic, tachypneic, or are unable to protect their airway from aspiration. Clinicians should use blood gases or oximetry to titrate oxygen flows to provide therapeutic levels on patients assessed to have moderate hypoxemia. Box 13-19 summarizes performance and clinical features of the nonreservoir mask.

BOX 13-19

SUMMARY OF CLINICAL CONSIDERATIONS FOR THE NONRESERVOIR MASK

FIO_2 range ≈ 0.3 to 0.6 at flows of 5 to 10 L/min

Advantages	Disadvantages
Higher FIO_2 than cannula	FIO_2 varies widely
Improved humidification versus cannula	Unable to measure FIO_2
	Potential for CO_2 rebreathing
	Mask limits speaking, eating/drinking
	Potential for aspiration

□ RESERVOIR MASKS

Incorporating some type of gas reservoir with a mask was a logical and early adaptation in mask equipment. Haldane and others developed fairly sophisticated-looking systems by the end of World War I.[7] The Boothby Lovelace and Bulbulian (BLB) oronasal mask (see Fig. 13-2E) was developed for World War II high-altitude aviation; it was also the clinical standard in the 1940s to 1960s.[15] The BLB mask and reservoir were made of nondisposable rubber. They had spring-loaded or foam expiratory valves. With adequate inlet flows, FIO_2s could approach 1.0.

Currently two types of reservoir mask are commonly used: the partial rebreathing mask and the nonrebreathing mask (Fig. 13-40A and B). Both are disposable, lightweight, transparent plastic under-the-chin reservoirs. The difference between the two relates to use of valves (Fig. 40 C and D). Mask reservoirs commonly hold approximately 600 mL or less.

The term partial rebreather refers to "part" of the expired air refilling the bag if empty. CO_2 in the initial expired gas is almost zero, as it is composed of upper airway deadspace. Refilling the bag with that gas should not result in patients rebreathing CO_2. The oxygen inlet is usually placed at the bag-mask connection or the neck.

The nonrebreather uses the same basic system as the partial rebreather but incorporates flap-type valves between the bag and mask and on at least one of the mask body exhalation ports. Oxygen is directed to the bag side of the mask valve connection by small-bore tubing. Some system must be provided to allow room air to enter in case of a failure of the oxygen supply. Manufacturers that have both exhalation ports valved have a spring-loaded valve at the neck of the bag that opens with subatmospheric pressure on the patient's side.

Placement

Both types of mask are placed on the patient's face with some attention to a good facial seal. A metallic strip allows a snug nose-bridge seal. Elastic straps hold the mask to the face. However, leaks are common, and room air will enter during brisk inspiratory flows, even when the bag contains gas.

Performance

Because of the lack of a good sealing system and a relatively small reservoir, both masks are considered variable performance devices. The key factor to successful application of the masks is to use sufficient flow of oxygen, so the reservoir bag is at least partially full during inspiration. Typical minimum flows are 10 to 12 L/min. Well-fitting partial rebreathing masks provide a range of FIO_2s from 0.35 to 0.60 with oxygen flows up to 10 L/min.[125] With inlet flows of 15 or more and ideal breathing conditions, FIO_2s may approach 1.0.

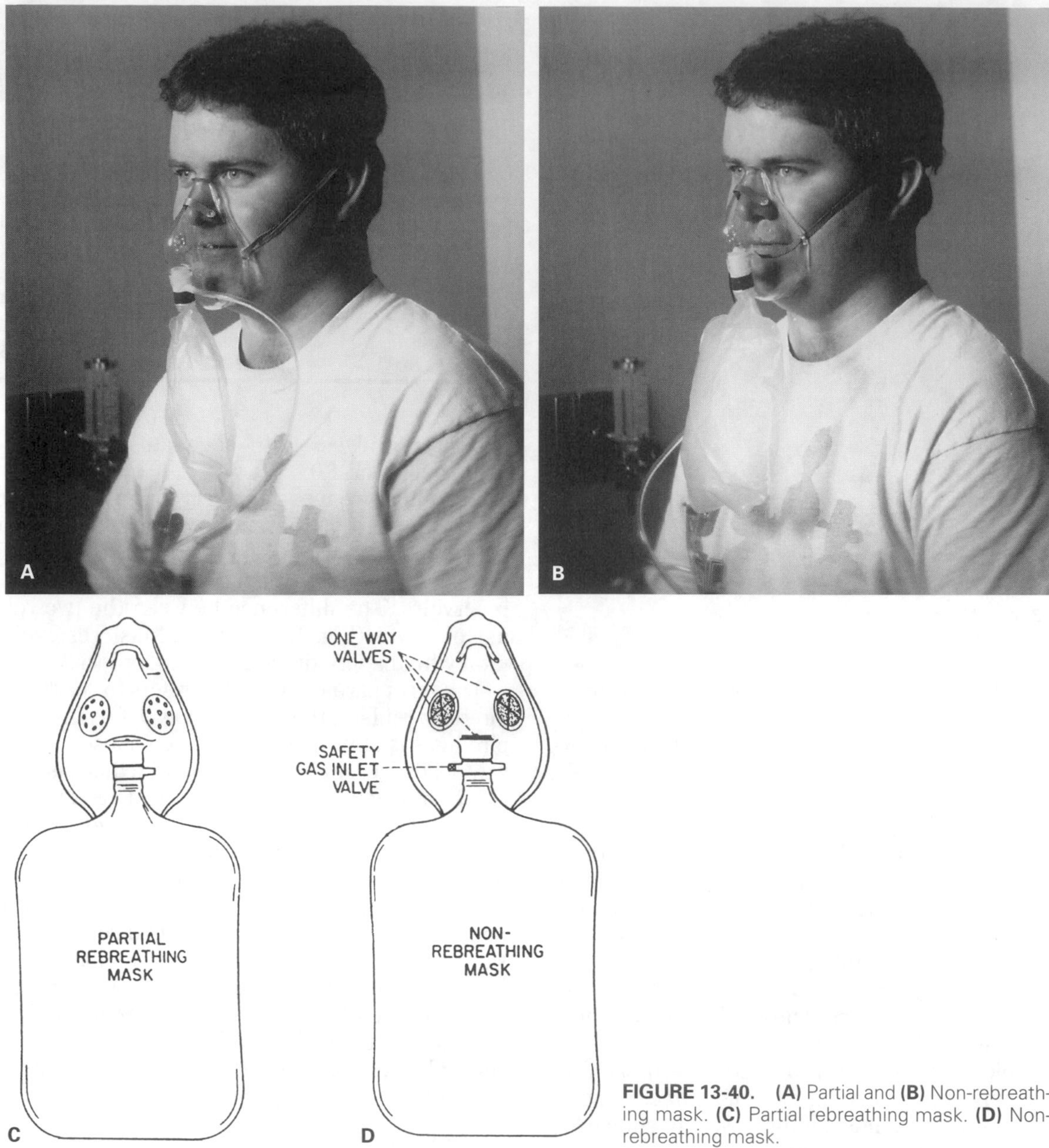

FIGURE 13-40. **(A)** Partial and **(B)** Non-rebreathing mask. **(C)** Partial rebreathing mask. **(D)** Non-rebreathing mask.

Nonrebreathing masks do not produce oxygen concentrations significantly higher than the unvalved version. Investigators have found that the highest FIO_2s range from 0.60 to 0.70 during normal breathing conditions.[129] There is a variable amount of room air dilution depending on mask valve function, mask seal, and ventilatory demand. Valves on these masks are simple rubber flaps and may not function perfectly, especially when wet. Both masks appear to be indicated for patients suspected of significant hypoxemia, with relatively normal spontaneous minute ventilation. Such patients may include victims of trauma, MI, or carbon monoxide exposure.

Troubleshooting

General problems of mask therapy have been mentioned. These masks are subject to those related to facial seals and aspiration. Blood gases or noninvasive oximetry are normally used to adjust flows to achieve therapeutic levels. However, profound changes in minute ventilation will require an adjustment of oxygen flow. Profoundly dyspneic patients with gasping respiration may be better suited with a fixed-performance, high-flow, oxygen system. Because of the high oxygen concentrations possible, clinicians must carefully observe those COPD patients who have a tendency to hypoventilate with a high FIO_2. Before placing masks on patients, the bag should be inflated by restricting its outlet. This will distend the folded plastic reservoir and ready it for patient use. Box 13-20 summarizes performance and clinical features of the reservoir masks.

Fixed Performance Devices

Although the following devices offer the potential for a constant FIO_2, it may not occur in all clinical situations. If these situations are not recognized, clinicians might be misled into thinking the patient is receiving a specific concentration of oxygen when the contrary is true. There are limits to the ability of each system to maintain its fixed-performance characteristics.

☐ BAG-MASK-VALVE OR ANESTHESIA BAG SYSTEMS

The basic design of this device is similar to the partial rebreathing and nonrebreathing oxygen masks previously reviewed. The difference deals with the more capable components. The self-inflating devices consist of a football-sized bladder often with some type of oxygen inlet reservoir (Fig. 13-41) or demand valve. Anesthesia bags are 1-, 2-, or 3-L non self-inflating reservoirs with a tail-piece gas inlet. The masks are those designed for ventilation purposes and have good facial sealing characteristics. In addition, most respiratory therapy and anesthesia departments have a supply of different styles and sizes to fit patients.

The inspiratory/expiratory valve systems may vary. Simple spring-loaded valves, if opened sufficiently, allow exhaust of exhaled carbon dioxide by the relatively high flows of inlet gas. The flow to the reservoir should be kept high so that the bags do not deflate substantially. When using an anesthesia bag, operators may have to frequently adjust the oxygen flow and exhaust valve spring tension to respond to changing breathing patterns or demands.

The most common system for disposable and permanent self-inflating resuscitation bags employ a unidirectional gas flow. A pair of one-way valves is used to prevent rebreathing, one directing reservoir gas to the mask and the other to exhaled gas from the mask.

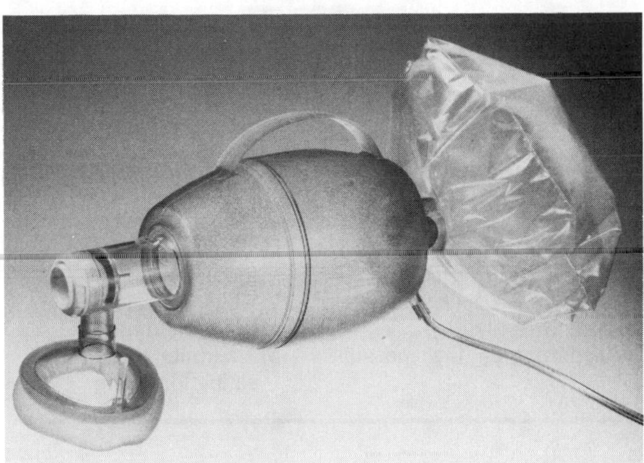

FIGURE 13-41. Self-inflating bag mask-valve.

BOX 13-20

SUMMARY OF CLINICAL CONSIDERATIONS FOR THE RESERVOIR MASK

Partial rebreathing: FIO_2 range ≈ 0.35 to 0.6 at flows of 10+ L/min
Nonrebreathing: FIO_2 range ≈ 0.6 to 0.7 at flows of 10 L/min

Advantages	Disadvantages
Higher FIO_2 than simple mask	FIO_2 varies widely
Improved humidification versus cannula	Unable to measure FIO_2
Easy to apply	Potential for CO_2 rebreathing
High oxygen flows possible	Mask limits speaking, eating/drinking
	Uncomfortable for extended periods

Placement

The face mask is carefully fitted to the patient's face to provide a comfortable leak-free seal. The mask is usually held on the patient's face by personnel providing care. This system is not to be used casually. There is a great risk of aspiration because of the mask seal. Straps to hold the mask on the face should be used only if there is low risk of aspiration in conscious cooperative patients. Spontaneously breathing patients who have an endotracheal or tracheostomy tube can breathe from this system by connecting the valve directly using the standard 15/22 mm inside diameter/outside diameter fittings.

Performance

FIO_2 that equal or approach 1.0 can be provided with both designs.[130] These type of devices can deliver oxygen or other specific gas mixtures such as heliox. Patients are allowed to breathe only the contents of the system if the mask seal is tight and reservoir maintained. Operators must adjust gas flow to the bag to accommodate for any increases in ventilation demand; patient and reservoir observation provide that information.

Troubleshooting

Although transparent masks allow inspection of the oropharynx, a primary concern for clinicians is aspiration. Patients who are receiving this therapy device are often quite ill. Operators must be able to immediately remove the mask. Nasogastric suction is helpful and minimizes the risk. However, sealing the mask with a nasogastric tube in place is more difficult.

Failure to maintain an adequate oxygen supply in the reservoir and inlet flow is another concern. Since room air breathing is prevented by some spring-loaded valve systems, anesthesia bag patients can suffocate if they exhaust the gas supply or if it is interrupted. When in doubt, increase the oxygen flow since any excess will pass out the valves. Remember to adjust the spring-

BOX 13-21

SUMMARY OF CLINICAL CONSIDERATIONS FOR SELF-INFLATING OR ANESTHESIA-BAG/MASK/VALVE SYSTEMS

F_{IO_2} range 0.9 to 1.0

Advantages	Disadvantages
High F_{IO_2}	Uncomfortable for extended periods
Can provide ventilation	Unable to measure F_{IO_2}
Good mask/face seal	Must be held in place
Easy to apply	Mask limits speaking, eating, drinking
High oxygen flows possible	

loaded valve properly. If the valve is not opened, the reservoir will pressurize, and the patient will be at risk for gastric insufflation or pneumothorax. Self-inflating bags do not look different when oxygen flow to the unit is lowered and more room air drawn into the bag, thus lowering the F_{IO_2}. Box 13-21 summarizes clinical features of these devices.

☐ AIR-ENTRAINMENT VENTURI MASKS

The concept in air-entrainment masks is somewhat different than the reservoir approach. The goal is to meet or exceed patient's inspiratory gas demand around the nose and mouth with high flows of fixed F_{IO_2} gas. Barach first used this type of device called the "Meter-Mask" in the early 1940s.[11] The gases premixed by a jet entraining a specific ratio of room air were held in a reservoir and made available to a mask (see Fig. 13-2C).

In 1960 Campbell developed an entrainment mask to provide low concentrations of oxygen with high flows to remove exhaled gas. The systems were designed to meet or exceed the patient's peak inspiratory flow with premixed gas. The original mask design had a hard plastic large volume enclosure with many small exhaust holes in a flexible shield.[20]

Masks based on Campbell's original design are used currently (Fig. 13-42). Commercially they are known as "Venturi" or "Venti-" masks or high air flow with oxygen-entrainment (HAFOE) systems.

High mask flows are required to match those of tachypneic and gasping patients. Therefore, formulas to estimate patient flows have been developed to assist the clinician (Table 13-10). Respiratory care practitioners should keep such calculations in perspective and not delay implementation and immediate assessment of effects.[131]

Placement

Entrainment masks are commonly lightweight disposable devices. The mask-face seal is loose-fitting, placed on the face in a similar fashion to other masks and attached by an elastic band. Oxygen is directed to the jet by small-bore tubing from flowmeter and optional bubble humidifier. Higher humidity may be needed because bubble humidifiers do not add much water to the total gas flow. An air-driven aerosol nebulizer can direct aerosol into a Venturi mask by attaching its wide-bore tubing to a cup-like adapter surrounding the entrainment ports. The masks are no less comfortable than those previously discussed and are not as good for long-term oxygen therapy as the cannula.

Performance

The oxygen concentration developed in an air-entrainment mask depends primarily on the oxygen flow and the mixing ratio of the jet system. Manufacturers

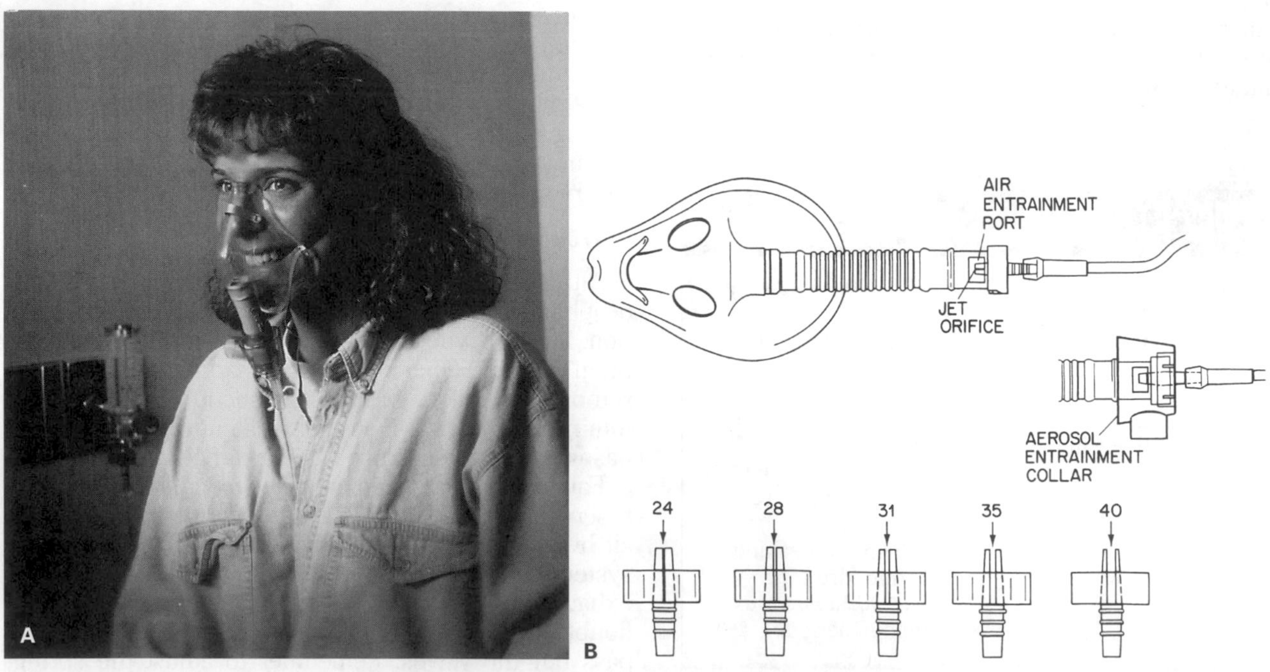

FIGURE 13-42. **(A)** Ventimask. **(B)** Schematic of ventimask.

TABLE 13-10. **Nomogram to Estimate Peak Inspiratory Flow Demand**

Tidal Volume (mL)	Breathing Frequency (breaths/min)				
	20	*25*	*30*	*35*	*40*
			Flow (L/min)		
200	19	24	28	33	38
400	38	47	57	67	75
600	57	71	85	99	115
800	76	94	113	130	150

Peak flow estimate (when the I:E ratio is 1:2) = $\frac{\pi \times Vt}{2\,T_I} \times 60$ sec/min

V_T = estimated tidal volume
T_I = estimated inspiratory time

have developed both fixed and adjustable selections over a large range. Most provide instructions for the operator to set a minimum flow of oxygen. Table 13-11 identifies total flow at various inlet flows and F_{IO_2}. However, they should be considered the low limits that can be exceeded if the patient requires higher flows.[132] Clinicians can run most masks on a wider range of flows and still maintain oxygen concentrations within a 1% to 2% range of accuracy. Despite of the high-flow concept, patient-received concentrations can vary up to 6%.[126,132–136] Some researchers have suggested the effect is caused by secondary dilution at the mask-face. The gas flows from the jet are subjected to high acceleration by patient's inspiration. Patients with short inspiratory times, larger I:E ratios, and larger tidal volumes will tend to have lower tracheal oxygen concentrations than found inside the mask. Oxygen flows that may have been appropriate to Campbell's larger volume-containing design may not be sufficient for the smaller masks, suggesting a minimum of 300 mL or higher flows.[137,138] Other clinicians have adapted secondary oxygen flow to the collar device around the Venturi intake ports. This technique allows increased flows and higher.[139] Clinicians must be aware that this mask may not perform as a high flow device at F_{IO_2}s greater than 0.35 to 0.4.

The air-entrainment masks are a logical choice for patients whose hypoxemia cannot be controlled on lower F_{IO_2} devices such as the cannula (because of increases in breathing frequency, tidal volume, or both). Patients with COPD who tend to hypoventilate with a moderate F_{IO_2} are candidates for the Venturi mask. Hypoventilation usually occurs when they have an exacerbation of their bronchitis and appear in the emergency room in distress.

Patients with asthma who are dyspneic may require supplemental oxygen beyond the oxygen delivery capabilities of a nasal cannula. Because of their tachypnea and rapid inspiratory efforts, an air-entrainment mask would be more appropriate. Venturi masks also operate without particulate water aerosol that can produce further bronchospasm by an irritant effect.

TABLE 13-11. **Air-Entrainment Mask Input Flow Versus Total Flow at Varying F_{IO_2}s**

F_{IO_2}	Input Flow (minimum)	Total Flow (L/min)
0.24	4	97
0.28	6	68
0.3	6	54
0.35	8	45
0.40	12	50
0.50	12	33

Troubleshooting

Clinicians providing oxygen therapy by air-entrainment mask therapy should be aware of the previously mentioned problems involving the mask itself. F_{IO_2} levels can increase if the entrainment ports are obstructed by the patient's hands, bed sheets, or water condensate. You should encourage the patient and caregivers to keep the mask on the face constantly. Interruption in the oxygen is a serious problem in unstable patients with hypoxemia and or hypercarbia.

Direct analysis of the F_{IO_2} during air-entrainment mask breathing is possible but difficult to do accurately. Correlating blood gases with some index of inspiratory flow demand, such as breathing rate, should allow clinicians to know when to suspect that the patient's demands may not be met by the mask's flow. Inlet oxygen flows may need to be increased or alternate device selected. Box 13-22 summarizes the entrainment mask.

□ AIR-ENTRAINMENT NEBULIZERS

Large-volume, high-output or "all-purpose" nebulizers have been used in respiratory therapy for many years to provide bland mist therapy with some control of the F_{IO_2} (Fig. 13-43). These units are discussed in detail in Chapter 15 for their aerosol-producing properties. Although commonly used because of their clinical adaptability there are several disadvantages that should be reviewed.

Both disposable and permanent nebulizers use an adjustable dilution setting device to vary F_{IO_2} at fixed setting points (eg, 0.3, 0.7, and 1.0) or are continuously adjustable from 0.3 to 1.0. Most commercial units have inlet orifice diameter that maximally allows only 15 L/min when the source pressure is 50 psig. This means that on the 100% setting with no air entrainment, the output flow is only 15 L/min. Only patients breathing at slow rates and small tidal volumes will receive 100% oxygen. In the typical device, as the F_{IO_2} is reduced, more room air is entrained, increasing the total flow output. Knowledge of the air/oxygen ratio and the input flow rate of oxygen allows the total outflow to be calculated, as shown in Equation Box 13-18.

To make matters more complex, air-entrainment nebulizers frequently are found to give a slightly higher F_{IO_2} than the indicated setting. The increased F_{IO_2} is the result of the resistance to the output flow caused by patient tubing. Thus, less room air is drawn into the system, the F_{IO_2} increases, and the total flow decreases. On a 40% setting, nebulizers may actually provide a F_{IO_2} of 0.45 to 0.5. With an increased F_{IO_2} comes a lower air/O_2 entrainment ratio, so the total flows would be lower than

BOX 13-22

SUMMARY OF CLINICAL CONSIDERATIONS FOR AIR-ENTRAINMENT MASKS

F_{IO_2} range 0.24 to 0.5

Advantages	Disadvantages
High flow and controlled F_{IO_2}	Uncomfortable for extended periods
	Unable to measure F_{IO_2}

EQUATION BOX 13-18

CALCULATION OF NEBULIZER OUTPUT FLOWS

Example: Given a large-volume nebulizer set on 40% and driven by an oxygen flow rate of 15 L/min. The patient has a respiratory rate of 25/min, the tidal volume and I:E ratio are estimated to be 600 mL and 1:2, respectively.

$$T = \frac{60\ \text{sec/min}}{25\ \text{breaths/min}} = 2.8\ \text{sec}$$

$$t_I = \frac{T}{I + E} = \frac{2.8}{3} = 0.8\ \text{sec}$$

Based on calculated data, is the total flow from the nebulizer sufficient for the inspiratory flow demand of the patient?

1. The flow from the nebulizer is:

$$\dot{V}_{tot} = \dot{V}O_2 + \dot{V}_{air}$$
$$= 15 + (3.17)15$$
$$\dot{V}_{tot} = 63\ \text{L/min}$$

2. The flow need of the patient is:

$$\dot{V}_{Imax\ (L/min)} = \frac{3.14 \times V_t}{2 \times t_I} \times 60\ \text{sec/min}$$

$$\dot{V}_{Imax} = \frac{(3.14 \times 0.6\ \text{L})}{2 \times 0.8\ \text{sec}} \times 60\ \text{sec/min}$$
$$= 70.5\ \text{L/min}$$

calculated. The settings for higher concentrations are severely flow limiting. When input flow is 15 L/min, the total flows at 0.6, 0.7, and 1.0 would be 30, 24.5, and 15 L/min, respectively. You should use high F_{IO_2} settings only with stable patients who have normal inspiratory flow demand. The problem with air-entrainment systems is that the most tachypneic and hypoxemic patients need the highest F_{IO_2} setting, but this results in the lowest total flow.

Placement

Nebulizer systems can be applied to the patient with many different devices. The aerosol mask (Fig. 13-44A), tracheostomy collar (Fig. 13-44B), face tent (Fig. 13-44C), and T-piece or Briggs adapter (Fig. 13-44D). These can all be used by attaching large-bore tubing to the nebulizer. All of these attachments provide an open system that freely vents inspiratory and expiratory gases around the patient's face or out a distal port of a Briggs adapter. Unfortunately the lack of any valves allows patients to easily breathe in room air. Although suffocation is unlikely, consistent delivery of gas is even less likely. Aerosol masks are placed on patients in a similar fashion to other masks. Tracheostomy collars are placed around patient's necks and loosely cover the tracheostomy. Face tents are placed with the lower edge under the chin with a head strap option. Briggs adapters can be simply attached to endotracheal tubes. It is common practice to use either a reservoir bag before the T or a reservoir tube on the distal side of the T to provide a larger volume of gas that can be available to match peak inspiratory flows. It has been proposed that up to 200 mL of distal reservoir may be added to 40% aerosol systems, run at 15 L/min, without risk of rebreathing carbon dioxide.[140]

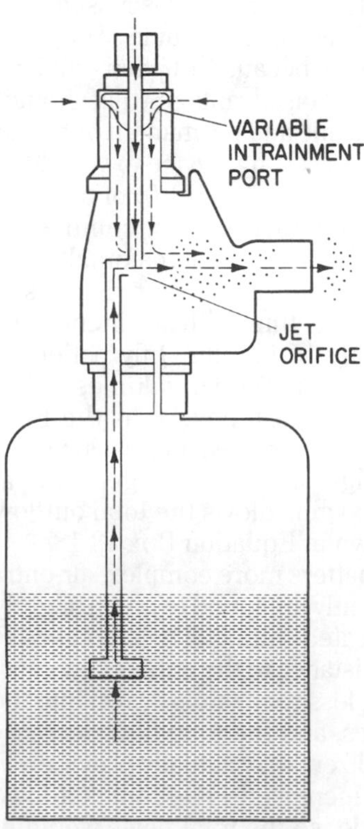

FIGURE 13-43. Aerosol nebulizer.

Performance

Performance of air-entrainment aerosol systems in providing consistent F_{IO_2} and adequate total flows have been studied. Investigators have documented variability of such systems.[141,142] At settings higher than 0.40, many air-entrainment devices cannot deliver ≥40 L/min and should not be considered low-flow systems.

In some clinical situations, severely dyspneic patients may not have their inspiratory needs met by nebulizer systems. To extended flow capabilities, there are several options:

- Increasing the nebulizer's inlet orifice, to provide "driving gas" flows higher than 15 L/min.

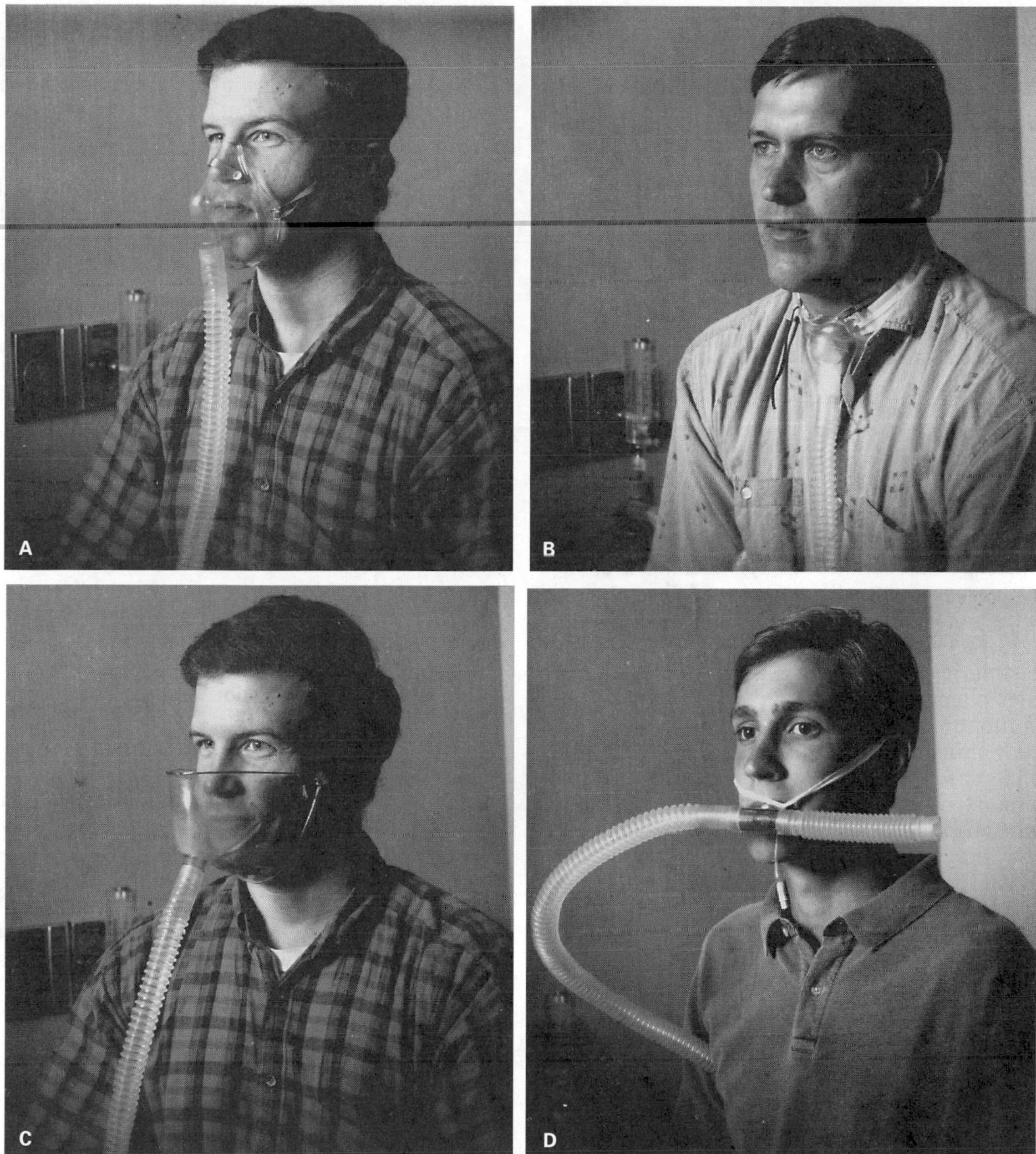

FIGURE 13-44. Aerosol nebulizer attachments. **(A)** Face mask, **(B)** Tracheostomy collar, **(C)** Face tent, and **(D)** Briggs adaptor "t-piece."

- Adding a second flow source (flowmeter)
- Adding a second large-volume nebulizer and "wye" that flow into the primary system

The first two options are commercially available. Misty Ox (Medical Molding Corp. of America) uses a larger inlet orifice found in the "High Flow-High FIO_2" model. When run at settings of 0.6 to 0.9, maximum flows are 60 to 50 L/min, respectively. The Gas Injection Nebulizer combines output flow with additional flow of either oxygen or air from a secondary flowmeter (see Fig. 13-22).[143] Noncommercial systems of this type have been described in the literature.[144]

Connecting two or three nebulizers in parallel can help in some patient situations but may not elevate the flow adequately. As additional nebulizers and tubing are added, the resistance to gas flow increases and there is interference with air entrainment. Thus, simply adding another nebulizer does not always double flow or guarantee the patient will receive the desired. Results of a recent study that measured hypopharyngeal oxygen concentrations during inspiration, when normal subjects breathed with an aerosol device and face tent, were similar to those of investigators who studied air-entrainment masks. Just supplying adequate flows may not

BOX 13-23

SUMMARY OF CLINICAL CONSIDERATIONS FOR HIGH-FLOW AEROSOL

F_{IO_2} range 0.35 to 1.0 (However, high flow will not likely be provided to adults when F_{IO_2} exceeds 0.6)

Advantages	Disadvantages
High flow and controlled F_{IO_2}	Uncomfortable for extended periods
High humidity	Limited flows at higher F_{IO_2}
Able to measure F_{IO_2}	Potential for bronchospasm
Adaptable, ie, mask, T-piece, etc.	

solve the problem if the positioning of the facial/airway attachment causes secondary dilution.

Troubleshooting

The major concern of those applying air-entrainment aerosol therapy with controlled oxygen concentration is that the system provides adequate flow. Clinicians should observe the mist like a tracer to determine adequacy of flow. In a T-piece, if the visible mist (exiting the distal port) disappears during inspiration, the flow is inadequate.

Another concern in clinical practice is that excess water in the tubing collects and can obstruct gas flow completely or offer increased resistance to flow. The latter may increase the F_{IO_2} above the desired setting.

Respiratory care practitioners should be alert to patients who worsen on an aerosol system. Tachypnea, chest discomfort, cough, and wheezing on auscultation are signs of bronchospasm. In such circumstances, a nonaerosol system should be substituted. Box 13-23 summarizes performance and clinical features of nebulizer systems.

High-Flow Air/Oxygen Systems

Dual air-oxygen flowmeters, air-oxygen blenders, or the Down's Flow Generator are commonly used for oxygen administration, or with CPAP and IMV systems. They have a major advantage in providing consistent F_{IO_2} delivery in contrast to air-entrainment nebulizer systems that are often flow limited at high F_{IO_2} settings. In addition, the total flow to the patient can be independently set to exceed patient needs, using a reservoir bag or constant flow up to 100 L/min.

Clinicians can use open masks, such as an aerosol mask, or well-fitted nonrebreathing system masks with blenders. Well-sealing mask systems can also be constructed but require a reservoir bag with a safety valve to allow breathing if the blender fails. The high flows of gas require use of heated humidifiers of the type commonly used on mechanical ventilators. Humidification offers an advantage for patients with airways hyperreactive to aerosol particle irritation. Figure 13-45 illustrates an air-oxygen blender with humidifier and reservoir bag.

The use of threshold positive pressure during exhalation is termed PEEP with mechanically ventilated patients, and CPAP with spontaneously breathing patients. Either technique is used to elevate functional residual capacity (FRC) if decreased, and decrease elevated intrapulmonary shunt. Use of PEEP or CPAP commonly elevates PaO_2 at the patient's current F_{IO_2}, which may allow subsequent reduction in oxygen concentration. This is a desirable technique in treating disorders like ARDS or RDS of the newborn, in which potentially harmful oxygen levels/duration may be reduced.

Oxygen Hoods

Although many of the devices previously described have pediatric-sized options, such as cannulas and masks, many young infants and neonates will not tolerate facial appliances. Oxygen hoods cover only the head, allowing access to the infant's lower body while still permiting use of a standard incubator or radiant warmer. The hood is ideal for relatively short-term oxygen therapy for newborns and inactive infants. However, for mobile infants requiring longer term therapy, for example, the nasal cannula, facemask, or full-bed enclosure affords greater mobility.

Normally oxygen and air are premixed by a blending device and passed through a heated humidifier, since

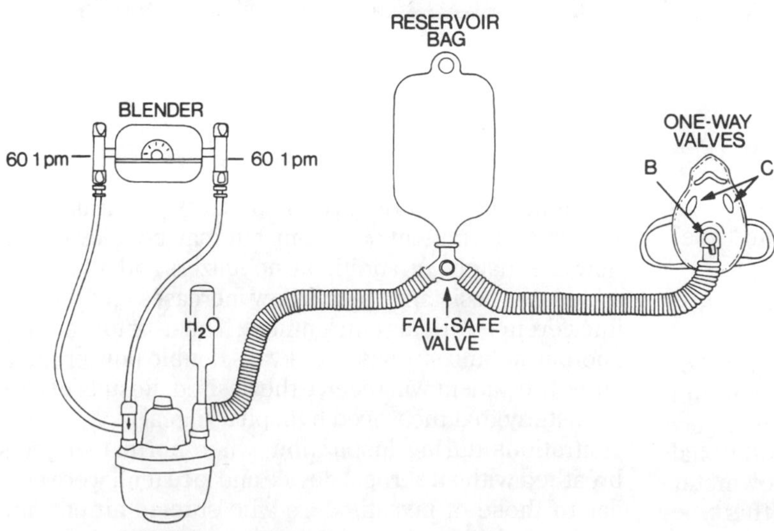

FIGURE 13-45. High-flow oxygen system using air–oxygen blender and mainstream humidifier. (From Foust GN, Potter WH, Wilson MD, Golden EB. Shortcomings of using two jet nebulizers in tandem with an aerosol face mask for optimal oxygen therapy. Chest 1991;99:1346. Reproduced with permission.)

many nebulizers approach dangerous limits for noise levels (65 dB) and cold gas can induce an increase in oxygen consumption.[18] Hoods come in different sizes to accommodate a variety of infants. Some are simple Plexiglas boxes; others have elaborate systems for sealing the neck opening. There is no attempt to completely seal the system, since a constant flow of gas is needed to remove carbon dioxide (minimum flow >7 L/min). Flow rates of 10 to 15 L/min are adequate for a majority of patients.[145]

Performance

The concentration of oxygen the infant will breathe is related to the device providing the oxygen. Normally dual air-oxygen flowmeters or blenders are used. Flow should be set to guarantee a flushing effect to remove carbon dioxide. When 100% oxygen is used, there can be a layering effect, with highest concentrations at the bottom of the hood depending on hood design and gas flows. Continuous oxygen analysis is required for hood systems. Analysis should be made at several different locations in the hood to evaluate if FIO_2 layering occurs.

Troubleshooting

Because of the simplicity of the device, there are no real problems if the hood is sized sufficiently large for the infant's head. The danger of hypoxemia or complications from oxygen justify the use of continuous alarm systems that can alert personnel to dangerously high or low FIO_2. Pulse oximetry is commonly used in combination to monitor the physiologic response to oxygen therapy.

Incubators

Incubators are commonly used to provide a humid, neutral thermal environment for infants, especially those born prematurely. Supplemental oxygen systems have been incorporated into incubators but often have difficulty maintaining a specific FIO_2. Because of the relatively large internal volume, maintaining a constant FIO_2 often cannot be achieved. Dilution of accumulated oxygen will occur if you open incubator access ports. A better system is to use a hood and incubator. After the "RLF epidemic" of the 1940s to 1950s, manufacturers of incubators installed systems to limit the flow of oxygen into the chamber. In theory, it was to prevent oxygen concentrations of more than 0.40, which was thought to prevent retrolental fibroplasia in sick babies. A red warning paddle on the back of the incubator was elevated to allow increased flows, reminding staff that high oxygen concentrations were possible.

Oxygen Tents and Aerosol Enclosures

In the 1920s there were developments to provide supplemental oxygen to the environment surrounding the patient similar to an incubator. Oxygen rooms with elaborate air conditioning systems were made in some hospitals. In 1926, Barach published information on an oxygen tent that had the ability to remove carbon dioxide (soda lime) and excess heat (ice) (see Fig. 13-2B).[8]

Tents continued to be used into the 1950s for oxygen administration. The major problems were difficulties in controlling the consistency of the FIO_2 and attaining levels higher than 0.50. Oxygen flow of 12 to 15 L/min were generally used with tents to deliver oxygen.

Tents are still commonly used in pediatric respiratory care for patients with problems such as croup and cystic fibrosis. Normally a high-output aerosol generator is used to provide a high humidity environment. A detailed discussion can be found in Chapter 15. Supplemental oxygen can be supplied to aerosol tents if the patient requires correction of hypoxemia in addition to bland mist therapy. The most common technique is to run the aerosol generators on oxygen and adjust the FIO_2 by manipulating the amount of room air that is entrained. Units can also be run on air with oxygen titrated into the system to produce a moderate FIO_2. Like the tent, it is difficult to consistently control the oxygen concentration.

Troubleshooting

The most publicized problem with oxygen tents or aerosol tents with supplemental oxygen is fire hazard. Static charge sparks, nurse call devices, and electric appliances are all potential fire starters if the spark generates enough heat energy above its flash or ignition temperature. Other problems deal with elimination of patient's body heat. Elaborate refrigeration systems have been developed along with open top tents that allow heat to rise. Finally, inadequate oxygen concentrations in aerosol enclosures will develop if children place teddy bears or other toys in the gas outlets or inlets that recirculate gas.

Air Travel and Oxygen Therapy

Patients who are at risk of developing arterial oxygen tensions below 50 mmHg (6.65 kPa) during air travel should receive supplemental oxygen in-flight. Commercial aircraft typically cruise at altitudes between 22,000 ft (6706 m) and 44,000 ft (13,411 m) where the barometric pressure is 141 mmHg, and the PIO_2 is 29 mmHg. However, cabin pressurization maintains a relative cabin altitude of 5000 ft (1529) and 8000 ft (2438 m), respectively. At that altitude, barometric pressure is 568 mmHg and PIO_2 108 mmHg. The Federal Aviation Administration requires aircraft to maintain an 8000-ft altitude at the highest operating level, but there are exemptions for temporary avoidance of adverse weather and variations among types of aircraft.[146]

Numerous practical, medicolegal, and airline policy issues confuse both patients and oxygen providers. Each carrier establishes his or her own guidelines, and this has led to frustrations and made generalized recommendations difficult. The potential flier should plan ahead and make inquiry with airline special services. Airlines in the United States do not permit personal oxygen systems. Those systems must be emptied to a pressure of less than 40 psig and carried as luggage.

U. S. carriers require a physician prescription stating the flow at 8000 ft and whether the oxygen should be used intermittently or continuously (several copies of the prescription should be carried by the patient). Equation Box 13-19 describes equations useful to clinicians for estimating FIO_2 needs or the possible effect of altitude on the patient's PaO_2.

Airlines charge a fee for providing in-flight oxygen service ranging from $40 to $150, based on the flight segments or number of O_2 cylinders used. Oxygen is available in either large compressed cylinders containing >3000 L or small cylinders containing 300 L. The former have adjustable flowmeters, yet small cylinders have only 2 or 4 L/min settings. Patients should have additional lengths of connecting tubing to allow ambulation or visits to the lavatory. Emergency oxygen is available if anyone has respiratory distress or if a passenger's purchased system runs out of gas. Most domestic flights can land an unstable patient at an airport in 30 to 40 minutes. You may want to enlist an oxygen vendor that can provide additional oxygen supplies for ground (terminal) use, that could continue at the final destination. If the new location is at a different altitude, measurement of oximetric data can allow adjustment of flow to a desirable level.[147,148]

HYPERBARIC OXYGEN THERAPY

Hyperbaric oxygen therapy (HBO) involves administration of gas at an increased atmospheric pressure. Patients are placed inside a chamber that can be pressurized to several times normal atmospheric pressure, 760 mmHg (101 kPa). HBO therapy has had a variable presence in medicine over the years. Currently it is receiving renewed enthusiasm for therapy.[58,149,150,151] Box 13-24 lists the medical and surgical indications for HBO.

An area of continuing controversy resides in the use of HBO to treat carbon monoxide (CO) toxicity. Biochemical and research complexity of CO poisoning and the advantage of HBO versus normobaric 100% oxygen therapy continue to be debated.[149,152] Treatment of recreational or occupational decompression sickness does not necessarily involve use of supplemental oxygen. The goal is to increase the oxygen dissolved in the blood, using Henry's law. Treatment of the bends (nitrogen coming out of solution in the joints of the body) has never been questioned. The reader is referred to Chapter 14 for a complete review of this topic.

HELIUM-OXYGEN THERAPY

Since Barach established the value of low-density gas therapy in 1934, helium-oxygen mixtures have a notable, yet limited, role in medicine.[13] Other than its uses in industry and deep sea diving, there are a number of medical uses for patients to breathe "heliox." Clinical indications are listed in Box 13-25.

Anesthesia: In anesthetic practice, pressures needed to ventilate patients with small diameter endotracheal tubes can be substantially reduced (halved) when an 80%/20% mixture is used.[153]

Airway Obstruction: Patients with upper airway lesions causing acute distress can have palliative therapy before definitive therapy, which is usually surgical correction.[154] Clinicians have reported benefit in chronic obstructive lung disease patients (emphysema, bronchitis). Reductions in their airway resistance can lead to a decrease in functional residual capacity and improved CO_2 removal.[155,156] Heliox's use in acute asthma has been poorly defined and anecdotal. Recent reports suggest its use may be a short-term alternative to immediate intubation and ventilation or in conjunction with ventiltion. It does not produce significant benefits in all patients.[157] The clinical acceptance and guidelines for this therapy are not firm. Some patients who require intubation also show improvement when receiving heliox via the mechanical ventilator.

Delivery Systems

Barach used a simple mouthpiece to administer heliox breathing mixtures as well as a tight-fitting mask. He also used heliox with continuous positive pressure breathing. In any breathing system, a tightly sealed closed system is required, because helium will easily leak through small holes.

Nonintubated patients may receive therapy via a well-fitting simple mask or a mask with reservoir bag. Nasal cannulas are ineffective and infant hoods are suboptimal.[158] Another option would be a demand valve or blender with a well-fitting mask.

EQUATION BOX 13-19

CALCULATIONS USEFUL FOR AIR TRAVEL[147]

$$FIO_2 \text{ (at altitude)} = \frac{\text{"usual" } FIO_2 \times \text{(ground level } P_B)}{P_B \text{ at altitude (eg, 8000 ft)}}$$

$$PaO_2 \text{ at altitude} = 22.8 - (2.74) \text{ altitude} + (0.68)\ PaO_2 \text{ ground}$$

BOX 13-24

INDICATIONS FOR HYPERBARIC OXYGEN THERAPY

Gas gangrene
Cyanide poisoning
Carbon monoxide poisoning
Chronic osteomyelitis
Body or inhalational burns
Ischemic tissue transplants
Severe anemia or hemorrhage
Decompression sickness
Air embolism

BOX 13-25

INDICATIONS FOR HELIOX THERAPY

- Anesthesia
- Short-term therapy for major airway obstruction
- Exacerbation of COPD (emphysema/bronchitis)
- Respiratory failure in acute asthma

Accurate flows are not required in administering He/O_2 mixtures. The objective when using a reservoir bag and mask is to keep the reservoir bag nearly full at all times. The precise flow is not ordered but the needle valve is adjusted to meet the breathing demands. Helium is premixed with oxygen in several standard mixtures. They are available in large-sized compressed gas cylinders. The most popular mixtures are the 80%/20% and 70%/30% helium-oxygen. The densities are 1.805 and 1.586 less dense, respectively, compared with pure oxygen.

For those needing accurate flow corrections, most companies who make calibration flowmeters will provide formulas or nomograms to allow accurate reading of low-density gases. Others may want to invest in flowmeters specifically designed to correctly indicate the accurate flow. You can estimate the actual flow by multiplying the level indicated on an oxygen flowmeter by a correction factor derived from the relative density of the heliox mixture compared with oxygen.

CARBON DIOXIDE GAS THERAPY

Historical Review

Thirty years ago, carbon dioxide therapy was commonly used for its pharmacologic effects. Today therapeutic applications are quite limited or controversial. This section functions as a historical review and provides examples of therapeutic applications for increased carbon dioxide fraction in the inspired gas. Carbon dioxide therapy has several dangerous side effects, and efficacy remains unproved in many of the following applications. Box 13-26 summarizes indications for carbogen.

☐ HISTORICAL INDICATIONS FOR O_2/CO_2 THERAPY

It was found that increasing inspired CO_2 levels could treat hysterical hyperventilation by lessening syncopal attacks due to hypocarbia. Five percent carbon dioxide in oxygen was used, or rebreathing into a paper bag or tubing reservoir. One advantage of the gas was its more rapid response.[58,160]

O_2–CO_2 mixtures stimulated spontaneous breathing of postoperative patients to hasten the removal of volatile anesthetics and to prevent atelectasis. It was an indirect approach to encourage patients to take deep breaths. Mechanical or nonmechanical methods to cause sustained inspiration with breath hold appear to attack the primary problem more directly; for example, IPPB, chest physical therapy maneuvers, incentive spirometry.

Treatment of hiccoughs (singultus) is occasionally successful, but the mechanisms are unknown. No more than 5% CO_2 is normally used.[11]

Seizures (petit mal) were terminated by decreasing brain excitability. Five percent carbon dioxide in oxygen was recommended.[161]

Treatment of carbon monoxide poisoning uses 3% to 7% carbon dioxide in oxygen. In theory, it increases the overall ventilation and facilitates the unloading of carbon monoxide from hemoglobin.[11] However, carbon dioxide can compound the acidosis if the victim has a significant lactic acidosis secondary to tissue hypoxia. Victims also often complain about headaches following therapy.

During cardiopulmonary bypass, low concentrations (3%) of CO_2 were used to prevent total body CO_2 washout.

CO_2 was used to improve regional blood flow by dilating vessels in the brain. Low concentrations (5% in oxygen) have been used to treat impending ophthalmic artery occlusion or prophylaxis for developing stroke. Although total blood flow may increase, perfusion to ischemic areas is probably not increased or may decrease.[162]

Treatment of neuropsychiatric disorders was accomplished by inducing seizure activity with 30% CO_2. This approach has been abandoned because of the side effect of significant acidosis.[11]

CO_2 has been used to facilitate uptake or elimination of potent volatile anesthetic agents. However, elimination of the drugs from the brain is not dependent on ventilation.[163]

BOX 13-26

INDICATIONS FOR CARBON DIOXIDE/OXYGEN BREATHING

- Hyperventilation
- Singultus
- Seizures
- Carbon monoxide poisoning
- Cardiopulmonary bypass
- Inducing seizure activity
- Augment elimination of volatile anesthetics

Delivery Systems

Because the expired air normally has an increased carbon dioxide fraction, rebreathing that gas can provide CO_2 gas therapy. The paper bag is the simplest device. The Adler Rebreather and Dale-Schwartz Tube have been commercial adaptations.

Administration of specific mixtures of carbon dioxide can be provided by premixed high-pressure gas cylinders. Regulators that attach to the cylinder valves must be specific for the concentration used. The most common are 5%/95% CO_2/O_2 and 7%/93% CO_2/O_2. Concentrations greater than 10% are available but are not used because of the risk of rapid development of side effects.

Administration devices for CO_2/O_2 gas therapy include the disposable nonrebreathing mask with reservoir and the well-fitted mask with reservoir. Administration times are normally limited to fairly short periods of 5 to 15 minutes.

Complications and Hazards

Toxic manifestations of carbon dioxide must be recognized by those administering therapy. Patients must be carefully monitored for pulse, respiratory rate, blood pressure, and mental state. Significant changes in any of the preceding items should prompt the discontinuance of the therapy. Higher concentrations cause more rapid onset and more severe symptoms and signs. Normally, pulse rate, frequency and depth of breathing all increase. Blood pressure usually increases, but the response is quite varied depending on the cardiovascular system and sympathetic nervous system response. CO_2 therapy may depress the mental state, ultimately resulting in convulsions, coma, and then death. When mask therapy is used, clinicians should be concerned with the potential for aspiration.

NITRIC OXIDE THERAPY

In 1987 it was found that nitric oxide was normally biosynthesized in vascular endothelial cells. It is an important mediator of physiologic function including vasodilation, neurotransmission, long-term memory, and immunologic defense.[24]

The molecule is highly diffusable and lipid soluble. Its half-life ranges from 3 to 50 seconds as its conversion to nitrates, nitrites, and higher oxides of nitrogen increases with higher oxygen tensions. The cation form (NO^+) reacts to produce metallo-nitrosyl compounds, which mediate physiologic responses such as vasodilation. This effect on the pulmonary vascular smooth muscle is seen when small concentrations are inhaled 18 to 36 parts per million (ppm).[25]

Uses of Nitric Oxide Therapy

Box 13-27 lists current research interests in therapeutic uses of nitric oxide.

□ PULMONARY VASODILATION

The greatest clinical research interest to date is in the use of nitric oxide for its relaxing effect on the pulmonary vascular bed.[26]

Inhaled NO has been reported to be successful as a selective vasodilator in treating persistent pulmonary hypertension of the neonate (PPPH).[164] This clinical syndrome does occur idiopathically or is associated with various neonatal cardiopulmonary diseases including meconium aspiration and group B streptococcal sepsis. Nitric oxide has been used to manage pulmonary hypertension following repair of congenital diaphragmatic hernia. Conventional treatment has included mechanical hyperventilation, invasive ECMO, and/or hyperoxia and pulmonary vasodilator drug therapy. All such therapies involve some complications; vasodilator therapy often results in systemic hypotension. In preliminary clinical trials, inhalation of 10 to 80 ppm of nitric oxide for 6 to 24 hours has proven therapeutic as a selective pulmonary vasodilator in PPHN.[165]

Infants and children with pulmonary hypertension-associated congenital heart lesions and mitral valve replacement have been successfully treated with nitric oxide as either a palliative measure or perioperatively.[165,166]

There is also interest in prolonged low concentration treatment of ARDS. Prolonged low concentration (5 to 20 ppm NO) has been shown to decrease the mean pulmonary artery pressure and improve arterial oxygen tension in selected patients. Pulmonary vasodilation was most dramatic in patients with the greatest degree of vasoconstriction (mean pulmonary artery pressure $\geq$30 mmHg).[167] Questions remain about effect on outcome, variability in response among patients, variability of response during the disease course, dosing strategies, and weaning from NO.

BOX 13-27

POSSIBLE CLINICAL USES FOR NITRIC OXIDE THERAPY

- Pulmonary vasodilation
  - Persistent pulmonary hypertension of the newborn
  - Following repair of congenital heart lesions
  - Adult respiratory distress syndrome
- Bronchodilation

□ BRONCHODILATION

Reversal of bronchoconstriction by inhaled nitric oxide has been shown to occur in canines challenged with histimine and methacholine.[168]

Complications and Hazards

Although there are only a few studies on the toxicity of nitric oxide, methemoglobinemia and nitrogen dioxide toxicity are potential hazards of inhaled nitric oxide. In the preseence of oxygen, nitric oxide rapidly oxidizes to nitrogen dioxide (NO_2), which in concentrations of 25 ppm can cause severe pneumonitis and at 5000 ppm can produce pulmonary edema and death. The rate of oxidation is directly proportional to the FIO_2, and to keep NO_2 production to a minimum, contact time with oxygen should be kept as brief as possible. Soda lime can remove NO_2 from anesthetic breathing circuits. Nitric oxide must be removed from the patient area by scavenger systems; safety limits of 5 ppm have been set by OSHA.[169] Some patients notice a metallic smell of nitric oxide. The threshold for NO's sharp-sweet odor is 0.3 to 1 ppm.

Application Systems

Systems to deliver and monitor inhaled nitric oxide have been described for adults and infants, breathing NO either spontaneously or via mechanical ventilation. The gas administration systems must be designed with capabilities to monitor both the potentially toxic nitrogen-based gases and FIO_2. Currently, chemiluminescence analyzers can accurately measure nitric oxide and nitrogen dioxide through a sampling port or the inspiratory circuit.

A circuit for nitric oxide inhalation for a spontaneously breathing patient is shown in Figure 13-46A. Pure nitric

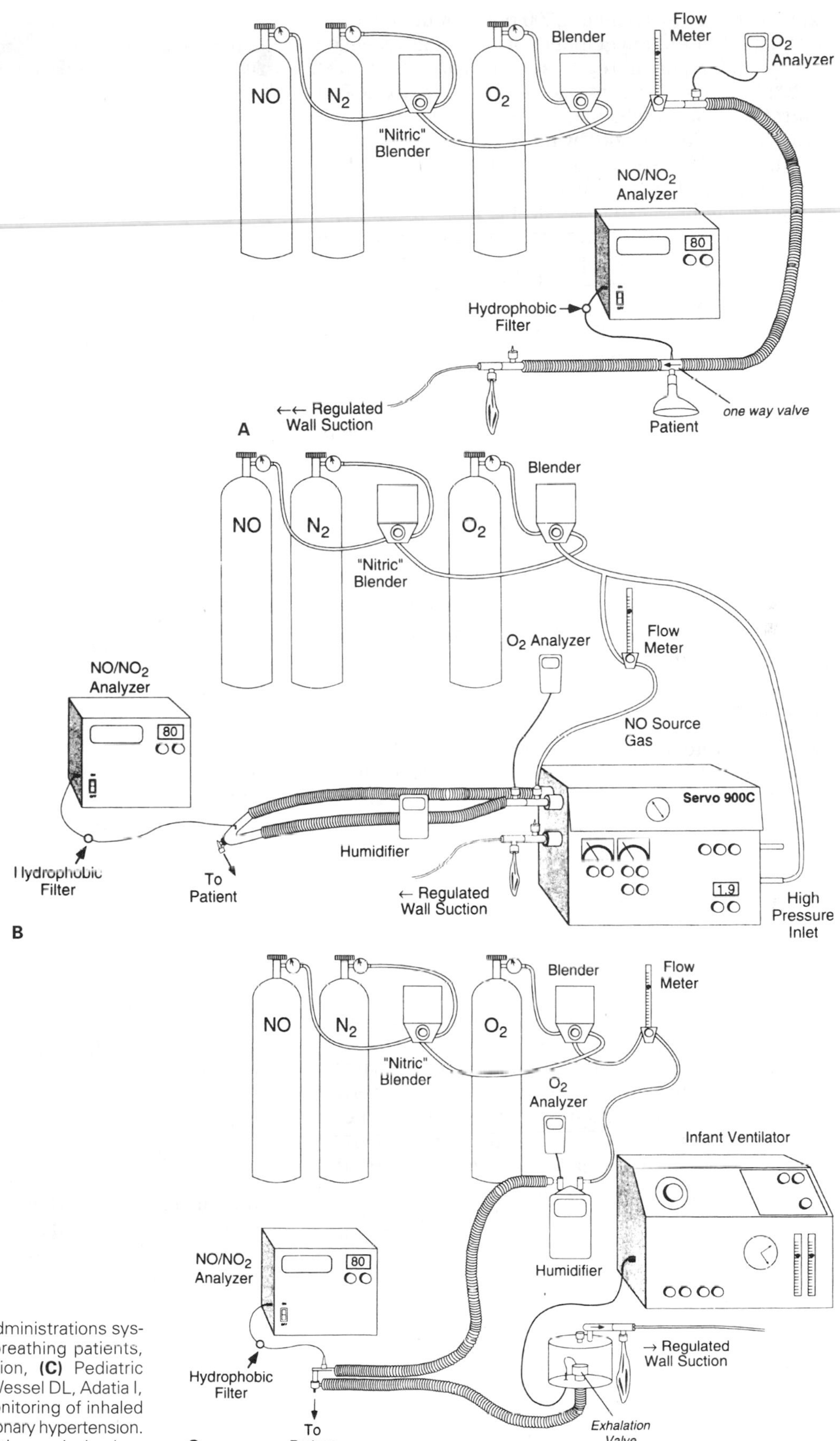

FIGURE 13-46. Nitric oxide administrations systems. **(A)** for spontaneously breathing patients, **(B)** Adult mechanical ventilation, **(C)** Pediatric time-cycled ventilation. (From Wessel DL, Adatia I, Thompson JE. Delivery and monitoring of inhaled nitric oxide in patients with pulmonary hypertension. Crit Care Med 1994;22:930. With permission.)

oxide, in either 800 ppm or 2200 ppm containing cylinders, is fed to the oxygen inlet of a standard low-flow 0_2/air blender; pure nitrogen is connected to its air inlet. This "nitric" blender controls the final nitric oxide concentration. The N_2/NO blend is fed into the air inlet of a second low-flow blender, with 50 psig oxygen directed to that inlet. This second blender allows control of the mixture's F_IO_2 using an in-line oxygen analyzer. Flow to the patient is adjusted with a standard flowmeter, to be set at two or three times the patient's minute ventilation. This minimizes formation of nitrogen dioxide. Expired gases from patient circuit are scavenged by wall suction. A one-way valve allows unidirectional flow. The system can be applied to the patient with a snug-fitting resuscitation-type mask or connection to an artificial airway.[169]

Mechanically ventilated adults and infants in the operating room or ICU can receive nitric oxide via ventilator circuit. The system previously described has been adapted to a "volume-preset" ventilator (Fig. 13-46B). Time-cycled, pressure-limited infant ventilators are arranged similarly (Figure 13-46C).

GASEOUS OXYGEN ANALYSIS AND NONINVASIVE OXYGEN MONITORING

Gaseous Analysis

When accurate analysis of oxygen concentrations can be performed, it should be done as part of safe therapy protocol. Analysis is routinely performed in infant oxygen hoods, incubators, mechanical ventilators, anesthetic circuits, and some fixed-performance oxygen administration devices (eg, aerosol-entrainment T-piece). Clinicians should check dual air-oxygen flowmeters and blenders to confirm desired oxygen concentrations. Monitoring can consist of spot sample, periodic, or continuous monitoring with high-low limit alarms.

Monitoring drug therapy is commonly done by comparing blood level and patient response to the amount given. This objective process allows a scientific approach. You should treat medical gas therapy patients in the same way. Gas analysis can often identify errors in gas concentrations and prevent harmful side effects. Some analyzers can document trends over long periods of time. Three methods have been commonly used to measure oxygen concentration. Only electrochemical cells continue to play a role in contemporary clinical care. They are described by terms that refer to their physical or chemical method of analysis. Box 13-28 identifies the types of gas analyzers. A complete review of the individual analyzers is found in Chapter 12.

BOX 13-28

TYPES OF GASEOUS OXYGEN ANALYZERS

- Paramagnetic analyzer (Pauling meter)
- Thermoconductivity analyzer (Wheatstone bridge)
- Electrochemical cells (electrodes)
  - Polarographic
  - Galvanic cell (fuel cell)

Patient Oxygen Monitoring

Monitoring clinical signs and results of arterial blood gas analysis are standards for documenting oxygenation, ventilation, and acid–base balance. Arterial blood gases and oxyhemoglobin saturation (SaO_2) measurements are intermittent samples, and there is usually some delay in analysis. In an attempt to overcome the periodic nature of oxygen analysis, other more continuous technologies have evolved. Transcutaneous and transconjunctival oxygen sensors measure oxygen tensions at the dermal or conjunctival surface and use technology similar to the polarographic Clark electrode. Their reliability and clinical related problems have reduced their popularity.[170,171]

Pulse oximetry has become the most common form to continuously monitor oxygen saturation (SpO_2). It has become the standard of care in the operating or recovery room, pulmonary function or sleep laboratory, intensive care unit, or emergency room, as well as other clinical areas throughout the hospital.[172,173] Clinicians can use oximetry to detect episodes of desaturation during patient transport, cardiac catheterization, bronchoscopy, or airway suctioning.[174] Its noninvasive approach, ease of use, and "real-time" feedback reflect its widespread acceptance in titrating oxygen levels to ventilated and spontaneously breathing patients. It may be used to "spot check" or in continuous measurement. Protocols must be developed to deal with desaturation episodes both in ICU and noncritical care settings (see Chapter 12).[175,176]

A detailed review of the technology is beyond the scope of this chapter. You should refer to definitive review articles.[173,174] Pulse oximetry combines technologic advances in light-emitting diodes (LEDs) and the microprocessor and the blending of optical plethysmography with spectrophotometry. A light source consisting of two known wavelengths (660 nm [red] and 940 nm [infrared]) is sent across a pulsating vascular bed. The light absorption at the two wavelengths identifies oxygenated and reduced hemoglobin. The ratio of pulsatile and baseline absorption (k) at the two wavelengths allows calculation of oxygen saturation.

The oximeter should not be used as the only monitor for critically ill patients since it does not provide information on acid–base status, ventilation, or electrocardiographic data. Limitations for clinical application of pulse oximeters are listed in Box 13-29.[87]

Equipment

Pulse oximeters come in a variety of configurations. Clinicians can select among such features such as portability, recording, memory for trend analysis,

BOX 13-29

LIMITATIONS OF PULSE OXIMETRY IN PATIENT CARE

- Probe motion artifact
- Hemoglobinopathies
- Intravascular dyes
- Probe exposure to ambient lighting
- Low tissue perfusion at probe site
- Skin pigmentation
- Nail polish (dark colors)
- Electrical interference

alarms, ECG synchronization, and probe styles, depending on their application and budget. Some units allow adjustment of averaging time of signals to allow for closer correlation in real time with the patient's data. Analyzers with faster response capabilities are also subject to greater effect from motion artifact.

Patient Probes

A variety of probe styles allows the clinician to collect data from the best patient site. The majority of pulse oximeters have probes that send light through the tissue of an extremity. The reflective type responds to light that is returned after "bouncing back" from a hard surface (skull). The best site location is one that provides the best local circulation and least motion. In adults, the earlobe, finger, thumb, nosebridge, and forehead are used. Because of the reduced thickness of a newborn's body tissue, the foot, hand, and heel are commonly chosen.

REFERENCES

1. Johnson CB: 1992 Respiratory care job analysis. NBRC Horizons 19:1, 1993
2. Fulmer JD, Snider GL (chrm): ACCP-NHLBI national conference on oxygen therapy. Chest 86:234, 1984
3. American Association for Respiratory Care: Clinical practice guideline oxygen therapy in the acute care hospital. Respir Care 36:1406, 1991
4. American Association for Respiratory Care: Clinical practice guideline oxygen therapy in the home or extended care facility. Respir Care 37:918, 1992
5. Cassebaum H, Schufle JA: Schelle's priority for the discovery of oxygen. J Chem Ed 52:442, 1975
6. Perkins JF: Historical development of respiratory physiology. In Fenn WO, Rahn H (eds): Handbook of Physiology, Vol 3. Respiration. Washington, DC, American Physiological Society, 1964, pp 1
7. Leigh JM: The evolution of the oxygen therapy apparatus. Anaesthesia 29:462, 1974
8. Barach AL: Symposium—inhalation therapy historical background. Anesthesiology 23:407, 1962
9. Smith JL: The pathological effects due to increase of oxygen tension in the air breathed. J Physiol (Lond) 24:19, 1899
10. Barach AL: New oxygen tent. JAMA 87:1213, 1926
11. Barach AL, Eckman M: A mask apparatus which provides high concentration with accurate control of the percentage of oxygen in the inspired air and without accumulation of carbon dioxide. Aviat Med 12:39, 1941
12. Barach AL, Eckman M: A physiologically controlled oxygen mask apparatus. Anesthesiology 2:421, 1941
13. Barach AL: Use of helium as a new therapeutic gas. Proc Soc Exp Biol Med 32:462, 1934
14. Barach AL: The therapeutic use of helium. JAMA 107:1273, 1936
15. Boothby WM, Lovelace WR, Bulbulian AH: I. Oxygen administration: The value of high concentration of oxygen for therapy. II. Oxygen for therapy and aviation: an apparatus for the administration of oxygen or oxygen and helium by inhalation. III. Design and construction of the masks for the oxygen inhalation apparatus. Proc Mayo Clin 13:641, 1938
16. Bean JW: Effects of oxygen at increased pressure. Physiol Rev 25:1, 1945
17. Severinghaus JW, Astrup PB: History of blood gas analysis: IV. Leland Clark's oxygen electrode. J Clin Monit 2:125, 1986
18. Millikan GA: The oximeter, an instrument for measuring continuously the oxygen saturation of arterial blood in man. Rev Sci Instr 13:434, 1942
19. Severinghaus JW, Astrup PB: History of blood gas analysis. J Clin Monit 3:135, 1987
20. Campbell EJM: A method of controlled oxygen administration which reduces the risk of CO_2 retention. Lancet 1:12, 1960
21. Nocturnal Oxygen Therapy Trial Group: Continuous and nocturnal oxygen therapy in hypoxic chronic obstructive lung disease: A clinical trial. Ann Intern Med 93:931, 1980
22. Health Care Financing Administration: Durable Medical Equipment Regional Carrier (DEMC) Supplier's Manual. Indianapolis, Adminastar, 1996, pp 13–87
23. Petty TL, O'Donahue WJ: Further recommendations for prescribing, reimbursement, technology development, and research in long-term oxygen therapy (Fourth Oxygen Consensus Conference). Am J Respir Crit Care Med 150:875, 1994
24. Palmer RMJ, Ferringe AG, Moncada S: Nitric oxide release accounts for the biological activity of endothelium-derived relaxing facture. Nature 327:524, 1987
25. Kam PCA, Govender G: Nitric oxide: Basic science and clinical applications. Anaesthesia 49:515, 1994
26. Zapol WM, Rimar S, Gillis N, Marletta M, Bosken C: Nitric oxide and the lung. Am J Respir Crit Care Med 149:1375, 1994
27. Pauling L, Wood RF, Sturdivent JH: An instrument for determining the partial pressure of oxygen in a gas. J Am Chem Soc 68:795, 1946
28. Chusid EL: Oxygen concentrators. Int Anesthesiol Clin 20:235, 1982
29. Bongard JP, Pahud C, DeHaller R: Insufficient oxygen concentration obtained at domiciliary controls of eighteen concentrators. Eur Respir J 2:280, 1989
30. Compressed Gas Association: Handbook of Compressed Gases, ed 2. New York, Van Nostrand Reinhold Co, 1990
31. Compressed Gas Association: Compressed Air for Human Respiration. Pamphlet G-7. Arlington, VA, Compressed Gas Association, 1976
32. Fink JB, Lopez A, Mahlmeister MJ: Blender and ventilator failure associated with hospital grade compressed air [abstract]. Respir Care 30:893, 1985
33. Compressed Gas Association: Compressed Air for Human Respiration. Pamphlet G-7. Arlington, VA, Compressed Gas Association, 1976
34. National Fire Protection Association: Respiratory Therapy, NFPA no 56B, Quincy, MA, National Fire Protection Association, 1973
35. Klein PE: Health Care Facilities Handbook, 4th ed. National Fire Protection Association, Quincy, MA, National Fire Protection Association, 1993
36. National Fire Protection Association: Storage of Liquid and Solid Oxidizing Materials, NFPA no 43A, Quincy, MA, National Fire Protection Association, 1980
37. Anderson WR, Brock-Utne JG: Oxygen pipeline supply failure: A coping strategy. J Clin Monit 7:39, 1991
38. Bancroft ML, du Moulin GC, Heldey-Whyte J: Hazards of hospital bulk oxygen delivery systems. Anesthesiology 52:504, 1980
39. Signoretti EC, Salvini R, Seghieri G: Liquid oxygen contaminants-increase in concentration during use of domiciliary liquid oxygen medical systems. J Clin Pharm Ther 16:367, 1991
40. Compressed Gas Association: Transfilling of high presure gaseous oxygen to be used for respiration Pamplet P-25. Arlington, VA, Compressed Gas Associaton, 1981

41. Feeley TW, Bancroft ML, Brooks, Hedley-White J: Potential hazards of compressed gas cylinders: A review. Anesthesiology 48: 72, 1978
42. Sawheney KK, Yoon YK: Erroneous labeling of a nitrous oxide cylinder. Anesthesiology 59:260, 1983
43. Menon MRB, Lett Z: Incorrectly filled cylinders. Anaesthesia 46:155, 1991
44. Jayasuriya JP: Another example of Murphy's law: Mix up of pin index valves. Anaesthesia 41:1164, 1986
45. Fischer and Porter Company: Theory of the Flowrater. FP no 98-A, Warminster, PA, Fischer and Porter Co., 1947
46. Fischer and Porter Company: Variable Area Flowmeter Handbook. Warminster, PA, Fischer and Porter Co., 1982 p 1021
47. Gilmont R, Mauer PW: A generalized equation for rotameters with special floats. Instruments Control Systems 34:40, 1961
48. Gilmont R, Roccanove BT: Low-flow rotameter coefficient. Instruments Control Systems 39:35, 1966
49. Yost LC, Barnhard WN, Kaiman A, Kaiman A, Paegle, RD: Oxygen air blending nomogram for medium and high flow rates. Respir Care 22:607, 1977
50. Emergency Care Research Institute: Oxygen-air proportioners. Health Devices 14:263, 1985
51. Fink JB, Lopez A, Mahlmeister MJ: Blender and ventilator failure associated with hospital grade compressed air [abstract]. Respir Care 30:893, 1985
52. Fried JL, Downs JB, Davis JE, Heenan TJ A new venturi device for administering continuous positive airway pressure. Respir Care 26:133, 1981
53. Fisher GC: The Down's adjustable flow generator. Anaesthesia 43:766, 1988
54. Vital signs: Product information. Totwana, NJ, Vital Signs 1983
55. Ward JJ, Awan ZI: Flow capabilities of the adjustable Down's flow generator [abstract]. Respir Care 32:906, 1987
56. Pasquale MD, Cipolle MD, Cerra FB, et al: Oxygen transport: Does incresasing supply improve outcome? Respir Care 38:800, 1993
57. Mellemgard K: $P(A - a)O_2$ in normal man. Acta Physiol Scand 67:10, 1966
58. Ziment I: Respiratory Pharmacology and Therapeutics. Philadelphia, WB Sanders Co, 1978, p 442
59. Mithoefer JC, Keighley JF, Karetzky MS: Response of the arterial PO_2 to oxygen administration in chronic pulmonary disease. Ann Intern Med 64:328, 1971
60. Helmholz HF Jr: The abbreviated alveolar air equation. Chest 75:748, 1979
61. Martin L: Abbreviating the alveolar gas equation: An argument for simplicity. Respir Care 30:964, 1985
62. Fisher AB, Dodia C: Lungs as a model for evaluation of critical intracellular PaO_2 and $PaCO_2$. Am J Physiol 241:47,1981
63. Kavanagh BP, Cheng DC, Sandler AN, Chung F, Lawson S, Ong D: Supplemental oxygen does not reduce myocardial oxygen ischemia in premedicated patients with critical coronary artery disease. Anesth Analg 76:950, 1993
64. Piantadosi CA: Carbon monoxide, oxygen transport and oxygen metabolism. J Hyperbaric Med 2:27, 1987
65. Tierney D: Conference on the scientific basis on in-hospital respiratory therapy-oxygen therapy: Final report summary. Am Rev Respir Dis 122:15, 1980
66. Petty TL, O'Donohue WJ: Further recommendations for perscribing reimbursement, technology development, and research in long-term oxygen therapy. Am J Respir Crit Care Med 150:875, 1994
67. Bunn HF, Forget BG: Carboxyhemoglobin and carboxyhemoglobinemia. In Bunn HF, Forget BG (eds): Hemoglobin: Molecular, Genetic and Clinical Aspects. Philadelphia, PA, WB Saunders, 1986
68. Burney RE, Wu SC, Nemiroff MJ: Mass carbon monoxide poisoning: Clinical effects and results of treatment in 184 victims. Ann Emerg Med 11:394, 1982
69. Segal D, Welch L: Carbon monoxide controversies: Neurophysiologic testing, mechanisms of toxicity and hyperbaric oxygenation. Ann Emerg Med 24:142, 1994
70. Didier EP: Some effects of anesthetics and the anesthetized state on the respiratory system. Respir Care 29:463, 1984
71. O'Donohue WJ: Effect of oxygen therapy on increasing arterial oxygen tension in hyporemic patients with stable chronic obstructive pulmonary disease while breathing ambient air. Chest 100:968, 1991
72. O'Donohue WJ: Prescribing home oxygen therapy: What the primary care physician needs to know. Arch Intern Med 152:746, 1992
73. Deneke SM, Fanberg BL: Normobaric oxygen toxicity of the lung. N Engl J Med 303:76, 1980
74. Durbin CG, Wallace KK: Oxygen toxicity in the critically ill patient. Respir Care 38:739, 1993
75. Fisher AB: Oxygen therapy: Side effects and toxicity. Am Rev Respir Dis 122:61, 1980
76. Ingrassia TS, Ryu JH, Trastek VF, Rosenow EC: Oxygen exacerbated bleomycin pulmonary toxicity. Mayo Clin Proc 66:173, 1991
77. LaManita KR, Glick JH, Marshall BE: Supplemental oxygen does not cause respiratory failure in bleomycin-treated surgical patients. Anesthesiology 60:65, 1984
78. Dunn WF, Nelson SB, Hubmayr RD: Oxygen induced hypercarbia in obstructive pulmonary disease. An Rev Respir Dis 144:526, 1991
79. Terry TL: Extreme prematurity and fibroblastic overgrowth of persistent vascular sheath behind each crystalline lense. Am J Opthalmol 25:203, 1942
80. Hoyt CS, Good W, Petersen R: Disorders of the eye. In Taeush HW, Ballerd RA, Avery ME (eds): Diseases of the Newborn, 6th ed. Philadelphia, PA, WB Saunders, 1991
81. Hoskins EM, Elliot E, Shennan AT, Skidmore MB, Keith E: Outcome of very low birth weight infants born at a perinatal center. Am J Obstet Gynecol 145:135, 1983
82. Silverman WA: Retinopathy of prematurity: Oxygen dogma challenged. Arch Dis Child 57:731, 1982
83. Hittner HM, Godio LB, Rudolph AJ, et al: Retrolental fibroplasia: Efficacy of vitamin E in a double-blind clinical study of preterm infants. N Engl J Med 305:1365, 1981
84. Lucey JF, Dangman B: A reexamination of the role of oxygen in retrolental fibroplasia. Pediatrics 73:82, 1984
85. McMurphy DM, Heyman MA, Rudolph AM, Melmon KL: Developmental changes in constriction of the ductus arterious: Response to oxygen and vasoactive agents in the isolated ductus arteriosis of the fetal lamb. Pediatr Res 6:31, 1972
86. Centers for Disease Control and Prevention: Guidelines for prevention of nosocomial pneumonia. Respir Care 39:1181, 1994
87. American Association for Respiratory Care: Clinical practice guideline: Pulse oximetry. Respir Care 36:1406, 1991
88. Hess D: Predictions of the change in [letter]. Crit Care Med 7:568, 1979
89. Hess D, Maxwell C: Which is the best index of oxygenation-$P(A\text{-}a)O_2$, PaO_2/PAO_2 or PaO_2/FiO_2 [editorial]? Respir Care 30:961, 1985
90. Don H: Decision Making in Critical Care. St. Louis, CV Mosby Co., 1985, p 102
91. Burton GG, Tietsort JA: Therapist-Driven Protocols: A Practitioner's Guide. Los Angeles, CA, Academy Medical Systems, Inc., 1993
92. Barach AL: Principles and Practices of Inhalation Therapy. Philadelphia, PA, JB Lippincott, 1944
93. Korey, RC, Bergmann JC, Sweet RD, et al: Comparative evaluation of oxygen therapy technique. JAMA 179:123, 1962
94. Kacmarek RM: Methods of oxygen delivery in the hospital. In Christopher KL (ed): The Current Status of Oxygen Therapy. Probl Respir Care 3:563, 1990
95. Ooi R, Joshi P, Soni N: An evaluation of oxygen delivery using nasal prongs. Anesthesia 47:591, 1992
96. Gibson RL, Comer PB, Beckham RW, et al: Actual tracheal oxygen concentrations with commonly used oxygen equipment. Anesthesiology 44:71, 1976
97. Schacter EN, Littner MR, Luddy P, Beck GJ: Monitoring of oxygen delivery systems in clinical practice. Crit Care Med 8:405, 1980
98. Dunlevy CL, Tyl SE: The effect of oral versus nasal breathing on oxygen concentrations received from nasal cannulas. Respir Care 37:357, 1992
99. Vain NE, Prudent LM, Stevens DP, Weeter MM, Maisels MJ: Regulation of oxygen concentration delivered to infants by nasal cannulas. Am J Dis Child 143:1458, 1989

100. Rotschild A, Schapira D, Kuyek N, Solimano A: Evaluation of nasal prongs of a new design for low-flow oxygen delivery to infants. Respir Care 34:801, 1989
101. Shigeoka JW, Bonekat HW: The current status of oxygen-conserving devices [editorial]. Respir Care 31:833, 1985
102. Shigeoka JW: Oxygen conservers, home oxygen prescriptions and the role of the respiratory care practitioner. Respir Care 36:178, 1991
103. Kerby GR, O'Donohue WJ, Romberger DJ, Hanson FN, Koenig GA: Clinical efficacy and cost benefit of pulse flow oxygen in hospitalized patients. Chest 97:369, 1990
104. Tiep BL, Lewis ML: Oxygen conservation and oxygen conserving devices in chronic lung disease: A review. Chest 92:263, 1987
105. Tiep BL, Belman M, Mittman C, et al: A new pendant storage oxygen-conserving nasal cannula. Chest 87:381, 1985
106. Tiep BL, Nicotra B, Carter R, Phillips R, Otsap B: Evaluation of low flow oxygen-conserving nasal cannula. Am Rev Respir Dis 130:500, 1984
107. Hoffman LA: Novel strategies for delivering oxygen: Reservoir cannula, demand flow, and trantracheal oxygen administration. Respir Care 39:363, 1994
108. Mecikalski M, Shigeoka JW: A demand valve conserves oxygen in subjects with chronic obstructive pulmonary disease. Chest 86:667, 1984
109. Tiep BL, Christopher KL, Spofford BT, Goodman JR, Worley PD, Macy SL: Pulsed nasal and transtracheal oxygen. Chest 97:364, 1990
110. Auerback D, Flick MR, Block AJ: A new oxygen cannula system using intermmittent-demand nasal flow. Chest 74:38, 1978
111. Anderson WM, Ryerson G, Block AJ: Evaluation of an intermittent demand nasal oxygen flow system with fluidic valve [abstract]. Chest 86:313, 1984
112. Block AJ: Intermittent flow oxygen devices—technically feasible, but rarely used [editorial]. Chest 86:657, 1984
113. Heimlich HJ: Respiratory rehabilitation with transtracheal oxygen system. Ann Otol Rhinol Laryngol 91:643, 1982
114. Reich D, Mingus M: Transtracheal oxygenation using simple equipment and a low-pressure oxygen source. Crit Care Med 18:664, 1990
115. Christopher KL, Spofford BT, Branin PK, Petty TL: Transtracheal oxygen therapy for refractory hypoxemia. JAMA 256:494, 1986
116. Hansen LA, Staats BA, Scanlon PD, Prakash UBS, Hepper NGG, Cummings KA: Transtracheal oxygen therapy: Long-term follow up [abstract]. Chest 94:325, 1988
117. Johnson JT, Ferson PF, Hoffman LA, Wesmiller SW, Mazzocco MC, Sciubra FC, Dauber JH: Transtracheal delivery of oxygen: Efficacy and safety for long-term continuous therapy. Ann Otol Laryngol 100:108, 1991
118. Johnson LP, Cary JM: The implanted intratracheal oxygen. Surg Gynecol Obstet 165:74, 1987
119. Wesmiller SW, Hoffman LA, Sciurba FC, Ferson PF, Johnson JT, Dauber JH: Exercise tolerance during nasal cannula and transtracheal oxygen delivery. Am Rev Respir Dis 141:789, 1990
120. Leger P, Gerard M, Mercatillo A, Robert D: Transtracheal catheter for oxygen therapy of patients requiring high oxygen flows [abstract]. Respiration 46(suppl 1):103, 1984
121. Couser JI, Make BJ: Respiratory tract infection complicating transtracheal oxygen therapy. Chest 101:273, 1992
122. Punzal P, Myers R, Ries AL, Harrell JH: Laser resection of granulation tissue secondary to transtracheal catheter. Chest 101: 269, 1992
123. Harvey JE, Schlecht BJ, Grant LJ, Tottle CR, Tanser AR: A new nasal oxygen mask. Br J Dis Chest 77:376, 1983
124. Ward JJ, Gracey DR: Arterial oxygen values achieved by COPD patients breathing oxygen alternately via nasal mask and nasal cannula. Respir Care 30:250, 1985
125. Jensen AG, Johnson A, Sandstedt S: Rebreathing during oxygen treatment with face mask: The effect of oxygen flow rates on ventilation. Acta Anaesthesiol Scand 35:289, 1991
126. Leigh JM: Variation in performance of oxygen therapy devices. Anaesthesia 25:210, 1970
127. Hudes ET, Marans HJ, Hirano GM, Scott AC, Ho K: Recovery room oxygenation: A comparison of nasal catheters and 40 percent oxygen masks. Can J Anaesth 36:20, 1989
128. Milross J, Young IH, Donnelly P: The oxygen delivery characteristics of the Hudson oxy-one face mask. Anaesth Intensive Care 17:180, 1989
129. Redding JS, McAfee DD, Parham AM: Oxygen concentrations received from commonly used delivery systems. South Med J 71:169, 1978
130. Emergency Care Research Institute: Pulmonary resuscitators. Health Devices 18:333, 1989
131. Bar ZG: Predictive equation for peak inspiratory flow. Respir Care 30:766, 1985
132. Spearman CB, Sanders HG, Feenstra L, Gee GN, Hodgkin JE: Effects of changing jet flows on O_2 concentrations in adjustable air entrainment masks [abstract]. Respir Care 25:1266, 1980
133. Hill SL, Barnes PK, Hollway T, Tennet R: Fixed performance oxygen masks: An evaluation. BMJ 288:1261, 1984
134. Klein EF, Mon BK, Mon MJ: Oxygen accuracy with Venturi nebulizer systems [abstract]. Crit Care Med 97:186, 1979
135. McPherson SP: Oxygen percentage accuracy of air-entrainment masks. Respir Care 19:658, 1974
136. Campbell EJM, Gebbie T: Masks and tent providing controlled oxygen concentrations. Lancet 1:468, 1966
137. Cox D, Gillbe C: Fixed performance oxygen masks. Anaesthesia 36:958, 1981
138. Hill SL, Barnes PK, Hollway T, Tennant R: Fixed performance oxygen masks: An evaluation. Anaesthesia 288:1261, 1984
139. Lyew MA, Holland AJ, Metcalf IR: Combined air and oxygen entrainment: Effect on the percentage output of fixed performance masks. Anaesthesia 45:732, 1990
140. Gura D, Saidman LJ: Alveolar oxygen and carbon dioxide concentrations during simulated breathing through a T-piece. Crit Care Med 2:11, 1974
141. Foust GN, Potter WH, Wilson MD, Golden EB: Shortcomings of using two jet nebulizers in tandem with an aerosol face mask for optimal oxygen therapy. Chest 99:1346, 1991
142. Schacter EN, Littner MR, Luddy P, Beck GJ: Monitoring of oxygen delivery systems in clinical practice. Crit Care Med 8:40, 1980
143. Quinn WW: MistyOx 441H in lieu of doubled-flow nebulizers: A bench study (abstract). Respir Care 37:1298, 1992
144. Durham M, Miller WF: Controlled oxygen administration with adequate humidification. Inhal Ther 14:87, 1969
145. Beckham RW, Mishoe SC: Sound levels inside incubators and oxygen hoods used with nebulizers and humidifiers. Respir Care 27:33, 1982
146. Stoller JK: Travel for the technology-dependent individual. Respir Care 39:347, 1994
147. Gong H: Air travel and oxygen therapy in cardiopulmonary patients. Chest 101:1104, 1992
148. Berg BW, Dillard TA, Rajagopal KR, Mehm WJ: Oxygen supplementation during air travel in patients with chronic obstructive lung disease. Chest 101:638, 1992
149. National Heart, Lung, Blood Institute: Hyperbaric oxygenation therapy. Am Rev Respir Dis 144:1411, 1991
150. Slack WK, Thomas DA, DeJode LR: Hyperbaric oxygen in treatment of trauma, ischemic disease of the limbs and varicose ulceration. In: Proceedings of the Third International Conference on Hyperbaric Medicine. Durham, NC, National Academy of Sciences, 1965, p 621
151. Sheffield PJ, Davis JC, Bell GC, Gallagher TJ: Hyperbaric chamber clinical support: Multiplace. In Davis JC, Hunt TK (eds): Hyperbaric Oxygen Therapy. Bethesda, Md: Undersea Medical Society, 1977:25.
152. Boutros AR, Hoyt JL: Management of carbon monoxide poisoning in the absence of a hyperbaric chamber. Crit Care Med 4: 144, 1976
153. Mathewson HS: Drug capsule. Helium—who needs it? Respir Care 27:1400, 1982
154. Lu TS, Ohmura A, Wong KC, Hodges MR: Helium-oxygen in treatment of upper airway obstruction. Anesthesiology 45:678, 1976
155. Chan-Yeung M, Abboud R, Tsao MS, Maclean L: Effect of helium on maximal expiratory flowrate in patients with asthma before and during induced bronchoconstriction. Am Rev Respir Dis 113:433, 1976
156. Ishilcawa S, Segal MS: Re-appraisal of helium-oxygen therapy on patients with chronic obstructive pulmonary disease. Ann Allergy 31:536, 1973

157. Swidwa DM, Montenegro HD, Goldman MD, Lutchen KR, Saidel GM: Helium-oxygen breathing in severe chronic obstruction pulmonary disease. Chest 87:790, 1985
158. Kass JE, Castriotta RJ: Heliox therapy in acute severe asthma. Chest 107:757, 1995
159. Stillwell PC, Quick JD, Munro PR, Mallory GB: Effectiveness of open-circuit and oxyhood delivery of helium-oxygen. Chest 95:1222, 1989
160. Meduna LJ: Alterations of neurotic pattern by use of CO_2 inhalation. J Nerv Ment Dis 108:373, 1948
161. Woodbury DM, Rollins LT, Gardner MD: Effect of carbon dioxide on brain excitability and electrolytes. Am J Physiol 192:79, 1958
162. Meyer JS, Fukuucni Y, Shimazu K: Abnormal hemispheric blood flow and metabolism in cerebrovascular disease: II. Therapeutic trials with 5% CO_2 inhalation, hyperventilation and intravenous infusion of THAM and mannitol. Stroke 3:157, 1972
163. Mathewson HS: Drug capsule: Carbon dioxide: Therapeutic for what? Respir Care 27:1272, 1982
164. Abman SH, Griebel JL, Parker DK, Schmidt JM, Swanton D, Kinsella JP: Inhaled nitric oxide in children with severe hypoxemic respiratory failure. J Petiatr 124:881, 1994
165. Roberts JD, Lang P, Bigatello LM, Vlahakes GJ, Zapol WM: Inhaled nitric oxide in congenital heart disease. Circulation 87:447, 1993
166. Girard C, Lehot J, Pannetier J, Filley S, French P, Estanove S: Inhaled nitric oxide after mitral valve replacement in patients with chronic pulmonary hypertension. Anesthesiology 77:880, 1992
167. Bigatello LM, Hurford WE, Kacmarek RM, Roberts JD, Zapol WM: Prolonged inhalation of low concentrations of nitric oxide in patients with severe adult respiratory distress syndrome. Anesthesiology 80:761, 1994
168. Brown RH, Zerhouni EA, Hirshman C: Reversal of bronchoconstriction by inhaled nitric oxide: Histamine vs. methacholine. Am J Respir Crit Care Med 150:233, 1994
169. Wessel DL, Adatia I, Thompson JE: Delivery and monitoring of inhaled nitric oxide in patients with pulmonary hypertension. Crit Care Med 22:930, 1994
170. New WJ: Pulse oximetry versus measurement of transcutaneous oxygen. J Clin Monit 1:126, 1985
171. Zaloga GP: Evaluation of bed-side testing options for the critical care unit. Chest 97:1755, 1990
172. Bowton DL, Scuderi PE, Harris L, Haponik EF: Pulse oximetry monitoring outside the intensive care unit: progress or problem? Ann Int Med 115:450, 1991
173. Kelleher JF: Pulmonary oximetry. J Clin Monit 5:37, 1989
174. Tremper KK, Barker SJ: Pulse oximetry. Anesthesiology 1989; 70:98, 1989
175. Smoker JM, Hess DR, Frey-Zeiler VL, Tangen MI, Rexrode WO: A protocol to assess oxygen therapy. Respir Care 31:35, 1986
176. King T, Simon RH: Pulse oximetry for tapering supplemental oxygen in hospitalized patients. Chest 92:713, 1987

14 Hyperbaric Oxygen Therapy

David A. Desautels

CLINICAL SKILLS

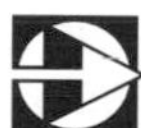

Upon completion of this chapter, the reader will:

- Define hyperbaric oxygen therapy
- List the disease processes acceptable for treatment in a hyperbaric chamber
- Describe the historic development of hyperbaric oxygen therapy
- Provide the basic gas laws pertinent to hyperbaric oxygen therapy
- Identify the physiologic response to hyperbaric oxygen therapy
- Explain how hyperbaric oxygen therapy supplements oxygen transport
- Relate effects of pressurization, pressure, and depressurization to human physiology
- Describe the construction of the two major types of hyperbaric chambers
- Name the fire protection precautions taken in each type of chamber
- Explain the major safety precautions taken in the delivery of hyperbaric oxygen therapy
- Describe the underlying methods of how hyperbaric oxygen therapy works
- Relate patient management under differing levels of chamber pressure
- List the absolute and relative contraindications for hyperbaric oxygen therapy
- Identify the different treatment schedules used for each acceptable hyperbaric oxygen therapy treatment

KEY TERMS

Absolute pressure
Arterial gas embolism
Carbon monoxide intoxication
Carbon monoxide poisoning
Cerebral oxygen toxicity
Crush injuries
Cyanide poisoning
Decompression illness
Gas gangrene
Hyperbaric
Monoplace chambers
Multiplace chambers
Osteomyelitis
Osteoradionecrosis
Pulmonary oxygen toxicity
Saturation treatment
Smoke inhalation
Wound healing

Hyperbaric oxygen (HBO) therapy is the systemic administration of oxygen at pressures greater than atmospheric. Patients are placed inside a pressure vessel known as a hyperbaric, recompression, or decompression chamber, and the pressure is increased. Delivery of oxygen to an isolated body part is *not* hyperbaric oxygen therapy. The pressure level to which the chamber is taken is prescribed by treatment schedules designed for each sanctioned disease. Many uses have been proposed, some with questionable scientific basis. To establish credibility within the medical community, the Hyperbaric Oxygen Committee of the Undersea and Hyperbaric Medical Society examines the scientific data and publishes the results every three years.[1] The disease entities identified are listed in Box 14-1.

The first concern of hyperbaric oxygen therapy in diving disorders is to reduce the bubble size of the intracorporeal oxygen and nitrogen. This is accomplished by increasing chamber pressure to the prescribed pressure of 60 to 165 feet of sea water (fsw) (Table 14-1). This function may be used for a disorder as benign as skin "bends" or as critical as arterial gas embolism. The secondary purpose of HBO therapy is to increase the nitrogen gradient to remove nitrogen from the tissue and to provide therapeutic oxygen to the ischemic areas caused by bubbles.

At increased pressures, the patient's physiology is altered and phenomena relative to increased pressure or increased oxygen tension, or both, can provide therapeutic results. In disorders for which the primary purpose is to provide increased pressure, HBO therapy is considered the primary mode of therapy. These disorders are *decompression illness* and *arterial gas embolism*.

In disorders treated primarily to increase oxygen concentration, HBO therapy is considered adjunctive. An exception to this is that of *carbon monoxide* and *cyanide poisoning* for which HBO therapy is considered the primary mode of therapy, but the purpose is still to provide increased oxygen tension at cellular level.

BOX 14-1

INDICATIONS FOR HYPERBARIC OXYGEN

Air or gas embolism
Carbon monoxide poisoning and smoke inhalation, carbon monoxide complicated by cyanide poisoning
Clostridial myonecrosis (gas gangrene)
Crush injury, compartment syndrome, and other acute traumatic ischemias
Decompression sickness
Enhancement of healing in selected problem wounds
Exceptional blood loss (anemia)
Necrotizing soft-tissue infections (subcutaneous tissue, muscle, fascia)
Osteomyelitis (refractory)
Radiation tissue damage (osteoradionecrosis)
Skin grafts and flaps (compromised)
Thermal burns

(From Hyperbaric Oxygen Therapy: A Committee Report, Revised 1992, Kensington, MD, Undersea and Hyperbaric Medical Society; with permission)

HBO therapy is a relatively new discipline for the respiratory care practitioner. It requires a firm background in gas laws, the mechanical aspects of respiratory care, and the nuances of medicine; thus the field is a "natural" for the respiratory care practitioner. In caring for a wide range of patients, from pediatric to geriatric ages and from quite healthy to critically ill, the hyperbaric technologist is unique, combining an industrial equipment orientation with that of a compassionate health care provider.

Despite controversy in the medical community, HBO therapy is increasing in popularity. With more chambers being installed, many respiratory care practitioners are becoming involved in this exciting and highly technical field.

HISTORY

The history of hyperbaric medicine was preceded by a long and tumultuous history in diving, linked more often than not to military triumphs. Aristotle writes of Alexander the Great using a diving bell at the siege of Tyre in 332 B.C. In peacetime, it was used as early as 1531 to raise the *Caligua*, sunk in the Lake of Nemi. In this recovery, Demarchi was able to stay underwater for 1 full hour. Sir Edmund Halley (1656 to 1742), astronomer of comet fame, dived in the Thames River for 1 hour in a barrel to a depth of 60 feet. He could stay underwater for the full hour because he used two barrels, one to observe from and the other to deliver fresh air to the diver at depth. (A brilliant young scientist, he was appointed to the Royal Society. Halley actually paid the cost of the publication of Sir Isaac Newton's famous *Principia*.[2])

It was not until 1662 that a British physician named Henshaw made a "domicilium," a chamber in which he used high pressure for acute diseases and low pressure for chronic diseases. This, of course, preceded Priestley's discovery of oxygen in 1775. However, Paul Bert is considered the "father of pressure physiology." Born in 1833 to well-to-do parents, he worked on such subjects as nitrous oxide/oxygen anesthesia under pressure, oxygen toxicity, and plant growth under pressure. His classic work, *La Pression Barometrique* is still considered the cornerstone of hyperbaric medicine. In the United States, HBO therapy began in Philadelphia, then "progressed" to Cunningham's Hotel, a five-story treatment facility built in Kansas City in 1928. Cunningham's rationale for the diseases he treated, such as hypertension, diabetes, and cancer, was based on his belief that these diseases had anaerobic origins. Despite attacks from the American Medical Association, Cunningham proceeded with construction. The "Hotel" eventually failed and was demolished. It was not until 1960 that HBO received a more scientific beginning, with its use in treating gas gangrene and supporting life without blood in anemic patients.[3]

Monoplace chambers were used for clinical therapy only after 1960. The first real clinical use of monoplace chambers was in radiation therapy. It had been demon-

TABLE 14-1. **Pressure Conversion Table**

The units of pressure preferred for manuscripts submitted to *Undersea Biomedical Research* are the pascal (Pa = Newton × meter^{-2}), kilopascal (kPa), or megapascal (MPa), defined by the International System of Units (SI). If the nature of the subject matter makes it appropriate to use non-SI units, such as fsw, msw, atm, or bar, a parenthetical conversion to pascals, kilopascals, or megapascals should accompany the first mention of a pressure value in the abstract and in the text.

Atmospheres absolute is a modified unit of pressure due to the appendage "absolute"; the symbol "atm abs" is preferred over "ATA" for the modified unit.

1 atm = 1.013247 bar	1 atm = 33.08 fsw	1 atm = 10.13 msw
1 atm = 101.3247 kPa	1 bar = 32.646 fsw†, §	1 bar = 10.00 msw
1 atm = 14.6959 psi	1 fsw = 3.063 kPa	1 msw = 10.000 kPa‡, §
1 atm = 760.000 mmHg*	1 fsw = 22.98 mmHg	1 msw = 1.450 psi
1 bar = 100.000 kPa	1 psi = 2.251 fsw	1 msw = 75.01 mmHg
1 bar = 100,000 Pa*		
1 bar = 14.50377 psi		
1 bar = 750.064 mmHg		
1 MPa = 10.000 bar		
1 psi = 6,894.76 Pa*		
1 psi = 51.7151 mmHg		
1 torr = 133.322 Pa*		

* Signifies a primary definition (1) from which the other equalities were derived.
† Primary definition for fsw; assumes a density for seawater of 1.02480 at 4°C (the value often used for depth gauge calibration).
‡ Primary definition for msw: assumes a density for seawater of 1.01972 at 4°C.
§ These primary definitions for fsw and msw are arbitrary because the pressure below a column of seawater depends on the density of the water, which varies from point to point in the ocean. These two definitions are consistent with each other if a density correction is applied. Units of fsw and msw should not be used to express partial pressures and should not be used when the nature of the subject matter requires precise evaluation of pressure; in these cases investigators should carefully ascertain how their pressure-measuring devices are calibrated in terms of a reliable standard, and pressures should be reported in pascals, kilopascals, or megapascals.
(From Standard Practice for Use of the International System of Units (SI). Document E380-89a, American Society for Testing and Materials. Philadelphia, PA, 1989; with permission.)

strated that some tissue was more radiosensitive under pressure; therefore, radiation therapy was delivered through acrylic hyperbaric chambers.

PHYSICS AND PHYSIOLOGY

As its name implies, HBO therapy is based on the principle of increased pressure and its effect on human physiologic function. The weight of a column of air, reaching from sea level to the outer reaches of space, constitutes the barometric pressure at sea level. Hyperbaric pressure is an extension of that sea level pressure, with 100% oxygen or air under pressure in the HBO chamber. In normal practice, when we view a pressure gauge we read its base pressure as zero. However, if we are to be accurate in our calculations we must use *absolute pressure*, which includes atmospheric pressure *and* the pressure read on the gauge. Because average atmospheric pressure is equal to 14.7 psi, to compute absolute pressure we add 14.7 psi to the pressure measured by a gauge (psig). For each additional one atmosphere increase, we add an additional 14.7 psi. Three atmospheres are equivalent to 44.1 psia or 29.4 psig (Table 14–2).

To explain the physics and physiologic principles involved in hyperbaric medicine we liken it to diving beneath the sea. The analogy of going beneath the sea is accurate even if we remain in a dry environment, such as a hyperbaric chamber. Progressing through a simulated "dive," we separate the treatment into three processes: the pressurization, the changes at pressure, and the depressurization. The pertinent physics and physiologic principles at each stage of the "dive" are described for clarity. The treatment from the perspective of the patient and what he or she will experience is discussed.

Pressurization

The patient begins the treatment by entering the hyperbaric chamber (with their attendant if in a multiplace chamber) and the door is closed. Gas added to this closed environment increases pressure. As the gas enters, noise is created from the turbulent motion of gas rushing into the chamber. Noise levels greater than 90

TABLE 14-2. **Pressure Equivalents (in feet of sea water [fsw])**

0 fsw	= 0 psig	= 14.7 psia	= 1 atm abs
33 fsw	= 14.7 psig	= 29.4 psia	= 2 atm abs
66 fsw	= 29.4 psig	= 44.1 psia	= 3 atm abs
99 fsw	= 44.1 psig	= 58.8 psia	= 4 atm abs
132 fsw	= 58.8 psig	= 73.5 psia	= 5 atm abs
165 fsw	= 73.5 psig	= 88.2 psia	= 6 atm abs

dB can be measured. Protection is provided by muffling the gas as it enters and by wearing ear protection devices. As gas rushes into the chamber, the addition of gas molecules into this closed space creates heat from the Joule-Thomson effect, or friction of molecules colliding. This heat buildup can be uncomfortable to the patient during compression. Slowing the rate of compression and increasing the amount of ventilation provided can make the temperature more comfortable for the patient. Once the pressure reaches about 8 to 10 feet of sea water (fsw), the pressure differential in any air-filled space in the body can cause barotrauma. The airspaces in the body, such as the lungs, sinuses, middle ears, and even teeth (if improperly filled) must all be pressurized at the same pressure or pain will result.

According to Boyle's law, if the temperature is held constant, the volume will vary inversely with the pressure. This means that if pressure surrounding the patient is doubled, the volume in any air space will be halved. This is the reason all body air spaces must communicate to the body surface for equilibration in HBO therapy. The middle ear communicates to the surrounding atmosphere by the eustachian tube. This flattened tube acts as a valve, requiring maneuvers such as a Valsalva (pinch nose and force air into middle ear), Frenzel (close mouth, nose, and glottis using tongue against roof of mouth to compress air into middle ear), Toynbee (swallowing with mouth and nose closed), or a yawn and swallow are used to open the eustachian tube and allow ambient pressure behind the tympanic membrane.

If pressure is not equalized, the eardrum will be flexed inward to try to fill the space with a volume to equalize the pressure, causing pain. Failure to equalize pressure can result in a rupture of the eardrum if pressurization is continued without equilibration. Unconscious patients who do not have the ability to communicate their discomfort on pressurization should receive myringotomies or have pressure equalization tubes placed to prevent eardrum tear. The same pressure effect applies to sinuses, lungs, or air spaces attached to the body (such as a tooth with a filling that has an air pocket beneath it). Failure to equalize pressure in these spaces can cause pain and damage from the body's attempt to reduce the volume by filling the space with body fluids.

As an example, if a diver swims down under water holding his breath, as he approaches 33 fsw (2 atm abs) lung volume will halve. Should he continue his pressurization to pressures greater than 132 fsw still holding his breath, the lung is compressed to one fifth its total volume, or roughly residual volume. Once residual volume is exceeded, pulmonary edema fluids will try to fill the lung. This sets a theoretical pressure limit to breath-holding dives; however, some divers can exceed this limit because of their increased total lung capacity to residual volume ratio (TLC:RV).

Additionally, all apparatus entering a hyperbaric chamber should be considered sources of potential danger, for the same pressure-volume principles apply. These might include sphygmomanometer cuffs, intravenous (IV) bottles (use only IV solutions in plastic bags), IV drip chambers, endotracheal tube cuffs, nasogastric tube cuffs, arterial line pressure bags, ventilation circuits, vials, syringes, medicine bottles, or any device with a closed air space.

Other interesting phenomena that occur at increased pressure relate to increased gas density. For example, sound travels faster in a dense medium: therefore the voice changes as pressure increases and breathing becomes more labored. Under extreme pressure of thousands of fsw, mitosis stops because cytokinesis cannot occur. In addition, cilia does not regenerate; red cells change shape; the peripheral platelet count decreases; and lactic acid increases, causing a rightward shift of the oxyhemoglobin dissociation curve.

At Pressure

At increased pressure, oxygen partial pressure is increased. This increased oxygen partial pressure will suppress the action of the carotid and aortic bodies; suppress respiratory sensitivity to carbon dioxide; decrease the "alveolar splinting effect" played by nitrogen; and vasoconstrict blood vessels, thereby decreasing blood flow to the brain, coronary arteries, and eyes, causing bradycardia. Once hemoglobin is fully saturated, the only increase in oxygen content that can occur is that of dissolved oxygen. Under *hyperbaric* conditions 2 mL of oxygen is added to each deciliter of blood (mL/dL) in a linear fashion, for each atmosphere of compression. Breathing 100% oxygen at 2.8 atm abs (60 fsw) a PaO_2 of 2059 mmHg or 6.4 mL/dL of physically dissolved oxygen will occur. In *carbon monoxide intoxication*, this physically dissolved oxygen can sustain life until the carbon monoxide unloads from the hemoglobin.

Oxygen under pressure is not without hazards. Like any drug, oxygen can be toxic at increased concentrations. Oxygen under pressure can be toxic in two ways by affecting the pulmonary system and the brain.

Pulmonary oxygen toxicity, known as the Lorrain-Smith effect, is caused by oxygen at concentrations greater than 40% for extended periods. HBO therapy patients are exposed to high-concentration oxygen therapy for short intervals on a daily basis: this exposure is dose-related and cumulative. Patients are observed on a daily basis for progressive symptoms, such as tickling cough, symptoms of carinal irritation and burning, uncontrollable cough, dyspnea, decreased tidal volume, tracheobronchitis, or atelectasis. Even attendants working in the hyperbaric chamber should be aware of the potential for diminishing vital capacity, (5% to 10% after 4.5 hours at 2 atm abs), diffusing capacity, compliance (15% after 6 hours at 2 atm abs), PaO_2 during exercise, and widening of $P(A\text{-}a)O_2$ (after 6 hours at 2 atm abs). Most symptoms return to normal after 12 hours at normobaric pressures. No treatment is required other than removal from the high-concentration oxygen environment.

Cerebral oxygen toxicity, known as the Paul Bert effect, is encountered any time 100% oxygen is breathed at pressures greater than 2 atm abs. Cerebral oxygen toxicity is dose related; therefore, as pressure increases, the time to onset of symptoms becomes shorter. Because the therapeutic effect of hyperbaric medicine is from high oxygen partial pressure and because most therapy schedules in multiplace chambers go to 2 to 3 atm abs, a solution for this problem is necessary. The solution is to use an oxygen/air-breathing schedule that allows the patient to breathe air every 20 minutes, so called "air breaks" (Fig. 14-1). After a 5-minute air-breathing period, another oxygen breathing cycle of 20 minutes is conducted. Any sign that the patient is becoming toxic is a signal to switch the patient from oxygen to air. Symptoms of cerebral oxygen toxicity include nausea, eye twitch, excitation, rigid tonic phase, unconsciousness, clonic contractions, amnesia, hiccups, headache, aphasia, weakness, and eventually grand mal seizure. To prevent oxygen toxicity, one should maintain body temperature, normal metabolic state, and decrease work. Treatment is not necessary, as symptoms cease as soon as the hyperbaric oxygen therapy is discontinued by removing the oxygen mask.

On occasion a patient is taken to pressures equivalent to 165 fsw. At this pressure, because of the toxic effects of oxygen, alternative gas mixtures such as air, nitrogen-oxygen (nitrox), or helium-oxygen (heliox) are breathed. These gas mixtures each create their own unique problems. The mixtures used most are air and nitrox (50/50). By Dalton's law, each gas exerts its own pressure proportional to the percentage of the total gas that it represents. In air, nitrogen exerts 80% of the partial pressure and in nitrox 50%.

This "inert" gas is not so inert at extreme pressures. In his book *The Silent World,* Cousteau popularized the term "l'ivresse des grandes profondres" or "rapture of the deep" to describe the narcotic effect of nitrogen at great pressures. According to the Meyer Overton hypothesis, this anesthetic effect of nitrogen, or any inert gas, is because narcotic potency is equal to the solubility of the agent in lipids. The inert gas gains access to the nervous system by virtue of lipid solubility. There is some evidence that carbon dioxide retention potentiates the onset of nitrogen narcosis. Varying the inert gas can occasionally reduce the potential for narcosis; however, complications of decompression can result from indiscriminate alteration of the inert gases. The effects of nitrogen or inert gas narcosis require only one circulation of blood through the system to affect the patient because of the vascular nature of the central nervous system. The greatest effects are noted within 2 minutes of reaching pressure and any detrimental symptoms will be no worse after 30 minutes. Symptoms

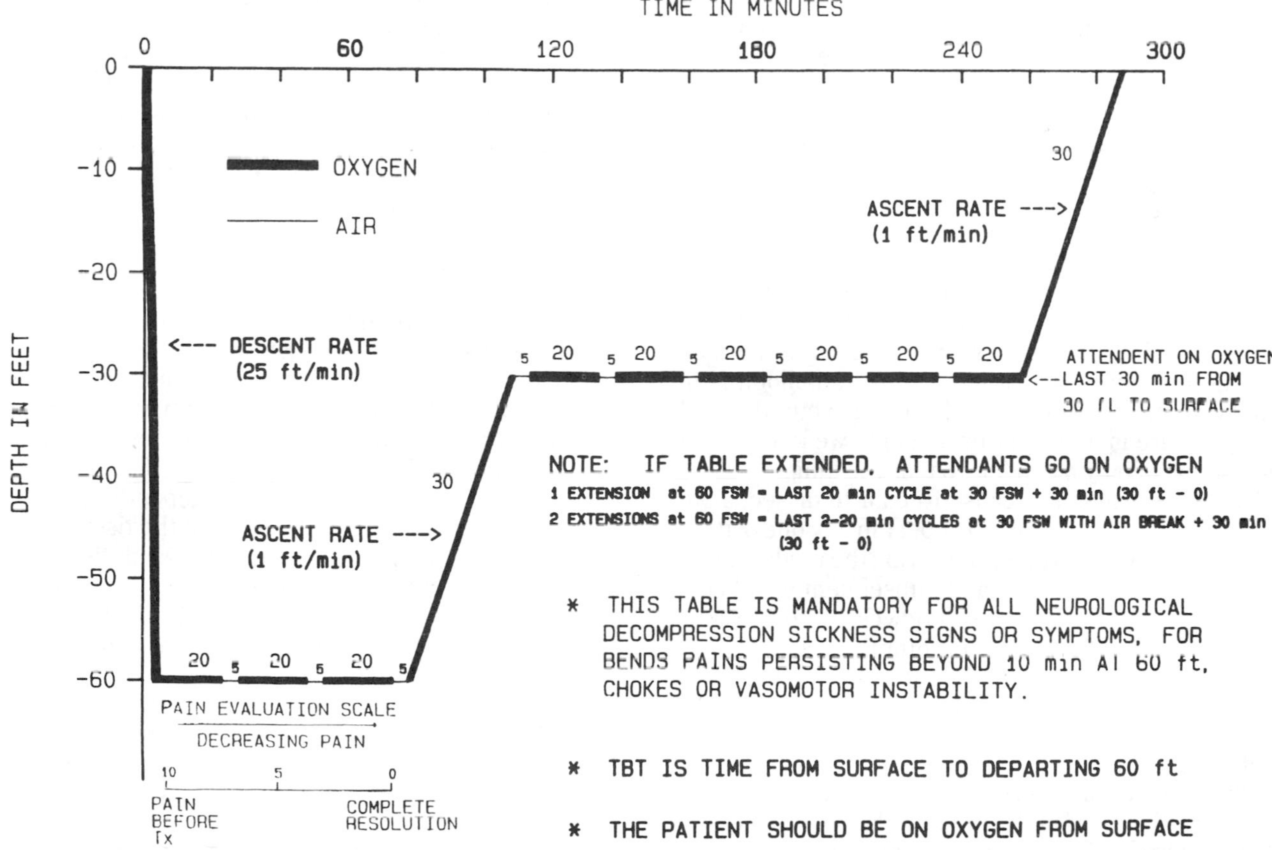

FIGURE 14-1. U.S. Navy Treatment Table 7. Time is indicated on X axis and pressure on Y axis. Oxygen breathing periods are represented by bold lines on X axis while air is represented by thin lines.

of inert gas narcosis include euphoria, a false sense of well-being, and paranoia.

Reasoning ability is affected the most, followed closely by a decrease in reaction time. The least affected ability is mechanical dexterity and motor skills. Emotionally stable individuals are better able to cope with nitrogen narcosis and once given a task, can carry it out. However, if the task should change, the individual is not able to think it through to a new solution.

This is why medical decisions should be made outside the chamber. Mistakes are easily made at hyperbaric pressure under the influence of nitrogen narcosis, and in fact, this may be an additive factor along with anxiety, fatigue, rapid pressurization, and carbon dioxide retention. Training for multiplace chamber attendants must include a deep dive to determine their ability to work at pressure. Recovery from symptoms is rapid and there are no ill effects.

Depressurization

The depressurization phase of a dive is the most dangerous part of the treatment. The patient is cautioned to breathe normally, and depressurization is carried out in a slow, controlled manner. Deviation from this can cause tragedy. As Boyle's law affects volume on pressurization, so also does it affect depressurization. If the patient has breathed compressed air in a hyperbaric oxygen environment, volume will increase at lesser atmospheres. Should the patient hold his or her breath, lock his or her glottis, have laryngospasm, or panic in any way during a rapid uncontrolled depressurization, there is a possibility of overdistending or stretching the lung until it tears. This is most acute as the patient nears the surface (atmospheric pressure), because this is the zone of greatest pressure change.

Depressurization of only 1 foot, while holding the breath, will increase the pressure in the lungs by 31 cmH_2O and its volume by 1/33. If volume expansion is allowed to inflate the lung without any splinting, the lung will tear. Think of a balloon held between the hands while inflating it. Pressure can get very high before the balloon bursts; however, if the balloon is inflated without being held, it will expand to bursting with little pressure in it. From this analogy, we know that it takes a rise of only 4 to 8 fsw to tear the lung.

A tear in the lung can cause free air to dissect along connective tissue lines and to appear in any one of three places: the pleura as a pneumothorax; the mediastinum, as a pneumomediastinum and subsequently, subcutaneous emphysema; or in the blood vessels to appear as arterial gas embolism. A pneumothorax will present as chest pain or dyspnea, or both. Should a pneumothorax occur at pressure in the multiplace chamber, pressure is increased in the chamber until the patient can breathe easily. The patient is placed on the affected side until a surgeon can insert a chest tube. In a multiplace chamber, treatment of the pneumothorax is necessary before depressurization can continue. Treatment of a pneumothorax that develops inside a monoplace chamber necessitates removal of the patient from the chamber. The chest tube is placed as soon as the patient is depressurized. The chest tube is attached to a one-way Heimlich valve to prevent air entry into the thorax when monoplace chamber therapy is resumed.

When air enters the mediastinum or subcutaneous tissue in the neck area, the symptoms will be crepitus, chest pain, difficulty swallowing, change in voice, or a combination thereof. Treatment is usually not necessary. However, the patient should be closely watched for a potential air embolism, which can often accompany this phenomenon.

On the other hand, when air gets into a blood vessel in the form of an *arterial gas embolism*, it is a true medical emergency that is treated immediately with compression to 165 fsw to shrink the bubble size. Immediate diagnosis and action are essential to survival. The first thing to be done for the patient is to place him or her flat; this will hopefully keep bubbles from rising to the brain. Symptoms of an arterial gas embolism include tunnel vision, acute loss of consciousness, respiratory distress, seizure, paralysis, convulsion, or death by coronary or cerebral occlusion. More objective signs that may be seen include air bubbles in retinal vessels, pallor of the tongue, marbling of skin, hemoptysis, focal or generalized convulsions, and neurologic abnormalities. Treatment by recompression (see Fig. 14-1) will usually reverse symptoms if treatment is immediate; any delay in beginning therapy reduces the chance of complete recovery.

Decompression illness is usually not a risk for patients undergoing HBO therapy because of the oxygen inhaled. The possibility of decompression illness occurs when one breathes an inert gas for an extended period at increased pressure. Attendants who accompany the patients in multiplace chambers are at risk because they breathe air during their pressure exposure.

According to Henry's Law, the solubility of gas in a liquid at a given temperature is proportional to the partial pressure of the gas above the solution. This defines only the relative quantity of gas entering solution, not the absolute amount in physical solution. The absolute amount of dissolved gas is determined by a solubility coefficient that varies with the gas. At increased pressures, tissues will receive increasing amounts of gas in an attempt to equilibrate with the gas tension in the blood owing to diffusion of gas from high to low. The equilibration takes a finite period, depending on the pressure differential and vascularity of the tissue.

Thus, when the patient is decompressed, tissue gas tensions will increase as ambient pressure is decreased if blood flow is not adequate to carry it off. The tissue pressure gradient increases to a point at which an excessive gas tension is created and gas (usually nitrogen) will come out of solution and cause a bubble. This is similar to opening a carbonated beverage quickly. The bubbles formed in this manner will press on nerve endings and cause symptoms known as *decompression illness* or "bends." Symptoms are graded into systems depending on the location of the bubble (Box 14-2).

First aid for decompression illness is to provide oxygen and fluids and to position the victim as though for

BOX 14-2

SYMPTOMS OF DECOMPRESSION ILLNESS

Skeletal: Bubbles in joints
Neurologic
Spinal cord: Paresthesia, paralysis, balance problems, incontinence, seizures, visual disturbances, headache
Brain: Unconsciousness, paralysis, visual disturbances
Lung: Dyspnea, substernal pain, nonproductive cough, cyanosis (called "chokes")
Vestibular: Bubbles in inner ear

arterial gas embolism, because the neurologic symptoms of one are indistinguishable from those of the other, and precautions must be taken against the potential for arterial gas embolism. Treatment is prompt recompression and then decompression according to prescribed treatment tables (see Fig. 14-1). Response to treatment in the hyperbaric chamber is subjective; therefore it is not advisable for the patient to take any analgesics before arrival and during treatment. The ability to detect the symptoms can dictate the course of his or her therapy.

The proper use of decompression tables removes most, but not all, risks inherent in hyperbaric exposures. The variability in human physiology can add risk to the process of decompression. It is known that age, temperature, fitness, obesity, trauma, smoking, fatigue, drugs (such as alcohol), dehydration, and female gender can increase the risk of decompression illness. It is also known that previous episodes of decompression illness predispose the patient to developing it again. Therefore, prevention is the cornerstone of proper decompression practices. Close supervision of all hyperbaric chamber treatments must be done in a professional manner to avoid subjecting patients or attendants to decompression illness. Adjustments in decompression schedules must be made for the amount of work, temperature, and rate of depressurization.

Any of the foregoing complications can occur, and each must be explained to the patient for informed consent. However, with proper precautions, training, quality controls, and procedure standards, HBO therapy is a routine procedure.

CHAMBERS

Hyperbaric chambers are of two general types: multiplace (more than one occupant) or monoplace (single occupant). Multiplace chambers may have one or more compartments that are interconnected. The National Fire Protection Association (NFPA) classifies chambers as follows:[4]

Class A—Human, multiple occupancy
Class B—Human, single occupancy
Class C—Nonhuman

Chambers are constructed from steel or acrylic according to the American Society of Mechanical Engineers—Pressure Vessels for Human Occupancy (ASME-PVHO-1) standards.[5] The ASME certifies pressure vessels that are stationary, whereas the Department of Transportation (DOT) certifies pressure vessels that cross state lines. Each must be hydrostatically tested upon manufacture. The DOT vessels are tested every 5 years thereafter. The ASME vessels are identified by the method of manufacture and the fact that they have a drain valve installed on them.

As in any enclosed space in which oxygen or compressed air is introduced, fire safety is a primary consideration. If any electricity is delivered into the chamber it must have explosion-proof connectors and lighting. For the most part, electricity is not provided inside chambers. If it is, any electrical connection made inside the chamber must be completed before the chamber is compressed and not disconnected during the treatment. Electrical and mechanical penetrations can be made for both multiplace and monoplace chambers, so that monitoring can be provided. Pressure transducers must be vented and calibrated before the door is closed.

Multiplace Chambers

Multiplace chambers (Fig. 14-2) are pressure vessels that may have more than one compartment, although not always (Fig. 14-3), which allow personnel to enter and leave the main treatment compartment at will. A multiplace chamber is large enough to accommodate one or more patients, plus an attendant. It has an additional compartment attached that serves as a lock through which additional personnel or supplies are compressed to the pressure of the patient. Hyperbaric chambers are used in the commercial diving industry as well as in medical industry. The major difference is the mode of use; most commercial diving chambers are closed-circuit systems (the chamber is sealed and only metabolic oxygen is added to the chamber as needed, while a CO_2 scrubber removes the CO_2). On the other hand, medical chambers are generally used as open-circuit systems (air ventilating the chamber is exhausted from the chamber).

Monoplace Chambers

Monoplace chambers (Fig. 14-4) resemble the "iron lungs" of yesteryear, which accommodate only one patient at a time. They have no additional compartment or direct access to the patient under pressure. However, with careful forethought and special devices, critical patients are treated in monoplace chambers, and one can monitor anything that can be monitored in a multiplace chamber. Because of the ease of installation, ease of operation, smaller space requirements, and expense considerations, use of monoplace chambers has proliferated.

Monoplace chambers are simple to operate and quite comfortable for the patient, unless he or she has confinement anxiety. The rate of pressurization and de-

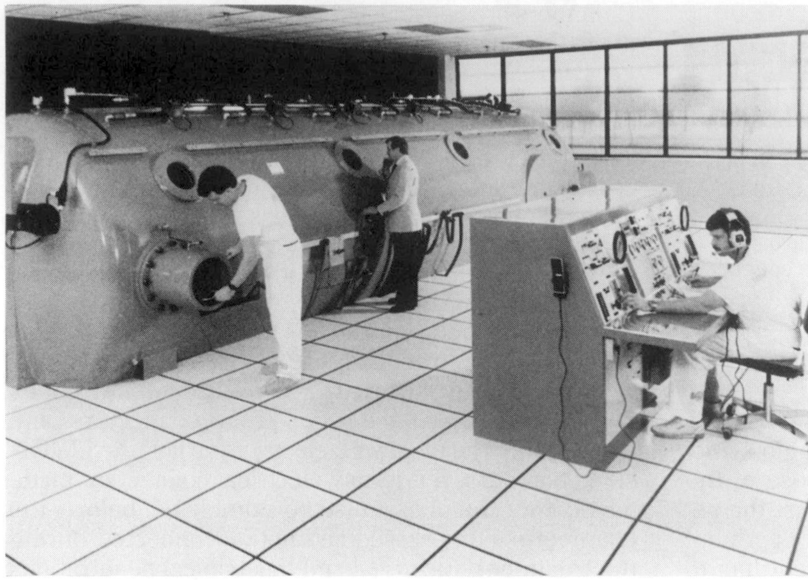

FIGURE 14-2. Photograph of a multiplace chamber.

pressurization is controlled and the patient is completely visible during operation. This allows the patient to see his or her surroundings, and in routine care, the patient can watch television, listen to the radio, and such. No electrical or battery-operated devices can be used inside a monoplace chamber. However, cables penetrating the chamber can measure ECG, temperature, respiration, pressure, and any other parameter that needs to be monitored. Transcutaneous oxygen should not be measured, because of the electrical voltage carried to the measurement site by the sensing electrode. The patient is grounded to the gurney, and all jewelry must be removed to avoid scratching the acrylic hull.

In a monoplace chamber a one-way valve is placed into the intravenous system as it enters the hull of the chamber to prevent exsanguination, and special pumps and high-pressure tubing are used. Should the patient need defibrillation, the patient is removed completely from the chamber and quickly moved to an area away from the chamber. All the patient's clothing is removed before placing the paddles and defibrillating the patient. In the event of seizure or cardiac arrest, the patient is vented to the surface by the emergency depressurization valve (button).

Chamber Systems

Materials, connecting piping, portholes, and electrical and support equipment must also meet the standards of ASME-PVHO-1, as well as NFPA 99, Compressed Gas Association (CGA)[6] (air purity), American National Standards Institute (ANSI), United States Coast Guard (USCG), Occupational Safety and Hazard Association (OSHA), and Joint Commission of Accreditation of Health Organizations (JCAHO) (Pending).

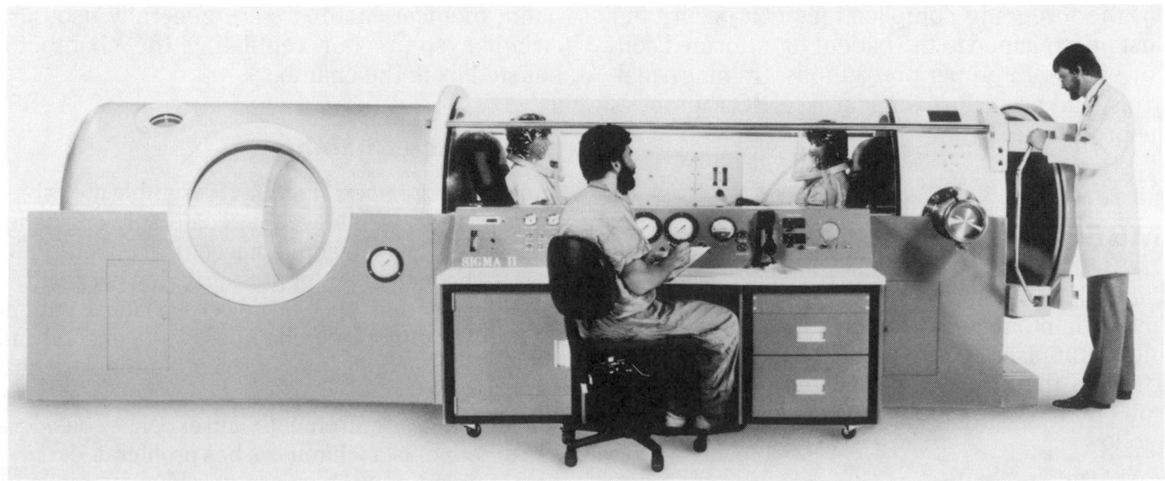

FIGURE 14-3. Photograph of a hybrid chamber.

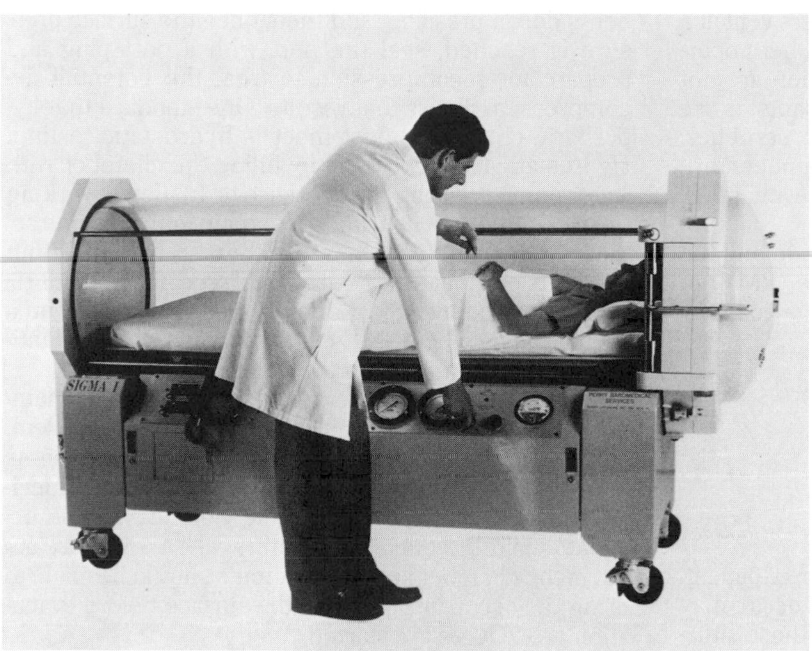

FIGURE 14-4. Photograph of a monoplace chamber.

CONSTRUCTION

The hyperbaric chamber is usually cylindrical, lying flat or on end, but it can be spherical. It must be constructed in accordance with the ASME-PVHO-1 Standards, grounded, and any pipe or fitting that attaches to the structure must be of compatible material. Metallic surfaces are painted with inorganic zinc or high-quality epoxy or an equivalent, which is flame-resistant, to prevent corrosion and deterioration. The multiplace chamber interior is fitted with bunks, a medical suction system, communication equipment, and breathing apparatus for all occupants.

An in-chamber ventilator is available for the patient who needs ventilation during HBO treatment.

Pressurization and Depressurization System

The pressurization-depressurization system encompasses ancillary equipment, such as the compressor system, receiver, and valves to pressurize or depressurize the chamber(s), which may consist of the main compartment, lock compartment, or medical lock in the multiplace system.

Breathing Gas System

The breathing apparatus delivers air, oxygen, or any gas mixture to the personnel inside the chamber. This system can also include compressors, booster pumps, cylinders, and oxygen administration systems such as flowmeters, masks, and hoods (see equipment section).

Fire Detection and Protection System

The fire detection-protection system is of prime importance. Only by always being on guard for fire can one avoid these catastrophic events. In the multiplace chamber, the fire system consists of a deluge system, fire detection system, fire hoses, and a pump to increase regular water pressure to that required by the increased pressure of the system. Manual backup systems are required for this essential system. Monoplace chambers do not usually have these fire suppression systems.

Electrical Systems

The electrical systems are for support services, outside the chamber. Electricity is usually not supplied inside; however, some chambers use explosion-proof connections and lights. Emergency electrical backup is required to maintain support during power failures; this may be as simple as a battery or as complex as the hospital emergency power-generating system.

Communication Systems

Communications must have open systems from inside to outside the chamber. To ensure that all conversations inside the chamber are heard, it must also have an emergency backup, even if this consists of a writing pad or previously agreed on set of hand signals.

Air-Conditioning Systems

Air-conditioning systems are required if a chamber is used in the saturation mode. Otherwise, a safe internal environment is maintained by periodic or continuous venting of the chamber (monoplace chambers vent at a rate of 200 to 400 L/min). Multiplace chambers operated in the closed-circuit mode for saturation are not vented. Oxygen consumed by the occupants is replaced, whereas CO_2 is absorbed with a CO_2 scrubber. In the open-circuit mode multiplace chambers are vented for high CO_2, high O_2 (multiplace chamber only), temperature, and comfort.

In an open-system chamber, carbon dioxide buildup is determined by the resting minute volume (RMV) of the occupants. The normal ventilation rate is given by the formula:

$$\text{Number of occupants} \times 12.5\ \text{ft}^3/\text{min}$$

SAFETY

Emergencies

Emergencies can involve the chamber system or patient. Virtually any medical emergency that can occur may happen inside a hyperbaric chamber. Only those situations unique to the hyperbaric chamber are discussed.

The most dreaded of all hyperbaric chamber emergencies is fire. In monoplace chambers, a fire is catastrophic; therefore, the only answer is prevention. Three factors must be present to cause a fire; burnable materials, proper oxygen concentration, and an ignition source. In hyperbaric chambers, especially the monoplace chamber, the oxygen concentration is high enough to cause just about any material to burn. Therefore, all burnable materials and ignition sources are removed. Close attention must be paid to all clothing that personnel wear inside the chamber (cotton or fire-retardant cloth, no nylon), dressings containing petroleum-based lubricants, and battery-operated or electrical systems inside unless they are contained in a unit that is nitrogen purged. The oxygen breathing systems must be scavenged to the outside.

In multiplace chambers, oxygen concentration is maintained at minimal levels to reduce the fire hazards by venting the chamber at regular intervals to maintain oxygen levels below 23.5% referenced to the surface. The NFPA 99 addresses hyperbaric chamber environments in Chapter 19 in that document and sets standards to avoid fire.

Because of these standards, personnel have survived multiplace fires in recent years. Fire burn is not the only hazard in multiplace chamber fires. The most acute hazard is inhalation of toxic fumes. Therefore, the procedure for a fire in a multiplace chamber would have the inside attendant first put a full face mask supplying air on himself or herself and then care for the patient. After that is accomplished, the sprinkler system is tripped or a hose is used. The outside operator may trip the sprinkler system, while the inside attendant is putting on the mask, and then turn off the oxygen supply. Halon 301 fire-extinguishing gas can also be used, as it does not harm chamber personnel.

Another feared accident in the multiplace chamber is an explosive decompression. The proper procedure here is to remain far away from the port while the chamber is decompressing, and then, once the surface pressure is reached, seal the port with a port plug and prepare for recompression to treat the potential decompression illness that results. One standard that hyperbaric chambers must meet is hydrostatic testing. Hydrostatic testing is done by filling the chamber with water and increasing the pressure to 1.5 times working pressure, then measuring the expansion and contraction of the chamber. The vessel must return to within 10% of its original size. Unlike DOT-certified cylinders, those certified by ASME do not have to be tested on a regular basis. The ASME-certified cylinders are identified by the drain valve on their ventral side.

A fire that occurs in the area surrounding the chamber while occupants are inside is also a critical problem. Codes require that sprinklers be installed in rooms housing hyperbaric chambers. However, difficult decisions must be made about the safety of the chamber occupants and the outside operators when a fire breaks out in the chamber area. All attempts should be made to bring the occupants safely to the surface before evacuation procedures are started.

Gas purity can also be a problem. If chamber air becomes fouled, a separate free-standing backup air-breathing system can be used, which is also always available for fires.

Occupational Safety

Occupational safety considerations are necessary to assure the health and safety of chamber personnel. Such workers are at risk for decompression illness and occupational accidents due to the difficult positioning while carrying patients through small hatches, lifting patients to cots when normal bed-transfer mechanisms do not work, high sound levels, infections related to high humidity in enclosed spaces, ear problems, and various hazards from devices that can explode or implode (eg, the LifePac portable defibrillator implodes at 100 fsw).

EQUIPMENT

Monoplace chambers are compressed with oxygen; therefore, the patient breathes chamber oxygen, unencumbered by any breathing device throughout the therapy period,unless ventilatory support is required. Multiplace chambers, on the other hand, are compressed with air; therefore, the patient must always breathe through some respiratory device to receive the therapeutic effect of oxygen.

In the multiplace chamber, the patient receives 100% oxygen delivered by a tightly fitting demand-valve oxygen mask, special hood, T-tube, or ventilator. Each of these devices must scavenge the exhaled gas and exhaust it outside the chamber to maintain low levels of oxygen concentration in the chamber environment. Aviator masks with demand-valve attached for inhalation and exhalation are the best type of oxygen delivery systems for patients who can tolerate them. There are two types of hoods, which can be more comfortable for patients with orofacial complications: one is taped to the chest, the other has a closure around the neck. Each has an inlet and outlet. The inlet is baffled for deflection of incoming gas; the outlet has holes in the adapter to protect against the scavenging system grabbing the patient's cheek.

Gas to the patient can be cooled by putting the delivery hose through an ice bucket or by placing ice in the nebulizer. Patients with tracheostomies, endotracheal tubes, and laryngectomies function well with a T-tube setup. However, the attendant must remember the effect of pressure changes on the cuff. Ventilators should be volume cycled,[7] and supplied pressure should be 50 psi above ambient. Exhaled gas must be scavenged to the outside of the chamber. Other respiratory devices used are a full face mask and gas mixture breathing devices.

Other equipment used inside multiplace hyperbaric chambers include diagnostic equipment such as stethoscopes, blood pressure cuffs, safety pins, reflex hammers, and monitoring equipment such as ECG and pressure recorders. Emergency equipment must be available inside the chamber or close by, including special trays for thoracentesis, minor procedures, vascular cut-downs, thoracotomies, chest tubes, lumbar punctures, tracheostomies, and cardiovascular procedures.

HYPERBARIC OXYGEN THERAPY

HBO therapy is used for primary and adjunctive care (Table 14-1). It is used as a primary mode of therapy in diving accidents (decompression illness and arterial gas embolism) because of the mechanical effect of bubble reduction from the increased pressure and, secondarily, for the therapeutic effects of hyperoxygenation. Hyperoxygenation increases the inert gas gradient for off gassing and repair of ischemic tissue. Tissues off-gas at a rate of 5 mL/sec, whereas the cardiac system off-gases at a rate of 1 mL/sec in the hyperbaric environment.

The rationale for the high-pressure oxygen used in hyperbaric oxygen is multifaceted. In *carbon monoxide intoxication* and *smoke inhalation*, the dissolved oxygen corrects cellular hypoxia while carbon monoxide is bound to hemoglobin, speeds carbon monoxide elimination, and thereby reduces cerebral and intercranial pressure. In *gas gangrene*, the high concentrations of oxygen shut down α toxin production and in high enough doses (1500 mmHg), are bacteriocidal. In *wound healing*, repair will not occur if the PO_2 is less than 30 mmHg. Therefore, oxygen enhances fibroblastic proliferation, improves collagen synthesis, and improves capillary budding in avascular areas. In *osteomyelitis* and *osteoradionecrosis*, oxygen stimulates osteogenesis and fibroblastic activity, as well as increases collagen production and neovascularization. In addition, oxygen affects microorganisms present by augmenting antibiotic action and improving phagocytic killing.

In *crush injuries* of the extremities, HBO therapy is used to produce vasoconstriction and is helpful in treating the edema associated with the injury. Tissue oxygenation is maintained and, indeed, improved by this technique, despite the vasoconstriction so induced.

TREATMENT PROTOCOLS

Each disease has a recommended therapy schedule that uses oxygen most effectively. In the multiplace chamber, the patient receives high-concentration oxygen through a demand-valve mask, hood, or T-tube. In monoplace chambers, the patient breathes the ambient chamber environment. Therefore, multiplace and monoplace chambers each have their own set of treatment schedules. Monoplace chambers use lower pressure without air-breathing cycles, for shorter duration, whereas multiplace chambers use higher pressure, with air-breathing cycles interspersed to reduce the oxygen toxicity potential. The disease entity being treated dictates the pressure, duration, and number of treatments. Most treatment schedules are empirical; however, many have a long history of success.

Special gas mixtures can be used for the treatment of patients with decompression illness or arterial gas embolism. This may even lead to a saturation treatment, in which the occupants of the chamber remain at the increased pressure long enough to bring their inert breathing-gas mixtures into equilibrium with the tissue. This might take many hours; however, it takes longer to surface from the decompression of a saturation treatment (usually 7 to 10 days). If a saturation treatment is performed, the logistics become extensive. At increased pressure, nitrogen is added to the system to decrease the oxygen tension to near atmospheric levels; otherwise the attendant inside the chamber will experience oxygen toxicity symptoms and will have significant decreases in vital capacity for extended periods.

Clinical Practice Guidelines, per se, have not been written for the field of hyperbaric medicine. However, Utilization Review Criteria are established for each of the disease modalities sanctioned by the Hyperbaric Oxygen Therapy Committee.[1] With these criteria, protocols may be developed in the field of hyperbaric medicine. An example of this would be HBO therapy for decompression sickness. The Utilization Review section of the Hyperbaric Oxygen Therapy Committee Report states: "The number and depth of treatments and the exposure times will vary depending on: 1) The elapsed interval between the onset of symptoms and the presentation for recompression care. 2) The confidence of the treating clinician as to the appropriate protocol to be applied. 3) Residual symptoms after the initial recompression. The treatment depths range between 60 and 165 feet of sea water (fsw) for time frames between 1.5 and 14 or more hours. Depending on the patient's initial response, there may be repetitive treatments. Patients should be treated until clinical examination reveals no further improvements in response to the HBO treatments."[1] A sample Therapist-Driven Protocol is presented (Table 14-3). Although the major decision-making must be by the hyperbaric physician, the therapist/technologist is often called on to give substantial input.

(text continues on page 418)

TABLE 14-3. **Hyperbaric Oxygen Therapy Protocol**

St. Joseph's Hospital
Wound & Hyperbaric Center
Tampa, FL

PROTOCOL

Decompression Sickness Treatment

Purpose: The certified hyperbaric technologist (CHT) will utilize the following protocol to provide the most efficient and effective care in initiating, evaluating, and eventual termination of recompression therapy.

Patient Type: Patients ordered to receive recompression therapy for decompression sickness.

Clinical Area: Hyperbaric facility.

Equipment Needed:
1. Evaluation form
2. Treatment algorithm
3. Treatment table

Laboratory Data Needed: Chest radiograph ECG for patients over 40 years of age

Overview: Flowchart diagram (see addendum A & B)

Protocol: The following guidelines will be followed when decompression sickness is suspected.

I. The following guidelines will be followed in determining the indications for recompression therapy.
   A. Patient assessment
      1. Neurologic examination
      2. Subjective pain level
      3. Risk factors
         a. age
         b. sex
         c. alcohol
         d. smoking
   B. Patient dive profile
      1. Decompression schedule for all dives on day of incident
      2. History of previous dives for last week
      3. Use of decompression tables or decompression computer
      4. Temperature of water
      5. Relative work performed

II. Upon receiving an order for treatment, the CHT will:
   A. Review patient's chart for all pertinent information including:
      1. Physician's order
      2. Patient history and physical examination
      3. Physician's progress note
      4. Vital signs sheet
      5. Nursing notes
      6. Laboratory data
      7. Diagnostic reports (eg, radiographs)
   B. Perform a physical assessment:
      1. General observations: color, pattern, and effort of breathing, chest expansion (symmetrical and bilateral).
      2. Neurologic observations: level of paralysis, strength, level of consciousness, and ability to ambulate.
      3. Auscultation: using the stethoscope, the CHT will listen and note quality of breath sounds, I:E ratio, and presence or absence of adventitious breath sounds in all lung fields, both anteriorly and posteriorly.
   C. Upon completion of the chart review and physical assessment, the CHT will orient the patient to hyperbaric oxygen therapy for the patient and have the patient sign an informed consent for therapy.

III. The following will determine the therapy protocol(s) to be followed (see diagram).
   A. Indications for decompression sickness protocol will include:
      1. Treatment with U.S. Navy Diving Manual Treatment Table 6
   B. Indications for arterial gas embolism protocol will include:
      1. Treatment with U.S. Navy Diving Manual Treatment Table 6A

Guidelines and Warning: Barotrauma may occur on compression and decompression of patient, observe for:
   A. Inability to equalize middle ear space, sinuses, and any air space attached to the patient
   B. Patient holding breath during decompression

Clinical Responsibilities:

I. The following will be adhered to in all decompression sickness patients at all times:
   A. Changes in patient condition must be communicated and coordinated with the hyperbaric physician at all times.
   B. Appropriate documentation should be placed in the patient chart in accordance with departmental policy.

Related Protocols:
   A. Air embolism
   B. Include forms and normal values
      1. Treatment tables
      2. Treatment algorithm

(Adapted from Kettering Medical Center Mechanical Ventilation Protocol; with permission.)

(continued)

TABLE 14-3. (Continued)

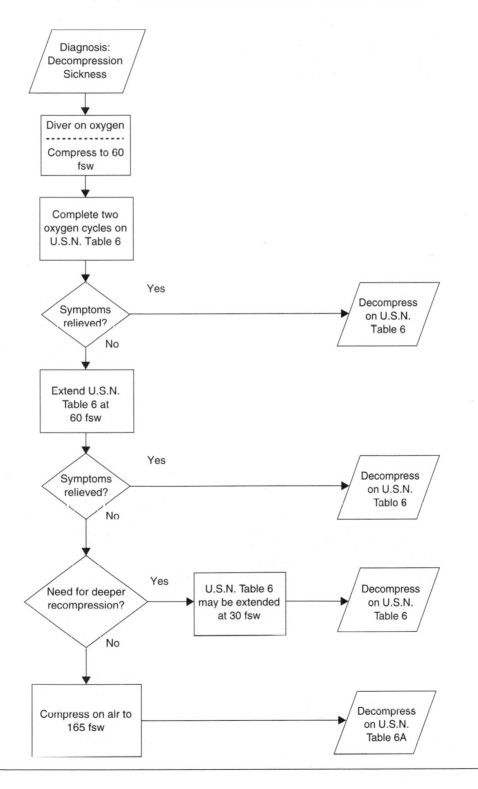

Addendum A

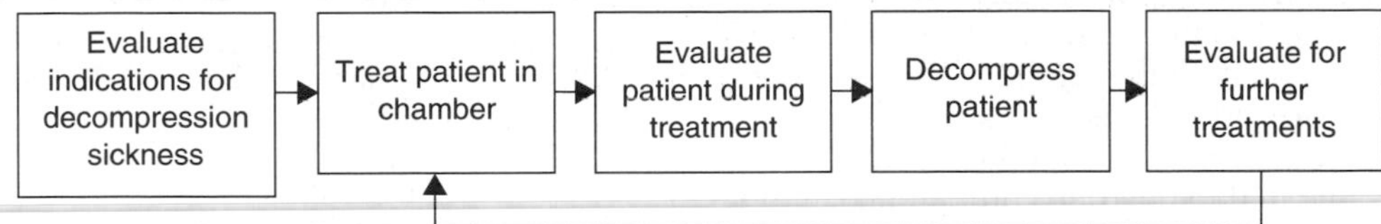

Addendum B

Diagnosis: Decompression Sickness

Diver on oxygen

Compress to 60 fsw

Complete two oxygen cycles on U.S.N. Table 6

Symptoms relieved?

Yes

Decompress on U.S.N. Table 6

No

Extend U.S.N. Table 6 at 60 fsw

Symptoms relieved?

Yes

Decompress on U.S.N. Tablo 6

No

Need for deeper recompression?

Yes

U.S.N. Table 6 may be extended at 30 fsw

Decompress on U.S.N. Table 6

No

Compress on air to 165 fsw

Decompress on U.S.N. Table 6A

STAFFING

A hyperbaric facility must be operated under the medical direction of a physician, preferably one who has hyperbaric medicine training and is interested in its growth and development. Staff members who function as chamber operators, attendants, and supervisors can be from many diverse areas of the medical community. They should be able to demonstrate competence in the technical aspects of HBO therapy, and they must maintain their skills through regularly scheduled training programs. A minimum number of personnel required to be in attendance should be defined for each treatment facility. For multiplace chambers a physician, operator, attendant, and supervisor should be the minimum. However, crew size can vary with condition of the patient. Additional personnel are helpful to serve as time keepers, recordkeepers, and messengers as cases warrant. These personnel can be on call until they are needed.

Nursing Care

Many aspects of hyperbaric nursing care are unique. We only consider these aspects in this section; it is not our intent to teach nursing practice.

Patients treated inside a hyperbaric chamber can be healthy young adults who have just made a mistake diving and now have "the bends," or they can be badly traumatized patients who will require the constant supervision of a critical care nurse, respiratory therapist, and physician inside the chamber with them. Alternately, they may be prepared and placed inside a monoplace chamber in which they are isolated until they reach the surface again. Any one of these patients, at any time, can have a crisis that requires extraordinary measures at a moment's notice.

Although there may be many relative contraindications to HBO therapy (Box 14-3) the only **absolute contraindication** is that of an untreated pneumothorax. It is important for the personnel treating these patients to be ever vigilant and prepared. The first treatment requires special instructions and patient preparation, including the removal of petroleum-based cosmetics and dressings, watches, nylon clothing, jewelry, burnable materials, devices that cause sparks, or any devices that trap air. All patients should sign an informed consent form concerning the potential hazards of HBO treatments, and attempts should be made to reduce their anxiety levels. The patient is then reinstructed on how to clear his or her ears. He or she should be told of the expected temperature changes (hot on pressurization, cold on depressurization), noise, and pressure changes and how to deal with them. Any untoward noises (such as venting, cylinder movement, or alarms) that might occur during the treatment should be announced to the patient before they occur. During changes in pressure, the attendant must change the air volume in all air-filled spaces such as endotracheal tubes, urinary bladder tubes, and gastric tubes. In monoplace chambers these balloons are filled with saline so that pressure changes do not affect them.

BOX 14-3

RELATIVE CONTRAINDICATIONS FOR COMPRESSION

1. Upper respiratory infection
2. Chronic obstructive pulmonary disease
3. Seizure disorder
4. Thoracic surgery
5. Spontaneous pneumothorax
6. Emphysema with CO_2 retention
7. Viral infection
8. Congenital spherocytosis
9. History of optic neuritis
10. History of spontaneous pneumothorax
11. Uncontrolled high fever
12. Chronic sinusitis
13. Pregnancy (?)
14. Medical history:
    - Epilepsy
    - Asthma
    - Prior decompression illness or other dive accident
    - Pneumothorax (untreated pneumothorax is only absolute contraindication)
    - Exercise wheezing
    - Heart attack
    - Diabetes
    - Problems with equalizing ear pressure

The attendant in a multiplace chamber should assure a good mask fit on the patient throughout the treatment and should be proficient in administering a neurologic examination. Talking should be minimized during therapy to assure proper oxygen concentration. On depressurization, air passages should be rechecked for patency.

In the hyperbaric environment, patient care is no different from that at the surface, except that access to assistance and equipment is limited. Only a few situations pose special problems inside the chamber; a little forethought can lessen these.

A quick depressurization to the surface can jeopardize the health of a normally healthy attendant working inside a multiplace chamber. Before any decision is made to bring occupants to the surface, all alternative methods should be considered and a decompression schedule should be carefully calculated.

SUMMARY

HBO therapy administered in either monoplace or multiplace chambers is a technical modality appropriate for the respiratory care practitioner's armamentarium. Although controlled studies of the efficacy of HBO therapy are still in progress, education in the physics and physiology of hyperbaric medicine should be basic to the field of respiratory care. The role of the respiratory care practitioner in the field of hyperbaric medicine should be firmly established in the basic tenants of quality patient care established by the Undersea and Hyperbaric Medical Society.

REFERENCES

1. Hyperbaric Oxygen Therapy: A committee report. Undersea and Hyperbaric Society, Kensington, MD, 1992
2. Jacobson JH, Morsch JHC, Randell-Baker L: The historical perspective of hyperbaric therapy. Ann N Y Acad Sci 117:651, 1991
3. Boerama I, Hoogendy KL: Treatment of clostridial infections with hyperbaric oxygen drenching: A report on 26 cases. Lancet 1:235–238, 1963
4. Standards for Health Care Facilities: NFPA 99 National Fire Protection Association, Quincy, MA, 1993
5. Safety Standards for Pressure Vessels for Human Occupancy: American Society of Mechanical Engineers, New York, 1993
6. Compressed Air for Human Respiration: Pamphlet G-7, Compresses Gas Association, New York, 1989
7. Blanch PB, Desautels DA, Gallagher TJ: Deviations in function of mechanical ventilators during hyperbaric compression. Respir Care 36:803–814, 1991
8. Burton GG, Tiersort JA (eds): Therapist-Driven Respiratory Care Protocols (TDP): A Practitioner's Guide. Los Angeles, Academy Medical Systems, 1993

BIBLIOGRAPHY

Bennett PB: The Aetiology of Compressed Air Intoxication and Inert Gas Narcosis. Pergamon Press, 1966

Bennett PB, Elliott DH (eds): The Physiology and Medicine of Diving and Compressed Air Work. New York, Williams and Wilkins, 1969

Bennett PB, Elliott DH (eds): The Physiology and Medicine of Diving and Compressed Air Work. London, Bailliere Tindall, 1975

Bert P: Barometric Pressure. Republished, Bethesda, MD, UHMS, 1978

Boycott AE, Damant GC, Haldane JS: The prevention of decompressed-air illness. J Hyg 8: 342, 1908

Brown JW, Cox B (eds): Proceedings of the Third International Conference on Hyperbaric Medicine. New York, National Academy of Sciences, 1966

Burton GG, Tietsort JA (eds): Therapist Driven Respiratory Care Protocols (TDP): A Practitioners Guide. Los Angeles, Academy Medical Systems, 1993

Cannan RK: Fundamentals of Hyperbaric Medicine. New York, National Academy of Sciences, 1966

Cousteau JY, Dumas F: The Silent World. New York, Harper and Row, 1953

Davis R: Deep Diving and Submarine Operations. London, Siebe Gorman, 1955

Davis JC (ed): Hyperbaric and Undersea Medicine. San Antonio, Medical Seminars, 1981

Davis JC (ed): Medical Examination of Sport Divers. San Antonio, Medical Seminars, 1986

Davis JC (ed): Treatment of Serious Decompression and Arterial Gas Embolism. 20th Undersea Medical Society Workshop, Duke University January, 11–14, 1979. Bethesda, MD, UHMS, 1979

Davis JC, Hunt TK: Hyperbaric and Undersea Medicine. Bethesda, MD, UHMS, 1977

Davis JC, Hunt TK (eds): Hyperbaric Oxygen Therapy. Bethesda, MD, UHMS, 1977

Davis JC, Hunt TK (eds): Problem Wounds: The Role of Oxygen. New York, Elsevier, 1988

Empleton BE, Lanphier EH, Young JE, Goff LG (eds): The New Science of Skin and SCUBA Diving. New York, Association Press, 1974

Freeman P, Edmonds C: Inner ear barotrauma. Arch Otolaryngol 95:556, 1972

Goff LG (ed): Underwater Physiology Symposium—First. New York, National Academy of Sciences, 1955

Hills BA: Decompression Illness: The Biophysical Basis of Prevention and Treatment. New York, Wiley and Sons, 1977

Hyperbaric Oxygen Therapy: A Committee Report. Kensington, MD, Undersea and Hyperbaric Medical Society, 1992

Lambertsen CJ (ed): Underwater Physiology, 3rd Symposium. New York, Williams and Wilkins, 1967

Lambertsen CJ (ed): Underwater Physiology V. Bethesda, MD, Publication Press, 1976

Lambertsen CJ, Greenbaum LJ (ed): Second Symposium on Underwater Physiology. New York, National Academy of Sciences, 1963

Miles S: Underwater Medicine. Philadelphia, JB Lippincott, 1962

Myers RAM (ed): Hyperbaric Oxygen Therapy: A Committee Report. Bethesda, MD, UHMS, 1986

NOAA Diving Manual: Diving for Science and Technology. Washington, DC, U.S. Government Printing Office, 1991

Safety Standards for Pressure Vessels for Human Occupancy. ASME, New York, 1988

Standards for Hyperbaric Facilities. NFPA-99, Boston, 1987

Standards for Hyperbaric Facilities intended for use in Medical Application. CGA, New York, 1966

U.S. Navy Diving Manual. NAVSHIPS 0994-001-9010, U.S. Government Printing Office, Washington, DC, Sept. 1973

15 Humidity and Aerosol Therapy

Jeffrey J. Ward
Dean Hess
H.F. Helmholz, Jr.

CLINICAL SKILLS

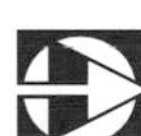

Upon completion of this chapter, the reader will be able to:

- Review patient records that may reveal history of secretion retention, bronchospasm, airway edema, or bacterial infection
- Assess the patient's need for humidity or aerosol therapy by inspection, auscultation, or interview
- Review the appropriateness of orders for humidity and aerosol therapy
- Select, assemble, and check humidifiers (bubble, pass-over, and cascade wick humidifiers and heat and moisture exchangers), aerosol generators (pneumatic and ultrasonic), and aerosolized medication administration systems (small-volume nebulizers, metered-dose inhalers, dry-powder inhalers, and aerosol [mist] tents) for proper function and cleanliness
- Explain therapy to patient and maintain records
- Provide adequate humidification to achieve maintenance of a patent airway
- Facilitate removal of bronchopulmonary secretions by use of aerosol therapy
- Modify therapeutic approach by changing one or more of the following: equipment, dilution of medication, temperature of aerosol or humidifier, patient breathing pattern, or aerosol output
- Recommend changes in aerosol drug dosage
- Recommend use of pharmacologic agents deliverable by means of aerosol: bronchodilators, vasoconstrictors, corticosteroids, antiasthma drugs (eg, cromolyn sodium), or antimicrobial agents

KEY TERMS

Absolute humidity
Aerosol
Bland aerosols
Body humidity
Boiling point
Breath-activated metered-dose inhaler
Cascade humidifier
Chlorofluorocarbons (CFC)
Critical pressure
Critical temperature
Dalton's law
Dead-space volume
Dew point
Diskhaler
Diskus inhaler
Dry-powder inhalers (DPI)
Freon
Goblet cells and submucosal glands
Gravitational sedimentation
Heat and moisture exchanger (HME)
Heat of vaporization
Heterodisperse and monodisperse
Humidity deficit
Hygroscopic property
Inertial impaction
Isothermic saturation boundary
Large-volume nebulizers
Mass median aerodynamic diameter (MMAD)
Metered-dose inhalers (MDI)
Pass-over humidifier
Pseudostratified ciliated columnar epithelium
Relative humidity
Rotahaler
Servo controlled (heat)
Small-volume nebulizers (SVN)
Small-particle aerosol generator (SPAG)
Specific heat
Spinhaler
Thermistor
Turbuhaler
Ultrasonic nebulizers (USN)
Vapor
Water vapor capacity
Wick humidifier

This chapter focuses on the clinical use of humidity and aerosols and briefly reviews related equipment. A background in science and technology is provided to allow the reader to better match therapeutic devices to patients' needs. In the past, there was a lack of a scientific basis for some forms of humidity and aerosol therapy. However, recent research has better defined the indications, limitations, and assessments to guide care and selection of therapy. Consensus conferences and clinical practice guidelines (CPGs) summarize current information to base therapy on a scientific approach and target future research.[1–6]

Humidification of inspired gases and application of bland mists are part of current respiratory care procedures. Medical gases for use in therapy and mechanical ventilation require humidification. Hydration of pulmonary secretions commonly precedes bronchial hygiene and volume-expansion therapy. Administration of aerosolized medications to airways or lung parenchyma is a primary medical treatment. The list of drugs that can be effectively delivered to the respiratory system continues to expand.

ANATOMY AND PHYSIOLOGY OF THE MUCOCILIARY SYSTEM

The airways of the respiratory system provide passage of gases to and from the alveoli. The upper airways (nasal, oral, pharyngeal, and bronchial) condition the inspired gas by warming and adding water in vapor, or molecular, form. Under normal room conditions, approximately one-sixth of the average adult daily heat output is required to condition inspiratory air. Inspired gas is usually 100% saturated with water vapor at 37°C by the time it reaches the tracheal carina. Mucosal surfaces also provide a complex system for clearing the airways of solids and substances that have dissolved in airway secretions.

The embryologic origin of the lungs is the primitive foregut. The airway-lining cells are epithelial and have some secretory function. These cells line the nasal passages to the terminal bronchioles (Fig. 15-1*A*,*B*). The cell type is *pseudostratified ciliated columnar epithelium,* attached to a basement membrane (Fig. 15-2). Within the alveolated respiratory bronchioles, the cells' shape changes to cuboidal. Each ciliated cell has approximately 200 *cilia.* These 6-μm long hairlike projections beat synchronously at about 1000 to 2000 strokes per minute to propel the mucous layer at 10 to 15 mm/min, from the terminal airways toward the pharynx (Fig. 15-3). The beating cilia are synchronized in a metachronal, wavelike fashion, similar to the "wave" cheer of fans at a sports stadium.

Bronchial secretions are produced by the *goblet cells* of the columnar epithelium and *glands* in the bronchial submucosa. Goblet cells lie in a 1:5 ratio among ciliated cells. In sustained states of irritation, such as chronic bronchitis and cystic fibrosis, increased numbers of submucosal glands and goblet cells develop. The glands have mucous- and serous-secreting cells and a network of tubules and ducts. They are innervated by parasympathetic branches of the autonomic nervous system, and they are affected by parasympathetic blocking agents (eg, atropine) that reduce secretions and by vagal stimulation that increases activity. Normally, secretion of mucus from all sites amounts to approximately 60 to 90 mL/day. The exact anatomical source of each layer is unclear.[7,8]

There are many pathologic conditions and environmental situations that cause disruption of the normal mucociliary transport system (Table 15-1). Inhaled substances, congenital disorders, and pathologic conditions can interfere with normal ciliary function. Awareness of such problems provides a rational basis for selecting candidates for humidity and aerosol therapy.[9–12]

Sputum (secretion from the lower respiratory tract) is a heterogeneous, proteinaceous material consisting mainly of glycoproteins and mucopolysaccharides, or mucins. The substance forms long, interconnected, fibrous molecules in a gel. Both viscous and elastic components of sputum can be modified by factors such as intermolecular charge and by the presence of other products such as DNA from polymorphonuclear neutrophils. Eosinophilic leukocyte breakdown results in cellular material in the form of Charcot-Leyden crystals and Curschmann's spirals. When desiccated, such material can lead to partial obstruction or complete mucous plugging. Airway epithelial ion transport plays a role in regulation of secretions. In cystic fibrosis, the genetic mutation in the CF transmembrane regulator protein (CFTR) alters chloride secretion and sodium absorption. The result is thick mucus that is difficult to clear, and recent therapy is targeted to correct the airway electrolyte imbalance.[13]

The Lucas-Douglas model of in vivo sputum proposes a two-layer system. The less viscous portion, next to the airway wall, is termed the sol layer; above that is the gel layer. Apparently, the tips of the cilia just touch the gel layer, which is propelled cephalad. During conditions of significant dehydration or when the normal physiologic "air-conditioning" system is bypassed, the lack of adequate humidity can lead to drying and disruption of the sol-gel system. In addition, cellular components and differing electrolyte concentrations can alter the viscosity and function of this protective system.[12] The temperature and moisture levels needed to preserve normal ciliary activity has been the focus of considerable research. A review of the background physics facilitates further discussion on these clinical aspects.

PHYSICAL PRINCIPLES OF HUMIDIFICATION

Temperature is the key factor in determining capacity of a gas to hold water vapor. Molecules of a substance are theoretically motionless (ie, there is no kinetic activity) at absolute zero on the Kelvin scale (or −273°K on the Celsius [centigrade] scale) (Table 15-2 gives a temperature conversion chart). *Critical temperature* is defined as the energy level of a substance above which the molecules can exist only as a gas. At or below the critical temperature, substances can be liquefied by compression. Above the critical temperature, additional compression cannot liquefy a gas.

Critical pressure is the vapor pressure of a substance at its critical temperature. It is the pressure required to liquefy a gas at its critical temperature, or that which is exerted by a liquid at its critical temperature. Box 15-1 provides a clinical example of the concept of critical temperature and pressure.

The *boiling point* of a substance is that temperature at which the escaping tendency of the molecules (kinetic energy) equals the confining pressure of 1 atmosphere. At boiling point, the substance changes completely to a gas (boils), although heat must be added. The boiling temperature rises when the total pressure rises, and it falls when the total pressure decreases.

Vapor pressure is the pressure at which a liquid boils at any given temperature; all liquid becomes a gas. A *vapor* is the molecular form of a substance below its boiling temperature, dispersed in a true gas (eg, water in molecular form in air). Vapor is present only if a true gas is also present. At a specific temperature, the vapor pressure of a liquid designates the escaping tendency of those molecules to produce an equal pressure of vapor in a gas phase, at equilibrium. Whenever ambient pressure is equal to or below a substance's vapor pressure, it boils, producing a gas.

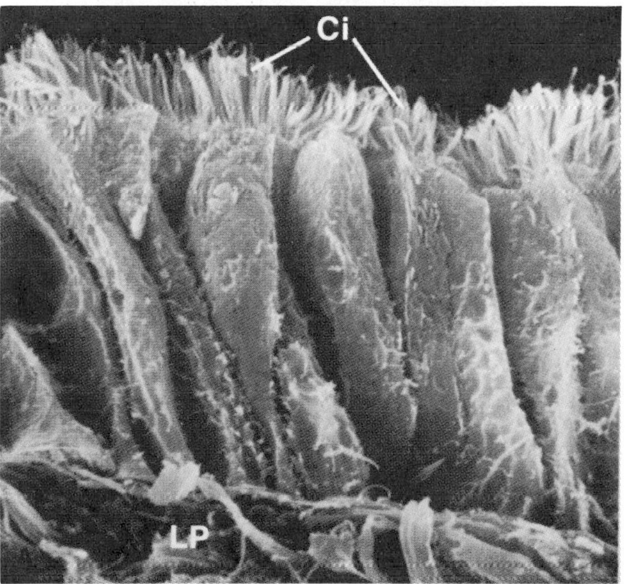

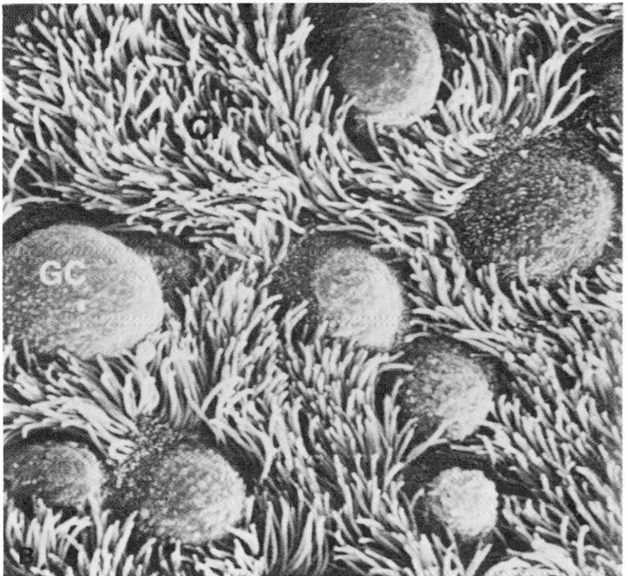

FIGURE 15-1. Scanning electron micrographs of the bronchial epithelium **(A)** Cross-sectional view: columnar epithelial cells with cilia (Ci) and lamina propria (LP). **(B)** Lower-power view from above: ciliated cells interspersed with goblet cells (Gc). (Kessel RG, Karoon RH: Tissues and Organs. A Text–Atlas of Scanning Electron Microscopy, p. 210. San Francisco, WH Freeman & Co, 1979. Reproduced with permission.)

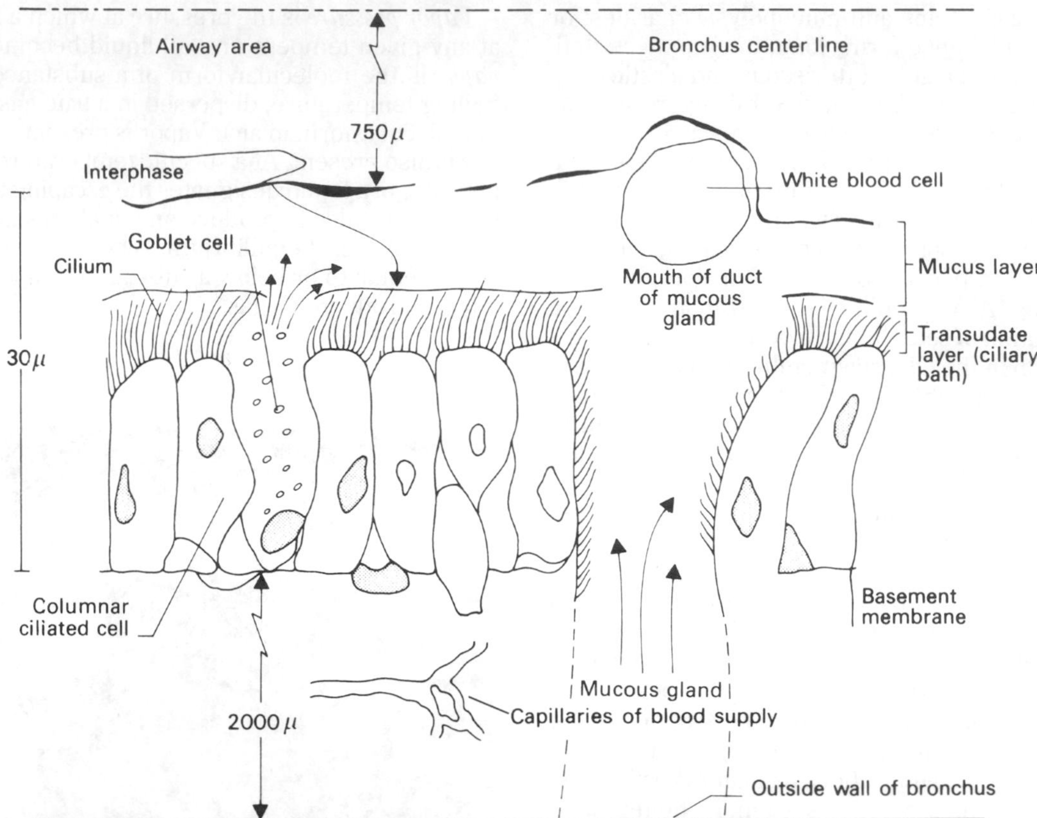

FIGURE 15-2. Drawing of surface of typical ciliated epithelium. (Adapted from Denton R, Hwang SH, Litt M: Chemical engineering aspects of obstructive lung disease. Chem Eng Progr 62:12, 1966. Reproduced with permission.)

Water vapor pressure designates the partial pressure effect exerted by water vapor in a gas sample. The pressures are presented in Table 15-2. Of note is the vapor pressure level at body temperature (37° C, 310° K), which is 47 mmHg (or 6.27 kPa). Because water vapor is not a true gas, when the partial pressure of humid gases are calculated, the water vapor pressure (PH_2O) must be subtracted from the barometric pressure before it is multiplied by the fraction of gas in a sample. *Dalton's law* describes the relationship of partial pressures of gases in a composite sample, with each gas exerting a partial pressure proportional to its concentration in the sample (FIO_2), and is dependent on the total barometric pressure (P_B). Water vapor can be thought of as a "contaminant," or nongas, yet it exerts a real pressure (PH_2O). Partial pressure of "moist" inspired oxygen is expressed as

$$(PIO_2) = (PB - PH_2O)\ FIO_2$$

Equation Box 15-1 provides an example of the calculation of the inspired oxygen pressure.

Humidity is the term used to describe water vapor in environmental gases. *Absolute humidity* refers to the mass (weight) of water vapor in a given volume of gas. The most common unit for this measurement in respiratory care is milligrams of water in 1 L of a gas-vapor mixture (mg/L). Temperature determines the amount of water that can be "held" in a volume of gas and the vapor pressure created. Gas containing this maximum is defined as *saturated.* Table 15-2 indicates these amounts and vapor pressures in saturated gas for a range of temperatures. Figure 15-4 depicts the same data in graphic form and identifies *body humidity,* or the content or partial pressure of saturated gas at normal body temperature. Box 15-2 reviews the calculation of body humidity.

Relative humidity is used to describe the actual content of water vapor compared with the potential amount that could be held, at the same temperature and at equi-

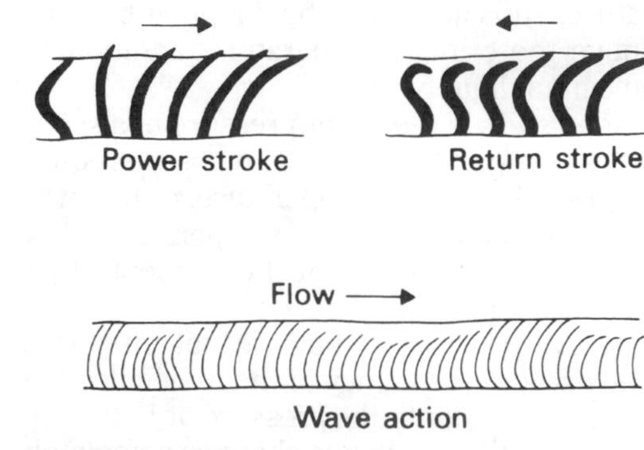

FIGURE 15-3. Drawing of cilium at each phase of beat cycle (metachronal movement). (Adapted from Denton R, Hwang SH, Litt M: Chemical engineering aspects of obstructive lung disease. Chem Eng Progr 62:12, 1966. Reproduced with permission.)

TABLE 15-1 **Factors That Affect Mucociliary Transport**

- Disorders that produce excessive or abnormal mucus
  - Cystic fibrosis
  - Acute and chronic bronchitis
  - Pneumonias (fungal, bacterial, and viral)
  - Bronchiectasis
  - Asthma
  - Airway burns
  - Pulmonary neoplasm (alveolar cell cancer)
- Disorders and causes of abnormal ciliary function
  - Dehydration
  - Chronic alcohol or other depressant drug intake
  - Aspirin and other prostaglandin inhibitors
  - Tobacco smoke
  - Trauma or defoliation (eg, tracheal suctioning)
  - Pulmonary oxygen toxicity
  - Nitrous oxide and sulfur dioxide
  - Local and general inhalational anesthetics

librium. This ratio is usually expressed as a percentage. Equation Box 15-2 describes the calculation of relative humidity.

Water vapor capacity is often used to describe the absolute humidity of a gas sample when saturated at a given temperature. This term would be consistent with maximum water content levels at specific temperatures (see Table 15-2).

Dew point defines the temperature to which a gas-vapor mixture must be cooled before "dew" condenses on the vessel containing the sample (ie, the temperature at which the content provides full saturation). High humidity levels correlate with higher dew-point temperatures. Accordingly, with high ambient humidity, condensation occurs more rapidly on an iced beverage glass than on one at room temperature. By looking at Table 15-2, one can see that if the dew point occurs at 37°C, the sample is maximally saturated and has a water content of 43.9 mg/L and a vapor pressure (PH_2O) of 47 mmHg.

Body humidity is a variant of relative humidity, but the temperature is specified as that of the patient (or assumed to be 37°C) and with full water saturation of the sample. Similar to relative humidity, it is expressed as the ratio (percentage) of absolute humidity and capacity at body temperature (normally 43.9 mg/L); therefore, it is 100% relative humidity at body conditions. Equation Box 15-3 describes an example of the calculation of body humidity.

Humidity deficit, as used for respiratory care, describes the condition of insufficient water to provide 100% body humidity (or to any other specified level). One can speak of a humidity deficit of any gas sample taken into the body that is not saturated at body temperature, even though it is saturated at a lower temperature. In theory, it is an index of how much water the mucosal surfaces of the upper airway must contribute to the inspired gas. Equation Box 15-4 continues the calculation, using data from the previous example.

Heat capacity, or *specific heat,* is that amount of heat energy required to raise a unit weight of a substance 1°C. The specific heat of water (commonly measured in calories per gram per degree Celsius [cal × g^{-1} × C^{-1}]) is considered to be 1.0.

The *heat of vaporization* is the heat energy required to change a unit mass of liquid to a gas at the same temperature. Figure 15-5 plots total calories added versus absolute temperature. From point *A* to *B,* a solid is

TABLE 15-2 **Relation of Temperature to Water Content and Vapor Pressure (in saturated gas)**

Temperature		Content		Vapor Pressure	
°C	*°F*	*mg/L*	*mmol/L*	*mmHg*	*kPa*
0	32	4.85	0.2694	4.58	0.6106
5	41	6.8	0.3777	6.54	0.8719
10	50	9.40	0.5222	9.20	1.2265
15	59	12.83	0.7127	12.79	1.7051
16	60.8	13.64	0.7578	13.62	1.8158
17	62.6	14.47	0.8039	14.51	1.9344
18	64.4	15.36	0.8534	15.46	2.0611
19	66.2	16.31	0.9061	16.45	2.1934
20	68.0	17.30	0.9611	17.51	2.3344
21	69.8	18.35	1.0194	18.62	2.4424
22	71.6	19.42	1.0789	19.79	2.6384
23	73.4	20.58	1.1433	21.02	2.8024
24	75.2	21.78	1.2100	22.32	2.9757
25	77.0	23.04	1.2800	23.69	3.1584
26	78.8	24.36	1.3533	25.13	3.3503
27	80.6	25.75	1.4305	26.65	3.5530
28	82.4	27.22	1.5122	28.25	3.7663
29	84.2	28.75	1.5972	29.94	3.9916
30	86.0	30.35	1.6861	31.71	4.2276
31	87.8	32.01	1.7783	33.58	4.4769
32	89.6	33.76	1.8755	35.53	4.7369
33	91.4	35.61	1.9783	37.59	5.0115
34	93.2	37.57	2.0872	39.75	5.2995
35	95.0	39.60	2.2000	42.02	5.6021
36	96.8	41.70	2.3167	44.40	5.9184
37	98.6	43.90	2.4389	46.90	6.2527
38	100.4	46.19	2.5611	49.51	6.6006
39	102.2	48.59	2.6994	52.26	6.9673
40	104.0	51.10	2.8389	55.13	7.3499
41	105.8	53.7	2.9833	58.14	7.7512
42	107.6	56.5	3.1500	61.30	8.1725
43	109.4	59.5	3.3056	64.59	8.6111
44	111.2	62.5	3.4722	68.05	9.0724
45	113.0	65.6	3.6444	71.66	9.5536
50	122.0	83.2	4.6222	92.30	12.3054
55	131.0	104.6	5.8111	117.85	15.7117
60	140.0	130.5	7.2500	149.19	19.8900
100	212.0	598.0	33.2222	760.0	101.3232
121	249.8	1156.0	64.2222	1530.0	203.9796*
374	705.2	400.0	22.2223	165,452.0	22,058.0†

* Autoclave conditions.
† Critical temperature.

BOX 15-1

EXAMPLE: CARBON DIOXIDE AND CRITICAL PRESSURE

Carbon dioxide has a critical temperature of 31.1°C (89.9°F, 304.1°K), with a corresponding critical pressure of 73 atmospheres (1071 psia). At temperatures above the critical temperature, CO_2 cannot be kept in liquid form regardless of pressure applied. Since that temperature is just above normal room temperature (eg, 21.5°C, 70.7°F, or 343.7°K), a compressed gas cylinder of CO_2 will contain a mixture of both liquid *and* gas. In clinical practice, the cylinder regulator's pressure gauge will read about 838 psig until all the liquid has vaporized. The gauge pressure will then rapidly drop as the remaining gas is used. Therefore, CO_2 cylinder contents must be regularly weighed to assess remaining contents.

heated to its melting point. Along *BC,* the solid is changed into a liquid. Line *CD* corresponds to the heating of a liquid to the boiling point. Along line *DE,* the liquid is changing to a gas at a constant temperature. The amount of heat needed to accomplish this is the heat of vaporization. At point *E,* only gas exists. Line *EF* corresponds to further gas heating. For water, it requires 539 calories to convert 1 g of water to 1 g of steam at 100°C (373°K). Water requires more heat in changing from liquid to vapor than does any other known substance.

The heat of vaporization is greater for water at temperatures below 100°C. The heat loss from the respiratory tract because of water evaporation is likewise significant at 579 cal/g H_2O. Under normal conditions, approximately 250 mL of water and 350 kcal of heat are lost from the lungs each day. Most of this heat loss is caused by heat of vaporization, not heating the air itself. No humidifier can produce 100% relative humidity at the temperature of the gas and water unless heat is also provided. The three major factors that influence this process are temperature, the area of contact between the water and gas, and the time allowed for gas-water contact. The rate at which an equilibrium (between vapor concentration and water) is approached depends on the amount of heat available. Equation Box 15-5 provides an example of heat needed in humidification.

EQUATION BOX 15-1

CALCULATION OF P_{IO_2}

The average barometric pressure is 760 mmHg (sea level). Water vapor exerts a pressure of 47 mmHg (normal body temperature). The fraction of oxygen in room air is 0.21. The following calculation illustrates the physical condition of gases after inspiration, being warmed and humidified by normal upper airways:

$$P_B = P_{H_2O} + P_{O_2} + P_{N_2}$$

$$760 = 47 + 149.73 + 563 \text{ (if no } CO_2 \text{ in inspired air)}$$

$$P_{IO_2} = (P_B - P_{H_2O})F_{IO_2}$$

$$P_{IO_2} = (760 - 47)0.21 = 149.73 \text{ mmHg (19.93 kPa)}$$

The *isothermic saturation boundary* (ISB) is a theoretical point in the airways at which inspired gases reach the 100% body humidity level. Some researchers specify this area to be just below the tracheal carina (assuming normal conditions).[14] Endotracheal intubation would shift the isothermic boundary deeper into the bronchial tree, as would inspiration of "bone-dry" medical gases through an endotracheal tube.[15] Above the ISB, the airway acts as a bidirectional heat and moisture exchanger facilitated by turbulent flow. Turbulence promotes rapid transfer of heat by convection.

RATIONALE FOR SUPPLEMENTAL HUMIDITY

Supplemental humidification is commonly indicated for patients when their natural airway is bypassed. This would apply to those breathing either spontaneously or by means of a mechanical ventilator. Patients receiving dry medical or anesthetic gases by facial mask or nasal appliance may require humidification depending on gas flow, humidity, and temperature of the ambient air, as well as minute ventilation. Mechanical ventilators are commonly equipped with humidifiers for anesthesia, ICU, or domiciliary use. (See Ch. 20, AARC Clinical Practice Guideline: Humidification During Mechanical Ventilation) Manufacturers have developed devices to humidify flows ranging from those needed for neonates to those for adults ventilated by high-frequency devices.

The respiratory tract can be used as a heat exchanger to allow active rewarming of hypothermic patients with heated and humidified systems. Patients with pathologic conditions of their mucociliary system or impaired cough may be helped with humidification. Box 15-3 summarizes indications for supplemental humidification.

The optimal humidification levels of heat and humidification for use with mechanical ventilators and other breathing systems (eg, high-flow CPAP system) have not been definitely determined for normal subjects. In the 1950s, Ingelsted found that the temperature in the subglottic space was normally between 32.2°C (inspiration) and 36.4°C (exhalation), with relative humidity for both at 98% to 99%.[16] Investigators have continued to work to determine the minimum humidity levels required in the airway,[14,17–19] and others have used electron microscopy to document the effect of overhydration on mucus and surfactant.[20] Besides consideration of the mucociliary function, prevention of crusting of mucus in the artificial airway is a concern.

Several organizations have published minimum standards for humidification during mechanical ventilation via an artificial airway.[1,21–24] Table 15-3 lists those recommendations identifying levels for the key variables; note that some groups specify only one condition. Temperature and absolute and relative humidity are interrelated; once any two of these three factors are set, the third is determined. Recent bench analysis of heated-wire humidifiers during mechanical ventilation demonstrated that inspissation of secretions can occur in spite

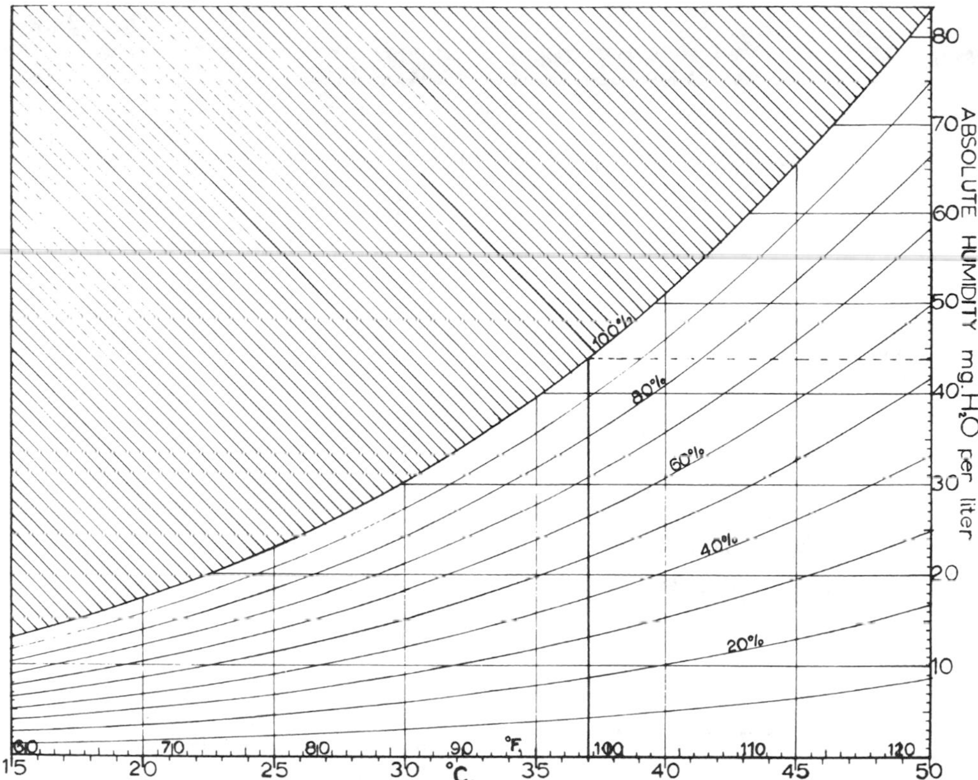

FIGURE 15-4. Nomogram demonstrating the water content of air over a range of temperatures. Temperature is displayed on the horizontal axis, water content (mg H_2O/L) on the vertical axis, and percentages of saturation as relative humidity on the curved isopleths. The bold vertical line arising from 98.6°F (37°C) identifies the water content at various levels of percentage (%) body humidity.

of meeting minimum absolute humidity standards. Miyao and co-workers noted that artificial airway occlusion occurred when absolute humidity was adequate but relative humidity was low because of the heated wire. Absolute humidity determines the total amount of humidity that needs to be added to the respiratory tract. Relative humidity determines where the water is added. Low relative humidity in inspired gas results in drawing water reserves from the proximal airway. In the intubated patient, this additional water is added at the level of the endotracheal tube. When humidification is inadequate, the result is crusting of secretions (with potential for occlusion) within tubes.[25] Apparently, adequate relative humidity is the dominant factor, and minimum criteria must be specified as part of standards. Box 15-4 summarizes humidification standards for clinicians and manufactures.[1,23,26]

It should be noted that the standard refers to the output at the humidifier, not at the patient entry point. Tubing that conducts gas to the patient is not always heated. This cooling decreases the temperature, lowers humidity levels, and causes condensation.

Humidity Added to Medical Gas: Applied to the Nose and Mouth

When completely dry medical gases are directed to the nose or nose and mouth, adding water can duplicate normal room air conditions (22°C at 50% relative humidity). This would include nasal oxygen masks, low-flow nasal cannulas, demand nasal cannulas, or oxygen enclosures (continuous high-flow oxygen cannulas may require a higher relative humidity). The moisture level of the room air is a major factor, as the patient significantly dilutes the oxygen with this environmental gas. Although an adequate level has not been defined for cannulas, some guidelines suggest that supplemental humidity not be required if the flows are 4 L/min or less.[27–29]

Gases directly entering the respiratory system at the oropharynx ideally should range from 29° to 32°C at

BOX 15-2

BODY HUMIDITY

Air we breathe at average "room" temperature (20°C or 293°K) has an absolute humidity of approximately 9 mg/L H_2O. This is less than the maximum 17.3 mg/L, as air is usually not maximally saturated, except during hot, humid weather. At body temperature (37°C or 310°K), air has an absolute humidity of 43.9 mg/L. The body's water content normally guarantees complete saturation of gas with water vapor in alveoli. **Under normal conditions, body humidity can be described as having the absolute humidity of 43.9 mg/L, which would provide vapor pressure of 47 mmHg (P_{H_2O}).**

EQUATION BOX 15-2

CALCULATION OF RELATIVE HUMIDITY

The room air described in the previous example, with an absolute humidity of 9 mg/L at 20°C (293°K), would then be compared with the content saturated at that temperature, or 17.3 mg/L (refer to Table 15-2).

$$\frac{\text{Water content in gas (measured)}}{\text{Water content in gas (capacity)}} \times 100 = \text{Relative humidity (\%)}$$

Note: Gas sample must be compared with capacity level at the same temperature.

$$\frac{9\ \text{mg/L}}{17.3\ \text{mg/L}} \times 100 = 52\%\ \text{Relative humidity (at 20°C)}$$

By algebraic manipulation, the content of a gas sample can be calculated, knowing the relative humidity and the capacity at that temperature (see Table 15-2).

$$\text{Water content} = \frac{\text{Water capacity} \times \text{relative humidity}}{100}$$

$$\frac{17.3\ \text{mg/L} \times 52}{100} = 9\ \text{mg/L}$$

EQUATION BOX 15-4

CALCULATION OF HUMIDITY DEFICIT

Example: The humidity deficit for each liter of gas with 9 mg/L or 21% body humidity is as follows:

Body "capacity"	43.9 mg/L
Ambient content	− 9.0 mg/L
Humidity deficit	**34.9 mg/L**

Another way of expressing humidity deficit is the percentage difference from 100% (from the previous example):

100%
− 21%
79% Humidity deficit

Humidity deficit can be extended to describe further situations. If the patient has a minute ventilation of 10 L/min, the total humidity deficit for 1 minute would be

34.9 mg/L
− 10 L/min
349.0 mg/min

If the subject continues to breathe for a 24-hour period, the total deficit would be

349 mg/min
× 1440 min/d
502,560 mg/d or 502.6 g/d

100% relative humidity. This applies to facial mask–type medical gas appliances, such as partial or nonrebreathing oxygen masks, in that the patient's own expired air humidifies incoming oxygen. The only exception is the Venturi mask. This device entrains most of the inspired gas from the room. The room ambient humidity is added to the dry medical gas, and humidification by an artificial device is usually unnecessary.

Special Applications for Humidity Therapy

The aforementioned approaches may need modification for patients with abnormal airway reactivity (ie, asthmatics), those with increased need for moisture in the upper airway (ie, laryngotracheobronchitis or croup), and those patients who have abnormalities in pulmonary secretions or their clearance. (Not following the foregoing plan may result in thickened secretions, and increased humidity will be required.) Some patients in the asthmatic population have documented increases in airway resistance when they hyperventilate, as with exercise, during sleep, or when breathing very cold air.[30–32] Breathing inspired air that is humidified to a water vapor content of 20 mg/L at 23°C blunts the obstructive response, and breathing gases at 100% body humidity (43.9 mg/L) can eliminate bronchospasm. Asthmatics who exercise when swimming do not show exercise-induced bronchospasm. It is suggested that there is less thermal stress by preventing heat loss in the form of latent heat of vaporization, preventing the shifting of the isothermic saturation boundary deeper into the airways. Local stimulation of mucosal mast cells is believed to be the cause of the bronchospasm.[32] Worsening of asthma in the nighttime hours may also operate on a similar scheme, in that airway cooling occurs as a result of total body temperature decrease.[30]

Supplemental humidification of inspired gas for nonintubated patients with upper airway pathology or secretion production or retention requires an analysis of the specific problem. Heated water humidification systems offer advantages of better temperature control and decreased risk of irritation or infection compared with bland aerosol systems. Patients with asthma or acute or chronic bronchitis do not need further irritation of hyperreactive airways. This is also true in patients with cystic fibrosis. Children with laryngotracheobronchitis (croup) may benefit from supplemental humidity that lessens airway resistance caused by topical irritation and mucosal crusting in the upper airway; this is most commonly provided by cool bland aerosol.[1,4]

EQUATION BOX 15-3

CALCULATION OF BODY HUMIDITY

The percentage body humidity of room-temperature air with a water vapor content of 9 mg/L (with a relative humidity of 52% at 20°C) is calculated as follows:

$$\%\ \text{Body humidity} = \frac{9\ \text{mg/L}}{43.9\ \text{mg/L}} \times 100 = 21\%$$

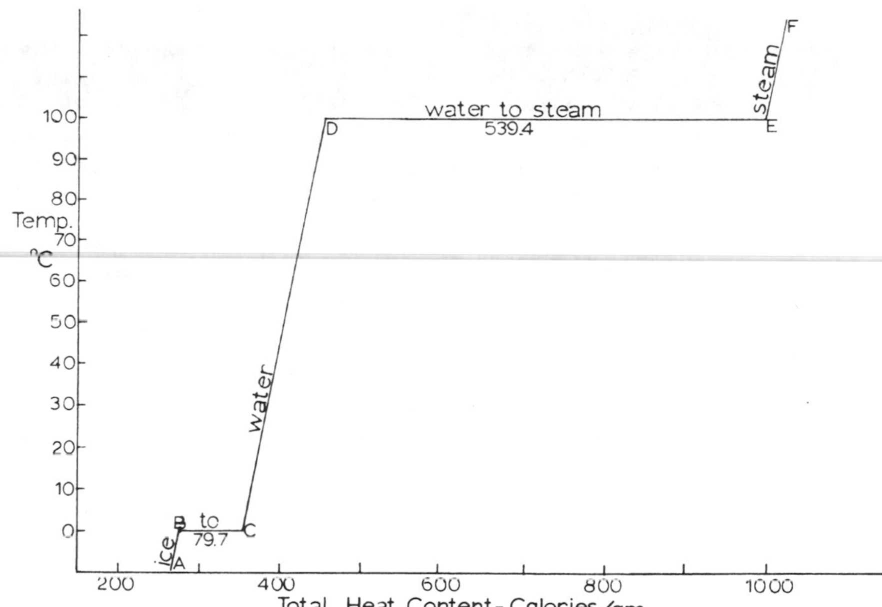

FIGURE 15-5. Behavior of a system for which temperature is plotted as a function of the total amount of heat added (refer to text for details).

Application of heated humidified breathing gases for victims of significant hypothermia has been advocated after CPR techniques have been effective. The respiratory system is less efficient as a heat exchanger for active core temperature rewarming, when compared with fluid lavage of body cavities or extracorporeal therapy. However, rewarming by means of this route is simple compared with other invasive techniques and can raise body temperature an average of 1 to 2°C per hour. Providing airway temperatures of 40 to 45°C has been recommended.[1,33]

EQUIPMENT TO PROVIDE HUMIDITY THERAPY

The purpose of these chapter sections on equipment is to review representative devices. For more comprehensive study, the reader is referred to specific texts or manufacturers' literature.[34–36] Classification of humidification equipment traditionally has been based on a description of the physical method or technique. Problems in classification arise because devices that produce aerosol normally produce humidity (water vapor). However, the reverse is less often true (ie, most humidifiers are intended to only generate water vapor). A general classification developed by Klein and co-workers is used in the following review.[37]

Humidity Generators

□ HEAT AND MOISTURE EXCHANGERS

The *heat and moisture exchanger (HME)* has also been termed "Swedish or artificial nose." Its operating principle is based on a mechanical replication of the body's anatomic humidification system. With this device, exhaled heat and moisture are collected and made available to warm and humidify the following inspiration. A scarf wrapped around the nose and mouth on a cold winter day is a nonmedical application of the HME used in respiratory care. The HMEs under discussion are primarily used with patients who are intubated or tracheostomized. Although used in Europe for some years, commercial HMEs have only seen increased use in United States hospitals since the early 1980s.

The method of operation applies basic physical principles. Expired gas at body temperature and fully saturated with water vapor exits the patient and enters the HME. As gas enters the device, water condenses on the inner surfaces, and the latent heat that has kept water in a vaporized state is released, causing warming (Fig. 15-6). This is inferior to the body's system in that the HME is passively heated and warmed, unlike actively heated mucosal tissues. During inspiration, the collected heat and moisture are transferred to the gas passing through. Dry inspired air progressively cools the HME; the cooling is essential for the surfaces to be able to condense the next breath of expired air. The temperature gradient across the HME, therefore, is an index of its efficiency or output. The higher the temperature of gas exiting an HME, the greater the level of humidification it can provide.[38] *Condenser-type* HMEs use metallic gauze or fine corrugated metal tubes that provide a surface for water to condense; they function at a 50% efficiency level.

When researchers studied certain animals, they were surprised to find that exhaled air was less than body temperature and below 100% saturation. When the camel is deprived of water, its nose becomes hygroscopic in that it can extract more water than would be collected from condensation alone.[39] This effect is said to hold water in a noncondensed state, which lessens evaporative cooling, thereby improving output. Surfaces of paper, wool, or foam have a low thermal

EQUATION BOX 15-5

EXAMPLE OF HEAT NEEDED IN HUMIDIFICATION

The heating and humidification of 10 L of dry oxygen in contact with water (all at 20°C or 293°K) require 342.8 calories (1,434.48 joules) to bring it to 100% body temperature:

$$10 \text{ L of } O_2 \text{ weighs } 13.31 \text{ g}$$

It has a heat capacity of 0.2178 cal/g/1°C (0.911 joules). Just to raise the gas temperature to 37°C requires

$$13.31 \times (37 - 20) \times 0.2178 = 49.28 \text{ cal } (206.24 \text{ joules})$$

However, the heating causes the volume to increase to 10.58 L, and addition of water vapor enlarges it to 11.28 L. The 43.9 mg H_2O/L (495.19 mg) from Box 15-2 will be required, and additional heat will be needed to raise this water to 37°C.

$$0.49508 \times 17 \times 1 = 8.42 \text{ cal } (35.22 \text{ joules})$$

The amount of heat required to change water at 37°C is given in the "steam tables" in handbooks of chemistry and physics to be 575.8 cal/g (2409.7 joules). The heat of vaporization is greater at temperatures below 100°C.

$$0.49508 \times 575.8 = 285.07 \ (1{,}193 \text{ joules})$$

In summary, the total energy needed is

$$\begin{array}{r} 49.28 \\ 8.42 \\ +\ 285.07 \\ \hline \end{array}$$

342.8 cal (1,434.48 joules)

If only the gas were to supply this energy, it would have to enter at 118.25°C above the 20°C, or 138.25°C. If only the water supplied the energy, it would have to be at 692.4°C above the 20°C, or 712°C. However, if a 100-mL reservoir of water were available, a temperature of only 40.26°C would be needed. One can see that this is the most efficient way to provide this energy. To some extent, the human airway functions to provide an efficient gas–water interface. The greater this area, the greater number of escaping molecules. If heat energy is available, the rapid escape continues; if not, the greater surface area increases the rate of temperature drop, decreasing molecular escape.

conductivity but are impregnated with various salts (calcium chloride or lithium chloride). The term *hygroscopic condenser* humidifier has appeared in the trade and medical literature to describe such units, which are approximately 70% efficient.[40]

Clinical Application and Performance

The purpose of heat and moisture exchangers is to humidify dry inspired gases for patients with artificial airways, who are either breathing room air or dry medical gas or being mechanically ventilated. All HMEs are supplied with inlet/outlet fittings (15/22 mm) to interconnect ventilator and airway. The HME is an alternative to heated-water humidifiers because of simplicity, safety (lack of electrical or thermal hazard), portability

BOX 15-3

INDICATIONS FOR SUPPLEMENTAL HUMIDIFICATION

- To replicate physiologic conditions when the normal upper airway is bypassed (eg, endo- or nasotracheal intubation and tracheostomy)
  - Spontaneous breathing (large minute ventilation, cold dry air, and dry medical gases)
  - Mechanical ventilation
- During medical gas therapy at high flows (>40 L/min)
- To prevent or correct hypothermia
- To improve conditions for mucociliary transport in patients with pathologic conditions involving mucus transport

(transport), and reduced cost. Some units may be useful for spontaneously breathing patients with permanent tracheostomy. A gauze pad "ascot" may be a simple system. Cold weather or problems with thick pulmonary secretions may present a need for a portable supplemental humidity device.

Performance standards for HMEs are the same as for heated-water devices when used with mechanical ventilators or anesthesia machines.[1] Laboratory testing of HME outputs shows values from 10 to 28 mg/L, with temperatures about 30°C (over the adult ranges of inspiratory flows and minute ventilation).[40–44] It appears that those using hygroscopic elements do perform better than HMEs without that design.

Box 15-5 summarizes factors that affect the clinical use of HMEs in patient application.

Limitations and Contraindications

Despite the apparent advantages of HMEs, their performance does pose limitations for humidification. Respiratory care practitioners should use HMEs with caution in the mechanical ventilation of patients with abnormal airway secretions or high minute volume requirements. Clinicians should monitor patients for signs of increased minute ventilation demand or greater work of breathing. This is of most concern when HMEs are used during weaning from mechanical ventilation. Large dead-space volume may lead to an increased minute ventilation requirement. This problem, coupled with added resistance through the devices, has the potential to negatively impact weaning. Box 15-6 summarizes contraindications for patient selection or problems that may occur with use.

Product Descriptions and Characteristics

Several examples of heat and moisture exchangers are pictured in Figure 15-7. Table 15-4 provides a composite to identify dimensions, element material, dead space, and moisture output. Advantages of convenience and cost should be considered with the knowledge that patients who are dehydrated, hypothermic, or have pulmonary abnormalities (that may lead to or result in retained secretions) are **not** ideal candidates for HMEs.[45–49] In addition, certain units with large internal dead space

TABLE 15-3 **Recommendations for Humidification Levels During Mechanical Ventilation**

	Temp. (°C)	AH* (mg/L)	RH* (%)
International Organization for Standardization (ISO)[21]	30	NS	NS
American National Standards Institute (ANSI)[22]	NS	30	NS
Emergency Care Research Institute (ECRI)[23]	34	37	NS
American Association for Respiratory Care (AARC)[1]	33 ± 2	30	NS
British Standards Institution[24]	>33		>75%

* AH, absolute humidity; RH, relative humidity.

may be contraindicated for perinatal and pediatric patients with small tidal volumes. Whether an HME can modify bacterial contamination during mechanical ventilation is controversial.[45] In summary, HMEs can be considered for routine use in transport and for anesthesia ventilation. They should be considered for short-term mechanical ventilation (< 72 hours) unless contraindicated by either patient pathology or development of the aforementioned problems.

☐ LOW-FLOW HUMIDIFIERS (UNHEATED)

Humidifiers can pass medical gases through a diffuser, "bubbler," or jet to increase the surface area for water-gas interface. By evaporation, humidity levels increase as gases rise in a vessel of water (Fig. 15-8). This kind of humidifier has been used to add water vapor to low-flow (< 10 L/min) medical gases. Various substances are used for the diffuser, including mesh, sintered metal, and plastic foam. The addition of water vapor is greatest if the bubbles are very small and the water container is tall; this allows maximum time for water-gas contact. Humidifiers of this type are not efficient but are best at low flows (eg, 1.5 to 5 L/min). Increasing flows cause evaporative cooling of the water, which lowers temperature and reduces water contact time, reducing the potential content of water vapor in the gas. These units typically are unable to humidify dry medical gas much beyond 40% body humidity, when operated at normal room temperature.[37]

Clinical Application and Performance

In the past, unheated low-flow humidifiers were traditionally used with low-flow medical gas administration systems such as nasal cannulas, simple (nonreservoir) masks, and reservoir masks (see Chap. 13). Over the last 10 years, there has been a clinical trend to eliminate the bubbler humidifier when providing low-flow oxygen. Consensus for deleting the device is based on its poor performance and efforts to further reduce hospital operating costs.

Although objective assessment of bubbler humidifiers has been sparse, two laboratory studies have produced similar results. Klein and co-workers found outputs to range from 38% to 48% body humidity when flows were 2.5 L/min. When flow was increased to 10 L/min, the percentage body humidity fell to 26% to 34% (Fig. 15-9).[37] Darin and associates reviewed prefilled (single-patient use) bubblers, with comparable results. At 2 L/min, units ranged from 39% to 46.6% body humidity, and decreased to 33% to 35% body humidity at 8 L/min. Bubblers reach their peak efficiency within 15 minutes of use, then decrease to a plateau level as the temperature decreases.[28] Both groups concluded that the two major factors determining performance are the design of the diffuser and the level of medical gas flow. Improved engineering design may increase vapor output.

Therapeutic gases delivered to the nose or mouth (eg, by nasal cannula or mask) should minimally match average room air conditions. (American National Standards Z-79.9 suggests 22°C at 50% relative humidity or 9.76 mg/L.[22]) However, meeting this level may not be necessary, as nasal cannula breathers inspire a large portion of ambient, humidified room air with the dry oxygen. Continuous nasal cannula breathers may find improved comfort if they need higher flows (> 4 to 5 L/min) and low ambient humidity.[27] Patients breathing with a nasal cannula or facial mask tend to warm and humidify gas with their expired air.

In clinical practice, a few technical problems can occur. Because small-bore tubing is used with bubblers, there is potential for blocking gas flow by kinking and compression by bed rails or wheelchair wheels. Water from the reservoir may spill into tubing or enter when high flows cause a churning action. Gas pressure will cause the water to spray into the patient's nose or face. Confirmation that connecting tubing is clear and that there is flow through the appliance should be part of the initial and ongoing check of patients using such systems. Bubbler humidifiers have gravity or spring-loaded pressure valves to vent off pressures that could rupture units if not relieved, which can alert operators to the problem. Because bubblers are water reservoirs, they can support the growth of *Pseudomonas aeruginosa*. Improperly handled humidi-

BOX 15-4

CONDITIONS TO PROVIDE ADEQUATE HUMIDITY DURING MECHANICAL VENTILATION

Absolute humidity	30 mg/L
Relative humidity	85–100%
Temperature	32–34°C

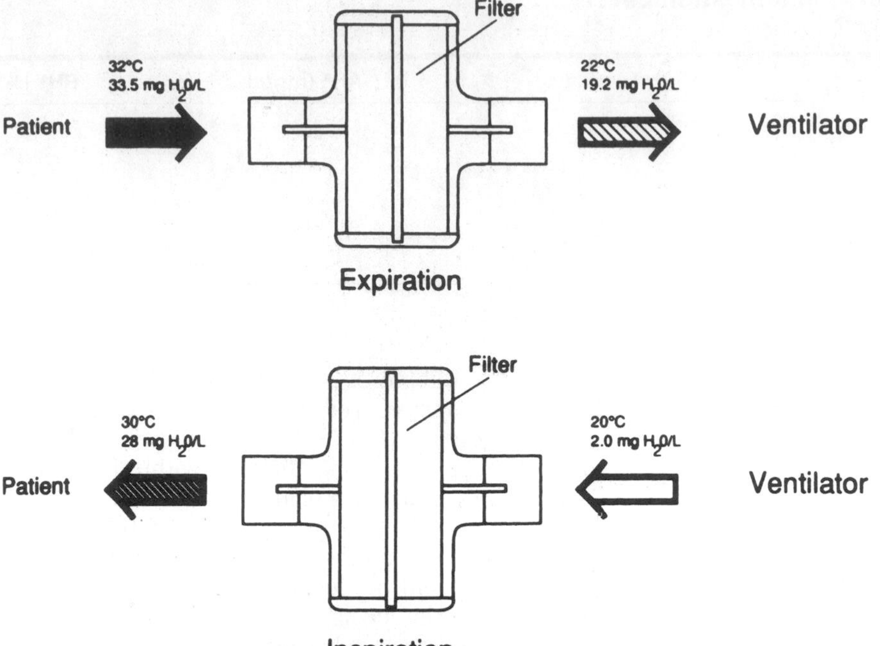

FIGURE 15-6. Diagram of a heat–moisture exchanger (HME).

fiers have been linked to nosocomial respiratory infections with this pathogen.[52]

□ HIGH-FLOW HUMIDIFIERS (HEATED)

Humidifiers using heated-water systems are used to condition dry inspired gases for patients who have artificial airways in place, are being mechanically ventilated, or are in oxygen hoods. By physically adding heat, these units can potentially replicate the heat and humidity levels that normal airways would provide. They are also termed *mainstream humidifiers* to indicate that the patient's entire source of inspired gas is conveyed through the humidifier.

Indications for clinical use and minimum performance conditions have been described earlier in this chapter (see Boxes 15-3 and 15-4).

Commercially available heated units have the capability of humidifying gas to 100% body humidity. They can be considered the standard device for mechanical ventilator–breathing circuits and for application of high-flow gas systems (eg, continuous positive airway pressure [CPAP]), medical gases for asthmatics, and delivery of gas to infant oxygen hoods. Some units have limits to the total flow that can be brought to 100% body humidity. Some units are stressed at high-flow conditions. Flows of 60 to 100 L/min may be required for continuous high-flow systems (eg, oxygen blender or Down's flow generator). Heated humidifiers must also be considered the devices of choice for patients with bypassed upper airway who have secretion problems. Patients with abnormal thickening of mucus, mucus plugs, or crusting of endotracheal or tracheostomy tubes can have their humidity deficit corrected. A history of lung disease that typically presents with secretion abnormalities may indicate that a heated humidifier be placed prophylactically, instead of a device (eg, HME) with less moisture capability.

Category Descriptions and Performance Classification of mainstream humidifiers is based on terms depicting the basic design. The following categories are based on those used by the Emergency Care Research Institute (ECRI).[23,53]

- Pass-over humidifier
- Diffuser or bubble-through (also referred to as "cascade") humidifier
- Pass-over or pass-through wick

BOX 15-5

CLINICAL FACTORS IN USE OF HMES

- Pressure: Units should be leak free or leak less than 30 mL/min when 30 cmH_2O pressure is applied. Units should withstand pressures of 100 cmH_2O.
- Resistance: The pressure drop across the HME is suggested to be less than 3 cmH_2O for flows of 50 L/min. Resistance has been noted to increase as HMEs absorb water.
- Compressible volume or dead space: Internal volumes should be as low as possible without compromising humidity output.
- Weight: Low weight is favored to reduce undue traction on artificial airways.
- Humidity output: Some units are superior to others.
- Cost: Individual unit cost may be high, but reduced expense for water and related equipment must be considered.
- Filter: Some devices serve as a filter as well as HME; the usefulness of this feature is not clear.

BOX 15-6

CONTRAINDICATIONS FOR USE OF HMES (DURING MECHANICAL VENTILATION)

- Thick, copious, or bloody secretions
- When exhaled tidal volumes are less than 70% of delivered tidal breaths (eg, bronchopleural fistulas or cuffless endotracheal or tracheostomy tubes)
- Hypothermic patients (body temperature <32°C)
- Excessively large tidal volumes (>1 L) or high spontaneous minute volumes (>10 L/min)
- During medicated aerosol therapy
- Small tidal volumes in HMEs with large internal dead space
- In conjunction with a heated humidifier or nebulizers

Adapted with permission from American Association for Respiratory Care: Clinical practice guideline: Humidification During Mechanical Ventilation. Respir Care 37:887, 1992

All three designs provide humidification by heating water and providing a water-gas interface for their contact. Units may also be described as *servo controlled* or non–servo controlled. This refers to some method of regulating the heating elements. Servo-controlled humidifiers have some type of *thermistor* (electronic thermometer) that works with a microprocessor to maintain a specific temperature. The thermistor probe is usually located in the inspiratory circuit near the patient connection. Some humidifiers have the option for *heated wires* to be added in the inspiratory-expiratory tubing, to reduce condensate. Manufacturers have also incorporated *continuous-feed* water systems for convenience, decreasing the likelihood of reservoirs running dry and reducing the potential for microbiological contamination.

Regardless of their physical design, heated humidifier systems must function over a wide range of clinical uses, accommodating both low and high gas flows. Adult ventilation with large minute ventilation and high inspiratory flows, and with high-frequency or jet ventilators, challenge humidifier performance. Box 15-7 describes ECRI's guidelines for design capabilities and safety features.

Pass-Over Humidifier The pass-over design of humidifier simply directs gas over a reservoir of heated water (Fig. 15-10*A*). Escaping molecules of water vapor are "scavenged" by the gas. Three clinical examples are available; original humidifiers are available with the Emerson 3-PV and 3-MV mechanical ventilators, the Bear VH-820 (Fig. 15-10*B* and 15-11*A*), and the Inspiron Vapor-Phase Plus (Fig 15-11*E*).

Emerson 3-PV ventilators were originally equipped with a modified kitchen pressure cooker filled with copper mesh in the proximal inspiratory tubing to enhance humidification. Heat was provided by an electric plate. Testing has shown that the Emerson pass-over humidifier is limited to water outputs less than 30 mg/L when used during mechanical ventilation.[54]

The Bear humidifier (Bear Medical Systems) uses spiral vanes that increase the pass-over surface area for water-gas contact, without a substantial increase in

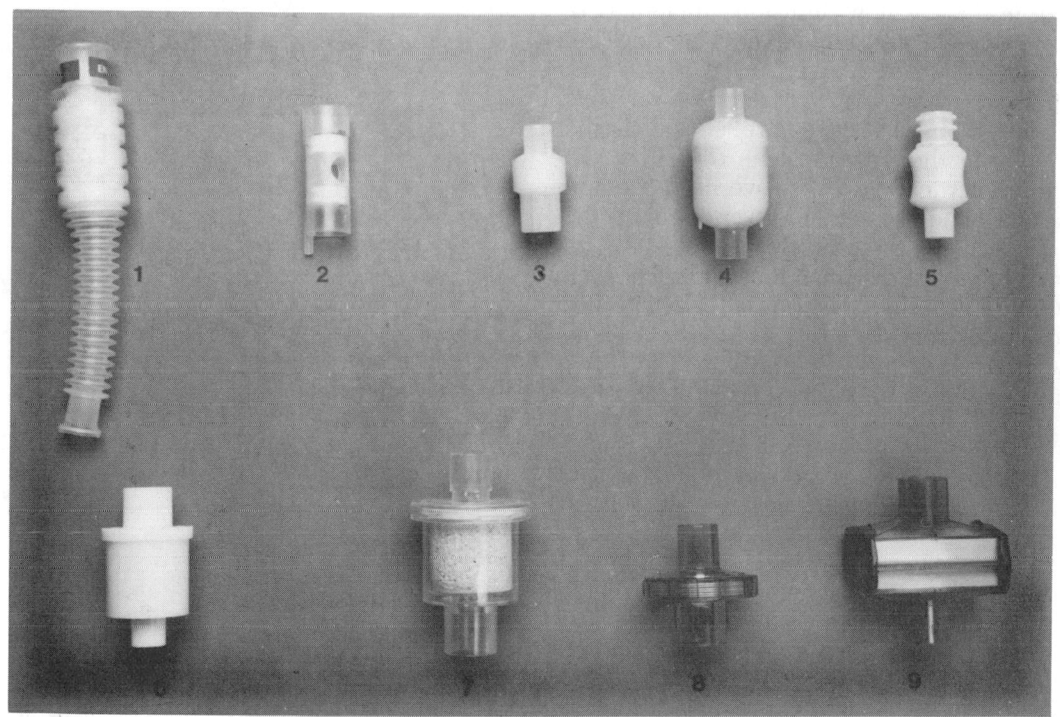

FIGURE 15-7. Commercially available heat–moisture exchangers. **(1)** Engstrom Edith, **(2)** Portex Humid-Vent, **(3)** Portex, **(4)** Mallinckrodt, **(5)** American Hospital Supply Humid-Air, **(6)** Siemens 152, **(7)** Siemens 150, **(8)** Vitalograph, **(9)** Pall Conserve.

TABLE 15-4 **Heat Moisture Exchangers***

Brand	Weight (g)	Vol. (mL)	Element	Compliance mL/cmH_2O	Output mg/L
Dameca	44	62	Corrugated aluminum	0.062	16
Portex Humid-Vent	9	10	Corrugated paper	0.01	21
Terumo Breath Aid	14	11.5	Aluminum and fabric disks	0.01	14
Airlife Humid Air	11.1	40.5	Synthetic felt	—	24
Siemens Servo 153	25	70	Cellulose sponge and felt	0.09	28
Engstrom Edith	18	89	Polypropylene fiber	—	27
Engstrom Edith 1000	9	28	Polypropylene fiber	—	27
Vitalograph	67	30	Stainless steel screens	0.03	16
Mallinckrodt	16	60.8	Plastic foam	—	21
Pall Conserve	47.2	98	Ceramic fiber	—	25
Gibeck Humid-Vent-2	18	25	Corrugated paper	—	26

* Data from references 43–48.

compliance or resistance (Figs. 15-10*B* and 15-11*A*). The VH-820 uses a servo-controlled system with the option for heated wire.

The pass-over design is slightly different in the Inspiron Vapor-Phase Plus (Inspiron) shown in Figure 15-11*E*. A hydrophobic filter separates the heated water and gas. Water is vaporized below the filter and is then removed by gas flow. This single-patient humidifier is available as a servo-controlled and continuous-feed system. The Fisher and Paykel 700 series is a servo-controlled humidification system using a pass-over design and has the potential for heated-wire use (Fig. 15-12).

Diffuser Cascade The *cascade* design is a more efficient design of the low-flow diffusion humidifier. Besides being heated, the area for gas-water interface is increased by use of a large diffuser tower (Figs. 15-11*F* and 15-13). The Puritan-Bennett Cascade I was developed in the late 1960s; a servo-controlled and alarmed unit followed with the Cascade II in the 1970s. The alarm functions alert care givers to overheated temperature at the sensor and sensor failure or disconnection. A continuous-feed water system can be used. In the tower of each humidifier, a small hole allows the ventilator to sense a pressure differential caused by the patient's inspiratory effort. In the past, it was assumed that no bacterial aerosol was emitted when using a cascade humidifier. A report of this occurring has been published.[55]

Bubble-Through Wick Several humidifiers use a submerged paper or composite (eg, Gore-tex®) wick through which the mainstream flow must pass. The saturated wicks may be vertical or horizontal and provide the surface for imparting water vapor to gas. Current designs using this principle include the Bird Wick (Figs. 15-11B and 15-14 (Bird Corp.), Conchatherm (Figs. 15-11G and 15-14) (Respiratory Care Inc.), Travenol-HLC-37S (Figs 15-11I) (American Pharmaseal), Fisher and Paykel MR-450 and MR600 (Figs. 15-C,D) (American Pharmaseal) and Saratoga SCT (Fig. 15-11H) (Marquest Products). All wick humidifiers use a servo-controlled thermostat, except the Bird. The Fisher and Paykel (model MR450 and MR600) and Saratoga units have capabilities for heated wires in the patient tubing.

These humidifiers have alarm systems that warn of overheated temperature, probe disconnection, and low temperature. Servo-controlled humidifiers tend to overheat if, during warm-up, the temperature probe is not placed in the breathing circuit. However, in most of the humidifiers, an alarm is activated. Non–servo-controlled units give overheated gas if the operator sets

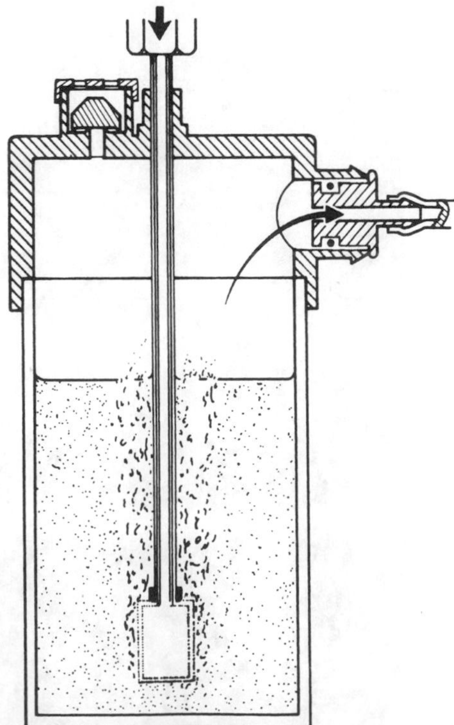

FIGURE 15-8. Section of a bubble humidifier. These devices are commonly used with low-flow oxygen appliances (eg, cannula, masks, and such). A weighted pressure pop-off is shown at the top of the housing.

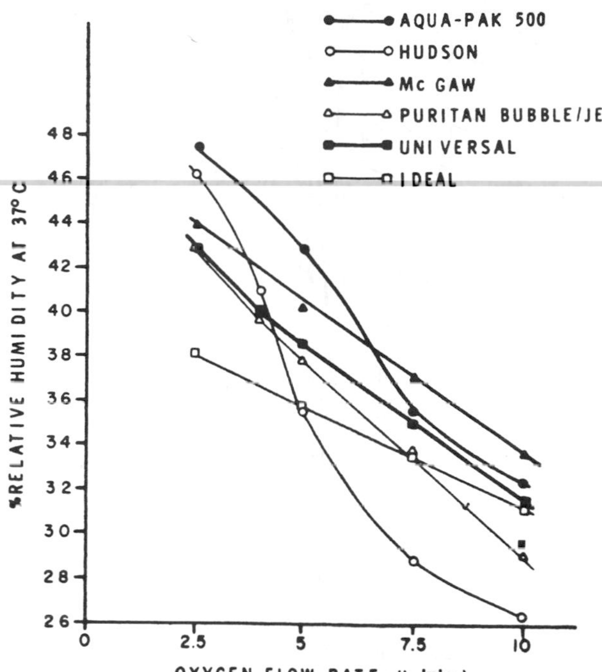

FIGURE 15-9. Humidity output (percentage body humidity) of six unheated bubbler humidifiers with increasing flow of oxygen. (Klein EF, Shah DA, Shah, NJ, Modell JH, Dasautels D: Performance characteristics of conventional and prototype humidifiers and nebulizers. Chest 64:690, 1973. Reproduced with permission.)

the temperature too high or if gas flow is substantially reduced.

The advantage of the heated-wire feature appears to be primarily convenience, in that, with reduced condensation, ventilator water traps need less maintenance. Dry circuits may eliminate aerosolized contaminants during water trap emptying or ventilator disconnection, reducing the potential for cross-contamination of neighboring patients and health care workers. Patients breathing on heated-wire humidifiers may not receive protection from nosocomial infection. However, if the wire heats gas higher than the temperature of gas in the tubing, relative humidity decreases, with a potential for inspissated secretions at the artificial airway.[20,25] A small level of condensate in the ventilator tubing is a reliable sign of achieving 100% relative humidity. Humidifiers without heated wires have acceptable output. Safety may also be a factor when using small tubing in breathing circuits (eg, neonatal ventilation) or when ventilator checks cannot be done reliably. Water collecting in low spots in the circuits can increase resistance to flow and, when in the expiratory limb, can create a PEEP-like effect.

The Bird humidifier is a non–servo-controlled unit that uses a vertical paper wick (see Fig. 15-13). It has a reusable chamber, which connects to the power module, and remote continuous water feed. Its alarm functions include probe disconnection, temperatures over 40°C, and humidification module disconnection.

The older Fisher and Paykel model is a servo-controlled unit with disposable wick and several options for the humidification chamber (see Fig. 15-11*C,D*). The MR600 can provide heated-wire operation. A continuous water feed system may be added to these humidifiers.

The Conchatherm III is a servo-controlled unit with some operator requirement (see Fig. 15-11*G*). It has relative, rather than specific, temperature controls. The system includes a remote continuous water feed but requires RCI-packaged sterile water.

The Saratoga SCT is a servo-controlled device with disposable heated wire and a humidification chamber (see Fig. 15-11*H*). A remote continuous feed is provided. Alarm functions include independently adjustable high and low temperature, probe or heated-wire disconnection, and power failure.

The Travenol HLC-37S is a servo-controlled humidifier with disposable heated-wire system (see Fig. 15-11*I*). A remote continuous feed is incorporated. The unit's alarm goes off at high and low temperatures, probe disconnection, and depletion of the water reservoir. Table 15-5 summarizes clinical heated humidifiers.

BOX 15-7

SUGGESTED HEATED-WATER HUMIDIFIER CAPABILITIES

Overtemperature protection: Temperatures should be set to be prevented to go above 40°C. Heaters should have power interrupted when temperature near the airway exceeds 40°C; visual and audible alarms should be activated.

Warm-up time: Humidifiers should reach operating temperature in an appropriate time and stabilize at the desired level.

Electromagnetic interference: Interference from adjacent electrical equipment should not affect humidifier function.

Electrical safety: Devices should not be affected by nor cause electrical hazard due to water spills.

Misassembly: It should not be possible to reassemble a humidifier system in a way that could lead to a hazardous situation for the patient. The direction for correct gas flow should be clearly indicated on the device.

Water level visibility: Water level in the humidifier or remote reservoir should be visible in typical ICU lighting.

Internal compliance and compressible volume (for mechanical ventilation): Compliance (volume and pressure) should be less than the compliance of the patient being ventilated. Neonatal application suggests a level of 1.0 mL/cmH_2O or less.

Resistance or pressure drop across a humidifier: The pressure caused by resistance to flow through a humidifier should be 5 cmH_2O or less with flows of 50 L/min.

Used with permission from Emergency Care Research Institute: Heated humidifiers. Health Devices 16:223, 1987

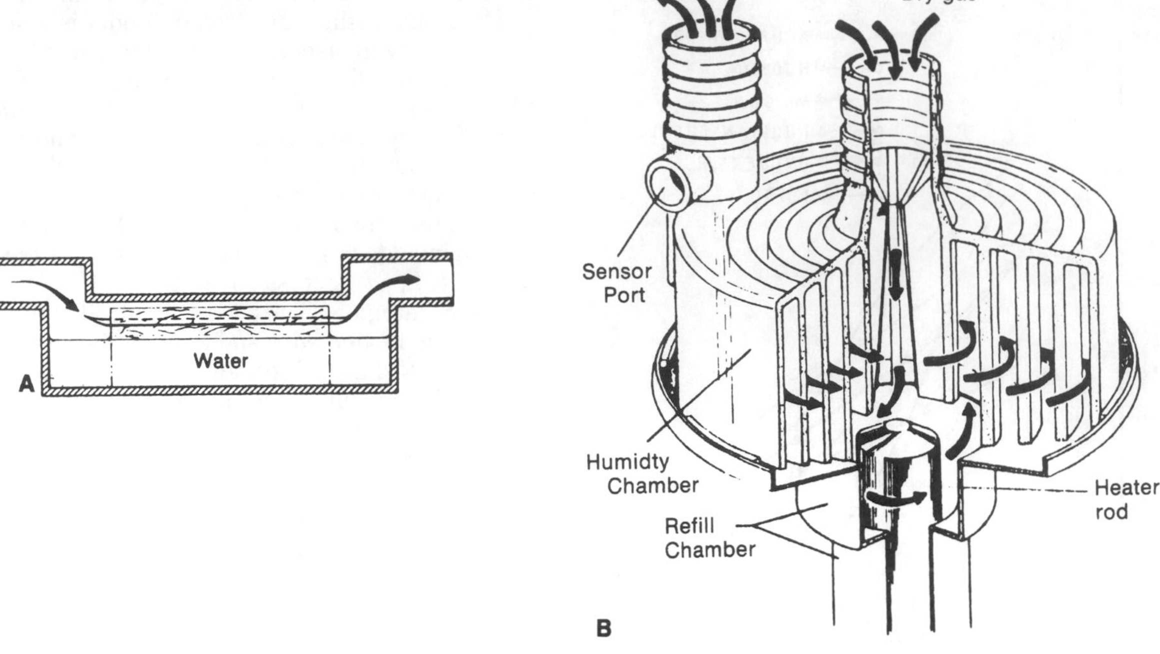

FIGURE 15-10. Pass-over humidifiers: **(A)** Section of generic "pass-over" humidifier; **(B)** Section of Bear VH-820 humidifier (Courtesy of Bear Medical Systems Inc., Riverside CA)

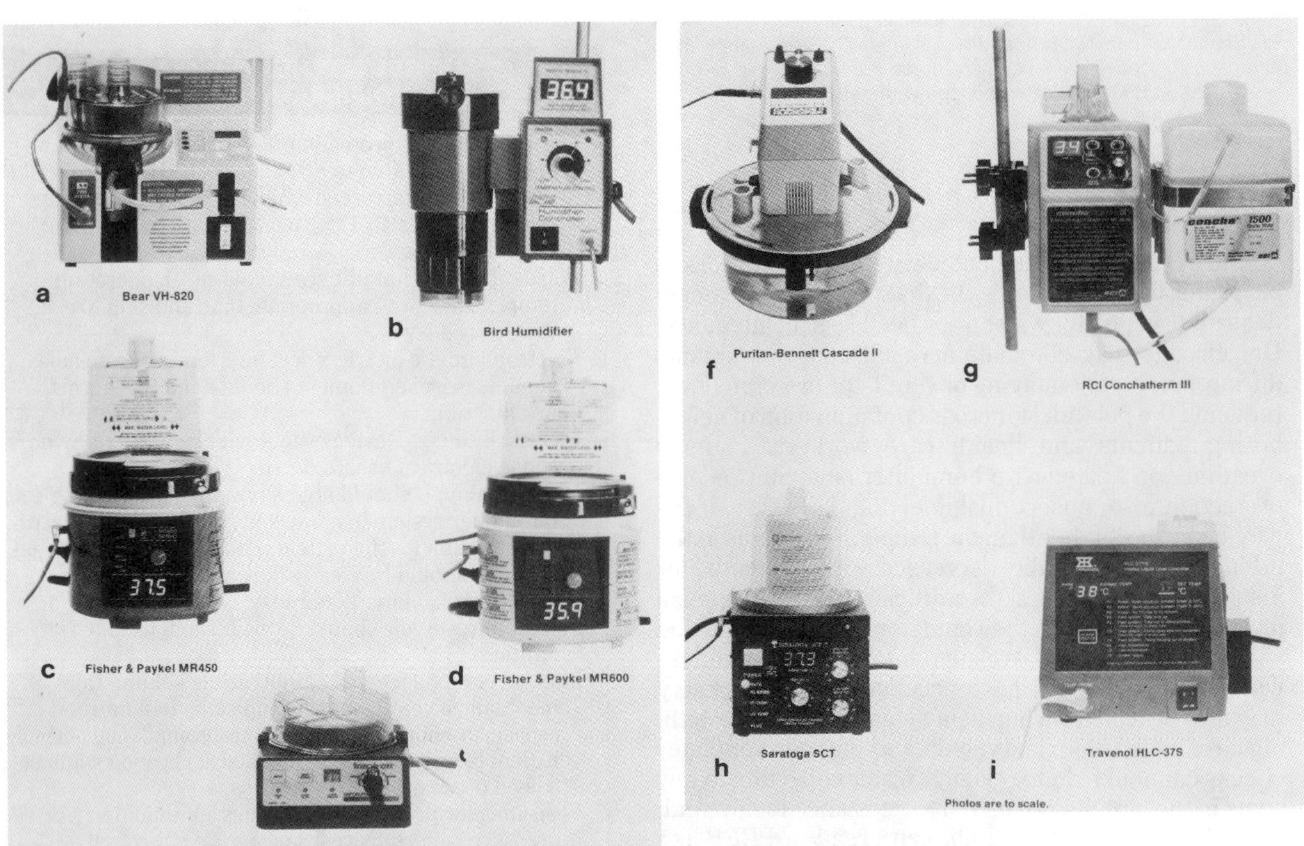

FIGURE 15-11. Commercially available heated humidifiers: **(A)** Bear VH–820, Bear Medical Systems, Inc.; **(B)** Bird, Bird Products; **(C)** Fisher & Paykel MR450 and **(D)** MR600, Fisher & Paykel/American Pharmaseal Co.; **(E)** Inspiron Vapor-Phase Plus, Inspiron Corp. Omnicare, Inc.; **(F)** Puritan-Bennett Cascade II, Puritan Bennett Corp.; **(G)** RCI Conchatherm III, Respiratory Care, Inc. **(H)** Saratoga SCT, Marquest Medical Products Inc.; **(I)** Travenol HLC-37S, Travenol/American Pharmaseal Co. (Courtesy ECRI from Health Devices 16:228–229, 1987.)

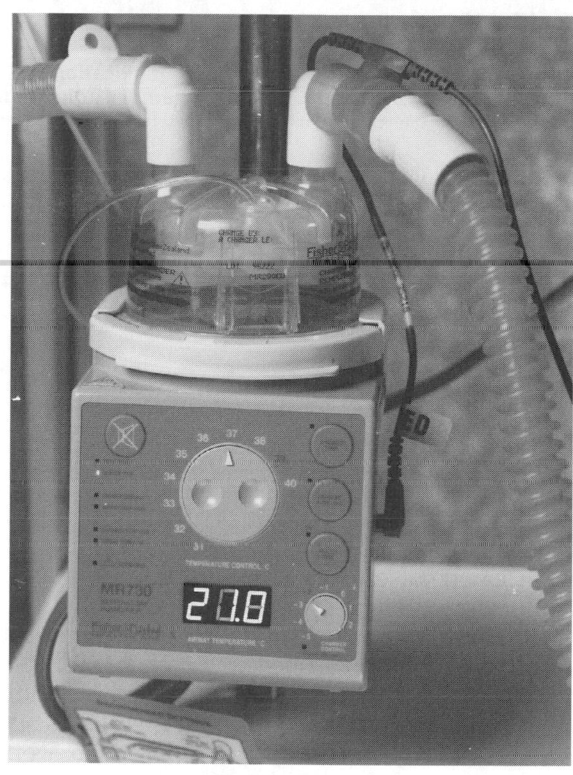

FIGURE 15-12. Fisher & Paykel MR 700 pass-over humidifier.

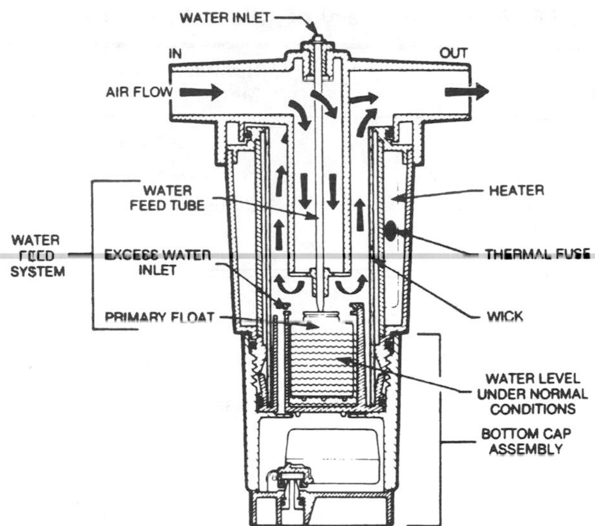

FIGURE 15-14. Section of a Bird Wick Humidifier. (Courtesy of Bird Products Corp., Palm Springs, CA)

COMPLICATIONS, HAZARDS, PATIENT ASSESSMENT, AND EQUIPMENT TROUBLESHOOTING

As each major type of humidity generator has been discussed, the rational and patient application have been reviewed. Although the practice of applying humidity to dry gases appears to be benign, there can be hazards and complications in clinical practice. Mucus plugging from ineffective humidification can result in hypoventilation, increased airway resistance, and gas trapping. All heated humidifiers heat water using AC electrical current. There is potential for electric shock; proper grounding and maintenance are required. Thermal injury to the airway or circuit meltdown can occur. Underventilation can occur during mechanical ventilation caused by volume loss due to gas compression within the humidifiers. Inappropriate choice of device, operator error, or malfunction may result in potential harm to the patient.

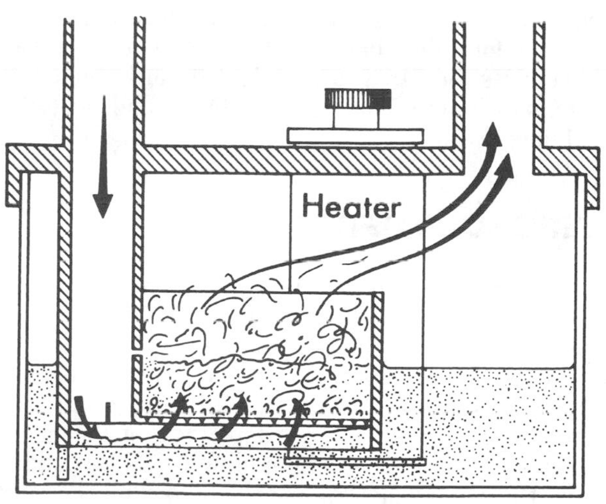

FIGURE 15-13. Section of a "cascade" humidifier.

Gas flows through humidifiers change with changing ventilation levels. Clinicians should monitor the ability of the humidifier to accommodate a patient's changing conditions. Figure 15-15 illustrates the effect of decreasing or increasing gas flow on patient gas temperature using servo and non–servo control. Falling or increasing airway temperature should alert respiratory care practitioners to significant change in inspiratory flows, minute ventilation, device malfunction, or limit of humidifier performance.

After a patient has been placed on some type of humidification system, the respiratory care practitioner should evaluate the effectiveness of maintaining the airway. Chest auscultation should alert one to increased retention of mucus (rhonchi) and to atelectatic lung zones (crackles).

Evaluating the character of the sputum after cough or suctioning can help assess whether there is adequate hydration of the airway. If the artificial airway frequently requires clearing because of crusting of mucus, the appropriateness of that system should be reevaluated. Patients without an artificial airway may also provide subjective information if poor humidification of nose or facial medical gas systems causes uncomfortable drying.

Respiratory care practitioners should constantly be attentive to condensate in breathing circuits. Water traps may not be completely effective. Mechanically ventilated patients commonly become colonized quite

TABLE 15-5. **Summary of Clinical Heated Humidifier Specifications**

Brand	Humidification Method	Servo Control	Heated Wire	Humidification Chamber Volume (mL)
Bear VH-820	Pass-over vanes	Yes	NA	5–10
Inspiron Vapor-phase	Pass-over filter	NA	NA	10
Puritan-Bennett Cascade	Diffuser	Yes	NA	900
Bird	Pass-over wick	NA	NA	20
Fisher-Paykel (MR600 & MR700 only)	Pass-over	Yes	Yes	280 Adult 210–230 Pediatric
RCI Conchatherm	Pass-over wick	Yes	NA	182 Adult 72 Pediatric
Saratoga SCT	Pass-over wick	Yes	Yes	300
Travenol HLC-37S	Pass-over wick	Yes	NA	75

rapidly with organisms found in the sputum. Changing circuits or removing condensate has been implicated as a cause of nosocomial pneumonia.[56,57] This potentially infected waste should be drained away from the patient to prevent inadvertent passage into the tracheobronchial tree. However, aspiration of the patient's own oral and gastrointestinal flora past leaks about artificial airway cuffs may be the most significant sources of nosocomial pneumonia. Bacteriocidal temperatures potentially allow humidifiers to remain sterile in spite of heavy circuit contamination near the patient. There is no current evidence that certain humidifier designs (eg, cascade-type vs. wick) or use of HME alters the incidence of ventilator-associated pneumonia. Closed-feed humidifier systems have not been shown to reduce nosocomial infections.

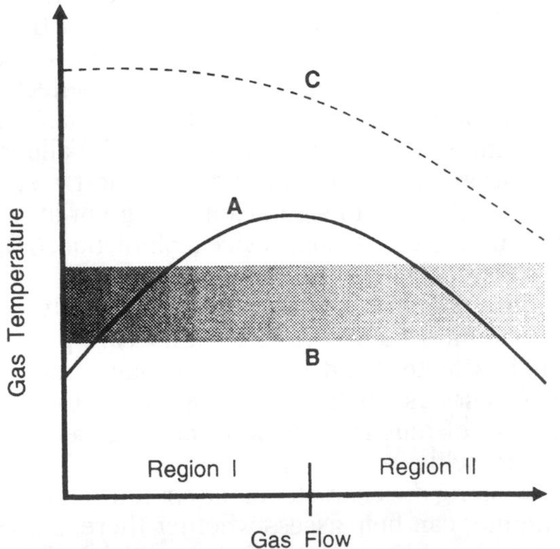

FIGURE 15-15. Gas temperature versus flow at a fixed setting of the humidifier heater. Line A refers to *patient gas temperature* using a non-servocontrolled humidifier. Shaded area B refers to *patient temperature variations* (some overshoot and some undershoot) produced by a servocontrolled humidifier. Line C represents temperature *at the humidifier outlet.* Region I demonstrates how patient temperatures increase as gas has less time to cool in the inspiratory tubing (nonservocontrolled). Region II shows how temperature falls because of heat transfer limitations of the humidifier. (From ECRI. An overview of heated humidifiers. Technology for Respiratory Therapy 1994;15:1. with permission.)

The length of time between routine ventilator-humidifier circuit changes has been a point of controversy and research interest.[58] A recent study suggests that ventilator circuits only need to be changed between patients.[59] Currently, national guidelines recommend no maximum time, but suggest that there is no advantage to changing breathing circuits less than every 48 hours.[60]

Circuit gas leaks in the humidifier portion of a breathing circuit may interfere with sufficient pressurization and lead to hypoventilation. Ventilators should be checked before patient use to confirm a leak-free system. Low-pressure or volume alarms should provide an ongoing clinical evaluation. Humidifiers with high resistance may prevent ventilator low-pressure alarms from detecting leaks or disconnection.

Malfunctions or misassembly of continuous water feed systems are potentially hazardous if the units flood the inspiratory circuit. Heated humidifiers that overheat can cause airway burns. The most common error that causes overheating is failure to place the servo probe in the circuit. It also can occur when gas flows are quite variable or with equipment malfunction. Recent sophistication of heater alarm systems reduces this hazard. However, operator error in non–servo-controlled systems can occur. Manufacturer's information should be available for individual humidifiers on troubleshooting procedures. Box 15-8 summarizes hazards and complications of humidification with HMEs and heated humidifiers.

AEROSOL THERAPY

Medical aerosols are used in the diagnosis and treatment of a variety of cardiopulmonary disorders. The size of aerosol particles is commonly targeted to a lung or airway region. Particle size is determined by the device, ambient conditions, and compound being aerosolized. Delivery often is dependent on the patient's inhalation technique and lung function. This section reviews the various factors that relate to clinical practice.

BOX 15-8

HAZARDS AND COMPLICATIONS OF HUMIDIFIERS

- Electrical shock
- Hypothermia (HME) and hyperthermia (heated humidifiers)
- Thermal injury to the airway and burns from hot surfaces
- Inspissation of airway secretions
- Hypoventilation caused by leaks or increased dead space or compressible volume
- Increased work of breathing from elevated gas flow resistance
- Ventilator- or humidifier-associated nosocomial pneumonia
- Increased airway pressures from pooled condensate in expiratory circuits
- Interfering with ventilator low-pressure or disconnect alarm function

Adapted with permission from American Association for Respiratory Care: Clinical practice guideline: Humidification During Mechanical Ventilation. Respir Care 37:887, 1992

A complete review of the background physics is beyond the scope of this chapter. However, respiratory care practitioners may be required to evaluate equipment and select devices for specific patient applications. Therefore, a brief introduction in terminology, physical characteristics, and methods of describing aerosols is provided.

Physical Principles

An *aerosol* is defined as a suspension of solid or liquid particles in gas. Particles may vary in shape, density, and size, all of which can affect their physical behavior. Such physical characteristics determine the depth of travel into the respiratory tract and tendency to be deposited.

In nature, smoke, dust, and fog are examples of aerosols. Box 15-9 gives approximate sizes of environmental aerosols.

Aerosols can be made by condensation of water vapor into the liquid state and by comminution of solid or liquid substances by *shattering* particles into a suspension. The latter method is frequently used in respiratory care. There are several techniques to accomplish the shattering effect, which will be examined later in this chapter.

BOX 15-9

DIMENSIONS OF AEROSOL PARTICLES IN NATURE (μM)

Sand grains	200–2000
Pollens	10–100
Fungal spores	0.5–100
Tobacco smoke	0.2–2
Viruses	.0028–0.2

Because the size of particles is critical to their distribution in the respiratory tract, scientists have devised a number of terms and techniques to help characterize the aerosol. Manufacturers often develop aerosol-generating devices that target a certain particle size. In reality, most therapeutic aerosols are composed of a range of particle sizes and are called *heterodisperse* aerosols. *Monodisperse* aerosols have a narrow range of diameters and are used for specific therapeutic or research applications.

During aerosol therapy, water or drugs are deposited into or on the respiratory tract surfaces. When the density is constant, the volume of substance in an aerosol particle is proportional to its size. Specifically, the *volume of a particle* is directly proportional to the cube of the radius:

$$\text{Aerosol volume} = 4/3 \times \pi \times \text{radius}^3$$

The implication of this relationship is significant to therapy. Many small particles must be deposited in the same area to equal one large particle. Particles below 1 μm have so little mass, hence volume, that they provide little deposition in the lung.[60] The surface area of an aerosol particle is related to its diameter by the following relationship:

$$\text{Particle surface area} = \pi \times \text{diameter}^2$$

The surface area–volume ratio increases as particles become smaller and their inertia becomes less. They tend to deposit less by impaction and to settle more slowly during breath holding.

The distribution of the aerosol-particle diameters can be characterized using statistics. The *mass median aerodynamic diameter (MMAD)* assists in describing size distribution. This concept is used to refer to an aerosol particle that has 50% of its fellow particles heavier and 50% lighter. (This assumes that the distribution follows a typical bell-shaped probability distribution.)

Some aerosol generators do not follow this distribution. Propellant-powered metered-dose inhalers have several peaks, and a number of clinical aerosols have a log-normal distribution. A plot of the latter giving mass mean diameter is provided in Figure 15-16. However, large particles constitute most of the mass.

Count median diameter (CMD) and *geometric mean diameter (GMD)* are both indexes used to reflect a "typical" particle, in that 50% of the other particles are larger and 50% smaller. The difference between the CMD and the MMAD is demonstrated in Figure 15-16. It is possible that about 1% of the large aerosol particles account for the difference between the two mean levels, in that it takes only a few large particles to increase the mass or volume exponentially.

The *aerodynamic mass diameter (AD)* is a measurement that helps correlate a particle's size with properties that would cause it to settle with gravity. An aerosol is assigned a particle diameter (spherical), with a specific density, that has a settling velocity identical with that of a reference particle. Therefore, size, shape, and density factors may differ, but if a particle settles out at a specific point, it is assigned that aerodynamic mass diameter.

Most therapeutic aerosols in clinical respiratory care applications have MMADs between 1 and 10 μm. This size range is sufficiently stable, and particles larger than

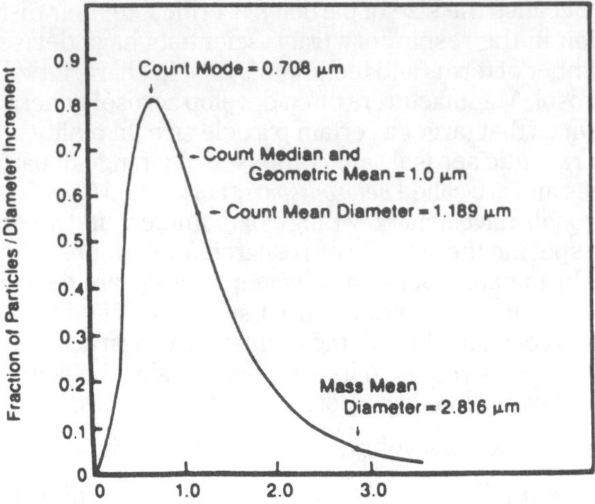

FIGURE 15-16. Log-normal distribution of aerosol particle diameter plotted against fraction of particles per increment in diameter. Because of the skewed nature of log-normal distribution, mode, median, and mean do not coincide. (Reproduced with permission, Lourenco RV, Cotromanes E: Clinical aerosols I: Characterization of aerosols and their diagnostic use. Arch Intern Med 142:2163, 1982.)

1 µm are large enough to carry sufficient volumes of water or drug. Particles of 0.01 to 1 µm diameter are so stable that they fail to deposit on lung surfaces and are exhaled.

Aerosol particles can either shrink through evaporation or grow in size as they travel. An increase in size by condensation of water vapor is termed *hygroscopic property.* The specific substance (ie, drug), water, and salinity, as well as the ambient humidity and temperature, influence this. The humidity level, in turn, is crucially dependent on the collective surface area of the gas-liquid interface. A 1-µm diameter aerosol particle is estimated to completely evaporate in 0.5 seconds, if warmed from 20° C to 37° C in transit from room to body temperature.[61,62]

The form of the aerosol relates to physical factors in delivery. Aerosolized drugs are available in both liquid and dry compounds. Dry-powder inhalers (DPI) allow inhalation of powders that are agglomerates or mixed with a lactose carrier. The deaggregation of the drug is favored by high turbulent flows (approximately 0.5 L/min) without necessity of breath holding. Liquid aerosols are better deposited with slow flows and breath holding.

Unfortunately, manufacturers and evaluators of aerosol equipment have not yet agreed on a uniform set of standards to allow easy assessment of performance. Recently, there has been more interest in research in small-volume medication nebulizers and their comparative performance. However, similar data on large-reservoir and disposable jet nebulizers have not always been made available.

FACTORS INFLUENCING PENETRATION AND DEPOSITION OF AEROSOLS IN THE LUNG

Three primary physical principles determine aerosol particle deposition: inertial impaction, sedimentation, and diffusion. *Inertial impaction* describes deposition of particles by collision with surfaces. This would most commonly occur as particles pass through the first 10 airway generations. Aerosols experience turbulent gas flows and abrupt airway bends, such as at bifurcations. With increased velocities from high inspiratory flows (> 30 L/min), particles tend to deposit in the upper airway zones. Finally, the size or mass of the particle affects the tendency for impaction. Particles in the 5- to 10-µm range tend to deposit before they reach bronchioles of 2-mm diameter.

Gravitational sedimentation is the term used to describe deposition of particles as they reach a velocity too slow to maintain travel. This time-dependent mechanism is believed to affect particles down to 1 µm in diameter. Deposition occurs in the last five or six airway generations. A patient's breath-holding time is the most significant factor in promoting deposition by sedimentation. A parallel physical mechanism that promotes deposition is that caused by *Brownian motion.* Random motion of aerosol particles by carrier gas molecules can cause fallout of the aerosol. This may be of only theoretical interest, as the particles are quite small (0.5 µm).

Actual measurements of penetration and deposition of aerosols in the lung zones have documented the combined effects of inertial impaction and sedimentation. There is some variation in the literature on specifics, but in general, a patient's breathing pattern and the particle size generated are the major factors. Figure 15-17

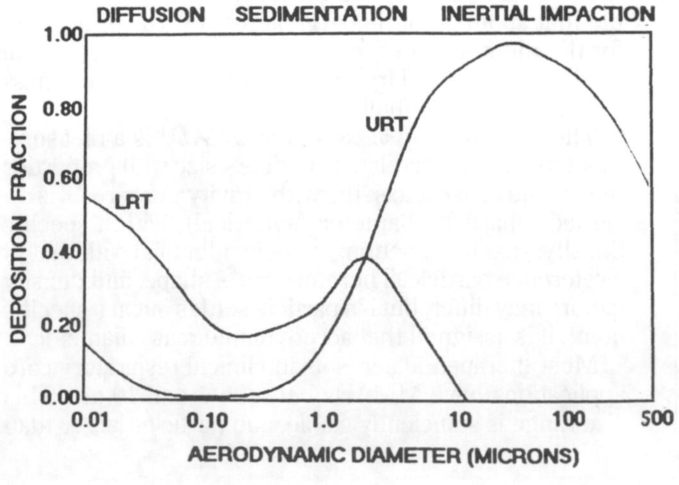

DIFFUSION SEDIMENTATION INERTIAL IMPACTION
DEPOSITION FRACTION
1.00
0.80
0.60
0.40
0.20
0.00
URT
LRT
0.01 0.10 1.0 10 100 500
AERODYNAMIC DIAMETER (MICRONS)

FIGURE 15-17. Proportions of aerosol deposition throughout the lung versus particle size (see text). (From Hess D. In: Dantzker DR, McIntyre NR, Bakow ED. (eds.) Comprehensive Respiratory Care. Philadelphia: W. B. Saunders, 1995. With permission.)

describes percentage of aerosol deposition in the upper (URT) and lower respiratory tract (LRT) versus particle diameter. Box 15-10 summarizes particle size with mean percentage of deposition, by general lung zone. In general, only 10% to 12% of particles from clinical nebulizers are retained in the lung.

The patient's *pattern of breathing* influences aerosol distribution and deposition. When using small-volume nebulizers (SVNs) and metered dose inhalers (MDIs), high inspiratory flows (> 1 L/sec) promote turbulence and particle deposition of large diameter particles on central airways. Conversely, slower inspiratory flows (< 0.5 L/sec) result in laminar flows and should produce greater delivery to peripheral bronchi.[62,63] *Technique and timing of device actuation* can be significant factors in deposition of aerosols, especially for MDIs. A 4- to 10-second breath hold following inhalation has a significant effect on increasing deposition of aerosols deliverd by MDIs and SVNs, though the effect is less significant for DPIs. Slow flow combined with breath holding is more important than the volume of the breath in determining favorable deposition patterns. Greater inspired volume does increase the volume of aerosol taken into the lung. There have been conflicting data on the effect of lung volume at which inhalation begins on deposition. It appears to be unimportant provided that a complete slow inhalation occurs. Teaching patients to actuate their MDIs as they slowly inhale from their functional residual capacity (FRC) appears reasonable.[64–66]

The *size and condition* of the conducting airways influence aerosol deposition. Aerosol penetration is more difficult through smaller anatomical, bronchospastic airways or endotracheal tubes.[65,67,68]

Aerosol *device performance* characteristics are determining in clinical practice. In general, only 10% to 12% of particles from medication nebulizers (MDIs, SVNs, and DPIs) are deposited in the lung of spontaneously breathing normal subjects. With endotracheal intubation, that figure drops to 4% to 5%.[65]

RATIONALE AND USE FOR CLINICAL AEROSOLS

History of Aerosol Therapy

There is a long record of aerosol therapy. Ancients began the practice of inhaling the smoke from various burning medicinal plants. Atropine-prepared cigarettes (Asmador) were first available in the early 1900s.[69] Steam vaporizers have been used with a variety of substances such as eucalyptus to treat viscid bronchial secretions. Aerosolized inhalation of epinephrine for bronchospasm and bronchial congestion was initiated in the United States in the mid-1930s. Alvan Barach promoted use of sympathomimetic agents including phenylephrine in the 1940s with devices such as the DeVilbiss and Vaponephrin nebulizers. The first reservoir nebulizers for mist therapy appeared in the early 1950s. Work by French physiologist Lucien Dautrebande extended the clinical knowledge of medicated aerosols through the 1960s. Aerosols were combined with intermittent positive-pressure breathing (IPPB) therapy in the 1960s to 1970s. Small-volume nebulizers became technically proficient, and bronchodilators more selective, in the 1980s and 1990s.

Aerosols are currently used for a variety of diagnostic tests and therapy. Box 15-11 summarizes the scope of practice.

Diagnostic and Therapeutic Aerosols

Diagnostic aerosols are used to evaluate a variety of pulmonary disorders. Mucociliary clearance of particles can be evaluated in disorders with ciliary dysfunction. Technetium 99m–labeled albumin (or sulfur colloid) and neutralized indium 133m chloride are agents that are used (clearance of agents demonstrates mucociliary activity). Bronchial provocation agents such as methacholine (Mecholyl) and histamine are used to determine if asymptomatic subjects demonstrate increased bronchial reactivity to the bronchospastic agents. A positive response would be defined as a 10% to 20% decrease from baseline of forced expiratory volume in 1 second (FEV_1).[70] Radioactively tagged aerosols (eg, xenon 133) can be inhaled to examine their lung distribution by τ-ray detectors. Xenon 133 is used in ventilation-perfusion lung scanning for suspected vascular disease or localized airway disorders.

Therapeutic aerosols are incorporated in the treatment of a variety of disorders. Table 15-6 lists major categories, with examples of drug groups and general usage. Box 15-12 summarizes the advantages of the aerosol route. (See AARC Clinical Practice Guideline: Delivery of Aerosols to the Upper Airway)

Aerosol therapy is one of the main forms of delivering drugs for prophylaxis or treatment of bronchospasm seen in asthma and other obstructive disorders, such as chronic bronchitis and cystic fibrosis.[71] The medication

BOX 15-10

MASS MEAN AERODYNAMIC DIAMETER (MMAD) AND DEPOSITION IN LUNG

MMAD (μm)	Lung Target Zone
0.8–2	Parenchyma
2–5	Lower airways
>5	Upper airways

BOX 15-11

SCOPE OF AEROSOLS IN DIAGNOSTIC TESTS AND THERAPEUTICS

- Diagnostic testing: Asthma challenge, $\dot{V}/\dot{Q}$ scanning
- Medical aerosols: Bronchodilators, anti-inflammatory agents, and antimicrobials
- Hydration of pulmonary secretions
- Sputum induction
- Humidification of medical gases

TABLE 15-6 **Major Categories of Medicated Aerosols and Clinical Use**

Drug Category	Generic (Trade) Examples	Disease Condition
Bronchodilators		
anticholinergic	ipratropium bromide (Atrovent)	Asthma or bronchospasm
sympathomimetic	albuterol (Ventolin)	Asthma or bronchospasm
Decongestant/vasoconstrictor		
sympathomimetic	racemic epinephrine (Vaponephrine)	Upper airway edema (eg, croup)
Antiasthmatic	cromolyn sodium (Intal)	Prophylaxis for bronchospasm
Anti-inflammatory corticosteroid	triamcinolone (Azmacort)	Asthma or inflammation
Mucoregulators		
mucolytic	acetylcysteine (Mucomyst)	Secretion retention
proteolytic	rhDNAse (Pulmozyme)	Infection (cystic fibrosis)
airway electrolyte	amiloride	Cystic fibrosis
Antimicrobial		Topical treatment of lung infections
antibacterial	gentamicin	*Pseudomonas*
antifungal	pentamidine isethionate (Nebupent)	*Pneumocystis*
antiviral	ribavirin (Virazol)	Respiratory syncytial virus (RSV)
Anesthetic	lidocaine (Xylocaine)	Preintubation and hiccups (singultus)
Surface tension–active	50% ethyl alcohol	Pulmonary edema

groups most frequently prescribed are the β_2 adrenergic agonist bronchodilators, corticosteroids, and cromolyn sodium. Therapy may be as simple as a self-administered MDI, on an as-needed basis, or before exercise. Aerosol therapy may also be involved in a complex medical regimen that includes parenteral medications. The emergency treatment of acute exacerbations of asthma involves an aerosol β-adrenergic agonist as the first drug of choice.[71,72] Parenteral sympathomimetics, corticosteroids, or methylxanthines are reserved for use in asthmatics whose initial response to inhaled medications is poor.[73] This signals the need for hospitalization and allows additional treatment beyond the emergency room.[72]

Aerosols of adrenergic agonists cause fewer untoward effects, such as tremor, tachycardia, palpitations, and the like, than equivalent doses of oral or intravenous medications. This is also true for the cholinergic-blocking drug ipratropium, reducing atropinelike effects.

Similarly, inhaled topical steroids act effectively in the lung. Aerosol preparations produce low serum levels, thus decreasing the risk of serious complications of long-term systemic steroid therapy.[74] Topical steroids are the preferred maintenance therapy for mild or moderate asthma.

Cromolyn sodium is a prophylactic aerosolized drug for asthma. However, it has no role in treatment and is contraindicated for urgent therapy.

BOX 15-12

ADVANTAGES OF THE AEROSOLIZED ROUTE FOR MEDICATIONS

Smaller dosage required than with systemic therapy
Usually has rapid therapeutic effect
Side effects are usually reduced (especially extrapulmonary ones)
Inhalational route normally is easily accessible
Administration is often simple (ie, patient self-administers)

Topical vasoconstriction delivered by aerosol therapy has been used in the treatment of tracheitis, laryngotracheobronchitis (croup), and before intubation or bronchoscopy.[3] In addition, nasal congestion caused by rhinitis is commonly treated with sympathomimetic agents with vasoconstricting properties. Aerosols in the 7- to 15-μm range are desirable to treat the upper airway.[75,76]

Results from administration of aerosolized antimicrobial agents for most pneumonias have generally been inferior to systemic administration. However, some controlled studies have shown value in controlling chronic pulmonary infections associated with cystic fibrosis.[77,78] Aerosol medications are FDA approved for use in therapy for respiratory syncytial virus (RSV) and prophylaxis and treatment of *Pneumocystis* pneumonia.[79,80] Topical treatment of pneumonia in alveoli requires aerosol particles to be in the 1- to 2-μm range.

Mucolytic drugs are used to aid the expectoration of mucus. Acetylcysteine acts to disrupt chemical bonds of mucoproteins.[81] Aerosolized recombinant deoxyribonuclease enzyme (rhDNase) reduces the viscoelasticity of purulent sputum laden with extracellular DNA from neutrophil breakdown. Patients with cystic fibrosis appear to benefit, as seen by reduced frequency of pneumonias and preservation of pulmonary function over time.[82]

Local anesthesia to the upper airway has been provided by aerosolized agents such as lidocaine for procedures such as laryngoscopy, bronchoscopy, and elective intubation.[3] Patient discomfort is aided as well as reduction in gag reflex and choking. Anesthetic aerosols may also be of value in cases of intractable hiccups (singultus), although the intravenous route is also effective.[83]

Aerosolized alcohol has a controversial role in the treatment of airway-obstruction foam in acute pulmonary edema. Ethyl alcohol (50%) denatures the surfactant and modifies the surface tension of the edema fluid, thus decreasing the tendency for frothing of the protein-rich secretions.[77]

AARC Clinical Practice Guideline

DELIVERY OF AEROSOLS TO THE UPPER AIRWAY

Indications: Upper airway inflammation (eg, to relieve inflammation due to laryngotracheobronchitis), anesthesia (eg, to control pain and gagging during endoscopic procedures), rhinitis (eg, to relieve inflammation and vascular congestion), systemic disease (eg, to deliver peptides such as insulin).

Contraindications: Known hypersensitivity to the medication being delivered.

Assessment of Need: ***In upper airway inflammation:*** stridor, brassy crouplike cough, hoarseness following extubation, diagnosis of laryngotracheobronchitis or croup, recent extubation, evidence of inflamed upper airway, soft-tissue radiograph suggesting edema, increased work of breathing. *For anesthesia:* severe localized pain in upper airway, impending invasive instrumentation of the upper airway. *In rhinitis:* diagnosis of allergic, nonallergic, or infectious rhinitis; symptomatic need such as nasal congestion, rhinorrhea, sneezing, or itching of nose, eyes, or palate. *In systemic disease:* presence of a systemic disease that warrants intranasal delivery of a therapeutic agent.

Assessment of Outcome: ***In upper airway inflammation:*** effectiveness of administration may be indicated by reduced stridor; reduced hoarseness; improvement in soft-tissue radiograph; decreased work of breathing, as evidenced by decreased use of accessory muscles. *For anesthesia:* effectiveness of administration is marked by reduced discomfort in the patient. *For rhinitis:* effectiveness of administration may be indicated by reduced nasal congestion; improved airflow through nose; reduced rhinorrhea; reduced sneezing; reduced itching of nose, eyes, or palate. *For systemic disease:* effectiveness of administration of agent is marked by the presence of the appropriate systemic therapeutic response.

Monitoring: The extent of patient monitoring should be determined on the basis of the stability and severity of the patient's condition: patient compliance and increase or decrease in symptoms, signs, and patient subjective response; heart rate and rhythm; blood pressure; change in indicators of therapeutic effect (eg, blood–glucose level with insulin).

From AARC Clinical Practice Guideline; see Respir Care 39:803, 1994, for complete text.

Hydration of Pulmonary Secretions and Sputum Induction

Bland aerosols of sterile water or isotonic saline have been administered with and without supplemental oxygen. There is no compelling scientific evidence to support the use of bland aerosols as mucoevacuants. However, periodic treatments with unheated bland aerosols of water or saline continue to be used in respiratory care.[4,84] (See AARC Clinical Practice Guideline: Bland Aerosol Administration) Bland aerosols are a poor substitute for appropriate systemic hydration (oral or parenteral). Indications for therapy include laryngotracheobronchitis (croup), subglottic edema, and postextubation edema. In addition, clinical practice also includes using aerosol generators instead of humidifiers when the upper airway is bypassed.[4] Studies show that only a small amount of water actually is deposited on the airways.[85] In objective studies, it is difficult to control variables such as cough, bronchial drainage, concomitant bronchodilator therapy, and type of disease. It is unclear whether clinical improvements are caused by just the liquefaction of mucus, stimulation of a vagally mediated production of mucus, or stimulation of cough receptors increasing expectoration.

AARC Clinical Practice Guideline

BLAND AEROSOL ADMINISTRATION

Indications: The presence of upper airway edema (cool bland aerosol—laryngotracheobronchitis, subglottic edema, postextubation edema, postoperative management of the upper airway); the presence of a bypassed upper airway; and the need for sputum specimens.

Contraindications: Bronchoconstriction and history of airway hyperresponsiveness.

Assessment of Need: The presence of one or more of the following may be an indication for administration of a water or isotonic or hypotonic saline aerosol: stridor; brassy, crouplike cough; hoarseness following extubation; diagnosis of laryngotracheobronchitis or croup; clinical history suggesting upper airway irritation and increased work of breathing (eg, smoke inhalation); and patient discomfort associated with airway instrumentation or insult. The presence of the need for sputum induction (eg, for diagnosis of *Pneumocystis carinii* pneumonia tuberculosis) is an indication for administration or hypertonic saline aerosol.

Assessment of Outcome: With administration of water or hypotonic or isotonic saline, the desired outcome is the presence of one or more of the following: decreased work of breathing, improved vital signs, decreased strider, decreased dyspnea, improved arterial blood gas values, and improved oxygen saturation as indicated by pulse oximetry. With administration of hypertonic saline, the desired outcome is a sputum sample adequate for analysis.

Monitoring: The extent of patient monitoring should be determined on the basis of the stability and severity of the patient's condition. Patient subjective response (pain, discomfort, dyspnea, restlessness); heart rate and rhythm; blood pressure; respiratory rate, pattern, mechanics, accessory muscle use; sputum quantity, color, consistency, odor; skin color; breath sounds; and pulse oximetry (if hypoxemia is suspected).

From AARC Clinical Practice Guideline: For complete text see Respir Care 38:1196–1200, 1993.

Aerosol therapy may be considered as supportive to more definitive methods of secretion mobilization through systemic hydration and chest physical therapy procedures, including effective coughing. Assessment of need includes stridor; brassy, crouplike cough; hoarseness or discomfort following extubation; and clinical history of upper airway irritation. Pediatric patients with croup and patients with postextubation laryngospasm have traditionally been treated with cool mist aerosols. The mist tent has been used for croup because of the difficulty with placement of masks on young children. However, its clinical value has been difficult to document.[81] In addition, some practitioners question a patient environment that might cause chilling, increases risk of bacterial contamination, offers poor visibility and poor access to the child. Use of topical aerosols such as racemic epinephrine for croup has an established role in treatment.[75]

There have been few clinical data to support the use of bland aerosols to treat postextubation laryngeal edema. Whether the high-humidity environment or the aerosol deposition on the upper airway produces a positive effect has not been clearly established.

In the past, children with cystic fibrosis were treated with mist tents while sleeping. This was abandoned after documentation of its ineffectiveness in delivering bland mists to the entire tracheobronchial tree. With nose breathing, at rest, deposition was localized to the upper airway.[81]

Sputum induction for microbiologic or cytologic examination is based on the empiric evidence that aerosols facilitate productive cough. Agents such as water, normal saline, or hypertonic saline mixtures may activate vagal pathways and augment production of mucus.[11] More likely, the irritant effects of the aerosol produce a profound stimulation to cough. Traditionally, ultrasonic or high-output pneumatic nebulizers have been used for this purpose.[81,86]

Humidification of Medical Gases

Before the availability of efficient heated humidifiers, both ultrasonic and cool or heated nebulizers were used to humidify medical gases. This included systems for both spontaneous breathing and mechanical ventilation. The rationale was to use devices that had the capability of adding enough water to oxygen or air to reach 100% body humidity levels. Currently, it is unusual to see nebulizers used as the primary humidifying device for mechanical ventilators. However, large-volume or mainstream nebulizers continue to be applied to humidify medical gases for patients with artificial airways or those breathing through the nose and mouth. The Briggs "T" piece, face mask or tent, and tracheostomy collars are frequently coupled with large-bore tubing and nebulizers.

This practice of using large-volume nebulizers with oxygen or air dilution appears to be based on tradition and reduced cost (compared with heated humidifiers and oxygen blender). Patients receiving oxygen by such systems may not always present an objective need for aerosol therapy (ie, hoarseness, stridor, and so forth). Although a relatively safe practice, such aerosol systems are not as effective as heated humidifiers or HMEs. Aerosol systems pose greater risks for microbial infection, overhydration, bronchoconstriction, and impairment of mucus transport.[4] Any aerosol particle is a potential bronchoconstrictive agent to asthmatics. It is prudent to recommend that this group, as well as others (eg, patients with bronchitis or cystic fibrosis) who exhibit increased airway resistance, be changed to humidification systems. The use of heated humidifiers appears to be the most desirable clinical method of delivering humidified high-flow medical gases for patients whose upper airway is bypassed. The primary benefits are that contamination is less of an issue and equipment needs to be changed infrequently (if at all).[3,59]

HAZARDS RELATED TO AEROSOL THERAPY

Although specific problems with each type of aerosol generator will be described, Box 15-13 lists major complications and hazards; a discussion follows.

Untoward Responses

Depending on the type of drug administered by aerosol methods, side effects can occur. Practitioners monitoring patients should be aware of the following side effects for the major categories of aerosolizable drug:

Bronchodilators
- Sympathomimetic (eg, epinephrine)—tachycardia, blood pressure changes, palpitations, central nervous system effects (headache, nervousness, irritability, anxiety, and insomnia), muscle tremor, nausea, increase in glucose, acute drop in arterial oxygen tension, and paroxysmal coughing with or without syncope
- Parasympatholytic (eg, atropine)—dryness of mouth and skin, tachycardia, blurred vision, dysphagia, dysphonia, difficulty with micturition, and mental confusion or excitement

Antiasthmatic (eg, cromolyn sodium)—bronchospasm, hoarseness, and dry mouth

Mucolytic (eg, acetylcysteine)—bronchospasm, bronchorrhea, and nausea

Corticosteroids (eg, triamcinolone)—upper airway fungal infections with *Candida* or *Aspergillus,* throat irritation, dry mouth, and coughing

Antimicrobial agents—anaphylactic sensitivity reactions and others specific to the drug

Bronchospasm and Nasal Irritation

Patients with hypersensitive airways have a tendency to develop increased airway resistance when aerosols are inspired. Certain substances are particularly irritating,

BOX 15-13

COMPLICATIONS AND HAZARDS OF AEROSOL THERAPY

- Drug-related untoward response
- Bronchospasm
- Nosocomial infection
- Airway burns
- Sound levels (newborns and infants only)
- Care-giver exposures (infectious and drug)
- Ineffective airway hydration

such as acetylcysteine, cromolyn sodium (powder), hypertonic saline, and antimicrobial agents. Paroxysms of coughing with or without syncope can occur. Pretreatment or simultaneous treatment with a rapid-acting β-adrenergic bronchodilating drug is often indicated. Aerosols of sterile water or normal saline have caused bronchospasm especially with high-output nebulizers.[4,87] Paradoxic response to inhaled bronchodilators does occur but is an uncommon finding.[4,88] Complications of α-adrenergic agonists include nasal irritation, burning sensation, sneezing attacks, and mucosal ulceration or bleeding. With extended use, patients risk nasal rebound (rhinitis medicamentosa).[3]

Infectious Contamination

Bacterial contamination of aerosol systems can occur as a result of cross-contamination or auto-infection. This was more of a problem in the 1960s before the use of ethylene oxide gas for sterilization procedures (for heat sensitive equipment). Large-volume nebulizers pose the greatest risk. Gram-negative bacteria appear to be the most common infecting agents. The hands of the workers changing water supplies, reflux of contaminated condensate, and contaminated water supplies have all been implicated.[3,4,89]

Airway Burns

Airway burns have occurred when immersion or bottom plate nebulizer heaters are improperly set or are defective and "run wild," or when reservoirs run out of water and heat inspired gas directly. Airway temperatures more than 44°C can potentially burn mucosal surfaces.[4]

Sound Levels

Sound levels of pneumatic nebulizers may cause hearing loss in newborns receiving humidified supplemental oxygen in enclosures such as hoods or incubators. The American Academy of Pediatrics Committee on Environmental Hazards recommends a level below 58 decibels (dB).[90] Such levels are exceeded by most mainstream nebulizers, even with 60 cm of tubing leading to the enclosure. Heated humidifiers are the preferred device.[1,91]

Overhydration and Excessive Salt Loads

Patients receiving long-duration or continuous aerosol therapy from high-output nebulizers may be subjected to fluid or sodium chloride overload. A positive water balance can occur with intubated and ventilated patients because of abolition of the normal exhaled water loss and increased antidiuretic hormone levels. Patients at greatest risk are in the neonatal or pediatric group and those with renal failure and congestive heart failure. Monitoring of urine output, body weight, electrolyte concentrations, and consistency of pulmonary secretions can indicate problems in this area.[4,92]

Care-Giver Exposure

Respiratory care practitioners are at risk for increased exposure to infections from droplet nuclei as a consequence of nebulization and patient coughing.[3] The respiratory care practitioner is also at risk to exposure from toxic aerosol exhausts, primarily antimicrobial drugs (eg, pentamidine and ribavirin). Patient enclosures, laminar hoods, exhalation filters, and wearing of efficient masks are prudent measures during drug therapy or sputum induction with bland aerosols.[93]

AEROSOL EQUIPMENT AND THERAPY

An array of aerosol-generating devices is currently available. The purpose of this section is to review general categories of equipment and key aspects of therapy. Major device groups include small-volume nebulizers (SVN), metered-dose inhalers (MDI), dry-powder inhalers (DPI), large-volume jet nebulizers, and ultrasonic nebulizers (USN). For details on specific models, the reader is referred to texts focusing on equipment and to manufacturers' literature.[34–36]

Small-Volume Nebulizers

Small-volume nebulizers (SVN) have been used to dispense medication since the 1940s. Early glass hand-bulb units were "baffled" versions of unbaffled atomizers (Figs. 15-18 and 15-19*A*). Today, there are a variety of contemporary devices that use the same principles, with various techniques and levels of sophistication of baffling. These "jet" nebulizers use the *Venturi application* of the *Bernoulli theorem.* A high-pressure gas source is passed through a constriction. The gas jet is positioned at an intersection of a tube that has the opposite end immersed in a fluid. The constriction increases gas velocity and decreases lateral pressure. Liquid is drawn up by the subatmospheric pressure and immediately shattered into small particles. The flow of

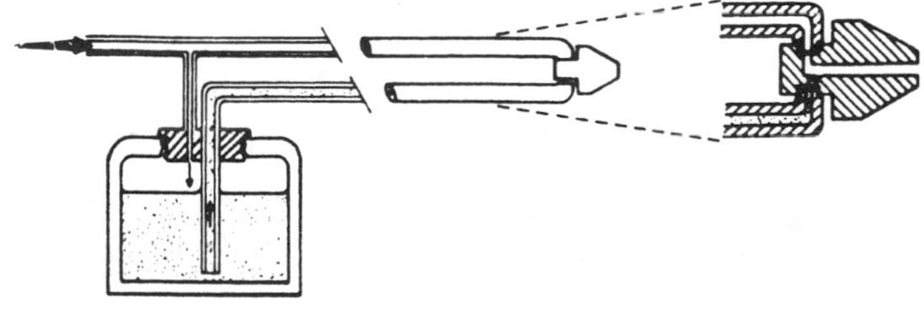

FIGURE 15-18. Sectional diagram of an atomizer. Pressurized air is applied at the point indicated by an arrow. This may be applied by a hand bulb. Common applications are administration of a local anesthetic for a tracheal intubation, endoscopy, or otolaryngology.

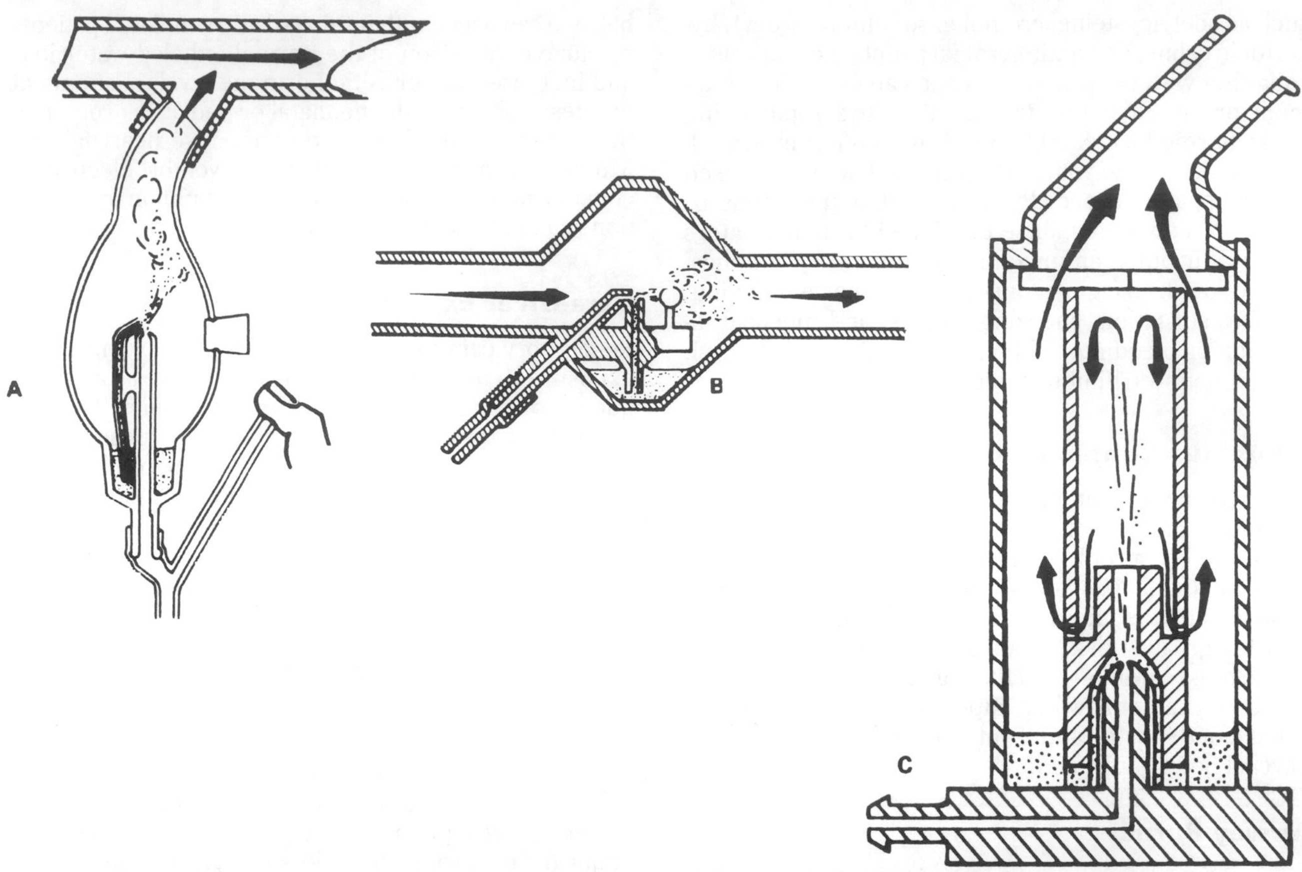

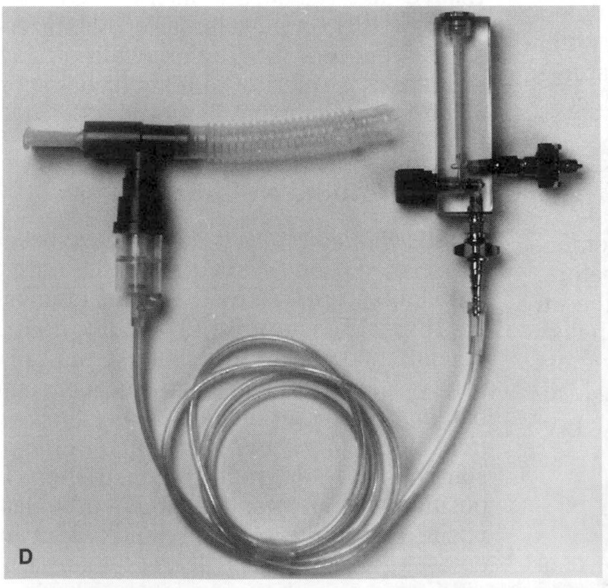

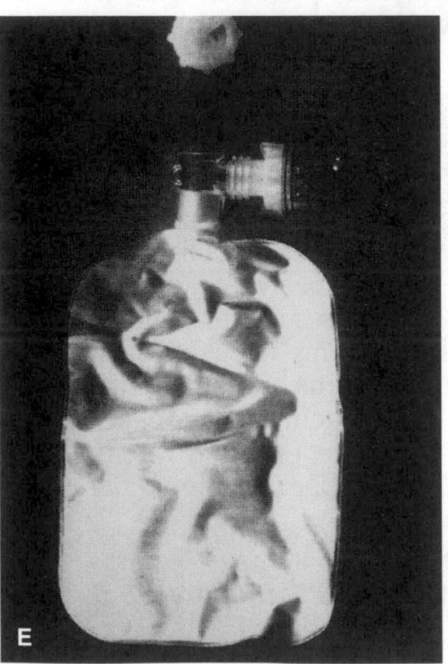

FIGURE 15-19. Sectional diagrams and photograph of medication nebulizers: **(A)** Vintage glass "sidestream" unit, with "wye" gas actuator; **(B)** Bird "mainstream" medication nebulizer; **(C)** Dautrebande design of baffling system used in contemporary medication nebulizer (R.E. Reynolds Co.); **(D)** Photograph of hand-held nebulizer, flowmeter, connecting tubing with thumb-operated gas port, and distal tubing reservoir; **(E)** Circulaire system combining a bag-reservoir with SVN. (From Mason JW, Miller WC, Small S: Comparison of aerosol delivery via Circulaire system vs. conventional small-volume nebulizer. Respir Care 1994;39:1157. With permission.)

gas and aerosols is directed at surfaces; hence, particles too large for therapeutic use impact and are retained in the liquid reservoir. Figure 15-19*A* illustrates nebulized medication being aerosolized in a side-stream design, and 15-19*B* shows a mainstream approach. Mainstream flow tends to carry larger particles to the patient. Dautrebande was known for his early work with sophisticated baffling systems, which can still be seen in contemporary nebulizers (Fig. 15-19*C*).

□ CLINICAL APPLICATION

Jet medication nebulizers are used as simple hand-held devices powered by either portable compressors or hospital gas supplies. Providing a compressed gas source is a high initial expense and an inconvenience for portable use, home, or work. However, SVNs do not rely on soon-to-be banned chlorofluorocarbon-containing compounds of MDIs and may gain in popularity. Small-volume nebulizers have been used extensively for administration of bronchodilators and other drugs, and they appear to be the device of choice for administration of β-adrenergic agonists in the initial phase of acute asthma.[72,94] The nebulizer may simply be placed in the vertical section of a breathing T-piece, with mouthpiece on one side and aerosol reservoir tubing on the other (Fig. 15-19*D*). Aerosol face masks allow fitting the upright nebulizer in the lower mask. Small-volume nebulizers have been incorporated into breathing circuits of intermittent positive-pressure breathing (IPPB) machines and mechanical ventilator circuits. Combining the SVN with a positive-pressure device facilitates aerosol delivery for patients incapable of adequate spontaneous inhalation (eg, vital capacity < 1.5 times the predicted tidal volume) or for synchronizing inspiration with nebulization.

□ PERFORMANCE AND FACTORS AFFECTING EFFICACY

Most small-volume nebulizers produce total fluid outputs of 1 to 2 mL/min. Aerosol particle diameters range from 1 to 5 μm (MMAD). In clinical practice, efficacy is based on several factors. Box 15-14 lists major factors to consider in care of spontaneously breathing patients.

Small-volume nebulizers are not efficient devices. With optimal conditions, only 8% to 12% of fluid in the medication cup is deposited in the lungs of spontaneously breathing patients. The majority of medication is lost in the nebulizer or exhaled (Fig. 15-20).[95] Doses

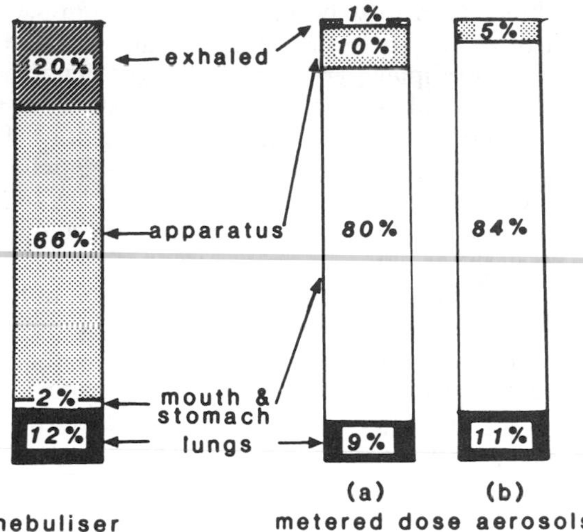

FIGURE 15-20. Fractional deposition of aerosol from small-volume (jet) nebulizer (SVN) and metered dose inhaler (MDI) (From Lewis RA, Fleming JS: Fractional deposition form a jet nebulizer: how it differs for a metered dose inhaler. Br J Dis Chest 1985; 79;361. Reproduced with permission.)

are larger by approximately 10-fold compared with those of MDIs. (The recommended dose of albuterol is 2.5 mg diluted in saline; 12% deposition would be 0.3 mg, or 300 μg. In contrast, the recommended MDI dose is 2 puffs, or 180 μg; 12% would be 21.6 μg.)

Many models of SVNs are commercially available, either disposable or reusable. Performance may vary considerably among brands and among nebulizers of the same model. A number of bench evaluations of commercial nebulizers with different types of medication have been published.[79,96–102] Both the time required for treatment and the percentage of particles in the respirable range (1 to 5 μm) should be considered by clinicians. Smaller particles would be required for treating parenchymal infections (0.8 to 3 μm) than for bronchodilator therapy (2 to 5 μm).[79] High delivery rates, not uniformity of particle size, is key in acute bronchodilator therapy. In other applications, time is less critical, and maximizing the percentage of respirable drug from the medication bowl is most important.[79,97]

Advantages of SVNs over MDIs include less patient coordination in technique, and ability to provide high doses and continuous nebulization. Clinical situations in which SVN therapy is preferable to an MDI include (1) patients incapable of performing the MDI maneuver (after appropriate instruction and attempt to incorporate auxiliary aids), and (2) adults who have a vital capacity <1.5 times their predicted tidal volume (7 mL/kg) **or** inspired flows <0.5 L/sec **or** breath hold <4 sec. Disadvantages to SVNs relate to the expense of a gas source, reduced portability, possibility for contamination if not cleaned properly, and nonavailability of medications.[6] In the United States, there are no currently FDA-approved nebulizable anticholinergic or corticosteroid solutions.

Use of distal tubing or bag *reservoirs* allows for improved performance (see Fig. 15-19*D,E*).[103,104] Small-vol-

BOX 15-14

FACTORS AFFECTING EFFICACY OF SVNS

- Performance of nebulizer design
- Use of reservoir
- Medication dead volume and flow of pressurized gas
- Temperature and humidity
- Patient technique and ventilatory pattern
- Dosing strategy

ume nebulizers can also be inserted into openings in the bottom of aerosol-type face masks that offer a small reservoir. Mouthpiece breathing is more efficient compared with face masks, which increase waste; however, there may be no difference in patient response. Less drug is wasted in nonreservoir systems by allowing patients to control the flow of gas to the nebulizer, so nebulization occurs only during inspiration by use of a finger-operated Y piece.

Regardless of design, a *dead volume* of solution (0.5 to 1 mL) can remain in SVNs after nebulization treatments. Frequent tapping of the nebulizer chamber should continue until dry. Bench testing has shown that optimal drug delivery occurs with large volumes of drug diluent (approximately 4 mL). Aerosol particle size is directly proportional to compressed gas flow. Flows of 8 mL/min (minimum of 6 L/min) are associated with reductions in both MMAD and dead-space volume.[102] Unfortunately, domiciliary use is frequently carried out with small-capacity compressors that cannot develop such flows with the resistance of the nebulizer jet. If flows of 8 L/min are used, medication diluent volumes can be increased from the often listed 2 mL up to 4 to 6 mL. The combination of high flows and larger volumes is recommended to ensure the highest output, smallest particle size, and reasonable treatment time.[65]

Gas flow driving the SVN causes a temperature reduction of the aerosol solution to about 8° to 12°F below ambient temperature. This is caused by evaporation and adiabatic expansion of the gas. This results in increased drug concentration of the remaining solution. Cool particles decrease their size as they rewarm. Temperature change of the solution can be minimized by having patients hold the medication cup in a closed hand.[65]

Correct aerosol inhalation technique should occur through an open mouth using a mask or mouthpiece. Respiratory care practitioners should match the aerosol mouth or face appliance to the patient's needs and preference. Intermittent nebulization by controlling flow by patient occlusion of a finger port results in improved drug delivery. Box 15-15 summarizes the steps in proper SVN technique for spontaneously breathing patients.[65]

BOX 15-15

SMALL-VOLUME NEBULIZER TECHNIQUE (SPONTANEOUSLY BREATHING PATIENT)

- Note pretreatment patient data such as pulse, breath sounds, and spirometry (eg, FEV_1 or peak expiratory flow rate [PEFR])
- Place drug in nebulizer cup; dilute with normal saline to 4 mL
- Connect to driving gas system with intermittent finger port control
- Set driving gas flow at 6–8 L/min; place medication cup in patient's hand
- Instruct patient to inspire through open mouth (mask) or with closed lips (around mouthpiece)
- Instruct patient to inhale (normal tidal volumes) slowly (<0.5 L/sec) from normal end-exhalation level
- Instruct patient to inspire to total lung capacity (TLC) periodically and perform breath hold for 4–10 seconds
- Have patient tap nebulizer cup to minimize dead volume
- Monitor for presence of side effects (eg, tachycardia, tremor, and nausea)
- Monitor posttreatment outcome measures (eg, pulse, breath sounds, and FEV_1 or PEFR)

☐ DOSE AND DOSING STRATEGY

The determinants of dose requirements and treatment intervals for optimal aerosol delivery with minimal effects is a complex issue. For bronchodilation therapy, dosing is affected by severity of illness, type (potency) of agent, frequency of administration, and the response characteristics of the patient. The underlying responsiveness of each patient depends on the type of disease (eg, asthma vs. chronic bronchitis), the baseline degree of obstruction, and the component of airway inflammation. Assessment is made by combining subjective and objective measures pre- and post-treatment. Measured response to bronchodilators is influenced by changes in lung volume, accuracy of testing outside a pulmonary function lab, and variable patient performance.

Small-volume nebulizer bronchodilator doses recommended by drug manufacturers are based on studies of chronic stable asthmatics (refer to Chap. 16). Furthermore, suggested treatment intervals are commonly 3 to 4 hours for many bronchodilators (eg, albuterol). Such recommendations may provide inadequate therapy for severe acute asthma. Therefore, titration regimens allow gradual increasing doses at specific time intervals, until maximal improvement is achieved or adverse side effects noted. Bedside measurement of FEV_1 and PEFR provide objective evidence of therapeutic drug effect.[105,106] To guide care, treatment algorithms have been developed.[72] This scientific approach requires high levels of attention and time. (See AARC Clinical Practice Guideline: Assessing Response to Bronchodilator Therapy at Point of Care)

☐ EQUIPMENT TROUBLESHOOTING

Small-volume jet nebulizers are technically simple devices. Failure to produce mist is usually caused by interruption in gas flow, clogged fluid pickup system, or clogged jet orifice. Most manufacturers of reusable nebulizers suggest cleaning and air drying between uses. Medication nebulizers are a source for circuit leaks in mechanical ventilators, as well as for microbial contamination.[57] Nebulizers using continuous flow of gas can alter the ability of the ventilator's sensitivity mechanism or demand valves to respond to patient inspiratory effort.

☐ SPECIAL PURPOSE SMALL-VOLUME NEBULIZERS

An alternative approach for acute asthma not responding to intermittent dosing is use of *continuous small-volume nebulization.* The Heart nebulizer (Vortran Medical Technology) is a commercial example of an

AARC Clinical Practice Guideline

ASSESSING RESPONSE TO BRONCHODILATOR THERAPY AT POINT OF CARE

Indications: Assessment of airflow and other clinical indicators are indicated when the need exists to confirm the appropriateness of therapy; to individualize the patient's medication dose per treatment or frequency of administration; to help determine patient status during acute and long-term pharmacologic therapy; to determine a need for change in therapy (dose, frequency, or type of medication).

Contraindications: When patients present in acute, severe distress, some assessment maneuvers may be contraindicated or should be postponed until therapy (eg, bronchodilator treatment) and supportive measures (eg, oxygen therapy) have been instituted.

Assessment of Need: Response to therapy should be evaluated in all patients receiving bronchodilator therapy. However, patients in severe distress may need immediate treatment that precludes establishing a quantitative baseline. Assessment of response must be made with due regard for the patient's history, clinical presentation, and results of physical exam.

Assessment of Outcome: Assessment of outcome answers the question, How did assessment of the effect of bronchodilator therapy impact on patient management? *Action based on results of assessment:* increase or decrease in dose or frequency, change medications, add medications, continue regimen, discontinue therapy. *To guide patient management:* baseline condition and changes from baseline must be determined prior to therapy to establish respiratory and cardiovascular baseline values, to establish presence of clinical indicators and need for therapy, to identify presence of contraindications. *During therapy:* adverse responses to medication, any clinical change from baseline. *Following therapy:* adverse responses, therapeutic responses (time course for peak varies with different medications), lack of therapeutic response. *For trend analysis:* change in patient baseline, need to modify dose, need to change therapy, need to discontinue therapy, direction of change in bronchial responsiveness. *Patient's progress:* ability to self-assess and to recognize the need for more aggressive therapy and when and how to communicate with health professional. Record of symptoms and concurrent PEFR measurements should be kept for or by the patient at home.

Monitoring: Monitoring seeks to establish baseline function and reveal the presence or absence of a desirable response to bronchodilator or other airway medication, and to identify changes in airway reactivity in response to allergens, exercise, infection, or other causes. *From observation of the patient:* general appearance is improved, use of accessory muscles is decreased, sputum expectoration is increased. *From auscultation:* breath sounds may be improved, with a decrease in wheezing or adventitious breath sounds and air movement increased; decreased wheezing (eg, the silent chest coupled with decreased volume of air moved can be an indication of a worsening condition rather than improvement); vital signs are more nearly normal; patient reports improvement (eg, less dyspneic). *From pulmonary function measurement:* It is important to note that although correlation is generally high between values obtained by conventional spirometry and measurement of PEFR, agreement may be poor for individual patients; FEV_1, FVC, or $FEF_{25-75\%}$ are improved; the ATS standards for a positive bronchodilator response in adults is 12% increase, calculated from the prebronchodilator response values; a 200-mL increase in either FVC or FEV_1; dynamic compression of the airways during forced maneuvers may mask bronchodilator response in some patients, and for these patients the additional measurement of airway resistance and calculation of specific conductance may provide more diagnostic evidence. Peak expiratory flow rate is increased (National Asthma Education and Prevention [NAEPP] Guidelines provide detailed directions for use of the PEFR in the asthmatic population). Values for SaO_2 (or SpO_2) and arterial blood gas are improved (effects of underlying chronic respiratory, metabolic, or other condition should be considered). Exercise performance is improved as reflected by a more normal PEFR during exercise or immediately following an increase in distance achieved during the 6-minute walking test. *Ventilator variables are improved:* lower PIP (during volume ventilation), lower plateau pressure, increased static lung compliance, decreased inspiratory and expiratory resistance, increased expiratory flow, improved flow-volume loop, decreased auto-PEEP.

From AARC Clinical Practice Guideline, see Respir Care 40:1300, 1995, for complete text.

SVN with large-volume medication cup (Fig. 15-21*A*). In theory, this approach can maintain more consistent biologic levels of drug yet may demand more careful monitoring than frequent intermittent SVN therapy.[107] The manufacturer indicates that the liquid output is 30 mL/hr with a driving gas flow of 10 L/min, and 50 mL/hr at a flow of 15 L/min. Noncommercial SVN devices have been developed using readily available oxygen delivery components (nonrebreathing oxygen mask and reservoir bag), continuous IV-drip feed, and standard SVNs (Fig. 15-21*B*).

Specialized SVNs such as the Respirguard II (Marquest) have been developed to target deposition of drug in alveolar zones, requiring particles with MMAD of 0.8 to 3 μm. Parenchymal deposition is favored by use of a "wye," with one-way valves allowing unidirectional patient gas flow (Fig. 15-22). One-way valves act as baffles to remove larger particles; the tubing reservoir makes a bolus of medication immediately available on inhalation. These and similar nebulizing systems have been used for topical administration of pentamidine isethionate (Pentam) for treatment or prophylaxis of *Pneumocystis carinii* pneumonia.[79,108] With normal inspiration, there is preferential distribution of gas particles to dependent lung zones. This has apparently resulted in relapses of pneumonia in the upper lobes. More homogeneous aerosol deposition may be achieved if patients initiate inspiration periodically from residual volume (RV), are recumbent, or breathe at higher frequencies.[79]

A continuous medication nebulizer specific for administration of the antiviral medication ribavirin (Virazole)

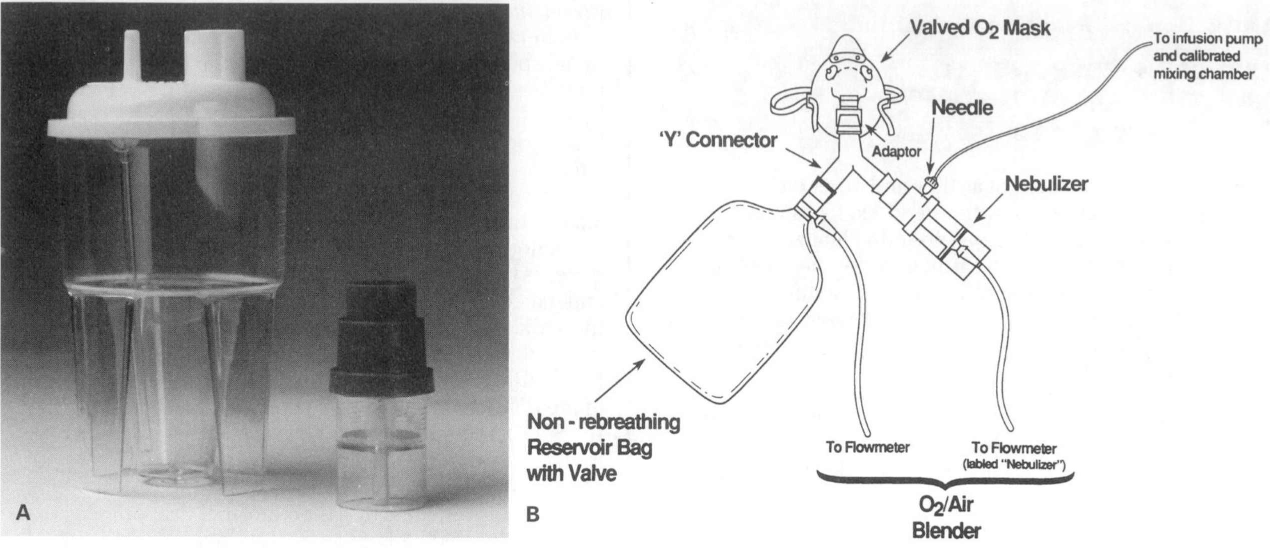

FIGURE 15-21. **(A)** Heart® nebulizer. An example of a SVN that can be administered continuously to either spontaneously or mechanically ventilated patients. **(B)** Non-commercial continuous aerosol device composed of a nonrebreathing oxygen mask with Y-adaptor and reservoir to administer continuous bronchodilator therapy. (From Moler FW, Johnson CE, Laanen CV, et al: Continuous versus intermittent nebulizer terbutaline: Plasma levels and effect. Am J Respir Crit Care Med. 1995;15:602.)

is commercially known as the *small-particle aerosol generator (SPAG)*. It was initially developed for treating selective groups of infants infected with respiratory syncytial virus (RSV). Most healthy infants can deal with this common infection. However, in children with congenital heart disease, immunodeficiency, or bronchopulmonary dysplasia, RSV can cause life-threatening pneumonia and bronchiolitis.[109] Ribavirin is also used to treat adults with RSV secondary to immunosupression (eg, posttransplant).

Ribavirin is supplied as a lyophilized crystalline powder that is reconstituted with sterile water. The aerosolizable solution's concentration is 20 mg/mL. The drug manufacturer provides the SPAG administration device (Fig. 15-23). The jet-type aerosol generator reduces 50 psig line pressure to 26 psig and allows regulation of flow to a nebulizer and drying chamber. The flow to the nebulizer should be 7 L/min and no less than 15 L/min total airflow, with use of the drying chamber flow meter. The particle diameter is nearly monodisperse, with aerosols in the 1.2- to 1.4-μm range.[110] Treatment with the medication proceeds over several consecutive days, depending on the severity of symptoms. The SPAG provides a retained dose of ribavirin of about 2.25 to 3 mg/kg of body weight when given for 18 to 24 hours.[111] The drug is poorly absorbed by the lung. High alveolar levels appear to interfere with viral replication. Administration through the SPAG can be performed using a head hood, aerosol mask, mist tent, or mechanical ventilator (Fig. 15-24). When a head hood is used, about 66% of the drug is delivered to the patient chamber.[110] Initially, there were problems with the ventilator route. However, with minor modification, appropriate attention to filtering exhaled air and pressure pop-off valves should prevent problems.[80,112]

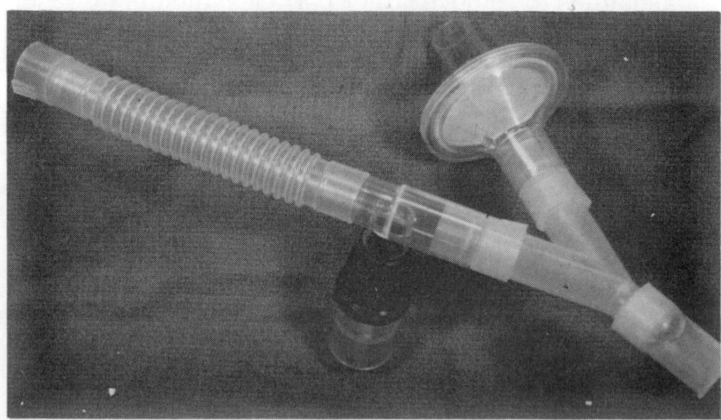

FIGURE 15-22. Respirguard II SVN medication nebulizer with one-way valves (for unidirectional gas flow), tubing reservoir, and expiratory particle filter.

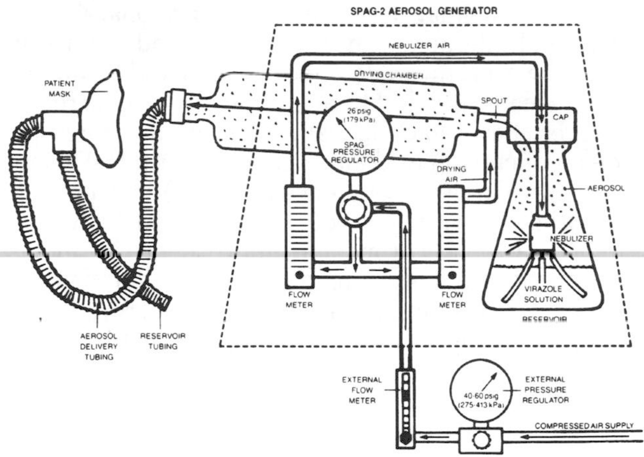

FIGURE 15-23. Sectional diagram of small-particle aerosol generator (SPAG) for administration of ribavarin aerosol. (Courtesy of ICN Pharmaceuticals, Inc.)

☐ SMALL-VOLUME NEBULIZER DELIVERY DURING MECHANICAL VENTILATION

Small-volume nebulizers have been adapted for use with mechanical ventilation since the 1960s as a likely carryover from their use with intermittent positive-pressure breathing (IPPB) devices. Small-volume nebulizers are placed in the inspiratory limb of the ventilator circuit, and side-stream aerosol is carried to the patient during tidal breathing. Some ventilators maintain constant tidal volume and F_{IO_2} by deferring part of the volume as the additional flow to the nebulizer during inspiration (only). Others require an auxiliary flow meter to power the SVN.

Recent studies have determined that aerosol deposition is significantly reduced in comparison with spontaneous breathing; reviews of that data are available.[65,113] Approximately 3% to 5% of therapeutic particles reach the lungs of ventilated adults. The endotracheal tube provides a significant barrier to aerosol penetration. Aerosol deposition to the lung is reduced as tube diameter decreases and with increasing inspiratory flow.[65]

Operation of SVNs for ventilator applications follow similar guidelines as for spontaneously breathing patients with regard to inlet flow, tapping medication cups, and so on. Deposition during ventilation can be enhanced by several techniques. The SVN should be positioned in the inspiratory circuit approximately 18 inches (46 cm) proximal to the ventilator Y piece. Heated humidifiers further decrease aerosol delivery and should be bypassed. Circuits with heated-wire hu-

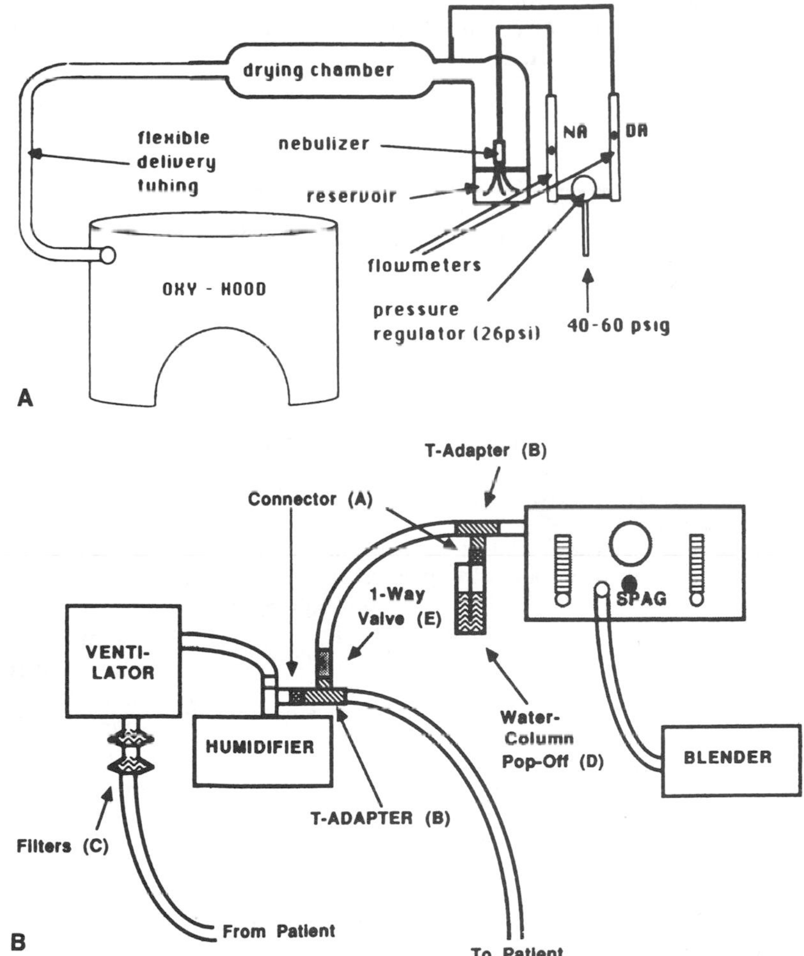

FIGURE 15-24. **(A)** Diagram of typical system for pediatric administration of ribavarin aerosol with SPAG and head hood. (Byron PR, Phillips EM, Kuhn R: Ribavarin administration by inhalation: Aerosol-generating factors controlling drug delivery to the lung. Respir Care 33:1011, 1988. Reproduced with permission); **(B)** Diagram of SPAG aerosol administration in combination with mechanical ventilation.

midifier systems make proper placement in the inspiratory limb difficult or impossible. They should be placed on their standby mode to prevent system malfunction during the treatment and also to avoid need to bypass the circuit. Heat and moisture exchangers must be removed for the duration of nebulization therapy to prevent filtering the medical aerosol before it reaches the lungs. Slow breathing frequencies and I:E ratios are adjusted to allow greater inspiratory time, favoring aerosol deposition. Inspiratory pause or hold time may be activated. When appropriate, tidal volumes for adults should be generous (12 mL/kg or greater). Intermittent nebulizer flow is desirable. When using continuous flow, tidal volumes (or flow) should be adjusted to preserve tidal or minute volume. Continuous flow can interfere with the subatmospheric pressure required to trigger mechanical ventilators in certain modes (eg, pressure support). In addition, the bias flow from the SVN may be interpreted as patient ventilation, resulting in failure of low minute ventilation alarms to detect apnea.[114,115] Nebulizers can deposit material on expiratory pneumotachygraphs and pressure sensors of some ventilators (eg, Siemens 900). Filters may be placed proximally to protect those devices. Box 15-16 summarizes SVN techniques applied in mechanical ventilation.

Titrating drug dose and evaluating effectiveness of SVN bronchodilator therapy in mechanically ventilated patients is not clear-cut. Airway changes caused by bronchodilation may be masked by the artificial airway, mechanical interaction by the patient, and ventilator mode. However, the effect may be evaluated by noting an increase in passive expiratory flows at specific recoil pressures. Favorable clinical response commonly includes reduction in peak pressures and auto-PEEP levels (when volume-preset modes are used).[116] Mechanical ventilators with microcomputer-interfaced visual graphics can display bronchodilator response by noting changes, in inspiratory-expiratory loops, of flow versus volume and pressure versus volume.[115] Figure 15-25 illustrates examples of the graphic display of bronchodilator response.

BOX 15-16

SMALL-VOLUME NEBULIZER TECHNIQUES (MECHANICAL VENTILATION)

- Note pretreatment patient data such as pulse, breath sounds, and ventilator parameters (eg, peak airway pressure and auto-PEEP levels)
- Heated-wire circuits should be placed in their standby function
- Remove HME from circuit
- Position side-stream nebulizer approximately 18 inches proximal to patient "wye"
- Use intermittent driving gas or continuous flow at 6–8 L/min
- With continuous flow, adjust flow to maintain pretreatment tidal volume or peak airway pressure
- Set tidal volume at 12 mL/kg or more unless contraindicated (volume-targeted modes)
- Set ventilator rate at 4–8 breaths/min unless contraindicated
- With pressure-support ventilation, add backup SIMV rate
- With pressure-limited infant ventilation, reduce ventilator flow to maintain constant total flow
- Tap nebulizer cup to minimize dead volume
- Monitor for presence of side effects (eg, tachycardia, tremor, and nausea)
- Monitor posttreatment outcome measures (eg, pulse, breath sounds, and other mechanical parameters)
- Return ventilator to pretreatment settings

Metered-Dose Inhalers

Metered-dose inhalers (MDIs) are glass, ceramic, or metal canisters containing drug in the form of a suspension of micronized crystals or in solution, with several propellants and dispersal agents. Metered-dose inhalers were first introduced in the mid-1950s and have become the most common administration device for topical respiratory medications (Fig. 15-26). Drugs are not soluble in propellants but can be dissolved in dispersal compounds. Manufacturers commonly employ soya lecithin, sorbitan trioleate, oleoyl alcohol, or oleic acid in volumes equal to that of the drug. *Chlorofluorocarbons (CFCs)*, such as Freon, or other propellants provide the positive pressure to activate the nebulization process and suspending medium. The vapor pressure of the propellants is high, approximately 3000 mmHg (400 kPa) being required to keep them as liquids at room temperature. When the device is actuated by pressing the nozzle down, the contents of a small metering chamber are released. Most MDIs have 50-µL size chambers that release 15 to 20 mL of gas on actuation. When the liquefied CFC gases exit the canister at temperatures above their boiling point, there is a flash boil, creating a fine aerosol of the dissolved or suspended drug. The propellant becomes a gas, leaving the drug suspended as droplets. The mass median aerodynamic diameter **at the orifice** is in the range of 35 µm or larger. However, particle size is reduced as the aerosol moves from the actuator orifice. Mass median aerodynamic diameter measured **at 10 cm from the orifice** ranges from 1.4 to 4.3 µm, but some particles may be as large as 40 µm. The weight of drug per "puff" varies among agents and ranges from 18 to 650 µg.[65,66,77,113,117,118]

International concern for the environment prompted the Montreal Protocol, which proposed a worldwide ban all CFC-based propellants beginning in 1978. However, medical aerosols were granted an extension until the year 2000.[119] Currently, pharmaceutical companies are investigating non-CFC gases and cosolvents that may provide suitable replacement.

□ CLINICAL APPLICATION

Over the past 15 years, the MDI has become the primary method of administering aerosolized drugs to patients. There is a variety of medications available

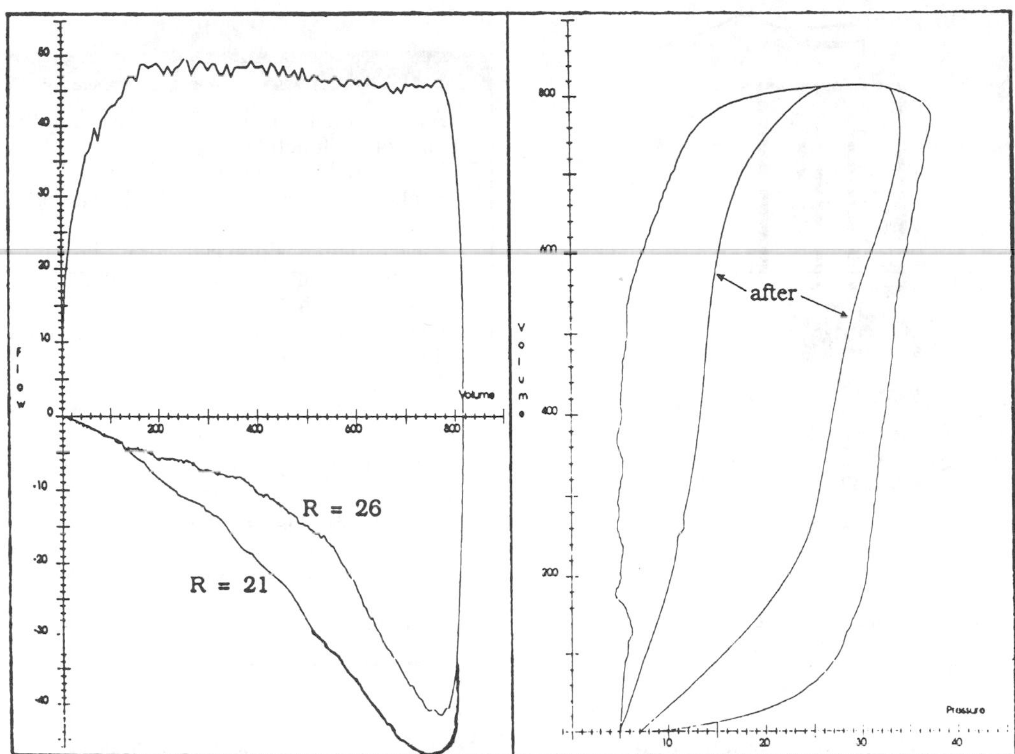

FIGURE 15-25. Examples of graphic displays of post-bronchodilator response during mechanical ventilation. *(left)* Flow vs. volume (expiratory flow is below the baseline) showing decreased airway resistance with increased flows at volume levels. *(right)* Pressure vs. volume loop demonstrating reduced airway pressures at volume levels labeled "after." (From Gross NJ, Jenne JW, Hess D: Bronchodilator Therapy. In Tobin MJ. ed. Principles and Practice of Mechanical Ventilation. New York: McGraw-Hill, 1994. With permission.)

including corticosteroids, bronchodilators, and antiasthma medications (eg, cromolyn sodium). Clinical acceptance has increased with the advent of adjunct devices such as self-actuating cartridges, connectors, spacers or holding chambers, and adapters for anesthesia or mechanical ventilation circuits.[2,65,66] Metered-dose inhalers have been used with increasing frequency in the hospital setting. Patients with stable asthma appear to obtain the same therapeutic effect from bronchodilators administered by MDIs as from those administered by small-volume jet nebulizers.[56,93,95,109] Metered-dose inhalers have been accepted for aerosol therapy in the ICU, emergency room, hospital wards, and pulmonary function lab as well as ambulatory practice.[120–124] There is also documentation of the potential cost savings of inhospital aerosol therapy by using MDIs as opposed to SVNs.[125,126]

□ PERFORMANCE AND FACTORS AFFECTING EFFICACY

MDI aerosol particle size is primarily dependent on the preparation of drug and condition of the propellant. The dimension of the nozzle plays a smaller role.[61] Most MDIs elaborate their contents in a fairly monodisperse pattern. There is a high level of variability in lung deposition because of technique-related issues. Under ideal conditions, between 9% and 11% of drug from MDIs (without adjuncts) is deposited in the lung (see Fig. 15-20). Unlike the SVN, which wastes drug in the apparatus (66%), the majority of drug wasted by MDIs (80%) is deposited in the oropharynx and stomach. However, the total dose (or amount wasted) is 4 to 10 times smaller than with the SVN. Metered-dose inhaler aerosol delivery to the patient involves additional effects that are summarized in Box 15-17.

Temperature affects the internal pressure of the propellant; with cooler-than-normal room temperatures, the lowered vapor pressure tends to produce larger particles. Patients living in cold climates should be instructed to carry MDIs close to their bodies and prewarm them before inhalation. Bench testing indicates that canisters at 37°C provide greatest deposition and smaller MMAD.[127] The first five puffs from a new MDI give variable doses and should be wasted. As the MDI canister is used, the remaining drug tends to concentrate as more propellant vaporizes to fill the canister's dead space. However, this effect is apparently balanced by the fact that most actuator valves decrease their dose through use. There is also a tendency for low doses to be emitted if the units are not used for several days. Shaking the canister and actuation once or twice is advocated.[65,66]

Lung deposition using MDIs is critically related to inhalation technique. The potential therapeutic drug dosage is relatively small, and delivering that dose to the

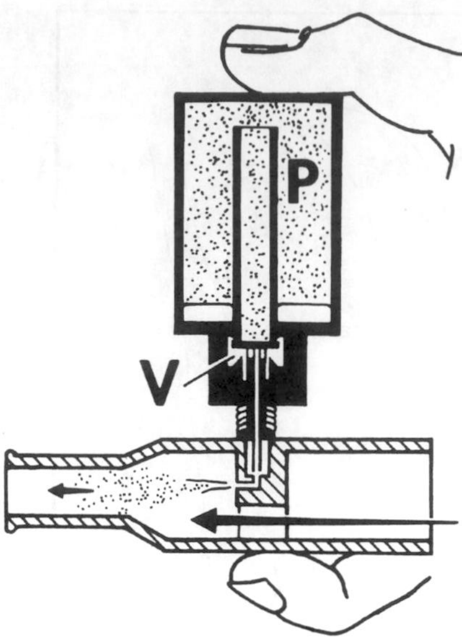

FIGURE 15-26. Sectional diagram of a gas-propelled hand nebulizer or metered-dose inhaler (MDI) for delivery of medication. (V) indicates the actuator valve, (P) is the fluid–vapor mixture containing the propellant and medication.

BOX 15-18

MDI TECHNIQUE

- Assess patient baseline data (pulse, breath sounds, and pulmonary function)
- Warm MDI to body temperature
- Shake vigorously (actuate if MDI has not been used in several days)
- Have patient position canister upright (nozzle down)
- Instruct patient to exhale to resting level
- Instruct patient to place mouthpiece 3 to 5 cm from the open mouth or place mouthpiece in mouth with open lips about mouthpiece
- Tell patient to:
  - Begin slow (<0.5 L/sec) inspiration to actuate inhaler as inhalation begins
  - Inspire deeply to total lung capacity
  - Hold breath for approximately 10 seconds (or, if less, as long as possible)
  - Wait 3–10 minutes before subsequent actuations
  - Repeat for subsequent doses
  - Rinse mouth or gargle
- Monitor patient for therapeutic and side effects

lung requires greater coordination with inspiration. Box 15-18 describes the proper MDI technique for spontaneously breathing patients without an artificial airway.

The major problem in clinical use is in proper patient education, coordination, and compliance. Even after appropriate education, some patients fail to master the skill or revert to incorrect technique.[123,128] It is estimated that 10% to 20% of patients fail to receive optimal aerosol deposition because of poor technique.[129] Most of this group are the very young and the elderly.[128] This has resulted in the development of a good deal of patient education literature, training effort, and inhalational aids.[64,66] The major problem relates to timing inhalation with canister actuation. Some patients just cannot perform the technique. Patients frequently stop inhalation when they feel the cold Freon on their pharynx. Alternately, they actuate the MDI after an inhalation has been completed. Other factors relate to aiming the device into mouth, placement in the mouth or tongue position, and failing to shake or clean the MDI.[66]

BOX 15-17

FACTORS AFFECTING EFFICACY OF MDIs (SPONTANEOUSLY BREATHING PATIENT)

- Temperature before actuation
- Technique
  - Lung volume at actuation
  - Inspiratory flow
  - Breath hold
  - MDI position
  - Timing of actuations
- Patient selection and instruction
- Dosing strategy

Current information does not clearly identify a superior MDI placement relative to the mouth. Although some studies identify a 3- to 4-cm distance as superior for its particle size effect, the problem of improperly aiming the MDI becomes much more clinically important. Placing the canister mouthpiece in the entrance of the open mouth is recommended.[65]

Greater bronchodilating effect of MDIs can occur with a delay between sequential actuations. It is likely that distribution of subsequent actuations is enhanced by the initial dose improving lung function. The ideal time is patient dependent and also based on practicality. Patients with episodic wheezing and poor control of symptoms derive greater benefit in delay than those with stable asthma.[130] There should be a minimum delay of 1 minute, with a 3- to 10-minute period recommended between doses.[65]

The respiratory care practitioner's role in patient education is emphasized in use of MDIs. Patients may require detailed individualized training initially and have their performance reevaluated. Respiratory care practitioners have been found to be the most proficient health care provider of in- and outpatient MDI instruction.[130–132]

□ DOSE AND DOSING STRATEGIES

Drug manufacturers do provide recommendations for MDI-administered drugs. Metered-dose inhaler canister valves regulate reasonably consistent doses per actuation, for example, 180 μg (90 μg/puff). Dose standards are based on care of patients with stable disease. It is likely that the typical β_2 agonist dose of two puffs may be conservative and suboptimal in bronchodilating effect in acutely ill patients. Up to 10 MDI actuations may be required to deliver the equivalent of a standard SVN dose of β_2 agonist.[71,106]

Those with severe acute asthma frequently cannot perform maneuvers required to deliver the MDI drug. Under these conditions, larger doses of aerosol medication are indicated because of the high inspiratory flows, low tidal volumes, and already narrowed peripheral airways.[68] Exhausted, dyspneic patients are unlikely to perform a breath hold. Switching from the MDI to SVN methods of bronchodilation is indicated in circumstances such as the acutely ill asthmatic. The number of actuations in a series and frequency of therapy should be based on patient response and tolerance of side effects.

□ INHALATIONAL ACCESSORIES FOR MDIs

Auxiliary aids for MDIs come in a variety of designs. They fall into three major categories: actuator aids (spring driven Autohaler and handles such as the VentEase), extension tubes (spacers), and extension tube chambers or bags with valves (Fig. 15-27*A–C*). *A breath-actuated MDI* (Autohaler) overcomes the patient coordination difficulties with regard to timing the start of actuation with inspiration. However, it does not aid sustaining inhalation. *Spacer tubes* provide both a partial reservoir for the bolus of the aerosol to be held for inhalation and a surface for large particle deposition. *One-way–valved MDI aids* act to hold the particles until the patient can evacuate them. Rigid or collapsible reservoirs are commercially available.

The goal of spacers and chambers is to eliminate the need for precise timing of MDI canister actuation with start of inhalation. They can also assist in the aiming of the MDI outlet in the mouth, optimize particle size, and promote low-flow inspiration. Spacers provide a distance for particles to evaporate and impact on internal walls. Particle shrinkage is related to the tube or chamber volume; impaction is relatively independent of volume or configuration of the device.[117,123,133,134]

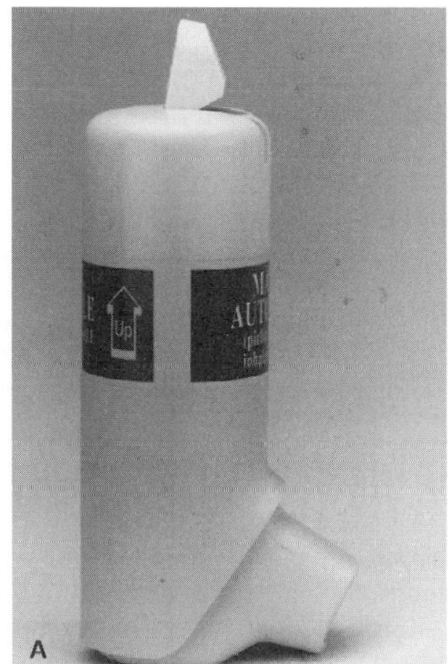

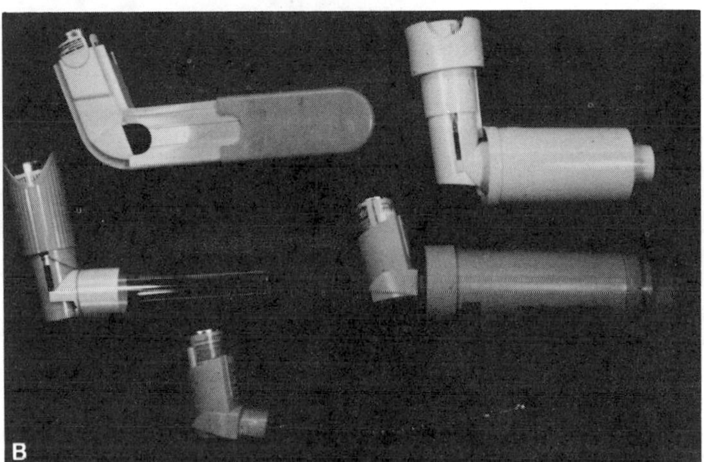

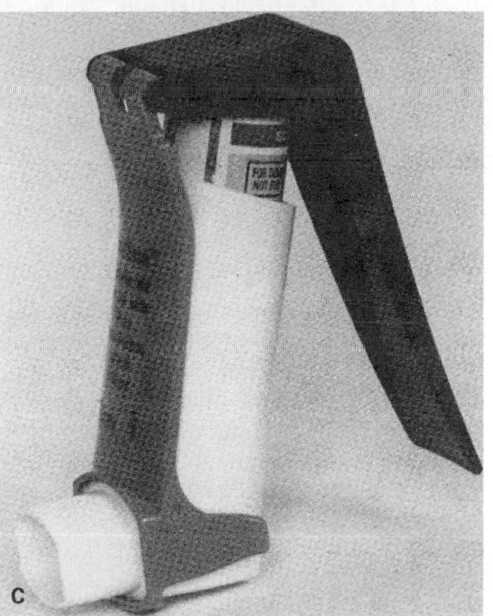

FIGURE 15-27. Metered-dose inhaler accessory administration devices for spontaneously breathing applications: **(A)** Autohaler and VentEase Actuator aids; **(B)** tube extensions/spacers; **(C)** chambers.

The MDI adjuncts appear to be of most benefit to children and elderly patients. Dyspneic asthmatic children tend to inhale rapidly and to have difficulty holding their breath. Ideally, inspiratory flows should be 10 to 20 L/min or less to better deposit aerosols in the 1- to 5-μm range.[135] Some MDI adjuncts are fitted with a reed valve as an audible "biofeedback" guide to inspiratory flow (eg, InspirEase, Aerochamber, and Aerosol Cloud Enhancer). It is reasonable to expect that MDI aids are effective when used properly. Some drug manufacturers supply a unit with the MDI; an example is a manufacturer-provided spacer to reduce oral cavity complications from topical corticosteroids. Lung deposition with a spacer is comparable to or greater than that from a correctly used MDI without a spacer. They do appear to help a standard MDI to be more effective if otherwise used poorly.[136] Some reservoir chambers may not provide adequate inspiratory volume for adults because they are limited to 600 to 700 mL. Inspired volumes should be larger than the tidal volume. Deposition increases directly with increased volumes; doubling the tidal volume results in approximately a 20% increase.[137] Volumes of tube spacers vary from 60 to 150 mL.

The efficacy of actuating multiple doses in valved chambers has been reviewed. After MDI activation into a chamber, particles do coalesce and deposit on surfaces. Inhaling puffs one at a time improves both the amount and delivery of smaller-diameter particles.[138] However, the use of two actuations in rapid succession (within seconds) gives an increase in total dose with some loss of efficiency. Increased numbers of rapid actuations give less increase in total dose and reduced efficiency of dose per puff.[139] The act of gargling after inhalation reduces side effects from pharyngeal absorption of sympathetic bronchodilators or topical corticosteroids.[74]

Some type of spacer is strongly recommended in several clinical situations. Oropharyngeal deposition with topical corticosteroid administration can be minimized. Children less than 3 to 4 years old commonly lack the ability to use an MDI effectively. Patients experienced in the used of their MDI may not need spacers. Commercial spacers cost $10 to $30. Their use does not assure proper administration technique. Patient compliance may not be aided by the bulky size of some units or by a reluctance to use them in public.

☐ METERED-DOSE INHALERS IN CIRCUITS OF MECHANICAL VENTILATORS

Metered-dose inhalers were used in anesthesia circuits in the 1960s and for intubated, mechanically ventilated patients by the 1980s. Their predominant application was for topical treatment of bronchospasm with minimal alteration of the ventilating system.[140,141] Like the use of SVNs, the endotracheal tube provides a significant barrier for aerosol penetration. Only 4% to 6% of the actuated aerosol traverses an adult-size tube. Most investigators have found that SVN- and MDI-generated aerosols are equivalent in efficacy for use in adult mechanical ventilation.[65,142] However, MDIs are the device of choice for most bronchodilator therapy in ventilated patients. The major advantage of MDIs over SVNs is negligible interference with a ventilator's cycling mechanism, airway pressure levels, and delivery (or monitoring) of tidal volume and minute ventilation.

As with SVNs, dosage adjustment for MDI use in ventilated patients is not clear. Because there is a 50% reduction in transendotracheal tube deposition, it is reasonable to expect that doubling the (nonintubated) dose would be equivalent.[114] Evaluation of patient bronchodilator response during mechanical ventilation was discussed previously in use of SVNs.

There are several types of *MDI adapters* that facilitate interfacing the cartridge nozzle into the ventilator circuit. They can be categorized as "ported" tracheal swivel adapters or elbows, inspiratory-limb adapters, and spacers or chambers for the inspiratory limb (Fig. 15-28*A,B*). Adapters vary in effectiveness, so the dose should be titrated.[143–145]

Bench studies have demonstrated that inspiratory-limb chambers are superior to in-line adapters or elbows.[146,147] Catheters to extend the tip of the MDI drug outlet beyond the endotracheal tube are under evaluation (Fig. 15-29).[65] Data regarding specific recommendations for MDIs and ventilator use are not complete. Preparation of the ventilator should proceed as it would with SVN therapy (see Box 15-16). However, it appears reasonable to time MDI actuation immediately after the beginning a mechanical breath, if an in-line adapter or elbow is used. With in-line chamber adapters, actuate 1 to 2 seconds before a mechanical breath.[65]

☐ COMPLICATIONS AND TECHNICAL PROBLEMS WITH MDIS

Temperature, shaking the canister, and positioning have been discussed. Soap-and-water cleaning of the actuator orifice should be done according to the manufacturer's recommendations. The remaining amount of drug can be approximated by observing an MDI canister placed in water. Full canisters remain submerged; those tending to float are approaching empty. Cross-contamination is not an issue, for this should be a single-patient item. There is a danger for aspiration of coins (eg, U.S. dime) or other purse or pocket articles that may get into uncapped or uncovered MDI mouthpieces.

High levels of Freon propellants can cause life-threatening cardiac dysrhythmias. However, blood levels of fluorocarbons with therapeutic nebulizers are too small to have any adverse effects.[148]

Dry-Powder Inhalers

In the early 1970s, the antiasthma drug cromolyn sodium was introduced using a solid particle administration device—the Spinhaler (Fisons). The drug was combined with lactose carrier particles to improve its aerosol penetration. The drug with lactose is contained in a gelatin capsule and is placed in a small cup (Fig.

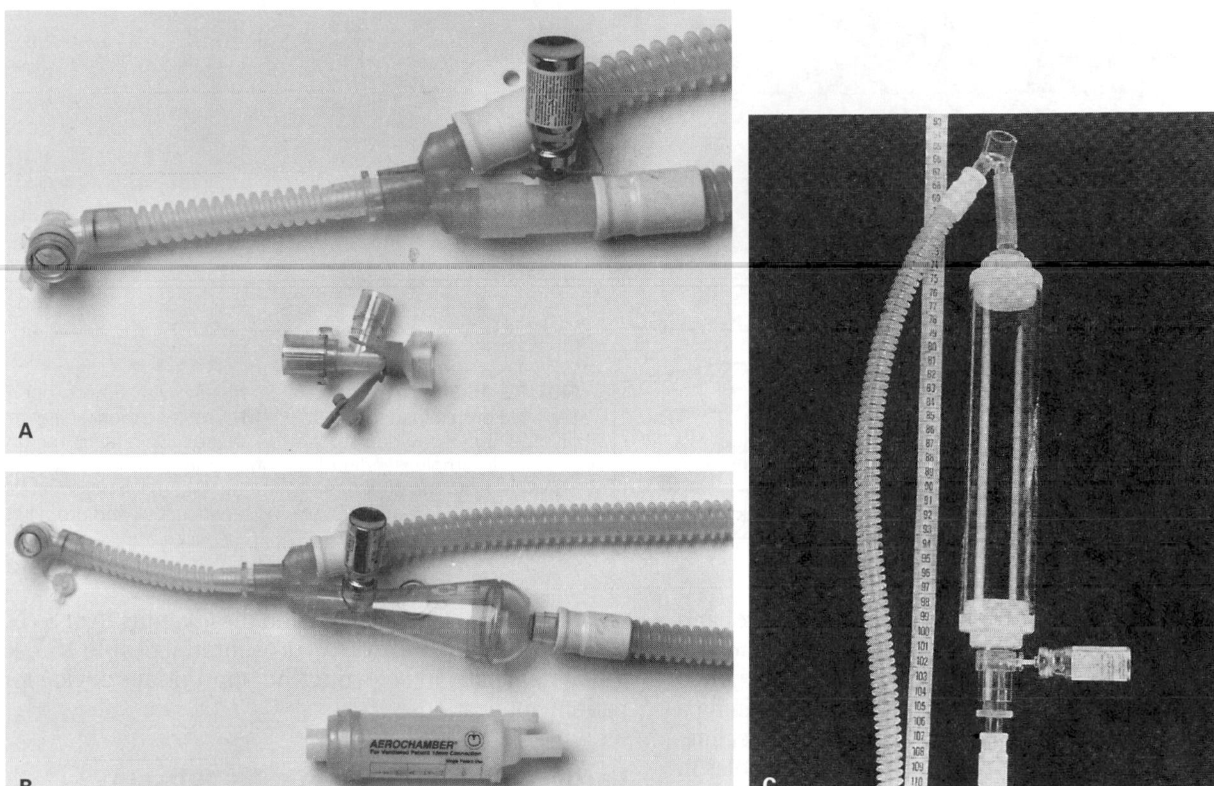

FIGURE 15-28. MDI adaptors for application with mechanical ventilator circuits. **(A)** Inspiratory limb and tracheal swivel adaptors; **(B and C)** Inspiratory limb chambers. (Reference No. 163 with permission)

15-30). A system allows piercing the capsule. This *dry-powder inhaler (DPI)* system is breath actuated as propellers, driven by subatmospheric pressure from the patient's inspiration, help disperse the medication. The spinhaler must be held with the barrel horizontal to aid in the capsule evacuation.[140]

Young children may find the device hard to technically operate, but there is no problem of timing the start of inspiration with actuation as in an MDI. Some patients may fail to follow instructions and exhale into the system, allowing moisture to collect powder and clog the system. Repeated capsule piercing can allow the

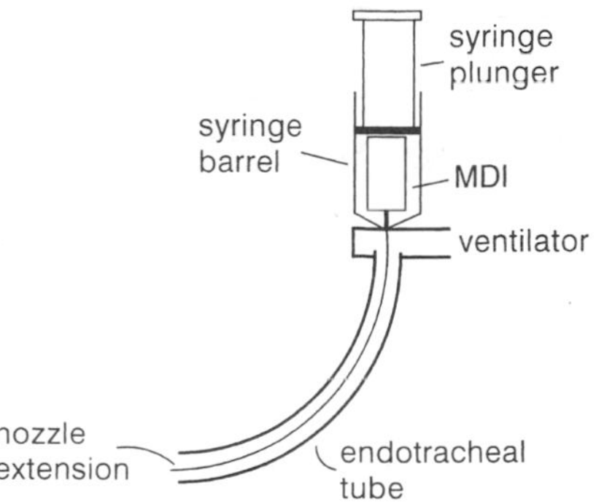

FIGURE 15-29. Nozzle extension for MDI application for patients with an endotracheal tube. (Reference No. 163 with permission)

gelatin capsule to break up and be aspirated. Such problems and the subsequent availability of cromolyn in liquid solution for both SVN and MDI has decreased the popularity of this aerosol medication nebulizer.

The Rotahaler (Glaxo) is a simpler device for administration of single-dose powdered albuterol and beclomethasone (Fig. 15-31). The drug capsule is placed in the end opposite the mouthpiece. The barrel is twisted, which shears the capsule, releasing the drug onto a plastic grid. The patient inhales the powder after several inhalations.

The principle advantages of the DPIs are avoidance of Freon or auxiliary compressed gas and requiring less timing coordination. The technique for using a dry powder differs from the SVN and MDI primarily in the need for rapid inspiratory flow and lack of need for breath hold. Box 15-19 describes the steps in DPI technique.

The main disadvantage of the first generation of DPIs related to their single-dose approach and limited selection of drugs. More recently, several devices have been developed that provide multiple dose capability. The Turbuhaler (Astra) is now available in the United States for administration of 200 doses of terbutaline sulfate (0.1 to 0.5 mg/puff) or budesonide (200 µg) (Fig. 15-32).[150] Two additional multidose DPIs are currently available in Europe. The Diskhaler (Glaxo) provides several days of drug therapy in a multidose unit, four or eight single-blister packs, called a Rotadisk (Fig. 15-33). Drugs available

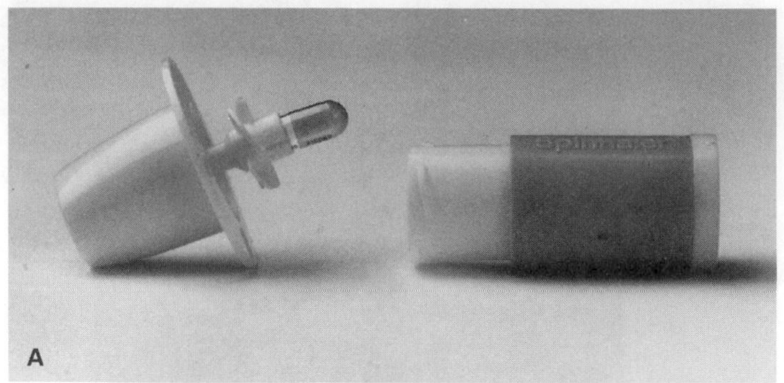

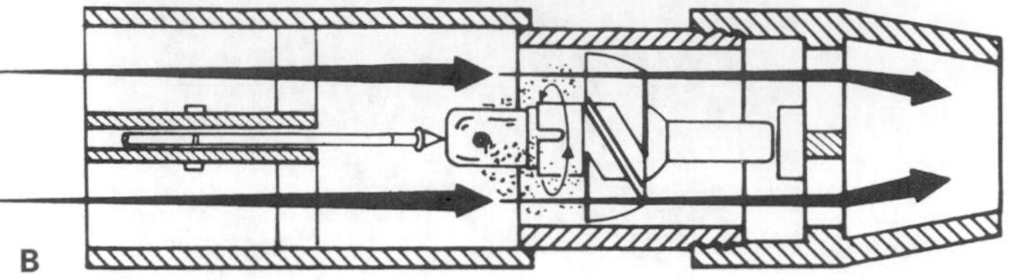

FIGURE 15-30. **(A)** Photo of Spinhaler with device open, showing drug capsule in position; **(B)** Cross-sectional diagram of a spinning powder aerosol dispenser (Spinhaler) for dry powder (cromolyn sodium) administration. Subatmospheric pressure from the patient's inspiration causes vanes to rotate and medication from a capsule to be evacuated and propelled to the airways.

in the Rotadisk include bronchodilators (albuterol and salmeterol) and corticosteroids (fluticasone and beclomethasone).[151] The Diskus Inhaler (Glaxo) extends the multidose capability by using a foil strip containing a 1-month supply (60-blister pack) of micronized salmeterol and lactose (Fig. 15-34).[152] In both designs, holes in the inhaler's plastic housing allow adequate flow of entrained inspired air without undue resistance. Newer DPI devices also provide dose-remaining counters, and small brushes allow cleaning of critical points in the inhaler.

□ CLINICAL APPLICATION

Dry-powder inhalers have gained greater acceptance in Europe than the United States. Dry-powder inhalers compare favorably when compared with either small-volume nebulizers or metered-dose inhalers in treatment of bronchodilation in asthmatic and COPD patients.[153,154] Bronchodilation appears to be equivalent to the MDI and SVN when proper technique is not a factor. Because of the eventual ban of Freon-driven MDIs, the DPI is likely to become the device of choice for aerosol drug therapy, unless patient cooperation is a problem. It should be noted that DPIs cannot be used in conjunction with mechanical ventilator circuits.

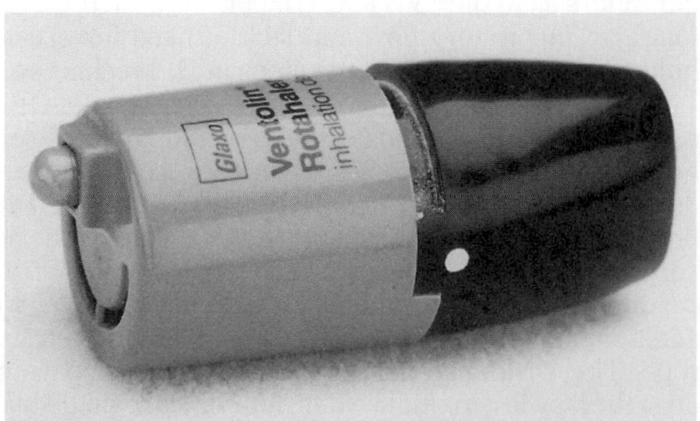

FIGURE 15-31. Photo of Rotohaler dry powder inhaler.

A summary of advantages and disadvantages of SVN, MDI, and DPI nebulizers is presented in Table 15-7 to guide clinicians in selecting the appropriate device for patient applications.

Large-Volume Pneumatic Nebulizers

Since the development of inhalation therapy, mainstream nebulizers have been used to aerosolize liquids, primarily water or physiologic saline solutions. The lack of objective evidence to guide their application has been documented.[2–4,155–157] A summary of nationally accepted indications for bland aerosol therapy with large-volume nebulizers is presented in Box 15-20. The use of bland aerosols for humidification purposes is not as efficient as heated humidifiers or HMEs, and it increases the potential risk of bronchospasm and infection and has greater difficulties in maintaining appropriate temperatures.

□ CATEGORY DESCRIPTIONS AND PERFORMANCE

Pneumatically driven large-volume nebulizers can be categorized by the physical technique of producing aerosol.

BOX 15-19

TECHNIQUE FOR DRY-POWDER INHALERS

- Note baseline patient data (pulse, breath sounds, and pulmonary function)
- Assemble apparatus and ready drug capsule or blister
- Tell patient to exhale to functional residual capacity
- Tell patient to place inhaler in mouth and seal lips around mouthpiece
- Instruct patient to inhale rapidly (>1 L/sec) through device (breath hold is not necessary)
- Have patient repeat process until capsule is evacuated
- Monitor patient for side effects and drug response

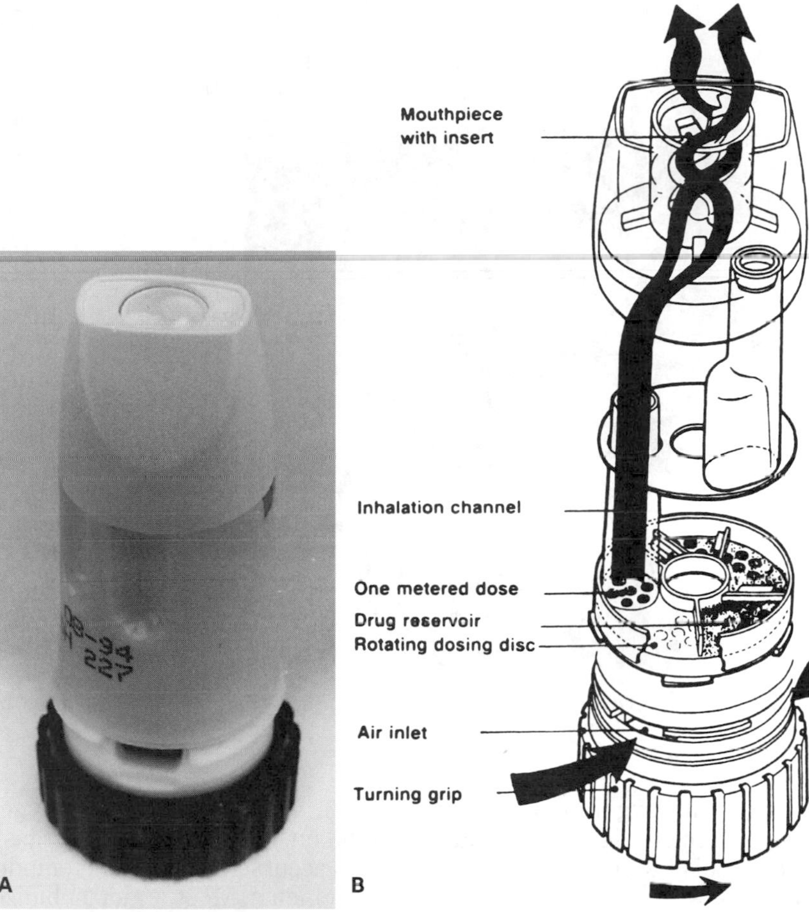

FIGURE 15-32. **(A)** Photo of the Turbuhaler DPI; **(B)** Cross-sectional diagram.

Large-volume nebulizers use the same principles as small-volume nebulizers but have greater capability of delivering moisture and flows to meet a patient's inspiratory needs (Fig. 15-35). Many nebulizers can dilute oxygen with room air to control FIO_2 but have relatively limited levels of driving gas flows (eg, ≤15 L/min). Respiratory care practitioners should be familiar with the gas output capabilities of pneumatic nebulizers at various FIO_2s. Besides the FIO_2 setting, the flow output must meet or exceed the patient's demands, to ensure

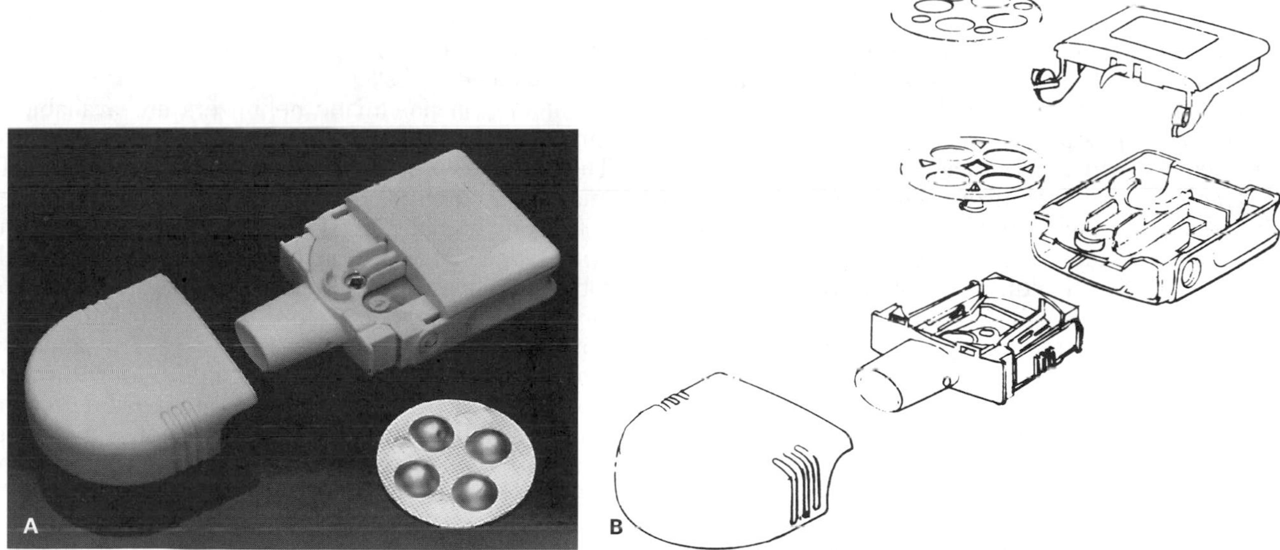

FIGURE 15-33. **(A)** Photo of Diskhaler, cover and drug rotadisk; **(B)** Cross-sectional diagram of Diskhaler (Courtesy of Glaxo).

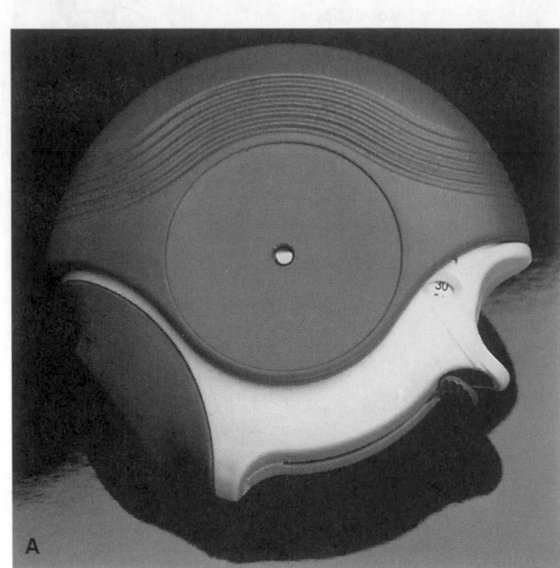

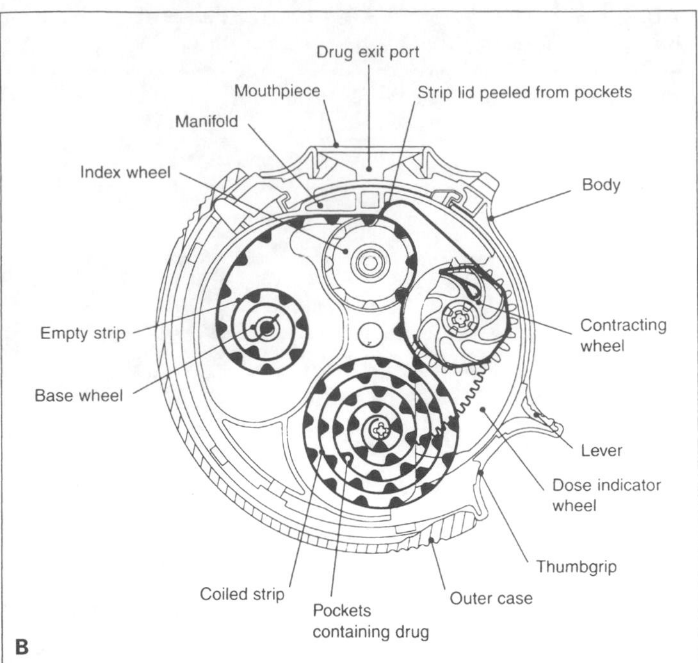

FIGURE 15-34. **(A)** Photo of Diskus inhaler; **(B)** Cross-sectional diagram of Diskus DPI (Courtesy of Glaxo.)

consistent oxygen levels. Large holes in masks and open-circuit design permit additional dilution by the patient. This lowers the F_{IO_2} and prevents accurate correlation with blood or oximetric measurements. Most manufacturers have limited the inlet orifice to allow about 15 L/min of source gas, which is the total output when set on the 100% mode. Severely dyspneic patients may require up to 60 to 90 L/min. By not having their inspiratory needs met, they inspire the necessary volume of room air. Sound decision making is impaired when a patient's blood oxygen levels are correlated to an incorrect F_{IO_2}. Recently, manufacturers have developed nebulizers that can provide approximately 40 L/min without entrainment or allowing additional flow from a second source (see Chap. 13).

Heating nebulizers can be accomplished by internal immersion rods, wrap-around or bottom plate heaters (which heat the water in a reservoir), or outlet "doughnut" heaters (which heat an aerosol).

Babbington-type nebulizers use a pneumatic pressure source, but instead of a jet, gas is directed into a glass sphere that is continuously coated with liquid (Fig. 15-36). Small aliquots of water are elevated to a drip chamber above the sphere by rising bubbles. A portion of the source gas is routed to a tube in the water reservoir and carries water between rising gas bubbles. Gas exits from a slit in the sphere, rupturing the water film and projecting aerosol particles toward an impactor.

During the aerosol-generating process, both jet and Babbington devices have the option of entraining room air. By governing the size of openings in the housings, an F_{IO_2} from 0.3 to 1.0 can be selected (if powered by pure oxygen). Most units can be connected directly to 50-psig gas sources or run from flow meters through diameter index safety system (DISS) fittings. Mainstream jet nebulizer water output (vapor and particulate) is most dependent on whether the units are heated or cool. The scientific literature is incomplete with respect to data for water output and aerosol particle size. Most units generate aerosols in the 1- to 10-μm range. Total water output ranges from 0.5 to 5 mL/min, but varies with manufacturer, temperature, gas flow, and length of tubing from the nebulizer. However, because these units are designed to deposit particles throughout the airways, particle size is not as significant as it is for medication nebulizers.[158] Levels of relative humidity or body humidity have been reviewed for commercial heated and unheated units.[34,37]

Babbington pneumatic nebulizers are available in three models: Solosphere, Hydrosphere, and Maxicool. These devices produce a dense aerosol of 3 to 5 μm with total water output of 60 to 70 mg/L, which can exceed 100% body humidity levels.[34,77] The Solosphere has the option for a clip-on bottom heater and is used clinically for face masks or tents, T-pieces, and tracheostomy collars. It can be connected to the source gas through a flow meter or run directly from 50 psig. The latter two models are high-output devices designed for aerosol enclosures (tents). All three have multiposition air entrainment attached to one arm of the housing to regulate F_{IO_2} when run on source oxygen. When run on 50 psig, the Hydrosphere and Maxicool units are used with closed or open-top croup tents. Their high-output flows can flush out heat and carbon dioxide from tents and commonly do not require a refrigeration unit to main-

TABLE 15-7 **Comparison of Advantages and Disadvantages of Medication Nebulizers**

Advantages	Disadvantages
■ Pneumatic small-volume nebulizers (SVN)	
Limited patient coordination required	Expensive compressed gas source
High dose levels possible	Inefficient
Continuous therapy available	Greater time required (expense)
	Contamination possible
No CFC release	Some medications not available (U.S.) (eg, corticosteroids and anticholinergics)
■ Ultrasonic small-volume nebulizers (USN)	
Less patient coordination	Expensive initial purchase
Small dead volume	Contamination possible
Fast delivery	Electrical or mechanical malfunction
No CFC release or compressed gas source required	Not portable
	Some medications not available
■ Metered-dose inhaler (MDI)	
Convenient	Requires significant patient coordination
Inexpensive	Requires patient actuation
Fewer problems in intubated or ventilated patient applications	Difficult to deliver high dose levels
—MDI with spacer, chamber, or self-actuation	CFC-based propellants
Less patient coordination required (some drugs available in breath-activated MDIs)	Not all medications available (U.S.)
	Greater cost and complexity
	Bulky, less portable
■ Dry-powder inhaler (DPI)	
Less patient coordination required (ie, breath activated)	Requires high inspiratory flows
	Limited medications
Breath hold not required	Cannot be used for intubated or ventilated patient administration
No CFC release	Difficult to deliver high dose levels

Adapted with permission from Kacmarek RM, Hess D: The interface between patient and aerosol generator. Respir Care 36:952, 1991.

tain an environment below ambient temperature. With lower driving gas flows (ie, from a flow meter), the Hydrosphere or Maxicool can be used for applications similar to an ultrasonic nebulizer (eg, sputum induction).

□ LARGE-VOLUME NEBULIZERS IN MIST TENT APPLICATIONS

Mist tents that use jet nebulizers commonly incorporate an adjunct cooling apparatus. By convention, most systems attempt to reduce the intratent temperature 5° to 15°F below room temperature. The Air-Shields Croupette uses ice to cool the aerosol. The Ohmeda Ohio Pediatric Aerosol Tent incorporates a Freon refrigeration unit, with fan, to cool tent contents. Mistogen's CAM-2 Tent uses a Freon refrigeration device to cool water that circulates in a radiatorlike cooling panel. That company's CAM-3 uses a thermoelectric system,

BOX 15-20

INDICATIONS FOR BLAND AEROSOL THERAPY

- Presence of upper airway edema
  - Secondary to laryngotracheobronchitis (croup)
  - Subglottic edema
  - Postextubation edema
  - Postoperative management of the upper airway
- Presence of a bypassed upper airway
- Sputum induction

Used with permission from American Association for Respiratory Care: Clinical practice guideline: Bland aerosol administration. Respir Care 38:1196, 1993

using the Peltier effect. Electric current passing through a semiconductor of dissimilar metals augments heat absorption and release. Warm air is circulated through the heat-transfer module, which returns cool air to the tent and exhausts warm air.

□ HAZARDS AND COMPLICATIONS OF PNEUMATIC NEBULIZERS

Airway burns have occurred with use of heated nebulizers. Most systems do not have sophisticated servo-controlled systems such as heated humidifiers. Heaters can be improperly set or become defective. It is less likely to produce burns with hot air, as it has a low specific heat. Hot water and steam have a higher specific heat and can cause burns easily. However, most heated nebulizers are not that efficient. Temperatures more than 44°C can potentially burn airway surfaces. Measurement of the gas temperature near the airway can be done to monitor safe operation.

Bronchospasm occurs as a response to aerosol particles irritating hyperreactive airways.[4] Hypertonic saline solutions, by design, are irritating. Respiratory care practitioners should note a patient's history of airway hyperresponsiveness. Switching patients to heated humidifiers or HME devices or pretreating patients with a bronchodilator, or both, are options to consider.

Sound levels of pneumatic nebulizers may cause hearing loss in infants when used with enclosures such as oxygen hoods or incubators. The American Academy of Pediatrics Committee on Environmental Hazards recommends a level below 58 dB. Such a level is exceeded by all mainstream nebulizers with up to 60 cm of large-bore tubing leading to the enclosure.[90]

Use of aerosol nebulization systems can be linked to nosocomial infections either by acting as a bacterial reservoir or by direct inoculation of microorganisms. Outbreaks of both pneumonia and sepsis caused by *Pseudomonas, Serratia, Legionella,* and other organisms have been documented in heated and cool pneumatic nebulizers.[159]

Overhydration and excessive salt loads are potential hazards, primarily to neonatal and pediatric patients receiving long-duration or continuous aerosol therapy.

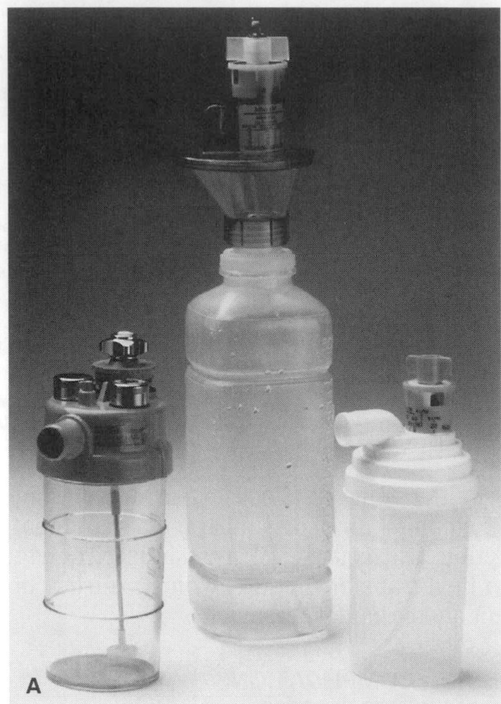

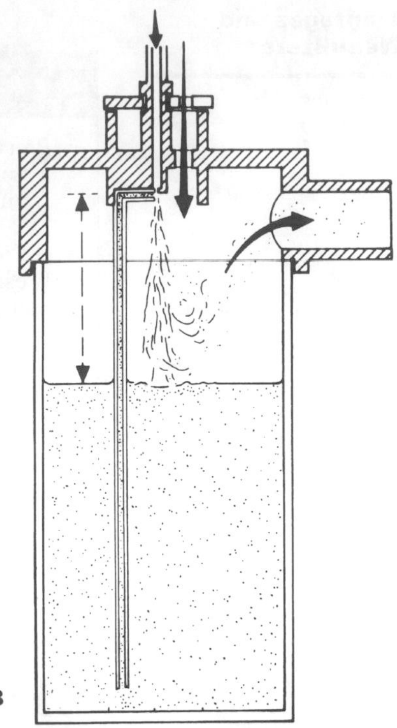

FIGURE 15-35. (A) Photograph of commercial large-volume nebulizers: (L→R) Puritan-Bennett "all-purpose," Misty-Ox Hi-F_IO_2 and Hudson-RCI single-use; **(B)** cross-sectional diagram of a large-volume "all-purpose" pneumatic jet nebulizer.

Ultrasonic Nebulizers

The *ultrasonic nebulizer (USN)* came into clinical practice in the United States during the 1960s. Although different from the pneumatic devices in nebulization mechanism, they are frequently used interchangeably for delivering bland mists, medications, and hypertonic solutions for sputum induction. Nebulization by these units is by application of vibrational energy to liquids. Electrical energy is first converted to sound waves of acoustic energy. This phenomenon, termed *piezoelectric effect,* involves vibrating planes of crystal material (quartz-barium titanate) and similar substances. When crystals are vibrated while placed in shallow depths of water, surface waves occur. The vibrational energy can be used to remove foreign material from jewelry and surgical instruments. At higher frequencies and greater energy levels, oscillation waves crest to form a liquid fountain. Aerosol particles form around the fountains as the vibrations rupture the fluid. The mass median aerodynamic diameter of droplets has been shown to be predictable, when the vibratory frequency or wavelength is known.[160] Auxiliary gas flow from a medical

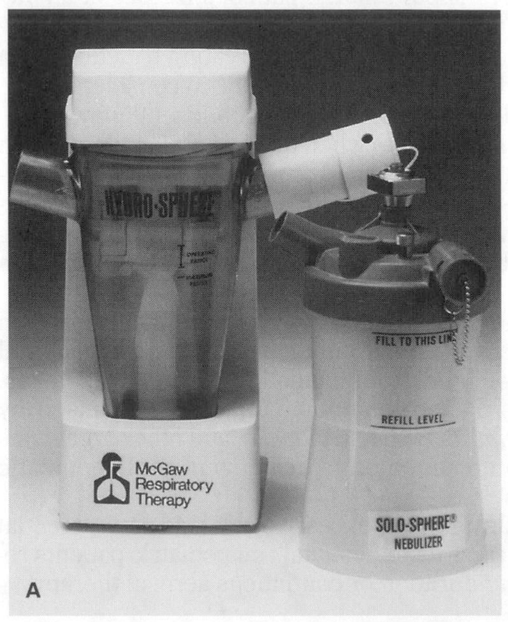

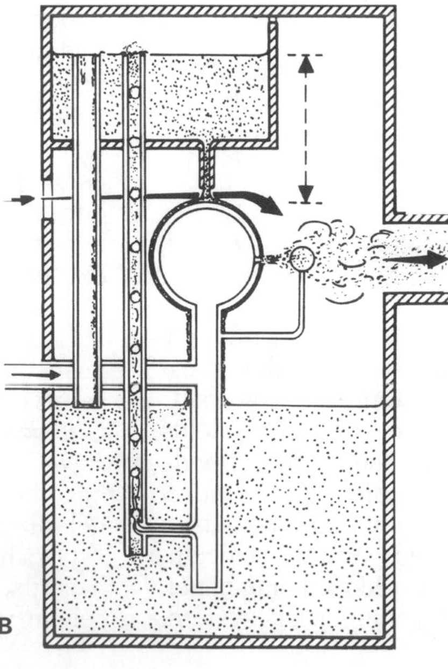

FIGURE 15-36. (A) Photograph of Babbington-type nebulizers, Hydrosphere *(left)* and Solosphere *(right)*; **(B)** Cross-sectional diagram of a "solosphere" nebulizer illustrating the Babbington principle.

gas flow meter or blower device evacuates the nebulizing chamber for delivery to the patient (Fig. 15-37).

□ CLINICAL APPLICATION

Manufacturers have created units for limited application of medicated aerosols and for uses similar to those of mainstream nebulizers. In addition, large-output ultrasonic nebulizers are also available to apply by mask, face tent, Briggs adapter, and so on. Mist tents may also be incorporated with ultrasonic devices. They have also been placed in breathing circuits of mechanical ventilators or IPPB devices. Ultrasonic nebulizers were touted as the device of choice to apply aerosols to distal airways of the lung by virtue of their high-density, small, and uniform particle size, as well as substantial water output. In theory, high-output deposition of sterile water or saline should aid therapy to mobilize thick, tenacious pulmonary secretions. Documentation of clinical improvement from such adjunctive treatment (ie, used with chest physical therapy, adequate hydration, and such) is not clear.

The ability to target a certain lung zone by delivering a particle size is quite dependent on the operating conditions of the nebulizer. Diameter and length of tubing, valves, and patient's breathing pattern are also significant variables. Most texts give a particle dimension of approximately 3 µm for ultrasonic nebulizers. The mass median aerodynamic diameters of commercial units can range from 0.93 to more than 10 µm. Clinical documentation for medication administration has been more abundant than for bland mist therapy. However, most clinically oriented in vitro studies demonstrate that ultrasonic medication nebulizers produce particles only slightly smaller than their pneumatic counterparts.[34,37,160] Advantages of these nebulizers include reduced sound levels compared to pneumatic units and greater porportion of aerosol particles smaller than 2 µm.[79] Other reports suggest there is little in vivo effect in distribution between particles with diameters of 1.4 or 5.5 µm when inhaled by stable asthmatic patients.[161] Some medications are not recommended for USN nebulization, for example, recombinant deoxyribonuclease (rDNase), because of the potential for chemical disruption.

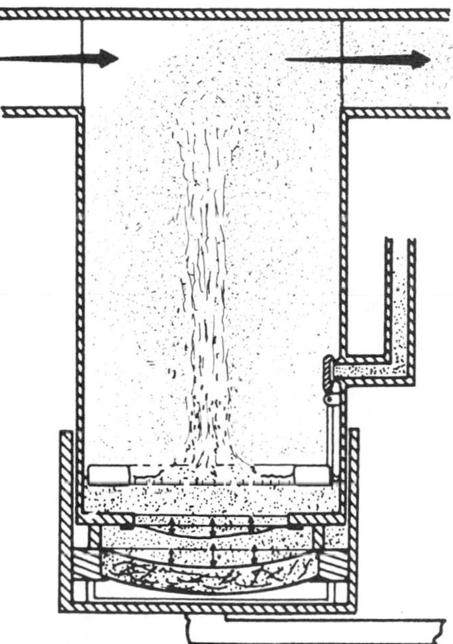

FIGURE 15-37. Sectional diagram of an ultrasonic nebulizer. The aerosol-producing geyser is formed by acoustic energy supplied by a vibrating crystal, shown at the bottom of the device.

To generate therapeutic aerosols, the frequency is increased above 800,000 cycles/sec (hertz, Hz) and the acoustic beam is focused on the fluid. Water couplant is commonly placed between the transducer and the substance being nebulized. Instead of crests, "ultrasonic fountains" are created. An aerosol is emitted adjacent to the bases and along the cylindrical column. The diameter of the fog formation area appears to be a function of frequency and acoustic energy density. Larger fountains, therefore greater output, can be created by increasing the power to the crystal, whereas the frequency remains in the 0.8 to 2.5 million hertz (MHz) range. However, there appears to be a plateau at which greater power fails to produce higher output. The physics tend to be complex and involve surface tension, liquid density, and viscosity, in addition to frequency and power.[160]

Another approach is used with a Swedish-designed nebulizer that drips water (by drop or up to 0.3 mL/min) on an unsubmerged transducer. The droplets explode in a high-intensity airborne field.

Unlike pneumatic aerosol generators that use their source gas to propel particles to the patient, ultrasonic nebulizers produce aerosols that must be evacuated from the transducer cup. Auxiliary oxygen flows or low-flow blowers (approximately 30 L/min) are used on commercial units. Ultrasonic nebulizers can also be connected to IPPB or mechanical ventilator circuits. Aerosol particle production is established by the USN's crystal function. The flow of gas evacuating the nebulizer chamber can affect the density of the generated aerosol, and mass median diameter of particles. Low-flow gases tend to produce dense mists of small particles; larger particles are forced back into the geyser. Higher flows produce lower-density mists with larger particles being carried.

□ DEVICE PERFORMANCE

Ultrasonic nebulizers can be grouped into two major categories: small-output units for medication administration (Fig. 15-38) and large-output nebulizers for bland mist therapy. Because the clinical setup and measuring procedures vary greatly, there is substantial variation in the literature on particle size output.

Current examples of ultrasonic medication units include the Pulmosonic (DeVilbiss Health Care Division), which has a "fluid" output of approximately 0.5 mL/min and with which an MMAD of 4.2 or 5.4 µm has been reported.[79,161] The device is designed for portable or home application. The Portosonic (DeVilbiss Health Care Division) is similar to the former unit, except that

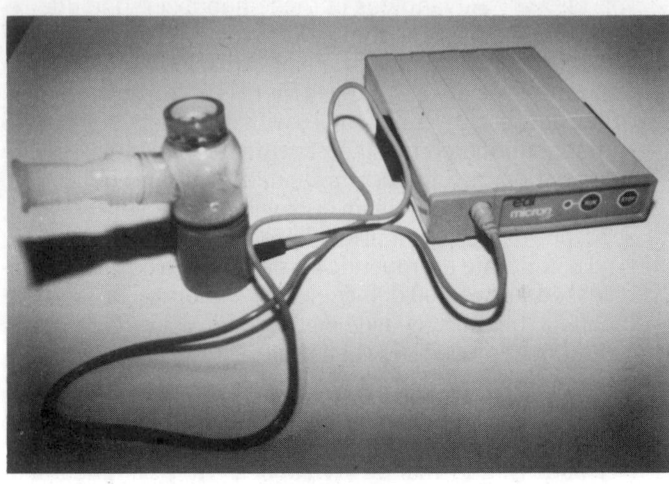

FIGURE 15-38. Example of ultrasonic medication nebulizer.

the mass median aerodynamic diameter is reported to be 1.6 μm. Both ultrasonic devices run on a continuous-flow mode. The Fisoneb (Fisons Corporation) produces particles by pressing a trigger. The mass median aerodynamic diameter of the particle is approximately 5 μm.[79] Ultrasonic medication nebulizers have advantages of less patient coordination requirements, small dead-space volume, no CFC or gas source required, and fast delivery. Disadvantages include relatively high initial expense, electrical or mechanical malfunction, and less convenience or portability (than MDI or DPI).[6] Table 15-7 summarizes advantages and disadvantages of USNs compared to other medication nebulizers.

Large-volume ultrasonic nebulizers typically have mist outputs of from 3 to 6 mL/min, depending on the power setting. This would provide body humidity levels of 100% for gas flows of 68 to 136 L/min.[37]

□ PATIENT COMPLICATIONS AND EQUIPMENT TROUBLESHOOTING WITH USNS

The most common untoward patient response from an ultrasonic nebulizer is some evidence of bronchospasm. Signs or symptoms include dyspnea, tachypnea, chest pain, or wheezing. This occurs more frequently when sterile water is used instead of normal saline or bronchodilator drugs. Other problems include overhydration or increased sodium loading. These side effects are of greatest concern when using large-volume devices with neonatal or pediatric patients and patients with renal disorders. If used with mist tents, ultrasonic nebulizers may best be used with open-top tents or auxiliary cooling devices. In contrast with pneumatic aerosol generators, ultrasonic nebulizers add heat.

Studies of ultrasonic nebulizers have shown that reservoirs rapidly become contaminated, which may lead to direct airway inoculation. The most common contaminating bacteria are *Bacillus, Staphylococcus, Pseudomonas,* and *Enterobacter* species. A high percentage of devices (33%) in intensive care units become contaminated by gram-negative microbes from background air.[4,97]

If ultrasonic nebulizers fail to produce mist during operation, several problems can occur that may be remedied at the bedside. Because of high-output capabilities, water can collect at bends or low spots in the tubing, causing blockage. Large-output units commonly have continuous-feed water supplies. Malfunction can flood

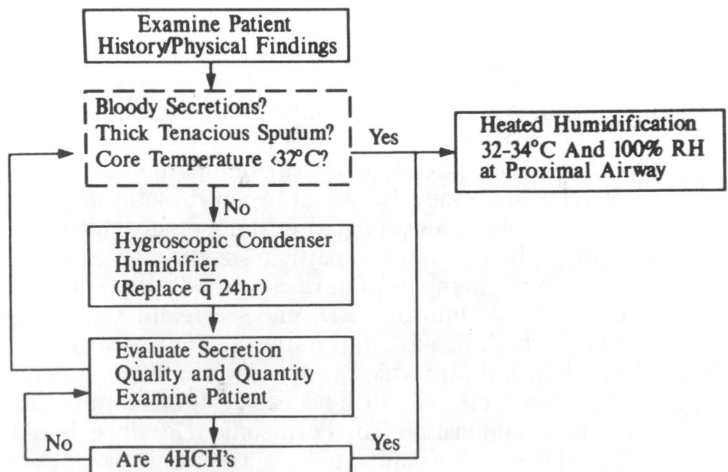

PROTOCOL 15-1. Alogrithm to direct use of HME and heated humidifiers for use in mechanically ventilated intensive care patients. (From Branson RD, Davis K, Campbell RS, Porembka DT. Humidification in the intensive care unit: Prospect study of a new protocol utilizing heated humidification and hygroscopic condenser humidifer, Chest 1993; 104:1800. With permission.)

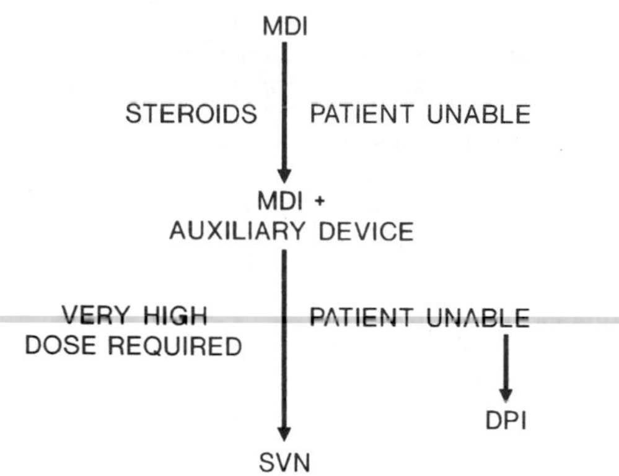

PROTOCOL 15-2. Decision tree to guide selection of aerosol delivery device. (From Hess DR. Aerosol therapy. Resp Care Clin NA 1995;1:235. With permission.)

out the geyser or allow too little water into the nebulization chamber. Other problems are unit specific and may involve water levels in the couplant chamber, blown fuses or circuit breakers, and vibrational frequency levels out of adjustment.

The possibility also exists for medication to undergo chemical breakdown. Increase in concentration of medication can also occur as solvent evaporates more rapidly than the solute. A prudent protocol involves periodically discarding the remaining nebulizer solutions of saline or medication during prolonged therapy and the addition of fresh solutions.

Clinical Practice Guidelines, Therapist-Driven Protocols, and Research in Humidity and Aerosol Therapy

Although humidity and aerosol therapy is at least 50 years old, exact physiologic needs for humidity and important aspects of delivery systems are only now being appreciated. The number and variety of aerosolizable drugs has continued to increase appreciably. Environmental concerns now affect future availability of the present Freon-based MDI devices. Our evolution in aerosol-generating technology continues. However, advances in patient care also require that respiratory care practitioners evaluate patients to recommend initial equipment selection and to modify therapy accordingly. Examples of this approach include protocols to direct use of either HME or heated humidifier (Protocol 15-1) and choice of device for aerosolized medication (Protocol 15-2).[2,162,163] Development of new equipment and rationale application of humidity and aerosol therapy can be guided by expert consensus and continued bench and clinical research.[164]

REFERENCES

1. American Association for Respiratory Care: Clinical practice guideline: Humidification during mechanical ventilation. Respir Care 37:887, 1992
2. American Association for Respiratory Care: Clinical practice guideline: Selection of aerosol delivery device. Respir Care 37:891, 1992
3. American Association for Respiratory Care: Clinical practice guideline: Delivery of aerosols to the upper airway. Respir Care 38:803, 1993
4. American Association for Respiratory Care: Clinical practice guideline: Bland aerosol administration. Respir Care 38:1196, 1993
5. MacIntyre NR, Brougher P, Hess DR, Newhouse MT, et al: Aerosol consensus statement—1991. Respir Care 36:916, 1991
6. O'Donahue WJ: Guidelines for the use of nebulizers in the home and domiciliary sites. Chest 109:814, 1996
7. Comroe JH: Physiology of Respiration, 2nd ed. Chicago, Year Book Medical, 1974
8. Gerrity TR, et al: The effect of aspirin on lung mucociliary clearance. N Engl J Med 308:139, 1983
9. Miller RD, Divertie MB: Kartagener's syndrome. Chest 62:130, 1972
10. Wilton LJ, Teichtahl H, Temple-Smith PD, de Kretser DM: Kartagener's syndrome with motile cilia and immotile spermatozoa: Axonemal ultrastructure and function. Am Rev Respir Dis 134:1233, 1986
11. Ziment I: Respiratory Pharmacology and Therapeutics. Philadelphia, WB Saunders, 1978
12. Chodosh S: Sputum Examination. In AF Fishman (ed) Pulmonary Diseases and Disorders, 2nd ed. New York, McGraw-Hill Book Co., 1988.
13. Knowles MR, Oliver KN, Honeker KW, et al: Pharmacologic treatment of abnormal ion transport in the airway epithelium in cystic fibrosis. Chest 107(suppl):71S, 1995
14. Dery R: The evolution of heat and moisture in the respiratory tract during anesthesia with a non-rebreathing system. Can Anaesth Soc J 20:296, 1973
15. Primiano FP Jr, Montague FW Jr, Saidel GM: Measurement system for water vapor and temperature dynamics. J Appl Physiol 56:1679, 1984
16. Ingelstedt S: Studies on the conditioning of air in the respiratory tract. Acta Otolaryngol 131(Suppl):7, 1956
17. Chanlon J, Loew D, Malbranche J: Effect of dry anesthetic gases on tracheobronchial epithelium. Anesthesiology 37:338, 1972
18. Forbes AR: Humidification and mucus flow in the intubated trachea. Br J Anaesth 45:874, 1973
19. McFadden ER, et al: Thermal mapping of the airways in humans. J Appl Physiol 2:564, 1985
20. Tsuda T, Noguchi H Takaumi Y, Aochi O: Optimum humidification of air administered to a tracheostomy in dogs: Scanning electron microscopy and surfactant studies. Br J Anaesth 49:965, 1977
21. Interntional Organization for Standardization: Humidifiers for medical use: Safety requirements. ISO 8185:1988(E) 60:14, 1988
22. American National Standards Institute: American National Standard for Humidifiers and Nebulizers for Medical Use, ANSI Z79.9-1979:8. New York, ANSI, 1979
23. ECRI: An overview of heated humidifiers. Technology for Respiratory Therapy 15:1, 1994
24. British Standards Institution: Specifications for humidifiers for use with breathing machines. Publications No. BS 4494. London, The Institution, 1970
25. Miyao H, Miyassaka K, Hirokawa T, Hawazoe T: Consideration of the international standard for airway humidification using simulated secretions and an artificial airway. Respir Care 41:43, 1996
26. Chatburn RL, Primiano FP: A rational basis for humidity therapy. Respir Care 32:249, 1987
27. American Association for Respiratory Care: Clinical practice guidelines: Oxygen therapy in the acute care hospital. Respir Care 36:1410, 1991
28. Darin JD, Broadwell J, MacDonell R: An evaluation of water-vapor output from four brands of unheated prefilled bubble humidifiers. Respir Care 27:41, 1982
29. Campbell E, Baker D, Crites-Silver P: Subjective effect of oxygen for delivery by nasal cannula: A prospective study. Chest 86:241, 1988
30. Chen WY, Horton DJ: Airway cooling and nocturnal asthma. Chest 81:675, 1982
31. Strauss RH, et al: Influence of heat and humidity on the airway obstruction induced by exercise in asthma. J Clin Invest 61:433, 1978

32. Wells RE, Walker JEC, Hickler RB: Effects of cold air on respiratory airflow resistance in patients with respiratory-tract disease. N Engl J Med 263:268, 1960
33. Danzl DF, Pozos RS: Accidental hypothermia. N Engl Med 331P:1756, 1994
34. Hess DR, Branson RD: Humidification: Humidifiers and Nebulizers. In RD Branson, DR Hess, RL Chataburn (eds): Respiratory Care Equipment. Philadelphia, JB Lippincott, 1995
35. McPherson SP: Respiratory Care Equipment. St. Louis, Mosby-Year Book, 1995
36. Op't Holt T: Aerosol Generators and Humidifiers. In TA Barnes (ed): St. Louis, Mosby-Year Book, 1994
37. Klein EF, Shah DA, Shah NJ, et al: Performance characteristics of conventional and prototype humidifiers and nebulizers. Chest 64:690, 1973
38. Revenas B, Lindholm CE: Temperature variations heat and moisture exchanges. Acta Anaesthesiol Scand 24:237, 1980
39. Schmidt-Nielsen K: Countercurrent systems in animals. Sci Am 244:118, 1981
40. Mebius C: A comparative evaluation of disposable humidifiers. Acta Anaesthesiol Scand 27:403, 1983
41. Walker AKY, Bethune DW: A comparative study of condenser humidifiers. Anaesthesia 31:1086, 1976
42. Weeks DB, Ramsey FM: Laboratory investigation of six artificial noses for use during endotracheal anesthesia. Anesth Analg 62:758, 1983
43. Emergency Care Research Institute: Heat moisture exchangers. Health Devices 12:155, 1983
44. Branson RD, Hurst JM: Laboratory evaluation of seven airway heat and moisture exchangers. Respir Care 32:741, 1987
45. Bygdeman D, von Euler C, Nystrom B: Moisture exchangers do not prevent patient contamination of ventilators. Acta Anaesthesiol Scand 28:591, 1984
46. Leigh JM, White MG: A new condenser humidifier. Anaesthesia 39:492, 1984
47. Weeks DB, Ramsey FM: Laboratory evaluation of six artificial noses during endotracheal anesthesia. Anesth Analg 62:753, 1983
48. Shelly M, Bethune DW, Latimer RD: A comparison of five heat moisture exchanges. Anaesthesia 41:527, 1986
49. MacIntyre NR, Anderson HR, Silver RM: Pulmonary function in mechanically ventilated patients during 24 hours use of a hygroscopic condenser humidifier. Chest 5:560, 1983
50. American College of Chest Physicians—National Heart, Lung, and Blood Institute: National conference on oxygen therapy. Respir Care 29:922, 1984
51. Estey W: Subjective effects of dry versus humidified low flow oxygen. Respir Care 25:1143, 1980
52. Goodison RR: Pseudomonas cross-infection due to contaminated humidifier water. Br Med J 281:1288, 1980
53. Emergency Care Research Institute: Heated humidifiers. Health Devices 16:223, 1987
54. Poulton TJ, Downs JB: Humidification of rapidly flowing gas. Crit Care Med 9:59, 1981
55. Rhame FS, Streifel A, McComb C, Boyle M: Bubbling humidifiers produce microaerosols which can carry bacteria. Infect Control 7:403, 1986
56. Craven DE, Goularte TA, Make BJ: Contaminated condensate in mechanical ventilator circuits: A risk factor for nosocomial pneumonia. Am Rev Respir Dis 129:625, 1984
57. Craven DE, Steger KA: Pathogenesis and prevention of nosocomial pneumonia in the mechanically ventilated patient. Respir Care 34:85, 1989
58. Hess D: Guideline for prevention of nosocomial pneumonia and ventilator circuits: Time for change? Respir Care 39:1149, 1994
59. Kollef MH, Shapiro SD, Fraser VJ, et al: Mechanical ventilation with or without 7-day circuit changes: A randomized controlled trial. Ann Intern Med 123:168, 1995
60. Tablan OC, Anderson LJ, Arden NH, et al: Guideline for prevention of nosocomial pneumonia. Respir Care 39:1191, 1994
61. Lourenco RV, Cotromanes E: Clinical aerosols I: Characterization of aerosols and their diagnostic use. Arch Intern Med 142:2163, 1982
62. Dolovich M: Clinical aspects of aerosol physics. Respir Care 36:931, 1991
63. Newman SP, Clarke SW: Therapeutic aerosols: Physical and practical considerations [Editorial]. Thorax 38:881, 1983
64. Newman SP, Clarke SW: Proper use of metered dose inhalers [Editorial]. Chest 86:342, 1984
65. Kacmarek RM, Hess D: The interface between patient and aerosol generator. Respir Care 36:952, 1991
66. Newman SP: Aerosol generators and delivery systems. Respir Care 36:939, 1991
67. Dolovich MB, Sanchis J, Rossmand C, Newhouse MT: Aerosol penetration: A sensitive index of peripheral airways obstruction. J Appl Physiol 40:486, 1976
68. Ruffin RE, Kenworthy MC, Newhouse MT: Response of asthmatic patients to fenoterol inhalation: A method of quantifying the airway bronchodilator dose. Clin Pharmacol Ther 23:338, 1978
69. Ziment I: Respiratory Pharmacology and Therapeutics. Philadelphia, WB Saunders, 1978
70. American Association for Respiratory Care: Clinical practice guideline: Bronchial provocation. Respir Care 37:902, 1992
71. Rossing TH, Fanta CH, McFadden ER: Effect of outpatient treatment of asthma with beta agonist on the response to sympathomimetics in an emergency room. Am J Med 75:781, 1983
72. National Asthma Education Program-Executive Summary: Guidelines for the Diagnosis and Management of Asthma. National Institute of Health Publication No. 91-3042A. Bethesda, MD; 1991
73. Williams S, Seaton A: Intravenous or inhaled salbutamol in severe acute asthma? Thorax 32:555, 1977
74. Li JT, Reed CE: Proper use of aerosol corticosteroids to control asthma. Mayo Clin Proc 64:205, 1989
75. Barker GA: Current management of croup and epiglottitis. Pediatr Clin North Am 26:565, 1979
76. Postma DS, Jones RO, Pillsbury HC: Severe hospitalized croup: Treatment trends and prognosis. Laryngoscope 94:1170, 1984
77. Lourenco RV, Cotromanes E: Clinical aerosols II: Therapeutic aerosols. Arch Intern Med 142:2299, 1982
78. Hodson ME: Antibiotic treatment-aerosol therapy. Chest 94: 156S, 1988
79. Corkery KJ, Luce JM, Montgomery AB: Aerosolized pentamidine for treatment and prophylaxis of *Pneumocystis carinii* pneumonia: An update. Respir Care 33:676, 1988
80. Demers RR, Parker J, Frankel LR, Smith DW: Administration of ribavirin to neonatal and pediatric patients during mechanical ventilation. Respir Care 31:1188, 1986
81. Wanner A, Rao A: Clinical indications for and effects of bland, mucolytic and antimicrobial aerosols. Am Rev Respir Dis 122:79, 1980
82. Shak S: Aerosolized recombinant human DNase I for the treatment of cystic fibrosis. Chest 107:65S, 1995
83. Dunst MN, Margolin K, Horak D: Lidocaine for severe hiccups (Letter). New Engl J Med 329:890, 1993
84. Hess D: The open forum: Reflections on unanswered questions about aerosol therapy delivery techniques [Editorial]. Respir Care 33:19, 1988
85. Dulfano MJ, Adler K, Wooten O: Physical properties of sputum IV: Effects of 100% humidity and water mist. Am Rev Respir Dis 107:130, 1973
86. Pavia D, Thomson ML, Clarke SW: Enhanced clearance of secretions from the human lung after the administration of hypertonic saline aerosol. Am Rev Respir Dis 117:199, 1978
87. Flick MR, Moody LE, Block AJ: Effect of ultrasonic nebulization on arterial oxygen saturation in chronic obstructive pulmonary disease. Chest 71:366, 1977
88. Shepherd KE, Johnson DC: Bronchodilator testing: An analysis of paradoxical responses. Respir Care 33:667, 1988
89. Craven DE, Lichtenberg DA, Goularte TA, et al: Contaminated medication nebulizers in mechanical ventilator circuits: A source of bacterial aerosols. Am J Med 77:834, 1984
90. American Academy of Pediatrics Committee on Environmental Hazards: Noise pollution neonatal aspects. Pediatrics 54:476, 1974
91. Beckham RW, Mishoe SC: Sound levels inside incubators and oxygen hoods used with nebulizers and humidifiers. Respir Care 27:33, 1982

92. Tamer MA, Model JH, Rieffel CN: Hyponatremia secondary to ultrasonic aerosol therapy in the newborn infant. J Pediatr 77:1051, 1970
93. Fallat RJ, Kandal K: Aerosol exhaust: Escape of aerosolized medication into the patient and caregiver's environment. Respir Care 36:1008, 1991
94. Morley TF, Marozsan E, Zappasodi SJ, et al: Comparison of β adrenergic agents delivered by nebulizer vs. metered dose inhaler with Inspirease in hospitalized asthmatic patients. Chest 94:1205, 1988
95. Lewis RA, Fleming JS: Fractional deposition from a jet nebulizer: How it differs for a metered dose inhaler. Br J Dis Chest 79:361, 1985
96. Loffert DT, Ikle D, Nelson HS: A comparison of commercial jet nebulizers. Chest 106:1788, 1994
97. Alvine GF, Rodgers P, Fitzsimmons KM, Ahrenns RC: Disposable jet nebulizers: How reliable are they? Chest 101:316, 1992
98. Loffert DT, Ikle D, Nelson HS: A comparison of commercial jet nebulizers. Chest 106:1788, 1994
99. Waldrep JC, Keyhani K, Black M, Knight VK: Operating characteristics of 18 different continuous-flow jet nebulizers with beclomethasone dipionate liposome aerosol. Chest 105:106, 1994
100. Fiel SB, Fuchs HJ, Johnson C, et al: Comparison of three jet nebulizer aerosol delivery systems used to administer recombinant human DNase I to patients with cystic fibrosis. Chest 108:153, 1995
101. Smith EC, Denyer J, Kendrick AH: Comparison of twenty three nebulizer/compressor combinations for domiciliary use. Eur Respir J 8:1214, 1995
102. Hess D, Horney D, Snyder T: Medication-delivery performance of eight small-volume, hand-held nebulizers: Effects of diluent volume, gas flow rate and nebulizer model. Respir Care 34:717, 1989
103. Puist FM: Comparison of medication delivery by T-nebulizer with inspiratory and expiratory reservoir. Respir Care 34:985, 1989
104. Mason JW, Miller WC, Small S: Comparison of aerosol delivery via Circulaire system versus conventional small volume nebulizer. Respir Care 39:1157, 1994
105. American Association for Respiratory Care: Clinical practice guideline: Assessing response to bronchodilator therapy at point of care. Respir Care 40:1300, 1995
106. Tashkin DP: Dosing strategies for bronchodilator aerosol delivery. Respir Care 36:977, 1991
107. Moler FW, Hurwitz ME, Custer JR: Improvement in clinical asthma score and $PaCO_2$ in children with severe asthma treated with continuously nebulized terbutaline. J Allergy Clin Immunol 81:1101, 1988
108. Montgomery AB, Debs RJ, Luce JM, et al: Selective delivery of pentamidine to the lung by aerosol. Am Rev Respir Dis 137:477, 1988
109. Hall CB, Powell KR, McDonald NE, et al: Respiratory syncytial viral infection in children with compromised immune function. N Engl J Med 315:77, 1986
110. Byron PR, Phillip EM, Kuhn R: Ribavirin administration by inhalation: Aerosol-generation factors controlling drug delivery to the lung. Respir Care 33:1011, 1988
111. Knight V, Wilson SZ, Wyde PR, et al: Small Particle Aerosols of Amantadine and Ribavirin in the Treatment of Influenza. In Ribavirin: A Broad Spectrum Antiviral Agent. London, Academic Press, 1980
112. Frankel LR, Wilson CW, Demers RR, et al: A technique for the administration of ribavirin to mechanically ventilated infants with severe respiratory syncytial virus infection. Crit Care Med 15:1051, 1987
113. Manthous C, Hall JB: Administration of therapeutic aerosols to mechanically ventilated patients. Chest 106:561, 1994
114. Gross NJ, Jenne JW, Hess D: Bronchodilator Therapy. In MJ Tobin (ed): Principles and Practice of Mechanical Ventilation. New York, McGraw-Hill, 1994
115. Beaty CD, Ritz RH, Benson MS: Continuous in-line nebulizers complicate pressure support ventilation. Chest 96:1360, 1989
116. Gay PC, Rodarte JR, Tayyab M, Hubmayr RD: Evaluation of bronchodilator responsiveness in mechanically ventilated patients. Am Rev Respir Dis 136:880, 1987
117. Eriksson NE, Haglind K, Hidinger KG: A new inhalation technique for Freon aerosols: Terbutaline aerosol with a tube extension in a 2-day cross-over comparison with salbutanol aerosol. Allergy 35:617, 1980
118. Hiller C: Aerodynamic size distribution of metered-dose bronchodilator aerosols. Am Rev Resp Dis 118:311, 1978
119. Balmes JR: Propellant gases in metered dose inhalers: Their impact on the global environment. Respir Care 36:1037, 1991
120. Jenkins SC, Heaton RW, Fulton TJ, Moxham J: Comparison of domiciliary nebulized salbutamol and salbutamol from a metered-dose inhaler in stable chronic airflow limitation. Chest 91:804, 1987
121. Rivlin J, Mindorff C, Reilly P, Levinson H: Pulmonary response to a bronchodilator delivered from three inhalation devices. J Pediatr 104:470, 1984
122. Ruffin RE, Montgomery JM, Newhouse MT: Site of β-adrenergic receptors in the respiratory tract: Use of fenoterol administered by two methods. Chest 74:256, 1978
123. Tobin MT, Jenouri G, Danta I, et al: Response to a bronchodilator drug administered by a new reservoir aerosol delivery system and review of the auxiliary delivery systems. Am Rev Respir Dis 126:670, 1982
124. Cissik JH, Bode FR, Smith JA: Double-blind crossover study of five bronchodilator medications and two delivery methods in stable asthma. Chest 90:489, 1986
125. Clausen JL: Self-administration of bronchodilators: Cost effective? [Editorial] Chest 91:475, 1987
126. Jasper AC, Mohsenifar Z, Kahan S, et al: Cost-benefit comparison of aerosol bronchodilator delivery methods in hospitalized patients. Chest 91:614, 1987
127. Wilson AF, Muki DS, Ahdout JJ: Effect of canister temperature on performance of mtered dose inhalers. Am Rev Respir Dis 143:1034, 1991
128. Shim C: Inhalation aids of metered dose inhalers. Chest 91:315, 1987
129. Crompton GK: Problems patients have using pressurized aerosol inhalers. Eur J Respir Dis 63(Suppl):119, 1982
130. Pedersen S: The importance of a pause between inhalation of two puffs of terbutaline from a pressurized aerosol with tube spacer. J Allergy Clin Immunol 77:505, 1986
131. Interiano B, Guntupalli K: Metered-dose inhalers: Do health care providers know what to teach? Arch Intern Med 153:81, 1993
132. Hanania NA, Wittman R, Kesten S, Chapman KR: Medical personnel's knowledge of and ability to use inhaling devices. Chest 105:111, 1994
133. Haesoon L, Evans HE: Evaluation of inhalation aids of metered dose inhalers in asthmatic children. Chest 91:366, 1987
134. Sakner MA, Kim CS: Auxiliary MDI aerosol delivery systems. Chest 885:161S, 1985
135. Dolovich MB, Ruffin RE, Roberts R, Newhouse MT: Optimal delivery of aerosols from metered dose inhalers. Chest 80(Suppl 6):911, 1981
136. Toogood JH, baskerville J, Jennings B, et al: Use of spacers to facilitate inhaled corticosteroids in treatment of asthma. Am Rev Respir Dis 129:723, 1984
137. Pavia D, Thompson M, Shannon HS: Aerosol inhalation and depth of deposition in the human lung: The effect of airway obstruction and tidal volume inhaled. Arch Environ Health 32:131, 1977
138. Clark AR, Rachelvsky G, Mason PL, et al: The use of reservoir devices for the simultaneous delivery of two metered dose aerosols. J Allergy Clin Immunol 85:75, 1990
139. Rau JL, Restrepo RD, Despande V: Inhalation of single vs. multiple metered-dose broncholator actuations from reservoir devices. Chest 109:969, 1996
140. Hess D, Beener C, Watson KK: An evaluation of the effectiveness of metered dose inhaler use with mechanical ventilation. Respir Care 33:910, 1988
141. Gutierrez CJ, Nelson R: Short-term bronchodilation in mechanically ventilated patients, patients receiving metaproterenol via small volume nebulizer or metered-dose inhaler: A pilot study. Respir Care 33:910, 1988
142. Gay PC, Patel HG, Nelson SB, et al: Metered dose inhalers for bronchodilator delivery in intubated, mechanically ventilated patients. Chest 99:66, 1991

143. Hess D: How should bronchodilator be administered to patients being mechanically ventilated? Respir Care 36:377, 1991
144. Newhouse MT, Fuller HD: Rose is a rose is a rose? Aerosol therapy in ventilated patients: Nebulizers versus metered dose inhalers—a continuing controversy. Am Rev Respir Dis 148:1444, 1993
145. Bishop MJ, Larson RP, Buschman DL: Metered dose inhaler aerosol characteristics are affected by the endotracheal tube actuator/adaptor used. Anesthesiology 73:1263, 1990
146. Rau JL, Harwood RJ, Groff JL: Evaluation of a reservoir device for metered-dose bronchodilator delivery to intubated adults: An in vitro study. Chest 102:924, 1992
147. Ebert J, Adams AA, Green-Eide B: An evaluation of MDI spacers and adaptors: Their effect on the respirable volume of medication. Respir Care 37:862, 1992
148. Hayton WL: Propellant-powered nebulizers. J Am Pharm Assoc 16:201, 1976
149. Nizami NP, Vakil DV, Lozynsky A, Nizami RM: Automatic piercing Spinhaler (Halermatic): A comparison study. Ann Allergy 60:399, 1988
150. Persson G, Gruvstad E, Stahl E: A new multiple dose powder inhaler (Turbuhaler), compared with a pressurized inhaler in a study of terbutaline in asthmatics. Eur Resp J 1:681, 1988
151. Sumby BS, Churcher KM, Smith IJ, et al: Dose reliability of the serevent Diskhaler system. Publication No. 0017. Pharmaceutical Technology, 1993
152. Brindley A, Sumby BS, Smith IJ, et al: Design, manufacture, and dose consistency of the serevent Diskus Inhaler. Publication No. PTE0053. Pharmaceutical Technology Europe J, 1995
153. Bronsky E, Bucholz GA, Buse WW, et al: Comparison of inhaled albuterol powder and aerosol in asthma. J Allergy Clin Immunol 79:741, 1987
154. Hindle M, Newton D, Chrystyn H: Dry powder inhalers are bioequivalent to metered-dose inhalers. Chest 107:629, 1995
155. American College of Chest Physicians—National Heart, Lung, and Blood Institute: National conference on oxygen therapy. Respir Care 29:922, 1984
156. Brain J: Aerosol and humidity therapy. Am Rev Respir Dis 122:17, 1980
157. Swift DL: Aerosols and humidity therapy: Generation and respiratory deposition. Am Rev Respir Dis 122(Suppl):71, 1980
158. Clay MM, Pavia D, Newman SP, et al: Assessment of jet nebulisers for lung aerosol therapy. Lancet 2:592, 1983
159. Rutala WA, Weber DJ: Environmental Issues and Nosocomial Infection. In BF Farber (ed): Infection Control in Intensive Care. New York, Churchill Livingstone, 1987
160. Boucher RM, Kreuter J: The fundamentals of the ultrasonic atomization of medicated solutions. Ann Allergy 26:591, 1968
161. Mitchell DM, Solomon MA, Tolfree SE, et al: Effect of particle size of bronchodilator aerosols on lung distribution and pulmonary function in patients with chronic asthma. Thorax 42:457, 1987
162. Branson RD, Davis K, Campbell RS, Porembka DT: Humidification in the intensive care unit: Prospective study of a new protocol utilizing heated humidification and hygroscopic condenser humidifier. Chest 104:1800, 1993
163. Hess DR: Aerosol therapy. Respir Care Clin North Am 1:235, 1995
164. Smaldone CG: Drug delivery by nebulization: "Reality testing." (Editorial). J Aerosol Med 7:213, 1994

16 Drugs Used in Respiratory Care

Irwin Ziment

CLINICAL SKILLS

Upon completion of this chapter, the reader will:

- Recount advantages and disadvantages of medication delivery via inhalation of aerosols
- Categorize respiratory medications according to functional purpose
- Identify the mode of action of commonly used respiratory medications
- Designate standard dosages of commonly used respiratory medications
- Identify major side effects of commonly used respiratory medications
- Evaluate the therapeutic response to medications delivered via inhalation
- Explain the importance of patient technique in maximizing the amount of aerosolized drug deposited in the respiratory tract

KEY TERMS

Adenyl cyclase
Administration of aerosol drugs
Anticholinergics
Antimicrobial drugs
Bronchodilator aerosol agents
Catecholamines
Corticosteroids
Drug dosage
Drugs for bronchospasm
Methylxanthines
Mucokinetic agents
Phosphodiesterase inhibitors
Prophylactic agents
Surfactants
Sympathomimetics
Tachyphylaxis

Many of the drugs used to treat disorders of the lungs can be administered by nebulization or by instillation into the respiratory tract. Drugs given directly are not always prescribed by physicians in precise dosages and concentrations. The actual administration of the medication is usually performed by a nurse or a respiratory therapist or by the patient. A ridiculous quibble occasionally is voiced, expressing doubts on the legal propriety of respiratory therapists mixing and delivering prescribed drugs. Because the patient obviously can be instructed in safe self-therapy, there can be no serious questioning of the trained therapist's capability as a provider of pharmacologic therapy in the hospital setting. Indeed, the educated therapist generally knows more about respiratory aerosol pharmacology than does the average physician or nurse; in fact, it would be reasonable to expect the nonspecialist physician to consult with a therapist about the details of aerosol drug administration.

Relatively few drugs are used in aerosol therapy, and it is essential for therapists to be completely familiar with the pharmacology of these agents and to know the indications and contraindications for their use, as well as the complications that may arise during their administration (see AARC Clinical Practice Guideline: Selection of Aerosol Delivery Device). The main emphasis herein will be placed on drugs commonly given by aerosolization, and less detail will be provided for the other drugs used to treat respiratory diseases. The well-educated respiratory therapist should maintain a strong interest in all respiratory pharmacologic preparations, not simply those given by nebulization.

AARC Clinical Practice Guideline

SELECTION OF AEROSOL DELIVERY DEVICE

Indications: The need to deliver—as an aerosol to the lower airways—a medication from one of the following drug classifications: β-adrenergic agents, anticholinergic agents (antimuscarinics), anti-inflammatory agents (eg, corticosteroids), mediator-modifying compounds (eg, cromolyn sodium), mucokinetics.

Contraindications: No contraindications exist to the administration of aerosols by inhalation. Contraindications related to the substances being delivered may exist. Consult the package insert for product-specific contraindications.

Assessment of Need: Based on proven therapeutic efficacy, variety of available medications, and cost-effectiveness, the MDI with accessory device should be the first method to consider for administration of aerosol to the airway. Lack of availability of prescribed drug in MDI, dry-powder, or solution form or inability of the patient to use device properly with coaching and instruction should lead to consideration of other devices. Patient preference for a given device that meets therapeutic objectives should be honored. When there is need for large doses, MDI, SVN, or LVN may be used. Clear superiority of any one method has not been established. Convenience and patient tolerance of procedure should be considered. When spontaneous ventilation is inadequate (eg, as in kyphoscoliosis or neuromuscular disorders, exacerbation of severe bronchospasm with impending respiratory failure that does not respond to other forms of therapy), delivery by a positive-pressure breathing device (IPPB) should be considered.

Assessment of Outcome: Proper technique applying device, patient response to or compliance with procedure, objectively measured improvement (eg, increased FEV_1 or peak flow).

Monitoring: Performance of the device, technique of device application, assessment of patient response including changes in vital signs.

From AARC Clinical Practice Guideline; See Respir Care 37:891, 1992, for complete text.

AEROSOL THERAPY

The use of inhalational drug therapy developed empirically, and numerous controversies about the value of such therapy still exist. Prescribers and providers of aerosols should recognize the advantages and limitations of aerosol therapy techniques.

Advantages (Box 16-1)

The main advantage of delivering a drug by aerosol is that relatively small quantities of the drug can be given, with maximal pulmonary effect and minimal extrapulmonary side effects. The onset of action usually is rapid, and repeated therapy with small doses can be given at relatively frequent intervals, according to the patient's needs, with little risk of toxicity. Certain drugs are specifically designed for aerosolization and cannot be given by other means.

Disadvantages (Box 16-2)

A major problem in inhalation treatment is that, unless the trachea is intubated, patients must be able to cooperate by breathing deeply in coordination with the administration of the aerosol by mouthpiece or mask. Oral therapy with a pill or liquid is usually much simpler because no expensive or cumbersome equipment is required. Domiciliary equipment suffers from dual disadvantages: difficulties in operation and maintenance may discourage patients from using the more expensive machines, whereas accessibility of ready relief from simple nebulizers may result in overuse of potent drugs; much money can be spent on domiciliary nebulization devices that are not indicated and are not used correctly by patients.

An additional concern about aerosol therapy is based on the experience of Great Britain in the 1960s: The death rate from asthma in children greatly increased because of overuse of metered aerosol bronchodilators.[1] However, a recent increase in many countries of deaths from asthma does not appear to be related to the proper use of prescribed drugs.[2] Aerosol therapy suffers from disadvantages that include overuse, underuse, and misuse of overprescribed medications. Furthermore, even if the drugs are administered appropriately, there is a lack of knowledge about what the appropriate dosage of

BOX 16-1

ADVANTAGES OF AEROSOL THERAPY

1. Topical administration results in a rapid therapeutic effect.
2. Only a small total dose of a potent drug need be nebulized into the lungs.
3. Minimal extrapulmonary side effects are produced.
4. Individual dosage titration is possible.
5. The respiratory route is always available for drug delivery.
6. Certain drugs (eg, cromolyn) cannot be given by other routes.
7. Humidification and bland droplet therapy are essential for tracheotomized and intubated patients.
8. Administration of aerosol therapy in the hospital involves the respiratory therapist, with the attendant benefits of skilled attention to the respiratory tract.
9. Patients develop faith in nebulizers and derive psychological benefits from their use.
10. Aerosol therapy may provide patients with an oral-inhalational substitute for smoking.

BOX 16-2

DISADVANTAGES OF AEROSOL THERAPY

1. Special, expensive equipment is often required.
2. Patients must be able to cooperate in taking synchronized deep breaths (unless intubated).
3. Precise drug dosage is usually not achieved; underdosage and overdosage are readily produced.
4. Only a small portion of a nebulized drug is deposited in the lung.
5. Oropharyngeal deposition of an aerosol may result in appreciable systemic absorption.
6. Oropharyngeal irritation by the aerosol can result in gagging, nausea, vomiting, or aerophagia.
7. Tracheobronchial irritation by the aerosol can result in bronchospasm, coughing (thus limiting the inhaled doses), and possibly tracheobronchitis.
8. The inhalational adjuvants may cause detrimental side effects (eg, oxygen, freon).
9. Nebulizers readily become dirty, thus losing effectiveness, and possibly become sources of infection.
10. Aerosol therapy can result in unreasonable complexity (involving patient, equipment, and personnel factors) compared with oral administration.

most inhalational agents should be. More precise dosing would be attained if clinicians prescribed drugs in milligrams, rather than in milliliters or in percentage strengths of solutions. Not only are drugs prescribed imprecisely, but many physicians and therapists fail to appreciate that the amount delivered can be extremely variable. The typical patient given an aerosol will deposit only 5% to 10% of the prescribed amount of the drug in the respiratory tract; with special effort, or with more efficient delivery systems, the amount delivered may reach 20% of the prescribed dose.

The problem of droplet size is a controversial topic, and it is difficult to know if any one of the conventional nebulizing units offers significant advantages over its competitors.[3] Less effective equipment delivers droplets of larger diameter, which are deposited mainly in the mouth and upper airways. The hypoxemic asthmatic may become even more hypoxemic after aerosolizing isoproterenol, because systemic absorption causes vasodilation of pulmonary vessels disproportionate to the bronchodilation achieved, resulting in an increased shunt through poorly ventilated areas of the lung.

There are other disadvantages to administering drugs as aerosols. Many patients find that the taste and the oropharyngeal irritation of the droplets cause gagging and nausea, whereas the irritant effect of the aerosol on reactive airways can cause deterioration in respiratory variables (eg, oxygen transport, dynamic compliance) and may result in bronchospasm. The latter problem is likely to arise with any nonbronchodilator aerosol, and consequently, incorporation of a bronchodilator drug with other classes of drugs may be appropriate. Unfortunately, bronchodilators are not entirely compatible with all other inhalational drugs; bronchodilators are acidic and undergo fairly rapid breakdown in an alkaline medium.

A further disadvantage of aerosol therapy is that the nebulizer readily becomes contaminated with microorganisms. Thus, inhalational apparatus is a potential source of serious nosocomial infections. This fact is so well known that elaborate precautions are taken, including the use of disposable equipment and the use of complex cleaning and sterilizing protocols in hospitals. The expense of such methods constitutes a major factor in the relatively poor cost-effectiveness of complex forms of aerosol therapy (Box 16-3).

PHARMACOLOGY OF RESPIRATORY DRUGS

The most important and frequently administered drugs in aerosol therapy are agents used to improve mucociliary clearance (mucokinetic agents) and agents used to relieve bronchospasm. Relatively few other categories of drugs are given by nebulization; they include antiasthmatic agents, mucosal vasoconstrictors, local anesthetics, and antimicrobial agents. The major drugs in these categories are reviewed in this chapter.

MUCOKINETIC AGENTS

Drugs in this category include mucolytics, expectorants, and other agents found in "cough medicines" (Table 16-1). The most important mucokinetic agent is often considered to be water. Factors involved in natural and abetted mucokinesis are outlined in Table 16-2.

The end result of successful mucokinetic therapy is usually seen in a sputum receptacle by the bedside or in the suction bottle in an intensive care unit. Sputum is a complex fluid consisting of mucoprotein (including mucopolysaccharides), electrolytes, water, cellular debris (including actin), and with expectorated specimens,

BOX 16-3

TROUBLESHOOTING TECHNIQUES

Delivery of Aerosol Drugs

- Ensure dosage, concentration/dilution of prescribed drugs are understood and appropriate for patient with respect to age, cardiac condition, and ability to cooperate in therapy.
- Ensure that patient has not experienced prior adverse reaction to the drug or the technique of delivery.
- Be aware that there is no "fixed dose," since patients will respond to a range of doses in individualistic fashion. Some do not tolerate average doses, whereas others tolerate and benefit from larger doses. Thus, any standard dose can be excessive, appropriate, or inadequate depending on individual patient factors.

Alternative Therapy

- Assess ability of patient to use a prescribed aerosol, and try to judge whether a nebulized wet aerosol or a metered dose inhalant with or without a spacer device is most appropriate. In some patients, an inhaled powder may be preferred.
- When an aerosol cannot be delivered effectively (eg, because of poor cooperation), special techniques such as breath-actuated delivery may be appropriate. In some patients, it may be best to give drugs orally if the inhaled route cannot be used effectively.

Adverse Effects

- Such effects may be exaggerated pharmacologic responses (eg, tachycardia after receiving a β_2 agonist), allergic (eg, a rash after receiving an antibiotic), idiosyncratic (eg, bronchospasm following administration of an aerosol bronchodilator), or toxic (eg, thrush after receiving an aerosol steroid). In all cases, a harmful or unexpected outcome should be carefully analyzed and documented. It should be reported in accord with local policy.
- Following an adverse effect, careful notation should be made indicating whether a drug or delivery technique should be avoided or whether a modified dosage or regimen would be appropriate. Alternative therapy should be considered as a possibility.

oropharyngeal secretions (ie, saliva, food particles, and bacteria).

The respiratory tract secretions originate from two major sources (Fig 16-1): the goblet cells that produce a gelatinous secretion, mainly in response to irritation; and the bronchial glands that secrete a more watery solution and are under vagal control. In addition, infected sputum contains DNA, which is liberated from polymorphonuclear (white) blood cells and bacteria. This material gives a yellow or green color to the secretions, which are rendered highly viscous.

The normal mucous blanket has two layers: the more watery sol layer in which the cilia beat, and the superficial viscous gel layer. The ciliary activity serves to waft the gel layer proximally up the respiratory tract against gravity. Problems with sputum expectoration occur when there is increased production of viscous secretions in airways having damaged cilia and impaired architecture, which interfere with effective coughing. The actions of mucokinetic agents are summarized in Table 16-3.

Although pharmacologic agents can alter the consistency of mucus, effective removal of the secretions, or mucokinesis, requires the presence of an effective cough. If a patient is unable or unwilling to cough, then postural drainage or, alternatively, tracheobronchial suctioning will be required. Thus, effective mucokinesis requires more than active drug therapy, and pharmacologic agents contribute only the first half of the process: physical therapy or coached coughing are equally or, at times, more important.[4]

Mucokinetic Drugs Suitable for Aerosolization

☐ WATER

The addition of water to mucus results in decreased viscosity of sputum. If relatively large quantities of water are added, the secretions are simply diluted; however, water can become incorporated into mucus to reduce the adhesiveness of gelatinous secretions. The ad-

TABLE 16-1. **Important Aerosol Mucokinetic Drugs**

Drug	Usual Aerosol Dosage	Comments
N-acetyl-L-cysteine (10%–20%) (Mucomyst, Mucosil)	2–5 mL every 6h	Breaks disulfide bonds, causes mucolysis. Malodorous and may cause bronchospasm. Solution should be diluted with an equal volume of isotonic saline or sodium bicarbonate because it is more active in an alkaline environment.
Sodium bicarbonate (2.1%–7.5%)	2–5 mL every 6h Range: 1–10 mL q2–8h	Surfactant in low concentrations, bronchorrheic in higher concentrations. May be combined with other drugs for immediate use.
Sodium chloride (0.45%–20%)	2–5 mL every 6h Range: 1–10 mL q2–8h	Hypotonic solution used for patients on sodium restriction. Hypertonic solutions stimulate cough and may have mucolytic effect; particularly useful for inducing sputum production. Normal saline is a standard diluting agent.
Propylene glycol (2%–25%)	2–5 mL every 4h Range: 1–10 mL q1–8h	Soothing demulcent for tracheobronchitis (2% solution). Stabilizes droplets; used with therapeutic aerosols to improve distal deposition. Effective for cough induction (15% or stronger solution). Rarely used.
Dornase alfa (0.1%) (Pulmozyme)	2.5 mg every 12–24h	Recombinant human deoxyribonuclease; digests purulent sputum. Of value in cystic fibrosis and possibly chronic obstructive airway disease.

TABLE 16-2. **Factors Involved in Mucokinesis**

Natural
Respiratory tract secretions of adequate amount and consistency
Maintenance of appropriate sol–gel relationship
Ciliary activity and coordination
Patent airways and adequate airflow
Muscular coordination with laryngeal activity and effective cough
Pharmacologic
Hypoviscosity agents and diluents
Bronchorrheics
Bronchomucotropic agents
Mucolytics and enzymes
Detergents and surfactants
Bronchodilators
Mucosal constrictors
Mechanical
Cough stimulation (eg, aerosols, pharyngeal catheter)
Postural drainage
Physical therapy (eg, percussion-vibration, rocking bed)
Suctioning
Psychic stimulation, encouragement, and teaching of patient

dition of water to a depleted sol layer allows the cilia to beat more effectively, thereby contributing to the proximal propulsion of the viscous gel layer.

There is still uncertainty as to whether water provided in the form of an aerosol, as humidity (eg, in "croup tents") or given orally has a significant effect on mucociliary clearance[5,6]; certainly, the nebulization of 2 mL of water (resulting in the actual deposition of less than 0.2 mL in the respiratory tract) may do no more than add an imperceptible amount of fluid to the gel layer coating the tracheobronchial tree.[7] In contrast, secretion of a watery fluid by the bronchial glands following systemic hydration may serve to replenish the sol layer from below and, thereby, to loosen adherent inspissated secretions.

Droplets that are aerosolized into the airways may rapidly evaporate to smaller sizes and may not deposit at all.[8] Consequently, plain water is not favored as a mucokinetic for nebulization therapy, although it does serve to prevent dehydration of the secretions in the upper airway during normal respiration. Plain water in inhalational therapy subserves a "demulcent," soothing effect, rather than acting as a mucokinetic; it is preferable to give it as humidification therapy or as hot or cold mists.

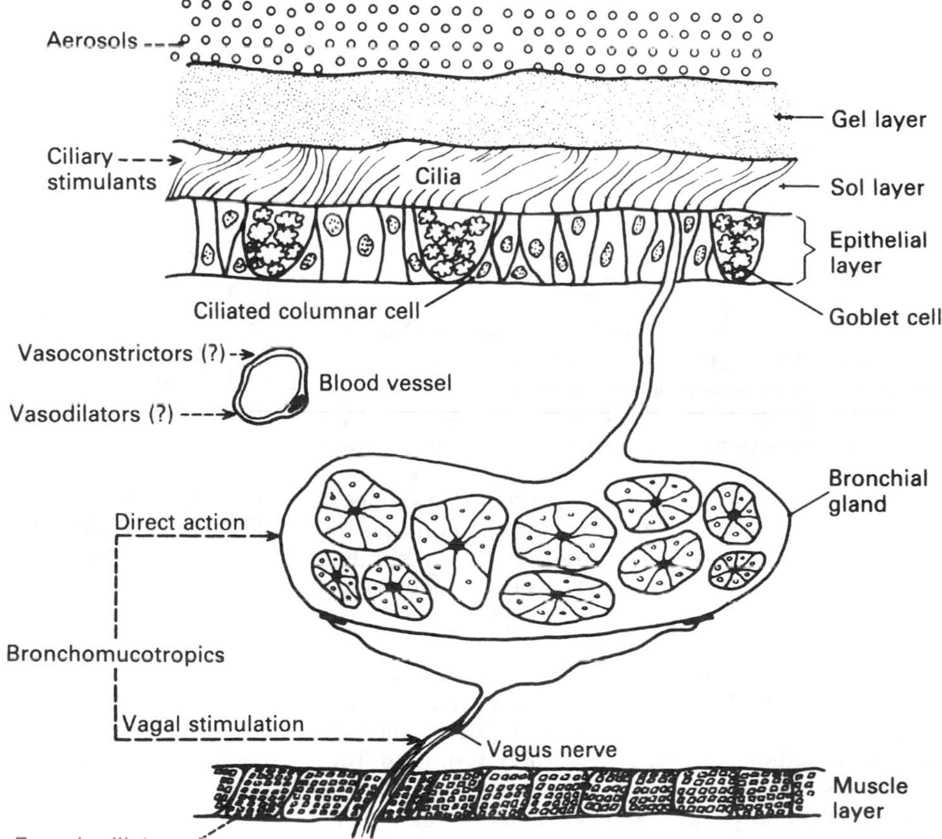

FIGURE 16-1. Schematic diagram illustrating the sites of action of various classes of pharmacologic agents within the wall and lumina of the respiratory tract.

TABLE 16-3. **Classification of Mucokinetic Drugs**

Class	Action	Examples
Drugs that increase the depth of the sol layer	Topical diluents	Hydrating agents (eg, water,* electrolyte solutions*)
	Stimulators of respiratory mucosa	Bronchorrheics
	Irritants	Smoke,* aromatic vapors,* ultrasonic particles,* alcohol*
	Hyperosmolar solutions	Hypertonic drug or salt solutions*
	Stimulators of mucous secretion	Bronchomucotropics (eg, iodide)
	Stimulators of gastropulmonary vagal reflex	Expectorants (eg, ipecac, guaifenesin)
Drugs that alter the consistency of the gel layer	Topical diluents	Hydrating agents (eg, water,* electrolyte solutions*)
	Breakdown (lyse) protein or DNA	True mucolytics
	Thiol (split disulfide bonds)	Acetylcysteine
	Decomplexing agents (break mucoprotein-DNA complexes)	Hypertonic salt solutions,* alkalis
	Enzymes (digest protein)	Proteases (eg, deoxyribonuclease)
	Activators of natural proteases	Iodides, electrolyte solutions*
	Reducing agents	Ascorbic acid,† copper*,†
	Amides	Urea*,†
	Calcium binders	l-Arginine*,† chelating agents, hypertonic saline*
	Normalize biochemical production of mucus:	
	Mucoregulators (alter mucoprotein synthesis)	Bromhexine,† ambroxol,† sobrerol,† stepronin,† S-carboxymethylcysteine†
	Antimicrobials (decrease DNA production)	Antibiotics
	Nonspecific	Glucocorticosteroids
	Thicken watery sputum	Mucospissics
		Anticholinergic agents (eg, atropine)
		Some antibiotics (eg, tetracycline*)
Drugs that decrease the adhesiveness of the gel layer	Wetting agents	Sodium ethasulfate,*,† water*
	Surfactant	Tyloxapol,*,† sodium bicarbonate,* glycerine,* propylene glycol,* natural surfactants
Agents that improve airway patency	Bronchodilators	Sympathomimetics,* methylxanthines
	Anti-inflammatory agents	Glucocorticosteroids
	Mucosal constrictors	Phenylephrine*
	Ciliary stimulants	Sympathomimetics*

* Usually given by inhalational route.
† Not available in the United States.

□ SALINE

Various concentrations of sodium chloride (NaCl) in water are used in aerosol therapy, either as primary drugs or as diluents or carriers for other drugs.

Normal saline (0.9% NaCl, which is isotonic with tissue fluids) is generally favored as a "bland" aerosol solution.

Half-normal saline (0.45% NaCl, hypotonic saline) is sometimes preferred, particularly for use in ultrasonic nebulization. The aerosol droplets of half-normal saline are thought to undergo some evaporative concentration in the respiratory tract; thus, the droplets that impact are almost isotonic.[9]

Hypertonic saline (eg, 1.8% to 15% NaCl) offers a theoretically more effective form of mucokinetic therapy. Deposition of hypertonic droplets on the respiratory mucosa results in the osmotic attraction of fluid from the mucosal blood vessels and tissues into the airway. Thus a "bronchorrhea" is induced, and the watery solution helps to dilute the respiratory tract secretions and to increase their bulk, thereby augmenting expectoration. Moreover, hypertonic saline has a direct effect on mucoprotein-DNA complexes, and by reducing the cohesive intramolecular forces the salt helps to decrease their viscous properties.

Hypertonic saline is most useful as a sputum-inducing agent. An aerosol of 3% to 15% sodium chloride is an effective stimulus to expectoration in patients who have little spontaneous sputum production, and such mixtures are recommended for inducing sputum specimens for cytologic and microbiologic studies. The delivery of hypertonic saline by ultrasonic nebulization can be very effective in inducing sputum for the diagnosis of *Pneumocystis carinii* infection.

For purposes of irrigation or instillation into the tracheobronchial tree, normal saline and half-normal saline are favored because they are relatively nonirritating to the airways. If hypertonic saline is used, no more than 10 mL/day should be given for a few days; excessive use is irritating and susceptible patients may develop edema, heart failure, or hypertension. Improved results may be obtained by using a heated aerosol, or perhaps, by adding 10% to 20% propylene glycol to the saline.

☐ SODIUM BICARBONATE

For many years, sodium bicarbonate ($NaHCO_3$) has been used as an irrigating fluid and for cleaning tracheostomy tubes. The mucokinetic aerosol Alevaire contained 2% sodium bicarbonate in combination with 0.125% tyloxapol (a "wetting" agent or "detergent") and 5% glycerin. There is no satisfactory evidence that Alevaire was more successful than hypertonic sodium bicarbonate alone; consequently, it is no longer marketed. However, tyloxapol is now included in the surfactant preparation, colfosceril. Bicarbonate solutions can be given by aerosolization or by direct instillation; higher concentrations may be irritating, but the 5% solution is probably optimal.

The success of sodium bicarbonate seems to be related partly to its alkaline pH (whereas sodium chloride is provided as an acidic solution), because sputum may be less adherent in an alkaline medium.[10] The hypertonic solutions also have a bronchorrheic effect and possibly a direct salt effect that helps disrupt some of the complex molecular bonds in mucus.

A minor disadvantage of sodium bicarbonate is that added bronchodilators (which have an acid pH) undergo more rapid breakdown in the alkaline solution, and the material that is subsequently expectorated or suctioned from the respiratory tract may be colored pink because of the presence of catecholamine breakdown products (adrenochromes). Sodium bicarbonate is the optimal diluent for acetylcysteine, which is more effective in an alkaline medium.

☐ ACETYLCYSTEINE

Acetylcysteine (*N*-acetyl-L-cysteine sodium salt; Mucomyst) is the most powerful mucolytic agent for general use in inhalational therapy. Like its parent compound, the amino acid cysteine, acetylcysteine contains a thiol group, and the free sulfhydryl radical of this group is a strong reducing agent that ruptures the disulfide bridges that give stability to the mucoprotein network of molecules in mucus. Agents that break down these disulfide bonds produce the most effective mucolysis in laboratory studies.[11] Interestingly, the main constituent of garlic, which is a traditional expectorant, is the compound *S*-allyl-L-cysteine sulfoxide (also known as alliin); however, this agent does not have the mucolytic properties of acetylcysteine.

It has not been clearly demonstrated that nebulization of thiol compounds in small amounts can produce the same degree of mucolysis as that seen in test tube experiments. Indeed, the acetylcysteine may simply induce bronchorrhea and stimulate coughing, thereby increasing expectoration. Acetylcysteine should be used as the 10% or 20% solution with the addition of an equal volume of normal sodium chloride or, preferably, 5% sodium bicarbonate. Once a bottle of the agent has been opened, it must be stored in a refrigerator; it should be used within a few days, as its potency rapidly declines at room temperature.

Acetylcysteine is an irritant to the respiratory tract and may induce bronchospasm. In addition, it can inhibit ciliary activity. These side effects may be obviated by pretreating with an aerosol bronchodilator, or by giving a systemic bronchodilator. Acetylcysteine has a sulfurous odor and an unpleasant taste, and on nebulization may induce gagging and nausea or vomiting. However, the drug has no serious toxicity and, indeed, can be given with a fair degree of safety orally or intravenously. In Europe and South America, oral acetylcysteine is a very popular mucolytic because the marketed product is odorless and flavored. Acetylcysteine by the oral or intravenous route is a specific antidote for the treatment of poisoning by acetaminophen. The drug provides cysteine, which is converted in the liver into glutathione, and this scavenger agent removes the toxic metabolites of acetaminophen. As a free-radical scavenger, regular administration of the drug may prevent pollutant damage to the lungs; it may also help if given in the early stage of adult respiratory distress syndrome (ARDS).

☐ ENZYMES

Until recently, enzymes were out of favor in respiratory therapy. Older formulations were irritating to the respiratory tract and induced bronchospasm; more prolonged use resulted in tracheobronchitis. Patients could develop hypersensitivity responses including rashes, asthma, pulmonary infiltrates, and fever.

Recently, the benefits of genetically engineered drugs have reached the respiratory tract. Recombinant human deoxyribonuclease (rhDNase, *dornase alfa*, Pulmozyme) has replaced pancreatic dornase as a proteolytic enzyme that breaks down DNA in purulent sputum. Formerly, bovine pancreatic dornase (Dornavac) was used to break up purulent secretions, but its liability to cause allergic reactions led to a decline in its use. The new agent is well-tolerated and has been studied in over 2000 patients; mild, transient voice alteration, pharyngitis, laryngitis, chest pain, conjunctivitis, and rash were recorded in some patients. The drug was released by the Food and Drug Administration (FDA) for the treatment of cystic fibrosis; it has been reported to produce a slight but significant improvement in pulmonary function accompanied by a marked improvement in quality of life.[12] The drug will probably be of use in patients with chronic obstructive pulmonary disease (COPD) who have viscous, purulent secretions, because early studies suggest it helps decrease mortality.

Trypsin has an antifibrin digestive effect. It was formerly used to treat fibropurulent exudates in the lung. The drug is no longer marketed.

Streptokinase and *streptodornase* were sometimes used in a combined preparation for inhalation. However, the use of these enzymes is no longer promoted for this purpose.

□ HYGROSCOPIC AGENTS

Several agents are incorporated into proprietary aerosols as soothing demulcents or as droplet-stabilizing adjuvants. *Propylene glycol* is probably the best of these agents; glycerol (glycerin) is more irritating and is not recommended.

□ ALCOHOL

Although alcohol may have mucokinetic properties, it is an irritant and results in bronchorrhea. Prolonged use of this drug causes tracheobronchitis and inhibits ciliary activity. One must not assume that the mucokinetic effect of an irritant agent is necessarily beneficial; after all, cigarette smoking is a prime means for stimulating mucus production, but obviously smoking is not beneficial. One established use for ethyl alcohol in respiratory therapy has been in managing foaming pulmonary edema. Alcohol, as a vapor or droplets, acts to reduce the stability of the edema bubbles and, thereby, results in rapid dispersion of the foam.[13] Alcohol has been used in the form of vodka diluted with one or two parts water; it is given by nebulization.

□ SURFACTANTS

The type II pneumocytes start to produce endogenous *surfactant* in the fetal lung at about the 34th week. This complex material serves to reduce the surface tension forces that would favor the sticking together of the air-liquid interfaces of the alveoli during expiration thus resulting in progressive atelectasis. The absolute or relative deficiency in surfactant in the premature neonate impairs the ability of normal inhalation to expand the lungs at birth, and progressive respiratory distress develops. The resulting advance of the problem, which culminates in the neonatal respiratory distress syndrome (RDS), can be seen in up to 60% of infants born before 30 weeks of gestation (see Chapter 25). During the development of RDS, progressive alveolar atelectasis is accompanied by leakage of plasma protein into the air space, a liability to pneumothorax, and shunting leading to increasing impairment of gas exchange. The condition can result in death or subsequent bronchopulmonary dysplasia in 60% to 70% of smaller premature infants. Supportive treatment with oxygen and ventilation does help, but provision of exogenous surfactant is required to maximize the chances of recovery.

Exogenous surfactants have been produced from natural sources and artificially. The natural products are those derived by lavage or whole organ extraction using the lungs of cattle, calves, and pigs, or human amniotic fluid. Artificial surfactants contain some of the synthesized component molecules of the natural materials with the addition of various adjuvants. Currently, human recombinant DNA is being used in cloned cells to produce a natural mix of surfactant compounds. The surfactants marketed in the United States include a synthesized product and a bovine product; a porcine-derived surfactant is available in some countries.

Beractant (surfactant TA, Survanta) is a lipoid extract of bovine minced lung with the addition of synthetic components. The extract contains phospholipids, neutral lipids, and fatty acids. Also present are surfactant protein B (SP-B) and SP-C, which facilitate the spreading and the absorption of the surfactant. The naturally occurring SP-A, which promotes recycling of surfactant, is destroyed in the processing of the extract. The lipid molecules include dipalmitoyl phosphatidylcholine (DPPC, also known as lecithin) and phosphatidylglycerol (PG); both of these, and especially DPPC, stabilize the air-alveolar interface. The effectiveness of the extracted molecular mixture is improved by the addition of synthetic DPPC, as well as palmitic acid and tripalmitin. The exogenous product is taken up by alveolar type II cells and is recycled; thus only one to four doses are usually needed in individual cases.

The product is made available as a suspension that is administered directly in the infant's trachea through a catheter. The technique to be used, which necessitates turning the neonate in different positions while administering increments of the dose, is detailed by the manufacturer in brochures and videos and in various reviews.

Colfosceril palmitate (Exosurf Neonatal) is synthetic DPPC in solution to which the following emulsifying agents are added: cetyl alcohol (a spreading agent) and tyloxapol (known as a wetting, detergent or dispersing agent; it was formerly marketed in the aerosol mucokinetic product, Alevaire). This synthetic product is theoretically safer than the natural product, which could contain sensitizing proteins or infectious agents. However, it appears that it is less likely to cause rapid improvement in oxygenation such as occurs with endotracheal instillation of natural surfactant. It is marketed as a powder that has to be reconstituted with sterile water before it can be instilled in one to three doses over 24 hours.

The value of surfactant therapy in leading to a rapid improvement of oxygenation in RDS is recognized, but its prophylactic value is more difficult to demonstrate.[14] The long-term benefit of these expensive drugs in preventing and treating RDS needs to be further defined, and their value in decreasing the incidence of bronchopulmonary dysplasia needs to be established. Different techniques of use, including aerosolization and continuous infusion, and the possible values of different products (such as Curosurf, Infasurf, Alveofact, and recombinant products) need to be studied. It is possible that larger doses and earlier administration in RDS may offer greater benefit, although some experts consider that two doses given 12 hours apart is sufficient. It is unlikely that surfactant therapy will be used in ARDS because the large amounts required would be extraordinarily expensive, and the results of initial studies have not been sufficiently encouraging.

Tergemist was formerly promoted in the United States. It contained 0.125% sodium ethasulfate (a "wetting" agent) and 0.1% potassium iodide.

Traditional household inhalational remedies such as menthol, eucalyptus, camphor, and benzoin are still popular. Years of apparently satisfactory experience suggest that steam, rendered aromatic by the addition of one of these essential volatile oils (eg, Vick's Vaporub and Friar's Balsam), may be an effective, inexpensive, and pleasant mucokinetic.[15] Menthol has been shown to have antitussive activity.

Noninhalational Mucokinetic Drugs

Most of the noninhalational drugs are given orally and are generally classified as expectorants. Boyd and others give evidence to suggest that these agents stimulate afferent receptors in the stomach.[16] These postulated receptors result in a vagal reflex that may relay through a "mucokinetic" medullary center, which possibly lies between the respiratory center and the vomiting center. The efferent arc of the reflex is thought to be provided by vagal fibers to the lungs. Strong stimulation of this reflex results in vomiting. A lesser stimulus by a subemetic dose of a vagal stimulant does not cause vomiting, but does result in increased expectoration, presumably by activating the bronchial glands (ie, the gastropulmonary mucokinetic vagal reflex). These glands are under vagal control, and an effective stimulus results in the output of a watery secretion.[17] Certain orally administered drugs are preferentially concentrated by the bronchial glands, which are then stimulated to secrete. Some agents, when secreted into the respiratory fluid, have a direct or indirect mucolytic effect on the mucoproteins.

In the following section, the more important oral mucokinetic drugs are discussed (Box 16-4/Table 16-4).

□ POTASSIUM IODIDE

For many years, a saturated solution of potassium iodide (SSKI) has been favored as a mucokinetic agent. There are several ways in which iodide may have an effect.

Iodide is usually administered as SSKI, 5 to 10 drops in a glass of water; as many as 20 to 30 drops may be given in this way three or four times a day. Iodide may cause an acneiform eruption or a rash. Long-term administration of the drug may affect thyroid function; therefore, TSH and T_4 tests should be checked after the first 2 or 3 months of therapy.

Organic iodide (iodinated glycerol) has been shown to be of some benefit in the management of chronic mucus stasis, but the evidence was not deemed adequate by the FDA, who asked for it to be withdrawn from the market. Sodium iodide was once given intravenously, but is no longer marketed.

□ SYRUP OF IPECAC

Syrup of ipecac is best known as an emetic agent. However, it has long been used, in small doses, as a mucokinetic agent. The appropriate dose for adults is 0.5 to 2 mL three to four times daily; at this dosage nausea should not occur.

□ SALTS

Various salt solutions are suitable for oral use as vagal stimulants. Thus, concentrated solutions of sodium chloride, ammonium chloride, and sodium citrate are used on their own or incorporated into proprietary expectorant mixtures. Each of these agents may be contraindicated in patients with electrolyte problems, particularly subjects who retain sodium.

□ GUAIFENESIN

Guaifenesin was formerly called glyceryl guaiacolate. It is still one of the most popular expectorants, being present in proprietary "cough medicines" such

TABLE 16-4 **Some Oral Mucokinetic Agents**

Agent	Usual Adult Dosage	Notes
Water	Variable	Essential
Potassium iodide (SSKI)	5–20 drops (500–2000 mg) 3 or 4 times a day	One of the most effective mucokinetics. Toxicity: rashes, metallic taste, parotid swelling, lacrimation, rhinorrhea, nausea, thyroid suppression
Iodinated glycerol	60–120 mg 2–4 times a day	Less toxicity than SSKI; no longer marketed
Syrup of ipecac	0.5–2 mL 3 times a day	Effective agent; may cause nausea and vomiting
Ammonium chloride	0.3–1 g 3 times a day	Probably effective; nauseating
Guaifenesin (glyceryl guaiacolate)	400 mg 4–6 times a day	Probably effective if more than 2400 mg/day is used. Toxicity: nausea, vomiting, drowsiness
Terpin hydrate	300 mg 4 times a day	Probably ineffective; no longer marketed
Bromhexine	8–16 mg 3 times a day	Not available in the United States
Ambroxol	0.5–1 g 2–3 times a day	Not available in the United States
S-Carboxymethylcysteine	375–750 mg 4 times a day	Not available in the United States
Acetylcysteine	200 mg 3 times a day	Oral form not available in the United States

BOX 16-4

MUCOKINETIC EFFECTS OF IODIDE-CONTAINING EXPECTORANTS

Iodide stimulates the gastropulmonary mucokinetic vagal reflex, thereby activating the submucosal bronchial glands.

The bronchial glands selectively concentrate circulating iodide, which then stimulates the glands to secrete. This is termed a "bronchomucotropic" effect.[6] The salivary, nasal, and lacrimal glands act similarly, and iodotherapy may cause salivation, rhinorrhea, and lacrimation; a metallic taste may be given to the secretions.

There is evidence that iodides stimulate natural proteolytic enzymes in the respiratory secretions, thereby enhancing the digestive breakdown of mucoprotein.[18]

There is some evidence that potassium iodide can stimulate ciliary activity.[19]

Iodide may have an anti-inflammatory effect, thus aiding in the resolution of conditions such as bronchitis, pneumonitis, and asthma.[20]

as Robitussin. The drug is derived from creosote, which was formerly used as an expectorant. There is evidence that guaifenesin acts both as a vagal stimulant and by direct stimulation of the bronchial glands. The drug is absorbed from the stomach and is concentrated by the bronchial glands, which rapidly secrete it into the respiratory tract. The usually recommended dose for adults is 100 to 200 mg four times daily, but it is doubtful whether this dosage is adequate.[21] The drug is also present in some bronchodilator mixtures, but the amount is less than 100 mg/dose, which is unlikely to have any mucokinetic effect. A more appropriate dosage would be 500 to 1000 mg; such amounts may produce vomiting and, rarely, may cause cerebral depression.

□ TERPIN HYDRATE

Terpin hydrate is a volatile oil derivative of turpentine, and it supposedly has similar actions to those of guaifenesin. However, in conventional dosages it is probably without effect. It is no longer marketed.

□ BROMHEXINE

Bromhexine (Bisolvon) is used in Europe, where it is one of several popular oral mucokinetic agents. Evidence suggests that bromhexine acts on the bronchial glands to increase their secretions, thereby causing an augmented volume of sputum of decreased viscosity in bronchitic patients. The drug may also have a mucolytic action. A derivative of bromhexine, *ambroxol*, appears to be a potent stimulator of surfactant production, and it has been used in the management of neonatal RDS as well as for its mucokinetic effect.

□ S-CARBOXYMETHYLCYSTEINE

S-Carboxymethylcysteine (Mucodyne) is an oral mucokinetic that is used in Europe. Although it is related to acetylcysteine, the molecular structure is such that its thiol group is not free (ie, it is "blocked"), and thus the molecule cannot directly rupture disulfide bonds. It is thought that this agent acts directly on the bronchial glands to induce secretion of an increased amount of sialomucins, thereby producing fluid of relatively low viscosity; this action has been called a mucoregulator effect. Interestingly, this drug is closely related to alliin, the basic compound in garlic, which is also believed to be a mucokinetic agent (Fig. 16-2).

□ MISCELLANEOUS ORAL MUCOKINETIC DRUGS

Other orally administered drugs are credited with mucokinetic properties, although substantiation is needed. Among the more popular agents are *anise, camphor, pine syrup, licorice, paregoric (camphorated tincture of opium), senega, squill, and tolu balsam. Menthol,* more than any other aromatic agent, may serve to suppress a distressing cough. Many of these agents are still incorporated into proprietary "cough medicines."[22]

Garlic has already been discussed, and this spice is credited with expectorant effects in several national pharmacopeias. Some evidence suggests that various foods and spices favored in folk medicine do have mucokinetic effect, as does chicken soup.[6] Agents such as pepper, mustard, and horseradish can cause lacrimation and rhinorrhea, and an appreciable augmentation of tracheobronchial secretions, presumably through stimulation of autonomic reflexes.

Parasympathomimetic drugs are powerful stimulants of the bronchial glands. However, although they can produce mucokinesis, they may also cause bronchospasm and other harmful parasympathetic effects. None are of practical therapeutic value.

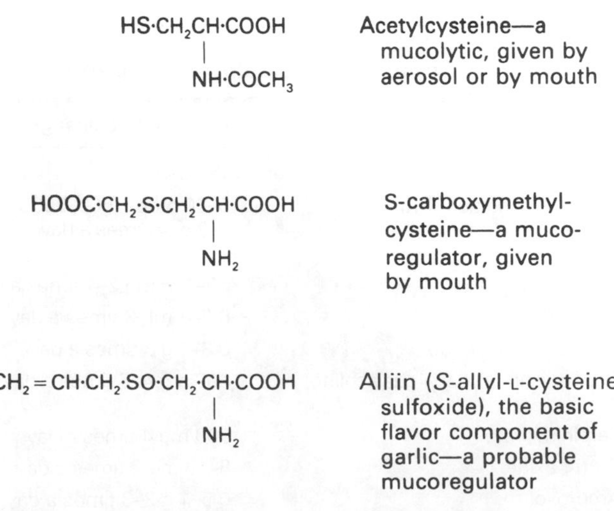

FIGURE 16-2. Chemistry of some related cysteine derivatives with mucokinetic properties.

BRONCHODILATORS AND ANTI-ASTHMA DRUGS

Most drugs used to manage bronchospasm act on the biochemical mechanisms that control bronchial muscle tone. A critical factor in the complex cascade is the "second messenger," cyclic 3',5'-adenosine monophosphate (cAMP), which serves to reverse bronchospasm. Intracellular levels of cAMP are increased by either of two mechanisms: Stimulation of the enzyme *adenyl cyclase* catalyzes the conversion of the precursor adenosine triphosphate (ATP) to form cAMP; and inhibition of the enzyme *phosphodiesterase* prevents the rapid breakdown of cAMP to inactive metabolites. The major bronchodilators have their effect on one or the other of these two mechanisms. *Catecholamines* and similar sympathomimetics stimulate adenyl cyclase, whereas *methylxanthines* are the best known phosphodiesterase inhibitors.

Bronchospasm is enhanced by cholinergic (ie, vagal) stimuli that may cause increased concentrations of intracellular cyclic 3',5'-guanosine monophosphate (3',5'-GMP); this is a further messenger, which, in effect, has an action opposite that of cAMP and results in bronchospasm. These mediators, in turn, control prostaglandin and leukotriene formation from arachidonic acid, and it is these products that modulate the biochemical processes involved in bronchospasm, mucosal inflammation, and mucus production. The inflammatory nature of chronic asthma emphasizes the need for anti-inflammatory drugs in more severe or persistent disease.

SYMPATHOMIMETIC DRUGS

The natural hormonal transmitters of the sympathetic nervous system are norepinephrine and epinephrine. These hormones are chemically related to catechol and are known as *catecholamines*; they are also classified as *sympathomimetic* agents, adrenergic agents, adrenoreceptor stimulators, or beta-agonists. These chemicals have various categories of effects on autonomic function, and these effects are subdivided into α, β_1, and β_2 properties, depending on the anatomic sites of the various receptors (Table 16-5). Stimulation of bronchial muscle β_2 receptors causes bronchodilation, whereas stimulation of β_2 receptors of the heart and blood vessels results in undesired side effects, including tachycardia, possible arrhythmias, and blood pressure changes. Blood vessel β_2 receptors mediate vasodilation in most organs. Many blood vessels, including those of the respiratory tree, are also supplied with α receptors, the stimulation of which causes vasoconstriction; this may be valuable in treating airway edema. A further β_2-sympathomimetic effect, which is unwanted, is stimulation of the nervous system, causing nervousness, sleeplessness, and tremor; this type of effect is inevitable with large doses of potent β_2 stimulators. The β_1 receptors are found mainly in heart muscle, and their stimulation results in tachycardia with the potential for arrhythmias.

Epinephrine is the prototype of the catecholamines. It has α, β_1, and β_2 effects; in addition to being a very effective bronchodilator, it has unwanted cardiovascular and nervous system side effects. Epinephrine also has the powerful β_2 effect of releasing glucose from the liver (glycogenolysis). The molecule of epinephrine contains hydroxyl groupings in the 3 and 4 positions of the benzene nucleus and, accordingly, is susceptible to degradation by at least two different enzyme systems. Enzymes that degrade by sulfatization are found in the bowel wall and the liver. Consequently, epinephrine and isoproterenol are relatively ineffective as bronchodilators when given orally. In various tissues, including the lungs, the enzyme catechol-*O*-methyltransferase (COMT) causes inactivation by *O*-methylation.

The amino group of the ethylamine side-chain is responsible for the α- and β-stimulatory properties of the catecholamines. The addition of alkyl substitution radicals in the amino group leads to a progressive increase in β_2 activity, with a corresponding decrease in β_1 and α potency.

Although the activities of the various catecholamines and derivatives used in therapeutics have been carefully evaluated, their effects are complex because their primary actions are complicated by reflex responses in the intact animal. Therefore, it is difficult to compare the bronchodilator potencies of the popular sympathomimetics and to determine their comparative β_2-receptor selectivity. The therapeutic response to an agent is also affected by the route of administration, with the best bronchodilator:side effect ratio being obtained by aerosolization rather than by oral administration.

In the following section, the various sympathomimetic agents best suited for respiratory therapy are described. Norepinephrine, which has an unsubstituted amino group, is a powerful α-receptor stimulator and also has strong β_1 effects; it is not a bronchodilator, although it is a potent pressor agent, and is not used as a respiratory tract drug.

Sympathomimetic Drugs Given by Aerosolization

Numerous individual products are available, with multiple formulations of the older bronchodilators epinephrine and isoproterenol.[23] For home use, almost all patients use metered-dose inhalers (MDI), but inhalant solutions for nebulizer delivery are often used in hospitals and for occasional outpatients. Currently, more reliance is being placed in MDI therapy, which is more economical than more complex aerosol delivery modalities. Most products no longer contain sulfites, because this preservative can induce bronchospasm in rare patients.

□ EPINEPHRINE

Epinephrine (adrenaline) is a natural sympathomimetic hormone that is rarely used in modern respiratory therapy because of its marked β_1 effects; it re-

TABLE 16-5. **Classification of Adrenergic Receptors**

	α	β_1	β_2
Distribution of Receptors			
Airways			
Muscle	Yes	No	Yes
Blood vessels	Yes	Yes	No
Heart	Yes	Yes	Few
Systemic blood vessels	No (?)	No (?)	Yes (?)
Central nervous system	?	?	Yes (?)
Result of Receptor Stimulation			
Bronchial muscle	Weak contraction	No effect	Relaxation
Bronchial glands	Stimulation (?)	Stimulation (?)	Stimulation
Cilia	?	?	Stimulation
Blood vessels (general)	Constriction	?	Dilation
Cardiac muscle	Excitation	Stimulation	Slight stimulation
Skeletal muscle	?	?	Excitation
Central nervous system	?	?	Excitation
Liver and muscle	Glycogenolysis	?	Glycogenolysis
Adipose tissue	?	Lipolysis	No effect
Uterus	Excitation	?	Inhibition
Physiologic Effects*			
Bronchospasm	Slight increase	No effect	Decrease
Respiratory tract secretions	Slight increase (?)	Slight increase (?)	Increase
Cough	?	No effect	Decrease
Airway resistance	Decrease (?)	No effect	Decrease
Heart rate	Reflex slowing (may cause ectopy)	Increase	No effect
Blood Pressure			
Weak stimulus	May increase	Varies	Varies
Strong stimulus	Increase	May decrease	Varies
Skeletal Muscle	No effect (?)	No effect (?)	Tremor
Pupils	Dilation	?	?
Central Nervous System	?	?	Stimulation
Uterus	Contraction	?	Tocolysis

* The effect on human adrenergic receptors depends on factors such as route of administration, total dose given, time at which measurement is made, and reflex responses, among other variables.

mains popular for self-therapy because it is available without a prescription. For inhalational therapy, a 1:100 solution is used; this is too high a concentration for subcutaneous administration (Tables 16-6, 16-7, and 16-8).

☐ RACEPINEPHRINE

Racemic epinephrine (Micronefrin, Vaponefrin) is obtained synthetically; it is a racemic mixture of *dextro-* and *levo-* epinephrine, whereas the natural hormone exists only in the *levo* form. The racemic mixture is claimed to have adequate β_2 potency, with less β_1 and α activity than epinephrine. Controlled comparisons of the two drugs do not show a significant difference in effectiveness or in toxicity, and racepinephrine is now becoming obsolescent.

The presence of α-receptor activity makes epinephrine a useful drug when mucosal congestion requires treatment. Both forms of epinephrine have been recommended for aerosolization in managing croup and epiglottitis as well as for asthma. Despite the ready availability of epinephrine without prescription, such use has not been shown to be dangerous.

☐ ISOPROTERENOL

Isoproterenol (isoprenaline, Isuprel) was once the most popular inhalational bronchodilator. The drug is a synthetic derivative and one of the most potent β_2 stimulators. The marked β_1 activity of isoproterenol can cause unwanted effects on the heart and blood pressure. Moreover, because the drug has no α effect (see Table 16-6), its unopposed β_2 effect causes vasodilata-

TABLE 16-6. **Structure and Actions of Common Bronchodilator Catecholamines and Derivatives Used As Aerosols**

ETHYLAMINE CHAIN: CH — CH — NH (β | R, α | R, | R)

BENZENE NUCLEUS (positions 1–6; R at 2, 3, 4, 5)

								Relative Effects on Adrenergic Receptors			
								Vasoconstriction	*Cardiac Stimulation*	*Bronchodilatation, Nervous System Stimulation, Vasodilatation*	*Persistence of Effect of Aerosol*
	2	**3**	**4**	**5**	**β**	**α**	**NH**	**α**	**β**	**β_2**	**Hours**
Epinephrine	H	OH	OH	H	OH	H	CH_3	+++	++++	+++	1–2
R-Epinephrine	H	OH	OH	H	OH	H	CH_3	++(+)	+++(+)	++(+)	1–2
Isoproterenol	H	OH	OH	H	OH	H	$CH(CH_3)_2$		++++	++++(+)	1–2
Isoetharine	H	OH	OH	H	OH	C_2H_5	$CH(CH_3)_2$		+(+)	−++(+)	2–4
Ethylnorepinephrine	H	OH	OH	H	OH	C_2H_5	H	++	++	++(+)	2–4
Metaproterenol	H	OH	H	OH	OH	H	$CH(CH_3)_2$		+(+)	−++(+)	3–5
Terbutaline	H	OH	H	OH	OH	H	$C(CH_3)_3$		+(+)	−++(+)	4–7
Colterol†	H	OH	OH	H	OH	H	$C(CH_3)_3$		+(+)	+++(+)	4–7
Albuterol	H	CH_2CH	OH	H	OH	H	$C(CH_3)_3$		+(+)	++++(+)	4–5
Pirbuterol	(N)	CH_2CH	OH	H	OH	H	$C(CH_3)_3$		+(+)	++++(+)	4–6
Fenoterol	H	OH	H	OH	OH	H	$(C_9H_{11}O)$		+(+)	++++(+)	5–8
Salmeterol	H	CH_2CH	OH	OH	OH	H	*		+(+)	+++++	8–18

Note. The relative effects are not established accurately, and therefore the above information is only approximate. The actual result obtained depends on the total dose given, the route and rate of administration, the presence of disease and other drugs, and factors such as tachyphylaxis. The measured response will also vary with time as initial pharmacologic effects result in reflex adjustments. Consequently, the actual findings at any time in a given patient may show major departures from this schema.

* $(CH_2)_6O(CH_2)_4C_6H_5$.

† Marketed as the prodrug bitolterol.

TABLE 16-7. **Metered Dose Inhaler Aerosol Bronchodilators**

Drug	Doses Per Cartridge (Approximate No.)	Amount of Drug Delivery Per Puff (mg)
Epinephrine		
Asthma Haler	300	0.160
Bronitin Mist	300, 400	0.160
Bronkaid Mist	300, 450	0.250
Bronkaid Mist Suspension	200	0.160
Medihaler-EPI	300	0.160
Primatene Mist	300, 450	0.220
Primatene Mist Suspension	200	0.160
Isoproterenol		
Isoproterenol	300	0.125
Isuprel Mistometer	200, 300	0.131
Medihaler-Iso	300, 450	0.080
Isoproterenol-Phenylephrine		
Duo-Medihaler (Isoproterenol and Phenylephrine)	300, 450	0.137 0.126
Isoetharine		
Bronkometer	200, 300	0.340
Metaproterenol		
Alupent	100, 200	0.650
Metaprel	200	0.650
Albuterol (Salbutamol)		
Proventil	200	0.090
Ventolin*	80, 200	0.090
Terbutaline		
Brethaire	300	0.200
Bitolterol		
Tornalate	300	0.370
Pirbuterol		
Maxair	400	0.200
Salmeterol		
Serevent	60, 120	0.021
Fenoterol†		
Berotect†		0.160

* Also available as a powdered preparation, 0.2 mg/capsule.
† Not marketed in the United States.

tion in the pulmonary vasculature; the increase in blood flow leads to rapid systemic absorption of the drug, with resulting shortening of the bronchodilator response and increased extrapulmonary side effects. Systemic absorption can cause pulmonary vasodilatation in poorly ventilated lung areas, which increases the shunt effect in the lungs, and this may be manifested as a fall in the PaO_2.

Isoproterenol is one of the shortest-acting bronchodilators. Patients with severe asthma frequently have to take inhalations of the drug every 1 to 2 hours and, by so doing, they run the risk of inducing *tachyphylaxis.* This is a phenomenon whereby responsiveness to the bronchodilating effects of a drug becomes progressively diminished, although β_1 effectiveness may be maintained. Overusing the aerosol may result in cardiac side effects, including tachyarrhythmias and even myocardial necrosis; large dosages are particularly hazardous when used for treating an asthmatic exacerbation.

When the drug is given by nebulizer, the therapist should watch for evidence of toxicity. The patient may complain of palpitations, anxiety, flushing, or tinnitus or may experience faintness or a throbbing headache. The pulse should be checked during and after therapy and, in patients at particular risk, monitoring of the electrocardiogram and blood pressure is advisable. Rinsing the mouth and throat may decrease systemic absorption through the oropharyngeal and gastric mucosa and may reduce the incidence of unwanted β_1 complications.

The main value of isoproterenol aerosol is in the pulmonary function laboratory to evaluate the reversibility of obstructive airway disease. It can be useful for treating occasional younger asthmatics with no cardiovascular abnormalities. The appropriate dosages of isoproterenol preparations are given in Tables 16-7 and 16-8.

□ ISOETHARINE

The catecholamine isoetharine is available as an aerosol. Isoetharine differs from isoproterenol in having an ethyl group on the α-carbon atom, and as a result, it has somewhat less of a β_2 effect than does isoproterenol, and much less β_1 activity (see Table 16-6).

Isoetharine was formerly very popular as a metered preparation (Bronkometer), as well as for nebulizer delivery (Bronkosol). In bronchospastic patients who are hypoxemic and who have tachycardia and underlying coronary artery disease, isoetharine is much less likely to cause serious cardiac side effects than is isoproterenol. Recommended dosages of isoetharine are provided in Tables 16-7 and 16-8.

□ METAPROTERENOL

Metaproterenol (orciprenaline, Alupent, Metaprel) is available as a metered aerosol and as an inhalant solution. It is chemically related to isoproterenol, but the hydroxy groups, which occupy the 3 and 4 positions in the benzene nucleus of isoproterenol, are in the 3 and 5 (meta) positions (see Table 16-6). This configuration renders metaproterenol immune to sulfatization in the bowel; therefore, it is effective when given orally. The molecule is not inactivated by COMT; consequently, the drug has a more sustained bronchodilator effect.

When used by aerosol, metaproterenol is far less likely to cause tachycardia than is isoproterenol. The effect of the aerosol usually lasts 3 to 4 hours or more, and

TABLE 16-8. **Bronchodilator Inhalant Solutions Available for Updraft Aerosolization Using Simple Jet Nebulizer, IPPB, or Compressor**

Drug	Concentration (%)	Initial Dosages*	
		Hand Nebulizer No. of Inhalations†	*Updraft or Compressor (mL)‡*
Epinephrine		2–3	
Adrenalin	1		0.25–0.7
Racemic Epinephrine		1–6	
Asthma Nephrin	2.25		0.4–0.8
Racepinephrine (various)	2.25		
Vaponefrin¶	2		0.,25–0.7
Isoproterenol§		6–12	
Dispos a Med	0.25, 0.5 (in 0.5 mL)	6–12	0.25–1
Isoproterenol (various)	0.25, 0.5 (in 0.5 mL)	6–12	0.5–1
Isuprel	0.5, 1	3–17	0.25–0.5
Isoetharine‡		3–7	
Arm-a-Med	0.062–0.25 (in 2.5–5 mL)		2–4
Bronkosol	1		0.25–1
Bronkosol Unit Dose	0.25		2
Isoetharine (various)	0.062–1		0.25–4
Metaproterenol		4–15	
Alupent	5		0.1–0.3
Alupent Unit Dose	0.4, 0.6 (in 2.5 mL)		2.5
Arm-a-Med	0.4, 0.6 (in 2.5 mL)		2.5
Metaprel	5		0.1–0.3
Metaproterenol (various)	5		0.1–0.3
Bitolterol			
Tornalate	0.2	1–6	0.5–1.75
Albuterol		4–15	
Albuterol (various)	0.083 (in 3 mL)		3
Proventil	0.5		0.25–0.5
Proventil Unit Dose	0.083 (in 3 mL)		3
Ventolin	0.5		0.25–0.5

* These dosages are based on manufacturers' recommendations and illustrate the imprecision in prescribing that exists.
† Dosages can vary considerably.
‡ The recommended amount can be diluted with 1 to 3 mL saline. Prepackaged unit-dose preparations are available with various diluents.
§ Generic preparations are marketed in various concentrations. Each manufacturer's information should be used in determining dosages.
¶ Available without prescription.

it is usually required four times daily. Dosages of the aerosol are listed in Tables 16-7 and 16-8.

□ TERBUTALINE

Terbutaline (Brethaire) is available as an MDI. The drug is long-lasting, but causes more tremor than other bronchodilators. Aerosol dosages are listed in Tables 16-7 and 16-8; there is little justification for giving the subcutaneous form by aerosol, because other authorized aerosol bronchodilators are preferred.

□ ALBUTEROL

Albuterol (salbutamol, Proventil, Ventolin) is available as an MDI and as an inhalant solution. Albuterol resembles terbutaline in having a tertiary butyl substitution in the amino group; therefore, it has similar β_2-selective properties. The drug is protected from sulfatization and from COMT, because the hydroxyl group in position 3 of the catechol nucleus has been replaced by a CH_2OH group that interferes with the activity of these enzymes. This drug is currently the favored aerosol bronchodilator.

□ BITOLTEROL

The only new bronchodilator developed in the United States was introduced as an MDI. The product is a prodrug, bitolterol (Tornalate), which is converted into the active drug colterol (see Table 16-6) in the body by esterases that are found in particularly large quantities in the lungs; conversion of the aerosol to colterol occurs within a few minutes. However, the resulting delayed onset of bronchodilation is unacceptable to many patients. The slow release of colterol from bitolterol can produce bronchodilation lasting 6 to 8 hours after a single dose. In structure, colterol is similar to terbutaline, and its effects and side effects appear to be similar.

☐ PIRBUTEROL

This drug is available as an MDI (Maxair). In structure it is related to albuterol, but carbon atom 2 of the benzene ring is replaced by a nitrogen atom in pirbuterol, which is thus a sympathomimetic pyridine derivative rather than a benzene derivative. It appears to be comparable to albuterol, although it may have a slightly slower onset of action and a more prolonged effect. Recently, it has been made available in a breath-activated inhaler unit (Autohaler).

☐ SALMETEROL

This is the first long-acting aerosol to be introduced into the United States; it is marketed as an MDI (Serevent) for use in asthma.[25] The basic molecule is that of albuterol with the ethylamine chain extending into a 10-carbon atom chain that terminates in a benzyl ring. This long chain enables the inactive terminal ring to become anchored to an exosite domain in the β_2 receptor, allowing the conventional active part of the agonist molecule to become recurrently detached and reattached to the receptor site. As a consequence of this anchoring effect, salmeterol has an action persisting for at least 12 hours in moderate asthma, with a range of about 8 to 20 hours. It is particularly valuable for providing prolonged prophylaxis against nocturnal or exercise-induced bronchospasm while its potent action may make it a preferred agent for asthma that responds inadequately to shorter-acting β_2 agonists. It can be given regularly as 1 to 2 puffs every 12 hours or just once at night; larger doses should be used with the greatest caution, if at all.

Although the drug may have some anti-inflammatory properties and tachyphylaxis does not seem to occur, it is advisable to give aerosol steroids concomitantly to patients with more severe degrees of asthma. Overdosage could cause prolonged tachycardia or arrhythmias. It is advisable to use minimal dosing in patients with heart disease or with liver disease since the drug is cleared by the liver.

Other long-acting aerosol agents, including formoterol, have been introduced in other countries.[25] Long-acting β agonists have to be used with care to avoid exceeding the stated dose, but in standard dosage they appear to be safe.[26] Concerns have been expressed about the potential danger of regular use of aerosol β_2 agonists in asthma, with particular concern about long-acting agents.[27] However, these fears appear to be exaggerated.[28]

☐ FENOTEROL

This agent is hydroxyphenylorciprenaline (orciprenaline is the European name for metaproterenol). It is claimed to be longer acting and to have a more selective effect on β_2-receptors than does metaproterenol. The drug's safety has been questioned,[25,27] and it is unlikely to be marketed in the United States.

Noninhalational Sympathomimetic Drugs

Several inhalational drugs for treating bronchospasm are also commonly given by alternative routes of administration. A few sympathomimetics are not suitable at all for inhalation, and these are also considered in this section.

☐ EPINEPHRINE

Epinephrine is available as the hydrochloride and as the bitartrate; there are no significant differences between these preparations. In status asthmaticus 0.1 to 0.5 mL of the 1:1000 aqueous solution can be given subcutaneously and repeated after half an hour if necessary. An aqueous solution for intramuscular administration (SusPhrine) has a longer persisting effect that lasts up to 8 hours. A 1:5000 solution in oil is available for intramuscular injection: 0.2 to 1.0 mL can be given and may have an appreciable effect for 8 to 16 hours. However, this route of delivery is not favored because it may cause local side effects. In some countries, epinephrine is given intravenously for status asthmaticus.

☐ ISOPROTERENOL

Isoproterenol is rarely given by the noninhalational route for the treatment of asthma. An oral preparation is available, but absorption is erratic. Sublingual tablets are effective, although it is difficult to regulate the dose when using this route of absorption. The drug has been given intravenously to adequately oxygenated young patients with status asthmaticus; adults are more susceptible to its cardiotoxicity and should not be treated with intravenous isoproterenol.

☐ METAPROTERENOL

This drug is only about 40% absorbed in the bowel, but effective bronchodilation usually lasts 3 to 4 hours, and as long as 6 hours or more. The dosage in adults is 10 to 20 mg every 4 to 8 hours. Generally, side effects are not severe, but nervousness, tremor, and palpitations may occur. Metaproterenol is available for oral intake as 10-mg and 20-mg tablets and as a syrup containing 10 mg of the drug per 5 mL.

☐ TERBUTALINE

This drug has an effect that may persist for 7 to 8 hours. However, this is accompanied by a relatively high incidence of side effects; tremor is the most troublesome complaint, particularly in older patients. Terbutaline is available as Brethine and Bricanyl, which are marketed as injectable solutions for subcutaneous use and as 2.5-mg and 5-mg tablets. The oral dose is 2.5 to 5 mg every 6 to 8 hours. The subcutaneous injection preparations contain 1 mg/mL of solution; the usual adult dose is 0.25 mg, which can be repeated if necessary in 15 to 30 minutes. Terbutaline injection causes equivalent side effects to those of epinephrine, although its bronchodilator action does not persist longer.

□ ALBUTEROL

Albuterol is available as rapidly acting tablets, a syrup, and as a slow-release oral tablet that need be given only twice a day. In some countries it is given intravenously, but this route is not approved in the United States. The available products are Proventil syrup and tablets (2 and 4 mg), slow-release tablets (4 and 8 mg), and Ventolin syrup and tablets. With its various formulations, albuterol currently is the most widely used bronchodilator.

□ EPHEDRINE

Ephedrine is the longest established oral agent for treating bronchospasm; it has not proved to be suitable for inhalational use. The drug is a strong stimulator of β_2 receptors, but also has a marked effect on β_1 and α receptors. The oral dose of 15 to 50 mg (given three or four times daily, according to individual needs of the bronchospastic patient) usually causes some stimulation of the central nervous system. Several proprietary preparations are marketed containing ephedrine and theophylline with a tranquilizer. Some of these are available without prescription; such use cannot, in general, be condoned. Ephedrine has other disadvantages: it can cause urinary retention in men with prostatic hypertrophy and is ineffective in severe asthma. Moreover, the long-term effectiveness of this drug cannot be relied on, since tachyphylaxis readily develops, apparently because ephedrine works in part by releasing catecholamines from neuronal storage vesicles, which eventually become depleted.

Other Sympathomimetic Bronchodilator Drugs

Several potentially useful bronchodilators have been described, including carbuterol, hexoprenaline, reproterol, clenbuterol, broxaterol, formoterol, bambuterol, tolubuterol, and procaterol. A number of these are marketed in other countries.

NONSYMPATHOMIMETIC BRONCHODILATORS AND ANTI-ASTHMA DRUGS

Several nonsympathomimetic drugs have been used to manage bronchospasm. These agents can be classified as phosphodiesterase inhibitors (methylxanthines); mucosal constrictors; anti-allergy agents; immunosuppressives; anticholinergics; and a miscellaneous group.

Methylxanthines

The methylxanthines are phosphodiesterase inhibitors; they increase the availability of cAMP by inhibiting its breakdown by the intracellular enzyme phosphodiesterase. Although tea, coffee, chocolate, and cola beverages all owe some of their characteristic taste and properties to their content of methylxanthines, they do not have any significant inhibitory effect on phosphodiesterase and, thus, are not of clinical value for treating bronchospasm. The exact mechanism of action of theophylline remains controversial, but recently it has been emphasized that the drug may control asthma through an immunomodulatory effect on T lymphocytes, which results in an anti-inflammatory effect.[29,30]

□ THEOPHYLLINE

Theophylline is a potent bronchodilator and has numerous less impressive, but generally beneficial, effects. Therapeutic doses can produce cardiac stimulation, resulting in an increased heart rate, and arrhythmias may occur with larger therapeutic doses. Cardiac performance and left ventricular output may be improved in patients with cor pulmonale, but in normal persons cardiac output is not significantly affected.

Generally, theophylline appears to be a vasodilator, and it may cause a useful decrease in vascular resistance in pulmonary and coronary arteries. However, the drug is believed to be a vasoconstrictor of the cerebrovascular supply and, indeed, theophylline was formerly used to treat hypertensive and migraine headaches. This is difficult to reconcile with the experience, particularly of pediatricians, that theophylline can cause headaches. An additional possible benefit of theophylline is its diuretic effect. Stimulation of the nervous system is produced by the methylxanthines, which accounts for their popularity in beverages. Normal serum levels of theophylline may produce anxiety and tremulousness in susceptible patients, whereas excessive levels may result in potentially lethal seizures.

Theophylline at therapeutic levels may cause increased gastric acid secretion that results in indigestion, vomiting, gastric irritation, reflux, abdominal pain, diarrhea, and even intestinal bleeding. The symptoms are related to the concentration of the drug in the blood rather than to the direct irritative effect of the preparation in the bowel.

A partial bronchodilator response may be produced by a serum level of theophylline of about 5 μg/mL (0.5 mg/dL), whereas a full response is usual with a serum level of 15 to 20 μg/mL. However, some patients require higher levels (20 to 25 μg/mL), and although such concentrations are potentially dangerous, there are patients who tolerate these levels without signs of toxicity. Thus, in practice, the therapeutic range for theophylline is 5 to 25 μg/mL (Table 16-9). However, the immunomodulatory benefit in asthma can occur with a level between 5 and 10 μg/mL, suggesting that this range may be appropriate in chronic therapy.[30,31]

Clearance of theophylline from the body occurs mainly as a result of enzymatic degradation in the liver.

TABLE 16-9. **Correlations of Serum Levels of Theophylline With Responses**

Serum Level (µg/mL)	Corresponding Bronchodilator Effect	Corresponding Possible Effects
5	Partial	Side effects unusual
10	Moderate	Vague discomfort
15	Usually optimal	Gastrointestinal problems
20	Usually maximal	Anxiety, tremors
25	This level is required for occasional patients	Tachycardia
30	This level is usually not tolerated	Arrhythmias
40+	This level is never therapeutic	Convulsions

Any condition that impairs hepatic function will decrease the clearance rate; hepatocellular failure, hypoxia, and venous congestion prolong the presence of the drug in the body. Stimulation of liver enzymes can increase the clearance rate, and this can result from the effects of constituents in cigarette smoke, smog, and barbecued protein. Certain drugs, such as phenytoin, barbiturates, and marijuana, also increase theophylline clearance. Generally, children clear theophylline more rapidly than do adults, and in very old patients clearance rates may be decreased. Dosages for theophylline depend on many factors,[32] and guidelines for achieving therapeutic serum levels are suggested in Table 16-10.

Numerous brand and generic preparations of theophylline have been marketed. In recent years, long-acting products have become extremely popular because they result in smoother bronchodilation and encourage better compliance. Slow-release products that need to be given only once a day are particularly useful for controlling nocturnal asthma. The main preparations are listed in Table 16-11. Combination products with ephedrine cannot be recommended, although very mild bronchospasm may respond adequately to such preparations. Currently, theophylline is one of the prime drugs for treating COPD and it is coming back into favor for use in unstable chronic asthma.[31]

□ AMINOPHYLLINE

A major disadvantage of theophylline is that it is relatively insoluble in water. This is why this hazardous drug is not suitable for inhalation; the solution would be too dilute to be of practical value. Theophylline is 20

TABLE 16-10. **Theophylline and Aminophylline Dosages**

		Theophylline (mg/kg)	Aminophylline (mg/kg)
Loading			
Initial			
Average		5	6
Range		2.5–7.5	3–9
Maintenance		***mg/kg/24h***	***mg/kg/h***
Average adult			
Nonsmoker		10	0.5
Smoker		15	0.9
Neonate		2.5	0.12
Young child		10–20	0.5–1.0
Geriatric		7.5–15	0.26–0.50
Adjustments	***Increase Dosage By (%)***	***Adjustments***	***Decrease Dosage By (%)***
Cigarette smoking	30–50	Liver failure	50
Marijuana smoking	20–50	Cimetidine	30–50
Phenytoin	20–50	Heart failure	20–50
Rifampin	20–50	Cor pulmonale	20–50
Carbamazepine	20–50	Quinolones*	20–50
Aminoglutethimide	20–50	Mexiletene	20–50
High-protein diet	10–20	Allopurinol (high dose)	25
Barbecued food	10–20	Propranolol	20–50
Smog exposure	10–20	Hypoxemia	10–30
Barbiturate	10–20	High-carbohydrate diet	10–30
Ketoconazole	10–20	Viral upper respiratory infection (children)	10–30
Isoniazid	10–20	Macrolide antibiotic therapy	25
		Oral contraceptives	25
		Verapamil, Nifedipine	10–20

* Ciprofloxacin, cinoxacin, enoxacin, and norfloxacin may cause a major decrease in theophylline clearance; ofloxacin has a minor effect, and lomefloxacin has little or no effect.

TABLE 16-11. **Examples of Theophylline and Derivatives**

Routes of Administration of Theophylline and Derivatives	Available Formulations	Range of Contents in Marketed Preparations
Theophylline 100%*		
Oral	Liquids, syrups, elixirs, suspension	80–150 mg/15 mL
	Immediate-release tablets, capsules	80–300 mg
	Slow-release tablets, capsules	50–500 mg
Rectal	No longer available	
Aerosol	No longer available	
Intravenous	In 5% dextrose	0.8–4 mg/mL
Aminophylline (Theophylline Ethylenediamine) 79%–84%*		
Injection	Intravenous	250 mg/10 mL
Oral	Tablets	100, 200 mg
	Slow-release tablets	225–300 mg
	Elixirs, liquids	100–315 mg/15 mL
Rectal	Solutions, suppositories	250–500 mg/U
Dyphylline (Hyphylline, Dihydroxypropyl Theophylline) 70%*		
Oral	Liquids, elixirs	100–300 mg/15 mL
	Tablets	200, 400 mg
	Slow-release tablets	400 mg
Injection	Intramuscular	250 mg/mL
Aerosol	Not approved	
Choline Theophyllinate (Oxtriphylline) 64%*		
Oral	Tablets	100, 200 mg
	Sustained-action tablet	400, 600 mg

* Content of theophylline.

times more soluble in the ammoniacal solvent ethylenediamine; the resulting solution is aminophylline. Ethylenediamine is not inert; one benefit is that it can stimulate the respiratory center and therefore correct some cases of Cheyne-Stokes breathing.

The average dosage of aminophylline is 5 to 7 mg/kg as a loading dose, to be given over 15 to 30 minutes intravenously; this is followed by 0.5 mg/kg per hour given as a continuous intravenous drip. A smaller loading dose is needed if the patient has recently taken a theophylline preparation. In contrast, some patients with status asthmaticus (particularly young smokers) need and tolerate a larger dose.[32] If in doubt as to the appropriate maintenance dosage, one should obtain a serum theophylline level for guidance.

Aminophylline has the same side effects as theophylline, as well as some individualistic ones. Although aminophylline is available for oral use as tablets, theophylline preparations seem to be better tolerated and are generally preferred. Rectal preparations of aminophylline should not be used because they irritate the mucosa and are unreliably absorbed. Inhalational aerosols of aminophylline may provoke bronchospasm; in practice, nebulization is not of therapeutic value. The ethylenediamine component of aminophylline is a potent sensitizing agent and, occasionally, results in skin reactions. Of greater concern is that, rarely, bronchospasm may be induced by ethylenediamine when the drug is given intravenously.

Intravenous administration of aminophylline has resulted in a number of deaths, usually caused by rapid infusion of the drug; hazards can be avoided by injecting the drug slowly or by giving it as a continuous infusion. Fatal hypotensive and hypertensive cardiac failure and arrhythmias have been reported. Deaths have occurred after the administration of excessive dosages of aminophylline per rectum (as suppositories or solutions) to young children.

□ DYPHYLLINE

Dyphylline (hyphylline, Dilor, Lufyllin, Neothylline) is the only substituted derivative of theophylline; it has only 70% of the effect of theophylline. It can be given intramuscularly because it is very soluble and does not cause tissue irritation. Dyphylline is available for oral administration. Of interest is the suggestion that the drug is suitable for intravenous use in acute asthma.[33] There is some evidence to suggest it could be a useful inhalational agent for treating bronchospasm.[34]

□ OXTRIPHYLLINE

Oxtriphylline (Choledyl) is the choline salt of theophylline, but claims that it is better absorbed in the gastrointestinal tract, with less irritation, are not convincing.

Mucosal Vasoconstrictors

Mucosal vasoconstrictors have α-receptor–stimulating properties. Drugs in this category are mainly used to treat the swollen nasal mucosa, but several of them have been used in inhalational therapy. Their main value in the respiratory tract is in decreasing vascular engorgement and the accompanying edema of the mucosa and also in delaying absorption and dispersion of topical bronchodilator drugs. Several agents are available, but the most important one is phenylephrine.

□ PHENYLEPHRINE

Phenylephrine (Neo-Synephrine) is the most popular nasal decongestant. It may be reasonable to administer 0.5 to 2 mL of 0.25% phenylephrine by nebulization into the tracheobronchial tree to manage conditions such as bronchitis, tracheobronchitis, or postextubation tracheitis. There is no evidence that rebound congestion occurs in the lung after use of phenylephrine, although this problem may arise in the nasal mucosa after treatment with nose drops or spray. The drug may be added to a bronchodilator for pulmonary aerosol therapy.

Anti-Allergy Agents

Because asthma is frequently caused by allergy, one would expect that antihistamines and other agents for treating allergic rhinitis would be valuable in managing asthma. However, the antihistamines are rarely beneficial in adult asthmatics, although they may be useful adjuvants in children.[35] Perhaps some of the newer drugs will be of greater value.

The main antiallergy drugs for asthma are the corticosteroids, cromolyn, and nedocromil. These drugs, and some less important ones, are discussed.

□ CORTICOSTEROIDS

The adrenal cortex secretes various natural hormones, including cortisol (hydrocortisone) and cortisone; the pharmaceutical industry has produced an additional bewildering array of synthetic *corticosteroids* (Table 16-12). These drugs have an extraordinary variety of effects and are used to treat innumerable diseases, even though the mechanism by which they help is not always understood. In respiratory medicine the corticosteroids are mainly used to manage allergic diseases, and they are of particular value in severe asthma.

The beneficial actions of corticosteroids in asthma include the following: inhibition of antibody formation, therby preventing antigen-antibody reactions; inhibition of formation or storage of messenger agents such as histamine, which are involved in the asthmatic response; and inhibition of various cellular mechanisms involved in bronchoconstriction by a nonspecific anti-inflammatory action. Additionally, there is evidence that corticosteroids potentiate sympathomimetic agents, probably by upgrading the responsiveness of β_2 receptors and by acting to increase the intracellular concentration of cAMP. Thus, the anti-inflammatory steroids (glucocorticoids) can be of value not only in preventing asthma, but also in managing status asthmaticus of any cause. The benefit of steroids in COPD is much less significant,[36] whereas their toxic effects may be more troublesome.

Unfortunately, the glucocorticoids can cause numerous long-term side effects that are dramatically serious.

TABLE 16-12. **"Older" Corticosteroid Preparations**

Generic Name	Trade Names	Topical Antiallergy Potency	Approximate Equivalent Dose (Oral) (mg)	Usual Dosage (Oral or IV) (mg/day)	Notes
Short-Acting (Plasma half-life less than 2 h)					Short-acting agents have more sodium-retaining potency
Hydrocortisone (cortisol)	Cortef, Solu-Cortef	1	20	80–120	Hydrocortisone has been given by inhalation in doses up to 30 mg/day; this is not recommended
Cortisone	Cortone	0.8	25	100–150	Used for replacement therapy in adrenal insufficiency
Intermediate-Acting (Plasma half-life 1–4 h)					
Prednisone	Meticorten, Deltasone	3.5	5	5–80	Standard oral drug
Prednisolone	Meticortelone, Delta-Cortef	4	5	5–80	Oral drug; may be indicated if patient has liver insufficiency
Methylprednisone	Medrol, Solu-Medrol	5	4	4–80	Parenteral alternative to hydrocortisone; may cause less electrolyte disturbance
Triamcinolone	Aristocort, Kenalog	5	4	4–80	Triamcinolone diacetate (Aristocort Forte has been given to prevent asthma) (eg, 3–48 mg IM every 1–4 weeks)

They may result in a constellation of bodily changes, known as cushingism. These unpleasant features include excessive weight gain, truncal obesity, hirsutism, acne, ecchymoses, striae, and edema. The more dangerous side effects include psychosis, hypertension, impairment of ability to fight infection, diabetes, cataracts, glaucoma, sodium retention, potassium loss, osteoporosis, avascular bone necrosis, and stunted growth; in some patients, peptic ulcer disease may be induced. Moreover, once a patient becomes dependent on steroid therapy, withdrawal of the drug may be difficult: the patient feels ill, and the disease exacerbates if dosage is lowered too quickly. Complications of inadequate adrenal and pituitary function may also appear.

Corticosteroid preparations are given intravenously in the treatment of severe asthma (status asthmaticus), and oral preparations are used for long-term therapy. MDI preparations of steroids have become important, but these drugs are not marketed for administration by aerosolization from a nebulizer (Table 16-13). Whenever steroid therapy is used, the dosage should be gradually reduced to the lowest that is effective, or an aerosol preparation should be substituted. However, systemic doses must not be changed rapidly to aerosol management because there is a danger of precipitating steroid-deficiency problems in a dependent patient.

Beclomethasone (Vanceril, Beclovent) is marketed as an MDI that delivers 50 µg per puff. Up to 2 mg/day may be given without significant adrenal gland suppression or other serious side effects, although the possibility of growth stunting in some children is a concern when unusually large doses are used. Steroid-dependent patients can be successfully transferred from oral preparations to the relative safety of beclomethasone aerosol therapy. Aerosolized steroids may produce oropharyngeal candidiasis in some patients; this is generally not severe and can be prevented by rinsing the mouth after inhaling an aerosol dose. Use of a spacer helps eliminate the risk of candidiasis.

For individual patients, it is uncertain how many administrations a day will be needed, but initially, the aerosol is used four times daily, two to four puffs at a time. Beclomethasone may be effective in milder asthma if it is administered only twice a day. A more concentrated formulation is available in Europe and can be given as two to four puffs twice a day when high doses are required.

Dexamethasone (Decadron) was the first metered preparation of a corticosteroid available for inhalation in the United States. The drug has lost popularity because effective dosages for asthmatic patients lead to appreciable systemic absorption with resultant side effects.

Triamcinolone (Aristocort, Kenalog) is available as an MDI with a built-in spacer (Azmacort): the usual dose is two to four inhalations three or four times a day. The long-acting depot preparation (Aristocort Forte) is sometimes given as a weekly intramuscular injection in the prophylaxis of asthma; the appropriate dosage and the overall benefit of this treatment require evaluation.

Flunisolide (AcroBid) is a fluorinated steroid that has a more prolonged action; therefore, it can be given twice a day, using two to four puffs of the MDI. The aerosol has an unpleasant taste; hence, it is advisable to use it with a spacer to decrease oral deposition. Recently, a mint-flavored preparation has been marketed.

Hydrocortisone (cortisol) is a valuable corticosteroid for general use in many diseases. It can be given orally and systemically and also as a cream and by injection into joints. The usual oral dose is 10 to 80 mg/day, and the intravenous dose for conditions such as status asthmaticus is 250 to 500 mg initially, followed by 100 to 250 mg every 3 hours. Hydrocortisone has been given as an inhalational aerosol to asthmatic patients, but it offers no advantage because considerable systemic absorption occurs.

Cortisone is occasionally used to treat asthma, but the drug is primarily of value in replacement therapy for patients with adrenocortical insufficiency. There is no reason for using this drug in respiratory therapy.

Prednisone and prednisolone are similar synthetic drugs that are suitable for oral maintenance therapy in asthma and in many other diseases. These two drugs

TABLE 16-13. **Corticosteroid Preparations Suitable for Aerosol Administration**

Generic Name	Trade Names	Topical Antiallergy Potency*	Dose Per Puff From Metered Cartridge (mg)	Aerosol Dosage (Adult) (mg/day)
Beclomethasone dipropionate	Beclovent, Vanceril	500	0.042	0.12–0.84
	Beconase,† Vancenase†			0.17–0.34†
Dexamethasone sodium phosphate	Decadron Respihaler	10	0.084	0.33 1
	Decadron Turbinaire†		0.084†	
Flunisolide	AeroBid, Nasalide†	30	0.25, 0.025†	1–2, 0.15–0.20†
Triamcinolone acetonide	Azmacort, Nasacort†	100	0.1	0.8–1.6
Budesonide	Rhinocort†	100	0.032	0.25†
Fluticasone propionate	Flovent, Flonase†	100	0.044, 0.110, 0.220	0.176–0.76

* Compared with hydrocortisone having a potency of 1.
† Nasal product.

are similar to hydrocortisone, but they are about four times as potent. The usual maintenance dose is 5 to 20 mg/day; cushingism can develop with prolonged use. Many asthmatic patients do well on alternate-day dosage; this markedly decreases the incidence of unwanted side effects.

Methylprednisolone (Solu-Medrol) is the favored intravenous preparation; it is also available for oral use (Medrol). It has less salt-retaining effect than prednisolone or prednisone.

Newer steroids have been developed. Budesonide was introduced in the United States for nasal topical therapy, and fluticasone marketed for nasal therapy and for asthma. Both offer advantages for aerosol therapy in asthma, since they are potent yet have a low incidence of side effects.

Phenobarbital increases the rate of steroid metabolism such as prednisone and dexamethasone. If an asthmatic patient being maintained on one of these drugs is started on a preparation that contains a barbiturate, the steroid dose may need to be increased. In contrast, the macrolide antibiotics, such as erythromycin, appear to potentiate steroids, and triacetyloleandomycin may act specifically to enhance the effect of oral methylprednisolone.

Antihistamines

Although antihistamines are of limited value in typical forms of asthma, cases accompanied by allergic rhinitis may respond. Some of the newer, long-acting nonsedating preparations may offer a modest benefit as adjuvants in asthma.[35] In Japan and some other countries, ketotifen (Zaditen) is an oral agent with antihistamine properties that has become popular in the treatment of asthma.

□ CROMOLYN

An old asthma remedy, khellin, was the source of a chromone derivative that was called disodium cromoglycate in England; it was subsequently introduced in the United States as cromolyn sodium (Aarane, Intal) but only Intal is currently marketed. Initially, it was packaged in capsules, and a special spinhaler was needed to release the powder when an inhalation was taken from the device. The content of cromolyn in each capsule was 20 mg. An MDI product has replaced the powder; each activation releases 0.8 mg. Inhalant solutions are marketed, which contain 20 mg/2 mL ampule, and can be given by updraft aerosolization. The drug is also available as an MDI.

Cromolyn is usually given as two to four puffs or one ampule of the inhalant solution four times daily for the first 2 to 3 weeks, and if a beneficial effect is obtained, the dosage may be reduced. Most asthmatics require two to four treatments a day. Several days or even weeks of therapy may be needed before the benefits of cromolyn become manifest. Prophylactic bronchodilator therapy may be needed before each inhalation of cromolyn to prevent reactive bronchospasm. The use of cromolyn in less severe asthma may be very effective. In more severe disease, the drug may allow the dosage of concomitant steroid therapy to be reduced.

Cromolyn is not a bronchodilator, and in fact, inhalation may cause reactive airways to develop bronchospasm. Cromolyn is of prophylactic value only and can be used instead of corticosteroids in some asthmatic patients who are steroid-dependent. Cromolyn is also effective in preventing exercise-induced bronchospasm. Patients must recognize that the drug will not relieve acute attacks of bronchospasm. Cromolyn is particularly valuable for the prevention and treatment of allergic rhinitis when given intranasally.

The drug is believed to act by interfering with the antigen-antibody effect on tissue mast cells (so-called stabilization of mast cells). The mechanism by which cromolyn prevents exercise-induced asthma has not been fully elucidated. The drug may also be of benefit in some types of cough, as it may inhibit the activity of nerves involved in the tussive reflex. Cromolyn may have a basic action on calcium flux. By interfering with the entry of calcium into the cell, subsequent reactions resulting in release of mediators are prevented.[37] Other drugs that interfere with calcium flux are of minor value in asthma, especially that induced by exercise—for example, verapamil and nifedipine.

□ NEDOCROMIL

Efforts to find drugs similar to cromolyn resulted in the marketing of nedocromil (Tilade) as an MDI for use in asthma. It is a pyranoquinoline and is unrelated to the chromones. However, it is similar to cromolyn in action: thus, it is not a bronchodilator and is used as an asthma prophylactic and for treating allergic rhinitis. It also has very few side effects and is usually very well tolerated. It offers the advantages of greater potency than cromolyn; thus, its effects may appear within a few days of initiating therapy, and although it should be first given as 2 inhalations four times a day, three-times-a-day dosing may suffice. After a few weeks of good control, maintenance with twice-a-day dosing may prove to be adequate.[38] The use of nedocromil may help some asthmatic patients reduce steroid dependency. The drug may have a limited role in asthmatic COPD.

Immunosuppressive Drugs

Many drugs, including corticosteroids, are used to suppress immunologic reactions, and such therapy is mandatory for patients with transplanted organs to prevent rejection reactions. Several of these drugs are also of value in immunologic diseases such as periarteritis or rheumatoid arthritis, and a number of these agents have been tried for asthmatics (eg, chloroquine, chlorambucil, 6-mercaptopurine, thioguanosine, azathioprine, and gold).[39] However, these immunosuppressive drugs do not seem to have been of major benefit in the treatment of asthma. It has been reported that methotrexate can be of considerable value for reducing the steroid requirements necessitated by severe asthma,[40] but the value of this toxic drug is limited.

Numerous other drugs are being investigated for treating asthma. One of the more promising is the 5-lipoxygenase inhibitor, zileuton.

Anticholinergic Agents.

The earliest drugs for the treatment of bronchospasm included plant sources of anticholinergic agents, such as Datura stramonium.[41] Cigarettes containing solanaceous plant materials were popular in the treatment of asthma in the nineteenth century, but were eventually replaced by aerosolized atropine. Several other agents are now preferred (Table 16-14).

□ ATROPINE

Atropine (*dl*-hyoscyamine) is a potent inhibitor of acetylcholine, which is released by parasympathetic postganglionic branches of the vagal nerves. Cholinergic stimulation is mimicked by muscarine, which is found in some poisonous mushrooms. The muscarinic activities mediated by vagal efferents to the lungs include bronchospasm and bronchial gland secretion; atropine, which is classified as an antimuscarinic drug, inhibits these actions. Thus, it is a bronchodilator and it can reduce mucus production. As a bronchodilator, it is more effective in the larger airways, which are the main site of obstruction in chronic obstructive airways disease (COPD).

Atropine sulfate is marketed in the United States and is available as a 1% inhalant solution. It is a tertiary ammonium compound, and it readily crosses membranes; thus, the aerosol can cause side effects such as dry mouth, tachycardia, and mental changes. Rarely, prostatic hypertrophy may be worsened, leading to urinary retention. If the aerosol enters the eye, the pupil dilates (the classic belladonna effect) and susceptible individuals may develop glaucoma. Although it can decrease airway secretions or increase their viscosity, the aerosol is usually well tolerated in bronchitis and does not appear to result in impaired mucokinesis.

□ IPRATROPIUM

Ipratropium (Atrovent) is a quaternary ammonium derivative of atropine. Unlike the tertiary derivatives such as atropine, it does not readily cross membranes, and therefore is much less likely to cause anticholinergic side effects.[42] However, direct deposition can cause drying of the nasal membrane, and thus it is of symptomatic value in rhinitis. In contrast, it does not significantly impair tracheobronchial mucociliary clearance.

Ipratropium is currently regarded as a primary drug for treating COPD, but it can also be effective in exacerbations of asthma that respond poorly to β_2 agonists.[36,43] Although there are reports that show it can act synergistically with β_2 agonists, this is not always the case. Nevertheless, when given in combination with albuterol (eg, as Combivent), it may be of special value in treating exacerbations of bronchospasm. Ipratropium is marketed as an MDI and as an inhalant solution. The usual dose is 2 to 4 puffs (each of 20 µg) of the inhaler three to four times a day; however, two to three times this dose may be required and is usually well tolerated. The standard dose of inhalant solution contains 500 µg, and is thus equivalent to about 25 puffs of the inhaler; one treatment can be given and repeated every 1 to 4 hours if tolerated. Ipratropium can also be used to treat rhinorrhea because it is a well-tolerated nasal drying agent; the MDI (two strengths) is used 2 to 4 times a day.[44]

□ OXITROPIUM

Oxitropium is a quaternary ammonium derivative of scopolamine with greater potency than ipratropium. It is available as an aerosol in Europe, but has not been introduced into the United States.

□ GLYCOPYRROLATE

Glycopyrrolate (Robinul) is a quaternary ammonium derivative of atropine. It has been used in anesthesia to help dry airway secretions and as an antispasmodic for

TABLE 16-14. **Anticholinergic Agents for Bronchospasm**

Drug	Aerosol Dose	Speed of Onset (min)	Peak Effect (min)	Duration (h)
Atropine Solution				
Sulfate (1%)	0.025–0.075 mg/kg	15–30	30–170	3–4
Methonitrate	1–1.5 mg	15–30	40–60	4–8
Ipratropium*				
Atrovent MDI, nasal sprays	20–120 µg, 42–84 µg†	3–30	90–120	4–8
Atrovent (0.1%)	500 µg	3–30	90–120	4–8
Scopolamine	(not by aerosol)	10–30	60–120	2
Glycopyrrolate Solution				
(Robinul)	500–2500 µg	15–30	30–45	2–12
Oxitropium	200–500 µg	15–30	90–120	6–10

* Also available in combination with albuterol in Combivent MDI.
†Nasal product

the bowel. It can be effective when given by aerosol in a dosage up to 1600 μg in the treatment of bronchospasm.

Miscellaneous Agents

Other agents have reportedly been effective in some cases of asthma.

Phentolamine is a blocker of α receptors and thus has a similar action to β_2 stimulators. This drug has been given orally and by inhalation and may prevent exercise-induced asthma. Other α blockers may have a similar effect in some patients with bronchospasm.

Ascorbic acid (vitamin C), the controversial agent advocated by some for the prevention of colds, does have definite effects on the respiratory tract. Ascorbic acid has been shown to inhibit histamine-induced bronchospasm. However, no convincing evidence justifies its use for the prevention or treatment of colds or asthma.

ANTIMICROBIALS

Antibiotics

Relatively little evidence suggests that the topical administration of antibiotics into the respiratory tract is of value in established infections, whereas there is an abundance of proof in favor of systemic therapy. There is a valid argument for giving small doses of antibiotics topically if the agents are very expensive or very toxic. However, there is no reason to give inexpensive or relatively safe antibiotics by this route; thus, agents such as penicillin, tetracycline, erythromycin, sulfonamides, and similar antimicrobics should not be given by inhalation. Inhalational administration of antibiotics carries risks of inducing hypersensitization and of causing bronchospasm and mucosal irritation.

Antibiotic drugs may be given by nebulization, although this is a relatively clumsy form of therapy; direct instillation may be preferable for localized lesions. In all cases, reactive bronchospasm must be guarded against by giving a bronchodilator. Some practitioners advocate nebulization or instillation of topical antibiotics to treat sinus or nasal infections, and topical antimicrobic treatment has been used to treat tracheostomy wounds that are colonized or infected.

Table 16-15 summarizes the available data on topical antimicrobial therapy for respiratory tract colonization or infection. The dosage ranges provided for most agents show a huge spread, reflecting the uncertainty about whether or not most of these drugs are truly effective.

TABLE 16-15. **Topical Antimicrobial Agents in Respiratory Therapy**

Agent	Antimicrobial Spectrum	Usual Dosage Range*
Amikacin	Gram-negative bacteria	Uncertain
Amphotericin B	Fungal infections	1–20 mg
Bacitracin	Staphylococci	5,000–20,000 U
Carbenicillin	*Pseudomonas* sp.	125–100 mg
Cephalosporin	Not recommended	
Colistin	Gram-negative bacteria	2–300 mg
Gentamicin	Gram-negative bacteria	5–120 mg
Kanamycin	Gram-negative bacteria†	25–300 mg
Macrolides	Not recommended	
Neomycin	Gram-negative bacteria	25–400 mg
Nystatin	*Candida, Aspergillus* spp.	25,000–50,000 U
Penicillin	Not recommended	
Pentamidine	*Pneumocystis carinii*	50–600 mg‡
Polymyxin	Gram-negative bacteria	5–50 mg
Tobramycin	Gram-negative bacteria	50 mg
Tuberculosis agents	Not recommended	
Viral agents	RCV	See text

* Dosages are poorly established. The drug should be dissolved in 2 mL of saline and each dose administered two to four times daily after initial bronchodilator therapy.

† Not suitable for *Pseudomonas*.

‡ Treatments given in large dosage daily for treatment, and in small dosage once every 1 to 2 weeks for prophylaxis.

□ PENTAMIDINE

The prophylaxis or treatment of *Pneumocystis carinii* pneumonia (PCP) has become all too common in hospitals in cities where AIDS is a significant problem. The standard prophylactic and therapeutic agent is the combined product, trimethoprim-sulfamethoxazole (TMP). Many patients cannot tolerate this medication, and inhaled pentamidine can be given as an alternative to prevent PCP.[45] The recommended dosages vary from 60 mg every 2 weeks when given by the more potent Fisone hand-held, patient-triggered, ultrasonic nebulizer to 300 mg once a month using the popular Respigard II nebulizer. Alternatively, 4 mg/kg given monthly by the Ultraneb 99 ultrasonic nebulizer has been recommended. Other useful nebulizers include the Portasonic and the AeroTech II.

The effectiveness of inhaled pentamidine as a prophylactic may depend on technique, but TMP appears to be more reliable. In the treatment of established PCP, TMP is more effective than inhaled pentamidine; in general, the latter drug is now given intravenously rather than by inhalation. The inhaled drug has the advantage of far lower systemic toxicity but it can cause bronchospasm, and susceptible patients should be pretreated with an aerosol bronchodilator. There is a concern that the caregiver who repeatedly inhales pentamidine is liable to develop toxic effects including conjunctivitis, pancreatitis, hypoglycemia, and possibly, teratogenicity; full precautions must be taken to prevent inadvertent breathing of the aerosol. Because the aerosolized drug is of secondary value, it is only used when other antipneumocystis agents cannot be tolerated.

□ RIBAVIRIN

The therapy of viral diseases remains an area of controversy with few successful agents and disputes as to their effectiveness. The one drug of interest in respiratory pharmacology is ribavirin (Virazole), which is known to inhibit the growth in tissue culture of influenza, respiratory syncytial, and herpes simplex viruses. The mechanism of its action is not fully understood, and its potential for toxicity is a concern. At present, ribavirin has only one major indication, respiratory syncytial virus (RSV) disease in infants. The drug is given by continuous inhalation for 12 to 18 hours a day, using a small-particle aerosol generator (SPAG), for 3 to 7 days. The daily dose is up to 300 mL of a solution containing 20 mg/mL, and the SPAG nebulizer delivers the medication in particles of about 1.3 μm MMD in a hood or an oxygen tent.

There is a danger that if given to an infant on ventilatory support, precipitated ribavirin could occlude the delivery lines and cause ventilator dysfunction. There is evidence that the drug is effective in very sick, high-risk infants, particularly those who also have congenital heart disease, but its value in less severe or in presumed but unproven cases of RSV infection is disputed.[46] Great care should be taken to protect the health care team from exposure to ribavirin because it may be teratogenic and, possibly, carcinogenic. When given to infants by aerosol, it is usually well tolerated, although conjunctivitis and rashes may occur.

Miscellaneous Antimicrobial Agents

Iodides are known to have an antifungal effect, and sodium iodide as a 1% to 2% solution has been used to treat pulmonary aspergilloma by means of an endobronchial drip. Whether nebulization therapy with sodium or potassium iodide would be valuable in treating other fungal problems in the lungs remains to be determined.

Acetic acid has been claimed to be a useful sterilizing agent for use in respiratory therapy. A solution of 0.25% acetic acid can be used as a decontaminating fluid for nebulizers; nebulization of 10 mL through the equipment can eliminate gram-negative bacterial contaminants. Some clinicians have nebulized 0.25% acetic acid into the lungs of patients with cystic fibrosis or bronchiactosis; apparently the agent is well tolerated and can kill colonizing bacteria.

LOCAL ANESTHETICS

To provide tracheobronchial anesthesia, various methods of drug administration are used, including direct application of the agent to the upper respiratory tract and ultrasonic nebulization or direct instillation into the larynx, trachea, and lower airways. Anesthesia can also be produced by injection, carefully placed to cause blockade of the glossopharyngeal nerve and its recurrent branch.

Local anesthetics may cause initial bronchospasm, and they may inhibit mucociliary activity, although low concentrations of some agents have allegedly improved ciliary action. Certain agents may have a bacteriostatic effect, and specimens of secretions taken for culture after exposure to local anesthetics may not yield their full microbial content. However, this does not seem to be a major concern in practice. Currently the only important inhaled anesthetic is lidocaine.

Lidocaine

Lidocaine (Xylocaine) is one of the safest of the local anesthetics and can be given in concentrations varying from 1% to 20%. It is usually given as a 4% solution by machine nebulization, as an ultrasonically generated aerosol, or by direct instillation, with a total dose of 10 to 20 mL. Epinephrine in concentrations of 1:250,000 to 1:50,000 may be added; this helps to prevent instrument-induced bronchospasm and constricts the mucosal vessels, thereby decreasing the systemic absorption of the lidocaine. Additionally, the presence of epinephrine may prevent or stop bleeding during instrumentation of friable mucosa.

Lidocaine may act as a bronchodilator in some asthmatic patients when given by aerosol or intravenously. The drug may also be valuable in some cases of intractable cough caused by damage to the tracheobronchial tree.

NICOTINE

The well-known addictive powers of tobacco products are largely attributable to nicotine; a smoked cigarette can deliver 0.05 to 2 mg in the body. Nicotine is an alkaloid, and is one of the rare natural ones that exists as a liquid. It has a "nicotinic" effect on autonomic ganglia, particularly at cholinergic receptor sites, causing either stimulation or depression, and thereby having complex actions. Typically, nicotine is a cerebral stimulant, but large doses cause depression. Its central action may relieve anxiety and improve concentration in people who become habituated or develop tolerance to it, but others who develop anxiety, depression, and nausea are unlikely to become dependent on nicotine. Among the potentially hazardous effects of nicotine are peripheral arteriolar and coronary artery spasm.

Many of the hazards as well as the satisfactions of smoking do not follow the intake of nicotine alone. Thus, nicotine in various forms can be used as a less-satisfying substitute for tobacco in the treatment of dependency. The most popular products are slow-release dermal patches and chewing gum; aerosols, vapors, sprays and special nontobacco cigarettes can also be used.[47]

☐ NICOTINE GUM

Therapy with nicotine gum may be favored for the opportunity it offers to the chewer to obtain multiple rapid doses of nicotine, thus serving as a substitute for cigarettes; however, blood levels increase more slowly and to a lower level with gum than is characteristically obtained with cigarette smoking. The gum has to be carefully and slowly chewed, and many patients find the product to be unacceptable.

☐ NICOTINE PATCHES

Slow-release patches are easier to use, but do not produce the same satisfaction of rapid increases in blood nicotine level that a smoker obtains. Thus, patches are regarded as a support for a smoker who quits, and they cannot be regarded as a substitute. Initially, larger dosage patches should be used on the day the patient quits, and then after a few weeks a reduction is made, using a smaller dosage patch. The commercial products contain 21 or 22 mg of nicotine in the large dosage patches; 10-, 11-, 14-, and 16-mg patches are available for intermediate dosages, and 5- and 7-mg patches for small dosages. Typically, patches of each of the three sizes may be used daily for 2 to 4 or 6 weeks, but some patients feel the need for them for several months. Patches could precipitate coronary ischemia, particularly if the patient continues to smoke. The major side effect is contact dermatitis.

☐ NICOTINE THERAPY

In hospitals, it may be appropriate in occasional cases to give nicotine gum as a cigarette substitute to a heavy smoker. For patients who have failed in attempts to stop smoking, patches are usually advised, but it is important to provide individual or group counseling with frequent reinforcement to reduce the high relapse rate. Overall, the results of nicotine gum or patches are appreciable, but failure to break the smoking habit can occur in 50% to 80% of patients.

ADMINISTRATION OF RESPIRATORY DRUGS

Physicians generally have greater familiarity and security with the administration of oral and intravenous drugs than they do with inhalational drugs. Accordingly, oral and intravenous drugs are prescribed with relative accuracy and appropriateness, whereas inhalational drugs do not receive the same consideration from most physicians. Respiratory therapists and nurses who administer therapy carry a considerable responsibility when they receive a physician's order, since the prescription must be interpreted and monitored with active awareness of the desired effects and the possible side effects (see Box 16-3 on page 472).

Dosages of Drugs

The appropriate dosages for inhalational drugs are, in fact, quite variable because many factors influence the effectiveness of the different agents. The reliability and efficiency of the equipment and the cooperation of the patient profoundly influence the amount of drug deposited in the lungs. The response to an individual dosage varies in each patient, particularly when catecholamines are given, because tachyphylaxis or converse effects may obviate the expected result. Side effects are variable and may be related to the gaseous vehicle, the diluent, or the droplets, rather than to the drug itself.

For all these reasons, therapists should not be overly surprised or concerned when a physician prescribes an "inappropriate," excessive amount of drug. If the physician, for some reason, is unwilling to change the prescription when the error is discussed, the therapist or nurse can administer the drug but should carefully monitor the patient for any adverse response; if evidence of toxicity appears, then the treatment can be stopped short before all the prescribed amount of the drug is given, and the fact should be recorded in the patient's chart. Similarly, when an "appropriate" recommended dosage is prescribed, the patient should be monitored for an idiosyncratic or individualistic adverse response.

Evaluation of Therapy

Unfortunately, the recognition of "adverse effects" is not cut and dried. Thus, when a bronchodilator is used, an increase in pulse rate from 70 to 110 may be tolerable, whereas an increase from 110 to 125 may not. Similarly, it is difficult to recognize a meaningful change in blood pressure, because observations are not easy to make and changes in systolic and diastolic values may vary independently. Thus, epinephrine in small doses may cause a small increase in diastolic pressure, whereas larger doses (such as those that probably are not attained with inhalational therapy) result in more marked changes in both values. Physicians expect the therapist to check blood pressure before, during, and after bronchodilator administration in those selected patients in whom these changes may be detrimental. However, it is unreasonable to expect a therapist to worry about the effect on the blood pressure in every patient who takes an aerosolized sympathomimetic.

Rational aerosol therapy requires a recognition of the therapeutic objectives, skillful administration of appropriate dosages, and accurate assessment of the effects of treatment. In most patients, bedside pulmonary function evaluations of vital capacity, peak flow rate, or forced expiratory volumes can be used to assess bronchodilator responsiveness. The patient's subjective feelings, volume of sputum production, and monitoring of the pulse and auscultatory findings in the lungs should be routinely evaluated to determine whether desired effects or undesired side effects have been obtained. The patient's subjective response is often the best indicator of adverse effects, and more objective measurements may be less helpful.

When a mucokinetic drug is given, it is the therapist's responsibility to ensure that a therapeutic response occurs. Thus, relying uncritically on the drug alone is inadequate; the patient must be encouraged to cough and to expectorate, and chest percussion, postural drainage, and even suctioning may be needed to facilitate the process. The therapist should record the amount of sputum produced and note the color and consistency.

Administration of Aerosolized Drugs

Whether bronchodilator therapy is given by means of a respirator or an air-driven nebulizer, much of the drug may be lost in the apparatus or in the air. Most studies suggest that aerosolization by means of a gas-driven nebulizer results in deposition of 5% to 10% of the drug in the lungs, whereas an equal amount might be deposited in the mouth and swallowed, thereby resulting in systemic effects. When the drug is nebulized through an endotracheal tube, a variable amount of the drug is deposited in the lungs, but none enters the gastrointestinal tract.

When an MDI is used, the amount deposited in the respiratory tract is extremely variable and is related to the competency of the patient's technique. With the best technique, it is unlikely that more than 20% to 30% of the "puff" of aerosol is deposited in the lungs, and the average patient is more likely to deposit closer to 10% of the metered dose. As shown in Table 16-16, manufacturers generally advise that about 10 times as much drug should be measured into a nebulizer as is released

TABLE 16-16. **Comparative Dosages Achieved Using Metered Dose Inhaler and Inhalant Solution Preparations of Bronchodilators**

	Metered Device		Inhalant Solution			
				Usual Dose		
	Dose per Puff (mg)	*Dose Delivered With Three Puffs (mg)*	*Potency of Solution (%)*	*(mL)*	*(mg)*	**Probable Amount Deposited in Lungs (ie, 10%) (mg)**
Epinephrine						
Medihaler-Epi	0.16	0.48				0.048
Primatene Mist	0.22	0.66				0.066
Vaponephrin			2.25	0.25	6	0.6
Isoetharine						
Bronkometer	0.34	1				0.1
Bronkosol solution			1	0.5	5	0.5
Bronkosol unit dose			0.25	2	5	0.5
Isoproterenol						
Medihaler-Iso	0.08	0.24				0.024
Isuprel Mistometer	0.13	0.39				0.039
Isuprel solution			1	0.5	5	0.5
Metaproterenol						
Alupent inhaler	0.65	2				0.20
Alupent solution			5	0.3	15	1.5
Alupent unit doses			0.4, 0.6	2.5	10, 15	1, 1.5
Albuterol						
Proventil inhaler	0.09	0.27				0.027
Ventolin inhaler	0.09	0.27				0.027
Ventolin solution			0.5	0.5	2.5	0.25
Proventil unit dose			0.083	3	2.5	0.25
Bitolterol						
Tornalate inhaler	0.37	1.11				0.1
Tornalate solution			0.2	1	2	0.2
Terbutaline						
Brethaire inhaler	0.20	0.60				0.06
Bricanyl solution*			0.1	2	2	0.2

Note: The probable amounts of each drug deposited varies considerably depending on whether a jet nebulizer or metered cartridge is used. The figures provided are based on typical recommended dosages.
* Marketed as a subcutaneous injection solution.

BOX 16-5

TECHNIQUE FOR USING METERED AEROSOL DEVICES

1. Shake the canister several times.
2. Hold upside down, with mouthpiece held either between closed lips or about ½ to 1 inch away from wide-open mouth. (The latter technique may be better, but most patients feel less comfortable using this method.)
3. Exhale normally but not forcefully.
4. Inspire deeply and release a puff of bronchodilator, breathing in the aerosol.
5. Hold breath for several seconds before exhaling. (*Note:* If an aerosol steroid is used, exhale through the nose to deposit steroid on the nasal mucosa, thereby treating any nasal allergy that may be present.)
6. Breathe normally. Waiting for up to 5 minutes to evaluate response would be desirable, but it is usually not practical.
7. Repeat with one, two, or three more inhalations over the next few minutes, if needed and if tolerated. Each time the canister should be shaken, then a single puff inhaled.
8. Rinse out mouth after each inhalation of drug to prevent oral absorption if side effects are a problem.
9. Do not overuse any drug; if more than 16 inhalations a day are needed, then a different treatment regimen or a change in drug is usually advisable.
10. Keep the dispensing unit clean by occasionally rinsing it in warm water or cleaning with a cotton-tipped stick.

by a standard treatment using the metered product. This results in a much larger dose being nebulized into the lungs than is obtained with the standard 2 to 4 puffs from an MDI.

Therapists should be very familiar with the appropriate technique to be used with each aerosol device, and the last day or two of a respiratory patient's stay in a hospital should be used to teach and to supervise the patient in the correct technique to be used following discharge home. In all cases, the patient must inhale the sprayed drug deeply and then hold the breath to encourage maximal deposition. If side effects are troublesome, then rinsing out the mouth and throat with water may help remove excess drug, the systemic absorption of which may add to the side effects. Further important concerns are that the patient should be instructed to keep the nebulizing unit clean and that overuse of aerosol should be avoided (see Box 16-5).

Multiple drugs are often prescribed in respiratory therapy; fortunately, most agents are compatible when mixed in the nebulizer. However, bronchodilators are relatively unstable, which is why they are stored in dark bottles and maintained at an acid pH. When the drugs are placed in a nebulizer and exposed to light and oxygen, they slowly breakdown to reddish-brown adrenochromes. Although these products are probably not harmful, their presence suggests that the mixture has diminished bronchodilator activity and thus should be discarded. Patients' secretions may be stained pink by a bronchodilator, and if recognized, this will not cause alarm.

Administration of Nonaerosolized Drugs

When given intravenously, the common respiratory agents can be mixed without any apparent adverse effects. Thus, saline, dextrose, aminophylline, and corticosteroids are all compatible. However, some antibiotics may be incompatible with various drugs, and they should be given through an independent setup.

Most oral drugs used in respiratory therapy are compatible with one another and are often administered in combination preparations. Alcoholic elixirs are potentially hazardous when given to alcoholics and are contraindicated if the patient is on disulfiram (Antabuse) or a similar type of drug. Epinephrine, when given subcutaneously (and perhaps when given by inhalation), may interact with various drugs (eg, with monoamine oxidase inhibitors) to cause hypertension and excitability; with digitalis glycosides to cause cardiac arrhythmias; or with hypotensive drugs to cause the reverse effect of hypertension. Epinephrine may also interfere with the action of insulin and oral antidiabetic agents, since catecholamines tend to cause an increase in blood sugar level. When theophylline is used, particular care is needed to avoid overdosage and toxic drug or metabolic interactions.

It is of interest that certain drugs can be administered by the intratracheal route, particularly in emergencies such as cardiac arrest. Naloxone, diazepam, lidocaine, epinephrine, and atropine are readily absorbed when given by this route in amounts similar to the standard intravenous dosage.[48]

APPENDIX: DOSAGES OF INHALATIONAL DRUGS

Volumes

The amount of solution delivered from an uncalibrated dropper is very variable and depends on the characteristics of the dropper, the method of use, and the nature of the solution. One drop approximates 1 minim of an aqueous solution, or 0.5 minim of an alcoholic solution, or 2 minims of a viscous solution. There are about 15 minims (or 15 drops of an aqueous solution) in 1 mL of water.

For practical purposes the following approximate conversion table can be used for dilute aqueous solutions.

1 minim = 1 drop
15 minims = 1 mL (1 cc) = 1 g
60 minims = 1 teaspoon = 4 mL (approximate)
240 minims = 1 tablespoon = 15 mL (approximate)
480 minims = 30 mL = 30 g = 1 oz

Abbreviations

mL = milliliter (1000 mL = 1 liter [L])
cc = cubic centimeter
mg = milligram (1000 mg = 1 gram)
g = gram (1000 g = 1 kilogram [kg])
1000 micrograms (μg or mcg) = 1 mg
1,000,000 micrograms = 1 g

Apothecary Versus Avoirdupois

Because these two systems of weights and measures differ, *pints* and *pounds* (lb) should not be used as pharmacologic units. The apothecary pint contains 16 oz, but there are only 12 oz to the pound in the apothecary scale, whereas there are 16 oz to the pound in the avoirdupois scale.

PERCENTAGES

Inhalational solutions are commonly labeled according to a percentage or ratio scale. The following scales may be used:

Weight-in-weight (w/w; eg, g/100 g)
Weight-in-volume (w/v; eg, g/100 mL)
Volume-in-volume (v/v; eg, mL/100 mL)

Most frequently, a w/v percentage is used:

1% = 1:100 = 1 g/100 mL = 1 g/dL (ie, 1000 mg/100 mL or 10 mg/mL)
5% = 5:100 = 5 g/100 mL (ie, 5000 mg/100 mL or 50 mg/mL)

Thus,

0.1% = 1:1000 = 0.1 g/100 mL (ie, 100 mg/100 mL or 1 mg/mL)

Various expressions can be used, for example:

0.5% = 5:1000 or 1:200
= 1 g/200 mL, or 0.5 g/100 mL, or 500 mg/100 mL, or 500 mg/dL, or 5 mg/mL, or 5 g/L.

Example: A mixture of 0.5 mL of 0.5% of albuterol in 2.5 mL of saline contains

0.5 mL of 0.5% albuterol
= 0.5 mL of a solution containing 1 g albuterol in 200 mL (or 5.0 mg/mL)
= 0.5 x 1000 mg = 2.5 mg

Thus, the mixture contains 2.5 mg (2500 μg) of isoproterenol in 3 mL solution. If this solution is nebulized, a maximum of about 10% will be retained in the lungs, providing about 0.25 mg (250 μg) of albuterol. In contrast, one activation of an MDI releases 0.09 mg (90 μg) of albuterol, of which about 10% (0.009 mg) is retained in the lungs. Thus, the mixed inhalant solution provides a standard dose that is equivalent to about 27 puffs of the MDI. In practice, much of the inhalant solution is wasted, thus giving perhaps the equivalent of 10 puffs of an MDI.

REFERENCES

1. Ernst P, Spitzer WO, Suissa S, Cockroft DW, Buist AS: Beta-agonists and asthma research: An international consultation. Eur Respir J 6:273, 1993
2. Kirn TF: Asthma mortality rate raises questions, emphasizes need to determine facts of situation. JAMA 260:455, 1988
3. Waldrep JC, Keyhani K, Black M, Knight V: Operating characteristics of 18 different continuous-flow jet nebulizers with beclomethasone dipropionate liposome aerosol. Chest 105:106, 1994
4. Miller WF: Aerosol therapy in acute and chronic respiratory disease. Arch Intern Med 131:148, 1973
5. Shim C, King M, Willians MH: Lack of effect of hydration on sputum production in chronic bronchitis. Chest 92:679, 1987
6. Ziment I: Hydration, humidification and mucokinetic therapy. In Weiss EB, Stein M (eds): Bronchial Asthma. Mechanisms and Therapeutics, 3rd ed, Chap 69. Boston, Little, Brown & Company, 1993
7. Parks CR, Woodrum DE, Graham CB: Effect of water nebulization on normal canine pulmonary mucociliary clearance. Am Rev Respir Dis 104:99, 1971
8. Morrow PE: Aerosol characterization and deposition. Am Rev Respir Dis 110(6 part 2):88, 1974
9. Newman SP: Delivery of drugs to the respiratory tract. In Chung KF, Barnes PJ (eds): Pharmacology of the Respiratory Tract, Chap 23. New York, Marcel Dekker, 1993
10. Lieberman J: Measurement of sputum viscosity in a coneplate viscometer. II. An evaluation of mucolytic agents in vitro. Am Rev Respir Dis 97:662, 1968
11. Hirsch SR, Zastrow JE, Kory RC: Sputum liquefying agents: A comparative in vitro study. J Lab Clin Med 74:346, 1969
12. Fuchs H, Borowitz DS, Christiansen DH, Morris EM, Nash ML, Ramsey BW, Rosenstein BJ, Smith AL, Wohl ME: Effect of aerosolized recombinant DNase on exacerbations of respiratory symptoms and on pulmonary function in patients with cystic fibrosis. N Engl J Med 331:637, 1994
13. Obenour RA, Saltzman HA, Sierer HO, Green JL: Effects of surface-active aerosols and pulmonary congestion on lung compliance and resistance. Circulation 27:888, 1963
14. Pramanik AK, Holtzman RB, Merritt TA: Surfactant replacement therapy for pulmonary diseases. Pediatr Clin North Am 40:913, 1993
15. Boyd EM, Sheppard EP: Friar's balsam and respiratory tract fluid. Am J Dis Child 111:630, 1966
16. Boyd EM: A review of studies on the pharmacology of the expectorants and inhalants. Int J Clin Pharmacol Ther Toxicol 3:55, 1970
17. Ziment I: What to expect from expectorants. JAMA 236:193, 1976
18. Lieberman J, Kurnick NB: The induction of proteolysis in purulent sputum by iodides. J Clin Invest 43:1892, 1964
19. Carson S, Goldhammer R: Mucus transport in the respiratory tract. Am Rev Respir Dis 98(2):86, 1966
20. Siegal S: The asthma-suppressive action of potassium iodide. J Allergy 35:252, 1964
21. Hirsch SR, Viernes PF, Kory RC: The expectorant effect of glyceryl guaiacolate in patients with chronic bronchitis. Chest 63:9, 1973
22. Ziment I: Cough. In Rakel R (ed): Conn's Current Therapy. Philadelphia, WB Saunders, 1991, p 23
23. Ziment I, Flaster H: Using bronchodilators effectively. Contemp Int Med 5:19, 1993
24. Lotvall J, Svedmyr N: Salmeterol: An inhaled β_2-agonist with prolonged duration of action. Lung 171:249, 1993
25. Boulet L-P: Long- versus short-acting β_2-agonists. Drugs 47:207, 1994
26. Castle W, Fuller R, Hall J, Palmer J: Serevent nationwide surveillance study: Comparison of salmeterol with salbutamol in asthmatic patients who require regular bronchodilator treatment. BMJ 306:1034, 1993
27. Taylor DR, Sears MR: Regular β-adrenergic agonists. Evidence, not reassurance, is what is needed. Chest 106:552, 1994

28. Ziment I: Beta-adrenergic agonist toxicity. Less of a problem, more of a perception. Chest 103:1591, 1993
29. Ward AJM, McKenniff M, Evans JM, Page CP, Costello JF: Theophylline—an immunomodulatory role in asthma? Am Rev Respir Dis 147:518, 1993
30. Sullivan P, Bekir S, Jaffar Z, Page CP, Jeffery P, Costello J: Anti-inflammatory effects of low-dose oral theophylline in atopic asthma. Lancet 343:1006, 1994
31. Barnes PJ, Pauwels RA: Theophylline in the management of asthma: Time for reappraisal? Eur Respir J 7:579, 1994
32. Hendeles L, Weinberger M: Theophylline, a "state of the art" review. Pharmacotherapy 3:2, 1983
33. Lawyer CH, Bardana EJ, Rodgers R, Gerber N: Utilization of intravenous dihydroxypropyltheophylline (dyphylline) in an aminophylline-sensitive patient, and its pharmokinetic comparison with theophylline. J Allergy Clin Immunol 65:353, 1980
34. Hirshman CA: Dyphylline aerosol attentuates antigen-induced bronchoconstriction in experimental canine asthma. Chest 78:420, 1981
35. Busse WW: Role of antihistamines in allergic disease. Ann Allergy 72:371, 1994
36. Ziment I: Pharmacologic therapy of obstructive airway disease. Clin Chest Med 11:461, 1990
37. Ahmed T, D'Brot J, Abraham W: The role of calcium antagonists in bronchial reactivity. J Allergy Clin Immunol 81:133, 1988
38. Edwards AM, Stevens MT: The clinical efficacy of inhaled nedrocromil sodium (Tilade) in the treatment of asthma. Eur Respir J 6:35, 1993
39. Ziment I: Unconventional therapy in asthma. In Gershwin ME, Halpern GM (eds): Bronchial Asthma. Principles of Diagnosis and Treatment, 3rd ed. Totowa, Humana, 1994, p 413
40. Mullarkey MF, Blumenstein BA, Andrade WP, Bailey GA, Olason I, Wetzel CE: Methotrexate in the treatment of corticosteroid-dependent asthma. N Engl J Med 318:603, 1988
41. Charpin D, Orehek J, Velardocchio JM: Bronchodilator effects of antiasthmatic cigarette smoke (*Datura stramonium*). Thorax 34:259, 1979
42. Gross NJ: Ipratropium bromide. N Engl J Med 319:486, 1988
43. Ferguson GT, Cherniack RM: Management of chronic obstructive pulmonary disease. N Engl J Med 328:1017, 1993
44. Borum P: Nasal disorders and anticholingeric therapy. Postgrad Med J 61(Suppl 1):61, 1987
45. Masur H: Prevention and treatment of pneumocystis pneumonia. N Engl J Med 327:1853, 1992
46. Wheeler G, Wolford J, Turner RB: Historical cohort evaluation of ribavirin efficacy in respiratory syncytial virus infection. Pediatr Infect Dis J 12:209, 1993
47. Sachs DPL, Leischow SJ: Pharmacologic approaches to smoking cessation. Clin Chest Med 12:769, 1991
48. Editorial: Intratracheal drugs. Lancet 1:743, 1988

BIBLIOGRAPHY

General Reviews of Drugs Used in Respiratory Therapy

AMA Drug Evaluations Annual, Chicago, American Medical Association, 1994

Barnes PJ, Rodger IW, Thomson NC (eds): Asthma: Basic Mechanisms and Clinical Management. London, Academic Press, 1988

Dautrebande L: Physiological and pharmacologic characteristics of liquid aerosols. Physiol Rev 32:214, 1952 (A classic account of aerosol therapy, with an extraordinary range of information.)

Gilman AG, Rall TW, Nies AS, Taylor P (eds): The Pharmacologic Basis of Therapeutics, 8th ed. New York, Macmillan, 1990 (The chapters on the autonomic nervous system and bronchodilators are extremely good.)

Page CP, Metzger WJ (eds): Drugs and the Lung. New York, Raven, 1994

Rau JL Jr, Reynolds JEF (eds): Respiratory Care Pharmacology, 4th ed. St. Louis, Mosby, 1994 (A good basic text.)

Reynolds JEF (ed): Martindale. The Extra Pharmacopoeia, 30th ed. London, The Pharmaceutical Press, 1993 (This compendium provides an extraordinary amount of information, including traditional and international drugs.)

Witek TJ Jr, Schacter EN: Pharmacology and Therapeutics in Respiratory Care. Philadelphia, WB Saunders, 1994 (An advanced text.)

Ziment I: Respiratory Pharmacology and Therapeutics. Philadelphia, WB Saunders, 1978 (A comprehensive practical guide to drugs used in inhalation therapy and pulmonary medicine.)

Ziment I, Popa V (eds): Respiratory Pharmacology. Clin Chest Med 7(3): 1986

Mucokinesis and Mucokinetic Agents

Braga PC, Allegra L (eds):. Drugs in Bronchial Mucology. New York, Raven, 1989 (A historical and current examination of mucokinetic drugs.)

Boyd EM: A review of studies on the pharmacology of the expectorants and inhalants. Int J Clin Pharmacol Ther Toxicol 3:55, 1970

Boyd EM: Respiratory Tract Fluid. Springfield, Charles C. Thomas, 1975 (A comprehensive review of Boyd's considerable research on agents affecting sputum.)

Dulfano MJ (ed): Sputum Fundamentals and Clinical Pathology. Springfield, Charles C. Thomas, 1973 (An encyclopedic account of sputum and its structure, examination, properties, and management.)

Gunn JA: The action of expectorants. BMJ 4:972, 1927 (A classic article.)

Lish PM, Salem H: Expectorants. In Salem H, Aviado DM (eds): International Encyclopedia of Pharmacology and Therapeutics, Vol 3, Sec 27. New York, Pergamon, 1970

Richardson PS, Phipps RH: The anatomy, physiology, pharmacology and pathology of tracheobronchial mucus secretion and the use of expectorant drugs in human disease. Pharmacol Ther B 3:441, 1978

Ziment I: Mucokinetic agents. In Hollinger MA (ed): Current Topics in Pulmonary Pharmacology and Toxicology, Vol 3, Chap 5. New York, Elsevier Science, 1987

Asthma

Barnes PJ: New drugs for asthma. Eur Respir J 5:1126, 1992

Chung KF, Barnes PJ (eds): Pharmacology of the Respiratory Tract. Experimental and Clinical Research. New York, Marcel Dekker, 1993

Jenne JW, Murphy S (eds): Drug Therapy for Asthma. Research and Clinical Practice. New York, Marcel Dekker, 1987

Middleton E, Reed CE, Ellis EF, Adkinson NF, Yunginger JW, Busse WW (eds): Allergy, Principles and Practice, 4th ed. St Louis, CV Mosby, 1993 (Volume I has excellent accounts on pharmacology.)

Weiss EB, Stein M (eds): Bronchial Asthma: Mechanisms and Therapeutics, 3rd ed. Boston, Little, Brown & Company, 1993

Sympathomimetic Agents

Clark TJH, Cochrane GM (eds): Bronchodilator Therapy. The Basis of Asthma and Chronic Obstructive Airways Disease Management. Auckland, ADIS Press, 1984

Howder C: Antimuscarinic and β_2-adrenoceptor bronchodilators in obstructive airways disease. Respir Care 38:1364, 1993

Svensson L-A: Development of β_2-adrenoceptor agonist bronchodilator prodrugs. In Hollinger MA (ed): Current Topics in Pulmonary Pharmacology and Toxicology, Vol 3, Chap 1. New York, Elsevier Science, 1987

Ziment I: Risk/benefit ratio of long-term treatment with β_2-adrenoceptor agonists. Lung 168(Suppl):168, 1990

Methylxanthines

Hendeles L, Massanari M, Weinberger M: Theophylline. In Middleton E, Reed CE, Ellis EF, Adkinson NF, Yunginger JW (eds): Allergy. Principles and Practice, 3rd ed, Chap 30. St. Louis, CV Mosby, 1988

Jenne JW (ed): Rationale for the use of theophylline in COPD: Bronchodilation and beyond. Chest 92(Suppl): 1987

Anticholinergics

Bergofsky EH (ed): Cholinergic pathway in obstructive airways disease. Am J Med 81(5A), 1986

Mann JS: Anticholinergic drugs in the treatment of airways disease. Rev J Dis Chest 79:209, 1985

Ziment I, Au JP: Anticholinergic agents. Clin Chest Med 7:355, 1986

Antibiotics

Corkery KJ, Luce JM, Montgomery AB: Aerosolized pentamidine for treatment and prophylaxis of *Pneumocystis carinii* pneumonia: An update. Respir Care 33:676, 1988

Hodson ME: Antibiotic treatment, aerosol therapy. Chest 94(Suppl): 156S, 1988

Newman SP, Woodman G, Clarke SW: Deposition of carbenicillin aerosols in cystic fibrosis: Effects of nebulizer system and breathing pattern. Thorax 43:318, 1988

Wanner A, Rao A: Clinical indications for and effects of bland mucolytic, and antimicrobial aerosols. Am Rev Respir Dis 122(5, Part 2):79, 1980

Corticosteroids

Clark TJH (ed): Steroids in asthma: A reappraisal in the light of inhalation therapy. Auckland, ADIS Press, 1983

Morris HG: Mechanism and action and therapeutic role of corticosteroids in asthma. J Allergy Clin Immunol 75:1, 1985

Ziment I: Steroids. Clin Chest Med 7:341, 1986

Cromolyn, Nedocromil

Altounyan REC: Review of clinical activity and mode of action of sodium cromoglycate. Clin Allergy 10:481, 1980

Wasserman SI (ed): Nedocromil sodium: A pyranoquinoline anti-inflammatory agent for the treatment of asthma. J Allergy Clin Immunol 92(part I, no. 2):143, 1993

17 Bronchial Hygiene Therapy

Dennis C. Sobush
Lana Hilling
Peter A. Southorn

CLINICAL SKILLS

Upon completion of this chapter, the reader will know how to:

- Determine how a patient's history is likely to contribute to secretion production, retention, or atelectasis
- Conduct a physical examination and recognize central nervous system, pulmonary, cardiovascular, or musculoskeletal signs of atelectasis, or likelihood of secretion retention related to impaired clearance
- Recognize values (PFTs, ABGs, CBC, oximetry, and/or sputum analysis) that are relevant to disease
- Read a chest radiograph to determine area(s) of infiltrate, heart size, diaphragm length, and excursion range
- Check function of positioning apparatus or devices (tilt tables, hospital beds, and positioning cushions/wedges) and monitoring equipment (blood pressure cuff, electrocardiogram, pulse oximeter, and stethoscope)
- Determine use of adjunctive equipment (mechanical percussors and vibrators, incentive spirometers, Flutter® valves, positive expiratory pressure [PEP] devices, and resuscitation bags), airway clearance resources (suctioning systems with appropriate solutions, catheters, gowns, gloves, and goggles), and humidity/aerosol equipment (humidifiers, bland and medicated aerosols)
- Explain planned therapy and goals to the patient (family) and obtain his or her consent to proceed
- Communicate and collaborate with other health care team members
- Conduct therapeutic procedures to achieve removal of bronchopulmonary secretions
- Recommend modifications in the respiratory care plan based on patient responses
- Document patient's response to treatment intervention

KEY TERMS

Air bronchogram
Atelectasis
Autogenic drainage
Bronchial hygiene therapy
Bronchiectasis
Chronic bronchitis
Cilia
Clearance
Consolidation
Cystic fibrosis
Directed cough
Huff cough
Hydration
Infiltration
Mucus plug
PEP therapy
Percussion
Postural drainage
Tactile fremitus
Sputum
Vibration
Viscosity

Bronchial hygiene therapy (BHT), often termed chest physical therapy (CPT) or chest physiotherapy, is an established area of respiratory care practice. The role of the respiratory care practitioner is to assess the need for therapy and apply appropriate techniques. These include the time-honored use of gravity-assisted bronchial or postural drainage, chest percussion, and/or vibration to clear bronchial secretions. Other modalities include assisted or directed cough (DC) and use of techniques to increase lung volumes. Chapter 18 follows with a detailed review of volume expansion therapy and related equipment. Box 17-1 lists the variety of airway clearance techniques with abbreviations, including newer terminology.[1]

The primary goals of all BHT methods are to remove excess airway secretions and to improve or prevent problems caused by obstruction, which include atelectasis, predisposition to infection, and disordered gas exchange.

The secondary goals include improving cardiopulmonary endurance for functional activity and preventing long-term effects of retained secretions on lung function.

BHT procedures consist of patient-positioning strategies to drain secretions with gravity assistance. Sometimes external manipulation of the chest is added with percussion or vibration (manual or mechanical) to help better mobilize pulmonary secretions. Airway hydration, administration of medical aerosols that promote mucokinesis, and mechanical aids to promote increased lung volume are commonly combined with BHT.

This chapter focuses on clinical indications, contraindications, hazards/complications, limitations, and assessment of both need for and outcome of BHT. Information is based on nationally accepted Clinical Practice Guidelines (CPG).[2–4] This chapter also describes controlled breathing exercises. Chapter 18 follows with a review of adjunctive procedures of positive expiratory pressure (PEP) therapy, mechanical aids to secretion removal, and devices to promote lung inflation.

The practitioner's role includes assessment using physical cardiopulmonary assessment and chest radiographic imaging skills in order to select types of BHT, as well as implementation of therapy. (The reader is referred to Chapters 6 [Assessment Skills] and 7 [Imaging Assessment] as prerequisite reading.) This chapter integrates areas of assessment and therapeutic techniques. The application of this approach is summarized by presentation of therapist-driven protocols (TDPs) for bronchial hygiene therapy. The Clinical Skills found at the beginning of this chapter are those needed to perform patient care related to BHT according to a published national survey.[5]

PAST AND FUTURE OF BRONCHIAL HYGIENE THERAPY

The beneficial effects of "bronchial drainage" for treatment of bronchiectasis were described in 1901. Winifred Linton, a physiotherapist at Brompton Hospital, London, England, introduced "localized breathing exercises" for thoracic surgery patients in the mid-1930s. Alvan Barach popularized the concept of "breathing exercises" in the United States during the 1940s. In 1953, Palmer and Sellick published pioneering work on the value of "chest physiotherapy" in postoperative surgical patients.[6] Although the techniques of BHT have been applied since the early 1900s, they have not always been applied with uniform scientific basis. The historic record traces the evolution of what the medical community defines as CPT. Current texts in respiratory care continue to vary in the definition of CPT. Some refer to maneuvers of postural drainage, percussion, and vibration.[7] Others consider it relaxation, breathing retraining, postural drainage, and exercise reconditioning.[8] The work force that provides CPT has also been di-

BOX 17-1

BRONCHIAL HYGIENE THERAPY/ AIRWAY CLEARANCE TECHNIQUES

- Bronchial/postural drainage therapy (PDT)
- Forced expiration technique (FET)
- Autogenic drainage (AD)
- Positive expiratory pressure (PEP)
- High-frequency chest-wall compression (HFCC) and high-frequency airway opening
- Flutter valve therapy
- Directed cough (DC)

verse. Physical therapists, respiratory therapists/technicians, and nurses may be the caregivers. Ambiguity in past definitions of therapy, less than rigorous scientific application of clinical research methodology, and imprecise or inappropriate referral for CPT has led to widespread confusion, abuse of therapy and suspicion of the exact benefits of BHT as we define it today.[9]

The two imperatives driving health care today are ensuring efficacious quality care is delivered and controlling its costs. The value of each intervention we as health care providers perform, including BHT, has come under increasing scrutiny.[10–12] Some of the questions being asked of us regarding BHT include the following:

- Does BHT improve clinical outcomes?
- What are the important clinical indicators for BHT?
- Can clinical situations be identified that suggest limited or prophylactic value of BHT?
- Which clinical situations suggest that BHT can be harmful?
- What are the frequencies and time intervals for effective BHT?
- What levels of training are needed for effective assessment and therapy?
- Can BHT be effectively applied in various medical environments: intensive care unit, skilled nursing (subacute) facility or home?

To improve the science and make quality practice more uniform, the American Association for Respiratory Care (AARC) has sponsored peer-reviewed CPGs.[2–4] In addition to scrutinizing the clinical practice, there has been interest in developing treatment algorithms, or clinical pathways, based on initial and continued assessment of the patient's condition. TDPs represent an effort to prescribe care based on valid indications and conservation of resources in its delivery.[13] With this outcome-oriented approach, the caregiver is required to operate in a problem-solving role. Both responsibility and discretion is exercised by the therapist or nurse according to the protocol's arrangement with the physician staff. The therapist or nurse initiates care based on referral and initial assessment. The patient's response is closely monitored and BHT procedures are modified or discontinued when judged to be no longer of benefit. The intent is to maximize clinical benefits while minimizing untoward effects and wasted resources.[14] Examples of TDPs for bronchial hygiene therapy are presented later in this chapter.

RATIONALE FOR BRONCHIAL HYGIENE THERAPY

Mucociliary Clearance

A functional mucociliary transport system normally mobilizes secretions within the 23 airway divisions (Fig. 17-1) of the tracheobronchial tree to a level where they

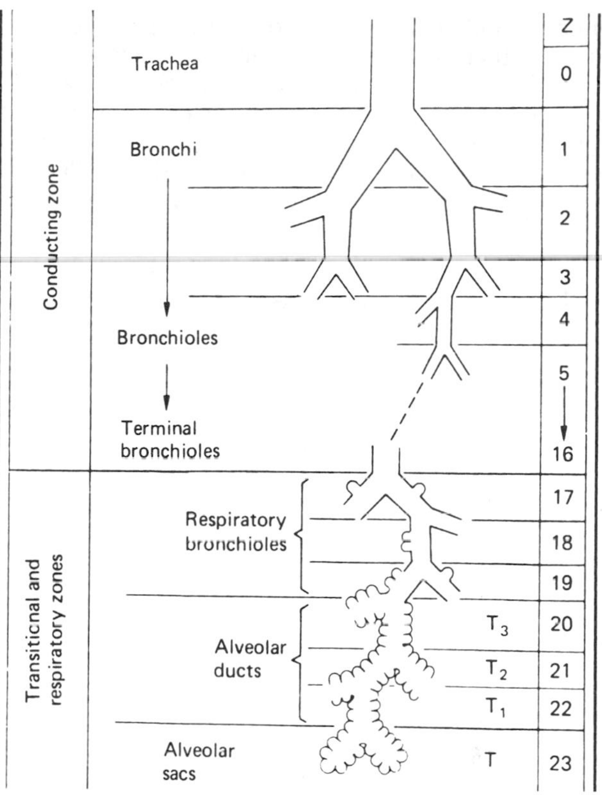

FIGURE 17-1. Generational structure of the human tracheobronchial tree. (From Weibel ER, Taylor CR: Design and structure of the human lung. (Fishman AP, ed. Pulmonary Diseases and Disorders, 2nd ed. New York: McGraw-Hill, 1988. With permission.)

can be expelled by coughing. Within these airway divisions, ciliary action, smooth muscle regulation of airway lumen size, mucus secretion from the goblet and serous cells lining the airway, and hydration status are important factors. When mucus cannot be cleared by the mucociliary transport system, gas exchange is impaired. Trauma (eg, smoke inhalation), environment (eg, ambient air temperature, air quality), medications (eg, bronchodilator), and emotional status (eg, anxiety) can individually or collectively impact on secretion retention and airway patency.

Airway secretions are driven toward the entrance of the larynx by metachronal (coordinated wave-like) movements of the cilia lining the respiratory tract. This is probably the single most important factor preventing the retention of secretions. These cilia normally are bathed in a mucus covering that consists of two layers: an outer layer of viscous mucus for trapping particulate matter such as dust, soot, or microorganisms; and an inner serous fluid that lubricates the ciliary mechanism. Abnormal sputum viscosity, whether too thick (eg, cystic fibrosis), too thin, as in bronchorrhic states (eg, pulmonary edema), or when mucus is desiccated (eg, breathing inadequately humidified gas through artificial airways), can impair ciliary activity and potentially cause sputum retention. This functional impairment of cilia can also occur in disease states such as chronic bronchitis when not only cilia are destroyed (by cigarette smoking), but there is also excess mucus production. In all these situations of impaired mucociliary clearance, the ability to mobilize secretions and expel/remove them from the airways becomes increasingly important and dependent on BHT intervention to restore defects in oxygen or carbon dioxide transport caused by secretion retention.[15,16]

Indications for Bronchial Hygiene Therapy

The exact value of BHT modalities (ie, postural drainage therapy, DC, autogenic drainage, positive airway pressure adjuncts) in different diseases/clinical conditions has been reviewed and reported. There remains a focus of intensive and ongoing research into the area of their efficacy.[15–17] Clinical indications that warrant a physician's referral for postural drainage therapy (PDT), or PEP adjuncts for airway clearance are summarized in Box 17-2. For details regarding BHT modalities see AARC Clinical Practice Guidelines: Postural Drainage Therapy; Directed Cough; and Use of Positive Airway Pressure Adjuncts to Bronchial Hygiene Therapy, pp. 505–507.[2–4]

Important Clinical Indicators

In addition to the indications specified for BHT under the CPG summaries, other relevant clinical indicators can be detected from the cardiopulmonary assessment and deserve highlighting.

☐ MEDICAL CHART REVIEW

The medical diagnosis should be identified first and foremost. Cystic fibrosis, asthma, chronic bronchitis, bronchiectasis, and atelectasis are examples of clinical entities, among others, that often indicate the need for and benefit from BHT.[1,17]

The medical history should identify conditions that have required radiation or chemotherapy, previous invasive surgery (eg, thoracotomy) or chest wall trauma (eg, rib fracture), or caused persistent or recurrent pulmonary infections, including opportunistic ones (eg, *pneumocystitis carinii)*.

A patient's history of present illness may reveal significant changes in weight loss or gains, or deterioration of activity tolerance, or if the patient's ventilation is being mechanically assisted. Another important detail is to determine how long he or she has been on assisted ventilation and on which mode (eg, control mode versus SIMV).

Arterial blood gas values should be reviewed serially for patterns of hypercapnia or hypoxemia. Close attention to change in pulmonary function, especially in forced expiratory volume in one second (FEV_1), and maximal inspiratory and expiratory mouth pressures would be enlightening, along with results from a 6-minute walk test.[20–23]

BOX 17-2

INDICATIONS FOR BRONCHIAL HYGIENE THERAPY ACCORDING TO CLINICAL PRACTICE GUIDELINES[2–4]

Postural Drainage Therapy (PDT)

- Excessive sputum production (eg, greater than 25–30 mL/day)
- Ineffective cough
- History of cystic fibrosis, bronchiectasis, lung abscess
- Evidence of retained secretions
  - Decreased breath sounds or crackles or rhonchi on auscultation
  - Change in vital signs (eg, fever, increased respiratory rate)
  - Abnormal chest radiograph consistent with atelectasis, mucus plugging, or infiltrates
  - Deterioration in arterial blood gas values (PaO_2, $PaCO_2$) and oxygen saturation (SaO_2 or SpO_2)

Directed Cough (DC)

- Spontaneous cough that fails to clear secretions from the airway
- Ineffective cough as judged by clinical observation, evidence of atelectasis, and/or results of pulmonary function testing (eg, maximal expiratory pressure)
- Postoperative care following upper abdominal or thoracic surgery
- Long-term care of patients displaying a tendency to retain airway secretions
- Cough not possible (eg, presence of endotracheal or tracheostomy tube)

Positive Airway Pressure Adjuncts (PAP)

- Sputum retention not responsive to spontaneous or directed coughing
- History of pulmonary problems treated successfully with postural drainage therapy
- Evidence of retained secretions
  - Decreased breath sounds or adventitious sounds
  - Change in vital signs (eg, tachypnea and tachycardia)
  - Abnormal chest radiograph consistent with atelectasis, mucus plugging, or infiltrates
  - Deterioration in arterial blood gas values or oxygen saturation

☐ SUBJECTIVE REPORT

Interviewing the patient and his or her family in order to determine the degree to which dyspnea limits activity is critical.[24,25] Use of a visual scale or analog can help to document any musculoskeletal pain he or she is experiencing.[26] The interviewer needs to inquire about the patient's daily productivity of sputum in terms of quality (eg, color, viscosity) and quantity (eg, ounces/day, mL/day). The degree to which sleep quality and quantity, nutritional intake patterns, and socialization events have been impaired should be evaluated.[27–29] The home environment, with respect to architecture (eg, stairs), equipment resources (eg, air conditioner and humidifier), and floor plan are important factors. The patient's own goals for physical activity should be determined.

AARC Clinical Practice Guideline

POSTURAL DRAINAGE THERAPY

Indications: ***Turning:*** inability or reluctance of patient to change body position (eg, mechanical ventilation, neuromuscular disease, drug-induced paralysis), poor oxygenation associated with position (eg, unilateral lung disease), potential for or presence of atelectasis, presence of artificial airway. *Postural Drainage:* evidence or suggestion of difficulty with secretion clearance; difficulty clearing secretions with expectorated sputum production greater than 25–30 mL/day (adult); evidence or suggestion of retained secretions in the presence of an artificial airway; presence of atelectasis caused by or suspected of being caused by mucous plugging; diagnosis of diseases such as cystic fibrosis, bronchiectasis, or cavitating lung disease, presence of foreign body in airway. *External Manipulation of the Thorax:* sputum volume or consistency suggesting a need for additional manipulation (eg, percussion and/or vibration) to assist movement of secretions by gravity in a patient receiving postural drainage.

Contraindications: The decision to use postural drainage therapy requires assessment of potential benefits versus potential risks. Therapy should be provided for no longer than necessary to obtain the desired therapeutic results. All positions are contraindicated for intracranial pressure (ICP) > 20 mmHg, head and neck injury until stabilized (absolute), active hemorrhage with hemodynamic instability (absolute), recent spinal surgery (eg, laminectomy) or acute spinal injury, active hemoptysis, empyema, bronchopleural fistula, pulmonary edema associated with congestive heart failure, large pleural effusions, pulmonary embolism, patients who do not tolerate position changes (aged, confused, or anxious), rib fracture (with or without flail chest), surgical wound or healing tissue. Trendelenburg position is contraindicated for ICP > 20 mmHg, patients in whom increased intracranial pressure is to be avoided (eg, neurosurgery, aneurysms, eye surgery), uncontrolled hypertension, distended abdomen, esophageal surgery, recent gross hemoptysis related to recent lung carcinoma treated surgically or with radiation therapy, uncontrolled airway at risk for aspiration (tube feeding or recent meal). Reverse Trendelenburg is contraindicated in the presence of hypotension or vasoactive medication. In addition to contraindications previously listed, external manipulation of the thorax is contraindicated for subcutaneous emphysema; recent epidural spinal infusion or spinal anesthesia; recent skin grafts or flaps on the thorax; burns, open wounds, and skin infections of the thorax; recently placed transvenous pacemaker or subcutaneous pacemaker (particularly if mechanical devices are to be used); suspected pulmonary tuberculosis; lung contusion; bronchospasm; osteomyelitis of the ribs; osteoporosis; coagulopathy; complaint of chest-wall pain.

Assessment of Need: Excessive sputum production, effectiveness of cough, history of pulmonary problems treated successfully with postural drainage therapy (eg, bronchiectasis, cystic fibrosis, lung abscess), decreased breath sounds or crackles or rhonchi suggesting secretions in the airway, change in vital signs, abnormal chest x-ray (consistent with atelectasis, mucous plugging, or infiltrates), deterioration in arterial blood gas values or oxygen saturation.

Assessment of Outcome: These represent individual criteria that indicate a positive response to therapy (and support continuation of therapy). Not all criteria are required to justify continuation of therapy (eg, a ventilated patient may not have sputum production > 30 mL/day, but have improvement in breath sounds, chest x-ray, or increased compliance or decreased resistance). If sputum production in an optimally hydrated patient is less than 25 mL/day with postural drainage therapy, the procedure is not justified. Some patients have productive coughs with sputum production from 15 to 30 mL/day (occasionally as high as 70 or 100 mL/day) without postural drainage. If postural drainage does not increase sputum in a patient who produces >30 mL/day of sputum without postural drainage, the continuation of the therapy is not indicated. Because sputum production is affected by systemic hydration, apparently ineffective postural drainage probably should be continued for at least 24 hours after optimal hydration has been judged to be present. Change in breath sounds of lung fields being drained; with effective therapy, breath sounds may worsen following the therapy as secretions move into the larger airways and increase rhonchi. An increase in adventitious breath sounds can be a marked improvement over absent or diminished breath sounds. Note any effect that coughing may have on breath sounds. One of the favorable effects of coughing is clearing of adventitious breath sounds. The caregiver should ask patient how he or she feels before, during, and after therapy. Feelings of pain, discomfort, shortness of breath, dizziness, and nausea should be considered in decisions to modify or stop therapy. Easier clearance of secretions and increased volume of secretions during and after treatments support continuation. Moderate changes in respiratory rate and/or pulse rate are expected. Bradycardia, tachycardia, or an increase in irregularity of pulse, or fall or dramatic increase in blood pressure are indications for stopping therapy. Resolution or improvement of atelectasis may be slow or dramatic. Oxygenation should improve as atelectasis resolves. Resolution of atelectasis and plugging reduces resistance and increases compliance.

Monitoring: Pain, discomfort, dyspnea, response to therapy; pulse rate, dysrhythmia, and ECG if available; breathing pattern and rate, symmetrical chest expansion, synchronous thoracoabdominal movement, flail chest; sputum production (quantity, color, consistency, odor) and cough effectiveness; mental function; skin color; breath sounds; blood pressure, oxygen saturation by pulse oximetry (if hypoxemia is suspected); intracranial pressure.

From AARC Clinical Practice Guideline, see Respir Care 36:1418–1426, 1991, for complete text.

□ INSPECTION

Watch for signs of ventilatory muscle pump fatigue. A triad of factors herald this condition whether occurring in singular or combined fashion. Tachypnea, active use of accessory muscle while at rest, and thoracoabdominal dyssynchrony occur when the load on breath-

AARC Clinical Practice Guideline

DIRECTED COUGH

Indications: The need to aid in the removal of retained secretions from central airways; the presence of atelectasis; as prophylaxis against postoperative pulmonary complications; as a routine part of bronchial hygiene in patients with cystic fibrosis, bronchiectasis, chronic bronchitis, necrotizing pulmonary infection, or spinal cord injury; as an integral part of other bronchial hygiene therapies such as postural drainage therapy, positive expiratory pressure therapy, and incentive spirometry; to obtain sputum specimens for diagnostic analysis.

Contraindications: Directed cough is rarely contraindicated. The contraindications listed must be weighed against potential benefit in deciding to eliminate cough from the care of the patient. Listed contraindications are relative: inability to control possible transmission of infection from patients suspected or known to have pathogens transmittable by droplet nuclei (eg, *M. tuberculosis*); presence of an elevated intracranial pressure or known intracranial aneurysm; presence of reduced coronary artery perfusion, such as in acute myocardial infarction; acute unstable head, neck, or spine injury. Manually assisted directed cough with pressure to the epigastrium may be contraindicated in presence of increased potential for regurgitation/aspiration (eg, unconscious patient with unprotected airway); acute abdominal pathology, abdominal aortic aneurysm, hiatal hernia, or pregnancy; a bleeding diathesis; untreated pneumothorax. Manually assisted directed cough with pressure to the thoracic cage may be contraindicated in presence of osteoporosis, flail chest.

Assessment of Need: Spontaneous cough that fails to clear secretions from the airway. Ineffective spontaneous cough as judged by clinical observation, evidence of atelectasis, results of pulmonary function testing, postoperative upper abdominal or thoracic surgery patient, long-term care of patients with tendency to retain airway secretions, presence of endotracheal or tracheostomy tube.

Assessment of Outcome: The presence of sputum specimen following a cough, clinical observation of improvement, patient's subjective response to therapy, stabilization of pulmonary hygiene in patients with chronic pulmonary disease and a history of secretion retention.

Monitoring: Patient response (pain, discomfort, dyspnea); sputum expectorated following cough (color consistency, odor, volume of sputum); breath sounds; presence of any adverse neurologic signs or symptoms following cough; presence of any cardiac dysrhythmias or alterations in hemodynamics following coughing; measures of pulmonary mechanics, when indicated, may include vital capacity, peak inspiratory pressure, peak expiratory pressure, peak expiratory flow, and airway resistance.

From AARC Clinical Practice Guideline; see Respir Care 38:495–499, 1993, for complete text.

ing muscles stresses their ability to perform.[21,30–33] Respiratory care practitioners should observe for discrepancies between movement of each hemithorax during spontaneous or mechanical ventilation. Observe whether the patient relies on postures that are forward leaning on supported upper extremities. Such positions allow recruitment of anterior chest wall muscles (pectoralis major and minor) to be used to augment upper rib cage movement.[34]

A posterior rib hump on forward bending may indicate an underlying restrictive, structural scoliosis. An increased anteroposterior (AP) chest configuration combined with inspiratory retraction of the lateral costal margin in paradoxical fashion could reflect a flattened, ineffective diaphragm caused by length-tension inappropriateness.[35]

Remove the patient's shoes and socks to determine whether dependent edema is displayed. Examine areas of exposed skin for petechiae or bruising as a result of abnormalities in blood coagulation or striae from chronic steroid use.

Observe how the patient is dressed and whether he or she is well groomed or not. Someone who spends the day in their pajamas (or hospital attire) may have a very poor activity tolerance, poor motivation, or both.

If the patient is confined to bed, observe for the circumstance and character of the immobility. Factors leading to immobilization include the following:

- Skeletal traction, casting, and splinting
- Drug administration: sedation, muscle relaxants
- Neurologic deficit: paralysis and central nervous system (CNS) depression
- Use of intensive care unit (ICU) monitoring equipment
- General debilitation
- Hemodynamic instability
- Mechanical ventilation

Identify invasive and noninvasive attachments to the patient for purposes of monitoring (eg, arterial and central venous catheters), treatment (eg, chest-tube drainage, Foley catheter, supplemental oxygen system, and intravenous infusions), or other appliances (eg, soft restraints).

☐ PALPATION, PERCUSSION, AND AUSCULTATION

Use *tactile fremitus* to document increased, decreased, or asymmetric vocal sound transmission. Lung zones with blocked bronchi will produce decreased fremitus; areas of consolidation or atelectasis will amplify normal vibrations. Hand placement on the chest during breathing can allow evaluation for symmetry of lateral costal expansion and to what degree the chest moves (eg, excursion range).

Palpate all areas of the chest wall firmly to discover musculoskeletal sources of discomfort versus those symptoms from cardiac or pleuritic origin. Percuss the anterior and posterior chest to evaluate symmetry of sound density of the underlying lung. Dullness may be associated with atelectasis, consolidation, or the patient's inability to inspire deeply.

Auscultate the chest to determine whether the location and character of lung sounds correspond to areas of suspected lung involvement. Absent breath sounds

AARC Clinical Practice Guideline

USE OF POSITIVE AIRWAY PRESSURE ADJUNCTS TO BRONCHIAL HYGIENE THERAPY

Indications: To reduce air trapping in asthma and COPD; to aid in mobilization of retained secretions (in cystic fibrosis and chronic bronchitis); to prevent or reverse atelectasis; to optimize delivery of bronchodilators in patients receiving bronchial hygiene therapy.

Contraindications: Although no absolute contraindications to the use of PEP, CPAP, or EPAP mask therapy have been reported, the following should be carefully evaluated before a decision is made to initiate PAP mask therapy. Listed contraindications include: Patients unable to tolerate the increased work of breathing (acute asthma, COPD); intracranial pressure (ICP) > 20 mmHg; hemodynamic instability; recent facial, oral, or skull surgery or trauma; acute sinusitis; epistaxis; esophageal surgery; active hemoptysis; nausea; known or suspected tympanic membrane rupture or other middle ear pathology; and untreated pneumothorax.

Assessment of Need: The following should be assessed together to establish a need for PAP therapy: Sputum retention not responsive to spontaneous or directed coughing; history of pulmonary problems treated successfully with postural drainage therapy; decreased breath sounds or adventitious sounds suggesting secretions in the airway; change in vital signs—increase in breathing frequency, tachycardia; abnormal chest radiograph consistent with atelectasis, mucus plugging, or infiltrates; deterioration in arterial blood gas values or oxygen saturation.

Assessment of Outcome: (1) *Change in sputum production*—if PEP does not increase sputum production in a patient who produces > 30 mL/day of sputum without PEP, the continued use of PEP may not be indicated; (2) *Change in breath sounds*—with effective therapy, breath sounds may clear or the movement of secretions into the larger airways may cause an increase in adventitious breath sounds. The increase in adventitious breath sounds is often a marked improvement over no (or diminished) breath sounds. Note any effect that coughing may have had on the breath sounds; (3) *Patient subjective response to therapy*—the caregiver should ask the patient how he or she feels before, during, and after therapy. Feelings of pain, discomfort, shortness of breath, dizziness, and nausea should be considered in modifying and stopping therapy. Improved ease of clearing secretions and increased volume of secretions during and after treatments support continuation; (4) *Change in vital signs*—moderate changes in respiratory rate and/or pulse rate are expected. Bradycardia, tachycardia, increasingly irregular pulse, or a drop or dramatic increase in blood pressure are indications for stopping therapy; (5) *Change in chest radiograph*—resolution or improvement of atelectasis and localized infiltrates may be slow or dramatic; and (6) *Change in arterial blood gas values or oxygen saturation*—normal oxygenation should return as atelectasis resolves.

Monitoring: Items from the following list should be chosen as is appropriate for monitoring a specific patient's response to PAP; Patient subjective response—pain, discomfort, dyspnea, response to therapy; pulse rate and cardiac rhythm (if EKG is available); breathing pattern and rate, symmetrical lateral costal expansion, synchronous thoracoabdominal movement; sputum production (quantity, color, consistency, and odor); mental function; skin color; breath sounds; blood pressure; pulse oximetry (if hypoxemia with procedure has been previously demonstrated or is suspected); blood gas analysis (if indicated); intracranial pressure (ICP) in patients for whom ICP is of critical importance.

From AARC Clinical Practice Guideline, see Reference #4.

may be associated with a misplaced endotracheal tube, blocked bronchi, pleural effusion, or pneumothorax. Bronchial breath sounds over lung zones where vesicular sounds should be heard warrant suspicion for atelectasis or consolidation. Describe any adventitious sounds you detect (eg, crackles, wheezes, rhonchi, or pleural friction rubs) by location to indicate such conditions as airway secretions, pulmonary parenchymal involvement, bronchospasm, and pleural involvement.

□ CHEST RADIOGRAPHY

Chest radiographic examination can either confirm signs elicited during the physical examination or reveal unexpected findings. The chest radiograph can be of major importance in identifying lung segments/lobes with most significant pulmonary involvement. These may then guide initial postural drainage positioning and assessment of therapeutic effect. Important radiographic skills include recognizing roentgenographic signs of atelectasis and infiltration.

Lobar collapse provides characteristic patterns of volume loss as the affected zone contracts. Respiratory care practitioners should note relative position of the diaphragm or mediastinum, which move to fill vacated lung volume. Figure 17-2 presents classic patterns of lobar collapse seen as areas of increased opacification. The silhouette sign refers to obliteration of normally seen differences in radiodensity of adjacent structures. Because the lung is normally air filled and radiolucent, atelectasis, consolidation, or infiltration will potentially eliminate a silhouette with the more radiopaque heart, diaphragm, and mediastinum. Anterior chest structures with obliterated borders indicate anterior lung involvement. Radiographic infiltration with preservation of these borders suggests that posterior lung zones are affected. Box 17-3 summarizes findings using the silhouette sign. The *air bronchogram* denotes differing radiographic density between air-filled bronchi and consolidated, edematous, or fibrosed lung. This is in contrast to well-aerated bronchi and lungs. A bronchial mucus plug will be apparent as a sharp cutoff of the air bronchogram.

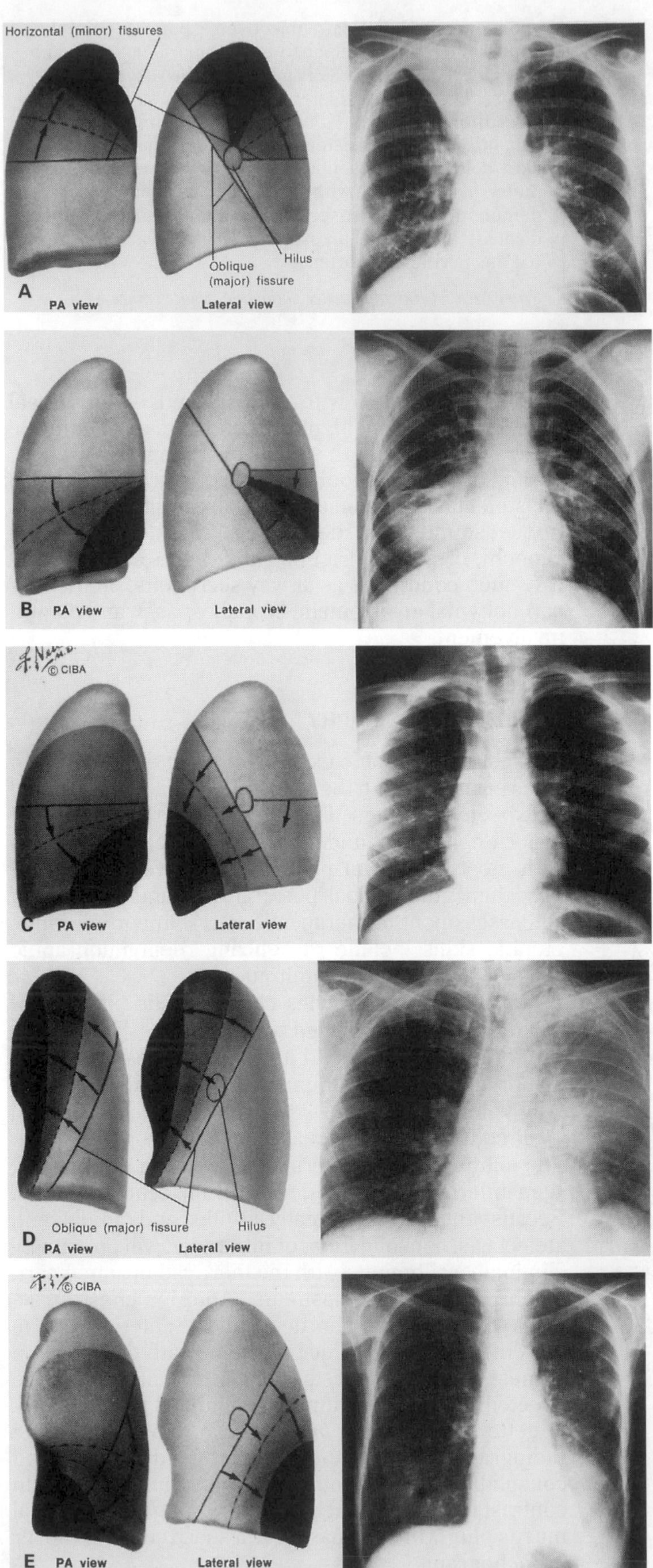

FIGURE 17-2. Radiographic examples of lobar collapse. **(A)** Right upper lobe collapse; **(B)** Right middle lobe collapse; note silhouette sign at right cardiac border/cardiophrenic angle; **(C)** Right lower lobe collapse; **(D)** Left upper lobe collapse; note silhouette sign at left mediastinum and cardiac border; **(E)** Left lower lobe collapse; note preservation of cardiac and diaphragmatic borders (From Netter FH: The Ciba Collection of Medical Illustrations. Summit, NJ: Ciba Pharmaceutical Company, 1980. With permission.)

BOX 17-3

SILHOUETTE SIGN PATTERNS

Normal Silhouette Lost	Affected Lung Zone
Superior mediastinum bilaterally	Right posterior and left apical posterior segments of upper lobes
Loss of the right and left heart borders	Middle lobe and lingula
Loss of diaphragmatic shadow	
Outer (lateral) third	Anterior segments of lower lobes
Middle third	Lateral segments of lower lobes
Inner (medial) third	Posterior segments of lower lobes

☐ SPECIAL TESTS

Gain insight into a patient's pulmonary performance by assessing diaphragmatic breathing, unilateral costal expansion, breathing at select lung volumes, whether 2-second inspiratory holds can be performed, and if controlled coughing or huffing is possible.

Obtain measurements of maximal inspiratory volume (eg, vital capacity) and/or maximal pressures (MIP and MEP) on a serial basis. Monitor for orthostatic hypotension and tachycardia in response to position change (eg, supine-sit-stand-Trendelenburg). Note how activity levels and position changes influence pulse oximetry values (Spo_2) compared with baseline.

A summary of these key clinical indicators that would support the need for BHT intervention to promote improved oxygenation and ventilation is provided in Box 17-4.

BOX 17-4

SUMMARY OF IMPORTANT CLINICAL INDICATORS FOR BRONCHIAL HYGIENE THERAPY

- Medical Chart
  - Diagnosis (eg, cystic fibrosis, chronic bronchitis, or bronchiectasis)
  - Previous medical history (eg, radiation and/or chemotherapy, previous surgery and chest wall trauma)
  - History of current illness (eg, mode and days on mechanical ventilation)
  - Blood gas or pulmonary laboratory data (eg, arterial blood gas values for hypoxemia or hypercapnia, decreased FEV_1)
- Subjective Report
  - Visual analog for pain (eg, 80 mm along a 0 to 100 mm line)
  - Sputum quantity and quality descriptors
  - Dyspnea as a limiting symptom
- Inspection
  - Presence of tachypnea, accessory muscle recruitment
  - Thoraco-abdominal asynchrony at rest or with minimal exertion
  - Presence of a posterior rib lump on forward bending
  - Inspiratory retraction of the lateral costal margin in a paradoxical fashion
  - Reliance on postures that are forward leaning on supported upper extremities
  - Posture
- Palpation and Auscultation
  - Tactile fremitus signs and pattern
  - Decreased chest excursion range is evident
  - Significant musculoskeletal chest wall pain is reproducible with palpation and/or movement
  - Breath sounds in corresponding lung segments are grossly distorted between right and left sides (eg, diminished, absent, or bronchial sounds over peripheral areas)
  - Adventitious sounds (eg, rales, wheezes, and rhonchi)
- Others
  - Chest radiographic interpretation: Collapse, "silhouette sign," air bronchogram, infiltrates suggesting presence and location of atelectasis, consolidation, effusion, or pneumothorax
  - Difficulty in controlling breathing with the diaphragm
  - Weak cough effort and/or poor expiratory control
  - Diminished maximal inspiratory volume
  - Oxyhemoglobin desaturation at rest and/or with minimal exertion or with changes in body position

CONTRAINDICATIONS, COMPLICATIONS, AND HAZARDS

Just as there are clinical indicators that justify the need for and appropriateness of physician referral for BHT, certain indicators and conditions require careful consideration before and during therapy. There are a number of relative contraindications. The desired outcomes of specific BHT techniques must be weighed against potential untoward effects. The precautions and relative contraindications to BHT techniques are summarized in Box 17-5.

SPECIFIC BRONCHIAL HYGIENE THERAPY TECHNIQUES AND PROCEDURES

Breathing Exercises

Adequate ventilation must occur in order to accomplish the BHT primary goals of removing excess airway secretions and preventing or improving atelectasis and disordered gas exchange. This can be accomplished therapeutically by a variety of breathing exercises. Box 17-6 provides a thorough but not exhaustive listing of breathing exercises, arranged by proposed categories according to treatment outcomes or therapeutic objectives:[36]

Certain breathing exercises (eg, controlled deep breathing) may accomplish more than one therapeutic objective as suggested in Box 17-6. Considerable redundancy also exists among the definitions for specific

BOX 17-5

PRECAUTIONS AND/OR CONTRAINDICATIONS FOR SPECIFIC POSTURAL DRAINAGE THERAPY TECHNIQUES[2,3]

- Intracranial pressure >20 mmHg
- Pulmonary embolism
- Rib fracture, with or without flail chest
- Empyema
- Head and/or neck injury until stabilized (A)*
- Osteoporosis
- Bronchospasm
- Coagulopathy
- Active hemorrhage with hemodynamic instability (A)
- Uncontrolled instability (A)
- Airway at risk for aspiration
- Pulmonary edema associated with congestive heart failure
- Open wounds and surgical incisions
- Large pleural effusions
- Complaint of chest wall pain or skin grafts
- Bronchopleural fistula, empyema
- Unstable arrhythmias
- Angina pectoris
- Uncontrolled hypertension
- Anoxic spells in premature infants

**(A):absolute contraindication*

BOX 17-6

BREATHING EXERCISES ACCORDING TO TREATMENT OBJECTIVE[36]

To Promote Chest Wall Mobility

Localized basal expansion	Controlled deep breathing
Posterior basal expansion	Lateral costal expansion
Apical expansion	Sustained maximal breathing
Segmental or localized breathing	IPPB
	Glossopharyngeal breathing

To Improve the Efficiency of Breathing

Diaphragmatic	Breathing retraining
Breathing control	Sustained maximal breathing
Relaxed breathing	Low-frequency breathing
Paced breathing	Deep breathing
Pursed-lip breathing	Controlled deep breathing
	Yogic practice (pranayama)

To Mobilize and Remove Excess Airway Secretions

Augmented abdominal breathing	Positive expiratory pressure (PEP) breathing
Forced expiration technique (FET)	Autogenic drainage (AD)
Segmental or localized breathing	Active cycle of breathing (ACB)
Controlled deep breathing	

To Recondition the Skeletal Muscles of Respiration for Improved Strength and/or Endurance

Resisted diaphragmatic breathing	Inspiratory muscle training
Resisted segmental or localized breathing	Inspiratory resistive training (fixed orifice versus threshold loading)
Resisted lateral costal expansion	

breathing exercise definitions as cited in the literature. For example, "diaphragmatic breathing,"[37] "breathing control,"[38] "relaxed breathing,"[39] or "breathing retraining"[37] appear to describe the same or similar breathing exercise maneuver. Until a CPG for "breathing exercises" is published, respiratory care practitioners should operationally define the breathing exercise(s) being used.

Controlled Deep Breathing

Controlled deep breathing refers to the ability of the patient to modulate his or her pattern, rate, and volume of breathing. A normal respiratory pattern primarily involves diaphragmatic movement, but individuals do have the ability to selectively change into a costosternal pattern at appropriate times. Elastic recoil of lung and chest wall allow exhalation during resting ventilation, yet patients must be able to recruit expiratory muscles actively on command. To promote alveolar-capillary gas exchange, it may be beneficial to pause 1 to 3 seconds at end inspiration before exhaling. The ability to alter inspiratory-to-expiratory ratios as desired in BHT techniques is quite important for some patients (eg, those with chronic obstructive pulmonary disease [COPD]). In addition, controlling the variable lung volumes at which therapeutic breathing is performed during BHT techniques (eg, low-lung, mid-lung, high-lung volumes) is also of value, theoretically. By altering the position of the equal pressure point, secretions are mobilized progressively from the more peripheral toward the more central airways.[38]

The equal pressure point (EPP) is defined as the point where the pressure within the airways is equal to the pleural pressure.[38] Forces during breathing, especially during exhalation, cause a dynamic compression or airway collapse downstream (toward the mouth) of the EPP. These "choke points" move upstream (toward the alveoli) as lung volume decreases. Breathing exercises that capitalize on altering the EPP and mobilizing secretions from peripheral toward central airways include the forced expiratory technique (FET) or huffing maneuver, which has been renamed the active cycle of breathing (ACB)[1,38] and autogenic drainage (AD).

Forced Expiration Technique and Active Cycle of Breathing

Described first by Pryor and Webber in 1979, the FET uses forced (but not violent) expirations or "huffs" through an opened mouth, which are produced by con-

BOX 17-7

ACTIVE CYCLE OF BREATHING (ACB) SET SEQUENCE[1,38]

- Breathing control
- Three to four thoracic expansion exercises with or without manual chest compressions or expiratory vibrations
- Breathing control
- Three to four thoracic expansion exercises with or without manual chest compressions or expiratory vibrations
- Breathing control
- FET or huffing attempts
- Breathing control

tracting abdominal and external intercostal muscles. Periods of "breathing control" (ie, gentle breathing using the lower chest with relaxation of the upper chest and shoulders) at mid-lung to low-lung volumes end with huffs or coughs at high-lung volumes to mobilize and expectorate excess bronchial secretions.

The fact that FET always incorporates "breathing control" with the forceful but controlled "huff" led to the terminology of ACB. That term denotes a set cycle of seven deliberate acts that can be subdivided into three component parts (ie, diaphragmatic or breathing control, thoracic expansion exercise, and the FET). The ACB cycle is outlined in Box 17-7.

At present, both the FET and ACB are considered adjuncts to the BHT technique of PDT and are used especially in patients with cystic fibrosis.[41]

Autogenic Drainage

Like the BHT techniques of FET and ACB, AD is a method initially developed in Belgium using breathing control in which the rate, location, and depth of respiration is voluntarily adjusted. It has proven valuable in treating patients who have diseases or conditions in which the nature or quantity of mucus is abnormal.[42,43] Figure 17-3 shows the three phases of this procedure. Phase 1 is intended to unstick mucus, phase 2 is collection, and phase 3 is the evacuation of secretions. Coughing must be suppressed while the breathing control of AD is performed. ACB is typically reserved for patients 4 years of age or older because of the learned skill that is required. It is generally performed with the patient seated in an upright position and requires no additional equipment so that once taught, the patient can perform it alone.[38,44]

In summary, the ability to control the rate and volume of spontaneous breaths during either the inspiratory or expiratory phases or both is essential for the techniques of FET, ACB, AD, as well as PEP and PDT, to move airway secretions toward the carina. Adequate ventilatory muscles must be functioning adequately for BHT techniques to be effective. Assessment considerations for determining the functional ability to deep breathe with control are offered in Box 17-8.

Postural Drainage Therapy

PDT has four component parts:

- Regular turning
- Use of specific postural drainage positions
- External manipulation of the thorax to mobilize secretions by percussion or vibration
- Cough or secretion removal by suctioning

The importance of regular turning is emphasized by the basic physiologic principle that various regions of the normal lung are neither ventilated nor perfused equally. During normal breathing, the inhaled tidal volume is preferentially distributed to dependent lung regions regardless of whether the patient is positioned upright, supine, sidelying, or even prone. Similarly, blood flow is greatest to the dependent regions.[10] Figure 17-4 illustrates this phenomenon of distribution of ventilation ($\dot{V}_A$) to pulmonary perfusion ($\dot{Q}$), respectively. The ratio of alveolar ventilation ($\dot{V}_A$) to pulmonary perfusion ($\dot{Q}$) is normally greater in the apices than at the bases in the upright patient. Positioning,

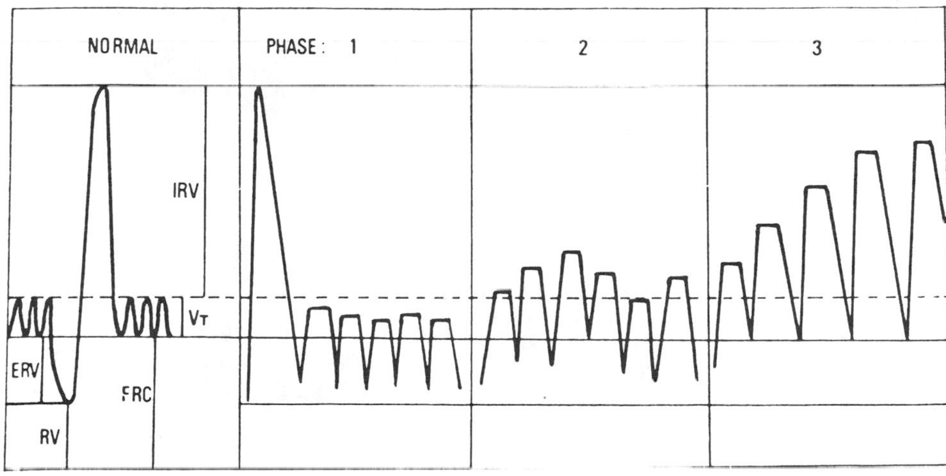

FIGURE 17-3. Spirogram of lung volumes during phases of autogenic drainage. (From Hardy KA: A review of airway clearance: new techniques, indications and recommendations. Respir Care 1994; 39:446 with permission.)

BOX 17-8

ASSESSMENT CONSIDERATIONS FOR DETERMINING ABILITY TO DEEP BREATHE WITH CONTROL*

- Is the patient's inspiratory capacity adequate based on gender, height, and age?
- Is symmetrical lateral costal expansion displayed?
- Is there thoraco-abdominal synchrony of movement? (eg, thoracic and abdominal movement occur in the same direction at the same time)
- Can the patient perform a 2-second inspiratory hold at the end of a maximal inspiration?
- Can the patient alter the durations of his or her inspiratory and expiratory phases as instructed?
- Is the patient's breathing pattern at rest primarily diaphragmatic?
- Can the patient regulate rate and depth of breathing as directed?

** Affirmative answers to each skill above is desirable for controlled deep-breathing ability.*

therefore, can influence the extent to which ventilation and perfusion are "matched." When attempting to maximize oxygenation, the "healthiest" lung should be in the dependent position.

The act of turning can be done by the patient, by a caregiver, or by a special bed or device (Fig. 17-5). A regular turning schedule can aid in mobilization of airway secretions, aid in prevention of decubitus ulcers (bed sores), provide an exercise/activity stimulus, help a patient's emotional outlook, promote joint and soft-tissue range of motion and flexibility, and facilitate basic nursing care.

Postural Drainage

Postural drainage is based on knowledge of the anatomy of the tracheobronchial tree. The patient is placed in one or more of the standard positions designed to place the involved segmental bronchi above and superior to the carina. The rationale behind this general rule of positioning with "bad side up, good side down" is to permit gravity to exert an influence in draining the retained secretions from the involved segments. Figure 17-6 shows these standard postural (bronchial) drainage positions.

When integrating information from the chest radiograph (eg, silhouette sign) together with physical examination findings (eg, increased tactile fremitus on palpation and crackles auscultated), the involved lung segments can be identified and the appropriate postural drainage position(s) can be selected.

External Manipulation of the Thorax

External manipulation of the thorax applies kinetic energy to the chest wall and lung by percussion (eg, chest clapping) and/or vibration. *Percussion* is accomplished

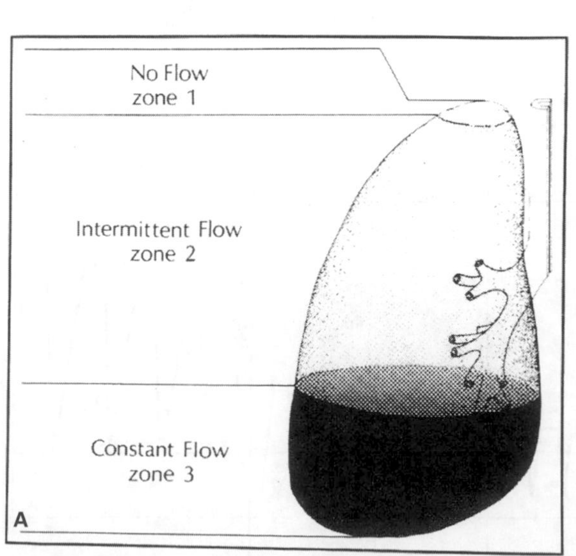

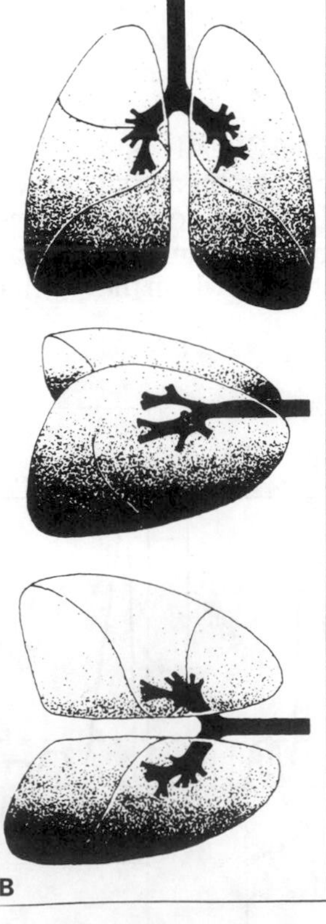

FIGURE 17-4. **(A)** Pulmonary perfusion distribution in an upright normal lung; **(B)** ventilation/perfusion relationships in the lungs with varying positions. (From Shapiro BA, Harrison RA, Cane RD, Templin RD: Clinical Application of Blood Gases. 4th ed. Chicago: Year Book Medical, 1989. With permission.)

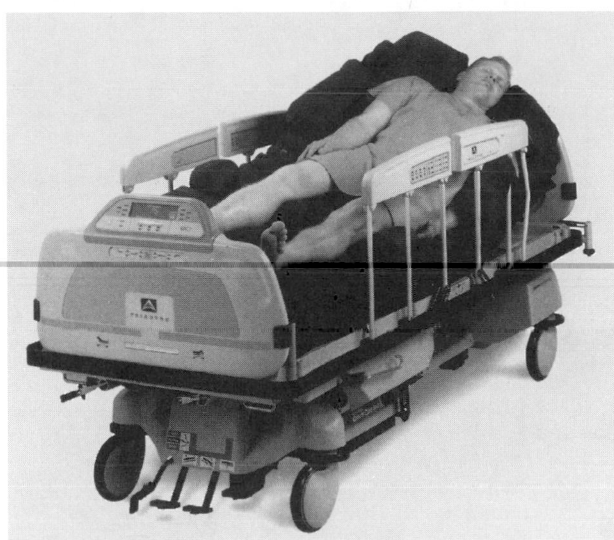

FIGURE 17-5. Special positioning/turning bed.

by rhythmically striking the thorax with cupped hand (eg, 3 to 5 Hz) or by using a mechanical device placed in contact with the thorax directly overlying the lung segment(s) to be drained (Fig. 17-7). Proper hand-cupping with closed fingers and thumb will result in a cushion of air that dampens the striking force. It may be applied over the bare skin or with a thin layer of cloth such as a patient gown or sheet. Thick towels should be avoided as they impair transmission of the kinetic energy. Hand motion should be rhythmic with wrists loose so a waiving motion is produced. Care must be taken not to clap over structures such as heart, kidneys, and breasts, as well as sites of trauma or surgery. Percussion over bony prominences should be avoided. To percuss the small chest wall of neonatal and pediatric patients, rubber bottle stoppers or commercially available cup devices are useful in limiting the area of an adult hand's percussive impact.

Vibration involves the manual application of fine tremorous action in the direction that the ribs and soft tissue of the chest move during exhalation (Fig. 17-8). It is often used with percussion. One hand is positioned over the involved lung zone. The second hand is placed on top. Following a deep breath, the practitioner presses down with the shaking vibratory action. Although hand-operated electrical or mechanical percussor/vibrators are available, there is no strong evidence to support their superiority over the manual techniques. Mechanical vests that replicate chest wall percussion/vibration are reviewed in Chapter 18. Such devices offer the patient independence from caregivers.

Shaking or rib springing is a vigorous form of vibration. It is an option used to treat unusually thick secretions. As with vibration, both hands of the clinician bear down on the chest after a deep breath, during the expiratory phase. The motion is more pumping in effect than vibratory. The patient can be asked to begin his or her next inspiration after a final downstroke. The resulting outward recoil forces of the lung and chest wall can augment the subsequent chest expansion.

A controlled or staged-cough attempt completes a typical sequence of turning into a postural drainage position, percussion over the segment being drained for at least 1 minute, or vibrating during several exhalation cycles. (Suctioning may be required to remove secretions in patients who cannot effectively cough.) This sequence is repeated as indicated and tolerated with a given position being treated for 3 to 15 minutes (longer in special situations).[2] In critically ill patients with retained bronchial secretions, such a treatment sequence is often performed every 4 to 6 hours with need for this referral to be re-evaluated at least every 48 hours, based on clinical indicators made before and following each treatment.

Directed Cough

Coughing can be initiated either voluntarily or by reflex. Examples of stimuli that can provoke coughing include the following: inflammation of the airways/lung parenchyma such as occurs in tracheitis or pneumonia, inhalation of dust particles, compression of the airway such as that produced by foreign bodies or bronchogenic carcinoma, chemical stimuli such as cigarette smoke or chemical fumes, and thermal stimuli including the inhalation of hot or cold air. The sequence of a cough comprises the following:

- Stimulus initiating a deep inspiration
- Glottic closure
- Contraction of the expiratory muscles against the closed glottis producing high, positive intrathoracic and intra-airway pressures
- Sudden glottic opening

The sequence of events creates large pressure gradients between the airways and the atmosphere which, when coupled with dynamic compression of the airways, produces high gas velocities and turbulent flow in the trachea and main bronchi. Shearing forces propel mucus and or foreign materials upward.

DC maneuvers are used when voluntary effective coughing is impaired or absent. Patients are taught how to obtain voluntary control over the various components of the cough reflex and how to compensate for those facets of their spontaneous coughing that limit its effectiveness. Common causes of such impaired spontaneous coughing include the following: reduced inspiratory or expiratory muscle strength or coordination, impaired glottic control, and lack of airway stability. Techniques for directed cough assistance include manually assisted cough and FET.[3]

Application of external mechanical pressure (eg, therapists' hands) to the epigastric region or thoracic cage coordinated with forced exhalation by the patient describes the manually assisted cough.[3] It is important that the therapist properly time the application of external pressure to the verbal command for the patient to

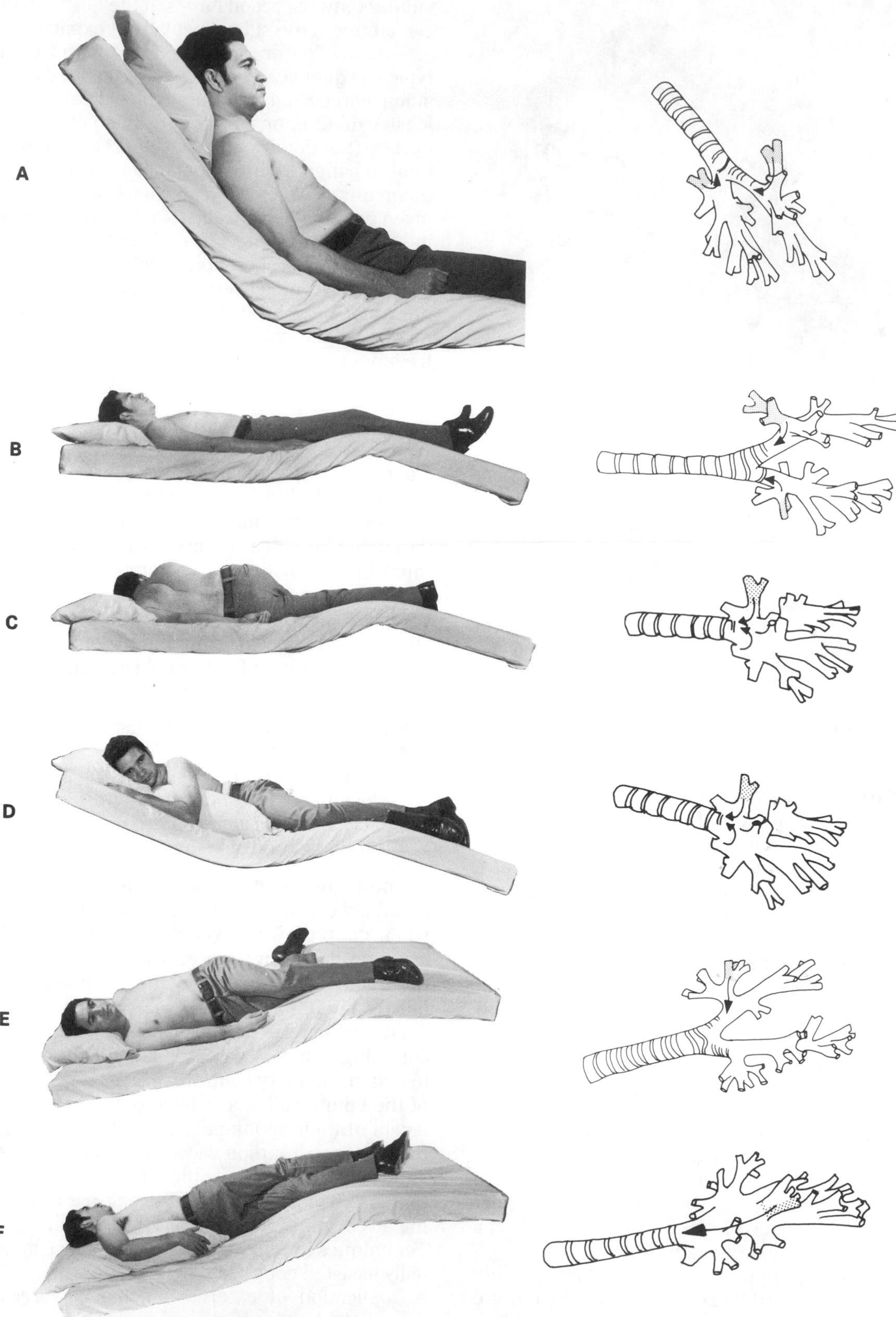

FIGURE 17-6. Bronchial drainage positions for specific pulmonary segments. **(A)** Left and right upper lobes (apical segment); **(B)** Left and right upper lobes (anterior segments); **(C)** Right upper lobe (posterior segment); **(D)** Left upper lobe (posterior segment); **(E)** Left upper lobe (lingular segment); **(F)** Middle lobe of right lung; **(G)** Lower lobes (superior segment); **(H)** Left lower lobe (lateral basal segment); **(I)** Left and right lower lobes (anterior basal segments; **(J)** Left and right lower lobes (anterior basal segments); **(K)** Left and right lower lobes (posterior basal segment).

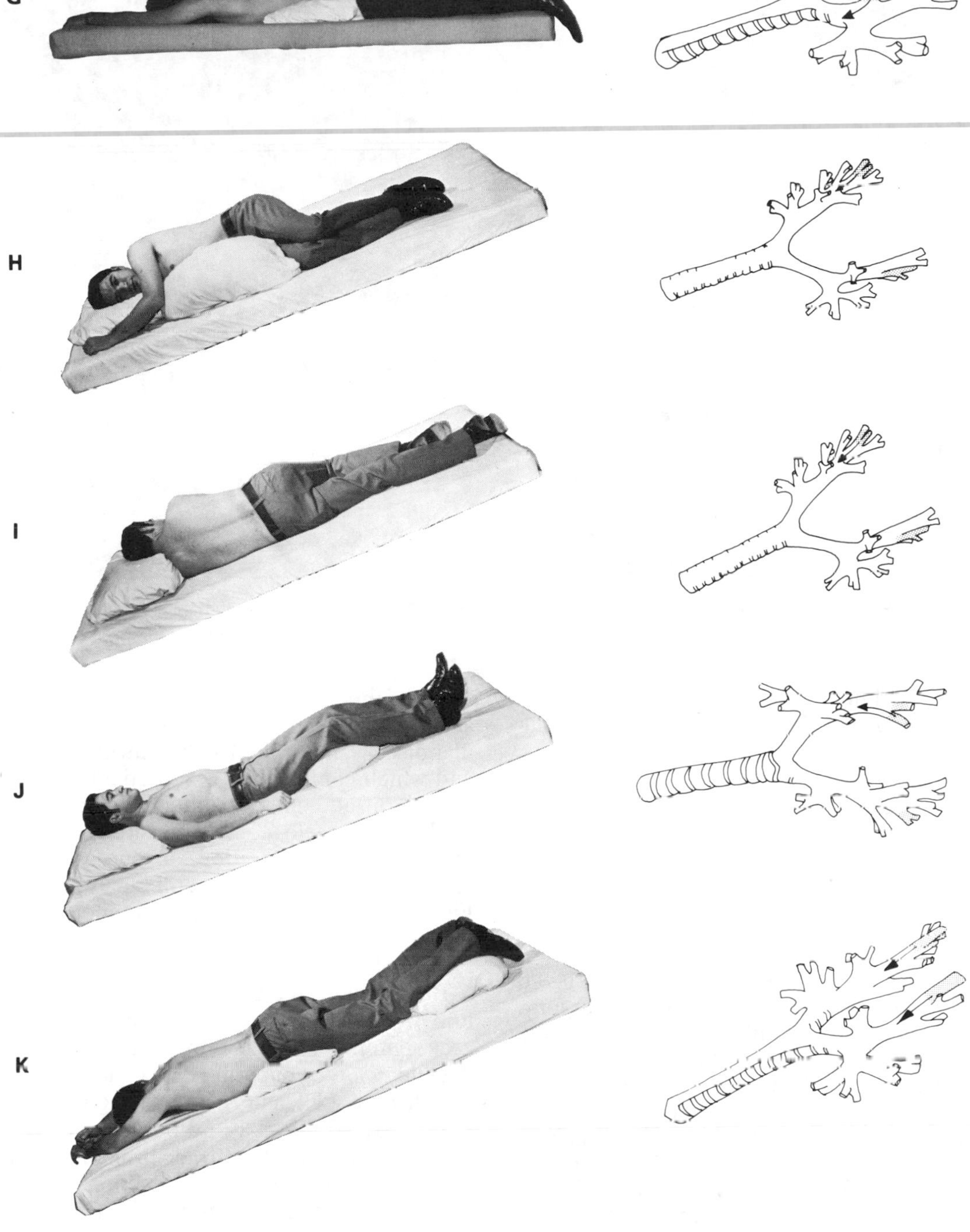

FIGURE 17-6. (continued).

"now cough." This technique is commonly used in patient conditions in which maximal expiratory pressures (MIP) are insufficient (eg, spinal cord injury, muscular dystrophy). Figure 17-9 shows the manually assisted cough being performed.

The FET has been described earlier in this chapter under breathing exercises. It is noteworthy that FET requires less patient effort than coughing and can be used effectively as a substitute for coughing in patients who have incisional pain (eg, thoracotomy, exploratory laparotomy). The FET cycle of combining "huffing" along with breathing control and thoracic expansion/compression will mobilize secretions from peripheral airways to the larger central airways. With the lungs in-

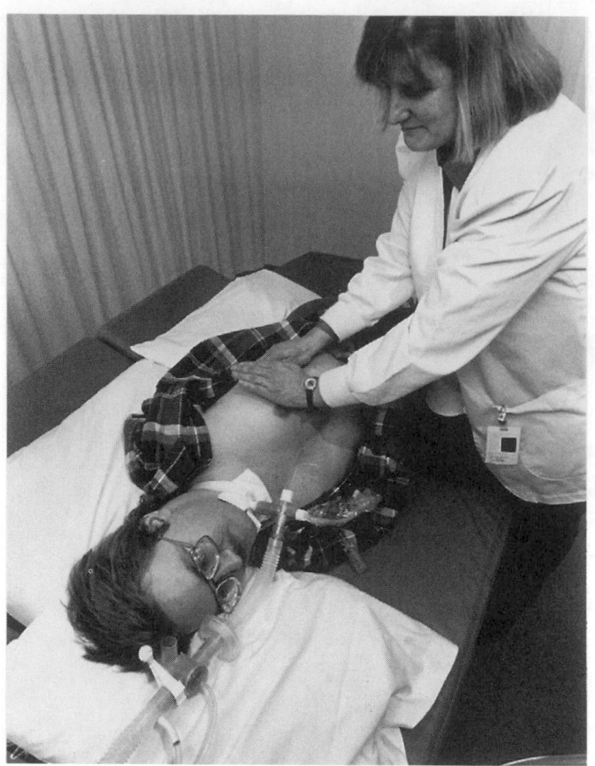

FIGURE 17-7. Application of manual percussion (chest clapping) during postural drainage positioning.

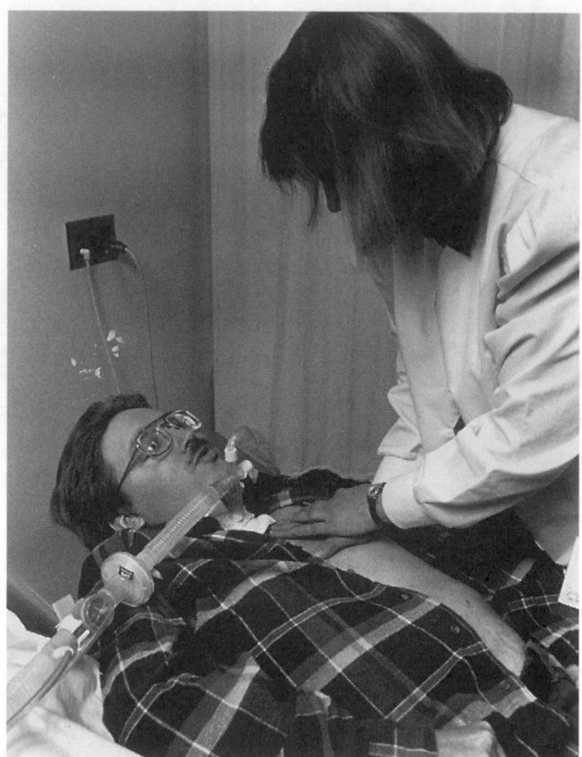

FIGURE 17-8. Application of manual vibration during exhalation to promote secretion mobilization.

flated to near total lung capacity, a single cough may then be more effective in clearing these centrally accumulated secretions.

Positive Expiratory Pressure

Positive expiratory pressure (PEP) is a positive airway pressure adjunct to BHT described in detail in Chapter 18. During *PEP therapy*, the patient exhales against a fixed-orifice resistor, generating positive pressures during expiration within the therapeutic range of 10 to 20 cmH_2O.[4] One-way valves allow for unobstructed inspiration, with the patient breathing in and out for a series of 5 to 20 breaths with ratios of inspiration to exhalation of 1:3 or 1:4 suggested.[1,46] This breathing series is followed by performing the FET (huff cough) and the overall sequence of PEP breathing, and FET is repeated until secretions are expelled.[1,46] This PEP effect (eg, positive pressure of 10 to 20 cmH_2O) can be accomplished by commercially made blow bottles or by exhaling a steady stream of bubbles through a 6-mm-diameter straw into a glass/cup of water.[47]

RECOMMENDATIONS FOR BHT TECHNIQUES IN SPECIFIC CONDITIONS

In the past, BHT was used in treating many different types of lung disease. More recently, the exact benefit, if any, of BHT in specific disease entities has been the focus of much scrutiny.[1,17] This research has also examined which BHT modality is best suited for a particular disease, how such treatments may best be applied, and which components of a particular treatment contribute to the benefit produced by that treatment. In PDT, for example, postural positioning appears more important than vibration or percussion, but such sputum mobilization may still be a useful adjunct.[48,49] Finally, other research has examined the potentially harmful effects of BHT and how these may be mitigated.

BHT is indicated to help patients with copious sputum production and to treat atelectasis secondary to excess sputum.[49] In cystic fibrosis, routine BHT slows the decline in forced expiratory flow rate over time.[19] With this disease, FET and AD are attractive alternatives to PDT because they can be performed by the patient without assistance. In chronic bronchitis or bronchiectasis with excess sputum production, BHT is likewise beneficial in helping sputum clearance and improving lung function. Humidification is a useful adjunct to BHT in bronchiectasis. When patients with chronic bronchitis do not have excess sputum production, BHT is not useful.[50] A similar lack of BHT benefit has also been documented in other lung diseases not associated with excess sputum production such as asthma[51] and primary pneumonia.[18]

Studies indicate that PDT is not valuable in patients undergoing upper abdominal or thoracic surgery if they do not have problems related to secretion retention or

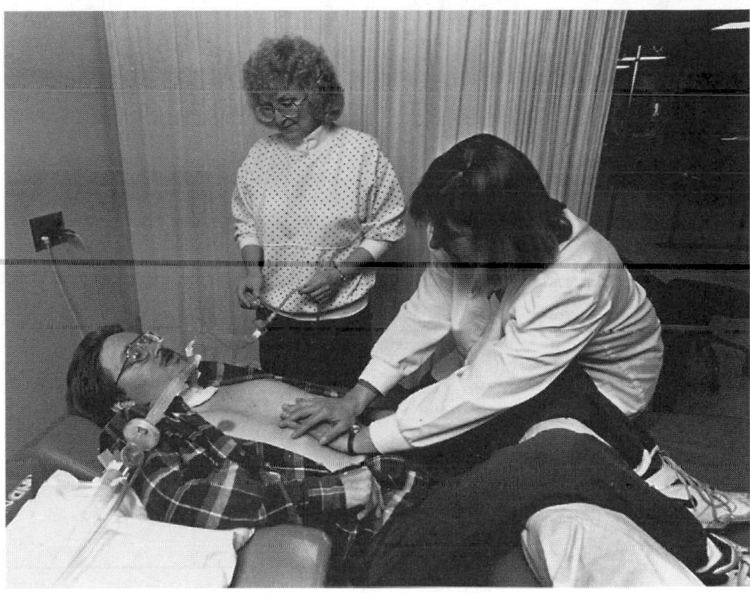

FIGURE 17-9. Manually assisting a directed cough.

atelectasis.[52] It can be beneficial for patients undergoing such surgery when they have chronic lung disease, particularly when combined with bronchodilator therapy. Otherwise it should be used selectively for patients with specific indications such as copious sputum or acute atelectasis. Such patients have the potential to develop hypoxemia during PDT, probably secondarily to atelectasis and the increased oxygen utilization that occurs during the treatment. Special care including monitoring arterial oxyhemoglobin saturation is required when providing BHT to such patients, particularly those who are already hypoxic.

THERAPIST-DRIVEN PROTOCOLS

Recently, "assess and treat" protocols have been supported by the American College of Chest Physicians (ACCP) in their position paper on "Respiratory Care Protocols." This position statement endorses CPGs, produced and published by the AARC, as "nationally referenced appropriateness indicators as practice standards and guides to rational respiratory care."[53]

CPGs take a scientific approach to cost-effective treatment. Careful scrutiny of the results obtained from randomized and controlled clinical investigations support or refute (eg, validate) the appropriateness of a given treatment to produce desired outcomes. The CPGs can be envisioned as a rationale for our current respiratory care practice as health care reform pushes for increased standardization of care using protocols aimed at improving outcomes and cutting costs.

Directed Cough

A common denominator contained in each of the BHT techniques described in this chapter is the voluntary attempt at using a forced expiratory maneuver (ie, DC) to expel obstructing secretions that have been mobilized. Efficient use of the ventilatory muscle pump to regulate volume of inspiration can enhance the effectiveness of DC by taking a prerequisite deep breath.

As the TDP for DC illustrates in Protocol 17-1, a diagnostic category that would compromise a patient's ability to take a prerequisite deep breath (eg, kyphoscoliosis) or generate inadequate muscle contractile force during exhalation (eg, spinal cord injury, C_3 Quadriplegia) would increase the likelihood of airway secretion retention. When clinical indicators identify that this is indeed the case, spontaneous (voluntary) cough ability should be assessed to determine whether or not further BHT treatment should be continued. That evaluation will determine whether DC or other BHT treatment options warrant application.

Postural Drainage Therapy

The initial and key phase of any protocol depends on patient assessment. This is shown in the two examples of postural drainage protocols illustrated in Protocols 17-2 and 17-3. Once the decision for PDT treatment is made, the clinician must then decide which PDT option(s) to apply (eg, DC, external manipulation of the thorax, postural drainage positioning, or regular turning schedule). It is quite common to combine PDT with other therapies. For example, while the patient is in a postural drainage position, percussion is typically administered manually with cupped hand(s) or mechanically with a commercial device. A series of deep breaths could then be encouraged, with manual vibrations applied during each expiratory phase overlying the lung segment(s) being drained by gravity. DC would then be applied to complete a PDT sequence, repeating as needed and tolerated.

With regard to the option of a regular turning schedule, a patient can be moved from a supine posture to ei-

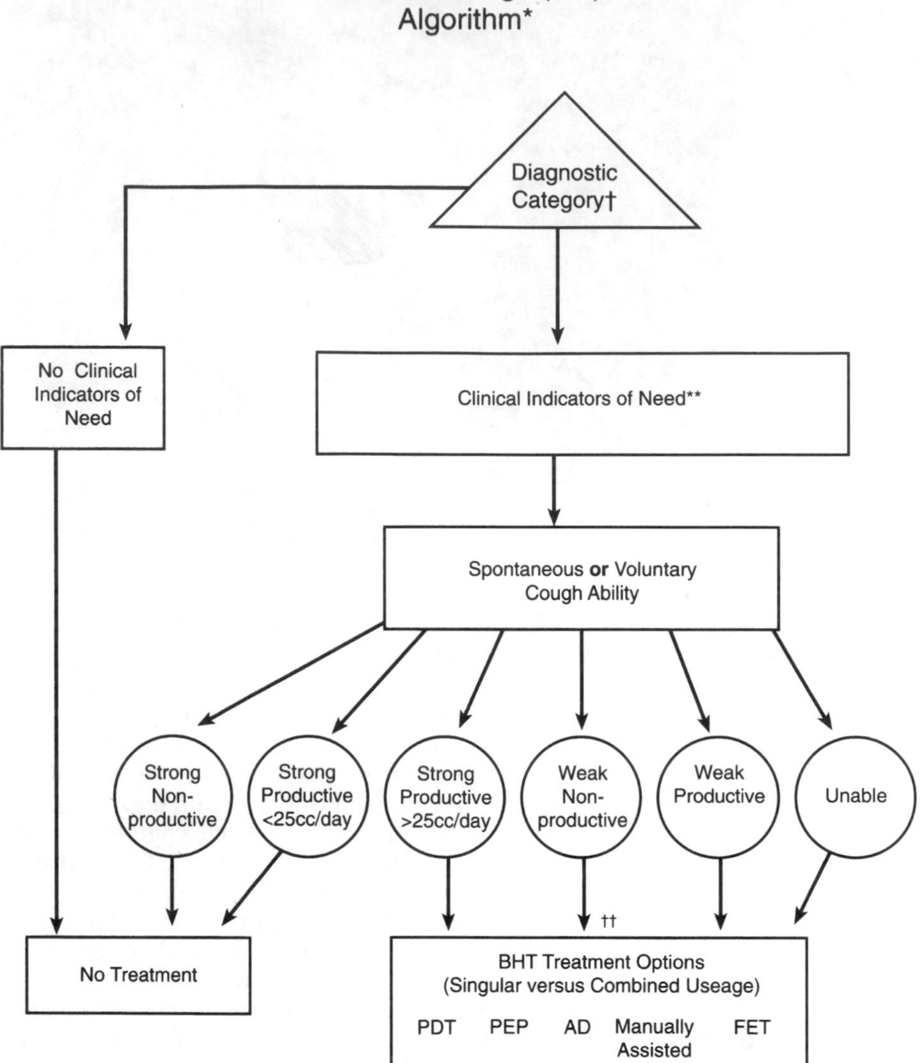

* Assume optimally hydrated patient
†Diagnostic categories include pulmonary, muscular disease, neuromuscular, musculo-skeletal, surgical, cardiac
**Clinical indicators of need include mechanical ventilation, sputum, decreased cognition, radiographic evidence, auscultation and palpation evidence, pain, impaired pulmonary function and/or spirometry tests
††If treatment does not produce more sputum than cough alone, discontinue

PROTOCOL 17-1. Therapist-driven protocol for directed cough.

ther sidelying position. The respiratory care practitioner can facilitate the move alone, with assistance or by an apparatus (Fig. 17-5). The degree of assistance required to turn the patient will depend on patient's weight, willingness and ability to assist, and the extent to which monitoring lines, treatment catheters, and so forth, limit mobility. For example, a patient with a very low Glasgow Coma score[37] secondary to neurologic insult or who is chemically paralyzed will require more assistance than a patient who has progressive return of motor control following a cerebral vascular accident with hemiparesis. In comparison, the patient who is alert and oriented and who has the motor ability and willingness may only require a reminder to turn frequently in bed.

Positive Expiratory Pressure

An example of a TDP for PEP Protocol 17-4 indicates that this therapy may be an option to include in the treatment plan when either clinical assessment warrants or a diagnosis exists in which airway secretions are clinically significant (eg, bronchiectasis or cystic fibrosis). PEP therapy is also indicated when airway closure occurs during forced expiration. Air trapping makes secretion removal difficult and may also be manifested in emphysema and symptomatic asthma.

When an appropriate diagnosis is identified along with clinical indicators of need, then PEP can be applied. Patients must demonstrate that controlled spontaneous breathing is possible. PEP requires the ability

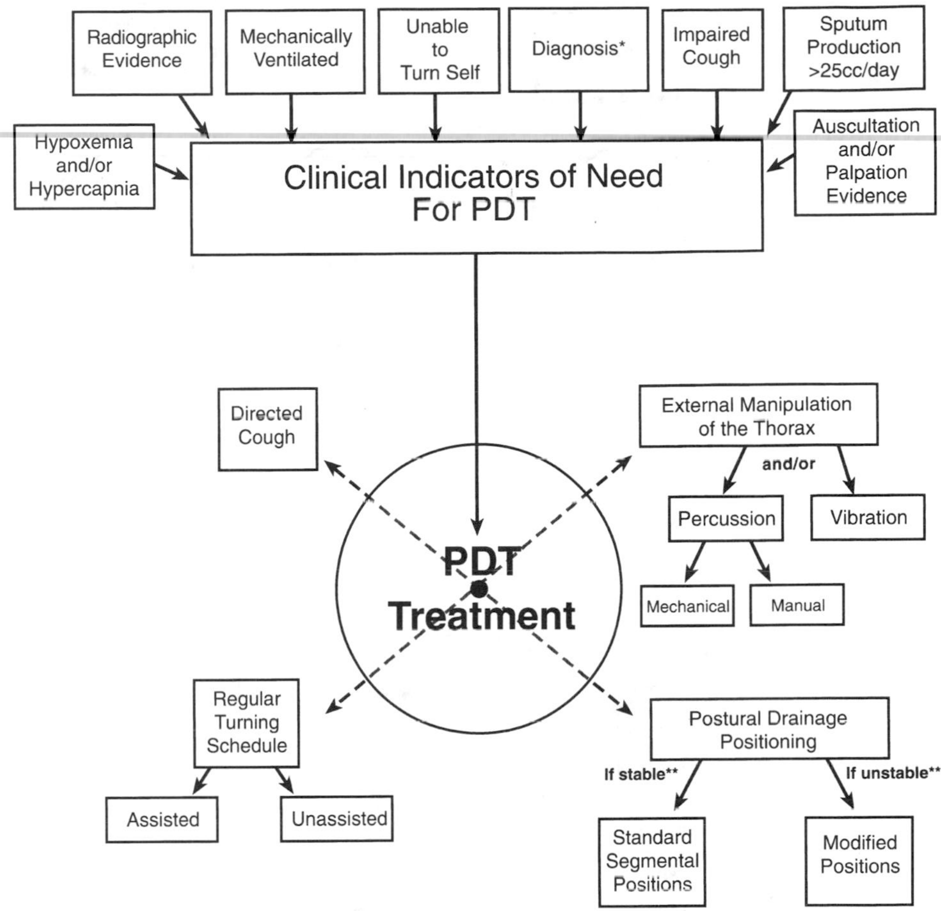

PROTOCOL 17-2. Therapist-driven protocol for bronchial hygiene techniques (Example 1).

* Diagnosis indicators include cystic fibrosis, bronchiectasis, lung abscess, necrotizing pneumonia, COPD, spinal cord injury, and others (MD, CVA, MS)

**Stability refers to neurologic (eg. intracranial pressure, aspiration risk, etc.) and hemodynamic (eg. EKG, central pressure monitoring, etc.) status

to use a controlled deep breath followed by an accentuated expiratory force (+10 to 20 cmH_2O) with a therapeutic inspiration to expiration ratio for effectiveness (eg, I:E ratio of 1:4). PEP is an option only when breathing control is exhibited. If not, then PDT is the likely treatment strategy to select.

Illustrative Case Scenario

The case scenario for KW, a 35-year-old male office worker who has cystic fibrosis, will demonstrate how the BHT techniques are used, often in a combined fashion, based on specific clinical indications.

At 70 inches (177 cm) and 133 pounds (60.5 kg), KW's clinical course displayed a progressive deterioration of cardiopulmonary performance over the past 5 years. The primary limiting symptom was dyspnea. In the past he had been an avid downhill skier and jogged regularly. However, 1 year ago he left his full-time job because of medical disability. Within the past few months he was essentially on bed rest, requiring continuous supplemental oxygen via nasal cannula at 2 L/min. He had been on chronic systemic corticosteroid therapy (prednisone 10 mg/day) and was also receiving combined topical aerosol therapy with steroid triamcinolone (Azmacort), plus bronchodilators metaproterenol (Alupent), ipratropium (Atrovent), and albuterol (Ventolin). He had become hypoxemic (PaO_2 = 61.4 mmHg on room air) and hypercapnic ($PaCO_2$ = 49.3 mmHg). His FEV_1 was 0.71 L (17% of predicted) and his total lung capacity (TLC) was 11.44 L (162% of predicted).

Inspection of his respiration revealed a forward-leaning posture with elbows propped on his thighs. He

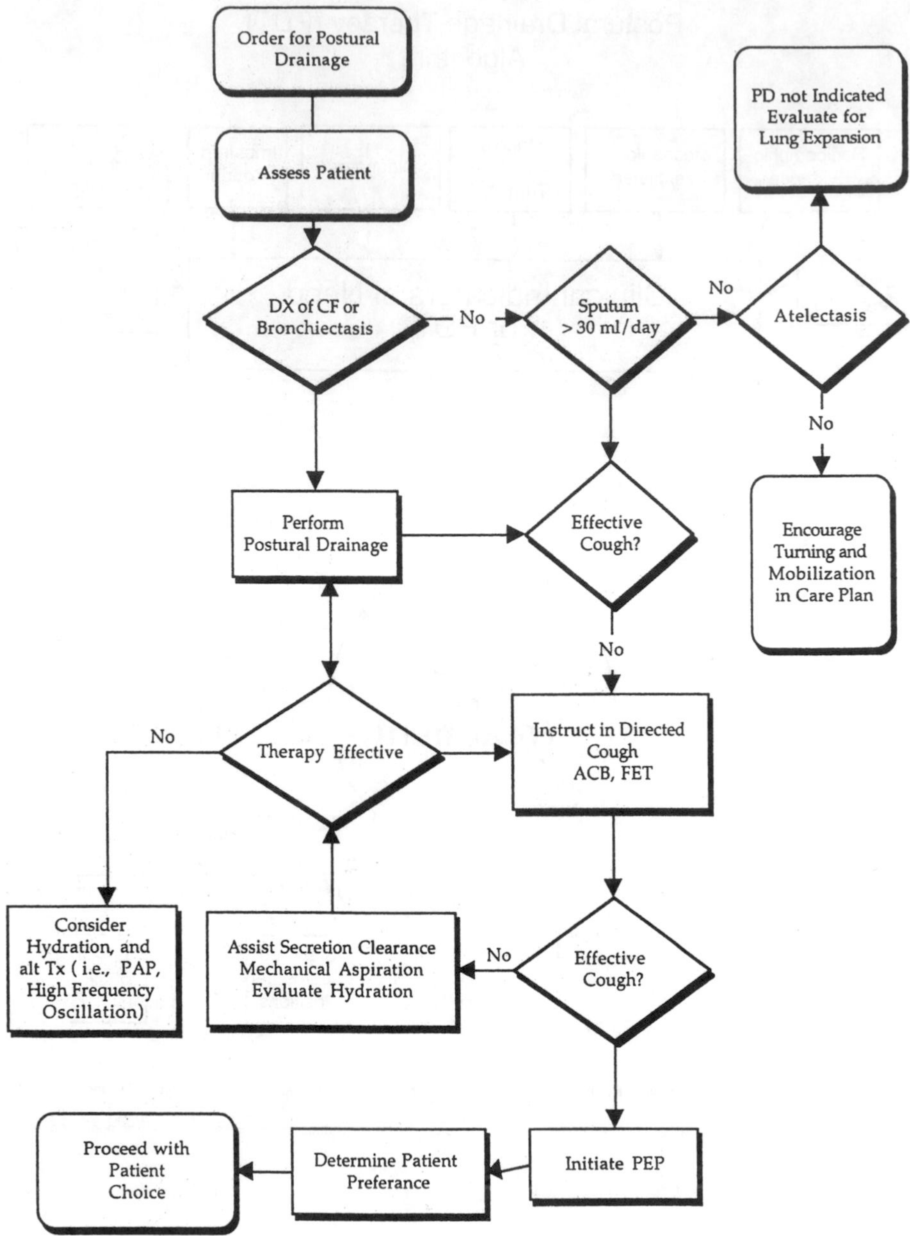

PROTOCOL 17-3. Therapist-driven protocol for bronchial hygiene techniques (Example 2).

was markedly kyphotic and his breathing pattern was dysynchronous for thoraco-abdominal motion and arrhythmical for inspiratory and expiratory phases. He appeared hyperinflated and displayed Hoover's sign of inward (paradoxical) lateral movement of costal rib margins of lower ribs on inspiration. He displayed a maximal inspiratory to expiratory excursion range of 1.5 cm at the level of the xiphoid. He was tachypneic at rest with a respiratory rate of 30/min (7 breaths during a count from 0 to 15). The degree of pulmonary hyperinflation is visualized in the posteroanterior and lateral chest radiographs shown in Figure 17-10A and B. Abnormal findings include bilateral diaphragmatic flattening, horizontal ribs, increased anterior-to-posterior dimension, and dorsal kyphosis of the thoracic spice. Abnormal pulmonary markings appear to be consistent with mucous plugging, bronchiectasis, and pneumonitis.

Palpation of his chest wall identified increased tactile fremitus over anterior and lateral regions. Coarse and moist inspiratory and expiratory sounds, with no apparent wheezing, were auscultated diffusely. He regularly produced approximately 4 ounces of tenacious yellow to yellow/green sputum each morning, through labored and exhaustive coughing. He was tachycardic at rest (122/min) and easily exceeded 160/min during coughing paroxysms. He had chest wall pain related to recent rib fractures (8th and 9th on the left, and 8th on the

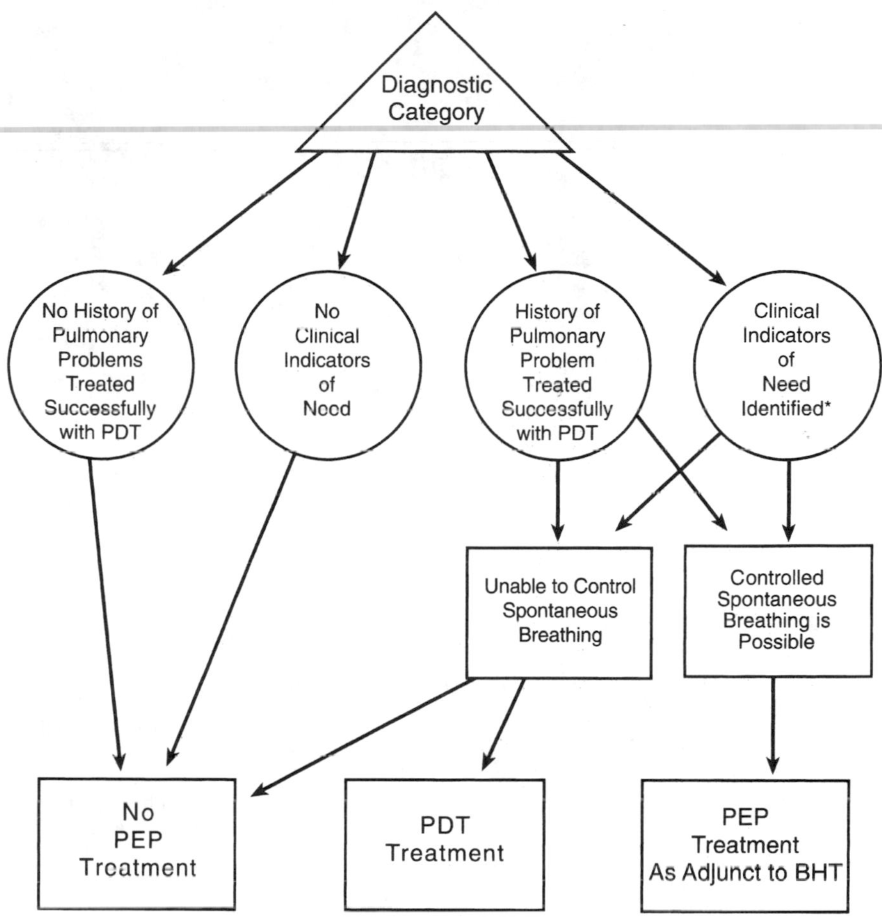

PROTOCOL 17-4. Therapist-driven protocol for positive expiratory pressure.

*Clinical indicators of need inlcude impaired cough, sputum production, decreased pulmonary function and/or spirometry, radiographic evidence of secretion retention and/or atelectasis, auscultation and/or palpation evidence for central airway secretions.

right) and coughing episodes. He had adequate maximum inspiratory pressure (MIP) of -95 cmH_2O and a maximum expiratory pressure (MEP) of $+235$ cmH_2O.

A functional 6-minute walk test in this motivated individual produced a distance of 1260 feet with one brief rest pause. While walking, his pulse oximetric oxygen saturation (SpO_2) decreased from 92% to 84% despite a 2 L/min supplemental O_2 via nasal cannula.

Multiple clinical indications for bronchial hygiene therapy are documented in the history, examination, radiograph, and pulmonary function data. KW has excessive sputum retention owing to cystic fibrosis; auscultation and palpation reveal evidence for central airway secretions. Pulmonary function tests were abnormal showing a predominant obstructed pattern. His stiff chest wall has assumed an inspiratory position; neuromuscular function was satisfactory as evidenced by the maximal inspiratory/expiratory pressures. He was hypoxemic and hypercapnic at rest.

The patient's diagnosis warrants chronic BHT as well as a history of successful use of PDT. He was able to tolerate the prone, Trendelenburg positions while a mechanical percussor was applied to his chest wall. The expulsive effort he generated with his strong cough narrowed the airway cephalad from the equal pressure point, making it more difficult for him to expectorate secretions.

Bronchial Hygiene Therapy Treatment Plan

KW was mature and able to demonstrate excellent voluntary control over his breathing rate, volume, and duration of inspiratory and expiratory phases. He was

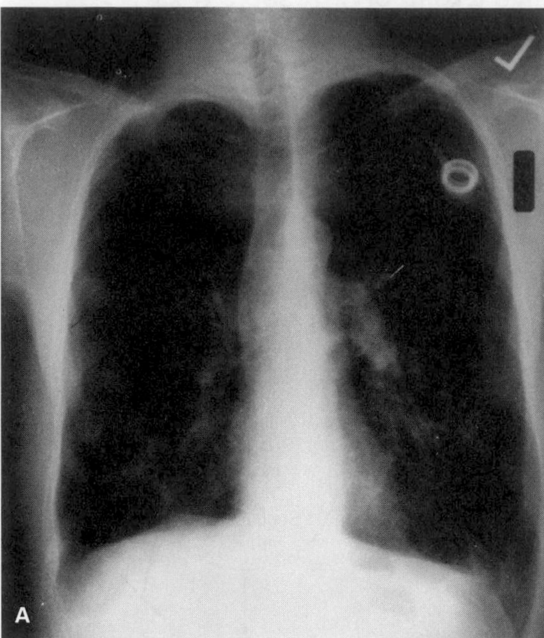

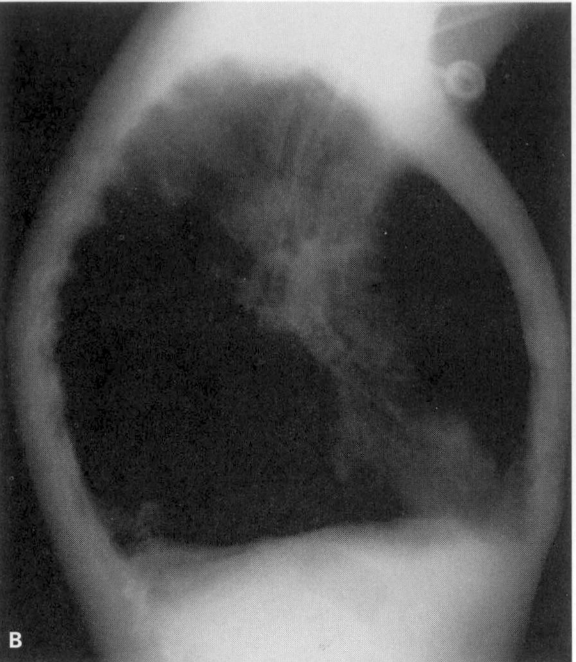

FIGURE 17-10. **(A)** Posteroanterior and lateral chest radiographs of cystic fibrosis patient KW in case scenario (see text).

placed in the DC protocol. His BHT also implemented options for PEP to follow his topical aerosol nebulization therapy. Through instruction he also became adept at AD to raise secretions so an FET could be used as needed. KW also was able to produce his own timed thoracic compression (ie, "chicken wing"), using glenohumeral adduction. His vital signs and arterial blood gases document the need for chronic oxygen therapy.

CONCLUSION

BHT combined with initial and ongoing patient assessment has evolved to become an established component of respiratory care. Effectiveness of individual and combined procedures such as bronchial drainage, chest percussion and vibration, along with DC, and various mechanical adjuncts, depends on matching therapy to the patient's changing needs. Improvements in BHT will rely on improved assessment skills, patient education, and providing care in a changing health care delivery system.

REFERENCES

1. Hardy KA: A review of airway clearance: New techniques, indications, and recommendations. Respir Care 39:4, 1994
2. American Association for Respiratory Care: AARC clinical practice guideline: Postural drainage therapy. Respir Care 36:1418, 1991
3. American Association for Respiratory Care: AARC clinical practice guideline: Directed cough. Respir Care 38:495, 1993
4. American Association for Respiratory Care: AARC clinical practice guideline: Use of positive airway pressure adjuncts to bronchial hygiene therapy. Respir Care 38:516, 1993
5. Johnson CB: 1992 Respiratory care job analysis. NBRC Horizons 19:1, 1993
6. Mackenzie CF: History and literature review of chest physiotherapy, ICU chest physiotherapy and respiratory care: Controversies and questions. In Mackenzie CF, Imle PC, Ciesla N (eds): Chest Physiotherapy in the Intensive Care Unit, 2nd ed. Baltimore, Williams & Wilkins, 1989
7. Shapiro BA: Chest physical therapy administered by respiratory therapists. Respir Care 26:655, 1981
8. Hodgkin JE: The scientific status of chest physiotherapy. Respir Care 26:657, 1981
9. Pierce AK, Saltzman HA: Conference on the scientific basis of respiratory therapy: Final report—physical therapy. Am Rev Respir Dis 110:12, 1974
10. Hillegass E, Sadowsky S: Essentials of Cardiopulmonary Physical Therapy. Philadelphia, WB Saunders, 1994
11. Zadai CC: Pulmonary Management in Physical Therapy. New York, Churchill Livingstone, 1992
12. Kinslay S, Olson LG: Patterns of use of chest physiotherapy in a teaching hospital. Australian Clin Rev 11:154, 1991
13. Bunch D: Therapist-driven protocols: saving costs and enhancing patient care. AARC Times 17:45, 1993
14. Stoller JK: Why therapist-driven protocols? a balanced view. Respir Care 39:706, 1994
15. Pasquale MD, Cipolle MD, Cerra FB: Oxygen transport: Does increasing supply improve outcome? Respir Care 38:800, 1993
16. Dean E, Ross J: Discordance between cardiopulmonary physiology and physical therapy. Chest 101:1694, 1992
17. Eid N, Buchheit J, Neuling M, Phelps H: Chest physiotherapy in review. Respir Care 36:270, 1991
18. Britton S, Bejstedt M, Vedin L: Chest physiotherapy in primary pneumonia. BMJ 290:1703, 1985
19. Thomas J, Cook DJ, Brooks D: Chest physical therapy management of patients with cystic fibrosis: A Meta-analysis. Am J Respir Crit Care Med 151:846, 1995
20. American Thoracic Society: Lung function testing: Selection of references values and interpretative strategies. Am Rev Respir Dis 144:1202, 1991
21. Rochester DF: Tests of respiratory muscle function. Clin Chest Med 9:249, 1988

22. Black LF, Hyatt RE: Maximal static respiratory pressures in generalized neuromuscular disease. Am Rev Respir Dis 103:641, 1971
23. Butland RJA, Pang J, Gross ER, Woodcock AA, Geddes DM: Two-, six-, and 12-minute walking tests in respiratory disease. BMJ 284:1607, 1982
24. Killian KJ, Jones NL: Respiratory muscles and dyspnea. Clin Chest Med 9:237, 1988
25. Mahler DA, Weinberg DH, Wells CK, Feinstein AR: The measurement of dyspnea. Chest 85:751, 1984
26. Bond MR, Pilowsky I: The subjective assessment of pain and its relationship to the administration of analgesics in patients with advanced cancer. J Psychosomat Res 10:203, 1966
27. McSweeny AJ, Grant I, Heaton RK, Adams KM, Timms RM: Life quality of patients with chronic obstructive pulmonary disease. Arch Intern Med 142:473, 1982
28. Prigatano GP, Wright EC, Levin D: Quality of life and its predictors in patients with mild hypoxemia and chronic obstructive pulmonary disease. Arch Intern Med 144:1613, 1984
29. Lewis MI, Belman MJ: Nutrition and the respiratory muscles. Clin Chest Med 9:337, 1988
30. Celli BR: Clinical and physiologic evaluation of respiratory muscle function. Clin Chest Med 10:199, 1989
31. Rochester DF, Braun NMT, Arora NS: Respiratory muscle strength in chronic obstructive pulmonary disease. Am Rev Respir Dis 119:151, 1979
32. Celli BR, Rassulo J, Make BJ: Dyssynchronous breathing during arm but not leg exercise in patients with chronic airflow obstruction. N Engl J Med 314:1485, 1986
33. Roussos C: Respiratory muscle fatigue and ventilatory failure. Chest 97:89S, 1990
34. Sharp JT, Drutz WS, Moisan T, Foster J, Machnoch W: Postural relief of dyspnea in severe chronic obstructive pulmonary disease. Am Rev Respir Dis 122:201, 1980
35. Tobin MJ: Respiratory muscles in disease. Clin Chest Med 9:263, 1988
36. Sobush DC: Breathing exercises: laying a foundation for a clinical practice guideline. Cardiopulmonary Physical Therapy 3:8, 1992
37. Irwin S, Tecklin JS: Cardiopulmonary Physical Therapy. St. Louis, CV Mosby, 1985, p 231
38. Pryor JA (ed): Respiratory Care. London, Churchill Livingstone, 1991, p 72
39. Downie PA (ed): Cash's Textbook of Chest, Heart, and Vascular Disorders for Physiotherapists, 4th ed. Philadelphia, JB Lippincott, 1987, p 333
40. Pryor JA, Webber BA: An evaluation of the forced expiration technique as an adjunct to postural drainage. Physiotherapy 65:304, 1979
41. Pryor JA, Webber BA, Hodson ME, Batten JC: Evaluation of the forced expiration technique as an adjunct to postural drainage in treatment of cystic fibrosis. BMJ 2:417, 1979
42. Schoni MH: Autogenic drainage: A modern approach to physiotherapy in cystic fibrosis. J R Soc Med 82(Suppl):32, 1989
43. Miller S, Hill DO, Clayton CB, Nelson R: Chest physiotherapy in cystic fibrosis—a comparative study of autogenic drainage and the active cycle of breathing techniques with postural drainage. Thorax 50:165, 1995
44. Pfeger A, Theissl B, Oberwaldner B, Zach MS: Self-administered chest physiotherapy in cystic fibrosis: A comparative study of high pressure PEP and autogenic drainage. Lung 170:323, 1992
45. Selsby D, Jones JG: Some physiological and clinical aspects of chest physiotherapy. Br J Anesth 64:621, 1990
46. Falk M, Andersen JB: Positive expiratory pressure (PEP) mask. In JA Pryor (ed): Respiratory Care. Edinburgh, Churchill Livingstone, 1991
47. Sobush DC, Dunning M, Schlueter D, Pauley K, Yesko J: Blowing bubbles: The therapeutic application of positive expiratory pressure (PEP) for bronchial hygiene [abstract]. Wisconsin Physical Therapy Association Newsletter 24:18, 1994
48. Sutton PP, Lopez-Vidriero MT, et al: Assessment of percussion, vibratory shaking and breathing exercises in chest physiotherapy. Eur J Respir Dis 66:147–152, 1985
49. Pavin D: The role of chest physiotherapy in mucus hypersecretion. Lung 168(Suppl):614, 1990
50. Mohsenifor Z, Rosenberg N, Goldberg HS, Koerner SK: Mechanical ventilation and conventional chest physiotherapy in outpatients with stable chronic obstructive lung disease. Chest 87:483, 1985
51. Asher MI, Douglas C, Airy M, Andrews D, Trendolme A: Effect of chest physical therapy on lung function in children recovering from acute severe asthma. Pediatr Pulmonology 9:146, 1990
52. Torrington KG, Sorenson DE, Sherwood LM: Postoperative chest percussion with bronchial drainage in obese patients following gastric stapling. Chest 86:891, 1984
53. American College of Chest Physicians: Respiratory Care Section Steering Committee. Respiratory care protocols: ACCP position paper. AARC Times 17:51, 1993

18 Volume Expansion Therapy

James B. Fink

CLINICAL SKILLS

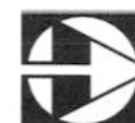

Upon completion of this chapter, the reader will:

- Determine the factors that contribute to the development of atelectasis
- Use and encourage patient positioning, deep breathing, and coughing techniques to enhance patient lung expansion
- Select equipment to aid in volume expansion therapy on the basis of patient assessment and device characteristics
- Effectively teach and administer incentive spirometry
- Describe the method and equipment used in the administration of IPPB therapy
- Discuss the value of positive airway pressure (PAP) to mobilize secretions and treat atelectasis
- Discuss alternative methods used to mobilize secretions, including high-frequency airway oscillation and high frequency chest wall compression
- Assess patients for outcome results of volume expansion therapy
- Identify contraindications and limitations of volume expansion therapy procedures

KEY TERMS

Atelectasis
Continuous positive airway pressure
Expiratory positive airway pressure
Fixed orifice resistor
Flow-oriented incentive device
Huff coughing
Hyperinflation therapy
Incentive spirometry
Intermittent positive pressure breathing
Magnetic valve resistor
Positive expiratory pressure
Spring-loaded resistor
Sustained maximal inspiration
Threshold resistor
Underwater seal resistor
Volume displacement
Water column resistor
Weighted ball resistor

Lung expansion is a subset of bronchial hygiene therapy, with the specific goal of assisting the patient to attain or maintain optimal lung volumes. This chapter reviews a range of techniques and mechanical devices to augment lung expansion and assist mobilizing airway secretions. There is an inherent overlap of content with Chapter 17 as lung volumes are directly related to expiratory flows, cough effectiveness, and the ability to clear secretions from the airways. Volume expansion therapy may be equipment oriented, but is frequently used in conjunction with postural drainage therapy (PDT), directed cough, and medical aerosols. The respiratory care practitioner's (RCP) role at the bedside is to document the need for therapy and implement appropriate technique(s).

Historically, the emphasis of lung expansion therapy focused on the treatment and prevention of pulmonary atelectasis. Therapeutic maneuvers for treating atelectasis include positioning (turning and mobilization), deep breathing, directed cough, incentive spirometry, intermittent positive pressure breathing (IPPB), positive airway pressure (PAP), manipulation of the thorax, bronchodilator administration, and mobilization and evacuation of secretions. More recently, the RCP must also provide documentation of initial assessment and ongoing need for therapy. Clinical skills needed in performing therapeutic services related to volume expansion are listed in Box 18-1.

Although most volume expansion techniques can be effective under a variety of circumstances, a majority of patients do not require any therapy to avoid or resolve atelectasis. Normal subjects only require instruction and reminders to perform periodic deep breathing preoperatively and postoperatively.[1,2]

Mechanical devices to provide pressurized inhalation were developed, starting in the late 1800s, to treat acute pulmonary edema and continued to be used for that purpose into the 1930s. Motley et al[3] popularized the use of IPPB to deliver bronchodilator aerosols in the late 1940s. There were scientific studies showing no advantage to using IPPB to administer aerosols in stable emphysema.[4,5] Failure to understand limitations, liberal medical reimbursement, and vigorous promotion by machine manufacturers combined to create unwarranted overuse. In the mid-1970s, the scientific basis of IPPB was reviewed at a conference sponsored by the National Heart and Lung Institute and the American Thoracic Society. The application of this therapy was rightly criticized, especially in stable chronic obstructive pulmonary disease (COPD) where a more comprehensive care regimen was more appropriate. There was lack of science to support its application and IPPB fell into disfavor in the early 1980s.[6] At the Second Conference on the Scientific Basis of In-hospital Respiratory Therapy, it was determined that IPPB had been largely replaced with less-than-scientific application of incentive spirometry, nebulizer treatments, and postural drainage. In some cases this had further escalated the cost of respiratory care.[7]

In 1985, O'Donohue conducted a national survey to evaluate national patterns of lung expansion therapies in the prevention and management of postoperative atelectasis associated with abdominal and thoracic surgery.[8] He reported that thoracic surgery was performed in 60% of hospitals with approximately 200 beds and in more than 95% of the hospitals with more than 200 beds. Thoracic surgical procedures ranged from 11 to 57 each month, and 32% of the cases had significant postoperative atelectasis. At that time, measurements of inspired lung volumes, such as tidal volume or inspiratory capacity, were performed at only 21% of hospitals as a means of objectively assessing the lung expansion maneuvers prescribed for the treatment of postoperative atelectasis. The treatments included incentive spirometry (95% of all hospitals for treatment of postoperative atelectasis, once it is diagnosed and judged to be clinically significant), chest physical therapy (83%), IPPB (82%), intermittent continuous positive airway pressure (CPAP) (25%), and blow bottles (17%).

In the decade following that survey, no substantial changes in the incidence of postoperative complications were reported, and many of the same treatment options are still used, often on a wholesale basis. As in many areas of respiratory care, the ordering patterns of physicians are all too often based on the practice they were exposed to

BOX 18-1

CLINICAL SKILLS NEEDED IN PERFORMING VOLUME EXPANSION THERAPY

Select, review, obtain, and interpret data relative to bronchial hygiene therapy.

- Review existing data in patient record:
  - *History*—childhood or adult disease likely to manifest in secretion retention or atelectasis
  - *Physical examination*—CNS, pulmonary, or cardiovascular signs of atelectasis or retained bronchial secretions
  - *Laboratory*—pulmonary function testing including arterial blood gas and pulse oximetry
- Recommend and perform procedures to obtain additional data
- Interview the patient to determine: sputum production, level of dyspnea, work of breathing, and ability to cooperate
- Review planned therapy to establish therapeutic goals, determine appropriateness of therapy, and recommend changes as indicated

Select, assemble, and check equipment for proper function, operation, and cleanliness.

- Incentive breathing devices
- IPPB, CPPB, and EPAP
- Percussors and vibrators
- PEP masks

Initiate, conduct, and modify prescribed therapeutic procedures.

- Explain planned therapy and goals to patient and communicate information regarding the patient's clinical status to health care team
- Position patient to minimize hypoxemia
- Conduct therapeutic procedures to achieve adequate ventilation
- Achieve volume expansion by removal of bronchopulmonary secretions
- Recommend modifications in the respiratory care plan based on patient response.

as students or residents, which were often specific strategies to protect every patient receiving upper abdominal or thoracic surgery from atelectasis and nosocomial pneumonias. However, as the health care industry evolves, no one appears to be willing to pay the bill for a "shot gun" approach for prevention of pulmonary complications.

Future care will likely limit reimbursement of therapy to patients who meet specific criteria. The role of the RCP will expand to identify patients at extreme risk. RCPs will recommend care or continued monitoring following a review of the history, laboratory/radiographic data, and physical examination. Efforts will be made to provide the best care at the lowest cost, with a critical reevaluation of each patient interaction or treatment throughout the course of care. To that end, this chapter examines the need for lung expansion therapies, with a detailed look at the available options in terms of efficacy, comfort, and cost. Clinical practice guidelines, recently published by the American Association for Respiratory Care (AARC), provide national consensus for issues of indications, hazards, contraindications, and limitations of therapy. Summaries of the guidelines for incentive spirometry, IPPB, and positive pressure adjuncts to bronchial hygiene therapy are presented.[9–11] The assessment-based approach is founded in therapist-driven protocols (TDPs) that direct intervention based on determined needs. An example of a TDP for volume expansion therapy concludes this chapter.

RATIONALE FOR VOLUME EXPANSION

Atelectasis

Atelectasis, or collapsed lung parenchyma, ranges from microatelectasis (invisible on radiograph) to macroatelectasis. Although macroatelectasis is estimated to occur in less than 6% of patients undergoing surgery, estimates range as high as 60% with upper abdominal procedures. Microatelectasis is probably quite common, but remains undetected, postoperatively. Microatelectasis may occur from alveolar tidal volume less than from net gas absorption. This leads to decreased alveolar size, reduced compliance, and further decrease in alveolar tidal volume. Microatelectasis may progress to involve subsegmental or larger areas and thus become visible on chest radiograph. The radiographic signs of atelectasis include localized increase in radiographic density, displacement of lobar fissures, elevation of the ipsilateral diaphragm, mediastinal shift, hilar displacement, regional approximation of ribs, and compensatory hyperinflation of the surrounding segments. Clinical features of atelectasis regress following relief of the obstruction without treatment with antibiotics, hence distinguishing atelectasis from a pulmonary infection. Atelectasis may cause pulmonary shunting and hypoxemia.[12] Engoren[13] found no correlation between fever and amount of atelectasis in 100 postoperative cardiac surgery patients. This contradicts "common textbook dogma" but agrees with previous human study and animal experiments. Box 18-2 identifies important factors that may cause atelectasis.

BOX 18-2

FACTORS CAUSING ATELECTASIS

- Retained secretions—Lobar, segmental, or subsegmental atelectasis can occur when an airway is obstructed, and the alveoli distal to it collapse as they absorb gas into the capillaries unless fresh gas enters via collateral channels.
- Altered patterns of breathing—The pattern of breathing is altered following surgery: there is a 20% decrease in tidal volume and a 26% increase in respiratory rate. In addition, the frequency of sighing (deep breaths, at least three times normal tidal volume) is decreased. This altered pattern of breathing causes a decrease in pulmonary compliance and an increase in small-airway closure. As we age, our frequency of sighs increases from about four times per hour (young adult) to 12 times per hour.[14]
- Pain associated with surgery or trauma (especially upper abdominal and thoracic) is associated with a breathing pattern consisting of relatively shallow breaths without sighs and splinting, which limits the motivation and effectiveness of cough efforts.
- Alterations in small-airway function—The postoperative state is associated with characteristic changes in small-airway functions. Closing volume (CV), the lung volume at which small bronchioles close during exhalation, is usually less than expiratory reserve volume (ERV), so small airways remain patent throughout the normal respiratory cycle. Postoperatively, ERV may be reduced to less than CV, so airways are closed or occluded during tidal breathing. CV is increased with cigarette smoking, COPD, and elderly patients. The greater the patient's CV, the greater their risk of atelectasis.
- Prolonged supine position—FRC is reduced in normal subjects while in the supine position. In 1956, Miller, Fowler, and Helmholz demonstrated that changing from supine to lateral decubitus (right or left) position causes a small volume reduction in the dependent lung and a larger increase in the superior lung, producing an overall increase in FRC.[15] In critically ill patients, the prone position has been shown to improve FRC and oxygenation.[16,17] Torres et al[18] demonstrated that the longer a ventilated patient remains in the supine position, the greater the incidence of aspiration of gastric contents and associated pulmonary complications, concluding that frequent position changes reduce risk.
- Increased abdominal pressure following laparotomy—Increased general pressure in the abdomen translates to pressure against the diaphragm and reduced volumes in the lung.
- Musculoskeletal or neurologic abnormalities such as muscular dystrophy, spinal muscular atrophy, myasthenia, poliomyelitis, or cerebral palsy may be associated with compromised bellows function and reduced lung volumes.
- Restrictive defects result in smaller vital capacities and reduced FRC.
- Surgical procedures such as open heart surgery, in which the left lung is deflated during the surgery, results in postoperative atelectasis that typically requires several days to resolve, with or without therapy.

GENERAL APPROACH TO THE PREVENTION OF ATELECTASIS

Patient Education

In patients with underlying pulmonary disease, aggressive preoperative preparation (ie, smoking cessation, bronchodilators, humidified air, aggressive coughing, and deep breathing) has been reported to result in a threefold reduction in postoperative complications. Preoperatively the patient is much more receptive to learning, practicing maneuvers, and consciously cooperating with the RCP. Postoperatively, pain and medication to treat or control that pain may inhibit cough, deep inspiration, early mobilization, attention span, and cooperation with respiratory care staff. Preoperative training is of particular importance in cigarette smokers, COPD, elderly, and obese (high-risk) patients.[19]

Without preoperative instruction, the patient (eg, who has undergone upper abdominal surgery), upon awaking from anesthesia, is instructed to take a deep breath and is rewarded with abdomen-splitting, gut-wrenching, and totally unexpected pain. Because patients (like people and small animals) tend to distrust people who surprise them with pain (and are too smart to be fooled into repeating painful maneuvers), they may be less than cooperative the next time someone asks them to cough. In contrast, preoperative instruction allows the patient to be forewarned that coughing will hurt, and that techniques such as splinting an abdominal incision with a pillow can minimize (not eliminate) the pain. The patient, who may be anxious before surgery, needs to understand that the consequences of not coughing includes possible pulmonary complications, a slower recovery, and even more discomfort. Deep breathing and coughing is one thing they can do that will help them speed their recovery. Forearmed with this knowledge, the patient wakes up from anesthesia realizing that coughing will hurt but must be done and is familiar with the previously taught maneuvers. When the RCP coaches the patient to cough, the pain is not a surprise, and the trust relationship (and further cooperation) is not compromised.

Patient Positioning

The first-line technique of choice for lung expansion is frequently turning patients from the supine to lateral or even prone positions. Patients should be encouraged to turn, or be turned, at least every 2 hours, while awake. Even better than turning is sitting up and getting out of bed. Early ambulation of patients (who can safely get out of bed) should be encouraged as soon as possible. These fundamental procedures are superb examples of how lung expansion therapy can be provided with minimal cost.[19] In critical care and postoperative situations, it is very convenient to keep the patient in the supine position for prolonged periods of time. Reasons often given include:

- Reduced risk of displacing tubes, leads, and lines
- Patient appears to be more comfortable on his or her back
- Less stress for the patient—stable vitals
- Less stress for the care provider.

The longer patients remain in the supine position, the greater the chance that lung volumes will be reduced and secretions as well as aspirated gastric contents and third space fluids will pool in gravity-dependent areas.[20,21]

Turning patients from supine to lateral, or to the prone position, results in increased functional residual capacity (FRC), and improved oxygenation.[15] Douglas et al[16] demonstrated that the use of the supported prone position results in greater increased in oxygen saturation than application the of CPAP. Just as changes in body position can improve distribution of ventilation and perfusion, it may have deleterious effects, so that each change in position should be evaluated for patient tolerance.[22–24] The use of rotating beds has been advocated in critically ill patients (continuously turning from side to side) with reported reductions in pulmonary complications[25–28]; however, further controlled studies are necessary to determine superiority over turning patients every 2 hours. Box 18-3 identifies the clinical procedure for patient positioning.

Deep Breathing and Coughing

The normal mechanism for lung expansion is spontaneous deep breathing (including yawn and sigh maneuvers) and an affective cough.[29] Instructing and encouraging the patient to take sustained deep breaths is among the safest, most effective, and least expensive strategies for keeping the lungs expanded (Box 18-4).[30]

BOX 18-3

PROCEDURE FOR POSITIONING

Turning (repositioning)/mobility (see Table 18-2 for indications, contraindications, complications, and recommended frequency for treatment)

1. Explain to the patient that the reason for frequent position changes and mobility is to promote lung expansion and to improve oxygenation of the blood.
2. Encourage patients to turn independently or assist them to change position as necessary. Optimal positions for lung expansion and secretion mobilization are oblique side-lying with the bed at any degree of inclination as tolerated by the patient, and prone. Sitting, dangling legs over the bedside, and ambulation are also effective in promoting lung expansion/secretion mobilization.
3. Repositioning frequency is determined in part by assessment of tissue tolerance. The reddened area marking the points of pressure should disappear within 30 minutes after the patient is repositioned. If the reddened area remains longer than 30 minutes, the turning frequency should be increased and/or the support surface changed. Positioning devices such as pillows should be used to keep bony prominences from direct contact with one another.
4. Document teaching accomplished, procedures performed, and patient response in the patient record.

BOX 18-4

PROCEDURES FOR DIRECTED COUGH

1. Explain to the patient that deep breathing and coughing will help to keep the lungs expanded and clear of secretions.
2. Assist the patient to a sitting position, or to a semi-Fowler's position if sitting position is not possible.
3. Standard directed cough procedure (see below for modifications):
   (a) Instruct patient to take a deep breath, then hold the breath, using abdominal muscles to force air against a closed glottis, then cough with a single exhalation.
   (b) Several relaxed breaths should be taken before the next cough effort.
   (c) Document teaching accomplished, procedures performed, and patient response in the patient record.
4. Alternate standard "huff" directed cough procedure
   (a) Instruct patient to take 3 to 5 slow deep breaths, inhaling through the nose, exhaling through pursed lips, using diaphragmatic breathing. Have patient take a deep breath, hold the breath for 1 to 3 seconds.
   (b) Exhale from mid-lung volumes to low-lung volumes (to clear secretions from peripheral airways). A normal breath is taken in and then squeezed out by contracting the abdominal and chest wall muscles, with the mouth (and glottis) open while whispering the word "huff" (sounds like a forced sigh) during exhalation. Repeat several times.
   (c) As secretions enter the larger airways, exhale from high- to mid-lung volumes to clear secretions from more proximal airways. Repeat maneuver two to three times.
   (d) Several relaxed diaphragmatic breaths should be taken before the next cough effort.
   (e) Document teaching accomplished, procedures performed, and patient response in the patient record.
5. Modified directed cough procedure for:
   (a) Patients who have had abdominal or thoracic surgery: Instruct patient to place hand or a pillow over the incisional site and to apply gentle pressure while coughing. Personnel may assist with incisional support during coughing. Support chest tubes as necessary.
   (b) Quadriplegic patients: Personnel place palms on the patient's abdomen, below the diaphragm, and instruct the patient to take three deep breaths. On exhalation of the third breath, push forcefully inward and upward as the patient coughs (similar to abdominal thrust maneuver performed on unconscious persons with an obstructed airway).

The negative intrathoracic pressure generated during spontaneous deep breathing tends to better inflate the less compliant, gravity-dependent areas of the lung than methods relying on lung inflation by application of positive airway pressure.

A deep breath is a key component for a normal effective cough. ACB, active cycle of breathing is comprised of a series of respiratory maneuvers including relaxed diaphragmatic breathing and mid-lung volume followed by FET or huff coughing, and has been shown to be more effective in mobilizing secretions and increasing lung volumes than postural drainage with percussion and vibration in both cystic fibrosis and chronic bronchitis patients.[31–34] An effective cough is a vital component of lung expansion therapy.

In the patient with COPD with unstable airways, high pressures and flow combine in the dynamic compression of the airways, trapping gas and secretions. For these patients, ACB with the FET or "huff" appears to be the maneuver of choice.[35–38] Huff coughing is a FET that is performed by exhaling from high to mid lung volumes through an open glottis. The individual takes in a slow, deep breath, followed by a 1- to 3-second breath hold, and then performs short, quick, forced exhalations with the glottis open. The subject may be instructed to say the word "huff" during exhalation. Small children can be taught to flap their arms to their lateral chest as they perform the huff cough, a technique referred to as the chicken (flapping wings) breath, to focus on the expiratory maneuver, associating positive reinforcement and play with the huff technique.[39]

SPECIFIC VOLUME EXPANSION TECHNIQUES AND DEVICES

Incentive Spirometry

Incentive spirometry (IS) is an equipment-oriented approach to coax patients to mimic natural sighing or yawning maneuvers. The RCP's role is to coach slow, deep breaths; the pattern is best described as *sustained maximal inspiration (SMI)*.[11,40] The spirometers can provide biofeedback and encouragement. Because patients often stop sighing and adopt rapid, shallow breathing patterns post surgery, they should be encouraged to take 5 to 10 deep breaths every hour. Incisional pain and splinting may make those breaths painful after upper abdominal surgery, so IS devices provide patients with sensory feedback to quantify how deep a breath they take. IS should provide patients with an objective comparison with the volumes (of flows) they were generating preoperatively, with the goal of attaining or returning to that preoperative volume, despite the pain experienced. In addition, the IS device instruction should include how long breaths should be held, how many times the breaths were attempted, and how many times the patient succeeded in meeting his or her volume goals.

Objectives of SI are to increase transpulmonary pressure and inspiratory volumes to near preoperative or "normal" vital capacity, improve inspiratory muscle performance, and re-establish or simulate the normal pattern of pulmonary hyperinflation. When the SMI maneuver is repeated on a regular basis, airway patency may be maintained and lung atelectasis prevented and reversed.[41–43]

Incentive spirometry is indicated for use as prophylactic treatment of conditions predisposing to the development of pulmonary atelectasis, including upper abdominal surgery and thoracic surgery in patients with COPD, obesity, and advanced age. Although IS is valuable in the treatment of pulmonary atelectasis, it should not be used as the sole treatment for major lung collapse or consolidation, but rather as a part of a more comprehensive program of lung re-expansion.

Because SMI requires patient cooperation, as well as the ability to understand and demonstrate proper use of the device, IS is not a viable therapeutic option for the obtunded, confused, or uncooperative patient. Incentive spirometry is not the therapeutic option of choice for the patient who cannot spontaneously generate a vital capacity (VC) greater than 10 mL/kg or inspiratory capacity (IC) more than one third of predicted (generally considered the level of lung volume or capacity required for an effective cough).[44] For these patients, options such as IPPB or PAP should be considered.

As with many therapeutic modalities in respiratory care, IS is ineffective unless properly performed at ordered frequencies, making compliance a critical issue. Many patients (especially the elderly) require one-on-one assistance to perform IS correctly. If the patient experiences significant pain during deep inspiratory efforts, pain management or alternative options such as PAP should be considered.

When patient compliance appears to be a problem, the IS device used should record the number of breaths attempted and the number of times volume and breath-hold goals were accomplished. While most IS devices are used with a mouthpiece, they may be adapted for use with an open tracheal stoma or artificial airway.

Evidence suggests that deep breathing and coughing, without mechanical aids, can be as beneficial as incentive spirometry in preventing or reversing pulmonary complications, and controversy exists concerning overuse of the procedure.[1,2,12,30,45–48] If patients can take deep breaths without the IS device, encourage them to do so at regular intervals. Deep breathing, coughing, and incentive spirometry, work best as shared tasks among all the patient care personnel in the surgical units and wards, with each individual providing frequent reminders to the patients.

Need assessment for IS should focus on factors including surgical procedures involving the upper abdomen or thorax, conditions predisposing to development of atelectasis (eg, immobility, poor pain control, and abdominal binders), and presence of neuromuscular disease involving respiratory musculature.[44] Outcome assessment should include absence of or improvement in signs of atelectasis (eg, decreased respiratory rate, improved breath sounds, normal chest radiograph, and improved PaO_2 and $P(A-a)O_2$). For the surgical patient, increased VC, peak expiratory flows, and return of functional residual capacity (FRC) or VC to preoperative values (in absence of lung resection) represent positive clinical outcomes. Improved inspiratory muscle performance and increased forced vital capacity (FVC) are desirable outcomes for patients with restrictive and neuromuscular problems.[44] (See AARC Clinical Practice Guidelines: Incentive Spirometry[11] for a summary of assessment.)

AARC Clinical Practice Guideline

INCENTIVE SPIROMETRY

Indications: Presence of conditions predisposing to the development of pulmonary atelectasis (upper abdominal surgery, thoracic surgery, surgery in patients with chronic obstructive pulmonary disease); presence of pulmonary atelectasis; and presence of a restrictive lung defect associated with quadriplegia or dysfunctional diaphragm.

Contraindications: Patient cannot be instructed or supervised to assure appropriate use of the device; patient cooperation is absent or patient is unable to understand or demonstrate proper use of the device. Incentive spirometry is contraindicated in patients unable to deep breathe effectively (eg, with vital capacity less than about 10 mL/kg or inspiratory capacity less than about one third of predicted). The presence of an open tracheal stoma is not a contraindication but requires adaptation of the spirometer.

Assessment of Need: Surgical procedure involving upper abdomen or thorax; conditions predisposing to development of atelectasis including immobility, poor pain control, and abdominal binders; and presence of neuromuscular disease involving respiratory musculature.

Assessment of Outcome: Absence of or improvement in signs of atelectasis, decreased respiratory rate, resolution of fever, normal pulse rate, absent crackles (rales) or presence of or improvement in previously absent or diminished breath sounds, normal chest x-ray, improved arterial oxygen tension (PaO_2) and decreased alveolar–arterial oxygen tension gradient, increased vital capacity and peak expiratory flows, return of functional residual capacity or vital capacity to preoperative values in absence of lung resection, improved inspiratory muscle performance, attainment of preoperative flow and volume levels, and increased forced vital capacity.

Monitoring: Direct supervision of every patient performance is not necessary once the patient has demonstrated mastery of technique. However, preoperative instruction, volume goals, and feedback are essential to optimal performance. Observation of patient performance and utilization: frequency of sessions, number of breaths/session, inspiratory volume or flow goals achieved and 3- to 5-second breath-hold maintained, effort/motivation, periodic observation of patient compliance with technique, with additional instruction as necessary, device within reach of patient and patient encouraged to perform independently, new and increasing inspiratory volumes established each day, and vital signs.

(From AARC Clinical Practice Guideline: For complete text see Respir Care 36:1402–1405, 1991.)

Incentive Spirometry Equipment

The original Bartlett-Edwards incentive spirometer (McGraw) was a *volume displacement* device (Fig. 18-1A). A piston-like plate rises as the patient inspires, and an indicator estimates the volume inspired while a battery-powered light flashes after a present volume goal is achieved. Other concepts in volume displacement in-

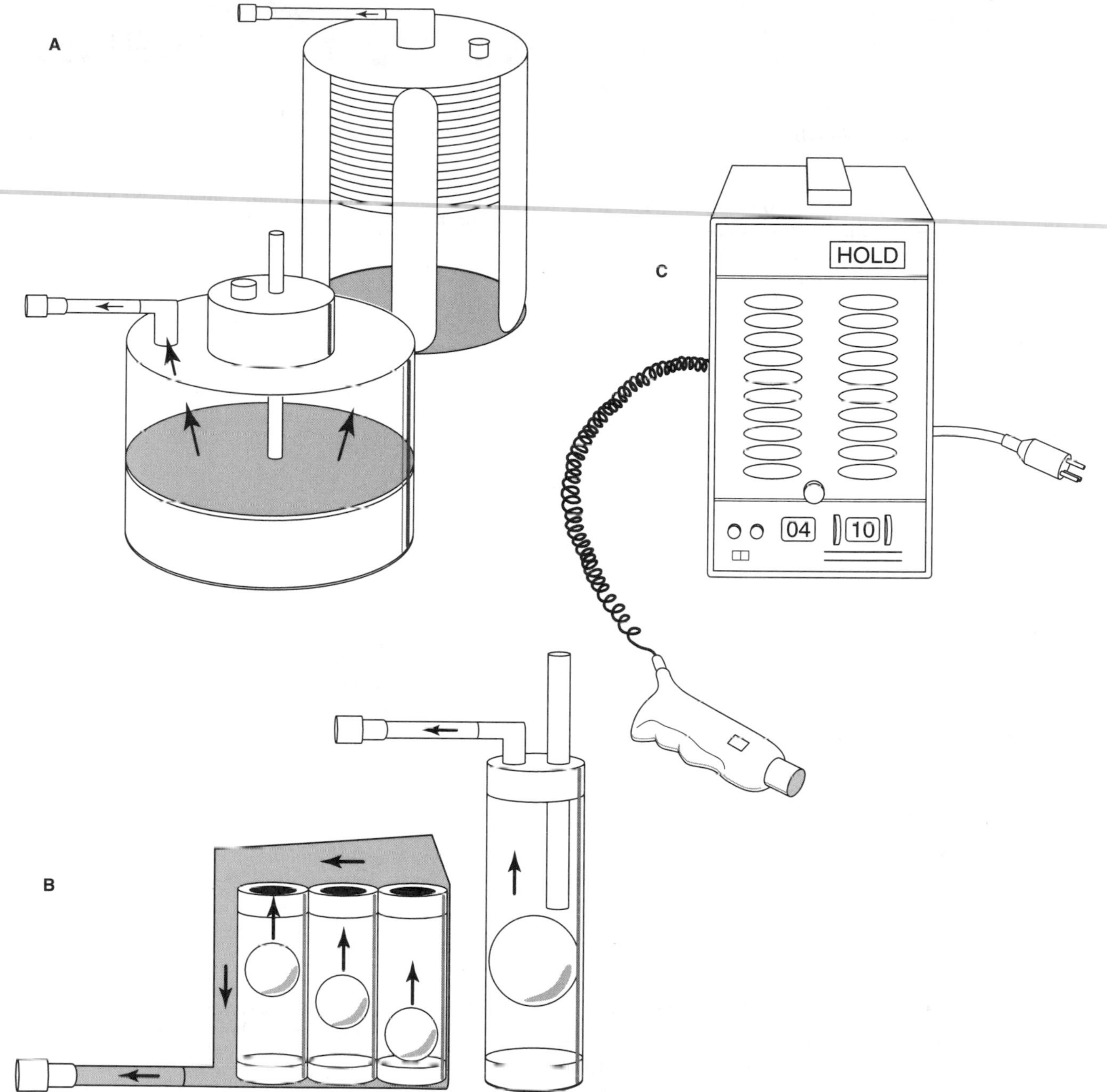

FIGURE 18-1. Three types of incentive spirometers. **(A)** volume displacement, **(B)** flow-based and **(C)** electronic pneumotachygraph.

clude a cylindrical bellows that is displaced upwards as the patient breathes in, with a scale on the side of the container with markers to indicate volume goals. These units do not record attempts or achieved goals and tend to be rather bulky, requiring a lot of space at the patient bedside and on the hospital supply shelves. The volumetric incentive spirometer combines a quasi volume displacement indicator (takes less space) and flow indicator (to encourage slow inspirations).

The other design of IS device is the *flow-oriented incentive device* (Fig. 18-1B). Although the underlying premise of IS is taking deep breaths with an inspiratory hold, a large number of institutions have adopted IS flow-oriented devices for space and cost reasons. These devices usually direct the patient's inspiratory flow through a tube to lift one or more light balls (or disks). The higher the patient's inspiratory flow rate, the greater number of balls that are raised. The longer the flow is maintained, the larger the volume, so the patient is encouraged to take deep, slow breaths. Unfortunately, high flows can be generated (with low volumes) to raise the flow indicator to target levels without the patient meeting therapeutic volume or breath-holding objectives. Although flow-oriented IS devices impose an additional work of breathing ranging from 0.33 to 0.66 J/L,[45] it is unclear whether this additional workload is deleterious or part of the therapy. Successful use of these IS devices depends on effective patient education and compliance.

Another type of flow-based IS device uses a flow pneumotachygraph to compute volumes based on flow and time (Fig. 18-1C). Increasing inhaled volumes results in lights on a scale ascending toward the level of a light on a parallel scale indicating the volume goal. When the goal is reached, a light goes on and stays on during the time that the patient should be holding his or her breath. Two digital counters indicate the number of attempts and number of times volume goal was achieved.

Lederer et al[46] compared the Bartlett Edwards Incentive Spirometer®, the Triflo II®, and the Spirocare® in 79 patients divided into three groups. Patients were instructed preoperatively to take deep breaths (from resting volume, with 2- to 3-second hold 10 times each hour while awake) with repeat instruction daily for 5 postoperative days. They concluded that when left at the bedside with only one daily reinforcement of instructions, the three devices showed no clinically important differences. It is not known whether a clinical difference would exist with more frequent coaching. Certainly a reduced frequency of use does not improve the relative efficacy of these devices.[47]

Independent of device, a number of researchers have demonstrated that IS is comparable in therapeutic effect to deep breathing exercises,[48,49] coughing,[50] early mobilization,[51] and IPPB[48] in the postoperative patient. Hall et al[52] demonstrated IS to be comparable to chest physical therapy after abdominal surgery,[52] while mounting evidence suggests that IS may not have a viable role in thoracic surgery for patients with healthy lungs.[49,50,53] Box 18-5 identifies key points in the IS administration.

BOX 18-5

PROCEDURES FOR INCENTIVE SPIROMETRY

1. Gather equipment.
2. Explain to the patient that taking deep breaths and coughing will keep the lungs expanded and that using the incentive spirometer will show them how big a breath is being taken, with the goal of returning to their normal volumes before surgery. Warn patients that taking deep breaths and coughing may be painful after surgery, but that deep breathing is essential for speedy recovery.
3. When possible, determine the patient's maximum lung volume achieved before surgery (or illness) and use that volume as the volume goal for incentive spirometry. If unable to assess preoperative volumes, set volume goal of 15 to 25 mL/kg of ideal body weight as a minimum, with their predicted VC as a maximum.
4. Assist the patient to a sitting position, or to a semi-Fowler's position.
5. Instruct or assist the patient to splint incision when appropriate.
6. Introduce the patient to the incentive spirometer, describing how it works per manufacturer's instruction. Instruct patient to:
   - (a) Place the spirometer on a flat surface or hold in an upright position.
   - (b) Place lips firmly around the mouthpiece.
   - (c) After a normal exhalation, inhale slowly through the mouthpiece, raising the volume indicator, taking as deep a breath as possible.
   - (d) Hold breath for 3 to 5 seconds.
   - (e) Remove mouthpiece and exhale normally (or through pursed lips).
   - (f) Relax and breathe normally for several breaths.
   - (g) Repeat the maneuver to a total of 10 breaths each session (encourage the patient to take progressively deeper breaths up to the maximum goal).
   - (h) Repeat series of breaths once each hour while awake.
7. Observe the patient's color, heart rate, respiratory rate, and degree of dyspnea before, during, and after the treatment. Care should be taken to avoid fatigue or dizziness.
8. Document procedures performed (including volume goals set, volume achieved, breaths per session and frequency), patient response and patient education in the patient medical record. Also document the ability of the patient to perform the maneuver without coaching.
9. Visit patient postoperatively to reinforce instruction and adjust volume goals as appropriate. Communicate with patient and nursing staff to determine compliance with self-administration; reassess or instruct as necessary.

Intermittent Positive Pressure Breathing

Intermittent positive pressure breathing (IPPB) is short-term or intermittent mechanical ventilation for the primary purpose of assisting ventilation and providing short duration *hyperinflation therapy*.[10] Although IPPB has historically been administered with a variety of pneumatically driven, pressure-triggered, and pressure-limited ventilators (often with significant inspiratory flow rate limitation capabilities), volume, pressure, time-limited, or flow-cycled ventilators may be used in the treatment of spontaneously breathing patients, with or without artificial airways.

In the 1950s, the use of IPPB began to gain popularity as a method to treat and later prevent postoperative atelectasis and other lung problems. Its use corresponded with a perceived decrease in postoperative nosocomial pneumonia in surgical patients across the country, but support for the use of IPPB was more anecdotal than empirically based. The 1960s became the decade of the "puffing parlor," outpatient areas where multiple patients with COPD and other disorders would come to receive their IPPB treatment with aerosol medications. In 1974, participants at the Sugarloaf Conference investigating the scientific basis for respiratory care concluded that there was little scientific basis for the use of IPPB.[5] This was soon followed by members of the U.S. Congress questioning the huge annual Medicare expenditure for IPPB therapy nationwide in light of the lack of evidence to support its use. IPPB soon became the "treatment non grata" of respiratory care departments, and the use of IPPB was abolished in many institutions.[7]

IPPB has been advocated as a method for administration of aerosolized medication, but has not been shown to provide any therapeutic advantage over the use of nebulizers or metered-dose inhalers for spontaneously breathing patients.[10] In fact, Dolovich et al[54] demonstrated that nebulized medication administered with IPPB results in 32% less drug deposited in the lung than spontaneous breathing with the same type of nebulizer. Consequently, IPPB should not be used for lung expansion or aerosol administration in spontaneously breathing patients when less expensive and less invasive therapies can reliably meet clinical objectives. A summary of indications, contraindications, hazards/complications, and assessment of IPPB can be found in AARC Clinical Practice Guidelines: Intermittent Positive Pressure Breathing.[10]

There are limitations of both the procedure and the devices. All of the mechanical effects of IPPB are short-lived, lasting an hour or less after the treatment. Efficacy of an IPPB device for ventilation and aerosol delivery is technique dependent (eg, coordination, breathing pattern, selection of appropriate inspiratory flow, peak pressure, and inspiratory hold). Efficacy is dependent on the design of the device (eg, flow, volume, pressure capability, aerosol output, and particle size).[47]

IPPB Equipment

IPPB may be provided with any device with assist mode or pressure-support: volume-, pressure-, or time-limited ventilator or manual resuscitation device. Manufacturers provide specific IPPB units for hospital (Fig. 18-2A & B) and home application (Fig. 18-2C). The basic IPPB machine functions (only) to assist the patient after he or she triggers inspiratory flow by creating a subatmospheric pressure at the mask or mouthpiece. However, some IPPB machines are equipped with inspiratory/expiratory timing devices so a controlled rate may be selected for short-term ventilation (eg, Bird MK-7 and Puritan-Bennett PR series).

Figure 18-3 illustrates airway pressure versus time for an IPPB breathing cycle. Following a subatmospheric deflection of the patients inspiratory trigger, flow begins and pressure increases until a preset level is reached. Common problems involve a leak in the patient-IPPB system, which prevents the device from either sensing inspiratory trigger, or cycling off at targeted pressure level that will produce volume expansion.

IPPB has not been shown to offer long-term or short-term benefit greater than other lung expansion therapeutic options in spontaneously breathing patients.[55–57] Like other lung expansion therapies, IPPB has been associated with increased work of breathing.[58] Its use for lung expansion should be considered only after all less invasive and expensive alternatives have been exhausted.[10] This should not be confused with the role of IPPB in the treatment of hypoventilation, as a form of noninvasive mechanical ventilation.[59–61]

AARC Clinical Practice Guideline

INTERMITTENT POSITIVE PRESSURE BREATHING

Indications: The need to improve lung expansion; the need for short-term ventilatory support for patients who are hyperventilated as an alternative to tracheal intubation and continuous ventilatory support; and the need to deliver aerosol medication.

Contraindications: Although no absolute contraindications to the use of IPPB therapy (except the oft-cited tension pneumothorax) have been reported, the patient with any of the following should be carefully evaluated before a decision is made to initiate IPPB therapy: intracranial pressure (ICP) > 20 mmHg; hemodynamic instability; recent facial, oral, or skull surgery; tracheoesophageal fistula; recent esophageal surgery; active hemoptysis; nausea; air swallowing; active untreated tuberculosis; radiographic evidence of bleb; and singulation (hiccups).

Asessment of Need: Presence of atelectasis; neuromuscular disorders or kyphoscoliosis with associated decreases in lung volumes and capacities; fatigue or muscle weakness with impending respiratory failure; presence of acute severe bronchospasm or exacerbated COPD that fails to respond to other therapy; with demonstrated effectiveness, the patient's preference for a positive pressure device should be honored.

Assessment of Outcome: Tidal volume during IPPB greater than during spontaneous breathing (by at least 25%); FEV_1 or peak flow increase; cough more effective with treatment; secretion clearance enhanced as a consequence of deep breathing and coughing; chest x-ray improved; breath sounds improved; and favorable patient subjective response.

Monitoring: Performance of machine trigger sensitivity, peak pressure, flow setting, FIO_2 inspiratory time, expiratory time; respiratory rate and volume; peak flow or FEV_1/FVC; pulse rate and rhythm from EKG if available; patient subjective response to therapy—pain, discomfort, dyspnea, sputum production—quantity, color, consistency, and odor; mental function; skin color; breath sounds; blood pressure; arterial hemoglobin saturation by pulse oximetry (if hypoxemia is suspected); ICP in patients for whom it is of critical importance; and chest radiograph.

(From AARC Clinical Practice Guideline: For complete text see Respir Care 38:1189–1195, 1993.)

POSITIVE AIRWAY PRESSURE

Positive airway pressure (PAP), as defined by the AARC Clinical Practice Guideline,[9] includes continuous positive airway pressure (CPAP), positive expiratory pres-

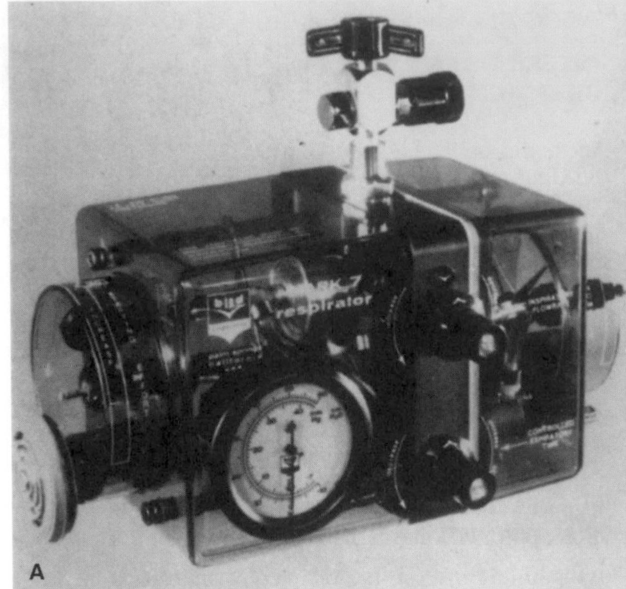

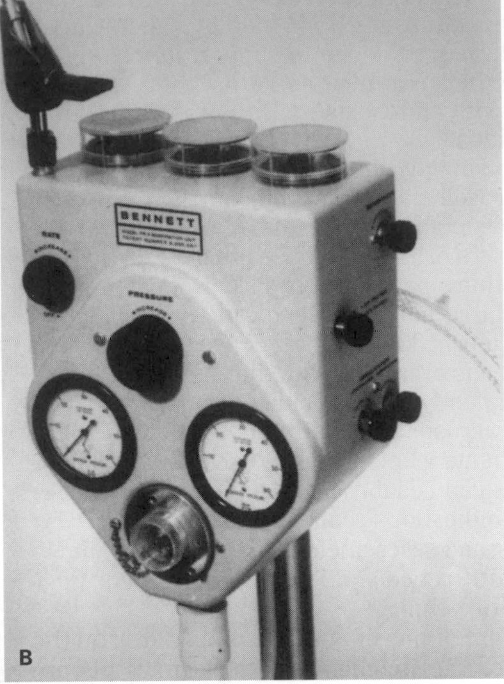

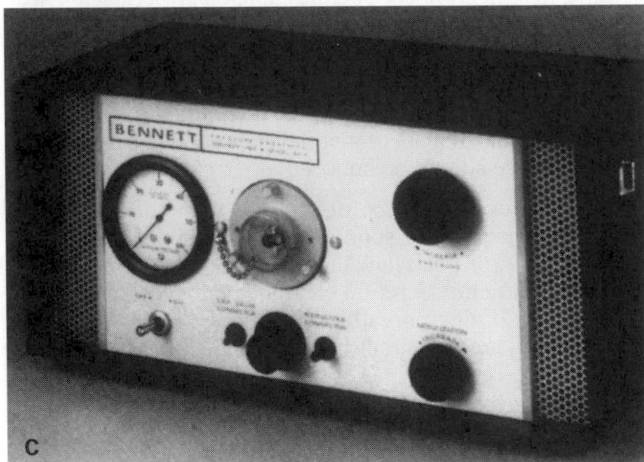

FIGURE 18-2. IPPB devices **(A)** Bird Mk-7 (Courtesy of Bird Corporation, Palm Springs, CA) [See Branson, Fig. 12-25], **(B)** Puritan-Bennett PR-1. (Courtesy of Puritan-Bennett Corporation, Kansas City, MO), **(C)** Puritan-Bennett AP-5. (Courtesy of Puritan-Bennett Corporation, Kansas City, MO).

sure (PEP), and expiratory positive airway pressure (EPAP) used to mobilize secretions and treat atelectasis. PAP bronchial hygiene techniques have proven to provide effective alternatives to chest physical therapy in expanding the lungs and mobilizing secretions. Evidence suggests that PAP therapy is more effective than incentive spirometry and IPPB in the management of postoperative atelectasis,[61–63] and as an adjunct to enhance the benefits of aerosol bronchodilator delivery.[64,65] Cough and other airway clearance techniques are essential components of PAP therapy.

CPAP is the application of a PAP to the spontaneously breathing patient during both inspiration and expiration. The patient breathes from a pressurized circuit with a *threshold resistor* (TR) on the expiratory limb of the breathing. CPAP maintains a consistent airway pressure (from 5 to 20 cmH_2O) throughout the respiratory cycle. CPAP requires a relatively high gas flow available to the patient's airway sufficient to maintain the desired PAP. *EPAP* applies positive pressure to the airway, much like CPAP, but only during expiration. During inspiration, patients with EPAP generate subatmospheric pressures and exhale against a threshold resistor, generating preset pressures of 5 to 20 cmH_2O (Fig. 18-4).

PEP consists of positive pressure generated as a patient exhales through a *fixed orifice resistor* generating pressures ranging from 10 to 20 cmH_2O (although pressures up to 60 cmH_2O have been reported). The fixed orifice resistor (which differentiates PEP from EPAP) only generates pressure when expired flows are high enough to generate pressure because of downstream resistance of the small orifice (Fig. 18-5). EPAP, using a threshold resistor, does not produce the same mechanical or physiologic effects that PEP does with a fixed orifice. Further study is required to determine how these differences affect clinical outcome.

In theory, threshold resistors exert a predictable, quantifiable, and constant force at the expiratory limb

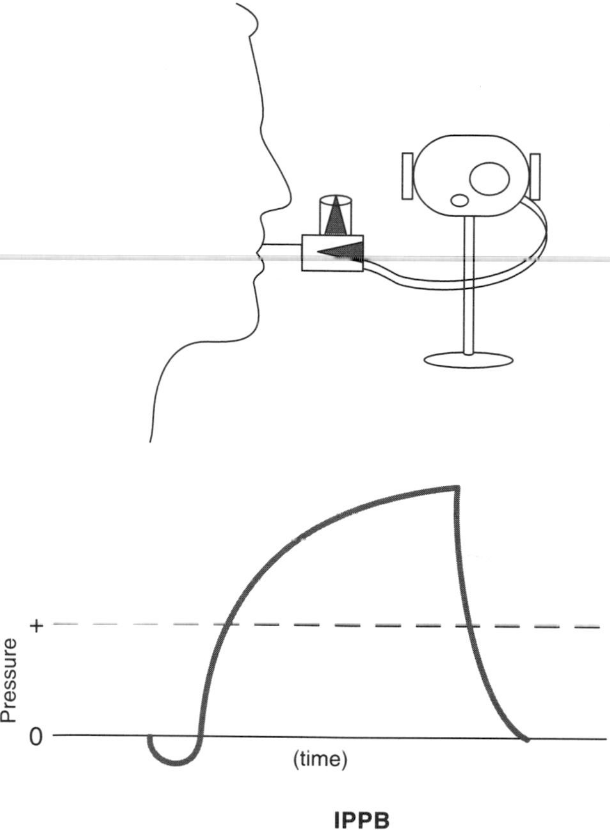

FIGURE 18-3. Airway pressure versus time tracing of intermittent positive pressure breathing (IPPB).

of a circuit. When the force is applied over a unit area, a constant threshold pressure is established. A pressure exceeding threshold opens the valve and allows expiration, while pressures below threshold close the valve, stopping the flow of gas. A true threshold resistor will maintain constant pressure in the circuit, independent of changing flow rates. Relatively few CPAP devices are *true* threshold resistors, in that they offer flow-dependent resistance once the valve is open so that pressure varies secondary to changes in flow rates, resulting in increased resistance and work of breathing.

Resistors vary in their physics and design. In *underwater seal* resistors, the expiratory limb of the circuit is submerged under water. The height of the water above the terminal end of the expiratory limb (cmH_2O) corresponds to the threshold pressure generated (Fig. 18-6A). In *water column resistors*, threshold pressure is generated from a column of water above a diaphragm directly above the expiratory limb of the circuit. Pressure in the circuit must be greater than the pressure of the water to raise the diaphragm and allow gas to exit. In this device, threshold pressure is a product of water column height and the surface area of the diaphragm. In *weighted ball* resistors, a precision ground ball of a specific weight sets above a calibrated orifice immediately above the expiratory limb of the circuit, in a housing with expiratory ports. (Fig. 18-6B). If the diameter of the orifice is not the narrowest point in the expiratory limb of the circuit, the weight of the ball determines the threshold pressure. Weighted ball systems require

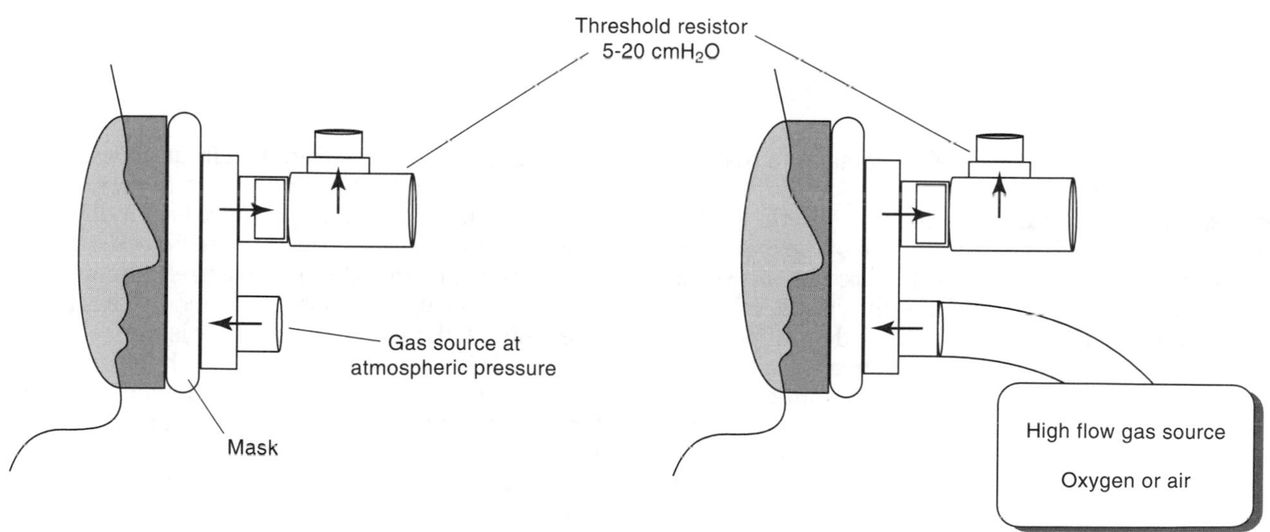

FIGURE 18-4. Diagram differentiating EPAP and CPAP systems. With EPAP, the inspiratory gas is at ambient pressure level. CPAP requires a high-flow gas source sufficient to maintain the desired airway pressure during inspiration.

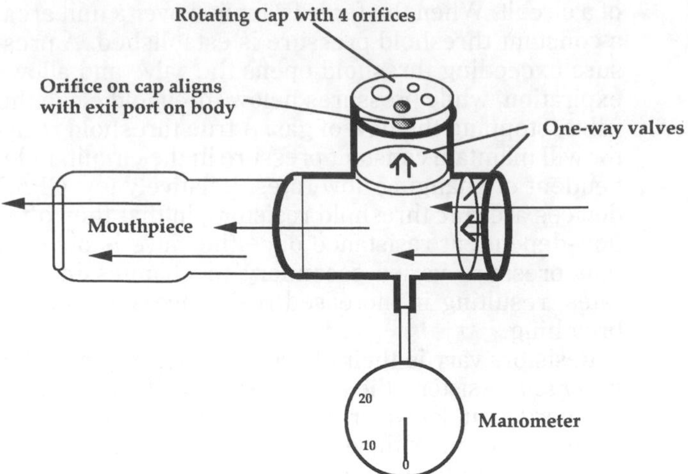

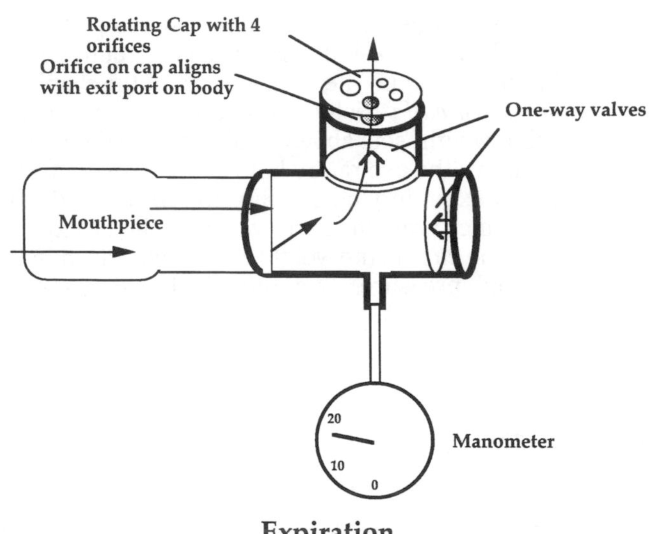

FIGURE 18-5. Diagram of Resistex® fixed orifice type resistor. On inspiration (*top*), gas enters through a one-way valve. During exhalation (*bottom*), gas is diverted through one of four orifices aligned with the exit port of the valve. A manometer may be attached to measure expiratory pressure levels.

meticulous attention to vertical orientation to maintain consistent pressures.

In *spring-loaded valve resistors*, a spring holds a disc or diaphragm down over the end of the expiratory limb of the circuit (Fig. 18-6C). Force of the spring must be overcome for gas to leave the circuit. Function of the spring-loaded valve is independent of position. In *magnetic valve resistors*, a bar magnet attracts a ferro magnetic disc to seat on the outlet orifice. As pressure exceeds the attraction of the magnet, the disc is displaced, allowing gas to exit the circuit. The greater the distance between the magnet and the disk, the lower the pressure required for gas to leave the circuit.

In *fixed orifice resistors*, a restricted opening of a fixed size is placed at the end of the expiratory limb of a breathing circuit (Fig. 18-6D). As gas reaches the restricted orifice, turbulence and airway resistance result in increased pressure within the circuit. For any given gas flow, the smaller the orifice, the higher the pressure generated. Expiratory pressure is flow dependent, so as flow decreases, pressure decreases. With this device there is no "threshold" pressure to be overcome before gas can exit the system. In fact, there is no pressure generated until expiratory flow is high enough to create turbulence upon exiting through the orifice. The fixed orifice resistor has long been a mainstay for producing CPAP (eg, the Gregory CPAP using a clamp to restrict the tail piece of a bag) for infants, but was considered to be less than desirable in the adult population, owing to the high pressure that might be generated with changing flows (ie, coughing). In reality, it appears that the pressures generated with the fixed orifice resistor during a cough are of no greater consequence than the normal cough with glottis closed. Figure 18-7 illustrates the differences in PAP devices by

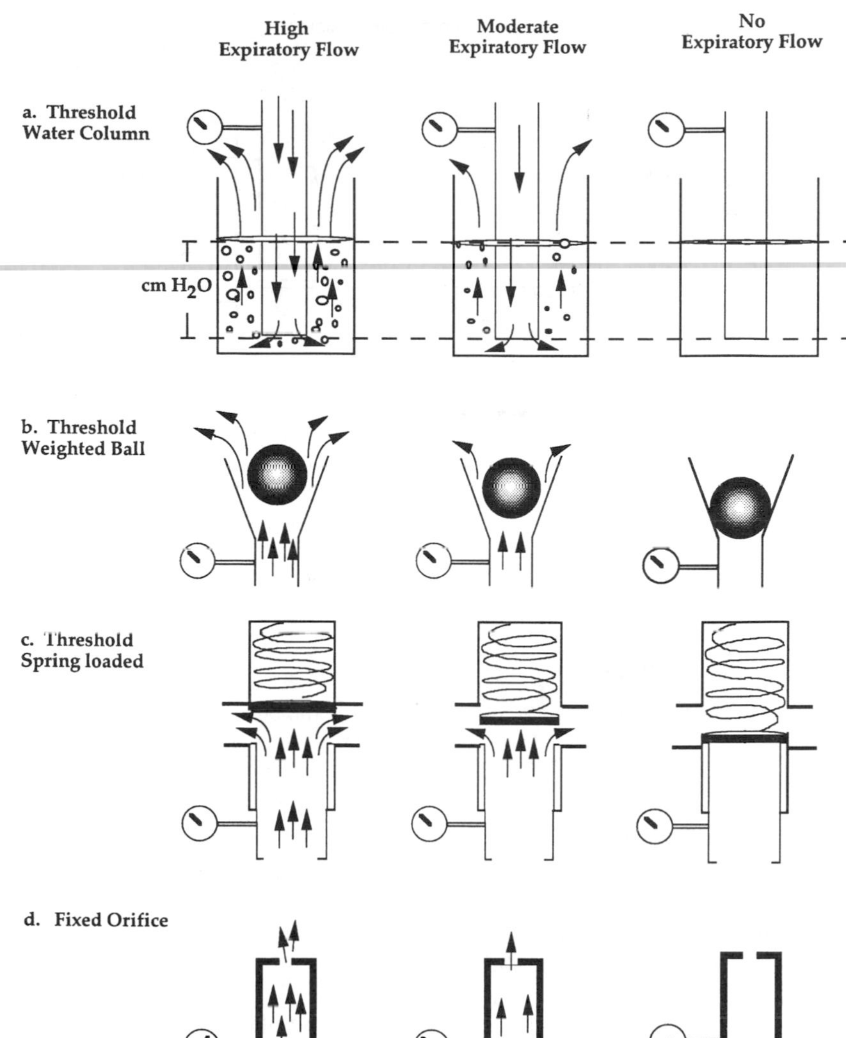

FIGURE 18-6. Four types of resistors used in positive airway pressure (PAP) devices. **(A)** water column, **(B)** weighted ball, **(C)** spring-loaded valve, and **(D)** fixed-resistor. Only the fixed orifice resistor **(D)** develops less pressure with reduced flow, and no pressure with no gas flow.

plotting the airway/mask PAP versus time during a breathing cycle.

Rationale for PAP

Pursed-lips breathing is a simple procedure that many patients with chronic obstructive lung disease have taught themselves to relieve air trapping caused by collapse of unstable airways during expiration. It is believed that the resistance at the mouth during a pursed-lips exhalation transmits back pressure to splint the airways open, preventing compression and premature closure (much like the fixed orifice resistor).[68,69] As an instinctive adaptation to disease, pursed-lips breathing represents a functional predecessor to many of our modern strategies of applying PEP to the airway.

In 1936, Poulton and Odon[70] described the use of the positive pressure mask for the treatment of congestive heart failure and cardiogenic pulmonary edema. One year later, Barach et al[71] reported the use of "continuous positive pressure breathing" (CPPB) by mask in patients suffering from respiratory obstruction and pulmonary edema. At that time, the positive pressure mask did not find application for the treatment or prophylaxis for postoperative pulmonary complications. Thirty years later, Cheney et al[72] described improvements in PaO_2 following the application of expiratory resistance in anesthetized patients on mechanical ventilation and speculated that this was caused by reversing alveolar collapse. In the late 1960s, articles by Ashbaugh et al[73] established the concept of positive end-expiratory pressure (PEEP) as a technique to improve oxygenation in acute respiratory failure and adult respiratory distress syndrome (ARDS). In 1971, Gregory et al[74] reported a significant reduction in mortality when CPAP was used to treat respiratory distress syndrome of the neonate, leading to its widespread application in the newborn population.

Further research[75–77] established that PEEP and CPAP can be effective in reducing the alveolar–arterial oxygen difference ($P(A-a)O_2$), and right-to-left intrapulmonary shunt (Qs/Qt), and increasing (FRC) in the intubated patient with acute respiratory failure (ARF)

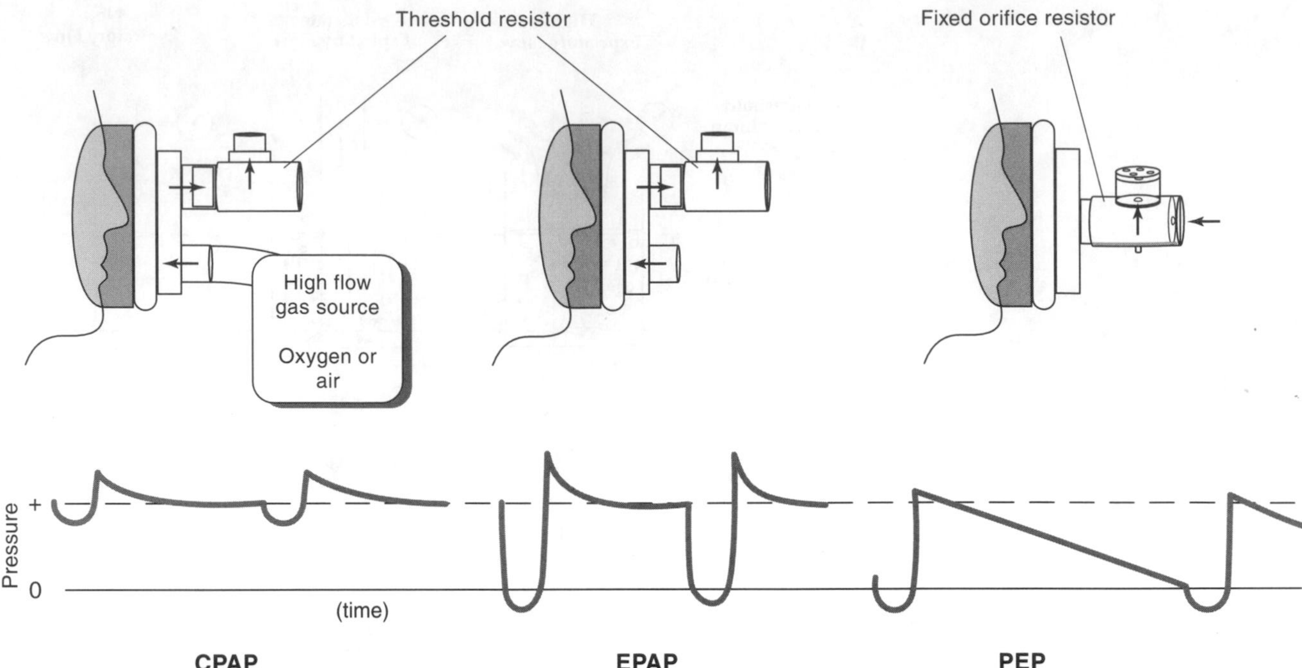

FIGURE 18-7. Comparison of three common methods of PAP with typical pressure versus time waveforms. CPAP consists of inspiration with a 1–2 cmH_2O pressure below baseline level and exhalation at the desired pressure threshold. EPAP and PEP show inspiratory pressures of 1–2 cmH_2O below ambient pressure. During exhalation both CPAP and EPAP generate a short pressure spike above baseline pressure, as exhaled gas overcomes inertia of opening the threshold resistor. The PEP valve generates highest pressure with beginning of expiration and decreases as expiratory flow decelerates towards ambient level.

with or without mechanical ventilation. In 1979, Andersen et al[78] showed that re-inflation of collapsed excised human lungs could be accomplished with CPAP by mechanisms involving collateral ventilation and noted that CPAP "has a potential secretion clearing effect in that pressure is built distal to an obstruction." The following year, Andersen and Jespersen[79] made castings of human lungs, identified communications between intersegmental respiratory bronchioles, and concluded that collateral ventilation might be important in normal lung function.

The prophylactic and therapeutic uses of CPAP and PEEP in nonintubated patients did not receive much attention until the early 1980s.[80,81] In 1980, Andersen et al[82] conducted a prospective, randomized, controlled clinical trial using a sequential analysis design to determine the effect of conventional therapy versus conventional therapy plus periodic CPAP by mask in the treatment of 24 surgical patients with atelectasis. CPAP was given each hour for 25 to 35 breaths with a pressure averaging 15 cmH_2O. At 12 hours, patients in the CPAP group exhibited significantly greater improvement (PaO_2 and radiographic findings) compared with the control group. This study prompted Pontoppidan et al[83] to consider periodic CPAP for treating postoperative pulmonary complications. Several studies during the early 1980s explored the application of PEEP and CPAP to nonintubated patients in different fashions with varying results,[2,84–89] including comparisons of mask CPAP to incentive spirometry, deep breathing and coughing, and IPPB. As more effective strategies were developed, Stock et al[88,89] concluded that intermittent mask CPAP was as effective as incentive spirometry or deep breathing and coughing in return of pulmonary function following thoracic or upper abdominal surgery. Additionally, the authors suggested that mask CPAP might be preferable, as it represented a more effortless, painless type of postoperative respiratory care.

Ricksten et al[63] performed a randomized comparative study of 43 upper-abdominal-surgery patients that looked at postoperative complications, $P(A-a)O_2$, PEF, and FVC in patients using either CPAP or PEP against a control group using incentive spirometry. All three groups took 30 breaths each hour while awake for 3 days postoperatively. Although peak flow did not change between groups, FVC was greater in the CPAP and PEP groups. $P(A-a)O_2$ increased uniformly for all groups for the first 24 hours, but then decreased in the CPAP and PEP groups (being insignificantly lower in the PEP group). Atelectasis was observed in 6 of 15 patients in the control group, 1 of 13 in the CPAP group, and 0 of 15 in the PEP group. The authors concluded that periodic PEP and CPAP are superior to deep-breathing exercises with respect to gas exchange, preservation of lung volumes, and prevention of postoperative atelectasis following upper abdominal surgery. They also concluded that "the simple and commercially available PEP mask is as effective as the more complicated CPAP system." A simple PEP system as described earlier certainly represents a cost savings over the use of a more complex CPAP system, which requires pressure monitor, oxygen analyzer, and gas flow that will not change FIO_2 in response to changes in downstream resistance.

Lindner et al,[90] in a randomized study of 34 upper-abdominal–surgery patients, compared postoperative physiotherapy with postoperative physiotherapy plus mask CPAP. Their findings indicated that the group treated with physiotherapy plus CPAP had a more rapid recovery of vital capacity and FRC with fewer pulmonary complications. Campbell et al[91] randomized 71 abdominal surgery patients into group 1 (breathing exercises and huff coughing) and group 2 (same as group 1 plus PAP using a water column threshold resistor adjusted to produce pressures of 5 to 15 cmH_2O with the patient exhaling through a mouthpiece). Differences in pulmonary function between the two groups, with incidence of respiratory complications of 31% in group 1 and 22% in group 2, were not statistically significant. The authors concluded that PEP could serve as an adjunct to routine chest physiotherapy, particularly with postoperative smokers, in that 43% of the smokers in their study developed respiratory complications, compared with none of the nonsmokers ($p < 0.01$).

By preventing expiratory collapse, PEP therapy is thought to facilitate a more homogenous distribution of ventilation throughout the lung, via these collateral inter bronchiolar channels.[67] Groth et al[93] measured lung function from the expiratory port of the PEP mask (in 12 patients with cystic fibrosis [CF]). They found a significant increase in FRC ($p < 0.02$), decrease in volume of trapped gas ($p < 0.05$), and decrease of washout volume ($p < 0.05$), compared with pretreatment measurements. The group concluded that changes were attributed to an improvement in the distribution of ventilation (more evenly within the lung) and the opening up of airways otherwise closed off during normal ventilation.

Because the patient must breathe down to subatmospheric pressures on inspiration, both EPAP and PEP are believed to require a higher work of breathing than CPAP. Van der Schans et al[94] examined the effect of EPAP with 5 cmH_2O using a threshold resistor (Vital Signs) in 8 COPD patients measuring work of breathing and myoelectrical activity of the scalene, parasternal, and abdominal muscles. During EPAP breathing at rest mean (SEM) work increased from 0.54 to 1.08 J/L. Expired minute volume decreased from 12.4 to 10.5 L/min, VD/VT decreased from 0.39 to 0.34. Phasic respiratory muscle activity was increased with EPAP. Dyspnea sensation during exercise test was higher than during the test with undisturbed breathing.

Indications, contraindications, hazards/complications, assessment of need, and outcome for PAP therapy can be found in AARC Clinical Practice Guideline: Use of Positive Airway Pressure Adjuncts to Bronchial Hygiene Therapy.

Limitations of PAP Therapy

PAP therapies for bronchial hygiene require spontaneously breathing patients. The level of cooperation depends on the device being used. CPAP and EPAP appear to require little or no patient coordination to be effective. In contrast, PEP works best when used by conscious cooperative patients. CPAP is an equipment-intensive procedure requiring an external gas source or compressor that will work in the face of back pressure and considerable training of personnel for proper setup and maintenance. These factors make CPAP more expensive and less portable than other PAP alternatives.

Procedure of Providing PEP Therapy

PEP therapy is performed with the subject seated comfortably, with elbows resting on a table. Equipment consists of a soft, transparent hand ventilation mask or mouthpiece, T-assembly with a one-way valve, a variety of fixed orifice resistors (or adjustable expiratory resistor), and a manometer. The mask is applied tightly but comfortably over the mouth and nose. The subject is instructed to relax while performing diaphragmatic breathing, inspiring a volume of air larger than normal tidal volume but not to total lung capacity, through the one-way valve. Exhalation to FRC is active but not forced through the resistor chosen to achieve a PAP between 10 and 20 cmH_2O (0.98 to 1.96 kPa) during exhalation.

A series of 10 to 20 breaths is performed with the mask or mouthpiece in place. The mask (or mouthpiece) is then removed, and the individual performs several coughs to raise secretions. This sequence of 10 to 20 PAP breaths, followed by huff coughing, is repeated 4 to 6 times per PEP therapy session. Each session for bronchial hygiene takes from 10 to 20 minutes, and may be performed one to four times per day as needed. For lung expansion, patients should be encouraged to take 10 to 20 breaths every hour while awake, and as needed.

Considerations During Therapy

Selection of a resistor with an appropriate orifice size is critical to proper technique. The therapeutic goal of exhalation is to achieve a PEP between 10 and 20 cmH_2O, with an I:E of 1:3 to 1:4. When using a fixed orifice, most adults achieve this pressure range using a flow-restricting orifice between 2.5 and 4.0 mm in diameter. Selection of the proper resistor also produces the desired inspiratory-to-expiratory ratio of 1:3 to 1:4. A manometer is placed in-line to measure the expiratory pressure while selecting the appropriate sized orifice. Once the proper resistor orifice has been determined, the manometer may be removed from the system. Selection of a resistor with too large an orifice produces a short exhalation, with failure to achieve the proper expiratory pressure. Too small an orifice prolongs the expiratory phase, elevates the pressure above 20 cm H_2O,

AARC Clinical Practice Guideline

USE OF POSITIVE AIRWAY PRESSURE ADJUNCTS TO BRONCHIAL HYGIENE THERAPY

Indications: To reduce air trapping in asthma and COPD, to aid in mobilization of retained secretions (in cystic fibrosis and chronic bronchitis), to prevent or reverse atelectasis, and to optimize delivery of bronchodilators in patients receiving bronchial hygiene therapy.

Contraindications: Although no absolute contraindications to the use of positive expiratory pressure (PEP) or continuous positive airway pressure (CPAP) therapy have been reported, the following should be carefully evaluated before a decision is made to initiate this therapy: patients unable to tolerate the increased work of breathing (acute asthma, COPD); intracranial pressure (ICP) >20 mmHg; hemodynamic instability; recent facial, oral, or skull surgery or trauma; acute sinusitis; epistaxis; esophageal surgery; active hemoptysis; nausea; known or suspected tympanic membrane rupture or other middle ear pathology; and untreated pneumothorax.

Assessment of Need: The following should be assessed to establish a need for PAP therapy: sputum retention not responsive to spontaneous or directed coughing; history of pulmonary problems treated successfully with postural drainage therapy; decreased breath sounds or adventitious sounds suggesting secretions in the airway; tachypnea and tachycardia; chest radiograph consistent with atelectasis, mucus plugging, or infiltrates; and deterioration in arterial blood gas values or oxygen saturation.

Assessment of Outcome: ***Change in sputum production:*** if PEP does not increase sputum production in a patient who produces >30 mL/day of sputum without PEP, the continued use of PEP may not be indicated. *Change in breath sounds:* with effective therapy, breath sounds may clear or the movement of secretions into the larger airways may cause an increase in adventitious breath sounds. The increase in adventitious breath sounds is often a marked improvement over diminished breath sounds. Note any effect that coughing may have had on the breath sounds. *Patient subjective response to therapy:* the caregiver should ask the patient how he or she feels before, during, and after therapy. Feelings of pain, discomfort, shortness of breath, dizziness, and nausea should be considered in modifying and stopping therapy. Improved ease of clearing secretions and increased volume of secretions during and after treatments support continuation. *Change in vital signs:* moderate changes in respiratory rate and/or pulse rate are expected. Bradycardia, tachycardia, increasingly irregular pulse, or a drop or dramatic increase in blood pressure are indications for stopping therapy. *Change in chest radiograph:* resolution or improvement of atelectasis and localized infiltrates may be slow or dramatic. *Change in arterial blood gas values or oxygen saturation:* normal oxygenation should return as atelectasis resolves.

Monitoring: Pain, discomfort, dyspnea, response to therapy; pulse rate and cardiac rhythm (if EKG is available); breathing pattern and rate, symmetrical lateral costal expansion, synchronous thoraco-abdominal movement; sputum production (quantity, color, consistency, and odor); mental function; skin color; breath sounds; blood pressure; pulse oximetry (if hypoxemia with procedure has been previously demonstrated or is suspected); blood gas analysis (if indicated); ICP in patients for whom ICP is of critical importance.

(From AARC Clinical Practice Guideline: For complete text see Respir Care, 38:516–521, 1993.)

and increases the work of breathing. Performing a PEP session for more than 20 minutes may lead to fatigue. During periods of exacerbation, individuals are encouraged to increase the frequency with which PEP is performed, rather than extending the length of individual sessions.

The equipment used to provide PAP mask therapy can be easily assembled from available parts in most respiratory care departments. The Food and Drug Administration (FDA) is now allowing manufacturers to market PEP devices with variable orifice resistors. Examples of commercially available fixed orifice resistors include the Resistex (Mercury Medical, Clearwater, FL) (see Fig. 18-5) and TheraPEP (DHD, Medical, Canastota, NY) (Fig. 18-8). Both models currently cost less than $10 and provide multiple fixed orifices to allow pressure adjustment. The TheraPEP valve can be ordered with an optional spring-loaded pressure indicator.

PAP and Aerosol Therapy

Aerosol therapy may be done simultaneously with or just before a PEP session, either by hand-held nebulizer or metered-dose inhaler (MDI). Andersen and Klausen[64] applied face mask PEEP while administering nebulized bronchodilators to eight patients with severe bronchospasm. A randomized crossover design was used, with each patient subjected to two PEEP treatments and two control treatments with zero end-expiratory pressure (ZEEP), at intervals of 3 hours between each treat-

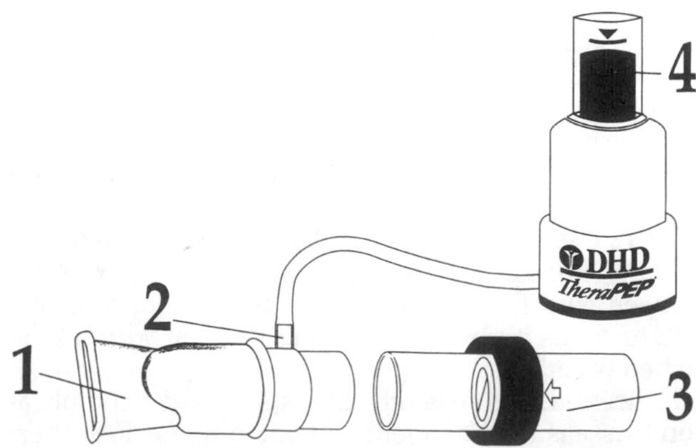

FIGURE 18-8. Diagram of DHD TheraPEP (Diemolding Healthcare Division). **(1)** mouthpiece, **(2)** pressure tap, **(3)** one-way inlet valve and **(4)** spring-loaded pressure device.

ment. FEV_1, FVC, and peak flow improved significantly following PEEP treatments ($p < 0.05$). They concluded that PEEP improved the efficacy of bronchodilator administration, probably mediated through a better distribution to the peripheral airways.

Frischknecht-Christensen et al[65] examined the effect of PEP mask applied in conjunction with β_2 agonists administered via MDI with spacer. In a randomized crossover study, 8 patients alternately received treatments of 2 puffs of terbutaline MDI without PEP, terbutaline MDI with PEP, and placebo MDI with PEP. Results showed statistically significant improvement ($p < 0.0001$) in peak expiratory flow when terbutaline was taken in conjunction with face-mask PEP of 10 to 15 cmH_2O. We described the use of an MDI and chamber-style adapter with the Resistex system (Mercury Medical, Clearwater, FL) (see Fig. 18-6), which accepts a spacer device on the distal inspiratory limb of the PEP assembly.[66,67]

Although no absolute contraindications to the use of PAP therapies have been reported, common sense dictates that patients with acute sinusitis, ear infection, epistaxis, or recent facial, oral, or skull injury or surgery should be carefully evaluated before a decision is made to initiate PEP mask therapy. Patients who are experiencing active hemoptysis or those with unresolved pneumothorax should avoid using PAP therapy until these acute pulmonary problems have resolved. Complications such as barotrauma or hemodynamic compromise are intuitive with the use of positive pressure; no complications have been reported when PEP mask therapy has been used for lung expansion or secretion clearance, in large part owing to the techniques involved in the therapy and the patient population.

In that some authors have used different terms to describe PAP options, Figure 18-4 shows the difference in pressure patterns generated with CPAP, EPAP (threshold resistors), and PEP with fixed orifice resistor. Further studies will be required to better understand the differences in effect of these three modalities. Box 18-6 summarizes the clinical procedure for PAP therapy.

BOX 18-6

PAP CLINICAL PROCEDURE

1. Respiratory care practitioner (RCP) will assess whether PAP therapy is indicated and design a treatment program designed to accomplish treatment objectives.
   (a) RCP will bring equipment to bedside and provide initial therapy to patient, adjusting pressure settings to meet patient need.
   (b) After initial patient treatment and/or training, RCP will communicate treatment plan to physician and nurse, and provide instruction to nursing staff if required.
2. Explain that PAP therapy is used to re-expand lung tissue and help mobilize secretions. Patients should also be taught to perform the "huff" directed-cough procedure.
3. Instruct the patient to:
   (a) Sit comfortably.
   (b) If using a mask, apply it tightly but comfortably over the nose and mouth. If mouthpiece is used, place lips firmly around it and breathe through mouth.
   (c) Take in a breath that is larger than normal, but don't fill lungs completely.
   (d) Exhale actively, but not forcefully, creating a positive airway pressure of 10 to 20 cmH_2O during exhalation (determined with manometer during initial therapy sessions). Length of inhalation should be approximately 1/3 of the total breathing cycle (I:E ratio of 1:3).
   (e) Perform 10 to 20 breaths.
   (f) Remove the mask or mouthpiece and perform two to three "huff" coughs, and rest as needed.
   (g) Repeat above cycle four to eight times, not to exceed 20 minutes.
4. Evaluate the patient for their ability to self-administer.
5. When appropriate, teach patient to self-administer. Observations on several occasions of proper technique uncoached should precede allowing the patient to self-administer without supervision.
6. When patients are also receiving bronchodilator aerosol, administer in conjunction with PAP therapy by placing a holding chamber/MDI or nebulizer at the inspiratory port of the PAP device.
7. When visibly soiled, rinse PAP device with sterile water and shake/air dry, leave within reach at patient bedside in a clear plastic bag.
8. Send the PAP device (if single-patient use) home with the patient or discard it on discharge. If nondisposable, send in-house for high-level disinfection.
9. Document procedures performed (including device, settings used, pressure developed, number of breaths per treatment, and frequency), patient response to therapy, patient teaching provided, and patient ability to self-administer in the patient's medical record.

Blow Bottles

Another procedure in vogue in the 1950s and 1960s was the blow bottle (Fig. 18-9). Two 1-L bottles were connected by a common conduit, with water filling one of the bottles. A tubing and mouth piece came from the top of each bottle. The patient is instructed to take a deep, sustained breath and blow into the tubing on the side of the full bottle, pushing water into the empty bottle.

Cogan et al[95] studied the effects of the Valsalva maneuver and blow bottles and sustained hyperinflation with a Elder Demand Valve Resuscitator. With blow bottles FRC increased significantly ($p = 0.04$) and shunt decreased slightly ($p = 0.07$). Inspiration resulted in airway pressures of -5 cmH_2O (-20 cmH_2O esophageal) with airway pressure rising to 32 cmH_2O (20 cmH_2O esophageal). The authors conclude that the efficacy of blow bottles depends on an initial large and sustained deep breath, with prolonged gradual transfer of water from one bottle to another, and that a single sustained deep breath offers the same favorable transpulmonary gradient that occurs with blow bottles, but some patients

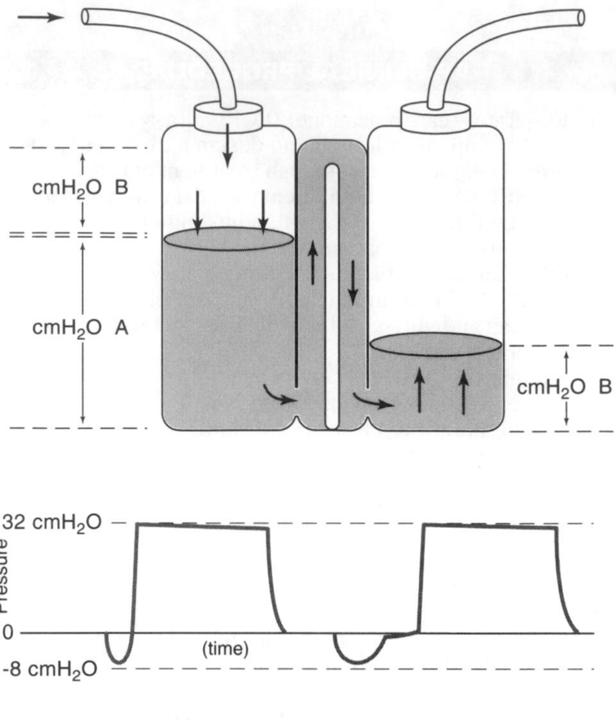

FIGURE 18-9. Blow-bottles (*top*) consisting of two 1 L bottles connected by tubing. Patients are instructed to perform a sustained maximum inspiration with inspiratory hold. Slow exhalation through the mouthpiece of the full bottle pushes water to the opposite bottle. Water in the two bottles act as a threshold resistor; the total pressure being equal to the sum of both heights. The pressure versus time tracing (*bottom-left*) shows incorrect use with sustained inspiration and high expiratory flows. The pressure versus time tracing (*bottom-right*) shows correct use with sustained inspiration and gradual exhalation producing positive expiratory pressure.

may benefit from the challenge offered by transfer of water as evidence of progressing therapy. Iverson et al[96] compared IPPB, IS, and blow bottles in 145 patients following cardiac surgery with 3 to 5 breaths every 3 hours. Pulmonary complications occurred in 30% (IPPB), 15% (IS), and 8% (blow bottles) of the patients in the respective groups ($p = 0.023$), with 20% of the IPPB patients complaining of gastrointestinal side effects.

Blow bottles have been criticized for emphasizing forced exhalation, rather than SMI. The theory is that the overzealous patient, to achieve the goal of moving all of the water from one bottle to the next, may continue forced exhalation beyond closing volume, precipitating airway closure and possibly reducing FRC. Although intuitively attractive, this criticism of blow bottles has taken the form of textbook dogma that has not been substantiated with empiric observation.

In defense of blow bottles, they do act as an expiratory resistor of the threshold variety, which may stabilize airways, splinting them open during a slow expiration (when dynamic compression tends to collapse airways) and improving homogenous emptying of the lung and improving distribution of ventilation. Blow bottles may be yet another valuable respiratory care technique driven to extinction before its time, which could provide real benefit when applied to the appropriate patient population with the proper instructions (ie, don't blow all the way out).

Figure 18-10 provides a summary of the PAP techniques. Typical airway/mask pressures (during both inhalation and exhalation) versus time are compared for the following: CPAP, EPAP, PEP, IPPB, and blow bottle breathing.

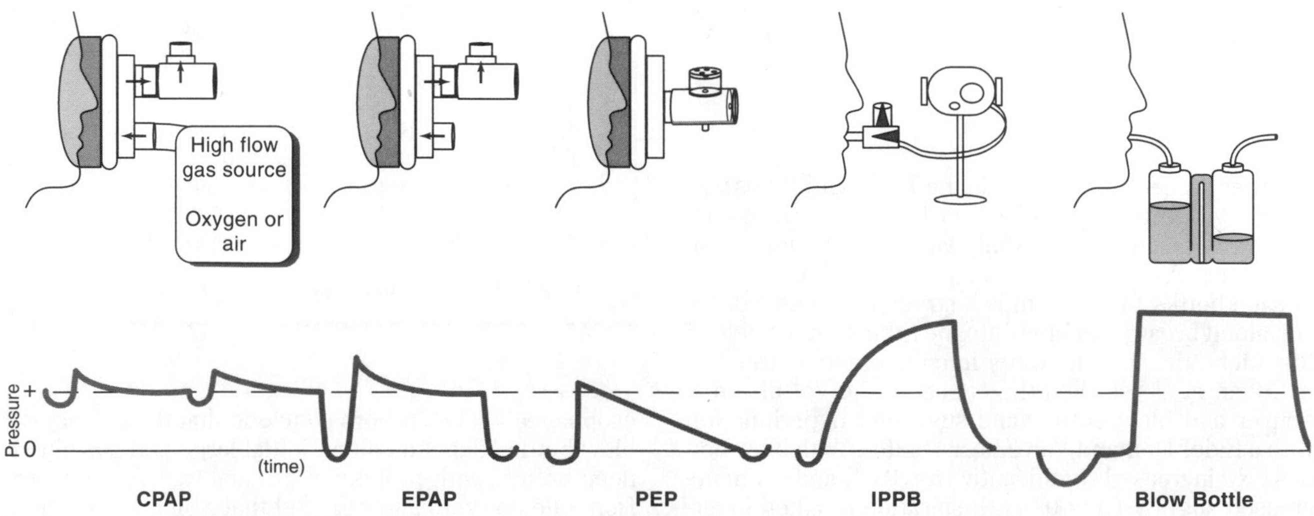

FIGURE 18-10. Airway pressure (during inspiration/exhalation) versus time comparing: CPAP, EPAP, PEP, IPPB, and blow bottles.

HIGH-FREQUENCY AIRWAY OSCILLATION OR INTRAPULMONARY PERCUSSIVE VENTILATION

Flutter Valve®

Developed in Switzerland, the Flutter mucus clearance device (VarioRaw SA, distributed by Scandipharm, Birmingham, AL), combines the techniques of PAP with high-frequency oscillations at the airway opening (HFao). A pipe-shaped device with a steel ball in the "bowl" is loosely covered by a perforated cap (Fig. 18-11). The weight of the ball serves as an EPAP device (at approximately 10 cmH_2O, whereas the internal shape of the bowl allows the ball to flutter, generating oscillations of about 15 Hz. In our laboratory, we found that the Flutter valve generated fluctuations in esophageal pressures quite similar to that generated during use of the ThAIRapy device (described below).

Although the Flutter has been available in Europe for several years, little has been published on its efficacy.[97] In 1994, Konstan et al[98] reported that the amount of sputum expectorated by 18 patients with cystic fibrosis was more than three times the amount expectorated with either voluntary cough (described as vigorous cough every 2 minutes for 15 minutes) or postural drainage (up to 10 positions in 15 minutes). It may be worthwhile to examine the study protocol from a more critical perspective than that of the FDA. Patients with CF and other types of airways obstruction tend to have airways close prematurely during vigorous cough (rather than FET, Huff, or ACB) resulting in trapped gas and secretions. National AARC guidelines suggest that effective postural drainage requires somewhere between 3 and 10 minutes per position[20] so those 10

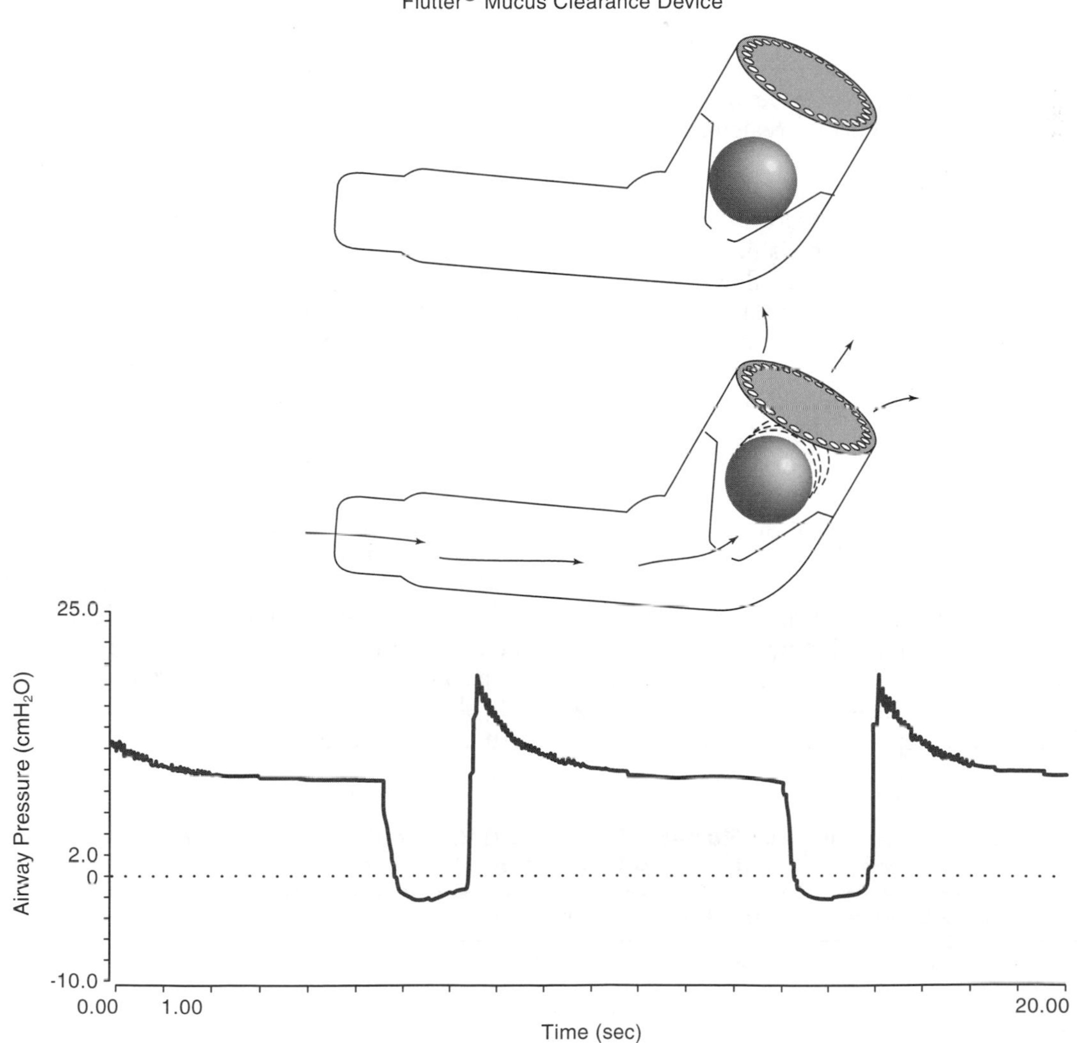

FIGURE 18-11. Diagram of the Flutter® mucus clearance device. A weighted ball seats in a ceramic pipe orifice. Exhalation causes the ball to vibrate as it lifts and reseats in the orifice. The diagram (*below*) traces airway pressure versus time as 0.8L is exhaled with a peak expiratory flow of 40L/min.

drainage positions would require between 30 and 100 minutes to provide effective results. It appears that neither the cough or postural drainage legs of the protocol were designed in light of available research to provide optimal results.

Later in 1994, Pryor et al[99] (who studied 24 patients with CF who averaged >11.9 g of sputum per day using active cycle of breathing as their standard bronchial hygiene), reported that active cycle of breathing alone resulted in significantly more sputum production than 10 minutes of flutter followed by ACB, expressing concern of the possibility of sputum retention when the Flutter was used.

To better understand how this device compares with other PAP devices, our laboratory[100] compared the Flutter valve with both threshold resistors and fixed orifice resistors to determine effects on the airway in vitro. Pressure patterns, peak expiratory flows (PEFR; L/min), peak expiratory pressure (P_{exp}; cmH_2O), mean airway pressures (MAP; cmH_2O), work of breathing (W_{pt}; Joule/L), and changes in residual volume (RV; mL above baseline) during passive exhalation (V_T 500 mL, PIF 40 L/min) were measured using a test lung with a compliance of 0.02 cmH_2O/L. The results with the Flutter valve, two levels of threshold resistor and two sizes of fixed orifice resistor are shown in Table 18-1.

The Flutter developed lower PEFR than the TH, but higher flows than fixed orifices. In all other respects the Flutter resembled the threshold resistor. The fixed orifice resistor developed lower peak flows, peak and mean airway pressures, work of breathing, and residual volume than either of the threshold resistors or the Flutter ($p < 0.001$).

EPAP requires greater work of breathing than CPAP.[101] In this bench study, both the Flutter and threshold resistors produced a greater work of breathing than the fixed orifice resistor. It is unclear what the effects of this increased patient work may be in the severely obstructed COPD patient. Clearly, CPAP has a role in reducing dyspnea,[102,103] even though EPAP may not (at least during exercise).[94] Further studies are definitely required to determine whether the relatively expensive Flutter device (≥$110) adds therapeutic benefit over other less expensive PAP ($6 to $20) or bronchial hygiene therapies (ie, ACB; free).

Percussionaire®

Intrapulmonary percussive ventilation (IPV) is a therapeutic form of chest physical therapy advanced by Dr. Forrest Bird for treatment of patients with COPD that consists of a pneumatic device called a Percussionator®. IPV was designed to treat diffuse patchy atelectasis, enhance the mobilization and clearance of retained secretions, and deliver nebulized medications and wetting agents to the distal airways.[104]

Patients breathe through a mouthpiece which delivers high flow "mini-bursts" at rates of more than 200 cycles/minute. During these percussive bursts of gas into the lungs, a continuous airway pressure is maintained while the pulsatile percussive intra-airway pressure rises progressively. Each percussive cycle is programmed by the patient or clinician by holding down a thumb button for 5 to 10 seconds for percussive inspiratory cycle and releasing the button for exhalation. Treatments of approximately 20 minutes are recommended by the manufacturer. Impaction pressures of 25 to 40 psig are delivered with a frequency from less than 100 to 225 percussive cycles/minute at 40 psig. The IPV-2 includes nonoscillatory demand CPAP or oscillatory demand CPAP with IMV.

Natale et al[105] reported that a single IPV treatment was as effective as standard chest physiotherapy in improving acute pulmonary function and enhancing sputum expectoration in nine CF patients. (Note: Directed coughing [huff], CPAP, PEP, and Flutter all have been shown to be *more* effective than standard chest physiotherapy in enhancing sputum expectoration). Further studies would be valuable in determining the relative merit of IPV in comparison to other lung expansion/secretion clearance techniques.

With so little information published on the use of IPV,[107,108] one might assume that contraindications and hazards are similar to those associated with other forms of mechanical ventilation. The manufacturer lists potential side effects to include sore ribs, fatigue, stress, and irritation. The role of airway oscillation of vibration on secretion clearance remains unclear. Van Henstum et al[109] reported no effect of oral high-frequency oscillation combined with forced expiration maneuvers on tracheobronchial clearance in chronic bronchitis. Further studies are warranted.

TABLE 18-1 **In Vitro Comparison of Flutter®, Threshold (TH), and Fixed Orifice (FO) Resistors (simulated passive exhalation of 0.5L and unrestricted expiratory flow)**

	PEFR L/Min	exp (cmH_2O)	EPAP (cmH_2O)	W_{pt} (Joule/L)	MAP (cmH_2O)	RV (mL)
Flutter®	27.1	18.8	8.4	1.406	7.5	450
TH 10 cmH_2O	39.0	15.5	7.5	1.255	6.6	450
TH 15 cmH_2O	40.0	20.6	12.5	1.694	9.9	700
FO 4.0 mm	23.7	9.5	0.3	0.738	0.8	0
FO 3.0 mm	13.4	10.2	0.3	0.714	1.6	0

High-Frequency Chest Wall Compression (HFCC)

High-frequency chest wall compression (HFCC) has been shown to increase tracheal mucus clearance rates and to correlate with improved ventilation in both animal and clinical studies.[110,111,112]

ThAIRapy Vest

ThAIRapy® (American Biosystems Inc., St. Paul, MN) was developed by Warwick et al at the University of Minnesota (Fig. 18-12). The device, designed for self-therapy, consists of a large-volume variable-frequency airpulse delivery system attached to a nonstretchable inflatable vest that is worn by the patient, extending over the entire torso down to the iliac crest. Pressure pulses that fill the vest and vibrate the chest wall are controlled by the patient (with a foot pedal) and applied during expiration. Pulse frequency is adjustable from 5 to 25 Hz, with pressure in the vest varying from 28 mmHg at 5 Hz to 39 mmHg at 25 Hz. Figure 18-13A illustrates an expiratory flow at lung volumes when the vest is vibrating at 14 Hz. In Figure 18-13B, airflow produced during several coughs is superimposed on the flow volume curve of HFCC at 10 Hz.

In theory, these vibrations to the chest wall cause transient increases in airflow in the lungs, to improve gas-liquid interactions and the movement of mucus. Animal and clinical studies demonstrated that the frequency of oscillations (cycles/second) and flow bias (inspiratory vs. expiratory) are important in determining effectiveness. Flow bias determines whether secretions move upstream or downstream.[111] Conjecture that this device has a role in lung expansion for patients other than those with CF in the acute care settings has not been empirically established.

ThAIRapy has been shown to be more effective than postural drainage in secretion clearance with CF patients[112], but there has been no comparison in a controlled manner with ACB, PEP, or other bronchial hygiene measures. It would seem that such comparisons would be vital to justify a device costing $500/month (current third-payer reimbursement rates).

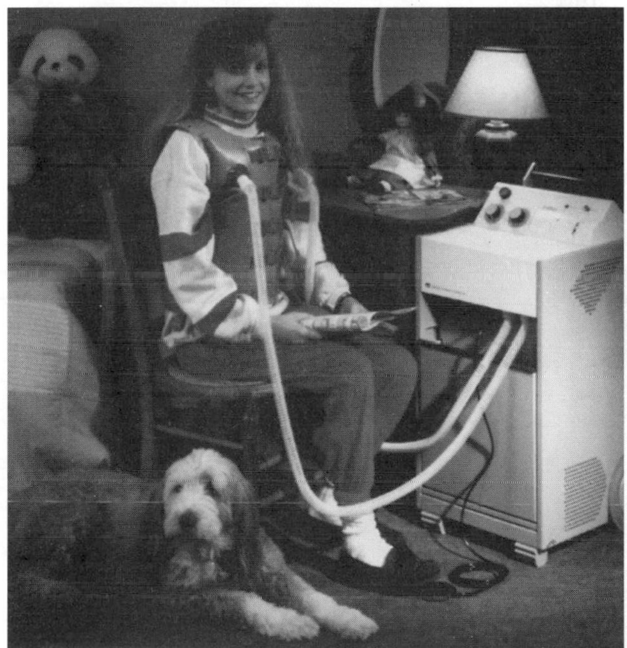

FIGURE 18-12. ThAIRapy® vest and air pulse delivery device. Actuation of a foot pedal engages the high-frequency chest compression (HFCC). (Courtesy American Biosystems, Inc., Stillwater, MN)

Hayek Oscillator

The Hayek Oscillator® (Breasy Medical Equipment, Stamford, CT) is an electrically powered, microprocessor-controlled noninvasive oscillator ventilator, which uses an external flexible chest enclosure (cuirass) to apply negative and positive pressure to the chest wall to deliver noninvasive oscillation to the lungs (Fig. 18-14). Subatmospheric pressure generated in the cuirass causes the chest wall to expand for inspiration, whereas positive pressure compresses the chest to produce a forced expiration. Both inspiratory and expiratory phases may be active and not reliant on passive recoil of the chest. Expiratory pressure can be positive, atmospheric, or negative, allowing ventilation to occur above, at or below the patient's normal FRC. Several groups have reported success in using this device as a method of ventilatory support.[113–115] Four adjustable parameters with the Hayek include frequency range (to 999 oscillations/minute), I:E ratio (6:1 to 1:6), inspiratory and pressure (-70 to $+70$ cmH_2O).

Anecdotal observations of "spontaneous expulsion of secretion"[116,117] during high-frequency ventilation have led to development of several discrete secretion management program recommendations in which the chest is oscillated through two sets of cycles: several minutes at a high frequency of up to 999 (usually 600/720) cycles per minute at an I:E ratio of 1:1 followed a 60/90 cycles/minutes at an I:E ratio of 5:1. Setting can be changed according to the patient's "need." Reports of efficacy of this or similar protocols for secretion management with the Hayek have yet to be published.

BRONCHODILATOR THERAPY WITH VOLUME EXPANSION

The β-adrenergic drugs are thought to improve mucociliary clearance in addition to its bronchodilator functions. This has formed the foundation for the argument to use sympathomimetics such as albuterol or terbutaline perioperatively to reduce incidence of pulmonary complications. Dilworth et al[118] performed a double-blind, placebo-controlled study with one group receiving

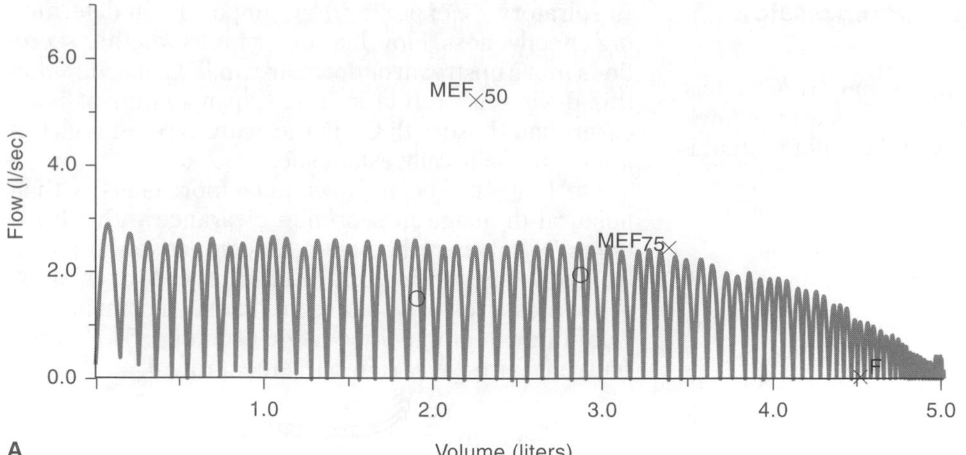

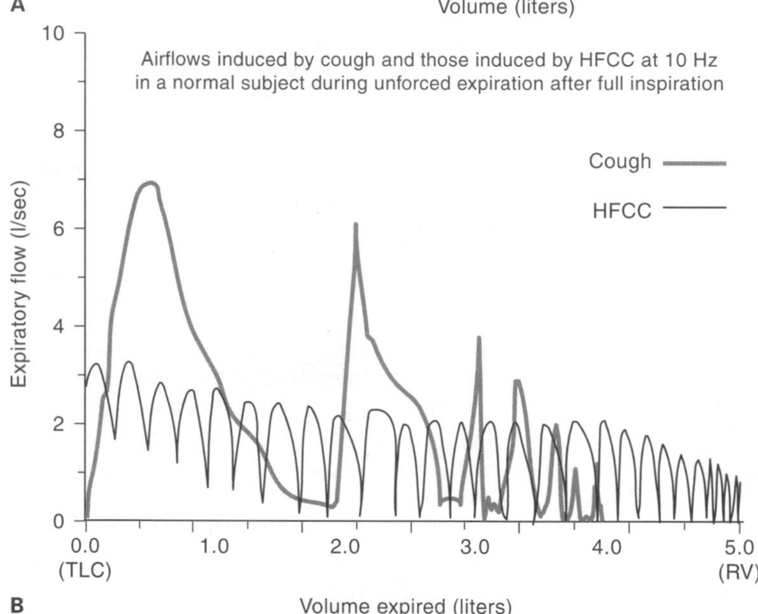

FIGURE 18-13. Tracing of expiratory flow versus volume curves with the ThAIRapy® system. The *top* curve represents the vent vibrating at 14 Hz. The *bottom* tracing shows an overlay of airflow induced by cough and flow produced by the HFCC device. (Courtesy American Biosystems, Inc., Stillwater, MN)

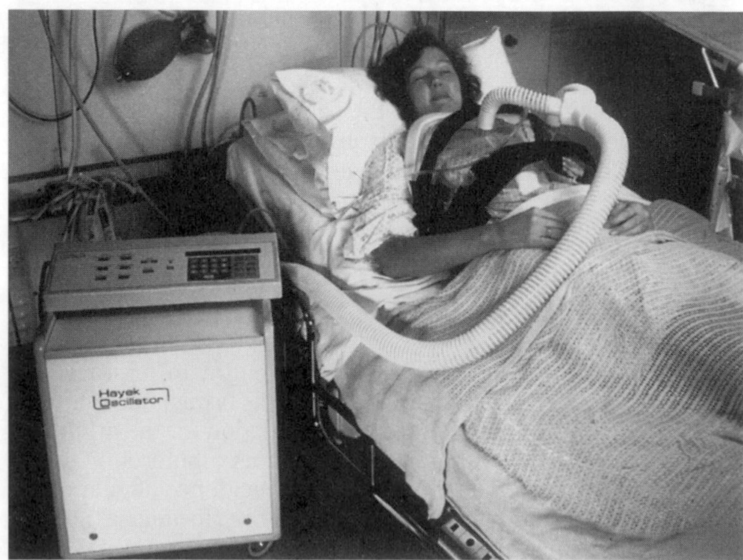

FIGURE 18-14. The Hayek Oscillator/ventilator connected to a chest cuirass. This device may be of value in both ventilation and secretion removal for patients unable to cooperate or without breath control needed to coordinate with other techniques. (Courtesy Breasy Medical Equipment, Stamford, CT)

5-mg salbutamol (albuterol), and the other group normal saline, every 6 hours for 2 days after abdominal surgery. They found no useful reduction in the incidence of pulmonary infections with high-dose bronchodilator therapy in the perioperative period and no reduction of postoperative chest infection in high-risk patients.

THE ROLE OF THE RCP IN RECOMMENDING LUNG EXPANSION THERAPY

Selecting the best volume expansion method or device is a difficult task. The key element is assessment of the patient, no matter what the initial order may be. Therapeutic objectives and alternatives that will reliably meet the therapeutic objectives must be reviewed. High among the considerations should be patient comfort and cost. Other factors include ability to learn procedures, need for attendant/assistants, and skill of the RCP as a teacher. Practitioners should start with the most comfortable, cost-effective option(s) available. Continuing assessment can gauge the patient's response to therapy as a re-evaluation of the current order's efficacy. Only with a balance of need and outcome assessment can the RCP fine tune a cost-effective program to meet each patient's needs.

Patient's age and primary pulmonary pathology may guide selection of specific techniques. Children older than 3 years of age can learn PEP therapy and can be fitted for HFCC chest appliances. Adolescents older than 12 years may appreciate the self-administered techniques that allow independence from parents or other caregivers. Box 18-7 summarizes personnel needs and roles.[119]

Table 18-2 provides a summary grid of the factors related to volume expansion therapy. This matrix compares indications, contraindications, and limitations of the major volume expansion therapies to guide initial orders and ongoing modification. The approach of using therapist-driven protocols lends itself to this theme. Protocol 18-1 diagrams a therapist-driven protocol for volume expansion therapy.

(text continues on page 551)

BOX 18-7

PERSONNEL NEEDS FOR VOLUME EXPANSION THERAPY

Staff initiating lung expansion therapy must be able to:

- Perform physical examination—auscultation, inspection, percussion, and vital signs
- Assess patient condition and response to therapy
  - Subjective response—pain, discomfort, response to therapy
  - Pulse rate and cardiac rhythm (if ECG is available)
  - Breathing pattern rate, symmetrical lateral rib expansion, and synchronous thoraco-abdominal movement
  - Sputum production
  - Mental function
  - Skin color
  - Breath sounds
  - Blood pressure
  - Pulse oximetry
  - Intracranial pressure
- Perform PEF, VC, spirometry, and ventilatory mechanics measurements
- Properly use and know limitations of IS, IPPB, PAP, and other equipment with ability to fit mask and/or identify best application device for a particular patient
- Recognize and respond to therapeutic changes, adverse response, and complications of techniques, equipment, and aerosol medications used
- Modify dose of medication/volume/pressure/flow rates and/or frequency of administration as prescribed in response to severity of symptoms
- Negotiate care plan and modifications with physician and health care team
- Identify the effects of increased pressure on ventilation, perfusion, and sputum mobilization
- Modify technique in response to adverse reactions
- Instruct patient/family/caregiver in the following:
  - Goals of therapy
  - Proper technique for administration
  - Proper use of equipment
  - Cleaning of equipment
  - Breathing patterns and cough techniques
  - Recognition—immediate response and follow-up to adverse reactions
  - Modification—response to severity of symptoms

TABLE 18-2 **Lung Expansion Therapy**

Therapy	Indications	Contraindications	Potential Complications	Frequency/Limitations/Costs
Turning/Repositioning/Mobility	Inability/reluctance of patient to change body position Poor oxygenation associated with position Potential for or development of atelectasis Presence of artificial airway Unprotected airway at risk for aspiration	All Positions ICP >20 mmHg Head/neck injury Active hemorrhage with hemodynamic instability Recent spinal surgery or acute spinal injury Reverse Trendelenburg Hypotension Vasoactive medication therapy	Hypoxemia Increased ICP Acute hypotension Injury/discomfort of muscles, bones Vomiting, aspiration Bronchospasm Dysrhythmias	Turn supine to lateral q 2 hr as tolerated Pain management may be required No additional costs beyond basic nursing care
Directed Cough	Removal of retained secretions Collection of sputum specimens Atelectasis Prophylactic use in surgical patients Routine for patients with bronchectasis and COPD	Elevated ICP or known intracranial aneurysm Acute unstable head, neck, spinal injury High risk for regurgitation/aspiration Acute abdominal pathology Flail chest	Reduced coronary artery perfusion Reduced cerebral perfusion Fatigue Headache Bronchospasm Chest/incisional pain, evisceration Rib or costochondral fracture Gastroesophageal reflux	As needed to expel secretions and prophylactically for postoperative patients (q 2 hr while awake) Limited value in paralyzed, obtunded, and uncooperative patient No additional costs beyond basic nursing care
Incentive Spirometry	Conditions predisposing to development of pulmonary atelectasis: Upper abdominal surgery Thoracic surgery Surgery on patients with COPD Atelectasis Restrictive lung deficit associated with quadriplegia and/or dysfunctional diaphragm	Patient cannot be instructed or supervised to insure appropriate use of device Patient cooperation is inconsistent Patient is unable to understand or demonstrate proper use of device Patient is unable to deep breathe effectively with this device	Hyperventilation Discomfort secondary to inadequate pain control Hypoxia Exacerbation of bronchospasm Fatigue	10 breaths per session every hour while awake No evidence that IS is more effective than deep breathing alone Concerns about overuse. Equipment <\$5–\$10 setup, minimum instruction and follow-up time.

Positive Airway Pressure Therapy (PAP)	To treat atelectasis To aid in mobilization of retained secretions To optimize delivery of bronchodilators in patients receiving bronchial hygiene therapy	Inability to tolerate the increased work of breathing ICP >20 mmHg Hemodynamic instability Recent facial, oral or skull surgery/trauma Active hemoptysis	Discomfort Hyperventilation, hypercarbia Increased ICP Skin breakdown/irritation Cardiovascular compromise	Frequency 1–6 hours (see text) Requires spontaneously breathing patient CPAP setup may cost >$100, requiring high flow gas source. Flutter <$120, EPAP <$25, and PEP <$10 Flutter may be less effective than active cycle of breathing (directed cough) in mobilizing secretions
Intermittent Positive Pressure Breathing (IPPB)	To improve lung expansion Ineffective cough Short-term ventilatory support for patients who are hypoventilating as an alternative to CMV To deliver aerosol medication (when other less expensive, invasive and complex options don't work)	Untreated pneumothorax ICP >15 mmHg Hemodynamic instability Recent facial, oral or skull surgery Uncontrolled hypertension Active hemoptysis Recent esophageal surgery Active hemoptysis Tracheoesophageal fistula Nausea or air swallowing Active untreated tuberculosis Singulation (hiccups)	Increased airway resistance Barotrauma, pneumothorax Nosocomial infection Hypocarbia/hypoventilation Hypoxemia/hyperoxia Increased ICP Gastric distension Impaction of secretions Psychological dependence Impedance of venous return Increased mismatch V/Q Air trapping, auto-PEEP	Frequency 1–6 hours (see text) All mechanical effects last ≤1 hour Less efficient for aerosol delivery than SVN or MDI Efficacy is technique (coordination, selection of inspiratory flow, peak pressure) and device (flow, volume, pressure capabilities) dependent Limited portability and convenience as aerosol delivery device Equipment and labor intensive Device costs >$500
Extrathoracic High Frequency Oscillation/Vibration	To aid in mobilization of retained secretions (when other less expensive, invasive, and complex options don't work)	Untreated pneumothorax ICP >15 mmHg Hemodynamic instability Uncontrolled hypertension Active hemoptysis Tracheoesophageal fistula Nausea or air swallowing Active untreated tuberculosis Singulation (hiccups)	Hypocarbia/hypoventilation Hypoxemia Increased ICP Impaction of secretions Psychological dependence Increased mismatch V/Q Air trapping, auto-PEEP Increased airway resistance	Frequency 1–6 hours (see text) Not shown to be more effective than active cycle of breathing (FET) or PAP Efficacy is technique (coordination, frequency, I:E ratio) and device dependent Limited portability and convenience Device cost >$10,000

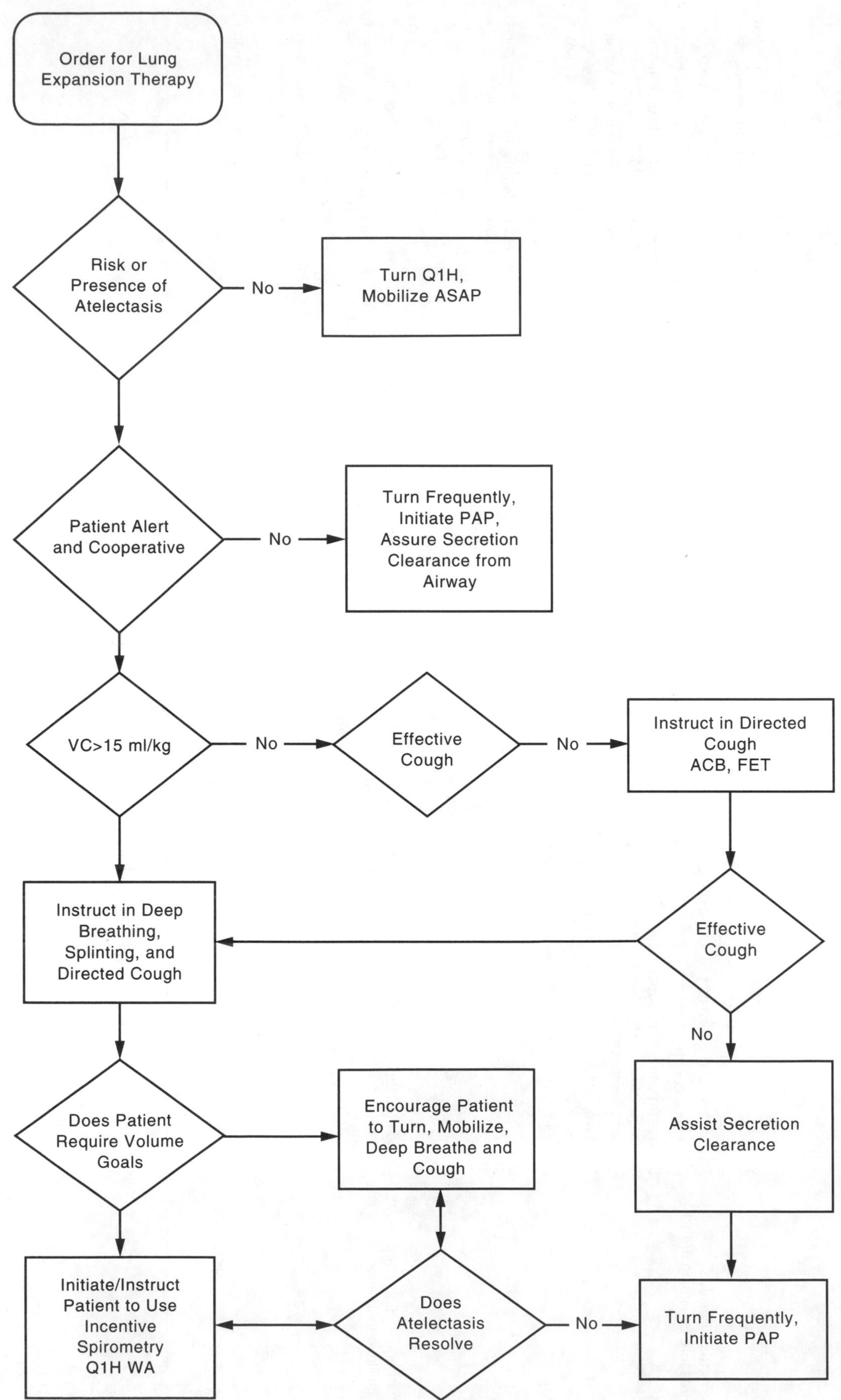

Protocol 18-1. Therapist-driven protocol for volume expansion therapy.

REFERENCES

1. O'Donohue WJ Jr: Postoperative pulmonary complications: When are preventative and therapeutic measures necessary? Postgrad Med 91:167–175, 1992
2. Pontoppidan H: Mechanical aids to lung expansion in non-intubated surgical patients. Am Rev Respir Dis 122 (5 pt 2):109–119, 1980
3. Motley HL, Lang LP, Gordon B: Use of intermittent positive pressure breathing combined with nebulization win pulmonary disease. Am J Med 5:853, 1948
4. Wu N, Miller WF, Cade RF, Richburg PR: Intermittent positive pressure breathing in patients with chronic bronchopulmonary disease. Am Rev Tuberc 71:693, 1955
5. Fowler WS, Helmholz HF, Miller RD: Treatment of emphysema with aerosolized bronchodilating drugs and intermittent positive pressure breathing. Proc Staff Mayo Clin 28:741, 1953
6. Murray JF: Review of the state of the art in intermittent positive pressure breathing therapy. Am Rev Respir Dis 110:193–199, 1974
7. Agency for Health Care Policy and Research (AHCPR) Health Technology Reports: Intermittent positive pressure breathing (IPPB) therapy. Bethesda MD: National Institutes of Health Number 1, 1991
8. O'Donohue WJ Jr: National survey of the usage of lung expansion modalities for the prevention and treatment of postoperative atelectasis following abdominal and thoracic surgery. Chest 87:76–80, 1985
9. American Association for Respiratory Care: Clinical Practice Guideline: Use of positive pressure adjuncts to bronchial hygiene therapy. Respir Care 38:516–5219, 1993
10. American Association for Respiratory Care: Clinical Practice Guideline: Intermittent positive pressure breathing. Respir Care 38:1189–1195, 1993
11. American Association for Respiratory Care: Clinical Practice Guideline: Incentive spirometry. Respir Care 37:1402–1405, 1992
12. Tobin MJ: Perioperative problems. In Essentials of Critical Care Medicine. Churchill-Livingston, New York, 1989, pp 515–528
13. Engoren N: Lack of association between atelectasis and fever. Chest 107:81–84, 1995
14. Meyers JR, Lembeck L, O'Kane H, Baue AE: Changes in residual capacity of the lung after operation. Arch Surg 110:567–583, 1975
15. Miller RD, Fowler WS, Helmholz F: Changes of relative volume and ventilation of the two lungs with changes to the lateral decubitus position. J Lab Clin Med 47:297–304, 1956
16. Douglas WW, Rehder K, Beynen FM, Sessler AD, Marsh HM Improved oxygenation in patients with acute respiratory failure: The prone position. Am Rev Respir Dis 115:559–566, 1977
17. Brussel T, Hachenberg T, Roos N, Lemzem H, Konertz W, Lawin P: Mechanical ventilation in the prone position for acute respiratory failure after cardiac surgery. J Cardiothorac Vasc Anesth 7:541–546, 1993
18. Torres A, Serra-Batlles J, Ros E, Picra C, Puig de la Bellacasa J, Cobos A, Lomena F, Rodriguez-Roisin R: Pulmonary aspiration of gastric contents inpatients receiving mechanical ventilation: The effect of body position. Ann Intern Med 116:540–543, 1992
19. Stein M, Cassara EL: Preoperative pulmonary evaluation and therapy for surgery patients. JAMA 211(5):787–790, 1970
20. Hilling L, Bakow E, Fink J, Kelly C, Sobush D, Southorn PA. AARC Clinical Practice Guideline: Postural Drainage Therapy. Respir Care 36:1418–1426, 1993
21. Zack MB, Pontoppidan H, Kazemi H. The effect of lateral positions on gas exchange in pulmonary disease: A prospective evaluation. Am Rev Respir Dis 110:49–55, 1974
22. Chulary M, Brown J, Summer W: Effect of postoperative immobilization after coronary artery bypass surgery. Crit Care Med 10:176–179, 1982
23. Piehl MA, Brown RS: Use of extreme position changes in acute respiratory failure. Crit Care Med 4:13–14, 1976
24. Coonan TJ, Hope CE: Cardio-respiratory effects of change of body position. Can Anaesth Soc J 30:424–437, 1983
25. Schimmel L, Civetta JM, Kirby RR: A new mechanical method to influence pulmonary perfusion in critically ill patients. Crit Care Med 5:277–279, 1977
26. Gentilello L, Thompson DA, Ronnesen AS, Hernandez D, Kapadia AS, Allen SJ, et al: Effect of a rotating bed on the incidence of pulmonary complications in critically ill patients. Crit Care Med 16:783–786, 1988
27. Summer WR, Curry P, Haponick EF, Nelson S, Elston R: Continuous mechanical turning of intensive care unit patients shortens length of stay in some diagnostic related groups. J Crit Care 4:45–53, 1989
28. Fink MP, Helsmoortel CM, Stein KL, Lee PC, Cohn SM: The efficacy of an oscillating bed in the prevention of lower respiratory tract infection in critically ill victims of blunt trauma: A prospective study. Chest 97:132–137, 1990
29. Hilling L, Bakow E, Fink J, Kelly C, Sobush D, Southorn PA: AARC Clinical Practice Guideline: Directed Cough. Respir Care 38:495–499, 1993
30. Roukema JA, Carol EJ, Prins JG: The prevention of pulmonary complications after upper abdominal surgery in patients with noncompromised pulmonary status. Arch Surg 123:30–34, 1988
31. Partridge C, Pryor J, Webber B: Characteristics of the forced expiratory technique. Physiotherapy 75(3):193–194, 1989
32. Pryor JA, Webber BA: An evaluation of the forced expiration technique as an adjunct to postural drainage. Physiotherapy 65:304–307, 1979
33. DeBoeck C, Zinman R: Cough versus chest physiotherapy: A comparison of the acute effects on pulmonary function in patients with cystic fibrosis. Am Rev Respir Dis 129:182, 1984
34. Webber BA, Hofmeyer JL, Morgan MDL, Hodson ME: Effects of postural drainage, incorporating the forced expiration technique, on pulmonary function in cystic fibrosis. Br J Dis Chest 80:353–359, 1986
35. Bain J, Bishop J, Olinsky A: Evaluation of directed coughing in cystic fibrosis. Br J Dis Chest 82:138–148, 1988
36. Hie T, Pas BG, Roth RD, Jensen WM: Huff coughing and airway patency. Respir Care 24:710–713, 1979
37. Oldenburg FA, Dolovich MD, Montgomery JM, Newhouse MT: Effects of postural drainage, exercise and cough on mucus clearance in chronic bronchitis. Am Rev Respir Dis 120:739–745, 1979
38. Sutton PP, Parker, Webber, Newman SP, Garland N, Lopez-Vidriero MT, Pavia D, Clark SW: Assessment of the forced expiration technique, postural drainage and directed coughing in chest physiotherapy. Eur J Respir Dis 64:62–68, 1983
39. Hardy KA: A review of airway clearance: New techniques, indications and recommendations. Respir Care 39:440–452, 1994
40. Bartlett RH, Krop P, Hanson EL, Moore FD: Physiology of yawning and its application to postoperative care. Surg Forum 21:223–224, 1970
41. Craven JL, Evans GA, Davenprot PJ, Wiolliam RHP: The evaluation of incentive spirometry in the management of postoperative pulmonary complications. Br J Surg 61:793–797, 1974
42. Scuderi J, Olsen GN: Respiratory therapy in the management of postoperative complications. Respir Care 34:281–291, 1989
43. Dohi S, Gold MI: Comparison of two methods of postoperative respiratory care. Chest 73:592–595, 1978
44. Walter J, Cooney M, Norton S: Improved pulmonary function in chronic quadriplegics after pulmonary therapy and arm ergometry. Paraplegia 27:278–283, 1989
45. Mang H, Obermayer A: Imposed work of breathing during sustained maximal inspiration: Comparison of six incentive spirometers. Respir Care 34:1122–1128, 1989
46. Lederer DH, Vandewater JM, Indech RB: Which breathing device should the postoperative patient use? Chest 77:610–613, 1980
47. Rau JL, Thomas L, Haynes RL: The effect of method of administering incentive spirometry on postoperative pulmonary complications in coronary bypass patients. Respir Care 33:771–778, 1988
48. Celli BR, Rodriguez KS, Snider GL: A controlled trial of intermittent positive pressure breathing, incentive spirometry, and deep breathing exercises in preventing pulmonary complication after abdominal surgery. Am Rev Respir Dis 130:12–15, 1984
49. Jenkins, SC, Soutar SA, Loukota JM, Johnson LC, Moxham M: Physiotherapy after coronary artery surgery: are breathing exercises necessary? Thorax 44:634–639, 1989
50. Stiller K, Montarello J, Wallace M, Daff M, Grant R, Jenkins S, Hall B, Yates H: Efficacy of breathing and coughing exercises in

the prevention of pulmonary complications after coronary artery surgery. Chest 105:741–747, 1994

51. Dull JL, Dull WL: Are maximal inspiratory breathing exercises better or incentive spirometry better than early mobilization after cardiopulmonary bypass? Phys Ther 63:655–659, 1983
52. Hall JC, Tarala R, Harris J, Tapper J, Christiansen K: Incentive spirometry versus routine chest physiotherapy for prevention of pulmonary complications after abdominal surgery. Lancet 337:953–956, 1991
53. Stiller K, Geake T, Taylor H, Grant R, Hall B: Acute lobar atelectasis: a comparison of two chest physiotherapy regimens. Chest 98:1336–1340, 1990
54. Dolovich MB, Killian D, Wolff RK, Obminski G, Newhouse MT: Pulmonary aerosol deposition in chronic bronchitis: Intermittent positive pressure breathing versus quiet breathing. Am Rev Respir Dis 115:397–402, 1977
55. The IPPB Trial Group: Intermittent positive pressure breathing therapy of chronic obstructive pulmonary disease: A clinical trial. Ann Intern Med 99:612–620, 1983
56. Pedersen JZ, Bundgaard A: Comparative efficacy of different methods of nebulizing terbutaline. Eur J Clin Pharmacol 25:739–742, 1983
57. Bartlett RH: Respiratory therapy to prevent pulmonary complications of surgery. Respir Care 29:667–669, 1984
58. DeTroyer A, Deisser P: The effects of intermittent positive pressure breathing on patients with respiratory muscle weakness. Am Rev Respir Dis 124:132–137, 1981
59. Moore RB, Cotton EK, Pinney MA: The effect of intermittent positive pressure breathing on airway resistance in normal and asthmatic children. J Allergy Clin Immunol 49:137–141, 1972
60. Rodenstien DO, Stanescu DC, Delguste P, Liistro G, Aubert-Tulkens G: Adaptation to intermittent positive pressure ventilation applied through the nose during day and night. Eur Respir J 2:473–478, 1989
61. Bach JR, Alba A, Mosher R, Delaubier A: Intermittent positive pressure ventilation via nasal access in the management of respiratory insufficiency. Chest 92:168–170, 1987
62. Paul WL, Downs JB: Postoperative atelectasis: Intermittent positive pressure breathing, incentive spirometry, and face-mask positive end-expiratory pressure. Arch Surg 116:861–863, 1981
63. Ricksten SE, Bengtsson A, Soderberg C, Thorden M, Kvist H: Effects of periodic positive airway pressure by mask on postoperative pulmonary function. Chest 89:774–781, 1986
64. Andersen JB, Klausen NO: A new mode of administration of nebulized bronchodilator in severe bronchospasm. Eur J Respir Dis 63(Suppl):119:97–100, 1982
65. Frischknecht-Christensen E, Norregaard O, Dahl R: Treatment of bronchial asthma with terbutaline inhaled by conespacer combined with positive expiratory pressure mask. Chest 100(2): 317–321, 1991
66. Kacmarek RM, Dimas S, Reynolds J, Shapiro B: Technical aspects of positive end expiratory pressure (PEEP): Part I. Physics of PEEP devices. Respir Care 27:1478–1489, 1982
67. Mahlmeister MJ, Fink JB, Hoffman GL, Fifer LF: Positive-expiratory-pressure mask therapy: Theoretical and practical considerations and a review of the literature. Respir Care 36: 1218–1230, 1991
68. Thoman RL, Stoker GL, Ross JC: The efficacy of pursed-lips breathing in patients with chronic obstructive pulmonary disease. Am Rev Respir Dis 93:100–106, 1968
69. Petty TL: Chronic obstructive pulmonary disease. New York, Marcel Dekker, 1978
70. Poulton EP, Odon DM:. Left-sided heart failure with pulmonary oedema: Its treatment with the "pulmonary plus pressure machine." Lancet 231:981–983, 1936
71. Barach AL, Martin J, Eckman L: Positive pressure respiration and its application to the treatment of acute pulmonary edema and respiratory obstruction. Proc Am Soc Clin Invest 16:664–680, 1937
72. Cheney FW, Hornbein TF, Crawford EW: The effect of expiratory resistance on the blood gas tensions of anesthetized patients. Anesthesiology 28(4):670–676, 1967
73. Ashbaugh DG, Petty TL, Bigelow DB, Harris TM: Continuous positive pressure breathing (CPPB) in adult respiratory distress syndrome. J Thorac Cardiovasc Surg 57:31–41, 1969
74. Gregory GA, Kitterman JA, Phibbs RH: Treatment of the idiopathic respiratory distress syndrome with continuous positive airway pressure. N Engl J Med 284:1333–1340, 1971
75. Pontoppidan H, Wilson RS, Rie MA, Schneider RC: Respiratory intensive care. Anesthesiology 47:96–116, 1977
76. Katz JA: PEEP and CPAP in perioperative respiratory care. Respir Care 29:6:614–623, 1984
77. Garrard CS, Shah M: The effects of expiratory positive airway pressure on functional residual capacity in normal subjects. Crit Care Med 6:320–332, 1978
78. Andersen JB, Qvist H, Kann T: Recruiting collapsed lung through collateral channels with positive end-expiratory pressure. Scand J Respir Dis 60:260–266, 1979
79. Andersen JB, Jespersen W: Demonstration of intersegmental respiratory bronchioles in normal lungs. Eur J Respir Dis 61:337–341, 1980
80. Branson RD, Hurst JM, DeHaven CB: Mask CPAP: State of the art. Respir Care 30:846–857, 1985
81. Branson RD: PEEP without endotracheal intubation. Respir Care 33:598–610, 1988
82. Andersen JB, Olesen KP, Eikard E, Jansen E, Qvist J: Periodic continuous positive airway pressure, CPAP, by mask in the treatment of atelectasis: A sequential analysis. Eur J Respir Dis 61:20–25, 1980
83. Pontoppidan H: Mechanical aids to lung expansion in nonintubated surgical patients. Am Rev Respir Dis 122:109–119, 1980
84. Carlsson C, Sonden B, Thylen U: Can postoperative continuous positive airway pressure (CPAP) prevent pulmonary complications after abdominal surgery? Intensive Care Med 7:225–229, 1981
85. Martin JG, Shore S, Engel LA: Effect of continuous positive pressure on respiratory mechanics and pattern of breathing in induced asthma. Am Rev Respir Dis 126:812–817, 1982
86. Stock MC, Downs JB: Administration of continuous positive airway pressure by mask. Acute Care 10:184–188, 1983
87. Stock MC, Downs JB, Corkran ML: Pulmonary function before and after prolonged positive airway pressure by mask. Crit Care Med 12:973–974, 1984
88. Stock MC, Downs JB, Cooper RB, Lebenson IM, Cleveland J, Weaver DE, Alster JM, Imrey PB: Comparison of continuous positive airway pressure, incentive spirometry, and conservative therapy after cardiac operations. Crit Care Med 12:969–972, 1984
89. Stock MC, Downs JB, Gauer PK, Alster JM, Imrey PB: Prevention of postoperative pulmonary complication with CPAP, incentive spirometry and conservative therapy. Chest 87:151–157, 1985
90. Lindner KH, Lotz P, Ahnefeld FW: Continuous positive airway pressure effect on functional residual capacity, vital capacity and its subdivisions. Chest 92(1):66–70, 1987
91. Campbell T, Ferguson N, McKinlay RGC: The use of a simple self-administered method of positive expiratory pressure (PEP) in chest physiotherapy after abdominal surgery. Physiotherapy 72:498–500, 1986
92. Frolund L, Madsen F: Self-administered prophylactic postoperative positive expiratory pressure in thoracic surgery. Acta Anaesthesiol Scand 30:381–385, 1986
93. Groth S, Stafanger G, Dirksen H, Andersen JB, Falk M, Kelstrup M: Positive expiratory pressure (PEP mask) physiotherapy improves ventilation and reduces volume of trapped gas in cystic fibrosis. Bull Eur Physiopathol Respir 21:339–343, 1985
94. van der Schans CP, de Jong W, de Vries G, Kaan WA, Postma DS, Koeter GH, van der Mrk TW: Effects of positive expiratory pressure breathing during exercise in patients with COPD. Chest 105:782–789, 1994
95. Colgan FJ, Mahoney PD, Fanning GL: Resistance breathing (blow bottles) and sustained hyperinflations in the treatment of atelectasis. Anesthesiology 32:543–550, 1970
96. Iverson LIG, Ecker RR, Fox HE, May IA: A comparative study of IPPB, the incentive spirometer, and blow bottles: The prevention of atelectasis following surgery. Ann Thorac Surg 35:197–200, 1978
97. Lindemann H: [The value of physical therapy with VRP 1—Desitin ("Flutter")] Pneumologie 46:626–630, 1992

98. Konstan MW, Stern RC, Doershuk CF: Efficacy of the flutter device for airway mucus clearance in patients with cystic fibrosis. J Pediatr 124:689–693, 1994
99. Pryor JA, Webber BA, Hodson, ME, Warner JO: The Flutter VRP1 as an adjunct to chest physiotherapy in cystic fibrosis. Respir Med 88:677–681, 1994
100. Fink JB: Pattern of pressure and work of breathing with flutter, threshold and fixed orifice resistors used for airway clearance. Chest
101. Schlobohm, RM, Fallrick RT, Quan SF, Katz JA: Lung volumes, mechanics and oxygenation during spontaneous positive pressure ventilation: The advantage of CPAP over EPAP. Anesthesiology 55:426–422, 1981
102. Petrof BJ, Calderini E, Gottfried SB: Effect of CPAP on respiratory effort and dyspnea during exercise in severe COPD. J Appl Physiol 69(1):179–188, 1990
103. Petrof BJ, Legare M, Godberg P, Milic-Emili J, Gottfried SB: Continuous positive airway pressure reduces work of breathing and dyspnea during weaning from mechanical ventilation in severe chronic obstructive pulm onary disease. Am Rev Respir Dis 141:281–289, 1990
104. McInturff SL, Shaw LI: Intrapulmonary percussive ventilation. Respir Care 30:884–885, 1985
105. Natale JE, Pfeifle J, Homnick DN: Comparison of intrapulmonary percussive ventilation and chest physiotherapy. Chest 105:1789–1793, 1994
106. Davis KJ, Hurst JM, Branson RD: High frequency percussive ventilation. Respir Care 34:39–47, 1989
107. Hurst JM, Branson RD: High-frequency percussive ventilation in the management of elevated intracranial pressure. J Trauma 28:1363–1367, 1988
108. Cioffi WG, Major MC: High frequency percussive ventilation in patients with inhalation injury. J Trauma 29:350–354, 1989
109. van Henstum M, Festen J, Buerskens C, Hankel M, van den Broek W, Corstens F: No effect of oral high frequency oscillation combined with forced expiration maneuvers on tracheobronchial clearance in chronic bronchitis. Eur Respir J 3:14–18, 1990
110. King M, Phillips DM, et al: Tracheal mucus clearance with high-frequency chest wall compression. Am Rev Resir Dis 128:511–515, 1983
111. King M, Zidulka A, Phillips DM, Wight D, Gross D, Chang HK: Tracheal mucus clearance in high-frequency oscillation: Effect of peak flow rate bias. Eur Respir J 3:6–13, 1990
112. Hansen L, Warwick W: High frequency chest compression system to aid in clearance of mucus from the lung. Biomed Instrum Technol 24:289–294, 1990
113. Spitzer SA, Fink G, Mittelman M: External high-frequency ventilation in severe chronic obstructive pulmonary disease. Chest 104:1698–1701, 1993
114. Soo Hoo GW, Ellison MJ, Zhang C, Williams AJ, Belman MJ: Effects of external chest wall oscillation in stable COPD patients. Am J Respir Crit Care Med 149: A637, 1994
115. Smithline HA, Rivers EP, Rady MY, Blake HC, Nowak RM: Biphasic extrathoracic pressure CPR: A human pilot study. Chest 105:842–846, 1994
116. Segawa J, Nakashima Y, et al: The efficacy of external high frequency oscillation: Experience in a quadriplegic patient with alveolar hypoventilation. Kokyu To Junkan 41:271–275, 1993
117. Gaitini L, Vaida S, Krimerman S, Werczberger A, Smorgik J, Naum M, Somri M: External high-frequency ventilation in patients with respiratory failure (external ventilation) [letter]. Intensive Care Medicine 21:191, 1995.
118. Dilworth JP, Warley RH, Dawe C, White RJ: The effect of nebulized salbutamol therapy on the incidence of postoperative chest infection in high risk patients. Respir Med 88:665–668, 1994
119. Hardy KA: A review of airway clearance: New techniques, indications and recommendations. Respir Care 39:440, 1994

19 Airway Management

David J. Plevak
Jeffrey J. Ward

CLINICAL SKILLS

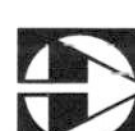

Upon completion of this chapter, the reader will:

- Identify anatomical structures in the adult; compare and contrast them with those of the infant
- Open an obstructed airway using manual techniques and mechanical adjuncts
- Identify basic features of various types of artificial airway appliances
- Take measures to reduce the hazards associated with tracheal tube cuffs
- Determine indications for specialized tracheal and tracheostomy tubes
- Perform nasal or oral intubations using appropriate equipment
- Evaluate the patient for correct tracheal tube placement
- Recommend sedatives and anesthetizing agents for the candidate for tracheal intubation
- Initiate alternative action when intubating the difficult-to-intubate patient
- Denote conditions that may precipitate pediatric airway emergencies
- Identify circumstances in which tracheostomy is advantageous over nasal or oral tracheal intubation
- List hazards and complications of various artificial airway appliances
- Perform safe tracheal suctioning procedures with consideration for patient's needs and outcome

KEY TERMS

Congenital craniofacial dysmorphologies
Laryngeal webs
Laryngomalacia
Laryngo/tracheoesophageal cleft
Stenosis
Subglottic stenosis
Tracheoesophageal fistula
Vocal cord paralysis

The goal of this chapter is to review the equipment and techniques necessary to manage the airway of critically ill patients, but also to include discussion of airway management for patients requiring long-term ventilatory support. Ensuring adequate ventilation and oxygenation is crucial. A brief interval of hypoxia can result in loss of consciousness, impairment of brain function, or death. The intent of this chapter is to provide the reader with information necessary to begin to master the art of airway management. Facility comes only after much practice in the laboratory and in controlled clinical settings. It is only after such training that certification is granted and unsupervised clinical performance allowed. The American Heart Association and the American Red Cross provide life support training and credentials. The National Board for Respiratory Care provides job-oriented tasks or matrices for the expected clinical skills needed for airway management. Those required for entry-level and advanced respiratory care practitioners (RCPs) are listed in Box 19-1.[1]

The chapter begins with a review of normal anatomy. Artificial airways and adjunct equipment are presented, including the indications and rationale for their use. Finally, the specific procedures of airway management, that is, suctioning, endotracheal intubation, tracheotomy, and tracheostomy care, are discussed. The potential complications associated with airway management are outlined so that they can be anticipated and avoided. Guidelines for clinical management developed by the American Heart Association (AHA)[2] American Association for Respiratory Care (AARC),[3–6] and American Society of Anesthesiologists (ASA)[7] are summarized. The reader may note that this chapter shares content similar to Chapter 22, which deals with airway management specific to cardiopulmonary resuscitation. Airways and airway care that are primarily used outside of hospital care are deferred to that chapter.

AIRWAY ANATOMY

A sound background in the anatomy of the upper airway is essential for respiratory care practitioners. Clinical situations arise when anatomic structures are not visible or are obscured, and the practitioner must rely on mental images of spatial relationships. When a patient develops an obstructed airway, a knowledge of upper airway anatomy encourages the application of proper head and neck maneuvers that result in airway patency. During a difficult intubation, the larynx may not be visible. The practitioner may have to rely on the relationships of adjacent structures to properly place the endotracheal tube. The airway of the adult is presented first, followed by a review of pediatric morphology to emphasize anatomic differences.

The nose, pharynx, and trachea function to warm, filter, and humidify inspired air. Figure 19-1*A* shows a sagittal section of the entire adult upper airway. Anatomically, the *pharynx* is divided into three major zones: the *nasopharynx, oropharynx,* and *laryngopharynx* or *hypopharynx.* These zones include several specialized structures that are individually reviewed.

The nose includes the external nose (which protrudes from the face) and the *nasal cavity,* or internal nose. The external orifices of the nose are the *nostrils,* or *nares.* The nasal cavity is divided into two chambers (fossae) by a cartilaginous septum. The floor is formed by the hard and soft palate. Each fossa has three *turbinates (conchae)* that project downward from the lateral surfaces to increase the air-tissue surface area. The nasal cavity opens into the *nasopharynx* through divided posterior choanae. Ciliated squamous columnar epithelial and secretory cells line the structure, which is highly innervated. Besides sensory capabilities, receptors evoke sneezing in response to irritating odors, chemicals, or particles (eg, smoke or pepper). The human nose can differentiate more than 4000 different odors.

Openings in the lateral and posterior nasal walls communicate with sinuses and the nasolacrimal duct. During normal breathing, the nose and nasopharynx account for approximately 50% of the total airway resistance. Access to this area may be made more difficult by a deviated septum, mucosal edema, nasal polyps, or trauma. Insertion of airways or catheters into the nasal cavity should be done in a horizontal direction following the floor of the nasal cavity. This will usually avoid painful trauma to the turbinates.

The nasopharynx begins at the posterior choana and reaches downward to the soft palate. The posterior wall is the location of the *pharyngeal tonsils (adenoids)*. The *eustachian tube* empties into the nasopharynx. Because the nasopharynx accepts drainage from the sinuses and the eustachian tube, the presence of an artificial airway (eg, nasopharyngeal airway) may lead to colonization or infection of adjacent structures. Otitis media and sinusitis may result.

The *oropharynx* begins at the distal tip of the uvula and extends past the tongue to the tip of the epiglottis. The *uvula* is a posterior extension of the soft palate and is a useful visual landmark. The *palatine tonsils* are located between the tissue folds of the palatoglossal and palatopharyngeal arches. The tonsils are collections of lymphoid tissue. The tongue occupies a large portion of the oral cavity. It is attached anteriorly to the hyoid

BOX 19-1

AIRWAY MANAGEMENT CLINICAL SKILLS

Select, review, obtain, and interpret data relative to airway management

- Review patient records and recommend diagnostic procedures to obtain additional data:
  - -History: Childhood or adult diseases, surgery or trauma likely to manifest in compromise of the airway or difficulty in securing an airway.
  - -Physical exam: Inspect the upper airway anatomy to note neck motion, ability to open mouth, anatomic variations, bleeding, and causes of pharyngeal obstruction. Assess evidence of chest or diaphragm motion, breathing pattern, and symmetry of chest movement. Auscultate the airway to determine presence of stridor, bilateral breath sounds, and leak around artificial airways.
- Perform and interpret diagnostic procedures: lateral neck radiograph, fiberoptic bronchoscopy, pulse oximetry, or arterial blood gas analysis.
- Participate in development of an airway management plan.

Select, assemble, and check equipment for proper function, operation, and cleanliness. Identify and correct malfunctions of equipment.

- Select equipment appropriate to the airway management plan. This would include:
  - -Resuscitation devices (manual and pneumatic)
  - -Exhaled CO_2 detection devices
  - -Intubation equipment (laryngoscope & blades)
  - -Artificial airways: oro/nasopharyngeal airways, oro/nasal endotracheal tubes, tracheostomy tubes and buttons
  - -Special aids for difficult intubation including fiberoptic bronchoscopes
  - -Suction systems
- Take actions to correct malfunctions of equipment.

Initiate, conduct, and modify prescribed therapeutic procedures.

- Evaluate, monitor, and record patient's response to airway management measures.
- Conduct therapeutic procedures to achieve maintenance of a patent airway. This would include mask-valve-bag ventilation, endotracheal intubation, tracheostomy tube changes, extubation, and suctioning.
- Conduct airway management maneuvers in an emergency setting.

bone and to the mandible, palate, and pharyngeal wall. It functions to provide speech, taste, and swallowing, and it also frequently causes obstruction of the pharynx. This occurs commonly in the unconscious patient, when the oropharyngeal musculature becomes relaxed. Motor innervation of the tongue includes the lingual, glossopharyngeal, and hypoglossal nerves.

The *larynx* is a group of specialized cartilaginous structures (Fig. 19-1*B*). They connect the lower part of the pharynx with the trachea and are about 5 cm long in the adult male (slightly shorter in the female). The adult larynx is located at the level of cervical vertebrae between C-3 through C-6. The cartilage skeleton consists of nine cartilages, three paired and three single.

The zone of the *hypopharynx* begins superiorly with the tip of the *epiglottic cartilage* and continues inferiorly to include the *cricoid cartilage*. It includes the area from the anterior larynx and base of the tongue to the cervical vertebra posteriorly. The epiglottis functions as a valve to guard the airway from fluids or food, especially during swallowing. The upper portion moves freely and is a well-known landmark for intubation. With a straight blade laryngoscope, the epiglottis is manipulated anteriorly to allow visualization of the glottis. The base of the *epiglottis* is attached to the thyroid cartilage near the *epiglottic vallecula*. The tip of a curved blade laryngoscope is placed in this space (vallecula), just below the tongue, during intubation. The epiglottis may become acutely inflamed and edematous. Acute epiglottitis is most frequently caused by *Haemophilus influenzae* and can be a life-threatening emergency.

The three sets of paired cartilages in the larynx are the *arytenoids* ("ladle"), *corniculates* ("horned"), and *cuneiforms* ("wedge-shaped"). The corniculates are superior to the pyramid-shaped arytenoids. These and the cuneiforms support the aryepiglottic and interarytenoid folds. These folds form the aditus, or entrance, of the larynx. Muscles and ligaments connect cartilages to interior vocal structures to allow movement of speech. Their value to the respiratory care practitioner is in the form of a visual landmark to the laryngeal opening.

The largest single cartilage in the larynx is the *thyroid*. It is a shield-shaped cartilage with hornlike cornua on its inferior and superior aspects. The anterior portion of the thyroid cartilage is known as the "Adam's apple" and is more pronounced in adult men. The *cricoid cartilage* articulates through the cricothyroid ligament with the thyroid cartilage. The cricoid is unique in that its cartilage forms a ring that provides a firm posterior border for the larynx at this level. Inferiorly, the cricoid cartilage is attached to the first tracheal ring. The cricoid is a signet ring–shaped structure, with the larger portion anterior to the esophagus.

Entering the interior cavity of the larynx would reveal the *glottis* or the opening between the *vestibular folds* or *false vocal cords*. When contracted, these folds allow breath holding against positive pressure, such as coughing or a Valsalva's maneuver. The laryngeal area above the true vocal cords is termed the vestibules, and below, the ventricles. The *true cords* lie just inferior to the false cords, and the zone below them is termed the infraglottic cavity. The vocal folds consist of a vocal ligament and the vocalis muscle. This is the narrowest part of the adult airway. These folds are readily moved aside by expired air, such as during speech, and resist inspiratory flow when opposed. Relative to surface anatomy, the vocal cords lie at midlevel of the thyroid cartilage.

The thyroid, cricoid, and most of the arytenoid cartilages are made of hyaline cartilage. These can benignly calcify at approximately 60 years of age. The remaining cartilages and the vocal processes of the arytenoids are made of elastic cartilage. Most of the interior surfaces of the larynx are lined with nonkeratinizing stratified

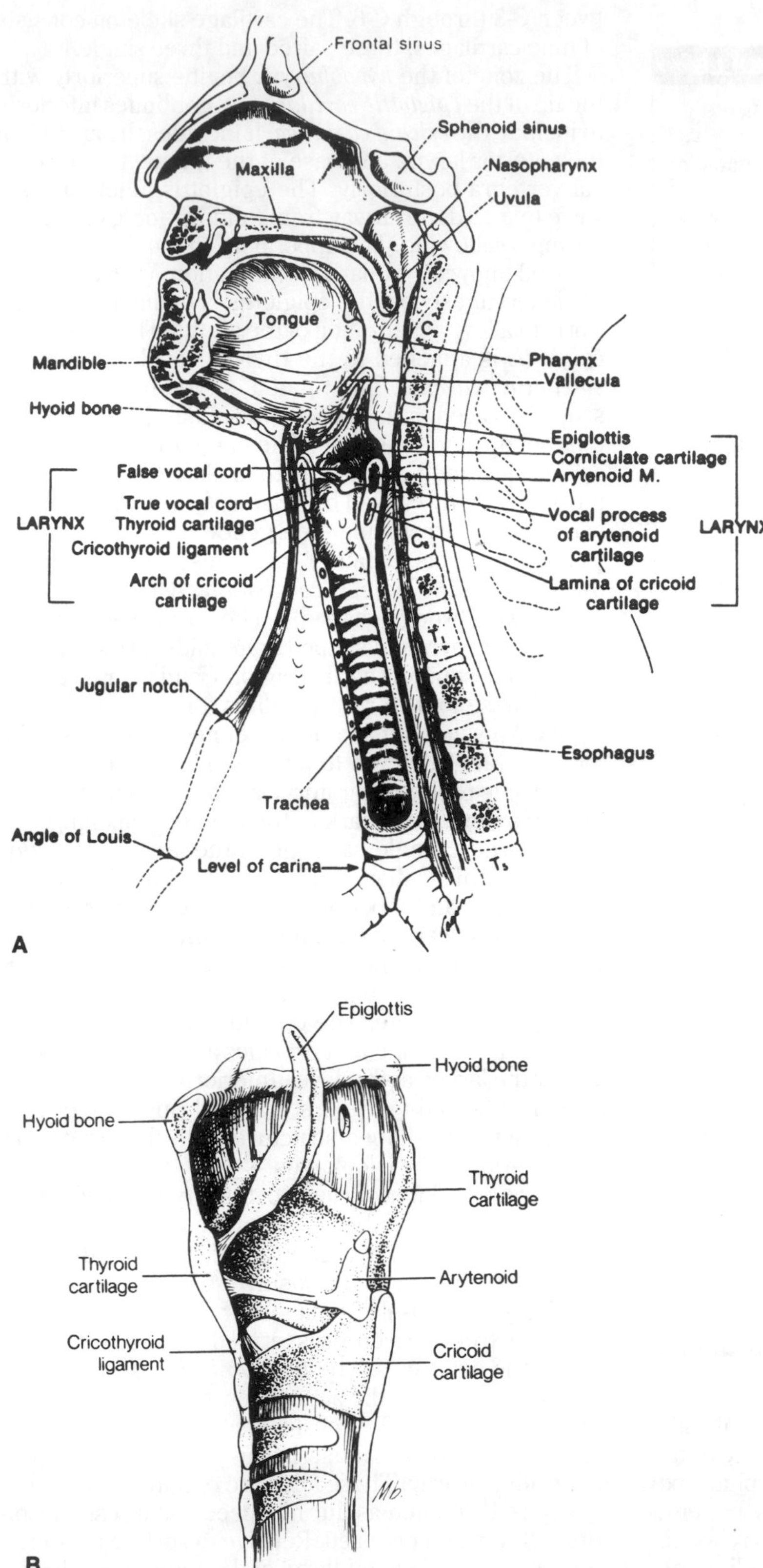

FIGURE 19-1. (A) Normal adult upper airway (sagittal section). (McCabe BF: Pathologic principles. In EW Wilkins (ed): MGH Textbook of Emergency Medicine, 2nd ed. Baltimore, Williams & Wilkins. © 1987, with permission) **(B)** Detailed view of the adult larynx. (BT Finucane, AH Santora (eds): Principles of Airway Management. Philadelphia, FA Davis, 1988, with permission)

squamous epithelium. The laryngeal ventricles and infraglottic areas are lined with ciliated pseudostratified columnar epithelium.

There is a complex system of musculature for the laryngeal structures. They can be separated into two groups: those that protect the airway by sphincteric contraction, and those that adjust the larynx and cords during breathing and phonation. Upper airway muscle tone may be compromised when patients are unconscious.

Innervation and blood supply to the larynx is provided by the superior and inferior laryngeal nerves and arteries. The superior laryngeal nerves arise from the vagus. They provide motor, sensory, and secretory innervation to small, widespread mucous glands in the larynx. The inferior laryngeal nerves are terminal branches of the recurrent laryngeal nerves that also arise from the vagus. The left-sided recurrent laryngeal nerve approaches the larynx after dipping below the aortic arch. On the right, connection is more direct, with the nerve looping around the subclavian artery. Both nerves innervate all of the intrinsic muscles, except the cricothyroid. Neoplasm, vascular disease, or surgery in the periaortic area can cause left-sided fold or cord dysfunction. At first, a paralyzed side of the vocal cords would bow outward and could not be abducted or adducted. The voice would sound different and hoarse because the two cords could not properly oppose. Over time, the paralyzed cord might gradually move closer to the midline with the aid of the still-innervated cricothyroid muscle.

The *trachea* is a D-shaped tubular structure with a flattened posterior surface. In the adult its length extends approximately 12 to 15 cm from the cricoid to the bronchial bifurcation. It is 1.8 to 2.5 cm in diameter. The anterior and lateral surfaces are supported by 16 to 22 C-shaped cartilage rings. The trachealis muscle forms the posterior wall of the trachea. During a cough, the latter area invaginates to decrease the cross-sectional area to 18%, allowing linear airflow velocities of up to 500 miles per hour. At approximately the level of the fourth or fifth thoracic vertebra, the trachea bifurcates into right and left main stem bronchi at the *carina*. In the adult, the right side's branching angle is more vertical, approximately 25° from midline. The left side angles about 45° from midline. Because of this configuration, aspiration of foreign bodies, liquids, and intubations are more likely to occur on the right.

Perinatal and Pediatric Anatomical Considerations

Structures of the airway in the newborn appear to facilitate feeding and breathing. The newborn's tongue is relatively larger, the entire larynx is located more cephalad, and the hyoid bone and thyroid cartilage lie closer together when compared with an adult (Fig. 19-2). The epiglottis is U shaped and stiff. The relative size of the infant's head is much larger than that of an adult, and the weight of the head can cause the cervical spine to assume a flexed position. This can precipitate airway obstruction. The vocal cords are more concave than an adult's and have an anteroinferior incline. The trachea of the newborn is short, and the narrowest part of the airway is at the level of the cricoid cartilage. Newborns are obligatory nose breathers for the first 3 to 6 months, reserving eating for the mouth. This allows them to breath and nurse simultaneously.[8]

Intubation is sometimes more difficult in the infant owing to a bulky tongue. In addition, the size of the epiglottis usually necessitates direct instrumentation with the laryngoscope blade. Passage of a tube through the larynx is sometimes difficult because the angle of the vocal cords may hinder its advance. Trauma to the

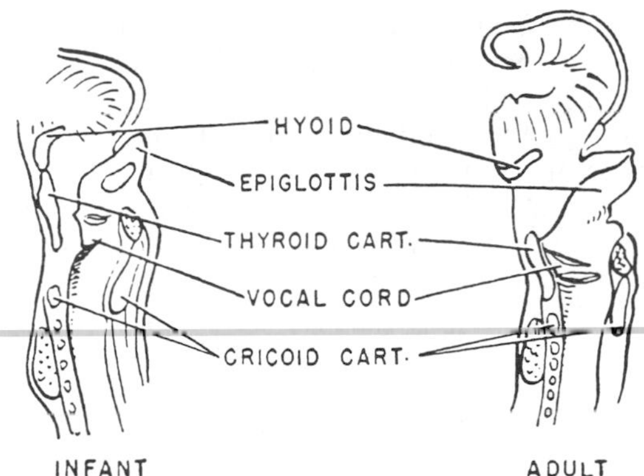

FIGURE 19-2. Anatomic comparison of infant (*left*) and adult (*right*) larynx. Refer to text for details. (Echenhoff JE: Some anatomic considerations of the infant larynx influencing endotracheal anesthesia. Anesthesiology 12:401, 1951, with permission)

mucosal tissue surrounded by the cricoid cartilage can result in edema and significant reduction in cross-sectional area. This may result in postextubation stridor. The shorter trachea provides a greater chance for unilateral endobronchial intubation.[8] The angle of the tracheal bifurcation in children totals approximately 80°. The right bronchial angle is 31° ± 5°, whereas the left bronchial angle is 49° ± 7°. Left bronchial intubations are more common in children than in adults.

Congenital anatomic airway abnormalities may result in respiratory distress for these obligate nose breathers and difficulties in airway management. Lesions of the nasopharynx include *stenosis* or *atresia of the choanae.* This rare lesion (1 in 8,000 births) can be diagnosed by the inability to pass a catheter through the nasopharynx. Distress oddly improves with crying. Radiographic examination can provide the definitive diagnosis. Obstructing lesions of the oropharynx that produce stridor involve abnormalities of the tongue and mandible. Macroglossia accompanies Beckwith-Wiedemann syndrome and Down syndrome. Practitioners must be aware of the potential for airway obstruction and provide close observation. A number of *congenital craniofacial dysmorphologies* can compromise the airway due to distortion of the normal anatomy. With Pierre Robin syndrome, the infant's tongue is displaced posteriorly due to mandibular hypoplasia. In Treacher Collins syndrome, there is hypoplastic maxilla and protrusion of the mandible.

Lesions of the larynx include *laryngomalacia, vocal cord paralysis, laryngeal webs or cysts, laryngo/tracheoesophageal cleft*, and *subglottic stenosis*. Instability of the trachea *(tracheomalacia)* and *tracheoesophageal fistula* are congenital abnormalities of the trachea. During a cough the walls of the trachea move back and forth, producing a harsh, barking cough.

AIRWAY MANAGEMENT

The American Heart Association (AHA) and the American Red Cross have been instrumental in training lay and medical personnel in techniques of airway management in situations requiring acute resuscitation.

Chapter 22 focuses on that aspect of care; however, these same techniques are also essential in the care of hospitalized patients.

Although the need to actively manage a patient's airway is often unexpected, the respiratory care practitioner must be aware of conditions that frequently lead to deterioration of vital signs and unconsciousness. Box 19-2 identifies conditions that predispose to resuscitation.[3]

MANUAL TECHNIQUES

Head-Tilt/Chin-Lift

Patients that are unconscious or unresponsive often have upper airways predisposed to lack of muscular tone and obstruction by pharyngeal structures. In addition, if the patient suffers an acute arrest, he or she may be in a body position that can compromise the airway. Of major importance to either resuscitation or manual ventilation is opening the airway. This basic technique is termed the "head-tilt/chin-lift" maneuver (Fig. 19-3). It is performed by placing the most cephalad hand on the victim's forehead and applying enough pressure with the palm to tilt the head back into the "sniffing" position (Fig. 19-4*A* and *B*). This posture of the head and neck provides a minimal angle between the pharyngeal and tracheal planes. The second component of this action is to use the first two fingers of the remaining hand to lift up the bony portion of the mandible near the chin (the thumb should not be used). This brings the tongue forward, preventing it from blocking the posterior oropharynx. The maneuver also supports the jaw and helps to hold the head-tilt positioning. The teeth may nearly occlude but be open enough for mouth-to-mouth ventilation to occur. Loose dentures should be supportive in this maneuver but should be removed if they prove to be obstacles in maintaining the airway.

Facial trauma may result in an inability to open the mouth or an inability to provide a leakproof mouth-to-mouth seal, which may require the rescuer to perform mouth-to-nose ventilation. The mouth is held closed with mouth-to-nose ventilation, but may need to be manually opened to permit exhalation.

Rescue breathing to all patients with a permanent tracheal stoma must occur by mouth-to-stoma ventilation. Patients who have received a laryngectomy cannot be ventilated in the standard fashion, as there is no longer a connection between trachea and mouth.

BOX 19-2

INDICATIONS FOR RESUSCITATION OR AIRWAY MANAGEMENT

- Airway obstruction
- Acute myocardial infarction with cardiodynamic instability
- Life-threatening dysrhythmias
- Hypovolemic shock
- Severe infections
- Spinal cord or head injury
- Drug overdose
- Pulmonary edema
- Anaphylaxis
- Pulmonary embolus
- Smoke inhalation
- High-risk delivery

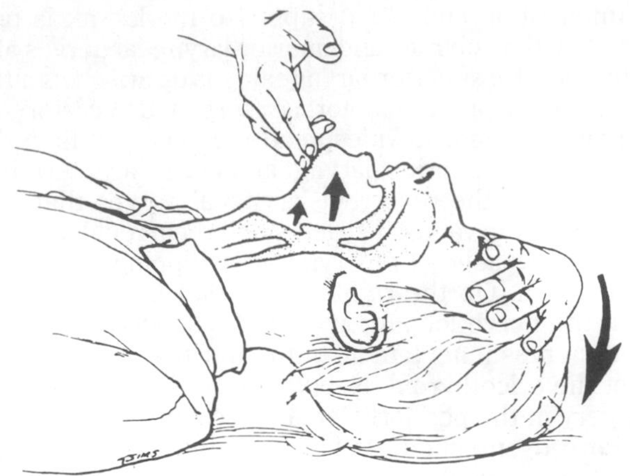

FIGURE 19-3. Manual opening of the adult airway using the head-tilt/head-lift. (Reproduced with permission. © Instructor's Manual for Basic Life Support. 1987. Copyright American Heart Association)

Jaw-Thrust/Head-Tilt

The "jaw-thrust/head-tilt" maneuver is a variant on the head-tilt/chin-lift maneuver (Fig. 19-5). It is recommended for use in opening the "difficult airway" and has also been termed the "triple airway maneuver." It can also be applied without the head tilt for suspected or confirmed neck injuries, in that it opens the airway without extension of the cervical spine.

To perform the jaw thrust, the rescuer positions both elbows on a surface, on either side of the victim's head. The fingers grasp the mandible at the angle and lift to displace the jaw forward. The thumbs are often employed to retract the victim's lower lip to allow mouth-to-mouth breathing. (This requires that the cheek be used to seal the nostrils of the victim.) The jaw thrust alone can be successful in opening the airway. To also incorporate the head tilt, the rescuer simply tilts the head backward. For the victim with suspected spinal trauma, the head should be supported and movement prevented. If the jaw thrust alone is not successful in opening the airway, the head should be tilted back slightly. Although the jaw-thrust maneuvers are difficult to perform and are fatiguing, they are quite effective.

Tongue-Jaw Lift

The tongue-jaw lift is recommended to visually check for foreign body obstruction in adults, children, and infants (Fig. 19-6). This mandibular displacement is also

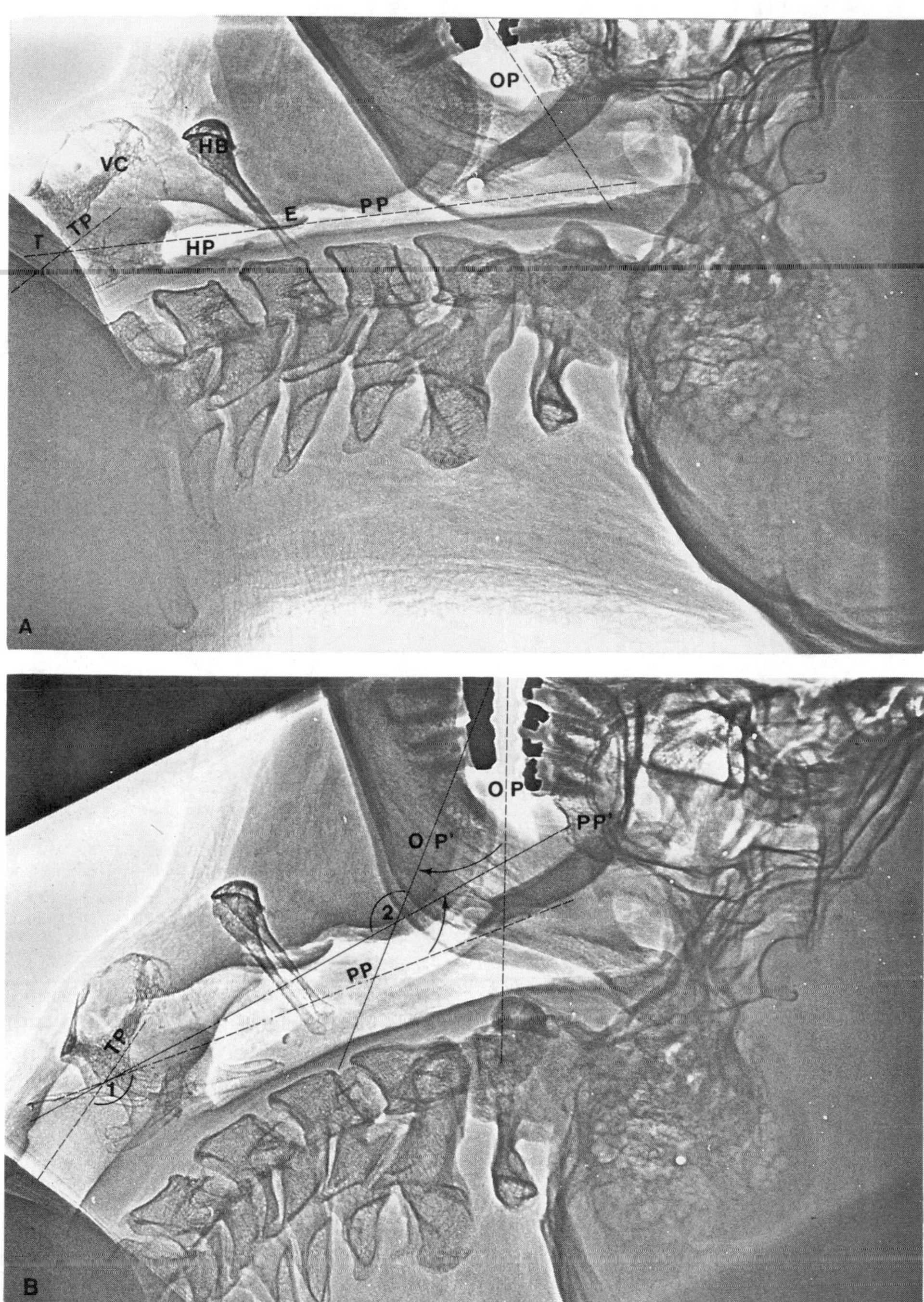

FIGURE 19-4. Xeroradiographs of the adult airway. **(A)** A supine posture neutral position, causing the tongue to obstruct the posterior pharyngeal plane (along line PP). **(B)** The "sniffing position" showing minimal angulation between pharyngeal and tracheal planes. This facilitates intubation: T, trachea; TP, tracheal plane; VC, vocal cords; HP, hypopharynx; HB, hyoid bone; E, epiglottis; PP, pharyngeal plane; PP′, pharyngeal plane with forward head tilt; OP, oral plane; OP′, oral plane in sniffing position.

very effective in providing an airway. However, the rescuer risks being bitten unless the victim remains unconscious or is edentulous. The thumb is placed in the mouth inside the lower incisors. The fingers grasp the chin, and the hand pulls upward. This position facilitates visual location of an obstructing substance or object and allows sweeping (clearing) of the airway with the fingers of the opposite hand.

Pediatric Considerations

The aforementioned techniques are also used for pediatric airway management. The head-tilt/chin-lift maneuver is employed, with special care taken to prevent overextension of the head or to prevent the soft parts of the underchin from occluding the airway (Fig. 19-7*A*). The jaw thrust, with or without head tilt, is performed

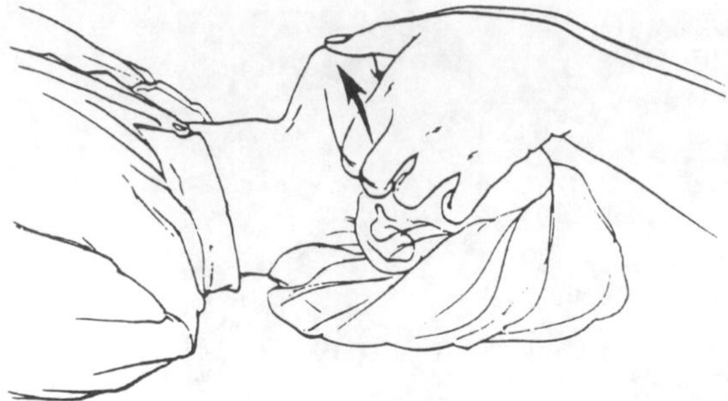

FIGURE 19-5. The jaw-thrust maneuver without head tilt. (Reproduced with permission, Instructors Manual for Basic Life Support. 1987. © American Heart Association)

as in the adult (Fig. 19-7*B*). The tongue-jaw lift is also used on unconscious children and infants who have complete airway obstruction. The AHA suggests it be combined with direct removal of a visualized object or "blind" sweeping of the posterior pharynx (in the adult and child only).

MANUAL METHODS TO CLEAR AN OBSTRUCTED AIRWAY

Even though manual techniques for airway opening are performed correctly, blockage of the upper airway may still prevent successful ventilation. An arrest victim or hospitalized patient who aspirates foreign materials, including food, toys, teeth, or other objects, should be encouraged to clear the object by coughing it up while he or she is conscious. Physical signs of hypoxia, increased dyspnea, and ineffective cough are signals for intervention. With complete obstruction, the victim is unable to breathe, speak, or cough. The universal distress signal for a conscious victim is the clutching of the neck between thumb and fingers. Unconscious victims will not respond to repeated attempts to ventilate if a foreign body is obstructing the airway. The rescuer will not see the chest rise upon mouth-to-mouth breathing or feel air freely move into the victim. This blockage will continue in spite of airway repositioning or altering the type of airway opening techniques. The reader is referred to Chapter 22 for a complete review of the techniques for relieving an obstructed airway.

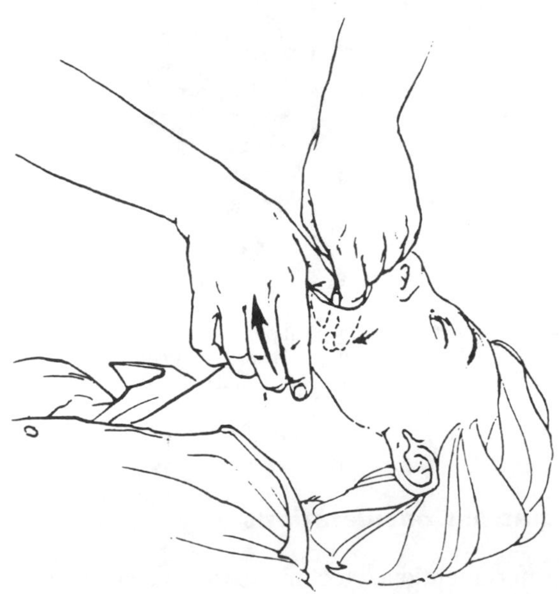

FIGURE 19-6. The tongue-jaw lift used in combination with a finger sweep maneuver performed on an unconscious victim of foreign body obstruction. (Reproduced with permission. Instructor's Manual for Basic Life Support, 1987. © American Heart Association)

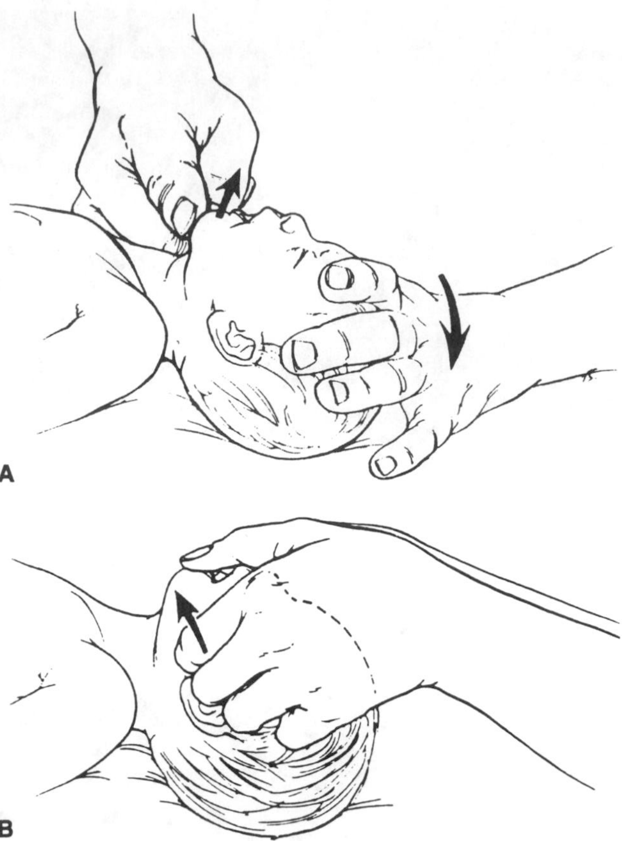

FIGURE 19-7. Infant airway maneuvers. **(A)** Head tilt/chin lift and **(B)** jaw thrust. (Reproduced with permission, Instructor's Manual for Basic Life Support, 1987. © American Heart Association)

ASSESSING BREATHLESSNESS AND RESCUE BREATHING

After successful opening of the airway, the rescuer must determine whether there is spontaneous respiration or whether rescue breathing is required. The AHA suggests the following:

1. Look for chest wall movement.
2. Listen for sounds of air movement.
3. Feel for exhaled air with the cheek.

The presence of all three indicate successful airway maintenance. When only chest wall movements (without air movements) are detected, an obstructed airway may be present. The rescuer should first reposition the airway or use an alternative manual technique of airway maintenance. If this is unsuccessful, alternative maneuvers (eg, the Heimlich) may be indicated.

Next, rescue breathing by mouth-to-mouth, mouth-to-nose, or mouth-to-stoma ventilation or by means of a mask-valve-bag device should be initiated with two breaths, each delivered in 1 to 1.5 seconds. For an average-sized adult, the volume should be between 0.8 L and 1.2 L. Children and infants require proportionally less volume. Exhaled air given with excessive pressure tends to inflate the stomach. Breathing can continue at 12 breaths per minute for an adult and 20 per minute for children and infants.

When possible, practitioners should take protective measures when performing airway maneuvers. Devices are available that act as a barrier to the patient's body secretions and blood; these include rubber gloves, eye shields, and valved or filtered face masks.

Summary

Figure 19-8 summarizes decision-making options for cardiopulmonary resuscitation (CPR), including obstructed airway protocol. Readers are urged to complete an AHA or Red Cross sponsored course with an opportunity to master techniques on manikins designed for such practice. A complete discussion of CPR procedures is found in Chapter 22.

MECHANICAL ADJUNCTS TO AIRWAY MANAGEMENT

Face Masks

The face mask enables CPR rescuers, respiratory care practitioners, or anesthesia personnel to effect a seal around the patient's airway, apply medical gases, and administer positive-pressure ventilation. Anesthesia-type face masks are commonly used in conjunction with an anesthesia bag or circuit or self-inflating resuscitators. Their purpose is to provide a leakproof interface between the patient and the gas source. Manufacturers have produced several sizes and styles of masks to allow fitting a variety of patients. Both permanent and disposable models are available (Fig. 19-9). A good mask fit is essential to ventilate the patient with positive pressure and to prevent dilution of inspired gases with room air in spontaneously breathing patients.

Masks are composed of three parts: the seal, the body, and the connector. Mask seals are commonly made of a cushion composed of covered foam or an inflatable rim. A rubber or plastic flange, which is an extension of the mask body and is not inflated, may also be used. The body of the mask provides it with a rigid structure. There is some effort made to keep the dead space of the mask body to a minimum. Average adult-sized masks have dead space volumes of 75 to 110 mL.[9] The smallest mask that fits properly minimizes dead space and is usually easier to hold on the patient's face. The mask seals rest on the nasal and maxillary bones; muscles in the cheeks help seal the area between the maxilla and mandible. Box 19-3 lists facial features that often present difficulty in achieving a tight mask-to-face fit.

Success with the aforementioned patients is increased by experimenting with a variety of mask shapes and styles. The vertical dimension of the face shortens in the edentulous patient. Insertion of an oral airway increases that distance by lowering the mandible.[9]

The connector in a mask allows fitting of a 22-mm (outside diameter) valve bag or other breathing device. Masks for anesthetic practice often have metal clips for attachment to a set of head straps. The use of such straps increases the risk of aspiration when emesis occurs. Consequently, patients who are at risk for regurgitation should not have masks applied in this manner.

The skill of holding a face mask and providing a tight seal must be combined with airway positioning, as discussed earlier. The most common method is using one hand and allowing the other to ventilate by bag device. Figure 19-10*A* illustrates hand placement. The thumb and forefinger grasp the body of the mask around the connector. The "ridge" of the mandible is grasped by the ring finger's distal phalanges. The little finger is placed under the angle of the mandible. As the head is held in the position of extension used in the jaw-lift/head-tilt maneuver, these fingers squeeze the mask to the face.

An alternate method is often reserved for the difficult airway and resembles the jaw-lift/head-tilt position, or triple airway maneuver (Fig. 19-10*B*). Both thumbs are placed on the body of the mask, on either side of the connector. The distal portions of the two index fingers grasp the under portion of the angle of the jaw. A second practitioner is then required if manual ventilation is necessary.

The construction and usage of masks as adjunct devices for ventilation have been reviewed by several organizations. The Emergency Care Research Institute (ECRI), American Society for Testing Materials (ASTM), and the International Standards Organization (ISO) publish recommendations on mask and other emergency ventilating devices.[10–12] Box 19-4 identifies characteristics of an ideal mask for mouth-to-mask or mask-valve-bag ventilation.[13]

Problems associated with mask usage include pressure damage to the eyes (eg, corneal abrasion) and facial nerves, contact or allergic dermatitis, and aspiration. Proper mask sizing, style, and holding technique should prevent pressure trauma. If sustained use of a mask is required, removal and readjustment will prevent pressure trauma. Use of positive-pressure ventilation increases the potential for gastric insufflation and regurgitation.

Face Shields and Barrier Devices

Face-shield CPR barrier devices have recently been developed as substitutes for direct mouth-to-mouth contact or use of mask-valve-bag device. This trend is

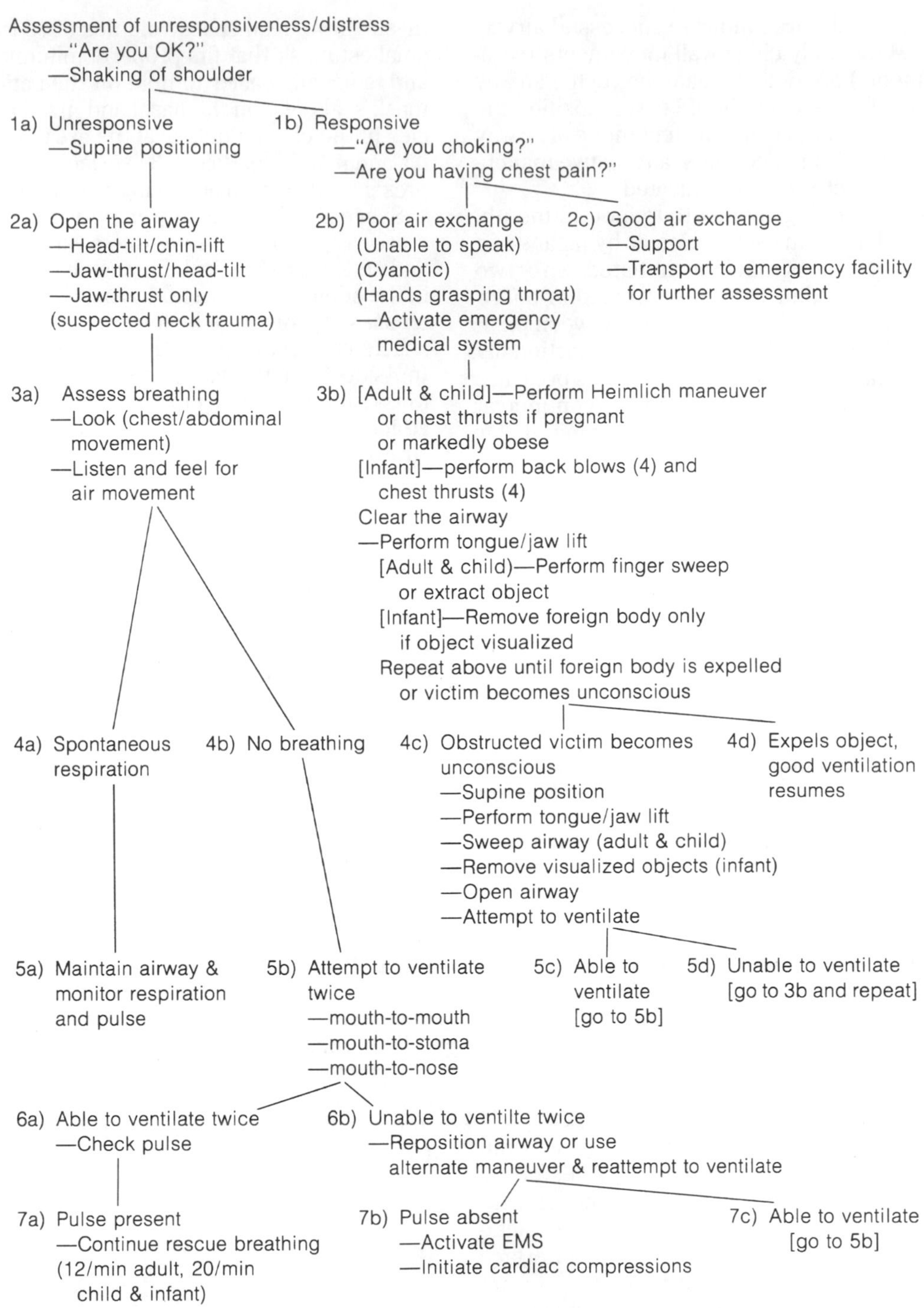
Assessment of unresponsiveness/distress
—"Are you OK?"
—Shaking of shoulder
1a) Unresponsive
—Supine positioning
1b) Responsive
—"Are you choking?"
—Are you having chest pain?"
2a) Open the airway
—Head-tilt/chin-lift
—Jaw-thrust/head-tilt
—Jaw-thrust only
(suspected neck trauma)
2b) Poor air exchange
(Unable to speak)
(Cyanotic)
(Hands grasping throat)
—Activate emergency
medical system
2c) Good air exchange
—Support
—Transport to emergency facility
for further assessment
3a) Assess breathing
—Look (chest/abdominal
movement)
—Listen and feel for
air movement
3b) [Adult & child]—Perform Heimlich maneuver
or chest thrusts if pregnant
or markedly obese
[Infant]—perform back blows (4) and
chest thrusts (4)
Clear the airway
—Perform tongue/jaw lift
[Adult & child)—Perform finger sweep
or extract object
[Infant]—Remove foreign body only
if object visualized
Repeat above until foreign body is expelled
or victim becomes unconscious
4a) Spontaneous
respiration
4b) No breathing
4c) Obstructed victim becomes
unconscious
—Supine position
—Perform tongue/jaw lift
—Sweep airway (adult & child)
—Remove visualized objects (infant)
—Open airway
—Attempt to ventilate
4d) Expels object,
good ventilation
resumes
5a) Maintain airway &
monitor respiration
and pulse
5b) Attempt to ventilate
twice
—mouth-to-mouth
—mouth-to-stoma
—mouth-to-nose
5c) Able to
ventilate
[go to 5b]
5d) Unable to ventilate
[go to 3b and repeat]
6a) Able to ventilate twice
—Check pulse
6b) Unable to ventilte twice
—Reposition airway or use
alternate maneuver & reattempt to ventilate
7a) Pulse present
—Continue rescue breathing
(12/min adult, 20/min
child & infant)
7b) Pulse absent
—Activate EMS
—Initiate cardiac compressions
7c) Able to ventilate
[go to 5b]

FIGURE 19-8. Decision-making flow sheet to deal with airway management, including foreign body obstruction.

largely related to the acquired immunodeficiency syndrome (AIDS) epidemic. The U. S. Centers for Disease Control and Prevention (CDC) currently recommends that a protective barrier be routinely used between rescuer and victim.[14,15]

The devices include mouth-to-mask devices (Fig. 19-11*A*) and face shields (Fig. 19-11*B*). The latter are also referred to as foils and barrier masks. Mouth-to-mask devices with masks similar to those used for anesthesia are available. Many of these devices have the added protection of a bacterial filter, in addition to a one-way valve. Typical barrier devices have a valved flange that is inserted into the patient's mouth or sits above the mouth. Plastic shields are held flush with the patient's lips. The airway is then manually positioned and the nares pinched closed under the mask. Clinical evaluation has shown that resistance and leakage result in slightly smaller volumes than comparable mouth-to-

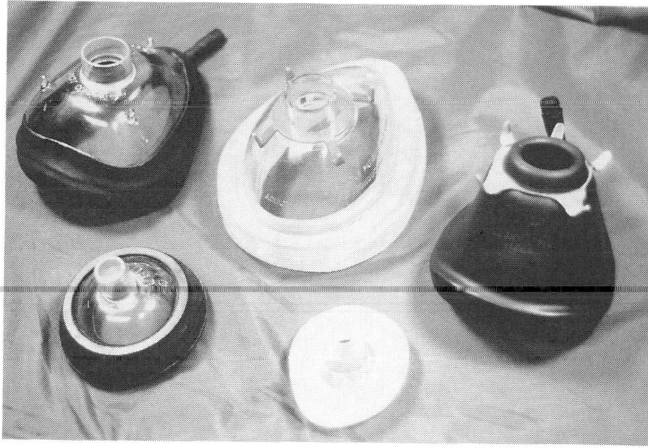

FIGURE 19-9. Assortment of mask styles and sizes to provide manual ventilation to adults and infants.

mouth ventilations.[16] Backward leakage can occur with some clinical models.[17]

Nasal Masks

Masks applied to the nose are used for nasal continuous positive airway pressure (CPAP) and for mechanical nasal ventilation. The CPAP mask acts as a pneumatic internal splint to maintain an open airway in patients with obstructive sleep apnea.[18] Nasal masks can serve as an alternative to tracheostomy in providing a means of mechanical ventilation to patients with neuromuscular weakness or restrictive lung or chest wall disorders. Commonly, these masks are custom-made with silicone rubber material.[19,20] A more detailed discussion on these topics can be found in Chapter 11 (Sleep-Disordered Breathing) and Chapter 24 (Respiratory Care in the Home and Alternate Sites). Nasal CPAP prongs are airway appliances used as alternatives to intubation in neonates (Fig. 19-12). A discussion of this device can be found in Chapter 25.

Manual Resuscitation Bags and Demand Valves

Manual resuscitation bags and demand valves provide medical gases under positive pressure to the sealed airway (ie, face mask, endotracheal tube, or tracheostomy). Manual resuscitators are available in a variety of sizes and styles, and many have the capability of providing positive end-expiratory pressure (PEEP). Because of their primary role in resuscitation, these devices are reviewed in detail in Chapter 22.

BOX 19-3

FEATURES MAKING MASK SEAL DIFFICULT

- Hawklike or flat noses
- Receding lower jaws (micrognathia) and other forms of maxillofacial dysmorphology
- Full beards
- Maxillofacial trauma
- Facial burns
- Edentulous patients
- Drainage tubes placed through the nose
- Patients with poor facial muscle tone or sagging cheeks

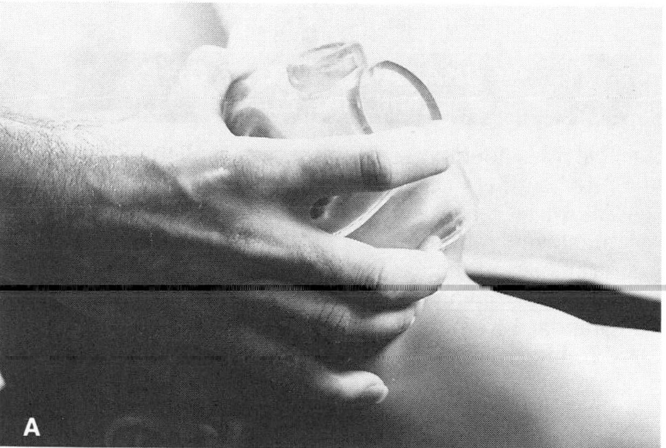

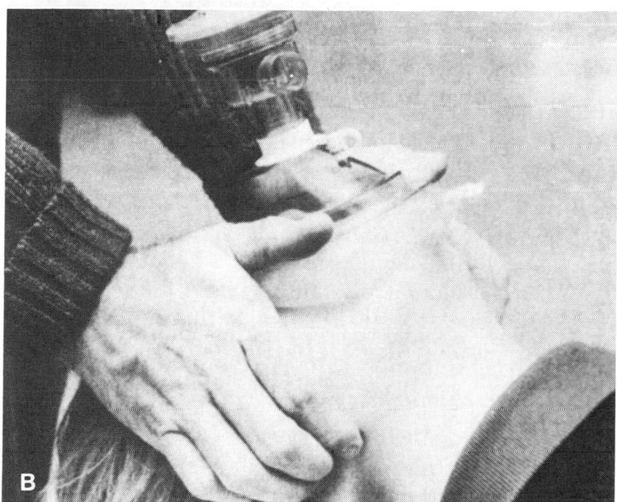

FIGURE 19-10. **(A)** One-handed technique to apply a mask to the airway. Notice placement of the fingers under the mandible and maintenance of head extension. **(B)** Two-handed technique. (From Hess D, Ness C, Oppel A, Rhoads K: Evaluation of mouth-to-mask ventilation devices. Respir Care 1989; 34:191, with permission)

Oropharyngeal Airways

The oral, or *oropharyngeal*, airway is a mechanical aid in mouth-to-mouth or mask ventilation. Box 19-5 summarizes indications for its use.

Placement of an oral airway is indicated when manual positioning of the airway must be interrupted or is limited, requiring a mechanical "splint." This device also facilitates suctioning of the airway. It can aid in preventing occlusion of an oral endotracheal tube or injury to fiberoptic bronchoscope by biting. When in place, the distal curved portion of the device lifts the posterior aspects of the tongue, elevating the epiglottis and adjacent tissue away from the pharyngeal wall.

Standards for the design of these airways have been provided by the American National Standards Institute

BOX 19-4

CHARACTERISTICS OF AN IDEAL MASK

- Provides adequate seal (often accomplished by an air-filled cuff)
- Allows increase in oxygen concentration (for mouth-to-mask ventilation, a mask nipple is provided)
- Transparent material to allow visualization of face and detection of vomitus
- Standard 15-mm/22-mm connectors
- Minimal resistance (>5 cm H_2O at 50 L/min) and dead space
- One-way valve or filter to protect rescuer from contamination for mouth-to-mask devices

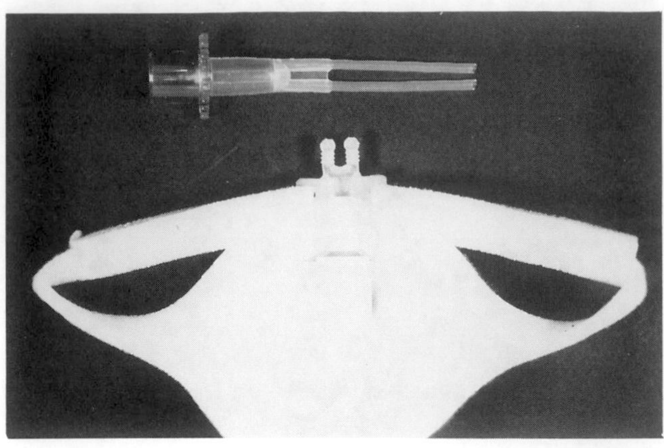

FIGURE 19-12. Nasal prongs to provide continuous positive airway pressure (CPAP) to neonatal patients.

(ANSI) and American Society for Testing and Materials (ASTM).[11,12] The basic design of the oral airway is quite simple, consisting of a flange, bite portion, and air channel. The flange prevents the airway from falling back into the mouth. The bite portion fits between the teeth. It, and the air channel, can be tubular (Guedel style, Fig. 19-13*A*) or open sided (Berman, computer-assisted design and Connell styles; Fig. 19-13*B*). The open-sided construction has the greatest potential for causing oral trauma because of its rigidity and relatively thin edges; however, it usually provides easier passage of a suction catheter. Whichever design is chosen, it must be firm enough that the patient cannot close the channel by biting and must provide a channel for passage of a suction catheter.

Manufacturers provide a variety of sizes to fit the anatomic sizes of all patients, from infant through adult. Other variants are the Ovassapian intubating airway, Williams airway intubator, and Berman intubation pharyngeal airway, which were originally devised to provide blind orotracheal intubation or for use during fiberoptic intubation.

Insertion of the airway may be accomplished by one of two methods. The practitioner should stand at the patient's head and separate the teeth with the crossed-finger technique previously discussed. Figure 19-14*A* shows the airway being inserted 180° from the final position. This avoids displacing the tongue backward and blocking the hypopharynx. Once the tip has passed the uvula, it is rotated 180°. This places the distal tip posterior to the tongue (Fig. 19-14*B*). An alternate method is to use a tongue depressor to move that structure forward so that the airway can be placed without rotation.

Problems are relatively few with use of this airway; Box 19-6 summarizes those concerns. Users must be aware that patients can traumatize the tongue and hard palate if adults chew or infants suckle the airway.[21]

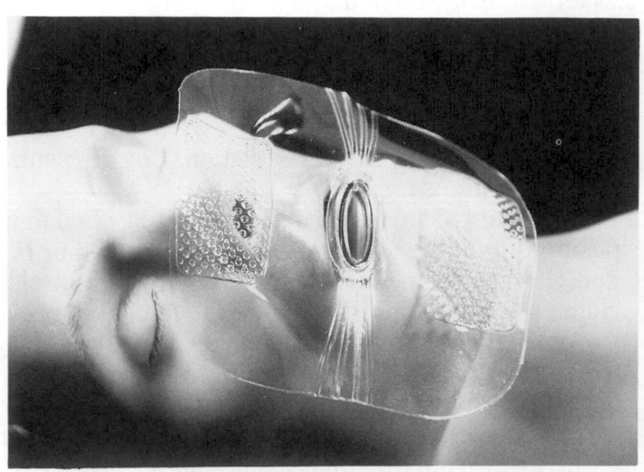

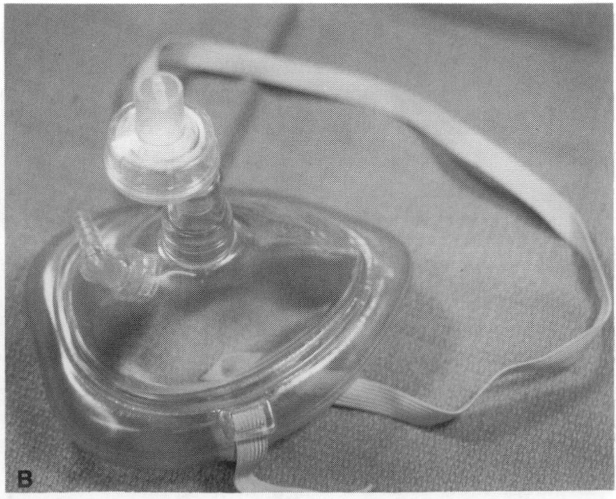

FIGURE 19-11. Protective barrier masks **(A)** Microshield mask with duckbill valve (not visible). **(B)** Pocket mask with valve.

BOX 19-5

INDICATIONS FOR USE OF THE ORAL AIRWAY

- Improves effectiveness or ease of maintaining a patent airway during manual positioning in patients who are unconscious or whose airway reflexes are diminished
- Enhances likelihood of a patent airway when the cervical spine cannot be manipulated
- Facilitates suctioning

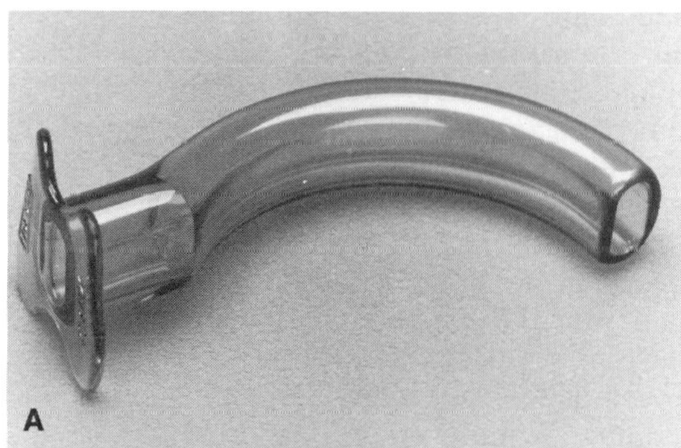

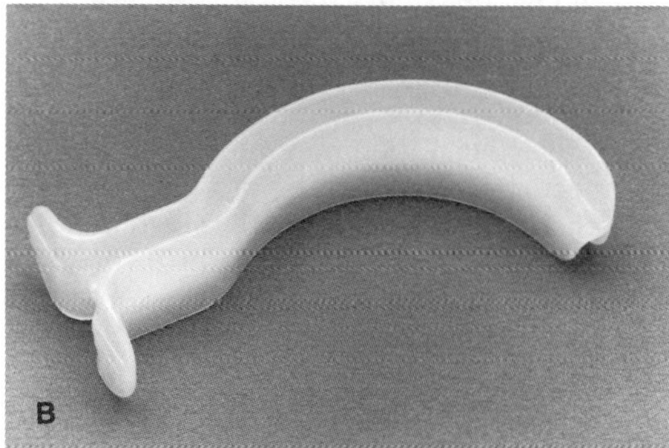

FIGURE 19-13. Oropharyngeal airways: **(A)** Guedel-style: **(B)** Connel style.

Therefore, the oral cavity should be periodically inspected. In such situations, a padded bite-block may be indicated to protect teeth and lips from trauma. Placement does not guarantee an open airway; the jaw lift may still be required.

Nasopharyngeal Airway

The *nasopharyngeal airway* is also known as the nasal airway and nasal trumpet. The tube extends from the nose to the pharynx with the distal tip just below the base of the tongue (Fig. 19-15). It is an alternative to the oral airway in that it provides similar functions. Box 19-7 lists indications for use of the nasal airway.

Insertion begins with lubrication of the entire tube with a water-soluble preparation (eg, lubricant jelly). The nasopharyngeal airway is held so the built-in curve follows the curvature of the anatomy (Fig. 19-16*A*).

The tube's tip should be advanced so it follows the floor of the nasopharynx, avoiding the nasal turbinates. The length for proper insertion can be estimated as the distance from the tragus of the ear to the nares plus 1 in., or from the meatus of the ear to the nares.[22,23] If resistance is encountered upon insertion, the opposite naris should be accessed. When properly positioned, the distal portion of the tube lies just above the epiglottis, protecting the posterior pharynx from obstruction (Fig. 19-16*B*).

Use of a nasopharyngeal airway is contraindicated in basilar skull fractures, pathologies that would result in hemorrhage (eg, anticoagulation or hemorrhagic disorders), and nasopharyngeal pathology. Major con-

BOX 19-6

PROBLEMS WITH THE ORAL AIRWAY

- Stimulation of the gag reflex (even when properly positioned)
- Ulceration or bleeding of the tongue and soft palate
- Ineffective airway patency

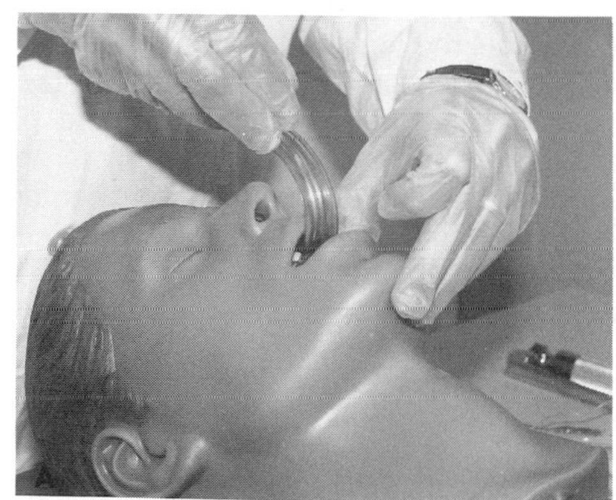

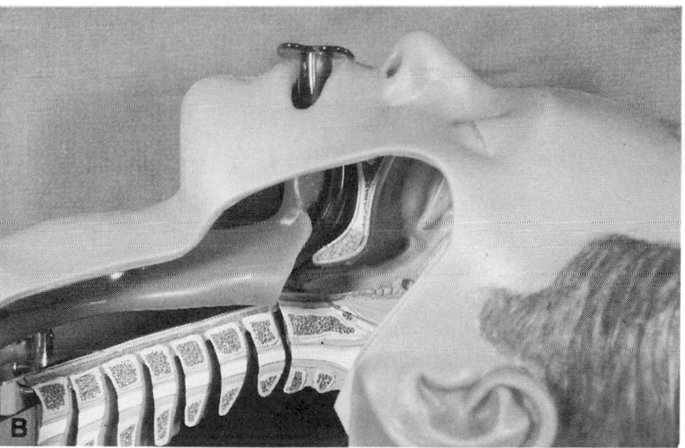

FIGURE 19-14. **(A)** Insertion of an oropharyngeal airway should be initiated in the "upside-down" position. As the airway is advanced, it is rotated so the distal portion supports the posterior pharynx. **(B)** Airway shown in position.

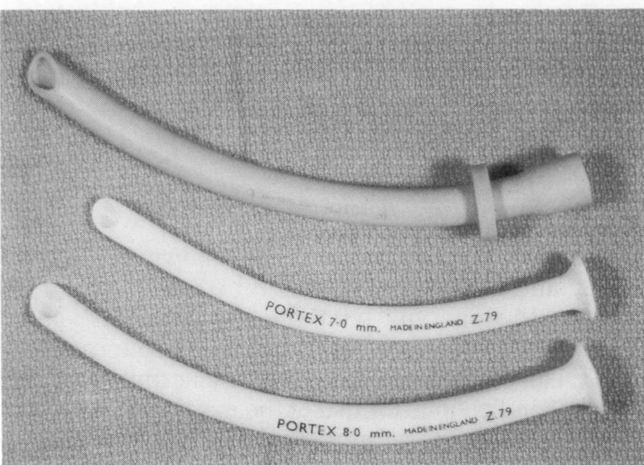

FIGURE 19-15. Nasopharyngeal airways.

cerns during use of the airway include bleeding; laryngospasm; aspiration of the airway; and occlusion caused by kinking, blood, or secretions. Box 19-8 summarizes problems with clinical use of the nasopharyngeal airway.

Esophageal Obturator Airway and Esophagogastric Airway

It has been estimated that approximately 70% of cardiac arrest victims in the field can be managed with oropharyngeal airway, head tilt, and mask-mask ventilation. Of the remaining 30%, approximately one-half are managed by direct tracheal intubation and the rest by esophageal intubation devices.[24] The *esophageal obturator airway* (EOA) and *esophagogastric tube airway* (EGTA) were originally developed for prehospital, or "field," airway management by emergency medical technicians and paramedics. Although the airway is not normally placed in the hospital setting, patients may present to the emergency room with the EOAs in place. Intubation should then occur before removal of the esophageal airway. The reader is referred to Chapter 22 for a detailed discussion of the use of this airway.

BOX 19-7

INDICATIONS FOR THE NASOPHARYNGEAL AIRWAY

- Provide a more tolerable and effective alternative to the oral airway in the conscious or semiconscious patient
- Facilitate reduced discomfort associated with nasotracheal suctioning
- Reduce trauma when passing a fiberoptic bronchoscopy (in nonintubated patients)
- Provide a patent airway when access to the oral cavity is limited (eg, mouth cannot be opened, facial trauma)
- Alternative to oral airway if the patient's teeth are loose or in poor condition
- Assist in management of Pierre Robin syndrome

Esophagotracheal Combitube and Pharyngotracheal Lumen Airway

The *esophagotracheal combitube* (ETC) and *pharyngotracheal lumen airway* (PTLA) are modifications of the esophageal obturator. Although initially developed for prehospital use, they may be alternate devices for in-hospital applications. Both propose to offer a solution to the problems of adequate face-mask seal and inadvertent tracheal intubation. The tracheal combitube (Fig. 19-17) is a double-lumen device: one channel resembles an esophageal obturator airway (with distal stopper), the other resembles an open tracheal tube. The tubes are separated by a partition wall, and the combined outer diameter is 13 mm. There are distal and proximal cuffs or balloons, each with pilot tubes for separate inflation. The distal balloon is designed to seal in the esophagus (intended location) or trachea if inadvertent placement occurs. The proximal or pharyngeal balloon replaces the mask of the EOA. When the ETC is inserted (blindly, until a printed ring mark lies at the teeth), the pharyngeal cuff seals the mouth and nose cavities. A group of holes are found in the esophageal tube between the two balloons[24] (see Fig. 19-17).

These newer designs allow the tube to provide tracheal ventilation regardless of esophageal or tracheal positioning. When properly placed in the esophagus, tracheal ventilation occurs through the perforations in the esophageal tube, much like an EOA. If the esophageal tube is placed in the trachea, there will be absence of breath sounds and gastric distension instead. The ventilator device can then be switched to the tracheal tube connector. Even if the rescuer does not realize a patient is being ventilated by a "false" lumen, spontaneously breathing patients can breathe through the unused lumen. In-hospital evaluation of the combitube has been favorable but limited.[24]

The PTLA is quite similar in purpose and design to the tracheal combitube (Fig. 19-18*A*). However, instead of dual tubes of similar length, the PTLA has a short tube (21 cm) and, passing through that, a long tube (31 cm). Both tubes have inflatable cuffs; the distal cuff seals the esophagus and the proximal cuff seals the pharynx. The latter cuff is applied at the end of the short tube, and the former midway down the long tube. Like the combitube, the long tube can provide ventilation if inadvertently placed in the trachea (Fig. 19-18*B*). An additional advantage of the combitube and pharyngotracheal airways is their apparent ability to protect the trachea from aspiration of upper airway hemorrhage.[25]

The PTLA is advanced blindly until the "teeth strap" is at the level of the incisors. A removable stylet provides rigidity for this process. Both cuffs are then inflated. The rescuer ventilates through the short tube and determines if the chest rises and bilateral breath sounds can be auscultated. If that is not the case, the trachea has been intubated. The stylet in the long tube is then removed and ventilation is applied to that tube connector. In this condition, the PTLA approximates an endotracheal tube. Limited animal and human simulation testing has shown this device to be a promising alter-

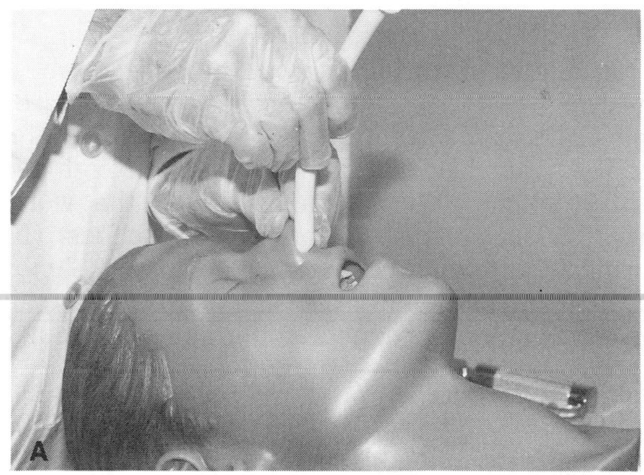

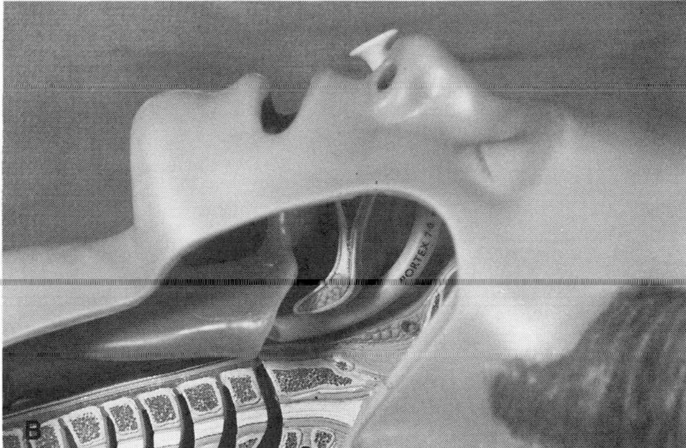

FIGURE 19-16. Placement of a nasopharyngeal airway. **(A)** Insertion showing the tip being inserted parallel to the floor of the nasal cavity; **(B)** Airway in position.

native to tracheal intubation in out-of-hospital airway management. The combitube and PTLA may have some advantage over the EOA and EGTA in patients for whom there is difficulty with face-mask seal or when airway hemorrhage is present.[26] However, if a patient does not display clinical signs of improvement with any of the aforementioned airways, the stomach should be decompressed and endotracheal intubation attempted. Intubation should be performed with an EOA or EGTA in place; the combitube and PTLA must be removed before that procedure.

Laryngeal Mask Airway

The *laryngeal mask airway* (LMA) provides a means of airway support that is potentially more secure than a face mask, yet less secure than endotracheal intubation[27] (Figs. 19-19 and 19-20). The LMA has recently become commercially available in the United States. It was conceived, developed, and refined by British anesthesiologist Archie Brain during the 1980s; it is also called the Brain mask or Brain mask airway. Box 19-9 lists clinical situations in which the LMA has been used successfully.

The laryngeal mask airway is constructed entirely of silicone rubber (latex free). The cuff is inflated with an air-filled syringe using a pilot valve–balloon system. When properly positioned, three fenestrated apertures sit directly above the patient's larynx. Size 4 is intended to fit a >70-kg adult. Four additional sizes are available. Size 1 for neonates and infants up to 6.5 kg; size 2 for infants from 6.5 to 20 kg; and size 3 for children over 30 kg and small adults (see Fig. 19-20).

Laryngeal mask insertion requires that patients have a depressed level of consciousness similar to that required for placement of an oropharyngeal airway. The "sniffing" position (neck flexed and head extended) best facilitates placement. The patient's mouth is opened and the tip of the cuff is firmly applied against the hard palate. The tube is then advanced using the forefinger until resistance is encountered. When the cuff is inflated, a characteristic upward movement of the tube occurs as the cuff is positioned over the patient's larynx (Fig. 19-21). With proper inflation of the cuff, a seal is formed around the laryngeal inlet that can remain competent with airway pressures up to approximately 25 cmH_2O.

BOX 19-8

PROBLEMS WITH THE USE OF A NASOPHARYNGEAL AIRWAY

- Bleeding of the nasopharynx (injury to turbinates)
- Occlusion of the laryngeal aperture
- Infection (otitis media and sinusitis)
- Laryngospasm and coughing
- Damage to adenoid tissue (children)
- "Swallowing" the airway

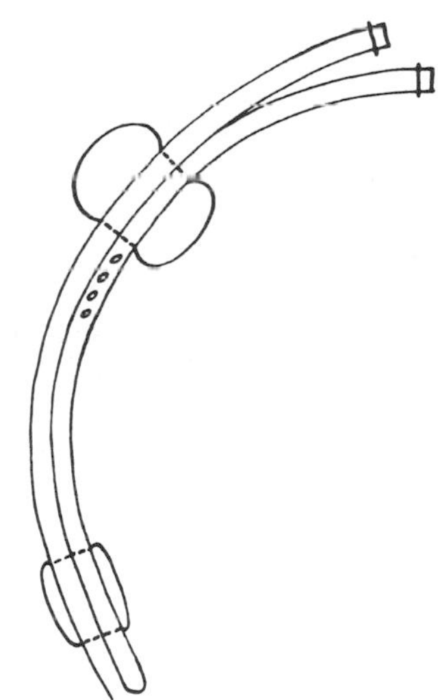

FIGURE 19-17. Esophagotracheal combitube. (Frass M, Frenzer R, Rauscha F, Weber H, Pacher R, Leithner C: Evaluation of esophageal combitube in cardiopulmonary resuscitation. Crit Care Med 15:609, 1986, © Williams & Wilkins, with permission)

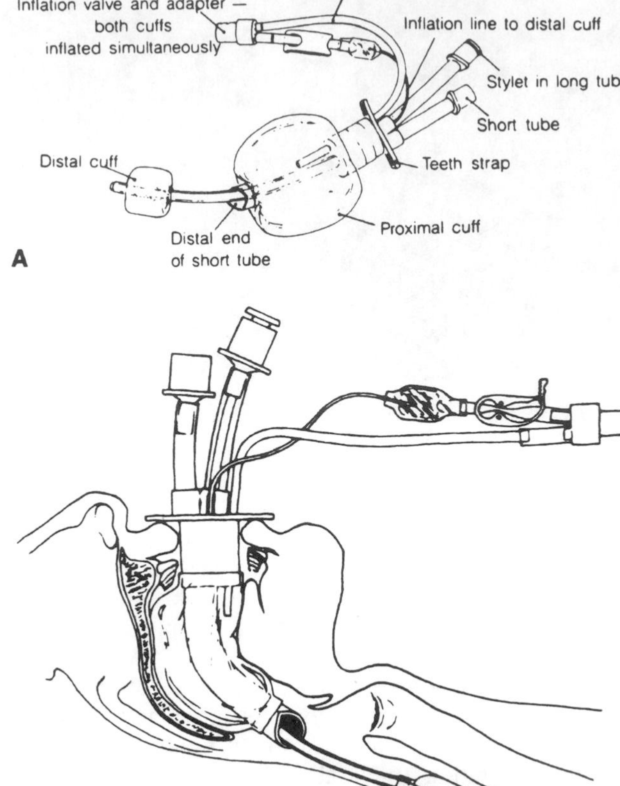

FIGURE 19-18. **(A)** Diagram of the pharyngotracheal lumen airway (PTL). **(B)** Representation of the PTL airway in position. (Niemann JT, Myers R. Scarberry EN: The pharyngotracheal lumen airway: preliminary investigation of a new adjunct. Ann Emerg Med 13:591, 1984. With permission)

The LMA provides an efficient means of airway management for the respiratory care practitioner. The blind insertion technique is readily mastered with formal training.[28] Contraindications to the use of the LMA include inability to extend the patient's neck or open the mouth, pharyngeal lesion, instances of low pulmonary compliance or high airway resistance, periods when patients are at increased risk for aspiration, and times when prolonged airway maintenance will be necessary.

Tracheal Tubes

The term *tracheal tube* is often used in this chapter to describe a tube placed through the larynx, either orally or nasally, that is positioned in the trachea. Synonyms are *endotracheal, intratracheal,* or *tracheal catheter.* This airway is considered to be the standard for definitive airway management in critical care or anesthesia applications.

□ BASIC DESIGN

Although there are numerous specialized tubes, the basic design of the tracheal tube has been standardized. The American Society for Testing and Materials (ASTM) provides voluntary standards through its F-29 subcommittee, a division subcommittee that works on airways, laryngoscopes, and bronchoscopes. **(Note:** Formerly, direction came from the ANSI Z-79.) Standardization can help those using airways by reducing variations among products from different manufacturers and eliminating inappropriate materials.[28,29]

The components of the endotracheal tube with standardizations of the ASTM are as follows (Fig. 19-22*A* and *B*).

Connector. A tapered fitting inserts into the tube's proximal end. The opposite end is a 15-mm (outside diameter) fitting that permits connection to a resuscitator bag, anesthesia device, or mechanical ventilator.

Tube Body. Tubes are made to have a curvature radius of 14 ± 2 cm. The internal diameters (ID) are used to size tubes of 6 mm (ID) or larger and are printed on the tube. Outside diameter marking is optional. Those that are smaller than 6 mm must have both the outside and inside diameter listed (ID/OD). The appropriate length is determined by the internal diameter. Tubes can be purchased either "precut" or in a longer form (with a minimum length). The latter tubes are then cut once in place so that the proximal end does not protrude extensively. Other markings include the length (measured from the patient end), whether it is intended for single use only, and "F29" if it meets ASTM standards. Radiopaque markers are placed the length of the tube or at the patient end. This helps locate the intratracheal position on a chest radiograph.

Tracheal Tube Cuff. A doughnut-shaped sleeve, when inflated, seals against the internal tracheal wall, permitting positive-pressure ventilation and preventing aspiration. When inflated, the cuff should not traumatize the adjacent tissue or herniate so as to block the distal tip. **(Note:** Tubes intended for perinatal or pediatric patients [prepubescent] are uncuffed.)

Inflating System. The cuff is inflated through a small-bore inflation tube. It lies within the wall of the endotracheal tube in the inserted portion, but diverges from the body of the tube. The take-off point varies with the tube length. An air-filled syringe is inserted into an inflation valve. Air cannot exit or enter unless a spring-loaded valve is actuated. The external pilot balloon indicates the general inflation state of the hidden cuff by allowing the operator to feel for air pressure. The intracuff pressure may be measured with an in-line manometer.

Distal Tip. The tip should be rounded with no sharp points or edges. The patient end of tracheal tubes has a bevel angle of 38° ± 8° from midline. Traditionally, oral tubes have had bevels facing left (when the concave aspect is up in the intubating position). Nasal tubes have had the bevel facing either direction.

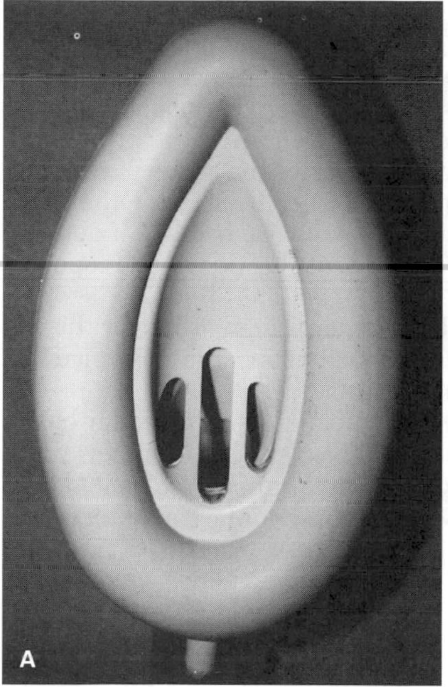

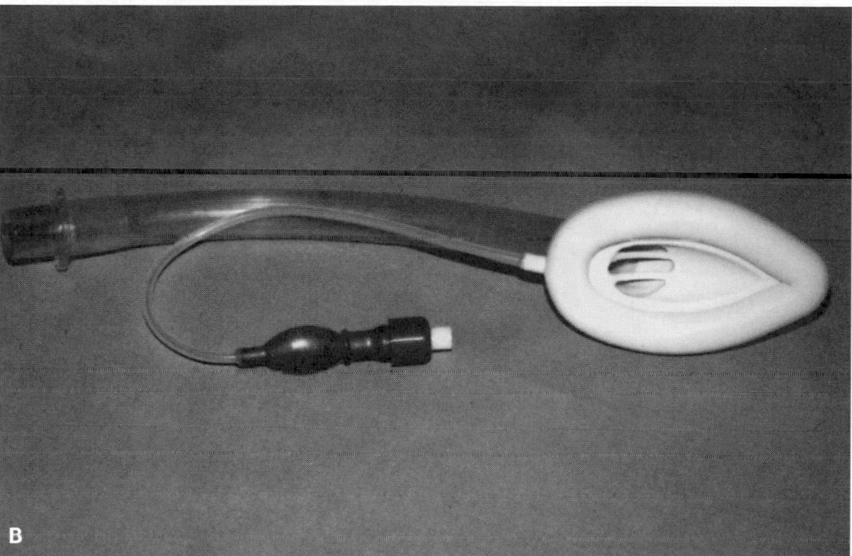

FIGURE 19-19. **(A)** Laryngeal mask airway. **(B)** Detail of mask ventilting orifices at the junction of the tube and the mask.

A *Magill-type tracheal tube* has only a distal opening in the tip. The *Murphy-type tracheal tube* also has a small hole opposite the bevel. The ASTM F-29 Committee specified that the eye must not be less than 80% of the cross-sectional area of the tube's lumen. This side port can allow ventilation if the tip becomes occluded by the tracheal wall, blood clots, sputum, or being advanced accidentally into a main stem bronchus.[30]

FIGURE 19-20. Diagram of laryngeal mask airway in place. The distal tip rests against the upper esophageal spincter; the mask's sides face the pyriform fossae. (From Dorsch JA, Dorsch SE: Understanding Anesthesia Equipment. 3rd ed. Baltimore: Williams & Wilkins, 1994 with permission)

□ ENDOTRACHEAL AND NASOTRACHEAL TUBE MATERIALS

Early endotracheal tubes were made of "natural" or synthetic rubber, with cuffs composed of latex. Several of the additives used in the manufacture of these tubes, or chemicals later absorbed, had the potential to be toxic to airway tissue. Currently, the ASTM recommends that materials be tested by *implantation testing,* or laboratory analysis of the material's effect on living tissue. Small slivers of the tube material are placed in the muscle of laboratory animals (rabbits). To validate

BOX 19-9

CLINICAL SITUATIONS IN WHICH THE LMA HAS PROVEN USEFUL[26]

- Outpatient surgery and short procedures in which intubation is unnecessary
- Difficult airway
- Fiberoptic bronchoscopy
- Obstetric patients
- Pediatric patients
- Head and neck surgery
- Burn patients
- Magnetic resonance imaging

(From Bartlett RL, Martin SD, Perina D, Raymond JI: The pharyngeo-tracheal lumen airway: An assessment of airway control in the setting of upper airway hemorrhage. Ann Emerg Med 16:343, 1987; with permission)

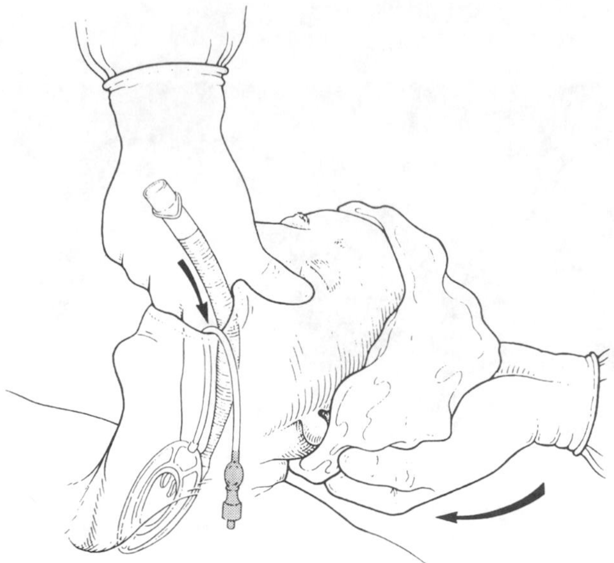

FIGURE 19-21. Insertion of laryngeal mask airway. (From Dorsch JA, Dorsch SE: Understanding Anesthesia Equipment. 3rd ed. Baltimore: Williams & Wilkins, 1994, with permission)

the test, known toxic and known tissue-inert materials are used as controls. The sites are inspected grossly and microscopically after 7 days. Tissue necrosis signals toxic problems. Those materials causing no damage are recommended for patient use. The printing of "F29" on a tracheal tube indicates that it has passed the ASTM implantation-testing specifications. Other test methods (eg, cell culture) may also be used if demonstrated to yield comparable results. Besides a response to chemical components, a reaction to the outer texture of the tube material can occur. The reasons for this effect are less well understood but apparently involve the roughness of the tube's surface.[30]

Currently, the following materials are used for endotracheal tubes: natural rubber, synthetic rubber, polyvinyl chloride (PVC), silicone rubber (polysiloxane), and polyethylene. Manufacturers use a variety of accelerators (catalysts), curing agents, plasticizers, stabilizers, antioxidants, fillers, and other additives. Each manufacturer may customize the material with various additives, altering the rigidity and slipperiness. Tubes are more rigid at room temperatures and quickly soften at body temperature. Exposure to temperatures below freezing can permanently alter materials.[31] Tracheos-

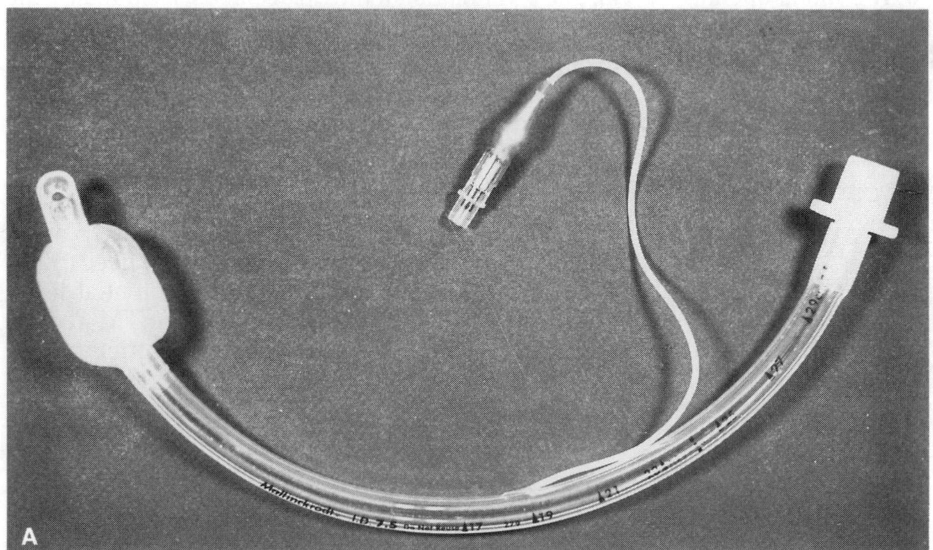

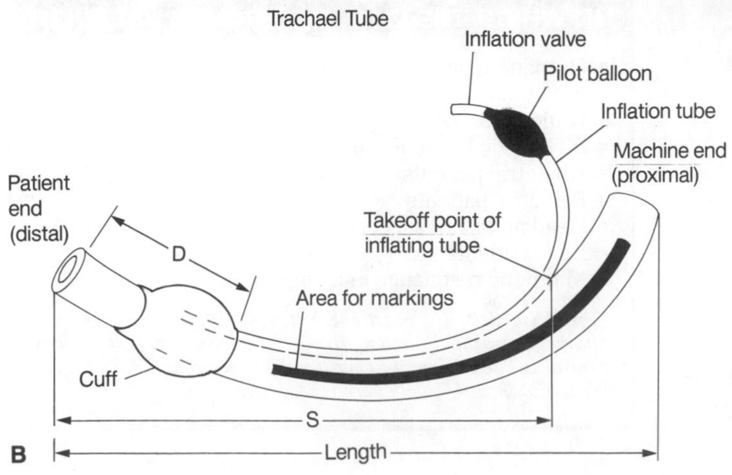

FIGURE 19-22. **(A)** A cuffed endotracheal tube. **(B)** Diagram illustrating basic design features and dimensional zones. (ASTM: Standards for cuffed and uncuffed tracheal tubes [F2290201] Philadelphia. © American Society for Testing and Materials, 1989, with permission.)

BOX 19-10

DESIRABLE FEATURES OF TRACHEAL TUBE MATERIALS

- Lack of tissue toxicity
- Transparency
- Disposable or easy to sterilize and durable with repeated sterilizations
- Slippery, smooth surfaces
- Sturdy to maintain shape on insertion and patency with kinking or external compression
- Thin wall to diameter ratio
- Thermoplasticity to allow bending at anatomical pressure points
- Nonreactive to lubricants or anesthetic agents
- Nonflammable

tomy tubes are also constructed of these materials. Tubes of other materials are reviewed later in this chapter.

An ideal material for tracheal tubes should be nontoxic, soft enough to allow conformation to anatomic pressure points, yet firm enough to resist kinking and permit insertion. The outer surfaces of tubes should be "microscopically" smooth to avoid tissue abrasion. Lastly, the materials used should resist surface bacterial adhesion.[32] Box 19-10 summarizes desirable features of tracheal tube materials and construction.

☐ TUBE SIZE

Manufacturers provide a range of outside diameters to accommodate differing sizes of upper airway structure. In adults, generally, the largest diameter tube that fits through the patient's glottis should be used. There is great variation in size and shapes of tracheas. Correlation between age, race, height, weight, and body surface area are poor. Recommended tube diameters (ID) for infants and adults appear in the literature and are summarized in Table 19-1.[2,33,34] Nasal intubation usually requires a tube one-half size smaller (or 2 mm), as it must pass through the nose and nasopharynx.

☐ GENERAL PHYSICAL PRINCIPLES: FLOW, DIAMETER, AND LENGTH

One of the major concerns in clinical care is the potential for airway tubes to increase the resistance to airflow. A greater pressure is required by the patient (or ventilating device) to breathe. As a result, the work of breathing is increased. The pressure gradient required to move air through a tube varies, depending on the type of flow conditions. Under laminar flow conditions, the pressure drop down a straight tube follows *Poiseuille's law:*

$$\text{pressure gradient } (\Delta P) = \frac{8 \times L \times \mu \times \dot{V}}{\pi r^4}$$

or

$$\text{resistance} = \frac{\Delta P}{\dot{V}} = \frac{8 \times L \times \mu}{\pi r^4}$$

It should be noted that, under laminar conditions, pressure gradient is linearly related to gas flow ($\dot{V}$), tube length (L), and viscosity (μ). Resistance is inversely related to and exponentially dependent on the fourth power of the tube's radius (r_4) or cross-sectional area.

Rohrer's equation also relates pressure drop to flow. Under laminar conditions, the following relationship exists:

$$\Delta P = K_1 \times \dot{V}$$

TABLE 19-1 **Recommended Sizes (ID) and Estimates for Tracheal Tubes**

Uncuffed Tubes (Based on age or body weight)		
Premature	2.5–3.0 mm	
below 1 kg	2.5 mm	
between 2–3 kg	3.5 mm	or $\frac{\text{Gestational age (in weeks)}}{10 + 0.5}$ = ID (mm)
1 to 6 months	3.0–4.00 mm	
over 3 kg	4.00 mm	or $\frac{3.5 + \text{age}}{3}$ = ID (mm)
6 months to 1 year	3.5–4.5 mm	or $\frac{4.5 + \text{age}}{4}$ = ID (mm)
Uncuffed Tubes (Based on body dimension)		
Choose a tube whose external diameter (OD) is the same width as the distal portion of the patient's little finger.		
Cuffed Tubes		
8 year old	6 mm	
12 year old	6.5 mm	
16 year old	7.0 mm	
average adult female	7.0–7.5 mm	
average adult male	8.0–8.5 mm	

K_1 refers to a constant of linear resistance. For Poiseuille's and Rohrer's relationships to best estimate clinical conditions, the tube must be long enough for the establishment of fully developed laminar flow. The distance from the entry point is termed the entrance length (Le), defined by the following equation:

$$\text{Le to develop laminar flow} = K_1 \times \text{Re} \times D$$

K_1 is a constant, (D) is tube diameter, and (Re) is the *Reynolds' number* for those clinical conditions. The Reynolds' number is a dimensionless number that compares inertial and viscous forces in flowing fluid. It can predict whether flow conditions would be laminar or turbulent; this is relevant because turbulent flows exist in clinical applications. Pressure gradient increases linearly as flow increases, until turbulent flow occurs. Reynolds' numbers reflect laminar flow if less than 2300, and turbulent flow if greater than 2500. The following equation defines the Reynolds' number:[35]

$$\text{Reynolds number (Re)} = \frac{4 \times \tau \times \dot{V}}{\pi \times \mu \times D}$$

where μ is viscosity, τ is density, (D) is the diameter, and $\dot{V}$ is flow.[35] The pressure gradient for fully developed turbulent conditions is described by the following equation:

$$\Delta P \text{ with turbulent flow} = \frac{8f \times (4D) \times \dot{V}^2}{\pi \times D^4}$$

The pressure drop is directly related to (f), a friction factor (which depends on the Reynolds' number and surface roughness), tube length/diameter (L/D), and flow squared ($\dot{V}^2$), but is inversely related to the fourth power of the diameter (D_2).

Rohrer's equation can include an estimate of pressure drop for turbulent flow conditions, as follows:

$$\Delta P = K_2 \times \dot{V}^2$$

K_2 is the coefficient of nonlinear resistance. It is suggested that under clinical conditions, laminar and turbulent flows coexist. An estimate of the pressure drop is better described by summing the two Rohrer equations:

$$\Delta P \text{ with mixed laminar \& turbulent flow} = (K_1 \text{ x } \dot{V}) + (K_2 \text{ x } \dot{V}^2)$$

Most bench tests on tracheal tubes indicate nonlinear flow patterns for breathing conditions that simulate clinical conditions.[36–38] Because tracheal tubes are not long enough to allow laminar conditions to fully develop, Poiseuille's law underestimates the pressure gradient.

Depending on tube size, gas flow, and experimental design, data for resistance or work of breathing vary. In general, data from in vitro studies indicate that resistance increases 25% to 100% for each 1-mm decrease in internal tube diameter.[35] Figure 19-23 demonstrates the effect of tube size on the pressure gradient at differing (constant) flows. Figure 19-24 illustrates the effect of changes in tube diameter on work of breathing at differing tidal volume and breathing frequencies.

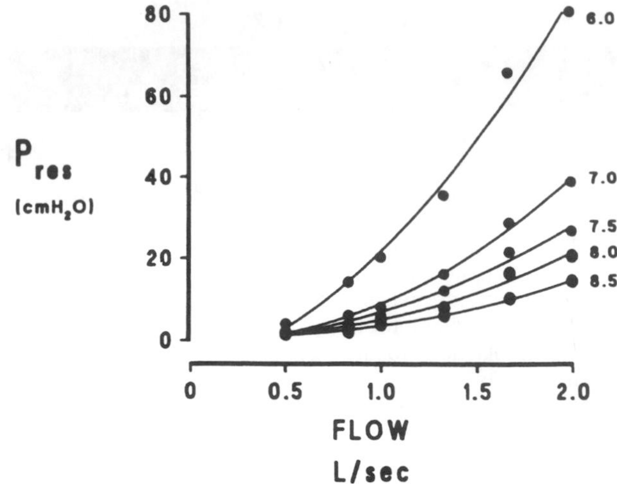

FIGURE 19-23. Graphic illustration of the pressure gradient or resistive pressure (P_{res}) required to maintain constant flows through varying diameter endotracheal tubes (Wright PE, Marini JJ, Bernard GR: In vitro versus in vivo comparison of endotracheal tube airflow resistance. Am Rev Respir Dis 140:10, 1989, with permission)

Patients seldom breathe at constant gas flows; rather, their flow patterns are oscillatory. The *Womersley number* predicts turbulent flow during oscillatory patterns and can be used like the Reynolds' number. The physics becomes more complex when tube curvature and internal surface roughness are also considered. The pressure gradient must increase to maintain flow if there is a bend in a tube. This becomes significant because tubes deform in the body, and the tracheostomy tube has its 90° bend. Secretions increase the *Moody friction factor,* which is an index of the roughness of the internal lumen.[33]

In vivo studies have demonstrated that airway resistance values are greater than when measured in vitro. All tubes contribute significantly to distortion of bedside measurements of pulmonary mechanics such as dynamic compliance and airway resistance.[39] In summary, artificial airways require a greater pressure gradient than natural airways, because resistance increases with smaller tubes, longer tubes, and increasing flow.

Clinicians should consider placing the largest tube possible to reduce work of breathing. In addition, larger-diameter tubes also increase the safety and ease of suctioning. Finally, with a larger outside diameter, the volume of air injected into the cuff can be reduced. If either very small volumes or excessively large volumes are required to produce a seal, there tends to be a change from the usual low-pressure cuff design to that of high pressure. Excessive pressure can lead to ischemic damage to the tracheal mucosa as well as cartilage erosion. In adults, the regions of the arytenoid and cricoid cartilages are particularly affected.

An empiric rule of thumb is to use an outside diameter (OD) of two-thirds the estimated tracheal diameter. Adult endotracheal tube diameters generally range from approximately 5 to 10 mm ID. Neonatal and pediatric anatomies require sizes in the 2.5 to 5.0 mm ID range.

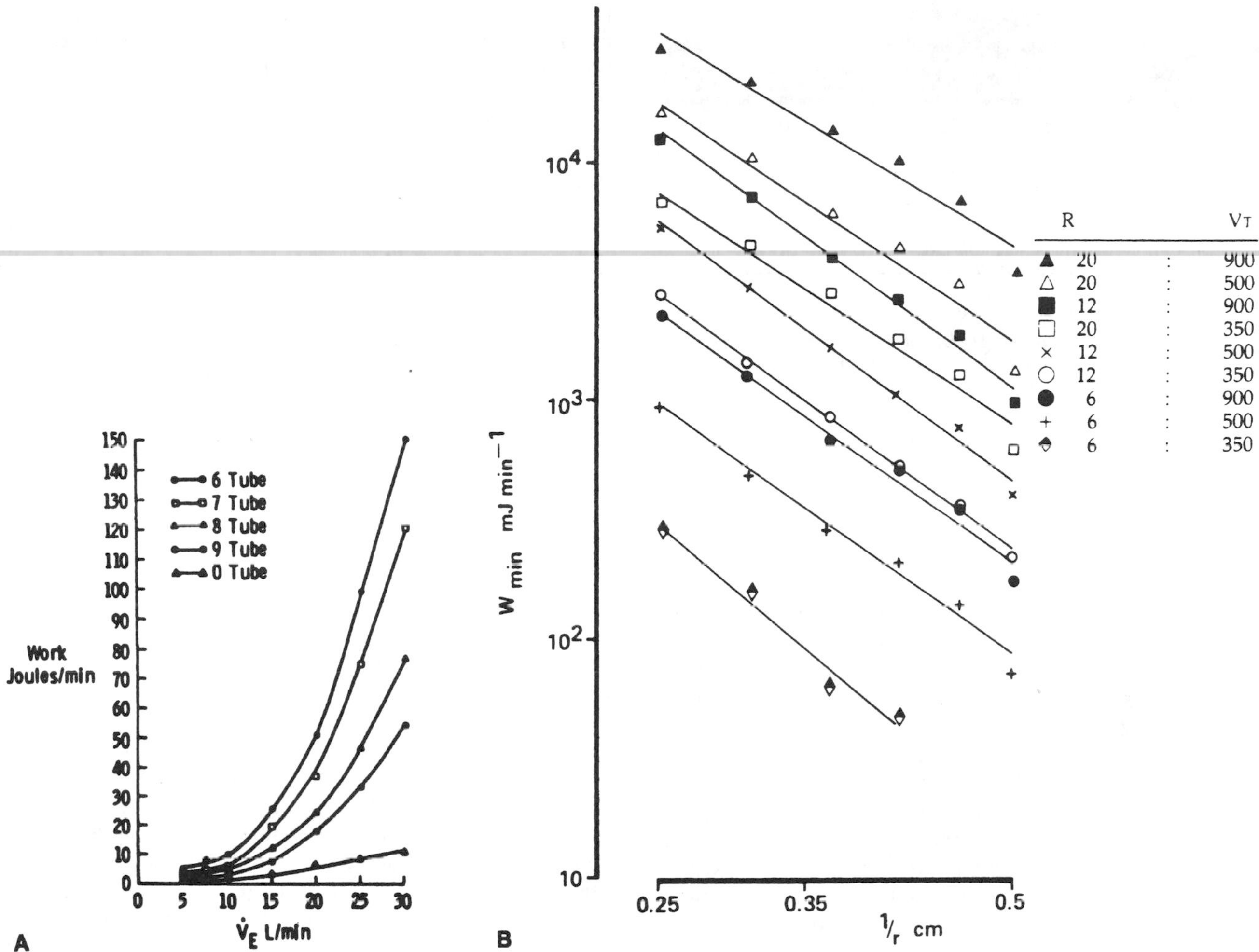

FIGURE 19-24. **(A)** Work of breathing through endotracheal tubes of varying diameters and at differing minute ventilation. (Shapiro M, Wilson RK, Gregorio C, Bloom K: Work of breathing through different-sized endotracheal tubes. Crit Care Med 14:1028, 1986, with permission) **(B)** Work of breathing for varying tidal volumes and respiratory frequencies, showing increase as the internal endotracheal tube diameter decreases. R, ventilatory rate; V_T, tidal volume. (Reprinted with permission from the International Anesthesia Research Society from Boulder AR, Beatty PC, Kay B: The extra work of breathing through adult endotracheal tubes. Anesth Analg 65:853, 1986)

Refer to Table 19-1 for age-based diameter estimates for adult and neonatal or pediatric use. Box 19-11 provides additional guidelines for assessing tube size in infants.

□ TUBE LENGTH

The length of tracheal tubes must be considered for proper placement. In pediatric patients, uncuffed tubes should be placed 1 cm past the cords in children under 6 months, no more than 2 cm in those up to 1 year, and no more than 3 to 4 cm in older children. The equation in Box 19-11 allows estimation of the optimal depth for nasal intubation in children.

Cuffed tubes should be positioned in the midtrachea or passed until the proximal cuff is 2.25 to 2.5 cm below the vocal cords.[40] In a normal adult, the average distance from the nose to midtrachea is approximately 25 cm. For oral tubes, distance from the incisors to the midtrachea averages 21 cm in adult females and 23 cm in males. This dimension is an important reference to avoid endobronchial intubation and should be noted in the patient record.[40] Auscultation and chest radiograph can determine placement location. Adult nasal tubes require an additional 2 to 4 cm in length over those used orally.

Manufacturers either provide tubes "uncut," with a minimum length recommended by the ASTM, or at a precut length (Table 19-2). The concern is to follow anatomic increases in the diameter dimension with appropriate increases in length. A tube that is too short cannot have the cuff placed below the vocal cords in the midtrachea; a tube that is too long is more likely to be accidentally advanced into a main stem bronchus.[41]

□ TRACHEAL TUBE CUFFS

Before the 1970s, cuffs for endotracheal and tracheostomy tubes were of the low-volume, high-pressure design, and use was limited to short-term, intraoperative

BOX 19-11

OPTIMAL (NASAL) TRACHEAL TUBE DIAMETER AND LENGTH FOR CHILDREN

Diameter (ID) = 18 + age (years)*

L(cm) = 0.16 – height (cm) + 4.5†

L(cm) = (3 – ID) + 2‡

* *Cuffed tubes should be one-half size smaller than calculated.*
† *From Mattila MK, Heikel PE, Suntarinen T, et al: Estimation of a suitable nasotracheal tube length for infants and children. Acta Anaesthesiol Scand 15:239, 1971*
‡ *From Yates AP, Harries AJ, Hatch DJ: Estimation of nasotracheal tube length in infants and children. Br J Anaesth 59:524, 1987*

application. Previously, rare tracheal and laryngeal lesions, such as tracheal stenosis, had begun to be reported in high numbers in the late 1960s.[42] This increase in problems paralleled the increase in the numbers of intensive care units and the acceptance of positive pressure as the method of ventilation (which required an artificial airway). To apply a softer seal to the tracheal wall, some clinicians learned to "prestretch" cuffs before their use. Manufacturers began producing tubes with a low-pressure design in the 1970s.

The beneficial sealing function of the tube's cuff is a threat to the inner tracheal tissue. The pressure applied to the wall can cause destruction of ciliated epithelium that interferes with mucus transport in the postextubation period. Continued high pressure may result in pressure necrosis of mucosal and deep tracheal wall tissue and dilatation and rupture of the trachea. Long-term problems include fibrous tracheal stenosis, tracheomalacia, and development of a tracheal zone with poor mucus transport.

It is currently accepted that high-pressure cuffs should not be considered for prolonged use. Cuff-to-tracheal wall pressures above 60 cmH_2O (8 kPa) destroy columnar epithelial tissue if sustained more than 15 minutes.[43,44] When a tracheal tube is properly sized within the trachea, intracuff pressure should approximate cuff-to-tracheal wall pressure. Pressure on the tracheal wall becomes excessive in low-pressure designs when the cuff has to be stretched to fill the trachea (ie, the tube is too small for the tracheal lumen). To prevent ischemic damage, the cuff-to-tracheal wall pressure should not exceed tissue capillary perfusion pressure. That pressure is estimated to be 20 to 30 mm Hg (27.2 to 40.8 cmH_2O, or 2.67 to 4.0 kPa), but it is lower with hypotension. When using low-pressure cuffs, the respiratory care practitioners should attempt to just seal the airway at pressures below those causing ischemic damage. Ideally, the peak intracuff pressures can be maintained at 25 to 27 cmH_2O (3.3 to 3.6 kPa) or less.[42–44] Local pressure points can develop, as the trachea is not circular in cross section. Normal anatomic variations include C-shaped, D-shaped, elliptic, and triangular-shaped tracheas.

Intracuff pressure can be determined using a three-way stopcock, syringe, and any pressure manometer (Fig. 19-25). Manufacturers also have developed devices to measure or control intracuff pressure, (eg, DHD CuffMate, InterMed Digital Cuff-Guage, and Posey cuff pressure measurement system). Pressure-relief valves, or large pilot balloon reservoirs, are also used to reduce the potential for high intracuff pressures. Respironics PressureEasy system allows airway pressure to better seal the cuff during the inspiratory phase of mechanical ventilation.

TABLE 19-2 **Tracheal Tube Internal Diameters and Lengths**

Nominal Size (mm)	Tolerance (mm)	Minimum Length (cm)	Precut Length (cm)
2.5	0.15	14	11
3.0	0.15	16	12
3.5	0.15	18	13
4.0	0.15	20	14
4.5	0.15	22	15
5.0	0.15	24	16
5.5	0.15	27	17
6.0	0.15	28	19
6.5	0.20	29	21
7.0	0.20	30	23
7.5	0.20	31	24
8.0	0.20	32	25
8.5	0.20	32	26
9.0	0.20	32	27
9.5	0.20	32	28
10	0.20	32	28

(Reproduced from American Society for Testing and Materials: Standards for cuffed and uncuffed tracheal tubes (F290201). Philadelphia, PA ASTM, 1989; with permission)

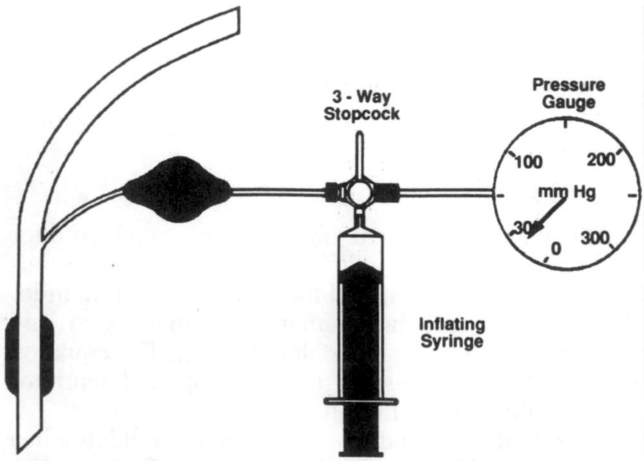

FIGURE 19-25. An aneroid pressure gauge and stopcock to monitor intracuff pressure. (From Fluck RR. Hess DR, Branson RD. Airway and suction equipment. In: Branson RD, Hess DR, Chatburn RL, eds. Respiratory Care Equipment. Philadelphia: JB Lippincott, 1995, with permission)

Clinicians using the *minimum-seal* or *just-seal technique* auscultate the area above the tracheal cuff for sounds of air movement around the cuff. The smallest amount of air that just limits airflow around the cuff is injected. Cuff location may move to larger-diameter parts of the trachea with head extension or flexion. This migration can be minimized with the use of tracheal tube stabilizer systems.[45,46]

Manufacturers produce a variety of cuff designs. Cuffs may be circular or cylindrical, large or small in diameter, long or short, of thin- or thick-walled materials, and air or foam filled. Thin-walled, large-diameter cuffs tend to form thin folds against tracheal mucosa. This allows minimal pressure to seal and reduces fluid aspiration through cuff folds. However, intubation and extubation may be more difficult with a cuff that has a "bulky" design when deflated (Fig. 19-26).[45] The ASTM recommends that the endotracheal tube lumen should resist compression from the inflated tube cuff. Nitrous oxide can diffuse into the closed gas space of a tracheal cuff. This results in an increase of intracuff volume and pressure.[47]

In spite of contemporary designs and materials, silent aspiration continues to be a problem.[43,48] Aspiration of gastrointestinal material occurs in approximately 30% to 40% of mechanically ventilated patients.[49] Endotracheal tubes bypass the natural defenses of the pharynx. This impairs ciliary activity, interferes with effective cough mechanics, and increases oropharyngeal colonization, which can lead to nosocomial pneumonia. Pneumonias of this type have a significant mortality (55%) in hospitalized, mechanically ventilated patients.[43,50]

□ SPECIALIZED TRACHEAL TUBES

Foam-cuffed or *Kamen-Wilkenson* endotracheal tubes differ from standard tubes only in the cuff design (Fig. 19-27). The sealing pressure relies on "recoil forces" of the covered internal foam. Unlike standard cuffs, the cuff self-inflates when the pilot tube is opened to the atmosphere. Active aspiration of air is required so that intubation or extubation can occur. The cuff is spacious and can seal at a low tracheal wall pressure, provided the relationship between the cuff and tracheal diameters is optimal.[51] Respiratory care practitioners must be alert to these differences. Injection of air can turn the device into a high-pressure system. Potential difficulties in using foam-cuffed tubes include air leak with positive airway pressures in excess of 45 to 50 cmH_2O (6.0 to 6.67 kPa). Also, cuffs can become soggy and resist complete deflation before extubation. Foam-cuffed tubes are an excellent choice for air transport, as they adapt to atmospheric pressure changes. In unpressurized aircraft or under loss of pressure, cuff volumes decrease with increased altitude. With descent, cuff volumes would increase according to Boyle's law (pressure is inversely related to volume).

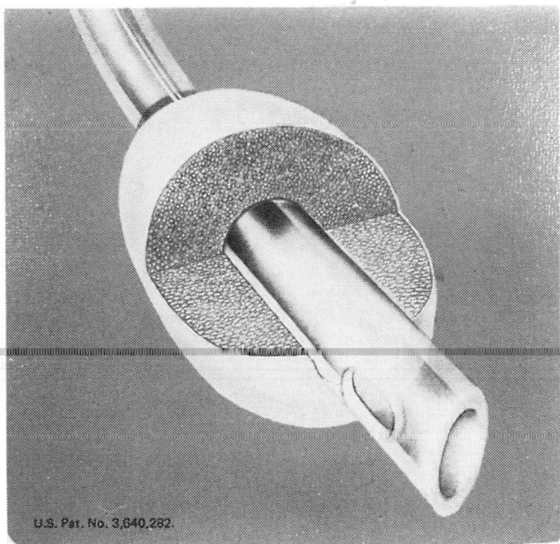

FIGURE 19-27. Diagram of the Bivona Fome-Cuff endotracheal tube. (Courtesy Bivona, Inc. Gary, Indiana)

The *Lindholm anatomic tube* was developed to better fit the curve angle into the trachea (Fig. 19-28). This

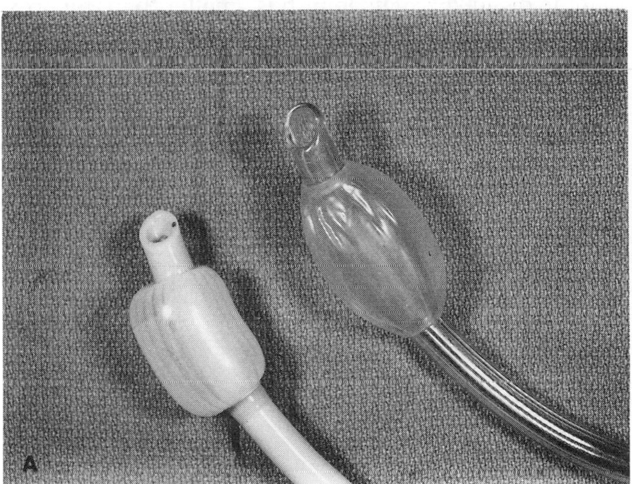

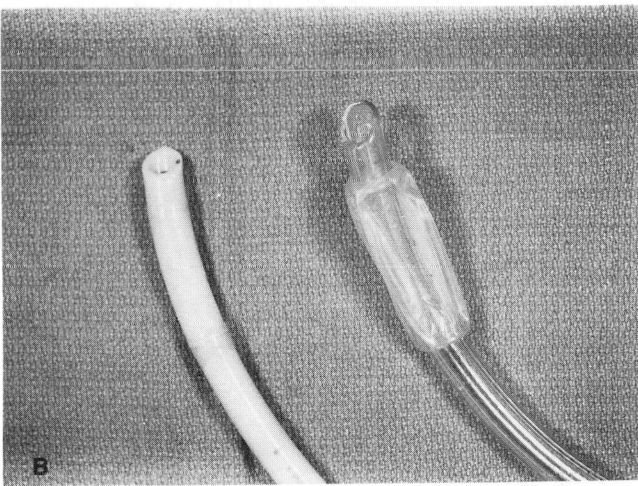

FIGURE 19-26. Endotracheal tube cuff designs demonstrating "trim" and "bulky" cuffs. **(A)** Tubes with cuffs inflated to therapeutic levels. **(B)** The same tubes with cuffs completely evacuated of air.

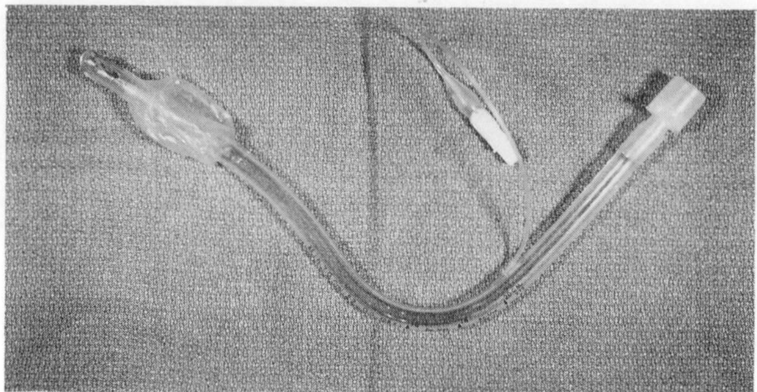

FIGURE 19-28. The anatomic-shaped Lindholm endotracheal tube.

BOX 19-12

INDICATIONS FOR DOUBLE-LUMEN BRONCHIAL TUBES

- One-lung anesthesia can be performed with the operative lung deflated
- Examination of the pleural space by means of thoracoscopy facilitated by deflation of the lung in that hemithorax
- Whole-lung lavage
- Control of contamination or hemorrhage
- Independent lung mechanical ventilation for bronchopleural fistula and unilateral disparity in lung compliance

tube appears to lessen tracheal damage at the cricoid cartilage area but does not spare the arytenoid and tracheal region from injury.[51,52]

Spiral-embedded tubes have the advantage of withstanding kinking and collapse from external pressure (Fig. 19-29). However, they have excessive flexibility in their longitudinal axis, similar to a long spring (like a Slinky). A stiffening guide wire or stylet is required for intubation.

Tubes with *monitoring lumen(s)* are useful for respiratory gas and pressure monitoring, and for injection of fluids or drugs.

Laser (protected) tubes offer protection from combustion during CO_2, KTP, and Nd:YAG laser use during bronchoscopy. Laser-resistant wrapping materials of aluminum foil or tape, copper tape, and moist cotton have also been used with standard tubes.

Double-lumen endobronchial tubes are used when it is desirable to isolate one lung from the other. Box 19-12 summarizes clinical situations that would indicate use of such tracheal tubes.

A left-sided double-lumen tube is normally used for right lung surgery. Right bronchial positioning is more difficult because of the immediate takeoff of the right upper lobe. Therefore, left-sided tubes are preferred by some for both left and right lung surgery. Older models such as the rubber Carlens tube have been replaced with contemporary, disposable plastic models (Fig. 19-30). Either the right or left main stem bronchus may be intubated, with use of tracheal and endobronchial cuffs. Flexible fiberoptic bronchoscopy makes tube location under direct vision possible. Care must be taken not to occlude either right or left segmental bronchi to the upper lobes. Ventilation occurs through two separate lumina.[53]

"Univent" bronchial-blocking tube (Fuji Systems Corporation) is a single-lumen tube with a separate, directable, bronchus-blocking cuff to isolate a lung (Fig. 19-31). The blocker cuff can be advanced or retracted on its separate tube, having both pilot and suction channels. This allows active lung deflation by syringe suction on the blocker lumen.[54]

□ PEDIATRIC TRACHEAL TUBES

Uncuffed oral and nasal endotracheal tubes are generally used in neonatal and pediatric practice (Fig. 19-32*A*). As the cricoid cartilage ring poses the narrowest point in the upper airway for prepubescent children (below the age of 8 years), an uncuffed tube of appropriate size should provide an adequate seal. Because the mucosa in this area is prone to trauma, a small leak is required. Table 19-1 and Box 19-11 provide estimates for tube diameter and length.

Endotracheal tubes have a black safety line that, if placed at the level of the vocal cords, ensures that the tip is in the midtracheal region. The Cole tube differs in that the distal 25% of its length is smaller than the proximal portion (Fig. 19-32*B*). The advantages are the increased proximal tube diameter and the fact that the

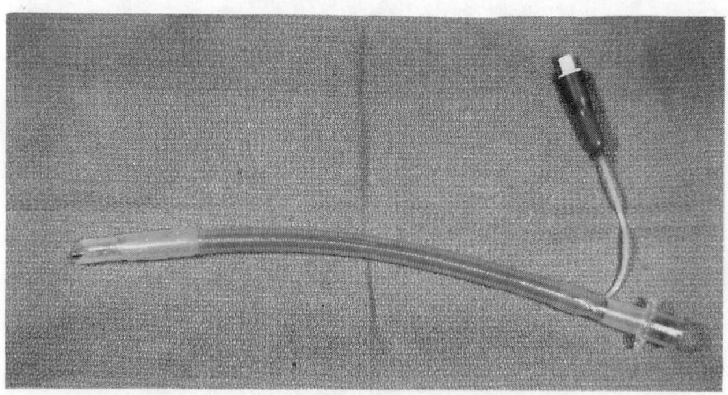

FIGURE 19-29. A metal spiral-embedded endotracheal tube.

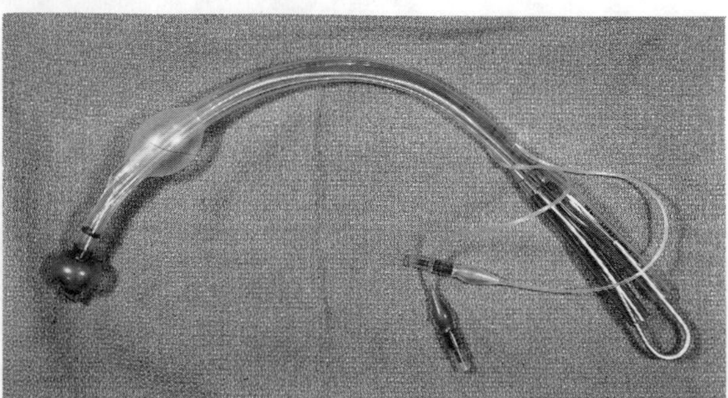

FIGURE 19-30. A double-lumen endotracheal tube. The distal tip with cuff is designed for left endobronchial intubation, and the proximal cuff seals the trachea above the carina. This system facilitates independent ventilation of right or left lung.

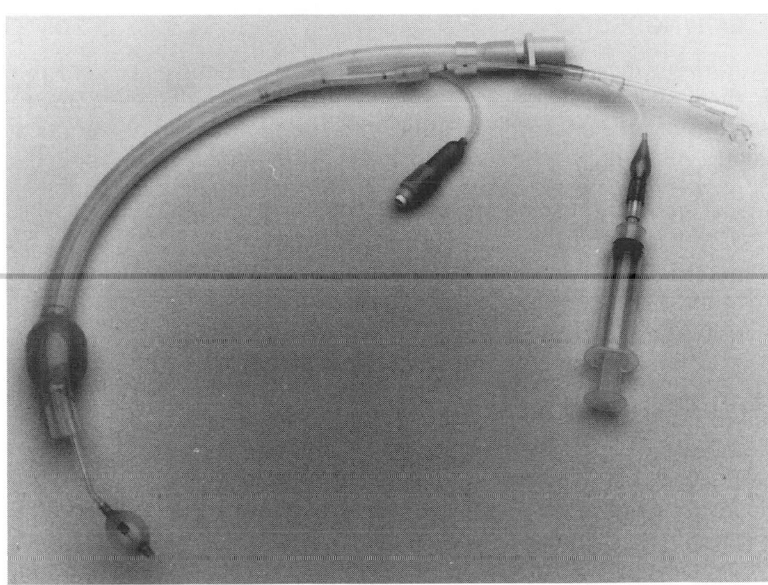

FIGURE 19-31. Univent bronchial-blocking tube.

"shoulder" area of narrowing abuts against the larynx, preventing accidental distal movement. However, pressure on glottic structures can result in necrosis.

High-frequency ventilation techniques for neonates has prompted the design of a specialized uncuffed tube. A jet delivery tube opens into the main lumen at a distance of 2 to 6 cm proximal to the end. In addition, a pressure monitoring channel opens 1 cm from the distal tube tip.[55]

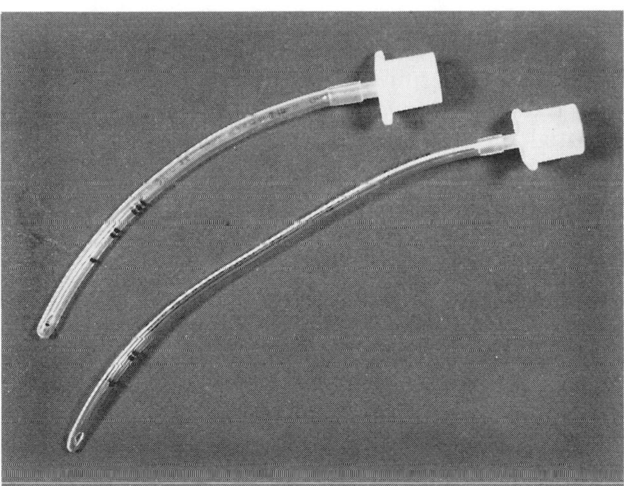

A

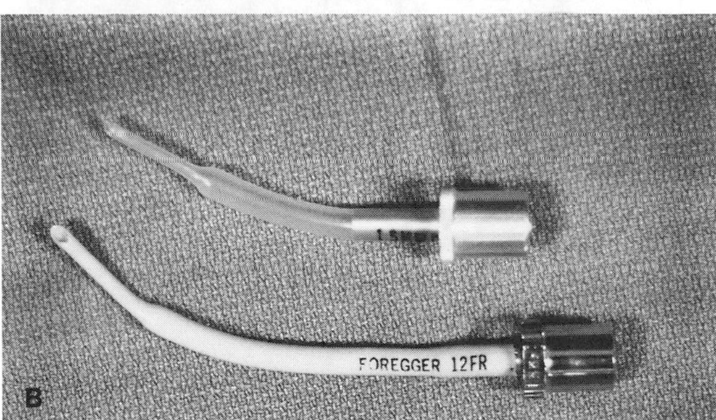

B

FIGURE 19-32. Pediatric endotracheal tubes. (A) Uncuffed. (B) Cole-style tubes.

□ STYLETS AND TUBE CHANGERS

Stylets are malleable metal wires that can be inserted through the ventilating lumen of oral endotracheal tubes. The wire provides internal support and allows alteration of the tube's natural curvature. Although not required for routine use, some manufacturers provide prepackaged stylets with each tube. Users should confirm that the wire does not extend beyond the distal tip of the tube. Stylets should be lightly lubricated with a water-soluble product. The stylet should be available for the more difficult intubation.

Tube Changers are also referred to as tube guides, bougies, endotracheal tube introducers, and elastic stylets. They can aid intubation when the clinician visualizes laryngeal landmarks but cannot direct the tip of the tracheal tube into the laryngeal inlet. Once the changer is in position, the tracheal tube is threaded over the device and into position. They can also facilitate removal and replacement of endotracheal tubes. They may be constructed of gum elastic or polyethylene tubing; the distal tip may be angled. Surface marks show the distance from the tip. Suction catheters, nasogastric tubes, and embolectomy catheters may can also function for this purpose. To act as an exchanger (changer), it is inserted through the existing endotracheal tube; the patient is extubated without removing the tube changer, and the new tube is then slipped over the changer using a rotating motion. A battery-powered lighted stylet ("light wand") is also available for intubation or changing tubes.[56] Hollow bougies allow placement of an adapter to the proximal end. This connection permits administration of oxygen, suction, or jet ventilation.[57]

□ LARYNGOSCOPES

A *laryngoscope* is used to manipulate the structures in the upper airway to permit direct visualization and insertion of an endotracheal tube into the glottis. The scope consists of a handle and blade with distal light (Fig. 19-33). The instruments are commonly made of plated metal, but disposable plastic laryngoscopes are also available. Batteries are contained inside the handle, which has an electrical contact point at the blade connection. Further discussion of laryngoscopes occurs later in this chapter when their use is detailed.

□ FORCEPS

A forceps can be used to direct a tracheal tube during intubation, insert pharyngeal packing, and retrieve objects from the upper airway. The *Magill forceps* is designed with a (right) offset handle. This permits handling without obstructing the line of site to the airway with laryngoscope in the left hand. The use of the forceps in nasotracheal intubation is reviewed later in this chapter.

Tracheostomy Tubes

Tracheostomy tubes provide an airway directly through the anterior neck into the tracheal lumen. Tracheostomy tube placement is generally indicated for long-term mechanical ventilation, chronic secretion management, and as an emergency airway. (A more complete discussion on the rationale and problems of tracheostomy care follows later in this chapter.) The tubes are available in a variety of sizes, styles, and materials. The standard clinical tracheostomy tube has a neck flange, tube body (extratracheal and intratracheal portions), and cuff (Fig. 19-34*A*). Tracheostomy tubes may also be uncuffed (Fig. 19-34*B*), have removable inner cannulas (Fig. 19-34*C*), and have fenestrations (openings) to allow ventilation through the larynx (Fig. 19-34*D*). A removable obturator permits easier insertion through the stoma.

□ DIMENSIONS

Table 19-3 lists dimensions for standard tracheostomy tubes. In contrast to the inside-diameter sizing of endotracheal tubes, several systems describe the outside diameter for tracheostomy tubes. Anatomic variations of neck length, location, and diameter of the tracheostomy incision are factors that affect tube sizing for patients. Surgeons hope to limit the damaged area in the trachea by avoiding large stoma sites and excessively large tubes. In general, 10-mm OD (approximately 7-mm ID) tubes are optimal for adult women and 11-mm OD (approximately 8-mm ID) for men. French sizing is based on the circumference of the outer surface of the tube. The following formula allows conversion to French sizing:

$$\text{Maximum diameter (Fr)} = \text{Inside diameter (mm)} \times 3$$

The lengths of tubes have been standardized, but extra-long tubes are available. These are helpful in morbidly obese patients. The intratracheal part of the tube should be straight and somewhat flexible. A desirable tube has a smooth curvature, with a small radius between intratracheal and extratracheal limbs. This permits an entrance of close to 90°, lessening pressure on the longitudinal aspect of the tracheal stoma. Once in the trachea, the tube sides or tip should not produce pressure points on the tracheal wall. In addition to the tracheal wall, the esophagus and major blood vessels are at risk for erosion. The flange should permit gentle yet firm fixation of the tube. Excessive movement of the tube increases the potential for lesions, especially at the stoma level. Some tubes have adjustable flanges to change the extratracheal dimension.[11]

□ MATERIALS

Contemporary, disposable tracheostomy tubes are composed of synthetic materials similar to endotracheal tubes. In addition, manufacturers produce

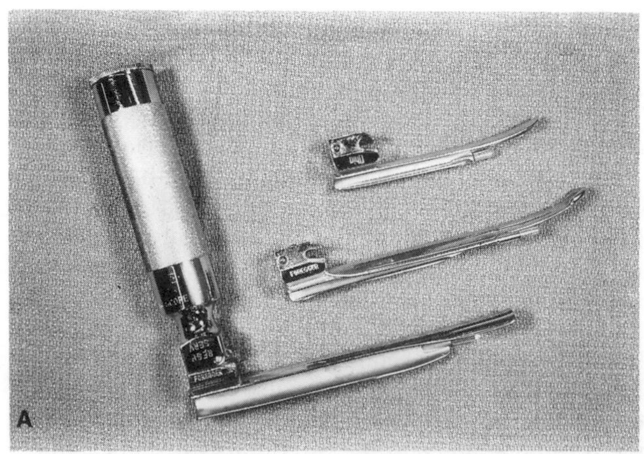

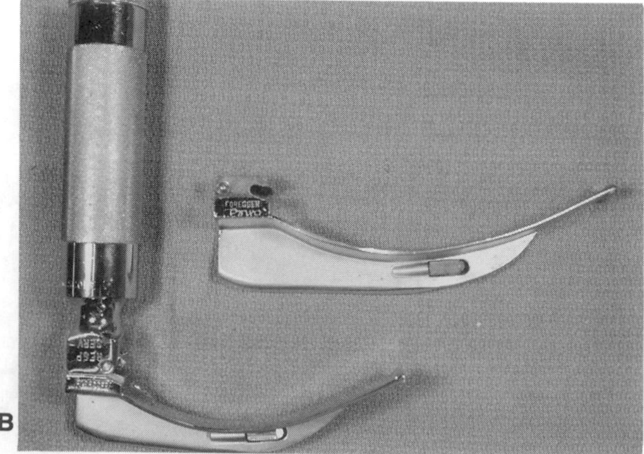

FIGURE 19-33. Laryngoscope handle and blades. **(A)** Straight blades; **(B)** Curved (McIntosh) blades.

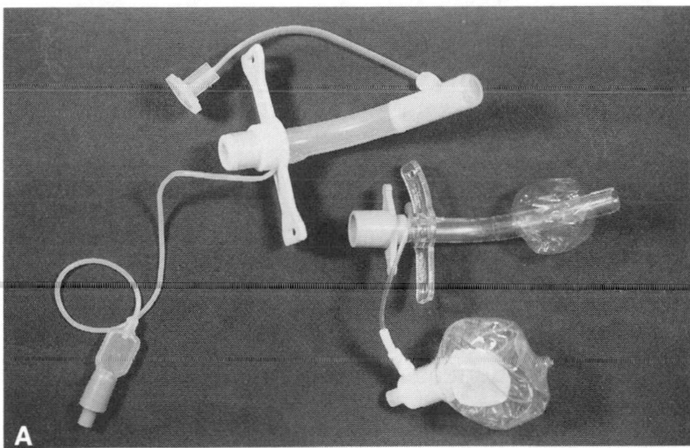

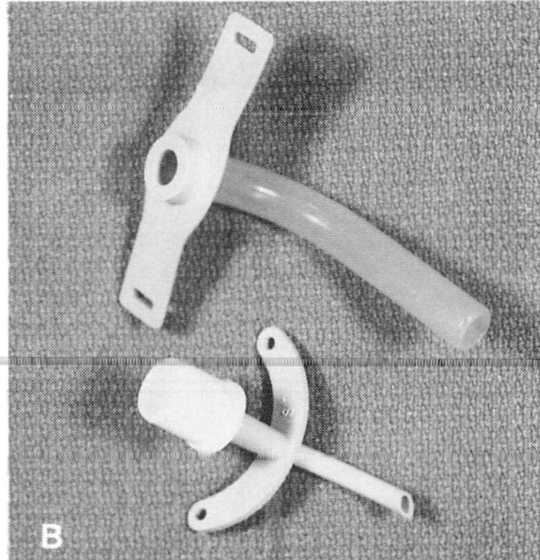

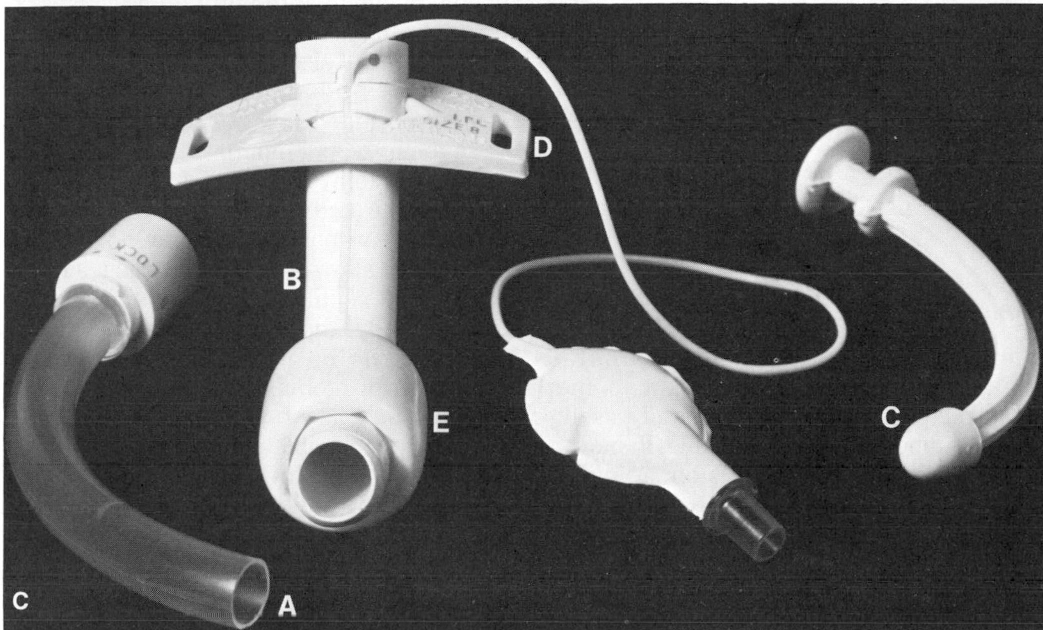

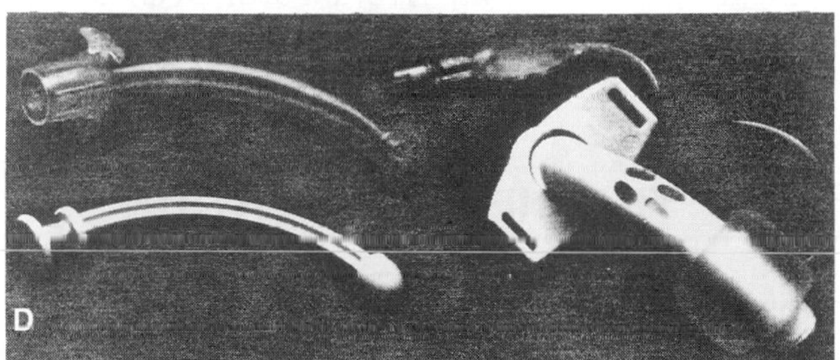

FIGURE 19-34. Tracheostomy tubes **(A)** Standard disposable cuffed tracheostomy tube; **(B)** Adult and pediatric uncuffed tracheostomy tubes; **(C)** Tracheostomy tube, with removable inner cannula (on left) and obturator (right); **(D)** Fenestrated tracheostomy tube, with inner cannula and obturator.

tracheostomy tubes made of silver (or silver plate), nylon, and Teflon. These materials are considered for permanent tracheostomy and are more rigid than rubber or synthetics. Their inability to flex with the trachea can cause pressure necrosis. Oxides from metal tubes tend to cause tissue irritation and increased mucus production. However, the advantage is the ability to be sterilized by boiling or autoclaving. Cuffs are less commonly used on these materials but can be applied. High-pressure cuffs generally have been replaced with high-compliance, low-pressure designs. Cuffs that are thin walled and that hug the tube when deflated are easier to insert or remove from a narrow stoma. The previously mentioned Kamen-Wilkinson Fome-Cuff is also available with tracheostomy tubes.

TABLE 19-3 **Tracheostomy Tube Size and Conversion**

Outside Diameter (mm)	French	Jackson	Approximate Inside Diameter (mm)
4.3	13	00	2.5
5.0	15	0	3.0
5.5	16.5	1	3.5
6.0	18	2	4.0
7.0	21	3	4.5–5.0
8.0	24	4	5.5
9.0	27	5	6.0–6.5
10.0	30	6	7.0
11.0	33	7	7.5–8.0
12.0	36	8	8.5
13.0	39	9	9.0–9.5
14.0	42	10	10.0
15.0	45	11	10.5–11.0
16.0	48	12	11.5

☐ SPECIAL PURPOSE TRACHEOSTOMY TUBES

Laryngectomy tubes are shorter than standard tracheostomy tubes from the outer neck skin to the trachea. Rigid, three-piece tubes are generally used, although synthetic rubber tubes are available. Removal of the larynx obviates the need for cuffs on laryngectomy tubes.

Armored wire, spiral-lined tubes are used to prevent compression from kinking in patients with short, bulky necks.

Fenestrated ("windowed") tracheostomy tubes allow selective opening of a channel to permit use of the natural airway above the tracheostomy tube (see Fig. 19-34*D*). Removal of an inner cannula gives access to a 6- to 8-mm by 8- to 10-mm orifice. The standard tracheal opening is plugged ("corked") and the cuff deflated, allowing air movement through the vocal cords. Patients who use this device should have fairly good control of their airway and adequate spontaneous ventilation. Patients who again require ventilation or protection from aspiration can have the inner cannula reinserted and cuff inflated. Although manufacturers produce precut fenestrations, only 50% of patients have an anatomic structure that can be accommodated. Patients with measured distances of 34 mm or more from skin to anterior trachea generally do not fit standard tubes; custom fenestrations may be created in both metal and plastic tubes.[58,59] The ASTM has adopted standards for pediatric tracheostomy tubes.[11]

Speaking tracheostomy tubes have a separate pilot tube that directs compressed gas to an exit point just above the cuff (Fig. 19-35*A,B*). With practice, the patient can coordinate speech. Being able to again vocalize is a delight for most patients, especially those who have long been ventilator dependent. Clinicians are required to set inlet flows to the patient's needs. Automated devices can synchronize gas flow to the talking port during the expiratory phase of mechanical ventilation.[60] This is necessary for use by patients unable to operate the gas flow Y-piece. Operators should not confuse the cuff and talking tubes, to avoid blowing up the cuff in situ. Special valves are also available for use with standard tubes with cuffs deflated (eg, Passy-Muir and Olympic Medical valves; Fig. 19-36*A,B*).

The *Montgomery tracheal T-tube* was developed to act as a flexible internal stent in supporting the tracheal wall (Fig. 19-37*A,B*). The upper limb of the T fits into the trachea; the remaining limb fits through the surgical opening. A stopper may be placed in its outer orifice. Placement is performed by manipulation of a curved hemostat, analogous to putting on trousers one leg at a time. The tube is made of silicone plastic and is available in a number of sizes. Emergency resuscitation of a patient with a T-tube should be attempted with the outer cannula occluded, using a mask-valve-bag device to ventilate the nose and mouth.[61]

Tracheostomy "buttons," and stoma cannulas, extend through the anterior neck to the tracheal wall (Fig. 19-38). The purpose of these devices is to prevent stoma closure and allow access to the trachea for suctioning or emergency ventilation. There is no intratracheal cannula. Usually, there is an internal structure made of plastic "petals" or "washers" to gently retain the tube at the posterior stoma wall. Units can be made of rigid Teflon, such as shown in Figure 19-38*A* (Olympic Medical), or flexible silicone rubber, as shown in Figure 19-38*B,C* (Kistner and Montgomery).[61,62] One-way valves may be added to allow inspiration through the tube, permitting vocalization on exhalation. Patient sizing requires measurement of distances from the neck to the posterior stoma; manufacturers make both standard and custom lengths.[63] In these patients, emergency access to the trachea can also be obtained by cricothyrotomy. A review of this technique can be found later in this chapter in the discussion of the difficult intubation.

TRACHEAL INTUBATION

Indications for Tracheal Intubation

Not all situations requiring airway management call for endotracheal intubation. In fact, less aggressive measures, such as those previously described, may result in an improved clinical condition in which airway support is no longer required. Even when the decision to intubate has been made, intelligent "preintubation" airway management permits a more controlled atmosphere in which tracheal intubation can take place.

Indications for intubation are not always clear-cut and should be made on an individual basis for each patient. Box 19-13 lists conditions for which emergency management of the airway is frequently indicated, according to AARC Clinical Practice Guidelines.[6]

To assure the patency of the airway in certain situations, a tracheal tube may need to be placed. Respira-

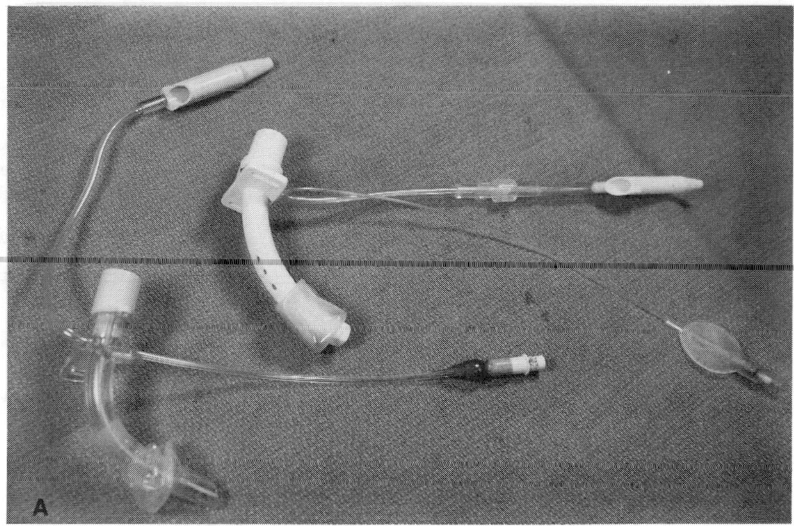

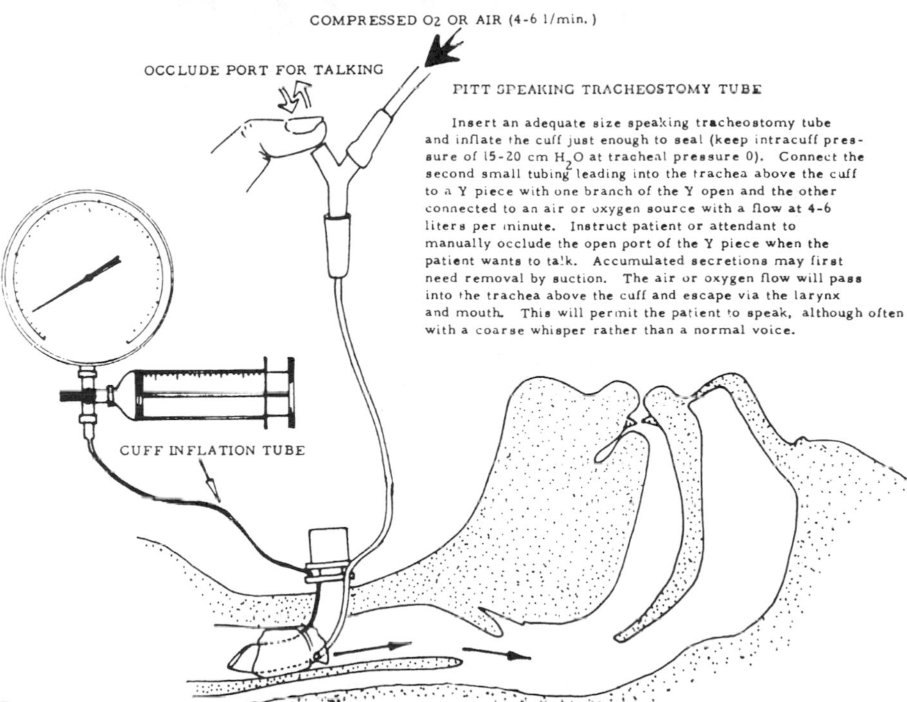

COMPRESSED O_2 OR AIR (4-6 l/min.)
OCCLUDE PORT FOR TALKING
PITT SPEAKING TRACHEOSTOMY TUBE
Insert an adequate size speaking tracheostomy tube and inflate the cuff just enough to seal (keep intracuff pressure of 15-20 cm H_2O at tracheal pressure 0). Connect the second small tubing leading into the trachea above the cuff to a Y piece with one branch of the Y open and the other connected to an air or oxygen source with a flow at 4-6 liters per minute. Instruct patient or attendant to manually occlude the open port of the Y piece when the patient wants to talk. Accumulated secretions may first need removal by suction. The air or oxygen flow will pass into the trachea above the cuff and escape via the larynx and mouth. This will permit the patient to speak, although often with a coarse whisper rather than a normal voice.
CUFF INFLATION TUBE
B

FIGURE 19-35. Speaking tracheostomy tubes **(A)** Two speaking tubes. **(B)** Diagram of airflow directed toward the vocal cords when the Y-tube is occluded. (Safar P, Grenvik A. Speaking cuffed tracheostomy tube. Crit Care Med 3:23, 1975, © Williams and Wilkins, with permission)

tory depression, a depressed gag reflex, depressed cough, and relaxation of the posterior pharynx can occur (eg, anesthesia, head trauma, and so on), and if the airway is not protected, can lead to aspiration. Anatomic abnormalities such as paralyzed vocal cords or external compression of the airway from hematoma or cervical tumor can also result in an inability to assure patency of the airway. Not only does the tracheal tube provide a conduit through which a patient can receive mechanical ventilatory support, it also allows the practitioner to institute various expiratory maneuvers, such as positive end-expiratory pressure (PEEP) or continuous positive airway pressure (CPAP). The tracheal tube provides a conduit for repeated suctioning of airway secretions in those patients who are producing copious quantities of sputum. Tracheal intubation is required during certain operative procedures, such as those in which the patients have either a full stomach or intestinal obstruction, intrathoracic procedures, operations in the prone position, and intracranial operations. Tracheal intubation should probably be performed whenever muscle relaxants are used, because these medications render the protective airway reflexes incapable of functioning.

Ethics

Intubation of some patients may not improve outcome because of the prognosis of the underlying disease. Identifying such patients is an important task facing the physician in charge. A decision not to intubate might be made after medical, legal, and ethical-religious issues

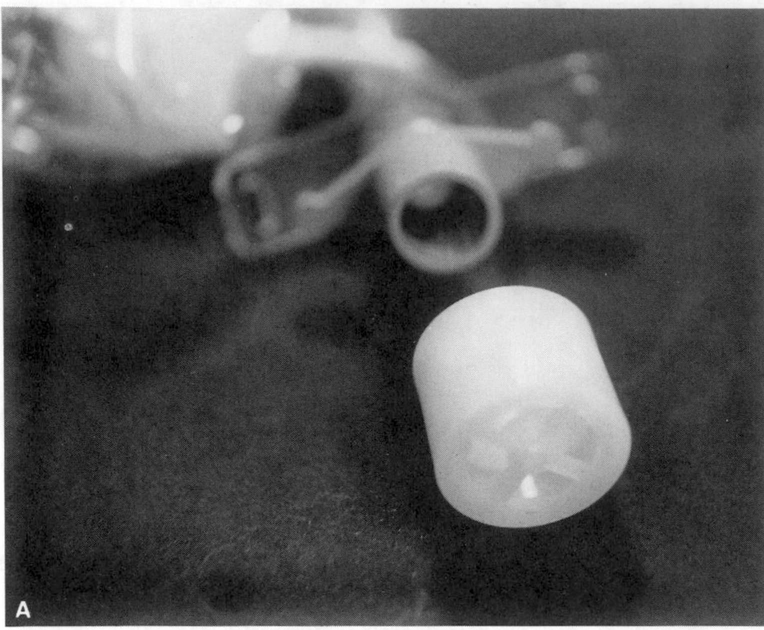

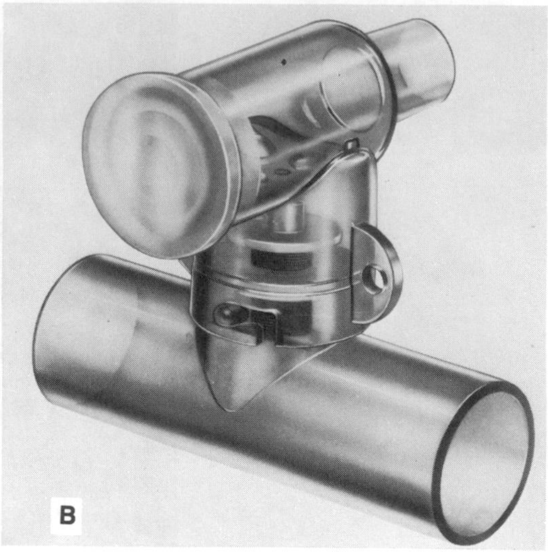

FIGURE 19-36. Valves to facilitate speech with tracheostomy tubes. **(A)** Passy-Muir valve; **(B)** An Olympic Trach-Talk valve.

have been addressed and the patient and responsible relatives have been given the opportunity to express their desires (see Chap. 2). To help resolve ethical questions related to the appropriateness of tracheal intubation, an institutional ethics committee may be of help in providing advice and support for the care providers, the patients, and their families.[64]

Credentialing

Because tracheal intubation is invasive and potentially associated with complications, only trained personnel should be allowed to perform the procedure. All health professionals who are members of resuscitation teams should have current basic life support (BLS) training. Those requiring skills in advanced management of airway emergencies should have advanced cardiac life support (ACLS), pediatric advanced life support (PALS), or neonatal resuscitation program (NRP) certification.[3,6] Institutions should credential personnel who perform intubation, with consideration given to formal training, on-the-job experience, and continued medical education.

Evaluation of the Patient

To predict the ease or difficulty of tracheal intubation, a thorough evaluation is necessary. Occasionally, despite evaluation, a patient may present unexpected problems; thus, a failed intubation attempt must always be anticipated even when the initial evaluation does not suggest potential difficulty. Any disease or anatomic defect (either acquired or congenital) that interferes with the mobility of the cervical spine or the mandible, or that alters the soft tissues of the nares, oral cavity, or neck, may create difficulties for the respiratory care practitioner who is attempting tracheal intubation.

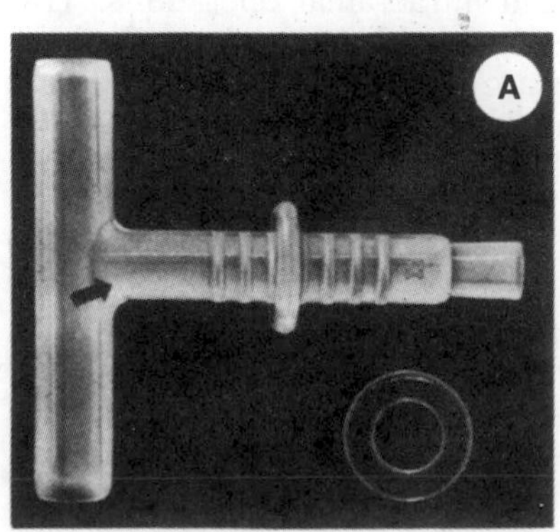

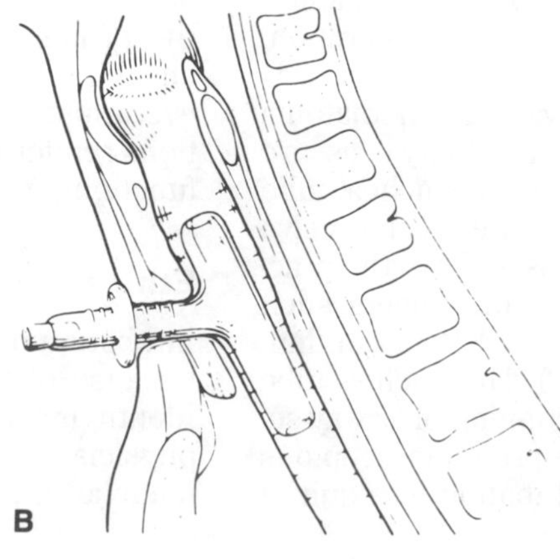

FIGURE 19-37. Montgomery T-tube. **(A)** Montgomery tracheal tube; **(B)** Montgomery tube in position. (Montgomery WW: Current modifications of the salivary bypass tube and tracheal tube. Ann Otol Rhinol Laryology 95:121, 1986; with permission)

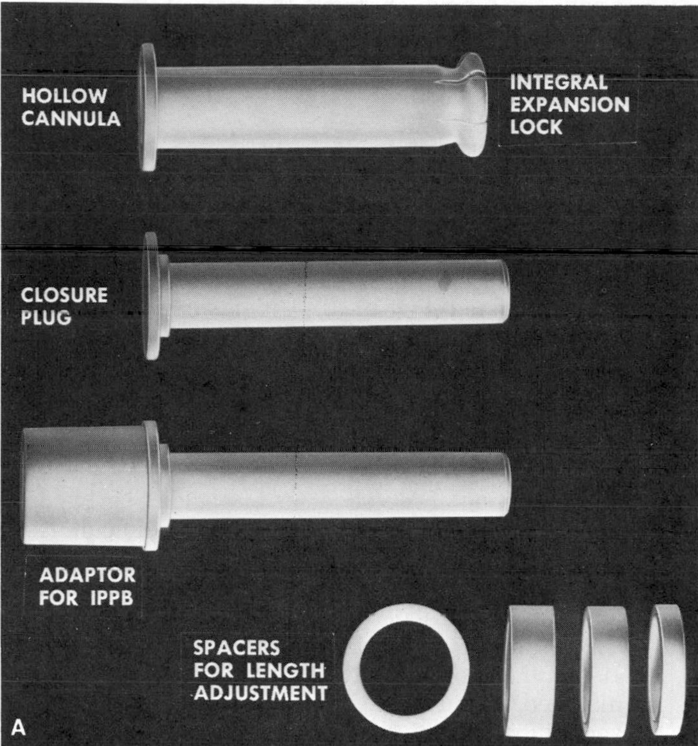

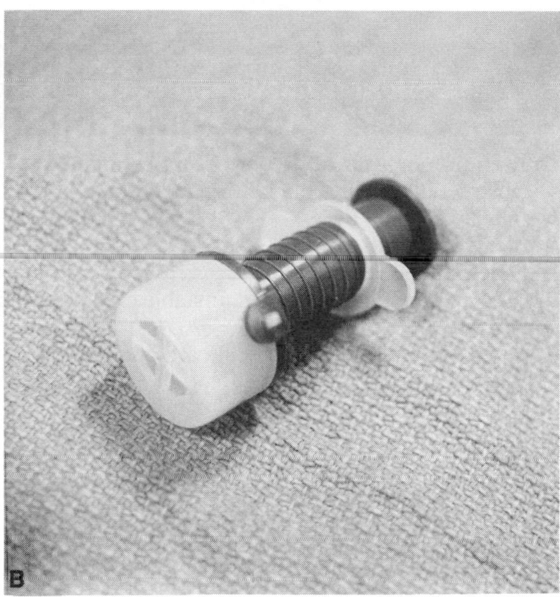

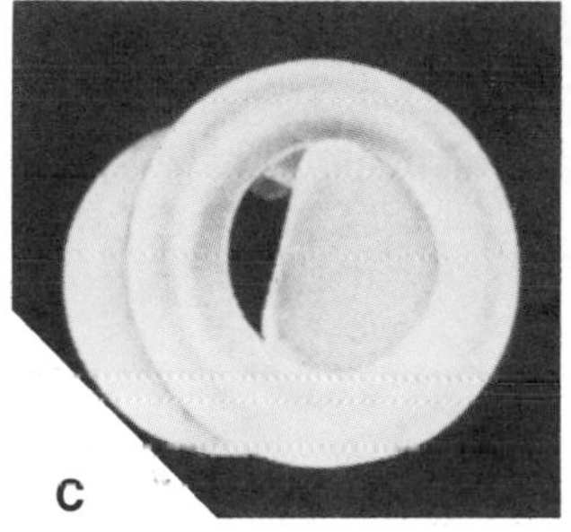

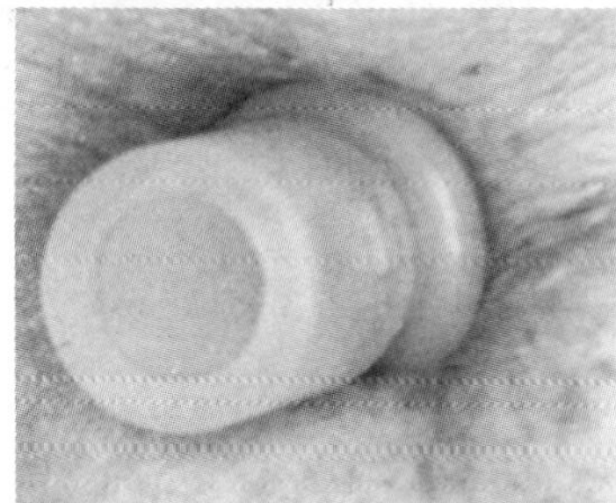

FIGURE 19-38. Tracheal stoma appliances. **(A)** Olympic tracheostomy button; **(B)** Kistner "valved" tracheostomy button; **(C)** Montgomery "valved" tracheostomy button. (Montgomery WW: Current modifications of the salivary bypass tube and tracheal tube. Ann Otol Rhinol Laryngol 95:121, 1986; with permission)

□ MEDICAL HISTORY

In addition to a thorough physical evaluation, an accurate history can be an indicator of a potential difficulty. Respiratory care practitioners should search the patient's history for documentation of previous intubations and whether these intubations were associated with difficulty. A medical history might alert the intubationist to potential difficulties if it includes certain congenital anatomic defects. These might include mandibular hypoplasia (eg, Pierre Robin and Treacher Collins syndromes), maxillary hypoplasia (eg, Apert's disease), a deficiency in number of cervical vertebrae (eg, Klippel-Feil syndrome), and macroglossia (eg, Beckwith-Wiedemann syndrome). In addition, certain acquired anatomic defects may suggest a potentially difficult intubation, including tracheal stenosis, retropharyngeal abscess, epiglottitis, and rheumatoid arthritis (which may affect mobility of the cervical spine, temporal mandibular joint, or the arytenoid cartilages). Patients should be questioned about recent food or liquid ingestion because pulmonary aspiration of gastric material is more likely in these patients. Patients should also be asked about dental appliances; these should be removed before intubation to avoid obstruction of the airway and aspiration. A history of blood-clotting disturbances or nasal polyps would be important information for the intubationist considering nasal intubation.

□ GLOBAL ASSESSMENT

A global assessment is a quick evaluation of the patient's level of consciousness, vital signs (blood pressure, pulse, respirations), and overall severity of illness. The patient who has lost consciousness or the ability to spontaneously breathe, or who is hemodynamically unstable, may require more immediate and special considerations when performing tracheal intubation.

BOX 19-13

CONDITIONS PREDISPOSING TO OR REQUIRING EMERGENCY AIRWAY MANAGEMENT

Impending or Actual Airway Compromise
- Obstruction of the artificial airway
- Apnea
- Acute traumatic coma
- Penetrating neck trauma
- Cardiopulmonary arrest and unstable dysrhythmias
- Severe bronchospasm
- Severe allergic reactions with cardiopulmonary compromise
- Pulmonary edema
- Sedative or narcotic drug effect
- Foreign body airway obstruction
- Choanal atresia in neonates
- Aspiration or risk of aspiration
- Severe laryngospasm

Requiring Emergency Tracheal Intubation
- Persistent apnea
- Traumatic upper airway obstruction (partial or complete)
- Accidental extubation of patients unable to maintain sponaneous ventilation
- Obstructive angioedema
- Massive uncontrolled upper airway bleeding
- Coma with potential for increased intracranial pressure
- Infection-related upper airway obstruction (eg, epiglottitis)
- Laryngeal and upper airway edema
- Neonatal or pediatric specific (eg, perinatal asphyxia, severe adenotonsillar hypertrophy, severe laryngomalacia, bacterial tracheitis, congenital diaphragmatic hernia, absence of protective reflexes, presence of thick or particulate meconium in amniotic fluid

Depending on the results of this global assessment, further evaluation may need to be abbreviated or particular aspects emphasized.

NASAL EXAMINATION

When nasotracheal intubation is being considered, each naris should be assessed for patency, and the nasal septum should be examined for deviation. The naris that allows the most unhindered approach should be used for tracheal tube introduction.

ORAL CAVITY

Before intubation, the oral cavity should be inspected for foreign bodies; if found, they should be removed. Any existing teeth are inspected. Long, protruding teeth may limit the opening of the oral cavity. Any loose teeth should be identified and possibly removed by trained dental personnel if time permits.[65]

TONGUE

A large tongue may present great difficulties to the intubationist, because this structure must be manipulated to directly view the larynx. If on inspection of the oral cavity, the tongue obstructs the view of the uvula, the patient should be asked to flatten the tongue by saying "ah." If the uvula still cannot be visualized, a difficult oral intubation should be anticipated (Fig. 19-39).[66,67]

TEMPOROMANDIBULAR JOINT

Temporomandibular joint function can be assessed by the insertion of adult fingers into the oral cavity. With fingers extended and placed into the oral cavity at its midline, three normal adult-sized fingers should be accommodated (Fig. 19-40). Patients capable of accommodating two or fewer fingers have some limitation of their temporomandibular joint and may be more difficult to intubate orally.

MANDIBLE

Recognition of severe forms of mandibular hypoplasia, as in Pierre Robin syndrome, is not difficult. However, more subtle hypoplasia may be identified by placing fingers horizontally beneath the chin. The distance from the hyoid bone to the mandibular symphysis is about three fingerbreadths in the normal adult (Fig. 19-41). If two or fewer adult fingerbreadths are accommodated, the mandible is considered to be hypoplastic, and intubation may be difficult.

CERVICAL SPINE

Patients with short and immobile necks are more difficult to intubate. Factors that limit neck (cervical spine)

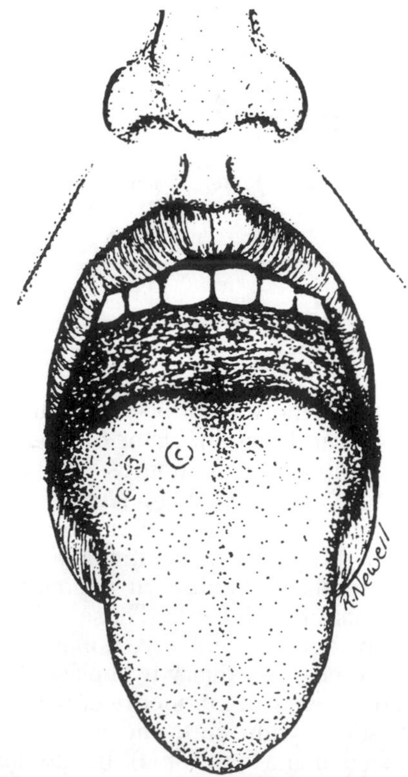

FIGURE 19-39. Inspection of the oral cavity showing obstructed view; uvula not visualized. (Mallampati SR, Gatt SP, Gugino LD, Sukumar PD, et al: A clinical sign to predict difficult intubation. Can J Anaesth 32:429, 1985; with permission)

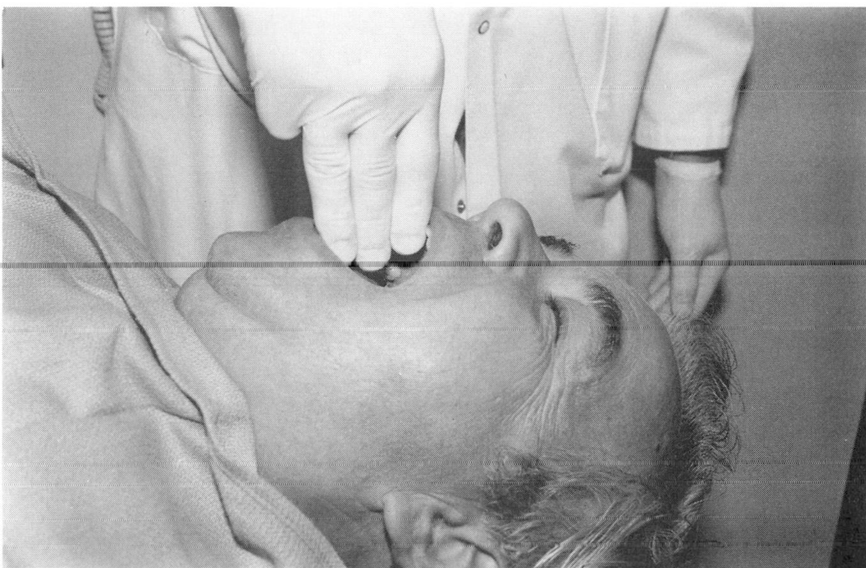

FIGURE 19-40. Accommodation of three fingerbreadths into the oral cavity, indicating adequate temporomandibular joint mobility.

mobility include obesity, cervical radiation therapy, previous cervical surgery, and other cervical deficiencies. Mobility of the cervical spine is assessed by measuring the distance from the lower border of the mandible to the thyroid notch at full neck extension; this distance should be greater than four fingerbreadths in the adult (Fig. 19-42).[68] With a thorough evaluation, potential intubation problems usually should be uncovered; however, there will always exist situations for which difficulty in intubation arises without good explanation. Accordingly, the intubationist should always be prepared for the unexpected.

Route for Intubation

Once a decision has been made to intubate a patient, the clinician must choose an appropriate route from which the tracheal tube is inserted into the trachea. The three main routes for tracheal intubation include the following:

- Oral
- Nasal
- Transtracheal (to be discussed under tracheostomy)

□ ORAL TRACHEAL ROUTE

In most instances, tracheal intubation can be accomplished most expediently through the oral route. Because the vocal cords are usually visualized during oral tracheal intubation, the tube can be placed with greater assurance. Oral tracheal tubes are less likely to kink than nasal tracheal tubes; this may result in less airflow resistance and, also, less obstruction to the passage of the suction catheter or fiberoptic bronchoscope. In addition, the oral route can usually accommodate a tube

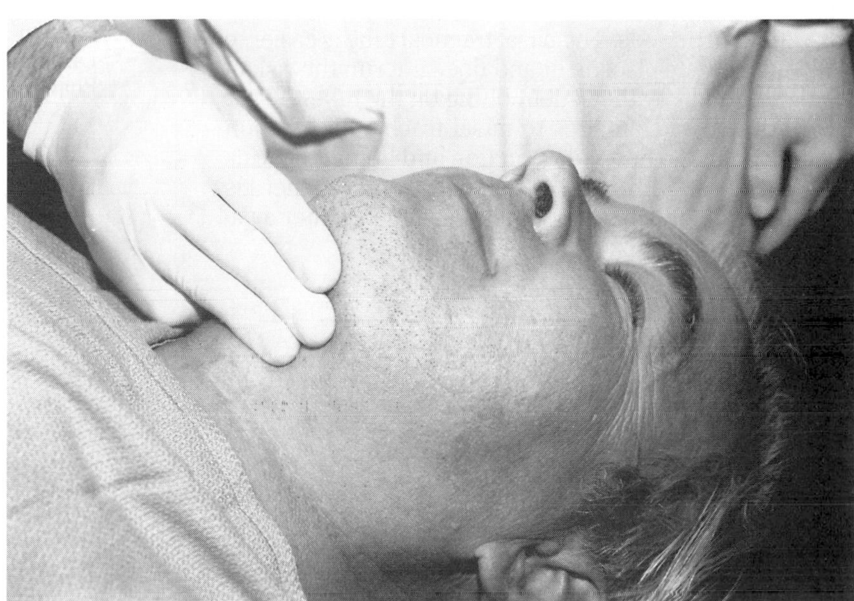

FIGURE 19-41. Adequate mandibular length is indicated by a three-fingerbreadth distance from the hyoid bone to the mandibular symphysis.

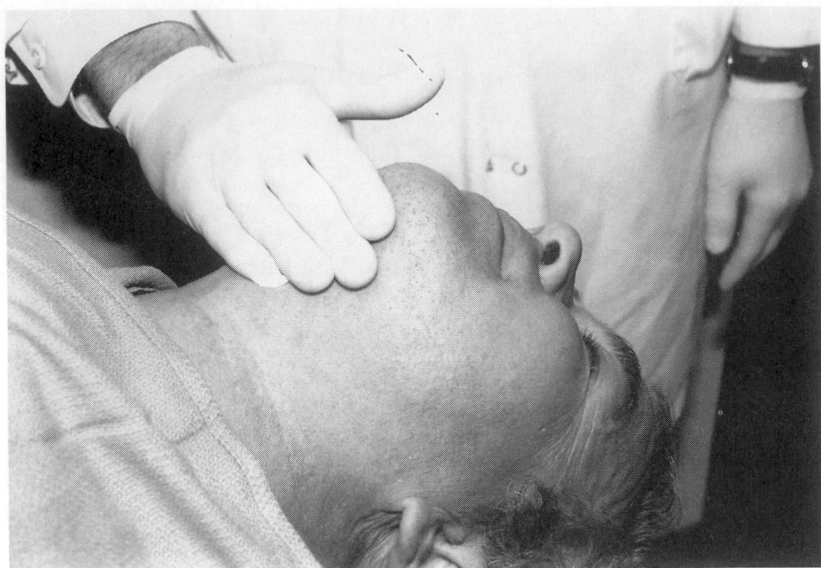

FIGURE 19-42. Adequate cervical spine mobility is indicated by a four-fingerbreadth distance from the mandibular symphysis to the thyroid notch at full neck extension.

0.5 to 1 mm wider than the nasal route and, for this reason, may lessen airflow resistance and facilitate suctioning.

Potential disadvantages of oral tracheal intubation include the activation of the gag reflex, which may require higher doses of sedatives for patient tolerance. Oral hygiene is more difficult to maintain with an oral tube, because the swallowing mechanism is interfered with and oral pharyngeal secretions are stimulated by the presence of the tube.

□ NASAL ROUTE

Possible advantages of the nasal route include situations in which access to the mouth is difficult or impossible, as when patients have mandibular trismus, status epilepticus, or a fractured mandible. In addition, certain oral surgical procedures require unhindered oral access. The nasal tracheal route is usually better tolerated by the patient, especially those who require tracheal intubation for extended periods. The nasal tracheal tube is easier to stabilize after its placement and does not run the risk of being occluded by the patient biting on the tube.

Possible disadvantages to nasal tracheal intubation include potential tissue destruction and hemorrhage as the tube passes through the nares. In addition, there is the potential for the development of sinusitis after a patient has been intubated for several days.

Equipment

Clinical practice guideline recommendations for equipment necessary for intubation are provided in Box 19-14.[3,6]

□ BLADES

There are two general types of laryngoscope blades, the straight blade and the curved blade (Fig. 19-43). Examples of the straight blade include the Miller, the Wis-Hipple, and the Flag. The primary example of the curved blade is the McIntosh. The curved blade (McIntosh) has a larger blade surface area for easier manipulation of the tongue; the larger blade also allows more room for passage of the tracheal tube. Because of the curved blade's placement in the vallecula during intubation, there is less stimulation of the highly innervated epiglottis and thus, at least potentially, less chance for laryngospasm. The straight blade (eg, Miller) allows

BOX 19-14

EQUIPMENT NEEDED FOR INTUBATION

- Ventilation devices
  - -Masks (variety of sizes)
  - -Manual resuscitation
- Airway management devices
  - -Oropharyngeal airways (variety of sizes)
  - -Nasopharyngeal airways (variety of sizes)
  - -Laryngeal mask airway
  - -Pharyngeotracheal lumen airway or esophageal tracheal combitude
  - -Intubation devices
    - Laryngoscope handles (2) with variety of curved and straight blades
    - Wire guide or stylet and introducer, changer, or bougie
    - Forceps
- Supplies and miscellany
  - -Lubricant
  - -Syringe
  - -12–16 gauge intravenous catheter-over-the-needle device for transcatheter ventilation
  - -Tape, endotracheal tube ties, or other method for tube stabilization
  - -Endotracheal tubes (variety of sizes)
  - -Eye shields and gloves
  - -Source of suction and suction catheters

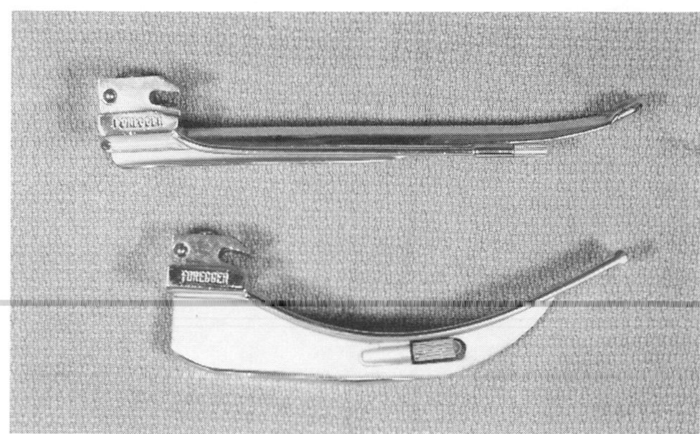

FIGURE 19-43. Miller (straight) blade (*top*) and McIntosh (curved) blade (*bottom*).

greater exposure of the glottic opening, thereby permitting visualization of the tube as it passes through the vocal cords and, consequently, greater assurance of proper tube placement.

☐ EQUIPMENT IN THE PEDIATRIC PATIENT

Equipment of varied shapes and sizes is necessary to accommodate the variety of patients seen in a pediatric practice. Suction catheters, laryngoscope blades, tracheal tubes, stylets, face masks, and so on must be selected in an appropriate size to accommodate the patient. Estimates of the sizes of the equipment to be used should be made before therapeutic intervention; however, a variety of sizes of all equipment should be available, in the event that initial estimations prove inaccurate. A laryngoscope of appropriate size and shape is important in the pediatric patient. When using a blade that is too long for a particular patient for tracheal intubation, the tendency is to use it as a lever and pry the mouth open, with potential injury to the upper teeth and lip. A straight, rather than a curved, laryngoscope blade is preferred in the pediatric patient, for it allows easier manipulation of the epiglottis and better exposure of the larynx.

☐ EQUIPMENT AND INFECTION CONTROL

Body secretions (blood, saliva, or other) of all patients should be treated as if they are contaminated. All contaminated equipment should be packaged in nonpenetrable bags and disposed of, if nonreusable, or transported to an area where cleaning of reusable equipment takes place. Reusable equipment is mechanically cleaned and then either gas sterilized with ethylene oxide, steam sterilized at 278°F for 10 minutes, or disinfected with 2% glutaraldehyde (a 45-minute soak in 2% glutaraldehyde is required to kill acid-fast bacilli; less time is required to kill viral organisms). To avoid the potential of contracting a transmissible disease, the practitioner should not come in contact with a patient's body secretions. Eye shields, rubber gloves, masks, and gowns may be necessary to avoid such exposure when performing endotracheal intubation.[14,15]

TRANSLARYNGEAL INTUBATION

Procedure

Translaryngeal intubation may be performed by several different approaches. The choice of approach depends on the patient's clinical condition and, hence, the immediacy of the required intubation, the skill and the preference of the respiratory care practitioner, and the availability and skills of the supporting staff. The following techniques of translaryngeal intubation are discussed:

- Awake oral intubation
- Intubation under sedation
- Intubation under general anesthesia
- Nasal intubation

Awake Oral Intubation

The awake oral intubation procedure is most appropriate for neonates and for patients who are unresponsive, who have recently ingested food, or in whom a preintubation evaluation has alerted one to the potential of a difficult intubation. A "first look" before the administration of sedative or anesthetic drugs is often desired in certain patients, such as patients with intestinal obstruction or trauma to the upper airway. In skillful hands, an awake intubation can be performed within a few seconds.

Despite the advantages of expediency, awake intubation is almost never ideal. In the patient who is not completely unconscious, awake intubation often provokes either vagal or sympathetic stimulation, with associated cardiac and bronchospastic effects. For the conscious patient, the experience of an awake intubation can be traumatic. If time permits, administration of local anesthesia to the oral cavity, plus intravenous sedative drugs, may render the procedure more tolerable. As in all procedures for endotracheal intubation, the first task to perform is an equipment check (see Box 19-14). Clinicians should administer 100% oxygen through a bag and mask for 3 minutes before intubation. The availability of a suction apparatus is essential. The laryngoscope should be checked for proper functioning, as should the competency of the cuff of the tracheal tube. The tracheal tube should not be removed from its sterile container until it is handed to the respiratory care practitioner at the time of the intubation. If lubrication jelly is applied to the distal end of the endotracheal tube, it should be done with sterile gauze, and then the endotracheal tube should be immediately replaced in its sterile container.

The patient is positioned supine; the neck is flexed to a moderate degree by placing a folded towel beneath the head. Next, the head is extended to achieve the sniff position. The three axes, those of the mouth, the pharynx, and the trachea, are then aligned to permit direct visualization of the larynx (see Fig. 19-4).

In patients with depressed levels of consciousness (especially those with recent food ingestion or intestinal obstruction), a *Sellick maneuver* should be performed. An assistant applies thumb and index finger pressure at

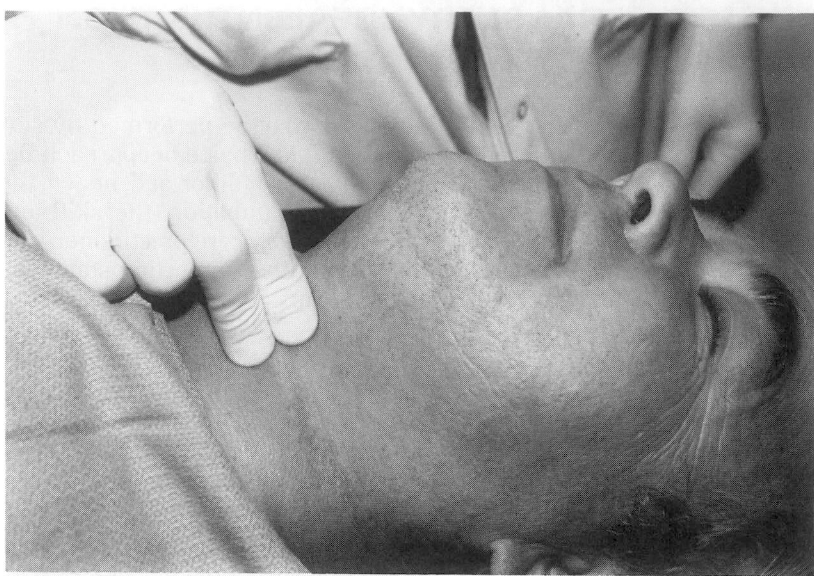

FIGURE 19-44. The Sellick maneuver is performed by having an assistant apply thumb and index finger pressure at the level of the cricoid ring.

the level of the cricoid cartilage to compress the esophagus and prevent any gastric contents from being regurgitated and aspirated (Fig. 19-44).[69] The cricoid cartilage is the best location for esophageal compression because it is at this point that a cartilaginous ring completely surrounds the airway.

The respiratory care practitioner uses eye shields and gloves for protection from potentially infectious body secretions. A gown is worn if splashing of contaminated material is possible.

The laryngoscope is held with the left hand and the blade is inserted to the right of the midline of the mouth (Figs. 19-45, 19-46). The tongue is elevated and moved to the left. As the blade is advanced, the epiglottis comes into view. When using a curved blade, its tip is placed in the vallecula; when using a straight blade, the tip is placed beneath the epiglottis. Elevation in the direction of the laryngoscope handle should bring the larynx into full view.

The laryngoscope should never be used as a lever against the upper teeth. The tracheal tube is next inserted with the right hand from the right corner of the mouth. The distal end of the tracheal tube is visualized as it passes between the vocal chords into the glottic opening.

Immediately after intubation, the location of the tracheal tube is verified by an assistant listening over the epigastrium for any gurgling as positive pressure is applied to the tracheal tube. Gurgling indicates an esophageal intubation. If gurgling is heard, the tracheal tube should be left in place, the cuff inflated, and the application of positive pressure to the proximal end of the tube discontinued. A second tracheal tube should then be obtained and placed under direct visualization

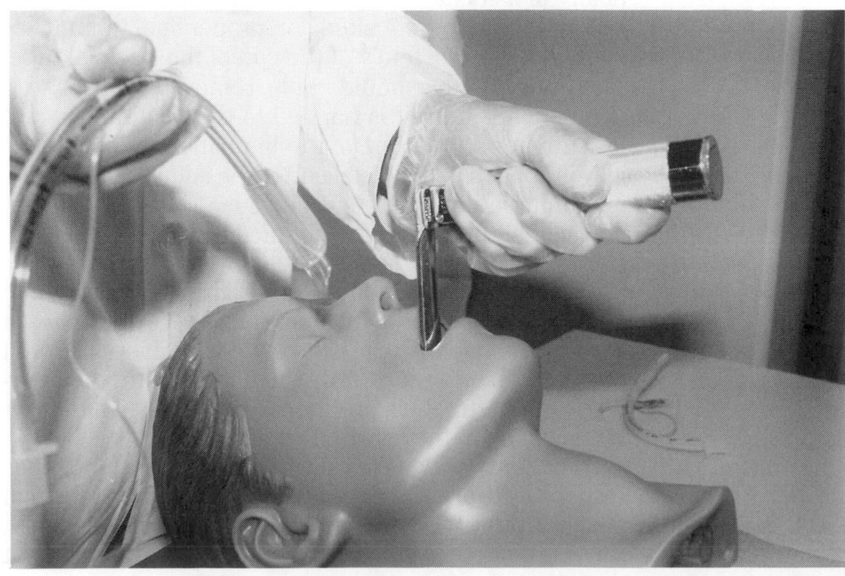

FIGURE 19-45. Intubation technique for oral tracheal intubation.

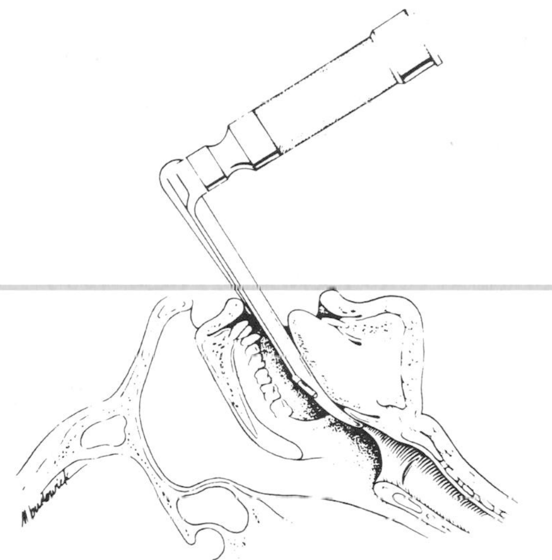

FIGURE 19-46. Direct oral laryngoscopy with a Miller (straight) blade (Finucane BT, Santora AH: Principles of Airway Management. Philadelphia, FA Davis, 1988, with permission)

into the trachea. An assistant listens to both lung apexes for breath sounds after a silent epigastrium has been verified.

The tracheal tube cuff is inflated to a volume that is required to just occlude any air leak around the endotracheal tube. After the endotracheal tube has been securely taped or tied into place, a chest radiograph is obtained to confirm that the tracheal tube tip lies in the middle portion of the trachea (near the level of the aortic knob). If the patient becomes hypoxic or if vital signs deteriorate immediately following tracheal intubation, one must strongly suspect misplacement of the tube and, under direct visualization with the use of a laryngoscope, establish that the tracheal tube traverses the glottic opening between the two vocal cords into the trachea.

Confirmation of tracheal intubation can also be obtained with use of a CO_2 monitor.[3,70] If a tracheal tube is correctly positioned in the trachea, the percentage of expired CO_2 should rise from almost 0% on inspiration to approximately 6% on expiration. If the endotracheal tube is placed in the esophagus, the percentage of CO_2 should rise and fall very little with respiration. Pulse oximetry is another useful monitoring device that may alert the respiratory care practitioner to the possibility of an esophageal or bronchial intubation by detecting hypoxemia.[71] However, the pulse oximeter is not as sensitive in detecting esophageal intubation as the CO_2 monitor, and will not alarm the practitioner until hypoxemia and possibly hypercarbic acidosis has occurred.

Intubation Under Sedation

The items discussed for awake oral intubation also apply to patients receiving tracheal intubation under sedation. Sedative drugs, when properly administered, usually allow a more relaxed atmosphere and a more pleasant intubation experience for both patient and practitioner. Because sedative drugs take time to administer and titrate to effect, their use may be inappropriate in certain emergency situations. In addition, sedative drugs may have undesirable side effects, such as cardiovascular and respiratory depression, that would be particularly disadvantageous in an emergency situation. Hence, sedative drugs are usually reserved for those situations for which the expediency of tracheal intubation is not paramount.

The most reliable way to administer sedative drugs is by the intravenous route. The infusion of two drugs (one benzodiazepine and one narcotic) is a popular means of achieving sedation. Numerous different combinations of these two classes of drugs are used. Benzodiazepines produce sedation along with sleepiness and anterograde amnesia, usually with minimal respiratory depression and a mild decrease in blood pressure. Benzodiazepines can sometimes have unpredictable sedative effects and, occasionally, a paradoxical central nervous system stimulation occurs. Special caution should be used when sedating elderly and debilitated patients with benzodiazepines, as such patients can be sensitive to the respiratory depressive, cardiovascular depressive, and sedative effects of the drug; also, the effects of the drug can be longer lasting.

Diazepam (Valium) is one of the most popular benzodiazepines and the one that, until recently, has been used most frequently. The anterograde amnestic effect of diazepam begins about 1 to 2 minutes after intravenous injection; however, the sedative effect is quite variable. In some patients, as little as 0.07 mg/kg given intravenously can produce unconsciousness; in others, as much as 1 mg/kg given intravenously produces little more than drowsiness. In adults, diazepam should be administered in incremental doses of 2.5 mg intravenously, with sedative, respiratory, and cardiovascular effects monitored carefully. The metabolites of diazepam (especially desmethyldiazepam) can accumulate after large or repeated doses and can cause prolonged effects of the drug.

Desmethyldiazepam is only slightly less potent than diazepam, and its plasma concentrations increase steadily over approximately the first 24 hours after injection of diazepam. This metabolite can contribute to a return of drowsiness after apparent recovery following diazepam administration.

Midazolam (Versed) is a newer benzodiazepine that has achieved recent popularity. This popularity results from the water-soluble nature of the drug, which causes less irritation and pain on intravenous injection. In addition, midazolam has a much shorter metabolic half-life (2 to 4 hours). However, as with diazepam, the effects of midazolam can be quite capricious and unpredictable. Midazolam is approximately two to four times more potent than diazepam; therefore, 0.5- to 1.0-mg increments of the drug should be used for sedation.

Opiates are often used in conjunction with benzodiazepines in preparing the patient for intubation. Opiates (narcotics) provide analgesia and also suppress the cough reflex. The side effects of opiates are primarily respiratory, but hypotension, bradycardia, nausea, and vomiting may also occur. The combination of benzodiazepines and narcotics can have a synergistic respiratory and cardiovascular depressive effect. Morphine is one of the most popular narcotics and has been used over the years for providing sedation. It is administered in incremental doses of 1 to 3 mg intravenously; its metabolic half-life is approximately 2 to 3 hours.

Fentanyl (Sublimaze) is a relatively new narcotic compound that has recently gained popularity. Fentanyl's possible advantage over morphine is that it is extremely lipid soluble and, therefore, has a more rapid onset and shorter duration of action unless it is given in anesthetic quantities (ie, greater than 500 µg/70 kg). Also, because of its lipid solubility, fentanyl has more sedative properties than morphine. It is usually associated with less hypotension than morphine. In an adult, 100 µg of fentanyl given slowly in combination with a benzodiazepine usually provides adequate sedation, amnesia, and analgesia for intubation purposes, especially when used in conjunction with topical local anesthesia.

During the administration of sedative drugs, all patients should be monitored continuously, with close attention being paid to the patient's vital signs (pulse, blood pressure, and respirations). Additional helpful monitoring devices might include a precordial stethoscope, an electrocardiogram, and a pulse oximeter. Sedation is usually adequate for intubation purposes when the patient appears to be sleeping quietly, yet is responsive to verbal stimulation. If a patient becomes unresponsive to verbal stimulation or exhibits signs of impending airway obstruction (snoring or retractions), he or she should be regarded as being oversedated and should receive intubation on a more emergent basis. Of note is that the narcotic effects of sedative overdose can be reversed by the opiate antagonist naloxone, 0.1 to 0.4 mg given intravenously. It is anticipated that a benzodiazepine antagonist will be on the American market in the near future.

All sedative medication should be prescribed by a physician and administered only by licensed personnel who are fully familiar with the properties, side effects, and dosages of sedative medication. Life-sustaining equipment, including cardiac defibrillator, airway management equipment, and cardiac resuscitative medications, should be immediately available.

As an adjunct to sedative medication, a topical local anesthetic may be applied to the mucous membranes of the nose, mouth, and larynx with a nebulizer, a spray, soaked pledgets, nose drops, or viscous jelly. When using a local anesthetic solution, one must pay particular attention to the total dose of anesthetic administered. When these anesthetics are applied directly to the mucous membranes, rapid circulatory uptake can occur, with resultant systemic toxicity.[72] This toxicity can be evidenced in the early stages by perioral paresthesias, a metallic taste in the mouth, light-headedness, and tinnitus, and can progress to muscle twitching, tremors, convulsions, respiratory depression, hypotension, and, ultimately cardiovascular collapse.[73] The local anesthetics most commonly used for topical application include lidocaine (2%, 4%, or 10% concentration), cocaine (4% concentration), and benzocaine (20% concentration). The dose of lidocaine, when administered alone, should not exceed 6.4 mg/kg.[74] The dose of cocaine, when used alone, should not exceed 200 mg in a 70-kg person.[73–75]

Intubation Under General Anesthesia

Only trained individuals should use general anesthetics to facilitate tracheal intubation. Excluding surgical patients, few patients require general anesthesia for intubation. In fact, if a patient needs to be restrained for intubation to the point of general anesthesia, then the need for intubation might need to be reexamined. However, there are certain circumstances in which it is necessary to call upon the skills of an anesthesiologist to afford translaryngeal intubation. These situations include intubation of the patient with cerebral or cervical spine injury, acute epiglottitis, and intubation of the patient who is totally uncooperative. All preintubation considerations as described in awake intubation are necessary to consider for patients receiving general anesthesia. Certain additional considerations are necessary when using this approach, including obtaining monitoring equipment (ie, electrocardiogram, blood pressure cuff, precordial stethoscope, pulse oximeter) and also anesthetic drugs or anesthetic-administration devices (volatile anesthetic vaporizers). The anesthetic drugs used to facilitate intubation can be categorized into three areas:

- Intravenous central nervous system (CNS) depressants
- Volatile general anesthetics
- Muscle relaxants

Thiopental sodium (Pentothal), the prototype intravenous CNS depressant, is an ultrashort-acting barbiturate. Its effects range from mild sedation to total loss of consciousness, depending on the dose and rate of administration. Thiopental has a rapid onset (approximately 30 seconds) and a short duration of action (approximately 5 minutes); consequently, it is ideal for short procedures such as intubation. It can significantly decrease blood pressure, especially in the critically ill and fluid-depleted patient. The average intubating dose is 2 to 5 mg/kg, depending on the size, age, and general physical status of a patient.

The prototype volatile anesthetic still in use today is halothane. Tracheal intubation following anesthetic induction with a volatile agent is performed routinely in pediatric anesthesia practice for which, because of patient noncooperation or lack of venous access sites, intravenous induction is not easily accomplished. In addition, there are certain circumstances in both children and adults during which a loss of spontaneous ventilation, such as would occur with a rapid bolus of intravenous medication, might lead to total airway obstruction (eg, acute epiglottitis). Under these circumstances, the patient is allowed to spontaneously breathe the volatile agent until anesthetized, at which time the anesthetist assumes control of ventilation. To achieve tracheal intubation with halothane anesthesia alone, one must approach drug doses that can cause cardiovascular depression (eg, bradycardia and hypotension). Hence, intravenous supplementation with sedative drugs and narcotics is sometimes used during volatile anesthetic induction to facilitate intubation. For halothane induction, the anesthetist begins with trace concentrations of the drug and gradually, over a 2- to 3-minute period, increases the inspired drug concentration to approximately 3%. Intubation is accomplished after the patient is apneic, there is a loss of eyelid reflex, and the pupils are centrally fixed.

The neuromuscular blocker most commonly used for intubation purposes is succinylcholine. This medication, like all muscle relaxants, is administered only after a patient is heavily sedated or anesthetized. Muscle relaxants provide no sedative or anesthetic effect. These drugs should never be prescribed for patients outside the operating room without close supervision by a physician who is familiar with their pharmacology and is capable of supporting the airway of a paralyzed patient. An intubating dose for succinylcholine is 1.5 mg/kg given intravenously. The onset of action is rapid (45 to 60 seconds), and the duration of effect is short (3 to 8 minutes), making it ideal for procedures such as intubation. Administration of succinylcholine to the infant and child can result in bradycardia. Atropine (0.01–0.02 mg/kg) should be given intravenously just before succinylcholine in all prepubertal children.

Nasal Intubation

Either naris may be chosen, depending on the history and examination, but the right naris is preferred because the bevel of most endotracheal tubes, when introduced through the right naris, faces the flat nasal septum, reducing damage to the turbinates. Topical anesthesia and vasoconstrictor drugs can be used to facilitate the passage of the tube through the nares, lessen the chance of hemorrhage, and make the procedure more comfortable for the patient. Two to three sprays of 0.25% to 0.50% phenylephrine can be used for vasoconstriction. When phenylephrine is dispensed by a plastic squeeze bottle, the bottle must be pointed upward when spraying; it is easy to overdose the patient with this sympathomimetic agent with the bottle pointing downward. Following administration of the vasoconstrictor, local anesthetic drugs can be applied to the nasal mucosa by means of soaked pledgets, spray, viscous jelly, or nose drops. The sequence of first administering the vasoconstrictor reduces the systemic uptake and the toxic manifestations of the local anesthetic.

The occiput of the head is elevated about 10 cm with a pillow, and a generously lubricated nasotracheal tube is introduced into the selected naris (Fig. 19-47). Extension of the head lifts the epiglottis from the posterior pharyngeal wall. The tube is then advanced along the floor of the nose into the oropharynx and aligned with the glottic opening by listening to the air passing through the tube in a spontaneously breathing patient (Fig. 19-48). The tube is advanced as long as breath sounds increase. If breath sounds diminish, the tube is withdrawn a few centimeters until breath sounds are maximal and then readvanced. Ideally, the tube is swiftly passed to the glottis at a time just before inspiration because the vocal cords are most open during inspiration. Nasotracheal intubation can be accomplished under direct vision by first inserting the tracheal tube through the nares and pharynx, holding the laryngoscope with the left hand, and advancing the tracheal tube with the right hand. If one cannot align the tracheal tube for introduction into the trachea, one can use a Magill forceps with the right hand while an assistant advances the nasotracheal tube at its entrance to the naris (Figs. 19-49 and 19-50).

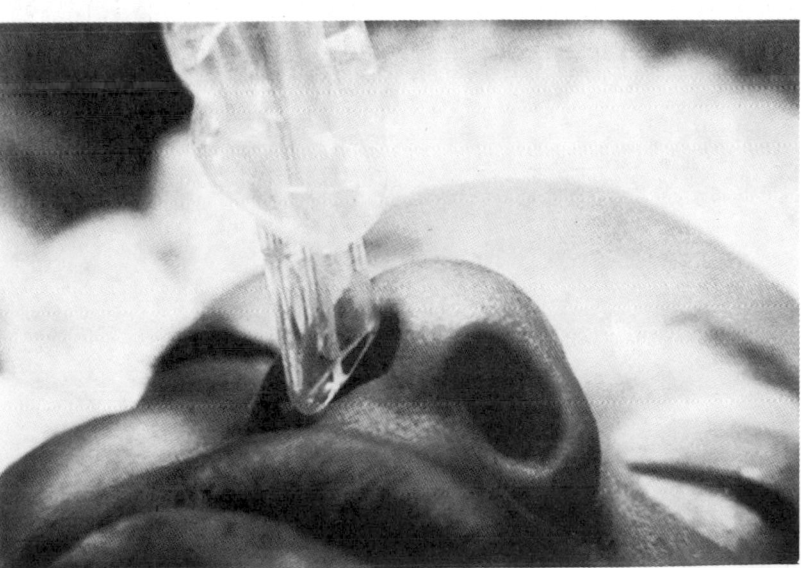

FIGURE 19-47. The head is positioned and a naris selected for nasal intubation. (Finucane BT, Santora AH: Principles of Airway Management. Philadelphia; FA Davis 1988, with permission)

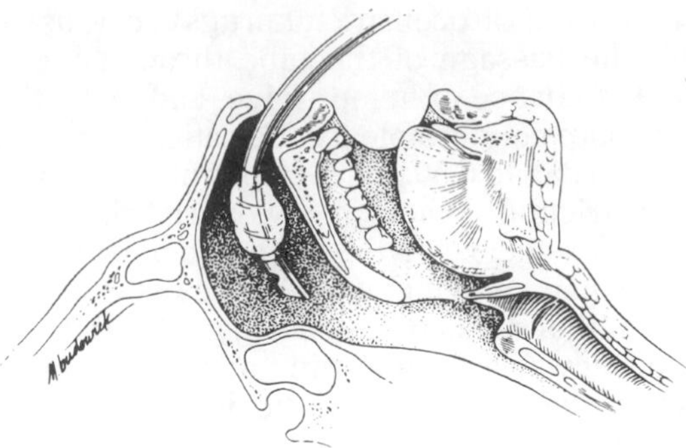

FIGURE 19-48. The endotracheal tube is passed through the nasopharynx during nasal intubation. (Finucane BT, Santora AH: Principles of Airway Management. Philadelphia, FA Davis, 1988, with permission)

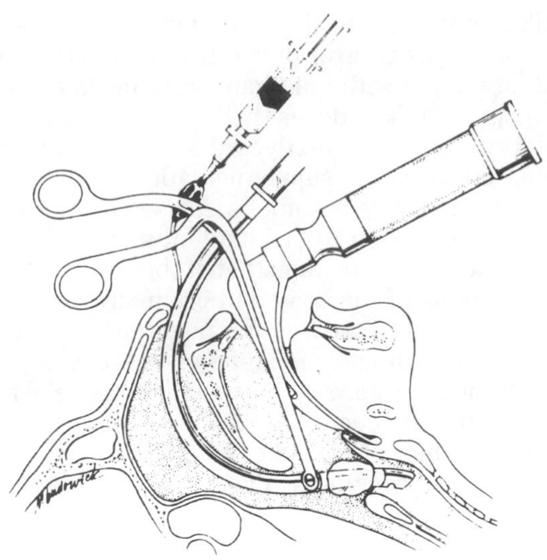

FIGURE 19-50. Nasotracheal intubation using a McIntosh (curved) blade and a Magill forceps (Finucane BT, Santora AH: Principles of Airway Management. Philadelphia, FA Davis, 1988, with permission)

INTUBATION OF THE PEDIATRIC PATIENT

Intubation of the pediatric patient is, in some ways, similar to that of the adult patient. Areas in which techniques may differ are emphasized here. Awake intubation is usually carried out in neonates and infants up to 6 weeks of age. Beyond this age, healthy infants are too vigorous, and consideration should be given to using sedative or anesthetic medication to afford patient cooperation. Nasal intubation is sometimes avoided in infants and children because adenoid hypertrophy can obstruct tube advancement in the nasopharynx and result in tissue obstruction and hemorrhage. Preoxygenation before intubation may be even more critical in the infant than in the adult because of several physiologic differences between infants and adults that predispose them to hypoxia. These differences include an increased oxygen consumption per kilogram of body weight, a reduced functional residual capacity, and a higher lung closing capacity.

It is important not to overextend the head when positioning for intubation, since this may contribute to complete airway obstruction in the infant. After passage of the tracheal tube and verification of tracheal intubation by maneuvers previously discussed, a main stem bronchus is intentionally intubated to document the position of the carina; the endotracheal tube is then retrieved to a position in the midtrachea. When the tube has been satisfactorily positioned, 20 to 25 cmH_2O positive pressure is applied to the proximal end of the endotracheal tube. At this pressure, an audible gas leak should occur. If there is no leak or if the leak is excessive, the tracheal tube should be replaced by one of a more appropriate size. Of note is that during the process of intubation in a neonate or infant, vagal stim-

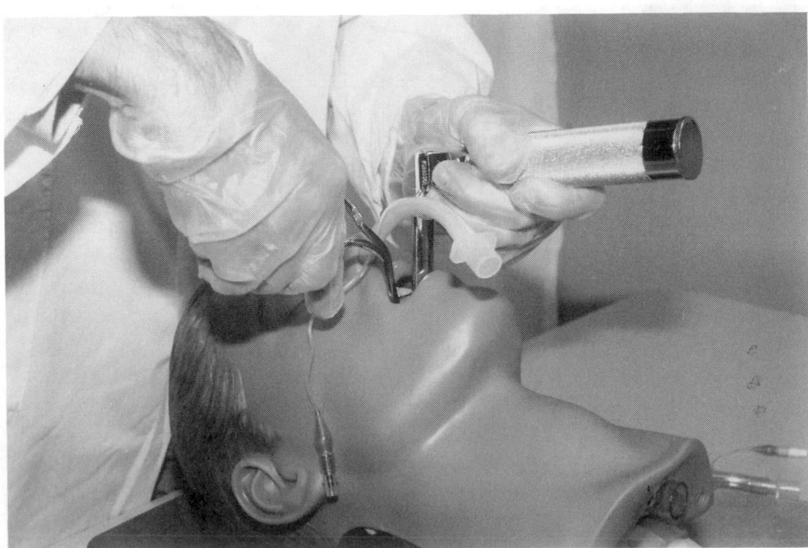

FIGURE 19-49. A Magill forceps is used to align the nasotracheal tube for introduction into the trachea.

ulation and bradycardia may occur; accordingly, intravenous atropine should be readily available for administration at an intravenous dose of 0.01 to 0.02 mg/kg.

DIFFICULT INTUBATION

Intubation difficulties may, sometimes, be anticipated by a preprocedural evaluation. Appropriate preparations can be made to obtain specialized equipment and to enlist the assistance of skilled colleagues. However, there are times when a difficult intubation is not anticipated and no good explanation for the difficulty can be found.

Difficult intubations can be divided into four categories:

- Limited access to the oropharynx
- Poor visualization of the larynx
- Diminished cross-sectional area of the pharynx or trachea
- Unexplained reasons

Access to the oropharynx can be obstructed by occluded nares, protruding teeth, a large tongue, temporomandibular joint disease, and so forth. Visualization of the larynx can be obstructed by cervical spine immobility from arthritis, obesity, soft-tissue masses, or other abnormalities. The cross-sectional area of the larynx or trachea can be limited by laryngeal or tracheal stenosis. Box 19-15 identifies conditions with potential for intubation difficulties.

When difficult intubations do occur, it is best from both medical and legal standpoints to rely on an established guideline or algorithm of clinical conduct.[6,7] One such algorithm is that which has been published by the American Society of Anesthesiologists (Fig. 19-51).[7] This approach includes options for intubation with fiberoptic bronchoscope, stylet or tube changer, light wand, and tracheostomy. The laryngeal mask airway, esophageal-tracheal combitube, and transtracheal jet are also given as options under the appropriate circumstances (Fig. 19-52). Other devices include specialized laryngoscope blades designed to facilitate difficult intubations. The Siker mirror blade may allow easier visualization of a more anterior larynx. The polio blade was designed for intubation at an obtuse angle, required for patients in iron lungs, body casts, or in those who have increased anteroposterior chest-wall dimensions.[76]

A stylet is an elongated metal or plastic rod that is inserted inside the tracheal tube to allow one to alter the natural curve of the tube. The stylet's purpose is to alter the shaft of the tube so that the tip can be maneuvered around structures that hinder direct vision of the larynx. A "tube changer" is an elongated hollow plastic tube that is usually used as a stent when changing endotracheal tubes in a previously intubated patient. This tube changer may also serve as a means of intubation when a difficulty is encountered, owing to its flexibility and ability to conform to different angles. After the trachea has been intubated with the tube changer, the endotracheal tube can be passed over it and the tube changer withdrawn. A light wand is a relatively new device that, like a tube changer, conforms to different angles to intubate the trachea. The advantage of the light wand is that a bright light at the tip transilluminates the trachea, verifying correct positioning.[77] The laryngeal mask airway has been used to support airways that are otherwise difficult to manage. Interestingly, Dr. Brain, the device's inventor, suggests that the LMA is actually easier to insert in situations where the larynx is located distantly anterior. In addition to it's use as an airway support device, the LMA can serve as a facilitator of fiberoptic tracheal intubation.[27]

A fiberoptic bronchoscope can serve as a stent over which a tracheal tube can be inserted into the trachea. The tip of the bronchoscope can be maneuvered under fiberoptic vision to allow tracheal insertion. Digital insertion of the endotracheal tube or the retrowire intubation technique can be considered if specialized equipment is not available or has proved unsuccessful with several attempts. During a difficult intubation, one should call for assistance early to allow for help in monitoring the patient, readying available equipment, obtaining more specialized equipment, and serving as an advisor or additional intubator. The excitement surrounding a difficult intubation occurs in an atmosphere in which professional egos are at risk. To avoid hazardous results for the patient, one should always be open to the advice of other practitioners. In the event that tracheal intubation cannot be accomplished and the airway cannot be maintained with mask ventilation, a *cricothyrotomy* should be considered. The purpose of the cricothyrotomy is to allow oxygen insufflation into the patient's airway to maintain oxygenation while further attempts at intubation are made or a tracheostomy is accomplished.

Cricothyrotomy does not allow for ventilation and carbon dioxide removal; hence, significant respiratory acidosis can occur when oxygen therapy is provided by this means alone. A catheter-needle combination (10 to

BOX 19-15

CONDITIONS WITH POTENTIAL FOR DIFFICULT INTUBATION

- Limited access to the oropharynx
  - Examples:
  - Occluding nares
  - Protruding teeth
  - Large tongue (macroglossia)
  - Temporomandibular joint immobility
- Poor visualization of the larynx
  - Examples:
  - Cervice spine immobility
  - Soft-tissue mass
  - Upper airway hemorrhage
- Limited cross-sectional area of the larynx or trachea
  - Examples:
  - Laryngeal stenosis
  - Tracheal stenosis
- Unexplained and unanticipated difficulties despite normal airway examination

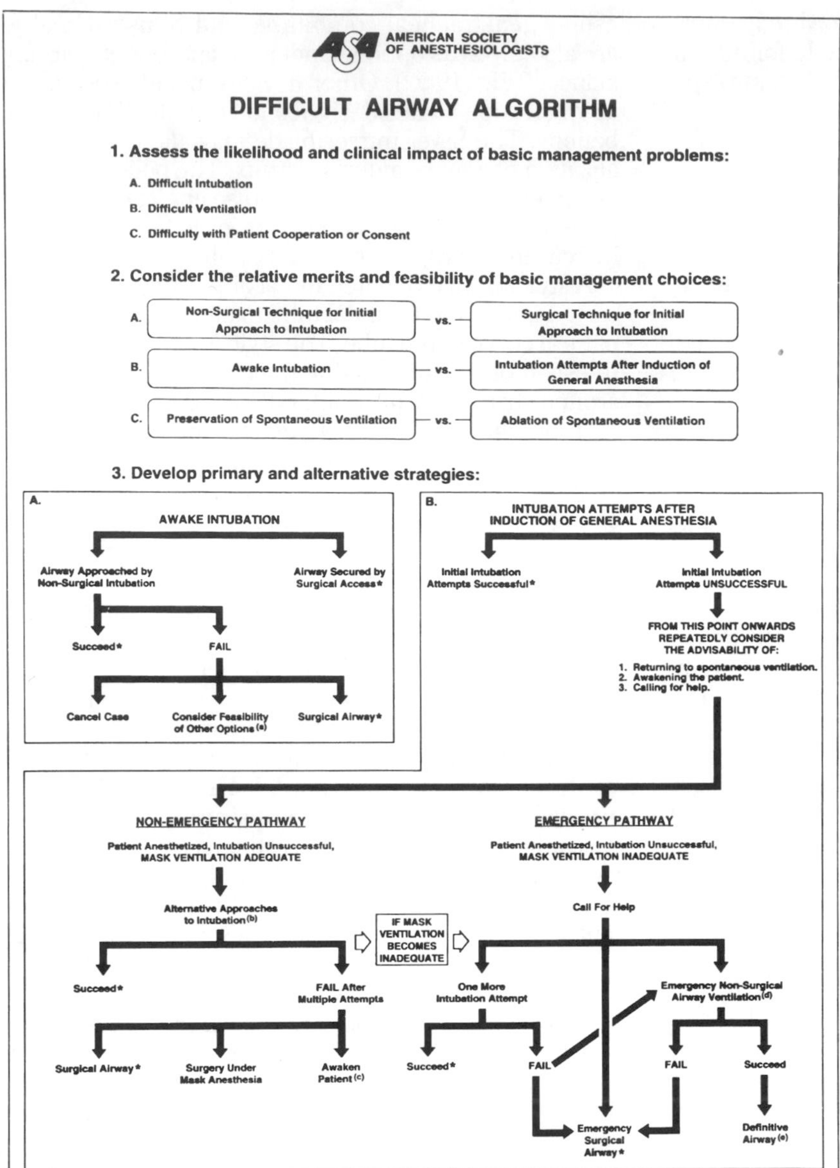

FIGURE 19-51. Algorithm for management of the difficult airway. (from American Society of Anesthesiologists. Practice guidelines for management of the difficult airway. Anesthesiology 1993;78:597, with permission)

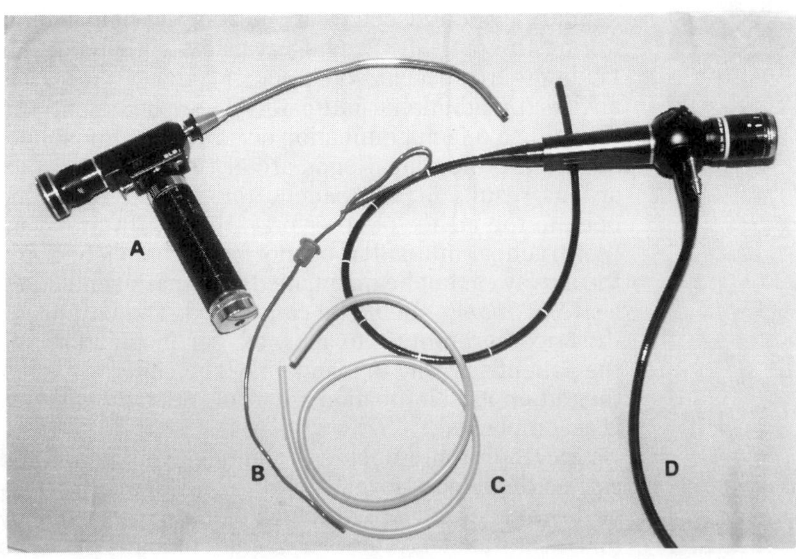

FIGURE 19-52. Equipment for difficult intubation. **(A)** Light wand; **(B)** Stylet; **(C)** Fiberoptic laryngoscope, **(D)** Fiberoptic bronchoscope.

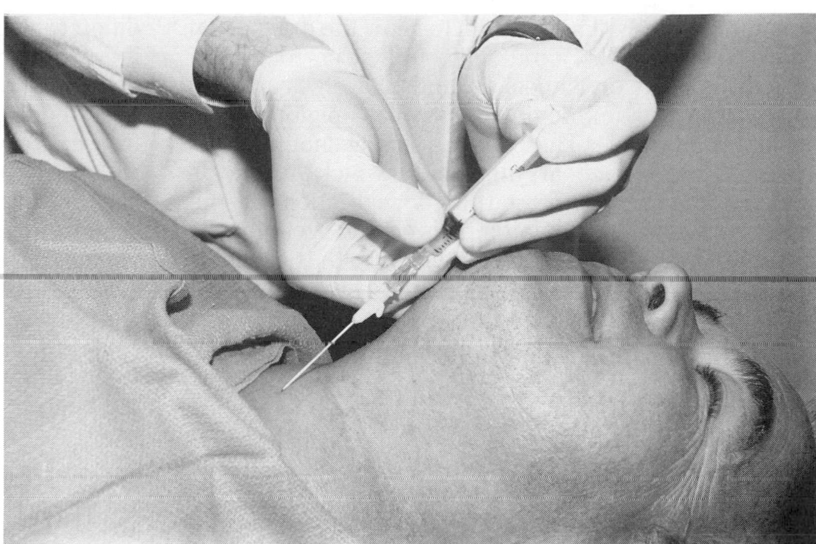

FIGURE 19-53. Cricothyrotomy being performed with an intravenous catheter.

14 gauge) is directed caudally at a 45° angle and inserted into the midline of the cricothyroid membrane. During insertion, negative pressure is applied to the syringe. The entrance of air within the syringe signifies that the needle is in the trachea (Fig. 19-53). The catheter is then advanced over the needle into the trachea. The hub of the catheter is connected to an oxygen source. If a jet ventilator is available, the Luer-Lok of the jet ventilator can be connected to the catheter; if airway obstruction is not complete, some ventilation will take place. The Nu-Trake (Armstrong Industries) is a sterile unit that combines a blade, needle, and cannula (Fig. 19-54). Potential complications of the placement and use of the cricothyrotomy include perforation of the esophagus, subcutaneous emphysema, pneumothorax, hemorrhage into the trachea, and infection.[78]

PEDIATRIC AIRWAY EMERGENCIES

Pediatric airway emergencies frequently present as upper airway obstruction. The signs and symptoms of upper airway obstruction are extremely variable and are dependent upon the etiology in the site of obstruction. Supraglottic lesions tend to cause inspiratory stridor, whereas subglottic lesions cause both inspiratory and expiratory stridor. The diagnosis of obstruction caused by a foreign body is made by the history of a previously healthy child (usually younger than 5 years of age) who becomes acutely short of breath after either sucking on small foreign objects or eating while exercising. If foreign body airway obstruction results in complete airway obstruction, back blows and chest thrusts are recommended as previously discussed. With incomplete airway obstruction, there may be time for x-ray confirmation and location of the object in the tracheobronchial tree. A bronchoscope can be used to retrieve the object.

Acute Epiglottitis

Acute epiglottitis results in supraglottic obstruction. It is caused by a bacterial infection (commonly *Haemophilus influenzae*) and is characterized by rapid onset (less than 24 hours), sore throat, and significant fever (higher than 39°C). Acute epiglottitis presents most commonly between the ages of 2 and 8 years. The child appears

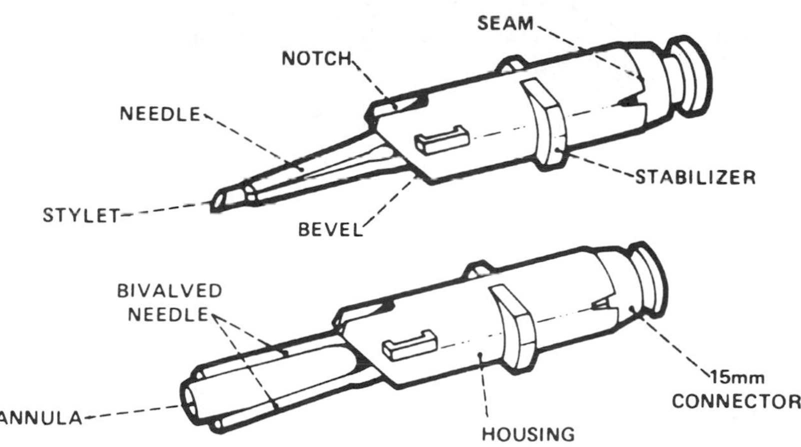

FIGURE 19-54. Nu-Trake cricothyrotomy device. (Bjoraker DG, Kumar NB, Brown AC: Evaluation of an emergency cricothyrotomy instrument. Crit Care Med 15:157, 1987; © Williams & Wilkins, with permission)

"toxic," adopts a sitting position to allow the drainage of saliva, and either has a muffled cough or no cough. Diagnosis is made on clinical grounds. Rarely is a lateral neck radiograph (exhibiting the swollen epiglottis) necessary or advisable. The patient's airway should be secured with endotracheal intubation, at which time the diagnosis can be confirmed by visualization of the cherry-red, swollen epiglottis. This should occur ideally in the operating room under general anesthesia (see intubation under general anesthesia). Any premature examination of the airway for diagnostic or other purposes may precipitate complete airway obstruction.

Croup

Croup, or viral laryngotracheobronchitis, is usually the result of an infection from parainfluenza or respiratory syncytial virus. It normally affects children under the age of 3 years, develops gradually over several days, is characterized by a "barking" cough, and results in only mild temperature elevation. As the airway narrowing occurs subglottically, both inspiratory and expiratory stridor can be heard. The diagnosis of croup is made on clinical grounds. The diagnosis can be supported by a neck x-ray film that shows subglottic narrowing ("steeple sign"; Fig. 19-55). Most children with this condition can be cared for at home with the aid of a humidifier. If hypoxia or signs of impending respiratory failure develop, the patient should be admitted to the hospital. Treatment consists of humidification with cool mist, oxygen, oral or intravenous fluids, and nebulized racemic epinephrine. Corticosteroid therapy is controversial, but, when used, dexamethasone is given at a dose of 4 mg intravenously. Endotracheal intubation is usually not necessary but should be considered if the patient shows signs of fatigue or remains hypoxic despite oxygen administration. Intubation in the operating room under general anesthesia is at times necessary, especially when the diagnosis of acute epiglottitis has not been completely excluded.

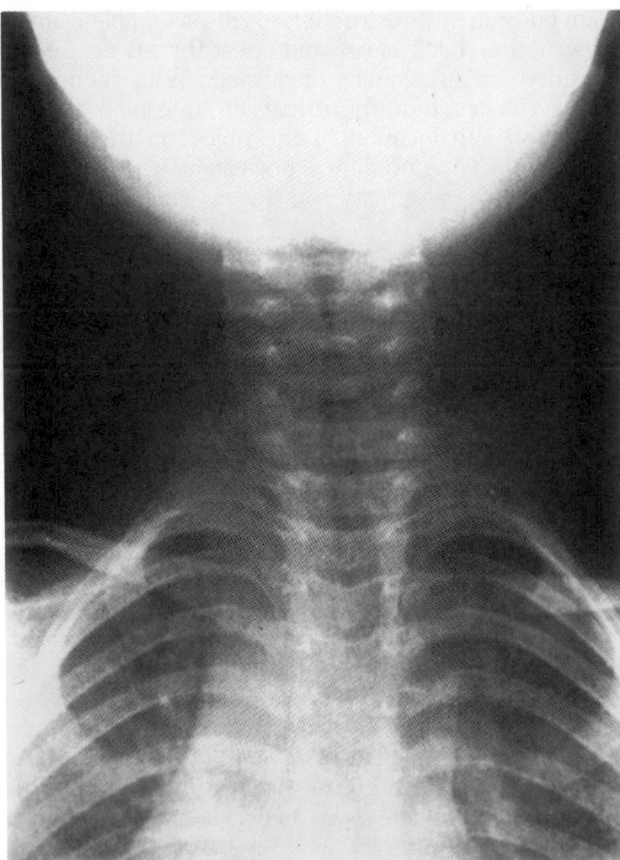

FIGURE 19-55. A neck radiograph showing subglottic narrowing (steeple sign). (Finucane BT, Santora AH: Principles of Airway Management. Philadelphia, FA Davis, 1988, with permission)

COMPLICATIONS OF TRACHEAL INTUBATION

The possible hazards and complications of tracheal intubation are numerous. Box 19-16 lists some of them according to the time frame of the intubation event.[6,79]

The frequency of complications associated with tracheal intubation can be reduced. The incidence of fascial

BOX 19-16

HAZARDS AND COMPLICATIONS OF TRACHEAL INTUBATION

- Complications during placement of the tracheal tube
  - -Failure to establish a patent airway by intubating the trachea
  - -Failure to recognize intubation of the esophagus
  - -Upper airway trauma: oral, nasal, pharyngeal, laryngeal, and esophageal
  - -Laryngospasm and bronchospasm
  - -Unrecognized endobronchial intubation
  - -Aspiration
  - -Dental and eye injuries
  - -Cardiac dysrhythmias
  - -Cervical spine and cord injuries
  - -Hypertension and tachycardia or hypotension and bradycardia
  - -Elevation of intracranial pressure
- Complications following placement of a tracheal tube
  - -Sinusitis or otitis media (nasal intubation)
  - -Laryngeal or tracheal injury leading to bleeding or stenosis
  - -Subglottic edema
  - -Secretion retention
  - -Patient discomfort
  - -Nosocomial colonization and infection
  - -Problems with the tube
    - Cuff perforation or herniation
    - Kinking or occlusion
    - Pilot-tube-valve incompetence
    - Inadvertent extubation
- Complications occurring as a result of extubation
  - -Laryngospasm
  - -Regurgitation and aspiration
  - -Sore throat
  - -Postextubation croup

and oral trauma can be diminished by appropriate training and credentialing. Endotracheal tube displacement can be limited by a compulsive postintubation physical examination and by the application of certain monitoring techniques used to verify tracheal intubation (ie, capnography). Tracheal injury may be reduced by adhering to established protocols for cuff inflation and by securing the endotracheal tube so that movement of the tube is minimized. Damage to the larynx may be reduced by placing appropriate limits on the duration of translaryngeal intubation. The risk of aspiration may be lowered by properly selecting a technique of tracheal intubation appropriate for the clinical situation (eg, use of the Sellick maneuver for a patient with a full stomach) and by close monitoring after endotracheal extubation (a time when laryngeal reflexes are depressed). Nosocomial infection may be reduced by observing clean intubation techniques with prepackaged, disposable equipment, and by following established cleaning practices when using reusable equipment. Hypoxemia during intubation may be limited by preoxygenation, observation of proper technique to allow expedient intubation, and the use of monitoring devices (pulse oximetry) that might detect a fall in arterial oxygen saturation. Patient discomfort may be avoided by the appropriate use of sedative and local anesthetic agents.

TRACHEOSTOMY

Tracheostomy provides access to the airway in patients with upper airway obstruction. It also provides an alternative route to tracheal intubation for the patient who requires long-term mechanical respiratory support. A tracheostomy offers several benefits to the patients receiving mechanical ventilatory support. Box 19-17 identifies advantages of this airway.

Some potential complications of tracheostomy also exist. Box 19-18 reviews problems that can be encountered following tracheotomy and with extended use of the tracheostomy.

BOX 19-17

ADVANTAGES OF TRACHEOSTOMY

- Spares direct laryngeal injury from a translaryngeal route
- Enhances patient comfort and patient mobility
- Facilitates airway maintenance, especially airway suctioning
- Facilitates transfer from the ICU setting
- Allows the patient to speak (with appropriate instrumentation)
- Facilitates mouth care and can permit oral nourishment
- Provides a psychological benefit that is difficult to quantitate, but at times can be substantial and can greatly assist in patient recovery
- Reduced airway resistance

BOX 19-18

COMPLICATIONS OF TRACHEOTOMY AND TRACHEOSTOMY

- Surgical complications
  - -Intraoperative and postoperative hemorrhage at the surgical site or as a result of erosion into the innominate vessels
  - -Injury to laryngeal nerves and thyroid gland
  - -Air leaks (pneumothorax and subcutaneous emphysema)
  - -Tracheoesophageal fistula
  - -Cardiac arrest
- Complications while tracheostomy is in place
  - -Tracheal injury (inflammation, hemorrhage, ulceration, cartilage and mucosal necrosis)
  - -Tracheal perforation
  - -Infection (sepsis, pneumonia, and mediastinitis)
  - -Displacement of the tracheostomy tube
  - -Reduction in mucociliary transport
  - -Air leak (pneumothorax and subcutaneous emphysema)
- Complications during and after decannulation
  - -Scar, granuloma, or keloid formation
  - -Persistent open stoma
  - -Dysphagia
  - -Tracheal stenosis
  - -Tracheomalacia
  - -Tracheal web formation

Ideally, the tracheostomy should be performed by an experienced surgeon, with an anesthesiologist in attendance in the operating room or in a fully equipped, intensive care setting. Ciaglia and colleagues have introduced a device and technique of ***percutaneous tracheostomy*** as an alternative to the conventional open surgical technique (Fig. 19-56*A*).[80] This percutaneous procedure is becoming more widely accepted due to advantages that potentially include performance at the ICU bedside, decreased operative time, and decreased cost. A large-bore needle enters the cricothyroid ligament, and a guide wire is introduced transtracheally. Dilatation of the entrance site is gradually accomplished by sequentially sized dilators, which range from 12 to 36 Fr (Figure 19-56*B*). The selected tracheostomy tube is fitted over the dilator and advanced into the trachea; the dilator and wire guide are then removed.

A decision to replace a translaryngeal endotracheal tube with a tracheostomy should be based on individual patient factors. The National Association of Medical Directors of Respiratory Care (NAMDRC) has recently published guidelines for the performance of tracheostomy.[81] They are summarized in Box 19-19.

Following tracheostomy, the trachea is cannulated with a tracheostomy tube. Most tracheostomy tubes are equipped with an inner cannula, an outer cannula, an obturator, and an inflatable cuff. The outer cannula contacts the stoma and maintains airway patency. The inner cannula allows cleaning of the airway, as it is easily removed from its position inside the outer cannula. The

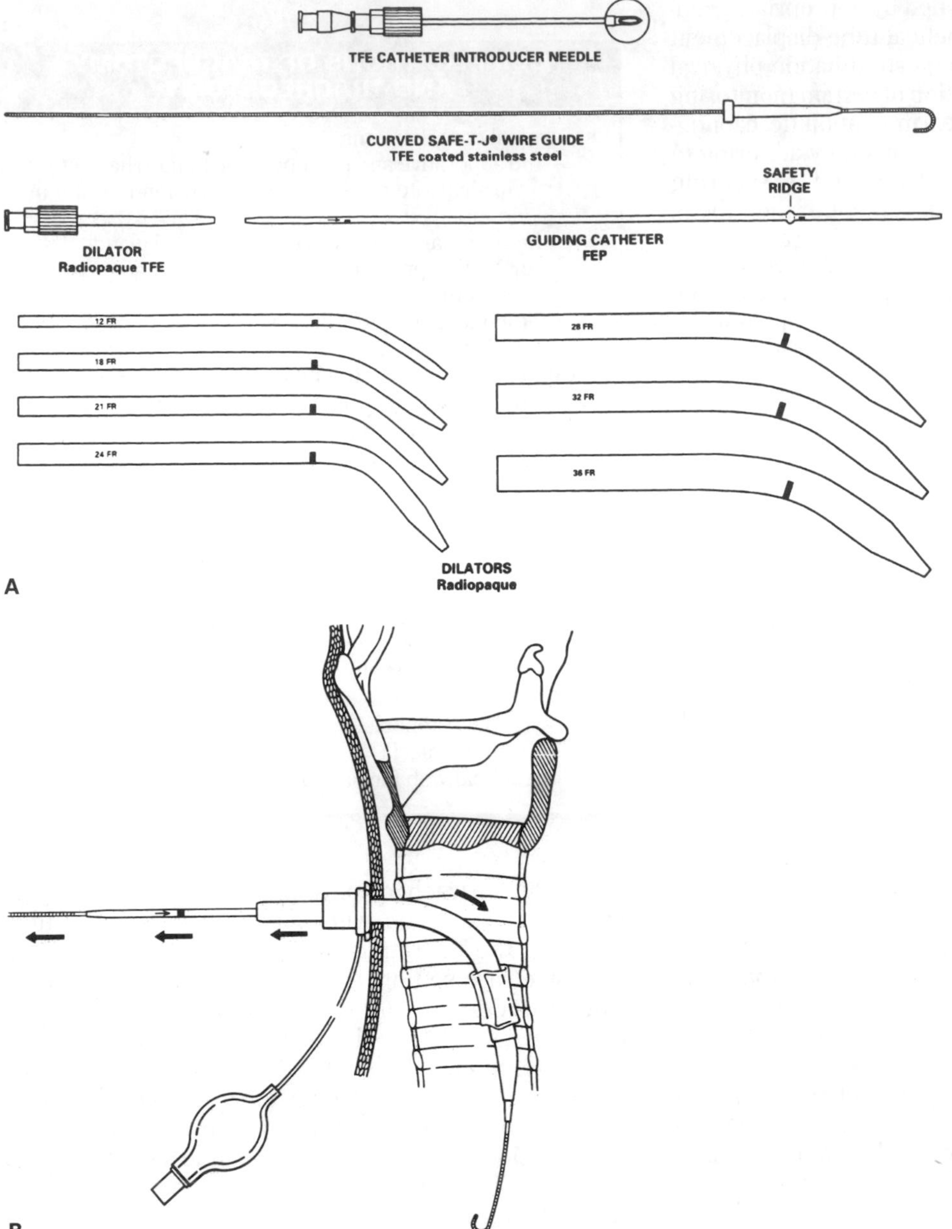

FIGURE 19-56. **(A)** Ciaglia percutaneous tracheostomy introducer set with various size dilators. **(B)** Cross-sectional diagram showing advancement of tracheostomy tube over guiding/dialator and wire guide. (Courtesy Cook Inc., Bloomington, IN)

obturator fills the lumen of the tube and aids during intubation of the stoma. After the tracheostomy tube is in place, the obturator is removed, and the cuff is inflated.

During the first 24 hours following tracheostomy, the inner cannula should be removed every 4 hours. It should be cleaned with a tracheostomy brush and hydrogen peroxide and rinsed in sterile water before it is replaced. Tracheostomy tubes should be changed regularly (approximately every week) to allow inspection of the stoma and the tracheostomy tube. The first tube change following a tracheostomy should be performed by a surgeon unless the tracheostomy has been allowed to fully mature (more than 7 days have elapsed since the operation). The obturator should be readily available for tube reintroduction in case an unanticipated dislodgment occurs.

SUCTIONING

Suctioning refers to mechanical aspiration of materials from the upper airway (mouth or nose, trachea, and main stem bronchi). This procedure may be required to remove saliva, pulmonary secretions, blood, or vomitus. It frequently provides a key role in clearing the airway to permit ventilation and oxygenation. Suctioning occurs when subatmospheric pressure (vacuum) is applied to a flexible catheter or rigid tube. Tracheal aspiration is frequently a component of resuscitation, bronchial hygiene therapy, and management of mechanically ventilated patients (see AARC Clinical Practice Guideline: Endotracheal Suctioning of Mechanically Ventilated Adults and Children With Artificial Airways). It is commonly performed in the hospital, ex-

BOX 19-19

NAMDRC GUIDELINES FOR IMPLEMENTING TRACHEOSTOMY

- For anticipated need of the artificial airway up to 10 days, the translaryngeal route is preferred
- For anticipated need of the artificial airway for longer than 21 days, tracheostomy is preferred
- In circumstances in which the time anticipated for maintenance of an artificial airway is not clear, daily assessment is required to determine if conversion to tracheostomy is indicated
- The decision for conversion to tracheostomy should be made as early in the course of management as possible to minimize the duration of translaryngeal intubation. Once the decision is made, the procedure should be done without undue delay except in conditions such as life-threatening cardiopulmonary instability, uncorrected coagulopathy, or other mitigating circumstances

tended care facility, home, field, or critical care setting. The term *nasotracheal suctioning* (NTS) refers to "blind insertion" of a flexible catheter through the nose and nasopharynx to access the trachea without a tracheal tube or tracheostomy appliance (although a nasopharyngeal airway may be used). Although a high-risk procedure, NTS can be implemented to avoid intubation solely provided for removal of secretions (see AARC Clinical Practice Guideline: Nasotracheal Suctioning).[4,5]

Indications for Suctioning

Normally, airway secretions are expectorated or swallowed. Loss of airway control, increased secretion production, inadequate cough, and lung pathologies that cause thickened secretions may, individually or combined, overwhelm a patient. Loss of consciousness or inability to control the airway, or both, results in an ineffective cough. This places patients at risk for secretion retention. Endotracheal or tracheostomy tubes also compromise both ciliary escalator and cough.

Suctioning may be performed in conjunction with chest physical therapy procedures, such as bronchial drainage, percussion, hyperinflation, and assisted coughing. Secretions must be mobilized from peripheral bronchi to the trachea and main stem bronchi for cough or suctioning to be effective. Instillation of sterile saline may be needed to help liquefy thick secretions. Suctioning is indicated based on clinical assessment. A common finding is rhonchi auscultated over the central airways, but suctioning has also been used prophylactically for ventilator and nonventilated patients to prevent secretion retention. In mechanically ventilated patients, there is frequently increased peak airway pressure (volume ventilation) due to narrowing or blockage of airway lumen. The difference between peak and plateau pressures may widen. Suctioning with an in-line trap is a method of sputum sampling for laboratory analysis.[82] Box 19-20 summarizes indications for suctioning.

AARC Clinical Practice Guideline

ENDOTRACHEAL SUCTIONING OF MECHANICALLY VENTILATED ADULTS AND CHILDREN WITH ARTIFICIAL AIRWAYS

Indications: The need to remove accumulated pulmonary secretions as evidenced by one of the following: coarse breath sounds by auscultation or noisy breathing, increased peak inspiratory pressures during volume-controlled mechanical ventilation or decreased tidal volume during pressure-controlled ventilation, patient's inability to generate an effective spontaneous cough, visible secretions in the airway, changes in monitored flow and pressure graphics, suspected aspiration of gastric or upper airway secretions, clinically apparent increased work of breathing, deterioration of arterial blood gas values, radiologic changes consistent with retention of pulmonary secretions, the need to obtain a sputum specimen to rule out or identify pneumonia or other pulmonary infection or for sputum cytology, the need to maintain the patency and integrity of the artificial airway, the need to simulate a cough in patients unable to cough effectively secondary to changes in mental status or the influence of medication, presence of pulmonary atelectasis or consolidation presumed to be associated with secretion retention.

Contraindications: Endotracheal suctioning is a necessary procedure for patients with artificial airways. Most contraindications are relative to the patient's risk of developing adverse reactions or worsening clinical condition as a result of the procedure. When indicated, there is no absolute contraindication to endotracheal suctioning because the decision to abstain from suctioning to avoid a possible adverse reaction may, in fact, be lethal.

Assessment of Need: Qualified personnel should assess the need for endotracheal suctioning as a routine part of a patient or ventilator system check.

Assessment of Outcome: Improvement in breath sounds, decreased peak inspiratory pressure (Paw) with narrowing of inspiratory plateau pressure (PIP); decreased airway resistance or increased dynamic compliance; increased tidal volume delivery during pressure-limited ventilation, improvement in arterial blood gas values or saturation as reflected by pulse oximetry (SpO_2), removal of pulmonary secretions.

Monitoring: The following should be monitored before, during, and after the procedure: breath sounds, skin color, pulse oximeter (if available), respiratory rate and pattern, hemodynamic parameters, pulse rate, blood pressure (if indicated and available), ECG (if indicated and available), sputum characteristics (color, volume, consistency, odor), cough effort, intracranial pressure (if indicated and available), ventilator parameters (peak inspiratory pressure and plateau pressure, tidal volume), ventilator waveform graphics (if available), arterial blood gases (if indicated and available).

From AARC Clinical Practice Guideline; see Respir Care 38:500, 1993, for complete text.

AARC Clinical Practice Guideline

NASOTRACHEAL SUCTIONING

Indications: The need to maintain a patent airway and remove secretions or foreign material from the trachea in the presence of inability to clear secretions; audible evidence of secretions in the large or central airways that persist in spite of patient's best cough effort.

Contraindications: Occluded nasal passages; nasal bleeding; epiglottitis or croup (absolute); acute head, facial, or neck injury; coagulopathy or bleeding disorder; laryngospasm; irritable airway; upper respiratory tract infection.

Assessment of Need: Auscultate chest for indications for nasotracheal suctioning and assess effectiveness of cough.

Assessment of Outcome: Effectiveness of nasotracheal suctioning should be reflected by improved breath sounds. Effectiveness of nasotracheal removal of secretions.

Monitoring: The following should be monitored during and following the procedure: breath sounds; skin color; breathing pattern and rate; pulse rate, dysrhythmia, ECG if available; color, consistency, and volume of secretions; presence of bleeding or evidence of physical trauma; subjective response including pain; cough, oxygenation (pulse oximeter if available); intracranial pressure, if equipment is available.

From AARC Clinical Practice Guideline; see Respir Care 37:898, 1992, for complete text.

Although a necessary and seemingly benign procedure, tracheal aspiration can be very uncomfortable and potentially hazardous to patients. Many of the side effects are the result of arterial desaturation. Arterial blood gas values provided the early documentation of the hypoxic effects.[83] Problems were most significant if the arterial oxygen tensions (PaO_2) decreased below 65 mmHg. The ear-finger probe oximeter provides an instant and continuous evaluation of oxyhemoglobin saturation (SpO_2). Saturations below 90% are of potential concern.[84] However, there are no absolute contraindications if failure to clear the airway may result in worsening of the patient's status or death.

Damage to the airway mucosa associated with suctioning has long been recognized at autopsy or after bronchoscopic study.[85,86] Microbial contamination is also a hazard to both patient and health care workers. Airway colonization and nosocomial pneumonia are linked to suctioning procedures, primarily from transmission by workers' hands.[87] Direct hand contact with infected tracheal secretions has been linked to outbreaks of herpes simplex virus types 1 and 2, causing a digital infection known as herpetic witlow.

Gloving of both hands is now part of standard suctioning protocol, a recent result of awareness that all body secretions may serve as vectors for the transmission of certain diseases (eg, AIDS or hepatitis). Centers for Disease Control guidelines should be followed.[14,15] Additional precautions, including eye shields, gowns, and masks, may be appropriate in instances in which splashing and aerosolization of secretions are possible.[88] Box 19-21 lists potential hazards and complications of suctioning.

BOX 19-20

INDICATIONS FOR SUCTIONING[4,5]

- Need to remove accumulated pulmonary secretions evidenced by one of the following:
  - -Visible secretions in the airway
  - -Inability to generate an effective spontaneous cough
  - -Chest auscultation of coarse, gurgling breath sounds or rhonchi
  - -Increased peak airway pressure (volume-controlled ventilation) or decreased tidal volume (pressure-controlled ventilation)
  - -Suspected aspiration of gastric or upper airway secretions
  - -Clinically apparent increased work of breathing
  - -Deterioration of arterial blood gas values suggesting hypoxemia or hypercarbia
  - -Chest radiographic evidence of retained secretions resulting in atelectasis or consolidation
- Need to maintain patency and integrity of an artificial airway
- To stimulate cough
- To obtain a sputum sample for microbiological or cytological analysis

Suctioning Equipment

All suctioning systems require a vacuum source with regulator, a trap bottle, connecting tubing, and a suction catheter. Wall vacuum is provided to hospital areas by a central pump and piping system (Fig. 19-57*A*). Hospi-

BOX 19-21

HAZARDS AND COMPLICATIONS OF SUCTIONING[4,5]

- Cardiac or respiratory arrest
- Laryngospasm, gagging, or vomiting (NTS only)
- Epiglottis or croup (NTS only)
- Cardiac dysrhythmias (tachycardia or bradycardia)
- Blood pressure changes (hypertension or hypotension)
- Mechanical trauma
  - -Mucosal hemorrhage
  - -Tracheitis
  - -Epistaxis from laceration of nasal turbinates (NTS only)
  - -Perforation of the pharynx (NTS only)
- Hypoxia or hypoxemia
- Increased intracranial pressure
- Discomfort and pain
- Bronchospasm
- Uncontrolled coughing
- Nosocomial infection

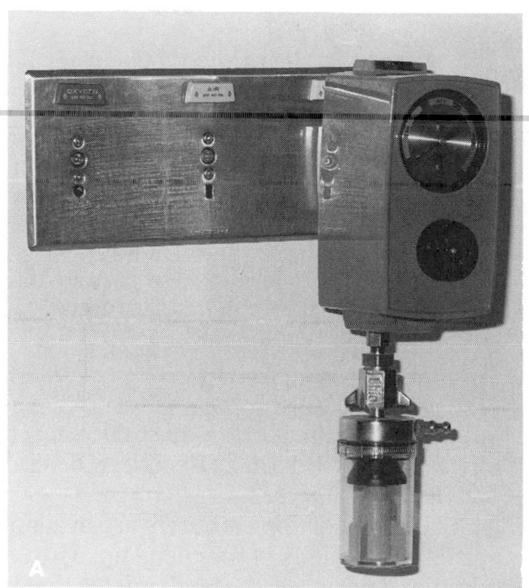
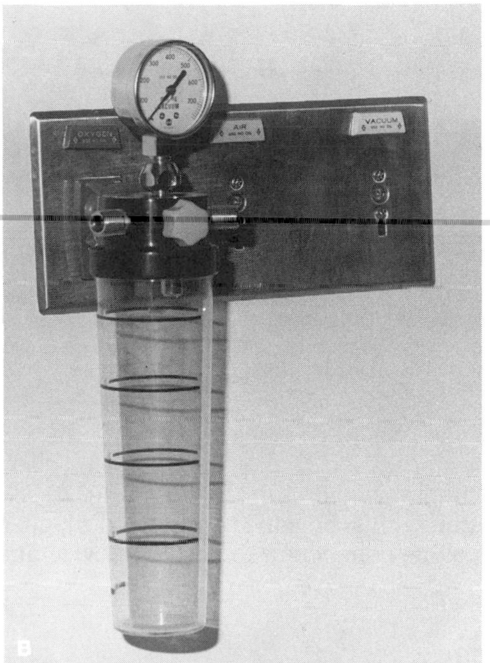
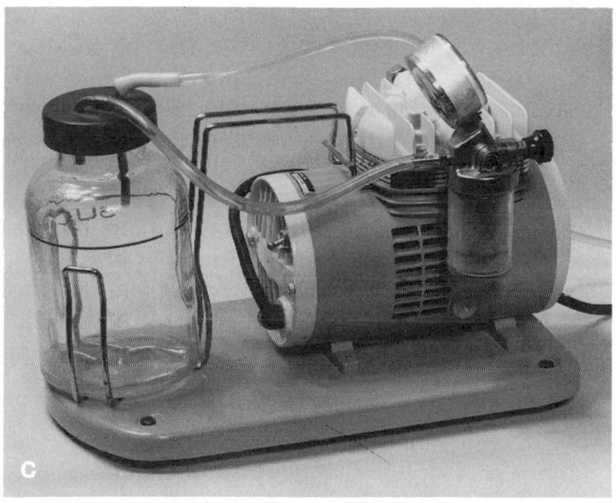
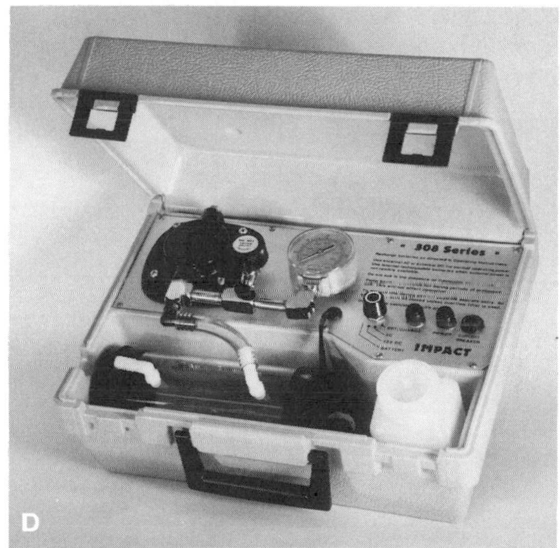

FIGURE 19-57. **(A)** Hospital pipeline vacuum outlet with regulator and collection bottle, **(B)** 50 PSIG gas source with venturi-generated suction system, **(C)** Electric-powered portable suction device, **(D)** Battery-powered portable suction system. (From Fluck RR, Hess DR, Branson RD. Airway and suction equipment. In: Branson RD, Hess DR, Chatburn RL, eds. Respiratory Care Equipment. Philadelphia: JB Lippincott, 1995, with permission)

tal pipeline 50-psig gas sources (oxygen or air) can produce suction by means of a venturi device (Fig. 19-57*B*). Portable electric, battery-powered, and manually operated devices are also available for field or transport use (Fig. 19-57*C* and *D*). Central vacuum pumps can generate subatmospheric pressures up to −25 in. Hg (−635 mmHg). Vacuum regulators reduce pressures to therapeutic levels; most are adjustable from a range of 0 to −200 mmHg. Suction regulators have both on-off controls and vacuum pressure–level controls. A subatmospheric pressure setting of −100 to −125 mmHg is recommended; higher levels do not enhance secretion recovery.[85] Maximum suction flows depend on the level of vacuum and on the diameter and length of the catheter and connecting tubing. Suction flows commonly range from 10 to 30 L/min, but research has not determined an ideal level. The suction flow is the main factor that influences the amount of gas removed from the lungs, which can lead to hypoxemia. *Trap-bottle reservoirs* collect suctioned materials, and valves protect the vacuum system from overflow. Specimen traps, such as the *Lukens trap*, can be placed between the suction

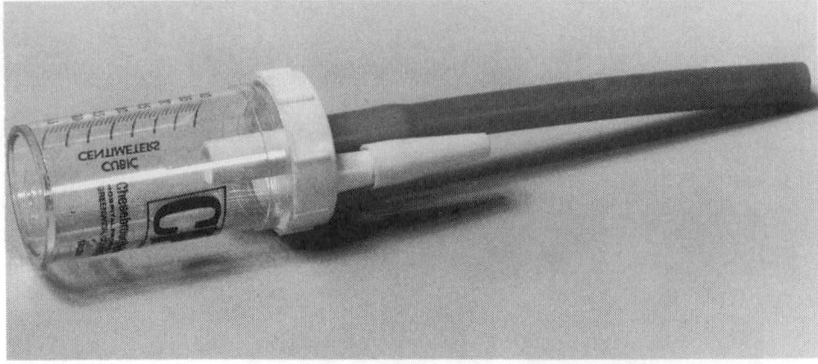

FIGURE 19-58. Lukens suction system specimine trap. (From Fluck RR, Hess DR, Branson RD. Airway and suction equipment. In: Branson RD, Hess DR, Chatburn RL, eds. Respiratory Care Equipment. Philadelphia: JB Lippincott, 1995, with permission)

catheter's thumb port and connecting tubing to collect suctioned sputum for laboratory analysis (Fig. 19-58). Connecting tubing must be noncompliant and supplied with ends to allow connection to vacuum device and catheter.

□ CATHETERS

The oropharynx may be suctioned using a nonflexible *tonsillar* or *Yankauer suction tip* (Fig. 19-59). Flexible catheters may be inserted directly into the nose and nasopharynx (nasotracheal suctioning) or through artificial airways. Box 19-22 describes desirable features for all flexible catheters.

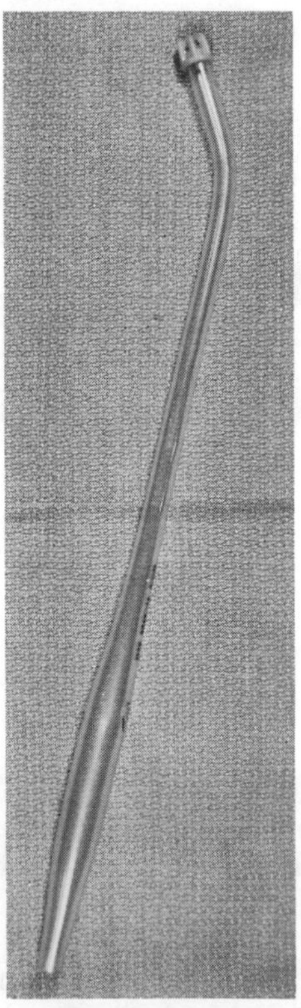

FIGURE 19-59. Yankaur rigid suction device. (From Fluck RR, Hess DR, Branson RD. Airway and suction equipment. In: Branson RD, Hess DR, Chatburn RL, eds. Respiratory Care Equipment. Philadelphia: JB Lippincott, 1995, with permission)

BOX 19-22

DESIRABLE FLEXIBLE SUCTION CATHETER FEATURES

- Sufficient length to enter the main stem bronchi [about 22 in. (55.9 cm)]
- A valve that allows interruption of vacuum. The majority have a thumb port. The diameter of that orifice should be larger than the catheter's internal diameter
- The catheter should be constructed to
  - remove mucus at pressures that do not damage tracheal tissue
  - possess minimal frictional resistance when passed through an artificial airway
  - retain its rigidity to allow passage through airways, yet be flexible enough to prevent airway damage on insertion

Standard suction catheters are available in a range of sizes and designs of the distal tip. Most authorities recommend using a catheter diameter that is less than one-half the inside diameter of an artificial airway. Larger diameter catheters increase the risk of atelectasis and hypoxemia. French (Fr) sizing is used by convention and determined by circumference [Fr= outside diameter × 3.14(p)] of the suction catheter. Box 19-23 provides the formula to estimate the proper outside diameter of suction catheter. Catheter length is more critical in care of neonates and infants. Some neonatal suction catheters have distance markings to prevent deep tracheal suction and associated complications.

Older catheters were made of red rubber with either an open end or a "whistle tip." Contemporary catheters are composed of polyvinyl chloride and silicone rubber. There is a variety of designs of either *straight-tipped* or *angle-tipped* (termed *coudé) catheters* (Fig. 19-60). The latter is designed to facilitate entrance to the left main stem bronchus. In clinical practice, coudé catheters increase the possibility of entering the left main bronchus, especially in tracheostomized versus intubated patients.[89] Although manufacturers suggest some tips that reduce the potential for trauma to mucosal surfaces, technique is probably a more important factor.[90] Trauma can occur when mucosa invaginates into the

BOX 19-23

FORMULAS TO ESTIMATE MAXIMUM (FRENCH) SUCTION CATHETER

$$\frac{\text{Inside diameter (ID)} \times 3}{2} = \text{Maximum diameter (Fr)}$$

For example, for a size 8.0 (ID) tracheal tube

$$\frac{8.0 \times 3}{2} = 12 \text{ Fr}$$

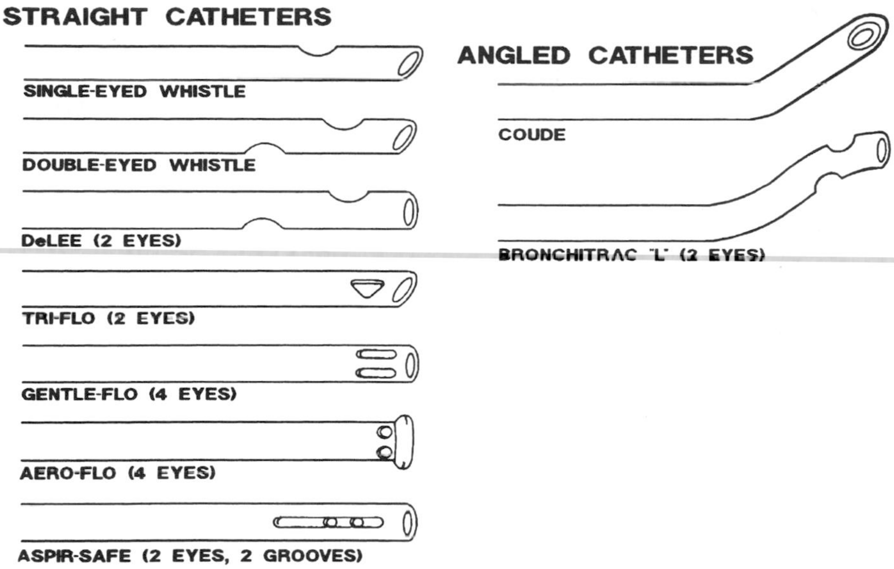

STRAIGHT CATHETERS
SINGLE-EYED WHISTLE
DOUBLE-EYED WHISTLE
DeLEE (2 EYES)
TRI-FLO (2 EYES)
GENTLE-FLO (4 EYES)
AERO-FLO (4 EYES)
ASPIR-SAFE (2 EYES, 2 GROOVES)
ANGLED CATHETERS
COUDE
BRONCHITRAC "L" (2 EYES)

FIGURE 19-60. Straight and curved-tip suction catheter tip designs. (From Fluck RR, Hess DR, Branson RD. Airway and suction equipment. In: Branson RD, Hess DR, Chatburn RL, eds. Respiratory Care Equipment. Philadelphia: JB Lippincott, 1995, with permission)

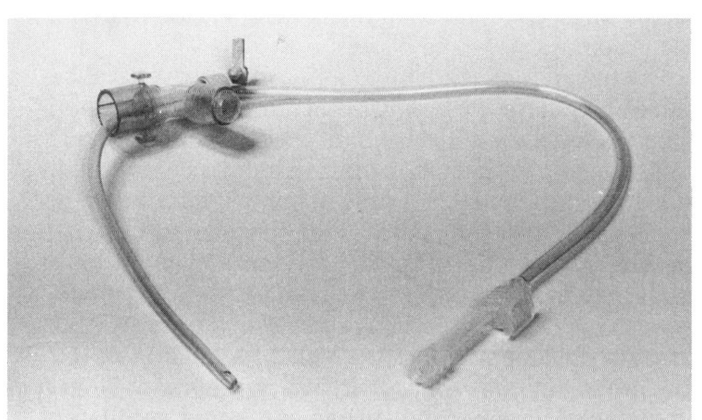

FIGURE 19-61. Artificial airway adaptor-swivel with port for suction. (From Fluck RR, Hess DR, Branson RD. Airway and suction equipment. In: Branson RD, Hess DR, Chatburn RL, eds. Respiratory Care Equipment. Philadelphia: JB Lippincott, 1995, with permission)

end and side hole(s) of the catheter. Mucosal surfaces are defoliated of cilia, and hemorrhagic erosion and edema result. Manufacturers offer single-use suction kits that include gloves, sterile field, and cup for water (sterile) to rinse the catheter.

Endotracheal or tracheostomy tube swivel adapters (eg, Bodai) have been developed to permit the catheter to pass through a side hole, while the patient is still connected to a mechanical ventilator (Fig. 19-61). This is advantageous for patients who have critical oxygenation and ventilation requirements.[91] This concept has evolved into *closed tracheal suction systems.* A plastic sleeve envelops the catheter to lessen catheter contamination when not in use; a separate irrigation port allows instillation of fluid (Fig. 19-62).[92] However, initial studies have not shown the closed system to have decreased rates of contamination when compared with single-use catheters.[92,93] The Jinotti oxygen insufflation catheter of-

IRRIGATION PORT
LOCK-UNLOCK CONTROL VALVE
LOCK
SUCTION CONNECTION
CATHETER IN SLEEVE
T-PIECE

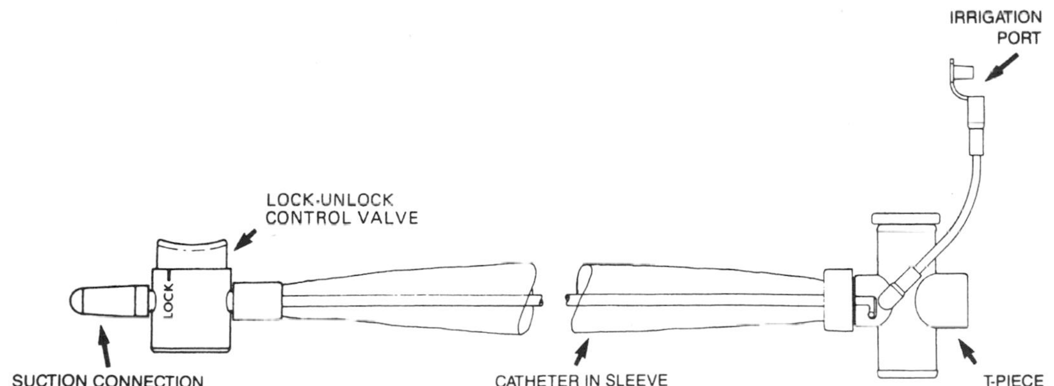

FIGURE 19-62. Diagram of closed suction catheter system (Ballard). (From Fluck RR, Hess DR, Branson RD. Airway and suction equipment. In: Branson RD, Hess DR, Chatburn RL, eds. Respiratory Care Equipment. Philadelphia: JB Lippincott, 1995, with permission)

To Suction: Valve tabs in closed position

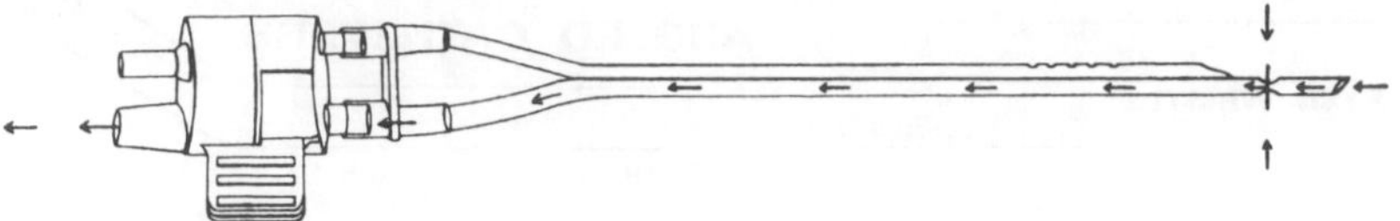

To Supply Oxygen: Valve tabs in open position

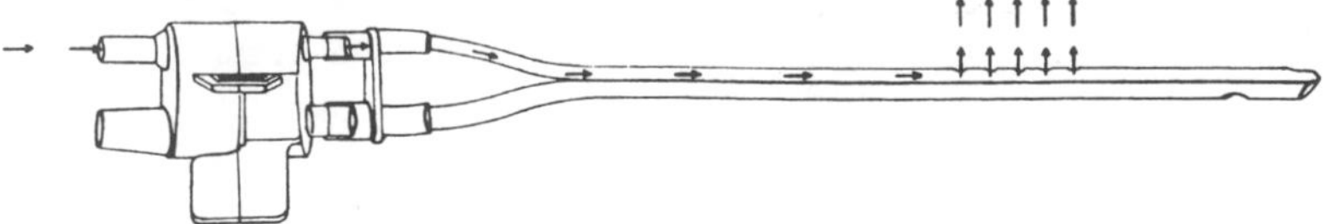

To Instill Tracheal Lavage Fluid: Inject fluid with luer tip syringe through oxygen tubing connection

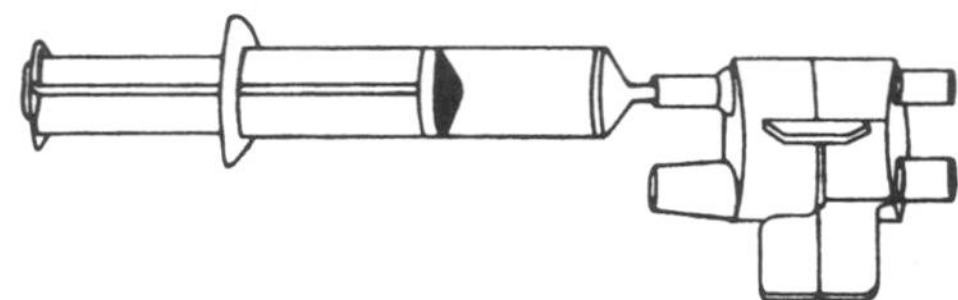

FIGURE 19-63. Jinotti oxygen insufflation/fluid instillation suction catheter. (Courtesy of American Pharmaseal Co. Valencia, CA)

fers a second lumen to provide either tracheal oxygen flow between suctioning procedures or fluid instillation (Fig. 19-63).[94]

Suctioning Protocol

Box 19-24 summarizes a general protocol for safe suctioning. Ideally the procedure should be performed by two health care workers, one to assure oxygenation and ventilation and the other to actually suction.

Current guidelines support the practice of hand washing and preoxygenation before beginning the suctioning.[4,5] Specific details as to numbers of breaths or time of preoxygenation depend on the condition of each patient. Many patients are protected from hypoxemia if given at least 30 seconds of 100% oxygen breathing.[95,96] The mechanical ventilator, self-inflating resuscitation bag, or high-concentration mask can provide hyperoxygenation.

The use of hyperinflation has been controversial because some hemodynamically unstable patients experience decreased cardiac output, increased intracranial pressure, and variations in arterial blood pressure with this technique.[97] Other researchers recommend increased volume of the breaths in the range of 1.5 times the size of the maintenance tidal volume of 12 to 14 mL/kg of lean body weight.[98,99] Delivery of the breaths may occur by anesthesia bag or self-inflating resuscitator. When a patient is on a mechanical ventilator, the airway pressure, tidal volume or sigh setting may be manipulated. The resetting of FIO_2 on some ventilators requires additional time to purge the internal reser-

BOX 19-24

SUMMARY OF SUCTIONING PROTOCOL

- Prepare and set up equipment
  - -Vacuum system: set pressure to −100 to −125 mmHg
  - -Suction catheter, water for instillation, and sterile water basin
  - -Protective equipment (gloves, mask, eye protection)
  - -Affix pulse oximeter
- Wash hands
- Prepare the patient
  - -Explain the procedure to alert patients
  - -Preoxygenate with 100% oxygen for more than 30 seconds (unless contraindicated)
  - -Hyperinflate with six or more breaths of approximately 1.5 times the baseline or estimated tidal volume (unless contraindicated)
  - -Note baseline pulse, ECG rhythm, and saturation by pulse oximeter
  - -Position neck in mild extension (adult)
- Prepare the catheter
  - -Glove both hands
  - -Moisten catheter in sterile water (artificial airway) or apply water-soluble lubricant (nasotracheal)
- Advance catheter (without suction)
  - -Nasotracheal: pass catheter through the nasopharynx. Suction any removable secretions. Advance catheter into hypopharynx, listening for tracheal breath sounds. Ask the patient to take a deep breath; advance the catheter through the vocal cords into the trachea until an obstruction is reached
  - -Artificial airway: advance catheter until an obstruction is felt
- Apply suction and gently withdraw the catheter
  - -Limit aspiration time to 10 to 15 seconds or less if SpO_2, ECG, or pulse indicate
- Provide rest, postoxygenation, and hyperinflation
- Repeat the procedure only as needed
  - -Artificial airway: suction the nares and mouth. Do not suction nose or trachea after oral use

voirs if the previous oxygen concentration was not 100%. Some ventilators have the ability to quickly flush gas from their systems. Operators must remember to return the oxygen concentration or volume settings to previous therapeutic levels.

Nasotracheal suctioning is technically more difficult because the catheter must be passed blindly into the trachea. A nasopharyngeal airway may be helpful in guiding the catheter and also decreasing bacterial colonization of the airway when repeated events are required. Airflow sounds may be heard from the proximal catheter. When sounds are at their loudest, cooperative patients can be asked to inspire as the catheter is advanced. Patients able to speak become hoarse, and speech becomes whisperlike. The catheter is then passed further into the trachea. Stimulation of cough receptors is likely to occur. A major concern with nasotracheal suction is laryngospasm. If that does occur, the suction catheter may be left in place to deliver an oxygen flow until the vocal cords relax spontaneously or by administration of a muscle relaxant.

Suctioning through a tracheal tube, tracheostomy tube, or stomal appliance is usually simpler, although not a benign procedure. After traversing the tube's lumen, the catheter should be gently advanced its full length (in adults), the desired depth (in neonates), or until an obstruction is encountered. Suction is then applied. There is no current research on whether suction should be intermittent or continuous as the catheter is withdrawn.[100] Some authors suggest twirling the catheter between thumb and forefinger to circumferentially contact secretions.[96] Suction should be applied for about 10 to 15 seconds or less.[4,5] The ECG, pulse oximetry, or clinical signs may indicate hypoxemia or cardiovascular stress at shorter time intervals. Animal research indicates that the lowest PaO_2 appears to occur in the first 5 seconds.[101] Postoxygenation and hyperinflation with 100% oxygen should follow. Nasotracheal, endotracheal, or tracheostomy suctioning should only be performed when clinically indicated. However, experience with individual patients may suggest a minimum frequency to maintain patency of the anatomical or artificial airway. Box 19-25 lists factors that when found suggest successful outcomes of suctioning.

Suctioning is a necessary procedure, especially for patients with artificial airways. Significant hazards do exist, though there are no absolute contraindications. Complications are relative to an individual patient's potential risk from the event, balanced by the grave consequence of failing to maintain a patent airway.

BOX 19-25

SUCTIONING: ASSESSMENT OF OUTCOME

- Successful retrieval of secretions
- Improved breath sounds
- Improved blood gas data or pulse oximetry
- Decreased spontaneous breathing frequency or patient dyspnea
- Reduced peak airway pressure or increased tidal volume (mechanically ventilated)

REFERENCES

1. Johnson CB: 1992 Respiratory care job analysis. NBRC Horizons 19:1, 1993
2. American Heart Association-Emergency Cardiac Care Committee and Subcommittee: Guidelines for cardiopulmonary resuscitation. JAMA 268:2171, 1992
3. American Association for Respiratory Care: Clinical practice guidelines: Resuscitation in acute care hospitals. Respir Care 38:1179, 1993
4. American Association for Respiratory Care: Clinical practice guidelines: Endotracheal suctioning of mechanically ventilated adults and children with artificial airways. Respir Care 38:500, 1993
5. American Association for Respiratory Care: Clinical practice guidelines: Nasotracheal suctioning. Respir Care 37:898, 1992
6. American Association for Respiratory Care: Clinical practice guidelines: Management of airway emergencies. Respir Care 40: 749, 1995
7. American Society of Anesthesiologists: Practice guidelines for management of the difficult airway. Anesthesiology 78:597, 1993
8. Eckenhoff JE: Some anatomic considerations of the infant larynx influencing endotracheal anesthesia. Anesthesiology 12:401, 1951
9. Dorsch JA, Dorsch SE: Understanding Anesthesia Equipment (3rd ed). Baltimore, Williams & Wilkins, 1994
10. Emergency Care Research Institute: Exhaled-air pulmonary resuscitators. Health Devices 18:333, 1989
11. American Society for Testing and Materials: Standard specifications for minimum performance and safely requirements for resuscitators intended for use with humans. (Designation: F920-85.) Philadelphia, ASTM, 1985
12. International Organization for Standardization: International Standard ISO 8382:1988 (E): Resuscitators Intended for Use with Humans. New York, American National Standards Institute, 1988
13. Hess DR: Manual and gas-powered resuscitators. In RD Branson, DR Hess, RL Chatburn (eds): Respiratory Care Equipment. Philadelphia, JB Lippincott, 1995
14. Centers for Disease Control: Recommendations for prevention of HIV transmission in health-care settings. MMWR Morb Mortal Wkly Rep 36:35, 1987
15. Centers for Disease Control: Guidelines for prevention of transmission of human immunodeficiency virus and hepatitis B virus to health care and public safety workers. MMWR Morb Mortal Wkly Rep 8(suppl 6):1, 1989
16. Hess D, Ness C, Oppel A, Rhoads K: Evaluation of mouth-to-mask ventilation devices. Respir Care 34:191, 1989
17. Simmons M, Deao D, Moon L, et al: Bench evaluation: Three face-shield CPR barrier devices. Respir Care 40:6518, 1995
18. Rapport DM, Sorkin B, Garay SM, et al: Reversal of the "Pickwickian syndrome" by long-term use of nocturnal nasal-airway pressure. N Engl J Med 307:931, 1982
19. Kerby GR, Mayer LS, Pingleton SK: Nocturnal positive pressure ventilation via nasal mask. Am Rev Respir Dis 135:738, 1987
20. Leger P, Jennequin JJ, Gerard M, Robert D: Home positive pressure ventilation via nasal mask for patients with neuromuscular weakness or restrictive lung or chest-wall disease. Respir Care 34:73, 1989
21. Stauffer JL, Petty TL: Cleft tongue and ulceration of hard palate: Complications of oral intubations. Chest 74:317, 1981
22. Collins VJ: Principles of Anesthesiology. Philadelphia, Lea & Febiger, 1969
23. Monheim LM: General Anesthesia in Dental Practice (3rd ed). St Louis, CV Mosby, 1968
24. Niemann JT, Rosborough JP, Myers R, Scarberry EN: The pharyngeo-tracheal lumen airway: Preliminary investigation of a new adjunct. Ann Emerg Med 13:591, 1984
25. Frass M, Frenzer R, Rauscha F, et al: Evaluation of esophageal tracheal combitube in cardiopulmonary resuscitation. Crit Care Med 15:609, 1986

26. Bartlett RL, Martin SD, Perina D, Raymond JI: The pharyngeotracheal lumen airway: An assessment of airway control in the setting of upper airway hemorrhage. Ann Emerg Med 16:343, 1987
27. Pennant JH, White PF: The laryngeal mask airway. Anesthesiology 79:144, 1993
28. Alexander R, Hodgson P, Lomax D, Bullen C: A comparison of the laryngeal mask airway and Guedel airway, bag and facemask for manual ventilation following formal training. Anaesthesia 48:231, 1993
29. American National Standards Institute: Standards for cuffed oral and tracheal tubes for prolonged use. New York, ANSI, 1983
30. American Society for Testing and Materials: Standards and specifications for cuffed and uncuffed tracheal tubes (ASTM F1242-89). Philadelphia, ASTM, 1989
31. Dahlgren BE, Nilsson HG, Viklund B: Tracheal tubes in cold stress. Anaesthesia 43:683, 1988
32. Sottile FD, Marrie TJ, Prouch DS, et al: Nosocomial pulmonary infection: Possible etiologic significance of bacterial adhesion to endotracheal tubes. Crit Care Med 14:265, 1986
33. Mattila MK, Heikel PE, Suutarinen T, et al: Estimation of a suitable nasotracheal tube length for infants and children. Acta Anaesthesiol Scand 15:239, 1971
34. Yates AP, Harries AJ, Hatch DJ: Estimation of nasotracheal tube length in infants and children. Br J Anaesth 59:524, 1987
35. Habib MP: Physiological implication of artificial airways. Chest 96:180, 1989
36. Bolder PM, Healy TE, Bolder AR, et al: The extra work of breathing through adult endotracheal tubes. Anesth Analg 65:853, 1986
37. Demers PR, Sullivan MJ, Paliotta J: Airflow resistance of endotracheal tubes. JAMA 237:1362, 1977
38. Wall MA: Infant endotracheal tube resistance: Effects of changing length, diameter, and gas density. Crit Care Med 8:38, 1980
39. Wright PE, Marini JJ, Bernard GR: In vitro versus in vivo comparison of endotracheal tube airflow resistance. Am Rev Respir Dis 140:10, 1989
40. Mehta S: Intubation guide marks for the correct tube placement. A clinical study. Anaesthesia 46:306, 1991
41. Owen RL, Cheney FW: Endobronchial intubation: A preventable complication. Anesthesiology 67:255, 1987
42. Lindholm CE, Grenvik A: Tracheal tube and cuff problems. Int Anestheol Clin 20:103, 1981
43. Bernhard WN, Cottrell JE, Sivakumaran C, et al: Adjustment of intracuff pressure to prevent aspiration. Anesthesiology 50:363, 1979
44. Bernhard WN, Yost L, Joynes D, et al: Intracuff pressure in endotracheal and tracheostomy cuffs. Chest 87:720, 1985
45. Badenhorst CH: Changes in tracheal cuff pressure during respiratory support. Crit Care Med 15:300, 1987
46. Conrardy PA, Goodman LR, Lainge F, Singer MM: Alteration of endotracheal tube position: Flexion and extension of the neck. Crit Care Med 4:8, 1976
47. Stanley TH: Nitrous oxide and pressure and volume of high and low pressure endotracheal tube cuffs in intubated patients. Anesthesiology 42:637, 1975
48. Petring OV, Adelhoj B, Jensen BN, et al: Prevention of silent aspiration due to leaks around cuffs of endotracheal tubes. Anesth Analg 65:777, 1986
49. Craven DE, Steger KA: Pathogenesis and prevention of nosocomial pneumonia in the mechanically ventilated patient. Respir Care 34:85, 1989
50. Craven DE, Kunches LM, Kilinsky V, et al: Risk factor for pneumonia and fatality in patients receiving continuous mechanical ventilation. Am Rev Respir Dis 133:792, 1986
51. Power KJ: Foam cuffed tracheal tubes: Clinical and laboratory assessment. Br J Anaesth 65:433, 1990
52. Eckerbom B, Lindholm CE, Alexopoulos C: Airway lesions caused by prolonged intubation with standard and with anatomically shaped tracheal tubes: A post-mortem study. Acta Anaesthesiol Scand 30:366, 1986
53. Burton NA, Watson DC, Brodsky JB, Mark JD: Advantages of a new polyvinyl chloride double-lumen tube in thoracic surgery. Ann Thorac Surg 36:78, 1983
54. Inoue H, Suzuki I, Iwasaki M, et al: Selective exclusion of the injured lung. J Trauma 34:496, 1993
55. Hamilton LH, Londino JM, Linehan JH, Neu J: Pediatric endotracheal tube designed for high-frequency ventilation. Crit Care Med 12:988, 1984
56. Rayburn RL: Light wand intubation. Anaesthesia 34:667, 1979
57. Bedger RC, Chang J: A jet-style endotracheal catheter for difficult airway management. Anesthesiology 66:221, 1987
58. Snyder GM: Individualized placement of tracheostomy tube fenestration and in situ examination with fiberoptic laryngoscope. Respir Care 28:1294, 1983
59. Cane RD, Woodward C, Shapiro BA: Customizing fenestrated tracheostomy tubes: A bedside technique. Crit Care Med 10:880, 1982
60. Honsinger MJ, Yorkston KM, Dowden PA: Communication options for intubated patients. Respir Manag 17:45, 1987
61. Montgomery WW: Current modifications of the salivary bypass tube and tracheal T-tube. Ann Otol Rhinol Laryngol 95:121, 1986
62. Petring OV, Adelhoj B, Jensen BN, et al: Prevention of silent aspiration due to leaks around cuffs of endotracheal tubes. Anesth Analg 65:777, 1986
63. Long J, West G: Evaluation of the Olympic Trach button as a precursor to tracheostomy removal. Respir Care 25:1242, 1980
64. Dustan HP: (Ad Hoc Committee on Medical Ethics). Ann Intern Med 101:129, 1984
65. Lockhart PB, Feldbau EV, Gabel RA, et al: Dental complications during and after tracheal intubation. JAMA 112:480, 1986
66. Mallampati SR, Gatt SP, Gugino LD, et al: A clinical sign to predict difficult tracheal intubation. Can J Anaesth 32:429, 1985
67. Samsoon GLT, Young JRB: Difficult tracheal intubation: A retrospective study. Anaesthesia 52:487, 1987
68. Patil VU, Stehling LC, Zauder HL: Predicting the difficulty of intubation utilizing an intubation gauge. Anesthesiol Rev 10:32, 1983
69. Sellick BA: Cricoid pressure to control regurgitation of stomach contents during induction of anesthesia. Lancet 2:404, 1962
70. MacLeod BA, Heller MB, Gerard J, et al: Verification of endotracheal tube placement with colorimetric end-tidal CO_2 detection. Ann Emerg Med 20:267, 1991
71. Yelderman M, New W: Evaluation of pulse oximetry. Anesthesiology 59:349, 1983
72. Sellers WFS, Dye A, Harvey J: Systemic absorption of lidocaine ointment from tracheal tubes. Anaesthesia 40:483, 1985
73. Raj PP, Winnie AP: Immediate reactions to local anesthetics. In FK Orlein, LH Cooperman (eds): Complications in Anesthesiology. Philadelphia, JB Lippincott, 1983
74. Covino BG, Vassallo HG: General pharmacological and toxicological aspects of local anesthetic agents. In BG Covino, HG Vassallo (eds): Local Anesthetics, Mechanisms of Action and Clinical Use. New York, Grune & Stratton, 1976
75. Scott DB, Cousins MJ: Clinical pharmacology of local anesthetic agents. In MJ Cousins, PO Bridenbaugh (eds): Neural Blockade. Philadelphia, JB Lippincott, 1980
76. Finucane BT, Santora AH: Difficult intubation. In BT Finucane, AH Santora (eds): Principles of Airway Management. Philadelphia, FA Davis, 1988
77. Yealy DM, Paris DM: Recent advances in airway management. Emerg Med Clin North Am 7:83, 1989
78. Bjoraker DG, Kumar NB, Brown AC: Evaluations of an emergency cricothyrotomy instrument. Crit Care Med 15:157, 1987
79. Stauffer JL, Silvestri RC: Complications of endotracheal intubation, tracheostomy, and artificial airways. Respir Care 27:417, 1982
80. Ciaglia P, Firshing R, Synico C: Elective percutaneous dilatational tracheostomy. A new simple bedside procedure: Preliminary report. Chest 87:715, 1985
81. Plummer AL, Gracey DR: Consensus conference on artificial airways in patients receiving mechanical ventilation. Chest 96:178, 1989
82. Larson RP, Ingalls-Severn KJ, Wright JR, et al: Diagnosis of *Pneumocystis carinii* suctioning method over sputum induction. Respir Care 34:249, 1989
83. Stone KS: Endotracheal suctioning in the critically ill. Crit Care Nurse Curr 7:5, 1989

84. Rosen IM, Hillard EK: The effects of negative pressure during tracheal suction. Anesth Analg 41:50, 1962
85. Plum F, Dunning MF: Techniques for minimizing trauma to the tracheobronchial tree after tracheostomy. N Engl J Med 254:193, 1956
86. Sackner MA, Landa JF, Greeneltch N, Robinson MJ: Pathogenesis and prevention of tracheobronchial damage with suction procedures. Chest 64:284, 1973
87. Craven DE, Steger KA: Pathogenesis and prevention of nosocomial pneumonia in the mechanically ventilated patient. Respir Care 34:85, 1989
88. Garner JG: Employee exposure and illnesses. In BF Farber (ed): Infection Control in Intensive Care. New York, Churchill Livingstone, 1987
89. Panacek EA, Albertson TE, Rutherford WF, Fisher CJ, Foulke GE: Selective left endobrachial suctioning in the intubated patient. Chest 95:885, 1989
90. Link Wj, Spaeth EE, Wahle WM, et al: The influence of suction catheter tip design on tracheobronchial trauma and fluid aspiration efficiency. Anaesth Analg 55:290, 1976
91. Bodai Bi, Briggs SW, Goldstein M, et al: Evaluation of the ability of the NeO_2 safe valve to minimize desaturation in neonates during suctioning. Respir Care 34:355, 1989
92. Carlon GC, Fox SJ, Ackerman NJ: Evaluation of a closed-tracheal suction system. Crit Care Med 15:522, 1987
93. Ritz R, Scott LR, Coyl MB, Pierson DJ: Contamination of a multiple-use suction catheter in a closed-circuit system compared to contamination of a disposable, single-use suction catheter. Respir Care 31:1086, 1986
94. Smith RM, Benson MS, Schoene RB: The efficacy of oxygen insufflation in preventing arterial oxygen desaturation during endotracheal suctioning of mechanically ventilated patients Respir Care 32:865, 1987
95. Brown SE, Stansbury DW, Merrill EJ, et al: Prevention of suctioning-related arterial oxygen desaturation: Comparison of off-ventilator and on ventilator suctioning. Chest 83:621, 1983
96. Riegel B, Forshee T: A review and critique of the literature on preoxygenation for endotracheal suctioning. Heart Lung 14:507, 1985
97. Wanner A, Zighelboim A, Sackner MA: Nasopharyngeal airway: A facilitated access to the trachea. Ann Intern Med 25:593, 1971
98. Preusser BA, Stone KS, Gonyon DS, et al: Effects of two methods of preoxygenation on arterial pressure, cardiac output, peak airway pressure and postsuctioning hypoxia. Heart Lung 17:290, 1988
99. Skelley B, Deeren S, Powaser M: The effectiveness of two preoxygenation methods to prevent endotracheal suction induced hypoxemia. Heart Lung 9:316, 1980
100. Fluck RR: Suctioning: Intermittent or continuous? (Editorial). Respir Care 30:837, 1985
101. Rindfleisch SH, Tyler ML: Duration of suctioning: An important variable. Respir Care 28:457, 1983

20 Mechanical Ventilation of the Adult Patient: Initiation, Management, and Weaning

Dean R. Hess

CLINICAL SKILLS

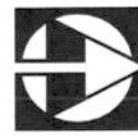

Upon completion of this chapter, the reader will know how to:

- Determine the need for mechanical ventilation and weaning based on the results of electrolytes, hemoglobin, and hematocrit, and chemistries; fluid balance; cardiovascular monitoring (eg, hemodynamic data and ECG); respiratory monitoring and derived values; physical examination (including cardiopulmonary signs of hypoxemia, hypercarbia, and increased work of breathing); and inspection of chest radiographs.
- Collect and perform all procedures to evaluate pertinent information in development of a respiratory care plan involving mechanical ventilation.
- Select, assemble, and check equipment for proper function, operation, and cleanliness, including ventilators, gas delivery systems and breathing circuits, respirometers, and monitoring systems.
- Perform quality control procedures for ventilator volume-flow-pressure settings and perform ventilator circuit checks and changes.
- Recommend initial ventilator settings based on patient data and modify ventilator settings or modes based on patient's response.
- Evaluate patient's response to initial ventilator settings or weaning parameters.
- Maintain records and communication using ventilator flow sheets.
- Recommend use (or discontinuance) of pharmacologic agents to facilitate mechanical ventilation.

KEY WORDS

Assist-control ventilation
Auto-PEEP
Compression volume
Continuous positive airway pressure
Controlled ventilation
Dys-synchrony
Extracorporeal life support
Flow trigger
High-frequency ventilation
Intermittent mandatory ventilation
Liquid ventilation
Mandatory minute ventilation
Mean airway pressure
Nitric oxide
Noninvasive positive pressure ventilation
Oxygen toxicity
Permissive hypercapnia
Positive end-expiratory pressure
Pressure augmentation
Pressure-regulated volume control
Pressure support ventilation
Pressure trigger
Pressure ventilation
Prone position
Respiratory muscle fatigue
Synchronized intermittent mandatory ventilation
T piece
Tracheal gas insufflation
Ventilator-associated acute lung injury
Ventilator-associated pneumonia
Volume-assured pressure support
Volume support
Volume ventilation
Volutrauma
Weaning

Care of the mechanically ventilated patient requires specialized knowledge and various skills on the part of respiratory care practitioners. The purpose of this chapter is to review the initiation, management, and weaning of patients requiring mechanical ventilation. The reader is referred to Chapter 1 to reflect on the history establishing the use of mechanical ventilators in the practice of contemporary critical care. Recent advancements in both technology and understanding of diseases and their treatment have extended the demands on respiratory care practitioners. Competent care requires abilities in medical science, patient assessment skills, technology, communications skills, troubleshooting, and human caring. The Clinical Skills section at the beginning of this chapter provides a partial list of necessary skills.

INDICATIONS AND COMPLICATIONS OF MECHANICAL VENTILATION

Indications

There are numerous indications for mechanical ventilation (Table 20-1).[1,2] These include gas exchange as well as mechanical indicators of acute respiratory failure. Although these criteria are useful in establishing the need for mechanical ventilation, clinical judgment may be as important as strict adherence to absolute guidelines. If acute respiratory failure appears imminent, it may be prudent to initiate mechanical ventilation (noninvasive or invasive), thereby avoiding overt respiratory failure and respiratory arrest.

Hyperventilation therapy and major surgery are indications for mechanical ventilation that may not involve primary respiratory failure. Although hyperventilation therapy is specifically used in the treatment of acute head injury, these patients often have associated respiratory failure. Short-term mechanical ventilation is also commonly used after major surgery such as open-heart surgery, major abdominal surgery, or thoracic surgery.

Complications

Although mechanical ventilation can be lifesaving, it is not a benign treatment, and it can have major effects on the homeostasis of the patient. Complications of mechanical ventilation are listed in Table 20-2.[3–5]

Mechanical ventilation for acute respiratory failure often includes placement of an artificial airway such as an endotracheal tube or tracheostomy. Thus, mechanically ventilated patients are at risk for all of the complications associated with the use of artificial airways (see Chap. 19). These include laryngeal trauma, tracheal mucosal trauma, contamination of the lower respiratory tract, and loss of the normal humidifying function of the upper respiratory tract. Adequate inspired gas humidification is necessary with intubated mechanically ventilated patients, and a humidification system is part of every ventilator system. Humidifiers (see Chap. 15) can actively heat and humidify the inspired gases, or the heat and humidity in the patient's exhaled gas can be trapped and returned to the patient during the next inhalation

TABLE 20-1. **Indications for Mechanical Ventilation**

Mechanical	
Respiratory rate	>35 breaths/min
Minute ventilation	>10 L/min
Maximal inspiratory subatmospheric pressure	<-20 cmH_2O
Vital capacity	<15 mL/kg
Respiratory muscle paradox	
Gas Exchange	
$P(A - a)O_2$	>300 mmHg on 100% oxygen
PaO_2	<60 mmHg on $FIO_2 > 0.60$
PaO_2/FIO_2	<200
VD/VT	>0.60
$PaCO_2$	>50 mmHg (acutely)
Hyperventilation Therapy	
Major Surgery	

TABLE 20-2. **Complications of Mechanical Ventilation**

Airway	Laryngeal edema, tracheal mucosal trauma, contamination of lower respiratory tract, loss of humidifying function of the upper airway
Mechanical	Accidental disconnection, leaks in ventilator circuit, loss of electrical power, loss of gas pressure
Pulmonary	Acute lung injury, barotrauma, oxygen toxicity, atelectasis, nosocomial pneumonia
Cardiovascular	Decreased venous return, decreased cardiac output, hypotension
Gastrointestinal and nutritional	Gastrointestinal bleeding, malnutrition
Renal	Decreased urine output, changes in ADH and ANP
Neurologic	Increased intracranial pressure
Acid-base	Respiratory alkalosis

(artificial nose)[6,7] (see AARC Clinical Practice Guidelines: Humidification During Mechanical Ventilation).

Numerous mechanical complications are associated with the use of continuous ventilation. The most serious of these is accidental disconnection, which can result in the death of an apneic patient. It is critically important that the ventilator disconnect alarm be correctly set and functional on all mechanically ventilated patients. Another common mechanical complication is leaks within the ventilator circuit. These must be detected and corrected promptly to prevent hypoventilation. Internal or external electrical and pneumatic failures can also occur, which can result in failure to ventilate the patient. A self-inflating manual ventilator should be at the bedside of all patients receiving continuous ventilation to be used in the event of a mechanical or electrical failure.

Ironically, mechanical ventilation can harm the lungs. Pulmonary barotrauma (pneumothorax, pneumomediastinum, subcutaneous emphysema) can result from excessive ventilation pressures and the associated overdistension.[8,9] Pulmonary barotrauma is also a problem when the expiratory time is too short and gas is trapped in the lungs at end-exhalation (auto-PEEP). Oxygen toxicity can occur if a high FIO_2 is used. Acute lung injury caused by overdistension (volutrauma) is now recognized as a complication of mechanical ventilation. Parenchymal overdistension can produce ARDS-like (high permeability pulmonary edema)[10,11] changes in the lungs. To avoid this injury, peak alveolar pressure (plateau pressure) ideally should be maintained < 35 cmH_2O during mechanical ventilation.[12]

Because mechanical ventilation increases intrathoracic pressure, it can decrease venous return, which may result in decreased cardiac output and decreased arterial blood pressure. Fluid and drug therapy (vasopressors and inotropes) may be necessary to maintain cardiac output, blood pressure, and urine output.

Ventilator-associated pneumonia is a common complication of mechanical ventilation, and it may occur at a

AARC Clinical Practice Guideline

HUMIDIFICATION DURING MECHANICAL VENTILATION

Indications: Humidification of inspired gas during mechanical ventilation is mandatory when an endotracheal or tracheostomy tube is present.

Contraindications: There are no contraindications to providing physiologic conditioning of inspired gas during mechanical ventilation. An HME is contraindicated under some circumstances: for patients with thick, copious, or bloody secretions; for patients with an expired tidal volume less than 70% of the delivered tidal volume (eg, those with large bronchopleurocutaneous fistulas or incompetent or absent endotracheal tube cuffs; for patients with body temperatures less than 32°C. Use of an HME may be contraindicated for patients with high spontaneous minute volumes (>10 L/min); an HME must be removed from the patient circuit during aerosol treatments when the nebulizer is placed in the patient circuit.

Assessment of Need: Humidification is needed by all patients requiring mechanical ventilation by means of an artificial airway. Conditioning of inspired gases should be instituted using either an HME or a heated humidifier: HMEs are better suited for short-term use (≤96 hours) and during transport; heated humidifiers should be used for patients requiring long-term mechanical ventilation (>96 hours) or for patients who exhibit contraindications for HME use.

Assessment of Outcome: Humidification is assumed to be appropriate if, on regular careful inspection, the patient exhibits none of the hazards or complications listed above.

Monitoring: The humidification device should be inspected visually during the patient-ventilator system check, and condensate should be removed from the patient circuit as necessary. HMEs should be inspected and replaced if secretions have contaminated the insert or filter. The following variables should be recorded during equipment inspection: (1) *humidifier setting* (temperature setting or numeric dial setting or both). During routine use on an intubated patient, a heated humidifier should be set to deliver an inspired gas temperature of 33 ± 2°C and should provide a minimum of 30 mg/L of water vapor; (2) *inspired gas temperature.* Temperature should be monitored as near the patient's airway opening as possible, if a heated humidifier is used: specific temperatures may vary with patient condition, but the inspiratory gas should not exceed 37°C at the airway threshold; when a heated-wire patient circuit is used (to prevent condensation) on an infant, the temperature probe should be located outside of the incubator or away from the direct heat of the radiant warmer; (3) *alarm settings* (if applicable). High temperature alarm should be set no higher than 37°C, and the low temperature alarm should be set no lower than 30°C; (4) *water level and function of automatic feed system* (if applicable); (5) *quantity and consistency of secretions.* Characteristics should be noted and recorded. When using an HME, if secretions become copious or appear increasingly tenacious, a heated humidifier should replace the HME.

rate as high as 15 cases per 1000 ventilator days.[13] It was commonly believed in the past that ventilator-associated pneumonia was associated with the ventilator tubing, and the circuit and humidification systems of ventilators were changed at frequent intervals (every 24 to 48 hours). It is now appreciated that the ventilator circuit is relatively unimportant in the development of pneumonia in mechanically ventilated patients, provided that reasonable infection control practices are followed. Pneumonia in a mechanically ventilated patient is usually caused by aspiration of oropharyngeal secretions (in spite of a cuffed endotracheal tube) and not the result of what is breathed through the endotracheal tube. Because ventilator-associated pneumonia is infrequently caused by the ventilator, breathing circuits can be changed infrequently (weekly or greater intervals).[14–16]

Patients who are mechanically ventilated are at risk for gastrointestinal bleeding. Many ventilated patients are treated with antacids or histamine$_2$ (H_2) blockers (eg, cimetidine) to avoid this complication. Although this treatment is controversial, there is evidence that raising the gastric pH with these medications leads to an increased risk of nosocomial pneumonia.[17] The use of oral sucralfate may reduce the risk of gastric mucosal bleeding without altering gastric pH, and thus may decrease the risk of ventilator-associated pneumonia.[18] If aspiration of stomach contents occurs during sucralfate therapy, the risk of lung injury may be greater secondary to a lower pH of the aspirate.[19]

It is also important to appreciate the nutritional needs of mechanically ventilated patients.[20] Undernourished patients are at risk for respiratory muscle weakness and pneumonia. On the other hand, excessive caloric intake can result in an increase in CO_2 production, which can markedly increase the patient's ventilatory requirements.

Mechanical ventilation can affect the patient's renal function and fluid balance. Elevations in plasma antidiuretic hormone (ADH) and reductions in atrial natriuretic peptide (ANP) can occur as a result of mechanical ventilation. The result of these alterations in ADH and ANP levels is a decrease in urine output and fluid retention.[21] Urine output may also decrease during mechanical ventilation as a result of decreased renal perfusion, caused by a decrease in cardiac output and blood pressure related to mechanical ventilation.

The increase in intrathoracic pressure from mechanical ventilation can result in an increase in intracranial pressure.[22] This may be particularly problematic when mechanical ventilation is used with positive end-expiratory pressure (PEEP) in closed-head-injured patients. In patients with head injury, it is prudent to keep the mean airway pressure ($\bar{P}aw$) as low as possible during mechanical ventilation. When a higher $\bar{P}aw$ is required in these patients, invasive monitoring of intracranial pressure and cerebral perfusion pressure are useful.

An acid–base disturbance frequently observed during mechanical ventilation is respiratory alkalosis. This may be desirable in the treatment of head-injured patients, but otherwise should be avoided because of its effects on the oxyhemoglobin dissociation curve, electrolyte balance, and cardiac function. Further, the increased ventilation associated with respiratory alkalosis increases the risk of acute lung injury and auto-PEEP.

VENTILATOR-ASSOCIATED ACUTE LUNG INJURY

It has become increasingly recognized in recent years that the process of mechanical ventilation can injure the lung. It has also been recognized that many forms of acute respiratory failure (eg, ARDS) are heterogeneous. That is, there are areas of the lung that are pathologic (eg, consolidated, collapsed) and other lung units that are relatively disease free (Figure 20-1).[23] Mechanical ventilation can result in overdistension and delivery of toxic O_2 concentrations to the relatively normal lung units of patients with ARDS.

Overdistension

Animal studies clearly demonstrate that alveolar overdistension results in acute lung injury (Figure 20-2).[10,11] Regional overdistension is a function of the pressure applied to the lung. Due to differences in regional compliance throughout the lungs, a high airway pressure preferentially delivers more of the tidal volume (VT) to high compliance lung units. The resultant overdistension results in acute lung injury similar to that which occurs with ARDS. The potential for overdistension is determined by airway pressure and not VT. Without use of extraordinary techniques (eg, computerized tomography), it is impossible to know how the VT will be distributed throughout the lungs.[23] However, a high peak alveolar pressure (Pplat) is transmitted to compliant alveoli, resulting in their overdistension.

Specifically, the risk of regional overdistension during mechanical ventilation is related to the peak alveolar pressure. Plateau pressure (the pressure during an end-inspiratory hold, see Chap. 12) is a good bedside indicator of peak alveolar pressure. To avoid acute lung injury during mechanical ventilation, plateau pressure should be maintained at less than 35 cmH_2O if chest wall compliance is normal.[12] This may result in a ventilatory strategy in which $PaCO_2$ is allowed to increase (permissive hypercapnia). It is important to appreciate that alveolar distension is determined by transpulmonary pressure and not Pplat per se. Thus, if chest wall compliance is reduced (eg, abdominal distension), a higher Pplat may be safe.

Oxygen Toxicity

The toxic effects of O_2 can also result in ARDS-like changes in the lungs.[24] Like overdistension, O_2 toxicity affects primarily normal lung units—these are the areas of the lung that receive most of the ventilation and are thus more likely to be injured. To avoid O_2 toxicity, the FIO_2 should be set no higher than that necessary to maintain adequate arterial oxygenation (> 90% arterial O_2 saturation). Ideally, the FIO_2 should be kept < 0.60.

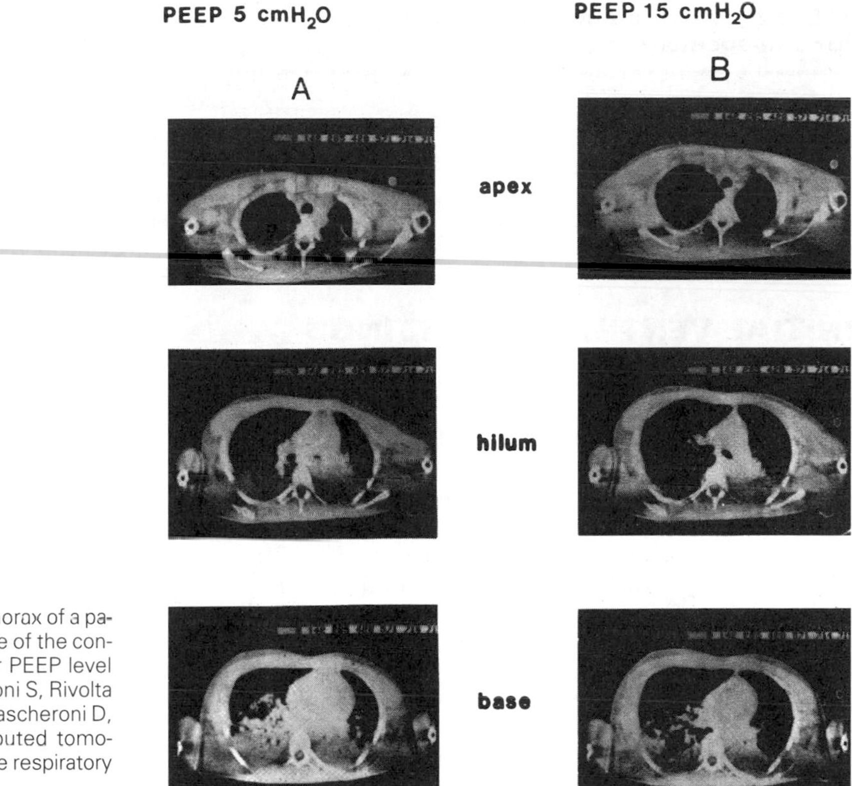

FIGURE 20-1. Computed tomography of the thorax of a patient with ARDS. Note the heterogeneous nature of the consolidation, with less consolidation at the higher PEEP level (From Gattinoni L, Pesenti A, Bombino M, Baglioni S, Rivolta M, Rossi F, Rossi G, Fumagalli R, Marcolin R, Mascheroni D, Torresin A: Relationships between lung computed tomographic density, gas exchange, and PEEP in acute respiratory failure. Anesthesiology 69:824, 1988).

Pressure or Oxygen?

Recommended priorities for management of oxygenation are listed in Table 20-3. Ideally, the plateau pressure should be kept < 35 cmH_2O, and the FIO_2 should be kept < 0.60. Many patients tolerate the elevated $PaCO_2$ that may occur with this strategy. However, this level of ventilation may not result in adequate oxygenation in some patients. The question is then whether the airway pressure or FIO_2 should be increased. Based on the current evidence, a higher FIO_2 may be preferable to a higher airway pressure, with the priority of keeping plateau pressure < 35 cmH_2O taking precedence over an FIO_2 < 0.60.

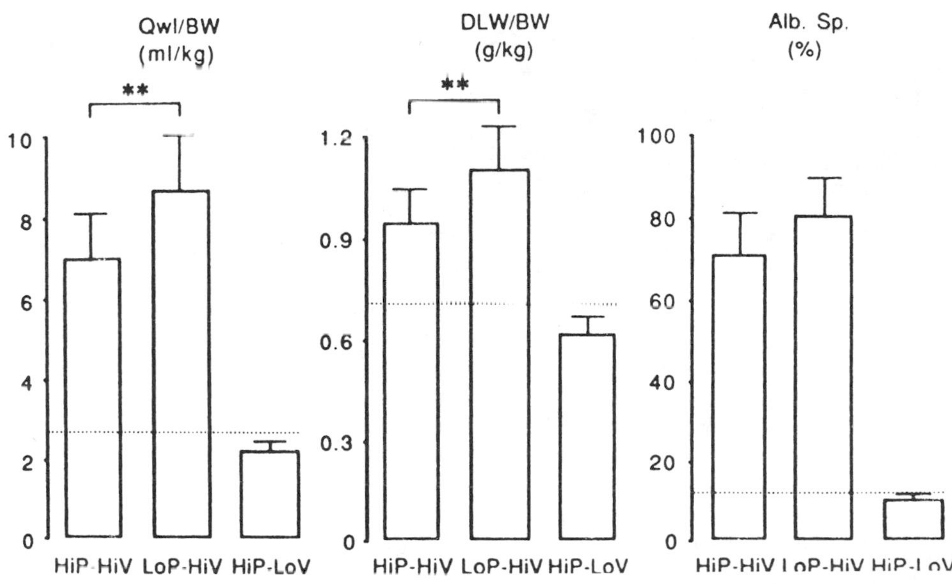

FIGURE 20-2. Comparison of the effects of high pressure (45 cm H_2O) positive inspiratory pressure high tidal volume (HiP–HiV) with those of negative inspiratory airway pressure-high tidal volume ventilation (iron lung, LoP–HiV) and high pressure positive pressure ventilation-low tidal volume ventilation (chest/abdomen strapping, HiP–LoV). Permeability pulmonary edema occurred in both groups receiving high volume ventilation. Qwl/BW = extravascular lung water, DLW/BW = bloodless dry lung weight, Alb space = albumin distribution in the lungs (From Dreyfuss D, Soler P, Basset G, Saumon G: High inflation pressure pulmonary edema: respective effects of high airway pressure, high tidal volume, and positive end-expiratory pressure. Am Rev Respir Dis 137:1159, 1988).

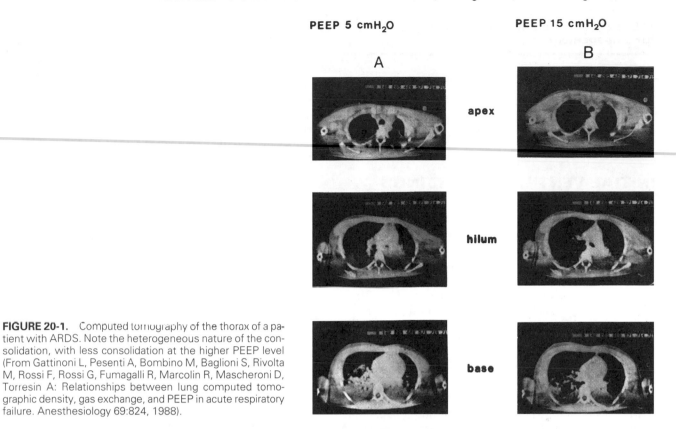

TABLE 20-3. **Recommended Priorities for Management of Oxygenation**

First priority: plateau pressure <35 cmH_2O
Second priority: PEEP 8 to 12 cmH_2O for ARDS; 3 to 5 cmH_2O for non-ARDS
Third priority: FIO_2 <0.60
Fourth priority: inspiratory time <1.5 sec

INITIAL VENTILATOR SETTINGS

Invasive versus Noninvasive Ventilation

Most patients are mechanically ventilated through an endotracheal tube or tracheostomy tube. It is now recognized that many patients can be noninvasively ventilated in both the acute care and long-term settings.[25] Noninvasive positive pressure ventilation (NIPPV) is achieved using either a nasal mask or a full face mask, and some ventilators have been designed specifically for mask ventilation.[26] NIPPV can be readily achieved in the acute care setting using a critical care ventilator and an anesthesia face mask (Figure 20-3).[27,28] With acute hypercapnic respiratory failure related to COPD, NIPPV may avoid intubation in > 50% of patients.[27–29]

Mask ventilation should not be attempted in patients who require an artificial airway. Thus, mask ventilation is a poor choice in patients with large volumes of secretions, in patients with upper airway obstruction (although some forms of upper airway obstruction are relieved by positive pressure, eg, obstructive sleep apnea), and in patients at risk for aspiration. Noninvasive ventilation is ideally suited to patients having acute exacerbations of chronic respiratory failure (obstructive or restrictive) in whom short-term ventilation is required. Noninvasive ventilation is also an option in patients with end-stage disease who do not desire intubation. Long-term noninvasive ventilation has also been used successfully.[30]

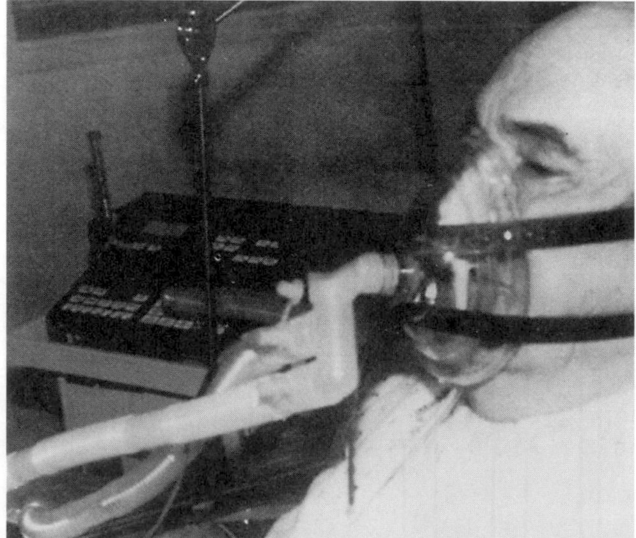

FIGURE 20-3. Noninvasive mask ventilation using a critical care ventilator (From Meduri GU, Abou-Shala N, Fox RC, Jones CB, Leeper KV, Wunderink RG: Noninvasive face mask mechanical ventilation in patients with acute hypercapnic respiratory failure. Chest 100:445, 1991).

Several key issues related to noninvasive ventilation must be appreciated when this form of ventilation is attempted. First, it is not always successful, and some patients will need to be intubated if noninvasive ventilation fails. Second, noninvasive ventilation is time consuming, and greater clinician time is needed to help the patient acclimate to noninvasive ventilation. Third, mask fit is very important to the success of the method—a poorly fitting mask usually results in failure of noninvasive ventilation. If nasal mask ventilation is unsuccessful, full face mask ventilation can be attempted. Finally, if a critical care ventilator is used for mask ventilation, a time-cycled mode should be selected (eg, pressure control). A flow-cycled mode (eg, pressure support) may be problematic because leaks that commonly occur during mask ventilation result in end-inspiration cycling problems.

Mode of Ventilation

Various options for breath delivery are referred to as modes of ventilation.[31] Common modes include control ventilation, assist-control ventilation (A-C),[32] intermittent mandatory ventilation (IMV),[33] synchronized intermittent mandatory ventilation (SIMV),[34] and pressure support ventilation (PSV).[35–37] Other newer modes include mandatory minute ventilation (MMV),[38] pressure-regulated volume control, volume support, and pressure augmentation (see Chap. 19). Breath delivery for some modes is illustrated in Figure 20-4 and compared in Table 20-4. The choice of the ventilation mode is often based on institutional policy or clinician bias, and there is no clear superiority of any single mode. When mechanical ventilation is initiated, it is often best to use either A-C or high-rate SIMV to produce nearly complete respiratory muscle rest (full ventilatory support). As the patient's condition improves, part of the ventilatory work load can be transferred to the patient using modes such as SIMV, PSV, or SIMV with PSV.

With controlled ventilation, the rate and V_T are set and cannot be altered by the patient. This mode is not desirable because the patient must be hyperventilated, sedated, or paralyzed to suppress the respiratory drive. A clinician-preset V_T at a clinician-preset minimum rate is delivered with A-C. With A-C, the patient can trigger additional breaths above the minimal rate, but the V_T (or pressure for pressure-limited ventilation) is constant at the preset level.

With IMV, the clinician sets a V_T (or pressure limit) and rate, but the patient determines the V_T and rate of the spontaneous breaths between the ventilator breaths. During IMV, the ventilator breaths may be delivered at regular intervals, or ventilator breaths may be synchronized with the patient's spontaneous efforts (SIMV). In practice, if the rate set on the ventilator is high enough to satisfy the patient's total ventilatory need, IMV and A-C ventilation are similar. Since its in-

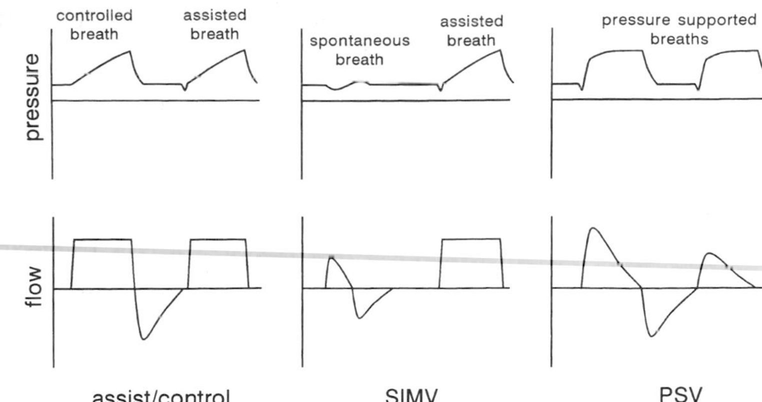

FIGURE 20-4. Pressure and flow waveforms for assist/control ventilation, SIMV, and PSV.

troduction in the early 1970s,[39] IMV and SIMV have become popular modes of ventilation. Although initially regarded as a weaning mode, SIMV is now commonly used as an alternative to A-C even when weaning per se is not occurring. Although IMV originally required a homemade add-on circuit to the existing ventilator circuit (with potentially disastrous mistakes in valve placement or disconnect alarm functions), most currently available ventilators feature built-in SIMV using either a demand valve or a continuous-flow system.

With PSV, patient effort is augmented by a clinician-determined level of pressure during inspiration. Although the clinician sets the level of pressure support, the patient sets the respiratory rate, inspiratory flow, and inspiratory time. The VT is determined by the level of pressure support, the amount of patient effort, and the resistance and compliance of the patient's lungs. At high levels of pressure support (> 20 cmH_2O), PSV is similar to pressure-limited assisted ventilation. PSV can be used with SIMV, in which case the spontaneous breaths between mandatory breaths are pressure supported. Low-level pressure support (with or without SIMV) can be used to overcome the resistance through the endotracheal tube or the unresponsiveness of demand valves in older-generation ventilators.

Continuous positive airway pressure (CPAP) is a spontaneous breathing mode. In this mode, airway pressure is usually (but not necessarily) elevated above atmospheric pressure. With older-generation ventilators, this mode was associated with an increased im-

TABLE 20-4. **Advantages and Disadvantages of A-C, SIMV, PSV, and CPAP**

	Advantages	Disadvantages
A-C	Guaranteed volume (or pressure) with each breath	High $\bar{P}aw$ and associated complications
	Low patient work if sensitivity and inspiratory flow set correctly	Respiratory alkalosis if patient assists at rapid rate
		Auto-PEEP if patient assists at rapid rate
		Respiratory muscle atrophy
SIMV	Avoids respiratory alkalosis	Fatigue and tachypnea if respiratory rate set too low
	Lowers $\bar{P}aw$	Hypercapnia if rate set too low
	Prevents respiratory muscle atrophy	High demand valve work of breathing for older ventilators
	Facilitates weaning	
PSV	Improved patient synchrony and comfort	Requires spontaneous respiratory effort
	Overcomes resistance to spontaneous breathing through endotracheal tube	Fatigue and tachypnea if PSV level set too low
		Activation of expiratory muscles if PSV level set too high
	Prevents respiratory muscle atrophy	
	Lowers $\bar{P}aw$	
	Facilitates weaning	
PSV + SIMV	Minimum guaranteed rate	Poor synchrony between SIMV and PSV breaths
	Low levels of PSV overcome endotracheal tube resistance	Respiratory alkalosis if SIMV rate or PSV level set too high
	Increased VT for spontaneous breaths	
CPAP	Allows spontaneous breathing at set FIO_2 and pressure levels	High demand valve work of breathing in older ventilators
		Fatigue
	Allows easy monitoring of ventilatory status	No ventilatory support

posed work of breathing, but this is no longer an issue with current-generation ventilators (and in particular with the use of low-level PSV). The CPAP mode is frequently used to evaluate a patient's spontaneous breathing ability before extubation. For long-term spontaneous breathing, low levels of pressure support are preferable to CPAP to lower the imposed work of breathing through the ventilator system and the endotracheal tube.

Mandatory minute ventilation, pressure-regulated volume control, volume support, and pressure augmentation are forms of closed-loop ventilation. Mandatory minute ventilation allows the patient to breathe spontaneously, but it ensures a minimal level of ventilation. The ventilator monitors $\dot{V}_E$ and increases the mandatory breath rate or pressure support level to increase $\dot{V}_E$ if it drops below a clinician-determined level. Mandatory minute ventilation is used primarily during weaning. With pressure-regulated volume control, the clinician sets a target V_T and maximum pressure level, and the ventilator attempts to achieve the volume target with the lowest airway pressure. Pressure-regulated volume control is intended for patients who are not spontaneously breathing, whereas volume support is intended for patients who are breathing spontaneously. Volume support combines volume-targeted ventilation with pressure support. Pressure augmentation (also called volume-assured pressure support or VAPS)[40,41] combines the benefits of pressure and volume ventilation to guarantee a minimal volume delivery, yet meeting high patient flow demands. The algorithms used for each of these forms of closed-loop ventilation vary among ventilator manufacturers.

Pressure versus Flow Trigger

Assisted or spontaneous breaths during mechanical ventilation can be either pressure or flow triggered. The effort required to trigger represents an imposed load for the patient. Pressure triggering occurs in response to a pressure drop in the system and ideally should be measured at the proximal airway. The pressure required to trigger is clinician determined and should be set so that trigger effort is minimal but autocycling is unlikely (typically -1 to -2 cmH_2O). With ideal conditions, the delay time with pressure triggering is 110 to 120 msec and can be much greater (> 200 msec) depending on the ventilator system and set trigger pressure.[42]

An alternative to pressure triggering is flow triggering. With flow triggering, the ventilator responds to inhaled flow rather than a pressure drop at the airway. This can be achieved in several ways. For some systems, a pneumotachometer is placed between the ventilator circuit and the patient to measure inspiratory flow. In other systems, a base flow and a flow sensitivity are set. When flow in the expiratory circuit decreases by the amount of the flow sensitivity, the ventilator is triggered. For example, if the base flow is set at 10 L/min and flow sensitivity is set at 3 L/min, the ventilator triggers when flow in the expiratory circuit drops to 7 L/min (the assumption is that the patient has inhaled at 3 L/min). Bench evaluations of flow triggering have found a delay of < 100 msec with this system, and flow triggering has been shown to result in a decreased work of breathing with CPAP.[43–45] However, flow triggering may not be superior to pressure triggering with pressure-supported breaths, SIMV mandatory breaths, or A-C breaths.[46,47] With the exception of CPAP, pressure triggering of 0.5 to 1.0 cmH_2O may be equivalent to flow triggering.

Neither pressure nor flow triggering may be effective if auto-PEEP is present. In the presence of auto-PEEP, the inspiratory effort of the patient must overcome the level of auto-PEEP before either a pressure or flow change is detected at the airway.

Volume versus Pressure Ventilation

Since the 1970s, volume-limited ventilation has been preferred in adult patients, and pressure-limited ventilation has been preferred in neonates. With volume ventilation, the clinician determines the V_T that is delivered with mandatory breaths. This V_T is then delivered regardless of resistance or compliance. With volume-limited ventilation, the proximal airway pressure is variable and dependent on those factors listed in Table 20-5. Volume ventilation should be used whenever a constant V_T is important to maintain a desired $PaCO_2$ (eg, iatrogenic hyperventilation with acute head injury). The principle disadvantage of volume-limited ventilation is that it can result in a high peak alveolar pressure and areas of overdistension in the lungs. Volume-limited ventilation is typically chosen when mechanical ventilation is initiated for adult patients.

With pressure-limited ventilation, airway pressure is set by the clinician and remains constant with changes in resistance and compliance. Factors affecting V_T with pressure-limited ventilation are listed in Table 20-6. The principle advantage of pressure-limited ventilation is that it prevents localized alveolar overdistension with changes in impedance (resistance and compliance) because the peak alveolar pressure cannot be greater than the set pressure limit. Pressure-limited ventilation has become increasingly popular in the ventilation of patients such as those with ARDS, in whom high airway pressures have been historically required.

TABLE 20-5. **Factors Affecting Airway Pressure With Volume-Limited Ventilation**

- Peak inspiratory flow setting: higher flow settings increase peak airway pressure
- Inspiratory flow pattern: peak airway pressure greatest with constant flow and least with decelerating ramp
- Tidal volume: higher V_T results in higher peak airway pressure
- Resistance: higher airway resistance results in higher peak airway pressure
- Compliance: lower compliance results in higher peak airway pressure

TABLE 20-6. **Factors Affecting Tidal Volume With Pressure-Limited Ventilation**

- Peak inspiratory pressure: higher PIP−PEEP(total) difference increases V_T
- PEEP: higher PIP−PEEP(total) difference increases V_T
- Auto-PEEP: higher PIP−PEEP(total) difference increases V_T
- Inspiratory time: increased inspiratory time increases V_T provided that active flow is occurring; after flow decelerates to zero, further increasing the flow does not affect V_T
- Compliance: decreased compliance decreases V_T
- Resistance: increased resistance decreases V_T provided that active flow is occurring; after flow decelerates to zero, resistance no longer affects delivered V_T

Pressure-control ventilation is now used as an alternative to volume ventilation for assisted mechanical ventilation. Inspiratory flow is fixed with volume ventilation, which may increase the inspiratory work of breathing during assisted ventilation. Inspiratory flow is variable with pressure ventilation, which decreases the inspiratory work during assisted breaths.[48] Pressure control may also be superior to PSV for some patients. During PSV, inspiration cycles to expiration when flow decelerates to a ventilator-specific level. In some cases, this results in a long inspiratory time, and the patient activates the expiratory muscles to terminate inspiration.[49] This problem can be corrected by using pressure control as an alternative to pressure support, because the inspiratory time is fixed during pressure control (the inspiratory time is variable during pressure support). In fact, the principle difference between pressure support and pressure assist control is the fixed inspiratory time with pressure control.

The use of volume- versus pressure-limited ventilation is often determined by clinician or institutional bias, and there are advantages and disadvantages of each (Table 20-7). Although much has been written about the potential benefits of pressure-limited ventilation in recent years,[50,51] improved outcome of one approach over the other has not yet been shown.[52] Most patients can be ventilated equally well with either pressure- or volume-limited ventilation if peak alveolar pressure (Pplat), $\dot{V}_E$, patient-ventilator synchrony, and arterial blood gases are monitored.[53,54]

Some ventilators are capable of providing periodic sigh volumes.[55] The use of sighs is controversial. The rationale for use of sighs is that the periodic hyperinflations decrease the risk of atelectasis. However, periodic sigh breaths can result in unacceptably high plateau pressures and are probably unnecessary if a correct PEEP level is set.

Inspiratory Time

For patients who are triggering assisted breaths, the inspiratory time should be short ($\leq$ 1 sec) to improve ventilator-patient synchrony. Increasing the inspiratory time increases $\bar{P}aw$, which may improve distribution of ventilation and oxygenation. A shorter inspiratory time requires a higher inspiratory flow, which increases peak airway pressure but should not greatly affect peak alveolar pressure. When long inspiratory times are used (> 1.5 sec), sedation or paralysis is frequently required. Long inspiratory times can also result in auto-PEEP; this must be monitored whenever long inspiratory times are used. Auto-PEEP is particularly likely with an inverse I:E ratio (ie, inspiratory time longer than expiratory time). Long inspiratory times can also cause hemodynamic instability, caused by either the associated elevated $\bar{P}aw$ or the auto-PEEP created. Although inverse-ratio ventilation has been advocated by some to improve oxygenation, this extreme (and potentially hazardous) form of ventilation is seldom necessary to achieve adequate oxygenation. When a long inspiratory time is useful to improve oxygenation, a lower respiratory rate (eg, longer expiratory time) is desirable to avoid auto-PEEP.

Inspiratory time can be set using one of several approaches. For volume-limited ventilation, the inspiratory flow setting is the principle determinant of inspiratory time and the I:E ratio. Other methods used to establish inspiratory time include setting inspiratory time directly, setting I:E ratio, or setting percent inspiratory time.

TABLE 20-7. **Advantages and Disadvantages of Volume- and Pressure-Limited Ventilation**

	Advantages	Disadvantages
Volume Ventilation	Constant V_T with changes in resistance and compliance Most clinicians are more familiar with this mode of ventilation	Increased plateau pressure with decreasing compliance; this could result in regional alveolar overdistension Fixed inspiratory flow during assisted mechanical ventilation
Pressure Ventilation	Decreased risk of overdistension with changes in resistance and compliance Decelerating flow waveform results in improved distribution of ventilation Square pressure waveform results in higher $\bar{P}aw$ Variable flow and improved synchrony during assisted mechanical ventilation	Changes in V_T with changes in resistance and compliance Many clinicians are less familiar with this mode of ventilation

Tidal Volume

Commonly recommended settings for VT during mechanical ventilation of patients with relatively normal lungs is 10 to 15 mL/kg ideal body weight. Patients are often mechanically ventilated at a VT greater than their spontaneous VT. However, high VT ventilation may produce localized overdistension, decrease cardiac output, and increase the risk of barotrauma. It has now become increasingly accepted to use a lower VT—particularly in patients with acute respiratory failure. Tidal volumes as low as 5 to 8 mL/kg may be appropriate in patients with acute lung injury to prevent injury associated with localized overdistension.[56–59] Rather than choose a VT based on body weight, it may be more appropriate to choose a VT based on the peak alveolar pressure (ie, Pplat). A VT should ideally be chosen that maintains a plateau pressure < 35 cmH_2O.[12]

Respiratory Rate

A respiratory rate (f) is chosen to provide an acceptable minute ventilation: $\dot{V}E = VT \times f$. A rate of 8 to 12 breaths/min is often used when mechanical ventilation is initiated. An acceptable $\dot{V}E$ may not produce a normal $PaCO_2$. For the patient with acute head injury, an acceptable $\dot{V}E$ is that required to produce a $PaCO_2$ of 25 to 30 mmHg. To avoid regional overdistension (Pplat < 35 cmH_2O), a higher respiratory rate (18 to 22 breaths/min) may be required. In patients with acute lung injury, a long inspiratory time is often desirable, and how high the respiratory rate can be set is limited by the creation of auto-PEEP. In such cases, a $\dot{V}E$ that produces a normal $PaCO_2$ may not be possible, and $PaCO_2$ may be allowed to rise (permissive hypercapnia).

Inspiratory Flow Pattern

For volume-limited ventilation, the most common inspiratory flow waveforms are constant flow (square wave), decelerating flow (ramp), and sine wave flow (Figure 20-5). Peak airway pressure is greater with constant flow than decelerating flow, $\bar{P}aw$ is greater with decelerating flow than constant flow, and gas distribution is better with a decelerating flow pattern. Because the flow is greater at the beginning of inspiration, patient-ventilator synchrony may be better with a decelerating flow pattern. Although the choice of flow pattern is often based on institutional bias or the capabilities of the specific ventilator that is used, decelerating flow may be desirable when compared to other inspiratory flow waveforms. An end-inspiratory pause can also be used and may improve distribution of ventilation. However, an inspiratory pause may have a deleterious effect on hemodynamics if it significantly prolongs inspiratory time. An end-inspiratory pause should not be used with patients who are triggering the ventilator because it results in significant dys-synchrony.

For pressure-limited ventilation, the inspiratory flow waveform is always exponentially decelerating. The rate of deceleration depends on the pressure limit and lung impedance. With high resistance, flow decelerates slowly. With a low compliance and long inspiratory time, flow decelerates more rapidly, and a period of zero flow may be present at end-inhalation (Figure 20-6). Some studies have shown improved oxygenation with pressure-limited ventilation,[40,41] which may be the result of the decelerating flow waveform and higher $\bar{P}aw$ with this form of ventilation.[43,44]

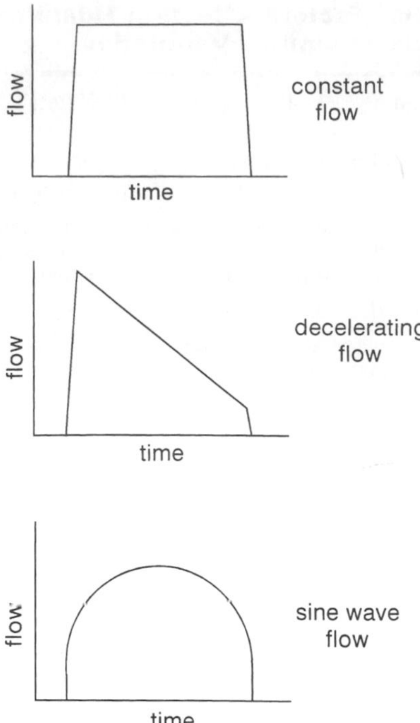

FIGURE 20-5. Waveforms for constant flow (square wave), decelerating flow (ramp), and sine wave flow.

Positive End-Expiratory Pressure

Positive end-expiratory pressure is commonly used in the care of patients with acute respiratory failure.[60] It is a common practice to use low-level PEEP (3 to 5 cmH_2O) with all mechanically ventilated patients.[61] Pos-

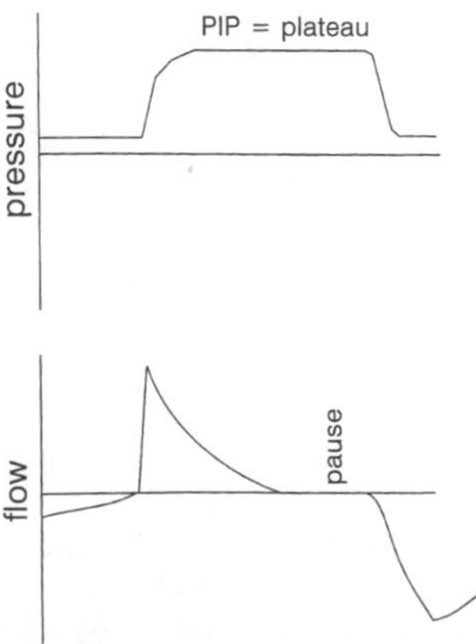

FIGURE 20-6. Pressure and flow waveforms for constant pressure ventilation.

itive end-expiratory pressure is used to increase functional residual capacity, decrease intrapulmonary shunting ($\dot{Q}s/\dot{Q}t$), improve lung compliance, and improve PaO_2. In patients with ARDS, a PEEP of 8 to 12 cmH_2O should be used to keep the PEEP level greater than the inflection point of the pressure-volume curve (see Chap. 12).[62] A PEEP level greater than 15 cmH_2O is seldom necessary and may be hazardous because high PEEP levels are associated with overdistension and altered hemodynamics. Positive end-expiratory pressure should also be used cautiously in patients with unilateral disease.[63] In this setting, PEEP may overdistend the more compliant lung, resulting in shunting of blood to the underventilated, less-compliant lung.

Positive end-expiratory pressure may also be useful to improve triggering by patients experiencing auto-PEEP.[64,65] Auto-PEEP is a threshold pressure that must be overcome before the pressure (or flow) will decrease at the airway to trigger the ventilator. By increasing the set PEEP to a level near the total PEEP (set PEEP + auto-PEEP), the ability of the patient to trigger may be improved (Figure 20-7).[66] Whenever PEEP is used to overcome the effect of auto-PEEP on triggering, the total PEEP level must be monitored to be certain that it does not increase when auto-PEEP is present. A set PEEP as much as 80% of the auto-PEEP can probably be used without elevating the total PEEP.[65]

Mean Airway Pressure

Many of the beneficial and deleterious effects of mechanical ventilation are related to $\bar{P}aw$. Factors effecting $\bar{P}aw$ during mechanical ventilation are listed in Table 20-8.[67] To avoid many of the complications of mechanical ventilation, a lower $\bar{P}aw$ is desirable. However, a $\bar{P}aw$ > 20 cmH_2O is often necessary for patients with ARDS to maintain adequate arterial oxygenation.

Inspired Oxygen Concentration

When instituting mechanical ventilation, it is usually best to begin with a high FIO_2. Hypoxia is more deleterious than hyperoxia. Some clinicians prefer to use 100% O_2 until the PaO_2 is known. After the first arterial blood gas measurement, the FIO_2 can be decreased to produce the desired PaO_2. Pulse oximetry is useful to guide titration of FIO_2,[68] provided that periodic blood gas analyses are obtained to confirm the pulse oximetry results. Although it has been common practice to wait 20 to 30 minutes before obtaining arterial blood gas measurements after an FIO_2 or other ventilator change, 10 minutes may be an adequate wait time, unless the patient has obstructive lung disease (which requires a longer equilibration time).[69]

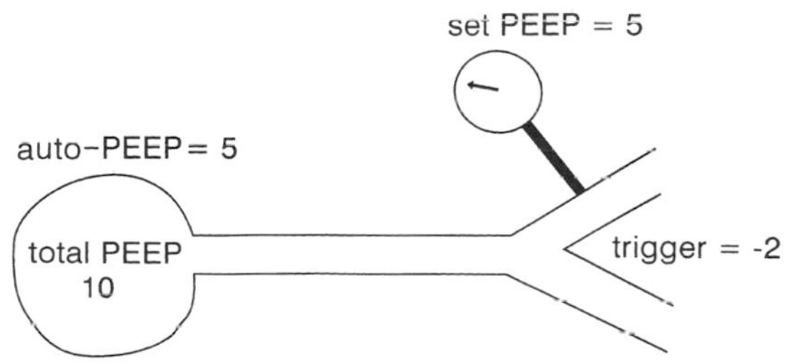

FIGURE 20-7. Trigger effort is increased when auto-PEEP is present. To trigger the ventilator, the patient's effort must first overcome the level of auto-PEEP that is present. Increasing the set PEEP level may raise the trigger level closer to the total PEEP, thus improving the ability of the patient to trigger the ventilator. However, this method should not be used if raising the set PEEP level results in an increase in the total PEEP.

TABLE 20-8. **Factors Effecting Mean Airway Pressure During Positive Pressure Ventilation**

- Peak inspiratory pressure
- Total PEEP level (set PEEP + auto-PEEP)
- I:E ratio (Ti/Ttot)
- Respiratory rate
- Inspiratory flow pattern

Alarms

It is particularly important that all alarms are correctly set on the ventilator. The most important alarm is the patient disconnect alarm, which can be a low-pressure alarm or a low exhaled volume alarm. A sensitive alarm should detect not only disconnection but also leaks in the system. Failure to properly set the disconnect alarm on the ventilator could result in serious harm to the patient should a disconnection or leak occur. The ability to detect a leak depends on the site at which the volume is measured (Figure 20-8). Other alarms set on the ventilator include high-pressure alarms, I:E ratio alarms, loss of PEEP alarms, and over-temperature alarms. The peak airway pressure alarm is important during volume-limited ventilation to detect changes in resistance and compliance, and the low exhaled volume alarm is important during pressure-limited ventilation.

Circuit

A technical consideration in the determination of an adequate VT for a mechanically ventilated patient is the effect of compressible volume loss.[70–73] Because of the gas compression within the ventilator circuit and the compliance (elasticity) of the ventilator circuit tubing, as much as 3 to 5 mL/cmH_2O can be "lost" in the ventilator circuitry. In other words, at a peak airway pressure of 40 cmH_2O, 120 to 200 mL of the gas delivered from the ventilator is not delivered to the patient. Thus, if the ventilator is set to deliver 800 mL, only 600 to 680 mL is delivered to the patient. For patients who are being ventilated with a small VT, compressible gas volume can greatly affect alveolar ventilation. Some ventilator systems (eg, Puritan-Bennett 7200) adjust for the effects of compressible volume such that the volume chosen by the clinician represents the actual delivered VT after correction for the effect of compressible volume. The ef-

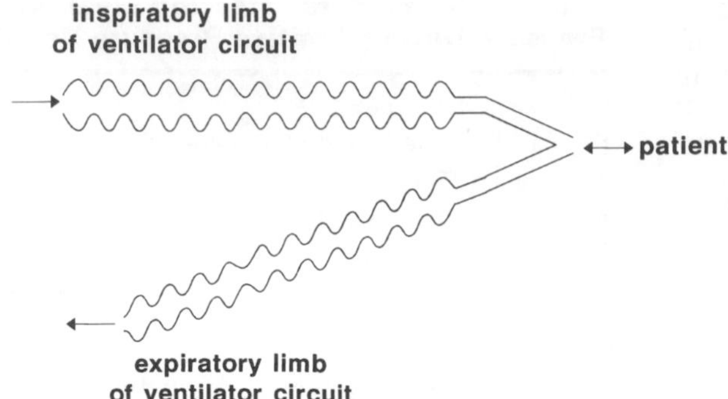

- **If volume on inspiratory limb > volume on expiratory limb, then there is a leak in the system (circuit or patient)**
- **If the inhaled volume at the patient is greater than the exhaled volume at the patient, then there is a leak in the patient (e.g., leak around airway cuff or bronchopleural fistula)**

FIGURE 20-8. The ability to detect a leak depends upon the site where volume is measured.

fect of compressible volume on delivered V_T can be expressed by the following relationship:

$$V_T\ (pt) = [1/(1 + Cpc/Crs)] \times V_T\ (vent)$$

where V_T (pt) is the V_T delivered to the patient, Cpc is the compliance of the ventilator circuit, Crs is the compliance of the respiratory system, and V_T (vent) is the V_T from the ventilator circuit.

Compressible volume also affects measurements of auto-PEEP and can be expressed by the following relationship:

$$\text{auto-PEEP} = (Crs + Cpc)/Crs \times \text{estimated auto-PEEP}$$

where estimated auto-PEEP is that measured (including the ventilator circuit).

The effect of compressible volume on mixed exhaled PCO_2 can be expressed by the following relationship:

$$P\bar{E}CO_2\ (pt) = P\bar{E}CO_2\ (pc) \times [V_T\ (vent)/V_T\ (pt)]$$

where $P\bar{E}CO_2$ (pt) is the patient's actual $P\bar{E}CO_2$, and $P\bar{E}CO_2$ (pc) is the mixed exhaled PCO_2 from the ventilator circuit.

Not only should the volume loss in the circuit be considered, but mechanical dead space should also be considered. Mechanical dead space is that part of the ventilator circuit through which the patient rebreathes and thus becomes an extension of the patient's anatomic dead space. Theoretically, V_A is zero if the sum of the volume loss in the circuit and the V_D is greater than the V_T set on the ventilator. Although in the past it was popular to use mechanical dead space to produce changes in $PaCO_2$, this therapy is now seldom used and is probably not effective.

MONITORING OF THE PATIENT ON A VENTILATOR

Critically ill patients on ventilators require the constant surveillance of the health care team. Frequent monitoring of physical findings, blood gases, lung mechanics, hemodynamics, and patient-ventilator synchrony are essential to good patient care (see AARC Clinical Practice Guidelines: Patient-Ventilator System Check). It is also important to frequently monitor the function of the mechanical ventilator, including checks of the correct ventilator settings, the ventilator alarm systems, the humidifier and circuitry, and the patient's airway (see AARC Clinical Practice Guidelines: Ventilator Circuit Changes). Flowsheet charting is often used at regular intervals to document the monitoring of patients on ventilators (Figure 20-9).

Physical Assessment

Much important information can be obtained by simply observing the patient. Cyanosis may be present in very hypoxemic patients. Asymmetric chest motion may indicate main stem (endobronchial) intubation, pneumothorax, or atelectasis. Paradoxical chest motion may be seen with flail chest or respiratory muscle fatigue. Retractions may be seen if the inspiratory flow and sensitivity are inappropriately set on the ventilator, or if the airway is obstructed. If the patient does not appear to be breathing in synchrony with the ventilator (ie, "bucking the ventilator"), this may indicate that the settings on the ventilator are not appropriate or that the patient may need sedation.

Palpation of the chest in conjunction with inspection can be used to assess symmetry of chest movement. Palpation to assess tracheal position can be useful; pneumothorax causes the trachea to be deviated away from the affected side, and atelectasis causes it to be deviated toward the affected side. Palpation of fremitus indicates the presence of secretions in the airways, and crepitation indicates subcutaneous emphysema.

Percussion can also be useful in the assessment of patients on ventilators. Unilateral hyperresonance or tympany may indicate the presence of a pneumothorax. Dullness may indicate consolidation, atelectasis, or pleural effusion.

The chest of a patient on a ventilator should be auscultated frequently. Unilateral decreased breath sounds

AARC Clinical Practice Guideline

PATIENT-VENTILATOR SYSTEM CHECKS

Indications: A patient-ventilator system check must be performed on a scheduled basis (which is institution-specific) for any patient requiring mechanical ventilation for life support. In addition, a check should be performed prior to obtaining blood samples for analysis of blood gases and pH; prior to obtaining hemodynamic or bedside pulmonary function data; following any change in ventilator settings; as soon as possible following an acute deterioration of the patient's condition (this may or may not be heralded by a violation of ventilator-alarm thresholds); any time that ventilator performance is questionable.

Contraindications: There are no absolute contraindications to performance of a patient-ventilator system check. If disruption of PEEP or F_{DO2} results in hypoxemia, bradycardia, or hypotension, portions of the check requiring disconnection of the patient from the ventilator may be contraindicated.

Assessment of Need: Because of the complexity of mechanical ventilators and the large number of factors that can adversely affect patient-ventilator interaction, routine checks of patient-ventilator system performance are mandatory.

Assessment of Outcome: Routine patient-ventilator system checks should prevent untoward incidents, warn of impending events, and assure that proper ventilator settings, according to physician's order, are maintained.

Monitoring: In order to assure that patient-ventilator system checks are being performed according to these guidelines, an indicator should be created to monitor this activity as part of the appropriate department's quality improvement program. Specific criteria for the indicator should at least include patient information and observations indicative of the ventilator's settings at the time of the check and a system check should be performed at regularly scheduled intervals.

From AARC Clinical Practice Guideline; see Respir Care 1992;37:882–886 for complete text.

may indicate bronchial intubation, pneumothorax, atelectasis, or pleural effusion. Decreased breath sounds and crackles at the lung bases usually indicates basilar atelectasis, which may be corrected with CPAP or PEEP or with chest physiotherapy. Bibasilar rales are heard with congestive heart failure, fluid overload, or basilar atelectasis. Coarse rales are heard with retained secretions, and wheezing usually indicates bronchospasm. An end-inspiratory squeak over the trachea usually indicates insufficient air in the artificial airway cuff.

AARC Clinical Practice Guideline

VENTILATOR CIRCUIT CHANGES

Indications: The decision to change a ventilator circuit should be governed by length of time the existing circuit has been in use; type of circuit and dehumidification device in use; circuit function (presence of a malfunctioning circuit or a circuit that leaks); appearance of ventilator circuit (circuits that are not clean in appearance should be replaced).

Contraindications: Contraindications to performing ventilator circuit changes are presence of conditions in the patient's cardiopulmonary or neurologic status that might make tolerance of disconnection from mechanical ventilation hazardous to the patient; inability to safely and effectively ventilate or maintain patient during the ventilator circuit change; absence of a clean and functional circuit to use as a replacement.

Assessment of Need: Limiting the transmission of infection: reliance on published Centers for Disease Control and Prevention (CDC) recommendations[25, 29] and reliance on institutional standards established by monitoring and surveillance and/or published research. To prevent malfunction and to maintain optimal performance: competency of the circuit should be monitored for tubing leaks; in-line filters should be assessed for increased resistance; equipment affected over time by water (eg, spirometers) should be monitored. To maintain a circuit clean in appearance: inspect appearance of circuit.

Assessment of Outcome: The following should be utilized to evaluate the benefit of the ventilator circuit change: an ongoing infectious disease surveillance program to include surveillance of incidence of nosocomial pneumonia in mechanically ventilated patients in the institution and surveillance of institutional compliance with stated institutional policy on infection control in mechanically ventilated patients; an ongoing equipment-malfunction surveillance program; an operational verification, as described in the AARC Patient-Ventilator System Check CPG, immediately following circuit change to assure physical integrity and proper function of system.

Monitoring: Monitoring of the ventilator circuit change should also include observation of and appropriate response to patient's hemodynamic values: blood pressure, heart rate, and rhythm; patient's oxygenation: S_{pO2}, and P_{aO2} and S_{aO2} (if available); patient's acid-base and ventilatory status: P_{CO2}, and pH and end-tidal CO_2 (if available); patient's chest excursion, color, appearance, comfort; stability of artificial airway and its placement; complete patient-ventilator system check.

From AARC Clinical Practice Guideline; see Respir Care 1994;39(8):797–802 for complete text.

Blood Gases

The earliest indicators of hypoxemia are often changes in the clinical status of the patient, which include restlessness and confusion, changes in level of consciousness, tachycardia or bradycardia, changes in blood pressure, tachypnea, bucking the ventilator, and cyanosis.

The most commonly used indicator of oxygenation is the PaO_2. A low PaO_2 indicates hypoxemia and a dysfunction in the ability of the lungs to oxygenate arterial blood. The PaO_2 must always be interpreted in relation to the FIO_2. This can be done by calculation of $P(A - a)O_2$, PaO_2/PAO_2, or PaO_2/FIO_2 (see Chap. 12). A $PaO_2/FIO_2 < 200$ is characteristic of patients with acute respiratory failure.

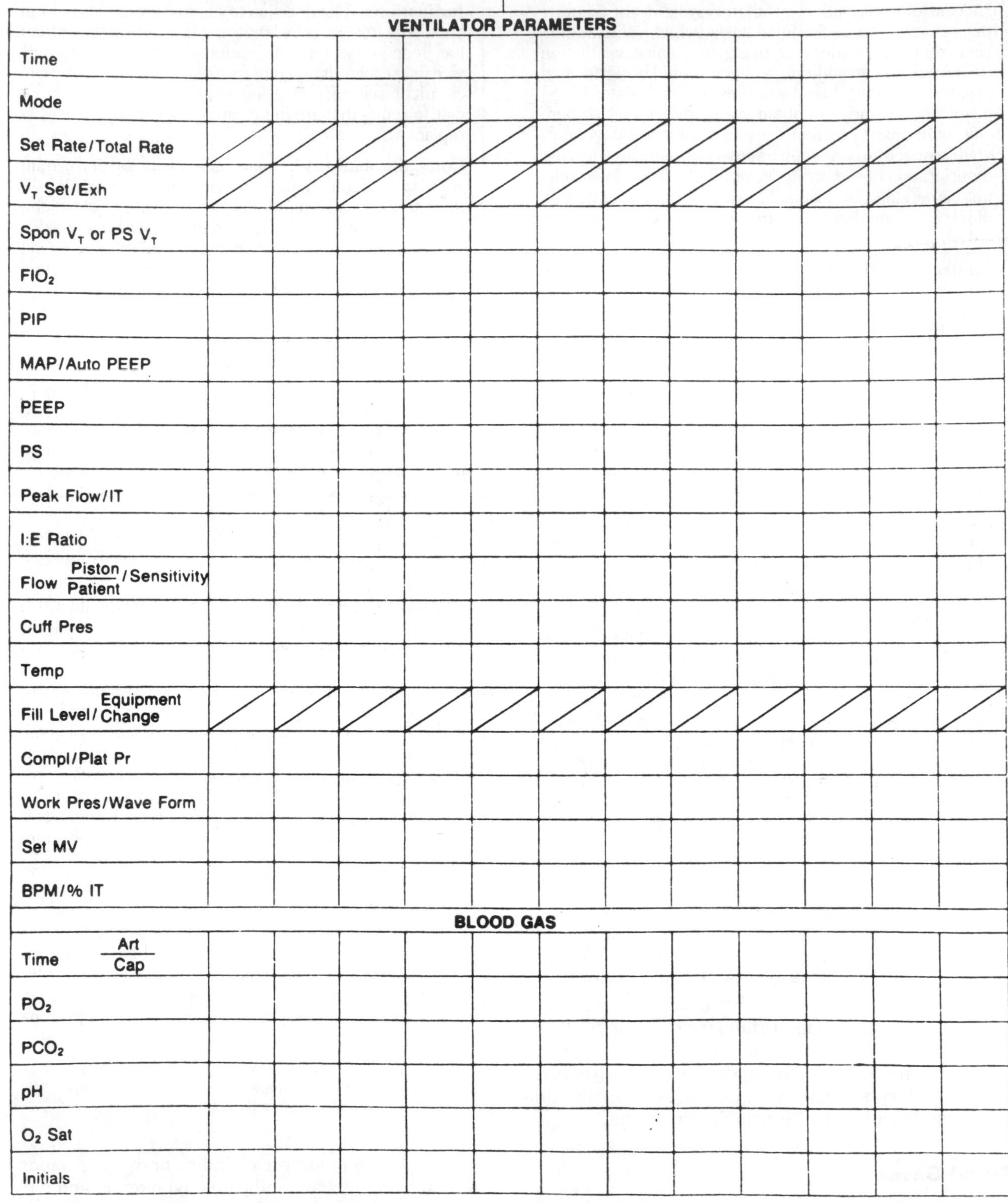

VENTILATOR RECORD

PAGE 2

VENTILATOR PARAMETERS												
Time												
Mode												
Set Rate/Total Rate												
V_T Set/Exh												
Spon V_T or PS V_T												
FIO_2												
PIP												
MAP/Auto PEEP												
PEEP												
PS												
Peak Flow/IT												
I:E Ratio												
Flow $\frac{\text{Piston}}{\text{Patient}}$/Sensitivity												
Cuff Pres												
Temp												
Fill Level/Equipment Change												
Compl/Plat Pr												
Work Pres/Wave Form												
Set MV												
BPM/% IT												
BLOOD GAS												
Time $\frac{\text{Art}}{\text{Cap}}$												
PO_2												
PCO_2												
pH												
O_2 Sat												
Initials												

FIGURE 20-9. Mechanical ventilation flow sheet used at the Massachusetts General Hospital.

In mechanically ventilated patients, a number of factors affect the PaO_2 (Table 20-9). A change in PaO_2 can be affected by changing the patient's lung function, FIO_2, and PEEP level. During mechanical ventilation, attempts should be made to improve the patient's lung function while using appropriate levels of FIO_2 and PEEP to avoid hypoxemia and hypoxia.

The PaO_2 is not necessarily a good indicator of tissue oxygenation (hypoxia). Mixed venous oxygenation ($P\bar{v}O_2$ or $S\bar{v}O_2$) is a better indicator of overall tissue oxygenation. A $P\bar{v}O_2 < 35$ mmHg (or an $S\bar{v}O_2 < 70\%$) indicates tissue hypoxia. The $P\bar{v}O_2$ may be decreased as the result of arterial hypoxemia, anemia, decreased cardiac output, or increased O_2 consumption. It is important to recognize that the PaO_2 may be normal, or even increased, but the patient may be hypoxic with a decreased $P\bar{v}O_2$. A pulmonary artery catheter (Swan-Ganz) must be present to obtain blood to measure $P\bar{v}O_2$ (see Chap. 12).

The $PaCO_2$ is determined by $\dot{V}CO_2$ and $\dot{V}A$. If $\dot{V}CO_2$ is constant, $PaCO_2$ varies inversely with $\dot{V}A$. The $\dot{V}A$ affects the $PaCO_2$ indirectly because of the relationship between $\dot{V}E$ and $\dot{V}A$. An increase in $\dot{V}E$ decreases $PaCO_2$, and a decrease in $\dot{V}E$ increases $PaCO_2$. This is illustrated by the following relationship:

$$PaCO_2 = (\dot{V}CO_2 \times 0.863) / [\dot{V}E \times (1 - VD/VT)]$$

Factors that determine $PaCO_2$ during mechanical ventilation are listed in Table 20-10.

The use of noninvasive monitors of oxygenation (see Chap. 12) may reduce the need for arterial blood gases and allows continuous assessment of arterial oxygenation between PaO_2 measurements.[74] Pulse oximetry can be used to titrate an appropriate FIO_2. Changes in oxygenation detected by noninvasive monitors signal the need to measure the PaO_2. In mechanically ventilated patients, continuous pulse oximetry has become a standard of care, although there is little scientific support for this practice. End-tidal PCO_2 is used to noninvasively monitor CO_2 levels.[74] In patients with normal lungs, the end-tidal PCO_2 closely approximates $PaCO_2$. However, in patients with an elevated VD/VT, as is common in many mechanically ventilated patients, there can be a large and inconsistent gradient between the $PaCO_2$ and end-tidal PCO_2 (see Chap. 12). For this reason, monitoring of end-tidal PCO_2 may be of limited usefulness to assess $PaCO_2$ during mechanical ventilation.

TABLE 20-9. **Factors That Affect PaO_2 During Mechanical Ventilation**

- Lung disease: secretions, infection, bronchospasm, atelectasis, ARDS, congestive heart failure, fluid overload
- Cardiac disease: decreased mixed venous oxygen
- Drugs: vasodilators (eg, nitroprusside)
- Mean airway pressure
- FIO_2

TABLE 20-10. **Factors That Affect $PaCO_2$ During Mechanical Ventilation**

- Dead space: pulmonary embolism, pulmonary hypoperfusion, positive airway pressure, high-rate and low-VT ventilation
- Carbon dioxide production: fever, sepsis, exercise, excessive caloric intake (especially carbohydrate), hyperthyroidism

Lung Mechanics

Breath-by-breath monitoring of airway pressure and VT is common during mechanical ventilation of adult patients. On current-generation ventilators, continuous waveforms of pressure, flow, and volume are available as well as pressure-volume and flow-volume loops. These are useful to evaluate lung mechanics during mechanical ventilation (see Chap. 12).

Peak pressure, plateau pressure, and auto-PEEP are particularly important to monitor. Factors affecting these are listed in Table 20-11. Plateau pressure is measured by applying an end-inspiratory pause of 0.5 to 1.5 sec, and auto-PEEP is determined by applying an end-expiratory pause of 0.5 to 1.5 sec. Both plateau pressure and auto-PEEP can only be accurately measured when the patient is relaxed and breathing in synchrony with the ventilator; these measurements are of limited value when the patient is triggering assisted breaths or breathing spontaneously. During pressure-limited ventilation, the inspiratory flow often decelerates to a no-flow period at end-inspiration. In this case, the peak pressure and plateau pressure are equivalent. As discussed previously in this chapter, plateau pressure represents the mean peak alveolar pressure and should ideally be kept < 35 cmH_2O to avoid overdistension and acute lung injury.

Hemodynamics

Because positive pressure ventilation can affect cardiac function, it is important to assess hemodynamics during mechanical ventilation.[75,76] At a minimum, arterial blood pressure and heart rate should be measured frequently. When a high $\bar{P}aw$ (> 20 cmH_2O) is used, invasive monitoring of arterial blood pressure, pulmonary artery pressure, and cardiac output is indicated. When the high airway pressures needed to support oxygenation adversely affect cardiac performance, hemodynamics

TABLE 20-11. **Factors That Affect Peak Pressure, Plateau Pressure, and Auto-PEEP During Mechanical Ventilation**

- Peak airway pressure: resistance, compliance, tidal volume, inspiratory flow, PEEP
- Plateau pressure: compliance, tidal volume, PEEP
- Auto-PEEP: expiratory time, tidal volume, resistance, compliance

may need to be supported with fluid, inotropes, and pressors.

It is important to appreciate the effect of positive pressure ventilation on hemodynamic assessments. During positive pressure ventilation, pleural pressure increases during inhalation by an amount determined by lung compliance and chest wall compliance:[77]

$$\Delta Ppl/\Delta Paw = C_L/(C_L + C_W)$$

where ΔPpl is the change in pleural pressure, ΔPaw is the change in airway (alveolar) pressure, C_L is lung compliance, and C_W is chest wall compliance. By convention, hemodynamic measurements are made at end-exhalation to account for the respiratory variation in pleural pressure. At end-exhalation, measurements such as pulmonary artery occlusion pressure (wedge pressure) are affected by the amount of PEEP transmitted to the pleural space, which is determined by lung compliance and chest wall compliance. In patients with normal chest wall compliance (150 mL/cmH_2O) and decreased lung compliance (50 mL/cmH_2O), about 1/4 of the alveolar pressure is transmitted to the pleural space.

Evaluation of Patient-Ventilator Synchrony

Dys-synchrony occurs when the patient is not breathing in phase with the ventilator. In its worst form, the patient is bucking the ventilator. However, many times dys-synchrony is much more subtle. Failure of the patient to breathe in synchrony with the ventilator decreases patient comfort, increases work of breathing, and increases O_2 cost of breathing. There are several causes of dys-synchrony during mechanical ventilation (Table 20-12).

It is commonly believed that patients relax their respiratory muscles during assisted breaths with A-C or SIMV. However, this is often not the case in either mode (Figures 20-10 and 20-11).[78–80] Lack of synchrony can be detected by evaluating the airway pressure waveform during volume ventilation and the flow waveform (Figure 20-12) during pressure ventilation. With dys-synchrony, the pressure waveform with each breath differs from every other, and there is breath-to-breath variability in peak airway pressure. Clinical signs of dys-synchrony include tachypnea, chest wall retractions, and chest-abdominal paradox.

Several things can be done to improve patient synchrony. The ventilator's trigger should be set as sensitive as possible without producing autocycling. Flow triggering may be tried if it is available. The inspiratory flow should be set high enough to meet the patient's peak inspiratory flow demands (this often results in an inspiratory time < 1 sec). A very common mistake is to set the inspiratory flow too low, and thus the inspiratory time is too long for patient comfort. A decelerating flow pattern may improve synchrony because the inspiratory flow is greatest at the beginning of inspiration when the patient's flow demands are greatest—this may be best achieved with pressure-control ventilation, which allows for variable inspiratory flow. With older-generation ventilators, patient effort to open the inspiratory demand valve with spontaneous breaths can be excessive. This can be corrected by adding a low level of pressure support.[72] Sometimes dys-synchrony can be corrected by increasing the respiratory rate to capture the patient's rate, thus decreasing the inspiratory efforts of the patient.

TABLE 20-12. **Factors That Affect Dys-Synchrony During Mechanical Ventilation**

Trigger sensitivity: increase trigger sensitivity or use flow triggering
Inspiratory flow: increase peak flow setting, try different inspiratory flow pattern, try pressure control or pressure support ventilation
Tidal volume: try higher or lower V_T
Respiratory rate: try higher or lower rate setting
Agitation: provide appropriate level of sedation

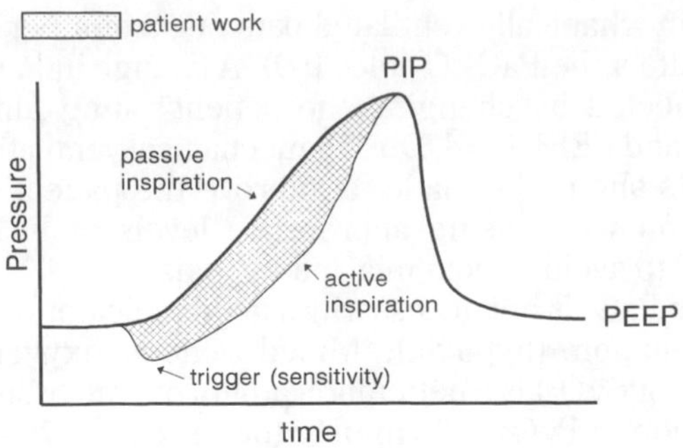

FIGURE 20-10. Effect of dys-synchrony on airway pressure waveform. The shaded area represents the increased work performed by the patient if the sensitivity and inspiratory flow are set incorrectly.

Anxiety is a common cause of failure to breathe in synchrony with the ventilator. In these cases, pharmacologic support may be necessary in the form of analgesics (narcotics such as morphine), sedatives (benzodiazepines such as midazolam or diazepam), and paralyzing agents (such as curare, pancuronium, or vecuronium). When short-term sedation is necessary to bring a patient into synchrony with the ventilator, propofol may be useful. When ventilation requires long inspiratory times and high airway pressures, pharmacologic control of the patient's breathing is almost always necessary. It must be remembered that all forms of respiratory suppression are associated with adverse side effects. It is most important that disconnect alarms be properly set when the patient's ability to spontaneously breathe is pharmacologically suppressed. Significant problems with pharmacologic suppression of respiration have recently been reported, such as long-term respiratory muscle weakness following use of paralyzing agents during mechanical ventilation.[81–83]

WEANING PATIENTS FROM MECHANICAL VENTILATION

Weaning from continuous ventilation can be a difficult, frustrating task for the patient and the health care team.[76–79] The weaning process is critical for the patient

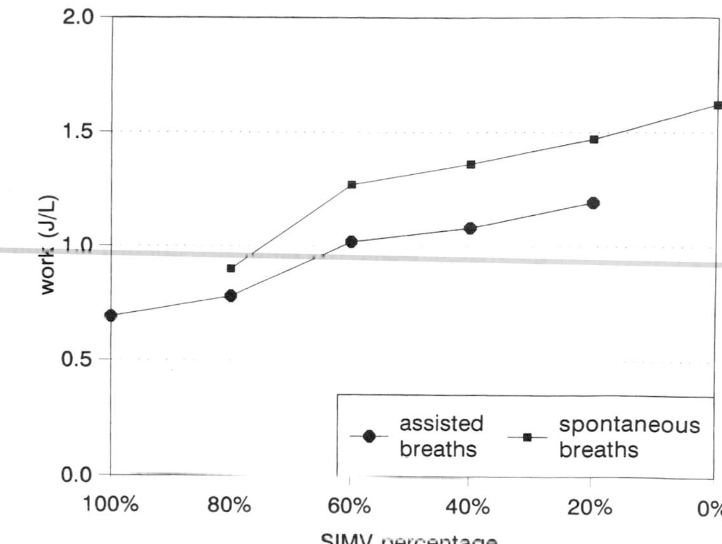

FIGURE 20-11. Work of breathing performed by the patient for assisted and spontaneous breaths during SIMV at varying levels of support. Note that decreasing the level of support results in increased work for both the assisted and spontaneous breaths (From Marini JJ, Smith TC, Lamb VJ: External work output and force generation during synchronized intermittent mechanical ventilation. Am Rev Respir Dis 138:1169, 1988).

both physiologically and psychologically. Many such patients have marginal respiratory reserve, and determining whether or not the patient can maintain adequate alveolar ventilation with spontaneous breathing may be challenging to the respiratory care team. The weaning process ranges from simple (as with the patient recovering from acute drug overdose) to complex (as with the patient recovering from ARDS). If proper guidelines are followed, weaning need not be a risky experience for the patient. One very important underlying principle during weaning is never to use any weaning strategy to the point of patient fatigue.

Factors to Be Improved Before Weaning

The patient's general condition must be evaluated, and any problems that are identified must be resolved or improved. As a general rule, patients who are homeostatically unstable are not good candidates for weaning from the ventilator. Patients with multisystem failure usually require continued mechanical ventilation. General factors to be optimized before weaning are listed in Table 20-13.[84-88] The condition that required initiation of mechanical ventilation should be resolved or resolving. In particular, issues such as bronchospasm, retained secretions, and fluid overload should be corrected. Left heart failure should be corrected before weaning is initiated, because transition from positive pressure breathing to spontaneous breathing can compromise left ventricular function.[89]

Acid-base abnormalities are commonly associated with mechanical ventilation. Both respiratory and metabolic alkalemia are common and physiologically troublesome. The normal compensatory mechanism for metabolic alkalemia is alveolar hypoventilation. Alkalemia also shifts the oxyhemoglobin dissociation curve to the left, resulting in an increased hemoglobin affinity for O_2 and, thereby, impaired release of O_2 to tissues. Metabolic acidemia may also interfere with weaning be-

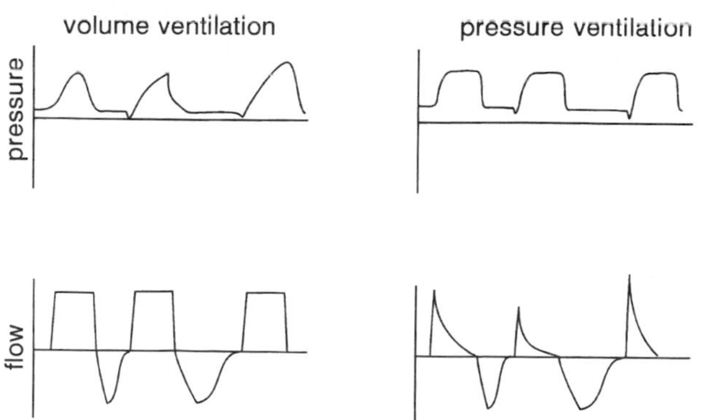

FIGURE 20-12. Effect of dys-synchrony on pressure waveform during volume ventilation and flow waveform during pressure ventilation.

TABLE 20-13. **General Factors To Be Optimized Before Weaning Is Begun**

Acid–base abnormalities (particularly metabolic alkalosis)
Anemia
Arrhythmias
Caloric depletion or excess
Electrolyte abnormalities
Fever
Fluid balance
Hyperglycemia
Infection
Protein loss
Reduced cardiac output (hemodynamic instability)
Renal failure
Sepsis
Shock
Sleep deprivation
Level of consciousness

cause it increases the ventilation requirement to compensate for the acidemia.

Hypocapnia often occurs during continuous ventilation. Respiratory alkalemia, if prolonged, may be compensated by renal mechanisms with renal loss of bicarbonate. When spontaneous ventilation resumes during weaning, the $PaCO_2$ may increase, resulting in acidosis. This is particularly a problem in patients who have chronic hypercapnia. It is useful to review the patient's past medical records to ascertain the pre–respiratory failure blood gas values because the ultimate goal is achievement of these values. A "relative" hypocapnia in a patient with chronic CO_2 retention must be corrected before weaning is initiated. Such patients may not be able to maintain a $PaCO_2$ lower than the pre–mechanical ventilation value once weaning is initiated. Unfortunately, the patient's baseline $PaCO_2$ value before the onset of mechanical ventilation is not always known.

Although clinicians frequently focus on the patient's PaO_2, there are multiple determinants of systemic O_2 transport. Because anemia results in a decreased O_2-carrying capacity, a hemoglobin of at least 10 g/dL is preferable for weaning. Cardiac output and blood pressure should be optimized to ensure adequate O_2 delivery to tissues. Cardiac arrhythmias should be controlled because they may decrease the cardiac output. Because of the life-threatening potential of arrhythmias, a cardiac monitor should be used on all patients during weaning. Arrhythmias may be aggravated by the hypoxemia, acidosis, and stress that may accompany weaning.

Hypokalemia may cause myocardial irritability and must be corrected. It can also lead to metabolic alkalemia. The combination of hypoxemia, alkalemia, and hypokalemia strongly predisposes patients to arrhythmias. Hyponatremia, hyperglycemia, and renal failure should all be treated and restored to normal if possible before weaning is begun. Hypophosphatemia should also be corrected because this can result in respiratory muscle weakness.[90–92] Hypocalcemia, hypomagnesemia, and hypermagnesemia should also be corrected.

Caloric and protein depletion may occur during mechanical ventilation in the patient being sustained solely by intravenous fluids. Respiratory muscles may atrophy from inactivity and may also be weakened by catabolism as a result of malnutrition. Therefore, proper nutrition and an exercise program should be started in advance of weaning in the patient who has spent a prolonged period on the ventilator.[92]

Fever should be controlled because it increases $\dot{V}O_2$ and $\dot{V}CO_2$. Its presence often signifies infection, which also increases O_2 demand. Thus, both fever and infection should be controlled, if possible, before weaning patients with minimal respiratory reserve. Septic patients usually cannot be successfully weaned.

Fluid balance can be critical, especially if borderline pulmonary edema is present. Continuous ventilation can promote fluid retention, which could further compromise the patient's respiratory reserve. This is particularly likely in malnourished patients with low colloid osmotic pressure secondary to hypoalbuminemia. Patients receiving inadequate fluids or diuretics may develop hypovolemia, which in turn can reduce the cardiac output and blood pressure. Fluid intake and output should be monitored carefully to prevent further compromise of the patient's reserve.

Sleep deprivation and pain are common in critically ill patients and interfere with the patient's ability to resume spontaneous ventilation. Narcotics and sedatives should be reduced or discontinued, if possible, to ensure alertness and to avoid respiratory center depression. However, a minimal analgesic dose is often useful in weaning the postoperative patient, because it dulls pain sufficiently to enable the patient to take deep breaths, optimizing alveolar ventilation and preventing atelectasis. Adequate rest enhances the patient's ability to cooperate. Therefore, sedatives should not be totally abandoned but should be used judiciously. Ideally, patients should be alert, conscious, and cooperative at the start of weaning, but this is not always possible. Following severe head injury or cerebral vascular accident, consciousness may be slow to return and may follow successful weaning by weeks or months.

Respiratory Muscles and Weaning

In recent years, there has been increasing interest in the role of respiratory muscles during acute respiratory failure, mechanical ventilation, and weaning from mechanical ventilation.[93–96] Respiratory muscle fatigue occurs if the load placed on the muscles is excessive, if the muscles are weak, or if the duty cycle (the inspiratory time relative to total cycle time) is too long. A fatiguing load can result from high airway resistance, low lung compliance, or high load imposed by the ventilator breathing circuit and endotracheal tube. Respiratory muscle function may be decreased by disease, disuse, malnutrition, hypoxia, or electrolyte imbalance. A long duty cycle may result from tachypnea. Respiratory muscle fatigue is clinically indicated by tachypnea; abnormal respiratory movements (respiratory alternans and abdominal paradox); and, finally, an increase in $PaCO_2$. Because maximal inspiratory pressure (MIP) is a good indicator of overall respiratory muscle strength, a low MIP may indicate respiratory muscle fatigue.

To avoid respiratory muscle weakness, appropriate amounts of O_2 and other nutrients must be supplied to these muscles. This requires both adequate tissue perfusion (cardiac output) and arterial O_2 content (CaO_2). Nutritional status is also important because inadequate caloric intake can result in catabolism of respiratory muscle protein.

Respiratory muscles must be rested if fatigue occurs. A period of rest for 24 hours or longer may be required.[97] Respiratory muscle rest is usually provided by a period of A-C or SIMV ventilation with a rate set high enough to eliminate spontaneous breathing. If respiratory muscle fatigue is the result of an excessive load, then that load should be reduced before attempts are made to wean the patient from the ventilator. This is done by increasing lung compliance and decreasing airway resistance. Patients with low compliance or high airway resistance are usually not good candidates for weaning because this high respiratory load may result in muscle fatigue.

Respiratory muscle performance, like that of other skeletal muscles, can be improved by training. Respiratory muscles can be trained for strength or endurance. High-tension–low-volume work tends to stimulate strength conditioning through the development of increased sarcomeres (Figure 20-13). Low-tension high volume work tends to stimulate endurance training through development of increased mitochondrial density. Spontaneous breathing during T-piece trials or SIMV may tend to promote respiratory muscle strengthening, whereas pressure support ventilation (PSV) may tend to promote respiratory muscle endurance. Inspiratory muscle training using isocapnic hyperpnea or a resistive training device has been used during difficult weaning, and a commercially available resistive-training device can be incorporated into the ventilator circuit for such training.[98]

The tension-time index has been used to predict diaphragmatic fatigue (Figure 20-14).[99] Tension-time index is calculated as the product of the contractile force ($P_{di}/P_{di\,max}$) and contraction duration (duty cycle, T_i/T_{tot}). This requires measurement of mean transdiaphragmatic pressure (P_{di}), transdiaphragmatic pressure with maximal inhalation ($P_{di\,max}$), inspiratory time (T_i), and total respiratory cycle time (T_{tot}). A tension-time index > 0.15 is predictive of respiratory muscle fatigue. Measurement of transdiaphragmatic pressure requires esophageal and gastric pressure measurements, which are almost never performed in mechanically ventilated patients. A simpler form of tension-time index is the pressure-time index (PTI),[100] which can be determined more readily using equipment available in the critical care unit:

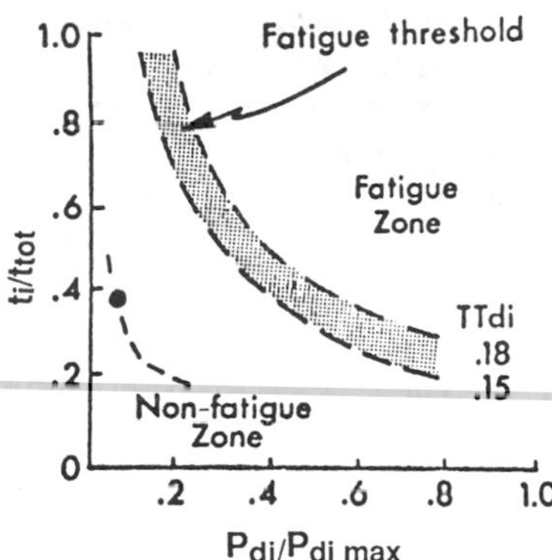

FIGURE 20-14. Tension-time index; note that the fatigue threshold is a tension time index of about 0.15–0.18 (From Grassino A, Macklom PT: Respiratory muscle fatigue and ventilatory failure. Ann Rev Med 35:625, 1984).

$$PTI = P_{breath}/MIP \times T_i/T_{tot}$$

where P_{breath} is the pressure required to generate a spontaneous breath. P_{breath} can be determined using esophageal balloon measurements during a short trial of spontaneous breathing (see Chap. 12). If an esophageal balloon is not present, P_{breath} can be estimated as:

$$P_{breath} = (PIP - PEEP) \times V_T\,sp/V_T\,mv$$

where PIP is peak airway pressure with a ventilator-delivered VT (VT mv), PEEP is the total PEEP level (including auto-PEEP), and VT sp is the patient's spontaneous VT.

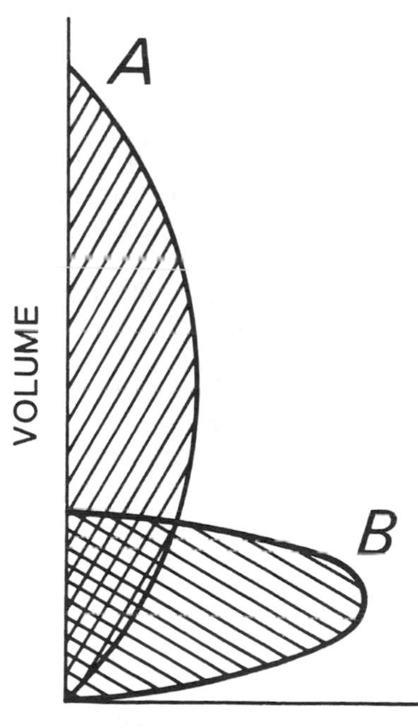

FIGURE 20-13. Low-tension/high-volume work **(A)** and high-tension/low-volume work **(B)**.

Determination of Adequate Pulmonary Function

This evaluation can be divided into two categories: the patient's mechanical or neuromuscular ability to breathe, and the lungs' ability to adequately oxygenate the arterial blood (eg, $\dot{V}/\dot{Q}$ inequality, diffusion defect, or shunt). The variables listed in Table 22-14 give the minimal values considered necessary to institute weaning.[101,102] Although these are a useful guide to weaning potential, they are less valuable in predicting weaning success or failure in patients requiring long-term ventilatory support than in those who have required mechanical ventilation for a shorter period.

A spontaneous VT of at least 5 mL/kg with a respiratory rate less than 30 breaths/min is considered acceptable for weaning. A patient who requires more than 10 L/min of ventilation while on the ventilator is not a good candidate for weaning because this is unlikely to be maintained during spontaneous breathing without fatigue. Tachypnea is often associated with failure to wean. Perhaps the best predictor of success or failure of weaning is the rapid shallow breathing index.[103,104] This index is calculated by dividing the respiratory rate by the VT (in liters). A rapid shallow breathing index > 100

TABLE 20-14. **Physiologic Parameters That Suggest Weaning Is Possible**

Tests of Mechanical Ability	
Maximal inspiratory pressure	>-20 cmH_2O
Vital capacity	>15 mL/kg
FEV_1	>10 mL/kg
Resting $\dot{V}E$	<10 L/min
Compliance on ventilator	>30 mL/cmH_2O
MVV	Twice spontaneous $\dot{V}E$
Spontaneous VT	>5 mL/kg
Spontaneous respiratory rate	<30 breaths/min and >6 breaths/min
Rate: VT ratio	<100
Tests of Gas Exchange	
PaO_2 on ≤40% O_2	≥60 mmHg
PaO_2/FIO_2	>200
PaO_2/PAO_2	>0.20
QS/QT	<0.15
VD/VT	<0.60

is predictive of weaning failure and < 100 is predictive of success.

Maximal inspiratory pressure is measured by attaching an aneroid manometer to the endotracheal or tracheostomy tube. The patient then forcibly inhales after maximal exhalation. When MIP is measured, it is recommended that a unidirectional valve be used, and that the airway is completely obstructed for 20 to 25 seconds (Figure 20-15).[105–108] An MIP greater than − 20 cmH_2O suggests adequate inspiratory muscle strength. However, if the patient has a high impedance (high resistance or low compliance), an MIP of − 20 cmH_2O may not be large enough to prevent fatigue. Serial MIP measurements may be useful during weaning to evaluate fatigue, and a drop in MIP indicates fatigue.

The vital capacity (VC) can be measured easily with any instrument that measures exhaled volume (eg, a Wright respirometer or portable electronic spirometer). The patient is instructed to take a maximal inspiration and then exhale maximally. The VC may be a better indicator of respiratory reserve than VT and is particularly useful in following the status of patients

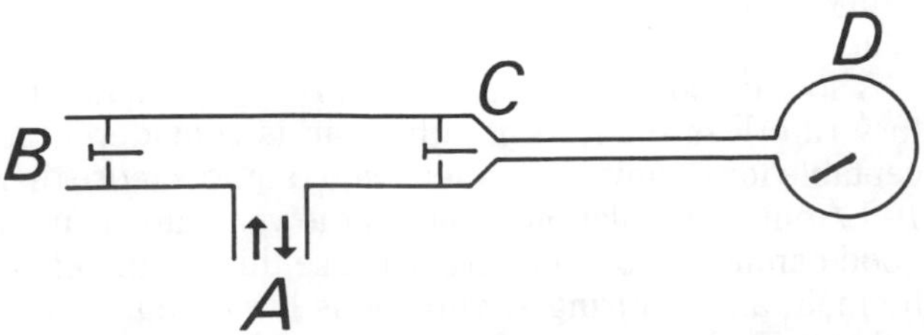

FIGURE 20-15. The one-way valve system used to measure maximal inspiratory pressure. The patient is connected at **(A)**, the manometer **(D)** is connected at **(C)**, and the patient exhales through **(B)**. In this way, maximal inspiratory pressure is measured at FRC.

with neuromuscular weakness (eg, Guillain-Barré syndrome or myasthenia gravis). The VC should be more than 15 mL/kg body weight for the patient to be able to sigh deeply enough to avoid atelectasis and to cough effectively.

The FEV_1 is considered by some practitioners to be a useful indicator of weaning ability in COPD patients. The vital capacity may be nearly normal if the patient slowly exhales. However, airway collapse may occur with forced exhalation. An FEV_1 of at least 10 mL/kg makes successful weaning more likely. However, FEV_1 is difficult to measure in intubated patients and is affected by the resistance of the endotracheal tube.

Although a patient may be able to produce an acceptable vital capacity when removed from the ventilator, his or her ability to sustain the muscular effort necessary for normal gas exchange is crucial. The maximal voluntary ventilation (MVV), although criticized because of its dependence on patient effort, is a test of this ability. The patient is a candidate for weaning if the spontaneous resting ventilation is < 10 L/min and can be doubled with an MVV maneuver.

The ability to measure spontaneous work of breathing at the bedside using an esophageal balloon has recently become commercially available (see Chap. 12).[109] Inspiratory work of breathing (W_I) measurements are probably not useful for most mechanically ventilated patients.[110] However, measurements of W_I may be useful in long-term mechanically ventilated patients who fail to wean from mechanical ventilation. In such patients, W_I/min ≤ 16 joules and W_I/L ≤ 1.4 joules are both necessary for successful weaning.[111] Other, more esoteric weaning parameters include measurements of O_2 cost of breathing and $P_{0.1}$.[88] These are difficult to accurately measure and are not commonly used.

A P(A − a)O_2 of less than 300 mmHg or a PaO_2 greater than 300 mmHg on 100% O_2 indicates adequate pulmonary oxygenation to allow weaning. However, because 100% O_2 predisposes patients to atelectasis, the use of 100% O_2 for the sole purpose of measuring P(A − a)O_2 should be avoided. If the PaO_2 is at least 60 mmHg on an FIO_2 of ≤ 0.40, the patient's oxygenation is acceptable to allow satisfactory weaning. In postoperative patients, the ability to maintain an arterial O_2 saturation > 90% during spontaneous breathing on room air and 5 cmH_2O CPAP has been shown to be predictive of successful extubation.[112]

The presence of significant intrapulmonary shunting interferes with the ability to adequately oxygenate arterial blood. Shunts greater than 20% make weaning difficult, with a shunt less than 15% being preferable. Frequent causes of intrapulmonary shunting in ventilator-dependent patients include retained secretions, bronchospasm, atelectasis, pulmonary edema, and pneumonia. These conditions can usually be corrected by use of suctioning, bronchodilators, chest physiotherapy, diuretics, and antibiotics. Infrequently, more invasive procedures such as bronchoscopy may be required.

The VD/VT should be < 0.55 before weaning is begun. Sometimes it is also useful to measure $\dot{V}CO_2$ and $\dot{V}O_2$ to assess weaning ability. An increase in $\dot{V}CO_2$ and

$\dot{V}O_2$ implies hypermetabolism, which results in an increased ventilatory requirement. An increase in V_D/V_T or $\dot{V}CO_2$ and $\dot{V}O_2$ increases the $\dot{V}_E$ requirement which can result in respiratory muscle fatigue.

Techniques for Weaning Patients From Mechanical Ventilation

Weaning a ventilator-dependent patient may involve one or a combination of several methods: T-piece trials of spontaneous breathing, IMV or SIMV, and PSV. Some clinicians also prefer to use PSV in combination with SIMV. As with many aspects of ventilator management, the choice of weaning technique is one of personal or institutional bias.

Psychologic preparation is very important and must begin before the patient has been disconnected from the ventilator. Before each weaning trial or weaning evaluation, the respiratory care practitioner or nurse should explain every detail of the procedure to the patient. The patient should be assured that there is continuous monitoring during weaning and a higher level of mechanical ventilation is provided, if necessary. Early in the weaning process, someone should always be with the patient for reassurance, to monitor the patient's tolerance of the weaning trial, and to check the equipment for malfunction. Frequent encouragement is needed because the success of weaning depends largely on the attitude and effort of the patient. The need for psychologic preparation appears to be directly proportional to the length of continuous mechanical ventilation. During weaning, setbacks are common, and the patient and staff must be prepared to accept this. Never wean to fatigue, and always provide adequate periods of rest between weaning trials.

T-piece Weaning

T-piece weaning allows spontaneous ventilation while providing supplemental O_2 as needed. The tubing from the gas source attaches to the T-piece, which in turn is connected to the endotracheal tube. While the patient is receiving humidified O_2 by a T-piece, care must be taken to prevent significant entrainment of room air. The application of a reservoir tubing distal to the patient's T-piece can prevent room air entrainment. With an adequate flow and reservoir, an F_{IO_2} of at least 0.5 can be delivered, if necessary. Patients with high inspiratory flow demand may require significantly higher gas flows, sometimes exceeding 70 to 90 L/min.

The design of the T-piece system should be simple. One way valves, reservoir bags, and elaborate systems can be hazardous. Valves can be inadvertently placed in the wrong direction, and reservoir bags can fill with water. A nebulizer is usually used for humidity, but a heated humidifier is preferred if the patient has reactive airways and is at risk for bronchospasm. A heated humidifier may also be needed when both high flow and a high F_{IO_2} are required.[113]

During periods of spontaneous breathing on the T-piece system, the cuff on the artificial airway may be deflated, removing pressure from the tracheal mucosa and allowing gas to pass around as well as through the tube. The cuff should not be deflated if there is a significant risk of aspirating upper airway secretions or gastric contents. The cuff must be inflated whenever ventilator-initiated breaths are being delivered.

Suctioning the patient before and during a T-piece weaning trial may help clear the airway, resulting in a reduced work of breathing and improved gas exchange. It is useful to hyperoxygenate the patient before and after suctioning to prevent hypoxemia and subsequent deterioration (see Chap. 19). Hyperinflation should also be used after suctioning to reverse suctioning-related atelectasis, but excessive airway pressures must be avoided.

Initially, spontaneous breathing may result in a decreased PaO_2. A smaller V_T may result in hypoventilation and hypoxemia. Therefore, the patient commonly needs a higher F_{IO_2} when initially off the ventilator. Increasing the F_{IO_2} by 0.1 above the ventilator setting is an acceptable rule of thumb to prevent hypoxemia. However, one should remember that some patients with chronic CO_2 retention may need a hypoxic drive to breathe, and raising the F_{IO_2} in these patients may be hazardous.

The patient should be as comfortable as possible before disconnection from the ventilator. A sitting or semirecumbent position is usually best tolerated during the weaning trial. Stress and blood gas changes during weaning may induce arrhythmias. An ECG monitor should be attached during weaning, because both early detection and early treatment of arrhythmias are essential.

The patient should be monitored closely during the T-piece trial. Indicators that the patient should be returned to the ventilator are listed in Table 20-15. These

TABLE 20-15. **Indicators That a Patient Should Be Returned to Mechanical Ventilation During Weaning**

Indicator	Magnitude
Blood pressure	Change >20 mmHg systolic or 10 mmHg diastolic
Pulse	Heart rate increase >20 beats/min
Respiratory rate	Increase of 10 breaths/min or rate >30/min
Tidal volume	<250 mL
Rate to tidal volume ratio	>100
MIP	A drop indicates respiratory muscle fatigue
Breathing pattern	Dyscoordinate breathing indicates respiratory muscle fatigue
PaO_2	<60 mmHg
$PaCO_2$	Increase greater than 10 mmHg from baseline
pH	Decrease greater than 0.10 from baseline
Pulse oximetry saturation	<90%
Significant ECG change	Increased ectopy

are guidelines and may not be applicable to all patients. For example, one may accept a lower PaO_2 or pH with a higher $PaCO_2$ in patients with chronic CO_2 retention. When the patient can tolerate being off the ventilator for 15 to 20 minutes, it may be useful to evaluate arterial blood gas values on the T-piece. However, evaluation of lung mechanics (ie, respiratory rate and VT) may be more useful than evaluation of blood gases. Pulse oximetry for monitoring of arterial oxygenation is useful during T-piece weaning. End-tidal PCO_2, however, is of limited value during weaning.

The patient should be monitored for signs of respiratory muscle fatigue during weaning trials. Early signs of fatigue include tachypnea and dyscoordinate breathing (respiratory alternans or respiratory paradox). A decrease in MIP during weaning also implies respiratory muscle fatigue. If fatigue occurs, the patient should be returned to full ventilatory support.

After each T-piece trial, the patient is returned to the ventilator for a period of rest. Ventilation during the rest periods is best provided by A-C mode or high SIMV rates. SIMV with a low rate or low-level PSV may not allow sufficient rest for the respiratory muscles. With T-piece weaning, the periods of spontaneous breathing become longer relative to the periods of ventilation until the patient is completely weaned from the ventilator.

A T-piece trial is not the same as a trial of spontaneous breathing with the patient attached to a ventilator in CPAP mode. In CPAP mode, most currently available ventilators supply spontaneous breaths from a demand valve. For older-generation ventilators, spontaneous breathing from a demand flow system increases the inspiratory work load imposed on the patient.[114–118] In some patients, this added work load may produce fatigue. However, this is not a problem with current-generation ventilators—particularly those with flow triggering. Advantages of CPAP mode over use of a T-piece for spontaneous breathing trials include convenience and the ability to better monitor the patient (eg, rate and VT) using the ventilator's monitoring and alarm systems.

Weaning may begin while the patient is still being ventilated with low levels of PEEP. In these patients, breathing by T-piece may result in a drop in functional residual capacity with deleterious effects on ventilatory mechanics and PaO_2.[119–121] In such cases, spontaneous breathing trials should be performed using a high-flow CPAP system or CPAP mode on the ventilator system rather than an ambient pressure T-piece.

Advantages of T-piece weaning include low cost and simplicity. The equipment is usually easy to assemble, with little risk of problems related to the equipment. The major disadvantage of T-piece weaning is that it requires the patient to abruptly resume complete spontaneous ventilatory support, thus requiring closer monitoring of the patient during T-piece weaning trials.

Weaning by SIMV

The use of SIMV involves gradually reducing the number of ventilator-delivered breaths, thereby allowing the patient to increase the amount of spontaneous breathing between the mandatory ventilator breaths.[122,123] Thus, ventilatory support is gradually withdrawn, allowing the patient to resume spontaneous breathing between ventilator-delivered breaths. As stated previously in this chapter, the patient may not relax the respiratory muscles during delivery of the mandatory breaths and may generate considerable effort during these breaths.

As with T-piece weaning, the patient should be closely monitored when SIMV weaning is begun (see Table 20-15). If the patient shows signs of fatigue during SIMV weaning, an increase in the mandatory rate is necessary, or the patient may need to be switched to A-C mode. During SIMV weaning, the patient may initially need rest periods of full ventilatory support.

An advantage of SIMV weaning is convenience. Simply changing the ventilator rate alters the patient's weaning progress. The patient's safety may be more readily ensured because ventilator-delivered breaths continue at the SIMV rate. By gradually decreasing the SIMV rate, the best $PaCO_2$ can be safely determined in those patients in whom the $PaCO_2$ before mechanical ventilation is unknown. This method may also be less stressful to the patient psychologically because of the gradual withdrawal of ventilatory support.

Although most currently available ventilators have a built-in SIMV mode, older ventilators require add-on circuitry to achieve IMV. This setup may be relatively complex, with the risk of incorrectly placed valves and disconnection of ventilator alarms. If add-on IMV circuits are used, extreme care must be taken to guarantee their correct assembly and function.

Virtually all commercially available ventilators deliver the spontaneous breaths during SIMV from a demand flow system. Although not an issue with current-generation ventilators,[124] there is an increased work of breathing from older ventilators.[114–118] The additional work imposed may be well tolerated by many patients, but there may be a substantial number of patients in whom this additional work results in fatigue. If fatigue occurs during demand-flow SIMV weaning, weaning may be successful if a continuous-flow system is used (eg, flow-by), or if T-piece weaning is used.

Although SIMV may be a convenient weaning technique, it does not necessarily reduce weaning time.[123] With a graded reduction in ventilator rate on SIMV, patients may remain intubated significantly longer than with T-piece weaning. The use of very low SIMV rates (ie, fewer than 4 breaths/min) can result in respiratory muscle fatigue and should be avoided.

Weaning by PSV

Several approaches can be used when weaning with PSV.[125] One of these involves choosing a level of pressure support that provides a targeted VT and respiratory rate, then decreasing the pressure support level in a stepwise fashion (provided that VT and rate remain adequate). The second approach involves a combination of SIMV and PSV, in which the patient's spontaneous breaths are supported by a low level of pressure. With this approach, the patient is weaned by decreasing the number of ventilator breaths (as in standard SIMV weaning). Low-level PSV may provide several beneficial effects. It eliminates the inspiratory work imposed by the ventilator and endotracheal tubes during spontaneous breathing.[126,127] It may be a more comfortable mode of ventilation than SIMV for some patients, and it promotes endurance training of respiratory muscles. It has been shown that PSV may improve the efficiency of breathing patterns in some difficult-to-wean patients (Figure 20-16).[128–130]

The appropriate level of PSV may be difficult to judge. A pressure support level set too high results in very little patient work, whereas too little PSV can result in fatigue. In difficult cases, measurements of esophageal pressure may be useful to titrate the PSV level.[131,132] Another concern with high levels of PSV is that it can result in expiratory muscle activation to terminate breath delivery. Because ventilators use flow deceleration to terminate inspiration during PSV, problems may occur during PSV with system leaks (eg, bronchopleural fistula).[133]

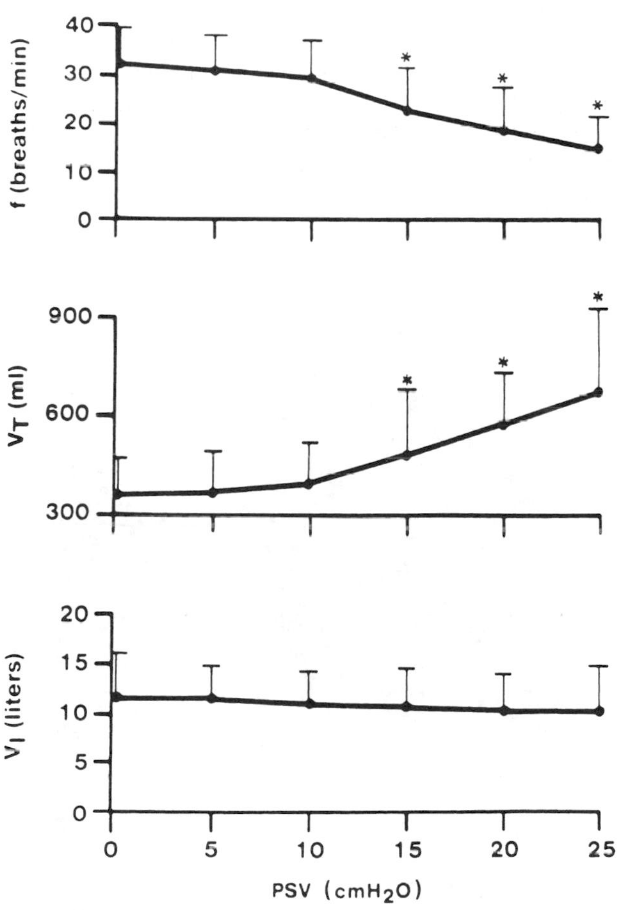

FIGURE 20-16. Effect of PSV on breathing pattern. Note the increase in tidal volume and decrease in respiratory rate with increasing levels of PSV. (Reprinted with permission from Ershowsky P, Krieger B: Changes in breathing pattern during pressure support ventilation. Respir Care 32:1011, 1987).

Which Weaning Technique Is Best?

A single, rigid approach to weaning is not appropriate for all patients, and most patients can be weaned by either T-piece, SIMV, or PSV. It is the occasional difficult-to-wean patient who presents a clinical dilemma. If a weaning attempt is not successful for a specific patient, it seems prudent to try another approach. With T-piece trials, SIMV, PSV, and variations and combinations, a successful weaning plan can be tailored to the needs of most patients. Large multi-institutional, randomized studies of weaning techniques have reported conflicting results.[134,135] The most successful approach to weaning is likely to be a strategy that alternates periods of work and rest that avoids respiratory muscle fatigue.

In a multi-institutional study,[134] 109 patients were randomized to PSV, SIMV, or T-piece weaning. These were difficult-to-wean patients who could not tolerate a 2-hour trial of spontaneous breathing. In the study, the probability of complete weaning from the ventilator at 21 days was greater in the group randomized to PSV weaning (Figure 20-17).

Another study compared IMV, PSV, intermittent trials of spontaneous breathing, and a once-daily trial of spontaneous breathing.[135] Patients assigned to the once-daily trial of spontaneous breathing were extubated if they tolerated a 2-hour breathing trial; otherwise they were returned to assist-control ventilation for a 24-hour period. A once-daily trial of spontaneous breathing led to extubation about three times more quickly than IMV and twice as quickly as PSV (Figure 20-18). Multiple daily trials of spontaneous breathing were as successful as a once-daily trial of spontaneous breathing.

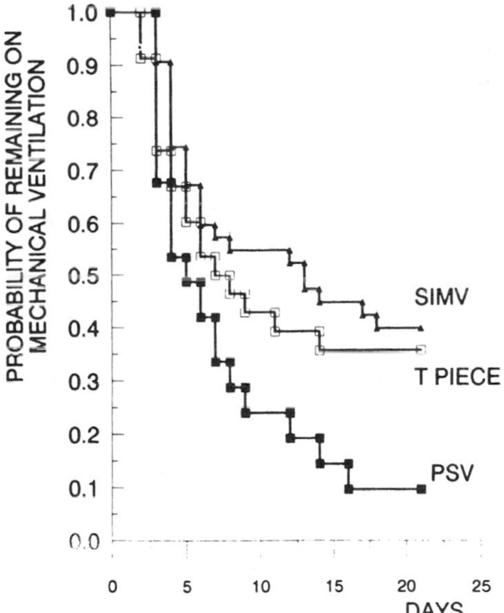

FIGURE 20-17. Probability of remaining on mechanical ventilation in patients with prolonged difficulty in tolerating spontaneous breathing. (From Brochard L, Rauss A, Benito S, Conti G, Mancebo J, Rekik N, Gasparetto A, & Lemaire F: Comparison of three methods of gradual withdrawal from ventilatory support during weaning from mechanical ventilation. Am J Respir Crit Care Med 150:896, 1994).

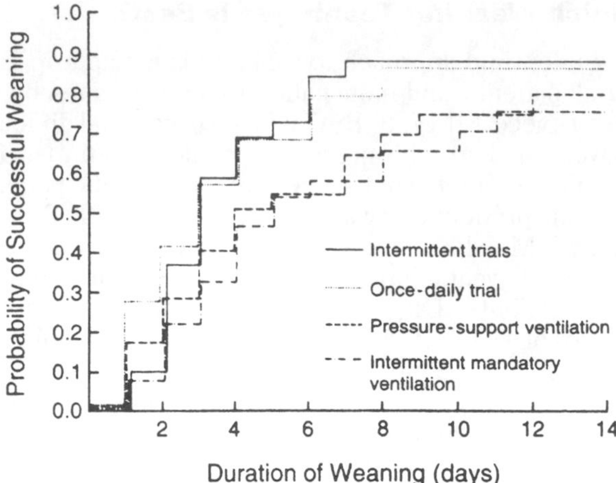

FIGURE 20-18. Probability of successful weaning using three weaning techniques. (From Estaban A, Frutos F, Tobin MJ, et al: A comparison of four methods of weaning patients from mechanical ventilation. N Engl J Med 332:345, 1995).

Weaning From the Artificial Airway

Although weaning and extubation are often closely related, they are technically separate events. For a patient to be extubated, not only does the patient need to be able to breathe spontaneously, but the patient must be able to protect the airway and adequately clear secretions. Prolonged spontaneous breathing before extubation is usually not desirable because of the high work of breathing imposed by the artificial airway (Figure 20-19),[136–138] and prolonged low-rate IMV may not be desirable because of the additional work imposed by the ventilator in addition to the airway. Consequently, some patients can be successfully extubated without a successful trial of spontaneous breathing.[121] However, it is usually best to evaluate the patient's ability to breathe spontaneously without any ventilatory support before extubation.

When weaning from a tracheostomy, a fenestrated tube may be useful (Figure 20-20).[139] With the cuff deflated and the inner cannula removed from this tube, the patient can breathe through the normal tube channel, through the fenestration in the posterior (superior) portion of the tube, and around the tube. This results in an increased V_T for the same amount of effort by reducing the resistance to airflow. This tube can also be plugged to evaluate the patient's ability to breathe through the upper airway. However, this tube should **never** be plugged unless the fenestration is open and the cuff is deflated; otherwise, the patient's airway may be totally obstructed! If the patient needs to be reconnected to the ventilator, the inner cannula must be inserted and the cuff inflated. Unfortunately, the fenestration in the tracheostomy tube is often not located in the lumen of the airway, but is occluded by tissue anterior to the trachea or by the posterior tracheal wall. Unless the fenestration is properly centered in the trachea, fenestrated tubes should not be used. A one-way valve (eg, Passey-Muir) can also be attached to a fenestrated tracheostomy tube. Such a valve allows inspiration through the tracheostomy tube and exhalation through the upper airway. This may allow the patient to speak and control exhalation (pursed lips). However, such a valve should only be used if the upper airway is unobstructed.

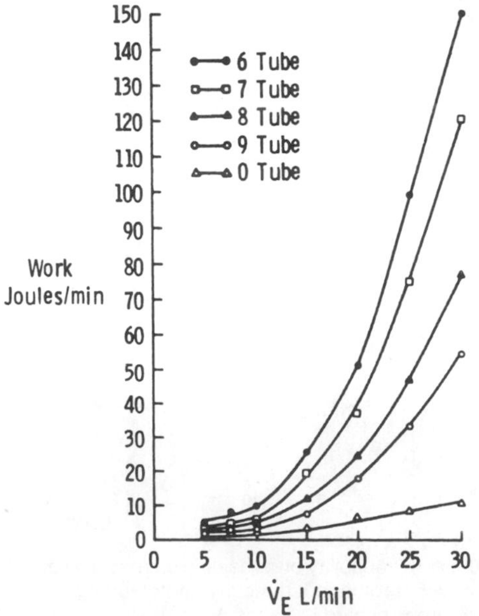

FIGURE 20-19. Effect of endotracheal tube size on work of breathing. (From Shapiro M, Wilson RK, Casar G et al: Work of breathing through different sized endotracheal tubes. Crit Care Med 14:1028, 1986)

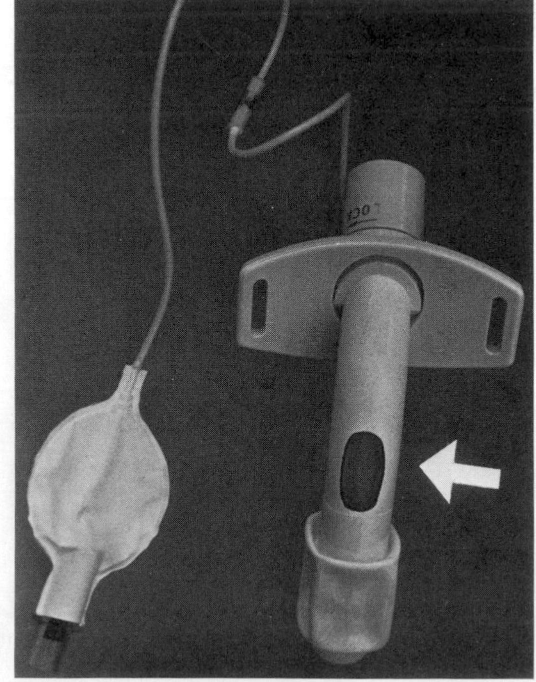

FIGURE 20-20. Fenestrated tracheostomy tube.

ADJUNCTIVE THERAPIES RELATED TO MECHANICAL VENTILATION

Permissive Hypercapnia

Permissive hypercapnia is a ventilatory strategy in which controlled mechanical hypoventilation is given priority over the potential deleterious effects of high alveolar pressure and overdistension.[140–143] As discussed previously in this chapter, the peak alveolar pressure during mechanical ventilation should ideally be kept < 35 cmH_2O. In addition, PEEP should be set at 8 to 12 cmH_2O during ventilation of patients with ARDS. The result is often a V_T of 5 to 8 mL/kg. Furthermore, long inspiratory times are often necessary to raise $\bar{P}aw$, which limits the respiratory rate at which auto-PEEP occurs.

Ventilator settings made to avoid alveolar overdistension during mechanical ventilation of patients with ARDS almost always result in hypercapnia. Uncontrolled studies have shown improved survival when overdistension is avoided and permissive hypercapnia is allowed.[144] What is unclear is the level of hypercapnia that can be safely tolerated. Anecdotal experience has shown that $PaCO_2$ levels as high as 60 mmHg are often well tolerated, and higher levels may be tolerated well if they do not occur acutely. The adverse effects of permissive hypercapnia are related to the resultant pH rather than the $PaCO_2$ **per se**. A pH > 7.25 is usually well tolerated, provided that the patient is hemodynamically stable and does not have closed head injury. Because CO_2 is a strong respiratory stimulant, appropriate sedation or paralysis is needed to allow permissive hypercapnia.

Positioning

In some patients with ARDS, there is an improvement in PaO_2 when they are turned from the supine to the prone position.[63,145–147] The effectiveness of this therapy is presumably related to an improvement in $\dot{V}/\dot{Q}$ in the prone position. This response tends to be greater for the first turn than for subsequent turns, and the effect is lost after 4 to 6 hours. Although this therapy is technically difficult, it is worthy of consideration in patients with severe hypoxemia in spite of a high FIO_2 and PEEP. To avoid airway dislodgement, a tracheostomy is preferable (but not absolutely required) for prone positioning. It should also be recognized that this therapy is not effective in 100% of cases and fails to improve PaO_2 in 1/4 of ARDS patients.

In patients with unilateral lung disease, positioning with the good lung down results in a higher PaO_2. This is caused by a greater blood flow to dependent lung zones, which presumably improves $\dot{V}/\dot{Q}$ by placing the more ventilated lung in the area of greatest blood flow. Positioning is often more effective than PEEP in patients with unilateral lung disease who are hypoxemic. Application of PEEP may shunt pulmonary blood flow away from the healthy lung to the diseased lung, thus increasing right-to-left shunt and decreasing PaO_2, so PEEP should be used judiciously in patients with unilateral lung disease.[63]

Turning patients at regular intervals can decrease the frequency of pulmonary complications in mechanically ventilated patients. Because frequent turning is labor intensive, there is interest in the use of beds that automatically turn the patient (Figure 20-21). Use of these beds for critically ill, mechanically ventilated patients has been shown to decrease the incidence of pulmonary complications, but their effect on overall outcome is unclear. Further, use of these beds is expensive, and their cost-effectiveness remains to be determined.

Inhaled Nitric Oxide

Inhaled nitric oxide is an experimental therapy that has been shown to improve PaO_2 in some ARDS patients.[148–150] Nitric oxide is a selective pulmonary vasodilator.[151] This means that it affects only that part of the pulmonary tissue that is ventilated, and it has minimal systemic effects. In the lungs of patients with ARDS, nitric oxide may improve blood flow to ventilated alveoli and thus improve pulmonary shunt and PaO_2. In patients with pulmonary hypertension, inhaled nitric oxide may decrease pulmonary vascular resistance without causing systemic hypotension. This is in marked contrast to agents such as nitroprusside (a nitric oxide donor), which produces systemic as well as pulmonary vasodilation and causes hypoxemia by increasing blood flow to underventilated areas of the lungs. Inhaled nitric oxide has a rapid onset of effect when initiated and a rapid loss of effect when discontinued (ie, within minutes).

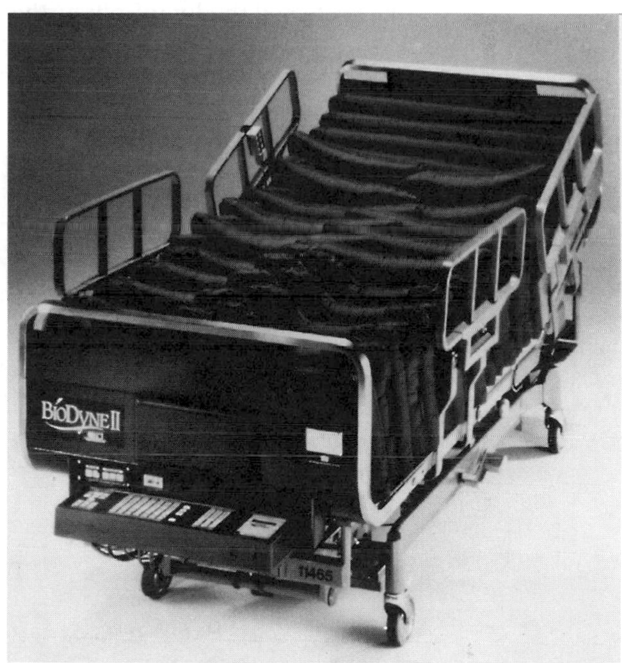

FIGURE 20-21. Kinetic bed designed to provide automatic continuous side-to-side rotation of the patient.

Due to its experimental nature, commercially available systems to administer inhaled nitric oxide to mechanically ventilated patients are not available. Nitric oxide is typically supplied in a high concentration cylinder (800 ppm), mixed with air or nitrogen in a blender to reduce its concentration, and delivered to the mechanical ventilator system (Figure 20-22). When used in the treatment of ARDS, nitric oxide concentrations < 20 ppm are typically used. The concentration of nitric oxide (and nitrogen dioxide) delivered is analyzed with either an electrochemical or chemiluminescence analyzer.

There are several significant potential complications of inhaled nitric oxide in mechanically ventilated ARDS patients. When mixed with O_2, nitric oxide is converted to nitrogen dioxide. Because nitrogen dioxide is toxic, levels < 2 ppm should be maintained. The conversion of nitric oxide to nitrogen dioxide depends on the nitric oxide concentration, F_{IO_2}, and residence time between nitric oxide and O_2.[152] Another complication of inhaled nitric oxide is methemoglobinemia, and methemoglobin levels should be determined frequently (daily, or less, depending on dose) during nitric oxide therapy. Finally, some patients have significant rebound when nitric oxide is discontinued, and for this reason care must be taken not to accidentally or prematurely discontinue the treatment.

Extracorporeal Techniques

Long-term extracorporeal support for acute respiratory failure was introduced in the 1970s. A multicenter trial of extracorporeal membrane oxygenation (ECMO) showed no difference in mortality between patients randomized to ECMO (with positive pressure ventilation) or positive pressure ventilation (without ECMO).[153] However, that study has been criticized because it did not use a strategy that protected the lung from further injury associated with mechanical ventilation during ECMO. More recently, venovenous techniques have been used for extracorporeal CO_2 removal.[154] These approaches combine extracorporeal techniques with strategies designed to rest the lungs during severe ARDS. Uncontrolled studies have demonstrated a high survival with this approach.[155] However, a randomized trial showed no difference in mortality between extracorporeal CO_2 removal (with ventilation designed to rest the lungs) and ventilation designed to avoid acute lung injury (without extracorporeal CO_2 removal). Because of its invasiveness, its expense, and the absence of randomized studies that demonstrate its effectiveness, extracorporeal methods in adult patients with ARDS have not been well accepted. However, ECMO has been shown to improve mortality in neonates with a variety of conditions, and it has been commonly accepted by clinicians in this population of patients.[156]

High-Frequency Ventilation

High-frequency ventilation is ventilatory support at rates greater than normal.[157,158] By using higher rates, the V_T and the associated peak airway pressure are both reduced. The rationale for use of high-frequency ventilation is to reduce airway pressure and the risk of barotrauma, and to improve $\dot{V}/\dot{Q}$ and gas exchange. In spite of periodic enthusiasm for this technique in the past, improvement in outcome with the use of high-frequency ventilation in adults is lacking. A commonly discussed potential application for high-frequency ventilation in adults is in the management of bronchopleural fistulas. However, high-frequency ventilation is probably no more effective than conventional methods to treat bronchopleural fistulas in adults.

In contrast to adult applications, high-frequency ventilation is a useful technique in neonates.[159,160] In this patient population, high-frequency ventilation may reduce the risk of air leaks, improve ventilation with preexisting air leaks, and decrease the incidence of ventilator-associated lung injury such as bronchopulmonary dys-

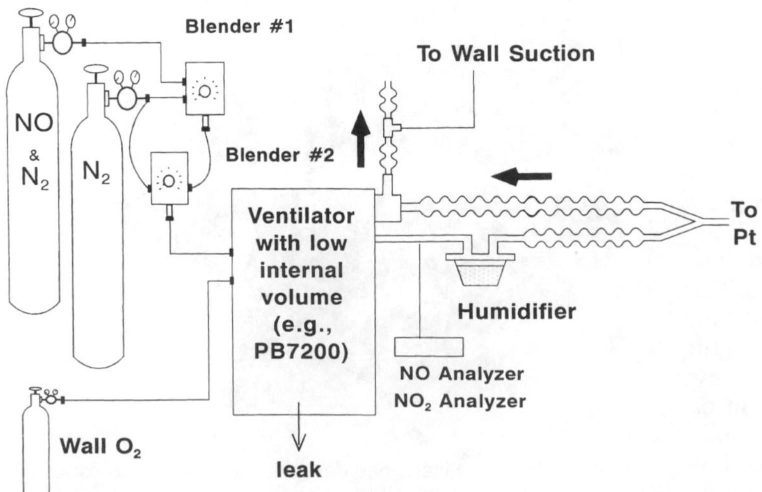

FIGURE 20-22. Schematic diagram of a system for inhaled nitric oxide delivery during mechanical ventilation.

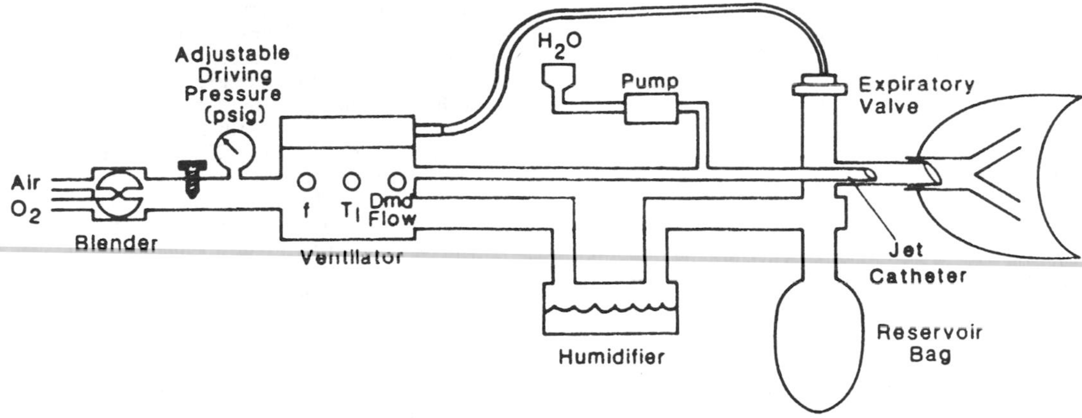

FIGURE 20-23. Schematic illustration of a system to provide high frequency jet ventilation (From Branson RD, Hess DR, Chatburn RL: Respiratory Care Equipment. Philadelphia, JB Lippincott, 1995).

plasia. These beneficial effects are likely due to the ability to provide an adequate $\bar{P}aw$, while limiting peak alveolar pressure.

The two most common approaches to high-frequency ventilation are high-frequency jet ventilation and high-frequency oscillation. High-frequency jet ventilators typically operate at rates of 110 to 400 breaths/min, and high-frequency oscillators operate at frequencies of 400 to 2400 breaths/min. High-frequency jet ventilation provides an intermittent flow of gas from a high-pressure source (20 to 50 psi) through a catheter placed into the endotracheal tube or tracheostomy tube (Figure 20-23). A solenoid controls the frequency and inspiratory time. As gas exits the catheter at high velocity, jet mixing drags additional flow into the airway. An auxiliary gas flow is necessary to supply the additional gas entrained by the jet effect. In some cases, the jet ventilator is designed to operate in tandem with a conventional ventilator (eg, Bunnell). Jet ventilators are commercially available for both neonatal and adult applications. The system to provide high-frequency oscillation can be a loudspeaker, diaphragm, or piston pump (Figure 20-24). To prevent CO_2 retention and to provide a supply of O_2, a bias flow is provided. A high frequency oscillator is currently available for infant and pediatric applications (Sensormedics).

Tracheal Gas Insufflation

Tracheal gas insufflation is a technique in which the anatomic dead space is flushed to decrease $PaCO_2$ or $\dot{V}_E$ requirements.[161–163] The technique involves placing a small catheter into the trachea (Figure 20-25). The central airways are then flushed by the catheter during either inhalation or exhalation, or throughout the respiratory cycle. Care must be taken to avoid augmentation of V_T, peak alveolar pressure, or PEEP during use of tracheal gas insufflation.[164] Most studies of this technique have been performed using animal models with normal lung function. The technique may be less useful with ARDS patients,[165–167] who have a high alveolar dead space and are ventilated with a short expiratory time (ie, long inspiratory time). Very little data is available regarding use of tracheal gas insufflation in patients, and it should be considered experimental at this time.

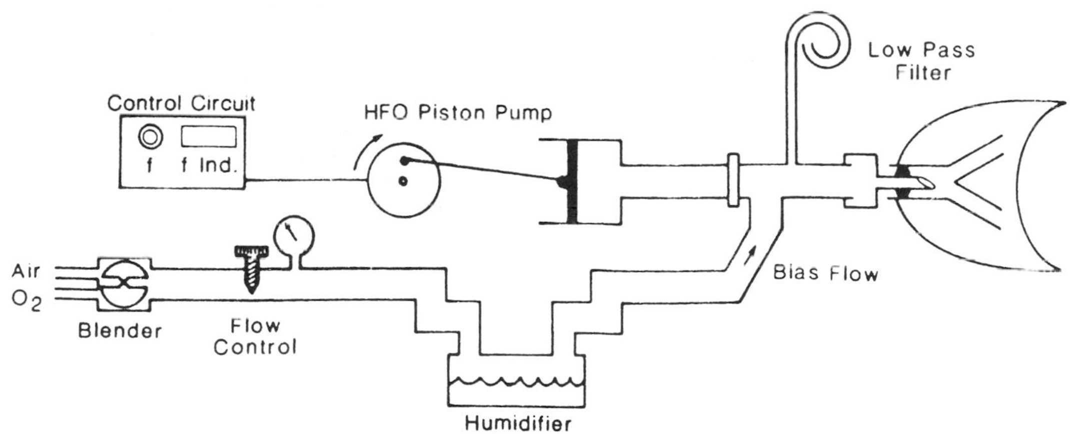

FIGURE 20-24. Schematic illustration of a system to provide high frequency oscillation (From Branson RD, Hess DR, Chatburn RL: Respiratory Care Equipment. Philadelphia, JB Lippincott, 1995).

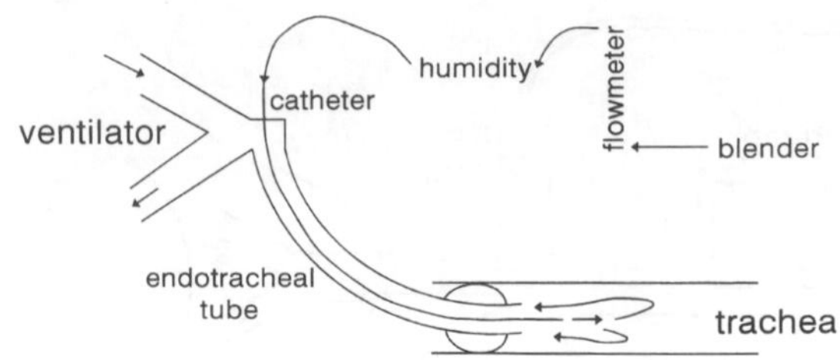

FIGURE 20-25. Schematic illustration of a system to provide tracheal gas insufflation.

Liquid Ventilation

Perfluorocarbon liquid ventilation is a promising technique in the treatment of infants and adults with acute respiratory failure. Animal studies and studies with newborn humans have been promising.[168–170] This technique has been shown to improve gas exchange, improve compliance, and reduce airway pressure requirements. Investigations in this technique have been underway for more than 20 years, and clinical trials with infants and adults are now underway. Most commonly, partial liquid ventilation is used. With this approach, the functional residual capacity is filled with perfluorocarbon, and the lungs are ventilated with conventional gas ventilation.[171]

REFERENCES

1. Pierson DJ: Indications for mechanical ventilation in acute respiratory failure. Respir Care 28:570, 1983
2. Aldrich TK, Prezant DJ: Indications for Mechanical Ventilation. In MJ Tobin: Principles and Practice of Mechanical Ventilation. New York, McGraw-Hill, 1994
3. Strieter RM, Lynch JP: Complications in the ventilated patient. Clin Chest Med 9:127, 1988
4. Zwillich CW, Pierson DJ, Creagh CE, et al: Complications of assisted ventilation: A prospective study of 356 consecutive cases. Am J Med 57:161, 1974
5. Pingleton SK: Complications Associated with Mechanical Ventilation. In MJ Tobin: Principles and Practice of Mechanical Ventilation. New York, McGraw-Hill, 1994
6. Shelly MP: Inspired gas conditioning. Respir Care 37:1070, 1992
7. Hess D, Kacmarek RM: Technical Aspects of the Patient-Ventilator Interface. In MJ Tobin: Principles and Practice of Mechanical Ventilation. New York, McGraw-Hill, 1994
8. Pierson DJ: Alveolar rupture during mechanical ventilation: Role of PEEP, peak airway pressure, and distending volume. Respir Care 33:472, 1988
9. Pierson DJ: Barotrauma and Bronchopleural Fistula. In MJ Tobin: Principles and Practice of Mechanical Ventilation. New York, McGraw-Hill, 1994
10. Dreyfuss D, Soler P, Basset G, Saumon G: High inflation pressure pulmonary edema: Respective effects of high airway pressure, high tidal volume, and positive end-expiratory pressure. Am Rev Respir Dis 137:1159, 1988
11. Dreyfuss D, Saumon G: Role of tidal volume, FRC, and end-inspiratory volume in the development of pulmonary edema following mechanical ventilation. Am Rev Respir Dis 148:1194, 1993
12. Slutsky AS: ACCP consensus conference: Mechanical ventilation. Chest 104:1833, 1993
13. George DL: Epidemiology of ventilator-associated pneumonia. Infect Control Hosp Epidemiol 14:163, 1993
14. Dreyfuss D, Djedanini K, Weber P, et al: Prospective study of nosocomial pneumonia and of patient and circuit colonization during mechanical ventilation with circuit changes every 48 hours versus no change. Am Rev Respir Dis 143:738, 1991
15. Hess D, Burns E, Romagnoli D, Kacmarek RM: Weekly ventilator circuit changes: A strategy to reduce costs without affecting pneumonia rates. Anesthesiology 82:903, 1995
16. Kollef MH, Shapiro SD, Fraser VJ, et al: Mechanical ventilation with or without 7-day circuit changes: A randomized controlled trial. Ann Intern Med 123:168, 1995
17. Cook DJ, Laine LA, Guyatt GH, Raffin TA: Nosocomial pneumonia and the role of gastric pH: A meta analysis. Chest 100:7, 1991
18. Rijan P, Dawson J, Teres D, et al: Continuous infusion of cimetidine versus sucralfate: Incidence of pneumonia and bleeding compared. Crit Care Med 18(suppl):253, 1990
19. Shepherd KE, Faulkner CS, Thal GD, Leiter JC: Acute, subacute, and chronic histologic effects of simulated aspiration of a 0.7% sucralfate suspension in rats. Crit Care Med 23:532, 1995
20. Pingleton SK: Nutritional support in the mechanically ventilated patient. Clin Chest Med 9:101, 1988
21. Perreault T, Gutkowska J: Role of atrial natriuretic factor in lung physiology and pathology. Am J Respir Crit Care Med 151:226, 1995
22. Borel C, Hanley D, Diringer MN, Rogers MC: Intensive management of severe head injury. Chest 98:180, 1990
23. Gattinoni L, Pesenti A, Bombino M, et al: Relationships between lung computed tomographic density, gas exchange, and PEEP in acute respiratory failure. Anesthesiology 69:824, 1988
24. Durbin CG, Wallace KK: Oxygen toxicity in the critically ill patient. Respir Care 38:739, 1993
25. Hill NS: Noninvasive ventilation: Does it work, for whom, and how? Am Rev Respir Dis 147:1050, 1993
26. Pennock BE, Crawshaw L, Kaplan PD: Noninvasive mask ventilation for acute respiratory failure: Institution of a new therapeutic technology for routine use in patients with respiratory failure. Chest 105:441, 1994
27. Meduri GU, Turner RE, Abou-Shala N, et al: Noninvasive positive pressure ventilation via face mask: First-line intervention in patients with acute hypercapnic and hypoxemic respiratory failure. Chest 109:179, 1996
28. Brochard L, Mancebo J, Wysocki M, et al: Noninvasive ventilation for acute exacerbations of chronic obstructive pulmonary disease. N Engl J Med 333:817, 1995
29. Kramer N, Meyer TJ, Mehareg J, et al: Randomized, prospective trial of noninvasive positive pressure ventilation in acute respiratory failure. Am J Respir Crit Care Med 151:1799, 1995
30. Bach JR, Saporito LR: Indications and criteria for decannulation and transition from invasive to noninvasive long-term ventilatory support. Respir Care 39:532, 1994
31. Kacmarek RM, Hess D: Basic Principles of Ventilator Machinery. In MJ Tobin: Principles and Practice of Mechanical Ventilation. New York, McGraw-Hill, 1994
32. Mador MJ: Assist-Control Ventilation. In MJ Tobin: Principles and Practice of Mechanical Ventilation. New York, McGraw-Hill, 1994
33. Weisman IM, Rinaldo JE, Rogers RM, Sanders MH: Intermittent mandatory ventilation. Am Rev Respir Dis 127:641, 1983
34. Sassoon CSH: Intermittent Mandatory Ventilation. In MJ Tobin: Principles and Practice of Mechanical Ventilation. New York, McGraw-Hill, 1994
35. MacIntyre NR: Respiratory support during pressure support ventilation. Chest 89:677, 1986
36. Kacmarek RM: The role of pressure support ventilation in reducing work of breathing. Respir Care 33:99, 1988
37. Brochard L: Pressure Support Ventilation. In MJ Tobin: Principles and Practice of Mechanical Ventilation. New York, McGraw-Hill, 1994
38. Quan SF, Parides GC, Knoper SR: Mandatory minute volume ventilation: An overview. Respir Care 35:898, 1990
39. Downs JB, Klein EF, Desautels D, et al: Intermittent mandatory ventilation: A new approach to weaning patients from mechanical ventilation. Chest 64:331, 1973
40. Amato MBP, Barbas CSV, Bonassa J, et al: Volume-assured pressure support ventilation (VAPSV): A new approach for reducing muscle workload during acute respiratory failure. Chest 102:1225, 1992
41. Branson RD, MacIntyre NR: Dual-control modes of mechanical ventilation. Respir Care 41:294, 1996

42. Sassoon CSH: Mechanical ventilator design and function: The trigger variable. Respir Care 37:1056, 1992
43. Sassoon CSH, Rosario ND, Fei R, et al: Influence of pressure- and flow-triggered synchronous intermittent mandatory ventilation on inspiratory muscle work. Crit Care Med 22:1933, 1994
44. Branson RD, Campbell RS, Davis D, Johnson DJ: Comparison of pressure and flow triggering systems during continuous positive airway pressure. Chest 106:540, 1994
45. Giuliani R, Mascia L, Recchia F, et al: Patient-ventilator interaction during synchronized intermittent mandatory ventilation: Effects of flow triggering. Am J Respir Crit Care Med 151:1, 1995
46. Goulet RL, Hess D, Kacmarek RM: Flow versus pressure triggering in mechanically ventilated adult patients. Respir Care 40:1205, 1995
47. Sassoon CSH, Gruer SE: Characteristics of the ventilator pressure and flow trigger variables. Intensive Care Med 21:159, 1995
48. Cinnella G, Conti G, Lofaso F, et al: Effects of assisted ventilation on the work of breathing: Volume-controlled versus pressure-controlled ventilation. Am J Respir Crit Care Med 153:1025, 1996
49. Jubran A, Van de Graaff WB, Tobin MJ: Variability of patient-ventilator interaction with pressure support ventilation in patients with chronic obstructive pulmonary disease. Am J Respir Crit Care Med 152:129, 1995
50. Abraham E, Yoshihara G: Cardiorespiratory effects of pressure-controlled ventilation in severe respiratory failure. Chest 98: 1445, 1990
51. Rappaport SH, Shpiner R, Yoshihara G, et al: Randomized, prospective trial of pressure-limited versus volume-controlled ventilation in severe respiratory failure. Crit Care Med 22:22, 1994
52. Kacmarek RM, Hess D: Pressure-controlled inverse-ratio ventilation: Panacea or auto-PEEP? (Editorial). Respir Care 100:494, 1991
53. Mang H, Kacmarek RM, Ritz R, et al: Cardiorespiratory effects of volume and pressure-controlled ventilation at various I:E ratios in an acute lung injury model. Am J Respir Crit Care Med 151:731, 1995
54. Lessard MR, Guerot E, Lorino F, et al: Effects of pressure control with different I:E ratios versus volume-controlled ventilation on respiratory mechanics, gas exchange, and hemodynamics in patients with adult respiratory distress. Anesthesiology 80:983, 1994
55. Branson RD, Campbell RS: Sighs: Wasted breath or breath of fresh air? Respir Care 37:462, 1992
56. Lee PC, Helsmoortel CM, Cohn SM, Fink MP: Are low tidal volumes safe? Chest 97:425, 1990
57. Leatherman JW, Lari RL, Iber C, Nwy AL: Tidal volume reduction in ARDS: Effect on cardiac output and arterial oxygenation. Chest 99:1227, 1991
58. Kiisk R, Takala J, Kari A, Milic-Emili J: Effect of tidal volume on gas exchange and oxygen transport in the adult respiratory distress syndrome. Am Rev Respir Dis 146:1131, 1992
59. Corbridge TC, Wood LDH, Crawford GP, et al: Adverse effects of large tidal volume and low PEEP in canine acid aspiration. Am Rev Respir Dis 142:311, 1990
60. Rossi A, Ranieri VM: Positive End-Expiratory Pressure. In MJ Tobin: Principles and Practice of Mechanical Ventilation. New York, McGraw-Hill, 1994
61. Smith RA: Physiologic PEEP. Respir Care 33:620, 1988
62. Muscedere JG, Mullen JBM, Gan K, Slutsky AS: Tidal ventilation at low airway pressures can augment lung injury. Am J Respir Crit Care Med 149:1327, 1994
63. Hess D, Agarwal NN, Myers CL: Positioning, lung function, and kinetic bed therapy. Respir Care 37:181, 1992
64. Smith TC, Marini JJ: Impact of PEEP on lung mechanics and work of breathing in severe airflow obstruction. J Appl Physiol 65:1488, 1988
65. Petrof BJ, Lagare M, Goldberg P, et al: Continuous positive airway pressure reduces work of breathing and dyspnea during weaning from mechanical ventilation in severe chronic obstructive pulmonary disease. Am Rev Respir Dis 141:281, 1990
66. Tobin MJ, Lodato RF: PEEP, auto-PEEP, and waterfalls (Editorial). Chest 96:449, 1989
67. Primiano FP, Chatburn RL, Lough MD: Mean airway pressure: Theoretical considerations. Crit Care Med 10:378, 1982
68. Jubran A, Tobin MJ: Reliability of pulse oximetry in titrating supplemental oxygen therapy in ventilator-dependent patients. Chest 97:1420, 1990
69. Hess D, Good C, Didyoung R, et al: The validity of assessing arterial blood gases 10 minutes after an FIO_2 change in mechanically ventilated patients without chronic pulmonary disease. Respir Care 30:1037, 1985
70. Forbat AF, Her C: Correction for gas compression in mechanical ventilators. Anesth Analg 59:488, 1980
71. Hess D, McCurty S, Simmons M: Compression volume in adult mechanical ventilator circuits: A comparison of five disposable circuits and a nondisposable circuit. Respir Care 36:1113, 1991
72. Valeri KL, Hill TV, Taft AA, et al: The effect of time and warming on breathing circuit compliance. Respir Care 39:793, 1994
73. Grootendorst AF, Lugtigheid G, van der Weygert EJ: Error in ventilator measurements of intrinsic PEEP: Cause and remedy. Respir Care 38:348, 1993
74. Hess D: Noninvasive respiratory monitoring during ventilator support. Crit Care Nurs Clin North Am 3:565, 1991
75. Van Hook CJ, Carilli AD, Haponik EF: Hemodynamic effects of positive end-expiratory pressure: Historical perspective. Am J Med 81:307, 1986
76. Miro AM, Pinsky MR: Heart-Lung Interactions. In MJ Tobin: Principles and Practice of Mechanical Ventilation. New York, McGraw-Hill, 1994
77. Marini JJ, Culver BN, Butler J: Mechanical effects of lung distension with positive pressure in cardiac function. Am Rev Respir Dis 124:382, 1981
78. Marini JJ, Rodriguiz M, Lamb V: The inspiratory workload of patient-initiated mechanical ventilation. Am Rev Respir Dis 134: 902, 1986
79. Marini JJ, Smith TC, Lamb VJ: External work output and force generation during synchronized intermittent mechanical ventilation. Am Rev Respir Dis 138:1169, 1988
80. Sassoon CSH, Light RW, Lodia R, et al: Pressure-time product on T-piece, continuous positive airway pressure and pressure support ventilation during weaning from mechanical ventilation. Am Rev Respir Dis 143:469, 1991
81. Segredo V, Caldwell JE, Matthay MA, et al: Persistent paralysis in critically ill patients after long-term administration of vecuronium. N Engl J Med 327:524, 1992
82. Kupfer Y, Namba T, Kaldawi E, Tessler S: Prolonged weakness after long-term infusion of vecuronium. Ann Intern Med 117:484, 1992
83. Hansen-Flaschen JH, Cowen J, Raps ED: Neuromuscular blockade in the ICU: More than we bargained for. Am Rev Respir Dis 147:234, 1993
84. Sporn PHS, Morganroth ML: Discontinuation of mechanical ventilation. Clin Chest Med 9:113, 1988
85. Menzies R, Gibbons W, Goldberg P: Determinants of weaning and survival among patients with COPD who require mechanical ventilation for acute respiratory failure. Chest 95:398, 1989
86. Morganroth ML, Morganroth JL, Nett LM, Petty TL: Criteria for weaning from prolonged mechanical ventilation. Arch Intern Med 144:1012, 1984
87. Hall JB, Wood LDH: Liberation of the patient from mechanical ventilation. JAMA 257:1621, 1987
88. Stoller JK: Establishing clinical unweanability. Respir Care 36: 186, 1991
89. Lemaire F, Teboul JL, Cinotti, et al: Acute left ventricular dysfunction during unsuccessful weaning from mechanical ventilation. Anesthesiology 69:171, 1988
90. Agusti AGN, Torres A, Estopa R, Agusti-Vidal A: Hypophosphatemia as a cause of failed weaning: The importance of metabolic factors. Crit Care Med 12:142, 1984
91. Aubier M, Murciano D, Lecocguic Y, et al: Effect of hypophosphatemia on diaphragmatic contractility in patients with acute respiratory failure. N Engl J Med 313:420, 1985
92. Benotti PN, Bistrian B: Metabolic and nutritional aspects of weaning from mechanical ventilation. Crit Care Med 17:181, 1989
93. Stoller JK: Physiologic rationale for resting the ventilatory muscles. Respir Care 36:290, 1991
94. Boysen PG: Respiratory muscle function and weaning from mechanical ventilation. Respir Care 32:572, 1987

95. Cohen CA, Zagelbaum G, Gross D, et al: Clinical manifestations of inspiratory muscle fatigue. Am J Med 73:308, 1982
96. Roussos C, Macklem PT: The respiratory muscles. N Engl J Med 307:786, 1982
97. Laghi F, N DA, Tobin MJ: Pattern of recovery from diaphragmatic fatigue over 24 hours. J Appl Physiol 79:539, 1995
98. Aldrich TK, Uhrlass RM: Weaning from mechanical ventilation: Successful use of modified inspiratory resistive training in muscular dystrophy. Crit Care Med 15:247, 1987
99. Grassino A, Macklem PT: Respiratory muscle fatigue and ventilatory failure. Ann Rev Med 35:625, 1984
100. Jabour ER, Rabil DM, Truwitt JD, Rochester DF: Evaluation of a new weaning index based on ventilatory endurance and the efficiency of gas exchange. Am Rev Respir Dis 144:531, 1991
101. Sahn SA, Lakshminarayan S: Bedside criteria for discontinuation of mechanical ventilation. Chest 63:1002, 1973
102. Sahn SA, Lakshminarayan S, Petty TL: Weaning from mechanical ventilation. JAMA 235:2208, 1976
103. Yang KL, Tobin MJ: A prospective study of indexes predicting the outcome of trials of weaning from mechanical ventilation. New Engl J Med 324:1445, 1991
104. Tobin MJ, Perez W, Guenther SM, et al: The pattern of breathing during successful and unsuccessful trials of weaning from mechanical ventilation. Am Rev Respir Dis 134:1111, 1986
105. Branson RD, Hurst JM, Davis K, Campbell R: Measurement of maximal inspiratory pressure: A comparison of three methods. Respir Care 34:789, 1989
106. Hess D: Measurement of maximal inspiratory pressure: A call for standardization (Editorial). Respir Care 34:857, 1989
107. Kacmarek RM, Cycyk-Chapman MC, Young PJ, Romagnoli DM: Determination of maximal inspiratory pressure: A clinical study literature review. Respir Care 34:868, 1989
108. Marini JJ, Smith TC, Lamb V: Estimation of inspiratory muscle strength in mechanically ventilated patients: The measurement of maximal inspiratory pressure. J Crit Care 1:32, 1986
109. Blanch PB, Banner MJ: A new respiratory monitor that enables accurate measurement of work of breathing: A validation study. Respir Care 39:897, 1994
110. Kacmarek RM, Hess D: Routine measurement of work of breathing: Is it necessary? (Editorial). Respir Care 39:881, 1994
111. Fiastro JF, Habib MP, Shon BY, Campbell SC: Comparison of standard weaning parameters and the mechanical work of breathing in mechanically ventilated patients. Chest 94:232, 1988
112. DeHaven CB, Hurst JM, Branson RD: Evaluation of two different extubation criteria: Attributes contributing to success. Crit Care Med 14:92, 1986
113. Foust GN, Potter WA, Wilons MD, Golden EB: Shortcomings of using two jet nebulizers in tandem with an aerosol face mask for optimal oxygen therapy. Chest 99:1346, 1991
114. Christopher KL, Neff RA, Bowman JL, et al: Demand and continuous flow intermittent mandatory ventilation systems. Chest 87:625, 1985
115. Gibney RTN, Wilson RD, Pontoppidan H: Comparison of work of breathing on high gas flow and demand valve continuous positive airway pressure systems. Chest 82:692, 1982
116. Henry WC, West GA, Wilson RS: A comparison of the oxygen cost of breathing between a continuous-flow CPAP system and a demand-flow CPAP system. Respir Care 28:1273, 1983
117. Katz JA, Kraemer RW, Gjerde GE: Inspiratory work and airway pressure with continuous positive airway pressure delivery system. Chest 88:519, 1985
118. Opt't Holt TB, Hall MW, Bass JB, Allison RC: Comparison of changes in airway pressure during continuous positive airway pressure (CPAP) between demand valve and continuous flow devices. Respir Care 27:1200, 1982
119. Quan SF, Falltrick RT, Schlobohm RM: Extubation from ambient or expiratory positive airway pressure in adults. Anesthesiology 55:53, 1981
120. Annest SJ, Gottlieb M, Paloski WH, et al: Detrimental effects of removing end-expiratory pressure prior to endotracheal extubation. Ann Surg 191:539, 1980
121. Gorbach MS, Kantor K: Extubation without a trial of spontaneous ventilation in the general surgical population. Respir Care 32:178, 1987
122. Hudson LD, Hurlow RS, Craig KC, Pierson DJ: Does intermittent mandatory ventilation correct respiratory alkalosis in patients receiving assisted mechanical ventilation? Am Rev Respir Dis 132:1071, 1985
123. Schachter EN, Tucker D, Beck GJ: Does intermittent mandatory ventilation accelerate weaning? JAMA 246:1210, 1981
124. Hirsch C, Kacmarek RM, Stanek K: Work of breathing during CPAP and PSV imposed by the new-generation mechanical ventilators: A lung model study. Respir Care 36:815, 1991
125. MacIntyre NR: Weaning from mechanical ventilatory support: Volume-assisting intermittent breaths versus pressure-assisting every breath. Respir Care 33:121, 1988
126. Fiastro JF, Habib MP, Quan SF: Pressure support compensation for inspiratory work due to endotracheal tubes and demand continuous positive airway pressure. Chest 93:499, 1988
127. Brochard L, Rua F, Lorino H, et al: Inspiratory pressure support compensates for the additional work of breathing caused by the endotracheal tube. Anesthesiology 75:739, 1991
128. Brochard L, Harf A, Lorino H, Lemaire F: Inspiratory pressure support prevents diaphragmatic fatigue during weaning from mechanical ventilation. Am Rev Respir Dis 139:513, 1989
129. Brochard L, Pluskwa F, Lemaire F: Improved efficiency of spontaneous breathing with inspiratory pressure support. Am Rev Respir Dis 136:411, 1987
130. Ershowsky P, Krieger B: Changes in breathing pattern during pressure support ventilation. Respir Care 32:1011, 1987
131. Banner MJ, Kirby RR, Garrielli A, et al: Partially and totally unloading respiratory muscles based on real-time measurements of work of breathing: A clinical approach. Chest 106:1835, 1994
132. Banner MJ, Kirby RR, Blanch PB, Layon AJ: Decreasing imposed work of breathing apparatus to zero using pressure support ventilation. Crit Care Med 21:1333, 1993
133. Black JW, Grover BS: A hazard of pressure support ventilation. Chest 93:333, 1988
134. Brochard L, Rauss A, Benito S, et al: Comparison of three methods of gradual withdrawal from ventilatory support during weaning from mechanical ventilation. Am J Respir Crit Care Med 150:896, 1994
135. Estaban A, Frutos F, Tobin MJ, et al: A comparison of four methods of weaning patients from mechanical ventilation. N Engl J Med 332:345, 1995
136. Shapiro M, Wilson K, Casar G, et al: Work of breathing through different sized endotracheal tubes. Crit Care Med 14:1028, 1986
137. Wright PE, Marini JJ, Bernard GR: In vitro versus in vivo comparison of endotracheal tube airflow resistance. Am Rev Respir Dis 140:10, 1989
138. Guttmann J, Eberhard L, Fabry B, et al: Continuous calculation of intratracheal pressure in tracheally intubated patients. Anesthesiology 79:503, 1993
139. Wilson DJ: Airway management of the ventilator-assisted individual. In ME Gilmartin, BJ Make: Mechanical ventilation in the home: Issues for health care providers. Prob Respir Care 1:192, 1988
140. Kacmarek RM, Hickling KG: Permissive hypercapnia. Respir Care 38:373, 1993
141. Bidani A, Tzouanakis AE, Cardena VJ, Zwischenberger JB: Permissive hypercapnia in acute respiratory failure. JAMA 272:957, 1994
142. Tuxen DV: Permissive hypercapnic ventilation. Am J Respir Crit Care Med 150:870, 1994
143. Feihl F, Perret C: Permissive hypercapnia: How permissive should we be? Am J Respir Crit Care Med 150:1722, 1994
144. Hickling KG, Walsh J, Henderson S, Jackson R: Low mortality rate in adult respiratory distress syndrome using low-volume, pressure-limited ventilation with permissive hypercapnia: A prospective study. Crit Care Med 22:1568, 1994
145. Douglas WW, Rehder K, Beynen FM, et al: Improved oxygenation in patients with acute respiratory failure: The prone position. Am Rev Respir Dis 115:559, 1977
146. Lamm WJE, Graham MM, Albert RK: Mechanism by which the prone position improves oxygenation in acute lung injury. Am J Respir Crit Care Med 150:184, 1994
147. Pappert D, Rossaint R, Slama K, et al: Influence of positioning on ventilation-perfusion relationships in severe adult respiratory distress syndrome. Chest 106:1511, 1994

148. Bigatello LM, Hurford WE, Kacmarek RM, et al: Prolonged inhalation of low concentrations of nitric oxide in patients with severe adult respiratory distress syndrome: Effects on pulmonary hemodynamics and oxygenation. Anesthesiology 80:761, 1994
149. Rossaint R, Falke KJ, Lopex F, et al: Inhaled nitric oxide for the adult respiratory distress syndrome. N Engl J Med 328:399, 1993
150. Hess D, Bigatello L, Kacmarek RM, Ritz R, Head CA, Hurford WE: Use of inhaled nitric oxide for treatment of patients with the acute respiratory distress syndrome. Respir Care (in press)
151. Zapol WM, Hurford WE: Inhaled nitric oxide in the adult respiratory distress syndrome and other lung diseases. New Horizons 1:638, 1993
152. Nishimura M, Hess D, Kacmarek RM, Ritz R, Hurford WE: Nitrogen dioxide production during adult mechanical ventilation with nitric oxide: Effects of ventilator internal volume, air versus nitrogen dilution, minute ventilation, and FIO_2. Anesthesiology 82:1246, 1995
153. Zapol WM, Snider MT, Hill JD, et al: Extracorporeal membrane oxygenation in severe acute respiratory failure. JAMA 242:2193, 1979
154. Gattinoni L, Pesenti A, Bombino M, Pelosi P, Brazzi L: Role of extracorporeal circulation in adult respiratory distress syndrome management. New Horizons 1:603, 1993
155. Gattinoni L, Pesenti A, Maschcroni D, et al: Low frequency positive pressure ventilation and extracorporeal CO_2 removal in severe acute respiratory failure. JAMA 256:881, 1986
156. Morris AH, Wallace CJ, Menlove RL, et al: Randomized clinical trial of pressure-controlled inverse ratio ventilation and extracorporeal CO_2 removal for adult respiratory distress syndrome. Am J Respir Crit Care Med 149:295, 1994
157. Bower LK, Betit P: Extracorporeal life support and high-frequency oscillatory ventilation: Alternatives for the neonate in severe respiratory failure. Respir Care 40:61, 1995
158. MacIntyre NR: High-Frequency Ventilation. In MJ Tobin: Principles and Practice of Mechanical Ventilation. New York, McGraw-Hill, 1994
159. Branson RD: High-Frequency Ventilators. In RD Branson, DR Hess, RL Chatburn: Respiratory Care Equipment. Philadelphia, JB Lippincott, 1995
160. HiFO Study Group: Randomized study of high-frequency oscillatory ventilation in infants with severe respiratory distress syndrome. J Pediatr 122:609, 1993
161. Naham A, Burke WC, Ravenscraft SA, et al: Lung mechanics and gas exchange during pressure control in dogs: Augmentation of CO_2 elimination by an intratracheal catheter. Am Rev Respir Dis 146:965, 1992
162. Adams AB: Tracheal gas insufflation (TGI). Respir Care 41:285, 1996
163. Naham A, Ravenscraft SA, Nakos G, et al: Tracheal gas insufflation during pressure-control ventilation: Effect of catheter position, diameter, and flow rate. Am Rev Respir Dis 146:1411, 1992
164. Imanaka H, Kacmarek RM, Ritz R, Hess D: Tracheal gas insufflation pressure control versus volume control ventilation: A lung model study. Am J Respir Crit Care Med 153:1019, 1996
165. Burke WC, Nahum A, Ravenscraft SA, et al: Modes of tracheal gas insufflation: Comparison of continuous and phase-specific gas injection in normal dogs. Am Rev Respir Dis 148:562, 1993
166. Ravenscraft SA, Burke WC, Naham A, et al: Intratracheal gas insufflation augments alveolar ventilation during volume cycled mechanical ventilation in patients. Am Rev Respir Dis 148:345, 1993
167. Naham A, Chandra A, Nikham J, et al: Effect of tracheal gas insufflation on gas exchange in canine oleic acid-induced lung injury. Crit Care Med 23:348, 1995
168. Shaffer TH, Wolfson MR, Clark LC: State of the art review: Liquid ventilation. Pediatr Pulmonol 14:102, 1992
169. Greenspan JS, Wolfson MR, Rubenstein D, et al: Liquid ventilation of human preterm neonates. J Pediatr 117:106, 1990
170. Hirschl RB, Merz SI, Montoya P, et al: Development and application of a simplified liquid ventilator. Crit Care Med 23:157, 1995
171. Hirschl RB, Pranikoff T, Gauger P, et al: Liquid ventilation in adults, children, and full-term neonates. Lancet 346:1201, 1995

21 Mechanical Ventilation

Susan P. Pilbeam

SECTION 1 Physical Characteristics of Mechanical Ventilators

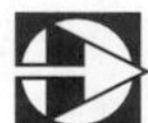

CLINICAL SKILLS

Upon completion of this chapter, the reader will:

- Collect and evaluate all pertinent patient data, including bedside procedures, to determine I:E ratio, maximum inspiratory pressure (MAP), and peak flow
- Explain the classification system of mechanical ventilators
- Select techniques or modes of mechanical ventilation, including ventilators (pneumatic, electric, microprocessor, high frequency, and BiPAP) and patient breathing circuits (mechanical ventilation, CPAP, and IMV pH-valve assembly)
- Troubleshoot common alarm situations that occur with mechanical ventilators
- Locate and use information regarding ventilator specification
- Operate specific ventilators described
- Identify ventilator modes and alarms for the specific ventilators described
- Troubleshoot and correct problems related to the ventilators or patient breathing circuits indicated
- Troubleshoot problems based on graphic data obtained during ventilation
- Initiate, evaluate, conduct, and modify therapeutic procedures based on patient's response

KEY TERMS

Alarm
Auto-PEEP
Chatburn's system of classification
Control panel
Control scheme
Cycling
Directly coupled stepper motor
Drive mechanism
Electromagnetically operated valves
Expiratory retard
Flow controller
Flow-cycled
Flow-triggered
Input power
Limiting
Manually triggered
Monitor
Output
Phase variables
Positive end expiratory pressure
Power conversion
Pressure controller
Pressure-cycled
Pressure-limited
Pressure-reducing valve
Pressure-triggering
Stepper motor-driven cam
Stepper motor with scissor valve
Thorpe tube
Time controller
Time-cycling
Time-triggered
Triggering
User interface
Ventilator parameters
Volume controller
Volume-cycled

An important aspect of caring for patients on mechanical ventilatory support is a thorough understanding of the equipment that is being used. A wide variety of ventilators is presently available for use in the practice of modern respiratory care. It would be extremely difficult for anyone to master all of these and their idiosyncrasies, therefore it is best to gain a basic understanding of how all ventilators function. With this base of knowledge, an individual can learn to operate the ventilators available at his or her institution in a more systematic fashion.

One of the best ways to gain an overview of ventilator function is to study their classification. A classification system is used to establish a systematic way of grouping ventilators based on how they operate. Classifying ventilators is similar to classifying cars as four cylinder versus six or eight cylinder, standard versus automatic transmission, and so on. The basic function of an automobile is transportation. The basic function of a ventilator is to substitute for the bellows action of the thoracic cage and diaphragm. Each ventilator does this with slightly different capabilities and options. The functional characteristics of many of the ventilators in use today, and the terminology used by manufacturers and by different authors varies considerably. How we describe the functions of these machines is increasingly important as they become more and more sophisticated and complex.

The earliest generation ventilators of the late 1960s and early 1970s such as the Post-op Emerson and the Bennett MA-1 were originally classified by a system used by Mushin et al.[1] Since that time, technology and the rapid development of the computer have drastically changed how ventilators work. These changes require a change in the way we classify and describe their function. Chatburn[2–4] has developed a system of ventilator classification that provides a fairly simple yet complete method for categorizing ventilator function (Table 21-1). Although both Mushin's and Chatburn's systems of classification each have advantages, Chatburn's system is more popular in current respiratory textbooks. For that reason, the basic components of *Chatburn's system of classification* are used in Parts I and II of this chapter.

BASIC OPERATION OF A VENTILATOR

For simplicity, a ventilator can be imagined as a "black box" that provides a way to deliver a breath of air to a patient. During inspiration a positive pressure gradient causes gas to flow from the ventilator to the patient's lungs. To accomplish what would seem like a fairly simple task, the ventilator has to be connected to a power source. The two most commonly used forms of power are electricity and high-pressure gas. This part of the classification system is termed the ***input power***, that is, the power that allows the ventilator to accomplish its tasks. This power must be either ***transmitted*** or ***converted*** to provide a breath of air to the patient. Another name for the device that converts or transmits the power is the ***drive mechanism***. Drive mechanisms can be high-pressure gas sources, compressors, or bellows. How this is done is controlled by a ***control scheme***. The control scheme determines if the ventilator will control pressure, volume, flow, or time during inspiration. In other words, a drive mechanism uses a power source that controls either the amount of pressure, the amount of flow, or the amount of volume provided in a certain time frame.

At the very least a mechanical ventilator must be able to provide a complete respiratory cycle; that is, both inspiration and expiration. To do this, it must mechanically be able to perform four functions or phases, which were first described by Mushin et al[1] (Fig. 21-1) and in-

TABLE 21-1 **Outline for Ventilator Classification System**

- I. Input
  - A. Pneumatic
  - B. Electric
    - 1. AC
    - 2. DC (battery)
- II. Regulation of inspiratory flow and flow waveform
  - A. External compressor
  - B. Internal compressor
  - C. Piston
    - 1. Electric motor/rotary wheel
    - 2. Electric motor/linear/rolling seal
  - D. Compressor bellows
  - E. Variable restriction
    - 1. Pressure-reducing valve
    - 2. Thorpe tube
    - 3. Stepper motor with scissors valve
  - F. Proportional solenoid
    - 1. Electromagnetic
    - 2. Directly coupled stepper motor
    - 3. Stepper motor-driven cam
  - G. Proportional manifold with digital valves
- III. Control scheme
  - A. Control circuit
    - 1. Mechanical
    - 2. Pneumatic
    - 3. Fluidic
    - 4. Electric
    - 5. Electronic
  - B. Control variables and waveforms
    - 1. Pressure
    - 2. Volume
    - 3. Flow
    - 4. Time
  - C. Phase variables
    - 1. Trigger variable
    - 2. Limit variable
    - 3. Cycle variable
    - 4. Baseline variable
  - D. Conditional variable(s)
- IV. Output
  - A. Pressure
    - 1. Rectangular
    - 2. Exponential
    - 3. Sinusoidal
    - 4. Oscillating
  - B. Volume
    - 1. Ramp
    - 2. Sinusoidal
  - C. Flow
    - 1. Rectangular
    - 2. Ramp
      - a. Ascending ramp
      - b. Descending ramp
    - 3. Sinusoidal
  - D. Effects of the patient circuit
- V. Alarm systems
  - A. Input power alarms
    - 1. Loss of electric power
    - 2. Loss of pneumatic power
  - B. Control circuit alarms
    - 1. General systems failure (ventilator inoperative)
    - 2. Incompatible ventilator settings
    - 3. Inverse inspiratory time/expiratory time (I/E) ratio
  - C. Output alarms
    - 1. Pressure
    - 2. Volume
    - 3. Flow
    - 4. Time
      - a. High and/or low ventilatory frequency
      - b. High and/or low inspiratory time
      - c. High and/or low expiratory time (high expiratory time = apnea)
    - 5. Inspired gas
      - a. High and/or low inspired gas temperature
      - b. High and/or low FiO_2

Adapted and reprinted with permission.[2, 6]

clude the following: (1) inspiratory phase; (2) change from inspiration to expiration; (3) expiratory phase; and (4) change from expiration to inspiration.

To accomplish the four phases of a complete breath, the operator selects certain functions and controls. These controls appear on the surface of the ventilator and are referred to as the *control panel* or the *user interface*. The control panel allows the operator to determine how breathing will be accomplished. For example, the control panel (user interface) may have buttons, knobs, or touch pads to control how deep a breath is (tidal volume), how fast it is delivered (gas flow and inspiratory time), how often the patient gets a breath (respiratory rate), and when the breath is delivered (triggering mechanism). *Phase variables* are those controls that determine the four phases of the breath, whereas the other values that are set are called *ventilator parameters*.

One of the problems with the user interface is that the names given to similar controls may actually be different depending on the manufacturer. For example, the knob or button that controls the maximum pressure during inspiration may be called "normal pressure limit" on one machine and "peak pressure limit" on another. This can lead to confusion, particularly if hospitals use a variety of ventilators.

The way the breath is delivered is called the *output* of the ventilator and can differ depending on how the ventilator is functioning. Finally, to be sure the breath has actually gone to the patient, the ventilator must *monitor* what is happening and sound an *alarm* if anything goes wrong. Each of these aspects of ventilator classification will now be reviewed.

INPUT POWER

As mentioned, the common power sources (input power) used to operate mechanical ventilators are electricity and high-pressure gas sources. Most American ventilators that use electrical power use normal electrical outlets (110 to 155 volts AC 50 to 60 Hz) to power the components that provide gas flow to the patient. Some infant and transport ventilators use rechargeable batteries as an alternative form of electrical power when they are not plugged into electric outlets. These are all referred to as electrically powered ventilators.

Other ventilators require a high-pressure gas source for power and are commonly referred to as pneumatically powered ventilators. In critical care areas of hospitals, high-pressure gas sources are available in the form of compressed air and oxygen at about 50 psig (range 35 to 100 psig) from a bulk gas supply system. Ventilators that use pressurized gas usually have internal reducing regulators that reduce the gas pressure to about 20 psig. Some ventilators have small built-in compressors that they can use as power sources when a high-pressure gas source is not available or fails, but electrical power is required to power these. An example is the Puritan Bennett 7200 ventilator.

Some of the earliest mechanical ventilators used only one of these power sources. For example, the Puritan Bennett PR series and the Bird Mark series are pneumatically powered. The Emerson 3MV and 3PV are electrically powered ventilators. Newer-generation ventilators are often driven by pneumatics; in other words, the power that provides the pressure gradient of gas flow to the patient is the pressurized gas itself. These newer-generation ventilators, however, are powered by electricity. The high-pressure gas sources are reduced in pressure, then blended, and their gas flow rate and pattern are controlled by electrically powered mechanical devices which, in turn, may be controlled by a microprocessor unit. Some sources refer to these as a combination of pneumatically and electrically powered because they cannot function unless both power sources are provided. Because many of these ventilators are computer controlled, they are referred to as microprocessor controlled.

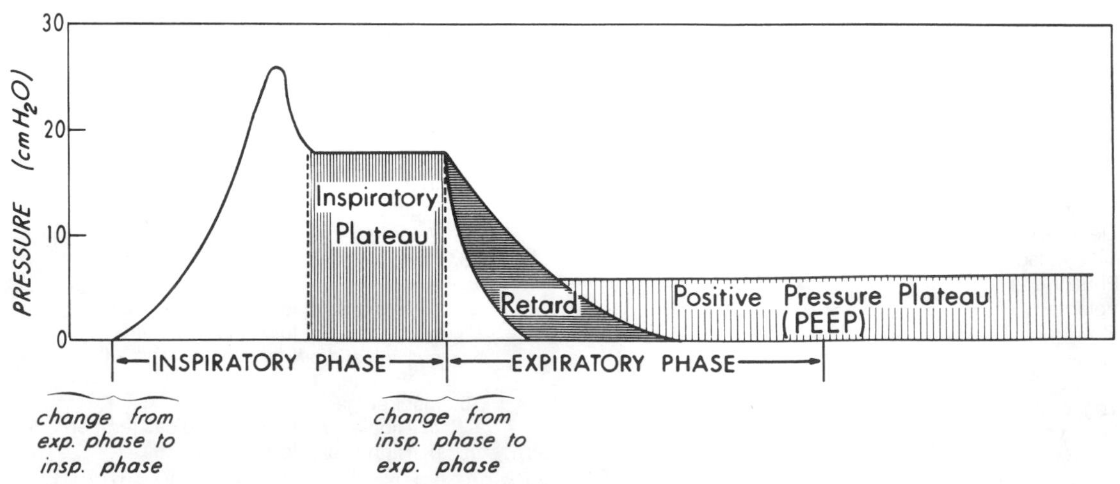

FIGURE 21-1. Phases of the mechanical ventilator cycle, with and without PEEP and retard.

POWER CONVERSION AND TRANSMISSION: THE DRIVE MECHANISM AND HOW FLOW AND PRESSURE ARE MANIPULATED TO DETERMINE INSPIRATORY FLOW PATTERN

The power transmission and conversion system, also called the drive mechanism, generates the force needed to make gas flow to the patient. It is the source that causes gas to flow to the patient.

High-Pressure Gas

Ventilators that require an external high-pressure gas source are pneumatically powered. As mentioned, the Puritan Bennett PR Series and the Bird Mark Series require a gas pressure source of about 50 psig to operate. Although these represent the first-generation ventilators, they are seldom used for continuous mechanical ventilatory support at present. They are most often connected to wall-outlet air or oxygen or a blender powered by air and oxygen when they are used for ventilation.

Compressors

Another example of a drive mechanism is a compressor. A compressor can be external to the ventilator or built into the ventilator.

□ EXTERNAL COMPRESSOR

Large external compressors are often used by hospitals to supply gas under high pressure (50 psig) to wall outlets in intensive care areas. When these outlets are used to power a ventilator, the ventilator is regarded as pneumatically powered using an external compressor. As the gas enters the ventilator, its pressure is reduced. In the case of the Newport Wave, for example, pressurized air and oxygen from wall outlets are connected to the ventilator by high-pressure gas hoses that attach to the ventilator. Gas from both sources is then reduced to equal pressure and sent to a metal cylinder called an accumulator. This stores the gas under pressure and also allows it to be mixed. Once the ventilator's controls are set into motion, they release some of the gas from the accumulator and send it to the patient.

In the case of the Servo 900C, high-pressure external gases are mixed by an air/oxygen blender before entering a spring-loaded bellows inside the ventilator. This bellows also acts as a type of accumulator or reservoir for the gases and keeps them at a pressure that can be controlled by the operator. This pressure control is located on the front of the ventilator and is called the "working pressure" control (Fig. 21-2).

□ INTERNAL COMPRESSOR

In an internal compressor system a bellows contains the gas that is to be delivered to the patient. The bellows is housed within a sealed chamber that is pressurized,

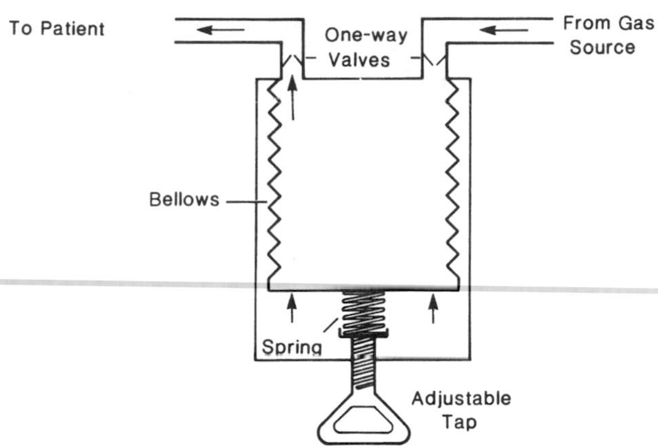

FIGURE 21-2. Drive mechanism consisting of a bellows under spring tension. (From Chatburn RL: Ventilator Classification in Branson RD, Chatburn RL, et al: Respiratory Care Equipment, Philadelphia, JB Lippincott Co, 1995, p 268)

causing the bellows to deliver inspiratory gas to the patient. The rate of compression and the amount of power available from the pressure source determine the rate of gas flow to the patient. Since the volume delivered is measured directly, these are called "volume controllers." Most anesthesia ventilators use this design. The Bennett MA-1 is another example. Few of the current-generation ventilators use this bellows system.

In the Bennett MA-1, a small built-in, electrically powered compressor creates a gas flow. The gas flow from the compressor travels to a cannister on the inside of the ventilator. The cannister contains a suspended bellows. Inside the bellows is the blended gas that eventually goes to the patient (Fig. 21-3). Air from the compressor enters the cannister through a hole in the bottom and creates pressure that causes the bellows to rise and the air in the bellows to be directed toward the patient. In this case, the MA-1 has an electrically powered internal compressor to power the ventilator.

Pistons

Another type of drive mechanism powered by electrical motors is pistons. The two common types are rotary crank pistons and linear drive pistons.

□ ROTARY CRANK

Rotary crank pistons are powered by an electrical motor and produce what resembles a sinusoidal motion, sometimes referred to as an "eccentric wheel" (Fig. 21-4). An example of a ventilator with this drive mechanism is the Emerson 3 MV.

□ LINEAR DRIVE PISTONS

An electric motor is connected by special rack and pinion to a piston rod or arm (Fig. 21-5). The rod moves a piston forward inside a cylinder. The air in front of and within the piston cylinder is the air directed toward the patient. It can move at either a constant rate or at a vari-

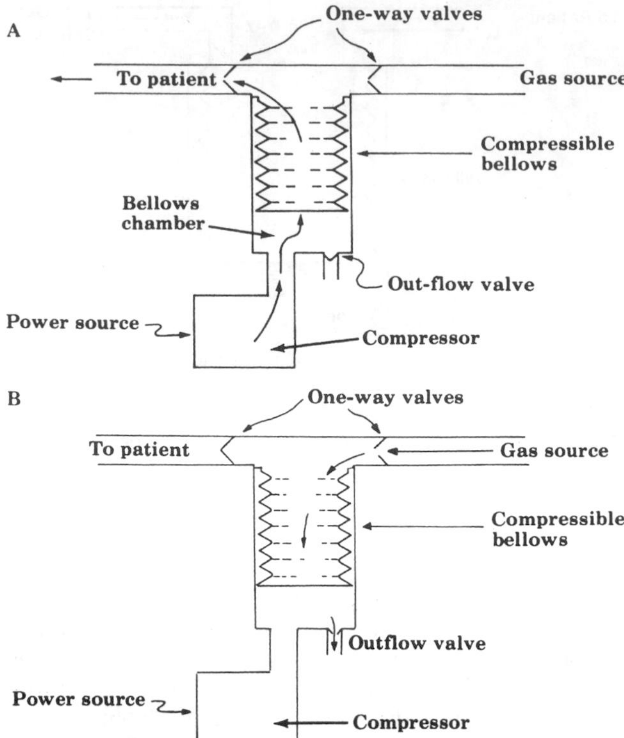

FIGURE 21-3. In this double-circuit ventilator, gas that goes to the patient is not in direct contact with the power source, as seen in this schematic representation of the Puritan-Bennett MA-1 in its simplest form. **(A)**, the compressor produces a high pressure gas source which is directed to a chamber. The chamber holds a collapsible bellows and the bellows contains the desired gas mixture which will go to the patient. The pressure in the chamber forces the bellows upward resulting in a positive pressure breath. **(B)**, After the inspiratory breath is delivered, the compressor no longer sends pressure to the chamber and exhalation occurs. The bellows drops to its original position and fills with the desired delivery gas in preparation for the next breath. (From Pilbeam SP: Mechanical Ventilation, Physiological and Clinical Applications (2nd ed.) Chicago, Mosby–Year Book, 1992, p 111)[5]

able rate depending on the control circuit.[4] An example is the Sechrist 2200B ventilator.

In either a rotary or linear drive, the piston draws air into the housing on the downstroke (return stroke) and pushes air out on the upstroke (forward stroke). The piston acts as the drive mechanism and controls the rate and pattern of delivery of the gas. The electrical motor powers the piston. The movement of the piston (linear or rotary) establishes the type of flow pattern or flow waveform that is delivered to the patient.

Output Control Valves

These valves or mechanical devices are what are used to manipulate the power source and produce a desired volume, pressure, and flow pattern during inspiration. They include devices such as variable restrictors, stepper motors with scissor valves, electromagnetic proportional solenoids (proportional valves), proportional manifolds with digital valves, and electromagnetic poppet valves.

□ VARIABLE RESTRICTION

Inspiratory gas flow is limited by a variable restriction that controls gas flow. Examples include the *pressure-reducing valve* in the Bear 1, 2, and 3; the *Thorpe Tube* in the Bear Cub and Sechrist ventilators. With this device the ventilator can be a flow controller if the pressure limit is set high enough. Volume delivery is determined by a preset inspiratory time and the flow setting (Fig. 21-6).[6] Another example of variable restriction is the *stepper motor with scissor valve* found in the Servo 900C and 300.

The scissor valve in the Siemens Servo 900C series is controlled by a stepper motor that moves in fixed steps or increments to determine the selected tidal volume or airway pressure. Using the ventilator to deliver a preset tidal volume allows a flow transducer to regulate the amount of flow, and the ventilator operates as a flow controller. When set up to deliver a preset inspiratory pressure it is a pressure controller and is controlled by a pressure transducer (Fig. 21-7).[6]

□ PROPORTIONAL SOLENOID (PROPORTIONAL VALVE)

In this type of valve, the flow of gas is controlled by either one (blended gas) or two (one for air and one for oxygen) proportional solenoids. These are *electromagnetically operated valves* that can shape the flow waveform during inspiration. This is accomplished by changing the diameter of the output orifice. For example, in Figure 21-8 the flowmetering aperture of the proportional solenoid is actuated by an armature moving linearly in a magnetic field.[6,7] Ventilators that include electromagnetically powered proportional valves are the Puritan-Bennett 7200, the Hamilton Veolar, the Amadeus, the Drager Evita, and the Servo 300.

An alternative design is the use of a stepper motor that is directly coupled to a flowmetering orifice (*directly coupled stepper motor)* or a *stepper motor-driven cam* pro-

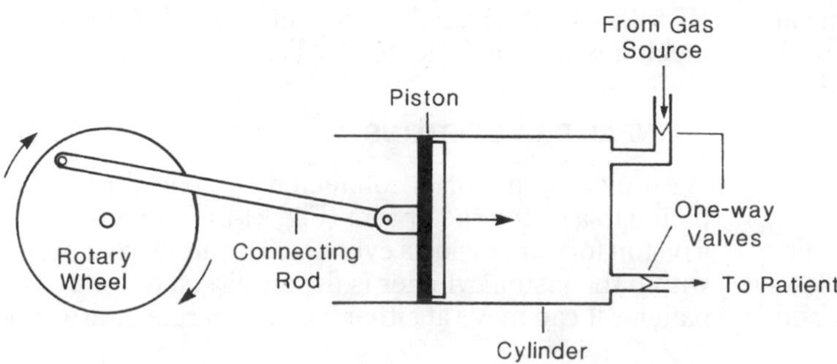

FIGURE 21-4. Drive mechanism consisting of eccentric wheel, piston connecting rod, and piston (From Chatburn RL: Ventilator Classification in Branson RD, Chatburn RL, et al: Respiratory Care Equipment, Philadelphia, JB Lippincott Co, 1995, p 267)[4]

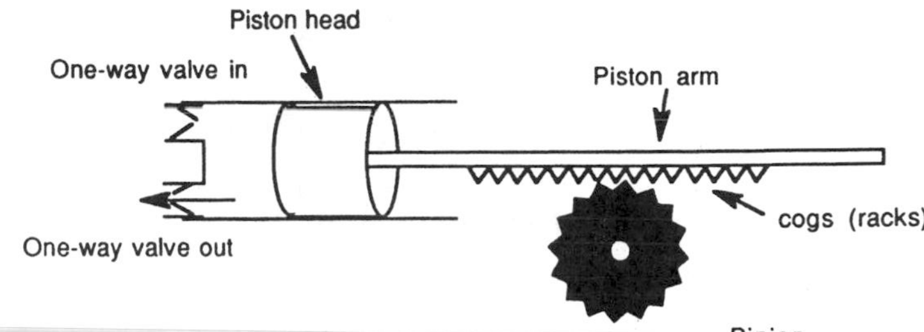

FIGURE 21-5. Linear drive piston with rack, pinion, piston rod and piston. The gears engage the cogs and move the piston arm forward in a linear motion. (From Pilbeam SP: Mechanical Ventilation, Physiological and Clinical Applications (2nd ed.) Chicago, Mosby–Year Book, 1992, p 105)

portioning solenoid as is used in the Bear 5 and Bear 1000, and the Bird 6400 and Bird 8400 (Fig. 21-9).[6,7] In these designs the position of the solenoid determines the flow pattern and the peak flow during inspiration.

☐ PROPORTIONAL MANIFOLD WITH DIGITAL VALVES

This design operates digital solenoid valves in a series in which each valve can be either opened or closed (Fig. 21-10).[7] Each valve offers one calibrated flow. The number of available flow steps depends on how many valves are available. The total flow is determined by the sum of the flow from each valve. The Infrasonics Infant Star is an example of a ventilator with this type of output control mechanism. This design can function either as a pressure or a flow controller.

☐ ELECTROMAGNETIC POPPET VALVE

This is an on/off type of valve that is operated with magnetic forces produced by electrical current. In the Infrasonics Infant Star ventilator, each of the digital valves operates in this manner. Other examples of ventilators using an electromagnetic poppet valve are the Bear Cub, which uses a plunger, and the Bunnell Life Pulse Jet Ventilator, which uses an electromagnetic pinch valve.[4]

☐ EXHALATION VALVES

A variety of methods can be used by manufacturers to control waveforms, as were discussed previously in this section. They can be as simple as the pistons or more complicated, such as stepper motors. Many ventilators have more than one device that controls gas flow as it leaves the ventilator and is delivered to the patient. For example, most ventilators have an exhalation valve located on the expiratory limb of a patient's circuit. Usually, some type of diaphragm or balloon valve or plunger closes the circuit during inspiration so that gas must flow to the patient. Technically, this valve does not affect the flow rate or pattern during inspiration. Without it, however, gas would not flow into the patient, so it is essential to the function of most ventilators. This diaphragm is activated either by a gas flow or a mechanical plunger. It can also be activated during exhalation to slow the rate of expired gas flow (*expiratory retard*) or it can maintain positive end-expiratory pressure (PEEP) (Fig. 21-11).[5]

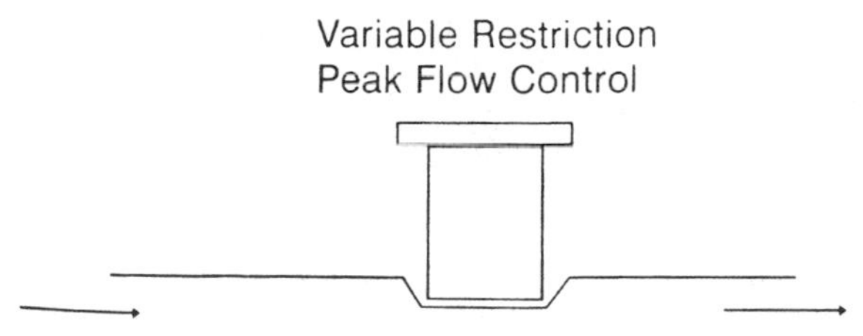

FIGURE 21-6. A variable restriction flow controller pneumatic system as used with the Sechrist infant ventilator. (From Kacmarek RM, Hess D: Basic principles of ventilator machinery. In Tobin, MJ: Principles and Practice of Mechanical Ventilation New York, McGraw-Hill, 1994 p 69)

CONTROL SCHEME—THE VARIABLE CONTROLLING INSPIRATION

There are basically four variables that can be controlled during ventilator operation: pressure, volume, flow, and time. The ventilator's control scheme is determined by what variable is being controlled. A ventilator is classi-

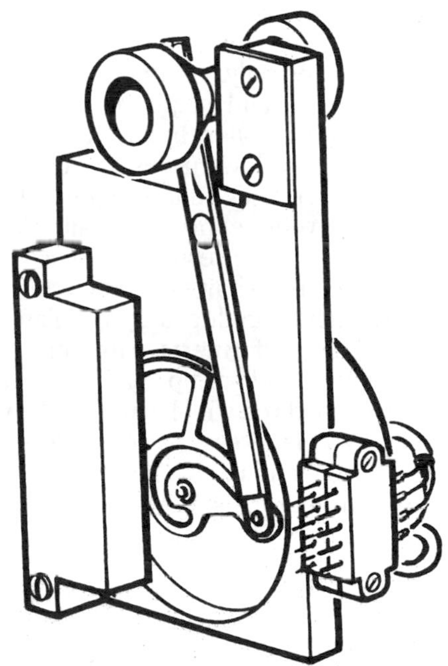

FIGURE 21-7. A stepper motor and scissor valve on the Siemens Servo 900C. On the motor is a cam that controls the moving arm. The valve is shown in the open position. (Courtesy of Siemens Life Support Systems, Schaumburg, Illinois).

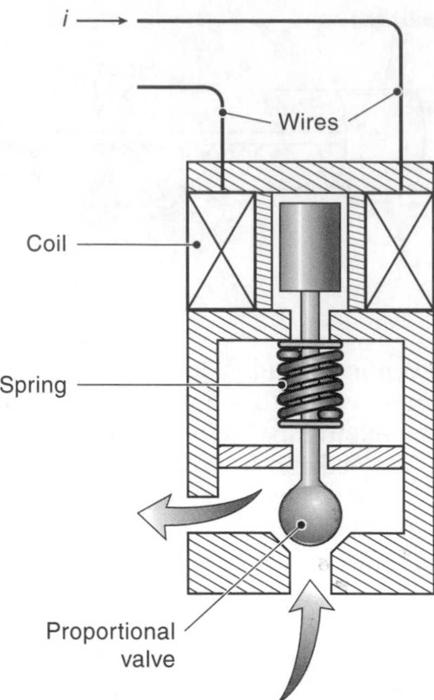

FIGURE 21-8. An example of a pneumatic valve used to control flow. This is one type of proportional solenoid valve. In this design, a controllable electrical current flows through the coil, resulting in a magnetic field. The strength of the magnetic field causes the armature to assume a specified position. With the armature and valve poppet physically connected, this assembly is the only moving part. The coil and armature designs vary, as do the strategies used to fix the position of the poppett. (From Sanborn WG. Microprocessor-based mechanical ventilation. Respiratory Care 38: 72–109, 1991, p 75)

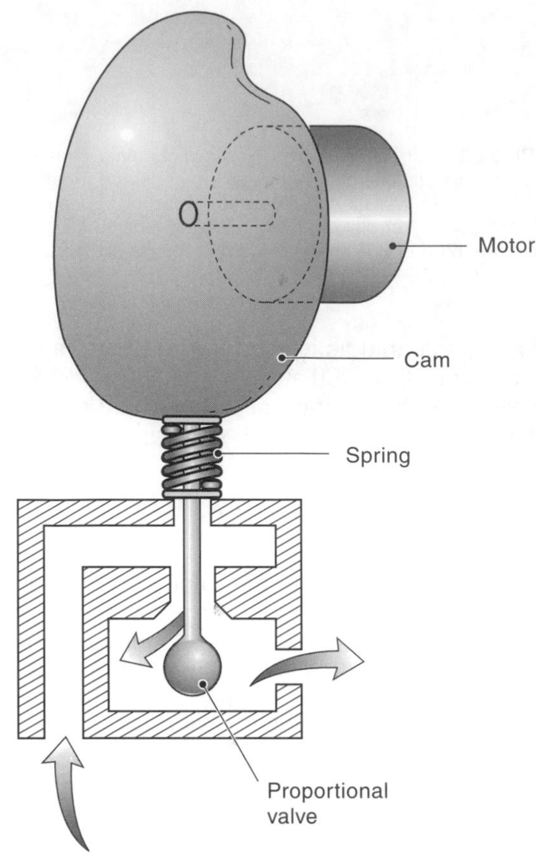

FIGURE 21-9. This is an example of an externally actuated proportional valve. Several different motor and cam schemes have been designed with which to control the position of the poppet. The stepper motor and scissor design implemented in the Siemens 900 series ventilators represents an early, highly successful strategy. (From Sanborn WG. Microprocessor-based mechanical ventilation. Respiratory Care 38:72–109, 1991, p 75)

fied as either a pressure, volume, flow, or time controller.[8] A *pressure controller* keeps the same pattern of pressure at the mouth regardless of changes in patient lung characteristics. A *volume controller* measures the volume and uses it to maintain a consistent volume waveform. Most commonly, volume delivery is a product of measured flow and inspiratory time, and the ventilator is a flow controller. In a time controller, the pressure, volume, and flow curves can change as the patient's lung characteristics change (Fig. 21-12).

The variables of volume, pressure, and flow can be graphed against time. The resulting shapes are called waveforms. Figure 21-13 shows the characteristic waveforms most commonly produced by ventilators during inspiration.[2] These waveforms have four basic patterns: rectangular, exponential, ramp, and sinusoidal. The type of pattern depends on which variable the ventilator controls. For example, pressure controllers have rectangular and exponential waveforms. Volume controllers have ramp and sinusoidal waveforms. Flow controllers have rectangular, sinusoidal, ramp (ascending and descending), and exponential decay waveforms.

A ventilator can directly control only one variable at a time: pressure, volume, or flow.[8] The ventilator either controls the airway pressure waveform, the inspiratory volume waveform, or the inspiratory flow waveform. These become the control variables; that is, pressure, volume, or flow are controlled, respectively. At the same time, when pressure is controlled, then volume and flow can vary with each breath, depending on the compliance and resistance characteristics of the patient's lungs.

Pressure Controller

When a ventilator is a pressure controller, the pressure waveform is unaffected by changes in patient lung characteristics (lung compliance and airway resistance). The ventilator can control pressure either at the airway or at the body surface. A positive pressure ventilator causes airway pressure to rise above body surface. When the ventilator controls the pressure on the body surface, making it fall below atmospheric during inspiration, it is a negative pressure ventilator. In this case, mouth pressure is usually at atmospheric.

Volume Controller

When a ventilator is a volume controller, the pressure waveform varies with changes in patient lung characteristics, but the observed volume waveform does not change. In addition, to be classified as a volume controller, the ventilator must measure volume and use the

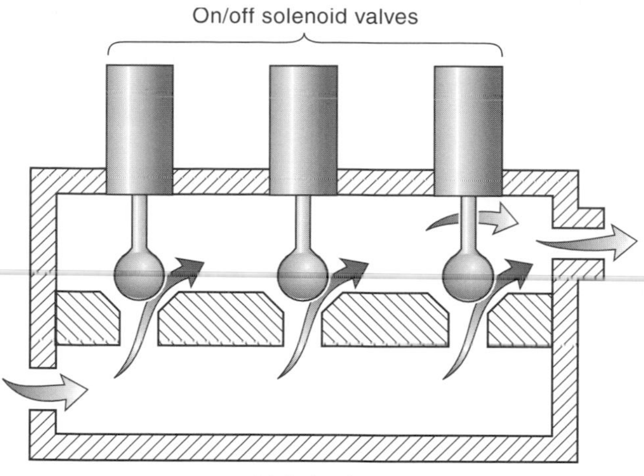

FIGURE 21-10. This is an example of a proportional manifold with a digital valves pneumatic system (the digital valve on-or-off concept). With each valve controlling a critical orifice and hence specified flow, the number of discrete flow steps (including zero) becomes 2^n (where N = number of valves). A 9-valve design, with 0.5 L/min flow increments between valves, yields a flow range of 0 to 255 L/min and a resolution of 0.5 L/min. (From Sanborn WG. Microprocessor-based mechanical ventilation. Respiratory Care 38: 72–109, 1991, p 75)

signal to control the volume waveform. The volume can be directly measured by using a piston or bellows or similar device. By controlling the excursion of a piston, for example, the ventilator automatically controls the volume waveform. Some ventilators, such as the Puritan-Bennett 7200, the Bear 1000, and the Servo 900C, display volume readings. They all measure and control flow, however, and only calculate the volume delivery. For this reason, they are functioning as flow controllers in modes where the operator selects a tidal volume, rate, and flow setting.

Flow Controller

A *flow controller* is one in which the volume change is unaffected by changes in lung characteristics and one in which volume change is not measured and used for controlling the ventilator.

When a ventilator is classified as a volume controller, one criteria is that the volume waveform does not change. But this alone is not a sufficient condition to classify a ventilator as a volume controller, because the same is true of a flow controller. The reason for this is that when the volume waveform is specified, the flow waveform is determined, since they are functions of each other. In other words, a volume delivered over a specified time defines a flow. For example, a volume of 1 L delivered in 1 second requires a flow of 1 L/sec. If changes in the patient's lung characteristics do not change the volume waveform, they will not change the flow waveform and vice versa.[4] For a ventilator to be classified as a volume controller it must meet both of the following criteria: (1) maintain the same volume waveform even when lung characteristics change, and (2) measure the volume and use the signal to control the volume waveform.

The most general terms used to describe ventilation are volume-controlled and pressure-controlled ventilation. Although the pressure-controlled description is pretty straightforward, the volume-controlled can be confusing. The previous discussion of volume-controlled ventilation and its distinction from flow-controlled ventilation is very specific. For the sake of simplicity, the term volume-controlled is acceptable for both volume-controlled and flow-controlled (volume/flow-controlled).[4] The reason for this is that any breath that is directly flow controlled is indirectly volume-controlled and vice versa.

In a situation where both pressure and volume waveforms are affected by changes in lung characteristics, the ventilator is a *time controller.* The only parameters being controlled would be inspiratory and expiratory times. Some high-frequency ventilators (HFVs) are time controllers. Even the distinction between inspiration and expiration can be difficult to make with all HFVs.[4]

Figure 21-12 shows the criteria that determine the control variable during a mechanical ventilator inspiratory phase. Table 21-2 shows the effects of changes in lung characteristics (respiratory system impedance) on actual waveform delivery in the two common types of ventilator functions (pressure controller and flow controller).

PHASE VARIABLES

The actual factors (variables) that provide the four components of a ventilator-delivered breath are called the phase variables. They are responsible for changing from one phase of the respiratory cycle into the next and for controlling what occurs during that portion of the breath. Again, the four parts of a breath are as follows: (1) inspiratory phase; (2) change from inspiration to expiration; (3) expiratory phase; (4) change from expiration to inspiration. In each of these four parts a certain variable (time, pressure, volume, or flow) is measured and used to begin, maintain, and end the phase. Figure 21-14 shows the criteria in determining the phase variable during a mechanical ventilator breath.[8]

There are three terms used to describe phase variables:

1. *Triggering* is the term applied to the variable that changes from expiration to inspiration.
2. *Cycling* is the term applied to the variable that changes from inspiration to expiration.
3. *Limiting* is a term used to describe which variables have a limited value during inspiration or expiration.

Triggering

When a variable such as time, pressure, volume, or flow reaches a preset value and causes the ventilator to change from expiration to inspiration, the ventilator is said to be *triggered* by that parameter. For example, suppose a preset rate is set on the ventilator at 12 breaths/min. A total respiratory cycle will equal 5

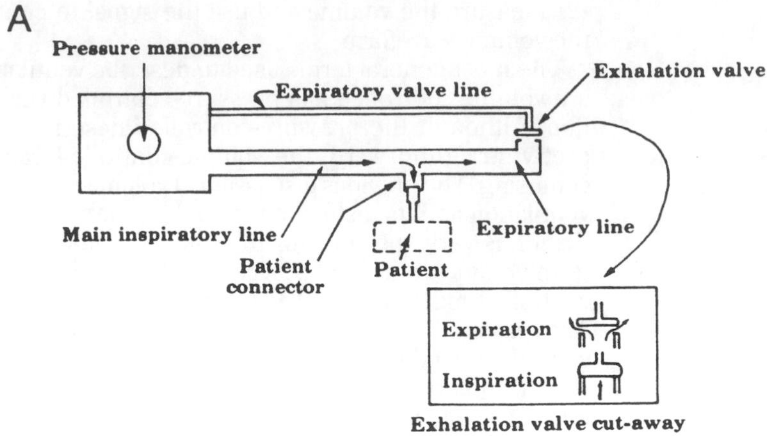

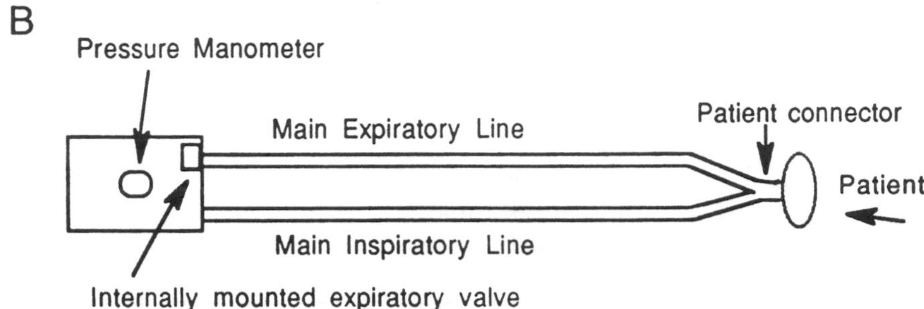

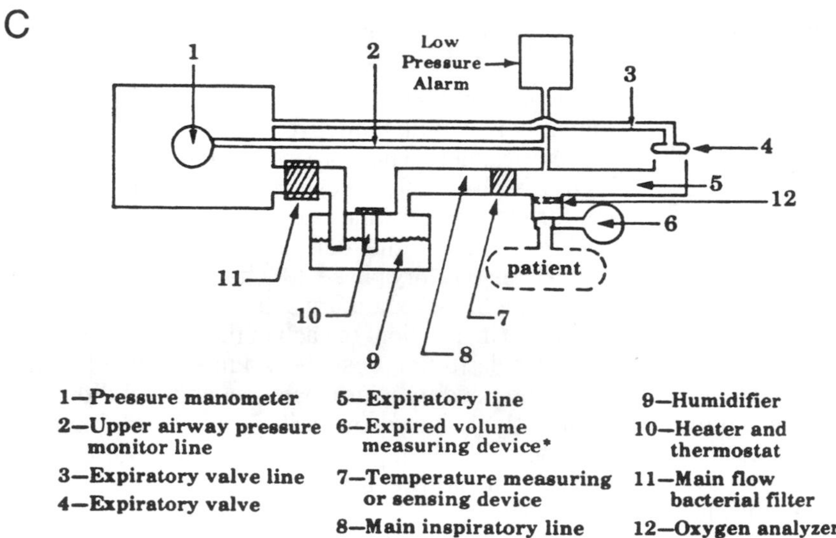

FIGURE 21-11. Basics of a patient circuit. **(A)**, the basic components of a patient circuit required to provide a positive pressure breath. The exhalation valve is mounted externally. **(B)**, an internally mounted exhalation valve. The expiratory valve line is not visible. It is inside the ventilator. **(C)**, a patient circuit containing additional components which are required for optimal functioning during continuous mechanical ventilation. (from: Pilbeam SP: Mechanical Ventilation, Physiological and Clinical Applications (2nd ed.) Chicago, Mosby–Year Book, 1992, p 113)

seconds (60/12 sec = 5 sec). Suppose the ventilator reaches the end of the 5 seconds and this causes the machine to start the next inspiration. The ventilator is then said to be *time-triggered.* Inspiration begins when a certain time has elapsed. This occurs independently from a patient's spontaneous effort.

When a ventilator has a sensitivity control (patient-triggering or patient effort control) on the user interface, this can be set to a preset pressure such as -1 cmH_2O. When the ventilator detects patient inspiratory effort sufficient to cause a drop in baseline pressure by -1 cmH_2O, it initiates inspiration. This is called *pressure-triggering.* This breath starts regardless of the set on the rate. It is essential that the operator sets the sensitivity for the individual patient's needs. If it is not set correctly and the machine is not sensitive to the patient, the patient must work harder to trigger a ventilator breath. If too sensitive, it can auto-trigger (start an inspiration on its own) when the patient is not actually making a significant inspiratory effort.

A ventilator is *flow-triggered* when the preset flow variable drops below the baseline flow. For example, suppose a baseline flow of 6 L/min is passing through the ventilator circuit. Assume the preset flow trigger is set at 3 L/min by the operator. When the ventilator detects the drop of 3 L/min from the baseline of 6 L/min as the

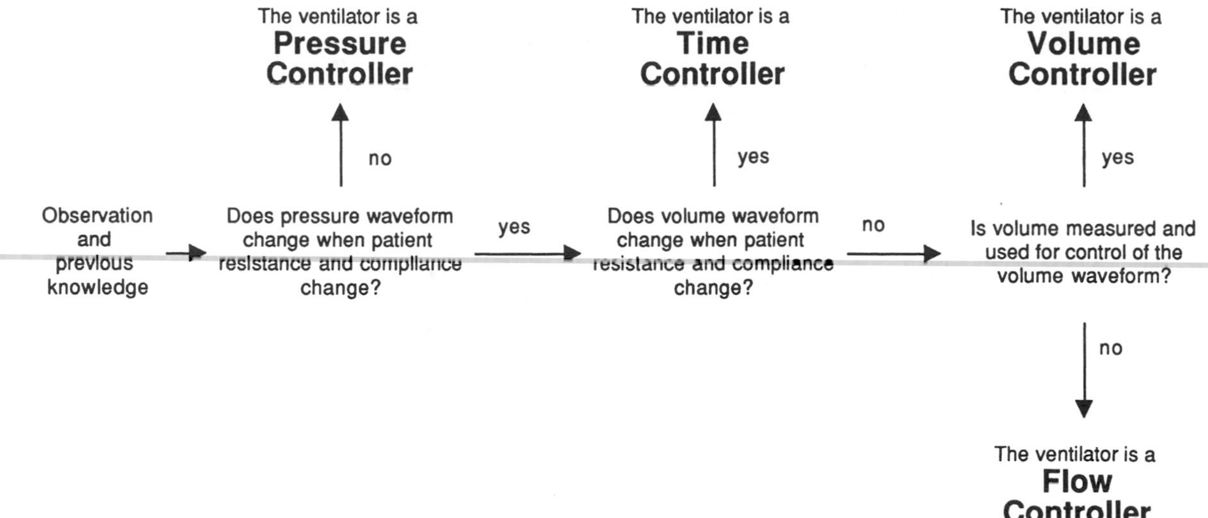

FIGURE 21-12. Criteria for determining the control variable during a ventilator supported inspiration. Beginning with observations and previous knowledge of this ventilator, decisions are based on the effect of load (patient lung characteristics, i.e. resistance and compliance) on ventilator output. (From Chatburn RL Ventilator Classification in Branson RD, Chatburn RL, et al: Respiratory Care Equipment, Philadelphia, JB Lippincott Co, 1995, p 271)

patient breathes in, it will initiate inspiration. Flow-triggering has been shown to require less inspiratory work of breathing (WOB) than pressure-triggering when set appropriately. The Puritan-Bennett 7200a and the Bird V.I.P. are examples of ventilators that provide flow-triggering.

Ventilators can also be *manually triggered* in most cases. This is accomplished by activating the "manual breath" button or control. They can even be set to trigger based on chest wall movement (Infrasonics Star Sync module on the Infant Star ventilator), although this is not a method commonly used.[4]

Inspiratory Phase and Limiting a Breath

The length of inspiration is the time from the beginning of inspiratory flow to the start of expiratory flow. During the inspiratory phase the ventilator can control pressure, volume, or flow as described previously in this section. In addition, the ventilator can also limit these variables. If one of these variables reaches but never goes higher than a preset value, then that variable is said to be *limited.* For example, suppose a ventilator was in a pressure control mode with a preset pressure of +20 cmH_2O. Imagine that it was set to cycle out of inspiration after 3 seconds of time had passed from the beginning of inspiratory flow. This breath would be described as pressure-limited and time-cycled. The pressure would not exceed the preset value, but reaching that pressure would not end inspiration. The preset time parameter would end inspiration in this example. It is important to remember that a limiting variable cannot exceed a certain value, but it is not by definition the variable that ends inspiration and begins expiration.

Maximum Safety Pressure

All commonly used mechanical ventilators have a maximum pressure capability. This limit may be incorporated into the basic design or added to the circuit in the form of a "pop-off" valve. Thus, whatever their primary cycling mechanism may be, ventilators are ultimately *pressure-limited,* whether or not they are also pressure-cycled. This feature is designed to protect the patient against possible excessive pressure buildup or tidal volume delivery that may occur inadvertently or through operator error.

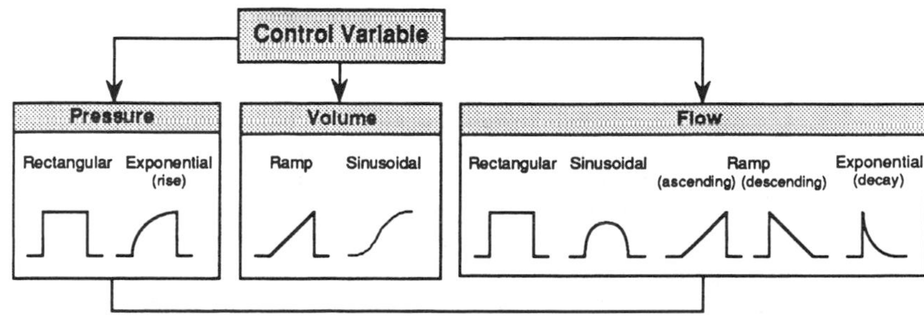

FIGURE 21-13. During inspiration, the ventilator is only able to control one of three variables, pressure, volume, or flow, during a breath. The common waveforms for each control variable are shown. (From Chatburn RL: A new system for understanding mechanical ventilators. Respiratory Care 36: 1132, 1991)

TABLE 21-2 **Idealized Load Effects for Pressure and Flow-Controllers**

Ventilator Type	Respiratory Parameters*	Load Effect	Desired Waveform	Actual Waveform
Pressure-controller	↑C, ↓R	Large	⊓	⊓
	↑C, ↑R	Medium	⊓	⊓
	↓C, ↓R	Medium	⊓	⊓
	↓C, ↑R	Small	⊓	⊓
Flow-controller	↑C, ↓R	Small	⊓	⊓
	↑C, ↑R	Medium	⊓	⊓
	↓C, ↓R	Medium	⊓	⊓
	↓C, ↑R	Large	⊓	⊓

* ↑ = high; ↓ = low; C = compliance; R = resistance.
From Chatburn RL: A new system for understanding mechanical ventilators. Respir Care 36:1132, 1991; with permission.

The pressure relief mechanism is adjustable in many ventilators, thereby adding to its protection effect. The relief valve is commonly set 10 cmH_2O higher than the pressure required to ventilate the patient in a volume control breath. The primary time-, flow-, or volume-cycling mechanism will then be operative, and slight to moderate decreases in compliance will be compensated for by the additional available pressure. Significant decreases in compliance or increases in resistance, or both, will cause a buildup in system pressure. The relief assembly is then activated and the excess gas flow and pressure, which might otherwise injure the patient, are vented from the circuit. An audible and/or visible alarm usually sounds at this time to alert persons caring for the patient that something has gone wrong. In some ventilators, when the maximum safety pressure is reached, it also cycles the ventilator into exhalation. In this case, however, the delivered tidal volume is not known and varies with pressure.

It is possible to remove or inactivate the pressure-limiting valve assembly and, thereby, develop a higher op-

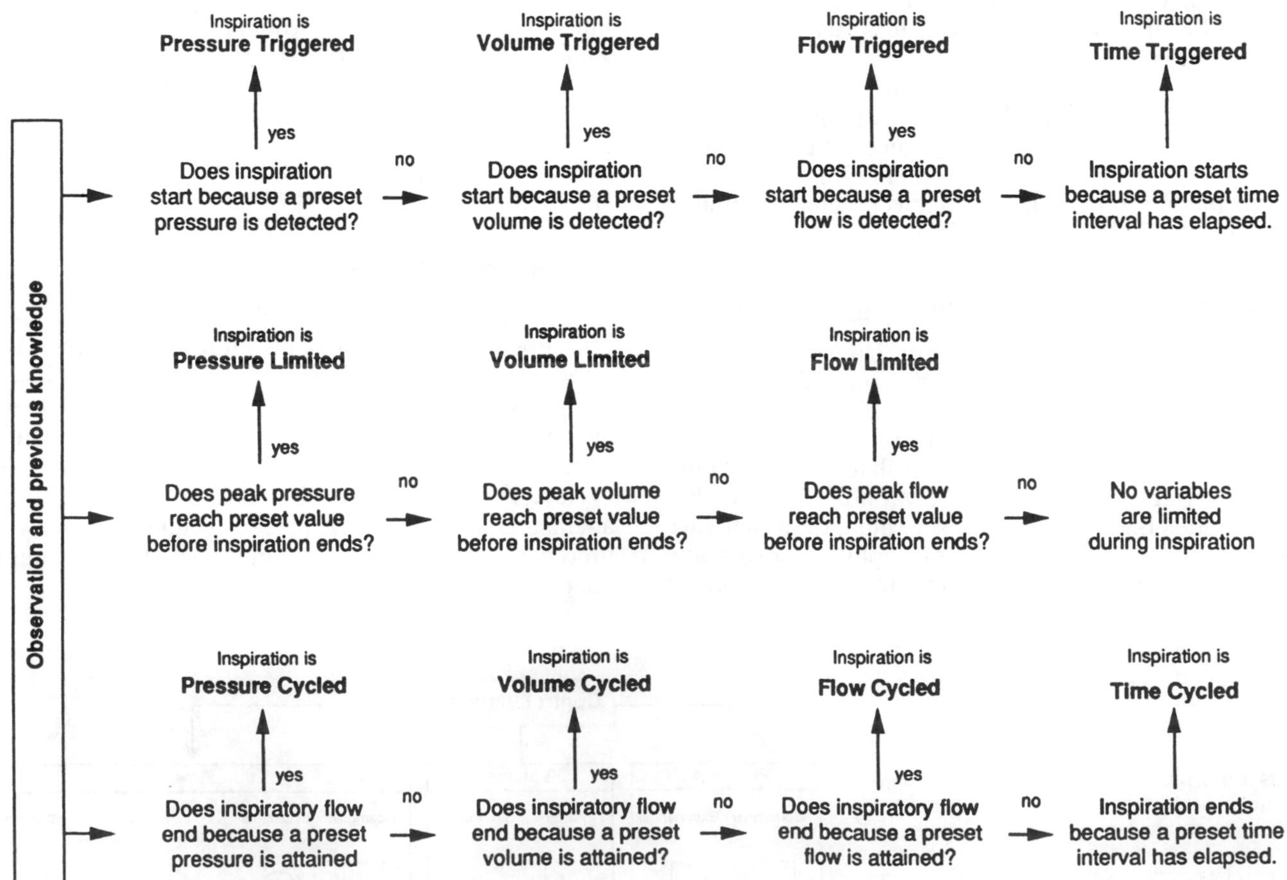

FIGURE 21-14. Criteria for determining the phase variables during a ventilator-supported breath. (From Chatburn RL: A new system for understanding mechanical ventilators. Respiratory Care 36:1135, 1991)

erational pressure. This temptation should be resisted because of the risk of injury to the patient and because ventilators generally are designed to operate efficiently within a preselected range of pressure.

CHANGEOVER FROM INSPIRATORY TO EXPIRATORY PHASE

Early classification systems were often confusing in the use of their terminology that described the changeover from inspiration to expiration.[9,10] Mapleson[11] introduced a system where the preset variable causing the ventilator to end the inspiratory phase was called the *cycling* mechanism. This included the categories of time-cycled, pressure-cycled, volume-cycled, and flow-cycled.

This system fits well into the ventilator classification scheme. The preset variable, time, pressure, volume, or flow are actually measured by the ventilator, and the information obtained from this measurement helps the ventilator to determine when to end the inspiratory flow. Table 21-3 lists the classifications of common ventilator modes and uses the control scheme and phase variables described in the section on classification in this chapter.[3,4,6,8,12]

Time-Cycled Ventilation

One of the common cycling mechanisms is time. *Time-cycling* terminates inspiratory gas flow and changes to the expiratory phase when a preselected time interval has elapsed after the start of inspiration. At the designated time, the exhalation valve opens (unless an inflation-hold is used), and the delivered tidal volume (V_T) is vented to the ambient atmosphere. If gas flow is constant and the time interval is precisely controlled, V_T can be predicted according to the following relationship:

$$\text{Volume} = \text{flow (volume/unit time)} \times \text{time}$$

In the United States, time-cycled ventilation has been used extensively to ventilate neonates. Several time-cycled ventilator models developed for older children and adults appear to be as versatile as volume-cycled ventilators in terms of pressure and flow capabilities.

In many of the third-generation ventilators, the ventilator can measure flow, compare it with the tidal volume setting, and calculate how much time would have to elapse to deliver that volume from the flow provided. Once this is calculated, it ends the breath after the calculated time has passed. For example, suppose the volume is set at 1 L and the flow is 60 L/min or 1 L/sec. By measuring and checking that the flow rate is 1 L/sec, the ventilator can then establish that the desired tidal volume (1 L) should have been delivered after 1 second, and ends inspiration. This volume, however, is delivered into the circuit, not necessarily into the patient. Changes in airway resistance and pulmonary or chest wall compliance may alter gas delivery to the patient and cause changes in airway pressure from one breath to the next. Volume delivery can be affected if there is a leak in the circuit as well. It should be noted that pressure-control ventilation is also time-cycled (see section on Pressure-Cycled Ventilation below).

Pressure-Cycled Ventilation

Pressure-cycled ventilation terminates the inspiratory phase when a preselected airway pressure has been achieved. The exhalation valve then opens, initiating the expiratory phase. If an inflation hold is used, expiration is delayed. A simple example of a pressure-cycled ventilator is the Bird Mark 7. Many other ventilators offer this feature, but many of them have alarms that come on when the pressure is reached. For example, if the pressure-limit control is set on the Bear 2, the ventilator will end inspiration when the pressure limit is reached, and this causes an alarm to sound and illuminate. In this example, the ventilator is actually pressure-cycled out of inspiration. To avoid the alarm going off if pressure cycling is desired, the alarm must be turned off or it will activate with each breath.

Tidal volume and the time of active flow delivery will vary in pressure-cycled ventilation according to airway resistance, pulmonary and chest wall compliance, and the integrity of the ventilator circuit. A significant decrease in the gas delivered to the patient may occur either because of leaks within the ventilator circuit, or increased resistance in the circuit or in the patient's airway. A large circuit leak prevents the buildup in pressure needed to terminate gas flow, but the gas does not reach the patient. In contrast, increased resistance, which may be caused by kinking of the circuit tubing or endotracheal tube or by mucus within the patient's airway, causes a rapid buildup in pressure, and premature cycling occurs before adequate V_T has been delivered.

Some pressure-cycled ventilators (such as the Bird Mark 14) incorporate an auxiliary flow augmentation device. This mechanism is activated at a preselected time during the inspiratory phase so that V_T is maintained and cycling pressure is reached even with significant leaks.

Because volume delivery is unpredictable with pressure cycling, this mode is seldom used in intensive care settings. Ventilators that are exclusively pressure-cycled usually lack a system to deliver precisely controlled levels of oxygen and PEEP. They are used predominately for intermittent positive pressure breathing (IPPB) and home therapy.

Volume-Cycled Ventilation

In *volume-cycled* ventilation the inspiratory phase ends when a preselected volume of gas has been delivered. As with pressure- and time-cycled ventilation, if an inflation hold is used, the expiratory phase will be delayed. Some volume-cycled ventilators are manufactured with pressure-limiting valves, some fixed and others adjustable, that prevent excessive pressure from developing within the system if airway obstruction occurs. Without this pressure-limiting valve, excessive pressure may lead to pulmonary barotrauma.

TABLE 21-3 **Suggested Terminology for Operational Modes, Their Classification, and Relationship to Old Terminology**

	Mandatory			
Mode	*Control*	*Trigger*	*Limit*	*Cycle*
Constant airway pressure (CAP)	—	—	—	—
Continuous spontaneous ventilation (CSV)	—	—	—	—
Continuous mandatory ventilation (CMV)	Pressure	Pressure, volume, flow, or time	Pressure	Time
	Volume/flow	Pressure, volume, flow, or time	Volume/flow	Volume, flow, or time
Intermittent mandatory ventilation (IMV)	Pressure	Pressure, volume, flow, or time	Pressure	Time
	Volume/flow	Pressure, volume, flow, or time	Volume or flow	Volume, flow, or time
Mandatory minute ventilation (MMV)	Volume/flow	Time	Volume or flow	Volume, flow, or time

One example of a ventilator that is volume-cycled is the MA-1. It measures the volume displacement of the internal bellows, and once the preset tidal volume has been reached, it ends inspiration, regardless of the time it may take.

Volume-cycled ventilators generally cannot compensate for a significant air leak. Gas delivery from a piston stroke or compressible bellows, the two most common mechanical devices used to deliver V_T, or flow from a proportioning valve (in one of the third-generation ventilators) continues unabated, even if the patient is disconnected from the circuit. A leak can be detected by monitoring the exhaled V_T. When the measured flow from the patient is substantially less than that delivered by the ventilator, a leak is present. Peak inspiratory pressure will usually be lower than previous values as well.

Physicians have been led to believe that volume-cycled ventilation maintains constant V_T delivery to the patient, regardless of changes in resistance and compliance. This alleged characteristic is largely responsible for the popularity of these devices in critical care settings. Actually, the volume of gas received by the patient may vary considerably with volume-cycled ventilation. When the ventilator triggers on, gas flows into both the circuit and the patient. How much is distributed to each depends on their relative compliance. If the patient's compliance decreases, a larger percentage of the volume is lost within the circuit due to expansion of the tubing and compression of the inspiratory gas within the humidifier or nebulizer, water traps, bellows or cylinder, connectors, and so forth. Conversely, if the patient's compliance improves, less inspiratory gas is retained within the circuit.

The compliance/compression factor of the circuit is variable, but a value of 4 mL/cmH_2O is representative for adult circuits. This means that 4 mL of gas is retained within the circuit for each cmH_2O of circuit pressure developed. If high airway pressures are used to maintain adequate ventilation, several hundred milliliters of the total volume may be retained in the circuit rather than delivered to the patient (Fig. 21-15). Personnel who are monitoring the patient and ventilator may be unaware of this discrepancy, however, because a monitor connected to the exhalation valve assembly records gas passing from both the patient and circuit. The sum of these is the volume that was delivered by the ventilator, but not necessarily to the patient. The latter can be determined only if exhaled gas is collected between the patient's airway and the Y-connector of the ventilator circuit, a technically difficult feat in some cases, or by interposing a respirometer in the same location.

Newer-generation ventilators can take this discrepancy into account. For example, the Puritan Bennett 7200 ventilator can measure the circuit compliance/compressibility during one of its start-up self-tests. From that point on, it can measure the peak pressure of a breath and estimate the volume that will be lost because of circuit compressibility. For the next breath it can add the volume to the target volume to compensate for this loss.

Flow-Cycled Ventilation

If a preset flow is obtained and reaching this flow ends inspiratory flow, the breath is *flow-cycled.* Flow-cycled ventilation is independent of airway pressure, V_T, or duration of inspiration. One example of a ventilator that uses flow-cycling is the Bennett PR-2 ventilator. Flow cycling is the most common form of cycling in the

Spontaneous				Control Logic			
Control	*Trigger*	*Limit*	*Cycle*	*Assisted?*	*Conditional Variable*	*Action*	*Prior Terms*
Pressure	Pressure, volume, or flow	Pressure	Pressure	No	—	—	CPAP
Pressure	Pressure, volume, or flow	Pressure	Volume	Yes	—	—	PSV
—	—	—	—	—	Time or patient effort	Machine-to-patient trigger	PC-CMV, PCIRV, PC-A/C
—	—	—	—	—	Time or patient effort	Machine-to-patient trigger	CMV, A/C
Pressure	Pressure, volume, or flow	Pressure	Pressure	No	Time or patient effort	Machine-to-patient trigger	PC-IMV, APRV, BiPAP, PC-SIMV
Pressure	Pressure, volume, or flow	Pressure	Pressure	No	Time or patient effort	Machine-to-patient trigger	IMV, SIMV
Pressure	Pressure, volume, or flow	Pressure	Pressure	Yes*	Minute volume or time	Spontaneous-to-mandatory breath	MMV, EMMV

* Optional.

CMV, continuous mandatory ventilation; A/C, assist/control; AMV, assisted mechanical ventilation; IMV, intermittent mandatory ventilation; SIMV, synchronized mandatory ventilation; CPAP, continuous positive airway pressure; PCV, pressure-controlled ventilation; PC-IMV, pressure-controlled IMV; PCIRV, PC inverse-ratio ventilation; APRV, airway pressure release ventilation; PSV, pressure support ventilation; MMV, mandatory minute ventilation; BiPAP, bilevel positive airway pressure.

From Branson RD, Chatburn RL: Technical description and classification of modes of ventilator operation. Respir Care 37:1026–1044, 1992; with permission.[12]

mode of ventilation called pressure support. In the pressure support mode, it is common for the ventilator to cycle into exhalation when the flow during inspiration has dropped to 25% of the peak flow measured during inspiration. This tells the ventilator that the patient's inspiratory effort is slowing and exhalation is about to begin.

Baseline

During exhalation, the variable that is controlled is called the baseline variable. Any variable of flow, volume, time, or pressure can theoretically be controlled. The most common variable that is monitored on current ventilators is pressure. The baseline pressure can be zero (atmospheric) and can also be positive or above atmospheric. This is commonly referred to as PEEP. During high-frequency oscillatory ventilation, the airway pressure goes through both positive and negative changes in relation to the mean airway pressure. In this situation, the baseline pressure is considered the mean airway pressure.

Flow can also be used as a baseline. It can be set at zero or above zero, such as 2 L/min. A continuous flow of 2 L/min is provided by the ventilator through the patient circuit. For example, on the Puritan-Bennett 7200 in the "flow-by" selection, a baseline flow is set by the operator. In this setting the ventilator is flow-triggered and the trigger sensitivity is a flow also selected by the operator.

EXPIRATORY PHASE

The expiratory phase begins when the exhalation valve opens or inspiratory flow ends. The expiratory valve may open immediately on cessation of inspiration or later if inflation hold is interposed. Ventilator control of expiratory events has become increasingly important.

Because exhalation is usually passive, a longer time is required than for inhalation. This ratio (I/E ratio), however, should be individualized, particularly when an inflation-hold is deemed necessary.

Expiratory Retardation

Observation of patients with chronic obstructive pulmonary disease (COPD) who use pursed-lip breathing, apparently to prevent premature airway collapse and air trapping, led to the design of systems that increase resistance or retardation to exhalation (see Fig. 21-1). More complete emptying of the lungs (decreased functional residual capacity [FRC]) occurs in contrast to PEEP, which characteristically increases FRC. At the termination of expiratory retardation, airway pressure returns to ambient before the next cycle.

All ventilator circuits produce a certain amount of retardation because of the intrinsic resistance to flow of the airway connectors, tubing, and the exhalation valve. The respiratory care practitioner must be aware of the normal expiratory flow pattern, so that undesirable increases in retardation can be detected. The easiest

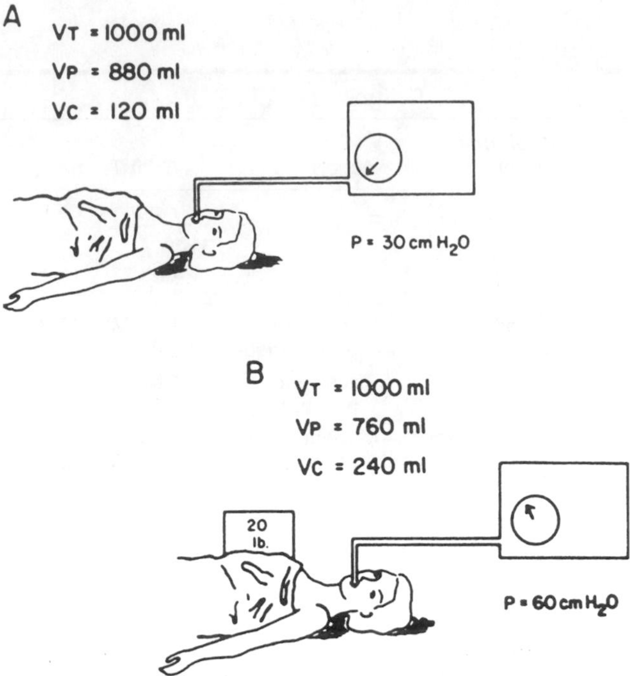

FIGURE 21-15. Effect of changing patient compliance on ventilation. **(A)** A pressure of 30 cmH_2O delivers a tidal volume of 1000 mL, of which 880 mL reaches the patient and 120 mL is retained in the ventilator circuit. **(B)** The ventilator again delivers the 1000 mL tidal volume, but because of decreased patient compliance a pressure of 60 cmH_2O is needed, and only 760 mL reaches her, whereas 240 mL is lost to the circuit. In this example, circuit compliance/compression is 4 mL/cmH_2O. (V_T = total volume delivered by ventilator; V_P = patient volume; V_c = retained circuit volume; P = airway pressure.)

method of detecting increased expiratory retardation is to note the rate at which the airway pressure manometer needle returns to baseline level from the peak after inflation. Another way is to view the graphics screen provided by the ventilator of pressure/time and observe the descent of the expiratory curve. To be most accurate, one should measure the airway pressure as close as possible to the junction of the ventilator circuit and patient; otherwise, the pressure measurements may be altered by resistance of the ventilator, tubing exhalation valve opening, and so forth.

The importance or desirability of the use of expiratory retard during mechanical ventilation of patients with COPD, acute asthmatic attacks, or the like is unknown. Some studies suggest that the importance attached to pursed-lip breathing has been exaggerated.

Subambient Pressure (Negative End-Expiratory Pressure)

The application of a subambient (negative) pressure to the ventilator circuit during the expiratory phase was at one time advocated for two primary purposes: to decrease mean airway pressure and, hence, mean intrathoracic pressure, in order to enhance venous return and improve cardiac output; and to offset the effects of excessive resistance that may result from an artificial airway.

Reduction of circuit pressure in this way increases the pressure gradient across the tube from the patient end to the circuit end, and, in theory, should enhance expiratory gas flow. How much practical importance should be attached to this maneuver is unclear. The use of subambient pressure fell from favor because it was difficult to determine whether the reduced pressure is transmitted to the patient's side of the airway. If this should occur, airway collapse and air trapping, the opposite of what is desired, would occur.

Positive End-Expiratory Pressure

Application of positive pressure to the airway during the expiratory phase (see Fig. 21-1) is a mainstay in the treatment of the adult respiratory distress syndrome (ARDS). The effects of this therapy presumably prevent terminal airway and alveolar collapse and improve overall ventilation–perfusion ratios, although some regional ventilation–perfusion relationships may actually worsen. Improvement in pulmonary compliance and arterial oxygenation is often significant and may allow a reduction of F_{IO_2}, a desirable goal to prevent absorption atelectasis and pulmonary oxygen toxicity.

Various techniques are used to generate PEEP. A simple method allows patient exhalation through tubing, the distal end of which is under water. The level of PEEP depends on the depth to which the tubing has been submerged. With other systems, the ventilator activates a valve assembly during exhalation. The valve closes when the desired expiratory positive pressure is reached, and any gas that has not been exhaled is held within the lungs and ventilator circuit. In some cases, the valve used to create PEEP also has a high internal resistance, which gives an expiratory retard effect. An elevated mean intrathoracic pressure above that produced by PEEP may result. This can produce unwanted reduction of venous return in the patient with marginal intravascular volume or cardiovascular performance.

The recommended maximum level of PEEP is usually 10 to 15 cmH_2O; however, some patients with severe ARDS do not respond with improved oxygenation and decreased shunting at these levels. In the late 1970s, studies suggested that increased PEEP (40 cmH_2O or more) was used successfully in selected patients, combined with intermittent mandatory ventilation (IMV) (see modes of ventilation).[13,14] A reduced mortality with no increase in ventilator-related morbidity was reported. However, this type of high PEEP therapy is controversial. Most persons who require PEEP respond adequately to the earlier recommended levels. For those who do not, however, alternative forms of ventilation may provide solutions. These might include pressure control ventilation (PCV), inverse ratio ventilation (IRV) (volume or pressure controlled), and HFV. More aggressive therapy may be life-saving. Current trends in ventilation suggest that using low tidal volumes as PEEP levels are increased is appropriate. Permitting $PaCO_2$ levels to rise (permissive hypercarbia) may be required by this maneuver. In addition, it is recommended that total alveolar pressures including total PEEP (PEEP + auto-PEEP) be kept at or below 35 cmH_2O to avoid lung damage associated with high ventilating pressure.[15] Chapter 20 provides some additional discussion on these alternative forms of ventilation.

MODES OF VENTILATION

On currently available ventilators there is usually a control called the "mode control." This may be a knob that can be turned to indicate a specific mode or it can be a touch pad or dial that can select a specific mode from a computer menu. Unfortunately, manufacturers are not consistent in naming, so trying to figure out what the actual mode "label" means can be confusing!

Up until this decade, respiratory care practitioners and pulmonary physicians learned a set of ventilator modes that constituted what was available on the various ventilators and how these modes operated. These included the following: control, assist/control, assist, IMV, synchronized intermittent mandatory ventilation (SIMV), pressure support, and pressure control. Explaining how a mode actually operated required a lengthy discussion. In 1991 Robert Chatburn proposed a new method of ventilator classification in an effort to remove some of the lengthy explanation required and to accommodate the development of new modes that no longer fit the old set of rules.[2] To assist in making the transition from the old terminology to the newer classification, the following discussion provides the original terms and then uses the newer system of description.

Modes are basically types of breaths that the ventilator can deliver in different patterns. Table 21-3 summarizes the classification of modes of ventilator operation. A mode should specify the control and phase variables for both mandatory and spontaneous breaths.[12] For example, the IMV plus pressure support would be described as follows: mandatory breaths are time-triggered, volume/flow controlled, flow-limited, and time-cycled; spontaneous breaths are pressure-triggered, pressure-limited, and flow-cycled.

Figure 21-16 shows some theoretical waveforms for pressure- and flow-controlled breaths that are associated with various modes of ventilation. These are es-

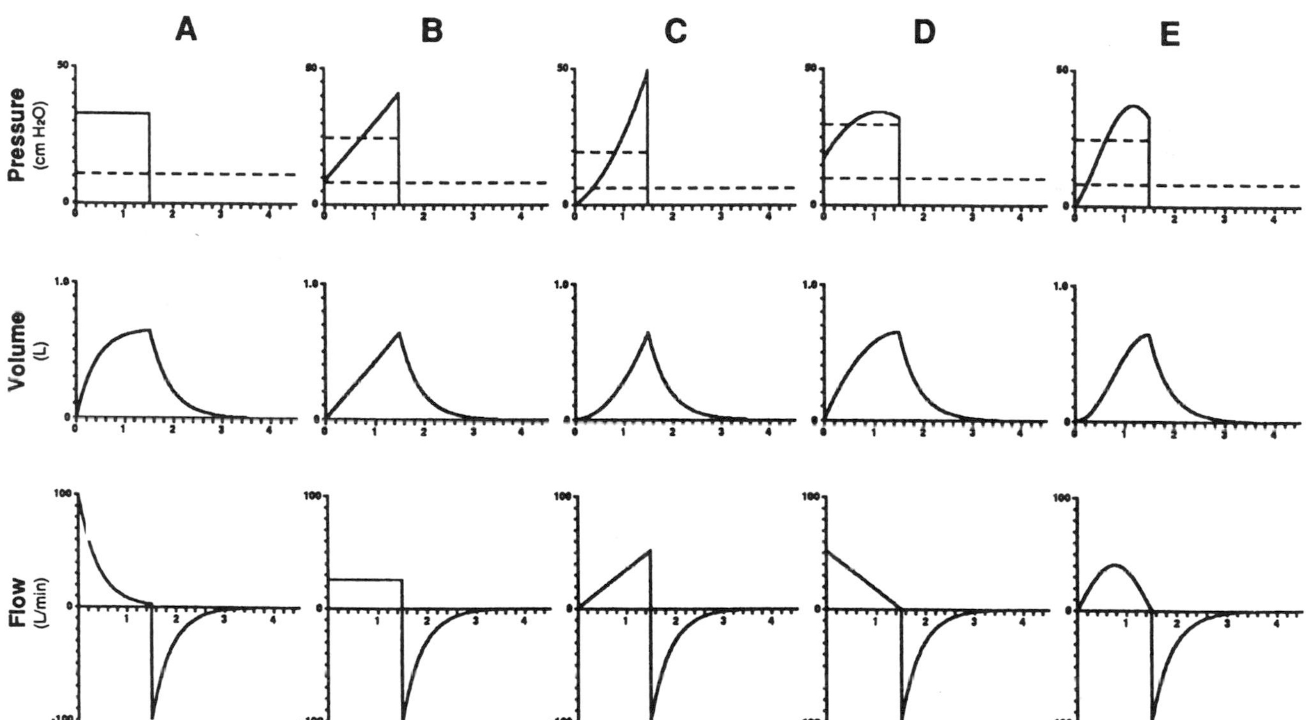

FIGURE 21-16. Theoretical output waveforms for **(A)** pressure controlled inspiration with rectangular pressure waveform, identical to flow controlled inspiration with an exponential-decay flow waveform; **(B)** flow-controlled inspiration with rectangular flow waveform, identical to volume controlled inspiration with an ascending-ramp volume waveform; **(C)** flow controlled inspiration with an ascending-ramp flow waveform; **(D)** flow controlled inspiration with descending-flow waveform; and **(E)** flow controlled inspiration with a sinusoidal flow waveform. The short dashed lines represent mean inspiratory pressure while the longer dashed lines denote mean airway pressure (assuming zero end-expiratory pressure). For the rectangular pressure waveform in **A**, the mean inspiratory pressure is the same as the peak inspiratory pressure. These output waveforms were created by (1) defining the control waveform (eg, an ascending-ramp flow waveform is specified as flow = constant × time) and specifying that the tidal volume equals 644 mL (about 9 mL/kg for a normal adult); (2) specifying the desired values for resistance and compliance (for these waveforms, compliance = 20 mL/cm H_2O and resistance = 20 cm H_2O/L/sec, according to American National Standards Institute (ANSI) recommendations); (3) substituting the above information into the equation of motion*; and (4) using a computer to solve the equation for pressure, volume, and flow, and plotting the results against time.

*muscle pressure + ventilator pressure = volume/compliance + (resistance × flow)

(From Chatburn RL: A new system for understanding mechanical ventilators. Respiratory Care 36:1143, 1991)

sentially selected by the ventilator's operator when he or she chooses a specific mode and flow waveform pattern to use with a particular patient.[2] Figure 21-17 shows typical pressure, flow, and volume waveforms for PCV and volume-controlled ventilation (VCV) and shows their application with the equation of motion.[2] The equation of motion is basically a mathematical way of describing the respiratory system and its behavior. In a simplified form the equation states:

$$\text{muscle pressure} + \text{ventilator pressure} = (\text{volume/compliance}) \times (\text{flow} \times \text{resistance})$$

where muscle pressure is the imaginary (not directly measurable) transrespiratory pressure (airway pressure minus body surface pressure), ventilator pressure is the transrespiratory pressure generated by the ventilator, and compliance and resistance are values for the patient's lung characteristics and are assumed to be constant.

Table 21-4 shows a variety of commercially available ventilators and the ventilator modes available with each.[6] Notice that in this table such terms as A/C (assist/control) and SIMV are used.

Pressure-Controlled (Targeted) Modes

Pressure-controlled modes (see Figs. 21-16 and 21-17) require that the operator set a peak inspiratory pressure. The ventilator's primary function is to achieve the target pressure. The beginning gas flow is rapid as the ventilator tries to achieve the pressure. Once the target pressure is reached, the flow usually tapers off in a slow descending fashion until the preset cycling mechanism, such as time, finally ends inspiratory flow and the pres-

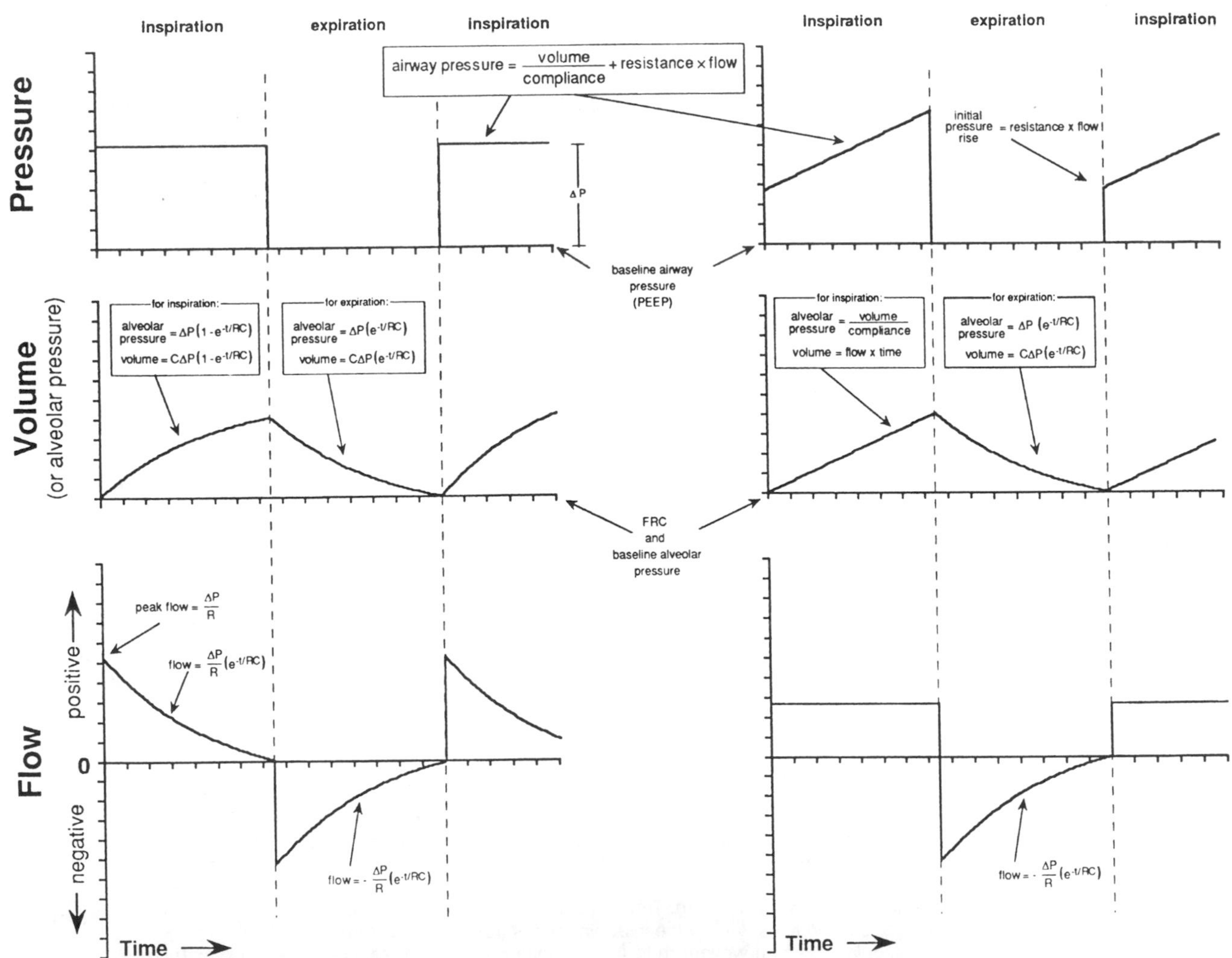

FIGURE 21-17. Typical pressure, volume, and flow waveforms for pressure controlled (rectangular pressure waveform) and volume controlled (rectangular flow waveform) ventilation. Pressure, volume, and flow are shown as functions of time in accordance with the equation of motion:

$$\text{muscle pressure} + \text{ventilator pressure} = \text{volume/compliance} + (\text{resistance} \times \text{flow})$$

(where muscle pressure = 0). Note that all variables are measured relative to their baseline, or end-expiratory values. P = change in airway pressure; R = resistance; C = compliance; t = time, e = base of natural logarithm (= 2.72), FRC = functional residual capacity. (From Chatburn RL: A new system for understanding mechanical ventilators. Respiratory Care 36: 1128, 1991)

TABLE 21-4 **Modes of Ventilation Available on Selected Mechanical Ventilators**

	CPAP	A/C	SIMV	MMV	PC	IRV	PC-IRV	BiPAP	PS	Continuous Flow	Apnea Ventilation
Bear 5	+	+	+	+					+	+	
Bird 6400ST	+	+	+						+		
Bird 8400ST	+	+	+						+		
Hamilton Veolar	+	+	+	+		+			+		+
Hamilton Amadeus	+	+	+						+		+
Infrasonics Adult Star	+	+	+			+			+		
Ohmeda Advent	+	+	+	+	+	+	+		+		+
PPG IRISA	+	+	+	+	+	+	+	+	+		+
Puritan-Bennett											
7200a	+	+	+			+			+	+	+
7200ae	+	+	+		+	+	+		+	+	+
7200sp	+	+				+			+		+
Siemens Servo 900E	+	+	+			+			+		
Siemens Servo 900C	+	+	+		+	+	+		+		

A/C: assist/control; BiPAP: bilevel positive airway pressure; IRV: inverse-ratio ventilation.
From Kacmarck RM, Hess D: Basic principles of ventilator machinery. In Tobin MJ (ed): Principles and Practices of Mechanical Ventilation. New York, McGraw-Hill, 1994, p 69; with permission.[6]

sure is released. When using modes that are pressure-controlled, the tidal volume varies based on several factors, mostly changes in the patient's lung characteristics.

PCV sometimes is used with inverse inspiratory-to-expiratory ratios and is referred to as pressure-control inverse-ratio ventilation (PCIRV). Figure 21-18 shows the pressure, flow, and volume curves during PCIRV.

Volume-Controlled (Targeted) Modes

Volume-controlled or volume-targeted modes (Fig. 21-19) require that the operator set a desired tidal volume. Usually the operator also sets the rate or inspiratory time and gas flow, including flow pattern. Using volume modes, the pressure varies depending on several factors, primarily patient's lung characteristics. But volume delivery usually stays constant.

Spontaneous and Mandatory Breaths

The terms spontaneous and mandatory are often used to describe the type of breath delivered during a particular mode of ventilation (Fig. 21-20). With spontaneous breaths, inspiration is initiated and ended by the patient. Sometimes flow, or pressure change, is based on patient lung characteristics. For example, during a pressure support breath, the ventilator ends inspiratory flow when the flow decreases to a certain value (flow-cycled). The reason that the flow slows in this instance is because the patient is coming to the end of inspiration. The patient's inspiratory flow is decreasing. The ventilator detects this and is programmed to shut off gas delivery to the patient. The programming is based on the idea that when flow is this slow, the patient must be at the end of his or her breath. As a result, the machine shuts off gas flow based on this internal programming. It is really the patient who terminates the breath. Thus, the pressure support breath is considered spontaneous.

Mandatory breaths are those that are either started or ended by the ventilator. For example, if a ventilator ends inspiratory flow when a preset volume is delivered (volume-cycled), then the breath is considered mandatory. If it starts a breath after a certain time has elapsed (time-triggered), it is considered a mandatory breath.

Assisted Ventilation

When the pressure curve for a breath rises above baseline during inspiration, the ventilator works on the patient. In this case the breath is said to be assisted, in that the ventilator is "assisting" the patient with the work of breathing. This terminology was first introduced by Chatburn[4] to describe any breath that fits this category. It will be easy to confuse the use of this term intended to describe any positive pressure breath, with the mode of ventilation sometimes called "assisted ventilation," where every breath is triggered by the patient (pressure-triggered) and the breath that follows is most commonly a volume-controlled breath.

Controlled Mechanical Ventilation

The term "controlled mechanical ventilation" (CMV) (Fig. 21-21) has been used to describe a volume-controlled, time-triggered form of ventilation. The patient is controlled by the ventilator. The patient cannot trigger the ventilator. Depending on the brand of ventilator used, the knob or dial may read "volume-controlled ventilation," "control mode," or "continuous mandatory ventilation." There is no consistency in how this is named on current ventilators. Controlled ventilation is volume-controlled, time-triggered continuous mandatory ventilation.

Controlled ventilation does not guarantee that patients will not attempt to initiate spontaneous ventilation. In such instances, the ventilator will not respond if

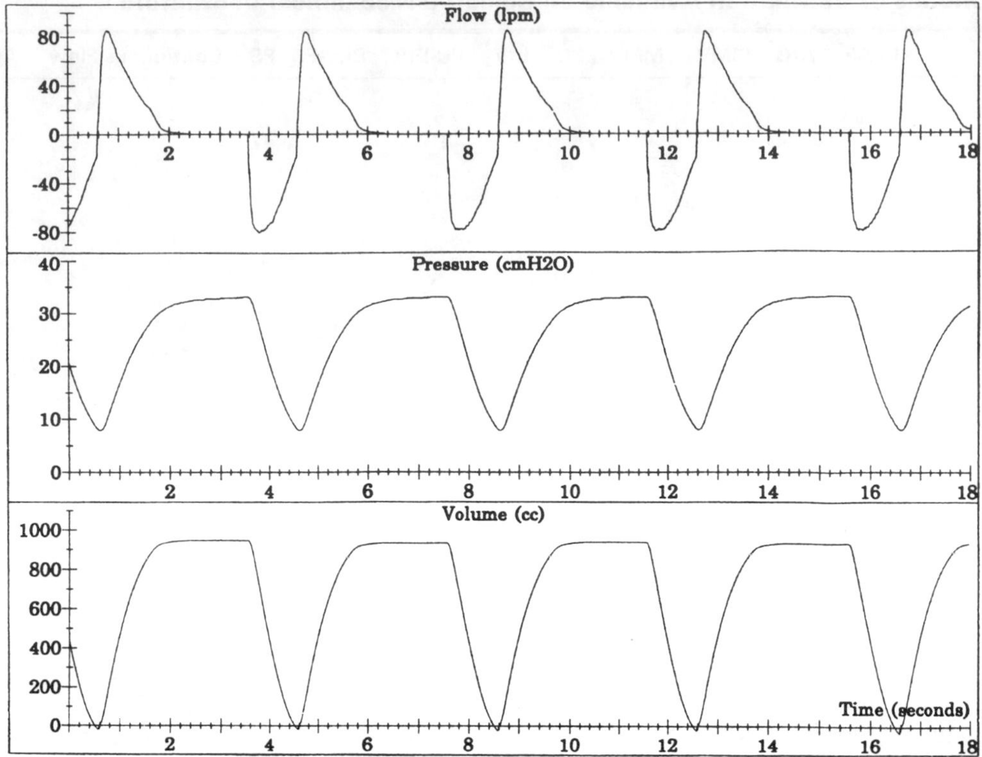

FIGURE 21-18. Pressure, flow and volume waveforms during pressure-control inverse-ratio ventilation (PCIRV), where the inspiratory-expiratory time ratio (I:E) is 3:1. Note that inspiratory flow has returned to zero before the end of the inspiratory phase, and an end-inspiratory hold is established. Volume is delivered into the patient's airway before half the inspiratory time is complete. As noted by the expiratory flow not returning to zero, some level of auto-PEEP is developed. (From Kacmarek RM, Hess D: Basic principles of ventilator machinery in Tobin, MJ: Principles and Practice of Mechanical Ventilation. New York, McGraw-Hill, 1994, p 82)[6]

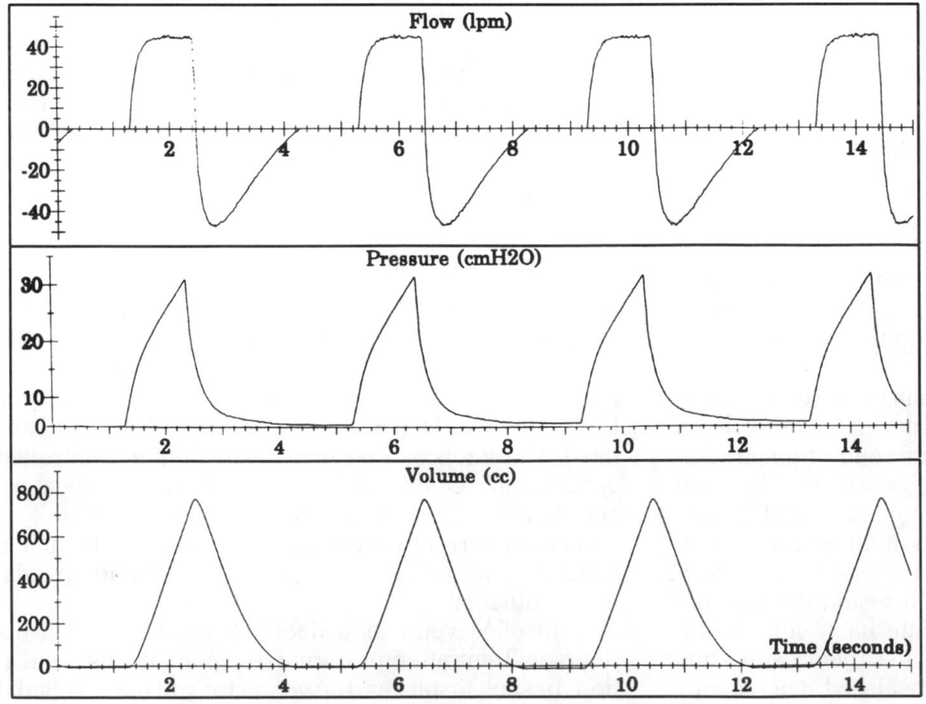

FIGURE 21-19. Pressure, flow, and volume waveforms during volume-targeted continuous mechanical ventilation (CMV) delivered with a rectangular waveform. Note no indication of patient triggering on the pressure waveform. (Modified from Kacmarek RM, Hess D: Basic principles of ventilator machinery in Tobin, MJ: Principles and Practice of Mechanical Ventilation. New York, McGraw-Hill, 1994, p 76)[6]

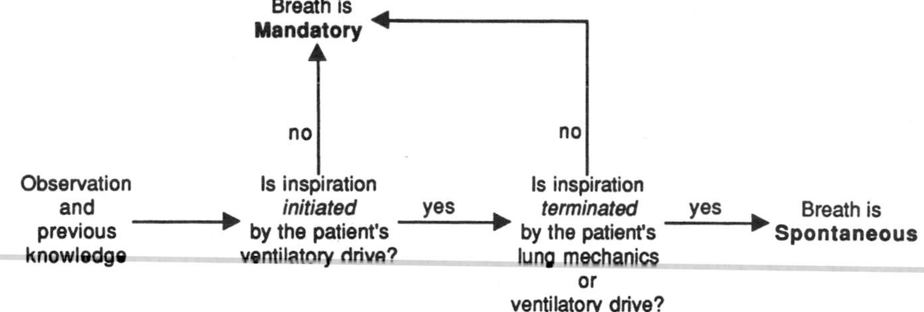

FIGURE 21-20. Algorithm defining spontaneous and mandatory breaths. If the breath is *triggered* according to a preset frequency or minimum minute ventilation or *cycled* according to a preset frequency or tidal volume, the breath is *mandatory*. All other breaths are *spontaneous*.

it is used strictly in a control mode (ventilator sensitivity "off") and the ventilatory pattern becomes assynchronous: the patient attempts to take more breaths than the ventilator will provide. Failure to obtain a breath on demand leads to patient apprehension and may result in carbon dioxide retention and increased work of breathing.

Assist-Control Ventilation

In this mode, a minimum acceptable rate and tidal volume is set by the operator (Fig. 21-22). The patient can pressure-trigger the ventilator at a higher rate and receive the preset volume with each effort. A/C can also be flow-triggered. The only real difference between control and A/C is that the operator must set a sensitivity setting. In newer terminology this would be considered volume-controlled, pressure-cycled, or time-cycled continuous mandatory ventilation.

If the pressure-trigger mechanism is not functioning properly, the patient expends considerable effort attempting to breathe. If the sensitivity is not correctly set or the flow rate is too low to meet patient demand, the patient may become agitated, hypoxic, hypercarbic, and may "fight the ventilator." This increases the patient's work of breathing.

The greatest difficulty with A/C ventilation is improper adjustment of the ventilator, leading to unreliability of many assist mechanisms. One frequently experiences situations in which the A/C mode is so sensitive that the ventilator autotriggers. In other instances, it is so insensitive that the ventilator does not respond to the patient's inspiratory effort. If patients are experiencing air-trapping (auto-PEEP), this impairs their ability to trigger the ventilator and increases the work of breathing.

Assisted Mechanical Ventilation

Historically, in assisted mechanical ventilation (AMV) (Fig. 21-23), all breaths were patient-triggered (pressure-triggered). Technically, there was no back-up rate set by the operator. Each breath that was triggered delivered the preset volume. This was basically a pressure-

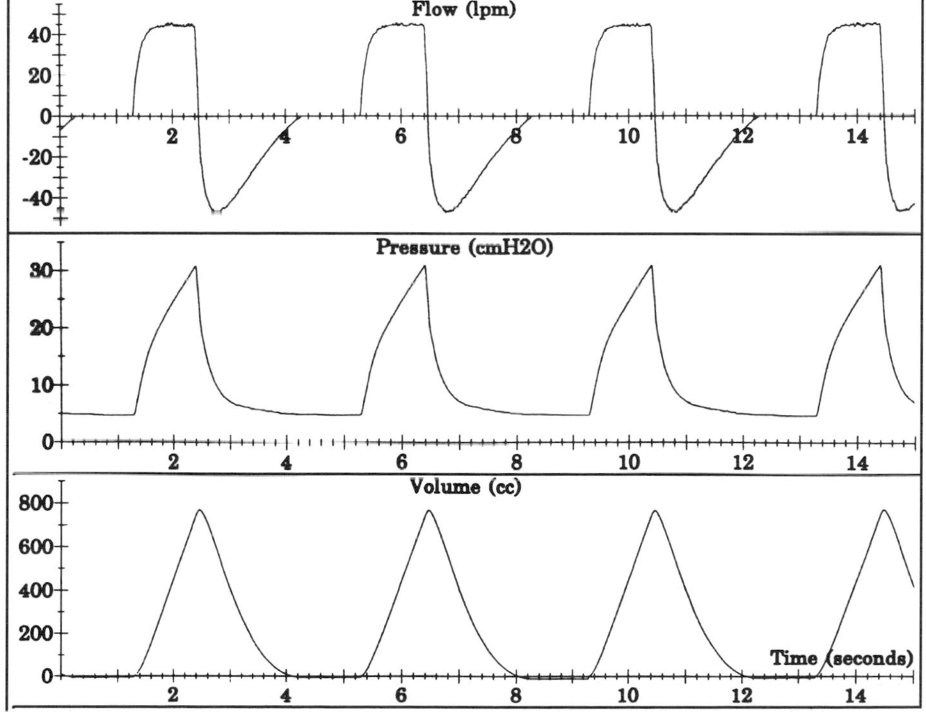

FIGURE 21-21. Pressure, flow and volume waveforms during volume-targeted continuous mechanical ventilation (CMV) delivered with a rectangular waveform. In addition, PEEP of 5 cmH_2O is present. Note no indication of patient triggering (pressure-triggering) on the pressure waveform. (From Kacmarek RM, Hess D: Basic principles of ventilator machinery in Tobin, MJ: Principles and Practice of Mechanical Ventilation. New York, McGraw-Hill, 1994, p 76)

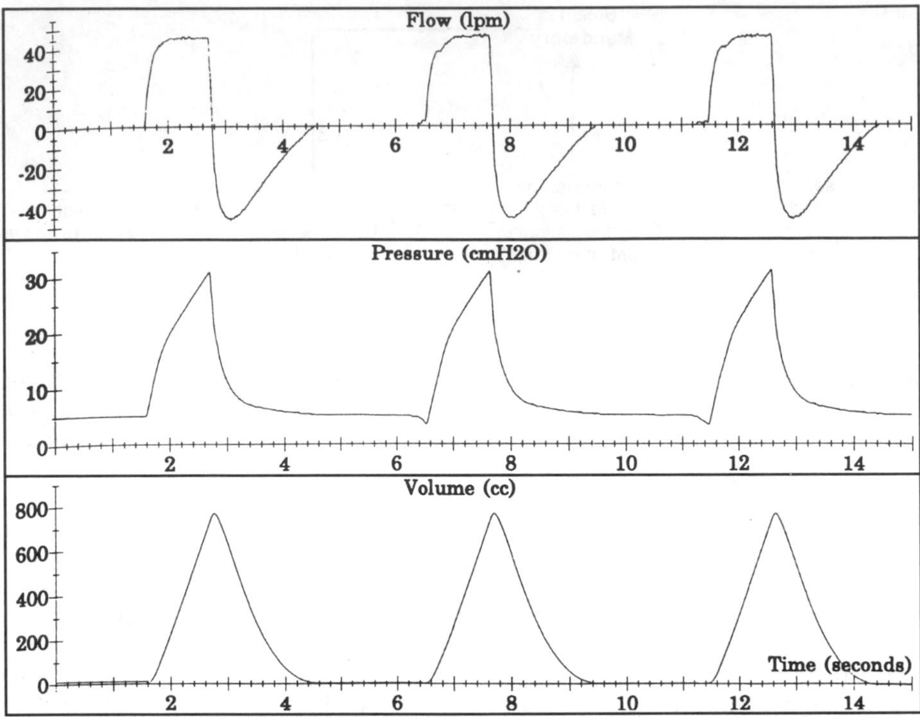

FIGURE 21-22. Pressure, flow and volume waveforms during volume-targeted assist-control mechanical ventilation delivered with a rectangular waveform. Note some breaths are patient triggered (pressure-triggering) on the pressure waveform (drop in airway pressure baseline prior to breath) while others are controlled breaths. (From Kacmarek RM, Hess D: Basic principles of ventilator machinery in Tobin, MJ: Principles and Practice of Mechanical Ventilation. New York, McGraw-Hill, 1994, p 77)[6]

triggered, volume-controlled, time-cycled mode of ventilation. This outdated mode is mentioned here only for completeness, but technically it is no longer used because individuals who manage ventilators now always set a back-up rate for patients (assist/control). In addition, the term "assisted ventilation" now has a new definition as stated in the previous section by that name.

Intermittent Mandatory Ventilation

Ventilators with IMV (Fig. 21-24) capability allow the patient to breathe spontaneously, usually through an independent gas supply, but periodically (at a preselected rate) give a "mandatory" breath. Thus, a combination of spontaneous and controlled breaths is provided for

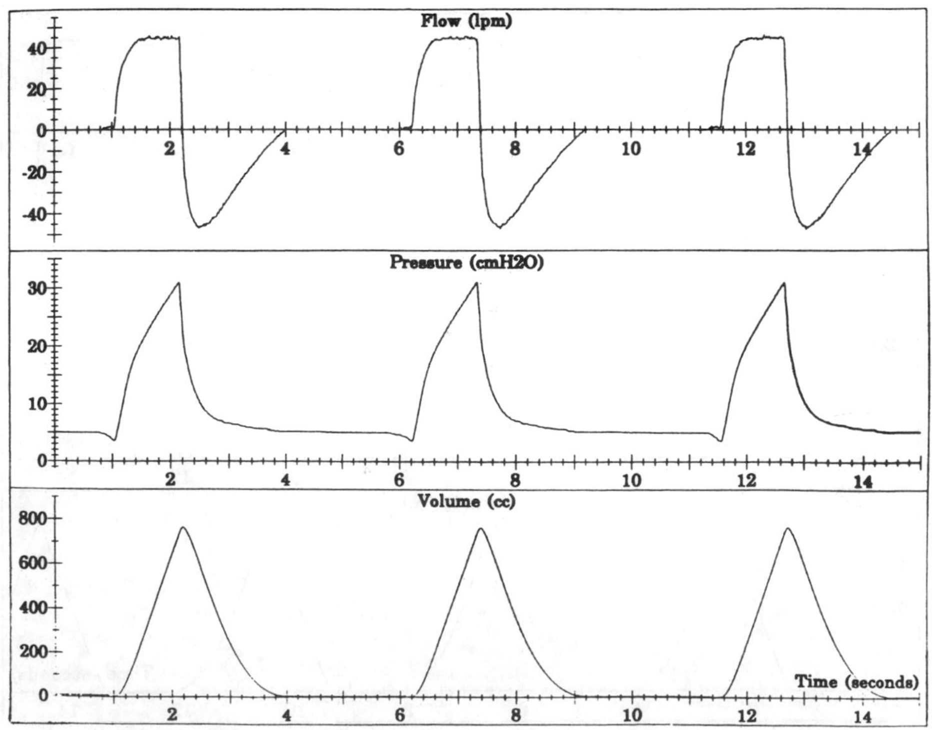

FIGURE 21-23. Pressure, flow and volume waveforms during volume-targeted assisted mechanical ventilation delivered with a rectangular waveform. Note that all breaths are patient triggered (pressure-triggering), that is the pressure drops on the airway pressure baseline prior to each breath (From Kacmarek RM, Hess D: Basic principles of ventilator machinery in Tobin, MJ: Principles and Practice of Mechanical Ventilation. New York, McGraw-Hill, 1994, p 77)[6]

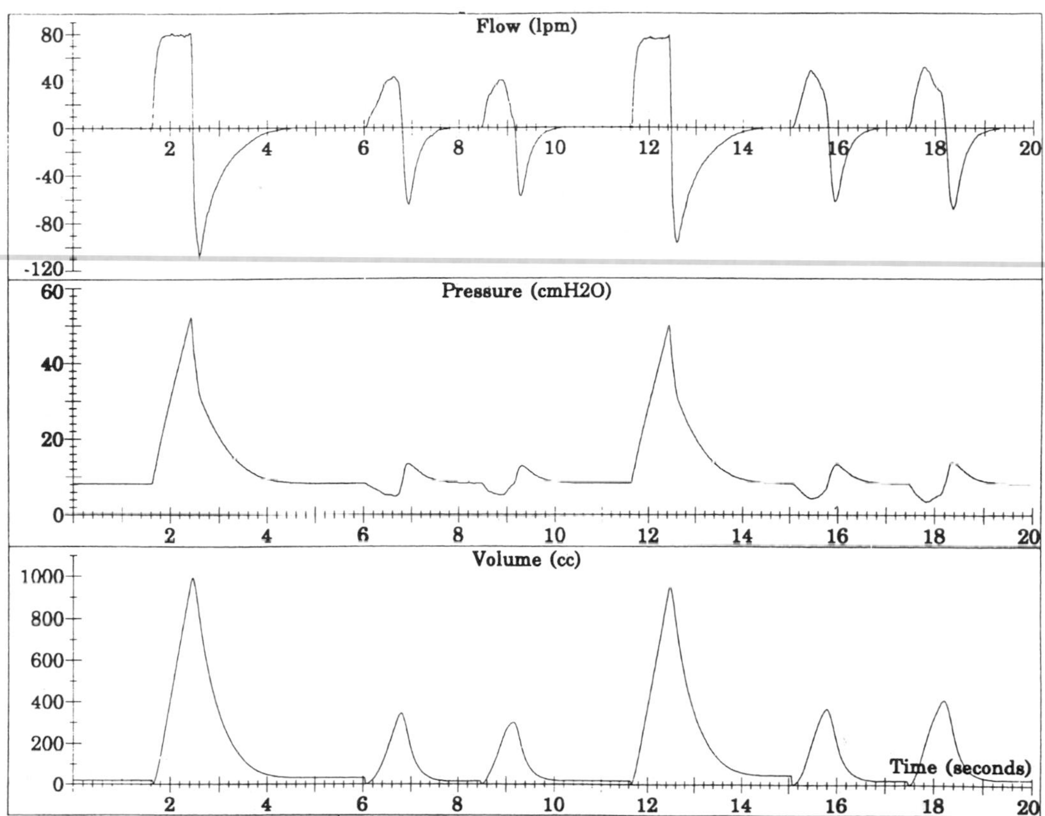

FIGURE 21-24. Pressure, flow, and volume waveforms during volume-targeted intermittent mandatory ventilation (IMV) with a continuous gas flow system. Note the spontaneous breaths interposed between the regularly spaced mandatory breaths. (From Kacmarek RM, Hess D: Basic principles of ventilator machinery in Tobin, MJ: Principles and Practice of Mechanical Ventilation. New York, McGraw-Hill, 1994, p 78)[6]

the best overall pattern of ventilation in the individual patient. With IMV a minimum amount of ventilatory support is provided. Mandatory breaths are volume-controlled, or pressure-controlled, time-triggered, and normally time-cycled. The spontaneous breaths are pressure-controlled, normally pressure- or flow-triggered, and pressure-cycled.

The earliest uses of IMV were achieved by setting the ventilator in the control mode (sensitivity off or low) and selecting a tidal volume and rate. Now, as described above, IMV can be set to use pressure-controlled breaths as well (Fig. 21-25). Various methods of administering IMV are available, both "home-made" and factory installed. Most of the early designs operated with a gas reservoir directed into the inspiratory limb of the ventilator circuit through a unidirectional valve (Fig. 21-26).[15] This IMV circuit was often located proximal to the system humidifier. In this design, when the patient inspires, the valve opens, admitting gas from the reservoir (5-L anesthesia bag); when the ventilator triggers into inspiration, the valve closes and machine breath delivery proceeds normally. Gas provided for spontaneous breathing may flow either continuously or from a demand regulator that is activated by the patient.

As with any system of ventilator support, certain potential mechanical disadvantages may be noted:

1. Many IMV devices are "homemade." Improper assembly, such as unidirectional valves installed backwards, may result in total malfunction and can be disastrous to the patient if not detected immediately. This problem is less frequent in manufactured units that incorporate IMV. Valves that "stick" open during switchover to the nonmandated mode are also an occasional problem.
2. The delivery of a mandated breath from the ventilator just as the patient finished spontaneous inspiration could lead to overdistention of the lung. Whether this concern is justified is debatable, particularly because a "sigh" mechanism has been used on many mechanical ventilators to achieve this very end: the delivery of a larger than normal V_T in the hope of preventing microatelectasis. In addition, if the ventilator's high pressure limit is set appropriately at +10 cmH_2O above the peak inspiratory pressure, then excessive pressures will not be delivered.
3. IMV devices are often associated with a high inspiratory work of breathing, especially if PEEP is being used. The system's flow must be at least four times the patient's minute ventilation and ideally more than about 60 to 90 L/min in order to satisfy peak inspiratory flow demands. A correctly de-

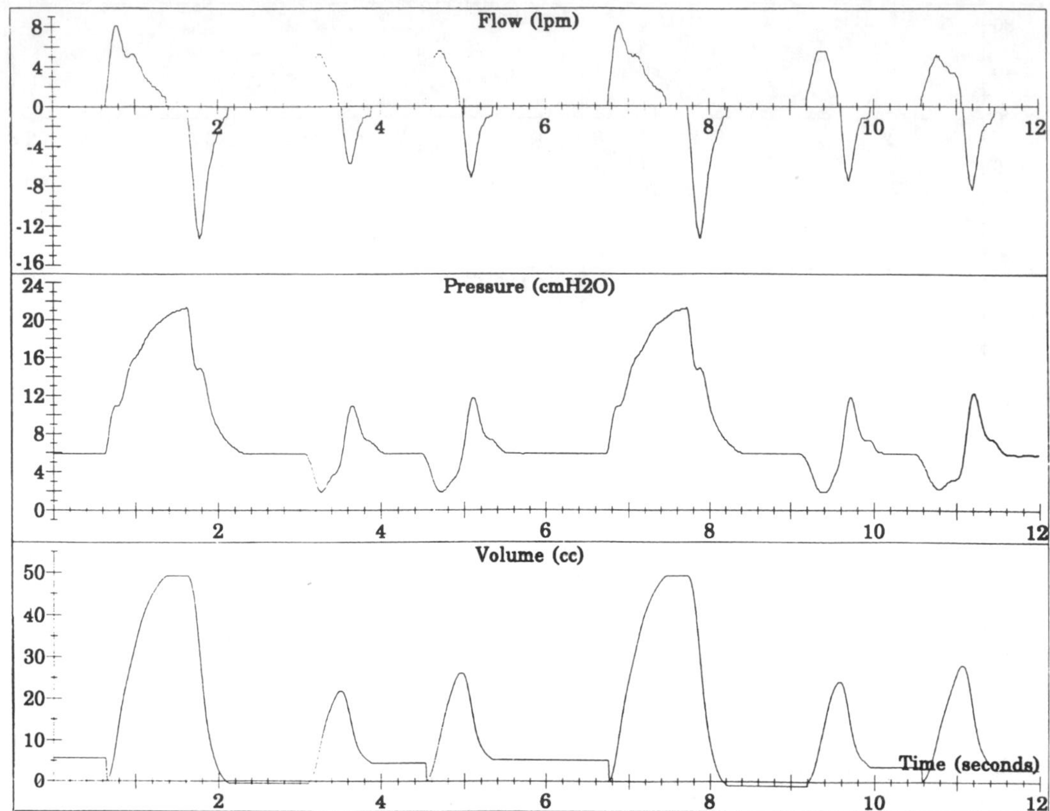

FIGURE 21-25. Pressure, flow and volume waveforms during pressure-targeted IMV with a continuous gas flow system. In this setting, the mandatory breath is delivered simply by closing the exhalation valve. Note the spontaneous breaths interposed between the regularly occurring mandatory breaths. (From Kacmarek RM, Hess D: Basic principles of ventilator machinery in Tobin, MJ: Principles and Practice of Mechanical Ventilation. New York, McGraw-Hill, 1994, p 78)

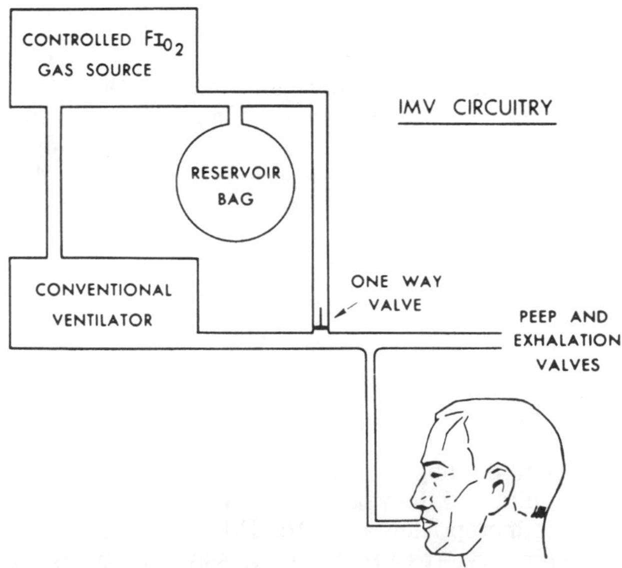

FIGURE 21-26. IMV circuitry. A demand regulator is substituted for the reservoir bag in some commercially available systems. Spontaneous ventilation is supported from the bag or regulator, while controlled breaths delivered intermittently from the ventilator close the unidirectional valve and are directed to the patient. (Reproduced with permission from Kirby RR: IMV held satisfactory alternative to assisted, controlled ventilation. Clin Trends Anesthesiol 6(4):14, 1976)

signed IMV continuous flow system shows only minor pressure fluctuations from baseline (±2 cmH_2O) during spontaneous breathing.

Synchronized Intermittent Mandatory Ventilation

Current ventilators are now available that deliver the mandated IMV breath only at the beginning of the patient's spontaneous inspiration. The manufacturers of ventilators that provide this modification of the basic IMV technique have termed it synchronized intermittent mandatory ventilation (SIMV). The ventilator breaths are usually pressure- or flow-triggered by the patient. If the patient fails to take a breath in the designated time frame, the ventilator will provide a time-triggered breath (Fig. 21-27). When this is delivered depends on how the manufacturer designs the machine. Consequently, the set rate may vary slightly depending on when the patient's effort occurs in relation to the time window. Gas is supplied during spontaneous breaths by a pressure-triggered demand system.

As with IMV, machine breaths can be either pressure (Fig. 21-28) or volume/flow-controlled (Fig. 21-29). In addition, pressure support ventilation can be provided during the spontaneous phase with either pressure- or volume/flow-controlled mandatory breaths.

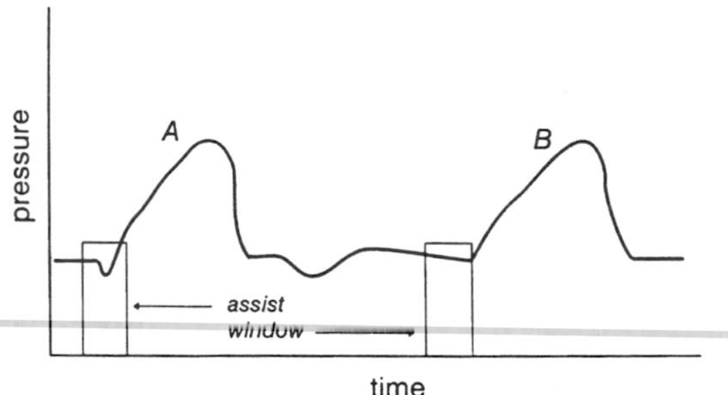

FIGURE 21-27. Depiction of the SIMV assist window. In assisted breaths **(A)**, the ventilator senses the patient's inspiratory effort and cycles the breath in synchrony with the patient's desires. In contrast, if patient effort is not sensed by the end of the assist time window **(B)**, a time-triggered breath is delivered. (From Kacmarek RM, Hess D: Basic principles of ventilator machinery in Tobin, MJ: Principles and Practice of Mechanical Ventilation. New York, McGraw-Hill, 1994, p 79)[6]

Pressure Support Ventilation

Pressure support ventilation (PSV) (Fig. 21-30) is a form of pressure-controlled ventilation. The concept of PSV should be considered in three phases: initiation of inspiration, inspiratory flow generation, and the cycling mechanism.

□ INITIATION OF INSPIRATION

The patient must initiate or trigger each breath by lowering airway pressure or flow to a predetermined level set by the pressure or flow sensitivity control on the ventilator. Patients with an unstable respiratory drive should not be considered candidates for PSV. Some, although not all, mechanical ventilators use backup modes of ventilation to assure ventilation during apneic episodes while on PSV or other ventilatory modes, depending on spontaneous ventilation.

□ INSPIRATORY FLOW

In pressure support the operator selects a pressure greater than the end-expiratory level. During inspiration, the ventilator will generate and maintain the selected pressure. Inspiratory flow generated by the ventilator depends on the selected pressure level, the flow-generating algorithm or drive pressure of the ventilator in use, and the lung–thorax compliance, inspiratory effort (muscle force), and airway resistance of the patient. The characteristic inspiratory flow pattern is a decaying exponential flow waveform and is the direct result of a reduced-pressure gradient across the ventilator circuit, which occurs concomitantly with filling of the lungs and the subsequent equilibration of pressure between the ventilator circuit and the pulmonary structures.

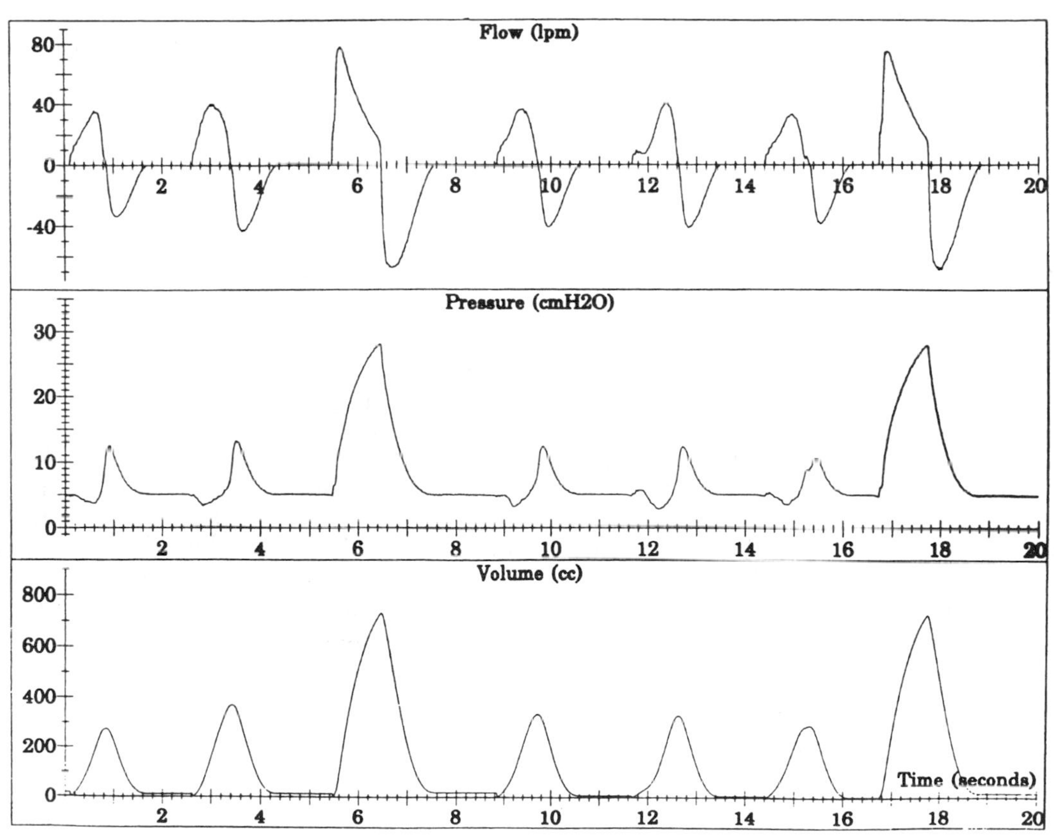

FIGURE 21-28. Pressure, flow, and volume waveforms during pressure-targeted SIMV. The positive pressure breath has the same configuration as any other pressure-targeted assisted breath. Between positive-pressure breaths, the patient breathes spontaneously from the demand system. (From Kacmarek RM, Hess D: Basic principles of ventilator machinery in Tobin, MJ: Principles and Practice of Mechanical Ventilation. New York, McGraw-Hill, 1994, p 80)[6]

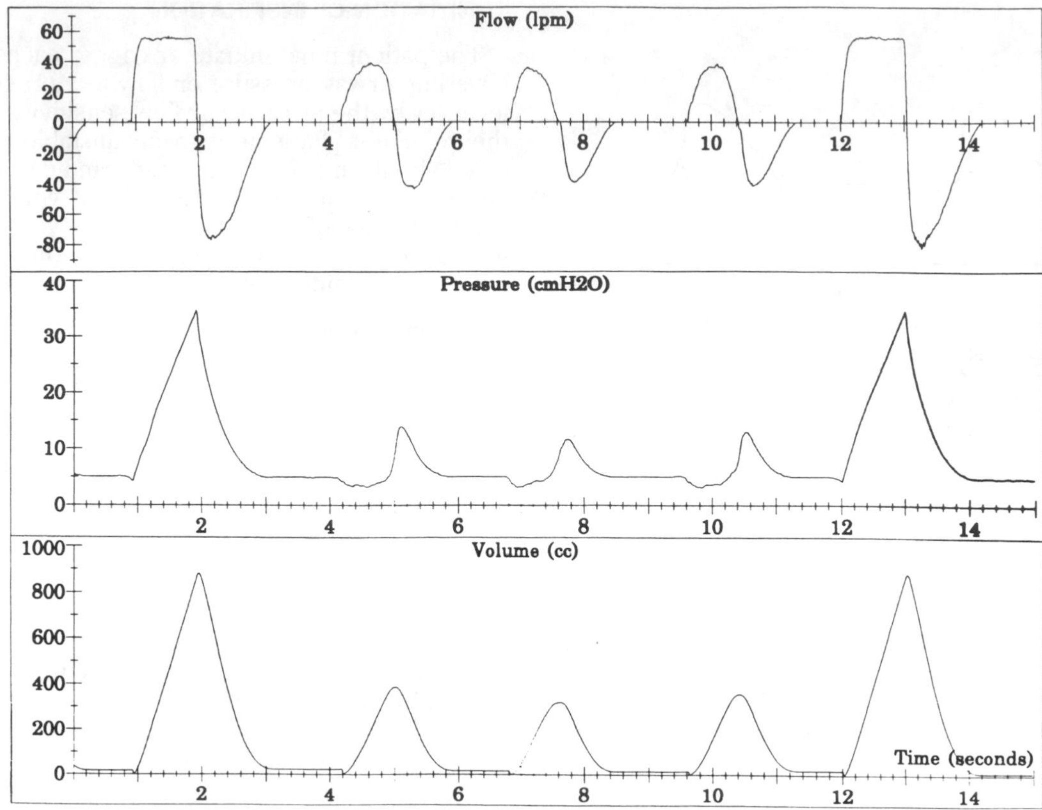

FIGURE 21-29. Pressure, flow, and volume waveforms during volume-targeted SIMV. The positive pressure breath has the same configuration as any other volume-targeted assisted breath. Various inspiratory waveforms may be selected (rectangular/constant, sine, descending ramp, etc). Between positive-pressure breaths, the patient breaths spontaneously from the demand system. (From Kacmarek RM, Hess D: Basic principles of ventilator machinery in Tobin, MJ: Principles and Practice of Mechanical Ventilation. New York, McGraw-Hill, 1994, p 80)[6]

□ CYCLING MECHANISM

As a pressure support breath begins, an initial high flow of gas is directed into the ventilator circuit, establishing the selected pressure support level. As the lung fills, airway pressure rises and the pressure gradient from airway opening to lung is reduced. At the same time, inspiratory flow decreases. With most ventilators, when inspiratory flow reaches approximately 25% of the initial flow, the pressure support breath is terminated. Although flow is the primary cycling mechanism in PSV, most ventilators incorporate several added back-up or safety-cycling mechanisms, such as time or pressure, or both. For example, if a patient on PSV developed an extensive leak around an artificial airway, it is possible that the ventilator might fail to cycle if the leak causes flow to stay above the critical value of 25% of the initial flow. A properly designed ventilator would terminate the pressure support breath after an appropriate time interval, generally 1 to 5 seconds. In addition, if for some reason pressure builds in the circuit during a pressure support breath, most ventilators will end inspiration when the airway pressure exceeds about 3 cmH_2O above the preset pressure level and baseline (PEEP).

□ TROUBLESHOOTING IN PSV

In many current ventilators, the initial flow of gas to the patient in PSV is the maximal flow for the ventilator. If this flow is too rapid, it can actually overshoot the preset pressure and cause a "ringing" in the circuit. This can prematurely end a breath and reduce volume delivery (Fig. 21-31).[17] Another problem can occur with PSV when an external nebulizer is added to deliver aerosolized medications to the patient. The flow from the external flowmeter can affect the ventilator's ability to detect a patient inspiratory effort. If the patient's effort is weak, this can prevent the triggering of a pressure support breath.[18] Because pressure support is flow-cycled, a large leak (eg, bronchopleural fistula) may result in a prolonged inspiratory phase.

Pressure-Control Ventilation

Pressure control ventilation (PCV) (Fig. 21-32) is a pressure-controlled mode of ventilation in which the operator sets a desired pressure, and delivered tidal volume changes as patient lung characteristics change. PCV has been available for many years and is used with IMV in neonatal ventilation.[6]

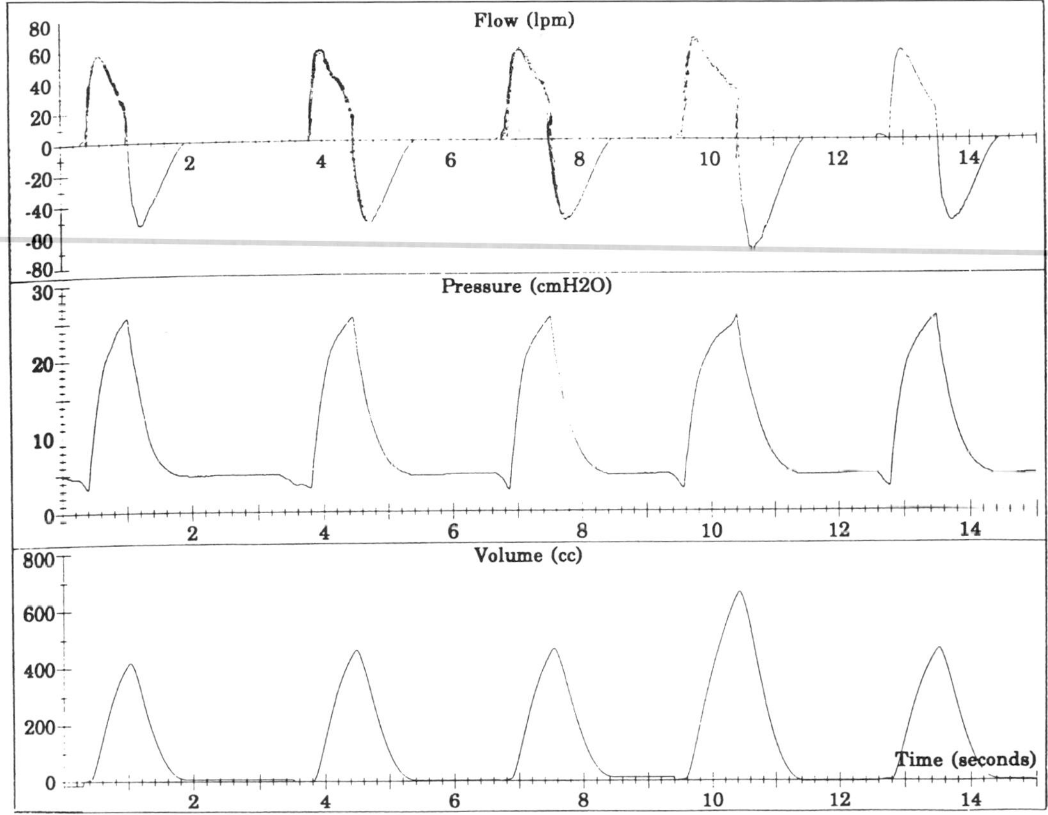

FIGURE 21-30. Pressure, flow and volume waveforms during pressure-support ventilation. Note that each breath is pressure-(patient-)triggered. In addition, inspiratory time and tidal volume vary with each breath. (From Kacmarek RM, Hess D: Basic principles of ventilator machinery in Tobin, MJ: Principles and Practice of Mechanical Ventilation. New York, McGraw Hill, 1994, p 83)[6]

The concept of PCV should be considered in three distinct phases: initiation of inspiration, inspiratory flow generation and pattern, and cycling mechanism.

□ INITIATION OF INSPIRATION

PCV can be set as either a time-, flow-, or pressure-triggered mode of ventilation, but it is most often time-triggered. It is also occasionally used with high I:E ratios (inverse ratio ventilation, IRV). Since this is a very uncomfortable breathing pattern for the patient, physicians often sedate and paralyze the patient. As a result, the ventilator is time-triggered. However, PCV can also be used in a pressure- or flow-triggered mode with normal I:E ratios. One advantage is that the patient can receive as high a flow as he or she demands, up to the flow limit capabilities of the ventilator (about 120 to 200 L/min). This is because in PCV the ventilator tries to maintain the preset pressure throughout inspiration (Fig. 21-33).

Until recently, ventilators offering PCV have provided the modality for use within the assist-control or control mode only. Newer ventilators, such as the Hamilton Veolar and the Servo 300, however, allow the operator to provide pressure-controlled, time- or pressure-triggered, and time-cycled breaths within the SIMV mode. Newer ventilators can also provide PCV in the SIMV mode with PSV for the spontaneous breaths.

□ INSPIRATORY FLOW

PCV, when selected, transforms ventilation into an operator-adjusted, pressure-limited breath. The operator selects a pressure above the end-expiratory level; then, during mechanical inspiration, the ventilator will generate and maintain the selected pressure. The inspiratory flow generated by the ventilator depends on several factors. One of these is the selected pressure level. The higher the selected pressure level, the greater the pressure gradient across the ventilator circuit and subsequently higher flow rates that result. Other factors include the flow-generating algorithm or drive pressure of the ventilator in use, as well as the lung–thorax compliance (C_{LT}) and airway resistance of the patient. The flow waveform is a decaying exponential flow pattern. This pattern is the result of a reduced pressure gradient from the upper airway to the lungs, which occurs concomitantly with filling of the lungs and equilibration of pressure between the ventilator circuit and the pulmonary structures.

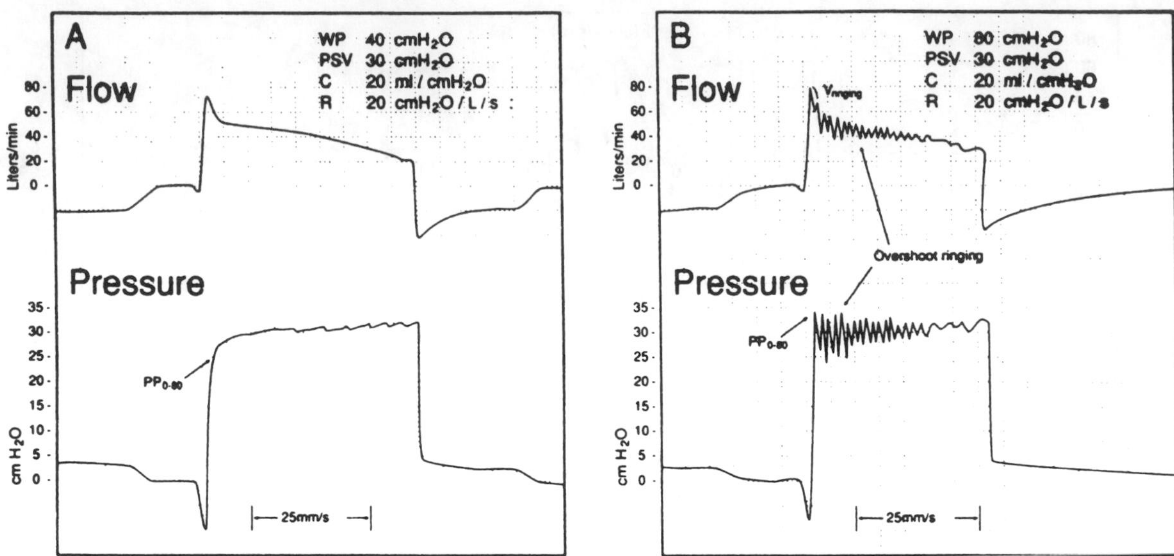

FIGURE 21-31. PSV delivered by the Siemens Servo 900C at a working pressure of 40 cmH_2O **(A)** and 80 cmH_2O **(B)**. Note the ringing that occurs with a working pressure set at the manufacturer's recommend 80 cmH_2O. (From Cohen IL, Bilen Z, Krishnamurthy S. The effects of ventilator working pressure during pressure support ventilation. Chest 103:588–592, 1993)

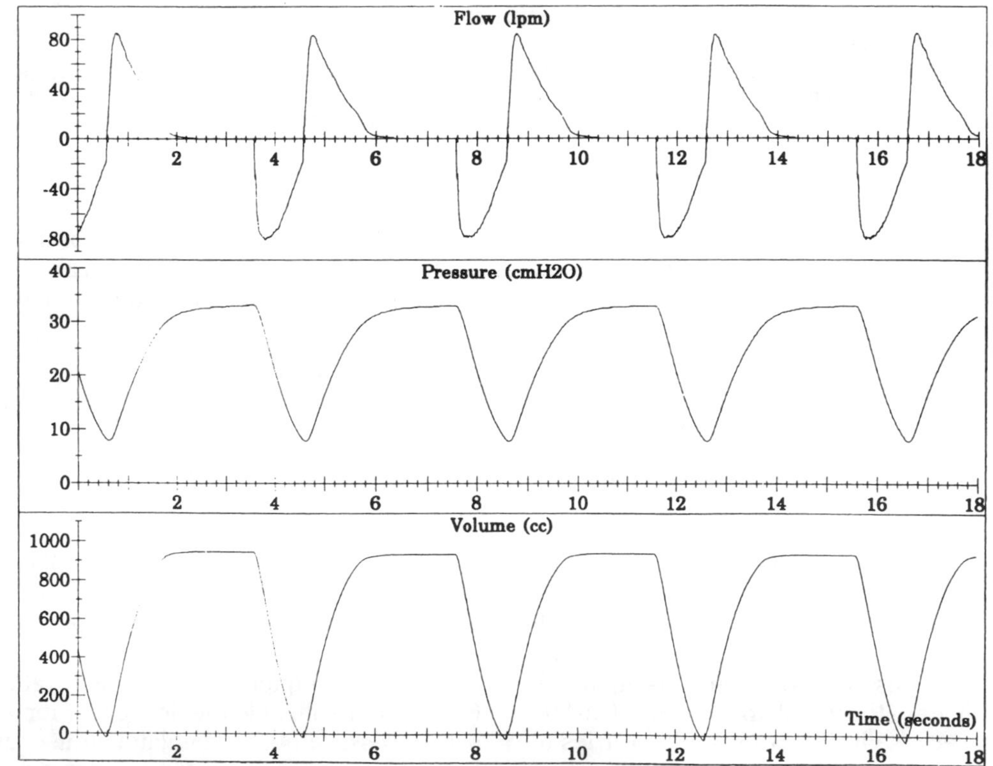

FIGURE 21-32. Pressure, flow, and volume waveforms during pressure-control inverse-ratio ventilation (PCIRV), where the inspiratory-expiratory time ratio (I:E) is 3:1. Note that inspiratory flow has returned to zero before the end of the inspiratory phase, and an end-inspiratory hold is established. Volume is delivered into the patient's airway before half the inspiratory time is completed, as noted by the expiratory flow not returning to zero; some level of auto-PEEP is developed. (From Kacmarek RM, Hess D: Basic principles of ventilator machinery in Tobin, MJ: Principles and Practice of Mechanical Ventilation. New York, McGraw-Hill, 1994, p 82)[6]

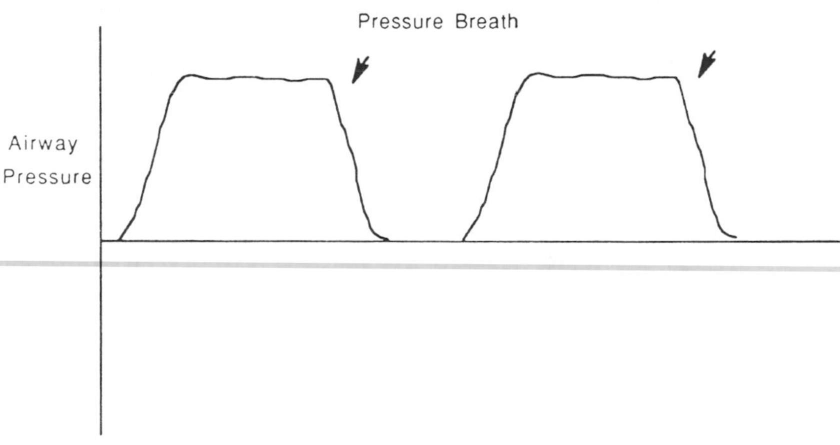

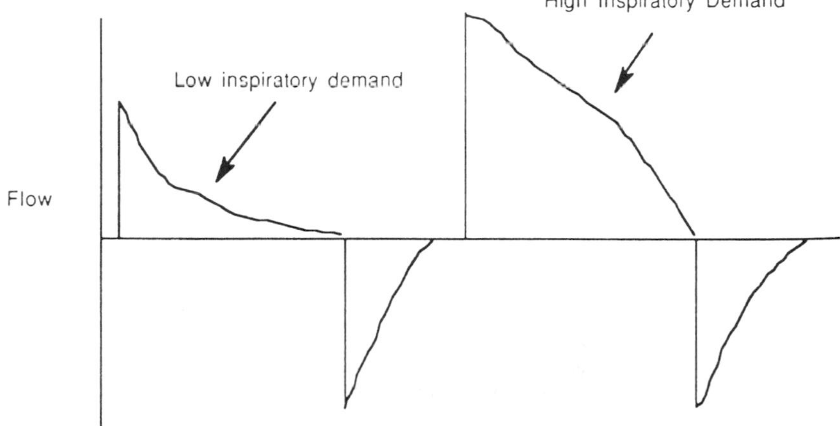

FIGURE 21-33. Pressure controlled ventilation showing low inspiratory flow demand on the left and high inspiratory flow demand on the right (From Pilbeam SP: Mechanical Ventilation, Physiological and Clinical Applications (2nd ed.) Chicago, Mosby–Year Book, 1992, p 176)

☐ CYCLING MECHANISM

The principal cycling mechanism for PCV is time. If the lung fills and flow terminates before the completion of the allotted inspiratory interval, an inspiratory pause will result. As a safety feature, premature cycling will occur if airway pressures in excess of about 2 cmH_2O (exact amount depends on the type of ventilator) above the selected PC level are sensed.

Continuous Positive Airway Pressure

Continuous positive airway pressure (CPAP) is a spontaneous mode of ventilation that is pressure-limited and pressure- or flow-triggered. That is, the spontaneous breath has a pressure limit that remains nearly the same, within a few centimeters of water pressure, during both inspiration and expiration. The patient's inspiratory effort causes the ventilator to increase flow to the patient to maintain the same pressure during inspiration. During expiration, flow out of the exhalation valve maintains the expiratory pressure at a fairly uniform level (Fig. 21-34). No mechanical positive pressure breaths are given. The operator sets the sensitivity of the demand valve system and the CPAP (preset pressure) level. This pressure level can be atmospheric (ambient) or above atmospheric, thus elevating the baseline.

PEEP and CPAP are often confused. CPAP is a mode of ventilation whereas PEEP is the pressure maintained above baseline during various modes of ventilation such as SIMV or CMV.

Airway Pressure-Release Ventilation

The acronym APRV (airway pressure-release ventilation) was coined by John B. Downs in 1987.[19] This is sometimes described as two levels of CPAP ventilation that allow spontaneous ventilation at both levels (Fig. 21-35)[6,20] Each level is time-cycled and time-triggered. The higher level pressure CPAP is usually longer than the lower level pressure CPAP and appears much like IRV. APRV is like PCV or PCIRV. When the patient is not breathing spontaneously, you cannot tell one from the other.

This mode is currently available on the Drager Evita and on most infant ventilators. Early investigations of this mode used a modified continuous-flow CPAP system with a release valve in the expiratory limb (Fig. 21-36).[21] In applying this technique, patients with acute lung injury are placed on a level of CPAP sufficient to re-

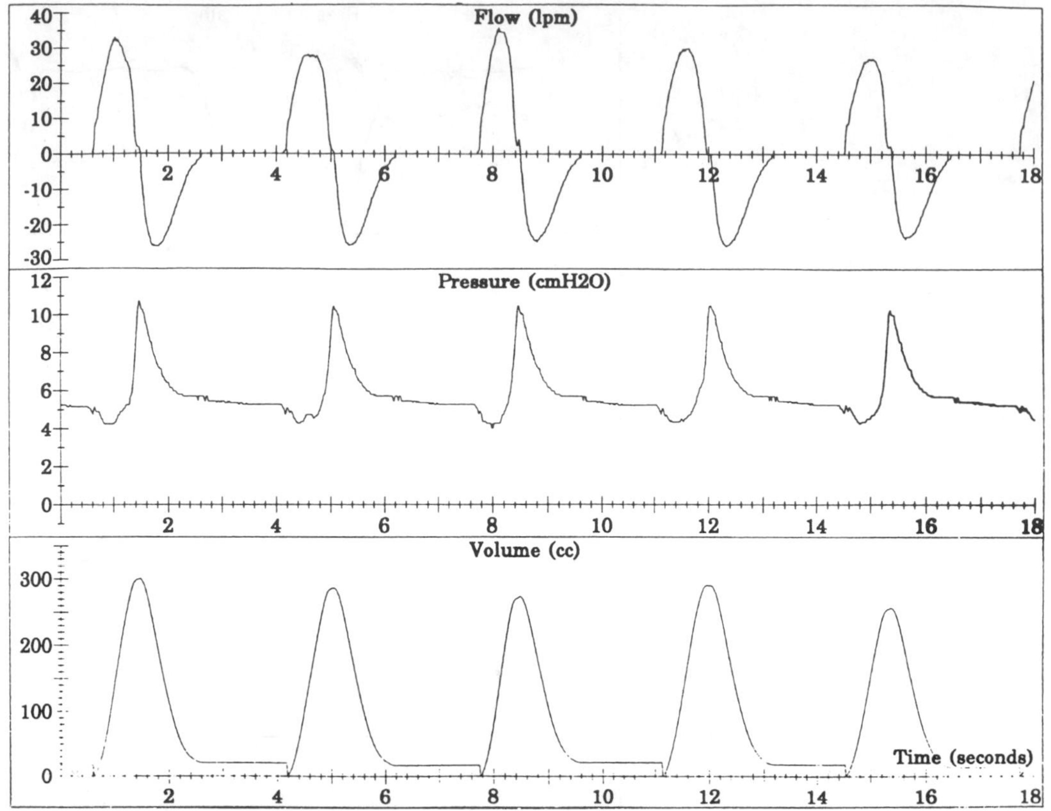

FIGURE 21-34. Pressure, flow and volume waveforms during continuous positive airway pressure (CPAP). All gas flow is provided by a patient-activated demand valve. (From Kacmarek RM, Hess D: Basic principles of ventilator machinery in Tobin, MJ: Principles and Practice of Mechanical Ventilation. New York, McGraw-Hill, 1994, p 81)[6]

store the FRC to a more normal physiologic level (higher level of CPAP). Spontaneous ventilation is allowed at all times. Should additional ventilation be required, however, airway pressure is periodically reduced to ambient or a lower level of CPAP. Removal of the airway pressure reduces the FRC, with a resultant patient exhalation and ventilation. At the moment exhalation is complete, the CPAP level is restored to its previous higher level. As a general rule, the exhalation phase is passive and dependent on the expiratory time constant of the lung and the ventilator system in use. Exhalation can be considered to be complete after five time-constant intervals. Time constants can be difficult to estimate at the bedside, and a flow-monitoring device might be useful in determining the appropriate expiratory interval. In the absence of such equipment, an expiratory interval of 1.5 to 2 seconds is recommended.[22,23]

Interestingly, because ventilation occurs by the removal of airway pressure, the more the ventilator rate is increased, the lower the mean airway pressure becomes. This has a distinct advantage when unstable cardiovascular patients require significant levels of mechanical ventilation.

At present, this modality is experimental and is not available on most ventilators. Ongoing research into APRV should help to verify its application and to determine how it compares with other forms of therapy.

Proportional-Assist Ventilation

Proportional-assist ventilation (PAV) is a new approach to ventilatory support in which pressure, flow, and volume delivery at the airway are in proportion to the patient's instantaneous, spontaneous effort (Fig. 21-37).[24,25] It is a form of PCV. The operation of this ventilator is based on the equation of motion described previously. Using a modified form of this equation will help explain the operation of this mode:

$$\text{Paw} = (K_1)(V) + (K_2)(\text{flow})$$

where K_1 = elastic load supported by the ventilator; K_2 = resistive load supported by the ventilator; V = volume; flow = gas flow; and Paw = pressure provided by the ventilator.

When the operator adjusts the amplification controls for elastance (K_1) and resistance (K_2), the amount of unloading by the ventilator is controlled. Setting K_1 and K_2 determines the amount of pressure generated by the ventilator, but as a percentage of ventilatory load and not as a specific pressure waveform.

For example, suppose the elastance of the patient is measured at 20 cmH_2O/L and the patient's airway resistance is 10 $cmH_2O/L/s$. The operator could set the ventilator to unload at 50% by setting the control for elastance at 20 cmH_2O/L and the control for resistance at 10 $cmH_2O/L/s$. Then all breaths are unloaded at this level

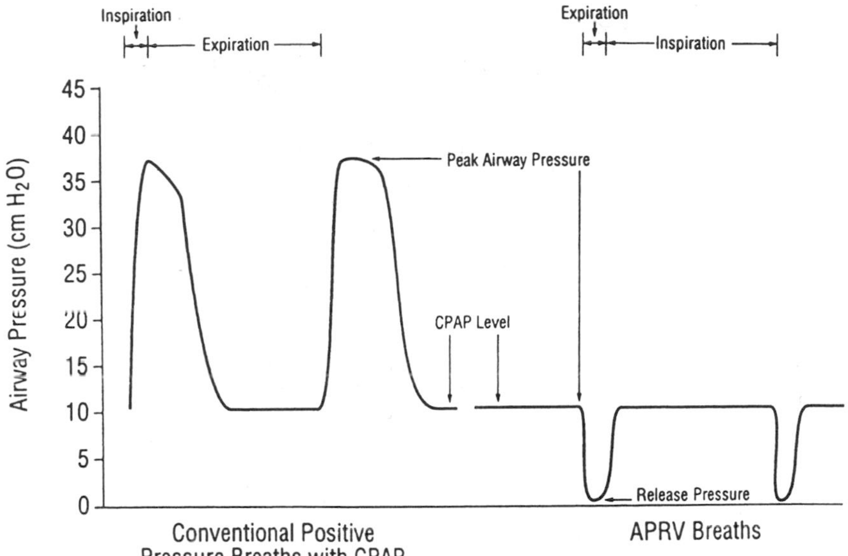

FIGURE 21-35. Typical airway pressure patterns of conventional positive pressure breaths with continuous positive airway pressure (CMV + CPAP) and of APRV breaths. In this example, the CPAP levels are identical during both modes of ventilation. During conventional volume-targeted ventilation, the positive pressure breath is delivered above the CPAP level, necessitating that mean airway pressure be greater than the CPAP level. In contrast, during APRV, expiration occurs by releasing airway pressure below the CPAP level, thus creating a situation where the mean airway pressure is necessarily less than the CPAP level. Further, the inspiratory-to-expiratory time ratio is reversed during APRV. During conventional positive pressure breaths, inspiration is shorter than or equal to expiration. During APRV breaths, expiratory time should not exceed 1.5 to 2.0 seconds, thus creating a situation where inspiratory time is longer than expiratory time when a mechanical ventilatory rate of less than 20 breaths/minute is employed. This figure also defines the CPAP and release pressure levels during APRV. The difference between CPAP and release pressure levels is the change in airway pressure and determines the mechanical tidal volume. Patients with lower lung compliance need a greater CPAP-release pressure gradient to obtain the same tidal volume compared to patients who have more normal (greater) lung compliance. (From Perel A, Stock MC Handbook of Mechanical Ventilatory Support, Williams & Wilkins, Baltimore, 1992, p 167)

no matter what the actual volume and flowrate are. In this example, Paw would be 10 cmH_2O to provide a tidal volume of 0.5 L at a flow of 0.5 L/s. Another 10 cmH_2O would be required from the respiratory muscles.

Ideally, this mode would provide for the patient's inspiratory effort and base its function on the patient's lung characteristics and the amount of unloading desired. This is still an experimental mode of ventilation but offers an attractive alternative to other modes of ventilation and warrants further study.

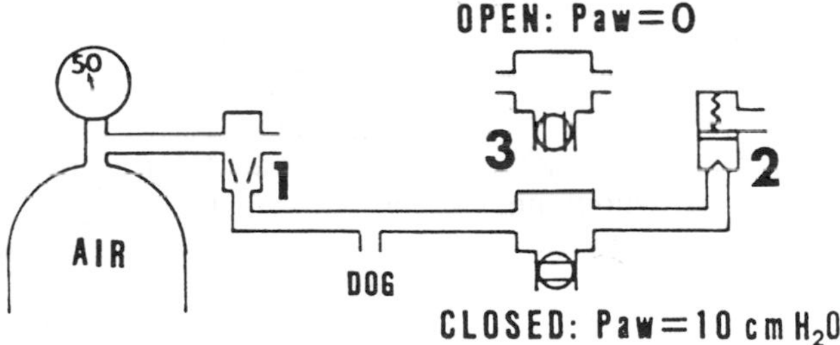

FIGURE 21-36. Airway pressure release ventilator schematically depicted. A 50-psi oxygen source drives a venturi device **(1)** capable of entraining enough room air to deliver 90–100 L/min. This high gas flow exceeds the peak inspiratory flow needs of the patient. When the switch in the expiratory limb **(3)** is closed, airway pressure (Paw) equals the pressure generated by the threshold resistor expiratory valve **(2)**. When the switch opens, gas escapes to the atmosphere at near-ambient pressure or to a predetermined, lower continuous positive airway pressure level. (From Stock MC, Downs JB, Frolicher DA Airway pressure release ventilation. Crit Care Med 15:462–466, 1987)

BiPAP

BiPAP is actually the name brand of a ventilator manufactured by the Respironics Corporation (Murraysville, PA). It is an electrically powered, compressor-blower-driven, microprocessor-controlled ventilator that uses a single gas flow delivery system. This system provides a constant pressure wave pattern and gas flow decreases during inspiration. It is time- or flow-triggered and flow- or time-cycled.

BiPAP is designed to provide CPAP in which both expiratory positive airway pressure (EPAP) and inspiratory positive airway pressure (IPAP) are adjustable. BiPAP was specifically designed to provide partial ventilatory support using a nasal or oronasal mask, particularly in patients with obstructive sleep apnea. It has a pressure-controlling valve to maintain the IPAP and EPAP levels. Inspiration is triggered when the patient's inspiratory flow is greater than 40 mL/s for more than 30 milliseconds. Expiratory flow is detected when the inspiratory flow decreases below a manufacturer-deter-

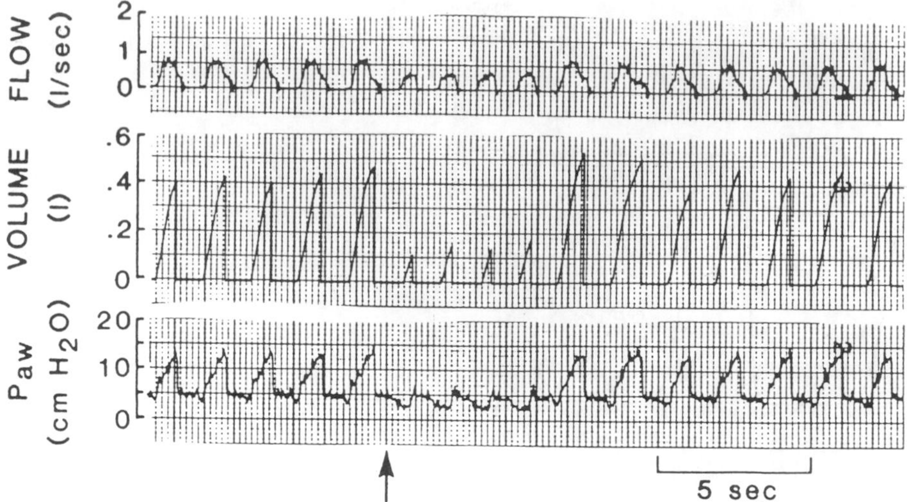

FIGURE 21-37. Inspiratory flow, tidal volume, and airway pressure in one patient before, during, and after temporary discontinuation of PAV *(arrow)*. Tidal volume is much smaller partly because of lower flow and partly because of shorter inspiration. (From Younes M, Puddy A, Roberts D, Light RB, Quesada A, Taylor D, Oppenheimer L, Cramp H: Proportional assist ventilation, results of an initial clinical trial. Am Rev Respir Dis 145:127, 1992)

mined threshold level (flow-cycled) or when IPAP is longer than 3 seconds (time-cycled).

Similar to BiPAP, there are now a number of bilevel pressure ventilators commercially available. These are similar in that they are controlled by a compressor blower and provide pressure support ventilation by mask. These ventilators are designed to function in the presence of a leak and do not have a true exhalation valve.

Mandatory Minute Ventilation

Mandatory minute ventilation (MMV) is a volume- or pressure-controlled mode of ventilation currently used for discontinuing ventilatory support. It guarantees a minimum level of ventilation in the presence of minute-to-minute changes in the patient's spontaneous ventilation. An MMV is set by the operator that is generally somewhat less than the anticipated patient's spontaneous minute volume. If the measured minute volume falls below the mandatory level, the ventilator supplements the patient's spontaneous efforts and guards against the ventilation going below the preset level.

MMV can be volume controlled as in the Ohmeda CPU-1. The ventilator compares the level of the patient's spontaneous breathing to the set MMV level. It then either increases, decreases, or maintains the frequency of machine breaths as needed by altering expiratory time. The tidal volume is preset. In the Hamilton Veolar, MMV is pressure controlled and the operator sets a pressure support level. With monitoring, the ventilator either increases, maintains, or decreases the pressure support level in increments of 1 to 2 cmH_2O to achieve the desired minute volume up to a pressure limit of 30 cmH_2O. The Bear 5 and Bear 1000, the Drager Evita, and the Engstrom Erica also provide methods of MMV ventilation.

The current problem with most methods of providing MMV is that the ventilator mandates only overall minute volume. It does not account for the possibility that spontaneous tidal volume may be dropping and spontaneous rate may be increasing to a level that may fatigue the patient, while this may actually maintain minute ventilation at or above the set level. For example, a V_T of 1.0 L and a rate of 10 has an equivalent minute ventilation of a V_T of 250 mL and a rate of 40 breaths/min. The latter parameters, however, would increase patient work of breathing. If the alveolar ventilation is compared in these two cases, assuming a deadspace of 150 mL, in the first example the alveolar ventilation would be 8.5 L/min, but it would only be 4.0 L/min in the second. The clinician using this mode must be careful to set a high rate and low tidal volume alarm to alert the clinician to this possibility.

Pressure-Regulated Volume Control Ventilation

Pressure-regulated volume control ventilation (PRVCV) is an attempt to provide both volume control and pressure control. The operator sets a target V_T and a maximum pressure. The operator also sets the inspiratory time, the I:E ratio, and the rate. The ventilator functions in PCV mode and monitors tidal volume delivery. It progressively increases pressure up to a preset maximum until the V_T is achieved or until the maximum pressure is reached, whichever occurs first. If the target volume is exceeded, the pressure limit is decreased. This mode of ventilation was designed to be used only in patients who are not spontaneously breathing. At present, it is available on the Servo 300 ventilator but has not been researched to clinically verify its benefits (Fig. 21-38).

Volume Support

Volume support, also currently available only on the Servo 300, uses PSV with volume targeting to ventilate spontaneously breathing patients (Fig. 21-39). The operator sets the pressure level. The inspiratory pressure is progressively increased until it achieves a target volume or reaches a maximum preset upper pressure limit. The difference between this and pressure-regulated vol-

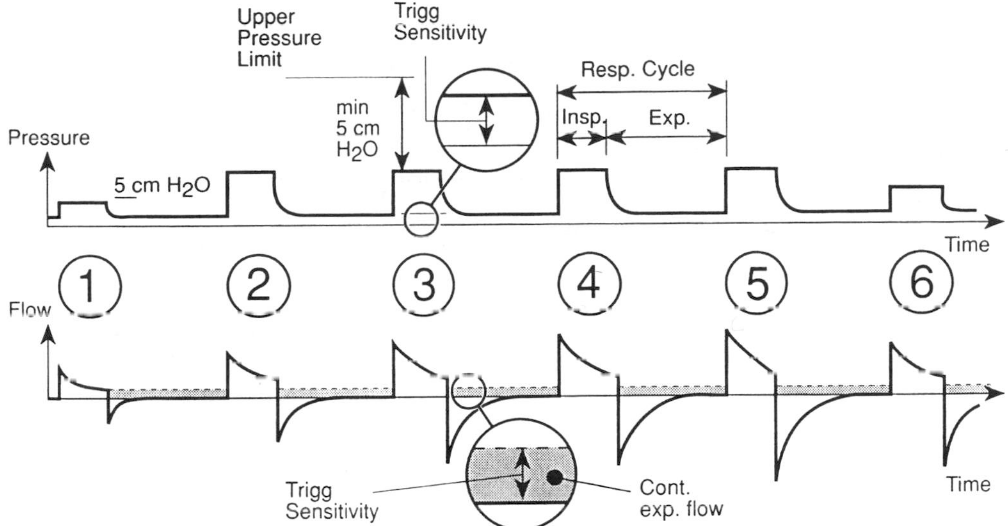

FIGURE 21-38. Pressure and flow waveforms during pressure-regulated volume control ventilation. (**1**) 5 cmH_2O test breath. (**2** and **3**) Adjustment of pressure target to ensure delivered tidal volume. (**4** and **5**) Pressure target constant. (**6**) Pressure target decreased because tidal volume is over target (see text for details) (Courtesy of Siemens Life Support Systems, Schaumburg, IL)

ume control is that the patient is spontaneously breathing. The patient pressure-triggers the breath and has control over the inspiratory phase just as in PSV. The inspiratory pressure is controlled automatically between PEEP and 5 cmH_2O below the set upper pressure limit.

Pressure Augmentation

In pressure augmentation (PA) the operator sets a pressure support level, a peak flow, and a tidal volume. In patients with high inspiratory flow and volume demands, the ventilator can guarantee tidal volume by monitoring volume delivery. The breath is delivered in a pressure support type of pattern with pressure-triggering and the ventilator providing an initial high gas flow. If the preset tidal volume is not reached, the pressure delivery increases, maintaining gas flow to the patient until the desired volume is reached (Fig. 21-40). This mode of ventilation is currently only available on the Bear 1000. It also augments volume delivery of the volume-targeted breaths only during SIMV + pressure support mode. The PSV breaths are not affected (Fig. 21-41).

The Bear 1000 also provides flow augmentation. This allows flow to be augmented (increased) to meet a patient's inspiratory demand to prevent inspiratory pressures from dropping below the set baseline (Fig. 21-42).

High-Frequency Ventilation

HFV represents a significant departure from conventional mechanical ventilation. In HFV ventilating rates are much higher than normal physiologic ventilatory

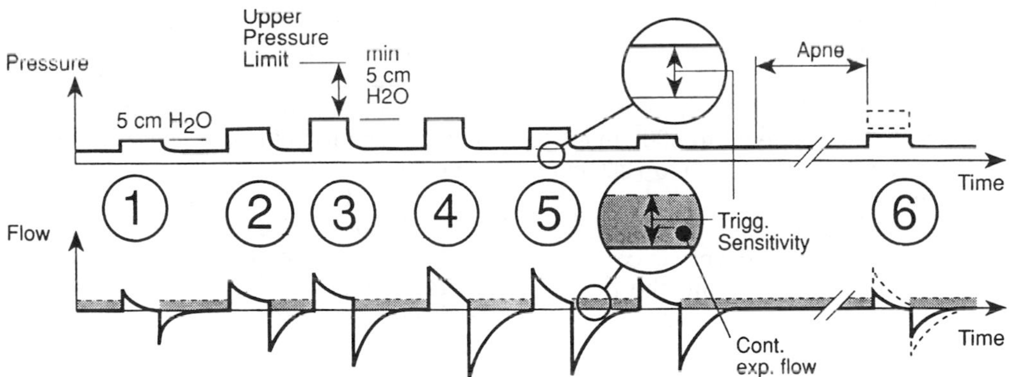

FIGURE 21-39. Pressure and flow waveforms during volume support. (**1**) test breath. (**2** to **5**) Adjustment of pressure target to ensure delivered tidal volume. (**5**) Pressure limit decreased to maintain tidal volume at target level. Note period of apneic ventilation where alarm is activated and PRVC begins. (Courtesy of Siemens Life Support Systems, Schaumburg, Illinois)

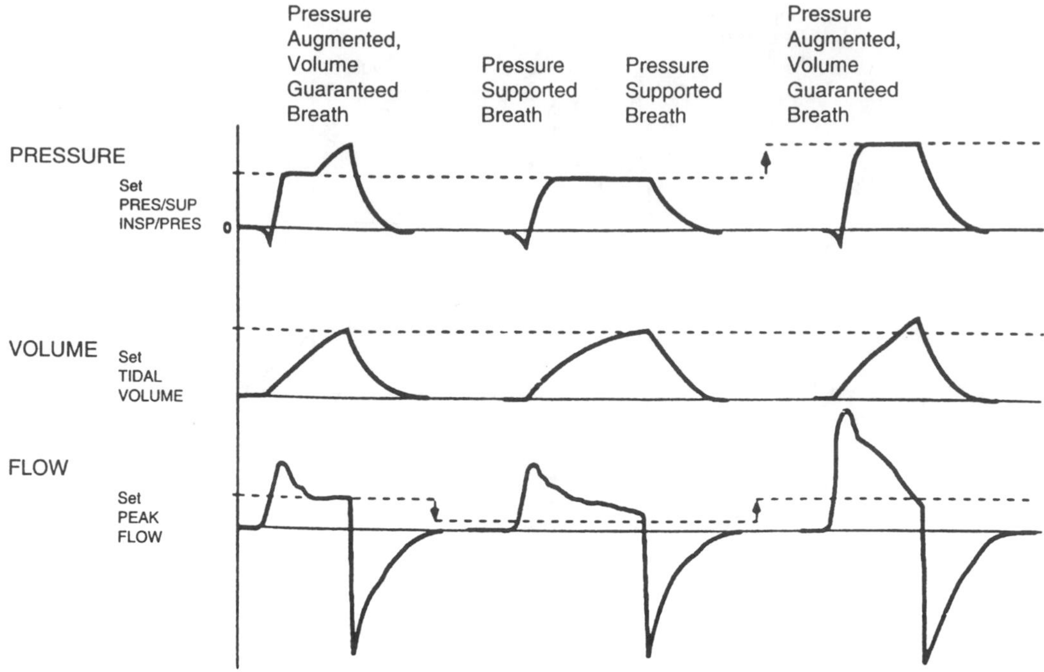

FIGURE 21-40. A minimum tidal volume is guaranteed during pressure augmentation. Note that the minimum tidal volume is delivered despite a decrease in patient demand or changes in resistance and compliance. With an increase in patient demand, the pressure and flow waveforms approximate those seen with pressure support ventilation. (Courtesy of Bear Medical Corp., Riverside, CA).

rates and tidal volumes are much lower than normal V_T. The idea of ventilating a patient at rates higher than normal is really not unusual, but supports the concept that it is not just the rhythmic movement of gas into and out of the lung that accomplishes ventilation.

There are three basic types of HFV. High-frequency positive pressure ventilation (HFPPV) is the one most similar to conventional positive pressure ventilation. Frequencies ranged from 60 to 100 cycles per minute (cpm; 1 to 1.7 Hz), and V_T, although reduced, still exceeded calculated dead space. Of major significance is that HFPPV reduces peak and mean airway pressure to the intrapleural space. High-frequency jet ventilation (HFJV) provides frequencies of about 100 to 600 cycles per minute (1.7 to 10 Hz) and tidal volumes often lower than dead space. It employs a ventilating mechanism comprised of a jet of gas that is directed into the lower airway at the set frequencies.

High-frequency oscillation (HFO) uses frequencies in the thousands-per-minute range up to 3000 to 4000 cpm (50 to 66.7 Hz) in clinical use and up to 7200 cpm (120 Hz) in experimental animals. To achieve the higher frequencies, amplifier-speaker assemblies or pistons can be used. Tidal volume delivery is considerably less than predicted dead space, and the mechanism by which alveolar ventilation is achieved is highly controversial. HFO is unique in that both inspiratory and expiratory phases are active.

The present and future roles of HFV are difficult to define. Many experimental studies have appeared in the published literature since 1967. However, clinical information has mostly been limited to case reports or series in which the small number of patients studied makes interpretation difficult. Nevertheless, most people involved in HFV research are optimistic that its proper role will eventually be defined, and that the technique, in its many forms, will contribute significantly to reduced ventilator-related morbidity. Its use in the neonatal population has gained a great deal of popularity and success. A recently developed HFV for adults (Infrasonics Adult Star 1010) has shown promise in the management of ARDS. HFV has been shown to be beneficial in the care of newborns with respiratory distress and has become a standard of care in many neonatal intensive care units.

ALARMS

Alarms are audible or visible signals or messages that alert the operator to possible events or conditions that require awareness or attention.[26] Technical events are those involving some change in the ventilator's performance. Patient events are those involving changes in the patient's condition that can be detected by the ventilator. Current ventilators are sophisticated enough and complicated enough to offer a variety of alarms. The clinician should remember to use alarms prudently, by setting alarm limits so they do not activate often enough that staff begins to ignore them and not so insensitively that they do not alert the staff to critical situations. Alarms should also be designed to alert people to critical and life-threatening circumstances and so they cannot be silenced or inactivated until the situation has been corrected.

The American Association for Respiratory Care has recommended that ventilator alarms be classified in three levels of priorities: Level 1 is an immediate life-

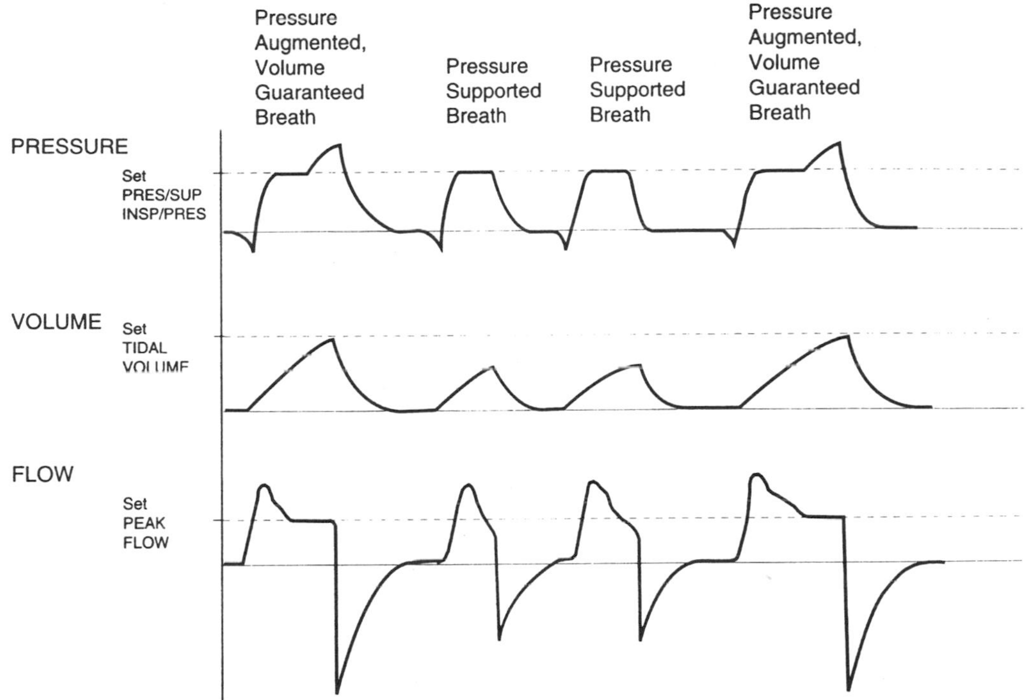

FIGURE 21-41. SIMV with pressure augmentation. Pressure-support breaths occur as usual, and mandatory breaths are augmented as needed. (Courtesy of Bear Medical Corp., Riverside, CA)

threatening situation; Level 2 is potentially life-threatening; and Level 3 is not life-threatening.[27]

Table 21-5 gives events that should be monitored and possible sites for monitoring each. Although Level 1 and 2 alarms are important, Level 3 alarms are probably not and perhaps need to be used as information that the ventilator can "report" to the clinician in a written format, but not one that requires audible or visible stimulation.

An alarm event should include the following specifications: (1) conditions that trigger the alarm; (2) the alarm response in the form of audible or visual messages; (3) any associated ventilator response such as termination of inspiration or failure to operate; and (4) whether the alarm is manually reset or self-reset when the alarm condition is corrected.[4]

Table 21-6 provides the different levels of alarm priority and includes alarm characteristics and alarm categories. The categories are based on the ventilator classification scheme and are discussed below.

Input Power Alarms

☐ LOSS OF ELECTRIC POWER

In the event of an electrical power failure, most electrically powered or electrically controlled ventilators have a battery-powered alarm that alerts staff to the loss of power. When the power switch is on and the ventilator is unplugged or loses electrical power, these conditions activate this alarm.

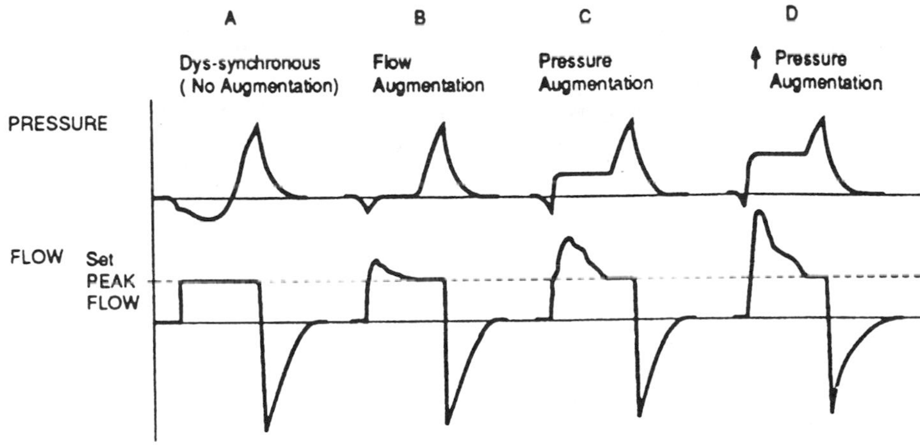

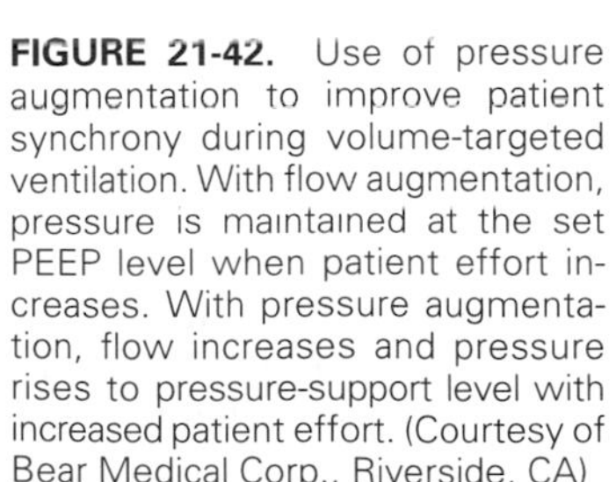

FIGURE 21-42. Use of pressure augmentation to improve patient synchrony during volume-targeted ventilation. With flow augmentation, pressure is maintained at the set PEEP level when patient effort increases. With pressure augmentation, flow increases and pressure rises to pressure-support level with increased patient effort. (Courtesy of Bear Medical Corp., Riverside, CA)

TABLE 21-5 **Events and Monitoring Sites for Ventilator Alarms**

Event	Possible Monitoring Site
Level 1	
Power failure (including when battery in use)	Electrical control system*
Absence of gas delivery (apnea)	Circuit pressure,* circuit flows, timing monitor, CO_2 analysis
Loss of gas source	Pneumatic control system*
Excessive gas delivery	Circuit pressures,* circuit flows, timing monitor
Exhalation valve failure	Circuit pressures, circuit flows, timing monitor
Timing failure	Circuit pressures, circuit flows, timing monitor
Level 2	
Battery power loss (not in use)	Electrical control system*
Circuit leak*	Circuit pressures,* circuit flows
Blender failure	F_IO_2 sensor
Circuit partially occluded	Circuit pressures, circuit flows
Heater/humidifier failure	Temperature probe in circuit
Loss of/or excessive PEEP	Circuit pressures
Autocycling	Circuit pressures, circuit flows
Other electrical or preventive subsystem out of limits without immediate overt gas delivery effects	Electrical and pneumatic systems monitor
Level 3	
Change in central nervous system drive	Circuit pressures, circuit flows, timing monitor
Change in impedances	Circuit pressures, circuit flows, timing monitor
Intrinsic (auto) PEEP >5 cmH_2O	Circuit pressures, circuit flows

* Alarms currently defined in the ISO and ASTM standards.
From AARC consensus statement on the essentials of mechanical ventilation. Respir Care 37:1007, 1992; with permission.

☐ LOSS OF PNEUMATIC POWER

Ventilators that require high-pressure gases (50 psig) usually have alarms that are activated if the oxygen or the air sources fall below a certain pressure. The alarms may be electrically operated as in the Bennett 7200 or may be pneumatically operated as in the blender on the Siemens Servo 900C.

Control Circuit Alarms

These alarms or indicators provide an alert or a message to the operator when a combination of incompatible control variables has been set on the ventilator. For example, the inspiratory time is longer than the expiratory time and the ventilator was not selected for inverse ratio ventilation. Another example is when a microprocessor ventilator runs a "self-test" and detects a problem and gives a warning such as "ventilator inoperative."

Output Alarms

These alarms alert for conditions connected to the ventilator's output capabilities. They include pressure, flow, volume, and time. These alarms activate when the value for the alarm set by the operator occurs outside of the anticipated range. The most common example is the high peak pressure alarm, also called the pressure limit. This is commonly set at a value of 10 cmH_2O above the peak pressure of an inspiration on a volume preset breath. If the pressure exceeds the pressure limit set, the high-pressure alarm sounds. Sometimes this event also terminates the inspiratory phase, depending on the manufacturer.

☐ PRESSURE

The following list includes some of the possible alarms available on various ventilators.

High and Low Inspiratory Pressure

The high-pressure alarm is described above. The low-pressure alarm may activate, for example, if the pressure in the airway fails to exceed the low-pressure alarm value, which might occur in the situation of a leak.

High and Low Mean Airway Pressure

As in the above examples, mean airway pressure alarms may indicate a possible leak in the system. They may also indicate a change in the ventilator's pattern that could affect a patient's oxygenation status. It is important to remember that mean airway pressure has an overall direct effect on oxygenation, in many circumstances.

High and Low Baseline Pressure

When PEEP or CPAP are used, these alarms indicate variation from the set baseline pressure. For example, a high baseline pressure might indicate that air is being trapped in the circuit or patient. The low alarm might indicate a leak in the system or a patient disconnection.

Failure of Pressure to Return to Baseline

If, for example, the patient circuit becomes obstructed or if the exhalation valve malfunctions, this alarm would be activated.

☐ VOLUME

High and Low Expired Volume

Low-volume alarms generally occur when there is a leak in the system on volume ventilation, or during pressure ventilation. They may indicate a change in the patient's condition resulting in a lower V_T. High-volume alarms can occur during pressure control ventilation if the patient's lung conditions improve and V_T increases for the set pressure. High- and low-volume alarms are also likely to occur during spontaneous ventilation with changes in the patient's V_T.

TABLE 21-6 **Classification of Ventilator Alarms**

	Priority			
	Level 1	*Level 2*	*Level 3*	*Level 4*
Event	Critical* ventilator malfunction	Noncritical† ventilator malfunction	Patient status change‡	Operator alert§
Alarm characteristics				
Mandatory	Yes	Yes	No	Yes
Redundant‖	Yes	No	No	No
Noncancelling¶	Yes	No	No	Yes
Audible	Yes	Yes	Yes	No
Visual	Yes	Yes	Yes	Yes
Automatic backup response#	Yes	No	No	No
Automatic reset				
Audible	Yes	Yes	Yes	—
Visual	No	Yes	Yes	Yes
Applicable Alarm Categories				
Input				
Electric power	Yes	No	No	No
Pneumatic power	Yes	No	No	No
Control circuit				
Inverse I:E ratio	No	Yes	No	Yes
Incompatible settings	No	No	No	Yes
Mechanical/electronic fault	Yes	No	No	No
Output				
Pressure**	Yes	Yes	Yes	Yes
Volume††	Yes	Yes	Yes	Yes
Flow‡‡	Yes	Yes	Yes	Yes
Minute ventilation	Yes	Yes	Yes	Yes
Time§§	Yes	Yes	Yes	Yes
Inspired gas ($F_{I}O_2$, temp)‖‖	Yes	Yes	No	Yes
Expired gas (FeO_2, $FeCO_2$)‖‖	No	No	Yes	No

* Immediately life-threatening.
† Not immediately life-threatening.
‡ Change in neurologic ventilatory drive, respiratory system mechanics, hemodynamic or metabolic status, etc.
§ Ventilator warns of potential danger (eg, control variable settings unusually high or low; alarm thresholds inappropriately set).
‖ Specific alarm mechanisms designed in duplicate or backed up by related alarm mechanisms.
¶ Operator cannot reset the alarm until the alarm condition has been corrected.
\# Backup ventilator mode or patient circuit opens to atmosphere.
** High/low peak, mean, and baseline pressure.
†† High/low inhaled and exhaled tidal volume. May also include alarm for leak (inhaled volume minus exhaled volume expressed as a percent of inhaled volume).
‡‡ Alarm triggered if expiratory flow rate does not fall below set threshold. Warns of alveolar gas trapping.
§§ Warns that inspiratory or expiratory times are too long/short.
‖‖ Analysis of inspired and expired gas may include other tracer gases that enable calculation of functional residual capacity.
From Branson RD, Hess DR, Chatburn RL: Respiratory Care Equipment. Philadelphia, Lippincott, 1995, p 292; with permission.

□ FLOW

High and Low Expired Minute Volume

These alarms may indicate conditions of hyperventilation (machine autotriggering) and possibly apnea, patient disconnect, or lower ventilation, respectively.

□ TIME

High and Low Ventilatory Frequency

As with minute volume alarms, these conditions may alarm to indicate higher respiratory rate (ventilator autotriggering), a higher patient ventilatory rate, or apnea or lower respiratory rates, respectively.

Inappropriate Inspiratory Time

This would alert the operator that the ventilator settings are making inspiratory time too long. This might be caused by airway obstruction or a malfunction in the expiratory manifold, for example.

Inappropriate Expiratory Time

This may indicate a period of apnea if the expiratory time is too long. If it is too short, it may indicate an inverse I:E ratio and the potential for air-trapping.

□ INSPIRED GAS

Alarms that might be activated for inspired gas conditions include excessively high or low gas temperatures, and high or low oxygen levels.

□ EXPIRED GAS

Exhaled Carbon Dioxide Tension

Use of exhaled CO_2 tensions (end-tidal carbon dioxide monitoring) may be useful in the assessment of patient ventilation, since this estimates arterial carbon dioxide pressures and can also give some reflection of changes in perfusion states, indirectly. Estimation of carbon dioxide production and respiratory exchange ratios can also be made with the use of "metabolic carts" during mechanical ventilation.

Exhaled Oxygen Tension

Evaluation of end-tidal oxygen levels and average (mean) expired oxygen pressures may be helpful in assessing gas exchange. This, along with CO_2 data can help evaluate the respiratory exchange ratio.

VENTILATOR TROUBLESHOOTING

Ventilator mechanical and operational problems are numerous (Table 21-7).[5] Failure of the device or failure of personnel to adequately monitor and care for the device are the main categories of problems encountered. It is important for respiratory care practitioners (RCPs) to be able to discover problems and solve them as quickly and safely as possible. Equipment troubleshooting is one of the most problematic content areas for respiratory care practitioner graduates. One of the most common difficulties faced by RCP during ventilator management is determining the cause of a problem when a ventilator alarm becomes activated or when an apparent problem occurs.

The purpose of this section is to describe some of the more common types of problems that occur during ventilator management. It describes potential problem situations related to ventilator equipment. It is not intended to cover problems related to the patient, which are addressed in Chapter 20.

Adequacy of Patient Ventilation

Whenever an alarm is activated or a problem seems to occur with a mechanically ventilated patient, it is essential that the practitioner evaluate the patient to be sure he or she is being ventilated. This generally requires that breath sounds be evaluated and, in some instances, that the patient be disconnected from the ventilator and manually ventilated with a resuscitation bag. The advantage of this later method is that it also gives the practitioner an opportunity to determine how easy or difficult ventilation is accomplished. This can indirectly provide information about patient lung compliance and airway resistance.

If the problem is more serious, as in the presence of asystole, critically low blood pressures, or oxygen desaturation as demonstrated by pulse oximetry, then the patient needs to be cared for immediately and until he or she is stable. In this situation, manually ventilating the patient for a short time is often both necessary and preferable.

Problems Related to Pressure Alarms

☐ LOW-PRESSURE ALARMS

Low-pressure alarms (Table 21-8) are commonly set 5 to 10 cmH_2O below the peak inspiratory pressure. They are generally used for detecting air leaks or patient disconnection from the ventilator. Low-pressure alarms are most often used in volume control modes, such as control, assist/control, and SIMV. The Servo 900C uses a low exhaled minute volume for the same purpose. If a low-pressure alarm becomes activated, one must make sure the patient is safely being ventilated before trying to determine the cause of the problem. If necessary, this can be accomplished by having someone manually ventilate the patient. The low-pressure alarm must be set correctly in relation to the patient's ventilator parameters.

A common cause of low-pressure alarms is disconnection of the patient's endotracheal tube from the ventilator circuit. The system must be reconnected and the

TABLE 21-7 **Potential Mechanical Failures With Mechanical Ventilation**

Disconnection from power source
Failure of power source
Failure of ventilator to function due to equipment manufacturing problems or improper maintenance
Failure of alarms to work due to mechanical failure or failure of personnel to turn them on or use them properly
Failure of heating or humidifying devices
Failure of pressure relief valve to open
Disconnection of patient wye connector
Leaks in the system resulting in inadequate pressure or tidal volume delivery
Failure of expiratory valve to function causing a large system leak or a closed system with no exit for exhaled air
Inappropriate assembly of patient circuit

From Pilbeam SP: Mechanical Ventilation: Physiological and Clinical Application, 2nd ed. St. Louis, Mosby–Yearbook, 1992, p 254; with permission.

TABLE 21-8 **Common Causes of Low-Pressure Alarm Situations**

Patient disconnect

Circuit leaks
- Mainline connections to
  - Humidifiers
  - Filters
  - Water traps
- In-line metered dose inhalers
- In-line nebulizers
- Proximal pressure monitors
- Flow monitoring lines
- Exhaled gas monitoring devices
- In-line closed suction catheters
- Temperature monitors
- Exhalation valve leaks: cracked or leaking valves, unseated valves, improperly connected valves

Airway leaks
- Use of minimum leak technique
- Inadequate cuff inflation
- Leak in pilot balloon
- Rupture of tube cuff

Chest tube leaks

low-pressure alarm set correctly. Another common cause of such alarms is leaks in the patient circuit. A simple leak test can help determine if this is the problem. To perform a leak test, be sure the ventilator is no longer connected to the patient. Change the mode to spontaneous or CPAP, tidal volume to 100 mL, the flow to 20 L/min, inspiratory pause to 2 seconds, and the peak pressure to maximum. Occlude the patient wye connector completely, using a sterile gauze. Manually cycle the ventilator and observe the airway pressure. The pressure should read high and should not fall more than about 10 cmH_2O during the 2-second pause. If it does, there is a leak in the circuit.

Common places for leaks in the ventilator system are listed in Table 21-8. These include connections to humidifiers, filters, water traps, in-line closed suction catheters, temperature probes, in-line metered dose inhalers, in-line nebulizers, proximal pressure or flow monitoring lines, or unseated or leaking exhalation valves. If it is still not possible to detect the leak, begin a systematic inspection of the circuit in the following manner. First, occlude the wye connector. Second, pinch closed the large-bore tubing of the patient circuit at the point where it leaves the ventilator. Third, manually cycle the ventilator. If the high-pressure alarm sounds, there is no large leak between the place the circuit is pinched closed and the output from the ventilator. Repeat this process, progressively pinching the circuit farther and farther from the main output connection. At the point where the high-pressure alarm does not sound, the leak can be isolated. This procedure can help pinpoint large leaks.

Another cause of low-pressure alarms is a leak in the airway. Common leaks can be associated with use of the minimum leak technique, an inadequately inflated endotracheal tube cuff, or a leak in the pilot balloon. Check the endotracheal tube cuff to see it if is providing an adequate seal. An air leak can be detected by listening to or palpating over the trachea. The cuff will need to be reinflated to an appropriate volume. Next check the pilot balloon. Sometimes a pilot balloon leak can be temporarily fixed by clamping the pilot balloon line. If a cuff leak cannot be corrected, the possibility exists that the tube cuff is ruptured and the endotracheal tube will need to be replaced.

Another potential leak source leading to a low-pressure alarm is the leaking of air from a bronchopleural fistula through a chest tube. Sometimes this cannot be corrected other than by increasing the volume delivery to compensate for the volume lost through the chest tube. This can help preserve adequate ventilation, but may not promote healing of the fistula.

TABLE 21-9 **Common Causes of High Pressure Alarm Situations**

Common causes
Patient coughing
Secretions or mucus in the airway
Patient biting tube (oral intubation)
Airway problems
Kinking of tube inside the mouth or in the back of the throat
Impinging of the tube on the carina
Change in the tube position
Cuff herniated over the end of the tube
Patient-related conditions
Reduced compliance, eg, pneumothorax or pleural effusion
Increased airway resistance, eg, secretions, mucosal edema, or bronchospasm
Patient "fighting" the ventilator, eg, dyssyncrony with ventilator settings
Ventilator circuit
Accumulation of water in the patient circuit
Kinking in the circuit
Ventilator's inspiratory or expiratory valves

☐ HIGH-PRESSURE ALARM/LIMIT

High-pressure alarms (Table 21-9) are usually set 10 cmH_2O above the peak inspiratory pressure reached during inspiration, for a volume-delivered breath. High-pressure alarms are used in volume control modes such as control, assist/control, and SIMV. Always be sure the alarm is set correctly in relation to patient ventilator parameters. Common causes of the high-pressure alarm sounding that can be checked quickly include patient coughing, secretions or mucus in the airway, and patient biting the tube (oral intubation). Check during the assessment of these to ensure adequate patient ventilation. In addition to listening to breath sounds, it is often helpful to disconnect the patient from the ventilator and manually ventilate him or her with a resuscitation bag. Other high-pressure alarm conditions generally fall into three categories: airway problems, patient-related problems, or problems with the ventilator.

Airway Problems

In addition to the common airway conditions mentioned previously (coughing, secretions or mucus plugging in the airway, the patient biting the airway), other common airway problems may exist. It is important to manually ventilate the patient to assess the airway. If you cannot ventilate the patient in this way, check the patency of the airway by trying to pass a suction catheter through the endotracheal tube. Be sure to select the correct size suction catheter. If the catheter will not pass and the patient is not biting on the airway, be sure that it is not kinking inside the mouth or in the back of the throat. In addition, sometimes the impinging of the tube on the carina or a change in the tube position may be the problem. One quick and easy maneuver to check tube position is to check the millimeter marking of the tube at the lips or incisor teeth to be sure it has not changed position. The tube may have slipped into the right main stem bronchus or may have moved above the vocal cords, activating the high-pressure alarm. Reposition the tube if necessary.

If the catheter still will not pass, deflate the endotracheal tube cuff. The cuff may have herniated over the end of the endotracheal tube. Deflating the cuff will allow a spontaneously breathing patient to move some air around the endotracheal tube if the tube itself is obstructed until the tube can be removed as needed. If this final effort does not clear the airway, the tube is obstructed and will need to be removed if the obstruction cannot be **immediately** cleared.

Patient-Related Conditions

Developments such as reduced compliance from a change in the patient's lung condition (such as pneumothorax or pleural effusion) or an increased airway resistance owing to secretions, mucosal edema, or bronchospasm may cause high-pressure alarms. Evaluation of breath sounds, percussion of the chest, and assessment of the chest radiograph can help determine the patient's problem. For example, the patient may have severe bronchospasm and air-trapping due to asthma. In this case, wheezing would likely be present. If scattered crackles are heard throughout, pulmonary edema may be present. If breath sounds are absent, percuss the affected site. A hyperresonant or tympanic note may indicate the presence of a pneumothorax. A dull percussion may indicate fluid in the pleural space or possibly a collapsed or consolidated area of lung. The patient may be in pain or "fighting" the ventilator (for example, breathing out of synchrony with ventilator settings) for a variety of reasons, such as inadequate gas flow settings or inappropriate sensitivity settings.

Finally, the ventilator circuit needs to be checked. Look for accumulation of water in the patient circuit. Water in the circuit is a common occurrence and is easily cleared. Sometimes when the ventilator forces air through the water as it cycles, bubbling of the water and movement of the water in the circuit result. This movement can cause fluctuations in the circuit pressure and can cause the ventilator to autocycle.

Kinking in the circuit is another cause of high-pressure alarm activation. A common site for this to occur is near a heated humidifier where warm air can sometimes soften the plastic of the circuit, rendering it more susceptible to kinking. In other instances, such as when patients are moved in bed, the ventilator circuits may become kinked during the move or blocked by the patient's body.

If these problems have been ruled out, another possible cause is malfunctioning of the ventilator's inspiratory or expiratory valves. If these valves become occluded, or closed, they may provide a source of the problem. For example, if aerosolized medications are given to the patients, the medication may accumulate on the exhalation valve or exhalation line filter and block the air from leaving the circuit. If the valves are malfunctioning, the ventilator will need to be replaced until the problem is corrected. During pressure ventilation, a high-pressure alarm may be the result of increased resistance or decreased compliance.

Although three different categories leading to high-pressure alarms have been reviewed, it is important to mention that the patient is the most important consideration in solving the problem. It is essential that an airway is correctly in place and the patient is being adequately ventilated at all times.

□ LOW PEEP/CPAP ALARM

Low PEEP/CPAP alarms are used when PEEP or CPAP are being used for patient ventilator management. The alarm is commonly set about 5 cmH_2O below the PEEP/CPAP level. First be sure the alarm is set appropriately. If the system manometer measures a different PEEP/CPAP level than what is actually set, then the ventilator may need to be repaired or recalibrated.

If the manometer indicates that the PEEP levels are not being maintained and the low PEEP/CPAP alarm is sounding, the patient may be actively inspiring (drawing off) the PEEP/CPAP settings. If the patient is actively inspiring and the ventilator is not sensing the patient's active inspiration, then the machine sensitivity may not be correctly set or the ventilator may not be providing adequate flow to meet patient inspiratory demand. Alternatively, the patient may have auto-PEEP (air-trapping). Check the patient and take corrective action depending on the cause of the problem in this situation. For example, readjust the triggering sensitivity, increase flow, or switch to a ventilator that is more responsive to patient inspiratory flow demand. If auto-PEEP is present, try to reduce its level by increasing inspiratory flow to shorten inspiratory time and lengthen expiratory time, or reduce minute ventilation. In some cases it is possible to adjust the PEEP level to nearly equal the auto-PEEP level so the patient can more easily trigger the ventilator.

Another possible problem exists with the use of heat moisture exchangers. If these devices become clogged with secretions, they may prevent the patient's inspiratory effort being detected by the ventilator. This would require changing the device.

When the manometer indicates that PEEP levels are not being maintained, but otherwise reads accurately and the patient is not actively inspiring, a possible system leak is present. Check to be sure that all circuit connections are tight. Systematically check the circuit and the patient's artificial airway as described for the low-pressure alarm problem described above. If all of these have been thoroughly checked and the problem still exists, then the problem is most likely in the ventilator. It may need to be recalibrated or changed.

Apnea Alarm

Apnea alarms are used to indicate absence of a detectable breath. Ventilators with this alarm usually are designed to measure both spontaneous and machine-delivered breaths. This alarm is commonly set at 20 seconds or at a time interval that does not allow a patient to miss more that two machine-delivered breaths. For example, if a patient has a control rate of 10 breaths per minute, each breath is 6 seconds long. Setting an apnea alarm of more than 6 but less than 12 seconds will allow the patient to miss one machine breath but not two.

A common cause of an apnea alarm is patient disconnect from the ventilator. This is often accompanied by a low-pressure alarm, which is often the first alarm to be activated. In some ventilators the presence of a low-pressure alarm activates the apnea alarm. If this is the problem, simply reconnect the patient.

If the patient is still connected to the ventilator, and the apnea alarm is sounding, the safest procedure is to disconnect the patient from the ventilator circuit and use a manual resuscitation bag until the cause of the activated apnea alarm is determined and corrected.

First, establish what mode of ventilation is in use. With control, or A/C, check the time interval of the apnea alarm. If it is set at less than the total cycle time of one breath, then set the time interval of the apnea alarm so it is longer than one total cycle time. For example, if the rate is set at six breaths, the total cycle time is 10 seconds. If the apnea alarm was set at 8 seconds, the apnea limit would be reached before a ventilator breath was again delivered.

Some ventilators have a volume as well as a time setting for the apnea alarm. If the time interval is set correctly, check the volume settings. The ventilator tidal volume setting or the patient's spontaneous tidal volume must be higher than the tidal volume set on the apnea alarm.

If the alarms are appropriately set and the patient is not apneic, then there may be a large leak in the circuit preventing the delivery of the tidal volume. Simply correct the leak. Again, however, this situation usually causes a low-pressure alarm.

Another possibility is that the working pressure of the ventilator is not adequate or the ventilator is for some reason not delivering the set tidal volume. Reset the working pressure or obtain another ventilator. Be sure that the ventilator circuit and flow detectors are correctly functioning and in place. If all this fails, change ventilators and call the manufacturer.

If you switch from control or A/C to the SIMV mode, there may be some lag time if the patient is not spontaneously breathing before a machine breath is delivered. This may activate the apnea alarm. To avoid this, be sure to give a manual breath when the switch is made to allow the normal cycle time to resume without activating the apnea alarm.

If the apnea alarm is activated while the patient has been on the SIMV mode, follow the procedure for control, A/C outlined above. Also, be sure to check that the patient's spontaneous tidal volumes are higher than the apnea alarm tidal volume setting. Otherwise, spontaneous volume breaths will be detected as below the desired setting and the alarm will activate.

Sometimes the apnea alarm is activated when the SIMV rate is set low, for example, two breaths/min. The common machine setting for the apnea alarm is usually a 20-second delay. Be sure the time interval and tidal volume on the alarm are set to detect the patient's spontaneous efforts. The patient may have no spontaneous respirations and this should be checked (see above, "Adequacy of Patient Ventilation"). It may be appropriate to at least temporarily increase the SIMV rate and to notify the physician of the patient's condition.

When the apnea alarm occurs in the pressure support mode, review the procedure for control, A/C as described above. Be sure the patient is being ventilated, that there are no leaks, and that the system is assembled correctly and working properly. Be sure the apnea parameters for time delay and volume are set correctly. Be sure sensitivity is set appropriately. If the apnea alarm is sounding and none of the above conditions are causing the problem, then the patient's spontaneous respiratory rate may be falling below acceptable levels. It may be necessary to switch to SIMV or A/C. Another possibility is that the preset pressure may be too low to deliver the tidal volume. This would require increasing the pressure setting on pressure support and evaluating the patient to determine what has caused a change in tidal volume, for example, reduced lung compliance or increased airway resistance. Some ventilators have apnea backup ventilation parameters. When an apnea alarm is detected, these ventilators automatically provide ventilation to the patient based on preset parameters.

Vent In-Operative Alarm

Most current generation ventilators are equipped with a ventilator in-operative alarm. This indicates that a major problem exists with the ventilator and it is not properly supporting the patient. Check to be sure the power source is connected. Be sure the inlet gases are connected and that they have adequate pressure. Check the exhalation valve assembly to be sure it is correctly assembled. If these are true and the ventilator is still giving the alarm, get another ventilator and contact the service agent.

Summary of Alarm Conditions

The above alarm conditions, low-pressure alarm, high-pressure alarm, low PEEP/CPAP alarm, apnea, and the ventilator inoperative alarm, are just a few of the more common types of alarms that are activated when changing events or conditions occur. The descriptions and algorithms with each are not intended to be exhaustive or to satisfy the needs of every individual situation. The practitioner must learn this as he or she becomes more familiar with the function of each ventilator used, and as he or she is faced with new patient situations to solve.

IDENTIFYING PROBLEMS FROM GRAPHIC MONITORING

During mechanical ventilation the ventilator settings that are established by the practitioner can actually interrupt the patient's natural breathing pattern. The resulting dyssynchronous pattern is not only uncomfortable for the patient, but can increase the work of breathing. In addition, if the patient's efforts are not properly detected or if the ventilator response is not rapid enough, this can result in hyperinflation of the lungs and possible barotrauma. In the past, clinicians have had to rely on patient assessment through evaluation of the use of accessory muscles, signs and symptoms of patient distress, and visualization of the ventilator pressure manometer to try and determine the cause of a patient's "fighting" the ventilator.

Fortunately, newer-generation ventilators offer graphic presentations of the waveforms for pressure, volume, and flow. With the use of this new aid, in addition to patient assessment, the clinician can now better adjust ventilator settings and modes to meet the patient's desired natural pattern of breathing. This section reviews how graphs can be used to detect problems with patient/ventilator dyssynchrony.

Patient Dyssynchrony During Volume-Targeted Ventilation

Figure 21-43 shows an example of volume-control ventilation with a constant flow pattern.[28] The inspiratory flow is inadequate for the patient. This can be identified by

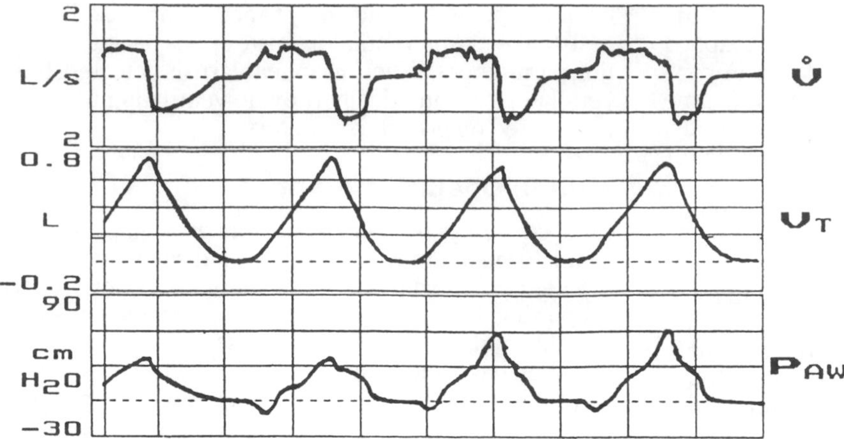

FIGURE 21-43. Airway pressure (Paw), flow ($\dot{V}$ and volume (V_T) waveforms during volume-targeted ventilation. Note the marked alterations in the airway pressure trace indicative of patient dyssynchrony. This patient's dyssynchrony is also reflected in the inability of the ventilator to maintain a constant flow pattern. (Waveforms recorded with a Bicore CP-100 monitor) (From Kacmarek, RM Management of the patient-mechanical ventilator system in Pierson DJ, Kacmarek RM. Foundations of Respiratory Care, Churchill Livingstone, New York, 1992)

looking at the airway pressure (Paw) waveform. The patient is trying to breathe in to gain gas flow but is unable to do so because the gas flow is fixed at a constant value.

Inadequate Gas Flow to Meet the Patient's Inspiratory Demand

Figure 21-44 shows a similar situation during A/C, volume-targeted ventilation using a constant (rectangular) gas flow.[28] In this mode of ventilation, the operator typically sets a tidal volume, gas flow, and respiratory rate. This fixes the gas flow to the patient at a certain flow rate. The flow waveform represents a situation of inadequate levels of inspiratory flow from the ventilator. The sustained sub-baseline airway pressure, which is less than zero in this example, provides the clue for the practitioner that flow is inadequate for the patient.

Inappropriate Ventilator Response to the Patient's Inspiratory Effort to Trigger a Breath

Figure 21-45 shows an example of an inadequate sensitivity setting.[28] This is another example of assisted ventilation in a volume-targeted mode using a constant flow waveform. Look at the pressure curve in the center of the figure. Notice how the curve deflects about −5 cmH_2O below baseline before the ventilator is triggered into inspiration. Notice that the flow curve on the top also has a negative deflection during this same time period. The sensitivity needs to be readjusted so the patient does not have to work so hard to trigger a breath.

Detection of Air-Trapping or Auto-PEEP

The airway pressure curve in this example shows variations in the curve when the patient is out of synchrony with the ventilator (Fig. 21-46).[42] Notice the variations in the airway pressure tracing. The arrows indicate points in the flow (top) and pressure (center) curves that mark the end of exhalation and the beginning of another ventilator breath. The patient in this situation has not completely exhaled. The expiratory flow at this point has not returned to zero. This is a common finding when air-trapping and auto-PEEP are present.

Evaluation of Response to Bronchodilator Therapy

Graphics can also be used to evaluate a patient's response to bronchodilator therapy (Fig. 21-47).[28] This example uses the A/C mode with volume-targeted venti-

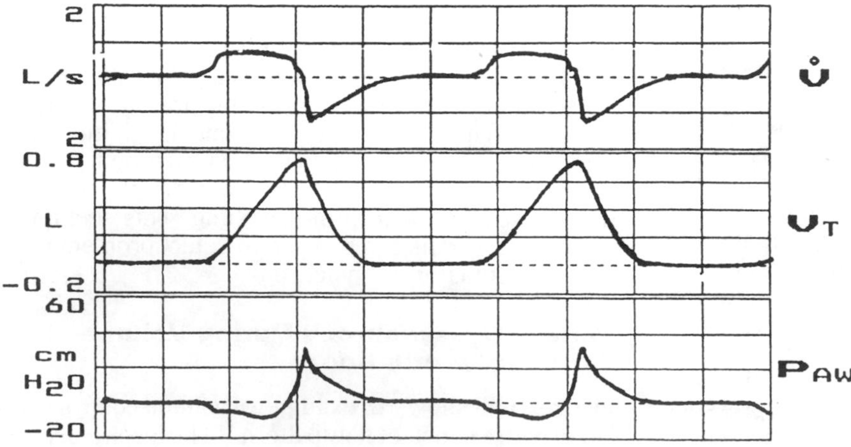

FIGURE 21-44. Airway pressure (Paw), flow ($\dot{V}$ and volume (V_T) waveforms during volume-targeted ventilation. The Paw illustrates grossly inadequate peak inspiratory flow. This patient's work of breathing is excessive, in spite of ventilatory assistance. (Waveforms recorded with a Bicore CP-100 monitor) (From Kacmarek, RM Management of the patient-mechanical ventilator system in Pierson DJ, Kacmarek RM. Foundations of Respiratory Care, Churchill Livingstone, New York, 1992)

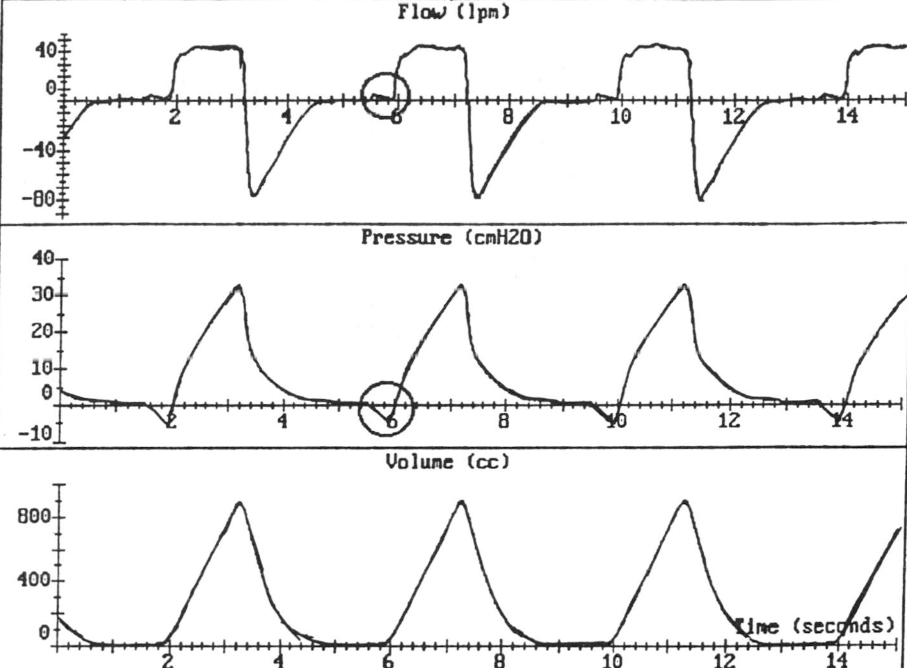

FIGURE 21-45. Flow, pressure, and volume waveforms in a patient for whom the trigger sensitivity is inappropriately set. A 5 to 6 cmH_2O pressure change is necessary to trigger the ventilator (circled area, pressure curve). Flow is measurable at the airway (circled area, flow curve) but the volume-targeted breath is not activated. (Waveforms recorded with a Ventrak monitor) (From Kacmarek, RM Management of the patient-mechanical ventilator system in Pierson DJ, Kacmarek RM. Foundations of Respiratory Care, Churchill Livingstone, New York, 1992)

lation and a constant flow waveform. Example A shows waveforms before therapy and example B shows waveforms after bronchodilator therapy. Notice how the expiratory flows improve following therapy, and also notice the decrease in peak airway pressure and expiratory time.

Inadequate Inspiratory Time During Pressure-Targeted Ventilation

Figure 21-48 illustrates the effects of changes in inspiratory time during pressure-control ventilation.[28] In example A the flow waveform does not return to the zero

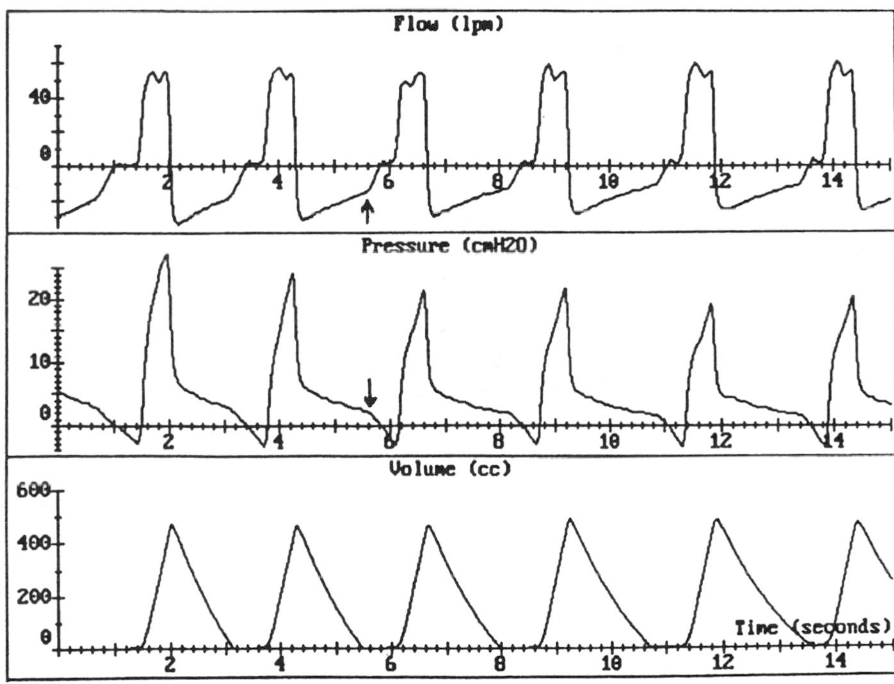

FIGURE 21-46. Flow, pressure and volume waveforms in a patient dyssynchronous with the mechanical ventilator (variable airway pressure curves) and with auto-PEEP present. *Arrow* on pressure and flow curves indicates end of exhalation. Note the considerable expiratory flow at this transition. Whenever expiratory flow does not return to zero, air trapping and auto-PEEP are present. (Waveforms recorded with a Ventrak monitor) (From Kacmarek, RM Management of the patient mechanical ventilator system in Pierson DJ, Kacmarek RM. Foundations of Respiratory Care, Churchill Livingstone, New York, 1992)

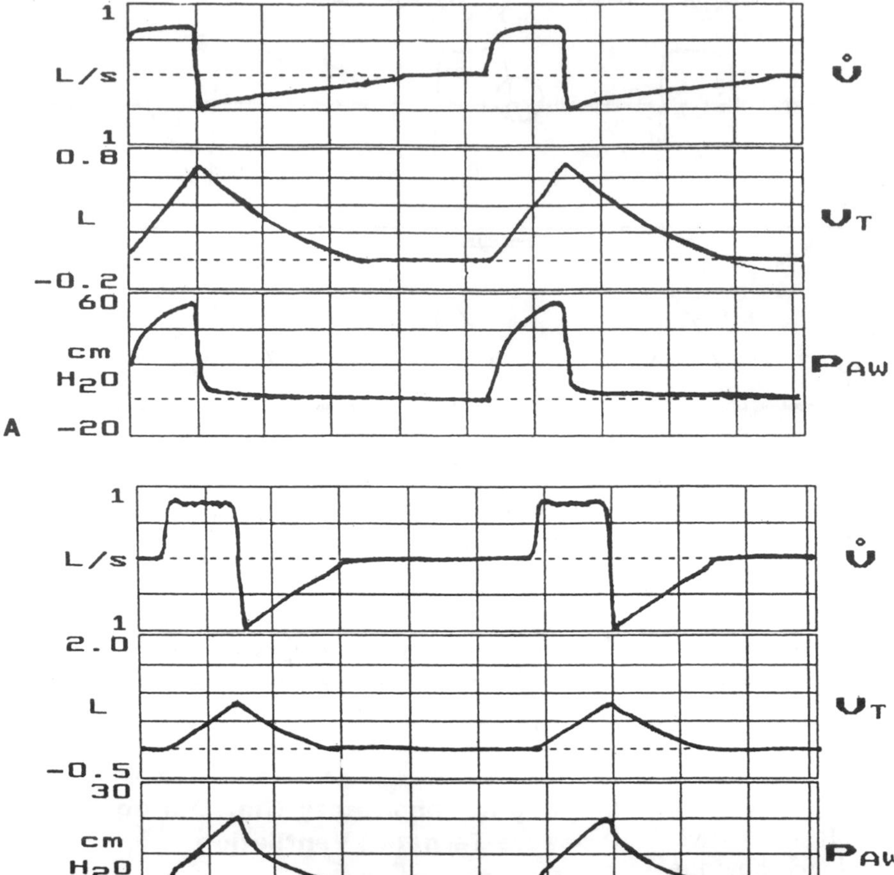

FIGURE 21-47. **(A)** Airway pressure (Paw), flow ($\dot{V}$ and volume (V_T) waveforms before bronchodilator therapy, during volume-control ventilation. Note the peak expiratory flow is 0.5 L/sec and the length of expiration is 3 seconds. **(B)** After bronchodilator therapy, peak expiratory flow increased to 1.0 L/sec and expiratory time decreased to 1.5 seconds. In addition, peak airway pressure dropped considerably, while peak inspiratory flow remained constant at 0.75 L/sec. (Waveforms recorded with a Bicore CP-100 monitor) (From Kacmarek, RM Management of the patient-mechanical ventilator system in Pierson DJ, Kacmarek RM. Foundations of Respiratory Care, Churchill Livingstone, New York, 1992)

baseline, which indicates a short inspiratory time. There is no period of zero flow (similar to an inflation hold). In example B, inspiratory time has been lengthened. There is a period of time of no flow. Notice how airway pressure has plateaued at the end of inspiration. This illustrates an end-inspiratory pause or inflation hold.

Patient and/or Circuit Air Leak

Figure 21-49 is an example of a large air leak.[28] When inspiration flow begins, the volume curve drops and there is a gap between the end of exhalation and the beginning of inspiratory flow. This represents the pneumotachograph zeroing itself before inspiratory flow begins.

These examples are just a few illustrations of the types of clinical situations that can be evaluated and identified using the graphic displays available on newer-generation ventilators.

UNEXPECTED VENTILATOR PROBLEMS ASSOCIATED WITH CURRENT-GENERATION VENTILATORS

Some of the problems that can occur with microprocessor-controlled ventilators stem from inappropriate use of the machine or from idiosyncrasies associated with the ventilator itself. These include such problems as excessive CPAP or PEEP levels, changes in sensitivity, unseating of the exhalation valve, inability to trigger a pressure support breath, inadequate flow, and low and high tidal volume delivery to name just a few.

Excessive CPAP or PEEP Levels

In certain situations, the level of PEEP/CPAP in the circuit will actually be above the set value. One such situation occurs with PSV. The potential problem is a sudden accidental delivery of high pressure and flow as the result of a leak in the circuit. For example, in the Bird 6400 ventilator during PSV, a gas leak, such as a leak around a tracheal cuff, can cause a rise in PEEP. The ventilator tries to correct for the leak by increasing the flow to the circuit. This sudden surge of flow can cause a rise in PEEP/CPAP levels above their set values. The patient may develop dyspnea, tachypnea, and tachycardia.[29] The problem can be managed by removing the leak.

Another situation occurs with the Puritan Bennett 7200 ventilator. Normally, the mechanism to end the inspiratory phase on this ventilator during PSV occurs when the flow drops to 5 L/min or lower. Sometimes leaks occur in a ventilator circuit or artificial airway.[29] If the leak is greater than the 5 L/min in this situation, the set PSV level is maintained throughout the cycle by an

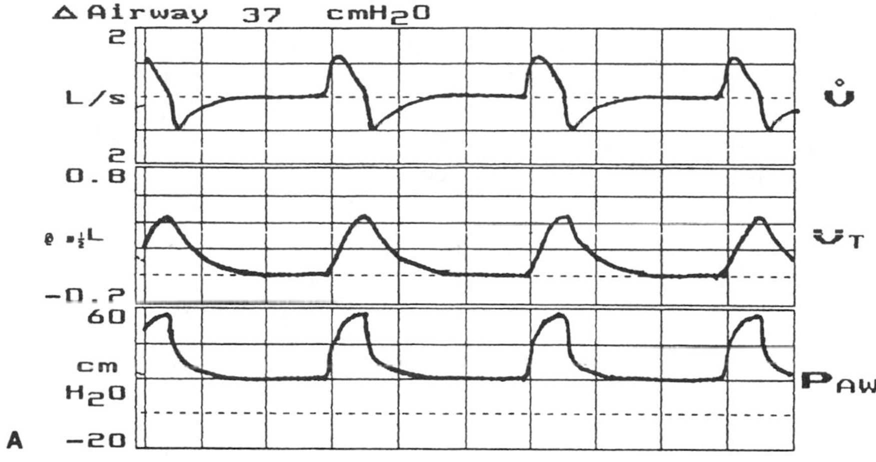

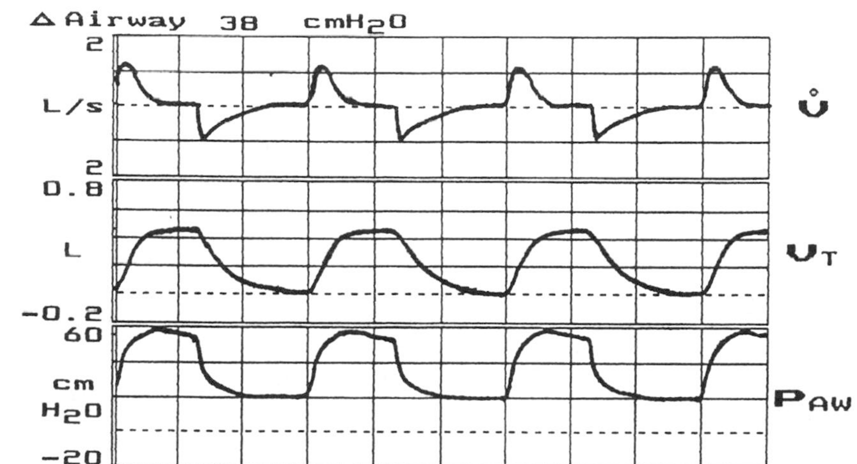

FIGURE 21-48. **(A)** Airway pressure (Paw), flow ($\dot{V}$ and volume (V_T) waveforms during pressure-control ventilation. Note, inspiratory time is inadequate; flow has not returned to zero, nor is an inflation hold (zero flow period) observed. **(B)** Results of increasing inspiratory time. Now flow returns to zero about midway through the inspiratory time period. The remaining inspiratory time illustrates an end-inspiratory hold. (Waveforms recorded with a Bicore CP-100 monitor) (From Kacmarek, RM Management of the patient-mechanical ventilator system in Pierson DJ, Kacmarek RM. Foundations of Respiratory Care, Churchill Livingstone, New York, 1992)

increase in the gas flow from the ventilator. This increased flow results in excessive CPAP in the circuit. The ventilator will finally end the inspiratory phase after a brief time interval or when pressure exceeds 1.5 cmH_2O of PSV + PEEP.

The Bear 3 ventilator has also been reported to cause excessive PEEP/CPAP levels. When the proximal line becomes disconnected during PEEP use, the ventilator tries to correct for the loss of PEEP by increasing flow.[30] An example of this occurs when the proximal airway pressure line is disconnected. The flow into the circuit can be large enough to cause pressure to be held in the circuit. The result is a rise in the baseline pressure. The next breath may result in a high enough pressure to cause the high-pressure limit to be reached, giving a high-pressure alarm. When this situation occurs, the

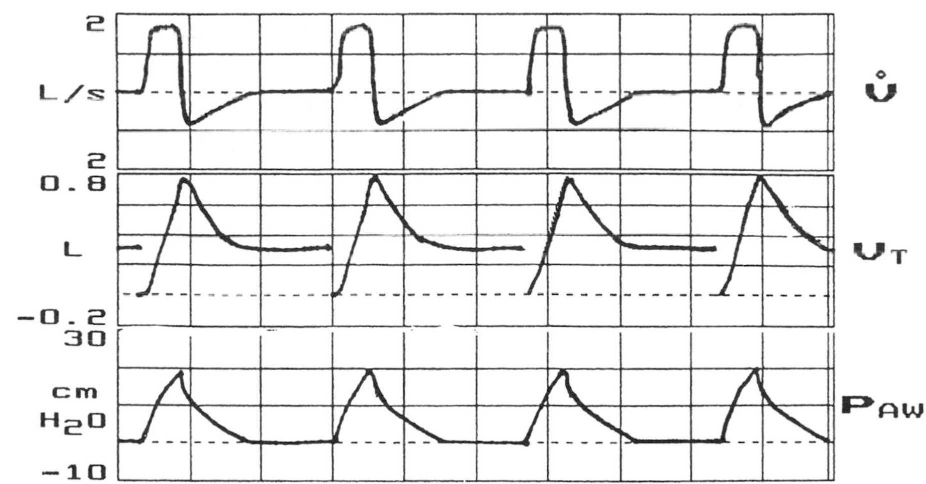

FIGURE 21-49. Airway pressure (Paw), flow ($\dot{V}$ and volume (V_T) waveforms in the presence of a large airleak. Note the pressure and flow waveforms provide little help in quantifying the airleak. However, one look at the volume waveform identifies a 300-mL airleak. The gap between end expiration and the next inspiration is a result of the pneumotachograph zeroing itself as inspiration begins. (Waveforms recorded with a Bicore CP-100 monitor) (From Kacmarek, RM: Management of the patient-mechanical ventilator system in Pierson DJ, Kacmarek RM. Foundations of Respiratory Care, Churchill Livingstone, New York, 1992)

proximal airway pressure display will be zero because the proximal line is disconnected. The problem is easily corrected by reconnecting the line.

Changes in Sensitivity: Trouble Triggering a Breath or Excessive Triggering

When a patient appears to be using accessory muscles to breathe during mechanical ventilation, but strong inspiratory efforts fail to trigger the ventilator, a few potential problems may exist. The most common is that the machine sensitivity is not correctly set. If the mode is a pressure-triggered mode, the machine should be sensitive enough to initiate a breath with a very slight effort, commonly -1 cmH_2O in adults. But it should not be so sensitive that the machine begins to self-cycle.

Self-cycling occurs when the machine is set at too sensitive a level. To correct this problem, simply reduce the sensitivity. Also check the circuit to be sure there is no water in the main line. Sometimes the movement of this water can cause triggering of the ventilator. This has been noted to occur in the pressure support mode and can interfere with adequate ventilation of the patient.

Another possibility that interferes with patient triggering of a breath occurs when the patient has air-trapping or auto-PEEP. The patient is unable to trigger the ventilator even though the sensitivity level is set appropriately and the patient is making an obvious effort. To trigger the ventilator in this setting, the patient's inspiratory effort must equal the sensitivity setting at end-expiration plus the auto-PEEP level in the lungs. To correct the problem, eliminate the auto-PEEP. If this is not possible, set an end-expiratory pressure slightly less than the measured auto-PEEP level. This helps keep airway pressure at or near pressure in the lungs and reduces the effort needed to trigger a breath.

If the patient is trapping air in the Bear 3 ventilator during PSV, the patient may not be able to trigger a ventilator breath. Apparently, when the inspiratory effort is weak and inspiratory flow is low, the internal demand valve will open but will not give a pressure support breath. Weak inspiratory flow demands or trapped air will result in an inability to meet the demand criteria to trigger a breath.

Besides the presence of air-trapping resulting in problems for patients triggering a breath, there is another problem that can occur. Sometimes small-volume nebulizers are used to deliver medication to ventilated patients. When an external flowmeter is used to provide continuous flow to the nebulizer, this adds additional volume and flow to the ventilator circuit. When the flow is placed between the patient and the sensing device, it makes it more difficult for the patient to generate enough negative pressure (inspiratory flow) to trigger a breath.[18] These sensing devices are usually on the inspiratory side of the ventilator. This is a possible problem for patients in a pressure-triggered mode. With use of A/C, the set back-up rate is usually enough to mask the presence of the problem. In the PSV mode, there is no back-up rate. To correct the problem, use only the nebulizer system provided by the ventilator or switch to a time-triggered mode such as A/C for the time of the treatment or use a metered-dose inhaler to deliver the treatment.

Inadequate Flow

During volume-controlled ventilation, the operator commonly sets the tidal volume, respiratory rate, inspiratory time, or gas flow. For example, when using the Hamilton Veolar in the SIMV mode, the patient's inspiratory flow is limited by these preset parameters. The preset flow may be inadequate to match the patient's inspiratory flow demands (see Fig. 21-44). Either in-

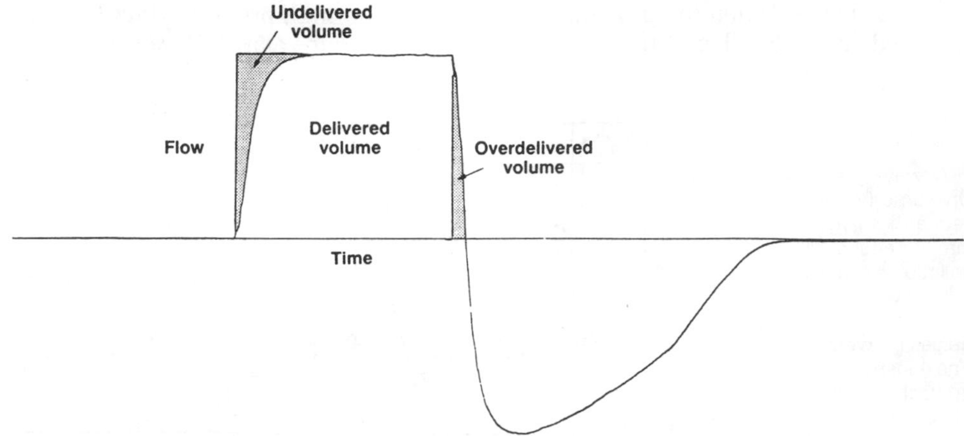

FIGURE 21-50. Graph shows how the left-hand of a constant flow curve can be "shaved off" with some ventilators when the tidal volume (V_T) is high and inspiratory time is short. This curve was produced with a 800-mL V_T at a flow of 40 L/min. The left-hand side of the curve shows a shaded portion of undelivered volume. This shows a rise of flow and its deviation from a true square shape. The *shaded portion* to the right of the curve shows a slightly overdelivered volume again since the flow does not stop in a perfect "rectangular" shape. (Courtesy of Warren Sanborn, PhD, Puritan-Bennett Corp., Carlsbad, CA)

creasing flow, reducing inspiratory time, or even switching flow patterns can improve inspiratory flow from the ventilator. Another possible solution is to switch to the pressure-control mode. This allows the patient to receive the amount of flow he or she needs up to the maximum capacity of the ventilator, but requires closer tidal volume monitoring.

Unseating of the Exhalation Valve

Clinicians often measure plateau pressure by occluding the exhalation valve with their hand at the peak of inspiration, before exhalation begins. In some ventilators this can unseat the exhalation valve. For example, this has been seen in the Bird 6400 ventilator. The occlusion of the valve causes a pressure buildup, occasionally causing the exhalation valve to disengage. This may cause a "vent in-op" alarm, a low-pressure alarm, or a low CPAP/PEEP alarm. If the patient is struggling to breathe in any of these situations, this may be the cause. The problem can be corrected by reseating the valve.

Low and High Tidal Volume Delivery

Sometimes the preset values used to control volume delivery and the digital display of volume delivery differ. This can occur under several circumstances, but the two most common are the use of externally powered nebulizers and the idiosyncrasy of certain microprocessor ventilators.

The use of externally powered nebulizers adds extra flow to the circuit. This can increase tidal volume and give high readings of exhaled minute volume. In most adult settings this is not clinically significant, but in neonatal patients it can be a problem.

Low tidal volume delivery can occur in the 7200ae and probably other microprocessor ventilators. The current programming in the 7200ae assumes that the delivery of flow is perfect. If you select the constant flow pattern, the ventilator assumes that the flow goes instantly from zero to the set flow. Of course, the flow cannot do this, so there is a slight lag where the flow is rapidly building up to the set value. Under most clinical settings, this amount is not important.[5]

When minute ventilation delivery is set for high volumes and high respiratory rates with a short inspiratory time, then a greater error occurs. The ventilator calculates its output assuming that it will give the perfect square flow. As seen in Figure 21-50,[5] the flow is not perfectly constant, so the actual output will be less than selected.

In this ventilator, the exhaled tidal volume is measured at the exhalation valve assembly. The ventilator's programs do not currently compare and correct the set value to the measured value. It is never "aware" that there is a difference. During delivery of high volume and rates, the exhaled volume reading will be lower than the set volume. To correct for this difference, the operator needs only to increase the volume setting or lengthen the inspiratory time until the exhaled volume reads at the desired value of gas exhaled from the patient's lungs.

ELECTROMAGNETIC INTERFERENCE

It has been common knowledge for some time that electrical devices that emit radio frequencies can interfere with the operation of clinical and other electronic equipment. More recently, with the boom in the cellular phone market, hospitals have been prohibiting cellular phones and similar devices that transmit radio frequencies, such as walkie-talkies, from being brought into the hospital environment. These types of devices have been known to interfere with infusion pumps, smoke detectors, mechanical ventilators, and telemetry equipment.[30] Early investigations suggest the following devices may also be affected: infant incubators, ECG, oxygen and apnea monitors, defibrillator/monitors, blood warmers, and dialysis units.[30]

Because many mechanical ventilators may be victim to radio frequency/electromagnetic interference, anyone operating a mechanical ventilator should contact the manufacturer to find out what safeguards have been built into the units and what precautions should be taken to prevent an accidental interference from causing jeopardy to a patient's life and safety.

SUMMARY

Each ventilator has its own idiosyncrasies. Practitioners using these machines become familiar with these characteristics and learn to correct situations as they occur. It is always important to be aware that events such as these can occur depending on the patient situation, the clinical setting, and the specific ventilator in use.

REFERENCES

1. Mushin MW, Rendell-Baker LL, Thompson PW, Mapleson WW: Automatic Ventilation of the Lungs. Oxford, Blackwell Scientific, 1980
2. Chatburn RL: A new system for understanding mechanical ventilators. Respir Care 36:1123–1155, 1991
3. Chatburn RL: Classification of mechanical ventilators. In Tobin MJ: Principles and Practice of Mechanical Ventilation. New York, McGraw-Hill, 1994
4. Chatburn RL: Classification of mechanical ventilators. In Branson RD, Hess DR, Chatburn RL (eds): Respiratory Care Equipment. Philadelphia, JB Lippincott, 1995
5. Pilbeam SP: Mechanical Ventilation, Physiological and Clinical Applications, 2nd ed. Chicago, Mosby Year Book, 1992
6. Kacmarek RM, Hess D: Basic principles of ventilator machinery In Tobin MJ: Principles and Practice of Mechanical Ventilation. New York, McGraw-Hill, 1994
7. Sanborn WG: Microprocessor-based mechanical ventilation. Respir Care 38:72–109, 1991
8. Chatburn RL: Classification of mechanical ventilators. Respir Care 37:1009–1025, 1992
9. Elam JO, Kerr JH, Janney CD: Performance of ventilators: Effect of changes in lung-thorax compliance. Anesthesiology 19:56, 1958
10. Hunter AR: The classification of respirators. Anaesthesia 16:231, 1961
11. Mapleson WW: The effect of changes of lung characteristics on the functioning of automatic ventilators. Anaesthesia 17:300, 1962
12. Branson RD, Chatburn RL: Technical description and classification of modes of ventilator operation. Respir Care 37:1026–1044, 1992

13. Kirby RR, Downs JB, Civetta JM, et al: High level positive end-expiratory pressure (PEEP) in acute respiratory insufficiency. Chest 67:156, 1975
14. Kirby RR, Perry JC, Calderwood HW, et al: Cardiorespiratory effects of high positive end-expiratory pressure. Anesthesiology 43:533, 1975
15. Kacmarek RM, Hickling KG: Permissive hypercarbia. Respir Care 38:373–387, 1993
16. Kirby RR: IMV held satisfactory alternative to controlled ventilation. Clin Trends Anesthesiol 6:14, 1976
17. Cohen IL, Bilen Z, Krishnamurthy S: The effects of ventilator working pressure during pressure support ventilation. Chest 103: 588–592, 1993
18. Beaty CD, Ritz RH, Benson MS: Continuous in-line nebulizers complicate pressure support ventilation. Chest 96:1360–1363, 1989
19. Downs JB: Airway pressure release ventilation: A new concept in ventilatory support [editorial]. Crit Care Med 15:459–461, 1987
20. Perel A, Stock MC:Handbook of Mechanical Ventilatory Support. Baltimore, Williams & Wilkins, 1992
21. Stock MC, Downs JB, Frolicher DA: Airway pressure release ventilation. Crit Care Med 15:462–466, 1987
22. Stock MC, Downs JB: Airway pressure release ventilation: A new approach to ventilatory support. Respir Care 32:517–524, 1987
23. Garner W, Downs JB, Stock CM, Rasanen J: Airway pressure release ventilation: A human trial. Chest 94:779–781, 1988
24. Younes M: Proportional assist ventilation, a new approach to ventilatory support. Am Rev Respir Dis 145:114–120, 1992
25. Younes M, Puddy A, Roberts D, Light RB, Quesada A, Taylor D, Oppenheimer L, Cramp H: Proportional assist ventilation, results of an initial clinical trial. Am Rev Respir Dis 145:121–129, 1992
26. Day S: Essentials for ventilator-alarm systems. Respir Care 37:1108–1112, 1992
27. AARC: Consensus statement on the essentials of ventilators. Respir Care 37:1000–1008, 1992
28. Kacmarek RM: Management of the patient-mechanical ventilator system. In Pierson DJ, Kacmarek RM (eds): Foundations of Respiratory Care. New York, Churchill Livingston, 1992, pp 973–997
29. Black JW, Grover BS: A hazard of pressure support ventilation. Chest 93:333–335, 1988
30. Monaco F, Goettel J: Increased airway pressures in Bear 2 and 3 circuits. Respir Care 36:132–143, 1991

Susan P. Pilbeam
F. Ross Payne

SECTION 2
Mechanical Ventilators

BEAR MEDICAL

Bear 1 Volume Ventilator*

☐ CLASSIFICATION

The Bear 1 (Table 21-10) (Fig. 21-51) adult volume ventilator is an electrically and pneumatically powered, electronically operated ventilator that may function as a pressure or volume controller. It can be triggered by time, pressure, or by manual operation. It is volume- or flow-limited and pressure- or volume-cycled. Inspiration may also be extended by a time-cycled plateau. End-expiratory pressure may be applied during mechanical or spontaneous (CPAP) breathing.

☐ SPECIFICATIONS

Table 21-11 provides a list of the specifications for the Bear 1.

☐ INPUT VARIABLES

The Bear 1 volume ventilator uses 115 volts AC at 60 Hz to power the electrical control circuit. The pneumatic circuit is powered by compressed gas sources, air, and oxy-

* Thanks to Ayres Mello, Greg Oliver, and Darryl L. Shelby of Bear Medical, Riverside, CA, for their technical assistance with Bear ventilators in this section

TABLE 21-10 **Classification of the Bear 1 Adult Volume Ventilator**

Power Source for Pneumatic Circuit	**Pressurized Gases (30–100 psig)**
Power source for control circuit	Electricity (115 volts AC at 60 Hz)
Control mechanism	Pressure, volume
Triggering	Time, pressure, manual
Limiting	Volume, flow
Cycling	Time, pressure

gen, at 25 to 100 psig and includes an integral air–oxygen blender. There is an internal compressor that can provide air at 11.2 psig. If a high-pressure air source is available, the ventilator compressor system is bypassed.

Operation

The type of ventilation desired is programmed by the mode selector knob (A) (Fig. 21-52). In the assist-control mode, a built-in safety feature prohibits the patient from initiating a breath until at least 100 ms after termination of the previous exhalation. If the patient becomes apneic, the ventilator will revert to a control mode at the frequency set on the normal rate control.

In the SIMV mode, gas flow increases as necessary to meet the patient's spontaneous ventilatory demand. When the appropriate time interval has elapsed, the IMV/SIMV breath is delivered in response to (and synchronous with) the spontaneous effort.

The mechanical tidal volume is adjusted with control (B), and the rate control (C) has a normal range of 5 to 60 breaths per minute; however, a "divisible by 10" toggle switch extends the range from 0.5 to 60 breaths per minute. The lower rates are used for SIMV. The pressure knob (D) adjusts the pressure limit (maximum safety pressure). In addition, the ventilator may be placed on standby by depressing button (E). In this mode, the patient may breathe spontaneously. A standby light remains illuminated until 60 seconds have elapsed, at which time an audible alarm sounds.

Single or multiple sigh breaths (F) may be programmed. A separate sigh volume (G) is selected from 150 to 3000 mL and may be delivered from 2 to 60 times per hour (H). The sigh breath has a separate pressure limit (I) identical in operation to the normal pressure limit control.

A minute volume accumulator (K) measures both ventilator and spontaneous breaths and displays them as exhaled minute volume. After 1 minute of display the indicator automatically reverts back to tidal volume display. The inspiratory flow pattern is altered by waveform control (L), which modifies the normal square wave by descending or tapering the flow as inspiration continues and as pressure in the circuit increases. A descending inspiratory flow from 120 down to 40 L/min is available.

The assist knob (M) adjusts the degree of patient effort required to trigger the machine to the inspiratory phase. A ratio limit control (N) provides an audible alarm if the I/E ratio is 1:1.

The oxygen percentage control (O) is adjustable from 21% to 100%. The inspiratory flow control (P) is adjustable from 20 to 120 L/min. Spontaneous ventilation is not affected by this control. An inspiratory pause control (Q) delays the opening of the exhalation valve from 0 to 2 seconds. This delay is part of the inspiratory time and, therefore, is included in the I/E calculation. If this control is used to generate inverse I/E ratios, the I/E ratio limit control must be turned off.

A nebulizer control (R) activates the medication nebulizer. The PEEP control (S) adjusts PEEP and is self-adjusting to compensate for minor leaks within the system.

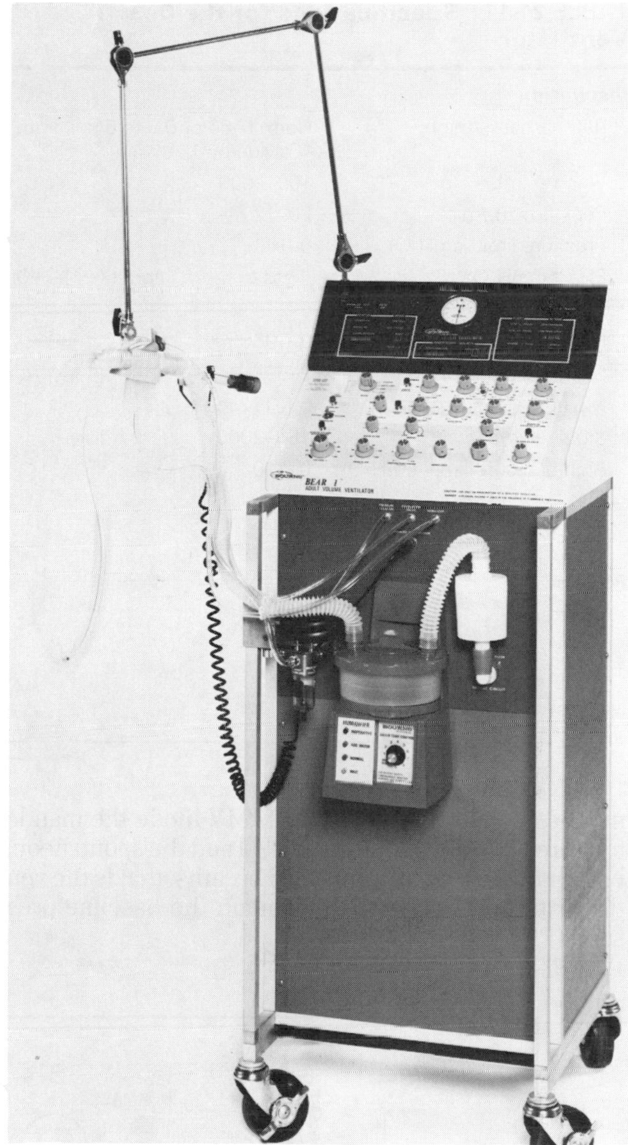

FIGURE 21-51. Bear 1 adult volume ventilator. (Courtesy of Bear Medical Systems, Riverside, CA)

☐ CONTROL VARIABLES

The Bear 1 controls inspiratory flow. In the CPAP mode it allows spontaneous breathing and controls the pressure. In the circuit and in the control and A/C

TABLE 21-11 **Specifications for the Bear 1 Ventilator**

Inspiration	
Rate (breaths/min)	Norm 5–60 or 0.5 to 6/min with divide-by-10 switch
Volume (mL)	100–2000
Peak flow (L/min)	20–120
Pressure limit (cmH_2O)	0–100
Effort (cmH_2O)	"less or more" about (−1)–(−6)
Hold (sec)	0–2
Demand flow (L/min)	0–100
Sigh rate (breaths/hour)	2–60
Multiple sighs	off, 1, 2, or 3
Sigh volume (mL)	150–3000
Sigh pressure limit (cmH_2O)	0–100
Expiration	
PEEP/CPAP (cmH_2O)	0–30
Modes	
Control	
Assist/control	
SIMV	
CPAP	

modes, it controls flow. In the SIMV mode the mandatory breaths are volume-controlled and the spontaneous breaths are pressure-controlled breaths, that is the ventilator targets pressure to maintain the baseline pressure (PEEP/CPAP).

Inspiratory Waveform

The inspiratory flow is continuously adjustable with the peak flow control (P, Fig. 21-52). Either the rectangular or descending ramp waveform can be selected (L, Fig. 21-52). In the rectangular setting the driving pressure for the peak flow valve (see below, Output Control Valve) is at 3.2 psig or approximately 225 cmH_2O). This is enough pressure to maintain a fairly constant inspiratory gas flow even with high workloads. When the descending ramp is selected, it actually provides a truncated exponential decay waveform. With this setting the driving pressure is 1.8 psig (about 125 cmH_2O). This low driving pressure is more affected by workloads in the clinical setting. When patient lung characteristics worsen, for example, increased airway resistance and reduced compliance, the flow rate decays more rapidly as tidal volume accumulates in the lungs. In this respect, a drop in peak flow rate as much as 50% can result.

□ PHASE VARIABLES

Triggering

Time-triggering occurs when no patient effort is sensed and is based on the ventilatory frequency set on the control panel. Time-triggering is also in effect when the sigh rate and multiple sigh dials are used. The sigh rate works in the control and A/C modes. Inspiration is pressure-triggered when the patient's inspiratory effort is sufficient to be detected by the ventilator. Trigger sensitivity is determined by the "assist" knob. For spontaneous breaths in the SIMV and CPAP modes, inspi-

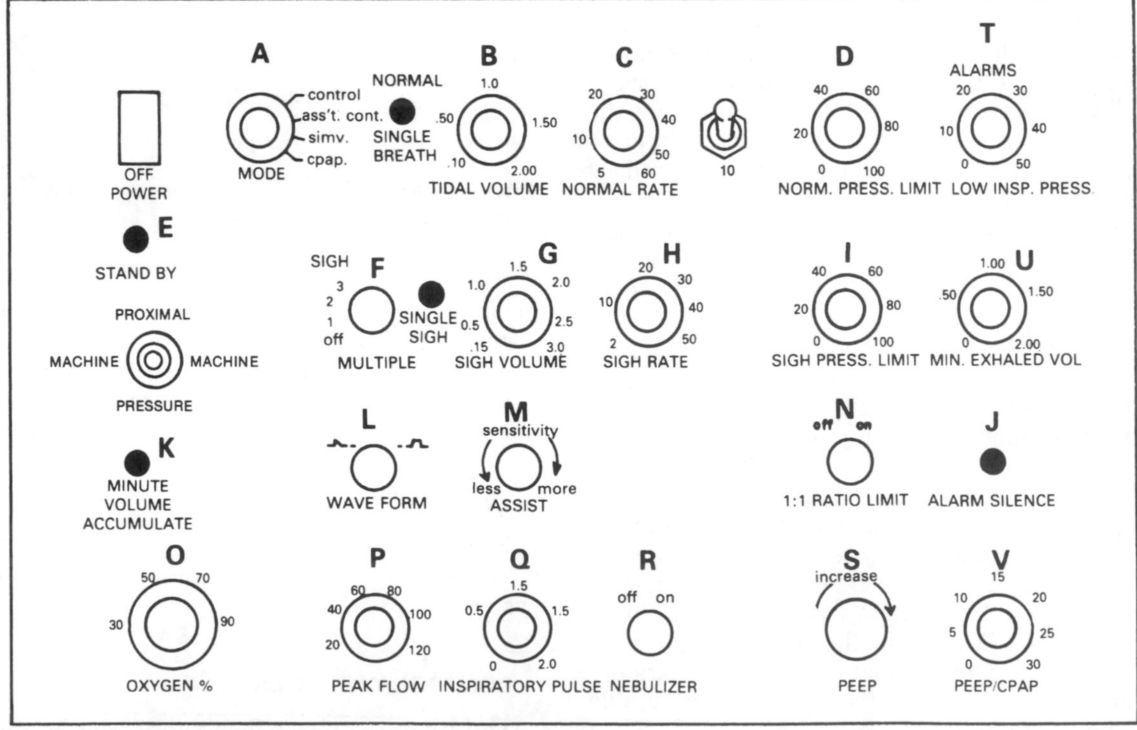

FIGURE 21-52. Control panel of the Bear 1 ventilator. See text for explanation.

ration is pressure-triggered when the patient receives all inspiratory flow from the demand valve. When the patient inspires fast enough from the demand valve to cross the triggering threshold (see Control Circuit below), then inspiration begins. Both normal and sigh breaths can also be manually triggered.

Limiting

Inspiration is flow-limited for volume-targeted breaths. It is pressure-limited during spontaneous breaths in both the SIMV and CPAP modes. A demand valve attempts to maintain the set PEEP level in these modes and, thus, controls inspiratory pressure. It may deliver a flow up to 100 L/min. In the inspiratory phase when inspiratory pause is selected higher than zero, inspiratory is volume-limited.

Cycling

Inspiration in volume-targeted modes is volume-cycled. The Bear 1 measures volume during inspiration by integrating the signal from the inspiratory flow transducer at the main flow control valve outlet. It can also be time-cycled in volume-targeted breaths when the inspiratory pause time has a value greater than zero.

Inspiration is pressure-cycled when the pressure reaches the value set on the normal pressure limit for normal volume breaths, or when it reaches the sigh pressure limit during a sigh breath. Spontaneous breaths in the SIMV and CPAP modes are also pressure-cycled, ending the flow from the demand valve.

Baseline Pressure

Baseline pressure is adjustable from 0 to 30 cmH_2O using the PEEP/CPAP control.

□ CONTROL SUBSYSTEMS

Control Circuit and Drive Mechanism

The ventilator is powered by 30- to 100-psig sources of air and oxygen. If a malfunction causes reduced pressure in either of the gases, a crossover solenoid (A) is activated so that the remaining functional gas continues ventilator operation (Fig. 21-53). If air pressure fails, a switchover valve (B) activates a compressor (C). This compressor also functions if the high-pressure line is not connected to an external source of compressed air. Both air and oxygen pressure are matched in the system and delivered to a gas-blending device (D). This mixed gas then passes to a solenoid valve (E), which functions as the main on/off switch. Some gas also bypasses the main solenoid valve to perform other functions described in "Output Control Valve" below.

An adjustable safety pop-off valve (I) limits the peak inspiratory pressure, and a subambient-pressure valve (J) allows the patient to inspire room air if a ventilator malfunction occurs. Humidification is provided by a cascade heated humidifier (K).

A secondary system bypasses the main patient supply flow. This system provides gas for breathing in the synchronized IMV (SIMV) mode of ventilation and in the CPAP mode. A patient-sensing pressure line (L) controls gas flow from a demand valve (M). The demand valve supplies gas flow to the patient distal to the main solenoid and waveform control valves.

For spontaneous breaths in the SIMV and CPAP modes, if the patient draws enough air from the circuit to decrease the pressure in the valve to a preset (unchangable) value of 1 cmH_2O below baseline pressure, the valve opens and flow goes to the patient. Once the pressure rises above the threshold, the flow stops.

For volume-targeted breaths in SIMV and A/C modes, the demand valve also plays a role. There is a flow transducer that measures the rate of change of inspiratory flow from the demand valve. If this transducer, the assist sensor (N), detects a large enough rate of change in the gas flow as the patient begins to breathe in, it provides a signal to the main solenoid valve. This triggers the delivery of a preset tidal volume or sigh volume, which is delivered through the main solenoid and flow modification valves. The magnitude of the flow change needed to trigger a volume-targeted inspiration is adjusted by the assist knob. The assist transducer is really more sensitive to the "suddenness" of a gas flow

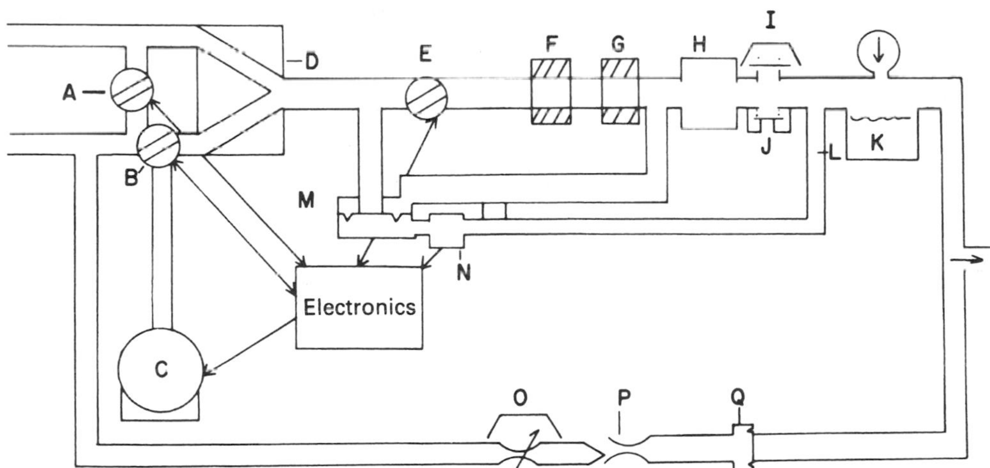

FIGURE 21-53. Schematic diagram of the Bear 1 ventilator. See text for explanation.

change than it is to actual flow or pressure change. If the patient breathes in very slowly in either SIMV or A/C, it is possible for the breath not to be detected, and the volume-targeted breath may not be triggered.

The assist transducer (assist sensor) is also used for monitoring. When flow from the demand valve is sensed by the transducer, it sends this information to (1) the rate display and counting circuit, (2) the expiratory volume display and counting circuit, (3) the apnea timing circuit, and (4) the "spontaneous" indicator display. For this reason, it is important that this sensor be adjusted properly even for spontaneous breathing modes like CPAP. For example, if the assist knob is set incorrectly during CPAP, the patient can still breathe from the demand valve, but the assist sensor may not detect the breaths. In this case, the exhaled volume would be zero or whatever the last counted breath was, and the rate would be zero. The apnea alarm would eventually activate. As another example, if, in the SIMV mode, the assist knob was not correctly set and ignored all spontaneous efforts, the ventilator would deliver time-triggered breaths (IMV) rather than pressure (patient)-triggered breaths (SIMV). All spontaneous efforts would be ignored by the assist sensor.

When the control mode is used, a "lockout solenoid" prevents gas from entering the demand valve. This, in effect, inactivates it.

PEEP is adjusted by a PEEP control valve (O) and a Venturi (P), which pressurizes the exhalation valve (Q) during the expiratory phase.

Output Control Valve

There are several output control valves that work together. Their function determines the shape of the inspiratory flow waveform.

As gas flows from the main solenoid valve, it is adjusted through a set of two controls. The first (F) modifies the waveform delivered to the patient; the second (G) determines the peak flow rate.

A vortex flow sensor (H) measures the volume of gas delivered to the patient. If the main solenoid-controlled time interval is not adequate to provide the preselected tidal volume, the flow transducer senses the discrepancy and signals the solenoid to remain open for an extended period until the volume has been delivered.

□ MODES OF OPERATION

Control

In the control mode, inspiration is volume controlled, and time-triggered based on the rate set on the "normal rate" knob. It is normally flow-limited, but volume-limited if the inspiratory pause control is used. With normal operation, it is volume-cycled but can be pressure-cycled if the pressure reaches the pressure limit setting.

Assist/Control

In A/C, the operation is similar to the control mode except that inspiration can also be pressure-triggered based on the value set on the assist knob and the patient's spontaneous inspiratory efforts.

SIMV

In the SIMV mode for mandatory breaths, the breaths are volume controlled and pressure-triggered (based on "assist" sensitivity and patient's spontaneous inspiratory effort) or time-triggered (based on the respiratory frequency set on the "normal rate" control). Mandatory breaths are normally volume-cycled. Spontaneous breaths that occur between mandatory breaths are pressure-controlled (flow varies to maintain baseline pressure, ie, set PEEP value), pressure-triggered, and pressure-cycled.

During SIMV, the SIMV rate is determined by the normal rate control. The synchronous period is equal to the rate control value divided into 60. For example, if the rate is set at 5 breaths/min, the synchronous period is 12 seconds (60 sec/5 breaths). A mandatory breath is triggered when a spontaneous effort is detected during each ventilatory period. Between the mandatory breath and the next rate signal, the patient can spontaneously breathe from the demand valve. If a breath is not detected in the next signal period, a mandatory breath will be delivered at the beginning of the next period. The ventilator continues to deliver breaths according to the rate setting until a spontaneous breath is detected. If no machine or mandatory breath is detected for a period of 20 seconds, an audiovisual alarm is activated.

CPAP

In the CPAP mode, spontaneous breaths are pressure controlled, pressure-triggered, and pressure-cycled.

□ OUTPUT DISPLAYS (MONITORS) AND ALARMS

The operating panel of the Bear 1 includes digital displays for exhaled tidal volume or minute volume, respiratory rate, and I:E ratio. Ventilatory pressures are displayed on an analog meter. A proximal airway pressure manometer is calibrated between 0 and 100 cmH_20. Later models have a -10 to 100 cmH_2O display that shows proximal airway pressure or system (machine) pressure depending on the position of this toggle switch.

Several light-emitting diodes (LEDs) provide information about ventilator status and alarm conditions. Ventilator status indicators include the following: power-on, standby, alarm silence, nebulizer-on, control mode, A/C mode, SIMV mode, CPAP mode, rate "divisible by 10," spontaneous breath, control breath, sigh breath, minute volume mode, exhaled volume liters, and rate of breaths per minute (breaths/min).

Power-on: This light indicates that the ventilator is plugged into an operative AC outlet and the power switch is on.

Standby: When this light indicator is flashing it means that the standby button has been depressed. The ventilator is put in the CPAP mode. All controls and alarms, with the exception of the "Vent. Inoperative" and the "Low Air Press." alarms are disabled. An audible alarm activates after 60 seconds. The ventilator can be returned to normal function by pushing the button again.

Alarm Silence: When illuminated, this indicates that this button has been depressed. All alarms, with the exception of the "Vent. Inoperative," the "Low Air Press," and "Standby" after 60 seconds has elapsed, are canceled for 60 seconds.

Nebulizer-on: Indicates visually that the nebulizer is on during mandatory inspirations.

Control Mode, A/C Mode, SIMV Mode, CPAP Mode: Visual indicators show which mode has been selected.

Rate "Divisible by 10": Light shows that the "normal rate" toggle switch has been set to the divide by 10 position. The number of mandatory breaths as indicated by the "normal rate" control is divided by 10.

Spontaneous Breath, Control Breath, Sigh Breath: These lights blink to indicate the type of breath delivered.

Minute Volume Mode: A flashing light shows the exhaled volume is being accumulated for 1 minute. A continuous light indicates that the minute volume is being displayed.

Exhaled Volume Liters: This digital display shows the breath-to-breath exhaled volume or minute volume.

Rate BPM: A digital display provides the breathing rate per minute based on the average of the last 20 seconds. The display is updated every second.

Input Power Alarms

The input power alarms include audible and visible alarms that are activated when either electric or pneumatic (low oxygen pressure, low air pressure) power supplies are interrupted.

When the oxygen inlet pressure is less than 30 psi with the oxygen % selector above 21%, the low O_2 pressure alarm will activate. When the air supply pressure is below 9.5 psi, the low air pressure alarm will activate.

A "Vent. Inoperative" alarm (visual and audible) will activate to indicate a total gas failure, AC power failure, or an electronic malfunction in the volume measuring circuit. It will also activate following a patient disconnect when PEEP/CPAP is used in the A/C, SIMV, and CPAP modes for models with an "A" following the serial number or serial numbers above 1100.

Control Variable Alarms

The alarm system has several controls and indicators on the main control panel (see Fig. 21-52). These include an indicator light for the normal pressure limit (0 to 100 cmH_2O). An audible and visual alarm sounds when the set value is exceeded. There is also a low inspiratory pressure alarm (T), which sets the lower limit of inspiratory positive pressure that must be generated by ventilator cycling (off to 50 cmH_2O). The minimum exhaled volume control (U) is adjustable from 150 to 2000 mL (less than 150 mL is off). It activates an audible and visual alarm when the exhaled volume that is monitored by the exhaled flow sensor does not exceed the control setting for three consecutive breaths, either mandatory or spontaneous.

A visual and audible alarm is activated when the PEEP or CPAP level falls below the control setting (off to 30 cmH_2O), and an apnea alarm is activated if neither spontaneous or mandatory breaths are detected for a period of 20 seconds.

Control Circuit Alarms

Control circuit alarms for the Bear 1 include the I:E ratio display. When the I:E ratio is off, this allows inverse I:E ratios. It will give a visual alert only, and the display panel light will show 1:1 ratio off. When the I:E ratio is on, it will give a visual and audible alarm if the I:E ratio is greater than 1:1 and it will terminate inspiration of mandatory breaths in the control and A/C modes. The display panel will give a digital display of the breath-to-breath ventilator inspiratory time to expiratory time ratio. A flashing display indicates that the expiratory portion of the ratio exceeds the inspiratory portion by at least 10.

Alarm Silence/Reset

All alarms can be silenced for 60 seconds by depressing the alarm silence button (J). It can be manually reset or it resets itself at the end of the 60 seconds.

□ TROUBLESHOOTING

Troubleshooting is simplified by the 28 lights and monitors that indicate problems as they develop.

Bear 2/3 Adult Volume Ventilator

□ CLASSIFICATION

The Bear 2/3 (Table 21-12) (Fig. 21-54) adult volume ventilator is electrically and pneumatically powered, electronically operated, and may function as a pressure or volume controller. Initiation of mechanical inspiration is either time- or pressure-triggered. Mechanical inspiration is terminated when a preselected tidal volume has been delivered (volume-cycled) and may be extended by a time-cycled plateau (time-cycled). Inspiration is also pressure-cycled if the pressure limit is reached. Inspiration is volume- or flow-limited. End-expiratory pressure may be applied during mechanical (PEEP) or spontaneous (CPAP) breathing. Pressure-supported ventilation is standard on the Bear 3; however, any Bear 2 can be updated to provide this modality.

TABLE 21-12 **Classification of the Bear 2/3 Adult Volume Ventilator**

Power Source for Pneumatic Circuit	Pressurized Gases (30–100 psig)
Power source for control circuit	Electricity (115 volts AC at 60 Hz)
Control mechanism	Pressure, volume/flow
Triggering	Time, pressure, manual
Limiting	Volume, flow
Cycling	Time, pressure

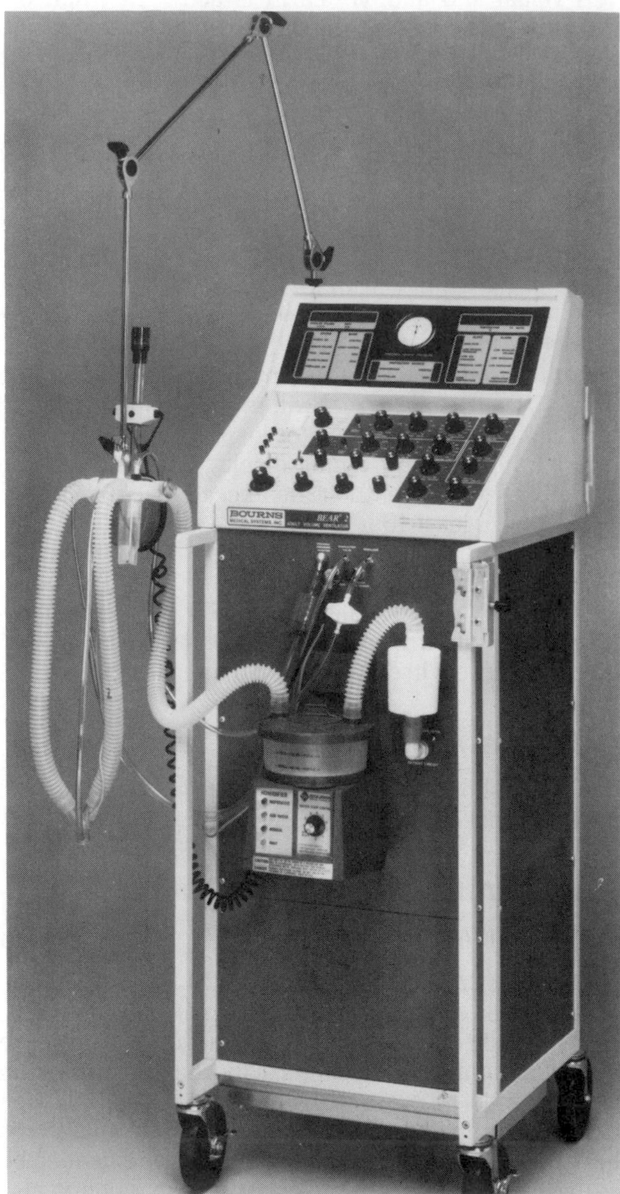

FIGURE 21-54. Bear 2/3 adult volume ventilator. (Courtesy of Bear Medical Systems, Riverside, CA)

□ SPECIFICATIONS

Table 21-13 lists specifications for the Bear 2/3.

□ OPERATION

The ventilator is connected to a 30- to 100-psi oxygen source and a 115-volt, 60-Hz electrical power source. If a 30- to 100-psi air source is available, the ventilator compressor system is bypassed. The type of ventilation desired is programmed by the mode selector knob (A) (Fig. 21-55). In the A/C mode, a built-in safety feature does not allow a patient to initiate a breath for at least 350 ms after termination of the previous exhalation. If the patient becomes apneic, the ventilator reverts to a control mode at the frequency set on the normal rate control (C).

TABLE 21-13 **Specifications for the Bear 2/3 Ventilator**

Inspiration	
Rate (breaths/min)	Norm 0.5–60
Volume (mL)	100–2000
Peak flow (L/min)	10–120
Pressure limit (cmH_2O)	0–120
Effort (cmH_2O)	"less or more" about (−1 at 2 L/min flow)
Hold (sec)	0–2
Demand flow (L/min)	0–120
Sigh rate (breaths/hour)	2–60
Multiple sighs	off, 1, 2, or 3
Sigh volume (mL)	150–3000
Sigh pressure limit (cmH_2O)	0–120
Expiration	
PEEP/CPAP (cmH_2O)	0–50
Modes	
Control	
Assist/control	
SIMV	
CPAP	
PSV (Bear 3)	

In the SIMV and CPAP mode the patient breathes spontaneously, setting his or her rate, V_T, and peak flow up to 120 L/min. When a mandatory breath is delivered, all machine settings are met for V_T, peak flow, and so forth. The SIMV is triggered by activating the A/C sensitivity after the designated spontaneous breathing period has elapsed. Should the patient not trigger a breath, one cycling period elapses, then the ventilator switches to control mode. The detection delay (U) may alarm during this period if the expiratory time exceeds the delay time and the patient is apneic.

The mechanical V_T is adjusted with control (B) mandatory (normal) rate with control (C), and the high pressure limit with control (D).

Single or multiple sigh breaths (E) may be programmed. A separate sigh volume is selected (F) from 150 to 3000 mL and may be delivered 2 to 60 times per hour (G). The sigh breath has a separate pressure limit (H) from zero to 120 cmH_2O.

The pressure can be measured from either a machine or a proximal tap. The pressure-sensing selector (I) can be directed to sample either source. There will be some difference between the two pressures because of system and humidifier resistance. A constant 100 mL/min bleed-in in the proximal pressure measuring line prevents humidity buildup. A piece of ¼-inch tubing should be used to connect the proximal tap to the proximal airway connector near the patient. The waveform selector (J) may be used to deliver a square wave flow pattern in which the flow will decrease only 15% as the V_T is attained or a tapered flow pattern that reduces the flow by 50%. The flow taper cannot be used when the peak flow is set below 20 L/min because the minimum flow is 10 L/min.

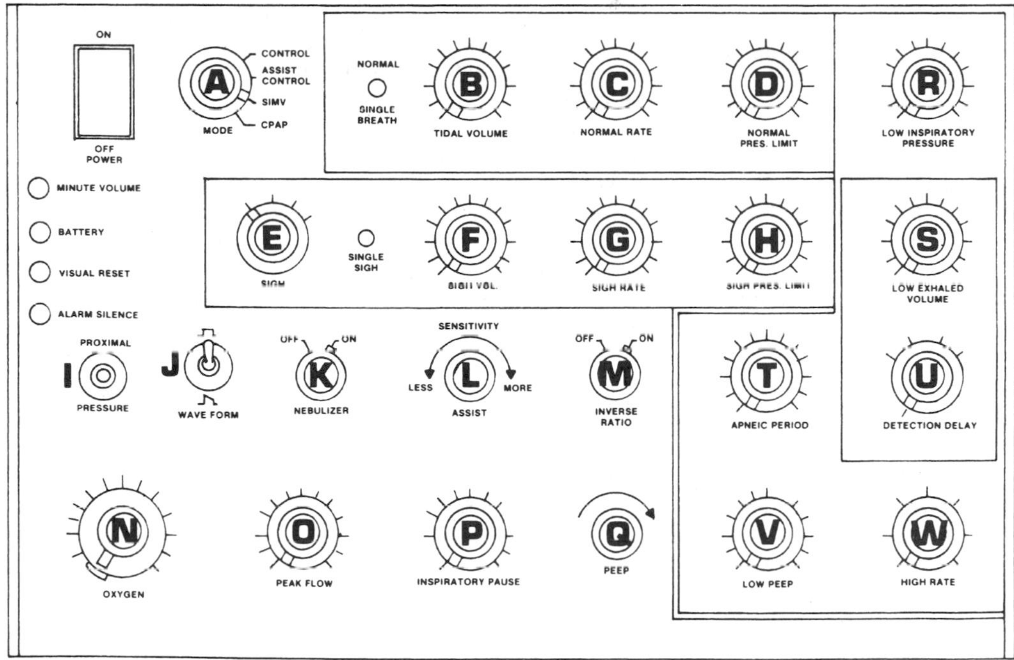

FIGURE 21-55. Control panel of the Bear 2/3 ventilator (see text). (Courtesy of Bear Medical Systems, Riverside, CA)

The nebulizer control (K) diverts a portion of the tidal volume through the nebulizer so that oxygen concentration and V_T are not altered during medication delivery. This nebulizer cannot be used if the peak flow (O) is set below 30 L/min. The assist control (L) adjusts the degree of patient effort required to trigger the machine. Turning the control toward "more" makes the system more sensitive both in the A/C mode and the spontaneous-breathing mode. The volume of gas added to the system by the patient's inspiratory efforts will be added to the V_T as measured by the V_T flow tube. A ratio-limit control (M) provides an audible alarm if the I/E ratio exceeds 1:1 and inspiration is terminated. If this control is turned to OFF, inverse I/E ratios may be attained. This control is inactivated in the A/C and SIMV modes.

The oxygen percentage control (N) is adjustable from 21% to 100%. The peak flow control (O) does not affect the spontaneous inspiratory flow but will affect the flow taper if it is set below 30 L/min. An inspiratory pause control (P) delays the opening of the exhalation valve from zero to 2 seconds once the V_T has been delivered. Only in this configuration is the ventilator considered a time-cycled ventilator. This pause period is included in the inspiratory time and, therefore, should be considered when setting appropriate I/E ratios. The PEEP control (Q) can maintain its calibrated pressure with leaks up to 25 L/min for 7 to 9 seconds. In the CPAP mode, the patient breathes from the demand valve with flows up to 100 L/min.

☐ CONTROL VARIABLES

The Bear 2/3 controls inspiratory pressure or flow. In the CPAP mode, it controls pressure, and in the control or A/C modes, it controls volume/flow. In the SIMV mode, spontaneous breaths are pressure controlled and mandatory breaths are volume controlled. In pressure support, ventilation is pressure controlled.

Inspiratory Waveforms

As with the Bear 1, the Bear 2/3 offers a rectangular or a descending ramp waveform (control J). When the rectangular waveform is selected, the waveform regulator samples the circuit pressure. As the pressure in the patient circuit increases, the regulator opens to maintain a constant pattern of flow by providing a higher driving pressure. The rectangular waveform gives the shortest inspiratory time for a given tidal volume.

When the descending ramp (a truncated exponential decay waveform) is selected, the waveform regulator changes its function and is shut off from the circuit pressure. The driving pressure is not much higher than the airway pressures commonly seen in the clinical setting. As the pressure in the patient circuit builds, the flow of gas decreases. At 120 cmH_2O of back pressure, the peak flow rate is reduced by about 50%, but the flow of gas will not drop below 10 L/min.

If the peak flow is set at 20 L/min, the waveform control system is bypassed and a rectangular waveform is provided.

☐ PHASE VARIABLES

The phase variables and baseline pressure are the same for the Bear 2/3 as they are for the Bear 1. With all Bear 3 ventilators, PSV is also provided. In pressure support, inspiration is pressure-triggered, pressure-limited, and normally flow-cycled. Inspiration ends when the flow to the patient circuit drops to 25% of the initial peak flow. PSV breaths can also be provided with SIMV between mandatory breaths.

□ CONTROL SUBSYSTEMS

Control Circuit and Drive Mechanism

The ventilator is powered by 30- to 100-psi sources of air and oxygen. If a malfunction causes reduced pressure of either gas, a crossover solenoid (A) is activated so that the remaining functional gas continues ventilator operation (Fig. 21-56). If external air pressure fails or if internal air pressure falls below 9.5 psi, a switchover valve (B) activates a compressor (C). This compressor also functions if the high-pressure line is not connected to an external source of compressed air. Both air and oxygen pressures are reduced to about 11 psi and mixed at calibrated rates as selected by the blender control (D). The mixed gas passes to a solenoid valve (E), which functions as the main on/off switch. Some gas also bypasses the main solenoid valve to perform other functions, as controlled by the bypass solenoid (R).

A constant or decelerating (tapered) inspiratory flow pattern waveform may be selected by a toggle switch (F), which regulates driving pressure to the peak flow control (G). In the square-wave position, driving pressure is 3.0 psi, and the ventilator outflow is equal to the peak flow adjustment. When flow taper is activated, driving pressure is reduced to 1.8 psi, and inspiratory flow decelerates as circuit pressure increases. Flow will decelerate at 50% of the peak flow at 120 cmH_2O back-pressure, to a minimum of 10 L/min.

When peak flow control (G) meters gas flow to the patient with the flow taper control set for square wave, there will be only a 15% drop in pressure shortly before termination of inspiration. Once the appropriate volume has passed through the flow transducer (H), a signal is sent through the electronic system to the main solenoid valve (E) to terminate inspiration, unless the pressure-limit control (I) has already cycled the ventilator to exhalation. Should an inspiratory pause be desired, the patient exhalation valve (Q) will remain closed for the extended pause period once the tidal volume has been delivered. It is during this phase that the ventilator is considered time-cycled. If all pneumatic and electronic systems fail, there is an anti-asphyxiation valve (J) through which a spontaneously breathing patient may inspire. Humidification is provided by an adjustable heated humidifier (K).

A secondary system bypasses the main patient supply flow. This system supplies gas for spontaneous breathing in synchronized IMV (SIMV) and CPAP modes. A sensing line (L) controls gas from the demand valve (M), which is activated in the A/C, SIMV, and CPAP modes. The demand valve system provides gas flow up to 120 L/min distal to the main solenoid valve (E) and waveform toggle (F). If the assist sensor (N) is activated, the SIMV is synchronized with the patient's inspiratory efforts, and the tidal volume is delivered through the main solenoid (E) and flow waveform toggle (F). PEEP is adjusted by the PEEP control valve (O) and a venturi (P), which pressurizes the exhalation valve (Q) during the expiratory phase. The compensation chamber (S) adjusts pressure on the exhalation valve during peak expiratory flow periods.

□ MODES OF OPERATION

Control

In the control mode, inspiration is volume controlled, and time-triggered based on the rate set on the normal rate knob. It is normally flow-limited, but volume-limited if the inspiratory pause control is used. With normal operation it is volume-cycled, but can be pressure-cycled if the pressure reaches the pressure limit setting.

Assist/Control

In A/C, the operation is similar to the control mode except that inspiration can also be pressure-triggered based on the value set on the assist knob and the patient's spontaneous inspiratory efforts.

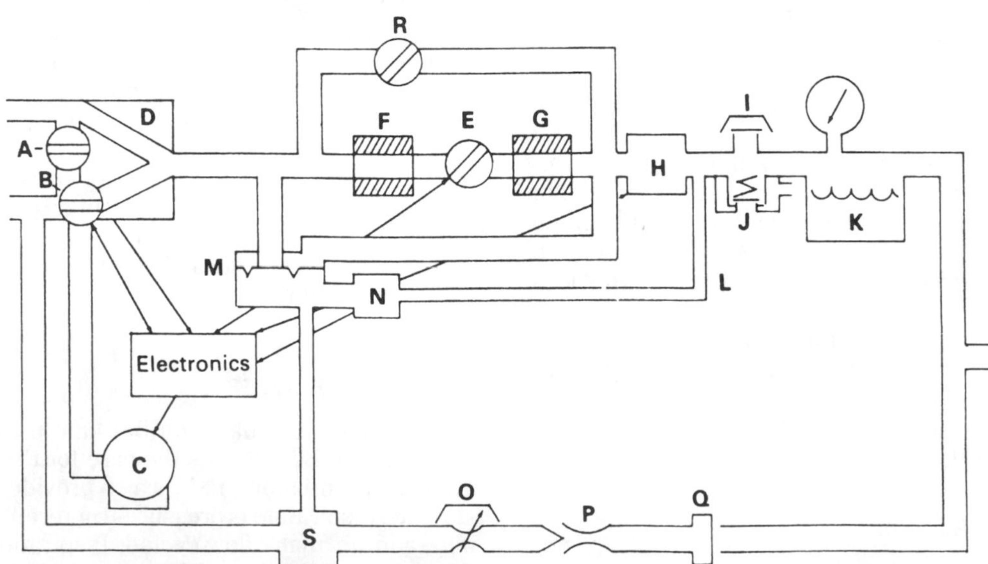

FIGURE 21-56. Schematic diagram of the Bear 2/3 ventilator. See text for explanation.

SIMV

In the SIMV mode for mandatory breaths, the breaths are volume controlled and flow-triggered (based on "assist" sensitivity and the patient's spontaneous inspiratory effort) or time-triggered (based on the respiratory frequency set on the normal rate control). Mandatory breaths are normally volume-cycled. Spontaneous breaths that occur between mandatory breaths are pressure controlled (flow varies to maintain baseline pressure, ie, set PEEP value), pressure-triggered, and pressure-cycled. When SIMV is used with PSV spontaneous breaths are normally flow-cycled rather than pressure-cycled.

During SIMV, the SIMV rate is determined by the normal rate control. The synchronous period is equal to the rate control value divided into 60. For example, if the rate is set at 5 breaths/min, the synchronous period is 12 seconds (60 sec/5). A mandatory breath is flow-triggered when a spontaneous effort is detected during each ventilatory period. Between the mandatory breath and the next rate signal, the patient can spontaneously breathe from the demand valve or receive pressure support breaths. If a breath is not detected in the next signal period, a mandatory breath will be delivered at the beginning of the next period. The ventilator continues to deliver breaths according to the rate setting until a spontaneous breath is detected. If no machine or mandatory breath is detected for a period of 20 seconds, an audiovisual alarm is activated.

Pressure Support Ventilation

PSV provides spontaneous breaths that are pressure controlled, pressure-triggered, and flow-cycled. It can be used alone or with SIMV or CPAP ventilation. All Bear 3 ventilators come with PSV and it may be added as an option to Bear 2 ventilators. It is adjustable up to 70 cmH_2O.

CPAP

In the CPAP mode, spontaneous breaths are pressure-controlled, pressure-triggered, and pressure-cycled.

□ OUTPUT DISPLAYS (MONITORS) AND ALARMS

The operating panel of the Bear 2/3 includes digital displays for exhaled tidal volume or minute volume, respiratory rate, temperature, and I:E ratio. Ventilator pressures are displayed on an analog meter. The proximal airway or machine pressure manometer is calibrated between −10 and 120 cmH_20. The meter shows proximal airway pressure or system (machine) pressure depending on the position of this toggle switch.

Several LEDs provide information about ventilator status and alarm conditions. Ventilator status indicators include the following: power-on, minute volume, tidal volume, alarm silence, and nebulizer-on; modes indicators include control mode, A/C mode, SIMV mode, CPAP mode, and PSV (Bear 3) spontaneous breath, control breath, sigh breath, minute volume mode, exhaled volume, and rate.

Power-on: This light indicates that the ventilator is plugged into an operative AC outlet and the power switch is on.

Minute Volume Mode: A flashing light shows the exhaled volume is being accumulated for 1 minute. A continuous light indicates that the minute volume is being displayed.

Tidal Volume: The exhaled volume displays the breath-to-breath tidal volume.

Alarm Silence: When illuminated, this indicates that this button has been depressed. All alarms, with the exception of the "Vent. Inoperative," the "Low Air Press.," and "Stand-by" after 60 seconds has elapsed, are canceled for 60 seconds.

Nebulizer-on: Indicates visually that the nebulizer is on during mandatory inspirations.

Control Mode, A/C Mode, SIMV Mode, CPAP Mode, and PSV Mode: Visual indicators show which mode has been selected. PSV can be on in the SIMV or CPAP modes. If PSV is activated in the control or A/C mode, the light will flash and no PSV breaths will be delivered. Spontaneous Breath, Control Breath, Assisted Breath, and Sigh Breath: Lights blink to indicate the type of breath delivered.

Exhaled Volume Liters: This digital display shows the breath-to-breath exhaled volume or minute volume.

Rate BPM: A digital display provides the breathing rate per minute based on the average of the last 20 seconds. The display is updated every second.

Temperature: This is a digital display of temperature at the patient wye connector.

I:E Ratio: This display of I:E ratio is on a breath-to-breath basis in control and A/C. A flashing display indicates that the expiratory portion of the ratio exceeds the inspiratory portion by at least 10 to 1.

Input Power Alarms

The input power alarms include audible and visible alarms that are activated when either electric or pneumatic (low oxygen pressure, low air pressure) power supplies are interrupted.

When the oxygen inlet pressure is less than 30 psi with the oxygen % selector above 21%, the low O_2 pressure alarm will activate. When the air supply pressure is below 9.5 psi, the low air pressure alarm will activate.

A "Vent. Inoperative" alarm (visual and audible) will activate to indicate a total gas failure, AC power failure, or an electronic malfunction.

Control Variable Alarms

The alert and alarm systems have eight adjustable controls on the face of the ventilator and multiple displays on the monitoring console (see Fig. 21-55). Maximum safety pressure limits are available for both normal mandatory breaths (D) and sigh breaths (H). A low inspiratory pressure alarm (R) sets the lower limit of the inspiratory positive pressure that must be generated by ventilator cycling (3 to 75 cm H_2O) The minimum exhaled volume control (S) is adjustable from 100 to 2000 mL (less than 100 mL is off). If the exhaled volume is less than the volume indicated on the detection delay control (U), the alarm is activated. The detection delay is adjustable from 2 to 5 breaths. When the selected number of breaths are of an undesirably low volume (set on low exhaled volume control), a visual and audible alarm is activated. Once the alarm has been activated, it can be deactivated within one breath with the appropriate tidal volume.

The apneic period alarm (T) is adjustable from 2 to 20 seconds; if the apneic interval exceeds the alarm setting, the alarm will activate. When using "Sigh Breaths," the apneic period should be set above the sigh interval, which is twice the normal breath interval. For example if the rate is set at 15, the normal breath interval is 4 seconds (60 seconds/15 breaths). The sigh interval should be set at 8 seconds. The apnea interval should be set above this.

The low PEEP/CPAP alarm (V) is adjustable from off, or 3 to 50 cmH_2O; should the PEEP level fall below the level set, the alarm will activate. The alarm will also activate when a constant flow of 25 L/min or more occurs for about 7 to 9 seconds, because of either a patient disconnect or a major system leak.

The high-rate alarm (W), adjustable from off, or 10 to 80 breaths per minute, is activated when respirations (spontaneous and mandatory) exceed the limit set.

All alarms have corresponding lights that are activated on the display console to alert the therapist when an alarm has been activated. Besides these indicator lights, there is a "ventilator inoperative" display. The ventilator must be turned off to correct this alarm. If turning the ventilator off and then on again does not remedy the ventilator inoperative condition, the unit should be repaired by appropriately trained service personnel.

Signal outputs provided on the back of the ventilator allow for remote nurse call, 9-volt DC outlet for accessories, pressure signal output, and flow signal output.

Control Circuit Alarms

Control circuit alarms for the Bear 2/3 include the "I:E Ratio" display. When "I:E Ratio" is off, this allows inverse I:E ratios. It will give a visual alert only and the display panel light will show 1:1 ratio off. When the "I:E Ratio" is on, it will give a visual and audible alarm if the I:E ratio is greater than 1:1 and it will terminate inspiration of mandatory breaths in the control and A/C modes. The display panel will give a digital display of breath-to-breath ventilator inspiratory time to expiratory time ratio. A flashing display indicates that the expiratory portion of the ratio exceeds the inspiratory portion by at least 10:1.

If inspiratory flow is greater than 20 L/min continuously for more than 9 to 12 seconds, a flow sensor malfunction will alarm (audible and visual—ventilator inoperative). This alarm cannot be silenced.

Alarm Silence/Reset

All other alarms can be silenced for 60 seconds by depressing the alarm silence button (J). It can be manually reset or it resets itself at the end of the 60 seconds.

TABLE 21-14 **Classification of the Bear 1000 Ventilator**

Power Source for Control Circuitry	**Electricity (95–135 volts AC at 60 Hz)**
Power source for pneumatic system	Air and oxygen (30 to 80 psig high-pressure gas sources)
Control circuit	Microprocessor
Control mechanism	Pressure, flow/volume
Triggering	Pressure, time, manual
Limiting	Pressure, volume, flow, time
Cycling	Volume, time, pressure, flow

□ TROUBLESHOOTING

Troubleshooting is simplified by the 24 indicator lights and four LED displays on the monitoring console. This is coupled with a rather complete troubleshooting guide in the instruction manual, which is provided with the purchase of this ventilator.

Bear 1000 Ventilator*

□ CLASSIFICATION

The Bear 1000 Ventilator (Table 21-14) (Fig. 21-57) is an electrically powered, microprocessor controlled ventilator that is designed for pediatric or adult use. It controls pressure or flow and may be pressure-, time- or manually triggered; pressure-, volume-, or flow-limited; and pressure-, volume-, flow-, or time-cycled. The Bear 1000 provides a pressure augmentation feature that replaces volume-targeted breaths with pressure supported breaths, thus guaranteeing delivery of at least the preset tidal volume. The demand system can be set to automatically augment flow and volume delivery during a volume-targeted breath, to meet patient demand. This ventilator is available in a variety of configurations. Currently, up to 11 configurable packages are available. A graphics package is also available with the Bear 1000 Ventilator.

□ SPECIFICATIONS

Specifications of the Bear 1000 Ventilator are listed in Table 21-15.

□ INPUT VARIABLES

The Bear 1000 Ventilator requires an electrical power source of 115 volts (95 to 135 with international voltage available) 60 Hz. Compressed oxygen and air between 30 to 80 psig are required for operation of the pneumatic control circuit. The pneumatic control circuit maintains an operating pressure of 27.5 psig. The control panel of the Bear 1000 is illustrated in Figure 21-58. The control

* Thanks to Ayres Mello of Bear Medical Systems, Riverside, CA, for his technical assistance with this section.

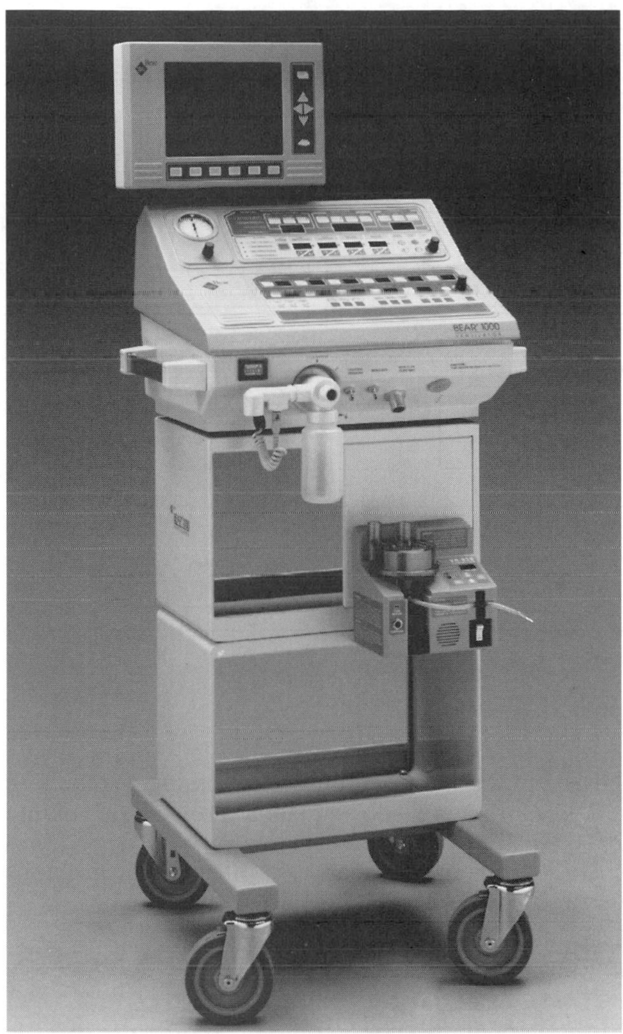

FIGURE 21-57. The Bear 1000 ventilator. (Courtesy of Bear Medical Systems, Riverside, CA)

panel is a large touch pad that provides a digital display of each variable to be adjusted, a selection key, and a single control knob for adjustment of the selected variable. Three groups of displays are available on the control panel. They are as follows: Controls, Monitors, and Alarms.

The control panel allows for operator selection of the mode of ventilation, pressure-triggering and pressure-limiting thresholds, pressure slope (waveforms), tidal volume, compliance compensation factor, inspiratory flow, inspiratory flow waveform, minimum minute volume (MMV), ventilatory frequency, inspiratory time, inspiratory pause time, and FIO_2. A separate knob located under the aneroid pressure gauge controls PEEP/CPAP.

Operation

Initial ventilator settings are obtained for all parameters by depressing the touch pad on the ventilator panel and adjusting the level of the desired parameter by rotating the set knob (see Figure 21-58). The three groups of displays on the front panel for controls, monitors, and alarms allow for efficient setting and adjustment of the ventilator. Adjustment of any parameter on the control panel is achieved by pressing the corresponding key on the touch pad, rotating the set knob to achieve the desired setting, and pressing the selected control on the touch pad again. This "sets" the parameter selected. The control panel allows for selection and adjustment of tidal volume, rate, peak flow, FIO_2, and mode of ventilation. Once the desired settings are made, activation of the "lock" prevents accidental loss of settings. Three operator-selected flow waveforms are available. They are constant, descending ramp, and sine waveforms. The sigh feature is available in any of the configurable versions of the Bear 1000 ventilator. Sighs are delivered at 1.5 times the tidal volume, every one hundredth breath. The FIO_2 is adjustable from 0.21 to 1.0 and is controlled through an internal blender.

TABLE 21-15 **Specifications for the Bear 1000 Ventilator**

Parameter	Range
Inspiration rate (breaths/min)	0, 0.5–120
Volume (mL)	10 (approximate) to 2000
Peak flow (L/min)	5–150 (mechanical) 200+ (spontaneous)
Inspiratory time (sec)	0.1–5.0
Inspiratory pause (sec)	0.0–2.0
High-pressure limit (cmH_2O)	120
Pressure augment (cmH_2O)	on/off
Effort (cmH_2O)	0.2–5
Pressure support (cmH_2O)	0–80
Expiratory hold (sec)	9 (max)
PEEP/CPAP (cmH_2O)	0–50
MMV (L/min)	0–50
Sigh	$1\frac{1}{2}$ times V_T

□ CONTROL VARIABLES

The Bear 1000 may be adjusted to control either inspiratory pressure, flow, or volume. Inspiratory pressure is controlled in CPAP, PSV, PCV, and pressure augment modes, and flow is controlled in the assist, CMV, SIMV, and MMV modes. An internal driving pressure of 18 psig is supplied to a flow control valve, which is positioned by a stepper motor, allowing rapid changes in flow when required. The microprocessor is a closed loop system that uses information from the monitors and the control panel to determine output flow from the valve. The microprocessor switches between pressure-targeted (spontaneous mode) and volume-targeted (mandatory breaths) in the SIMV (PSV) and MMV modes. When "Pressure Augment" is activated for the Assist CMV and SIMV modes, the microprocessor switches between pressure-targeted ventilation and volume-targeted ventilation within a single breath. Delivered flow is dependent on input from volume and pressure logic. At the flow control valve, two input sig-

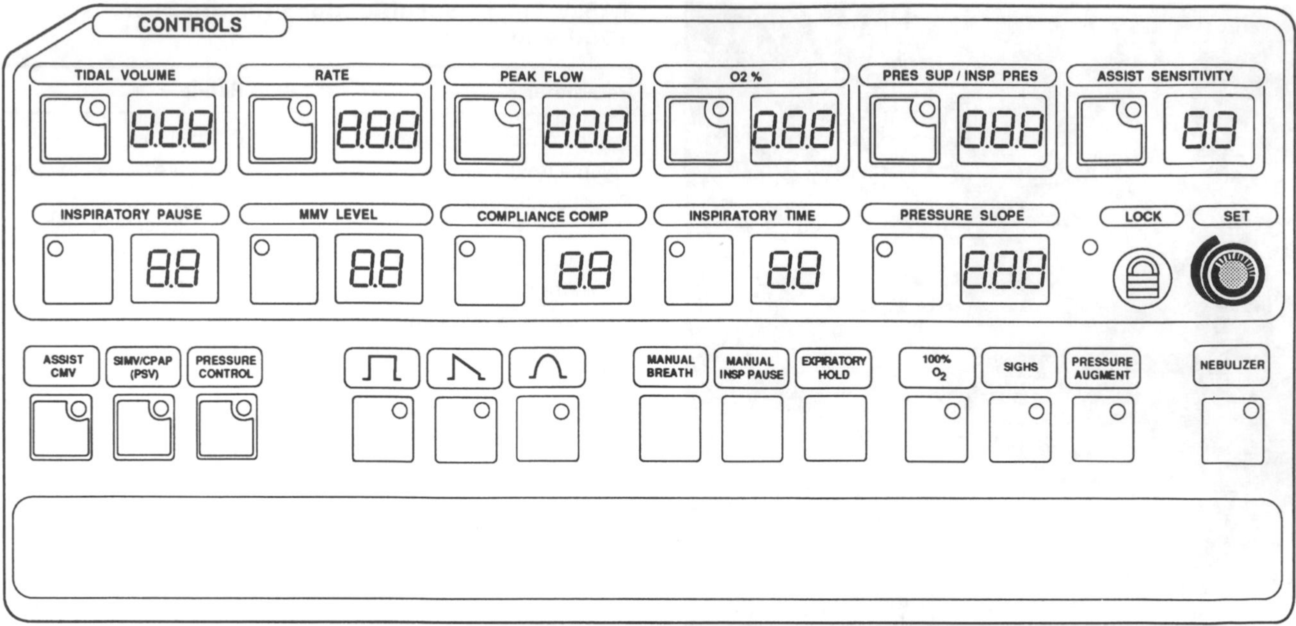

FIGURE 21-58. The control panel and monitor panel of the Bear 1000 ventilator. (Courtesy of Bear Medical Systems, Riverside, CA)

nals for flow are compared and the greater signal determines flow released from the valve.

Input from all pressure settings is processed by the pressure logic that monitors the proximal airway pressure for feedback. The same mechanism is applied by the volume logic for volume delivery and monitoring. The pressure processor is responsible for delivery of demand breaths during spontaneous and pressure support breathing. In these modes, breaths are delivered when the proximal airway pressure drops below the trigger level. In the pressure support mode, when delivered flow drops to 30% of the peak inspiratory flow, the pressure processor stops the flow.

A pressure slope control is available for all pressure breaths. This control allows for adjustments in the pressure-time relation for pressure-limited breaths. This means that the pressure can be made to increase slowly or quickly to the preset limit, as required by patient demand and patient circuit mechanics.

Another feature of the Bear 1000 is flow and volume augmentation. During mandatory, volume-targeted breaths in the CMV mode, if the patient's inspiratory demand exceeds the preset peak flow or tidal volume, volume-targeted breaths are augmented. Augmentation is operator-selected by depression of the augment key (see Fig. 21-58). This means that volume-cycling may be overridden if pressure augment is active and the patient demands more than the set tidal volume. Pressure augmentation is also available for volume-targeted breaths in the A/C and SIMV modes by setting the inspiratory pressure level and pressing the "Pressure Augment" key. Volume-targeted SIMV breaths are the only breaths in this mode that will be pressure augmented. Pressure augmentation guarantees that the set volume in pressure-controlled ventilation is delivered to the patient when the required flow continues, resulting in a pressure increase adequate to provide the volume that the patient requires.

All versions of the Bear 1000 offer a Bear graphics display for pressure and flow waveforms.

Inspiratory Waveform

The Bear 1000 provides three inspiratory flow waveforms with variable inspiratory pressure. The inspiratory flow waveform may be operator selected for constant, descending ramp or sine wave configuration. With the constant inspiratory flow waveform, gas delivery is relatively constant at the peak flow setting. When the descending ramp inspiratory flow waveform is selected, flow begins at the peak flow value and decreases in a linear fashion to 50% of peak flow by the end of inspiration. With selection of the sinusoidal flow waveform, inspiratory flow progresses from zero to peak and back to zero in a sinusoidal waveform.

□ PHASE VARIABLES

Triggering

Inspiration is ordinarily pressure-triggered, with sensitivity adjustable from 0.2 to 5 cmH_2O below baseline when a patient's inspiratory effort is detected. Sensitivity is PEEP compensated. Spontaneous inspiratory effort producing a pressure drop of as little as 0.2 cmH_2O accesses demand flow.

As a function of the ventilator frequency, or rate, inspiration can be time-triggered and is adjustable from 0 to 120 breaths/min. Time-triggering remains in effect when a sigh is activated. A sigh is delivered as a single breath each one hundredth mandatory breath. The

Bear 1000 may also be manually triggered by pressing the manual breath button. Depression of the expiratory hold key allows for manual override of time and pressure-triggering and will assist in the measurement of auto-PEEP.

The manufacturer is currently developing a flow-triggering feature.

Limiting

Pressure-Targeted Ventilation: In pressure-targeted ventilation, inspiration is pressure-limited for mandatory breaths and for all spontaneous breaths. Inspiratory pressure is controlled by a demand flow delivery system that is designed to maintain the set PEEP/CPAP level. PEEP/CPAP is adjustable from 0 to 50 cmH_2O. Although the Bear 1000 has no specific mode selection for pressure-support, when PRES SUP/INSP PRES is set at a value above zero, spontaneous breaths are pressure-supported. The pressure range for this setting is 0–80 cmH_2O above baseline. When PRES SUP/INSP PRES is adjusted at a value greater than zero and the pressure augment function is active, a segment of volume-targeted breaths may be pressure-limited.

Volume-Targeted Ventilation: In volume-targeted ventilation, inspiration can be time- or pressure-cycled. If the patient's inspiratory demand causes airway pressure to fall below the set PEEP level (inadequate set inspiratory flow), the ventilator will switch to pressure-targeting, providing increased flow to maintain the set PEEP level. Volume-limiting of inspiration occurs any time the inspiratory pause time is greater than zero. Inspiration is flow-limited when the ventilator is volume targeted. The range of flow available for peak inspiratory flow is 10 to 150 L/min, and through activation of pressure augment, peak flow for mandatory pressure controlled or spontaneous breaths may reach 200 L/min.

Cycling

With the Bear 1000, one of four variables will determine termination of inspiration: pressure, volume, flow, or time.

Pressure-Cycling

There are two cases in which inspiration may be pressure-cycled. The first is when the peak inspiratory pressure alarm threshold is violated. The second is when spontaneous breaths occur when PRES SUP/INSP PRES is not used.

Volume-Cycling

Volume-cycling of inspiration occurs in the assist CMV and SIMV modes. Volume is not directly measured; however, the microprocessor takes feedback from the flow control valve and ends inspiration when tidal volume and the optional compliance "comp volume" have both been delivered. The range of adjustment for tidal volume is from 30 mL to 2000 mL and is corrected to STPD, with sigh volume automatically adjusted to 150% of the set tidal volume. When pressure augment is activated in a volume-targeted mode, (eg, assist, CMV, and SIMV), volume-cycling may be overridden in response to patient demand for increased tidal volume when the ventilator provides increased flow and increased pressure to the patient.

Flow-Cycling

Flow-cycling occurs in two instances: First, inspiration may be flow-cycled in PRES SUP/INSP PRES (pressure-supported) spontaneous ventilation when the inspiratory flow rate falls below 30% of the set peak inspiratory flow rate. The second instance in which flow-cycling may occur is in the assist CMV and SIMV modes when pressure augment is activated. In this setting, flow-cycling occurs when the patient produces a prolonged inspiration that exceeds the set tidal volume.

Time-Cycling

The fourth variable terminating inspiration is inspiratory time. Time-cycling for mandatory breaths occurs with the PCV mode. Inspiratory time may be set from 0.1 to 5.0 seconds.

In all cases, when the inspiratory pause time is set at any value greater than zero, inspiration is time-cycled. Inspiratory pause is adjustable from 0 to 2.0 seconds. When the time/I:E limit alarm is activated, inspiration is also time-cycled.

Baseline Pressure

Baseline pressure is adjusted from 0 to +50 cmH_2O in PEEP/CPAP mode using the PEEP/CPAP knob.

□ CONTROL SUBSYSTEMS

Control Circuit

The control circuit of the Bear 1000 requires pneumatic and electronic control signals (Fig. 21-59). The following six pressure transducers provide input to a microprocessor: (1) proximal airway pressure, (2) machine pressure, (3) proximal/PEEP differential pressure, (4) flow control valve pressure, (5) air, and (6) oxygen supply pressure. Additional input to the microprocessor comes from a temperature sensor and from the external flow sensor. These measure, respectively, delivered gas temperature and exhaled flow. The primary output control signals are to the air-oxygen blender, the flow-control valve, the nebulizer solenoid valve, and to the exhalation solenoid valve. Control of peak inspiratory and baseline pressures is allowed through pneumatic signals to the exhalation valve from the exhalation solenoid valve.

Drive Mechanism

Gas is supplied to the Bear 1000 either through external compressed gas (air and oxygen) or from a combination of an electric motor and air compressor with a pressure regulator (Fig. 21-59). The initial gas pressure is regulated at about 18 psig, before reaching the air–oxygen blender. Mixed gases are directed from the blender to a rigid-walled vessel (accumulator), which has a volume of approximately 3.5 L. Pressure from the accumulator drives the flow-control system. Accumulator pressure varies from 10 to 18 psig. When increased flow is required, the stored accumulator volume is immediately available. This diminishes the demand re-

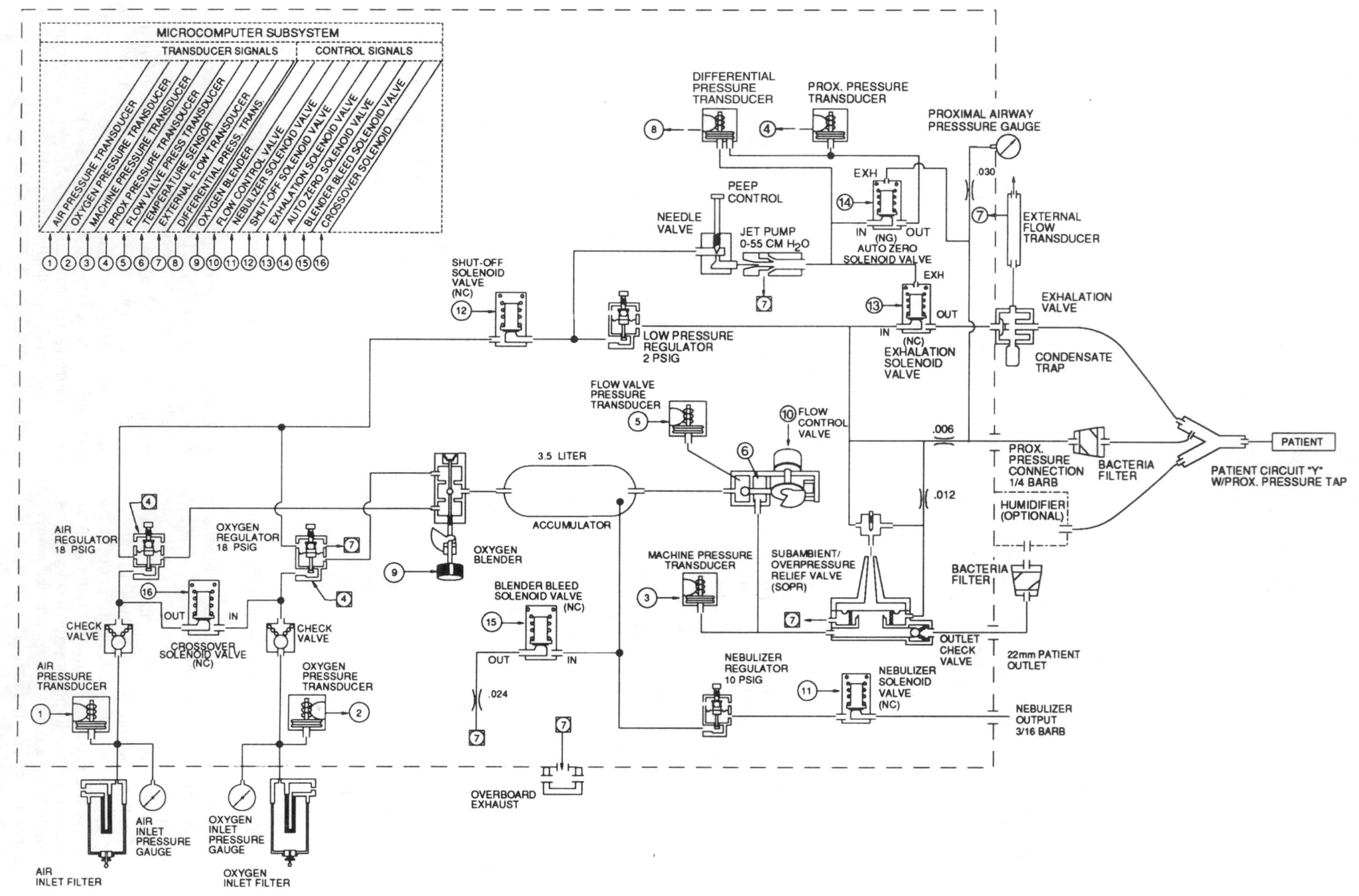

FIGURE 21-59. Internal components of the Bear 1000 ventilator control panel (Courtesy of Bear Medical Systems, Riverside, CA)

quired of the blending system and of the upstream pressure regulating system. This system is highly efficient in providing for a wide range of peak flow settings and in reducing the flow required from the compressed gas supply. In addition, response time is greatly improved. The accumulator provides the additional benefit of serving as a mixing chamber, thus assuring stability of the delivered FIO_2 within a given breath.

Output Control Valves

The pneumatic main flow control valve, which is connected to a stepper motor, regulates all gas flow to the patient. The exhalation valve receives two pneumatic signals. The first is from a 2-psig pressure regulator, which keeps a diaphragm-type exhalation manifold closed for assisted breaths. The second is a jet venturi generating an adjustable pressure signal controlling baseline pressure (ie, PEEP/CPAP). The action of the two valves is coordinated by the microprocessor to assure that the exhalation valve closes as the flow control valve delivers flow to the patient's circuit.

☐ MODES OF OPERATION AND ADDITIONAL FEATURES

The Bear 1000 names the following modes on its control panel: Assist CMV, SIMV/CPAP (PSV), MMV, Pressure Control Ventilation, Pressure Augment (Table 21-16). An additional feature is the flow or volume augmentation.

Assist CMV

When Assist CMV is selected, inspiration is pressure-triggered or time-triggered. Pressure-triggering is determined by the presence of spontaneous breathing efforts and adjustment of the assist sensitivity setting. Time-triggering is determined by the rate setting. Inspiration is volume-targeted. When inspiration is time-triggered and inspiratory pause is set above zero, inspiration may be volume-limited. Inspiration is flow-limited and volume-cycled in accordance with the tidal volume setting. Inspiration is time-cycled when inspiratory pause is set above zero.

TABLE 21-16 **Modes and Features of Ventilation Available with the Bear 1000 Ventilator**

Modes
Assist CMV
SIMV/CPAP (PSV)
Pressure control ventilation
Pressure support ventilation
Mandatory minute ventilation (MMV)
Sigh
Features
Pressure augmentation of volume- or flow-targeted breaths
Pressure slope
Pressure augmentation with volume guaranteed
Flow or volume augmentation

SIMV/CPAP (PSV)

In SIMV, mandatory breaths are volume-targeted and/or pressure- or time-triggered. Mandatory breaths may be volume- or flow-limited and volume-, time-, or pressure-cycled. Volume-targeted, pressure-triggered breaths occur when there are spontaneous breathing efforts and assist sensitivity is set. Time-triggering is determined by the rate setting. Volume-limiting occurs when inspiratory pause is set above zero. Flow-limiting and volume cycling is determined by the tidal volume setting. Time-cycling occurs when inspiratory pause is set above zero.

To initiate CPAP, rate and PRES SUP/INSP PRES settings are zero and the PEEP/CPAP control is set at a value greater than zero. In CPAP, spontaneous breaths can be pressure supported by setting PRES SUP/INSP PRES greater than zero.

When spontaneous inspirations occur between mandatory breaths, they are pressure-triggered, pressure-limited, and pressure-cycled. When PRES SUP/INSP PRES is set greater than zero, spontaneous inspirations occurring between mandatory breaths are flow-cycled and assisted by pressure support.

MMV

MMV differs from SIMV in that the average exhaled minute volume must exceed the threshold as determined by the operator-selected MMV level setting. If the MMV threshold setting is not exceeded by the patient's average exhaled minute volume, a new backup rate is initiated. The new backup rate is established by the following equation:

$$\text{Backup rate (cycles/min)} = \text{MMV level (L/min)} / \text{Tidal volume (L/breath)}$$

When the average exhaled minute volume meets or exceeds the MMV level setting, the ventilator resumes operation at the rate set.

Pressure Control Ventilation

Mandatory breaths are pressure-targeted and pressure- or time-triggered. They are pressure-triggered when spontaneous breathing efforts are present and assist sensitivity is set. Mandatory breaths are time-triggered in accordance with the rate setting. Pressure limiting of mandatory breaths is determined by the PRES SUP/INSP PRES setting. Time-cycling of mandatory breaths is determined by the inspiratory time setting.

Pressure Augment With Volume Guarantee

The pressure augment control logic feature of the Bear 1000 allows the ventilator to combine pressure-targeted ventilation and volume-targeted ventilation within a single breath (see Fig. 21-41). The intent of this design is to provide a flow that more closely matches the patient's inspiratory demand with the assurance of guaranteed volume provided by volume control.

Activation of pressure augment causes inspiration to begin under pressure support, whereas the pressure limit is determined by PRES SUP/INSP PRES. In this mode, pressure slope may be used to adjust the pressure rise time. The initial peak flow value, which is determined by the PRES SUP/INSP PRES setting and the resistance of the patient's respiratory system decays from its initial peak value. When the targeted tidal volume is achieved, pressure support continues until flow decays to 30% of the initial peak value. At this point, inspiration is terminated. Should tidal volume not be achieved, inspiration continues under volume control at the set flow rate to assure delivery of tidal volume. At this point, inspiration is terminated. If the patient's inspiratory effort causes the circuit pressure to drop below the PRES SUP/INSP PRES setting, inspiration may switch from volume-targeting back to pressure-targeting. Pressure and volume settings in conjunction with patient inspiratory demand may cause pressure, volume, and flow curves during pressure augment to vary considerably.

Flow and Volume Augmentation

Volume-targeted breaths are automatically augmented because of the way the flow control system functions (Fig. 21-60). If a patient's inspiratory demand exceeds the peak flow setting or the tidal volume setting, the pressure processor will signal for more flow. This occurs because the proximal airway pressure falls below baseline (flow augmentation). Even when the tidal volume has been delivered as preset and the volume processor stops the signal for flow, the ventilator will continue flow to the patient if the patient's inspiratory demand keeps the proximal airway pressure below baseline (volume augmentation).

In Figure 21-60, example 1, the curve on the left shows a situation where augmentation is not in use and the ventilator is set for volume-targeted ventilation with a constant flow rate. The ventilator delivers a constant flow regardless of whether the patient is demanding flow in excess of what is being delivered. This can be seen on the pressure manometer where the pressure drops below baseline during inspiration. With pressure augmentation active, even though patient demand is high (see Fig. 21-60, example 1, right-hand curves), the pressure curve remains at baseline and flow rises above set flow to meet patient demand. As demand drops the flow returns to the set value and the remainder of the tidal volume is delivered.

In Figure 21-60, example 2, the curve on the left shows the patient demanding both extra flow and extra volume. During one volume-targeted breath, the ventilator has ended flow, but the patient continues to actively breathe in. This triggers a second breath (autocycle triggered). In the right-hand curves using the augmentation feature, the patient has a flow demand higher than the set flow value and a volume demand higher than the set tidal volume. With augmentation, the patient receives both more flow and more volume and is not limited by the ventilator settings.

□ OUTPUT DISPLAYS (MONITORS) AND ALARMS

The front panel of the Bear 1000 is divided into three groups of displays: Controls, Monitors, and Alarms (Tables 21-17 and 21-18). An aneroid pressure gauge is also provided. Indicator lights are present in the monitor panel for the following: controlled breaths (lit when mandatory breath is delivered), sigh breaths (lit when sigh is delivered), patient effort (lit to indicate inspiratory effort sufficient to drop the pressure greater than the set assist sensitivity), and MMV active (lit when MMV backup rate is activated).

Three keypads are available that control one digital readout and that can be selected to show peak, mean, or plateau pressures. PEEP/CPAP (baseline pressure) is read from the aneroid pressure manometer.

Three keypads and one digital display are used to display exhaled tidal volume, total minute ventilation, and spontaneous minute ventilation. All expired volumes are corrected to STPD to provide consistency with the set tidal volume display.

Four keypads with a single digital display are used to display total ventilatory rate, spontaneous ventilatory rate, I:E ratio, and MMV%. MMV% indicates the percentage of time over the last half hour that the MMV backup rate has been used instead of the normal breath rate control.

Input Power Alarms

Audible and visual alarms are activated when electrical power fails or when the pneumatic power supply falls below 27.5 psig.

Control Variable Alarms

Peak Inspiratory Pressure

A low and high peak inspiratory pressure alarm threshold can be set. The low pressure threshold ranges from 3 to 99 cmH_2O, and the high alarm threshold ranges from 0 to 120 cmH_2O. Inspiration is terminated when the high pressure alarm is activated. Both low and high alarm thresholds can be set for baseline pressure.

A proximal disconnect alarm is also present. This alarm is activated in the event that proximal pressure measures less than 3 cmH_2O, whereas machine pressure measures greater than the high peak inspiratory pressure alarm plus 10 cmH_2O. The most likely cause of this alarm is a disconnected proximal pressure line. A very large leak can also activate this alarm. When the alarm is activated, "PRO" is displayed in the peak inspiratory pressure readout.

Alarms for low and for high total minute volume also are present. The range available for low minute volume is 0 to 50 L/min and for high minute volume is 0 to 80 L/min. Alarms also are present for total breath rate. The low rate alarm may be set in the range of 3 to 99 breaths per minute and the high rate alarm may be set in the range of 0 to 155 breaths per minute.

Control Circuit Alarms

Audible and visual alarms are activated if the ventilator fails because of an internal or external malfunction. "Failure to cycle" indicates that the ventilator is not providing any mechanical breaths or that demand flow and PEEP are not maintained.

Should inspiratory time exceed the sum of 5 seconds plus the inspiratory pause setting or if the I:E ratio

NO AUGMENTATION CAPABILITY

WITH AUGMENTATION CAPABILITY

EXAMPLE 1: Patient demands extra flow.

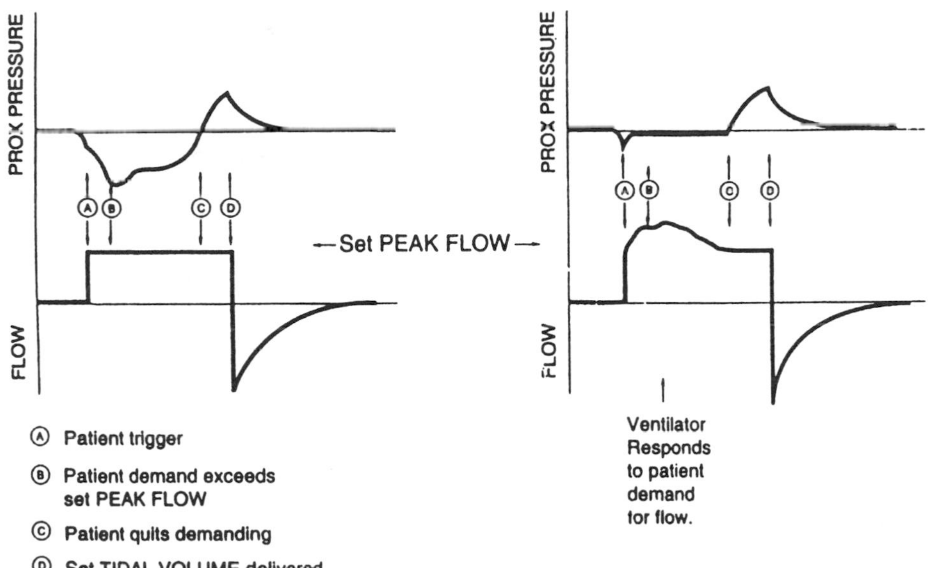

EXAMPLE 2: Patient demands both extra flow and extra volume.

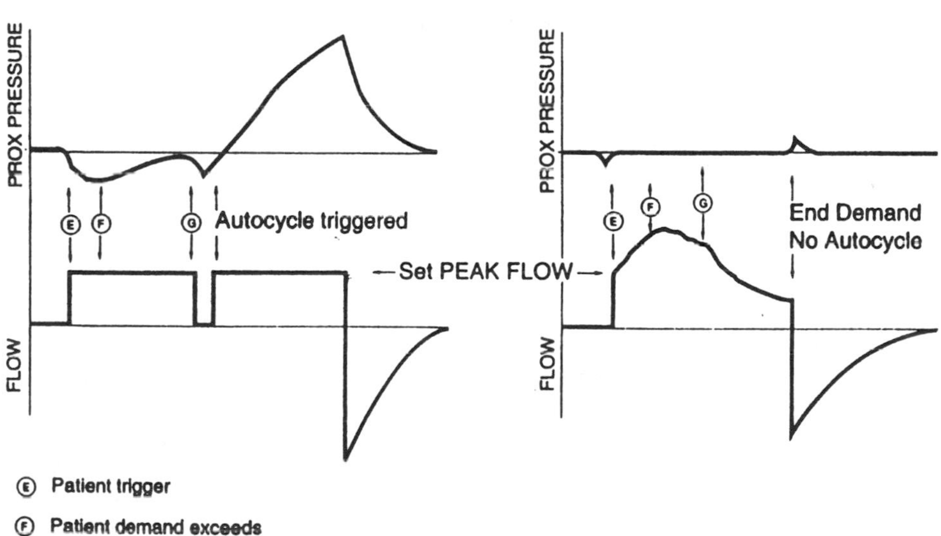

FLOW & VOLUME AUGMENTATION

FIGURE 21-60. Graphs of flow and volume augmentation for the Bear 1000 ventilator. See text for explanation. (Courtesy of Bear Medical Systems, Riverside, CA)

reaches the set limit for mandatory breath, audible and visual alarms are activated and inspiration terminates. The set limit for I:E ratio is normally 1:1. The clinician may override this default value through activation of the I:E override setting. When activated, this allows for a new default I:E ratio of 4:1.

☐ TROUBLESHOOTING

Troubleshooting instructions are available in the Operator's Manual provided by the manufacturer. Radio frequency interference (RFI)/electromagnetic frequency interference (EFI) can affect the operation of the Bear

TABLE 21-17 **Monitors and Displays Available on the Bear 1000 Ventilator**

Monitors	
Breath type indicators	
Controlled breath	LED on/off
Sigh breath	LED on/off
Patient effort	LED on/off
MMV active	LED on/off
Tidal volume	0.00–9.99
Total minute volume	0.0–99.9
Spontaneous minute volume	0.0–99.9
Total rate (breaths/min)	0–155
Spontaneous rate (breaths/min)	0–155
I:E ratio	1:0.2–1:99
MMV%	0–100%
Peak pressure (cmH_2O)	0–140
Mean pressure (cmH_2O)	0–140
Plateau pressure (cmH_2O)	0–140
Built-In Alarms	
Time/I:E limit	
Run diagnostics	
Gas supply failure	
Failed to cycle	

1000. In accordance with a clinical application bulletin issued by the manufacturer, it is best not to operate walkie-talkies or cellular telephones in close proximity to the Bear 1000. It is possible for EMI/RFI to cause the Bear 1000 to alarm or to go into an inoperative condition even though all Bear Medical products are in voluntary compliance with the International Electrotechnical Commission (IEC) standard (IEC601-1-2). In the event that alarms or inoperative conditions are displayed, any transmitting devices in close proximity to the Bear 1000 should be removed. If the Bear 1000 does not self-correct or reset, the ventilator should be restarted and re-evaluation of the settings and of the patient should be pursued.

Although the phenomenon of RFI with Bear Medical products can occur, it is rare. Bear Medical Systems, Inc., discourages the use of walkie-talkies or cellular phone devices from being used in the immediate vicinity of its products.

TABLE 21-18 **Alarms on the Bear 1000 Ventilator**

Alarm	Range or Setting
Time/I:E limit	LED on/off
Run diagnostics	LED on/off
Gas supply failure	LED on/off
Failed to cycle	LED on/off
I:E override	LED on/off
Total minute volume (LPM)	
High	0–80
Low	0–50
Total breath rate (breaths/min)	
High	0–155
Low	3–99
Peak inspiratory pressure (cmH_2O)	
High	0–120
Low	3–99
Proximal airway disconnect	<3 with machine Pressure = PIP + 10
Baseline pressure (cmH_2O)	
High	0–55
Low	0–55

Bear Cub 2001 Infant Ventilator

□ CLASSIFICATION

The Bear Cub 2001 infant ventilator (Table 21-19) (Fig. 21-61), which is electrically and pneumatically powered and electronically operated, functions as a pressure or flow controller. Initiation of a mandatory breath is time- or manually-triggered and time-cycled. End-expiratory pressure may be applied during mechanical (PEEP) or spontaneous (CPAP) breathing.

□ SPECIFICATIONS

Table 21-20 provides a list of ventilator specifications.

□ INPUT VARIABLES

The Bear Cub 2001 infant ventilator requires an electrical power source of 117 volts 60 Hz. Activating the ventilator is accomplished by moving the power switch from the off position to CPAP or CMV/IMV position. This ventilator requires external compressed gas to power its pneumatic circuit. Medical grade air and oxygen at 30 to 75 psig are supplied to the blender. FIO_2 is selected by positioning the oxygen control knob on the front panel. This ventilator has no internal compressor.

Operation

The Bear Cub 2001 infant ventilator functions as a continuous flow, time-cycled infant ventilator. Gas flows continuously through the ventilator circuit and is periodically diverted to the patient by closure of the exhalation valve. Figure 21-62 illustrates the control panel of the Bear Cub ventilator. The control panel is well organized with all pressure alarms and adjustments placed beneath the pressure manometer. Alarms may be adjusted for loss of PEEP/CPAP or low inspiratory pressure. The

TABLE 21-19 **Classification for Bear Cub 2001 Infant Ventilator**

Power Source for Control Circuitry	Electricity (117 volts AC at 60 Hz)
Power source for pneumatic system	Air and oxygen (30–75 psig)
Control mechanism	Pressure, flow
Triggering	Pressure, time, manual
Limiting	Pressure, time, flow
Cycling	Time

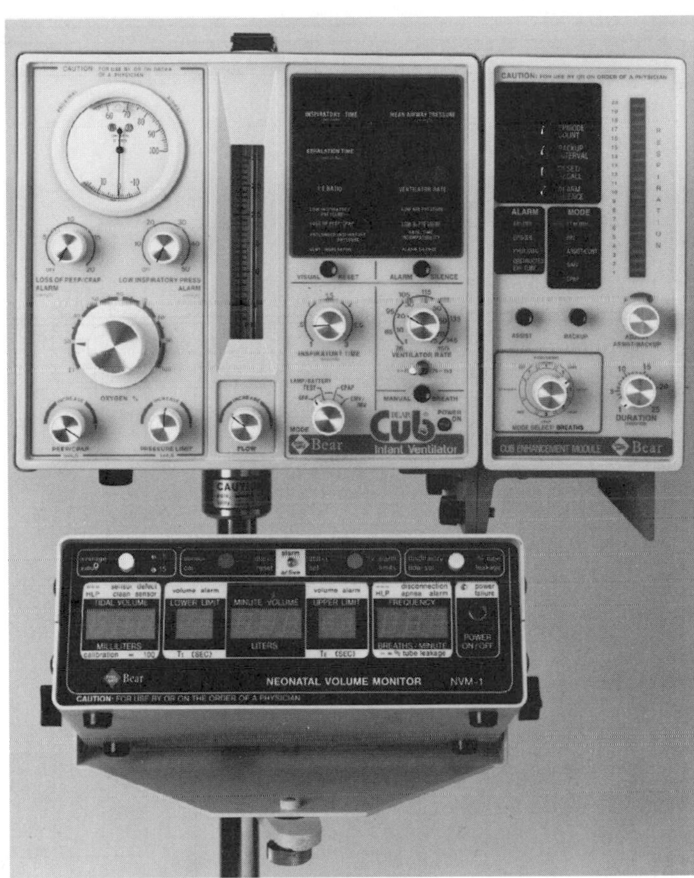

FIGURE 21-61. The Bear Cub 2001 ventilator. (Courtesy of Bear Medical Corp, Riverside, CA)

PEEP/CPAP level and peak inspiratory pressure adjustments also are available. The ventilator provides a detailed digital displal of inspiratory time, exhalation time, I:E ratio, mean airway pressure, and ventilation rate. LED's light indicates low inspiratory pressure, loss of PEEP/CPAP, prolonged inspiratory pressure, ventilator inoperative, low air pressure, low oxygen pressure, rate/time incompatibility, and alarm silence.

Flow and inspiratory time determine tidal volume. Two ranges of respiratory rate are available with the ventilator rate adjustment and are selected by positioning a toggle switch. When the toggle switch is in the left position, the range of ventilator rate is from 1 to 75 breaths per minute, and when the toggle switch is in the right position, the range of rate is from 76 to 150 breaths per minute. Manual breaths may be delivered by depression of the manual breath button. Their volume is determined by flow and inspiratory time. The mode selector switch provides for selection of CPAP or CMV/IMV modes. The ventilator can operate in CMV, IMV, IMV/CPAP, or CPAP alone.

TABLE 21-20 **Specifications for the Bear Cub 2001 Infant Ventilator**

Parameter	Range
Rate (breaths/min)	1–150
Flow (L/min)	3–30
Inspiratory time (sec)	0.1–3.0
Pressure limits (cmH_2O)	0–72
PEEP/CPAP (cmH_2O)	0–20
Modes of Ventilation	
CMV/IMV	
CPAP	

□ CONTROL VARIABLES

The Bear Cub 2001 infant ventilator controls flow and pressure. Gas that is delivered to the patient comes from the blender at a continuous flow selected by the flowmeter adjustment on the front panel (see Fig. 21-62). The design of the Bear Cub allows it more to limit instead of control inspiratory pressure. The pressure limit control knob is not calibrated, and the peak inspiratory flow rate is always limited to the value indicated on the flow meter. It is possible that for a given inspiratory time, there may be insufficient flow to produce the targeted inspiratory pressure limit within the inspiratory time provided. The compliance and resistance of the patient's respiratory system has marked impact here. The Bear Cub is best viewed as a flow controller.

Inspiratory Waveform

The inspiratory pressure and flow waveforms are rectangular (constant under normal circumstances). The ventilator will pressure-limit but will not pressure-cycle.

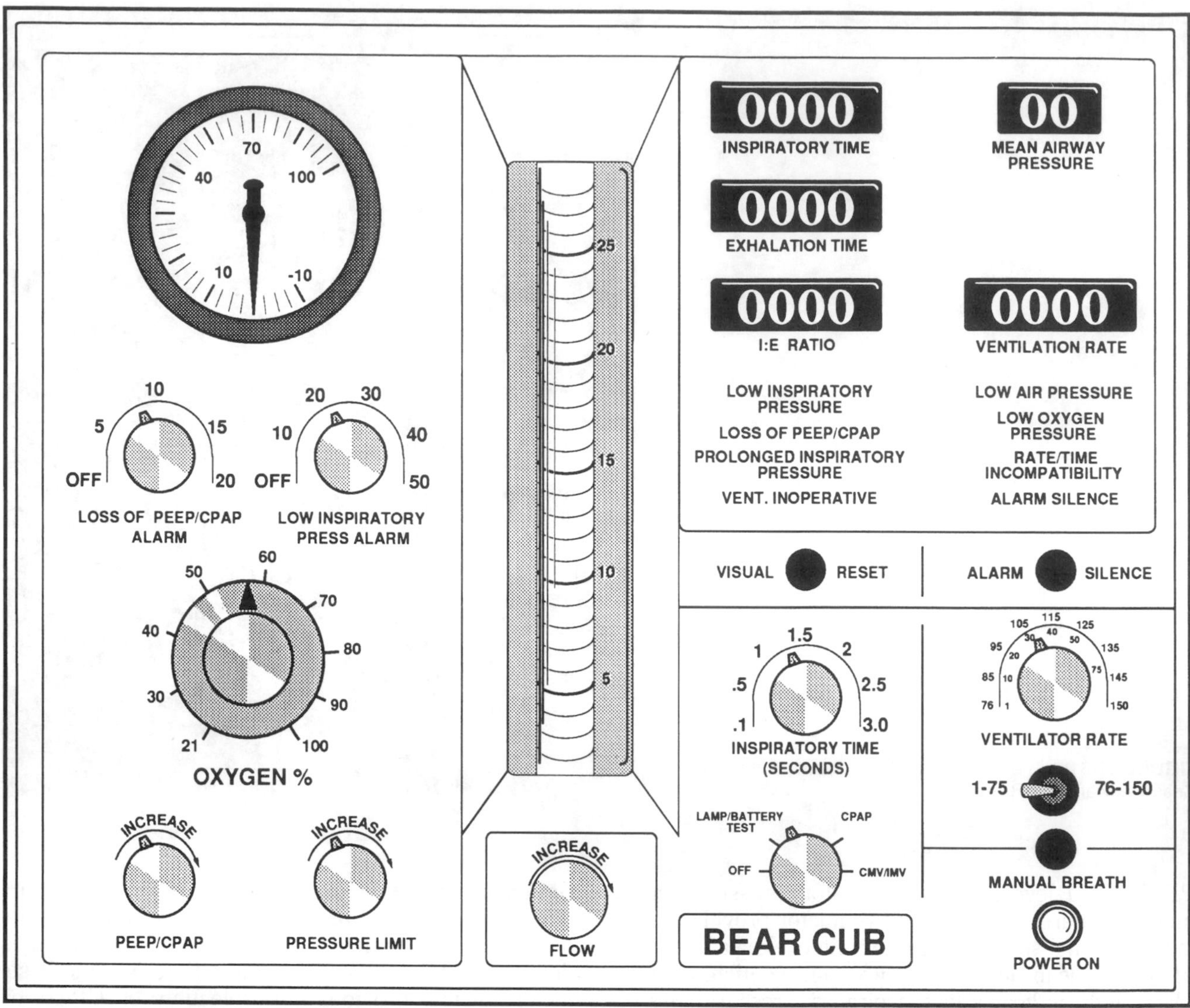

FIGURE 21-62. The control panel of the Bear Cub ventilator. (From Branson, R.D., Hess, D.R., and Chatburn, R.L., Respiratory Care Equipment, J.B. Lippincott Co., Philadelphia, 1995, p 319, permission requested)

The Bear Cub continually produces a semirectangular pressure waveform in pressure controlled (pressure-limited) operation. When peak inspiratory pressure is set high enough to achieve flow control, a rectangular flow waveform results.

□ PHASE VARIABLES

Triggering

Spontaneous inspiration is pressure-triggered in the CPAP mode. The patient's inspired gas flow is provided by the continuous flow of the circuit. In the CMV/IMV mode, mandatory breaths are time- or manually-triggered.

The ventilator rate is determined by adjustment of the ventilator rate knob. Manual breaths may be initiated by pressing the manual breath button. Manual breaths are available in IMV and CPAP and the inspiratory time and mean airway pressure during the manual breath is displayed.

Limiting

Volume delivered to the patient is limited with respect to the flow setting and inspiratory time. Inspiration is pressure-limited based on the preset pressure limit. When pressure-limiting of inspiration occurs, tidal volume is determined by inspiratory time, respiratory system resistance and compliance, and the inspiratory pressure waveform. When flow-limiting of inspiration occurs, estimated tidal volume is the product of the set flow rate and the inspiratory time minus any compressed gas volume.

Cycling

Normally, the Bear Cub 2001 infant ventilator ends inspiration in accordance with the inspiratory time selected. The machine does pressure-limit based on the pressure limit adjustment, but does not pressure-cycle.

Inspiratory and expiratory timing signals are sent by the control circuit to the three-way solenoid, which switches the source of the exhalation manifold's pneumatic signal from the pressure limit control or from the PEEP control valve. The airway opening pressure sensing line carries its pneumatic signal to the pressure limit control system. This system provides for control of the inspiratory pressure and results in production of an exponential pressure waveform.

Baseline Pressure

To achieve a baseline pressure above zero, the PEEP/CPAP control is adjusted. This uncalibrated control allows for adjustment of PEEP/CPAP from 0 to +20 cmH_2O.

□ CONTROL SUBSYSTEMS

Control Circuit

The Bear Cub 2001 infant ventilator is electrically controlled and pneumatically powered (Fig. 21-63). The electronic control circuit sends its inspiratory and expiratory signals to the three-way solenoid. An external pneumatic power source is required for operation of the Bear Cub. An external gas source powers the internal blender. Compressed air is required at 35 to 75 psig, and oxygen is required at 35 to 75 psig. The blender delivers its gas to the flow meter, which then sends a continuous flow to the patient's circuit.

Drive Mechanism

The Bear Cub 2001 infant ventilator is primarily pneumatic in design, with a three-way electronic solenoid responsible for changing ventilatory phases (Fig. 21-64). High pressure gases (air and oxygen) and a 115 volt 60 Hz AC electrical source are required. Each gas is filtered before being reduced to 17 psig by precision regulators (A and B) to ensure that gas is blended accurately. Output pressures of the air and oxygen regulator must be within ±2 cmH_2O of each other; the gases are delivered to the dual orifice blender (C). At the operator-selected FIO_2, flow through the flow control (D) and the flowmeter (E). Gases entering the breathing circuit are regulated by an overpressure relief valve (F), factory-adjusted to crack open at approximately 87 cmH_2O, and an anti-suffocation valve (G), which opens at −2 cmH_2O.

The oxygen regulator (B) also powers two venturi devices: the peak inspiratory pressure (PIP) venturi (H) and the PEEP venturi (I), both of which are operator controlled (J or K). The air regulator (A) also includes a nonadjustable, expiratory venturi (L) that reduces inadvertent CPAP generated by the movement of gas across the breathing circuit. The three-way solenoid (M) delivers pressure from the PEEP venturi to the exhalation valve (N) and diaphragm during the expiratory phase. Mechanical inspiration begins with an electronic signal that actuates the three-way solenoid, which terminates flow from the PEEP venturi, delivers pressure from the PIP venturi to the diaphragm of the exhalation valve, and diverts gas at a set flow rate to the patient's lungs. Airway pressure is monitored simultaneously with a pressure transducer (O) and a mechanical, aneroid manometer (P).

Output Control Valve

The output control valve of the Bear Cub 2001 infant ventilator regulates the transmission of the inspiratory control pressure to the exhalation valve diaphragm and also regulates the speed with which pressure may rise within the patient circuit. The output control valve functions as a metering valve that results in an inspiratory pressure waveform, which tends to be exponential rather than rectangular in form. This is especially true at low inspiratory flows. Consequently, the flow and volume waveforms are also exponential. When used as a flow-controller, the pressure and volume outputs produce ascending ramp waveforms and the flow waveform is essentially rectangular.

In inspiration, pressure from the pressure limit control is transmitted through to the exhalation valve through the metering valve. As a result, pressure builds in the patient circuit. In expiration, the PEEP valve venturi transmits its pressure through the three-way solenoid through the exhalation valve. This allows for maintenance of the PEEP level in the patient circuit.

An oxygen-powered venturi, which is controlled by the pressure limit control, determines inspiratory pressure limit. Clockwise rotation of the pressure limit control produces occlusion of the venturi outflow. As a result, increased pressure transmits through the metering valve, the check valve, and three-way solenoid to the exhalation valve in inspiration. When inspiratory pressure exceeds the preset pressure limit, inspiratory plateau results as gases are vented out the outlet manifold.

When low inspiratory flows are required, the metering valve pressurizes the exhalation valve, which results in creation of increased back pressure. This pressure is applied to the bleed regulator and the metering valve. As a result, the metering valve is depressed, producing resistance to gas flow leaving the pressure limit control. As the three-way solenoid is positioned for inspiration, there is a momentary delay in pressure delivery through the exhalation valve. This creates a relatively slow occlusion of the exhalation valve and the patient experiences a rather slow increase in pressure within the circuit.

When higher continuous flows are required, the flow control is opened more widely. As a result, the pressure applied to the metering valve is diminished. This allows the pressure limit control to close the exhalation valve more rapidly, which results in more rapid pressure increases in the patient circuit during inspiration. Additionally, an external spring-loaded pressure-relief valve is used to provide an adjustable pop-off system. This is located in the inspiratory limb of the patient circuit and provides an adjustable safety mechanism that protects the patient from exposure to high pressures should the expiratory tubing become obstructed.

□ MODES OF OPERATION

The control panel of the Bear Cub 2001 infant ventilator allows operator selection of the following modes:

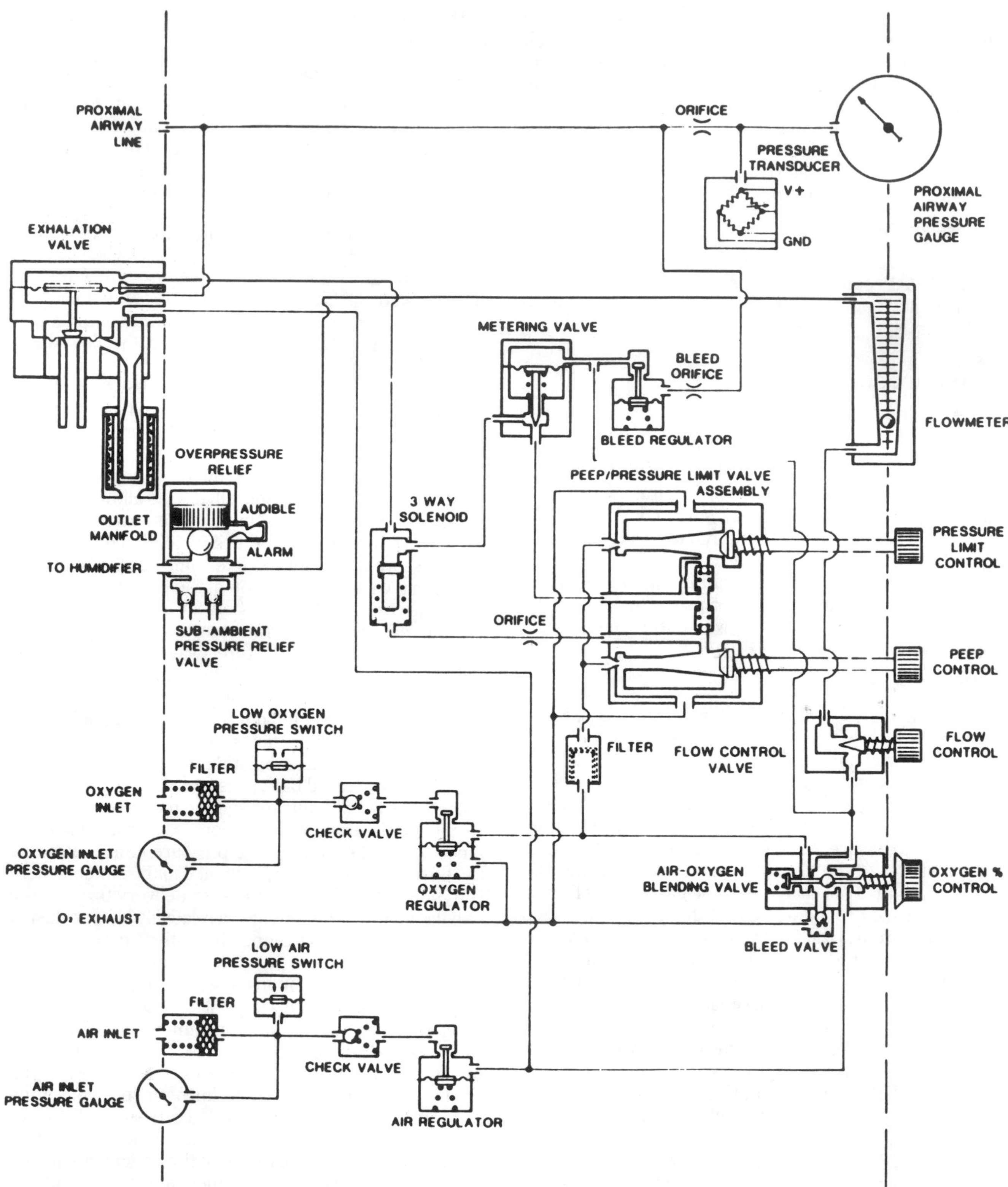

FIGURE 21-63. The internal components of the Bear Cub ventilator control circuit. (Courtesy of Bear Medical Corp, Riverside, CA)

CMV/IMV

In normal operation, inspiration is time-triggered (determined by the set ventilator rate), pressure-limited, and time-cycled (determined by inspiratory time). A continuous flow of gas is directed to the pneumatic circuit of the ventilator as set by the flow control knob, which allows for spontaneous breathing between mandatory breaths. In the event that inspiratory time or inspiratory flow is insufficient, inspiration is not pressure-limited but it is time-triggered, flow-limited, and time-cycled.

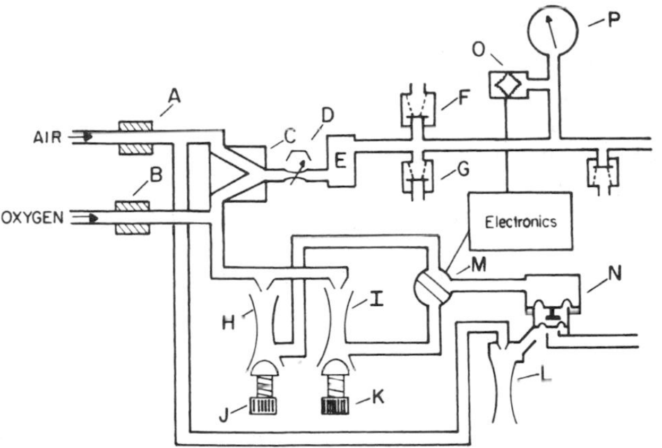

FIGURE 21-64. A simplified schematic diagram of the Bear Cub ventilator (see text).

TABLE 21-22 **Monitors and Displays Available on the Bear Cub 2001 Infant Ventilator**

Power on	
Inspiratory time (sec)	0–9.99
Expiratory time (sec)	0–99.9
I:E ratio	1:0.0–1:9.99
Mean airway pressure (cmH_2O)	0–99
Proximal airway pressure (cmH_2O)	0–99
Ventilator rate (bpm)	1 150
Alarm silence	30 seconds
Battery/lamp test	off/on
FIO_2	21%–100% (internal blender)
Flow rate (L/min)	3–30

The Bear Cub 2001 infant ventilator is incapable of providing a variable flow to meet situations in which the patient's inspiratory flow demand exceeds that delivered by the ventilator. When this condition exists to the extent that negative airway pressure is generated below (less than) baseline, it is essential that the operator make appropriate increases in the continuous flow rate.

CPAP

In the CPAP mode, inspiration is not controlled. All ventilatory needs of the patient are provided by the continuous flow of gas from the flow meter. Surplus inspiratory flow and to a greater extent the PEEP/CPAP setting produces the typical pattern of pressure fluctuation for the CPAP mode.

□ OUTPUT DISPLAYS (MONITORS AND ALARMS)

An array of five digital display windows provides a continuous display of monitored settings including inspiratory time, expiratory time, ventilator rate, I/E ratio, and mean airway pressure (see Fig. 21-62 and Tables 21-21 and 21-22). There are two operator-controlled alarms and five factory-adjusted alarms. To assist the operator in rapidly recognizing alarm conditions, each alarm consists of an audible alarm and a visual LED indicator and is listed in the display area. In the event that an alarm condition remits, the visual indicator remains lighted until the operator is able to determine which alarm limit was exceeded and resets the display ("visual reset" control). Audible alarms, with the exception of that indicating that the ventilator is inoperative, may be silenced for a period of 30 seconds ("alarm silence" control).

TABLE 21-21 **Alarms on the Bear Cub 2001 Infant Ventilator**

Low inspiratory pressure
Loss of PEEP/CPAP
Prolonged inspiratory pressure
Ventilator inoperative
Low air pressure
Low O_2 pressure
I:E ratio > 3:1
Rate/time incompatibility

Adjustable alarms consist of the following:

- Low PEEP/CPAP alarm. Audible and visual alarms are activated if the instant proximal airway pressure exceeds the limit of PEEP/CPAP set.
- Low inspiratory pressure alarm, which provides a second pressure threshold that must be exceeded with each mechanical breath or audible and visual alarms are activated. If subsequent breaths return the airway pressure to proper limits, the audible alarms cease.

An additional alarm condition associated with the low PEEP/CPAP setting is referred to as prolonged inspiratory pressure. This audible and visual alarm activates if the airway pressure remains above the set low PEEP/CPAP setting plus 10 cmH_2O for 3.5 seconds or more. Therefore, the low PEEP/CPAP setting must be appropriately adjusted, particularly when elevated levels of PEEP or CPAP are required. Factory-adjusted alarms consist of an I:E ratio alarm, which alerts the operator to inverse ratios in excess of 3:1 (expressed as 1:0.3); rate/time incompatibility, which warns that the rate and inspiratory time settings are such that the mandatory 0.25-second expiratory time has been violated; and the low air and oxygen pressure alarms, which sound when the inlet pressure of either gas falls below 22.5 psig.

The ventilator-inoperative alarm can be activated for several reasons: failure of the ventilator to cycle, loss of electric power, disconnection, control panel problems, timing-circuit failure, prolonged expiratory cycle, or excessive inspiratory time (±24% of programmed). This alarm interrupts all electronic functions and cannot be silenced until the problem is corrected. Gas flow and end-expiratory pressure are maintained during the alarm.

□ TROUBLESHOOTING

The Bear Cub 2001 infant ventilator has proved to be extremely reliable. The most frequently encountered problems are breathing circuit leaks and problems as-

TABLE 21-23 **Classification of the Bear Medical Systems BP-200 Infant Pressure Ventilator**

Power Source for Control Circuitry	Electricity (117 volts AC at 60 Hz)
Power source for pneumatic system	Air 15–75 psig and oxygen 30–75 psig
Control mechanism	Pressure, flow
Triggering	Pressure, time, manual
Limiting	Pressure, time, flow
Cycling	Time

sociated with the exhalation valve. In earlier models, the plunger within the exhalation valve sometimes would stick, which prevented cycling and resulted in a ventilator-inoperative alarm; these valves have been redesigned. The administration of nebulized medications to patients being ventilated on a Bear Cub 2001 may also lead to problems related to the exhalation valve. The saline mixture used to dilute pharmaceutical solutions can leave a salt crust around the exhalation valve that may occlude the expiratory venturi, and thereby, prevent the ventilator from cycling. A warm, damp rag can remove the crust, unless it is extremely thick and totally occluding the venturi orifice. For this, the venturi will need to be cleaned with a tool, which requires extreme care not to dilate or damage the orifice.

Many institutions install an external pressure relief valve, which adds an additional margin of safety if conditions prevail that cause the internal pressure relief system to fail.

Since this ventilator is microprocessor controlled, concern exists for the effects of EFI and RFI with the operation of this ventilator. The respiratory care practitioner should ensure that walkie-talkies, cellular telephones, and other types of devices that may emit an EFI or RFI are not operated in close proximity to the Bear Cub 2001 infant ventilator.

BP-200 Infant Pressure Ventilator*

□ CLASSIFICATION

The Bear Medical Systems BP-200 infant pressure ventilator (Table 21-23) (Fig. 21-65) is electrically and pneumatically powered, electronically operated, and functions as a pressure or flow controller. Mandatory inspiration is time- or manually-triggered and time-cycled. Inspiration is pressure-, flow-, or time-limited. End-expiratory pressure may be applied during mandatory (IMV/PEEP) or spontaneous (CPAP) breathing.

□ SPECIFICATIONS

Specifications for this ventilator are listed in Table 21-24.

□ INPUT VARIABLES

The BP-200 pressure ventilator requires an electrical power source of 117 volts 60 Hz to power the control circuit. It also requires a compressed gas source for oxygen and for air at pressure ranges specified on the back of the ventilator. Activating the ventilator (Fig. 21-66) is accomplished by setting the power switch (A) to the "On" position. This ventilator has an integral air-oxygen blender, but has no internal compressor.

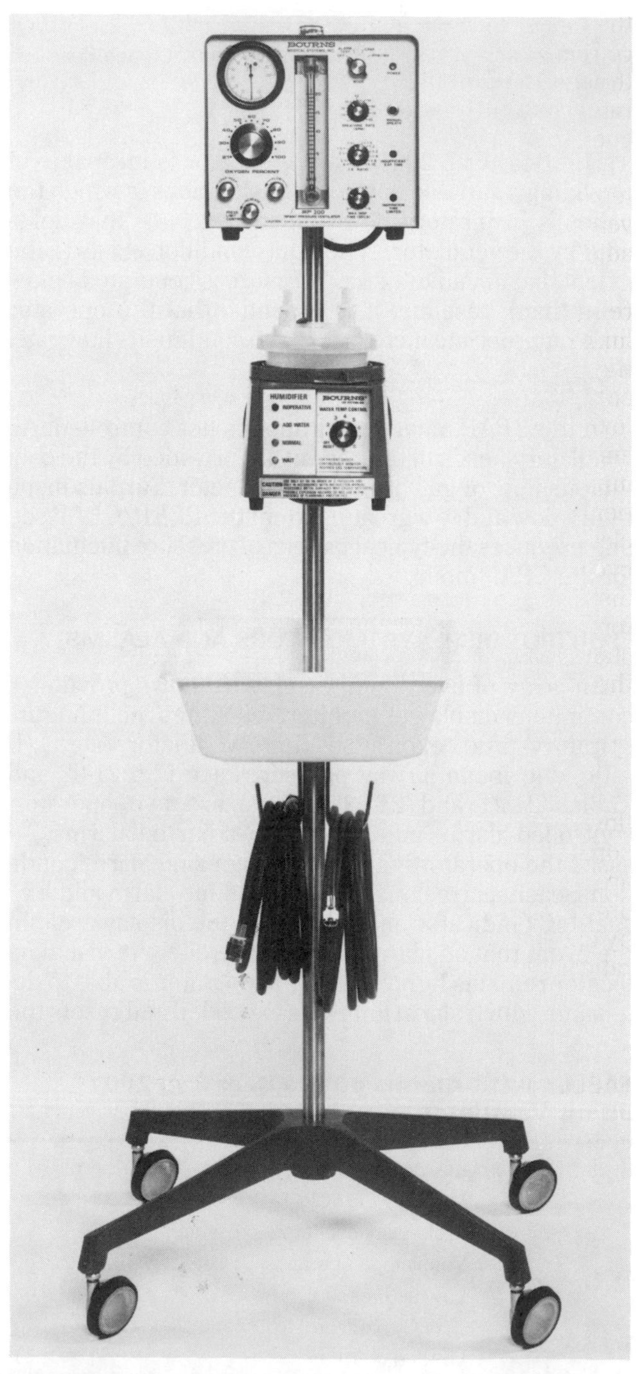

FIGURE 21-65. Bear Medical Systems BP-200 infant pressure ventilator. (Courtesy of Bear Medical Systems)

* Thanks to Ayres Mello of Bear Medical Systems, Riverside, CA, for his technical assistance in preparation of this section.

Operation

Ventilator function and settings are adjusted on a compact control panel (see Fig. 21-66). A four-position control knob (A) serves as an electric power switch, alarm test, and ventilatory mode selector (IPPB/IMV or CPAP). In the alarm test position, an audible alarm buzzer sounds. When CPAP is selected, the pneumatic and electrical alarm circuit is activated. If air or oxygen inlet pressure decreases below 15 or 20 psig, respectively, or an electrical power interruption occurs, an audible alarm, powered by a "D" cell battery (9 volts in older models) is activated. If IPPB/IMV is selected, the ventilator will time-trigger in addition to engaging the electronic and pneumatic power loss surveillance alarm system. When the mode selection is in any position but off, an amber-colored power light (B) is illuminated. Mechanical V_T is the result of an adjusted breathing rate control (C), I/E ratio control (D), and continuous flow control (E). The continuous flow is indicated by means of a calibrated Thorpe tube (F). A manual breath (J) may be administered only in the CPAP mode and is determined by the ventilator settings similar to IMV/IPPB V_T. The F_{IO_2} is adjustable (N) from 0.21 to 1.0 (center of left panel)

If the preset circuit pressure reaches the set pressure relief value, gas exits the circuit through a pressure limit valve. The inspiratory pressure limit is adjusted by the uncalibrated pressure limit control. During the resulting inspiratory plateau, gas flow to the patient's lungs becomes a function of the patient's lung compliance and airway resistance. Gas flows into the patient's lungs until pressure in the ventilator circuit and the patient's lungs equilibrate or until the ventilator time-cycles. In this situation, the ventilator does not pressure-cycle, but pressure-limits and may produce an inspiratory pressure plateau for the duration of inspiratory time. The flow remains essentially linear in a constant (rectangular) wave pattern in instances in which the preset pressure limit is never reached.

□ CONTROL VARIABLES

As determined by the operator, the BP-200 controls flow and pressure. All gas that is delivered to the patient comes through a continuous flow circuit. Tidal volumes are delivered to the patient by closure of the expiratory limb of the circuit by a solenoid valve. Expiration occurs by opening the solenoid valve. Inspiratory time and I/E ratio is controlled by the function of the solenoid valve.

Inspiratory Waveform

The inspiratory waveform is rectangular (constant) under normal circumstances. A prolonged inspiratory plateau may be produced when the pressure relief valve opens during inspiration. High peak inspiratory pressures and prolonged inspiratory times will produce this pattern.

□ PHASE VARIABLES

Triggering

In the IPPB/IMV mode, inspiration is time-triggered. In the CPAP mode, inspiration is pressure-triggered. During mechanical expiration or CPAP, the patient breathes spontaneously from a continuous flow of gas.

TABLE 21-24 **Specifications for the Bear Medical Systems BP-200 Infant Pressure Ventilator**

Rate (breaths/min)	1–60
New units	1–150
Flow rate (L/min)	0–20
Pressure limit (cmH_2O)	10–80 (approximate)
Time (sec)	0.5–5
New units	0.2–5
I:E ratio control	4:1–1:10
Maximal expiratory time (sec)	
Internally preset	0.5
New units	0.2
Oxygen concentration	21%–100%
Pressure manometer (cmH_2O)	0–100
PEEP/CPAP (cmH_2O)	0–100
Modes of ventilation	
CPAP	
IPPB/IMV	

Breathing rate is controlled by the rate adjustment (C). Manual breaths may be delivered only when the ventilator is set in the CPAP mode. Depressing the manual breath button (J) results in the delivery of a tidal volume, which is determined by the ventilator flow and inspiratory time settings.

Limiting

The BP-200 infant pressure ventilator will pressure-limit but will not pressure-cycle. In the event that high inspiratory pressures and prolonged inspiratory times occur, an inspiratory plateau is produced.

Cycling

Inspiration is time-cycled as determined by the I/E ratio set by the I/E ratio knob (D).

Baseline Pressure

To achieve a baseline pressure above zero, the CPAP/PEEP pressure limit control (L) is adjusted. PEEP/CPAP is produced by activation of a venturi, which generates a pressure against the expiratory valve. PEEP/CPAP of 0 to +20 cmH_2O is available with the BP-200 Infant Pressure Ventilator.

□ CONTROL SUBSYSTEMS

Control Circuit

The BP-200 uses electrical control components to power and regulate most of its functions. Gas flow is regulated by the flow meter.

By design, the BP-200 infant pressure ventilator is to be used as a time-limited, pressure or flow controller. When the inspiratory pressure limit is reached for a given breath, delivered tidal volume is determined primarily by flow, pressure limit, and inspiratory time. Volume also is influenced by the resistance and compliance of the patient's respiratory system. The following formula allows for calculation of the optimal available tidal volume:

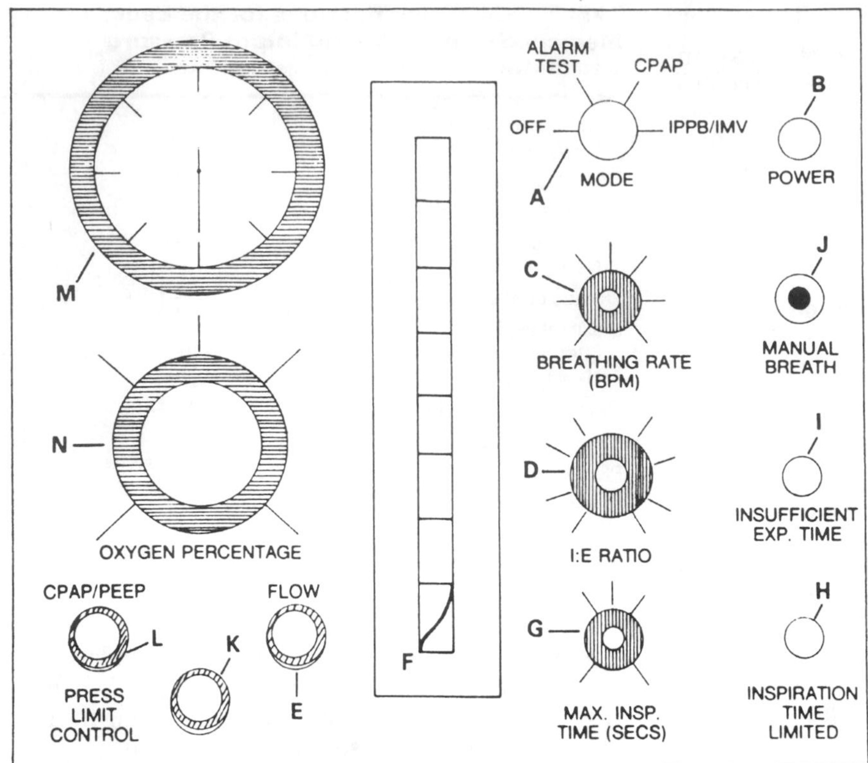

FIGURE 21-66. Control Panel of the Bear Medical Systems BP-200 infant pressure ventilator (see text).

$$\text{Targeted Tidal Volume} = \text{Inspiratory Time (sec)} \times \text{Flow (L/Min)}/60$$

It is important to note that the results of this calculation are not indicative of the actual volume the patient receives, especially when the ventilator pressure limits before determination of inspiration. This calculation is useful, however, in determination of the targeted tidal volume.

Drive Mechanism

Gas is provided to the BP-200 infant pressure ventilator through the air-oxygen blender (Fig. 21-67). Gas is directed past a spring-loaded pressure relief valve through the humidifier and out to the inspiratory limb of the circuit. The electronics operate the solenoid valve, which determines breathing rate and I/E ratio. PEEP/CPAP is maintained by a venturi system. Air and oxygen at 15 to 75 psig and 30 to 75 psig, respectively, are pressure-equilibrated and mixed (A) to the desired FIO_2.

Output Control Valve

A continuous flow of blended gas is metered (B) into a calibrated Thorpe tube and directed past a spring-tension pressure-relief valve (C). The gas is warmed and humidified (D) before it enters the breathing circuit. During mandatory inspiration a solenoid valve (E) closes,

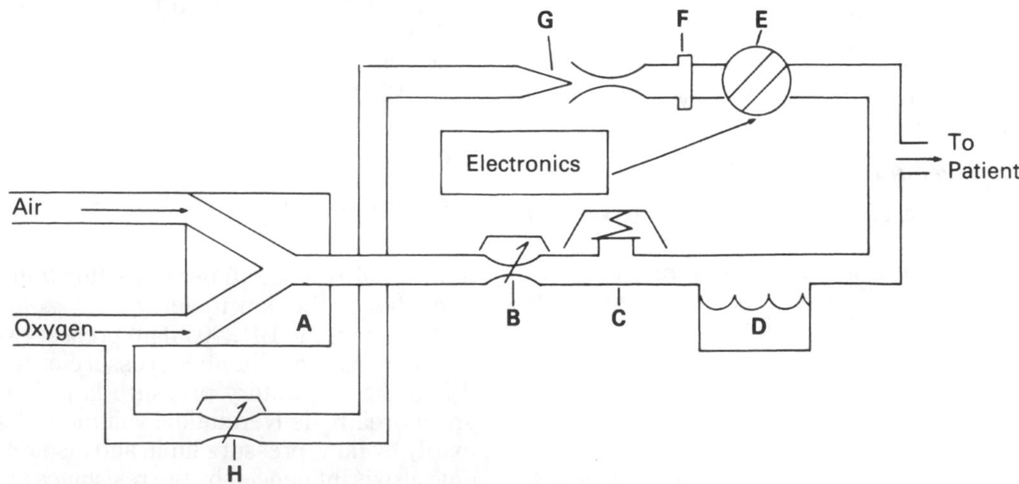

FIGURE 21-67. Schematic diagram of the Bear Medical Systems BP-200 infant pressure ventilator (see text).

interrupting the continuous flow vent, thus diverting gas into the infant's airway. During mechanical expiration or CPAP, the patient breathes spontaneously from the continuous flow of gas. Gas flow may be opposed by a pressurized expiratory check-leaf valve (F). The amount of threshold expiratory generated depends on jet venturi flow (G) metered by the PEEP/CPAP control (H).

Peak inspiratory pressure (K) (see Fig. 21-66) and threshold expiratory pressure (L) may be regulated from 12 cmH_2O at 2 L/min to >80 cmH_2O at 20 L/min, and zero to 20 cmH_2O at >45 psi oxygen inlet pressure, respectively. Each is adjusted by an uncalibrated control; consequently, the pressure limit must be observed on an aneroid manometer (M), while the proximal airway connection is occluded.

□ MODES OF OPERATION

There are essentially two modes of operation for the BP-200 infant pressure ventilator: IPPB/IMV and CPAP. These are selected by the mode selector (A) (see Fig. 21-66). Ventilator functions and settings are adjusted on the compact control panel. A four-position control knob (A) serves as an electric power switch, alarm test, and ventilatory mode selector (IPPB/IMV or CPAP).

CPAP

When CPAP is selected, the pneumatic and electrical alarm circuit is activated. If air or oxygen inlet pressures decrease below 15 or 30 psig, respectively, or an electrical power interruption occurs, an audible battery-powered alarm is activated. A manual breath (J) may be administered only in the CPAP mode and is determined by the ventilator settings similar to IMV/IPPB V_T. The FIO_2 is adjustable (N) from 0.21 to 1.0.

IPPB/IMV

When IPPB/IMV is selected, the ventilator will time-trigger in addition to engaging the electronic and pneumatic power loss surveillance alarm system. When the mode selection is in any position but off, the amber-colored power light (B) is illuminated. Mechanical V_T is the result of an adjusted breathing rate control (C), I/E ratio control (D), and continuous flow control (E). The continuous flow is indicated by means of a calibrated Thorpe tube (F).

TABLE 21-25 **Monitors and Displays Available on the Bear Medical Systems BP-200 Infant Pressure Ventilator**

Visual indicators
Power light
Inspiration time limited
Insufficient expiratory time (sec)
Air inlet pressure gauge (rear panel)
Oxygen inlet pressure gauge (rear panel)
FIO_2
Flow
Pressure

TABLE 21-26 **Alarms on the Bear Medical Systems BP-200 Infant Pressure Ventilator**

Audible alarms
Electric power failure
Inadequate air and/or oxygen pressures

Output Displays (Monitors and Alarms)

Monitored and alarm settings are mixed in with the patient controls (Tables 21-25 and 21-26). At low IMV rates the maximum inspiratory time control may be used to override I/E control, obviating prolonged inspiratory time. When maximum inspiratory time has been reached, a red indicator light (H) (see Fig. 21-66) illuminates. If the electronic timer allows adjusted mechanical expiratory times less than 0.22 to 0.28 seconds, a red insufficient expiratory time indicator (I) illuminates.

□ TROUBLESHOOTING

The simplicity of this ventilator facilitates rapid recognition of problems. An audible alarm indicates either pneumatic or electrical power loss. If this occurs, gas inlet pressure gauges on the rear panel, the electrical connection, or the circuit breaker should be checked. Failure to develop circuit pressure during IPPB/IMV is usually caused by circuit leaks or a low-pressure limit adjustment.

BIRD MEDICAL TECHNOLOGIES*

Bird 6400ST Volume Ventilator

□ CLASSIFICATION

The Bird 6400ST volume ventilator (Fig. 21-68) is electrically and pneumatically powered, microprocessor operated, and may function to control pressure or flow/volume. Initiation of mechanical inspiration is either time- or pressure-triggered. The inspiratory phase is flow- or pressure-limited. Termination of mechanical inspiration is time-cycled; however, inspiratory flow becomes the cycling mechanism in pressure support (Table 21-27). End-expiratory pressure may be applied during mechanical (PEEP) or spontaneous (CPAP) breathing.

□ SPECIFICATIONS

Table 21-28 provides the specifications for the Bird 6400ST.

□ INPUT VARIABLES

The Bird 6400ST uses 120-volt AC (at 60 Hz) to power the control circuitry. Two high-pressure compressed gas sources, air and oxygen at 30 to 70 psig, power the

* Thanks to Becky Mabry and Fritz Westerhout of Bird Medical Technologies, Inc, Palm Springs, CA, for their technical assistance with the Bird ventilators.

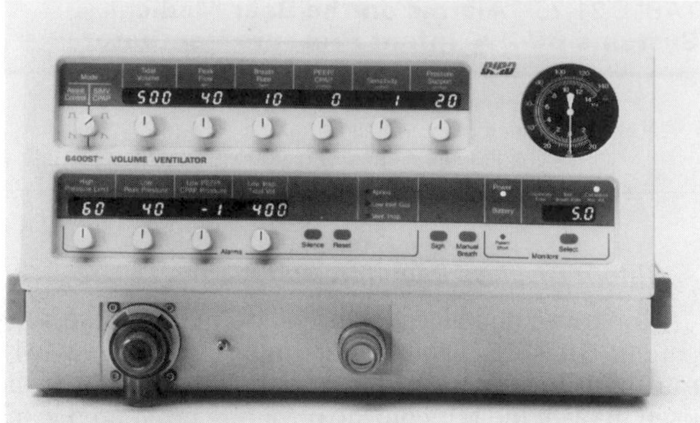

FIGURE 21-68. The Bird 6400ST volume ventilator (Courtesy of Bird Products Corp., Palm Springs, CA)

pneumatic circuit. These are connected to an external Bird 3800 Microblender. Operation of the 6400ST is facilitated by a compact, easily understood control panel (Fig. 21-69). The top half of the panel is used for ventilatory settings, and the bottom is reserved for alarms and monitors.

□ CONTROL VARIABLES

High-pressure (30 to 70 psi) blended gas and 120 volt AC electricity should be provided through the appropriate receptacles on the rear panel of the 6400ST ventilator. The 6400ST requires an external blender capable of mixing 120 L/min at 50 psi. It is possible to substitute blenders, if they are capable of blending sufficient quantities of gas at 50 psig.

□ PHASE VARIABLES

Triggering

Inspiration is pressure-triggered when a patient's inspiratory effort is enough to drop the system pressure to the level set on the sensitivity control. Inspiration is time-triggered when the breath rate is set. It can also be manually triggered

Limiting

Inspiration is flow-limited during flow/volume-controlled breaths and pressure-limited during spontaneous breaths in SIMV and CPAP. It is also pressure-limited in PSV. Inspiration is manually volume-limited if the inflation hold control button is pressed.

TABLE 21-27 **Classification of the Bird 6400ST**

Power Source for Control Circuitry	Electricity (120 volts AC at 60 Hz)
Power source for pneumatic system	Air and oxygen (30–70 psi)
Control mechanism	Flow/volume and pressure
Triggering	Pressure, manual, time
Limiting	Pressure, volume, flow
Cycling	Pressure, flow, time

TABLE 21-28 **Specifications for the Bird 6400ST**

Inspiration	
Rate (bpm)	0–80
Volume (mL)	50–2000
Flow (L/min)	10–120
Demand flow (L/min)	0–110
I/E ratio	not controlled
Pressure (cmH_2O)	1–140
Effort (cmH_2O)	1–20 below PEEP
Hold (pause) (sec)	not controlled
Pressure support (cmH_2O)	0–50 above PEEP
Sigh volume	1.5 × set tidal volume (3000 mL max)
Sigh rate	on/off, 1 every 100 breaths
Expiration	
PEEP/CPAP (cmH_2O)	0–30
Retard (L/min)	not controlled

Cycling

The end of inspiration is pressure-cycled when the maximum high-pressure limit is reached. It is also pressure-cycled during spontaneous ventilation when PSV is not used. This occurs when airway pressures rise above the PEEP setting as a spontaneous exhalation begins. Inspiration is flow-cycled during pressure support when the flow drops to 25% of peak flow. Inspiration is time-cycled for volume-targeted mandatory breaths when inspiratory time reaches the value dictated by the volume and flow settings. Inspiration will also time-cycle in PSV if the inspiratory time reaches 3 seconds before flow has decreased to 25% of peak.

Operation

The operator must first select a mode and flow pattern by placing the four-position mode selector switch (A) (see Fig. 21-69) in the desired combination. Selections include A/C with square flow pattern, A/C with descending flow pattern, SIMV/CPAP with square flow pattern, and SIMV/CPAP with descending flow pattern. Selection of the patient ventilator setting is monitored by a window, positioned above each control, that displays each selected value and changes as they are made. Ventilator settings with associated display windows include mechanical tidal volume (B), peak flow rate (C), breath rate (D), PEEP/CPAP (E), assist sensitivity (F), and pressure support (G). Pressure support is available in the SIMV/CPAP mode only and is not available in the A/C mode.

Inspiratory Waveform

The flow waveforms available include a constant or a descending ramp flow pattern. When the constant waveform is selected, the inspiratory gas flow is delivered at

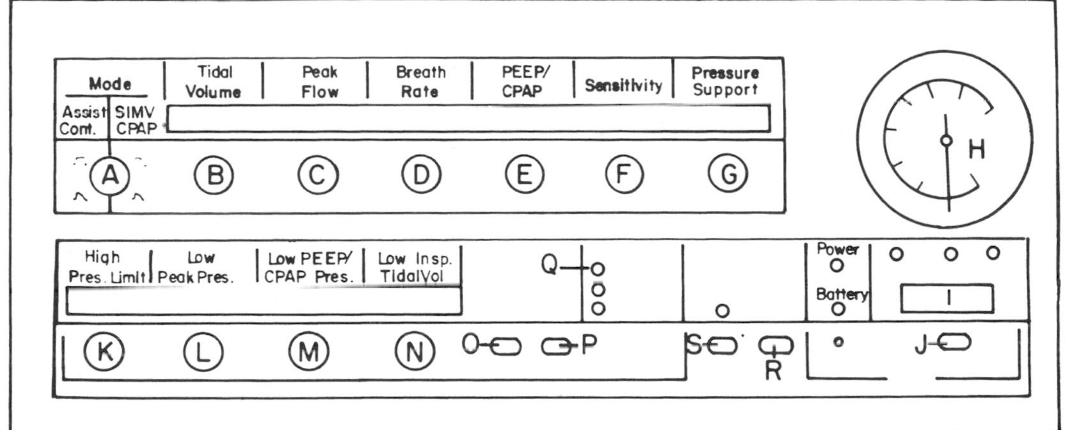

FIGURE 21-69. Control panel for the Bird 6400ST ventilator (see text). (Courtesy of Bird Products Corp., Palm Springs, CA)

a constant rate based on the peak flow rate setting. In the descending ramp waveform, the flow peaks at the value preset on the peak flow setting and decreases to 50% of the peak flow by the end of the breath.

Baseline

Baseline pressure is adjustable from 0 to 30 cmH_2O using the PEEP/CPAP control.

□ CONTROL SUBSYSTEMS

The Bird 6400ST uses electric control components. There is a pneumatically driven safety valve that permits the patient to breathe from room air in the event of an electrical power loss or in a ventilator-inoperative situation.

Control Circuit

The internal microprocessor reads input signals relating to airway pressure and control variable settings and sends control signals to the output control valves. Airway pressure is measured at the proximal airway port and inside the ventilator. Feedback from the airway pressure transducer provides information to determine triggering, cycling, and alarm signals and to control airway pressure waveforms during pressure-controlled modes such as PSV.

Information about flow is determined by sensing the position of the stepper motor inside the flow control valve (see Output Control Valve below). The signals from the flow control valve are used to determine the shape of the flow waveform and for volume adjustment. There is a flow transducer connected to the exhalation valve that is used to measure exhaled tidal volume and minute volume through the optional monitoring module.

The Pneumatic System: The Drive Mechanism

Blended gas at the selected F_{IO_2} is filtered and regulated to 20 psi (A) and delivered to a high-pressure 1.1 L reservoir (B) (Fig. 21-70). The output pressure of (B) is monitored by transducer (C), which alerts the operator of potential regulator problems or low blended gas inlet pressure. The reservoir stores pressurized gas for augmenting the blender flow during high inspiratory flow demands. The blender can deliver up to about 75 L/min with inlet and outlet pressures of 50 and 35 psig, respectively. The reservoir allows the ventilator to deliver up to 120 L/min flow. The extra flow is provided from gas stored in the reservoir during exhalation.

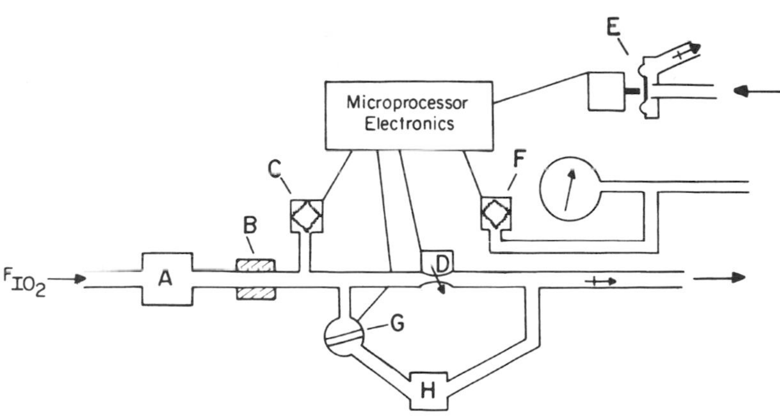

FIGURE 21-70. Schematic diagram of the Bird 6400ST ventilator (see text). (Courtesy of Bird Products Corp., Palm Springs, CA)

Output Control Valve

The flow-control valve (D) receives blended gas from (B) and is responsible for the delivery of all breathing gases to the patient. The flow-control valve is defined as an *electromechanical* stepper valve. Such valves convert rotary motion into linear motion. Precise electrical signals from the microprocessor cause a motor to rotate a shaft. Rotation of the shaft occurs as a series of steps, each step opening or closing a poppet-type orifice located within the inspiratory flow valve. Resolution of flow through the orifice is claimed to be approximately 1 L per rotational step. The relationship between valve position and inspiratory flow rate is programmed into memory. This information allows the microprocessor to move the flow control valve in a sequence that will deliver the tidal volume, peak flow, and flow waveform selected by the operator. The exhalation valve (E) is also under microprocessor control and functions in a manner nearly identical with the flow control valve, except the rotating shaft applies pressure to the exhalation diaphragm rather than modulating an orifice.

To provide for spontaneous breathing, the microprocessor refers to information it receives from the proximal airway transducer (F). As the airway pressure falls during a spontaneous breath, the microprocessor opens the flow-control valve in an effort to maintain the CPAP level. The microprocessor then regulates flow to simultaneously meet patient demand and hold the CPAP at the selected level. As the flow required to meet these demands approaches zero, the breath ends, and the exhalation valve opens.

Pressure support breaths are delivered in a fashion similar to a spontaneous breath. The only difference is that the microprocessor attempts to maintain the selected pressure support level instead of the CPAP level.

The safety solenoid (G) can be opened during emergency alarm conditions, allowing the patient access to room air through the ambient valve (H), until appropriate action can be undertaken.

□ MODES OF OPERATION

The Bird 6400ST provides several modes of ventilation (Table 21-29).

Control

In the control mode, inspiration is flow/volume-controlled, time-triggered based on breath rate, flow-limited, and time-cycled.

TABLE 21-29 **Modes of Ventilation Available for the Bird 6400ST**

Control, assist/control
SIMV
Pressure support
Spontaneous (CPAP)

Assist/Control

A/C is the same as the control mode except inspiration can also be pressure-triggered by a patient effort as long as the sensitivity is appropriately set.

SIMV

The mandatory breaths in SIMV are flow/volume-controlled, flow-limited, time-triggered (according to the breath rate if patient effort does not start a breath), pressure-triggered when patient effort drops the circuit pressure to the sensitivity setting value, time-cycled, or pressure-cycled (if maximum safety pressure is reached). Spontaneous breaths between mandatory breaths are pressure-controlled (pressure-targeted); that is, the flow varies to maintain the pressure at the set PEEP/CPAP level. The spontaneous breaths are pressure-triggered and normally pressure-cycled. Inspiration for spontaneous breaths is flow-cycled in the PSV mode used with SIMV when flow drops to 25% of peak.

A mandatory breath is pressure-triggered the first time a patient effort is detected during the ventilatory period. After that, spontaneous breaths will not trigger a mandatory breath until the next ventilatory period. If a patient effort is not detected during the next ventilatory period, a mandatory breath is then given.

Spontaneous (Pressure Support and CPAP)

All spontaneous breaths are pressure controlled. The inspiratory flow varies to maintain pressure above the set baseline (PEEP/CPAP) or PSV level selected. They are pressure-triggered and pressure-cycled (normally) or flow-cycled (during PSV).

Sigh

A sigh volume is delivered at 150% of the set tidal volume every 100 breaths if the sigh is selected. The pressure limit threshold is automatically increased to 150% immediately before each sigh breath and returned to normal after the sigh has been delivered.

□ OUTPUT DISPLAYS AND ALARMS

The 6400ST provides monitoring with an airway pressure manometer (H) and a message window (I) located on the front control panel (Table 21-30) (see Fig. 21-69). The message window is used to alert the operator to potential problems, or it can be used to select (J) one of the following for display: inspiratory time (seconds), total breath rate (breaths per minute), which includes both spontaneous and mechanical breaths; and calculated minute volume (L/min), which is simply the product of the tidal volume and breath rate settings. LEDs adjacent to the message window indicate use of battery power (not internal), or AC power, and any patient effort that meets the sensitivity setting. The 6400ST does not measure exhaled tidal volume; however, an external, optional monitor may be purchased to accompany the ventilator.

There are four primary patient alarms, each with a control knob and window to display the established

TABLE 21-30 **Alarms on the Bird 6400ST Ventilator**

High pressure (cmH_2O)	Exceeds set limit
Low peak pressure (cmH_2O)	When prox. airway pressure transducer does not reach set limit during I
Low PEEP/CPAP (cmH_2O)	Pressure below set value (range, −20–30)
Low insp tidal volume (mL)	20–2000
	When inspired volume less than set for four consecutive breaths
Apnea	No breaths for 20 seconds
Low inlet gas	Pressure less than 17 psig
Vent. inoper.	Loss of power, low gas inlet pressure (<16 psig for 1 sec), system failure, or exhalation valve improperly installed
Circuit alarm	Disconnected, kinked, occluded proximal sensing line; occluded or kinked inspiratory limb or pressure transducer failure

value. The high-pressure limit control (K) establishes a pressure threshold that, when violated, terminates inspiration and activates an audible and visual alarm. If the airway pressure returns to the PEEP level within 3 seconds, normal ventilation resumes, and the audible alarm is cancelled. Should the airway pressure remain above the pressure limit setting or not return to the PEEP level, the internal safety solenoid will open. Airway pressure will then bleed to the PEEP level through an orifice in the main flow isolation valve. On reaching the PEEP level, the system will reset and attempt to deliver another breath. If the problem is not resolved, the scenario will repeat itself, and operator intervention will be necessary to rectify the situation.

The pressure limit threshold is automatically increased to 150% immediately before each sigh breath and returned to normal after the sigh has been delivered. However, the pressure limit cannot exceed 140 cmH_2O. The low peak pressure control (L) activates an alarm if the airway pressure fails to exceed the selected value during the inspiratory phase of any mandatory breath tidal volume. The low PEEP/CPAP control (M) is activated if the proximal airway pressure falls below the selected value for longer than 0.5 seconds.

The low inspiratory tidal volume control (N) establishes a volume threshold that must be exceeded by both spontaneous and mechanical breaths. If four consecutive breaths fall below this setting, an alarm is activated. The alarm silence button (N) will disable the audible alarm for 60 seconds, and the alarm reset (P) functions to reset the visual indicator for any alarm conditions that no longer exist. The ventilator-inoperative alarm cannot be silenced or reset.

Additional alarm conditions are listed with adjacent LED (Q). An apnea alarm occurs any time 20 seconds elapse without a mandatory or spontaneous breath. The low inlet alarm alerts the operator that the internal gas pressure has fallen below 17 psi and may be the result of low inlet pressure, internal regulator malfunction, or transducer error or malfunction.

The ventilator-inoperative alarm terminates all ventilator functions, opens the safety solenoid, providing the patient access to room air, and activates audible and visual alarms. Conditions that will precipitate a ventilator-inoperative alarm include loss of electrical power, extended high or low system pressure, electrical or mechanical failure detected by the microprocessor, and improper installation of the exhalation valve housing.

A manual breath (R) may be administered during any mode, provided that the patient is neither actively inhaling (mechanical or spontaneous) or exhaling. The sigh button (S) activates the automatic sigh function in all available modes.

☐ TROUBLESHOOTING

Troubleshooting is made easy through the judicious use of alarms and display windows. Potential patient circuit problems result in an audible alarm and the message "CIRC." The following conditions should be investigated as possible causes of the condition: disconnected proximal airway line, occluded or kinked proximal airway line, occluded or kinked inspiratory or expiratory limb of the breathing circuit, and transducer failure (either proximal or machine pressure transducer). Several problems can be avoided by ensuring that the exhalation valve diaphragm is properly engaged on the shaft of the valve-actuating motor and that the valve housing is securely latched. This is a complex pneumatic and electronic ventilator, and attempts to repair this ventilator should not be undertaken unless the operator is properly trained or qualified to make the repairs.

Bird 8400STi Volume Ventilator*

☐ CLASSIFICATION

The Bird 8400STi volume ventilator (Fig. 21-71) is electrically and pneumatically powered, microprocessor operated, and may function to control pressure or flow/volume. Initiation of mechanical inspiration is either time, flow-, or pressure-triggered. The inspiratory phase is flow- or pressure-limited. Termination of mechanical inspiration is time-, pressure-, or flow-cycled (Table 21-31). A software upgrade is available for flow-triggering. End-expiratory pressure may be applied during mechanical (PEEP) or spontaneous (CPAP) breathing. The blender has a gas outlet port that will power a nebulizer during inspiration. The ventilator requires the use of a blender.

☐ SPECIFICATIONS

Table 21-32 provides the specifications for the Bird 8400STi volume ventilator.

The Bird 8400STi is similar in design to the 6400, with a few exceptions. Airway pressure is measured at the

* Thanks to Fritz Westerhout and Rebecca A. Mabry of Bird Products Corp., Palm Springs, CA, for their technical assistance with Bird ventilators.

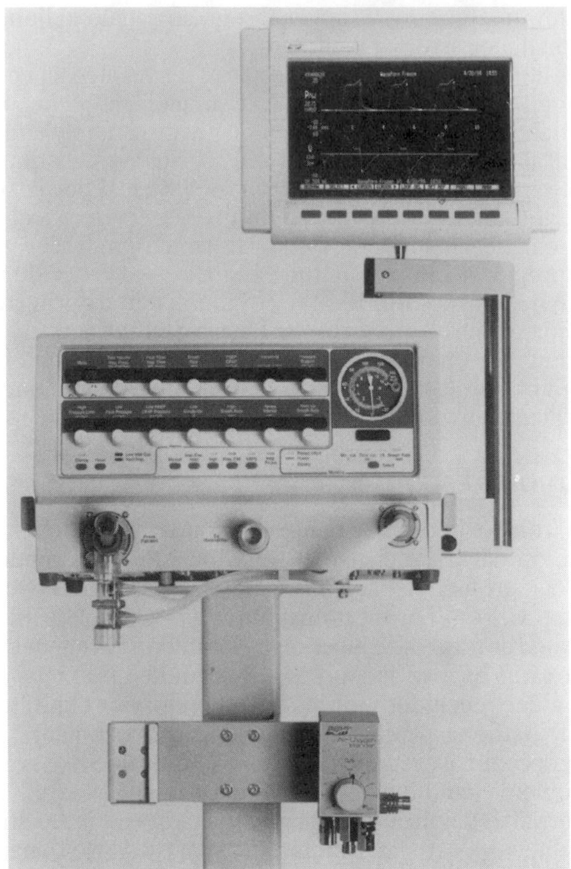

FIGURE 21-71. The Bird 8400 STi volume ventilator (Courtesy of Bird Products Corp., Palm Springs, CA)

exhalation valve, not at the proximal airway. A flow transducer (differential pressure transducer) at the exhalation valve measures exhaled tidal volume and minute volume. The electrical system has a separate display/exhalation valve control microprocessor. Special purge valves allow gas flow, every 60 seconds during exhalation, through the flow transducer and the differential pressure transducer lines to prevent moisture accumulation. During the purge event, the exhalation valve microprocessor calibrates the differential pressure transducer to keep accuracy in the exhaled tidal volume measurement. Otherwise, the gas delivery system is the same as in the 6400ST.

TABLE 21-31 **Classification of the Bird 8400STi**

Power Source for Control Circuitry	**Electricity (120 volts AC at 60 Hz)**
Power source for pneumatic system	Air and oxygen (30–70 psi)
Control mechanism	Flow/volume and pressure
Triggering	Pressure, manual, time, flow
Limiting	Pressure, volume, flow
Cycling	Pressure, flow, time

TABLE 21-32 **Specifications for the Bird 8400STi**

Inspiration	
Rate (breaths/min)	0–80
Volume (mL)	50–2000
Flow (L/min)	10–120
Demand flow (L/min)	0–110
I/E ratio	not controlled
Pressure (cmH_2O)	0–140
Effort (cmH_2O)	0–20 below PEEP
Flow trigger (option) (L/min)	1–10
Hold (pause) (sec)	not controlled
Pressure support (cmH_2O)	0–50 above PEEP
Sigh volume	1.5 x set tidal volume
Sigh rate	1 every 100 breaths
Pressure control (cmH_2O)	off, 5–100
Expiration	
PEEP/CPAP (cmH_2O)	0–30
Retard (L/min)	not controlled

□ INPUT VARIABLES

The Bird 8400STi uses 120 volts AC at 60 Hz to power the control circuitry. Two high-pressure compressed gas sources, air and oxygen, at 30 to 70 psig power the pneumatic circuit. Operation of the 8400 is facilitated by a compact, easily understood control panel (Fig. 21-72). The top half of the panel is used for ventilatory settings, and the bottom is reserved for alarms and monitors.

□ CONTROL VARIABLES

High-pressure (30 to 70 psi) blended gas and 120-volt AC electricity should be provided through the appropriate receptacles on the rear panel of the 8400STi ventilator. The 8400STi requires an external blender capable of mixing 120 L/min at 50 psig. It is possible to substitute blenders, if they are capable of blending sufficient quantities of gas at 50 psig.

□ PHASE VARIABLES

Triggering

Inspiration is pressure-triggered when a patient's inspiratory effort is enough to drop the system pressure to the level set on the sensitivity control. Inspiration is time-triggered when the rate is set. It can also be manually triggered. When the flow-triggering option is available and activated, the sensitivity window will display "Fxx," where "F" indicates activation of the flow-trigger option. The "xx" indicates the flow-trigger level in L/min. This is available in a range of 1 to 10 L/min. Inspiration is then flow-triggered. A "Back-up Breath Rate" becomes active if the apnea alarm is triggered. This control cannot be set lower than the "breath rate" control.

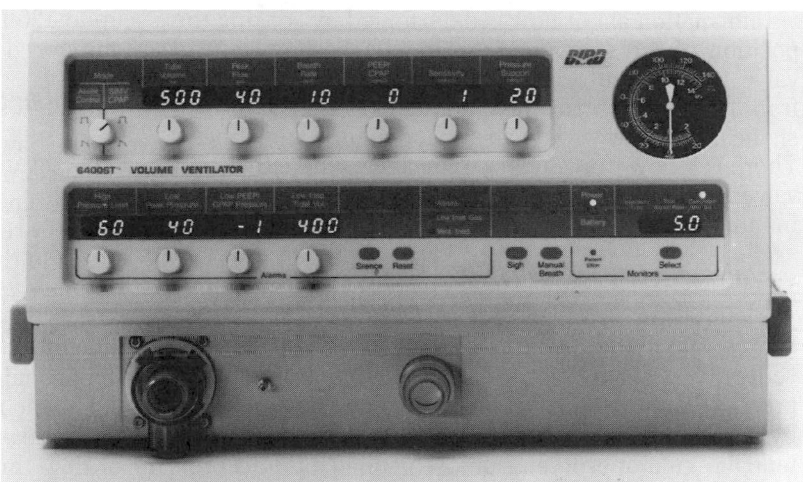

FIGURE 21-72. Control panel for the Bird 8400STi ventilator (Courtesy of Bird Products Corp., Palm Springs, CA)

Limiting

Inspiration is flow-limited during flow/volume-controlled breaths, pressure-limited during spontaneous breaths in SIMV and CPAP and is also pressure-limited in PSV. Inspiration is manually volume-limited if the inflation hold control button is pressed.

Cycling

Inspiration is time-cycled for mandatory breaths when inspiratory time reaches the value dictated by the volume and flow settings. The end of inspiration is pressure-cycled when the maximum pressure threshold is reached. It is also pressure-cycled during spontaneous ventilation when PSV is not used. This occurs when airway pressures rise above the PEEP setting as a spontaneous exhalation begins. Inspiration is flow-cycled during pressure support when the flow drops to 25% of peak flow. Inspiration will also be flow-cycled in the CPAP mode when the flow support option is selected. It will time-cycle in PSV if the inspiratory time reaches 3 seconds before flow has decreased to 25% of peak.

Operation

The operator must first select a mode and flow pattern by placing the four-position mode selector switch (see Fig. 21-72) to the desired combination. Selections include A/C with square flow pattern, A/C with descending flow pattern, SIMV/CPAP with square flow pattern, and SIMV/ CPAP with descending flow pattern. Selection of the patient ventilator setting is monitored by a window, positioned above each control, that displays each selected value and changes as they are made. Ventilator settings with associated display window include mechanical tidal volume, peak flow rate, breath rate, PEEP/CPAP, sensitivity, and pressure support. Pressure support is available in the SIMV/CPAP mode only and cannot be adjusted in A/C.

When the flow-support option is selected, a bias flow of 10 L/min flows through the patient circuit. The patient's flow during inspiration and expiration is calculated by comparing the flow through the flow control valve with the flow measured at the exhalation manifold. This calculation is based on the following equation:

$$F(pt) = F(vlv) - F(trn)$$

where F(pt) is the patient flow; F(vlv) is flow leaving the main flow control valve; and F(trn) is flow measured at the exhalation manifold transducer.

During inspiration, flow through the exhalation transducer falls below the 10 L/min constant value as patient flow (F(pt)) increases. The exhalation manifold closes and the inspiratory flow valve opens to provide flow to equal patient demand to bring exhalation transducer flow back to 10 L/min. Near the end of inhalation, as patient flow demand drops, F(vlv) and F(trn) become closer to being equal, F(pt) drops to zero and inspiration ends.

Inspiratory Waveform

The flow waveforms available include a constant or a descending ramp flow pattern. When the constant waveform is selected, the inspiratory gas flow is delivered at a constant rate based on the peak flow rate setting. In the descending ramp waveform, the flow peaks at the value preset on the peak flow setting and decreases to 50% of the peak flow by the end of the breath.

Baseline

Baseline pressure is adjustable from 0 to 30 cmH_2O using the PEEP/CPAP control.

□ CONTROL SUBSYSTEMS

The Bird 8400STi uses electric control components. There is a pneumatically driven safety valve that permits the patient to breathe from room air in the event of an electrical power loss or in a ventilator-inoperative situation.

Control Circuit

The internal microprocessor reads input signals relating to airway pressure and control variable settings and sends control signals to the output control valves. Feedback from the airway pressure transducer provides information to determine triggering, cycling, and alarm signals and to control airway pressure waveforms during pressure-controlled modes such as PSV.

Information about flow is determined by sensing the position of the stepper motor inside the flow control valve (see Output Control Valve below). The signals from the flow control valve are used to determine the shape of the flow waveform and for volume adjustment. There is a flow transducer connected to the exhalation valve that is used to measure exhaled tidal volume and minute volume.

The Pneumatic System: The Drive Mechanism

Blended gas at the selected FIO_2 is filtered (2) and delivered to a high-pressure 1.1 L reservoir (4) and, subsequently, regulated to 20 psig (Fig. 21-73). The output pressure of the reservoir or accumulator is monitored by a transducer (13), which alerts the operator of potential regulator problems or low blended gas inlet pressure. The reservoir stores pressurized gas for augmenting the blender flow during high inspiratory flow demands. The blender can deliver up to about 75 L/min with inlet and outlet pressures of 50 and 35 psig, respectively. The reservoir allows the ventilator to deliver up to 120 L/min flow. The extra flow is provided from gas stored in the reservoir during exhalation.

Output Control Valve

The flow-control valve (7) receives blended gas from the accumulator by way of a pulsation dampener, which buffers pressure fluctuations. The flow-control valve is responsible for the delivery of all breathing gases to the patient. The flow-control valve is defined as an *electromechanical stepper valve*. Such valves convert rotary motion into linear motion. Precise electrical signals from the microprocessor cause a motor to rotate a shaft. Rotation of the shaft occurs as a series of steps, each step opening or closing a poppet-type orifice located within the inspiratory flow valve. Resolution of flow through the orifice is claimed to be approximately 1 L/min per rotational step. The relationship between valve position and inspiratory flow rate is programmed into memory. This information allows the microprocessor to move the flow control valve in a sequence that will deliver the tidal volume, peak flow, and

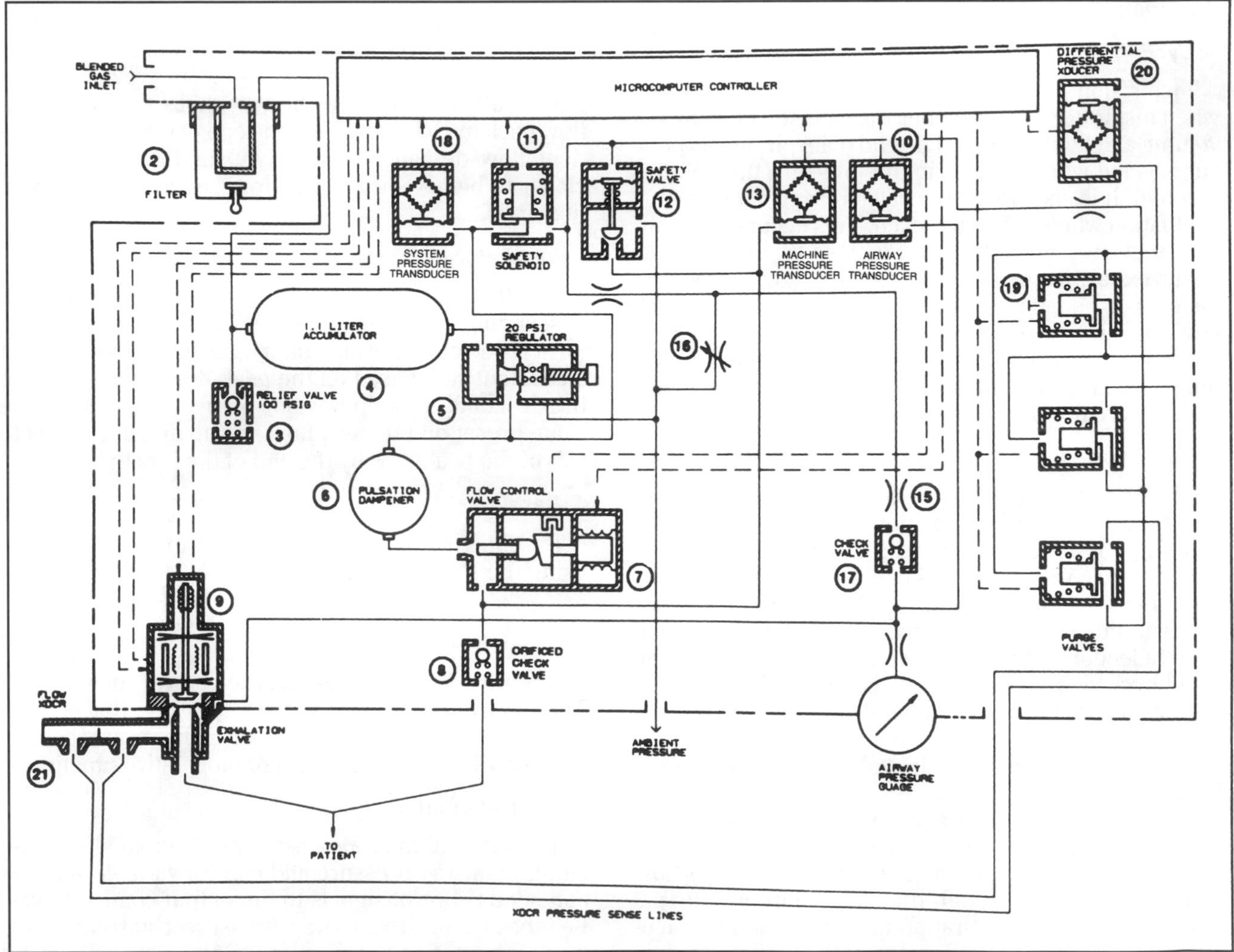

FIGURE 21-73. Schematic diagram of the 8400STi ventilator (Courtesy of Bird Products Corp., Palm Springs, CA)

flow waveform selected by the operator. The exhalation valve (9) is also under microprocessor control and functions as a linear actuator electromagnetic valve. To provide for spontaneous breathing, the microprocessor refers to information it receives from the proximal airway transducer (10). As the pressure falls during a spontaneous breath, the microprocessor opens the flow-control valve in an effort to maintain the CPAP level. The microprocessor then regulates flow to simultaneously meet patient demand and hold the CPAP at the selected level. As the flow required to meet these demands approaches zero, the breath ends, and the exhalation valve opens.

Pressure-support breaths are delivered in a fashion similar to a spontaneous breath. The only difference is that the microprocessor attempts to maintain the selected pressure-support level instead of the CPAP level.

The safety solenoid (11) can be opened during emergency alarm conditions, allowing the patient access to room air through the ambient valve (12) until appropriate action can be undertaken.

□ MODES OF OPERATION

The Bird 8400STi provides several modes of ventilation (Table 21-33).

Control

In the control mode, inspiration is flow/volume-controlled, time-triggered based on breath rate, flow-limited, and time-cycled.

Assist/Control

A/C is the same as the control mode except inspiration can also be pressure- or flow-triggered by a patient effort as long as the sensitivity is appropriately set.

SIMV

The mandatory breaths in SIMV are flow/volume-controlled, flow-limited, time-triggered (according to the breath rate if patient effort does not start a breath), pressure-triggered when patient effort drops the circuit pressure to the sensitivity setting value, and flow-triggered with the flow support option. Inspiration is time-cycled or pressure-cycled (if maximum safety pressure is reached).

Spontaneous breaths between mandatory breaths are pressure-controlled; that is, the flow varies to maintain the pressure at the set PEEP/CPAP level. The spontaneous breaths are pressure-triggered and can be flow-triggered when the flow support option is used. Spontaneous breaths are normally pressure-cycled. Inspiration for spontaneous breaths is flow-cycled in the PSV mode used with SIMV when flow drops to 25% of peak.

A mandatory breath is pressure-triggered the first time a patient effort is detected during the ventilatory period. After that, spontaneous breaths will not trigger a mandatory breath until the next ventilatory period. If a patient effort is not detected during the next ventilatory period, a mandatory breath is then given.

TABLE 21-33 Modes of Ventilation Available on the Bird 8400STi

Control, assist/control
SIMV
Pressure support
Spontaneous (CPAP)
Pressure control

Spontaneous (Pressure Support and CPAP)

All spontaneous breaths are pressure-controlled. The inspiratory flow varies to maintain pressure above the set baseline (PEEP/CPAP) or PSV level selected. They are pressure-triggered or flow-triggered with the flow support option. Spontaneous breaths are pressure-cycled (normally) or flow-cycled (during PSV).

Pressure Control

Pressure control is an available option for the Bird 8400STi. It provides pressure-targeted breaths that are time-cycled. It can be time-, pressure-, or flow-triggered (if "Flow Support" option has been added). Inspiratory pressure is available from 5 to 100 cmH_2O. Maximum inspiratory pressure is PEEP plus an inspiratory pressure of 100 cmH_2O. It is operational in A/C, SIMV, or SIMV + PS. The flow waveform in pressure support starts high at the beginning of inspiration and decreases to baseline as the breath is delivered. Flow pattern will vary depending on the patient's lung characteristics and active inspiratory effort.

Sigh

A sigh volume is delivered at 150% of the set tidal volume every 100 breaths if the sigh is selected. The pressure limit threshold is automatically increased to 150% immediately before each sigh breath and returned to normal after the sigh has been delivered.

□ OUTPUT DISPLAYS AND ALARMS

The 8400STi provides monitoring with an airway pressure manometer and a message window located on the front control panel (Tables 21-34) (see Fig. 21-72). The message window is used to alert the operator to potential problems, or it can be used to select one of the following for display: I:E ratio, measured tidal volume, measured minute volume, and total respiratory rate. LEDs adjacent to the message window indicate use of battery power (not internal), or AC power, and any patient effort that surpasses the sensitivity setting.

There are four primary patient alarms, each with a control knob and window to display the established value. The high-pressure limit control establishes a pressure threshold that, when violated, terminates inspiration and activates an audible and visual alarm. If the airway pressure returns to the PEEP level within 3 seconds, normal ventilation resumes, and the audible alarm is cancelled. Should the airway pressure remain above the pressure limit setting or not return to the PEEP level, the internal safety solenoid will open. Air-

TABLE 21-34 **Alarms on the Bird 8400STi Ventilator**

High pressure (cmH_2O)	1–140
Low pressure (cmH_2O)	off, 2–140
Low PEEP/CPAP (cmH_2O)	−20 to +30, below set value
Low minute volume (L)	0–99.9, below set level
High breath rate (bpm)	3–150, total rate above setting
Apnea interval (sec)	No breaths for 10–60
Flow trans. disconn.	Flow transducer disconnect during operation
I:E ratio	Indicator when I > E (flashing display)
Low inlet gas	Pressure less than 17 psig
Vent. inoper.	Loss of power, extended low or high gas inlet pressure (<16 or >24 psig, for 1 sec) system failure, or exhalation valve improperly installed
Circuit alarm	If inspiratory pressure >29 cmH_2O or <9 cmH_2O below airway pressure for >100 msec. Same pressures for exhalation but time is 1 sec.

way pressure will then bleed to the PEEP level through an orifice in the main flow isolation valve. On reaching the PEEP level, the system will reset and attempt to deliver another breath. If the problem is not resolved, the scenario will repeat itself, and operator intervention will be necessary to rectify the situation.

The pressure limit threshold is automatically increased to 150% immediately before each sigh breath and returned to normal after the sigh has been delivered. However, the pressure limit cannot exceed 140 cmH_2O. The low peak pressure control activates an alarm if the airway pressure fails to exceed the selected value during the inspiratory phase of any mandatory tidal volume. The low PEEP/CPAP control (adjustable from −20 to 30 cmH_2O) is activated if the proximal airway pressure falls below the selected value for longer than 0.5 seconds.

The low inspiratory tidal volume control on the 6400 is replaced with a low minute volume alarm on the 8400STi. An alarm is activated if the exhaled minute volume of all breaths does not exceed the alarm setting. There is a backup rate used during apnea ventilation. This rate cannot be set lower than the control breath rate. It can be set on zero. The alarm silence button will disable the audible alarm for 60 seconds, and the alarm reset functions to reset the visual indicator for any alarm conditions that no longer exist. (The apnea alarm condition can also be reset by the patient.) The ventilator-inoperative alarm cannot be silenced or reset.

A high breath rate alarm is activated if the total respiratory rate (spontaneous and mandatory) exceeds the alarm setting (available range is 3 to 150 breaths/min).

Additional alarm conditions are listed with adjacent LED. An apnea alarm occurs any time a selected interval (range 10 to 60 seconds) elapses without a mandatory or spontaneous breath. Audible and visual alarms are activated, and the apnea backup ventilation is started. The ventilator will automatically set the A/C mode and begin ventilation based on the settings for tidal volume, peak flow, waveform, PEEP, and backup rate controls. The ventilator will resume its previous operation under two conditions: First, if the patient initiates two consecutive breaths and exhales at least 50% of the set tidal volume, and second, if the operator pushes the alarm reset button.

The low inlet alarm alerts the operator that the internal gas pressure has fallen below 17 psig as a result of either low inlet pressure, internal regulator malfunction, or transducer error/malfunction.

The ventilator-inoperative alarm terminates all ventilator functions; opens the safety solenoid, providing the patient access to room air; and activates audible and visual alarms. Conditions that will precipitate a ventilator-inoperative alarm include loss of electrical power, extended high or low system pressure, electrical or mechanical failure detected by the microprocessor, and improper installation of the exhalation valve housing.

A manual breath may be administered during any mode, provided that the patient is neither actively inhaling (mechanical or spontaneous) or exhaling. The sigh button activates the automatic sigh function in all available modes.

□ TROUBLESHOOTING

Troubleshooting is made easy through the judicious use of alarms and display windows. Potential patient circuit problems result in an audible alarm and the message "CIRC." The following conditions should be investigated as possible causes of the condition: disconnected proximal airway line, occluded or kinked proximal airway line, occluded or kinked inspiratory or expiratory limb of the breathing circuit, and transducer failure (either proximal or machine pressure transducer). Several problems can be avoided by ensuring that the exhalation valve diaphragm is properly engaged on the shaft of the valve-actuating motor and that the valve housing is securely latched. This is a complex pneumatic and electronic ventilator, and attempts to repair this ventilator should not be undertaken unless the operator is properly trained or qualified to make the repairs.

Bird V.I.P. Infant Pediatric Ventilator

□ CLASSIFICATION

The V.I.P. Bird (Table 21-35) (Fig. 21-74) is a new-generation ventilator that is marketed as a neonatal and pediatric ventilator that can treat newborns and infants weighing up to 50 kg. It is a pressure- or flow/volume-controller. It can be pressure-, time-, or manually-triggered. Inspiration is pressure- or flow-limited and pressure-, time-, or volume-cycled. It can be flow-cycled with the flow synchronization upgrade. When the Bird Partner volume monitor is added, flow-triggering is also available. Mixed gas is provided by an air/oxygen blender. An auxillary port is available to provide power for a nebulizer.

TABLE 21-35 **Classification of the V.I.P. Bird**

Power Source for Control Circuitry	**Electricity (120 volts AC at 50/60 Hz)**
Power source for pneumatic system	Air and oxygen (40–75 psig)
Control mechanism	Flow/volume and pressure
Triggering	Pressure, manual, time
Limiting	Pressure, flow
Cycling	Pressure, time, volume (flow as add-on with Bird Partner)

□ SPECIFICATIONS

Table 21-36 lists the ventilator specifications.

□ INPUT VARIABLES

The V.I.P. Bird uses 115 volts AC 60 Hz to power the control circuit. External compressed gas sources (air/oxygen) at 40 to 75 psig are used to power the pneumatic circuit. The front control panel (Fig. 21-75) allows the operator to select the mode of ventilation. The ventilator modes are divided into two specific categories by the manufacturer. One section labeled "Volume Cycled" includes A/C and SIMV/CPAP (mandatory breaths pressure- or time-triggered). The section labeled "Time Cycled" includes IMV/CPAP (mandatory breaths time- or flow-triggered). As the mode selector switch (A) is turned, the ventilator brightens the digital display for each control functional for the selected mode. Those that are not functional remain dimmed.

There are also controls for tidal volume (B), inspiratory time (C), respiratory rate (D), flow (E), high-pressure limit (F), PEEP/CPAP level (G) sensitivity (H), and pressure support (I). If the Bird Partner volume monitor is also attached, then flow-cycling thresholds can also be set. Settings are adjustable using dials while the value of the parameter is displayed on a small LED screen above the dial.

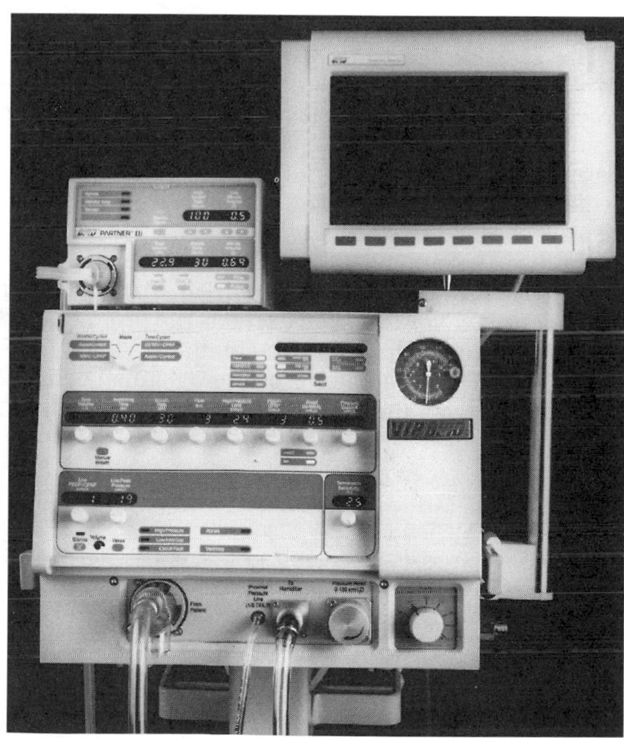

FIGURE 21-74. The V.I.P. Bird ventilator (Courtesy of Bird Products Corp., Palm Springs, CA)

TABLE 21-36 **Specifications for the V.I.P. Bird**

Inspiration	
Rate (breaths/min)	0–150
Volume (mL)	20–995
Peak flow (L/min)	
IMV/CPAP TCPL	3–40
SIMV/CPAP TCPL	3–40
Assist/Control VCV	3–100
SIMV/CPAP VCV	3–100
Inspiratory time (sec)	0.1–3.0
High-pressure limit (cmH_2O)	
Time-triggered	3–80
Volume-triggered	3–120
Effort (cmH_2O)	1–20 below PEEP, off
Flow synchrony (L/min)	0.2–5.0
Pressure support (cmH_2O)	0–50 above PEEP, off
Over-pressure relief (cmH_2O)	0–130 (±10)
Expiration	
PEEP/CPAP (cmH_2O)	0–24
Retard (L/min)	not controlled

TCPL, time-cycled, pressure-limited (manufacturer's terminology); VCV, volume-cycled (targeted) ventilation (manufacturer's terminology).

□ CONTROL VARIABLES

The V.I.P. Bird controls either pressure or flow/volume during inspiration. It controls inspiratory pressure in the "Time Cycled" setting for the IMV/CPAP mode.

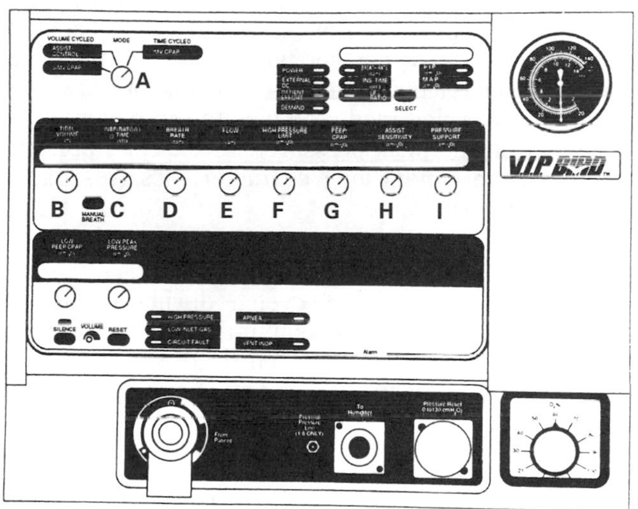

FIGURE 21-75. Control panel for the V.I.P. Bird ventilator (Courtesy of Bird Products Corp., Palm Springs, CA)

Inspiration is flow/volume controlled in the volume-cycled A/C and SIMV/CPAP modes. It is pressure controlled for spontaneous breaths in the volume-cycled SIMV/CPAP mode while mandatory breaths are flow/volume controlled in this mode.

□ PHASE VARIABLES

Triggering

Inspiration is time-triggered as a function of the "breaths/min" dial (0 to 150 breaths/min). Inspiration is pressure-triggered for spontaneous ventilatory efforts when the patient's effort drops the pressure below the pre-set sensitivity level (1.0 to 20.0 cmH_2O below PEEP/CPAP). In the "Time-Cycled" IMV/CPAP mode, the sensitivity is preset at 1.0 cmH_2O.

When the Bird Partner volume monitor is used, two indicators are added below the "Assist Sensitivity" control. These identify the trigger source and the calibration of the control and allow for flow-triggering. In the volume cycled modes, the "H_2O" indicator illuminates (1.0 to 20.0 below baseline). In the "Time-Cycled" mode the "lpm" indicator illuminates (0.2 to 5.0 L/min; increments of 0.1 L/min up to 2.0 L/min and 0.2 L/min above 2.0 L/min). When the breaths/min dial is set on zero in the IMV/CPAP, the display dims because it is not functional.

Limiting

In all modes during spontaneous breathing, inspiration is pressure-limited. An internal demand flow system controls inspiration pressure. It attempts to maintain the set baseline (PEEP/CPAP) level (0 to 24 cmH_2O). In the pressure support function, the pressure limit range is 0 to 50 cmH_2O above baseline pressure.

In time-cycled modes, inspiratory pressure is limited to 3 to 80 cmH_2O. A mechanical pressure relief control can be used to adjust the pressure relief from 0 to 130 cmH_2O in any mode.

Inspiration is flow-limited in all volume-cycled modes. Peak inspiratory flow rate can be adjusted from 3 to 100 L/min. Spontaneous inspiratory flow is not affected by this control. The demand flow during a spontaneous inspiration has a maximum flow available of 120 L/min. In the time-cycled mode the flow to the patient is dependent on the peak pressure and baseline pressure settings, the patient lung characteristics (resistance, compliance), and time.

Cycling

Inspiration is pressure-cycled during mandatory breaths when the preset maximum inspiratory pressure threshold is reached (3 to 120 cmH_2O). When pressure support is not in use, all spontaneous breaths are pressure-cycled.

The manufacturer notes in its literature that the ventilator is volume-cycled. Technically, this is a time-cycling function because the ventilator monitors flow and time by monitoring the flow control valve position and the flow of gas to move the valve in a predetermined sequence to achieve the preset tidal volume and flow settings. It does not actually measure volume. However, we will refer to this as volume-cycling to avoid confusion.

During pressure support, inspiration is flow-cycled when flow drops to 25% of the peak flow setting. Also, in pressure support, inspiration will be time-cycled if a leak prevents the ventilator from dropping flow to the 25% preset value and ends inspiration after 3 seconds or two breath periods (based on breath rate setting), whichever comes first. In a new software upgrade, an inspiratory time display will become functional when the pressure support control is set to something other than the off position. When activated, this control ends a breath if the inspiratory flow does not drop to the predetermined percentage of peak flow. Thus the breath becomes time-cycled. This can help when a large leak occurs, but the minute volume may not be guaranteed.

When the Bird Partner IIi volume monitor is available, there is a "Termination Sensitivity" control that can be used in the time-cycled modes. This permits pressure-limited mandatory breaths to be flow-cycled out of inspiration. This flow-cycling is based on a percentage of peak flow (range 5% to 25% in 5% increments). If the flow of gas to the patient does not drop below the set percent (in situations such as leaks or with the low settings), inspiration is then time-cycled based on the Inspiratory Time control setting.

Inspiration is time-cycled in the time-cycled mode depending upon the Inspiratory Time setting.

Baseline

The baseline pressure can be adjusted using the PEEP/CPAP dial (0 to 24 cmH_2O).

Operation

The V.I.P. Bird uses three microprocessors that help provide speed and safety for its operation. The microprocessors, transducers, and safety valves allow the ventilator to use a variety of algorithms, integrated alarms, and safety features not found in many infant and pediatric ventilators (Table 21-37). The monitors and displays that are available are shown in Table 21-38.

There are several features available in the V.I.P. Bird that help to reduce the patient's work of breathing. For example, when flow demand exceeds the programmed continuous flow setting in the continuous-flow, time-cycled mode, the ventilator provides a parallel demand valve that can augment flow of gas up to 120 L/min.

TABLE 21-37 **Modes of Ventilation Available for the V.I.P. Bird**

Modes
Assist/control (TCPL & VC)
IMV/CPAP (TCPL)
SIMV/CPAP (TCPL)
Spontaneous (CPAP) (TCPL & VC)
Pressure support (SIMV VC only)

TCPL, time-cycled, pressure-limited (manufacturer's terminology); VC, volume-cycled (manufacturer's terminology).

TABLE 21-38 **Alarms on the V.I.P. Bird Ventilator**

High-pressure limit	3–120 (cmH_2O)
Low peak pressure	When airway pressure does not reach set limit during I (3–120 cmH_2O, off)
Low PEEP/CPAP	Pressure below set value (range, −9 to +24 cmH_2O)
High pressure	
Time cycled	High-pressure limit +10 (cmH_2O)
All modes	PEEP/CPAP +6 (cmH_2O)
Apnea (Vol. trig)	20, 40, 60 seconds
Low inlet gas	Pressure $<$22.5 psig or $>$27.5 psig
Vent. inoper.	Red indicator lamp
Circuit fault	Red indicator lamp

During volume-cycled SIMV mode, the ventilator provides pressure support ventilation for spontaneous breaths to overcome the work of breathing imposed by the ventilator circuit, endotracheal tube, humidifier, and demand valve. Further titration of the pressure support level can be used to reduce the muscle work even further as desired by the operator.

The termination of a pressure support breath on the V.I.P. Bird is actually based on the tidal volume delivery to the patient and the gas flow. When tidal volume is between 0 and 50 mL, the pressure support breath ends when the ventilator measures a decrease in inspiratory flow to 5% of the peak inspiratory flow. When volume is 50 to 200 mL, the breath ends between 5% and 25% of peak inspiratory flow, and the percent increases linearly as the tidal volume delivery increases. When the tidal volume is more than 200 mL, the pressure support breath ends when the inspiratory flow drops to 25% of peak inspiratory pressure. This feature allows for better volume delivery in PSV with very small infants who have low tidal volumes.

□ CONTROL SUBSYSTEMS

Control Circuit

The V.I.P. Bird uses only electronic control components. It does, however, have a pneumatically driven safety valve that opens the patient circuit to room air in the event of an electrical power failure or a ventilator inoperative state. The microprocessors accept input signals for airway pressure and control variable settings and output control signals to the output control valves.

Pressure is measured at the airway opening, inside the ventilator, and at the exhalation valve. During pressure-controlled breaths, information from the proximal airway pressure transducer is used to provide triggering, cycling, alarm and display functions, and to provide control for airway pressure waveform. The proximal air way pressure is also measured using a redundant aneroid pressure gauge. Machine outlet pressure is monitored by a machine pressure transducer and is compared with the proximal airway pressure and also with the exhalation valve transducer. If the signals do not agree within certain preset tolerance limits, the circuit fault alarm is activated.

The Pneumatic System: The Drive Mechanism

The V.I.P. Bird uses either compressed gases (air and oxygen) or an electrically powered air compressor along with a pressure regulator for powering the pneumatic system. There is an internally mounted Bird 3800 Micro Blender built into the ventilator. Compressed gas from this blender passes into a 1.1 L rigid chamber that acts as an accumulator. This accumulator is used to store pressurized gas for times of high flow demand to augment the available gas flow from the blender itself. The blender can deliver 75 L/min with 50-psig inlet pressures and a 35-psig outlet pressure. The accumulator allows a total gas delivery of up to 120 L/min. Storage of gas in the accumulator occurs during the expiratory phase.

Gas from the accumulator chamber flows through a regulator that adjusts the driving pressure of the flow control valve to 25 psig. There is another accumulator located between the regulator and the flow control valve called the pulsation dampener. It has a volume of 200 mL. The pulsation dampener compensates for transient pressure fluctuations that occur because of the regulator's slow response time in relation to the change in gas flow during a ventilator cycle. It thus helps to keep a constant driving pressure to the flow control valve. This constant pressure assures the accuracy of the delivered gas flows and the tidal volumes.

Output Control Valves

There are two electromechanical valves that control the gas flow to the patient. The main flow control valve is a stepper motor where rotary motion is converted to linear motion. This is required for controlling gas flow through a variable poppet-type orifice.

One valve controls the instantaneous gas flow during inspiration. It is designed to maintain a known relationship between position and orifice opening. The flow range is 0 to 120 L/min. It is designed to maintain a fixed flow through the orifice with a system pressure of 25 psig. This flow is unaffected by patient circuit pressures up to 350 cmH_2O.

The second valve is used to occlude the expiratory path (closes expiratory valve) of the gas during inspiration and with PEEP/CPAP in use. The expiratory valve is controlled by the microprocessor based on feedback from the proximal airway pressure line and the expiratory valve pressure monitor. This information is used to govern the position of the valve against the exhalation valve housing. This helps prevent rapid rises in airway pressures that can occur in situations such as a cough or hiccup. Microprocessor function also coordinates the action of both the inspiration and expiratory valves.

There is a jet solenoid that is used to power the expiratory valve jet venturi. This solenoid is only in operation during the time-cycled mode. It functions to overcome the inadvertent PEEP caused by the continuous flow of gas through the expiratory line of the circuit.

□ MODES OF OPERATION

Volume Cycled Section

The Bird VIP mode selection switch provides the A/C and SIMV/CPAP when the "Volume Cycled" section is chosen (Table 21-39).

Assist/Control

During A/C mode, inspiration is flow/volume controlled, pressure-triggered (based on sensitivity setting) or time-triggered (based on breaths/minute setting), and flow-limited (based on peak flow setting). It is volume-cycled out of inspiration (based on tidal volume setting).

SIMV/CPAP

During SIMV/CPAP mode, mandatory breaths are flow/volume controlled. Inspiration is pressure-triggered (depending on the presence of spontaneous efforts and the sensitivity setting) or time-triggered (when no spontaneous effort occurs according to the breaths/min setting). Inspiration for mandatory breaths is volume-cycled.

For spontaneous breaths, inspiration is pressure controlled, pressure-triggered, and pressure-cycled. Inspiratory flow varies to maintain the set baseline level for PEEP/CPAP. When pressure support is set above zero for spontaneous breaths, inspiration is flow-cycled.

During this mode, a mandatory breath is normally pressure-triggered when a patient's effort drops the pressure at the preset sensitivity level. After that, spontaneous efforts do not trigger a mandatory breath. However, if a spontaneous inspiratory effort is not detected for a given ventilatory period, the ventilator will deliver a mandatory breath at the beginning of the next ventilator period.

When the breath rate control is set at zero, the patient can spontaneously breathe at the baseline pressure that is set.

Time-Cycled, Pressure-Limited Section

When the "Pressure Cycled" section is chosen, the Bird VIP mode selection switch provides the IMV/CPAP mode.

IMV/CPAP

In this mode, mandatory breaths are pressure controlled. The pressure limit control determines a plateau pressure during IMV/CPAP (range 0 to 80 cmH_2O). Inspiration is normally time-triggered based on the breath rate setting. Inspiration can be set from 0.1 to 3.0 sec, provided that it allows at least 250 msec (0.25 sec) for exhalation. If expiratory time would exceed this value based on respiratory rate and flow, the ventilator will not let exhalation be less than 250 msec. The ventilator automatically limits the inspiratory time to permit this minimum expiratory time and the "inspiratory time" display flashes to alert the operator.

Inspiration is pressure-limited as determined by the high pressure limit setting and time-cycled based on the inspiratory time setting. Minute volume is determined by the set flow, inspiratory time and rate. The flow control operates differently in this mode. If the set flow is less than 15 L/min, the continuous flow during inspiration and the baseline flow during exhalation are identical. The inspiratory flow can be adjusted up to 40 L/min. However, when the flow is greater than 15 L/min, the expiratory baseline flow remains at 15 L/min.

Spontaneous breaths are supported by a continuous flow of gas from the demand flow system. The continuous flow is determined by the flow rate setting. If spontaneous inspiratory flow exceeds the set value and airway pressure drops 1 cmH_2O below baseline, the demand flow system provides the additional flow. Those breaths that activate the demand flow are pressure-triggered, pressure-limited, and pressure-cycled.

When the Bird Partner IIi volume monitor option is used in this mode, mandatory breaths are pressure controlled, flow-triggered (based on the assist sensitivity setting and the patient's spontaneous effort), pressure-limited, and time-cycled. In other words, the first spontaneous effort in a ventilatory cycle (cycle based on breath rate setting) will be a flow-triggered breath that is also pressure-limited and flow-cycled. All spontaneous breaths during that period are supported by either the continuous flow or the demand system.

TABLE 21-39 **Monitors and Displays Available on the V.I.P. Bird Ventilator**

Peak inspiratory pressure
Mean airway pressure
Respiratory rate (mandatory + spontaneous)
Inspiratory time
I:E ratio
Patient effort
Flow demand exceeding flow setting

□ OUTPUT DISPLAYS AND ALARMS

Input Power Alarms

If the power supply fails or if the inlet gas pressure is too high or too low (Pressure <22.5 psig or >27.5 psig; "Low Inlet Gas Alarm"), alarms are activated (see Tables 21-38 and 21-39). Whenever the pressure difference between the input air pressure and the input oxygen pressure is more than 20 cmH_2O, an audible blender input gas alarm is activated. Whenever this alarm is activated, whichever of the two gas pressures is the highest, that gas is "bypassed" through to the ventilator and it becomes the gas source to power the pneumatic circuit. The FIO_2 will vary accordingly (0.21 to 1.0).

Control Variable Alarms

High Pressure Limit (3 to 120 cmH2O)

The high pressure limit serves as an alarm parameter in the volume-cycled mode. When the airway pressure exceeds the set high pressure limit, the display flashes, an audible alarm is heard, and inspiration is pressure-cycled. This also occurs when the machine outlet pressure is higher than the alarm setting plus 30 cmH_2O.

In the event that the pressure in the circuit does not fall below PEEP plus 3 cmH_2O within 3 seconds during exhalation, the exhalation valve and the safety valve are opened. This allows the patient to breathe room air. During this event, if the pressure does finally fall below PEEP plus 3 cmH_2O within 3 seconds, the ventilator resumes its normal operation.

Low Peak Pressure (3 to 120 cmH2O, off)
The low peak pressure alarm is activated when airway pressure does not exceed the alarm set limit during a mandatory breath (3 to 120 cmH_2O, off).

Low PEEP/CPAP
The low PEEP/CPAP alarm is activated whenever the proximal airway pressure falls below the set value (range −9 to +24 cmH_2O) for more than 0.5 second during the ventilator cycle.

High Pressure Alarm
The high prolonged pressure alarm is functional during both "Time-Cycled" and "Volume-Cycled" modes. In the "Time-Cycled" mode, the alarm is activated when the peak inspiratory pressure exceeds the level set on the high pressure limit by 10 cmH_2O. Under these conditions, inspiration ends (pressure-cycled).

In the volume-cycled modes, just as with the high pressure limit alarm, the high pressure alarm ends flow to the patient and results in the expiratory and safety valves opening and allows pressure to drop to ambient. If the pressure falls to PEEP plus 3 cmH_2O, the ventilator resets and resumes normal operation.

In all modes, the high pressure alarm will activate if the proximal pressures exceeds PEEP plus 6 cmH_2O for 250 msec (0.25 sec), but no action is taken. This time period starts 500 msec (0.5 sec) from the beginning of expiratory phase.

Apnea
The apnea alarm is activated whenever no inspiratory effort is detected for the set time interval during volume-cycled modes. The alarm is not functional in the IMV/CPAP mode. The range is 20, 40, and 60 seconds and it is set internally.

Control Circuit Alarms

Ventilator Inoperative
The ventilator inoperative alarm will activate under three conditions:

1. Electrical power supply voltage is out of range.
2. System gas pressure is <20 psig or >30 psig for more than 1 second.
3. Software determination of an unacceptable condition (out-of-tolerance).

The ventilator inoperative alarm causes the ventilator to stop its normal function, open the patient circuit, and allows the patient to breathe room air. When electrical or gas power resumes within normal levels, the ventilator will run a self-test and resume normal operation. For the third condition, the operator must turn the power switch off and then on again to reset the ventilator.

Circuit Fault
The circuit fault alarm warns the clinician of a possible transducer or patient circuit malfunction. The ventilator compares the values for the proximal airway and exhalation pressure transducers during inspiration and expiration, and the proximal and machine transducers during expiration. If the proximal airway-to-machine outlet (exhalation valve) pressure difference or the proximal airway-to-exhalation valve pressure difference is out of tolerance, the alarm will activate. Once it is activated, the ventilator cycles out of inspiration. The higher of the two pressures is fed to the exhalation valve to control the PEEP level. If the condition continues for more than 8 seconds, the expiratory and safety valves open to room air. This alarm does not function during the inspiratory phase of PSV but is active during all other modes

Leak Compensation
A recent upgrade of the V.I.P. Bird provides for leak compensation. With air leaks around artificial airways, leak compensation helps to stabilize the baseline and allows the "Assist Sensitivity" to function optimally without autotriggering. The ventilator automatically defaults to the leak compensation being on, whenever the ventilator is powered down and up again. The monitor display window alerts the operator with the message "LK ON" when leak compensation is on and "LK OFF" when it is off. The maximum amount of leak compensation with an "Assist Sensitivity" of 1 cmH_2O is 5 L/min, and with an "Assist Sensitivity" of 2 to 5 cmH_2O it is 10 L/min.

□ TROUBLESHOOTING

The various alarm and monitoring functions allow for easy troubleshooting with the V.I.P. Bird infant-pediatric ventilator. Manufacturer's literature also provides a comprehensive troubleshooting section.

HAMILTON MEDICAL*

Hamilton Amadeus Ventilator

□ CLASSIFICATION

The Hamilton Amadeus[FT] ventilator (Table 21-40) (Fig. 21-76) is electrically and pneumatically powered, and microprocessor operated. Inspiration is flow/volume- or pressure-controlled. Inspiration can be time-triggered when the rate is set and pressure- or flow-triggered when the sensitivity is appropriately set in the spontaneously breathing patient. It can also be manually triggered. Termination of mechanical inspiration is time-cycled and may be extended by a plateau. Inspiratory flow becomes the cycling mechanism in pressure support. Pressure becomes the cycling mechanism if the safety pressure limit is reached during inspiration

* Thanks to David Thompson of Hamilton Medical, Reno, NV, for his technical assistance with the Hamilton ventilators.

TABLE 21-40 **Classification of the Hamilton Amadeus[FT]**

Power Source for Control Circuitry	**Electricity (115 volts AC at 60 Hz)**
Power source for pneumatic system	Air and oxygen (29–86 psig)
Control mechanism	Flow/volume and pressure
Triggering	Pressure, flow, manual, time
Limiting	Pressure, volume, flow
Cycling	Pressure, flow, time

TABLE 21-41 **Specifications for the Hamilton Amadeus[FT]**

Inspiration	
Rate (breaths/min)	CMV 0.5 to 120
Volume (mL)	20–2000
Flow (L/min)	Up to 180 (indirectly adjusted)
I/E ratio (% cycle time)	1:9–4:1
Pressure (cmH_2O)	0–110
Pressure trigger (cmH_2O)	off, 1–10 below PEEP
Flow trigger (L/min)	off, 3–5
Pressure control (cmH_2O)	5–100
Hold (pause) (sec)	Varies*
Pressure support (cmH_2O)	0–100
Safety pressure (cmH_2O)	120
Sigh (every 100 breaths)	50% of V_T
Expiration	
PEEP/CPAP (cmH_2O)	0–50
Retard (L/min)	Not controlled

* Adjusted as function of Total Cycle Time with I/E controls.

during a flow/volume or pressure controlled breath. Inspiration is flow- or pressure-limited and can be volume-limited with the use of inspiratory pause. End-expiratory pressure may be applied during mechanical (PEEP) or spontaneous (CPAP) breathing.

□ SPECIFICATIONS

See Table 21-41 for specifications of this ventilator.

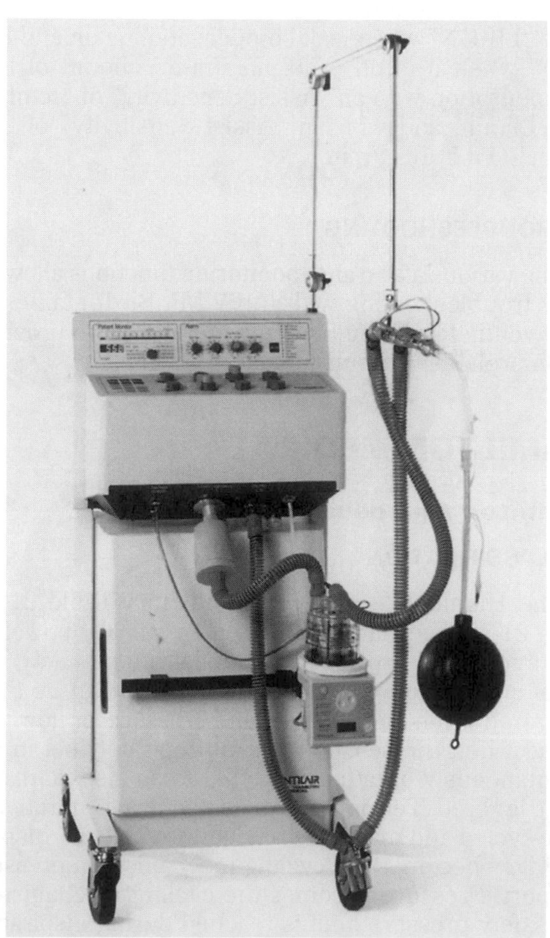

FIGURE 21-76. Hamilton Amadeus[FT] ventilator (Courtesy of Hamilton Medical Corp., Reno, NV)

□ INPUT VARIABLES

The Hamilton Amadeus[FT] uses 115 volts AC at 60 Hz electrical power source to power the control circuit. The pneumatic circuit includes an air-oxygen blender and operates using external high pressure gas sources (air and oxygen) at 29 to 86 psig (see Table 21-41).

□ CONTROL VARIABLES

The Amadeus[FT] acts as a pressure or flow/volume controller during inspiration. It controls pressure in pressure-controlled CMV, pressure-controlled SIMV, and spontaneous and pressure support modes. It controls flow/volume during CMV ventilation. In SIMV, mandatory breaths can be pressure- or flow/volume-controlled, whereas spontaneous breaths are pressure-controlled.

□ PHASE VARIABLES

Triggering

Inspiration is time-triggered in the CMV and SIMV modes when the frequency is set and the patient is not spontaneously breathing. It is pressure- or flow-triggered when the patient makes an inspiratory effort during CMV, SIMV for both mandatory and spontaneous breaths, and in the PSV mode. Sensitivity must be set appropriately for patient-triggering with CMV, SIMV, PCV, and PSV.

The ventilator provides gas flow that is pressure- or flow-triggered for spontaneous breaths in SIMV/IMV and the CPAP mode. To overcome the lag time and reduce the inspiratory work, the ventilator gives a pressure support breath at 10 cmH_2O for the first 50 msec for all pressure-triggered spontaneous breaths. After this period, the preselected CPAP level is maintained for the remainder of the breath.

The front panel of the Amadeus[FT] ventilator (Fig. 21-77) is subdivided into three distinct sections: patient monitoring, alarm, and control subsections. All ventilator settings, except the pressure-limit, are located in the control subsection.

Limiting

Inspiration is flow-limited in CMV and mandatory breaths for SIMV/IMV. It is pressure-limited in pressure control, pressure support, and CPAP modes. If inspiratory pause (inspiratory hold) is used, inspiration is volume-limited.

Cycling

Inspiration ends after a preset time in the CMV, PCV, and SIMV modes for mandatory breaths. It is pressure-cycled if the preset pressure limit is reached during these mandatory breaths. Inspiration is flow-cycled in the PSV mode.

Operation

To begin operation, the operator must select a mode by depressing the desired touchpad (see Fig. 21-77) on the control panel. To prevent accidental selection of settings, touchpads must be depressed for a minimum of 2 seconds before changes occur. The settings include the mode controls that are in the upper left-hand corner of the control panel. The operator can select A/C, which is either time-triggered or may be patient-triggered; SIMV, which provides access to fresh gas for spontaneous ventilation and periodic SIMV timing windows during which a mandatory breath may be pressure-triggered in lieu of a mandatory breath at the end of the window; and spontaneous breathing, with or without CPAP. In addition, there are two pressure-controlled modes, PCV-CMV, a pressure-controlled, time-, flow-, or pressure-triggered mandatory breath; or PCV-SIMV, which is similar to SIMV except that the mandatory breaths are pressure controlled.

When a mode is selected, only the controls requisite to that mode are activated. Green LEDs beside each control are used to indicate when a control is active (LED on) or not (LED off). The control knob labeled "rate" is used to determine ventilator frequency; however, for the purpose of determining inspiratory and expiratory time, the total cycle time (TCT) remains at 4 seconds at ventilator rates lower than 15 breaths per minute. In the SIMV mode, the maximum frequency is limited to 60 breaths per minute. The mechanical tidal volume is active in both SIMV and CMV modes and is regulated by a single control marked "Tidal Volume." The operator may select from either a constant or a descending flow pattern.

Inline (DIP) switches (found on the back of the ventilator) are used to access optional ventilator routines. Option switch number 9 controls the waveform: *off* will yield a constant flow pattern and *on* a 50% descending pattern. The microprocessor "consults" the position of the DIP switches only once during the first second after the ventilator is turned on. After this time, changing the position of the switch will have no effect on ventilator operation.

The inspiratory and expiratory time controls are contained together in the dual-control knob marked "Insp. Pause." The frequency control predetermines the TCT, and the inspiratory and expiratory time controls divide this time on a percentage basis. The expiratory time is set by a small, lighter-colored control and inspiratory

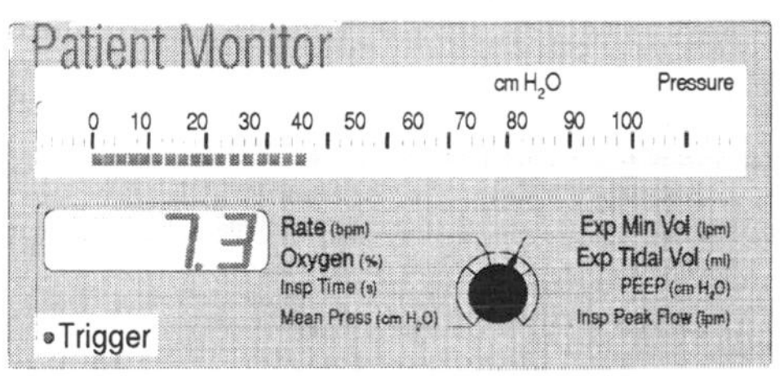

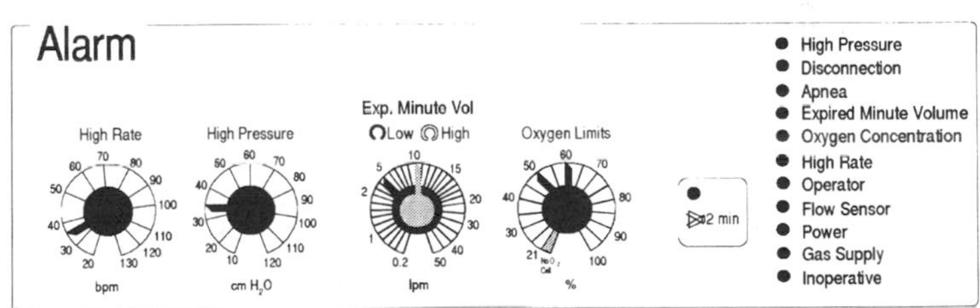

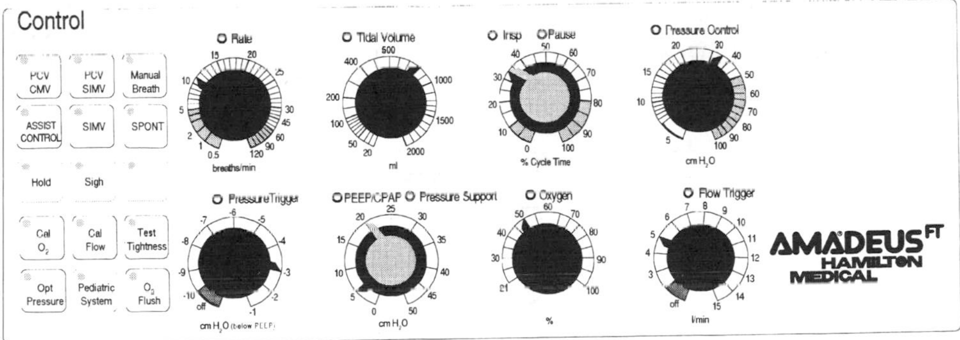

FIGURE 21-77. Control panel for the Hamilton Amadeus[FT] ventilator (see text). (Courtesy of Hamilton Medical Corp., Reno, NV)

time by the larger, darker-colored control. If the two controls are separated, an inspiratory plateau or pause will result. Pause time is considered part of the inspiratory time; therefore, the sum of the pause and the inspiratory time may not exceed 80% of the TCT.

The trigger or sensitivity control, marked "Pressure Trigger," is active in all modes and is used to determine the reduction in breathing circuit pressure required to initiate the inspiratory phase cycling mechanism. The magnitude of pressure deflections is continuously adjustable and is referenced to the baseline circuit pressure (ie, end-expiratory pressure). At the maximum counterclockwise position, the mechanism is off and will not permit patient initiation of breaths.

The trigger or sensitivity control, marked "Flow Trigger," is active in all modes and is used to determine the reduction in baseline flow required to initiate the inspiratory phase cycling mechanism. The flow sensor is located at the proximal airway. The magnitude of flow deflections is continuously adjustable and is referenced to the base flow. A flow trigger level of 5 to 6 L/min is recommended by the manufacturer for most patients. Patients that have high flow demands may benefit from a higher flow trigger such as 8 or more L/min. On the other hand, patients with minimal inspiratory effort or those with low generated flow rates, such as pediatric patients, may benefit from a flow trigger of 3 to 4 L/min. A base flow is used during the expiratory phase. This acts as a leak compensator, helps stabilize PEEP, and also provides immediate flow in response to a patient's inspiratory effort, which helps reduce the work of breathing. Base flow is delayed at the beginning of exhalation to allow the patient to exhale without added resistance. During flow-triggering, the base flow value is twice the Flow Trigger setting. During inspiration, when inspiratory effort is detected at the patient's airway, the ventilator triggers a breath.

A second dual-function control, "PEEP/CPAP; Pressure Support," regulates the level of CPAP and inspiratory pressure support (range, 0 to 100 cmH_2O). Pressure support may be used in any spontaneous-breathing mode. During PSV, a rapid gas flow is directed into the breathing circuit and produces the desired pressure level. As the lungs fill and inspiratory demand decreases, flow decelerates, but the inspiratory pressure is maintained. When flow drops to approximately 25% of the initial flow rate, pressure support is terminated and baseline circuit pressure is restored. The small, lighter-colored inner knob adjusts the CPAP and the outer, darker-colored knob adjusts the inspiratory pressure support level above the CPAP. It should be pointed out that when using pressure support and CPAP, any adjustments made to the CPAP level will require concomitant readjustment of the inspiratory pressure support level to maintain the equivalent level above CPAP.

The Pressure Control knob adjusts the preset level of pressure that is provided during pressure control breaths in the PCV CMV mode and PCV SIMV mode.

Inspiratory Waveform

Constant or 50% descending flow waveforms may be selected. Normally, the constant flow waveform is provided. The descending flow waveform is operational when the "on" switch on the rear panel of the ventilator is selected. A higher peak inspiratory flow relative to the constant flow occurs when this waveform is selected. When the flow decreases to 33% of the peak flow, the preselected tidal volume will have been delivered and inspiration ends.

A constant or rectangular pressure waveform is available with pressure control and pressure support.

Baseline

Baseline can be ambient (zero), or above ambient (PEEP/CPAP) if the CPAP control is used.

Other Available Options

Oxygen concentration is infinitely adjustable between 21% and 100%. The operator may depress one of four touchpads to facilitate calibration, testing, and temporary 100% oxygen delivery. The O_2 FLUSH key pad in the lower left hand area of the control panel (see Fig. 21-77) allows the operator to provide 100% oxygen for 5 minutes, with an automatic return to the selected F_{IO_2}. In this same area of the control panel, the operator can depress the "CAL O_2" touchpad, and the oxygen sensor is automatically calibrated. The "CAL FLOW" and "TEST TIGHTNESS" touchpads permit the operator to calibrate the flow sensor and test the breathing circuit for leaks.

□ CONTROL SUBSYSTEMS

Control Circuit

Mechanical operation (Fig. 21-78) is accomplished by three separate, but interconnected, microprocessor-controlled subsystems: the front panel, valve control,

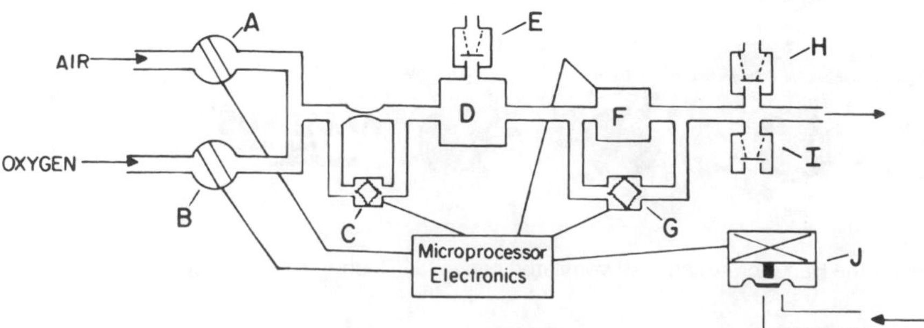

FIGURE 21-78. Schematic diagram of the Amadeus[FT] ventilator (see text).

and the oxygen-mixing system. The front panel processor is responsible for interpreting the input of all physiologic data and controlling alarms and displays. The valve control processor integrates signals from the front panel into the appropriate mechanical function of the servovalve. The oxygen-mixing microprocessor is responsible for mixing air and oxygen in the proper quantities, providing gas flow to the servovalve during ventilatory maneuvers, and maintaining the reservoir in a full state. Each of the three microprocessors continuously monitors the operation of the other two, ensuring proper operation at all times, as well as facilitating the rapid diagnosis and subsequent termination of any unpredictable or errant behavior.

The Pneumatic System: The Drive Mechanism

The Amadeus^{FT} should be supplied with sources of medical-grade air and oxygen (29 to 86 psig) and 115 volts AC through the provided receptacles on the rear panel. The gases are filtered and then delivered to separate electronic solenoids (A) and (B). On demand or depletion of the reservoir, the oxygen processor opens and closes the solenoids as required to produce the operator-selected FIO_2. A differential pressure transducer (C) monitors the flow generated by the mixer and terminates blender operation when the flow required to maintain the operational reservoir pressure approachs zero. The mixer is capable of blending approximately 90 L/min at an accuracy of +3%. After being blended, the gas mixture either flows directly to the patient or fills the large, cast aluminum reservoir (D), which, when pressurized to 350 cmH_2O, holds nearly 8 L of blended gas. An overpressure relief valve (E) ensures that the tank pressure does not exceed 400 cmH_2O, in the event of failure of the gas-mixing system. The large volume of compressed gas in this reservoir permits the Amadeus^{FT} to achieve momentary peak inspiratory flow rates of nearly double the maximal mixing rate of the flow system.

Output Control Valve

The delivery of gas from the reservoir into the breathing circuit is accomplished by the servocontrolled flow valve (F), which separates the reservoir from the patient-breathing circuit. The entire process is under the coordination of the control microprocessor; however, the actual electronic servocontrol circuitry is analog. The flow valve comprises an electromagnetically actuated plunger (not illustrated), position sensor (not illustrated), and differential pressure transducer (G) coupled into a single unit. At the base of the plunger is an orifice configured as an isosceles triangle. During the delivery of a mechanical tidal volume, electric signals from the front panel and front panel processor are used to predict the flow required to meet requirements of the programmed settings. The control processor then raises the plunger in the flow valve to the desired height, creating an orifice of sufficient size to produce the requisite flow. The desired height and consequent orifice size are accurately verified by the position sensor

Gas begins to flow from the reservoir into the breathing circuit. Transducer (G) measures the flow and compares the actual flow signal against the desired flow signal. If the actual flow signal is more or less than desired, the analog circuitry closes or opens the servovalve appropriately until the measured flow and desired flow signals are equivalent. This flow adjustment loop may be repeated as many as 10 times per second, if necessary, and ensures extreme accuracy in the delivery of the selected flow and tidal volume. After leaving the flow valve, the gas passes a mechanical overpressure relief valve (H), which is factory set to relieve at 120 cmH_2O; the oxygen-sensing fuel cell (not illustrated); and the ambient (antisuffocation) valve (I), which allows the patient access to room air in the event of ventilator failure

The exhalation valve (J) comprises a large silicon diaphragm, stabilized in the center with a metal plate. The diaphragm is seated during mechanical inspiration by an electromagnetic plunger. The same electromagnetic plunger produces an extremely predictable threshold resistance and is responsible for generating CPAP.

□ MODES OF OPERATION

CMV

CMV is either time-, flow- or patient-triggered (pressure-triggered) (Table 21-42). Flow- or pressure-triggering requires the setting of their respective sensitivity controls. CMV is flow/volume controlled (volume-targeted), and flow-limited. Inspiration is time-cycled. The tidal volume delivery is fairly constant and is established by the tidal volume setting.

SIMV

SIMV provides access to fresh gas for spontaneous ventilation and periodic SIMV timing windows during which a mandatory breath may be patient-triggered (pressure-triggered) or flow-triggered in lieu of a mandatory breath at the end of the window (time-triggered). Sensitivity must be set to allow patient-triggering. Mandatory breaths are flow/volume-controlled and flow-limited. Spontaneous breathing can occur with or without CPAP and between the mandatory breaths. Spontaneous breaths are pressure-controlled. The ventilator varies the flow to keep the pressure at the set PEEP level. Spontaneous breaths are usually pressure-triggered and pressure-cycled. If pressure support is used (SIMV + PSV), these breaths will be flow-cycled.

TABLE 21-42 **Modes of Ventilation Available for the Hamilton Amadeus^{FT}**

Control, assist/control
SIMV
Pressure support
Spontaneous (CPAP)
Pressure control CMV
Pressure control SIMV

Pressure Controlled Ventilation

PCV (PCV CMV) provides pressure preset mandatory breaths that can be time-, pressure-, or flow-triggered and are pressure-limited and time-cycled. Tidal volume varies based on preset pressure, patient lung characteristics, and patient spontaneous effort if it is present.

PCV SIMV

This mode is similar to SIMV except the mandatory breaths are pressure-targeted and similar to the mandatory breaths in PCV CMV.

Pressure Support

During pressure support, which may be used in any spontaneous-breathing mode, a rapid gas flow is directed into the breathing circuit to produce the set pressure level. As the lungs fill and inspiratory demand decreases, flow decreases, but inspiratory pressure is maintained. When flow drops to approximately 25% of the initial flow rate, inspiration is cycled into exhalation and baseline circuit pressure is restored. When CPAP (small, dark inner knob) and pressure support (outer knob) are used together, adjusting CPAP requires concomitant adjustment of PS to keep it at the same level above CPAP.

Spontaneous

Spontaneous breaths are pressure-controlled. The flow of gas from the ventilator will change to maintain the set CPAP level or the pressure support level if this mode is selected. Breaths are pressure-triggered and normally pressure-cycled. In the PSV mode, spontaneous breaths are flow-cycled.

□ OUTPUT DISPLAYS AND ALARMS

Output displays and alarms are shown in Tables 21-43 and 21-44.The patient monitor subsection of the control panel (see Fig. 21-77) of the Amadeus[FT] contains a dynamic bar graph located at the top of this section. The bar graph provides a visual indication of airway pressure; an eight-position selector switch and accompanying display window are located just below the bar graph.

TABLE 21-43 **Patient Monitoring Information on the Hamilton Amadeus[FT]**

Peak flow: L/min
Rate (breaths/min) breaths per minute, total: spontaneous + machine-cycled
Tidal volume: Expired mL/breath
Expired minute volume: L/min
PEEP/CPAP: cmH_2O
Static lung–thorax compliance: mL/cmH_2O
Inspiratory airflow resistance: $cmH_2O/L/sec$
Inspired oxygen concentration: %
Mean airway pressure cmH_2O
Inspiratory time (sec)

TABLE 21-44 **Alarms on the Hamilton Amadeus[FT] Ventilator**

Operator Adjustable Alarms	
High rate (breaths/min)	20–130
High pressure (cmH_2O)	10–110
Low/high minute volume (L/min)	11–40 or 0.2–50
Oxygen limit (%)	±5% of selected F_{IO_2}
Apnea (sec)	20–40
Nonadjustable Alarms	
Power	loss of electrical power
Ventilator inoperative	microprocessor detected
Disconnection	2 breaths
Gas supply	29 psig
Flow sensor/user	check flow sensor position, or operational error

There is also a trigger LED in this section of the panel, which is illuminated to indicate patient-initiated breaths.

The Amadeus[FT] monitors in "real time" and each setting available for display has been measured. Information for display is gathered primarily from a miniature pneumotachograph located at the patient airway and pressure transducers within the ventilator. Location of the flow-sensing pneumotachograph at the airway allows the measurement of exhaled tidal volume without being affected by compressed gas trapped in the ventilator circuit. This location also prevents the erroneously high tidal volume readings that can result when the pneumotachograph is positioned distal to the exhalation valve.

The selector may be rotated and situated to display PEEP/CPAP (cmH_2O), Rate (breaths per minute), total (spontaneous + machine-cycled), Exp Tidal Vol (mL), Exp Min Vol (L/min), Compliance (static; mL/cmH_2O), Insp Resistance ($cmH_2O/L/sec$), Insp. Peak Flow (L/min), and oxygen concentration (%). For estimation of compliance and resistance, the Amadeus[FT] requires that the operator provide an inspiratory pause before the measurements of compliance and resistance can be made. The equations used are as follows:

$$C_{static} = V_{Texp}/(P_{plateau} - PEEP)$$

$$R_{insp} = (P_{end\text{-}insp} - P_{plateau})/FLOW_{end\text{-}insp}$$

The dynamic bar graph illuminates one segment for each 2 cmH_2O airway pressure, and the highest pressure segment remains lighted, providing the peak inflation pressure, until the next successive mechanical inspiration. The alarm section includes 5 operator-adjustable alarms; 11 indicator LEDs with adjoining alarm description; and 1 alarm-silence touchpad. The operator must appropriately position each alarm control: high rate, high pressure, high/low minute volume dual control knobs, and the oxygen limit (range, ±5% of selected F_{IO_2} or off).

Alarm indicator LEDs (see Table 21-44) provide nearby clinicians with immediate visual information to indicate which alarm or alarms have been violated. In addition to the adjustable alarm conditions, the Amadeus^{FT} also monitors for APNEA, which is defined as no patient exhalation measured at the flow sensor for 15 consecutive seconds; POWER, which alerts the operator to a loss of electric power; DISCONNECTION, which indicates the patient has become detached from the ventilator; GAS SUPPLY, which signals a high-pressure gas (air or oxygen) source failure; FLOW SENSOR/USER, which alerts the operator that the flow sensor has been inserted backward or that there has been operator error in setting patient controls; and VENTILATOR INOPERATIVE, which signals that the internal diagnostics carried out by the microprocessors have detected a dysfunction. The ventilator-inoperative condition also terminates all ventilator function, opens the exhalation valve, and allows the patient to breathe spontaneously through the internal safety (antisuffocation) valve. All alarm conditions provoke both audible and visual alarms. The audible portion of all alarms with the exception of the ventilator-inoperative may be silenced for 2 minutes by depressing the alarm silence touchpad.

□ TROUBLESHOOTING

Internal, electronic, or pneumatic problems are quickly diagnosed by the three microprocessors, which watch each other constantly and abort operation as soon as any errant behavior is diagnosed. A series of tests, stored in the software, can be accessed with the aid of a service manual and will help an interested operator or service technician quickly troubleshoot virtually any problem.

External or breathing circuit–related problems include tears or small holes in the silicon exhalation valve diaphragm and problems with the miniature pneumotachograph. Inability to calibrate the Amadeus^{FT} is most frequently remedied by replacing the pneumotachograph.

Hamilton VeolarFT Ventilator

□ CLASSIFICATION

The Hamilton Veolar^{FT} ventilator (Table 21-45) (Fig. 21-79) is an electrically and pneumatically powered, microprocessor-controlled ventilator. It is flow/volume or pressure-controlled. Inspiration can be flow- pressure-, time-, or manually-triggered. It is pressure-, volume-, or flow-limited and time-, pressure-, or flow-cycled out of inspiration. When inspiration is time-cycled, it may be extended by a plateau. End-expiratory pressure may be applied during mechanical (PEEP) or spontaneous (CPAP) breathing.

TABLE 21-45 **Classification of the Hamilton Veolar^{FT}**

Power Source for Control Circuitry	Electricity (115 volts AC at 60 Hz)
Power source for pneumatic system	Air and oxygen (29–116 psig)
Control mechanism	Flow/volume and pressure
Triggering	Pressure, manual, time, flow
Limiting	Pressure, volume, flow
Cycling	Time, pressure, flow

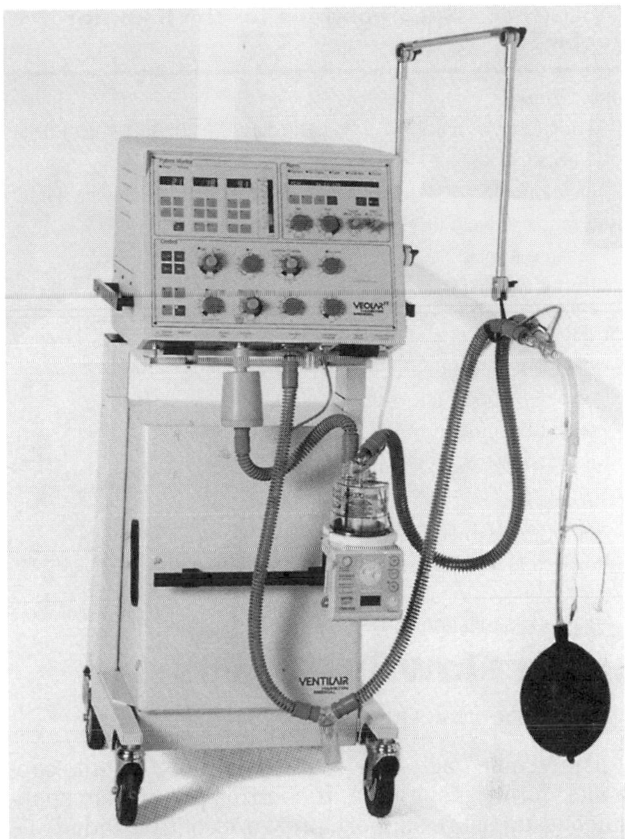

FIGURE 21-79. Hamilton Veolar^{FT} ventilator (Courtesy of Hamilton Medical Corp., Reno, NV)

□ SPECIFICATIONS

Table 21-46 provides specifications of the Hamilton Veolar^{FT} Ventilator.

□ INPUT VARIABLES

The Hamilton Veolar^{FT} uses 115 volts AC at 60 Hz electrical power source to power the control circuit. The pneumatic circuit includes an air-oxygen blender and operates using external high pressure gas sources (air and oxygen) at 29 to 116 psig (see Table 21-46).

The control panel of the Veolar^{FT} ventilator (Fig. 21-80) is subdivided into three distinct subsections: patient monitoring, alarm, and control. All ventilatory settings, except the pressure limit, are located in the control subsection.

When the Veolar^{FT} is turned on (push button on the rear panel), a 31-character alpha numeric display in the upper right-hand section prompts the operator to select a mode. The mode-selection switch is in the bottom section on the left side.

TABLE 21-46 **Specifications for the Hamilton Veolar[FT]**

Inspiration	
Rate (breaths/min)	CMV 5–120; SIMV 0.5–60
Volume (mL)	20–2000
Flow (L/min)	up to 180 (indirectly adjusted)
I/E ratio (% cycle time)	1:9–4:1
Pressure (cmH_2O)	10–110
Effort (sensitivity)	
Pressure (cmH_2O)	0–15 below PEEP
Flow (L/min)	3–15 peak inspiratory flow
Hold (pause) (sec)	0–8*
Pressure support (cmH_2O)	0–100
Pressure control (cmH_2O)	up to 99
MMV (L/min)	1–25
Expiration	
PEEP/CPAP (cmH_2O)	0–50
Retard (L/min)	not controlled

* Adjusted as function of TCT with I/E controls.

☐ CONTROL VARIABLES

The Veolar[FT] acts as a pressure- or flow/volume-controller during inspiration. It controls pressure in spontaneous, pressure support, pressure control, and MMV modes. It controls flow/volume during CMV ventilation. In SIMV, mandatory breaths can be pressure- or flow/volume controlled, while spontaneous breaths are pressure controlled.

☐ PHASE VARIABLES

Triggering

For spontaneous ventilatory efforts, inspiration is flow- or pressure-triggered. The patient must drop the pressure in the circuit below the trigger threshold set (adjustable from 1.0 to 15 cmH_2O below baseline) when the pressure trigger setting is used. When flow trigger sensitivity is used, the patient must generate an inspiratory flow of 3 to 15 L/min based on the set value. Sensitivity can also be turned off. In the CMV and SIMV modes, inspiration can be time-, flow-, or pressure-triggered.

Limiting

Inspiration is pressure-limited during spontaneous breaths in SIMV, MMV, and during spontaneous modes (eg, CPAP). A demand flow system tries to maintain the set PEEP/CPAP level (range, 0 to 50 cmH_2O) during inspiration in response to inspiratory flow demand if pressure support is not used. When pressure support is used, the pressure range is 0 to 50 cmH_2O above PEEP/CPAP level.

Inspiration is volume-limited when inspiratory pause is greater than zero. Inspiration is flow-limited for mandatory breaths. A peak flow of up to 180 L/min is available.

Cycling

Inspiration is pressure-cycled when the maximum inspiratory pressure setting (range, 10 to 110 cmH_2O) is exceeded. Active inspiration is also pressure- or flow-cycled in spontaneous breath.

Inspiration is flow-cycled during pressure support. Inspiration ends with PSV when the flow drops to 25% of peak flow rate for the breath. PSV has two safety backup cycling mechansims. If inspiration exceeds 3 seconds, pressure support is time-cycled. If the pressure exceeds the high pressure limit, then the breath is pressure-cycled.

Inspiration is time-cycled during mandatory breaths based on the frequency setting and the percent cycle time setting (% inspiration is adjustable from 10% to 80%). Use of the pause time extends inspiratory time. Inspiratory pause time is set as a percentage of total cycle time. For example, if the inspiratory dial is set at 20% and the expiratory dial for 30%, there will be a 10% pause time and inspiratory time will be 30% of the total cycle time.

Operation

When a mode is selected, only the controls requisite to that mode are activated. Green LEDs beside each control are used to indicate when a control is active (LED on) or not (LED off).

Ventilator frequency can be set for SIMV (small dark knob) or CMV (larger, light-colored knob). In addition, the CMV control serves as the primary control to determine the TCT of mandatory breaths in either the SIMV or CMV modes. The expiratory time is set as a percentage of the TCT (small, dark knob). If the inspiratory (larger, light-colored knob) and expiratory controls are separated, an inspiratory plateau or pause will result. Pause time is considered part of the inspiratory phase, and therefore, the sum of the pause and the inspiratory time may not exceed 80% of the TCT.

Mandatory tidal volume is active during both SIMV and CMV and is regulated by a single control. Mandatory tidal volume may be delivered with any of seven possible flow waveforms, which are described below under Waveforms.

The trigger or sensitivity controls are active in all modes and are used to determine the reduction in pressure or flow from a spontaneous effort required to initiate the inspiratory triggering mechanism. The magnitude of pressure deflection is continuously adjustable and is referenced to the baseline circuit pressure (ie, end-expiratory pressure; maximum counterclockwise position is off and will not permit patient initiation of breaths in the A/C or PCV CMV mode).

The magnitude of flow deflections is continuously adjustable and is referenced to the base flow. The flow sensor is located at the proximal airway. A flow trigger level of 5 to 6 L/min is recommended by the manufacturer for most patients. Patients who have high flow demands may benefit from a higher flow trigger such as 8 or more L/min. On the other hand, patients with minimal inspiratory effort or those with low generated flow

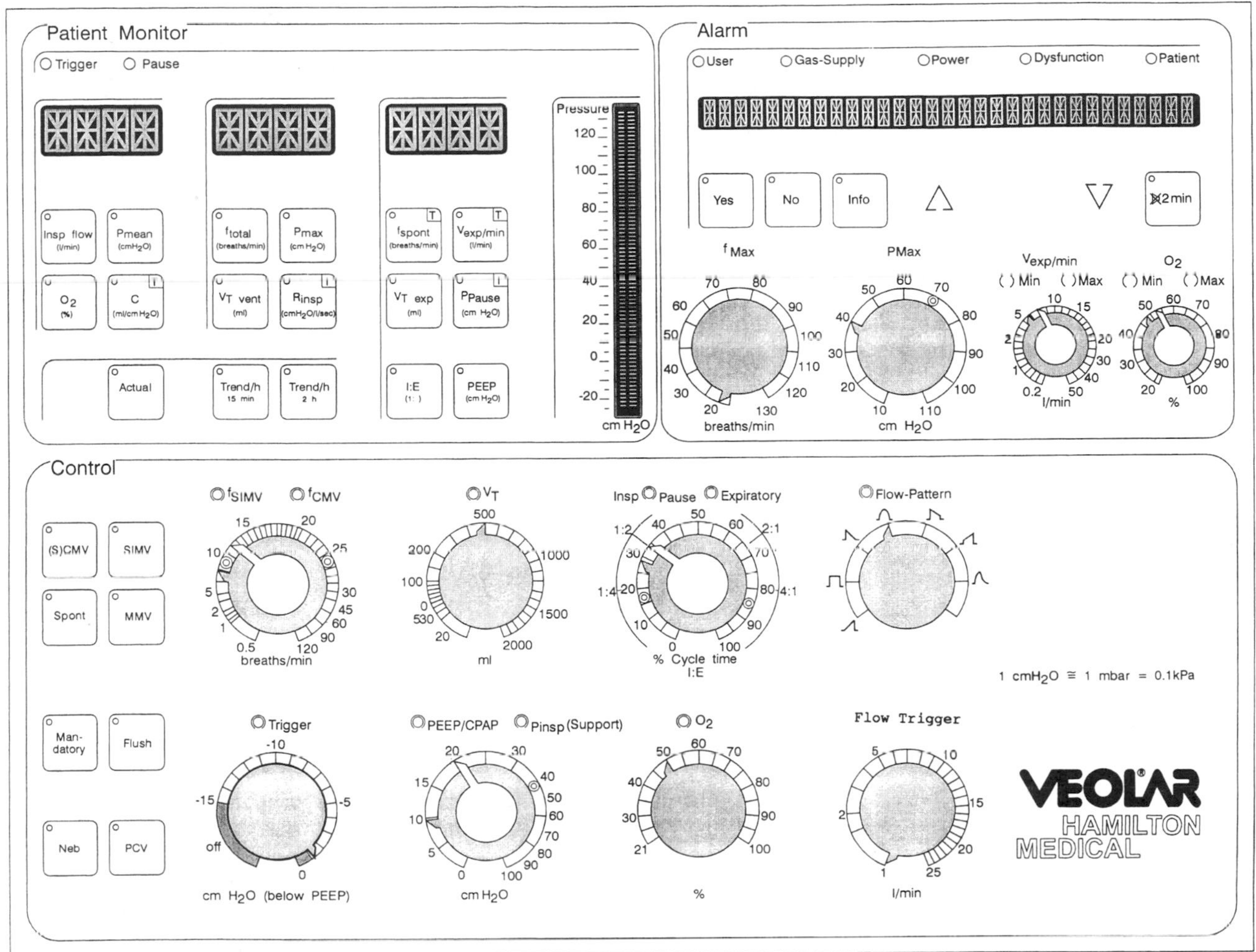

FIGURE 21-80. Control panel for the Hamilton Veolar[FT] ventilator (Courtesy of Yvon DuPuis, Ilderton, Ontario, Canada)

rates, such as pediatric patients, may benefit from a flow trigger of 3 to 4 L/min.

A base flow is used during the expiratory phase. This acts as a leak compensator, helps to stabilize PEEP, and provides immediate flow in response to a patient's inspiratory effort, which helps reduce the work of breathing. Base flow is delayed at the beginning of exhalation to allow the patient to exhale without added resistance. During flow-triggering, the base flow value is twice the Flow Trigger setting. During inspiration, when a patient's inspiratory efforts are detected at the patient's airway, the ventilator triggers a breath.

Inspiratory Waveform

The Veolar[FT] currently offers one inspiratory pressure waveform and seven different flow waveforms. The pressure waveform is rectangular (constant) in pressure control modes and pressure support modes. The seven inspiratory flow waveforms include ascending and descending ramps, modified ascending and descending ramps, constant (rectangular), sine, and modified sine. Inspiratory time is not altered when flow pattern is changed; consequently, the microprocessor must adjust peak flow for the appropriate tidal volume to be delivered. For example, as a point of reference, at any given tidal volume and inspiratory time, peak flow of the sinusoidal waveform is 57% higher than the constant-flow pattern, whereas the ascending or descending patterns are 100% higher than constant flow. The monitoring section of the front panel can provide information about the peak inspiratory flow if selected.

Baseline

In regulating the level of CPAP, pressure support (range, 0 to 100 cmH_2O), and pressure control (range, 0 to 99 cmH_2O), the combined pressure levels cannot exceed 100 cmH_2O.

Other Available Options

Oxygen concentration is continuously adjustable from 21% to 100%. Manual breaths at a set tidal volume or set pressure control levels may be administered during mechanical exhalation using the mandatory breath control. The reservoir tank and breathing circuit can be flushed with 60 L/min of fresh gas by selecting the "flush" control. This allows rapid changes in F_{IO_2}.

Bronchodilator and other pharmaceutic solutions may be administered using the nebulizer control in the lower left corner by a nebulizer placed into the inspiratory limb of the breathing circuit; mandatory tidal volume is increased by the volume of gas required to power the nebulizer. A hinged panel, located just below the control panel on the right side of the Veolar[FT], contains several additional controls: an audible alarm volume control; a calibration button, which initiates calibration; a lamp test; a hold, which stops the ventilator and keeps the exhalation valve closed as long as the button is depressed; and option switches (a series of eight, on or off, dual inline package [DIP] switches).

On all ventilators, all but switch 1 are reserved for options or future ventilatory enhancements. When switch number 1 is on, backup ventilation is activated, which provides mechanical ventilation in the event of patient apnea. The apnea alarm is adjustable from 20 to 40 seconds and backup ventilation is activated when no exhaled gas passes the expiratory flow sensor for the apnea alarm period. The backup ventilation mode also requires switching to CMV or SIMV; therefore, these settings should be adjusted when activating backup ventilation. The microprocessor detects the position of this switch only once during the first second after the ventilator is turned on; after that time, changing the position of the switch has no effect on ventilator operation.

□ CONTROL SUBSYSTEMS

Control Circuit

Mechanical operation (Fig. 21-81) is accomplished by two separate but interconnected subsystems: the pneumatic gas-blending and the flow system and the electronic control system. These are described below.

The Pneumatic System: The Drive Mechanism

The pneumatic system uses two precision regulators (A and B), which accept medical-grade air and oxygen between 29 and 116 psig and reduce their pressure to 22 psig. These gases then enter the mechanical gas mixer (C), where they are blended to set F_{IO_2}; maximal blending approaches 90 L/min. The blended gases are routed into a large, cast-aluminum reservoir, or surge tank (D), compressed to 350 cmH_2O that holds nearly 8 L of blended gas. An overpressure relief valve (E) ensures that the tank pressure does not exceed 400 cmH_2O. The large volume of compressed gas in this reservoir permits the Veolar[FT] to achieve momentary peak inspiratory flow rates of nearly double the maximal mixing rate of the flow system.

Output Control Valve

The delivery of gas from the reservoir into the breathing circuit is accomplished by a servocontrolled flow valve (F) (Fig. 21-82) under the coordination of a microprocessor; however, the actual electronic servocontrol circuitry is analog. The flow valve comprises an electromagnetically actuated plunger position sensor and differential pressure transducer (G) coupled into a single unit. At the base of the plunger is an orifice shaped like an isosceles triangle. During the delivery of a mandatory breath, electric signals from the front panel and front panel processor are used to predict the flow required to meet requirements of the programmed physiologic variables.

The control processor then raises the plunger within the flow valve to a set height, which opens the orifice to a size sufficient to produce the requisite flow; the height and size of the orifice are verified by the position sensor. Subsequently, the gas begins to flow into the breathing circuit.

The transducer (G) measures the flow and compares the actual flow signal with the flow-setting signal. If the actual flow signal is more or less than the setting, the analog circuitry closes or opens the servovalve as needed. This flow adjustment loop may be repeated as many as ten times per second, if necessary, and ensures extreme accuracy in the delivery flow and volume. After leaving the flow valve, the gases pass a mechanical overpressure relief valve (H), which is directly linked to the maximum pressure (Pmax) control. A set Pmax simultaneously sets the mechanical overpressure valve to approximately 10 cmH_2O higher than the Pmax setting.

The gas also passes the oxygen-sensing fuel cell (not illustrated) and the ambient valve (I), which gives access to room air in the event of ventilator failure. The exhalation valve (J), a large silicon diaphragm, is stabilized in the center with a metal plate (see Fig. 21-82 and Fig. 21-83). The diaphragm is seated during mechanical inspiration by an

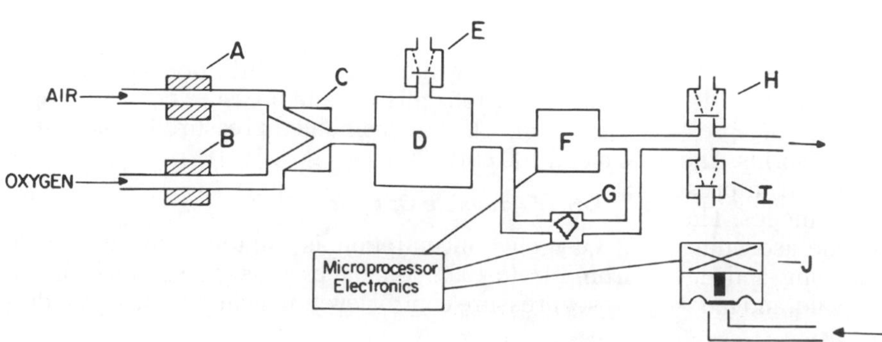

FIGURE 21-81. Schematic diagram of the Veolar[FT] ventilator (see text).

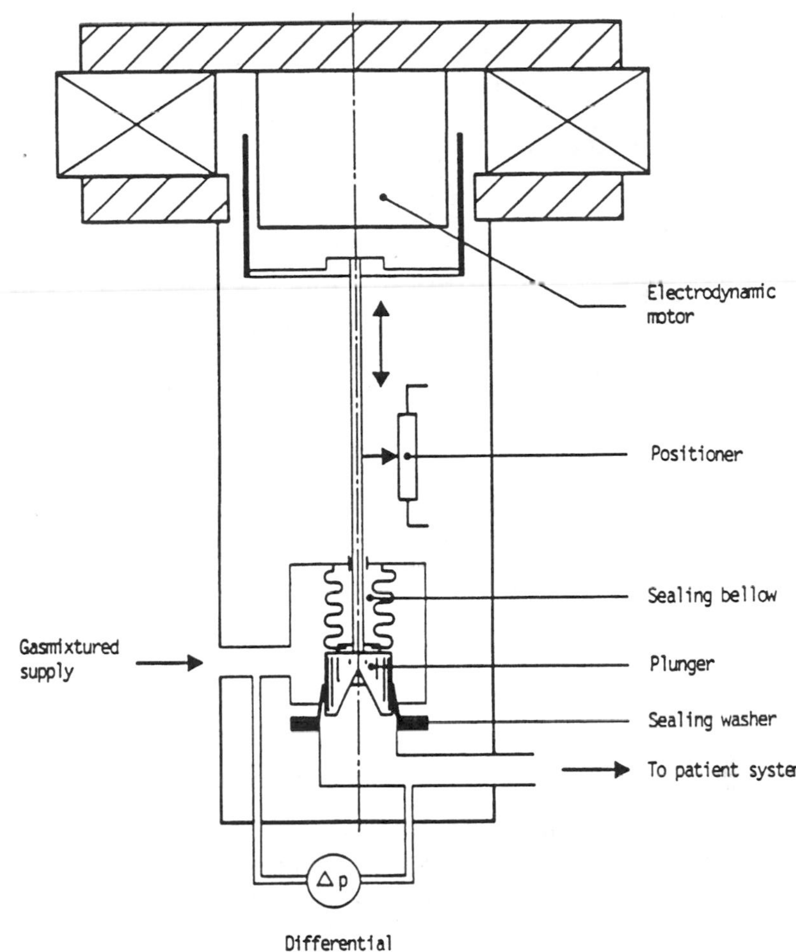

FIGURE 21-82. The servo controlled flow valve in the Hamilton Veolar Ventilator[FT] (Courtesy of Hamilton Medical Corp., Reno, NV)

electromagnetic plunger (see Fig. 21-82). The same electromagnetic plunger produces an extremely predictable threshold resistance force and generates CPAP.

□ MODES OF OPERATION

CMV

CMV is either time-, flow-, or patient-triggered (pressure- and flow-triggered require appropriate sensitivity setting) (Table 21-47). It is flow/volume controlled (volume-targeted), and flow-limited. Inspiration is time-cycled. The tidal volume delivery is fairly constant and is established by the tidal volume setting.

SIMV

SIMV provides access to fresh gas for spontaneous ventilation and periodic SIMV timing windows during which a mandatory breath may be patient-triggered (pressure or flow-triggered) in lieu of a mandatory breath at the end of the window (time-triggered). Sensitivity must be set to allow patient-triggering. Mandatory breaths are flow/volume-controlled and flow-limited. Spontaneous breathing can occur with or without CPAP and between the mandatory breaths. Spontaneous breaths are pressure-controlled. The ventilator varies the flow to keep the pressure at the set PEEP level. Spontaneous breaths are usually pressure-triggered and pressure-cycled. If pressure support is used (SIMV + PSV), these breaths will be flow-cycled.

Pressure Support

The control marked "SPONT" in the upper left portion of the control panel allows for spontaneous ventilation with or without CPAP and/or pressure support. During pressure support, which may be used in any spontaneous-breathing mode, a rapid gas flow is directed into the breathing circuit to produce the set pressure level. As the lungs fill and inspiratory demand decreases, flow decreases but inspiratory pressure is maintained. When flow drops to approximately 25% of the initial flow rate, inspiration is cycled into exhalation, and baseline circuit pressure is restored. When CPAP (dark, outer knob) and pressure support (inner knob) are used together, adjusting CPAP requires concomitant adjustment of pressure support. PSV is added by rotating the pressure support control to the desired level above PEEP. For example, in Figure 21-80, the PEEP/CPAP control is at 10 cmH_2O and the pressure support control is at 20. This indicates the pressure support level is 10 cmH_2O above PEEP.

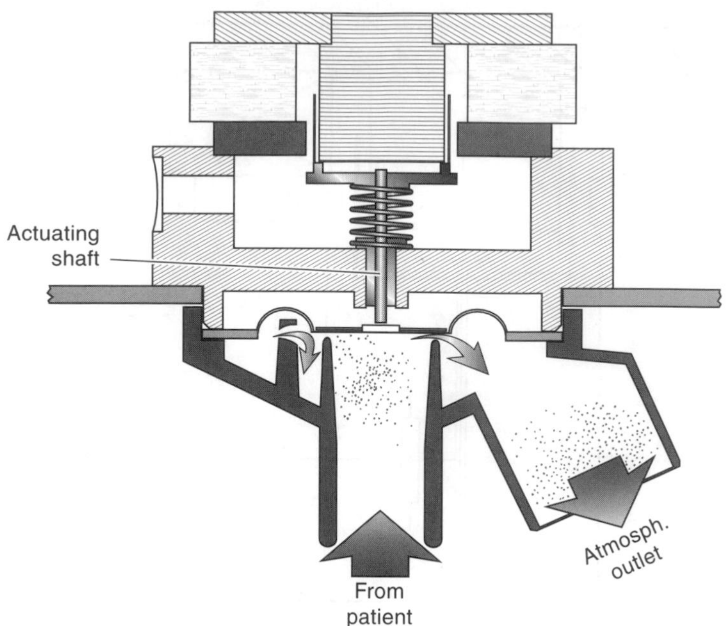

FIGURE 21-83. The exhalation valve in the Hamilton Veolar ventilator[FT] (Courtesy of Hamilton Medical Corp., Reno, NV)

Pressure Control

The pressure control mode can be used during pressure-, flow-, or time-triggered CMV ventilation. It can also be used with SIMV and provides the mandatory breaths in this mode. In PCV SIMV, as in SIMV, spontaneous breaths can be set for PSV. Pressure control breaths are pressure controlled, pressure-limited, and time-cycled. PCV can also be used with PEEP. Available pressure range is from 0 to 99 cmH_2O. Flow varies during inspiration to maintain the preselected pressure.

Minimum Minute Ventilation

MMV provides microprocessor-titrated pressure support of spontaneous inspiration to ensure delivery of the selected minute ventilation. The ventilator determines the level of pressure support based on the exhaled minute ventilation. Pressure support is automatically added to the patient's spontaneous breaths when the exhaled minute volume is less than the preset MMV level. MMV may be selected from 1 to 25 L/min. The MMV mode is selected by pressing the touch pad in the control panel. The alpha numeric window in the alarm panel will shows MMV level. The operator programs the desired level using the increase (arrow up) or decrease (arrow down) keys. The baseline pressure support will be automatically titrated upward in increments of 1 to 2 cmH_2O at a time if the minute volume estimated from eight breaths is less than the selected MMV. If minute volume equals MMV, pressure support remains constant; when minute volume exceeds MMV, pressure support is progressively reduced toward the set baseline.

The maximum-allowed increase in pressure support can be selected by using the high pressure control in the following manner: Determine the peak inspiratory pressure (PIP) at the initial MMV setting. Set the high pressure control to the desired level above the PIP. For example, if the pressure is 8 cmH_2O at the initiation of MMV and the operator sets the high pressure control to 20 cmH_2O, the ventilator can add an additional 12 cmH_2O of pressure support.

The maximum pressure support that can occur is 30 cmH_2O plus the set pressure support level. For example, if the set pressure control is 10 cmH_2O, the maximum pressure support that can occur is 40 cmH_2O.

To monitor MMV, the operator watches the peak pressure displayed in the patient monitor section. For example, suppose a peak pressure of 8 cmH_2O is present when MMV is initiated and later the pressure reads 16 cmH_2O. In this configuration, the ventilator has added 8 cmH_2O of pressure support.

TABLE 21-47 **Modes of Ventilation Available for the Hamilton Veolar[FT]**

Control, assist/control
Pressure control CMV
Pressure control SIMV
SIMV (volume- or pressure-targeted mandatory breaths)
Pressure support
Spontaneous (CPAP)
MMV (minimum minute ventilation)

Spontaneous

Spontaneous breaths are pressure controlled. The flow of gas from the ventilator will change to maintain the set CPAP level or the pressure support level if this mode is selected. Breaths are pressure-triggered and normally pressure-cycled. In the PSV mode, spontaneous breaths are flow-cycled.

Apnea Backup Ventilation

Apnea backup ventilation is an emergency mode to be sure that the patient is being ventilated when apnea is detected. Apnea backup ventilation is available in all modes. How the ventilator operates in this mode depends on the original mode of ventilation selected for the patient. For this mode to work, the operator must select this option immediately after the ventilator is started up. If the SIMV mode was selected, the ventilator switches to CMV. If the patient was in a spontaneous mode (PSV or CPAP) or in MMV mode, the ventilator switches to SIMV. The ventilator will operate in all situations with the current operator-selected parameters for frequency, tidal volume, inspiratory time, and flow pattern.

□ OUTPUT DISPLAYS (MONITORS) AND ALARMS

The monitoring section comprises a vertical airway pressure bar graph (see Fig. 21-80) and three small alphanumeric display windows. A miniature, variable-orifice pneumotachograph (Fig. 21-84), located at the patient airway, and pressure transducers within the ventilator, gather information for display. With the flow-sensing pneumotachograph at the airway, exhaled tidal volume can be measured without being affected by compressed gas trapped in the ventilator circuit, which prevents the erroneously high tidal volume readings that can result when the pneumotachograph is positioned distal to the exhalation valve.

Three of fourteen possible variables may be displayed (Table 21-48). Normally, these variables are displayed on a breath-by-breath basis; however, the measurements are stored in random access memory (RAM). To display trends, a 15-minute or 2-hour time frame must be selected; the trend is displayed for 10 seconds and then the display returns to breath-to-breath monitoring. The 15-minute trend represents the most recent 15 consecutive minutes, and the 2-hour trend is the mean of the previous eight 15-minute trends. Alarms are conveniently grouped together in the control panel, and a series of LEDs at the top identify the source of the problem: user, gas supply, power, dysfunction, and patient. Self-limited alarm conditions are stored in RAM but may be recalled and displayed. Alarms may be silenced for 2 minutes.

Adjustable alarms (Table 21-49) consist of maximum respiratory frequency; maximum airway pressure, maximum and minimum minute exhaled volume, and maximum and minimum oxygen percentage.

TABLE 21-48 **Patient Monitoring Information on the Hamilton Veolar^{FT}**

Inspiratory peak flow (or patient expiratory time) and I:E ratio
Rate: Total and spontaneous
Tidal volume: Delivered and expired at airway
Expired minute volume*
Pressure: maximum, mean, PEEP, on-line
Static lung-thorax compliance*
Inspiratory airflow resistance*
Plateau pressure (or expiratory resistance)*
Inspired oxygen concentration

* Trended over 15 minutes and 2 hours.

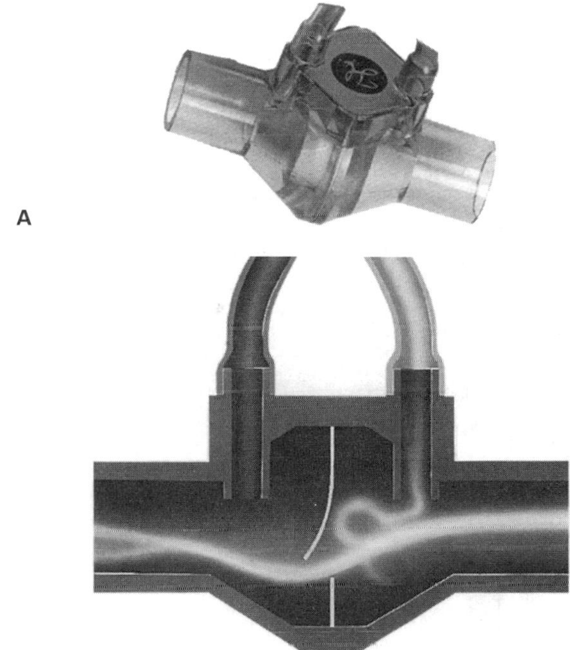

FIGURE 21-84. **(A)** The variable orifice pneumotachograph used as the flow sensor in the Hamilton Veolar^{FT} Ventilator. **(B)** A cross section of the pneumotachograph. (Courtesy of Hamilton Medical Corp., Reno, NV)

□ TROUBLESHOOTING

Internal, electronic, or pneumatic problems are quickly diagnosed by the two microprocessors that sense each other constantly and abort ventilation as soon as any problem is detected. A series of tests stored in the software help troubleshoot virtually any problem.

TABLE 21-49 **Alarms on the Hamilton Veolar^{FT} Ventilator**

Operator Adjustable Alarms	
High rate (breaths/min)	20–130
High pressure (cmH_2O)	10–110
Low minute volume (L/min)	0.2–50
High minute volume (L/min)	0.2–50
Low oxygen concentration (%)	18–103
High oxygen concentration (%)	18–103
Apnea (sec)	20–40
Nonadjustable Alarms	
Fail to cycle (sec)	25–45
Disconnection (breaths)	2
Loss of PEEP (sec)	10
Flow out of range (L/min)	>180
Gas supply (psig)	<29

TABLE 21-50 **Classification of the Infrasonics Infant Star Ventilator**

Power Source for Pneumatic Circuit	**Pressurized Gases (45–90 psig)**
Power source for control circuit	Electricity (105–123 volts AC at 50 to 60 Hz)
Control mechanism	Pressure, flow
Triggering	Time, manual
Limiting	Pressure, flow
Cycling	Time, pressure

External or breathing circuit-related problems include tears or small holes in the silicon exhalation valve diaphragm and problems with the minature pneumotach. Inability to calibrate the Hamilton is most frequently remedied by replacing the pneumotach. Current reports on the Veolar[FT] indicate it is an extremely reliable and trouble-free ventilator.

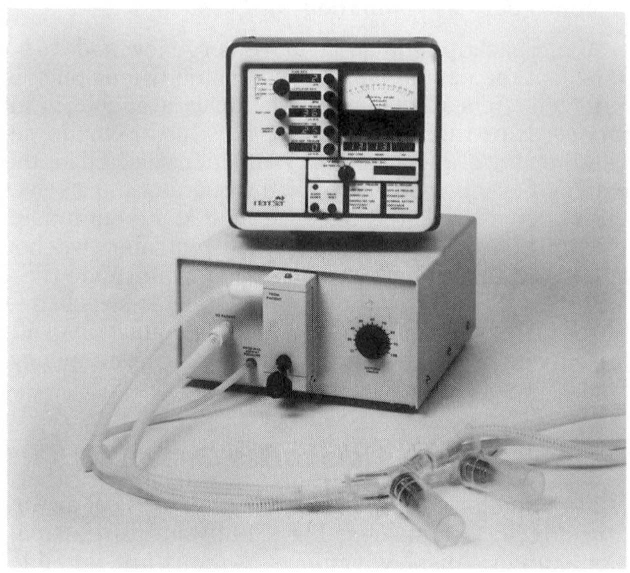

FIGURE 21-85. Infrasonics Infant Star ventilator (Courtesy of Infrasonics, San Diego, CA)

INFRASONICS, INC.

Infrasonics Infant Star Ventilator*

□ CLASSIFICATION

The Infrasonics Infant Star ventilator (Table 21-50) (Fig. 21-85) is a pressure or flow controller. Mandatory breaths are time- or manually triggered, pressure- or flow-limited, and pressure- or time-cycled. Mandatory breaths can be pressure-triggered via an abdominal capsule by a patient's inspiratory effort with the addition of the Star Sync Patient Triggered Interface. Spontaneous breaths are pressure-triggered, pressure-limited, and pressure-cycled. Continuous gas flow is available through the circuit for spontaneous breathing. It has an internal air-oxygen blending system. There is no internal compressor.

□ SPECIFICATIONS

Table 21-51 lists the specifications of the Infant Star ventilator.

□ INPUT VARIABLES

The Infant Star consists of two modules. The upper electronic module contains the microprocessors and electronic controls, and the lower module contains the pneumatic circuit along with the internal oxygen blending device. The ventilator's electrical control circuit is powered by 105 to 123 volts AC at 50 to 60 Hz. Two separate high pressure gas sources (45 to 90 psig, air/oxygen) power the pneumatic circuit providing gas flows up to 40 L/min.

* Thanks to Terry Ailport, John Denny, and Roger McWilliams of Infrasonics, Inc., San Diego, CA, for their technical assistance with the Star ventilators.

Operation

Fig. 21-86 shows the control panel for the Infant Star. The operator can select one of four modes available: CPAP/CONTINUOUS FLOW, CPAP/DEMAND FLOW, IMV/CONTINUOUS FLOW, and IMV/DEMAND FLOW. He or she then selects peak inspiratory pressure, gas flow, ventilatory rate, inspiratory time, and baseline pressure. The ventilator then adjusts the I:E ratio, expiratory time, tidal volume, and minute volume.

TABLE 21-51 **Specifications for the Infrasonics Infant Star Ventilator**

Inspiration	
Rate (breaths/min)	norm 1–150
One-breath increments	from 1–60
Two-breath increments	from 61–130
Five-breath increments	from 131–150
Peak flow (L/min)	4–40
Peak inspir. press. (cmH_2O)	8–90
Pressure limit (cmH_2O)	5–90
Inspiratory time (sec)	0.1–3.0
0.01 increments	from 0.1–0.6
0.02 increments	from 0.61–1.0
0.10 increments	from 1.1–3.0
Expiration	
PEEP/CPAP (cmH_2O)	0–24
Modes	
Continuous flow IMV	
Demand flow IMV	
Continuous flow CPAP	
Demand flow CPAP	

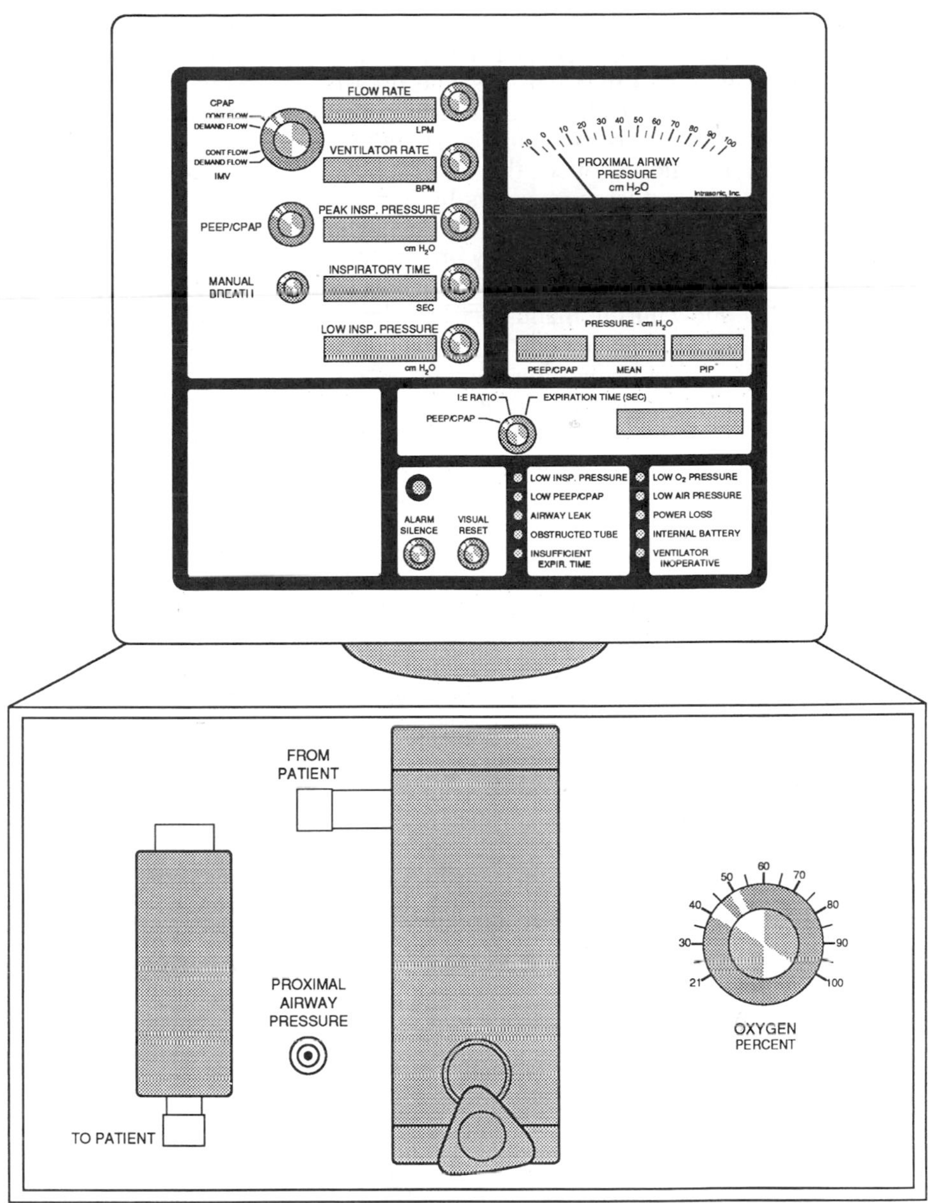

FIGURE 21-86. Control panel of the Infant Star ventilator (From Branson, R.D., Hess, D.R., and Chatburn, R.L.: Respiratory Care Equipment, J.B. Lippincott Co., Philadelphia, 1995, p 340)

□ CONTROL VARIABLES

The Infant Star normally operates to control inspiratory pressure. The operator selects the PIP desired for a mandatory breath. During inspiration, as the pressure approaches the set level of peak inspiratory pressure, the microprocessor starts to reduce some of the flow from the flow solenoid valves until PIP is reached. From the time that PIP is reached and the time inspiration ends, only the amount of flow that is necessary to maintain PIP is provided to the circuit in a pressure-hold manner. This actually reduces gas usage during a mechanical breath.

As with most infant ventilators, however, the Infant Star is really designed to limit rather than control inspiratory pressure. This is because the inspiratory flow is limited to the value set on the flowmeter. For a set inspiratory time, this flow setting may not be enough to achieve the set PIP in the time provided. This depends, in part, on the compliance and resistance of the patient's respiratory system. Therefore, in this situation, the Infant Star actually becomes a flow controller rather than a pressure controller.

The ventilator provides both demand and continuous gas flow in both CPAP and IMV/SIMV modes. In the continous flow modes, the Infant Star is similar to conventional continuous flow, time-triggered infant ventilation until the patient's spontaneous peak inspiratory flow demand exceeds the ventilator set flow. With some other infant ventilators this might increase the work of breathing. The negative airway pressure generated by the patient results in the Infant Star ventilator increasing the gas flow incrementally, by activating its demand valve system until the airway pressure returns to the set baseline. This helps reduce the inspiratory work of breathing and eliminates the need for the operator to increase flow.

In the demand flow modes (CPAP and IMV), a continuous bias flow of 4 L/min is available for spontaneous breaths and functions to maintain baseline pressure, even when small system leaks or leaks around an uncuffed endotracheal tube are present. If a patient's spontaneous inspiratory effort reduces the circuit pressure by -1 cmH_2O, the ventilator responds by increasing flow to the patient in incremental steps of 2 L/min up to a total flow of 40 L/min. For mandatory breaths in DEMAND FLOW/IMV mode, breaths are time-triggered and time-cycled. Flow during mandatory breaths is established by the operator-selected value on the flow control knob. At the end of inspiration, the flow again returns to 4 L/min. The same is true of mandatory breaths in the CONTINUOUS FLOW/IMV mode, with the exception that the flow returns to the flow rate setting at the end of inspiration.

Inspiratory Waveform

The *pressure* waveform provided by the Infant Star during a mandatory breath is primarily a rectangular (constant) curve. In relation to the flow waveform, if the PIP is set high enough that PIP is not limited, the ventilator can then operate as a flow controller, where the *flow* waveform is approximately rectangular.

□ PHASE VARIABLES

Triggering

Mandatory inspiration is time-triggered. This is a function of the ventilator rate set by the operator. It can also be manually triggered by pressing the manual breath button.

Limiting

Inspiration is pressure-limited (5 to 90 cmH_2O). Under conditions where inspiration is not pressure limited, then it is flow-limited (adjustable from 4 to 40 L/min).

Cycling

The ventilator time-cycles out of inspiration for a mandatory breath, depending on the inspiratory time set on the control panel. Inspiration is pressure-cycled if the measured peak airway pressure is greater than the control setting for PIP by more than 5 cmH_2O. This not only ends inspiration, but activates an audible and visual alarm. Normal operation then continues with the next ventilator cycle. This function can be overridden by the mechnical pressure-limiting pop-off valve.

Baseline Pressure

Baseline pressure (PEEP/CPAP) is adjustable from 0 to 24 cmH_2O.

□ CONTROL SUBSYSTEMS

Control Circuit

Figure 21-87 shows a schematic diagram of the ventilator's internal components. The Infant Star uses two Intel 8085 microprocessors that provide an RS-232 serial output connector. This allows the ventilator to be linked to a personal computer. In this way ventilator parameters can be recorded. It contains an erasable, programmable, read-only memory (EPROM), which allows the manufacturer to update the function of the ventilator without costly changes.

Drive Mechanism

Compressed air and oxygen (45 to 90 psig) are required to power the pneumatic system. Its internal blender is fed by these two gases and provides oxygen concentrations from 21% to 100%. Pressure regulators take the incoming air and oxygen high pressure gases and reduce and match the gas pressures to 38 psig for mixing in the oxygen blender. The blender uses a storage system and an electronic snap-acting regulator that turns the blender on and off. The blended gas is stored in the accumulator and is then further reduced to 18 psig by another regulator before entering the flow-proportioning manifold.

Output Control Valves

The proportioning manifold consists of an arrangement of six individual solenoids. Each can open and each is designed to give a specific and discrete amount of gas flow. By opening these solenoids in various combinations, a gas flow range of 4 to 40 L/min is available in 2 L/min increments. Three valves are preset to deliver 16 L/min: one is set at 8 L/min, one at 4 L/min, and one at 2 L/min. Gas from the manifold flows past a pressure transducer and pressure relief valve to the patient circuit. During inspiration for a mandatory breath, as gas flows to the patient, the pressure in the patient circuit builds. The pressure will increase until it matches the pressure set on the PIP control. The pressure is held at this level until inspiration is time-cycled into exhalation.

During a mandatory inspiration the gas flow from the expiratory line of the patient circuit is controlled by a pneumatic diaphragm expiratory valve. Another internal solenoid valve directs a pneumatic (gas) signal to one side of the diaphragm of this expiratory valve. When the expiratory valve diaphragm receives this gas signal, the valve closes and gas flow is directed to the patient. The diaphragm is pressurized by gas from the PEEP regulator during exhalation in order to maintain the set baseline (PEEP/CPAP) pressure in the patient circuit. The microprocessor determines which of the pressures is applied to the diaphragm and uses a selector valve to control the gas flow to the diaphragm. There is a servoregulated jet venturi in the expiratory manifold that creates a negative pressure. It is designed to reduce the resistance to exhalation through the expiratory valve, which can cause inadvertent PEEP in the patient circuit.

□ MODES OF OPERATION

The Infant Star provides four modes of ventilation including the following: CPAP/CONTINUOUS FLOW, CPAP/DEMAND FLOW, IMV/CONTINUOUS FLOW, and IMV/DEMAND FLOW.

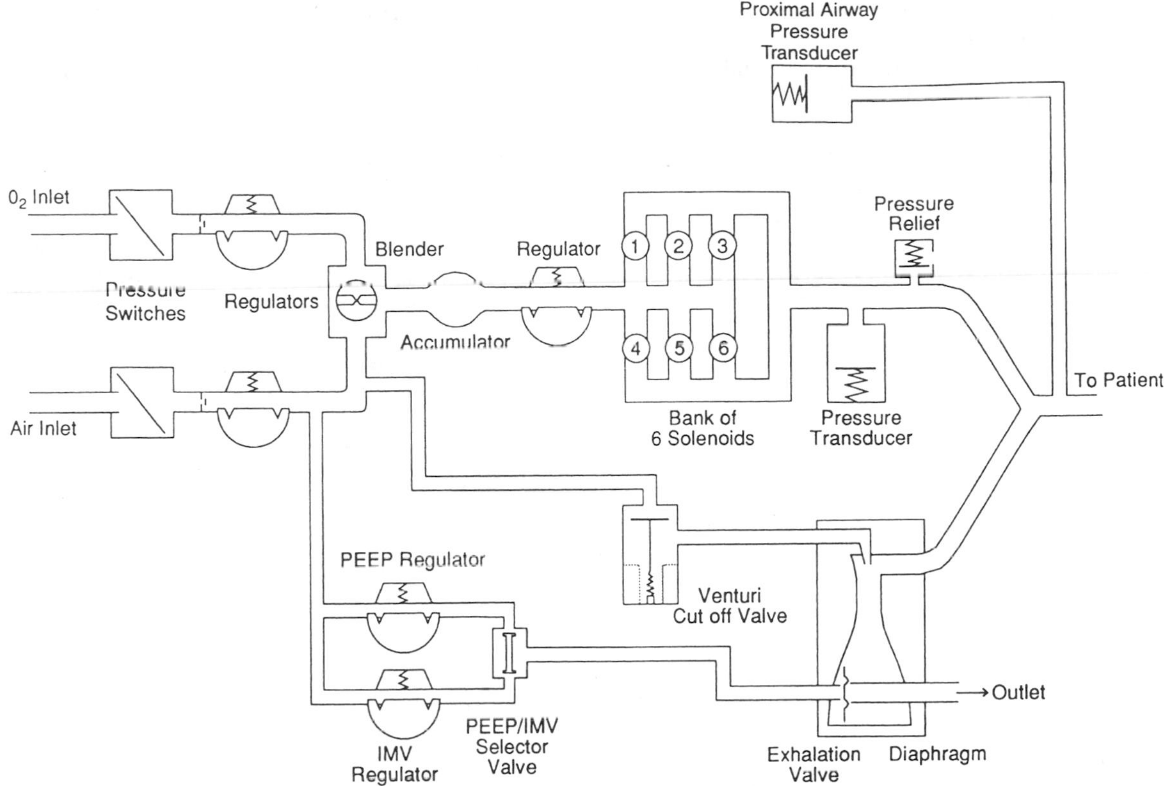

FIGURE 21-87. Internal components of the Infant Star ventilator control circuit. (From Branson, R.D., Hess, D.R., and Chatburn, R.L.: Respiratory Care Equipment, J.B. Lippincott Co., Philadelphia, 1995, p 342)

During spontaneous breathing in any mode, if the patient's inspiratory flow exceeds that provided and the circuit pressure drops to −1 cmH_2O below the set PEEP/CPAP (baseline) level, the flow from the ventilator will increase in increments of 2 L/min to supply the flow needed to maintain the baseline.

CPAP/Continuous Flow

In this mode, the ventilator provides gas through the patient circuit in a flow-by fashion at a constant rate that is based on the flow rate control. The flow varies to maintain the baseline pressure.

CPAP/Demand Flow

In demand flow CPAP, the baseline flow is 4 L/min and is preset by the manufacturer. This amount varies to maintain the selected PEEP/CPAP level. In this mode, the patient also exhales into this 4 L/min flow.

IMV/Continuous Flow

In continuous flow IMV, the continuous gas flow is set by the flow rate control. Spontaneous breathing occurs as described in the CPAP/Continuous Flow section. Mandatory breaths are time-triggered based on the ventilator rate set on the control panel. Inspiration is time-cycled, based on the inspiratory time setting. If inspiration is not pressure-limited as a result of insufficient gas flow or inspiratory time, then it is time-triggered, flow-limited, and time-cycled.

IMV/Demand Flow

In demand flow IMV, the baseline gas flow is 4 L/min between mandatory breaths. Spontaneous breaths occur as described in the CPAP/Demand Flow section. During a mandatory breath the exhalation valve closes during inspiration. Gas flow for the mandatory breath starts at the level set on the flow rate control. It then decreases as the PIP level is approached, to whatever is needed to maintain the PIP level until the inspiratory time setting ends inspiration. When the mandatory breath ends, the exhalation valve opens, flow through the circuit returns to 4 L/min, and the patient exhales into this flow.

□ OUTPUT DISPLAYS (MONITORS) AND ALARMS

Output Displays

Digital displays are available for the following control settings: flow rate, ventilator rate, PIP, inspiratory time, low inspiratory pressure, and PEEP/CPAP (see Fig. 21-86). Also available are digital displays of the following measured parameters: I:E ratio (calculated), expiratory time (seconds calculated), PEEP/CPAP, mean airway pressure, and PIP. There is an analog meter for display of pressures measured at the proximal airway line.

Input Power Alarms

Electrical Power Failure

In the event of an electrical failure, the ventilator can continue operation by switching to the internal battery. Fully charged, this battery can provide up to 30 minutes of operating time, depending on the ventilator settings and the condition of the battery. When this occurs, a visual indicator illuminates to signal the operator that the internal battery is in use. When only 5 to 10 minutes of battery power remain, audible and visual alarms activate. Flashing light indicators and a continual beeping alarm notify of both internal battery and external power loss. The Vent. Inop. and power loss indicators illuminate. Flow is stopped and the internal safety valve and the expiratory valve open to allow the spontaneously breathing patient to breathe from room air.

Pneumatic Power Failure

If oxygen inlet pressure falls to less than 45 psig, an audible and visible alarm activates (low O_2 pressure). The ventilator can continue to operate if air is still available, but the FIO_2 will be 0.21. If the set FIO_2 is more than 0.8, the ventilator performance may be compromised.

If air inlet pressure is less than 45 psig, an audible and visible alarm activates showing "low air pressure." The ventilator will fail to cycle as this model has no crossover network capability.

If both pressures are low, both indicators illuminate and an audible alarm sounds. The internal safety valve and the expiratory valve open to allow the spontaneously breathing patient to breathe from room air.

Control Variable Alarms

Low Inspiratory Pressure

This alarm activates if the set pressure is not exceeded for each mandatory breath. Range available is 3 to 60 cmH_2O.

Low PEEP/CPAP

This alarm occurs if the measured pressure is less than the set value. The alarm condition is based on a 25-second average measurement of PEEP/CPAP. The threshold for this alarm is set by the microprocessor. The microprocessor compares the set value with the measured PEEP level as follows:

IF PEEP/CPAP IS SET AT:	MEASURED PEEP MUST DROP BY AT LEAST:
0–5 cmH_2O	2 cmH_2O
6–8 cmH_2O	3 cmH_2O
9–12 cmH_2O	4 cmH_2O
13–24 cmH_2O	5 cmH_2O

Airway Leak

The airway leak alarm is for detecting gross leaks in the system. If the flow through the circuit (4 L/min in demand modes and set flow rate for continuous flow modes) exceeds the continuous flow rate by at least 8 L/min for at least 4 seconds, then this audible and visual alarm activates.

Obstructed Tube

This alarm is completely automatic and alerts the clinician immediately in the following five circumstances:

1. When airway pressures rise by 5 cmH_2O above the set PIP for a mandatory breath (message window reads "HI-PP-AO1"). Inspiration ends when pressure equals PIP + 5 cmH_2O.
2. When airway pressures rise by 10 cmH_2O or more above the set PIP for a mandatory breath (message window reads "HI-PP-AO2"). Inspiration ends and both the exhalation valve and the internal safety valve open to atmospheric pressure.
3. If anything interferes with active exhalation (message window reads "HI-PP-AO3"). For example, this can occur when the expiratory tube is blocked. The flow solenoid valves stop flow and the internal safety valve opens.
4. When PEEP/CPAP level is 6 cmH_2O above the set baseline for more than 5 seconds (message window reads "HI-PP-AO4"). The flow solenoids stop flow and the internal safety valve opens.
5. When the pressure readings by the internal transducers are higher than the readings at the proximal airway by more than 15 cmH_2O (message window reads "HI-PP-AO5"). Both the expiratory and internal safety valves open.

Insufficient Expiratory Time

This alarm occurs when the inspiratory time and ventilator rate settings are not set correctly and result in expiratory times that are too short. For rates of 1 to 98, the minimum acceptable expiratory time is 0.3 seconds. For rates of 100 to 150, the minimum time is 0.2 seconds. If these parameters are violated, the ventilator automatically decreases the respiratory rate until the minimum allowable time is achieved. In addition to the insufficient expiratory time alarm, the ventilator rate display will flash, indicating that the set rate is not being delivered.

Alarm Silence

When this is pressed, the audible alarms silence for 60 seconds and then reactivate after 60 seconds. If it is pushed a second time (in the 60 seconds), it is cancelled. The ventilator inoperative and power loss alarms cannot be silenced.

Control Circuit Alarms

Ventilator Inoperative

This audible and visual alarm cannot be silenced. When it occurs, the gas flow from the ventilator stops and the internal safety valve opens, as does the expiratory valve. It can occur under the following circumstances:

- The exhalation valve stays closed 3.5 seconds or more.
- The exhalation valve did not close for a period of 66 seconds in an IMV mode.
- The internal battery is completely discharged.
- A microprocessor failure or data disagreement has occurred between two microprocessors.
- Other electrical failures.

The Infant Star also provides an operator-adjustable, spring-loaded, mechanical relief valve. It is part of the gas flow outlet. It is recommended that this be set approximately 20 cmH_2O above the PIP setting. When its set value is reached, this valve opens to vent excess gas to the atmosphere.

☐ **TROUBLESHOOTING**

The available alarms and indicators and the computer functioning capability provide quick evaluation and solution to most of the common problems that occur.

Infrasonics Infant Star 500 Ventilator

☐ **CLASSIFICATION**

The Infrasonics Infant Star 500 ventilator (Table 21-52) (Fig. 21-88) is a pressure or flow controller. It was designed for neonatal and pediatric patient use (less than 40 lbs). Mandatory breaths are time- or manually triggered, pressure- or flow-limited, and pressure- or time-cycled. Mandatory breaths can be pressure-triggered via an abdominal capsule by a patient's inspiratory effort with the addition of the Star Sync Patient Trigger Interface. Spontaneous breaths are pressure-triggered, pressure-limited, and pressure-cycled. Continuous background gas flow is available through the circuit for spontaneous breathing at a flow of 2 to 30 L/min. It has an internal air-oxygen blending system. There is no internal compressor.

☐ **SPECIFICATIONS**

Table 21-53 shows a list of the ventilator's specifications.

☐ **INPUT VARIABLES**

The Infant Star 500 consists of two modules. The upper electronic module contains the microprocessors and electronic controls, and the lower module contains the pneumatic circuit along with the internal oxygen blending device. The ventilator's electrical control circuit is powered by 105 to 127 volts AC at 50 to 60 Hz. Two separate high pressure gas sources (45 to 90 psig, air/oxygen) power the pneumatic circuit, providing gas flows up to 40 L/min.

Operation

Figure 21-89 shows the control panel for the Infant Star 500. Operators can select one of two modes available: IMV or CPAP. They then select peak inspiratory pressure, gas flow rate, ventilatory rate, inspiratory time, PEEP/CPAP, and background flow. The ventilator then automatically adjusts the I:E ratio, expiratory time, tidal volume, and minute volume.

TABLE 21-52 **Classification of the Infrasonics Infant Star 500 Ventilator**

Power Source for Pneumatic Circuit	**Pressurized Gases (45–90 psig)**
Power source for control circuit	Electricity (105–127 volts AC at 60 Hz)
Control mechanism	Pressure, flow
Triggering	Time, manual
Limiting	Pressure, flow
Cycling	Time, pressure

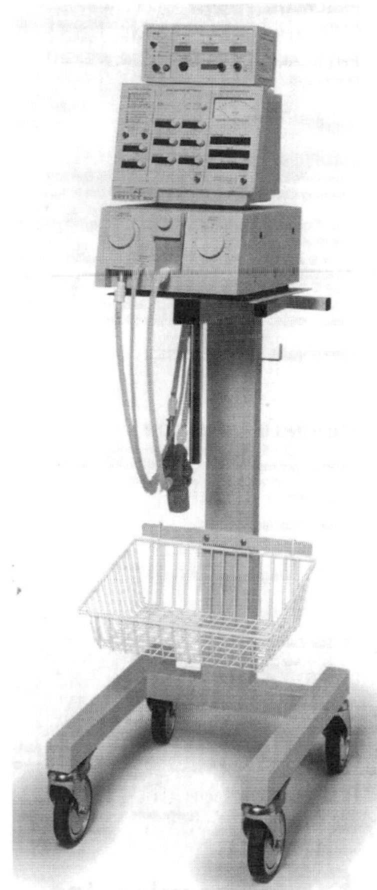

FIGURE 21-88. Infrasonics Infant Star 500 ventilator with Star Synch on Star Cart (Courtesy of Infrasonics, San Diego, CA).

☐ **CONTROL VARIABLES**

The Infant Star 500 normally operates to control inspiratory pressure. The operator selects the PIP desired for a mandatory breath. During inspiration, as the pressure approaches the set level of PIP, the microprocessor starts to reduce some of the flow from the flow solenoid valves until PIP is reached. From the time that PIP is reached and the time inspiration ends, only the amount of flow that is necessary to maintain PIP is provided to the circuit in a pressure-hold manner. This actually reduces gas usage during a mechanical breath.

As with most infant ventilators, however, the Infant Star 500 is really designed to limit rather than control inspiratory pressure. PIP is set by the operator, and this value is not exceeded during inspiration. The inspiratory flow is limited to the value set on the control panel. For a set inspiratory time, this flow setting may not be enough to achieve the set PIP in the time provided. This depends, in part, on the compliance and resistance of the patient's respiratory system. Therefore, in this situation, the Infant Star 500 actually becomes a flow controller rather than a pressure controller.

TABLE 21-53 **Specifications for the Infrasonics Infant Star 500 Ventilator**

Inspiration	
Rate (breaths/min)	norm 1–150
One-breath increments	from 1–60
Two-breath increments	from 61–130
Five-breath increments	from 130–150
Peak flow (L/min)	4–40
Background flow (spont.) (L/min)	2–30
Peak inspir. press. (cmH_2O)	5–90
Inspiratory time (sec)	0.1–3.0
0.01 increments	from 0.1–0.6
0.02 increments	from 0.61–1.0
0.10 increments	from 1.1–3.0
Expiration	
PEEP/CPAP (cmH_2O)	0–24
Modes	
IMV	
CPAP	

The ventilator provides both demand and continuous gas flow in both CPAP and IMV/SIMV modes. When a continous background flow is selected, the Infant Star 500 is similar to conventional continuous flow, time-triggered infant ventilation until the patient's spontaneous peak inspiratory flow demand exceeds the ventilator set flow. With some other infant ventilators this might increase the work of breathing. The negative airway pressure generated by the patient results in the Star ventilator increasing the gas flow incrementally by activating its demand valve system until the airway pressure returns to the set baseline. This helps reduce the inspiratory work of breathing and eliminates the need for the operator to increase flow.

When the background flow is not being used, the ventilator provides flow through its demand valve system. If a patient's spontaneous inspiratory effort reduces the circuit pressure by -1 cmH_2O, the ventilator responds by increasing flow to the patient in incremental steps of 2 L/min, up to a total flow of 40 L/min. Mandatory breaths in this operation are time-triggered and time-cycled. Flow during mandatory breaths is established by the operator-selected value on the flow control.

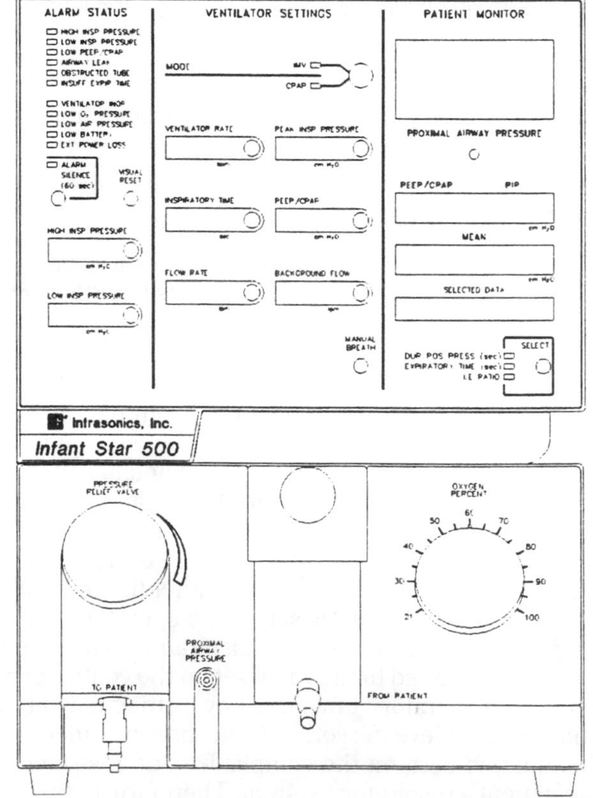

FIGURE 21-89. Control panel of the Infant Star 500 ventilator (Courtesy of Infrasonics, San Diego, CA).

Inspiratory Waveform

The pressure waveform provided by the Infant Star 500 during a mandatory breath is primarily a rectangular (constant) curve. In relation to the flow waveform, if the PIP is set high enough that PIP is not limited, then the ventilator can operate as a flow controller where the flow waveform is approximately rectangular.

□ PHASE VARIABLES

Triggering

Mandatory inspiration is time-triggered. This is a function of the ventilator rate set by the operator. Inspiration can also be manually triggered by pressing the manual breath button.

Limiting

Inspiration is pressure-limited (5 to 90 cmH_2O). Under conditions where inspiration is not pressure-limited, then it is flow-limited (adjustable from 4 to 40 L/min).

Cycling

The ventilator time-cycles out of inspiration for a mandatory breath depending on the inspiratory time set on the control panel. Inspiration is pressure-cycled if the measured peak airway pressure meets or exceeds the high inspiratory pressure alarm setting. This not only ends inspiration but activates an audible and visual alarm. Normal operation then continues with the next ventilator cycle. This function can be overridden by the mechnical pressure-limiting pop-off valve.

Baseline Pressure

Baseline pressure (PEEP/CPAP) is adjustable from 0 to 24 cmH_2O.

□ CONTROL SUBSYSTEMS

Control Circuit

The Infant Star 500 uses two Intel 8032 microprocessors, which provide an RS-232 serial output connector. This allows the ventilator to be linked to a personal computer. In this way ventilator parameters can be recorded. It contains an EPROM, which allows the manufacturer to update the function of the ventilator without costly changes.

Drive Mechanism

Compressed air and oxygen (45 to 90 psig) are required to power the pneumatic system. Its internal blender is fed by these two gases and provides oxygen delivery from 21% to 100%. Pressure regulators take the incoming air and oxygen high pressure gases and reduce and match the gas pressures to 38 psig for mixing in the oxygen blender. The blender uses a storage system and an electronic snap-acting regulator that turns the blender on and off. The blended gas is stored in the accumulator and is then further reduced to 18 psig by another regulator before entering the flow-proportioning manifold.

Output Control Valves

The proportioning manifold consists of an arrangement of six individual solenoids. Each can open and each is designed to give a specific and discrete amount of gas flow. By opening these solenoids in various combinations, a gas flow range of 4 to 40 L/min is available in 2 L/min increments. Three valves are preset to deliver 16 L/min: one is set at 8 L/min, one at 4 L/min, and one at 2 L/min. Gas from the manifold flows past a pressure transducer and pressure relief valve to the patient circuit. During inspiration for a mandatory breath, as gas flows to the patient the pressure in the patient circuit builds. The pressure will increase until it matches the pressure set on the PIP control. The pressure is held at this level until inspiratory is time-cycled into exhalation.

During a mandatory inspiration, the gas flow from the expiratory line of the patient circuit is controlled by a pneumatic diaphragm expiratory valve. Another internal solenoid valve directs a pneumatic (gas) signal to one side of the diaphragm of this expiratory valve. When the expiratory valve diaphragm receives this gas signal, the valve closes and gas flow is directed to the patient. The diaphragm is pressurized by gas from the PEEP regulator during exhalation to maintain the set baseline (PEEP/CPAP) pressure in the patient circuit. The microprocessor determines which of the pressures is applied to the diaphragm and uses a selector valve to control the gas flow to the diaphragm. There is a servoregulated jet venturi in the expiratory manifold that creates a negative pressure. It is designed to reduce the resistance to exhalation through the expiratory valve that can cause inadvertent PEEP in the patient circuit.

□ MODES OF OPERATION

The Infant Star 500 provides two modes of ventilation, IMV and CPAP.

CPAP

In this mode, the ventilator provides background flow through the patient circuit in a flow-by fashion at a constant rate that is based on the background flow knob. The level of PEEP/CPAP selected on the control panel adjusts the baseline pressure. If the patient's inspiratory flow exceeds the flow provided and the pressure drops to −1 cmH_2O below the set PEEP/CPAP (baseline) level, the demand system automatically supplies additional flow.

IMV

In IMV mode, mandatory breaths are time-triggered based on the ventilator rate set on the control panel. Inspiration is time-cycled based on the inspiratory time setting. If inspiration is not pressure-limited as a result of insufficient gas flow or inspiratory time, then it is time-triggered, flow-limited, and time-cycled. The background flow sets the amount of flow through the circuit during exhalation. This flow is also available for spontaneous breathing. During a spontaneous breath, if the pressure in the circuit drops to −1 cmH_2O because of inadequate flow to meet a patient's inspiratory demand, the demand system will automatically supply additional flow.

□ OUTPUT DISPLAYS (MONITORS) AND ALARMS

Output Displays

In the patient monitoring section of the front panel, there are displays for proximal airway pressure (an analog meter for display of pressure measured at the proximal airway line) with a range from −10 to 120 cmH_2O, PEEP/CPAP, PIP, mean airway pressure (0 to 99.9 cmH_2O), and selected data including duration of positive pressure (0.2 to 5.0 sec), expiratory time (0.2 to 59.9 sec), and I:E ratio (1:0.1 to 1:99.9).

Input Power Alarms

Electrical Power Failure

In the event of an electrical failure, the ventilator can continue operation by switching to the internal battery. Fully charged, this can provide up to 30 minutes of operating time depending on the ventilator settings and the condition of the battery. When an electrical failure occurs, a visual indicator illuminates to signal the operator that the internal battery is in use. When only 5 to 10 minutes of battery power remain, audible and visual alarms activate. Flashing light indicators and a continual beeping alarm notify of both internal battery and external power loss. The "Low Battery" and "Ext. Power Loss" indicators illuminate. Flow is stopped and the internal safety valve and the expiratory valve open to allow the spontaneously breathing patient to breathe from room air.

Pneumatic Power Failure

If oxygen inlet pressure falls to less than 45 psig, an audible and visible alarm activates (low O_2 pressure). The ventilator can continue to operate if air is still available, but the FIO_2 will be 0.21. If the set FIO_2 is more than 0.8, the ventilator performance may be compromised.

If air inlet pressure is less than 45 psig, an audible and visible alarm activates showing "low air pressure." The ventilator can continue to operate but provides an FIO_2

of 1.0. For FIO_2 values set less than 0.30, the ventilator performance may be compromised.

If both pressures are low, both indicators illuminate and an audible alarm sounds. The internal safety valve and the expiratory valve open to allow the spontaneously breathing patient to breathe from room air.

Control Variable Alarms

High Inspiratory Pressure

This alarm is activated if the established pressure limit is exceeded (range 5 to 105 cmH_2O). When this occurs, the ventilator opens the expiratory valve, gas flow stops, an audible alarm sounds, and the "High Insp. Pressure" LED illuminates and the display reads "HI PIP AO1" in the PEEP/CPAP, PIP, and SELECTED DATA displays. To ensure patient safety, the maximum high inspiratory pressure alarm is 15 cmH_2O above the PIP. If the operator sets the high inspiratory pressure alarm more than 15 cmH_2O, the alarm display flashes and the microprocessor automatically sets the value to 15 cmH_2O above PIP.

Low Inspiratory Pressure

This alarm activates if the set pressure is not exceeded for each mandatory breath. Range available is 3 to 60 cmH_2O. This alarm will be activated if there is a breathing circuit leak, if the control settings are inappropriate, or if an incorrect pressure relief valve setting is used.

Low PEEP/CPAP

This alarm occurs if the measured pressure is less than the set value. The alarm condition is based on a 25-second average measurement of PEEP/CPAP. The threshold for this alarm is set by the microprocessor. The microprocessor compares the set value to the measured PEEP level as follows:

IF PEEP/CPAP IS SET AT:	PRESSURE DIFFERENCE BETWEEN SETTING AND AIRWAY REQUIRED TO ACTIVATE ALARM:
0–5 cmH_2O	2 cmH_2O
6–8 cmH_2O	3 cmH_2O
9–12 cmH_2O	4 cmH_2O
13–24 cmH_2O	5 cmH_2O

Airway Leak

The airway leak alarm is for detecting gross leaks in the patient circuit connections for PEEP/CPAP settings of 3 cmH_2O or more. It most commonly occurs when low background flow rates are used and when increased flow exceeds background flow by 13 L/min for 4 seconds or more.

Obstructed Tube

This alarm is completely automatic and alerts the clinician immediately in the following circumstances:

1. When airway pressures rise by 5 cmH_2O above the set high inspiratory pressure alarm for a mandatory breath. Inspiration ends when pressure equals HIP + 5 cmH_2O. Message displayed on the "Selected Data" screen is HI PIP, AO2.
2. If anything interferes with active exhalation. This can occur when the expiratory tube is blocked (message window reads "HI-PP-AO3"). The flow solenoids stop flow and the internal safety valve opens.
3. When PEEP/CPAP pressure rises 6 cmH_2O above the set value for more than 5 seconds. Message displayed on the "Selected Data" screen is HI PIP, AO4.
4. When the pressure readings by the internal transducers are higher than the readings at the proximal airway by more than 10 cmH_2O above HIP alarm (message window reads "HI-PP-AO5"). Both the expiratory and internal safety valves open.

Insufficient Expiratory Time

This alarm occurs when the inspiratory time and ventilator rate settings are not set correctly and result in expiratory times that are too short. For rates of 1 to 98, the minimum acceptable expiratory time is 0.3 seconds. For rates of 100 to 150, the minimum time is 0.2 seconds. If these parameters are violated, the ventilator automatically decreases the respiratory rate until the minimum allowable time is achieved. In addition to the insufficient expiratory time alarm, the ventilator rate display will flash, indicating that the set rate is not being delivered.

Alarm Silence

When this is pressed, the audible alarms silence for 60 seconds and then reactivate after 60 seconds. If it is pushed a second time (in the 60 seconds), it is cancelled. The ventilator inoperative and low battery alarms cannot be silenced.

Control Circuit Alarms

Ventilator Inoperative

This audible and visual alarm cannot be silenced. When it occurs, the gas flow from the ventilator stops and the internal safety valve opens, as does the expiratory valve. It can occur under the following circumstances:

- The exhalation valve stays closed 3.5 seconds or more.
- The exhalation valve did not close for a period of 66 seconds in an IMV mode.
- The internal battery is completely discharged.
- A microprocessor failure or data disagreement has occurred between two microprocessors.
- Other electrical failures.

The Infant Star 500 also provides an operator-adjustable, spring-loaded, mechanical relief valve. It is part of the gas flow outlet. It is recommended that this be set 10 to 15 cmH_2O above the high inspiratory pressure alarm setting. When its set value is reached, this valve opens to vent excess gas to the atmosphere.

☐ TROUBLESHOOTING

The available alarms and indicators and the computer functioning capability provide quick evaluation and solution to most of the common problems that occur. The operating manual provides a table listing common problems that may require troubleshooting.

TABLE 21-54 **Classification of the Infrasonics Adult Star Ventilator**

Power Source for Pneumatic Circuit	**Pressurized Gases (30–90 psig)**
Power source for control circuit	Electricity (115 volts AC at 50–60 Hz)
Control mechanism	Pressure, flow
Triggering	Pressure, time, manual
Limiting	Pressure, volume, flow
Cycling	Time, pressure, flow

Infrasonics Adult Star Ventilator*

□ CLASSIFICATION

The Infrasonics Adult Star ventilator is a pressure or flow controller (Table 21-54) (Fig. 21-90). Inspiration can be pressure-, time-, or manually triggered. It can be pressure-, volume-, or flow-limited and is pressure-, flow-, or time-cycled. It has an internal air-oxygen blending system and a built-in internal compressor.

A separate nebulizer outlet port provides a means to power a micronebulizer without altering volume or oxygen delivery. The nebulizer is supplied by a 10-psig gas source, which provides an 8-L/min gas flow. The nebulizer gas volume (flow) is removed from the set tidal volume prior to leaving the ventilator outlet. This volume of gas is returned to the patient through the nebulizer. As a result, set tidal volume and FIO_2 are not changed. The nebulizer automatically shuts off after 30 minutes or when its control button is pressed a second time.

□ SPECIFICATIONS

Table 21-55 shows a list of the ventilator's specifications. The Adult Star can be used for pediatric or adult patients.

□ INPUT VARIABLES

The Adult Star's electrical control circuit is powered by 107 to 132 volts AC at 60 Hz. It is a fully microprocessor-operated system. Two separate high pressure gas sources (30 to 90 psig, air/oxygen) power the pneumatic control circuit, providing gas flows up to 160 L/min. An optional air compressor housed in an enclosed, wheeled base is available and replaces the wheeled stand.

Operation

The front control panel (Fig. 21-91) allows the operator to communicate with any of three computer screens that are displayed on a cathode ray tube (CRT). Through these screens, the operator can select the mode of ventilation, desired control variables, monitoring functions, and alarm settings. Selections are chosen using the front control panel while viewing the appropriate display screen.

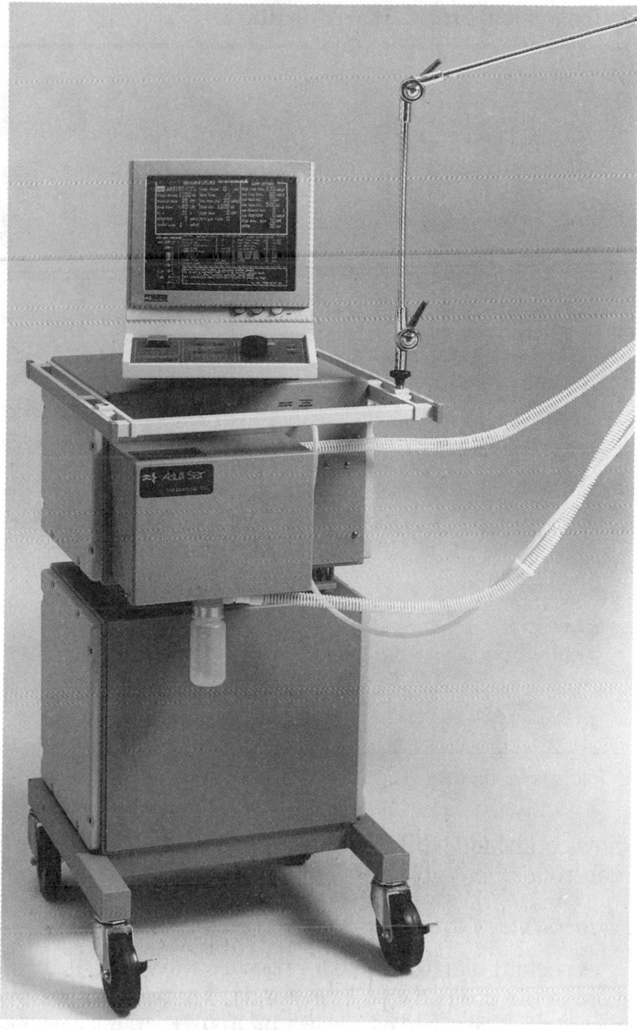

FIGURE 21-90. Infrasonics Adult Star ventilator (Courtesy of Infrasonics, San Diego, CA).

The control panel contains a large rotary knob (optical encoder) that functions similarly to a mouse that is used with a personal computer. This knob allows the operator to highlight (inverse video) various ventilator parameters as they appear on the CRT screen. Once the desired parameter is highlighted, it can be selected by pushing the enter button. The cursor then highlights the current numeric value of the parameter (variable) chosen. By rotating the select knob, the operator can then highlight a new desired value for this parameter. Pushing the enter button a second time on this value allows the new value to become activated as the new setting for that parameter. Alarm settings can also be selected in this manner.

□ CONTROL VARIABLES

The Adult Star controls inspiratory pressure in PSV and CPAP modes and controls inspiratory flow in the A/C and SIMV modes. In SIMV, mandatory breaths are

* Thanks to Roger McWilliams and John Denny of Infrasonics, Inc., San Diego, CA, for their technical assistance with the Adult Star ventilators.

TABLE 21-55 **Specifications for the Infrasonics Adult Star Ventilator**

Inspiration	
Rate (breaths/min)	0.5–80 (to 120*)
Volume (mL)	100–2500 (50–2500*)
Peak flow (L/min)	10–120 (machine) 10–160 (spontaneous)
Pressure limit (cmH_2O)	10–120
Pressure support (cmH_2O)	0–70
Inspiratory time (sec)	0.1–3.0 (variable*)
Effort (cmH_2O)	0.5–20 below baseline
Hold (sec)	0–2.0
Sigh rate (breaths/h)	0–20
Sigh frequency (multiple)	off, 1, 2, or 3
Sigh volume (mL)	100–2500
Expiration	
PEEP/CPAP (cmH_2O)	0–30 (0 to 50 option)
Modes	
Assist/control	
SIMV	
SIMV + PPS	
CPAP	
CPAP + PPS	

* Pediatric option

flow controlled while spontaneous breaths are pressure controlled.

Inspiratory Waveform

A rectangular (constant) pressure waveform is available in the pressure support mode. There are four flow waveforms available. These include rectangular, ascending ramp, descending ramp, and sine waves. For the rectangular waveform the flow is nearly constant at the peak flow setting. In the ascending ramp, inspiratory flow starts at 30% of the peak flow setting and increases linearly to the peak flow value. In the descending ramp pattern, flow starts at the peak flow setting and decreases linearly to 30% of the peak flow setting. In the sine flow waveform, inspiratory flow starts at 30%, builds to set peak flow, and decreases to 30% of the peak flow during inspiration in a sinusoidal manner.

□ PHASE VARIABLES

Triggering

Inspiration can be time-triggered and is a function of the ventilator rate set by the operator. It is also affected by the sigh rate and multiple sigh selections. The sigh rate works in all modes except CPAP. A sigh breath can be manually triggered in CPAP. When it is pressure-triggered, it is a function of the sensitivity setting and the patient's inspiratory effort. It can also be manually-triggered.

Limiting

Inspiration is flow-limited for mandatory volume-targeted breaths. It is pressure-limited during PSV breaths and PEEP/CPAP (spontaneous modes). An internal demand valve controls the inspiration pressure by trying to maintain the set baseline value (PEEP/CPAP). If an inflation hold is used (inspiratory pause), the ventilator is volume-limited.

Cycling

The ventilator time-cycles out of inspiration for flow-controlled mandatory volume-targeted breaths depending on the respiratory rate and peak flow setting set on the control panel. Technically, the Adult Star does not measure volume, so it is not a volume-cycled ventilator, but it calculates volume from flow and time.

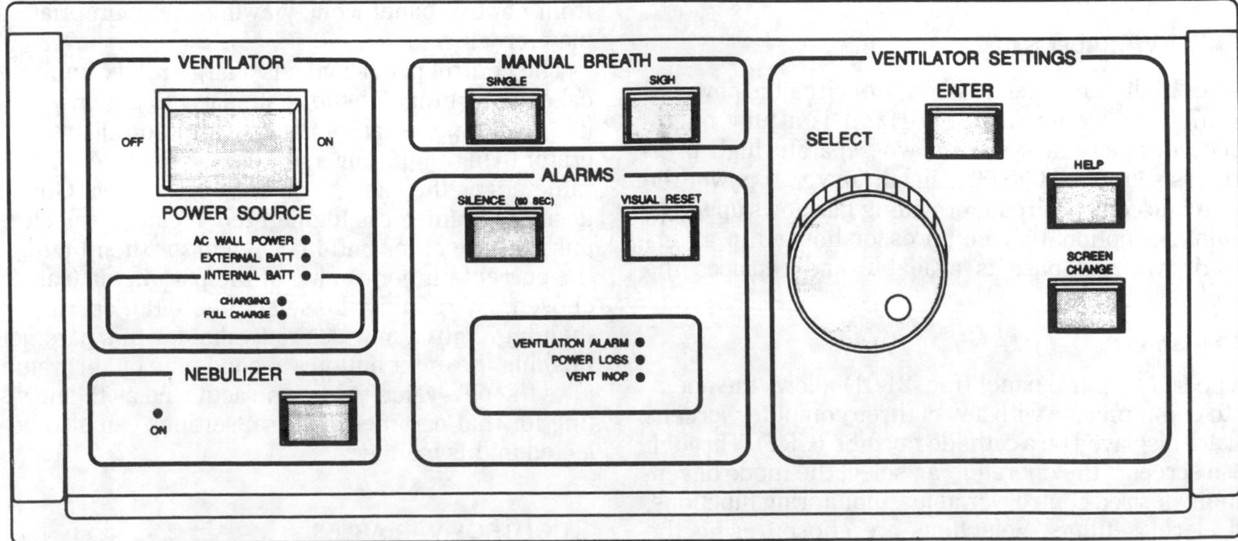

FIGURE 21-91. Control panel of the Adult Star ventilator. (From Branson, R.D., Hess, D.R., and Chatburn, R.L.: Respiratory Care Equipment, J.B. Lippincott Co., Philadelphia, 1995, p 346).

Use of the inspiratory pause extends the inspiratory time. Inspiration is pressure-cycled if the measured peak airway pressure is greater than the control setting for maximum safety pressure limit for a mandatory volume-targeted breath. This not only ends inspiration but activates an audible and visual alarm. Inspiration is also pressure-cycled for spontaneous breaths (except for PSV breaths). The ventilator tries to maintain the baseline pressure (PEEP/CPAP).

Baseline Pressure

Baseline pressure (PEEP/CPAP) is adjustable from 0 to 30 cmH_2O and a range of 0 to 50 cmH_2O is optional as an add-on feature.

□ CONTROL SUBSYSTEMS

Control Circuit

Figure 21-92 shows a schematic diagram of the ventilator's internal components. There are actually five microprocessors that provide both control and display functions. They include the main processor, a graphics processor, an A/D processor, and two stepper motor processors.

The main processor is responsible for the control of the pneumatic system. It does this by direct I/O interface with the valve driver board and by a serial interface with the two stepper motor-controlled proportioning valve. It accepts information (input) from several pressure and flow transducers along with the control variable settings on the control panel, as well as the output control signals to the output control valves. With this information, it controls such processes as ventilator triggering, cycling, pressure and flow waveform generation, and alarm functions.

The graphics processor board operates the video display (CRT) and the user interface. The A/D processor converts analog to digital signals for use by the other processors.

Should a major problem occur with the microprocessors, the ventilator is placed in a fail-safe mode called "Vent. Inop." or ventilator inoperative. If this occurs, both audio and visual alarms are activated. The audible alarm cannot be silenced. Both the expiratory valve and the internal safety vent valve open to allow a spontaneously breathing patient to breathe room air.

Drive Mechanism

Compressed air and oxygen (30 to 90 psig) are used to power the pneumatic system. An integral, electric motor and piston-type compressor with regulator can be purchased to provide an air source if wall air is not available. Gas sources are regulated to 6.5 to 7.5 psig before entering the internal air and oxygen proportional valves.

Output Control Valve

The air and oxygen proportional valves, which are driven by stepper motors, regulate the gas flow to the patient. They adjust the waveform, flow, oxygen con-

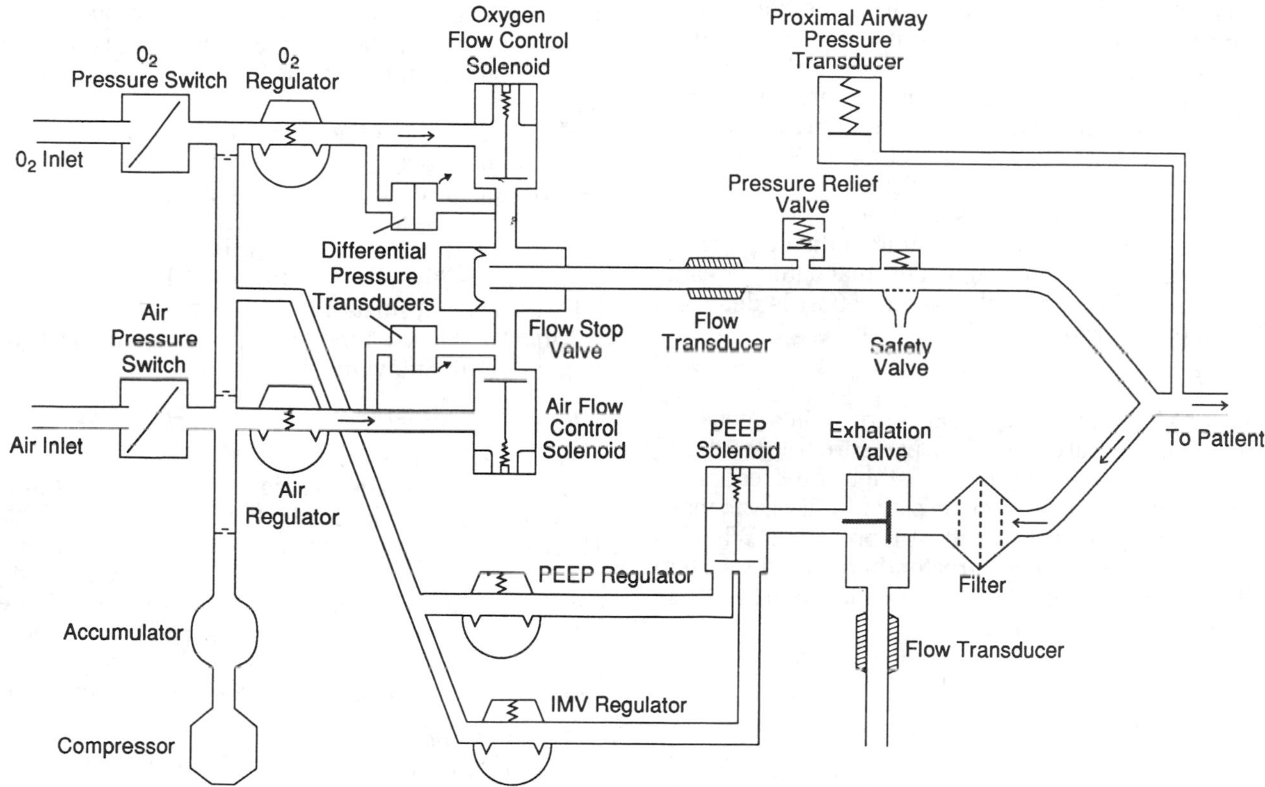

FIGURE 21-92. Internal components of the Adult Star ventilator control circuit.

centration, and volume under microprocessor control. There is also a pneumatic signal that is directed to the pneumatic, diaghragm-type, exhalation valve. This pneumatic signal comes from a pilot pressure control valve that is connected to the pneumatic interface valve.

□ MODES OF OPERATION

Assist/Control

The A/C mode is flow controlled, pressure- or time-triggered, flow-limited, and time-cycled. It can be volume-limited when the inspiratory pause is set higher than zero. The mandatory breaths in this mode are volume-targeted, with volumes staying constant from breath to breath, based on the tidal volume and sigh volume settings.

SIMV

The SIMV mode provides volume-targeted, flow controlled, mandatory breaths that are pressure- or time-triggered, flow-limited, and time-cycled. Spontaneous breaths between mandatory breaths are pressure controlled, that is, the flow to the patient will vary to maintain the baseline (PEEP/CPAP) pressure. Spontaneous breaths are pressure-triggered and pressure-cycled for CPAP breaths, while they are normally flow-cycled for PSV breaths. PSV can also be pressure-cycled at 3 cmH_2O over the target pressure, or time-cycled at 3.5 seconds as a back-up cycling mechanism in case of leaks.

In SIMV, a synchronized mandatory breath is commonly pressure-triggered when a patient makes an inspiratory effort adequate to trigger the ventilator. Triggering effort is based on the sensitivity setting and the patient's actual effort. The volume-targeted breath is then delivered to the patient. Following the synchronized mandatory breath, a patient can breathe spontaneously without triggering a mandatory breath until the next ventilator breath occurs in the preset ventilatory period. If the ventilator does not detect an inspiratory effort during the next ventilatory period, a mandatory breath is delivered at the beginning of the next period. The ventilator continues to deliver mandatory breaths at the set SIMV rate until a patient effort is detected. Then the cycle repeats itself.

CPAP

In the CPAP mode, all breaths are spontaneous. Inspiration is pressure controlled, pressure-triggered, and pressure-cycled. If PSV is used, then the breaths are flow-cycled. The gas flow to the patient will vary to maintain the baseline (PEEP/CPAP) pressure. When in PEEP/CPAP at a baseline greater than zero, the system will automatically compensate for leaks up to 22 L/min (7 L/min with the pediatric ventilator option). When a leak exceeds 6 L/min, this activates an alarm system to alert the operator to the problem.

Pressure Support

Positive pressure support, as it is termed by the manufacturer, is like PSV on other ventilators. It is used to assist spontaneous breaths in the SIMV (SIMV + PPS) and CPAP (CPAP + PPS) modes. For a pressure support breath, when a patient's spontaneous inspiratory effort drops airway pressure to the set sensitivity level, inspiration is then provided to the pressure support level set by the operator plus the baseline pressure. It then cycles out of inspiration when inspiratory gas flow drops to a rate of less than 4 L/min. PSV can also be pressure-cycled or time-cycled as backup cycling mechanisms.

□ OUTPUT DISPLAYS (MONITORS) AND ALARMS

Output Displays

There are three different screens of information available on the CRT. Screen one is for ventilator settings. It displays mode, pressure, volume, gas flow, respiratory rate, FIO_2, sensitivity settings and so on. It also provides information on ventilator alarm settings and alarms status such as apnea, pressure, volume, and respiratory rate alarms. There is also a panel on this screen that gives information on patient status. In addition, there is a representation of airway pressure in a dynamic analog bar graph on this screen, which also shows high and low inspiratory pressure and low PEEP/CPAP alarm settings.

Screen two is for patient monitoring information and gives measured values for exhaled tidal and minute volumes, spontaneous minute volume, and breath type (ie, spontaneous, controlled). In addition, it provides digital displays for measured peak, mean, PEEP/CPAP, and plateau pressures, measured respiratory rate, I:E ratio, and inspiratory time. Screen two provides a summary of other alarm limits and ventilator settings and also displays the analog pressure graph.

Screen three is a graphics monitor that shows real-time graphs of pressure, volume, and flow over time in a waveform display. As in screen two, this screen also provides summary information of other alarm limits and ventilator settings.

The operator of the Adult Star can get information on any screen display parameter by simply pushing the help button when the parameter in question is highlighted. In addition, for alarm variables the screen displays information about possible causes that would have activated the alarm. In this way, the ventilator provides its own information booklet right at the bedside.

Table 21-56 shows monitoring information available with the Adult Star ventilator.

Input Power Alarms

Electrical Power Failure

Both visual and audible signals are activated in the event of a power failure (less than 104 volts available). There is also a low-battery alarm that activates when the internal battery is low and can only be expected to power the ventilator for less than 5 more minutes. When the battery is maximally charged, it can be expected to provide power for about 20 minutes of ventilator operation should the external power source fail.

Pneumatic Power Failure

If air or oxygen inlet pressure is less than 30 psig for 1 second, an audible and visible alarm activates. There are separate indicators for either air or oxygen supply. If the oxygen source fails, the low oxygen inlet alarm

TABLE 21-56 **Available Monitoring Information on the Adult Star Ventilator**

Parameter	Range
Exhaled tidal volume (mL)	0–2500
Minute volume (L/min)	0–99.9
Spontaneous minute volume (L/min)	0–99.9
Breath type monitor	assist, control, spontaneous, sigh
Peak pressure (cmH_2O)	0–120
Mean airway pressure (cmH_2O)	0–120
PEEP/CPAP pressure (cmH_2O)	0–30
Plateau pressure (cmH_2O)	0–120
Breath rate (breaths/min)	0–120
I:E ratio	1:0.1–1:99.9
Inspiratory time (sec)	0–99.9 (mandatory only)

will activate (O_2 pressure <30 psig for 1 sec and FIO_2 set >0.21) and the ventilator will continue to operate with compressed air.

If the external air source fails, the integral compressor will activate if it is available and no alarm condition will occur. If there is no external air source and the compressor fails (<16 psig with FIO_2 <1.0) or is not available, the ventilator will activate the low air inlet alarm and will continue to operate from the 100% oxygen source.

When both gas sources fail, about 3 to 4 minutes of gas volume remains in the internal accumulator tanks under normal operating conditions (23 to 25 L). Once this volume is depleted, the safety vent valve and the exhalation valve open allowing the patient to spontaneously breathe from room air. A "Vent. Inop." message will appear on the CRT and audible and visual alarms occur.

Control Variable Alarms

The four available pressure alarms are as follows:

High Inspiratory Pressure (cmH_2O) 10 to 120
Low Inspiratory Pressure (cmH_2O) 3 to 60
Low PEEP/CPAP (cmH_2O) 0 to 25
High PEEP/CPAP (cmH_2O) *Automatically activated if baseline pressure is 10 cmH_2O higher than the set PEEP/CPAP level for 2 seconds or if the baseline pressure fluctuates between 5 and 10 cmH_2O above the set PEEP/CPAP level for more than 5 seconds.

The four available volume and rate alarms are as follows:

Low mandatory (mechanical) volume (mL) 0 to 2500
Low spontaneous volume (mL) 0 to 2500
Low minute volume (L/min) 0 to 60
Low respiratory rate (breaths/min) 0 to 90

Control Circuit Alarms

Control circuit alarms available on the Adult Star ventilator are listed in Table 21-57.

TABLE 21-57 **Control Circuit Alarms Available With the Adult Star Ventilator**

Insufficient inspiratory and expiratory times*
Inverse I:E ratio indicated by inverse video on screen
Apnea alarm (5–60 sec)*
Expiratory valve leak (activated if the expiratory flow transducer measures flow more than 10% of the inspiratory flow **and** that flow is more than 4 L/min for 60 min during the time when the expiratory valve is closed)
Obstructed tube: a condition exists that may be obstructing flow to the patient, or airway line is obstructed. This activates in three possible conditions:
The internal pressure transducer is reading a pressure greater than the pressure-support setting and CPAP (CPAP + PPS) for a mechanical breath.
The internal pressure transducer is reading a pressure greater than the set high inspiratory pressure limit for a mechanical breath.
During a spontaneous breath, the airway pressure is greater than 10 cmH_2O above PEEP/CPAP baseline for more than 3 seconds.
Alarm silence quiets the audible alarms for 60 seconds except for "vent. inop" and "power loss."

* Visual and audible indicators.

☐ TROUBLESHOOTING

The available alarms and indicators and the computer functioning capability provide quick evaluation and solution to most of the common problems that occur. For troubleshooting, the manufacturer's operating manual also provides a chart of ventilator symptoms, how they are indicated, possible causes, and corrective actions.

As with all microprocessor-based medical equipment, caution must be taken with transmitting devices such as cellular phones and walkie-talkies, because they can adversely influence the computer function of the ventilator.

Infrasonics Adult Star 2000 Ventilator*

☐ CLASSIFICATION

The Infrasonics Adult Star 2000 ventilator is a pressure or flow controller (Table 21-58) (Fig. 21-93). Inspiration can be pressure-, time-, or manually-triggered. It can be pressure-, volume-, or flow-limited and is pressure-, flow-, or time-cycled. It has an internal air-oxygen blending system and a built-in internal compressor.

A separate nebulizer outlet port provides a means to power a micronebulizer without altering volume or oxygen delivery. The nebulizer is supplied by a 10-psig gas source that provides an 8 L/min gas flow. The nebulizer gas volume (flow) is removed from the set tidal volume before leaving the ventilator outlet. This volume of gas is returned to the patient through the nebulizer. As a result, set tidal volume and FIO_2 are not changed. The nebulizer automatically shuts off after 30 minutes or when its control button is pressed a second time.

* Thanks to Roger McWilliams and John Denney of Infrasonics, Inc., San Diego, CA, for their technical assistance with the Adult Star ventilators.

TABLE 21-58 **Classification of the Infrasonics Adult Star 2000 Ventilator**

Power Source for Pneumatic Circuit	**Pressurized Gases (30–90 psig)**
Power source for control circuit	Electricity (108–132 volts AC at 60 Hz)
Control mechanism	Pressure, flow
Triggering	Pressure, time, manual
Limiting	Pressure, volume, flow
Cycling	Time, pressure, flow

□ SPECIFICATIONS

Table 21-59 shows a list of the ventilator's specifications. The Adult Star 2000 can be used for pediatric (pediatric ventilation option) or adult patients.

□ INPUT VARIABLES

The Adult Star's electrical control circuit is powered by 108 to 132 volts AC at 60 Hz. It is a fully microprocessor-operated system. Two separate high pressure gas sources (30 to 90 psig, air/oxygen) power the pneumatic control circuit, providing gas flows up to 160 L/min. An optional air compressor can be purchased separately and replaces the wheeled base.

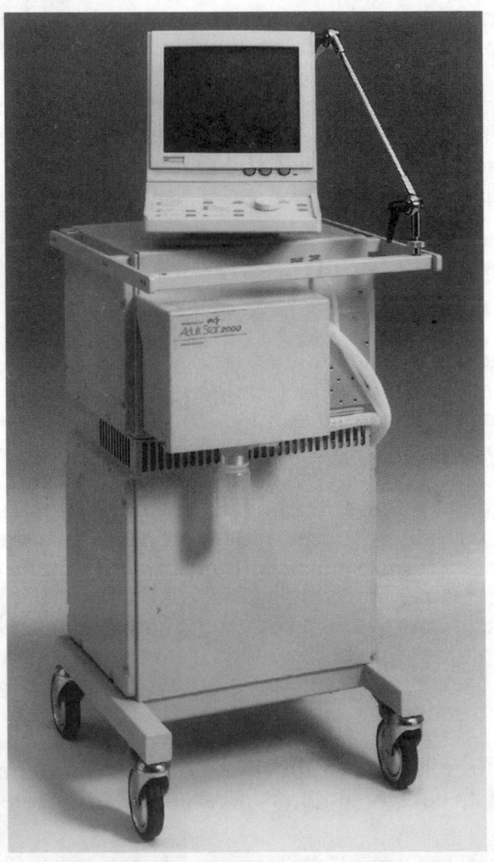

FIGURE 21-93. Infrasonics Adult Star 2000 ventilator. (Courtesy of Infrasonics, San Diego, CA

TABLE 21-59 **Specifications for the Infrasonics Adult Star 2000 Ventilator**

Inspiration	
Rate (breaths/min)	0.5–80
Volume (mL)	100–2500
Peak flow (L/min)	10–120 (machine) 10–160 (spontaneous)
Pressure limit (cmH_2O)	10–120
Pressure support (cmH_2O)	0–70
Inspiratory time (sec)	0.1–3.0
Effort (cmH_2O)	0.5–20 below baseline
Hold (sec)	0–2.0
Sigh rate (breaths/h)	0–20
Sigh frequency (multiple)	off, 1, 2, or 3
Sigh volume (mL)	100–2500
Apnea rate (breaths/min)	0.5–80
Expiration	
PEEP/CPAP (cmH_2O)	0–30 (0–50 option)
Modes	
A/C	
SIMV	
SIMV + PPS	
CPAP	
CPAP + PPS	
PCV (option) (time-cycled; I:E cycled)	

Operation

The front control panel (Fig. 21-94) allows the operator to communicate with any of three computer screens that are displayed on a CRT. These are Ventilator Settings (Screen 1), Patient Status (Screen 2), and Graphic Monitoring (Screen 3). Through these screens the operator can select the mode of ventilation, desired control variables, monitoring functions, and alarm settings. Selections are chosen using the front control panel while viewing the appropriate display screen.

The control panel contains a large rotary knob (optical encoder) that functions similarly to a mouse that is used with a personal computer. This knob allows the operator to highlight various ventilator parameters with reverse video as they appear on the CRT screen. Once the desired parameter is highlighted, it can be selected by pushing the enter button. The cursor then highlights the current numerical value of the parameter (variable) chosen. By rotating the select knob, the operator can then highlight a new desired value for this parameter. Pushing the enter button a second time on this value allows the new value to become activated as the new setting for that parameter. Alarm settings can also be selected in this manner.

□ CONTROL VARIABLES

The Adult Star controls inspiratory pressure in PCV (option), PSV, and CPAP modes and controls inspiratory flow in the A/C and SIMV modes. In SIMV, mandatory breaths are flow controlled while spontaneous breaths are pressure controlled.

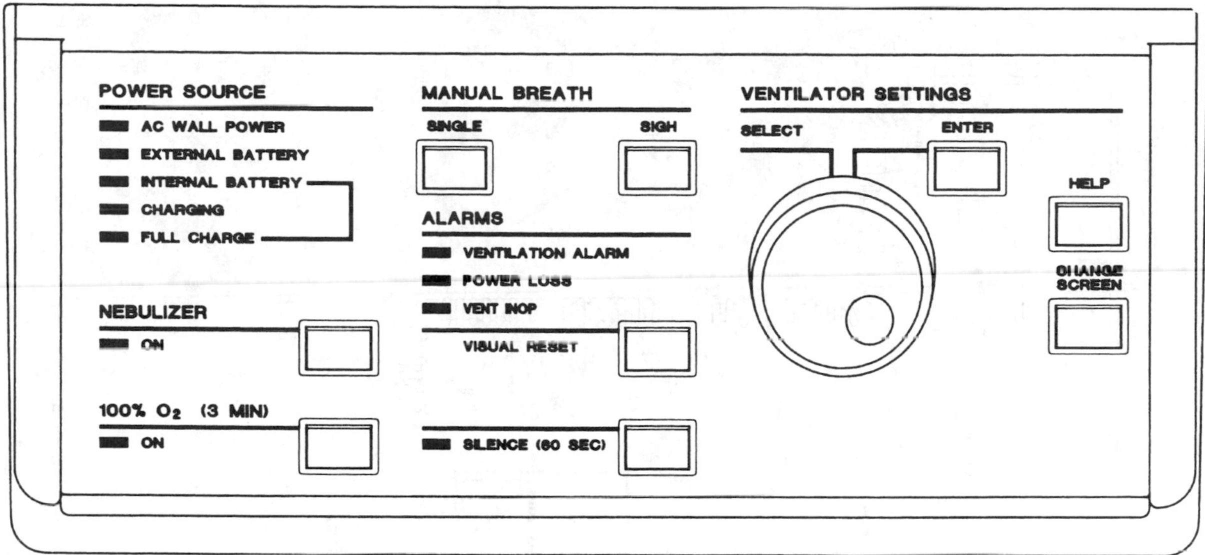

FIGURE 21-94. Control panel of the Adult Star 2000 ventilator. (Courtesy of Infrasonics, San Diego, CA)

Inspiratory Waveform

A rectangular (constant) pressure waveform is available in the pressure controlled modes. There are four flow waveforms available. These include rectangular, ascending ramp, descending ramp, and sine waves. For the rectangular waveform, the flow is nearly constant at the peak flow setting. In the ascending ramp, inspiratory flow starts at 30% of the peak flow setting and increases linearly to the peak flow value. In the descending ramp pattern, flow starts at the peak flow setting and decreases linearly to 30% of the peak flow setting. In the sine flow waveform, inspiratory flow starts at 30%, builds to set peak flow, and decreases to 30% of the peak flow during inspiration in a sinusoidal manner.

□ PHASE VARIABLES

Triggering

Inspiration can be time-triggered and is a function of the ventilator rate set by the operator. In the PCV I:E ratio-cycled mode, the ventilator is time-triggered and only the A/C mode is allowed for this setting. The patient cannot pressure-trigger inspiration in this mode.

Time-triggering is also affected by the sigh rate and multiple sigh selections. The sigh rate works in all modes except CPAP, but a sigh breath can be manually triggered in CPAP. When it is pressure-triggered it is a function of the sensitivity setting and the patient's inspiratory effort. It can also be manually triggered.

Limiting

Inspiration is flow-limited for mandatory volume-targeted breaths. It is pressure-limited during PCV (option), PSV breaths, and PEEP/CPAP (spontaneous modes). An internal demand valve controls the inspiration pressure by trying to maintain the set baseline value (PEEP/CPAP). If an inflation hold is used (inspiratory pause), the ventilator is volume-limited.

Cycling

The ventilator time-cycles out of inspiration for flow controlled mandatory (volume-targeted) breaths depending on the respiratory rate and peak flow setting set on the control panel. Technically, the Adult Star 2000 does not measure volume, so it is not a volume-cycled ventilator, but it calculates volume from flow and time.

Use of the inspiratory pause extends the inspiratory time. Inspiration is pressure-cycled if the measured peak airway pressure is greater than the control setting for maximum safety pressure limit for a mandatory volume-targeted breath. This not only ends inspiration but activates an audible and visual alarm. Inspiration is also pressure-cycled for spontaneous breaths (except for PSV breaths). The ventilator tries to maintain the set baseline pressure (PEEP/CPAP).

In the PCV option, there are two selected ways to cycle the ventilator. In the PCV time-cycled ventilation mode, inspiration ends when the preset inspiratory time has elapsed. In the PCV I:E ratio cycled ventilation mode, inspiration ends when the inspiratory time has elapsed. This is based on the machine rate and I:E ratio setting. I and E are the numeric values of the I:E ratio setting.

Baseline Pressure

Baseline pressure (PEEP/CPAP) is adjustable from 0 to 30 cmH_2O. A 0 to 50 cmH_2O option is available for PEEP/CPAP.

□ CONTROL SUBSYSTEMS

Control Circuit

Figure 21-95 shows a schematic diagram of this complex ventilator's internal components. There are actually five microprocessors that provide both control and display functions. They include the main processor, a

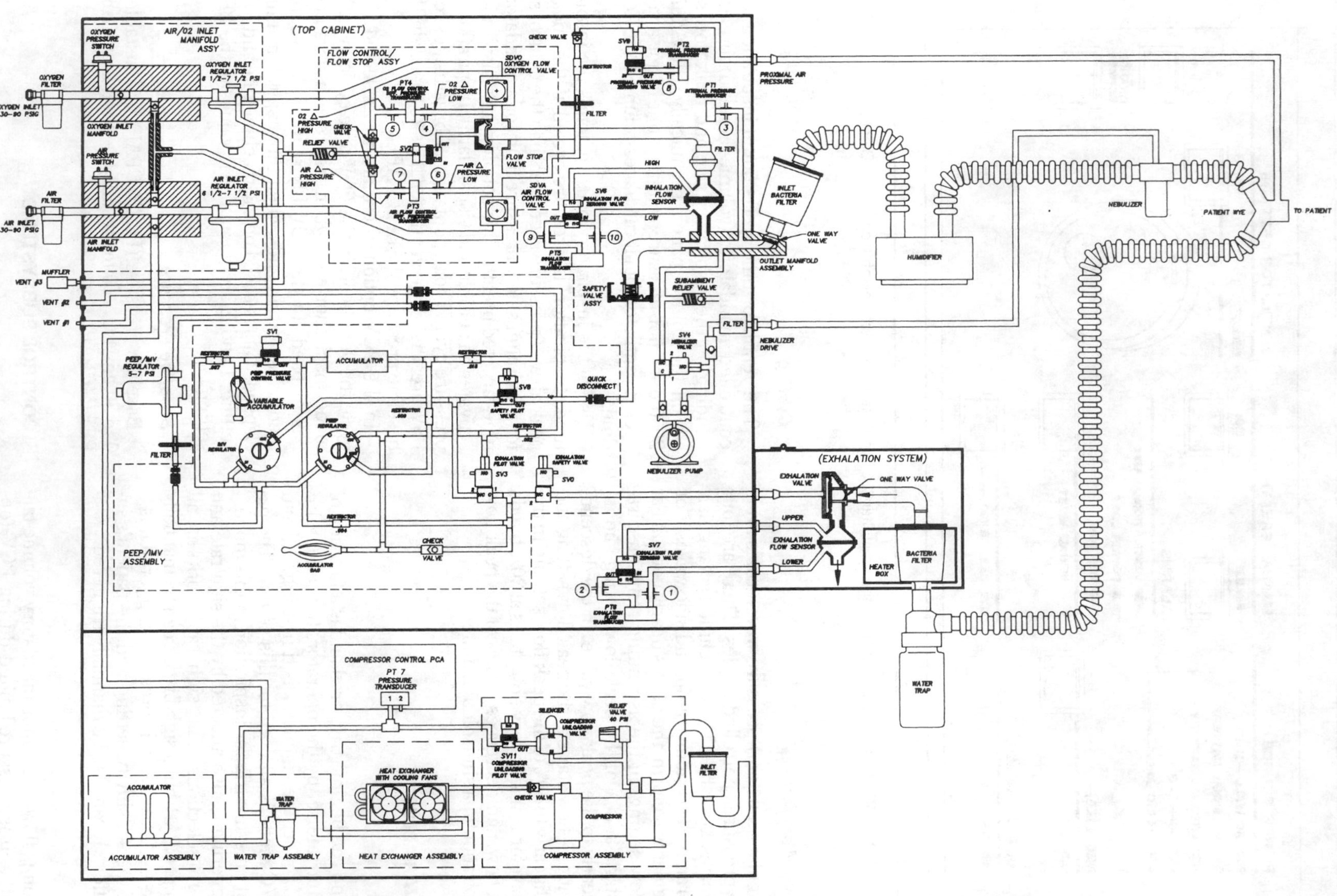

FIGURE 21-95. Schematic of the pneumatic circuit of the Adult Star 2000 ventilator. (Courtesy of Infrasonics, San Diego, CA)

graphics processor, an analog/digital processor, and two stepper motor processors.

The main processor is responsible for the control of the pneumatic system. It does this by direct interface with the valve driver board and by a serial interface with the two stepper motor controlled proportioning valves. It accepts information (input) from several pressure and flow transducers along with the control variable settings on the control panel, as well as the output control signals to the output control valves. With this information, it controls such processes as ventilator triggering, cycling, pressure and flow waveform generation, and alarm functions.

The graphics processor board operates the video display (CRT) and the user interface. The A/D processor converts analog to digital signals for use by the other processors

Should a major problem occur with the microprocessors, the ventilator is placed in the fail-safe mode, Vent. Inop., or ventilator inoperative. If this occurs, both audio and visual alarms are activated. The audible alarm cannot be silenced. Both the expiratory valve and the internal safety vent valve open to allow a spontaneously breathing patient to breathe room air.

Drive Mechanism

Compressed air and oxygen (30 to 90 psig) are used to power the pneumatic system. An integral, electric motor and piston-type compressor with regulator can be purchased to provide an air source if wall air is not available. Gas sources are regulated to 6.5 to 7.5 psig before entering the internal air and oxygen proportional valves.

Output Control Valve

The air and oxygen proportional valves, which are driven by stepper motors, regulate the gas flow to the patient. They adjust the waveform, flow, oxygen concentration, and volume under microprocessor control. There is also a pneumatic signal that is directed to the pneumatic, diaphragm-type, exhalation valve. This pneumatic signal comes from a pilot pressure control valve, which is connected to the pneumatic interface valve.

□ MODES OF OPERATION

Assist/Control

The A/C mode is flow controlled, pressure- or time-triggered, flow-limited, and time-cycled. It can be volume-limited when the inspiratory pause is set higher than zero. The mandatory breaths in this mode are volume-targeted, with volumes staying fairly constant from breath to breath, based on the tidal volume and sigh volume settings.

SIMV

The SIMV mode provides volume-targeted, flow controlled, mandatory breaths that are pressure- or time-triggered, flow-limited and time-cycled. Spontaneous breaths between mandatory breaths are pressure controlled, that is, the flow to the patient will vary to maintain the baseline (PEEP/CPAP) pressure. Spontaneous breaths are pressure-triggered and pressure-cycled for CPAP breaths, while they are normally flow-cycled for PSV breaths. PSV breaths can also be pressure-cycled if the pressure exceeds target pressure by 3 cmH_2O. PSV breaths are time-cycled at 3.5 seconds as a backup in case of leaks.

In SIMV, a synchronized mandatory breath is commonly pressure-triggered when a patient makes an inspiratory effort adequate to trigger the ventilator. Triggering effort is based on the sensitivity setting and the patient's actual effort. The volume-targeted breath is then delivered to the patient. Following the mandatory breath, a patient can breathe spontaneously without triggering a mandatory breath until the next ventilator breath occurs in the preset ventilatory period. If the ventilator does not detect an inspiratory effort during the next ventilatory period, a mandatory breath is delivered at the beginning of the next period. The ventilator continues to deliver mandatory breaths at the set SIMV rate until a patient effort is detected. Then the cycle repeats itself.

CPAP

In the CPAP mode, all breaths are spontaneous. Inspiration is pressure controlled, pressure-triggered, and pressure-cycled. If PSV is used, then the breaths are flow-cycled. The gas flow to the patient will vary to maintain the baseline (PEEP/CPAP) pressure. When in PEEP/CPAP at a baseline greater than zero, the system will automatically compensate for leaks up to 22 L/min (7 L/min with the pediatric ventilation option). When a leak exceeds 6 L/min this activates an alarm system to alert the operator to the problem.

Pressure Support

"Positive pressure support," as it is termed by the manufacturer, is like PSV on most ventilators. It is used to assist spontaneous breaths in the SIMV (SIMV + PPS) and CPAP (CPAP + PPS) modes. For a pressure support breath, when a patient's spontaneous inspiratory effort drops airway pressure to the set sensitivity level, then inspiration is provided to the pressure support level set by the operator plus baseline pressure. It then cycles out of inspiration when inspiratory gas flow drops to a rate of less than 4 L/min. It can also be pressure- or time-cycled out of inspiration in the event of problems.

Pressure Control

There is a pressure control option that can be added to the Adult Star 2000. It provides two methods of giving PCV: PCV time-cycled, and PCV I:E ratio-cycled. During PCV in either mode, the ventilator is pressure-controlled and flow varies to maintain preset pressure. During PCV, the control pressure is equal to the PEEP level plus the value for PCV pressure. If the high pressure alarm limit is reached, the breath is pressure-cycled out of inspiration.

PCV in the time-cycled mode can be used with the following ventilation modes: A/C, CPAP, CPAP + PSV, SIMV, and SIMV + PSV. When CPAP or CPAP + PSV are selected, PCV only operates during the apnea backup mode of ventilation or when a manual breath is delivered. In A/C and SIMV modes the mandatory breaths are pressure controlled, time- or pressure-triggered into inspiration, and time-cycled. The range of inspiratory time is 0.24 to 5.0 seconds. I:E is limited to 4:1. If expiratory time is less than 200 msec, the "insufficient exhalation time" alarm will activate. The delivered machine rate will not agree with the set machine rate. This mode will also pressure-cycle if the high pressure limit is reached.

PCV I:E ratio-cycled can ONLY be used in the A/C mode. The ventilator in this mode is time-triggered, pressure-limited, and time-cycled. This mode will also pressure-cycle if the high pressure limit is reached. Inspiratory time is a function of the machine rate and the I:E ratio settings such that:

$$Ti = (60/f)[I/(I + E)]$$

where Ti is inspiratory time, f is machine rate setting, and I and E are the numeric values of the I:E ratio setting. The range of I:E is 4:1 to 1:499. If the expiratory time is less than 200 msec, the insufficient exhalation time alarm will activate and the delivered machine rate will be less than the set rate.

□ OUTPUT DISPLAYS (MONITORS) AND ALARMS

Output Displays

There are three different screens of information available on the CRT. Screen one is for ventilator settings (Fig. 21-96). It displays mode, pressure, volume, gas flow, respiratory rate, FIO_2, PEEP/CPAP, and sensitivity settings. It also provides information on ventilator alarm settings and alarms status such as apnea, pressures, volumes, and respiratory rate alarms. There is also a panel on this screen that gives information on patient status. In addition, there is a representation of airway pressure in a dynamic analog bar graph on this screen which also shows high and low inspiratory pressure and low PEEP/CPAP alarm settings.

Screen two (Fig. 21-97) is for patient monitoring information and gives measured values for exhaled tidal and minute volumes, spontaneous minute volume, and breath type (ie, spontaneous, controlled). In addition, it provides digital displays for measured peak, mean, PEEP/CPAP, and plateau pressures, measured respiratory rate, I:E ratio, and inspiratory time. Screen two also provides a summary of other alarm limits and ventilator settings and also displays the analog pressure graph.

Screen three (Fig. 21-98) is a graphics monitor that shows real-time graphs of pressure, volume, and flow over time in a waveform display. As in screen two, this screen also provides summary information of other alarm limits and ventilator settings.

The operator of the Adult Star can get information on any screen display parameter by simply pushing the help button when the parameter in question is highlighted. In addition, the screen displays information about possible causes that would have activated various alarms. In this way the ventilator provides its own information booklet right at the bedside.

Monitoring information available on the Adult Star 2000 ventilator is listed on Table 21-60.

Input Power Alarms

Electrical Power Failure

Both visual and audible signals are activated in the event of a power failure (less than 104 volts available). There is also a low-battery alarm that activates when the

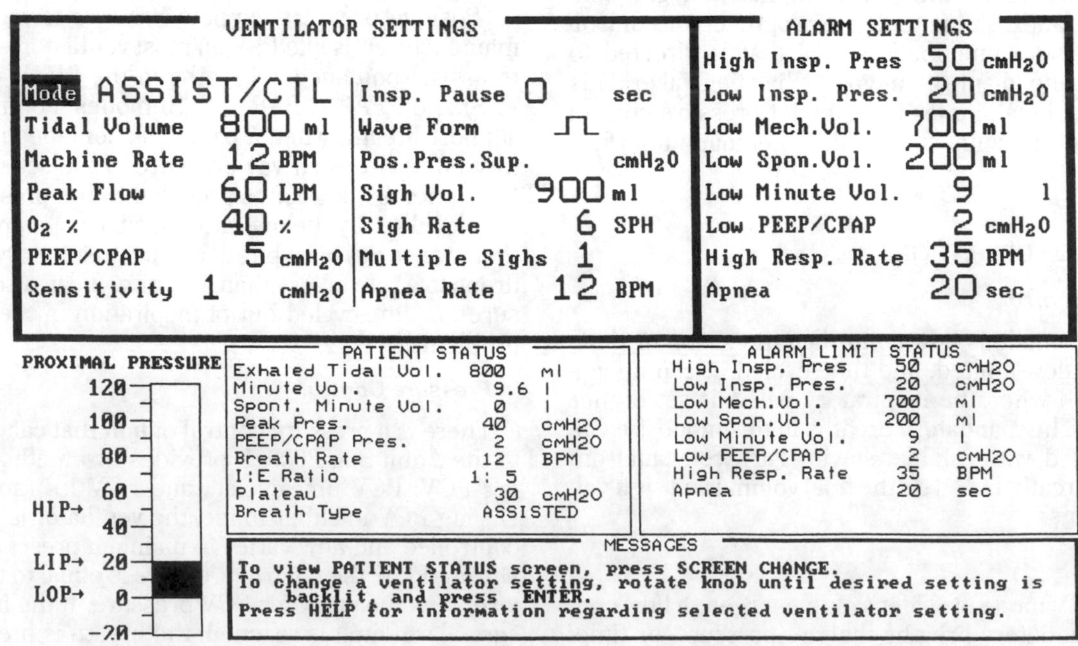

FIGURE 21-96. View of Screen 1, the Ventilator Settings screen for the Adult Star 2000. (Courtesy of Infrasonics, San Diego, CA)

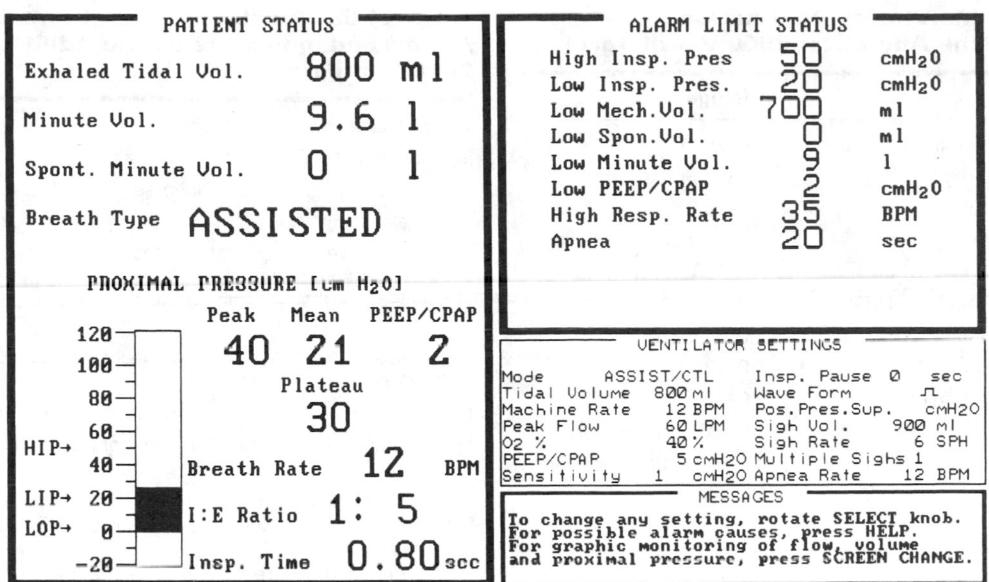

FIGURE 21-97. View of Screen 2, Patient Status screen for the Adult Star 2000. (Courtesy of Infrasonics, San Diego, CA)

internal battery is low and can only be expected to power the ventilator for less than 5 minutes. When the battery is maximally charged, it can be expected to provide power for about 20 minutes of ventilator operation should the external power source fail.

Pneumatic Power Failure

If air or oxygen inlet pressure is less than 30 psig for 1 second, an audible and visible alarm activates. There are separate indicators for air and oxygen supply. If the oxygen source fails, the low oxygen inlet alarm will activate (O_2 pressure <30 psig for 1 sec and FIO_2 set >0.21) and the ventilator will continue to operate with compressed air.

If the external air source fails, the integral compressor will activate and no alarm condition will occur. If there is no external air source and the compressor fails (<16 psig with FIO_2 <1.0) or is not available, the ventilator will activate the low air inlet alarm and will continue to operate from the 100% oxygen source.

When both gas sources fail, about 3 to 4 minutes of gas volume remains in the internal accumulator tanks under normal operating conditions (23 to 25 L). Once

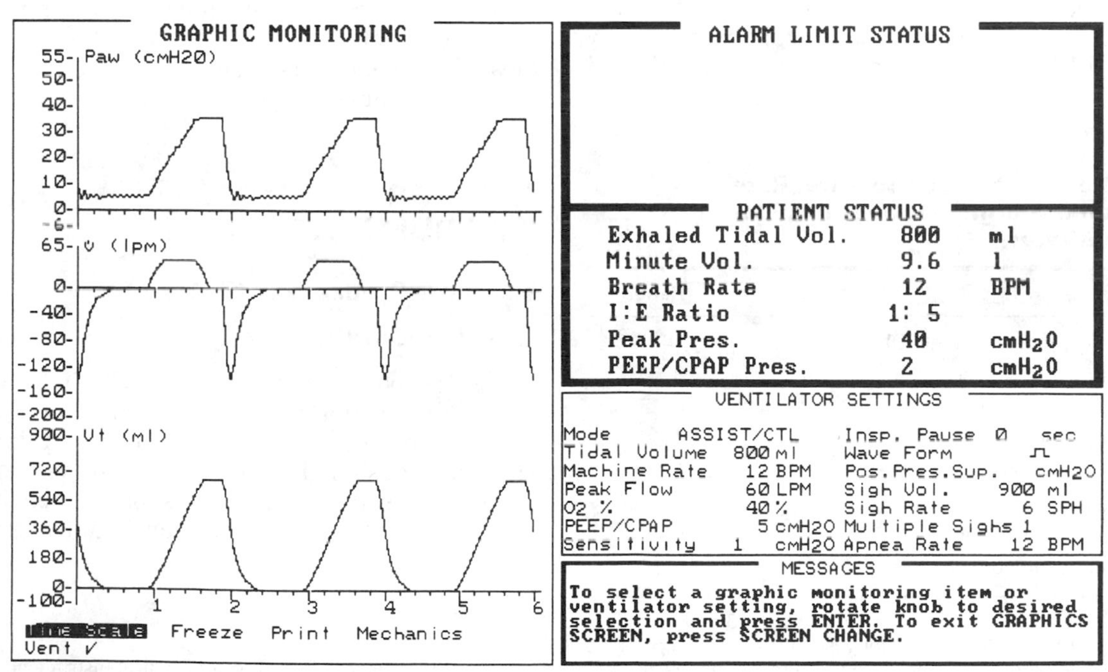

FIGURE 21-98. View of Screen 3, Graphic Display for the Adult Star 2000. (Courtesy of Infrasonics, San Diego, CA)

TABLE 21-60 **Monitoring Information Available on the Adult Star 2000 Ventilator**

Parameter	Range
Exhaled tidal volume (mL)	0–2500
Minute volume (L/min)	0–99.9
Spontaneous minute volume (L/min)	0–99.9
Breath type monitor	A/C, spontaneous, sigh
Peak pressure (cmH_2O)	0–120
Mean airway pressure (cmH_2O)	0–120
PEEP/CPAP pressure (cmH_2O)	0–30 (0–50 option)
Plateau pressure (cmH_2O)	0–120
Breath rate (breaths/min)	0–120
I:E ratio	99.9:1–1:99.9
Inspiratory time (sec)	0–99.9 (mandatory only)
Proximal airway pressure (cmH_2O) (bar graph)	(−) 20 to 120

this volume is depleted, the safety vent valve and the exhalation valve open, allowing the patient to spontaneously breathe from room air. A Vent. Inop. message will appear on the CRT and audible and visual alarms occur.

Control Variable Alarms

Table 21-61 lists the available pressure, rate, and volume alarms.

Control Circuit Alarms and Indicators

Table 21-62 lists the available control circuit alarms and indicators.

An option for Respiratory Mechanics Alarms is also available. The ventilator can provide information of auto-PEEP levels with this added option, as well as provide information on such patient lung mechanics variables as resistance, compliance, maximum inspiratory pressure (MIP), or negative inspiratory force (NIF) and vital capacity.

TABLE 21-61 **Available Pressure, Rate, and Volume Alarms on the Adult Star 2000 Ventilator**

Parameter	Range
High inspiratory pressure (cmH_2O)	10–120
Low inspiratory pressure (cmH_2O)	3–60
Low PEEP/CPAP (cmH_2O)	0–25
High PEEP/CPAP (cmH_2O)	*
Low mandatory (mechanical) volume (mL)	0–2500
Low spontaneous volume (mL)	0–2500
Low minute volume (L/min)	0–60
High respiratory rate (breaths/min)	0–90

* Automatically activated if baseline pressure is 10 cmH_2O higher than the set PEEP/CPAP level for 2 seconds or if the baseline pressure fluctuates between 5 and 10 cmH_2O above the set PEEP/CPAP level for more than 5 seconds.

TABLE 21-62 **Available Control Circuit Alarms and Indicators on the Adult Star 2000 Ventilator**

Airway leak alarm; leak >6 L/min

Insufficient inspiratory and expiratory times*

Inverse I:E ratio indicated by inverse video on screen

Apnea alarm (5 to 60 sec)*

Expiratory valve leak (activated if the expiratory flow transducer measures flow more than 10% of the inspiratory flow **and** that flow is more than 4 L/min for 60 ms during the time when the expiratory valve is closed)

Low pressure oxygen alarm: oxygen inlet pressure is low (range, 28–32 psig)

Low pressure air alarm: air inlet pressure is low (range, 28–32 psig)

Low internal battery alarm: 4 minutes or less remain on the internal battery

Obstructed tube (a condition exists that may be obstructing flow to the patient, or airway line is obstructed. This activates in three possible conditions:
- The internal pressure transducer is reading a pressure greater than the pressure-support setting and CPAP (CPAP + PPS) for a PSV breath.
- For a mandatory breath, the internal pressure transducer is reading a pressure greater than the set high inspiratory pressure limit.
- During a spontaneous breath, the airway pressure is greater than 10 cmH_2O above PEEP/CPAP baseline for more than 3 seconds.

Alarm silence quiets the audible alarms for 60 seconds except for "vent. inop" and "power loss"

* Visual and audible indicators.

□ TROUBLESHOOTING

The available alarms and indicators and the computer functioning capability provide quick evaluation and solution to most of the common problems that occur. For troubleshooting, the manufacturer also provides a chart of ventilator symptoms, how they are indicated, possible causes and corrective actions in its operating manual.

NEWPORT MEDICAL INSTRUMENTS*

Newport Breeze Ventilator

□ CLASSIFICATION

The Newport Breeze ventilator (Table 21-63) (Fig. 21-99) can function as a flow/volume-controlled, or a pressure-controlled, time-cycled, constant flow ventilator. It is designed as a general purpose ventilator that can be used for ventilatory support of infants, children, or adults. The ventilator is microprocessor controlled.

* Thanks to Duane Sell of Newport Medical Instruments, Newport Beach, CA, for his technical assistance with this material.

TABLE 21-63 **Classification of the Newport Breeze Ventilator**

Power Source for Control Circuitry	Electricity (100–120 volts AC at 47 to 63 Hz)
Power source for pneumatic system	Air 35–70 psig and oxygen 35–70 psig
Battery power (internal) battery rechargeable	Minimum 1 hour to maximum 18 hours
Control mechanism	Pressure, flow
Triggering	Pressure, time, manual
Limiting	Pressure, time, flow
Cycling	Time, pressure

☐ SPECIFICATIONS

Specifications are listed in Table 21-64.

TABLE 21-64 **Specifications for the Newport Breeze Ventilator**

FIO_2	0.21–1.0 ± 3%
Flow (L/min)	3–120
Inspiratory time (sec)	0.1–3.0
Rate (breaths/min)	1–150
Tidal volume (mL)	30–2000
Peak inspiratory pressure (cmH_2O)	0–60
PEEP/CPAP (cmH_2O)	0–60
Spontaneous flow (L/min)	0–50+
Trigger level (cmH_2O)	−9–+60
Maximum inverse I:E	4:1
Pneumatic pressure relief (cmH_2O)	0–120
Manometer range (cmH_2O)	−10–120
Emergency power supply (internal battery)	1 hour

☐ INPUT VARIABLES

The Newport Breeze ventilator requires 100 to 120 volts AC at 60 Hz to power the microprocessor-controlled electronic circuit. Additionally, the ventilator requires external compressed air and oxygen at 35 to 70 psig for pneumatic power. Although this ventilator has an internal air-oxygen blender, it has no internal compressor. The front panel (Fig. 21-100) allows for easy operator selection of ventilator mode, pressure limit (PIP), baseline pressure (PEEP), trigger threshold, inspiratory time, ventilatory rate, FIO_2, a separate flow rate for mechanical breaths and one for spontaneous breaths, and settings for airway pressure alarms.

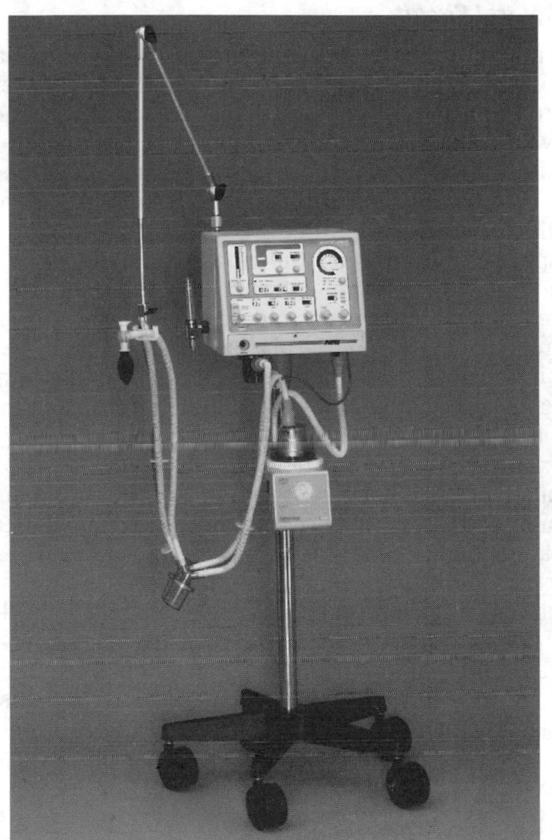

FIGURE 21-99. The Newport Breeze ventilator (Courtesy of Newport Medical, Newport CA).

Operation

Following attachment of appropriate compressed gas and electrical supply sources, activation of the ventilator is accomplished by setting the Off/On switch to the On position. At this time, a temporary audible alarm sounds and all lights on the front panel are illuminated for 2 seconds. This indicates that the system is functional and that the self-testing of the ventilator is completed. When the Off/On switch is in the Off position, all electronically operated ventilator functions are deactivated.

☐ CONTROL VARIABLES

The Newport Breeze ventilator can operate as a flow control or pressure control ventilator. Inspiratory time may be adjusted from 0.1 to 3.0 seconds and flow may be adjusted from 3 to 120 L/min. Maximal peak inspiratory pressure is 60 cmH_2O and maximal tidal volume is 2000 mL. A pneumatic pressure relief valve allows the machine to vent at pressures as high as 120 cmH_2O. Separate flow rates are set for mechanical inspiration and for spontaneous inspiration. Mechanical flow is calibrated from 3 to 120 L/min in increments of 1 L/min. This setting determines the flow delivered to the patient during mechanical or manual breaths. Spontaneous flow is calibrated from a minimal value of 28 L/min to a maximal value of approximately 58 L/min when the flow meter is set at "flush." In the event that the patient's inspiratory flow rate exceeds that available in accordance with the spontaneous flow setting, the patient may draw mixed gas from the reservoir bag. In volume-targeted modes of operation, tidal volume is the product of flow and inspiratory time. Tidal volume is digitally displayed as "set tidal volume" in the data display panel.

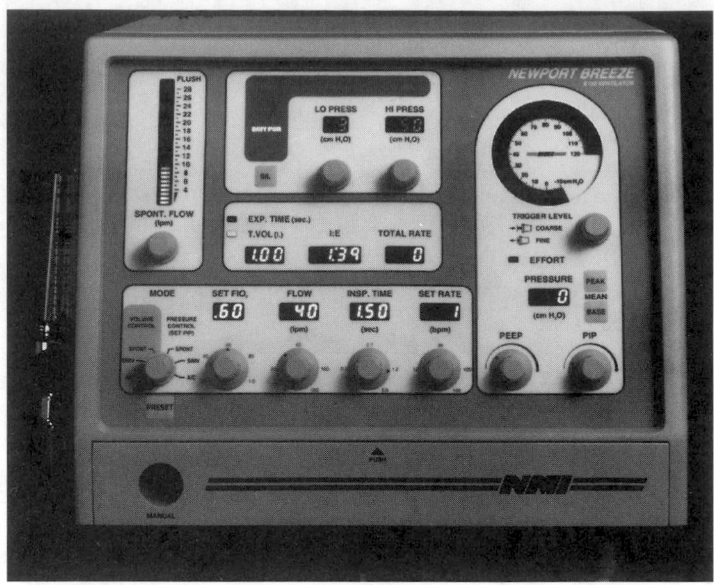

FIGURE 21-100. The control panel of the Newport Breeze ventilator. (Courtesy of Wave Medical Instruments, Newport Beach, CA)

In pressure-targeted modes, a positive pressure breath is delivered with each spontaneous inspiratory effort (that meets the trigger level) by the patient. Peak pressure is determined by the PIP setting.

Inspiratory Waveform

In ordinary operation, the Newport Breeze produces a rectangular pressure waveform in pressure controlled modes. It also produces a rectangular flow waveform in volume-targeted modes.

□ PHASE VARIABLES

Triggering

Inspiration is time-triggered as a function of the ventilatory frequency, which is operator determined by adjustment of the "set rate" adjustment. Rate is adjustable from 1 to 150 cycles/min.

Limiting

Pressure-triggering of inspiration is also possible when the airway pressure falls below the set trigger level. The set trigger level is adjustable from approximately −9 to +60 cmH_2O. Manual triggering of inspiration is also available. Pressure-limiting of inspiration from 0 to 60 cmH_2O is available. Inspiration is flow-limited in cases in which it is not pressure-limited. The inspiratory flow rate is adjustable from 1 to 120 L/min. The constant flow directed through the patient's circuit (throughout expiratory time) is adjustable from 0 to 50 L/m. The calibrated flow range for this adjustment is 0 to 28 L/m.

Cycling

Adjustment of the inspiratory time from 0.1 to 3.0 seconds determines time-cycling of inspiration. Inspiration time-cycles at 2 seconds when manually triggered. Inspiration may be pressure-cycled if the airway pressure is detected as greater than the set high pressure alarm threshold (adjustable from 10 to 120 cmH_2O).

The uncalibrated PEEP knob may be used for adjustment of baseline pressure. The range of adjustment available is from 0 to 60 cmH_2O.

□ CONTROL SUBSYSTEMS

Control Circuit

The Newport Breeze ventilator uses electronic and pneumatic components. The Duoflow system allows operator control of mechanical flow and of spontaneous flow separately. Mechanical flow is delivered to the patient during mandatory breaths only, and spontaneous flow is directed through the patient's circuit between mandatory breaths.

Spontaneous flow on the front panel serves as the source gas for spontaneous breathing and to stabilize baseline pressure between mechanical breaths. This system also provides a source of gas for spontaneous breathing in the unlikely event of an electronic ventilator malfunction. Spontaneous flow is calibrated from a minimum value of 28 L/min and will deliver a maximal flow of approximately 58 L/min when turned to "Flush." Spontaneous flow should be set to meet the patient's spontaneous inspiratory flow demands during spontaneous breathing in the SIMV or spontaneous modes. A reservoir bag containing mixed gas is available should the patient's inspiratory effort exceed the set spontaneous flow. If it is noted that the manometer displays a significant negative pressure swing during spontaneous inspiration, spontaneous flow should be increased to offset this increased demand. During exhalation, if the manometer displays a significant positive pressure swing, the spontaneous flow setting should be diminished.

The expiratory drive line outlet delivers pressure to the mushroom diaphragm of the exhalation valve. This is essential to maintenance of positive pressure and to the addition of PEEP or CPAP.

The microprocessor directs timing signals to a series of solenoid valves, which use pneumatic signals to activate flow and pressure control valves as well as the exhalation manifold. Airway pressure is monitored by an internal pressure transducer. This component generates signals for the high and low airway pressure alarms.

Drive Mechanism

An external pneumatic gas source that powers the air-oxygen blender is required for operation of the Breeze ventilator (Fig. 21-101). The blender delivers pressurized gas to the flow meter, which then directs a continuous flow of gas into the patient circuit.

Mechanical flow is calibrated from 3 to 120 L/min in increments of 1 L/min. This setting determines the delivered flow rate to the patient during mandatory or manual breaths. Mandatory tidal volume is a product of mechanical flow and inspiratory time. In the volume-targeted modes, set tidal volume is digitally displayed in the data display panel above the flow and FIO_2 displays. Accuracy is guaranteed only above 30 mL even though digital display of volumes below 30 mL may occur.

Inspiratory time is adjustable from 0.1 to 3.0 seconds and is graduated in increments of 0.01 second from 0.1 to 1 seconds and in increments of 0.1 second from 1 second to 3 seconds. The inspiratory phase is terminated when the selected time is reached and the Newport

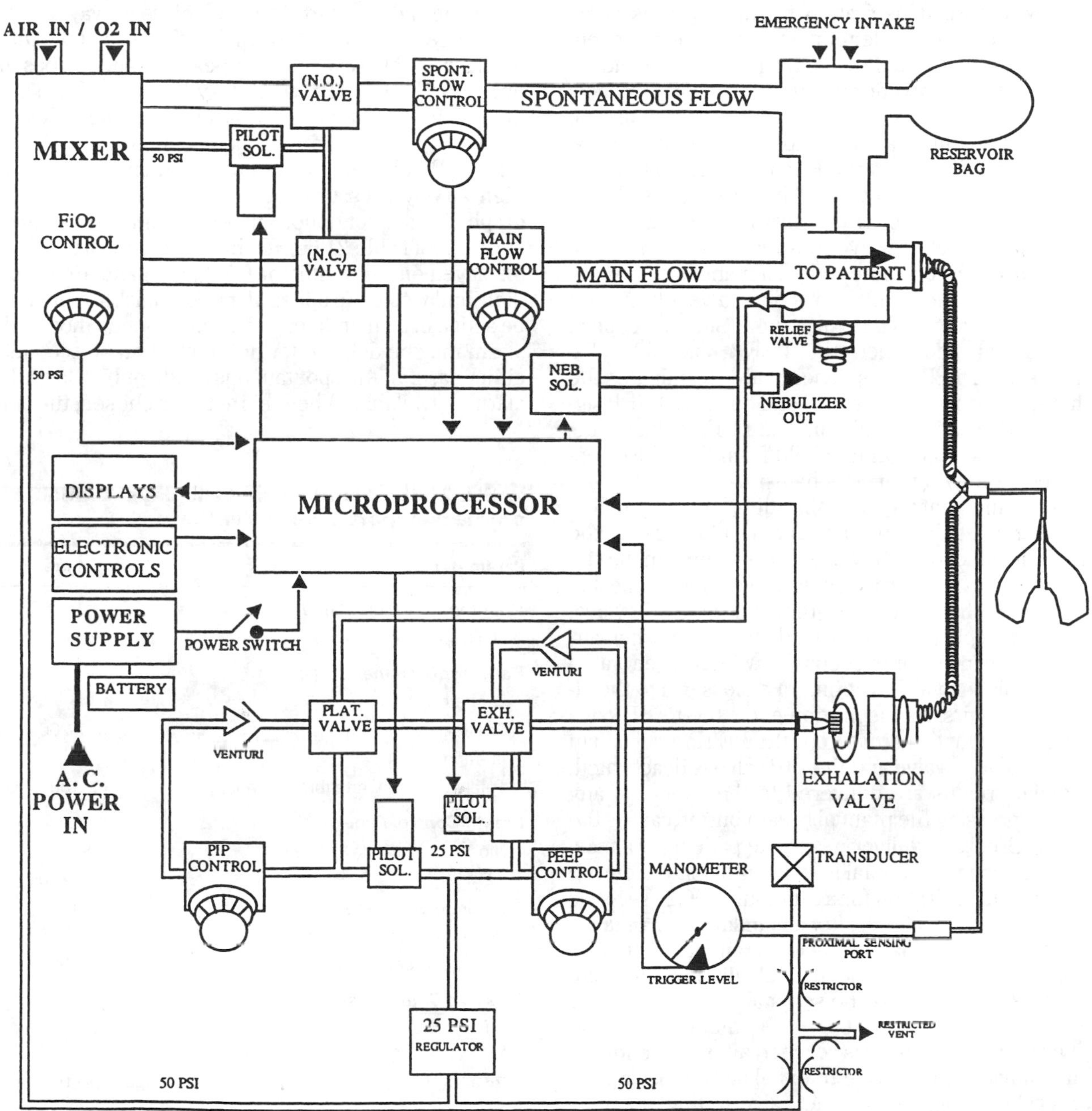

FIGURE 21-101. The internal schematic diagram of the Newport Breeze ventilator. (Courtesy of Wave Medical Instruments, Newport Beach, CA)

Breeze cycles into the expiratory phase. In the event that inverse I:E ratio is set to be delivered, the colon flashes in this display. In the event that at the maximal inverse I:E ratio is exceeded, the entire inspiratory time display flashes. The maximal inverse I:E ratio is 4:1.

Output Control Valves

A series of components comprises the output control valves of the Newport Breeze ventilator (see Fig. 21-101). They include the following: (1) control valves for spontaneous and for mandatory inspiration, (2) flow-switching valves, (3) flow-regulating needle valves, (4) inspiratory and expiratory pressure-switching valves, (5) pressure-regulating needle valves, and (6) a diaphragm exhalation valve. Inspiration is either flow controlled or pressure controlled.

In flow-controlled inspiration, the microprocessor activates the flow pilot solenoid. This generates a pneumatic signal that opens the master flow valve and directs gas from the blender through the inspiratory flow controlled needle valve. Simultaneously, a pneumatic signal from the internal inspiratory limb of the ventilator is generated through the PIP and PEEP valves and is sent to the exhalation valve. This pressure is always greater than pressure at the airway opening, which causes the exhalation valve to remain closed until the end of the inspiratory time. When a mandatory inspiration terminates, the spontaneous flow valve is turned on and the main flow valve is turned off. Simultaneously, PEEP is activated when the PEEP solenoid valve switches on. The PEEP solenoid valve terminates the high pressure pneumatic signal and directs a PEEP signal to the exhalation manifold. The PEEP signal is delivered to the exhalation manifold from the PEEP control needle valve/venturi mechanism.

In pressure-controlled inspiration, the main flow valve is activated; however, under influence of the plateau solenoid, the PIP valve directs a pneumatic signal from the PIP control needle valve/venturi mechanism to the exhalation valves through the PEEP valve. As a result, in pressure-controlled inspiration when airway pressure meets or exceeds that which is generated in the exhalation valve, venting of excess gas to the atmosphere occurs. As inspiration ends, the PEEP valve directs a pneumatic signal from the PEEP mechanism to the exhalation valve and the PIP valve is deactivated.

Manual breaths are delivered to the patient in any mode. Depressing the manual breath button causes the Newport Breeze to deliver gas to the patient for a maximum of 2 seconds. Manual inflation is displayed during a mechanical inspiration for a minimum of 0.24 seconds of the set inspiratory time, after a mandatory/manual inspiration. The maximal number of manual inflations is 150 breaths per minute. The manual inflation will create an inspiratory plateau at the set peak inspiratory pressure level in the pressure-controlled mode only. If the high pressure alarm limit is reached after 2 seconds, all manual inflations will cycle to exhalation. If peak pressure reaches the pressure relief valve setting, the pressure will plateau. In all modes, F_{IO_2} and flow of the manual inflation are delivered as set, and inspiratory time and rate are operator determined.

The pressure relief valve is positioned in the upper left corner of the rear panel of the Newport Breeze. This valve determines the maximal pressure that can be delivered in the patient circuit during spontaneous, mandatory, and manual ventilation. This valve may be adjusted from 0 to 120 cmH_2O. The pressure relief value is increased by clockwise rotation of the blue knurled knob and decreased by counterclockwise rotation. In all cases, the pressure relief valve should be set slightly above the high pressure alarm setting so that it will function as a safety pop-off. The pressure relief valve is factory preset at zero.

Output Displays

An aneroid pressure gauge displays airway pressure in a range of −10 to +120 cmH_2O (Table 21-65). Digital displays are also available for peak, mean, and baseline pressure; F_{IO_2}; peak inspiratory flow rate; inspiratory time; expiratory time (in pressure control modes); set frequency; calculated (set) tidal volume (V_T= flow × I time); I:E ratio; total respiratory frequency; and low and high airway pressure alarm thresholds. An LED bar graph displays continuous flow for spontaneous breaths.

Alarms (Table 21-66) for high and low pressure are displayed on the ventilator front panel and are both audible and visual. An apnea alarm is available, which may be active in all mandatory and spontaneous modes. The alarm may be delayed for not more than 60 seconds in either case. In the spontaneous mode only, a low CPAP alarm is available. When this alarm is chosen, the apnea

TABLE 21-65 **Monitors and Displays Available on the Newport Breeze Ventilator**

Parameter	Range
Spontaneous Flow Panel	
Digital display (L/min)	0–40 (+)
Data Display Panel	
Expiratory time	
Set tidal volume (mL)	30–2000
I:E ratio	
Total respiratory rate (breaths/min)	1–150
Breath Control Panel	
Mode	
F_{IO_2}	.21–1.00
Inspiratory flow mechanical (L/min)	3–120
Inspiratory time (sec)	0.1–3.0
Set rate (breaths/min)	1–150
Pressure Control Panel	
PIP (cmH_2O)	0–60
Mean (cmH_2O)	
Baseline (PEEP/CPAP) (cmH_2O)	0–60
Trigger level (cmH_2O)	−9–+60

TABLE 21-66 **Alarms for the Newport Breeze Ventilator**

Audible and Visible	
High pressure (cmH_2O)	10–120
Low pressure (cmH_2O)	3–99
Apnea (seconds delay)	5, 10, 15, 30, 60
Low CPAP (seconds delay)	4
Low battery (remaining operational time—minutes)	15
Audible only	
Source gas supply failure	Immediate
Adjustment of alarm loudness	72–82 dBA
Alarm silence (sec)	60

alarm delay knob may be placed in first position. This inactivates the apnea alarm and activates the low CPAP alarm. The low pressure alarm limit should be set just below the CPAP level. In the event that pressure within the circuit drops below the low pressure alarm limit for 4 seconds, the low pressure alarm will sound. The alarm silence may be activated before an alarm infraction such as suctioning. The alarm silence can be deactivated by pressing alarm silence a second time. System failure is indicated by a continuous alarm indicating electrical or mechanical failure. A continuous alarm also indicates low gas pressure for either air or oxygen entering the blender. A low battery alarm is indicated by a quick pulse alarm with a short interrupt that indicates that the backup battery is weak.

□ MODES OF OPERATION

The mode selector knob allows for operator selection of the appropriate ventilator mode (Table 21-67). Controlled modes include A/C, A/C plus Sigh, SIMV, and spontaneous, and the pressure controlled modes include spontaneous, SIMV, and A/C. FIO_2 is adjusted by movement of the FIO_2 selector and FIO_2 in the range of 0.21 to 1.0 is displayed digitally. The operator may check existing settings in the spontaneous mode by pushing "preset." This causes digital displays to indicate existing settings. Rate is adjustable in one breath per minute increments from 1 to 150 breaths per minute. Mandatory breaths are available to the patient in all mechanical modes. In the spontaneous mode, the respiratory rate is determined by the patient. The pressure manometer displays pressures in the range of −10 to +120 cmH_2O.

Pressure is displayed on the analog manometer (see Fig. 21-100). The pressure display window provides a continuous readout of mean airway pressure. Mean airway pressure is monitored by a integral pressure transducer through the proximal pressure inlet. Peak or baseline pressure readings can be displayed for 30 seconds by depressing either momentary push button. The display always returns to mean airway pressure after 30 seconds or when preset is pushed. The trigger level sensor is activated by the manometer needle. This sensor detects the patient's spontaneous inspiratory effort. The trigger level should be set just below baseline pressure so that in all modes the patient effort indicator lights when minimal inspiratory effort is exerted. In an assisted mode, each time the manometer needle passes the trigger level sensor, the Newport Breeze indicates an assisted mandatory breath.

The apnea alarm receives its input from the patient effort indicator in all modes. In the spontaneous mode, the apnea alarm delay may be set in the first or low CPAP alarm position. When this is done, the trigger level indicator no longer monitors spontaneous breathing efforts; instead, the low pressure alarm acts as a disconnect alarm. Patient effort is indicated by the patient effort indicator, which functions in all modes to indicate the patient's inspiratory effort. This indicator lights each time the manometer needle passes the trigger level sensor.

The nebulizer outlet provides a gas supply to a nebulizer, which is placed in line within the ventilator circuit. This allows for efficient delivery of aerosolized medications during mechanical ventilation. The nebulizer outlet provides a gas flow of approximately 6 L/min. It is important to note that this flow is additive to the set flow. The type of nebulizer used in the circuit influences the actual quantity of flow entering the patient's circuit. This is because different designs of nebulizers provide different levels of flow restriction. In the volume controlled mode, the approximate gas volume delivered through the nebulizer outlet is automatically added to and displayed in "SET TIDAL VOLUME." When inspiratory times are less than 0.4 seconds, it may be necessary to use an auxiliary flow meter to assure delivery of the medication. This should be done in place of and not in addition to the flow from the nebulizer outlet.

TABLE 21-67 **Modes of Ventilation for the Newport Breeze Ventilator**

Volume Modes	Pressure Modes
Assist CMV	Assist CMV
Assist CMV plus sigh	SIMV
SIMV	Spontaneous
Spontaneous	

□ TROUBLESHOOTING

A comprehensive troubleshooting chart is provided by the manufacturer in the Newport Breeze Ventilator Operating Manual.

Since this ventilator is microprocessor controlled, the respiratory care practitioner should exercise caution when operating devices that may emit electromagnetic interference or radiofrequency interference (such as cellular phones) in near proximity to the machine.

TABLE 21-68 **Classification of the Newport Wave Ventilator**

Power Source for Control Circuitry	**Electricity (100–115 volts AC at 60 Hz)**
Power source for pneumatic system	Air and oxygen (40–70 psig) High pressure gas sources
Control circuit	Microprocessor
Control mechanism	Pressure, flow/volume
Triggering	Pressure, time, manual
Limiting	Pressure, flow, volume, time
Cycling	Time, pressure, flow

Newport Wave Ventilator

☐ CLASSIFICATION

The Newport Wave Ventilator (Table 21-68) (Fig. 21-102) is a microprocessor based, servo feedback, pressure-triggered, flow/volume, or pressure-controlled ventilator for ventilatory support of neonates, children, or adults. The device features a predictive learning logic, bias flow, unique PSV breath ending criteria, and peak flow monitoring. Synchronized (Master/Slave) ventilation for independent lung ventilation is available.

☐ SPECIFICATIONS

Table 21-69 lists the specifications for the Newport Wave ventilator.

☐ INPUT VARIABLES

The Newport Wave ventilator requires 100 to 110 volts AC at 60 Hz for operation of its electronic controlled circuitry (see Table 21-68). Its pneumatic control circuit is operated by external compressed gas sources at 40 to 70 psig for both air and oxygen. As illustrated on the front panel of the Newport Wave (Fig. 21-103), the operator may select the mode of ventilation; pressure-limiting and pressure-cycling thresholds; PEEP/CPAP; peak inspiratory flow rate; inspiratory time; ventilatory rate; bias flow; and FIO_2.

Expiratory gas in the expiratory limb of the patient's circuit is controlled by a pneumatic exhalation valve that uses a balloon diaphragm to operate the valve opening. The internal pressure of the balloon is determined by gas from the main flow outlet manifold or by a flow of gas regulated by the PEEP control valve. Pressure in the exhalation valve is monitored by an electronic pressure transducer.

Operation

Operation of the Newport Wave is divided into two major ventilatory functions: mandatory and spontaneous (see Fig. 21-103 and Fig. 21-104). Mandatory functions include flow/volume controlled (volume-targeted) ventilation, pressure-controlled (pressure-targeted) ventilation, and Slave/Master ventilation involving the use of two Newport Wave ventilators for independent lung ventilation. Spontaneous ventilatory modes allow for the following: (1) bias flow, (2) demand flow, (3) pressure support ventilation, (4) bias flow plus demand flow, and (5) bias flow plus PSV.

When the Newport Wave is operated in volume-targeted ventilation, mandatory tidal volume (see Fig. 21-104) is set by adjusting flow (b) and inspiratory time (c). Tidal volume is displayed in the set tidal volume display (q). When volume-controlled ventilation is selected, the pressure control knob (h) must be in the "Off" position.

When the Newport Wave is operated in the SIMV or A/C mode with volume-targeted, mandatory breaths, the pressure control knob (h) must be rotated clockwise to the "Off" position. The mode, SIMV or A/C, is then selected.

Spontaneous ventilation is also available and pressure support may be used to augment spontaneous breaths when SIMV and spontaneous modes are selected.

At the set-flow rate (1 to 100 L/min) volume preset mandatory breaths are flow-limited and time-cycled at the end of the set inspiratory time interval (0.1 to 3 seconds). The set tidal volume ranges from 30 mL to 2000 mL and is calculated as the product of flow rate and the inspiratory time settings and is displayed digitally. Signals from the inspiratory flow sensor are used by the microprocessor to adjust the flow-control valve as necessary, throughout the inspiratory phase, to guarantee that the set flow rate is maintained. An inspiratory pause

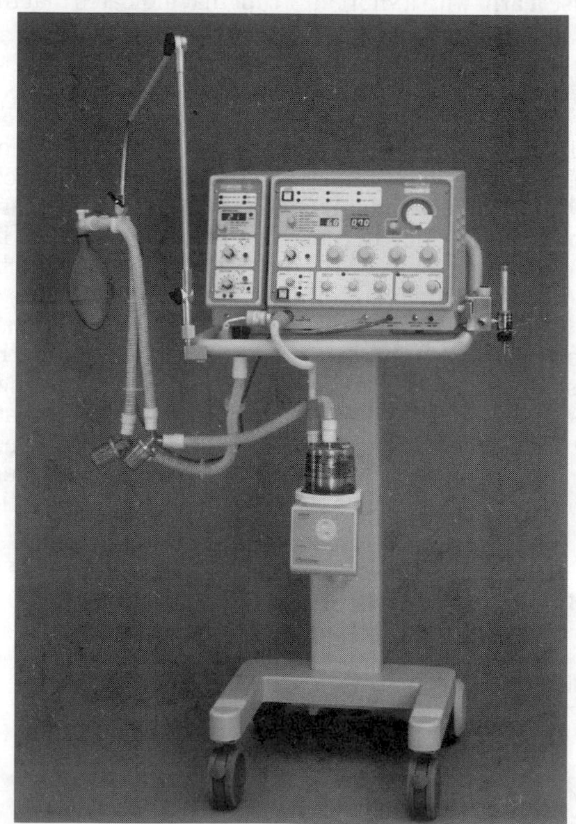

FIGURE 21-102. The Newport Wave ventilator. (Courtesy of Wave Medical Instruments, Newport Beach, CA)

TABLE 21-69 **Specifications for the Newport Wave Ventilator**

FIO_2	0.21–1.0
Gas flow (L/min)	1–100
Inspiratory time (sec)	0.1–3.0
Inspiratory pause (% Ti)	0, 10, 20, and 30
Rate (breaths/min)	1–100
Tidal volume (L)	10–2000
Pressure control level (cmH_2O)	0–75
Pressure support level (cmH_2O)	0–60
PEEP/CPAP (cmH_2O)	0–45
Bias flow (L/min)	0–30
Spont/demand flow (L/min)	0–160
Sensitivity (cmH_2O)	0–−5
Maximum inverse I:E	3:1
Manometer range (cmH_2O)	−10–+120
Pneumatic pressure relief (cmH_2O)	0–120
Nebulizer power source	On/off
Sigh	1.5 × tidal volume every 100 breaths
Manual breath	Operator controlled: volume or pressure breath

(10%, 20%, 30% of set inspiratory time) can volume-limit volume-targeted breaths.

In the pressure-control mode, mandatory breaths are pressure-limited at the level determined by the pressure control setting (0 to 80 cmH_2O) and time-cycled at the end of the set inspiratory time interval. The microprocessor, as a closed loop, regulates the inspiratory flow rate so that it will not exceed the set flow rate. If airway pressure reaches the high pressure alarm setting, pressure-targeted and volume-targeted mandatory breaths are pressure cycled before the end of the set inspiratory time interval. No plateau occurs.

In the spontaneous and SIMV modes, breaths may be supported with demand flow or continuous flow (set as bias flow: 0 to 30 L/min) or as a combination of the two.

Mandatory breaths can be pressure-triggered. As the inspiratory effort drops the proximal pressure, by an amount equal to the set sensitivity (0 to −5 cmH_2O), inspiration begins. Mandatory breaths are pressure-triggered with each spontaneous effort meeting the sensitivity criteria in the assist mode or time-triggered at a frequency set by the respiratory rate setting (0 to 100 breaths per minute). Mandatory breaths (flow/volume or pressure controlled) are pressure- or time-triggered at the set respiratory rate when in the SIMV mode.

Pressure support is available from 0 to 60 cmH_2O plus PEEP. Pressure support is pressure-triggered by the patient's inspiratory effort. The microprocessor initiates flow cycling when the inspiratory flow falls below a predetermined threshold based on the peak flow required to reach the pressure limit and elapsed inspiratory time. Pressure support is pressure cycled if airway pressure exceeds 2 cmH_2O above the set pressure support. Pressure support is time cycled if patient generated flow does not fall to the required flow-cycling threshold.

Mandatory breaths can be manually triggered in all modes. In SIMV and A/C modes, sigh breaths may be set. Sighs are pressure- or flow-limited and are time cycled at the end of a time interval equal to 1.5 × the set inspiratory time. Sighs are triggered each hundredth breath.

The baseline pressure is adjustable in a range of 0 to 45 cmH_2O. The FIO_2 is determined by the FIO_2 control setting (0.21 to 1.00). The nebulizer "On/Off" button controls flow to a micronebulizer. A safety pop-off valve is available through an adjustable pressure relief valve (0 to 120 cmH_2O).

□ CONTROL VARIABLES

Inspiratory pressure or flow is controlled by the Newport Wave. In the spontaneous mode, the ventilator controls inspiratory pressure at the limit set by the operator using the pressure control knob. In all other cases the unit controls flow.

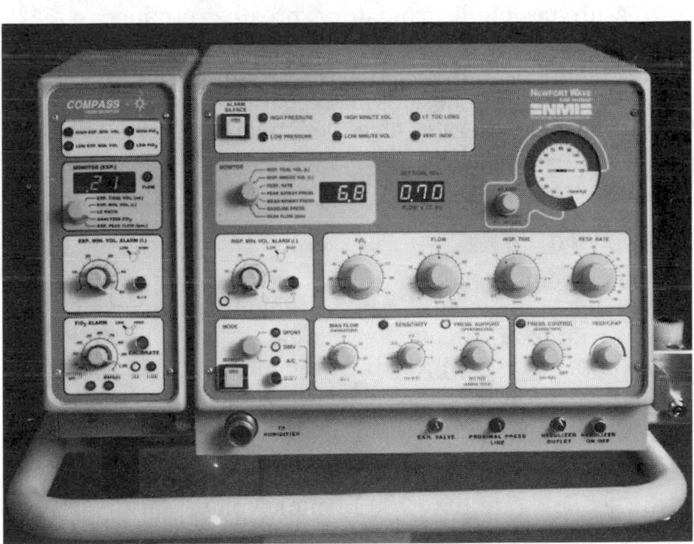

FIGURE 21-103. Portion of the control panel of the Newport Wave ventilator. (Courtesy of Wave Medical Instruments, Newport Beach, CA)

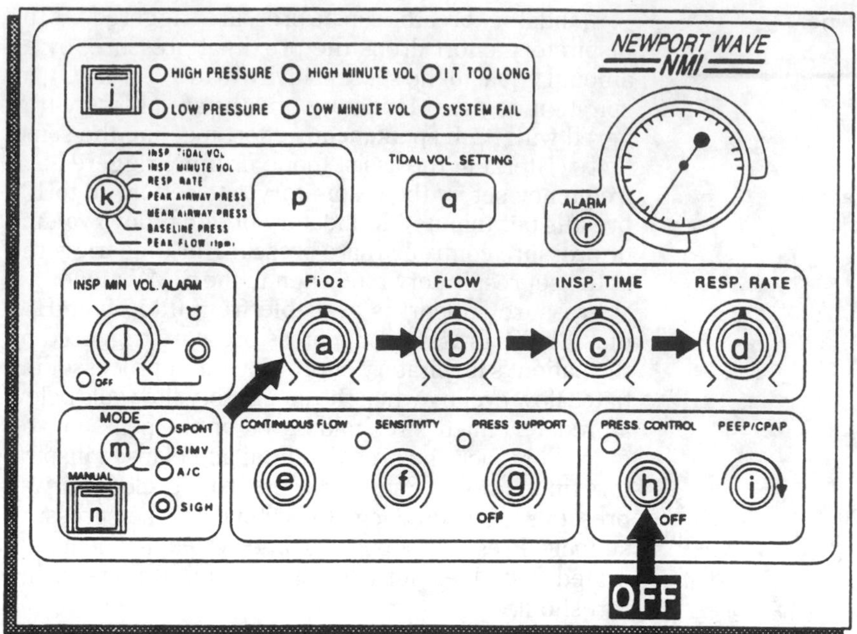

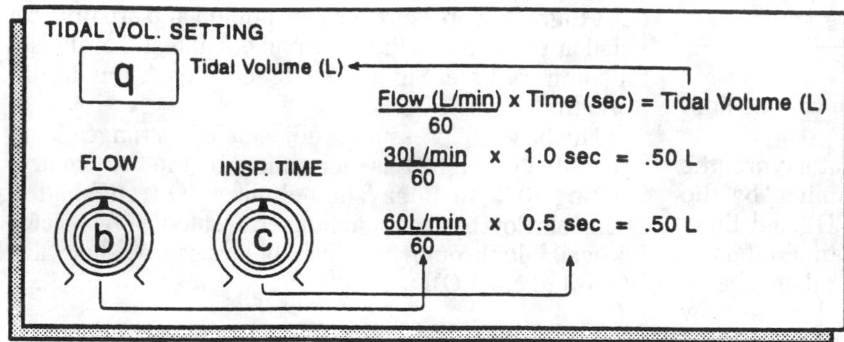

FIGURE 21-104. Labeled control panel of the Newport Wave ventilator. See text for explanation. (Courtesy of Wave Medical Instruments, Newport Beach, CA).

Inspiratory Waveform

The inspiratory flow waveform is essentially rectangular because volume-targeted breaths are delivered at a constant inspiratory flow rate. As a result, the volume and pressure waveforms are ramp-shaped.

Pressure-targeted mandatory breaths produce a nearly rectangular or exponential pressure waveform, which is influenced by the inspiratory flow setting. The volume waveform generates an exponential rise and the flow waveform generates an exponential decay.

□ PHASE VARIABLES

Triggering

Spontaneous breaths are pressure-triggered in the SIMV and spontaneous modes. Volume-targeted or pressure-targeted mandatory breaths are initiated (time- or pressure-triggered) by the microprocessor in both the assist control and SIMV modes.

Limiting

Volume-targeted mandatory breaths are flow limited at the set flow rate (0 to 100 L/min). Volume-targeted breaths may be volume-limited with the inspiratory pause set at zero. Mandatory, pressure-targeted breaths may be pressure-limited as determined by the pressure control setting.

Cycling

Mandatory breaths are pressure- or time-cycled. Spontaneous breaths are flow- or pressure-cycled. For spontaneous breathing, continuous flow is also available.

□ CONTROL SUBSYSTEMS

Control Circuit

The Newport Wave uses a closed loop microprocessor to control and power functions of the ventilator (Fig. 21-105). Pneumatic and electronic controlled components comprise the control circuit of the ventilator. Input is accepted by the electronic control circuit for triggering and cycling signals from the inspiratory time and ventilatory rate settings and from the airway pressure transducer. Flow is controlled by four transducers. Two of these are pressure transducers and two are flow transducers. Two pressure transducers monitor airway pressure and pressure in the exhalation valve. The flow transducers monitor output from the master control valve. Control of the exhalation manifold is pneumatic.

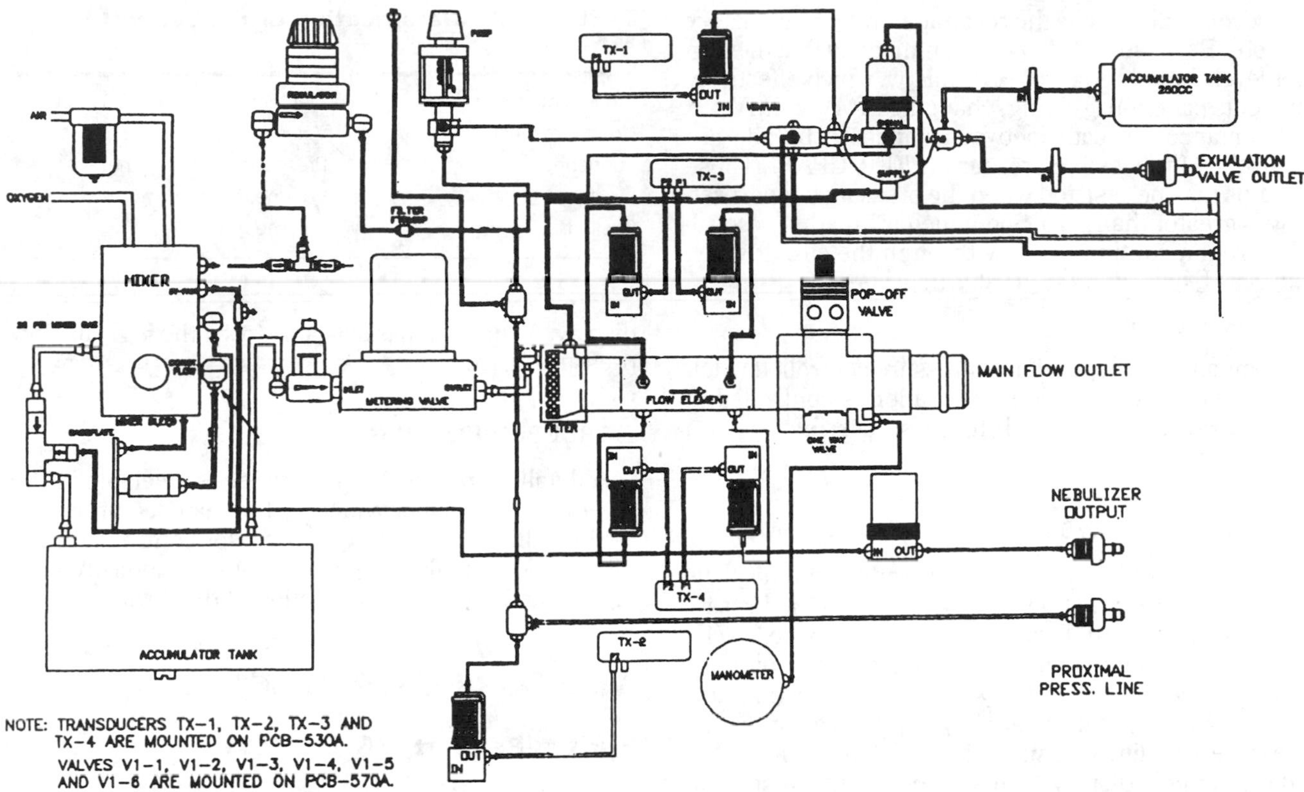

FIGURE 21-105. Internal circuit of the Newport Wave ventilator. (Courtesy of Wave Medical Instruments, Newport Beach, CA)

An electromagnetic coil and plunger regulate gas flow through the valve opening of the flow control valve. The position of the plunger is determined by the amount of electric current applied to the coil. Gas from the flow control valve is monitored by a differential pressure flow sensor and a mechanical pressure manometer before entering the inspiratory limb of the patient's circuit.

Drive Mechanism

Compressed air and oxygen are supplied to the oxygen air blender. The mixed gas leaving the blender at 28 psig enters a rigid-walled vessel referred to as "the accumulator," from which it is provided to the high-speed servo control valve. The high-speed servo control valve is microprocessor controlled. This valve directs its gas flow to two independent flow sensors, which in turn direct their gas flow to the patient. Flow (volume) is sequentially monitored by the microprocessor with input to the alarm module. This system improves response time, reduces the flow required of the compressed gas supply system, and provides for a wide range of peak flow settings.

□ MODES OF OPERATION

Operating modes are selected through adjustment of the Mode Selector on the front panel of the ventilator (Table 21-70) (see Fig. 21-103). Modes available are spontaneous, SIMV, and A/C (with or without sigh).

Assist/Control

In the A/C mode, inspiration is pressure-triggered, given that inspiratory effort is made and that sensitivity is appropriately set. Inspiration may also be time-triggered in accordance with adjustment of the respiratory rate setting. Also in A/C, inspiration may be pressure- or flow-limited and is normally time-cycled.

SIMV

In SIMV mode, all synchronized mandatory breaths are pressure-triggered, given that spontaneous breathing efforts are made and that the sensitivity adjustment is appropriate. Inspiration may also be time-triggered in accordance with the rate setting on the ventilator. Inspiration is pressure- or flow-limited and time-cycled.

It should be noted that when SIMV rates are in excess of 20 breaths/min, some mandatory breaths may be asynchronous with the patient's. The triggering mechanism in the Newport Wave delivers a mandatory breath to the patient when spontaneous breathing effort is sensed during the last 25% of each ventilatory period

TABLE 21-70 **Modes of Ventilation Available on the Newport Wave Ventilator**

A/C
SIMV
Spontaneous

(60 seconds divided by the respiratory rate = ventilatory period). Because of this, it is recommended that the trigger level should be set at −10 cmH_2O, which effectively prevents patient-triggering, changing SIMV to IMV.

Spontaneous breaths between mandatory breaths are controlled for baseline pressure (PEEP/CPAP). These breaths may be assisted when the pressure support setting is greater than zero. Spontaneous breaths are available from a continuous flow through the circuit when the Bias Flow setting is greater than zero.

Spontaneous

Spontaneous inspiration is pressure controlled when in the spontaneous mode. Inspiration is controlled at the set PEEP/CPAP level. It is also possible to set a pressure support level.

□ OUTPUT DISPLAYS (MONITORS AND ALARMS)

The Newport Wave ventilator monitors and displays seven ventilator functions and set tidal volume for safe monitoring of gas delivery to the patient (Table 21-71). Monitored functions include the following: inspiratory tidal volume (L), inspiratory minute volume (L/min), respiratory rate, peak inspiratory pressure, mean airway pressure, baseline pressure, and peak flow (L/min). Set tidal volume is displayed in a second digital display in the same panel as the monitored functions. Key parameters included in the alarm section are high pressure, low pressure, high minute volume, low minute volume, excessive inspiratory time, ventilator inoperative, and system failure. There is also a 60-second alarm silence. Ventilator outlet pressure is monitored with an analog display. A pull switch is available to set the high and low pressure alarm.

TABLE 21-71 **Monitors and Alarms Available on the Newport Wave Ventilator**

Monitors	
Inspiratory tidal volume (L)	0–99.9
Set tidal volume (L)	0–99.9
Inspiratory minute volume (L)	0–99.9
Respiratory rate (breaths/min)	0–999
Peak pressure (cmH_2O)	0–120
Mean airway pressure (cmH_2O)	0–120
Baseline pressure (cmH_2O)	0–120
Peak flow (L/min)	0–160
Alarms	
Audible and visual	
High pressure (cmH_2O)	10–120
Low pressure (cmH_2O)	0–110
High minute volume (L)	1–50 or 0.1–5
Low minute volume (L)	0–49 or 0–4.9
Inspiratory time too long	
Ventilator inop	
System failure	
Audible only	
Gas supply source failure	
Power failure	
Alarm silence	60 sec

TABLE 21-72 **Classification of the Bennett MA-1**

Power source	Electricity (115 volts AC at 60 Hz)
Control mechanism	Volume
Triggering	Pressure, manual, time
Limiting	Volume, flow
Cycling	Volume, pressure

□ TROUBLESHOOTING

A detailed troubleshooting guide is available in the Operator's Manual provided by the manufacturer.

Since this device is microprocessor controlled, careful attention should be given to considerations regarding EFI and RFI during operation of the device.

NELLCOR PURITAN-BENNETT

Puritan-Bennett MA-1*

□ CLASSIFICATION

The Bennett MA-1 ventilator (Nellcor Puritan-Bennett Corporation, Carlsbad, CA) (Table 21-72) (Fig. 21-106) is electrically powered and is a volume controller. It can be pressure-triggered (patient effort), time-triggered, or manually triggered into inspiration. The inspiratory phase is volume- or flow-limited. The inspiratory waveform is a descending ramp. Inspiration ends when the preset volume is reached (volume-cycled) or when the preset pressure limit is reached (pressure-cycled). It has a built-in air compressor,and a connection for a 50 psig oxygen source that allows oxygen delivery to the internal blending device. A wall air option allows the system to use hospital air in place of the main compressor.

The Bennett MA-1 has a gas outlet port that can power a micronebulizer during inspiration. There is also an expiratory retard control. The MA-1 may be modified to provide IMV, PEEP, or spontaneous CPAP.

□ SPECIFICATIONS

Table 21-73 lists specifications for the MA-1 ventilator.

□ INPUT VARIABLES

The Bennett MA-1 ventilator requires an electrical power source of 115 volts 60 Hz. The Bennett MA-1B uses 230 volts 50 Hz. Activating the ventilator is accomplished through turning the power switch (A) to the on position (Fig. 21-107). To access oxygen, a hose is plugged into a 50-psig oxygen outlet

* Thanks to John Canfield of Nellcor Puritan-Bennett, Carlsbad, CA, for his technical assistance with the MA-1.

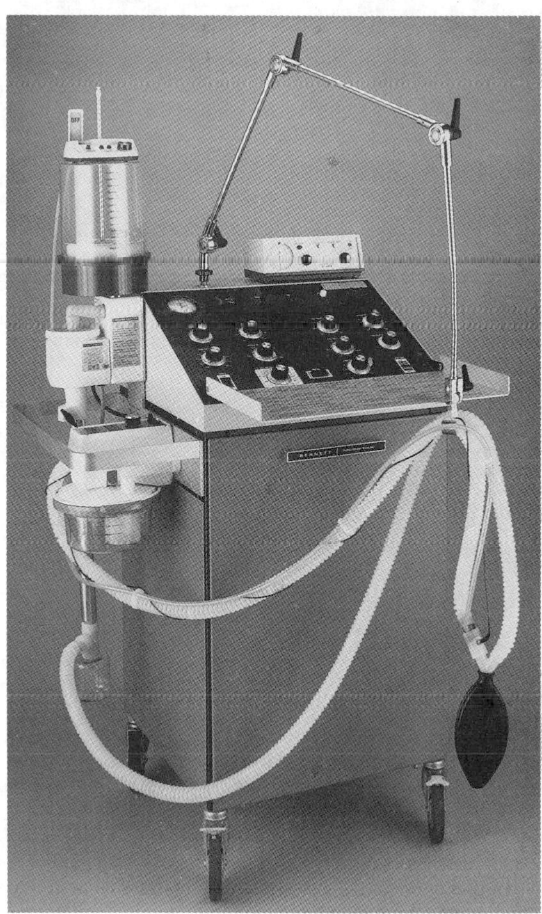

FIGURE 21-106. Bennett MA-1 ventilator. (Courtesy of Nellcor Puritan Bennett Corp., Carlsbad, CA)

TABLE 21-73 **Specifications for the Bennett MA-1 Ventilator**

Inspiration	
Rate (breaths/min)	Min (approx 0.5)–60
Volume (mL)	Min (approx 50)–2200
Flow rate (L/min)	Min (approx 15)–100
Pressure (cmH_2O)	20–80
Time (sec)	NC
Effort (cmH_2O)	−9–+10 (and lockout)
Hold (sec)	NC (see retard)
Demand flow (L/min)	NC
Safety pressure (cmH_2O)	85
Pressure support (cmH_2O)	NC
MMV (L/min)	NC
Expiration	
Time (sec)	NC
PEEP/CPAP (cmH_2O)	Optional
Retard (sec)	5–20*
I/E ratio	NC
Modes	
Assist	
Control	
A/C	
*IMV (Optional)	

* See text for explanation.
NC = not controlled.

Operation

The humidifier should be filled and adjusted to the proper temperature at least 20 minutes before use so it will preheat while the ventilator is on standby. The ventilator sensitivity (B) must be adjusted for pressure triggering. Peak flow (C), mechanical ventilatory breathing rates (D), V_T up to 2200 mL (E), and normal high-pressure limit (F) must be set. Pressure-cycled ventilation can be used, but at the end of each inspiration, the pressure-limit alarm (P) will sound unless it is silenced (switch just below front panel, inside cabinet). For sighs, the pressure limit (G) and the volume limit (H) function exactly as the normal pressure, volume limits, and rate, but at greater intervals; the sigh has its own volume and pressure that are independent of the ventilator breath. Up to three sighs may be administered (I). Manual breaths may be selected (normal or sigh) with button (J).

The control for oxygen concentration is adjustable from 21% to 100% (K) and accurate to within plus or minus 2.5%. This is pneumatically powered with any high-pressure oxygen source. Thus, careful attention to the oxygen connection is essential. The amount of expiratory retard is controlled by the expiratory resistance control (L). The expiratory resistance control varies the rate at which the air leaves the circuit during exhalation, but it does not change the total cycle time, which is based on the rate setting. At a pressure of 20 cmH_2O, with the expiratory resistance knob set at maximum, an inspiratory plateau will occur, which lasts approximately 0.75 to 1.0 seconds. As the pressure increases, the plateau becomes longer. In theory, the plateau period can be present when another breath is triggered, thus the ventilator might never allow for exhalation.

Medication is nebulized by filling a nebulizer cup and activating the switch (M). PEEP is adjusted by an optional control on the side of the ventilator, and the level is registered on the ventilator system pressure gauge (N).

□ CONTROL VARIABLES

The MA-1 controls volume. The gas that is delivered to the patient comes from an internal bellows. This bellows empties its gas when the internal compressor (drive mechanism) forces air into the bellows chamber causing the bellows to rise (see Drive Mechanism below).

Inspiratory Waveform

The waveform generated is rectangular (constant) when no load is present and becomes a descending ramp when a load is present (see "Troubleshooting" section below).

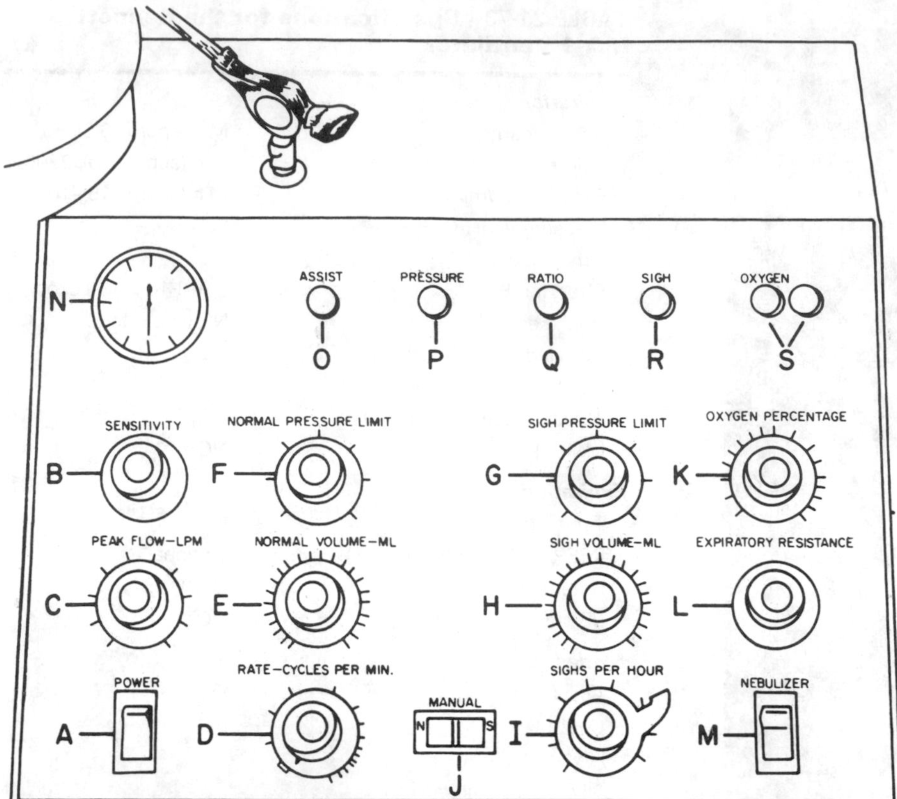

FIGURE 21-107. Control panel of the Puritan-Bennett MA-1 (see text).

☐ PHASE VARIABLES

Triggering

Inspiration is commonly pressure triggered. The sensitivity knob, which is uncalibrated, can be increased or decreased. The patient draws air out of the circuit during inspiration, causing the circuit pressure to drop, triggering the ventilator to deliver a breath. Sensitivity is usually adjusted so that the patient need only drop the pressure about -1 to -2 cmH_2O for the ventilator to trigger.

The ventilator is time-triggered when the patient's respiratory rate is established by the ventilator. This is controlled by the rate knob. Time-triggering also functions during the sigh mode. Manual triggering occurs when the manual breath button is pushed and the preset tidal volume is delivered. The same is true of the sigh breath manual button, in which case a sigh volume is delivered.

Limiting

The volume is limited in the respect that the volume contained in the bellows is predetermined and cannot exceed that set amount. Since the volume cannot rise higher than this value, it is limited. In general use, the moment the volume is reached, the ventilator generally cycles into exhalation. So, technically, it volume-cycles out of inspiration during normal operation. However, if the expiratory resistance knob is turned to its maximum value, a slight pause occurs at the end of inspiration before exhalation begins. In this instance, the ventilator is volume-limited but not volume-cycled.

The ventilator can also be flow-limited in the sense that the flow value is set by the operator and this is never exceeded.

Cycling

Normally, the MA-1 ends inspiration and begins expiration when the preset volume is achieved. It can be pressure cycled if the pressure reached during inspiration exceeds the pressure set on the pressure limit control.

Baseline Pressure

To achieve a baseline pressure above zero, a special PEEP attachment must be added to the side of the ventilator. This uncalibrated control provides a PEEP range of 0 to about 15 cmH_2O. Historically (1970s), another attachment was available for negative pressures during exhalation from about -9 to 0 cmH_2O. This is now obsolete.

☐ CONTROL SUBSYSTEMS

Control Circuit

The MA-1 uses electrical control components to power and control most functions of the ventilator, along with pneumatic and mechanical components.

Drive Mechanism

Air is drawn into the MA-1 (Fig. 21-108) through an air filter (A) to an oxygen blender (C) by the descending bellows. From a compressor (B), air is pumped into

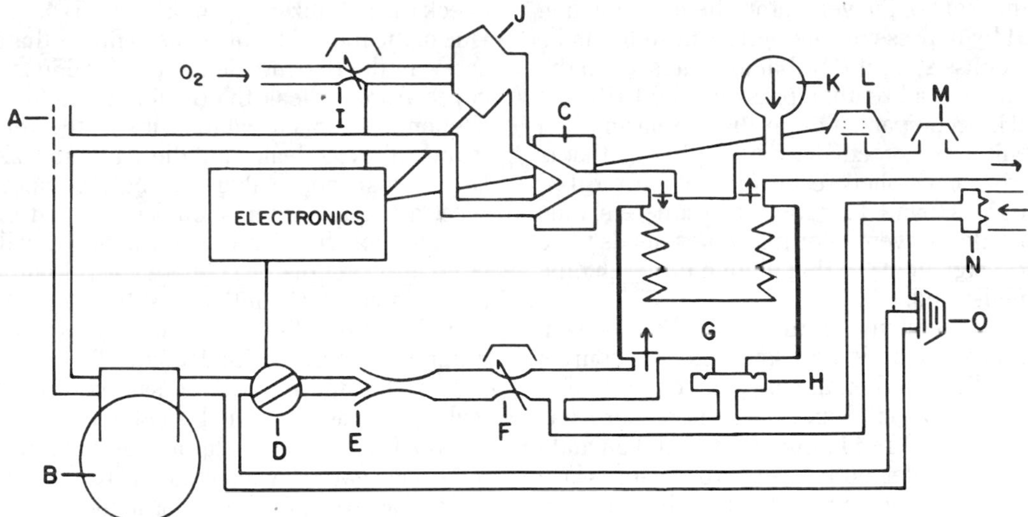

FIGURE 21-108. Schematic diagram of the MA-1 ventilator (see text for explanation).

the power drive system, which causes the bellows to ascend. A solenoid valve (D) cycles the ventilator according to the logic of the electronic circuit and produces inspiratory and expiratory phases. The compressed gas passes through a jet venturi (E) and flow control valve (F). The jet venturi is designed to boost the flow and to provide a descending waveform for flow. The slope of the ramp depends on the load. The higher the load, for example, the higher the patient's airway resistance and the lower the compliance, the more the flow decreases and extends inspiratory time. Pressure here is up to a maximum of 1.8 psig (127 cmH_2O). Distal to the venturi booster is the peak-flow control knob (F), which regulates the inspiratory flow rate by the rate of compression of the bellows. The peak flow valve operates as a variable restrictor. As the flow is reduced, the amount of pressure is reduced.

After passing the flow rate control, the major portion of gas flows into the bellows compression canister (G) through a one-way valve, and the remainder flows to a mushroom valve and compresses it (H). Gas is exhausted from the bellows compression chamber once inspiration is complete.

In the patient intake circuit, air is drawn in through a filter (A), delivered to a blending chamber (C), and mixed with oxygen according to the proportion set on the oxygen-control knob (I). Oxygen flow to the blending chamber is switched electronically and coupled mechanically and proportioned by an oxygen delivery bellows (J) (oxygen accumulator). The oxygen–air mixture then enters the bellows through a one-way valve as it begins to descend (expiration). When the bellows (G) begins to ascend, a second one-way valve opens, and the bellows gas is discharged into the patient circuit. Pressure is monitored by the ventilator system pressure gauge (K) and is limited by a pressure-relief control (L). When the assist mode is used, sensitivity can be adjusted (M). The patient system bifurcates to allow flow from the internal compressor to also send gas to the mushroom (exhalation) valve (N). This mushroom valve inflates during inspiration and seals the system, forcing the gas into the patient's airway. Flow to this mushroom valve can also be controlled independently to obtain PEEP using a special PEEP attachment.

Output Control Valve

The basic operating components that help determine the shape of the inspiratory flow waveform are the main solenoid valve, which turns the breath on and off by supplying gas flow to the peak flow valve, and the jet venturi system. These all interact with the internal bellows, which supplies the gas to the patient. In addition, during inspiration, gas flows to the mushroom valve in the exhalation line and this seals the patient circuit.

□ MODES OF OPERATION

There is no switch to control the modes on the MA-1. They are controlled by using the sensitivity and rate knobs. Control mode (volume-controlled, time-triggered, flow-limited, and volume-cycled) means all breaths are timed by the ventilator. The patient is usually apneic. If the sensitivity is turned completely off, the patient cannot trigger a machine breath and technically this would be control mode, but clinically this is not a good idea.

Assist mode (volume-controlled, pressure-triggered, flow-limited, and volume-cycled) means all breaths are triggered by a patient effort. The rate would be set at zero and sensitivity would detect the patient's inspiratory effort.

A/C is a combination of the control and assist modes where a minimum rate is set on the rate knob and inspiration can be pressure- or time-triggered, whichever comes first.

□ OUTPUT DISPLAYS (MONITORS) AND ALARMS

The ventilating pressures are monitored with an analog meter, which displays pressure in cmH_2O (see Fig. 21-107 [N]). The monitoring and alarm systems consist of lights on the front of the ventilator; the bulb function can be tested by depressing the light. These lights include an amber assist light (O) that indicates when the patient has initiated a breath; a pressure light (P) that turns red and is accompanied by an audible alarm when the pressure limit is exceeded; a ratio light (Q) that is activated during controlled respiration when the I/E ratio becomes less than 1:1 for the set parameters, thus the inspiratory flow or ventilator frequency needs to be adjusted; and a sigh light (R) that illuminates each time a sigh is administered.

An oxygen light system (S) functions when the ventilator is connected to a high-pressure oxygen source; a green light indicates when the oxygen concentration is set at greater than 21% and a high-pressure gas source is connected. A red light activates and an audible alarm sounds under both high- and low-pressure conditions in the oxygen accumulator. If the pressure in the accumulator is >3 or <1 cmH_2O, this alarm will activate. In the event that the pressure is >7 cmH_2O, the accumulator will actually pop-off from the seating edge. This was designed as a safety measure to prevent pressures inside the bag from becoming too high. One example of the alarm condition is when a high-pressure gas source has not been connected to the ventilator and when the oxygen control knob (K) is turned to some value other than 21%.

Use of the exhaled gas-collecting spirometer can assist the operator to ensure the delivery of adequate V_T and that the patient is connected to the ventilator. Optional modes such as IMV that require constant flow for spontaneous breathing, however, interfere with the spirometer and will require the clinician to provide additional monitoring to prevent accidental patient disconnection.

□ TROUBLESHOOTING

Because electronic components form a major part of this ventilator, most major malfunctions should be repaired by a manufacturer's representative.

If the ventilator will not develop pressure, look for leaks at circuit connecting points. For example, check the connection of the patient circuit to the humidifier or check the nebulizer cup to be sure it is screwed on tight. One of the most difficult leaks to find is that from a loose screw in the heating element housed in the humidifier cover. Another leak that is difficult to find is a disconnection of the bacterial filter inside the ventilator door. If you check for leaks and there are no leaks, the exhalation mushroom valve may be incompetent or torn. Also, a thermometer should be placed in the orifice provided for this purpose or the orifice will leak. Similarly, if the ventilator is operated without the spirometer, the spirometer outlet must be plugged.

If the humidifier does not heat satisfactorily, the water level may be inadequate, the heating element may be burned out, or the safety switch may not be making contact with the humidifier cover.

If the I:E ratio alarm illuminates, but the ventilator settings have not been changed, the problem may have developed as a result of problems in the patient's lung characteristics. Because of low driving pressure (only 127 cmH_2O) available on the MA-1, if the patient's lung compliance is low and the airway resistance is high, a constant flow pattern cannot be maintained. This is caused by a decrease in the pressure gradient between the ventilator and the alveoli. When the drive mechanism cannot maintain a pressure at least five times the airway pressure needed for the patient, the ventilator flow begins to taper off. Since this is a volume-cycled ventilator, the ventilator will not cycle off as soon as it would under normal lung conditions. Because flow tapers off or slows (Fig. 21-109) inspiratory time gets longer. However, the MA-1 normally time-triggers. That means that the total time for one breath is fixed to a constant value when the operator selects a specific rate.

For example, let the rate be 12 breaths/min. The time for one breath is 5 seconds (60 seconds/12). If the inspiratory time gets longer, then the expiratory time must get shorter. Only volume or pressure can cycle the ventilator out of inspiration. This changes the I:E ratio. When the I:E ratio exceeds 1:1 based on the frequency setting, the ratio light will illuminate and give this warning. To correct the situation without changing the minute ventilation, try increasing the inspiratory flow of gas. But remember, the flow pattern will still be tapered.

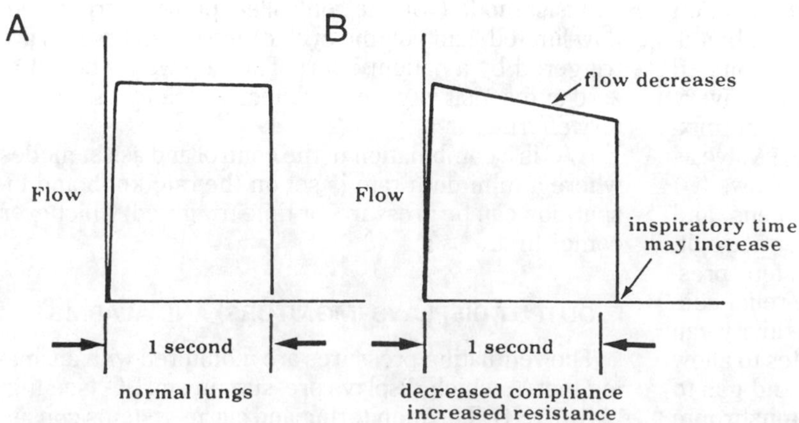

FIGURE 21-109. Inspiratory curves represent the changes in flow that occur using a constant flow ventilator with a low working pressure. Under normal conditions, flow is constant **(A)**. As compliance decreases significantly and resistance increases, the flow decreases slightly **(B)**. This type of curve is a tapered or modified square wave and resembles a descending ramp. If the ventilator is volume-cycled, the volume will be delivered, but inspiratory time may increase **(B)**. This can affect the inspiratory-expiratory ratio. (From Pilbeam, S.P., "Mechanical Ventilation: Physiological and Clinical Applications," Mosby–Year Book, St. Louis, 1992, p 135, with permission)

TABLE 21-74 **Classification of the Bennett 7200**

Power source for gas delivery	Electricity (115 volts AC at 60 hz), High pressure gas sources
Control circuit	Microprocessor
Control mechanism	Pressure, flow/volume
Triggering	Pressure, flow, time, manual
Limiting	Pressure, volume, flow
Cycling	Volume, time, pressure, flow

Nellcor Puritan-Bennett 7200 Microprocessor Ventilator*

☐ CLASSIFICATION

The Nellcor Puritan Bennett 7200 ventilator (Table 21-74) (Fig. 21-110) is electrically and pneumatically powered and microprocessor operated. It is a pressure or flow controller. Triggering can be accomplished by pressure, time, flow, or manual operation. It is pressure-, volume-, or flow-limited and pressure-, time-, or flow-cycled. Pressure supported and pressure control ventilation and numerous special functions are optional and may be purchased separately and installed at any time.

☐ SPECIFICATIONS

Table 21-75 lists the specifications for the 7200 and Table 21-76 lists some of its special functions.

☐ INPUT VARIABLES

The electrical system of the ventilator is powered by common current of 115 volts AC 60 Hz. The primary elements of the pneumatic system are two proportional solenoid valves (PSOLS), one for air and one for oxygen, that both mix and meter breathing gas. Source gas can range between 35 and 100 psig.

Operation

On receiving electrical power, the microprocessor of the 7200 ventilator initiates a series of tests known by the acronym POST (power on self-test) designed to verify the proper function of the microprocessor and associated circuitry. This test lasts 10 to 15 seconds in the 7200a version and nominally 5 seconds in the 7200ae version. All ventilator functions are disabled during this interval. After the POST, all previous ventilatory settings are recalled from memory and reset. This RAM receives power from an internal set of batteries, which prevent loss of data in the event of a power disruption. If batteries are absent or fail, the 7200 uses a set of default settings stored in a read-only memory (ROM). Failure to complete POST requires the attention of appropriately trained personnel.

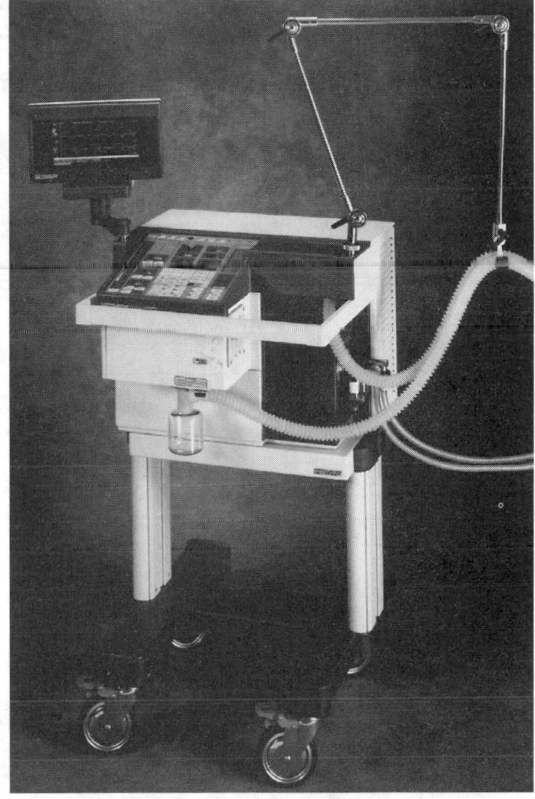

FIGURE 21-110. Nellcor Puritan-Bennett 7200 Series microprocessor ventilator. (Courtesy of Puritan Bennett Corp., Carlsbad, CA)

The ventilator is operated from the front panel (Figs. 21-111, 21-112, and 21-113), which is partitioned into three sections: ventilator settings, patient data, and ventilator status. To change any settings except PEEP/CPAP, there is a function key within the ventilator settings section that causes the preexisting value for that setting to be displayed in the message display window. This preexisting value is changed by sequentially pressing keys on the numeric touchpad keys; the new setting is stored in RAM by touching the ENTER key, which is confirmed by two beeps. If a setting lies outside of its specified range, the microprocessor rejects the entry with four beeps, and the message INVALID ENTRY is displayed. Pressing CLEAR redisplays the function to facilitate entry of an acceptable value. If the operator neglects to touch the ENTER key for a specific time frame, the display reverts to the previously selected value. The interval lasts between 10 and 18 seconds for the 7200a version and 30 seconds for the 7200ae version. PEEP/CPAP is adjusted by a control knob that regulates the relief pressure of the expiratory valve.

The ventilatory modes are selected by individual mode keys, including CMV, SIMV, and CPAP. Additional breathing functions like PSV and PCV and special functions like respiratory mechanics testing are accessed by the "++" key in older models and discrete membrane keys in the newest models. Values for mechanical tidal volume, respiratory rate, peak inspiratory flow rate, oxygen percentage, from 21% to 100%, and the

* Thanks to Warren Sanborn, Nellcor Puritan-Bennett Corp., Carlsbad, CA, for his technical assistance with the 7200 ventilator.

TABLE 21-75. **Specifications for the Nellcor Puritan-Bennett 7200 Microprocessor Ventilator**

Modes

- A/C (CMV) (volume control)
- A/C (CMV) (pressure control)
- SIMV (volume control)
- SIMV (pressure control)
- SIMV (volume control) + PSV
- SIMV (pressure control) + PSV
- CPAP (with PSV)
- CPAP (without PSV)

Breath Type	**Range**
Breath type—mandatory	
Volume control	
Volume (mL)	100–2500
Rate (breaths/min)	
A/C (CMV)	0.5–70
SIMV	0.5–70
Peak inspiratory flow (L/sec)	10–120
Flow waveform	Square, descending ramp
Plateau (sec)	0–2.0
Inspiratory hold (sec)	0.0–2.0
Pressure control	
Inspiratory pressure (above PEEP) (cmH_2O)	5–100
Inspiratory time (sec)	0.2–5
Rate (breaths/min)	
A/C (CMV)	0.5–70
SIMV	0.5–70
I:E ratio	1:9.0–4:1
Breath type—spontaneous	
Pressure support (cmH_2O)	10–70
PEEP/CPAP (cmH_2O)	0–45
Common Parameters	
Oxygen percentage	21–100
Inspiratory trigger	
Pressure (below PEEP, cmH_2O)	0.5–20
Flow (L/min)	1–15

Other Featured Parameters/Functions

- Manual inspiration
- Manual sigh
- Automatic sigh
- 100% oxygen suction (2 min)
- Nebulizer
- Apnea interval and ventilation
- Flow-by (flow-triggering)
- Clock/calendar set
- Auto-PEEP
- Digital communications interface
- Respiratory mechanics
- Graphics
- Trending
- Pulse oximeter
- Display screen
- Metabolics (integrated)

Alarm Indicators

- High and low pressure
- Apnea
- I:E ratio
- Power loss
- Exhalation valve leak
- Low volume
- Low exhaled minute volume
- Ventilator inoperative
- Low pressure oxygen/air inlet
- High rate
- Low CPAP/PEEP
- Low battery

desired waveform (constant, descending, or sinusoidal) are sequentially entered into RAM. Pressure during all types of inspiration may be limited up to 120 cmH_2O, using the high-pressure limit key. If the PIP threshold is equaled or exceeded, the inspiratory phase is terminated. Pressure sensitivity, for patient-initiated breaths, whether mechanical or spontaneous, is adjustable from 0.5 to 20 cmH_2O below the baseline pressure in the breathing circuit. Likewise, flow-triggering may be selected and can be set between 1 and 15 L/min. A plateau of up to 2.0 seconds extends mandatory, volume-targeted inspirations. Other submodes and keys include the following: 100% O_2 suction, manual inspiration, manual sigh, automatic sigh, and nebulizer. A small LED on the touchpad indicates when the function is active.

During CMV (also known as A/C), all breaths are mandatory and are either volume-targeted or pressure-targeted. Individual breaths are either ventilator initiated (ie, triggered as a result of the rate setting) or patient initiated (ie, the patient effort causes circuit pressure or inspiratory flow to equal the trigger threshold) depending on which trigger method is set. During CPAP, all breaths are spontaneous and may or may not be pressure supported, depending on the value of the support pressure setting.

With SIMV selected, both mandatory (VC or PC) and spontaneous breaths (with or without PS) may be delivered. Each SIMV interval, as defined by the SIMV rate setting, contains one mandatory breath. This breath is either ventilator initiated or patient initiated. The mandatory breath could also be operator initiated by using the manual control. Triggering for all breaths can be by pressure or flow depending on the trigger type selected. The mandatory breath may be followed by one or more spontaneous breaths with or without pressure support and is/are always patient initiated as long as the patient generates spontaneous efforts before the beginning of the next SIMV interval. Each new SIMV interval always begins with the ventilator poised to deliver a

TABLE 21-76 **Listing of Options/Functions for the Bennett 7200 Microprocessor Ventilator**

Option/Function Number	Description	Option/Function Number	Description
1	Apnea parameters*	30/40	Respiratory mechanics
2	Clock reset	50	Flow-by (flow trigger)
3	Patient data	60	Graphics
4	Auto-PEEP	80	Pressure control
10	Pressure support	90	Pulse oximetry
20	Digital communications		

* When the mandatory breath type is pressure control (function 80), pressure-targeted parameters can be set with function 81.

mandatory breath triggered by the patient's first inspiratory effort. If the patient fails to initiate an inspiratory effort before the end of the SIMV cycle interval, a ventilator-initiated mandatory breath is delivered.

Nebulization may be activated during each mechanical breath, but cannot function when peak flow is set at less than 20 L/min. Nebulizer function automatically ends after 30 minutes. Sigh volume is adjustable from 0.1 to 2.5 L and may not exceed twice the value of the set V_T or be less than the set V_T. The automatic sigh mechanism is active only with CMV and SIMV and allows 1 to 15 sighs per hour in lieu of normally scheduled mechanical or patient-triggered breaths. One, two, or three consecutive sigh breaths can be delivered and the PIP for each sigh can be adjusted up to 120 cmH_2O. End-expiratory pressure (PEEP/CPAP) is continuously adjustable up to 45 cmH_2O with a rotary control. Rotating the knob updates the targeted value of PEEP/CPAP displayed in the patient data section.

With the individual option/function keys on the Enhanced-Plus Keyboard, introduced in 1994, or with the "++" option-menu-selection key on earlier versions, a series of messages and prompts are presented to the operator through the alpha numeric window and settings are keyed, as with ventilation settings (see Table 21-75).

During pressure support ventilation and pressure control ventilation, the 7200 becomes a pressure controller (pressure-targeted). Pressure support may be set with any spontaneous breathing mode. Pressure-control ventilation can be set with CMV or with SIMV. A rapid flow of gas directed into the breathing circuit generates the pressure level. As the airway pressure rises, flow decreases until airway pressure and the preset pressure level are equivalent. In PCV, inspiration ends depending on inspiratory time, whether selected directly through the T_i parameter or indirectly through the I:E parameter. In PSV mode, inspiration is terminated when flow has decelerated to 5 L/min and baseline circuit pressure is

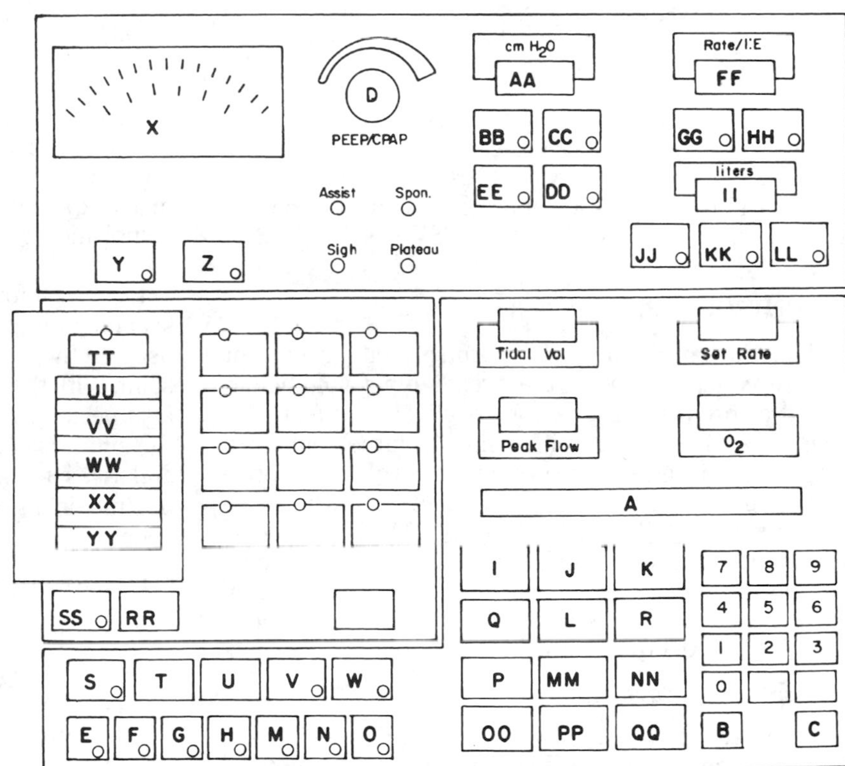

FIGURE 21-111. Nellcor Puritan-Bennett 7200 Series Microprocessor ventilator basic control panel (see text). (Courtesy of Puritan-Bennett Corp., Carlsbad, CA)

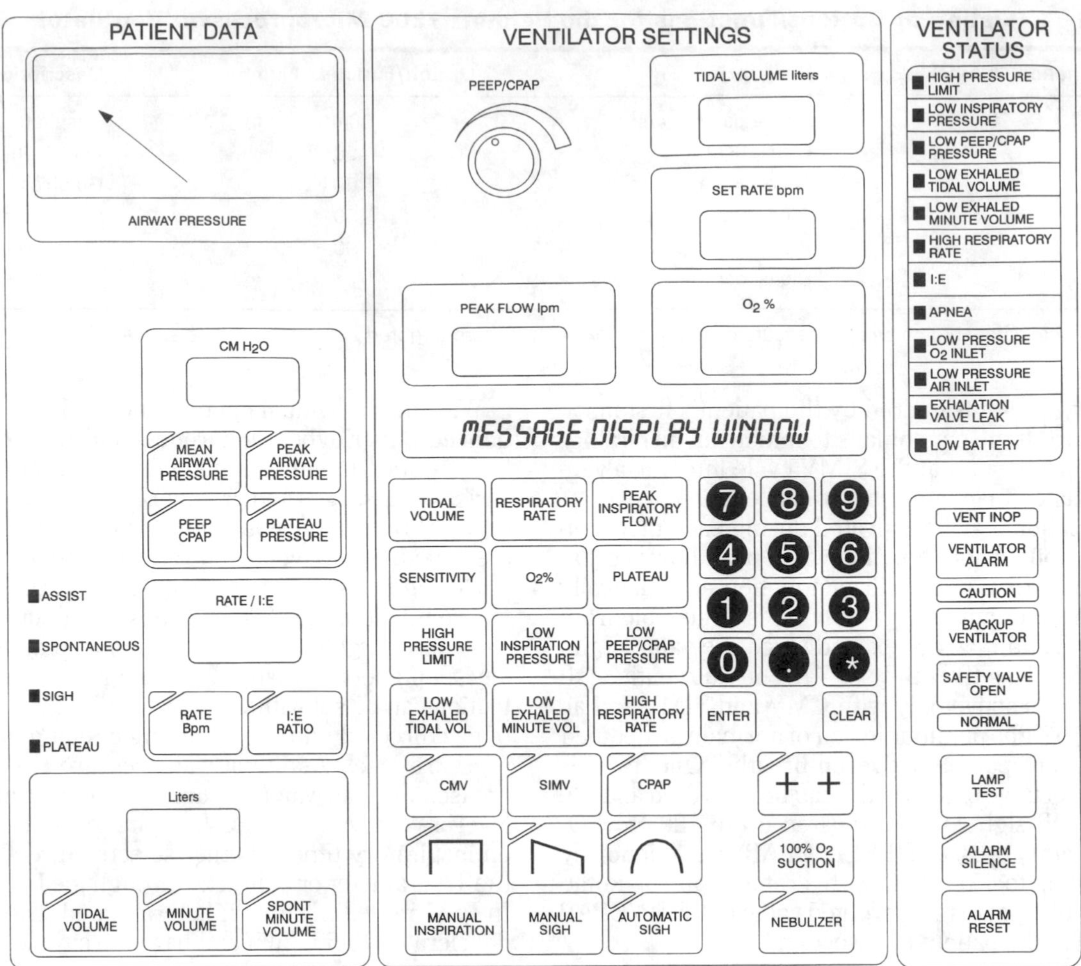

FIGURE 21-112. Nellcor Puritan-Bennett 7200 Series Microprocessor ventilator enhanced control panel. (Courtesy of Yvon G. Dupuis, Ilderton, Ontario, Canada)

then restored. If the breathing circuit has a leak, inspiratory flow may not decelerate to 5 L/min, which will prolong inspiratory intervals. Pressure support would then terminate after 5 seconds. PSV will also terminate if pressure rises 1.5 cmH_2O above PSV + PEEP/CPAP.

□ CONTROL VARIABLES

The Puritan-Bennett 7200 controls either flow or pressure depending on the breath type: volume-targeted or pressure-targeted, respectively. Thus, CMV, mandatory breaths are either flow/volume controlled (ie, volume-targeted) or pressure controlled (ie, pressure-targeted). CPAP breaths are always pressure controlled, that is, CPAP or PSV. Since SIMV is defined as a mixed mode, the mandatory breaths are flow controlled if they are volume-targeted and pressure controlled if they are pressure-targeted. The spontaneous breaths (CPAP or PSV) are always pressure controlled.

Inspiratory Waveform

There are one inspiratory pressure and three inspiratory flow waveforms available. During pressure control and pressure support ventilation, the 7200 targets a constant pressure equal to PEEP/CPAP plus the setting for PCV or PSV. The pressure curve is nearly rectangular (constant). The actual pressure rise to the target is a quasi-exponential trajectory. The lower the lung-thorax compliance and the higher the airways resistance, the more rapid the rise of circuit pressure to the target.

Flow waveforms include rectangular (constant), descending ramp, and sine. When the peak flow setting is used on the rectangular waveform, gas delivery is constant. With the descending ramp, inspiratory flow starts at at peak flow and descends linearly to 5 L/min. With the sine waveform, inspiratory flow begins at 5 L/min and rises to peak flow and then descends again to 5 L/min in a sinusoidal pattern.

□ PHASE VARIABLES

Triggering

Pressure-triggering occurs when a patient's spontaneous inspiratory effort drops the pressure in the patient circuit enough to reach the sensitivity threshold. The sensitivity setting can be adjusted from 0.5 to 20.0 cmH_2O below baseline pressure.

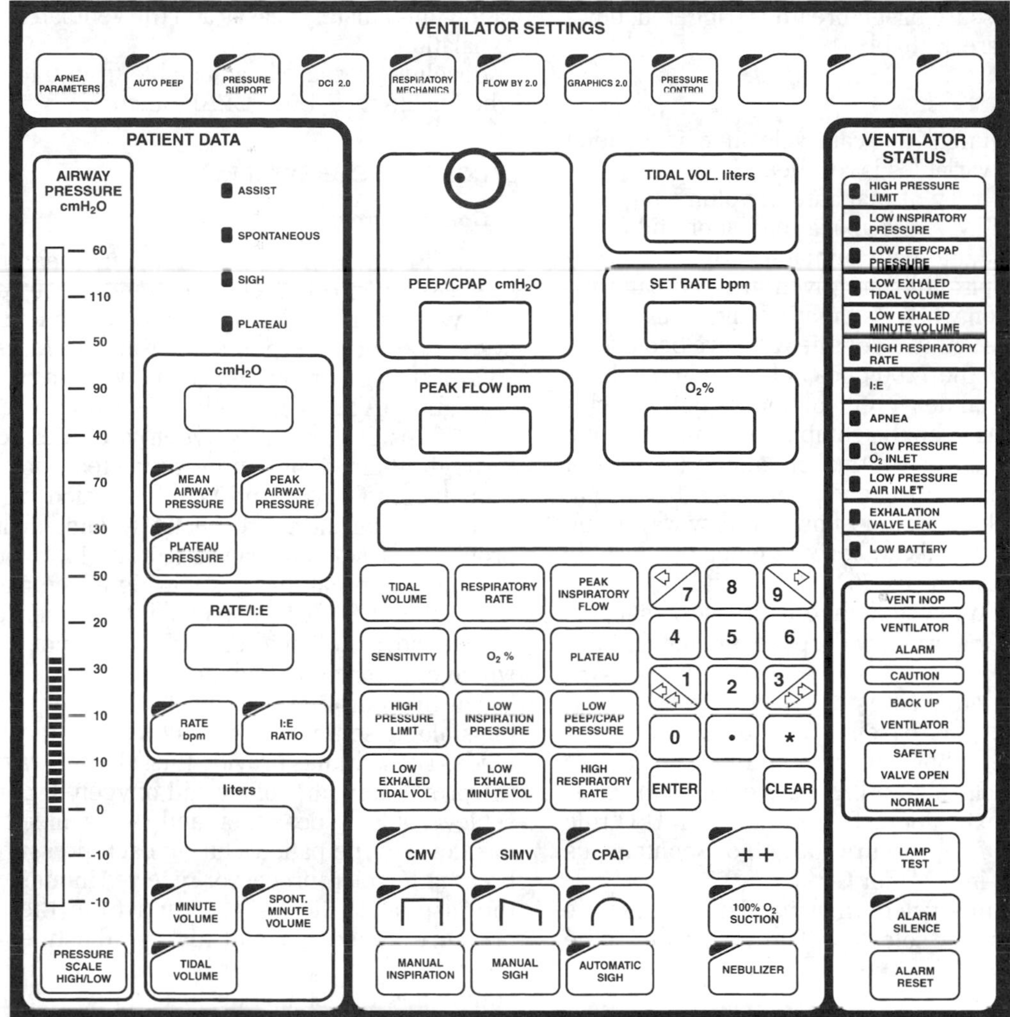

FIGURE 21-113. Nellcor Puritan-Bennett 7200 Series Microprocessor ventilator enhanced *(PLUS)* control panel. (Courtesy of Puritan-Bennett Corp., Carlsbad, CA)

Flow-triggering occurs in the "Flow-by" setting when a patient's inspiratory effort reduces the flow through the expiratory flow sensor by an amount equal to the set flow-triggering level (1 to 10 L/min in Flow-by 1.0, and 1 to 15 L/min in Flow-by 2.0) below base flow. Flow-by provides a continuous base flow from which a patient may trigger a spontaneous or a mandatory breath.

Inspiration may also be time-triggered and will be a function of the frequency or respiratory rate setting. Rate can be adjusted from 0.5 to 70 breaths/min. Time triggering is also operating when the sigh rate and multiple sigh functions are set. The sigh rate is adjustable from 1 to 15 sighs per hour. The multiple sigh function allows one, two, or three sighs to occur in a row. Each set of multiple sighs is delivered at the frequency set by the sigh rate.

The 7200 can also be manually triggered using the manual-inspiration key.

Limiting

Pressure-limiting is present during spontaneous breaths in the pressure support, pressure control, and CPAP modes. In pressure support, pressure is set from 0 to 70 cmH_2O above PEEP/CPAP. In pressure control, pressure is set from 5 to 100 cmH_2O above PEEP/CPAP. In the SIMV and CPAP modes when PSV is not active, a servocontrolled flow system controls inspiratory flow by attempting to maintain a pressure target equal to the set PEEP/CPAP minus the setting for pressure sensitivity (pressure-triggering) or to PEEP/CPAP +0.5 cmH_2O (flow-triggering).

Inspiration is volume-limited whenever the inspiratory pause time is set to a value greater than 0 seconds.

Inspiration is flow-limited during volume-targeted breaths when any of three preset waveforms are selected. Flow can be set over a range of 10 to 120 L/min. Peak flow for a pressure-targeted breath (PCV or PSV) can be as high as 180 L/min. In the Flow-by option, the flow can be set from 5 to 20 L/min. Because base flow has no purpose other than providing background flow from which the patient inhales to generate the inspiratory (flow) trigger signal or providing extra flow to offset a circuit leak, lower base flows and lower trigger settings offer the optimum conditions for minimal trigger work. Once a pressure-based breath is triggered, flows up to 180 L/min are available.

Cycling

The Puritan-Bennett 7200 can cycle out of inspiration when one of four variables is reached.

During the delivery of mandatory, volume-targeted breaths in CMV, SIMV, and apnea ventilation and whenever sigh breaths (automatic or manual) or manual, volume-targeted inspirations are given, the ventilator cycles into exhalation when its breath-delivery algorithm computes that the set tidal volume will have been delivered. Technically, the 7200 does not cycle into exhalation based on actual delivered volume; rather, it cycles into exhalation based on the computed inspiratory time required for the delivery of the set volume (in units of BTPS—body, temperature, and pressure, saturated) at the specified peak inspiratory flow and flow waveform. The inspiratory interval can be lengthened by the addition of an inspiratory pause (0 to 2.0 seconds).

The 7200 is flow-cycled in the pressure support mode. When inspiratory flow drops to 5 L/min in PSV, inspiration ends.

Pressure-targeted breaths can also be pressure-cycled. If pressure plus baseline in the patient circuit reaches 1.5 cmH_2O above the target pressure before inspiratory flow declines to 5 L/min, the ventilator pressure cycles into exhalation. This same 1.5 cmH_2O rule also applies to nonpressure targeted spontaneous breaths, whether in SIMV or CPAP.

Inspiration is time-cycled when mandatory, pressure-targeted breaths are selected. The inspiratory time is specified either with the T_i parameter or the I:E parameter

The 7200 can be pressure-cycled if the high-pressure limit is reached before the end of a normal, volume-, or pressure-targeted, mandatory breath. The high-pressure limit range is from 10 to 120 cmH_2O and is used in CMV, SIMV, and CPAP (although less likely here), regardless of breath type. By setting a reasonable value for high-pressure limit, the operator specifies that pressure in the patient circuit shall not exceed the set value. If circuit pressure reaches the limit value, inspiration immediately ceases and the ventilator cycles into exhalation.

Baseline pressure is adjustable from 0 to 45 cmH_2O when using the PEEP/CPAP function.

□ CONTROL SUBSYSTEMS

Control Circuit

The Bennett 7200 series ventilator features microprocessor control of electrical and electropneumatic subsystems (Fig. 21-114). The electropneumatic subsystem requires oxygen and air at pressures between 35 to 100 psig. Air and oxygen flow through filters into regulators (A and B), which reduce pressure to a nominal 10 psig. Air and oxygen are then conducted through their temperature-corrected, hot-film, flow transducers Q1 (D) and Q2 (E), which measure the flow of oxygen and air, respectively, and, finally, to their proportional solenoid valves (F1 and F2), which meter and mix the breathing gas flowing to the patient. Normally, the PEEP/CPAP is generated by air taken from the crossover solenoid (C) unless it is not available, in which case oxygen is substituted.

The microprocessor, using the operator-programmed physiologic settings, controls the air and oxygen solenoids. These values provide the selected waveform and the proper amounts of air and oxygen to generate the set level of FIO_2, peak flow, and V_T. As mixed breathing gas flows to the patient during each pressure-targeted breath, the microprocessor receives input signals from the inspiratory flow sensor and from the expiratory pressure transducer and makes adjustments accordingly. If, for example, flow is insufficient, the processor commands the solenoids to open wider, thereby increasing flow. As mixed breathing gas is delivered to the patient circuit, it passes a pressure transducer (G) that functions as an internal barometer and through a safety/check valve that functions as both an overpressure relief valve (H) and an antisuffocation valve (I). The overpressure valve, which is mechanical, vents circuit pressures in excess of 140 cmH2O. The electronic antisuffocation valve opens in the event of gas or electric power loss and during POST.

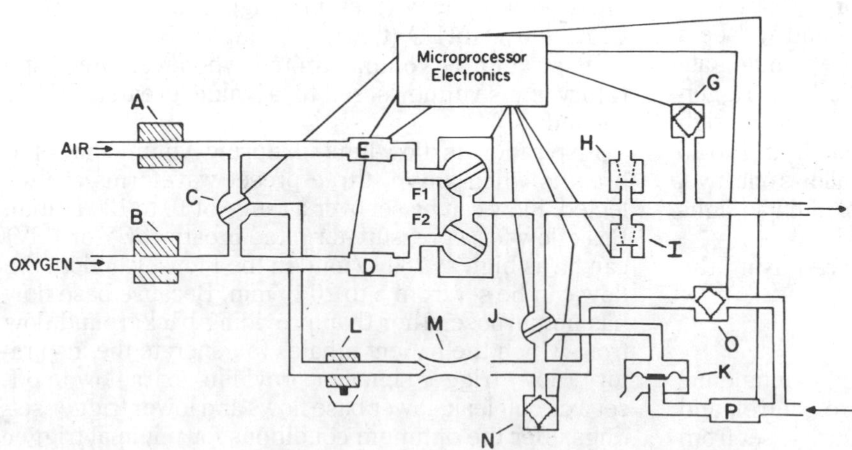

FIGURE 21-114. Schematic diagram of the Puritan-Bennett 7200 ventilator (see text).

The ventilator automatically adjusts the delivered volume to correct for BTPS. This correction assumes that the gas delivered to the patient becomes 100% saturated at normal body temperature (37° C) in the lungs.

Gas pressure to the exhalation valve is controlled by a three-way solenoid (J). During mechanical inspiration, the solenoid opens and allows pressure from the proportional solenoid to close the exhalation valve (K). At the onset of exhalation, the solenoid closes and directs flow from the PEEP regulator (L) and PEEP venturi (M) into the space behind the diaphragm of the exhalation valve, which produces the set level of end-expiratory pressure (PEEP/CPAP). A differential pressure transducer (N) measures the output pressure of the PEEP venturi and a second differential pressure transducer (O) is used to measure airway pressure, referenced to the output pressure of the PEEP venturi. (Note that in this implementation, circuit pressure equals O − N). Once each hour the microprocessor opens a solenoid connected to each pressure transducer to ambient (not illustrated) and reestablishes the zero point. This ensures accuracy, because only the zero point is subject to drift. It also serves as a critical operational verification. Failure of a transducer to zero will necessitate the termination of normal ventilation and require that the ventilator be serviced before further use. Exhaled patient gas is directed through the temperature-compensated, expiratory, flow transducer (P) referred to as Q3. Signals from this flow transducer are integrated and displayed, providing the data for V_T and minute ventilation measurements (converted to BTPS). The measurements of V_T made at the expiratory flow transducer are constantly referenced against those made by the air and oxygen flow transducers coupled to the proportional solenoid. In the event that these two measurements disagree by more than 25%, normal operation is immediately discontinued and appropriate servicing is recommended.

The Puritan Bennett 7200 compensates for the volume that is compressed in the patient circuit (compressible volume). It does this in the following manner: During an EST test, the ventilator determines the compliance of the patient circuit being used. While delivering volume targeted breaths, the 7200 measures the end-inspiratory pressure of each breath and increments or decrements the delivered volume of the next inspiration to ensure that the volume delivered to the lungs equals the set tidal volume. The ventilator adds volume by increasing the flow by an amount determined by the patient circuit compliance. During compensation, the inspiratory time, which is determined by the set tidal volume, set flow, and flow waveform, is held constant. In a similar manner, every exhaled volume is corrected for the compressed circuit volume that did not come from the patient's lungs. This simple subtraction routine allows the ventilator to display the best estimate of the patient's true lung volume. It should be pointed out that the expiratory flow transducer, hot-film anemometer, Q3, used to measure exhaled volumes for display, is also monitored and used for alarm functions.

7200 ventilators are fitted with one of three control panels (user interfaces): The original basic interface (see Fig. 21-111), the enhanced interface introduced in 1991 (see Fig. 21-112), and the enhanced plus interface introduced in 1994 (see Fig. 21-113). With ventilators having the original basic interface, one of two exhaled volumes could be selected for display. Specifying "exhaled volume" meant that all flow integrated by the expiratory flow sensor (measured in STP-standard temperature and pressure) was displayed by the analog meter. In addition, the total exhaled volume was corrected for circuit compliance volume, corrected to BTPS, and displayed in a digital display in the patient data section. Ventilators fitted with the enhanced and enhanced plus interfaces only retain the BTPS estimate of volume exhaled from the patient.

Drive Mechanism

The 7200 uses external pressurized gas sources for air and oxygen to provide the mixed gas to the patient. Alternately, wall air may be replaced by air supplied by an integral, rotary vane compressor. The compressor outputs air at 11 psig, which is internally reduced to about 10 psig. At this pressure, the air from the compressor simply substitutes for wall air.

Output Control Valve

The gas flow to the patient is controlled by two proportional metering valves, one for air and one for oxygen. During a breath these valves operate singly or together to achieve the desired F_{IO_2} setting. Another solenoid valve gates pressure from the patient outlet of the pneumatic system to the exhalation valve, causing it to close during inspiration when the proportional valves are open.

□ MODES OF OPERATION

The Puritan-Bennett 7200 offers five modes of ventilation: CMV (also know as assist/control), SIMV, pressure control, pressure support, and CPAP (also known as spontaneous, SPONT). Each of these primary modes is a mix of the 7200's two breath types, mandatory and spontaneous.

Mandatory breaths may be pressure-triggered, flow-triggered (by selecting the flow-by option), time-triggered, or operator-triggered by pressing manual inspiration. Mandatory breaths will be either volume-targeted or pressure-targeted. Volume-targeted breaths are defined by the specified tidal volume, peak inspiratory flow, and the waveform. Pressure-targeted breaths are defined by the specified inspiratory pressure and the inspiratory time, using the T_i parameter or the I:E parameter. CPAP or spontaneous breaths are pressure supported by selecting option 10, the pressure support option, or are not pressure supported by selecting zero pressure support (ie, zero pressure support = traditional CPAP). CPAP breaths are only pressure- or flow-triggered.

The Puritan-Bennett 7200 names the following modes on its control panel:

CMV (Assist/Control)

In volume-targeted CMV, the operator sets the tidal volume, rate, flow, and sensitivity. Inspiration is flow-controlled (volume-targeted) and will be time-triggered if patient effort is absent or pressure- or flow-triggered depending on the selection of trigger type. It is volume-limited if an inspiratory pause is used. Three flow-limited waveforms are available, in the rectangular or constant waveform, descending ramp, and sine. The ventilator is time-cycled out of inspiration based on the flow, tidal volume, and waveform selections.

PCV

In pressure-targeted CMV ventilation (PCV), the operator selects a pressure setting, respiratory rate and inspiratory time (T_i) or I:E parameter. The inspiratory phase is pressure-controlled and time-, flow-, or pressure-triggered. It is pressure-limited and time-cycled (determined by set inspiratory time or by a combination of rate and I:E setting).

SIMV

SIMV is called a mixed mode because both mandatory and spontaneous breaths can be delivered. Given the rules by which SIMV operates, each SIMV interval will contain at least one mandatory breath, and, if sufficient time remains after the mandatory breath and before the beginning of the next SIMV interval, further patient effort yields spontaneous breaths.

In volume-targeted SIMV, the SIMV rate is set for mandatory breaths as is tidal volume, sensitivity and peak flow. Inspiration during mandatory breaths is flow-controlled (volume-targeted). In pressure-controlled SIMV, the mandatory breaths also require setting the SIMV rate. The operator must also select pre-set pressure, rate and T_i or the I:E parameter.

Depending on the type of breath, mandatory or spontaneous, triggering results from time, patient effort, or operator action. The mandatory breath is initiated by patient effort or failing that, time. The mandatory breath can also be operator initiated. Operator action yields a single mandatory breath, which, if delivered before the normal SIMV, substitutes for that breath. Once the normal SIMV mandatory breath has been delivered, each manual inspiration yields an additional mandatory breath. Spontaneous breaths are only initiated by patient effort. In triggering, the operator has the choice of selecting either pressure- or flow-triggering (with Flow-by 2.0, all breaths resulting from patient effort, regardless of type, are flow-triggered).

The SIMV algorithm dictates that each SIMV interval normally receives a mandatory breath and that this breath precedes the spontaneous breath. Thus, at high SIMV rates most breaths will be mandatory, and at low SIMV rates a substantial percentage of the breaths can be spontaneous. Each new SIMV interval begins with the ventilator poised to synchronize a mandatory breath with the first-recognized patient effort. Lacking patient effort, the ventilator delivers a time-triggered, mandatory breath at the beginning of the next SIMV interval. If no patient effort is generated, mandatory breaths follow at the beginning of each new SIMV interval. By triggering a mandatory breath within the SIMV interval, the ventilator responds to all subsequent patient efforts in the remainder of the interval by delivering spontaneous breaths. These breaths are pressure-targeted. That is, the inspiratory flow of gas varies to maintain any set PEEP/CPAP plus pressure support level selected. Spontaneous breaths are pressure- or flow-triggered. It should be noted that Flow-by and PSV cannot be used at the same time unless version 2.0 of Flow-by has been installed.

CPAP

In this mode, all patient-initiated breaths are spontaneous, that is, they can be pressure supported (yielding PSV) or not (yielding CPAP). Operator action (manual inspiration) causes the ventilator to deliver a single mandatory breath. Breath initiation will be triggered by the currently active selection of pressure or flow.

Flow-by

The initial introduction of Flow-by (Flow-by version 1.0) was conceptualized as a smart version of continuous flow. With its flow-triggering feature, flow-by could be activated in CPAP and SIMV, but only if pressure support was off. Flow-by version 1.0 provided a continuous flow of gas through the patient circuit from the inspiratory side of the ventilator, past the airway to the exhalation valve.

With the introduction of Flow-by version 2.0, flow-triggering became available in all modes and for all patient-triggered breaths.

The operation of Flow-by 2.0 means that flow-triggering and pressure-triggering are seen as two methods by which a patient can trigger the ventilator to deliver a breath. In flow-triggering, the base flow functions as a stable background of flow from which the patient inhales at the beginning of an inspiratory effort. The key parameter is the flow sensitivity. Too great a value prolongs the inspiratory effort necessary to generate the triggering level of inspiratory flow. Base flow need only be large enough to prevent flow starvation during trigger detection. The manufacturer has designed the algorithm to force baseflow to be at least twice the setting for flow sensitivity. The minimum flow sensitivity is 1 L/min, and the maximum is 10 L/min for Flow-by 1.0 and 15 L/min for Flow-by 2.0. The minimum base flow is 5 L/min and the maximum is 20 L/min. Lower selections for flow sensitivity require less trigger work. The manufacturer recommends 1 L/min for patients weighing less than 25 kg. For weights between 25 and 50 kg, 2 L/min is recommended, and above 50 kg, 3 L/min is recommended.

As a patient's lung–thorax compliance moves toward normal values, the rhythmic contraction of the heart can cause a sinusoidal-like flow oscillation. With very sensitive triggering values, autotriggering can result (as it can during pressure-triggering). When this problem arises, the monitored respiratory rate will equal the heart rate. By increasing the value for the flow sensitivity, the autotriggering will disappear.

The following provides an example of how the Flow-by option is set. Imagine the baseline (continuous) flow was set at 5 L/min and the "sensitivity" flow was set at 2 L/min. Flow through the circuit is measured by the expiratory flow sensor. When the ventilator detects a flow of 3 L/min or less (5 − 2 = 3), the mode-specific breath is triggered.

With spontaneous inspirations, flow-cycling into exhalation may occur if the ventilator senses a flow through the expiratory flow sensor equal to at least 2 L/min greater than the measured value for inspiratory flow or when end inspiratory pressure equals 1.5 cmH_2O above the pressure target. At the beginning of exhalation (by whatever method), the base flow is reduced to 5 L/min for a brief interval (the lesser of .5 seconds or 50% of the average of the last three expiratory intervals), then restored to the set value. This action helps reduce resistance during exhalation.

Flow-by is not operational during nebulization. With the older version of Flow-by, flow-triggering must be turned off until nebulization is finished. With Flow-by version 2.0, the switch to pressure-triggering is automatic, but operator action is required to restart Flow-by after nebulization is finished.

Manual Breaths

Manual inspirations and manual sighs may be delivered at any time (except during inspiration) by pressing the appropriate key.

Emergency Operation States

Under certain problem conditions detected by the ventilator, one of three modes of ventilation or methods of operation become active to support the patient: apnea ventilation, disconnect ventilation, and backup ventilation.

Apnea Ventilation

During ventilator set-up, the operator selects an apnea interval, which places a limit on the maximum allowable breath-to-breath period. The default interval is 20 seconds. When apnea is detected and no low pressure alarm exists, the ventilator will begin apnea ventilation and activate audible and visual alarms. Depending on the current status of PCV (function 80), apnea ventilation will deliver volume or pressure-targeted breaths. If function 80 (option 80) is off, apnea ventilation will be volume-targeted. If function 80 has been set up (ie, values for the PCV parameters have been selected) and, in addition, values for function 81, PC apnea ventilation, also have been selected, then apnea ventilation will deliver pressure-controlled mandatory breaths. With function 80 set-up but function 81 inactive, apnea ventilation will consist of volume-targeted, mandatory breaths. Table 21-77 shows the parameter ranges for volume-targeted and pressure-targeted apnea ventilation.

Apnea ventilation can be reset under two standard conditions: (1) when the patient triggers two consecutive breaths and each exhaled volume is at least 50% of the delivered volume as measured by the inspiratory flow sensor, and (2) when apnea ventilation is cancelled by pressing "Alarm Reset." Once reset, the ventilator automatically resumes ventilation using the previous mode and settings.

TABLE 21-77 **The Parameter Ranges for Volume-Targeted and Pressure-Targeted Apnea Ventilation in the Nellcor Puritan-Bennett 7200 Ventilator**

	Ranges of Selection	Default Value
Volume Controlled (Function 1)		
Apnea interval (sec)	10–60	20
Breath rate (breaths/min)	0.5–70	12
Tidal volume (L)	0.1–2.5	0.5
Peak flow (L/min)	10–120	45
Oxygen percentage	21–100	100
Pressure Controlled (Function 80 Set-Up and Function 81 (Active)		
Apnea interval (sec)	10–60	
Breath rate (beats/min)	0.5–70	
Inspiratory pressure (cmH_2O)	5–100	
Inspiratory time (sec)	0.5–50	
I:E ratio	1:9–4:1	
Oxygen percentage	21–100	

Airway Pressure Disconnect

Airway pressure disconnect (APD) is an emergency mode designed to protect the patient when pressure on the inspiratory side of the patient circuit is detected as unreasonably higher than that on the expiratory side. An audible alarm sounds and the message display window reads "AIRWAY PRESS DISCONN." This mode ignores spontaneous breathing from the patient to avoid autotriggering. It also assumes preset (default) parameters that are the same as those in apnea ventilation. APD can be deactivated by correcting the problem. The operator should check for an obstruction in the patient circuit or a disconnected or obstructed pressure line. After correcting the problem, the operator must press the "alarm reset" key since airway pressure disconnect does not automatically reset.

Backup Ventilation

This mode, which is completely separate from microprocessor controls, is activated by a background fault detection system only if the pneumatic delivery systems are functioning correctly. Backup ventilation (BUV) provides emergency ventilation in the event that this becomes questionable. It is also activated if the AC voltage falls to less than 90% of the rated input voltage. In this mode, the ventilator defaults to preset parameters as listed in Table 21-78.

The red BUV lights up when the ventilator is in this emergency ventilatory mode. To restore normal operation, the 7200a must be repaired or, at the very least, must successfully pass the extended self-test (EST) procedure.

TABLE 21-78 Preset Parameters for Backup Ventilation (BUV) in the Nellcor Puritan-Bennett 7200 Microprocessor Ventilator

Parameter	Values
Peak flow (L/min)	45
V_T (L)	0.5 (uncorrected)
Rate (breaths/min)	12
O_2 percentage	100 (if available, or 21%)
Pressure limit cmH_2O	30 above PEEP*
Peak CMV (sensitivity ignored)	

* Note that because the high pressure limit is set to PEEP + 30 cmH_2O, the breath will pressure-cycle if the pressure limit is reached before the 0.5 L is delivered.

□ OUTPUT DISPLAYS (MONITORS) AND ALARMS

The 7200's user interface (UI) has been upgraded twice since the introduction of the product. The patient data section of the original, "basic" interface featured an analog meter that could be commanded to display either circuit pressure or exhaled volume. In the early 1990s the basic UI was replaced by the "enhanced" interface. It retained the analog meter but lost the exhaled volume reading feature. Finally, beginning in 1994, Puritan-Bennett replaced the enhanced UI with the "enhanced plus" interface. Instead of an analog meter, the new UI featured a dual-scale, pressure-reading bar graph.

All patient data displays contain three digital display windows (see Figs. 21-111, 21-112, and 21-113). Under each data display is a cluster of touch pads by which the operator can select the variable to be viewed. Specific components of airway pressure, which are displayed in the "cmH_20" window, are mean airway pressure, peak airway pressure, plateau pressure, and PEEP/CPAP level.

A second digital display window can be keyed to read the actual respiratory rate (all breaths) or the actual I:E ratio. The third digital display, the "Liters" window, can be keyed to read exhaled patient tidal volume (corrected to BTPS), total minute ventilation (mandatory plus spontaneous breaths or only spontaneous minute ventilation).

Each of the monitored parameters is calculated by a unique algorithm. The analog meter on the basic and enhanced interfaces is damped to prevent "needle bounce," and hence the displayed airway (or circuit) pressures may lag behind the actual, real-time values. [Note: the dual-scale bar graph on the enhanced-plus interface did not require damping.] This is because at end exhalation, airway pressure generally changes slowly. A pressure reading at this moment represents the best estimate of the actual PEEP/CPAP pressure. It is important to read the actual end-expiratory pressure because too brief an expiratory interval could yield a higher-than-expected value due to insufficient expiratory time. Only on the basic interface can total exhaled volume be selected. As stated earlier, this selection causes the analog meter to display the integration of all flow through the expiratory flow sensor (ie, patient plus compressed circuit volume, in standard liters).

In the pressure cluster of the UI, main airway pressure is the breath-by-breath average of all pressures (sampled every 20 min) from beginning inspiration to the next beginning inspiration regardless of breath type. Peak airway pressure is monitored only on mandatory inspirations and represents the maximum value detected. Plateau pressure is displayed only when an inspiratory pause has been added to a mandatory, volume-targeted breath. The displayed value is the average of the last four 20-min pressure samples before the plateau times out. PEEP/CPAP represents the pressure the expiratory value is attempting to maintain at end exhalation. Only if the area ratio is correct will the targeted PEEP/CPAP value be accurate.

Since the mid 1980s all original and new 7200s have been equipped with a precision-designed, permanent exhalation valve. The area ratio of this device is computed every time a self-test program is run. From test to test the value of the area ratio changes little or none. Thus, the operator-set target for PEEP/CPAP, which requires the area-ratio value for accuracy, is a good representation of the actual PEEP/CPAP that will be maintained under stable conditions. Insufficient expiratory time or circuit leaks will cause the actual end-expiratory pressures to read high or low, respectively.

In the "rate/I:E ratio" cluster of the user interface, the rate selection yields the average respiratory rate for all breaths (mandatory and spontaneous) measured over the last 10 breaths or 1 minute (whichever occurs first) expressed as breaths per minute. The I:E ratio is calculated for mandatory breaths only and represents the actual value. Note that a set value for I:E ratio (whether the result of specifying a volume-targeted breath, flow, and respiratory rate; or from a pressure-targeted breath, inspiratory time, and respiratory rate) may not equal the actual value if the patient is successful in triggering extra mandatory or spontaneous breaths.

In the "liters" cluster, selection of tidal volume causes the display of the estimated volume, expressed in BTPS liters, exhaled from the patient's lungs. This means the volume contained within the pressurized patient circuit at end inspiration has been subtracted. When the just-delivered breath was a mandatory one, the displayed value represents the average of an eight-breath (all mandatory) running sample. If an individual mandatory volume differs by more than 50 mL from the running average, the displayed value applies only to the current breath. When the just-delivered breath was a spontaneous one, the displayed value applies only to the current breath and spontaneous tidal volumes are not averaged. With minute volume selected, the displayed value represents the average minute ventilation for all mandatory and spontaneous breath over an eight-breath running sample or 1 minute, whichever occurs first. The selection of spontaneous minute volume means that the running eight-breath sample, or 1 minute, whichever occurs first, applies only to spontaneous breaths.

A series of four LEDs appear next to the rate display window, representing assist, spontaneous, sigh, and plateau events. Each light illuminates after each breath to identify it, except where a mandatory breath was not patient-triggered, in which case no light illuminates.

In the ventilator settings panel there are alarm setting keys for high pressure limit; low inspiratory pressure, which detects ventilator-patient circuit leaks during mechanical inspiration; low PEEP/CPAP pressure, which facilitates detection of breathing circuit leaks, disconnection, or insufficient gas flow to meet spontaneous inspiratory requirements; low exhaled V_T; low exhaled minute volume; and high respiratory rate. Alarms are programmed in a manner identical with the procedure for programming ventilator settings. When limits are violated, an audible alarm is activated and a visual indicator illuminated along with an associated message describing the conditions presented in the message display window. The audible alarm automatically cancels if the alarm condition does not occur on the next breath. The LED indicator remains on, however, until the alarm has been reset; thus, if the clinician is away from the patient, data from the event is retained for later reference.

The Ventilator Status panel on the right side of the enhanced plus interface (left side on the basic interface) contains two rectangular groupings. Arranged in vertical order in the top grouping are all of the 7200's alarmed events, including LEDs for all of the alarm conditions discussed above plus I:E ratio, apnea, low-pressure O_2 inlet, low-pressure air inlet, exhalation valve leak and low battery (named "low internal power" on the enhanced plus interface). Grouped in the lower rectangle, in descending order (new enhanced plus display panel) are LEDs for vent inop, ventilator alarm, caution, backup ventilation, safety valve open, and normal. As their names suggest, these indicators illuminate, as appropriate, to identify the overall status of the ventilator. An alarm silence key in the lower portion gives a 2-minute period without audible alarms to permit undisturbed bedside procedures. There are also touchpads to control lamp test and alarm reset in this section.

The general activation plan for all individual alarmed events is the same. When an alarm threshold is reached, the ventilator turns off the normal display, activates the audible sound generator, and concurrently flashes both the red "Ventilator Alarm" display and LED for the offending event. For events that can auto-reset and then do so, the red "Ventilator Alarm" display turns off, the "Caution" display turns on (steady); the individual-alarm LED changes from flashing to steady; and the audible sound ceases. This scheme allows the operator to view events that were active but have since reset. To clear the autoreset indication, the operator presses the "Alarm Reset" key, which turns back on the Normal indicator.

"Low Battery" and "I:E" alarms differ slightly from the above scheme. They do not autoreset. When these events are detected, there is no audible sound and no flashing ventilator alarm display. Instead, the LED of the offending event illuminates steadily. When the offending condition is corrected, the event LED turns off and the normal indicator again illuminates.

Events that deprive the ventilator of its gas supplies, render it inoperable, or severely compromise its ability to operate normally trigger additional alarms and operational states. If the ventilator is otherwise operable but both gas supplies are lost, the "Safety Valve Open" (SVO) illuminates along with the activation of the audible alarm sound. Note that in this specific case both the individual low-pressure air and oxygen outlet alarms would activate concurrently with the flashing of ventilator alarm. A major fault, sufficient to prevent safe ventilator operation, would cause the illumination of the two red alarm indicators, "Ventilator Inoperative" and "Safety Valve Open." If the gas delivery system is operable but the electronics are not, the red "Backup Ventilator" (BUV) indicator would illuminate, indicating the activation of the backup ventilator function while the audible alarm sounded. When no active alarms exist and all autoreset alarms have been cleared, the green "Normal" indicator illuminates.

The Puritan-Bennett 7200 also measures, calculates, and displays static and dynamic mechanics as well as other parameters of the respiratory system, such as negative inspiratory pressure, vital capacity, and rapid shallow breathing index (f/V_T). It uses two different algorithms to calculate resistance and compliance. The static mechanics are calculated using tidal volume and inspiratory flow as well as peak, plateau, and baseline pressures. The necessary data are captured during a constant-flow, volume-targeted breath followed by a plateau.

Dynamic mechanics are determined by sampling the instantaneous values of pressure, volume, and flow at many intervals during inspiration. These data are then massaged using the equation of motion, which is a mathematical model of the form: $P_{tr} = V/C + R \times \text{flow}$, where P_{tr} is transrespiratory system pressure (ie, airway pressure) relative to baseline pressure, V is tidal volume, C is respiratory system compliance, R is resistance of the respiratory system and endotracheal tube, and "flow" is the inspiratory gas flow.

□ TROUBLESHOOTING

Troubleshooting potential internal problems or failures with the 7200a is facilitated by the extended self-test (EST) procedure. This extensive battery of tests, performed in sequence, verifies the functional readiness of virtually every subsystem of the ventilator, including microprocessor and associated electronics checked during POST program, each pressure transducer and flow transducer, the exhalation valve and the patient-breathing circuit, the PEEP regulator, BUV, and the safety valve with associated overpressure relief. The test takes approximately 5 minutes to complete and must **not** be performed while the ventilator is on a patient. Each test sequence is given a code number, and if the test does not meet specifications, the code number is displayed in the message display window. The Puritan-Bennett Corporation suggests that the EST procedure be used to troubleshoot ventilator malfunctions and that a shortened version—quick extended self-test (QUEST)—be used to verify day-to-day readiness for use.

Problems during routine use are minimized by a "simplified" circuit and by ease of operation. One problem that is frequently encountered and not well understood is *"autotriggering."*

Notwithstanding this general statement, the operator needs to be aware of the interaction among finite values for pressure-trigger sensitivity, low SIMV rates, and the setting for apnea interval. As with many critical-care ventilators, severely sensitive settings for pressure-triggering can lead to autotriggering, particularly with leaky patient circuits or low lung–thorax compliance relative to the size of the endotracheal tube coupled with significant levels of PEEP. When PEEP is set to values several cmH_20 above atmospheric pressure, any event that leads to momentary pressure dips below PEEP during exhalation can trigger an unwanted or autotriggering inspiration. The proper selection for triggering (pressure as well as flow) always represents a tradeoff between the factors that enhance the chance of autotriggering and the factors that eliminate autotriggering, but at the expense of excessive effort.

When setting the apnea interval in the 7200, one needs to be aware of its impact on apnea ventilation with low SIMV breath rates. The SIMV algorithm dictates that the patient receive one mandatory breath (either patient or ventilator initiated) during each SIMV interval. Each SIMV interval begins with the ventilator poised to deliver this mandatory breath, synchronized to the first patient effort. If no such effort is detected by the end of the SIMV interval, the ventilator initiates a mandatory breath just before the new SIMV interval is due to begin.

At very low SIMV rates, a patient may trigger a mandatory breath at the initial part of a new SIMV interval and therafter fail to initiate any further effort. In this case, the next SIMV interval would begin and proceed to the near end of the interval, at which time the ventilator would initiate with mandatory breath. In this situation, the interval between the patient-initiated mandatory breath and the ventilator-initiated mandatory breath approaches twice the SIMV interval. If the duration of the currently set apnea interval was less than twice the current SIMV interval, apnea ventilation would initiate. Note, however, that should the patient's lapse of inspiratory effort be the cause of apnea ventilation, two successive patient-initiated efforts will reset the ventilator to the currently set mode of ventilation.

As with any medical equipment that is microprocessor controlled, care must be taken to avoid electromagnetic interference from devices such as portable cellular phones, walkie-talkies, and other transmitting devices.

SECHRIST INDUSTRIES, INC.*

Sechrist IV 100B Infant Ventilator

□ CLASSIFICATION

The Sechrist IV 100B infant ventilator (Table 21-79) (Fig. 21-115) is designed for neonatal and pediatric use. It is electronically and pneumatically powered, fluidically and electronically operated, and microprocessor controlled. It is time-cycled. It may provide end-expiratory pressure during mechanical (PEEP) and spontaneous (CPAP) breathing. Mechanical inspiration is time- or manually triggered. It is not pressure-triggered.

* Thanks to Steve Jenkins of Sechrist Industries, Inc., Medical Products Div., Anaheim, CA, for his technical assistance with the Sechrist ventilator.

TABLE 21-79 **Classification of the Sechrist IV 100B Infant Ventilator**

Power Source for Control Circuitry	Electricity (117 volts AC at 50 Hz)
Power source for pneumatic system	Air and Oxygen (30–80 psig) High pressure gas sources
Control mechanism	Pressure, flow/volume
Triggering	Time, manual
Limiting	Pressure, volume, flow, time
Cycling	Time

□ SPECIFICATIONS

Specifications for this device are listed in Table 21-80.

□ INPUT VARIABLES

The Sechrist IV 100B requires 117 volts AC 50/60 Hz electrical power source. As a transport ventilator, it requires a 12V DC 1.2 amps power source. This ventilator requires external air and oxygen at 11 to 100 psig. There is no internal compressor.

Operation

The Sechrist IV 100B ventilator (Fig. 21-116) is a compact neonatal ventilator that can be easily used for transport or long-term ventilation. Flow from the flow indicator (A) is blended in the air-oxygen mixer (B) to the desired concentration. The inspiratory time (C) is adjustable from 0.10 to 2.90 seconds. The time selected is indicated on the LED display for inspiratory time (D). This real-time display forms the basis for the microprocessor's determination of "inspiratory time." When the time-based generator has indicated the time dialed on the inspiratory time control (C), the microprocessor terminates the inspiratory phase. The expiratory time control (E) and the expiratory time display (F) are similar to the inspiratory functions. Once the inspiratory time (C) and the expiratory time (E) have been programmed into the unit, the microprocessor can calculate the I:E ratio (G), and rate (H), which may be adjusted up to 150 breaths/minute.

The inspiratory pressure limit (I) is adjustable from 5 to 70 cmH_2O, and the expiratory pressure (PEEP/CPAP) (J) is adjustable up to 20 cmH_2O. A manual button (K) allows a single breath at any time. This breath will be limited to the inspiratory pressure limit (I), as set, but will continue as long as the button is held down. The mode selector switch (L) provides the choice of IMV or CPAP.

□ CONTROL VARIABLES

The Sechrist IV 100B ventilator controls inspiratory and expiratory flow and limits inspiratory pressure. Inspiratory pressure is set with the pressure limit control, which

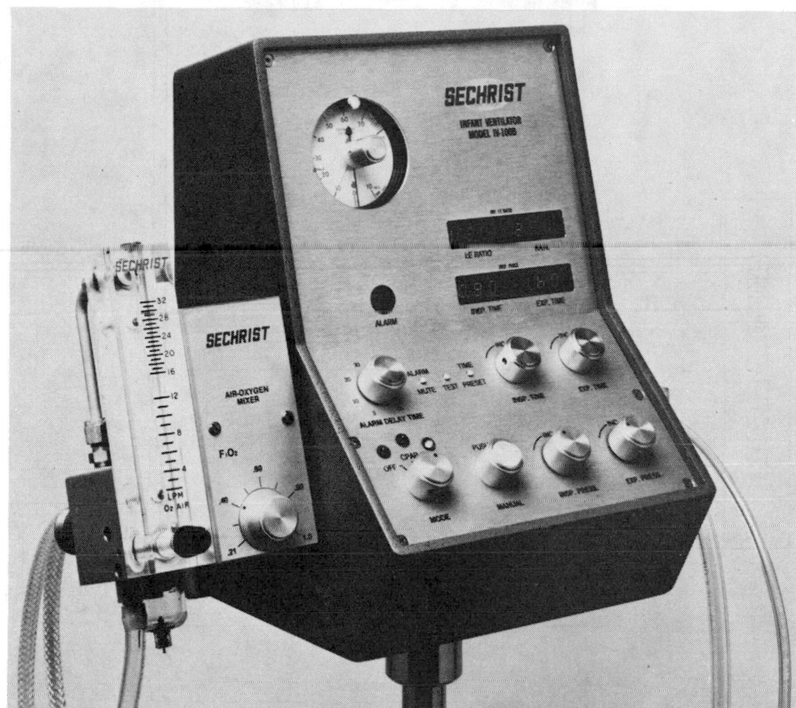

FIGURE 21-115. The Sechrist IV 100B ventilator. (Courtesy of Sechrist Industries, Inc., Medical Products Division, Anaheim, CA)

is uncalibrated. In every case, the peak inspiratory flow is limited to the value set by the flow meter. For any selected inspiratory time, the set flow rate may be insufficient to produce the targeted inspiratory pressure limit within the allotted inspiratory time. As with most infant ventilators, this condition is affected by compliance and resistance of the patient's respiratory system. When these conditions prevail, the Sechrist IV 100B functions as a flow controller.

Inspiratory Waveforms

The pressure or flow waveform is variable from rectangular to a modified sine pattern, independent from adjusting flow, time, or pressure limits (Fig. 21-117). Ordinarily, this ventilator operates with a rectangular pressure waveform and performs like a pressure targeted ventilator. When the rectangular pressure waveform is produced, the volume waveform exhibits an exponential rise and the flow waveform an exponential decay. The waveform modifier determines the shape of the waveforms. If fully opened, the waveform modifier opens and closes the exhalation valve abruptly, providing a rectangular (constant flow) waveform pattern. If the waveform modifier decreases the gas flow to the exhalation valve, the flow will tend toward a sine flow pattern. When a sinusoidal pressure waveform is produced, the volume and flow waveforms are also sinusoidal. When the ventilator functions as a flow controller, the inspiratory flow waveform is nearly rectangular and the pressure and volume waveforms are ascending and ramp-shaped.

TABLE 21-80 **Specifications for the Sechrist IV 100B Infant Ventilator**

Inspiration	
Rate (breaths/min)	1–150
Flow rate (L/min)	0–32 (flush 40)
Pressure (cmH_2O)	5–70
Time (sec)	0.1–2.9
Hold (sec)	NC
Expiration	
Time (sec)	0.3–60.0
PEEP/CPAP (cmH_2O)	2–20
Retard (L/min)	NC
I/E ratio	10:1–1:600
Modes of Ventilation	
Ventilation	
CPAP	

NC = not controlled.

□ PHASE VARIABLES

Triggering

Inspiration is time-triggered or manually triggered. In ordinary operation, inspiration is time-triggered as a function of the set inspiratory time and the set expiratory time. Inspiratory time is adjustable from 0.1 to 2.9 seconds and the expiratory time is adjustable from 0.3 to 60.0 seconds. As a result, the ventilator can operate at a ventilatory frequency ranging from 1 to 150 cycles/min.

Limiting

Inspiration is pressure-limited from 5 to 70 cmH_2O. In the event that inspiration does not pressure-limit, it becomes flow-limited. The range of adjustment available for the inspiratory flow rate is from 0 to 32 L/min. The volume is limited with respect to the inspiratory flow rate and the inspiratory time selected.

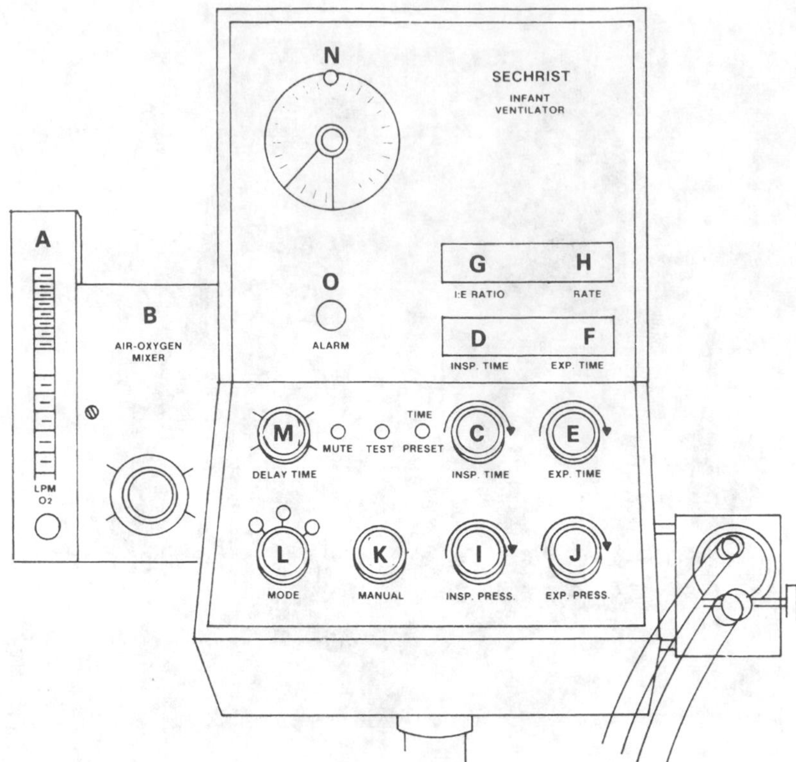

FIGURE 21-116. The control panel of the Sechrist IV 100B ventilator (see text). (Courtesy of Sechrist Industries, Inc., Medical Products Division, Anaheim, CA)

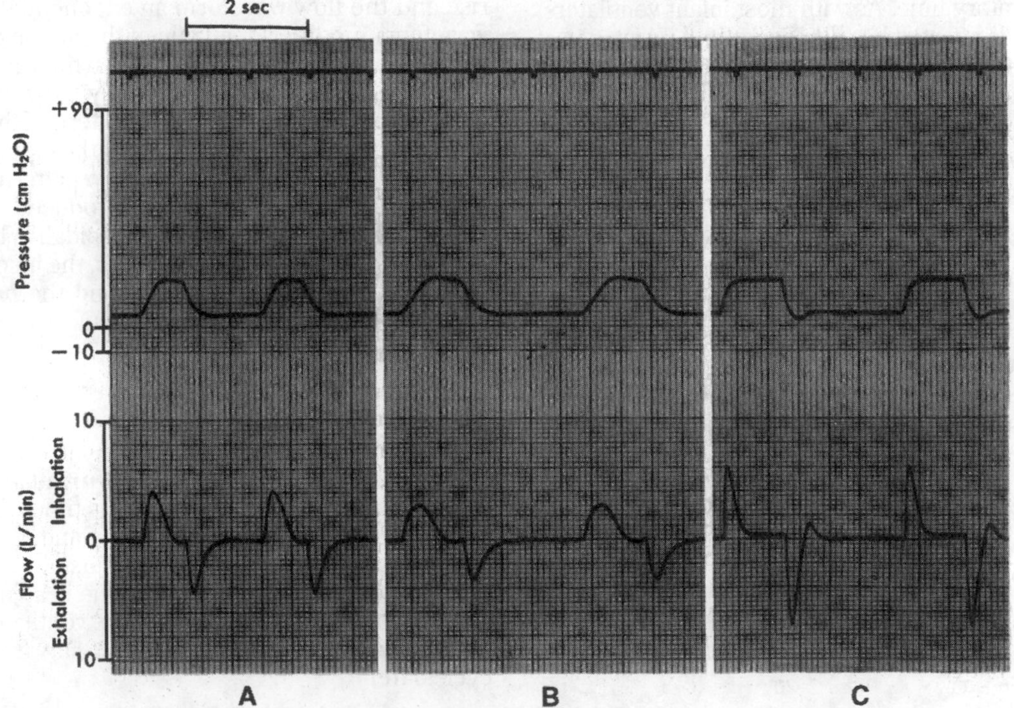

FIGURE 21-117. Flow and pressure waveforms for the Sechrist IV 100 ventilating a lung simulator set at a compliance of 2 ml/cmH_2O and an approximate resistance of 50 cmH_2O/L/sec. **(A)** The waveform control as set by the manufacturer **(B)**. The waveform control set for maximum dampening of pressure **(C)**. The waveform control set for minimum dampening of pressure rise. All graphs show use of the pressure relief set near 20 cmH_2O pressure. (From McPherson, S.P., Respiratory Care Equipment (5th ed.) Mosby–Year Book Chicago, 1995, p 345, Courtesy of Sechrist Industries, Inc. Medical Products Division, Anaheim, CA)

Cycling

In accordance with the set inspiratory time, inspiration is time-cycled.

Baseline Pressure

The uncalibrated expiratory pressure knob allows for adjustment of the baseline pressure. The range available is 2 to 20 cmH_2O.

□ CONTROL SUBSYSTEMS

Control Circuit

The control circuit of the Sechrist IV 100B combines the use of electronic, pneumatic, and fluidic components controlled by a microprocessor (Fig. 21-118). The microprocessor transmits timing signals to a solenoid valve, which in turn, operates two fluidic components,

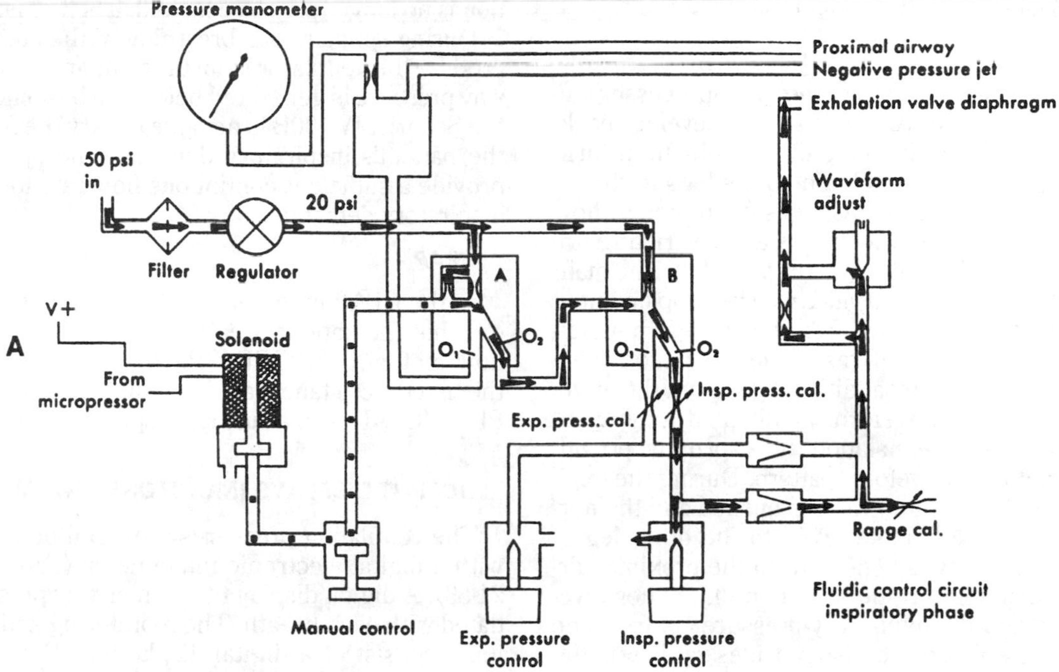

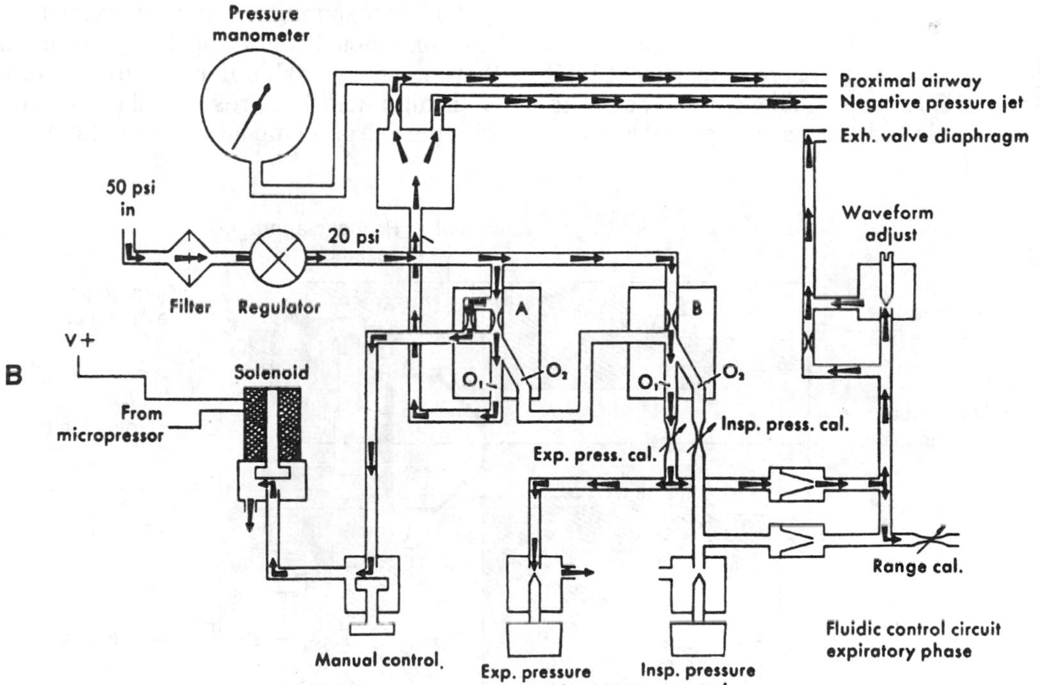

FIGURE 21-118. The functional flow diagram for the Sechrist IV 100B ventilator. **(A)** Inspiratory phase. **(B)** Expiratory and CPAP phases. (Courtesy of Sechrist Industries, Inc., Medical Products Division, Anaheim, CA)

and/or a gate and a back-pressure switch. The fluidic component transmits a pneumatic signal, which drives a diaphragm-type valve in the exhalation manifolds (Fig. 21-119).

Drive Mechanism

The Sechrist IV 100B ventilator requires external air and oxygen to drive the blender. The blender delivers pressurized gas to a flow meter, which then delivers its continuous gas flow to the patient's circuit.

Output Control Valves

When inspiration is desired, the microprocessor signals the solenoid valve (D) to close; this develops back-pressure through the fluidic unit (E), which, in turn, sends pressure through only one of its legs to the inspiratory pressure control (G); gas continues to flow through a series of one-way valves and restricting orifices to the exhalation valve (C) (Fig. 21-120). The main flow of gas to the exhalation valve may be supplemented by additional gas (bias flow) from the waveform modifier (H). The main flow of gas to the exhalation valve may be supplemented by additional gas from the waveform modifier. The waveform modifier, if fully open, opens and closes the exhalation valve abruptly, providing a constant flow waveform pattern. During the expiratory phase, the solenoid valve is opened and the normal route of gas flow is switched to the other leg of fluidic unit; this provides gas flow to the proximal airway tap (as a purge to remove humidity), the negative-pressure jet, and the expiratory pressure control. The expiratory pressure control also provides gas flow to the exhalation valve to provide PEEP/CPAP when needed.

□ MODES OF OPERATION

The control panel allows the operator to select CPAP or ventilation (VENT) mode (Table 21-81). When the ventilation mode is selected, the machine provides either CMV or IMV with normal or inverse I:E ratios. PEEP also may be selected. In normal operation, inspiration is time-triggered (in accordance with ventilatory rate); pressure-, time-, flow-, or volume-limited; and time-cycled (in accordance with set inspiratory time). The flow control knob on the front panel of the ventilator allows the operator to set the continuous flow of gas for spontaneous breathing between mandatory breaths. When inspiratory time or inspiratory flow is insufficient, inspiration is no longer pressure-limited, it is flow-limited.

During spontaneous breathing, if the gas flow delivered by the ventilator is insufficient and a negative airway pressure is generated below the baseline pressure, the Sechrist IV 100B is not able to vary the flow to meet the patient's inspiratory demand. The operator must provide a sufficient continuous flow rate for all patient inspiratory demands.

CPAP

In the CPAP mode, inspiration is not controlled. All gas that the patient breathes is provided through the flow meter. The PEEP/CPAP level is determined by the fixed resistance at the exhalation manifold (set PEEP/CPAP) and a surplus inspiratory flow.

□ OUTPUT DISPLAYS (MONITORS AND ALARMS)

The ventilating pressures are monitored constantly with a digital electronic manometer (Table 21-82 and 21-83). A digital display of mean airway pressure is updated with each breath. The monitoring and alarm systems consist of a digital display of I:E ratio (10:2 to 1:600) (see Fig. 21-116) (G), readout (1:0.1 to 1:99), rate (1 to 150 bpm) (H), inspiratory time (0.1 to 2.90 seconds) (D), expiratory time (0.30 to 60.0 seconds), and (F) continuously. For the low-pressure limit alarm, there is an adjustable delay of from 3 to 60 seconds. Both high- and low-pressure alarms can be adjusted with the use of the up and down buttons on the control

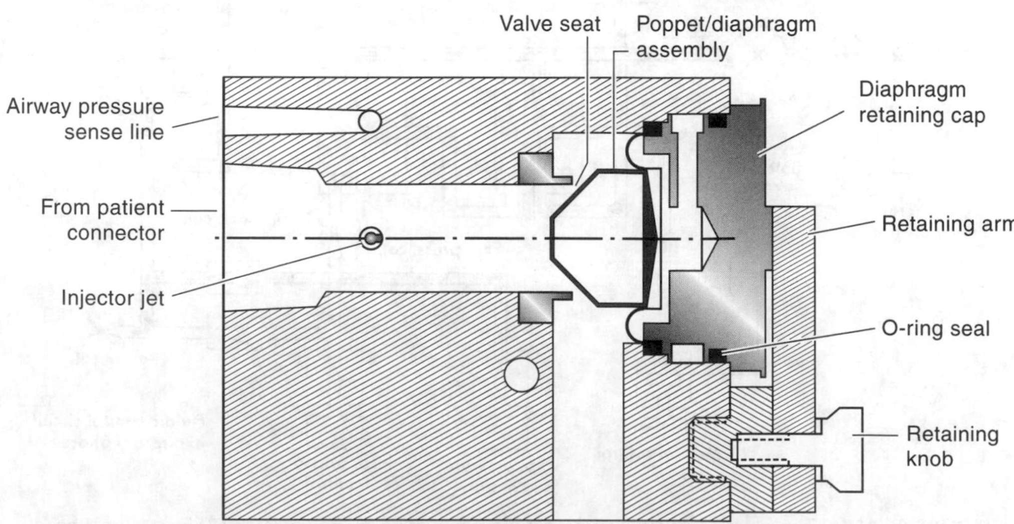

FIGURE 21-119. The exhalation valve of the Sechrist IV 100B ventilator. (Courtesy of Sechrist Industries, Inc., Medical Products Division, Anaheim, CA)

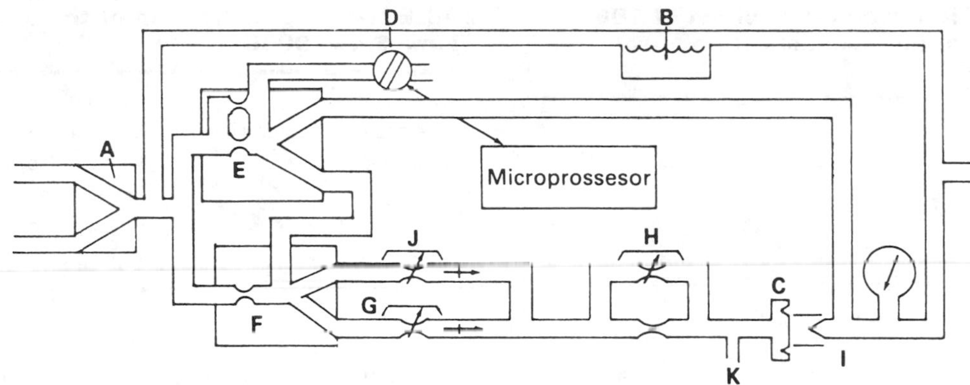

FIGURE 21-120. The schematic diagram of the Sechrist IV 100B ventilator (see text).

panel. An alarm mute is also available and activates for 30 seconds. Alarms are also available that are independent from the microprocessor (see Tables 21-82 and 21-83). These are low airway pressure, leaks, patient disconnect, failed to cycle, source gas failure, power failure (battery backup), apnea, prolonged inspiration, and microprocessor failure.

The electronic pressure manometer provides a bar graph display of proximal airway pressure. The mean airway pressure is displayed digitally and updated per breath.

□ TROUBLESHOOTING

A comprehensive troubleshooting chart is included in the operator's manual. A thorough review of the operator's manual will further simplify operation of this ventilator. The Sechrist IV-100B should not be used for transport aboard aircraft. High frequency digital circuitry emits small amounts of RFI, which may interfere with the sensitive navigational radio receivers used by the aircraft.

SIEMENS MEDICAL SYSTEMS

Siemens-Elema Servo 900C*

□ CLASSIFICATION

The Servo 900C (Table 21-84) (Fig. 21-121) is an electrically controlled and pneumatically powered ventilator. It can be a pressure or flow controller that is pressure-, time-, or manually triggered. It is pressure-, volume-, or flow-limited. The termination of mechanical inspiration is time-, pressure-, or flow-cycled. Inspiration may be extended by using a plateau. A separate blender is attached to control the FIO_2 and provide high-pressure gas to power it pneumatically. End-expiratory pressure may be applied during mechanical (PEEP) or spontaneous (CPAP) breathing.

* Thanks to Bruce Dammann with Siemens Medical Systems, Danvers, MA, for his technical assistance with the Siemens Servo ventilators.

□ SPECIFICATIONS

Table 21-85 lists the specifications for the Servo 900C.

□ INPUT VARIABLES

The electronic control circuit is powered by standard 115 volts AC current at 60 Hz. The pneumatic circuit has two input connecting ports. Both can be used simultaneously. Normal ventilator operation uses a high-pressure port that is usually powered by a blender attached to the unit, such as the Bird blender. This provides approximately 50 psig of pressure. The second port is for low-pressure gas and can be used in the delivery of anesthetic gases.

Operation

Ventilator function and variables are adjusted and displayed on a compact control panel (Fig. 21-122). Mechanical V_T is the result of an adjusted minute volume, "PRESET INSP. MIN VOL," and rate, "BREATHS/MIN" (tidal volume = minute volume/breaths per min). The inspiratory time, "INSP. TIME %," and pause time, "PAUSE TIME %," are regulated as a percentage of the total ventilator cycle and are cumulative. If the inspiratory time exceeds 80% of the total ventilatory cycle, the pause time is automatically reduced. Inspiratory time is adjustable at 20%, 25%, 33%, 50%, 67%, and 80% of the ventilatory cycle. There are five pause times: 0%, 5%, 10%, 20%, and 30%.

A simulated sine or constant-flow inspiratory pattern may be selected, by the flow control switch. A descending inspiratory flow pattern can be used by adjusting the ventilator working pressure "PRESET WORKING PRESSURE" to a level equal to, or slightly higher than peak airway pressure during volume-targeted ventilation. The desired ventilator mode is se-

TABLE 21-81. **Modes of Ventilation on the Sechrist IV 100B Ventilator**

Modes of ventilation
Ventilation
CPAP

TABLE 21-82 **Alarms on the Sechrist IV 100B Infant Ventilator (independent from microprocessor)**

Low airway pressure	
Leaks	
Patient disconnect	
Failed to cycle	
Source gas failure	
Power failure (battery backup)	
Apnea (during certain CPAP conditions)	
Prolonged inspiration	
Alarm delay time (sec)	3–60 (±10%)
Alarm mute (sec)	25 (±5)

lected by an eight-position rotary knob, the "mode control knob."

Airway pressure during mechanical or spontaneous breathing modes is manipulated by the following control knobs located in the second panel from the left: "PEEP," "TRIG SENSITIVITY BELOW PEEP," "INSP PRESS LEVEL ABOVE PEEP," and "UPPER PRESS LIMIT." The airway pressure (range, −20 to 120 cmH_2O) is indicated on an analog meter at the top of this same panel.

PEEP is adjustable, up to 50 cmH_2O, with a safety catch at 20 cmH_2O. Inspiratory effort (below PEEP) necessary for patient-triggered breaths is adjustable from zero to 20 cmH_2O subatmospheric. Each patient-triggered breath activates an indicator light near the trigger sensitivity control. During "PRESS SUPPORT," "PRESS CONTR," and "SIMV and PRESS SUPPORT" modes, the constant airway pressure above PEEP is adjustable from zero to 100 cmH_2O, with a safety catch at 30 cmH_2O. Peak airway pressure may be limited from 20 to 120 cmH_2O. When the upper pressure limit is exceeded, the ventilator cycles to exhalation.

TABLE 21-83 **Monitors and Displays Available on the Sechrist IV 100B Infant Ventilator**

Power	On/off
FiO_2	0.21–1.00
Flow	Single or double flow meter system
Mode selector	Off/CPAP/vent
Inspiratory pressure (cmH_2O)	5–70
Expiratory pressure (cmH_2O)	−2–15
Expiratory time (sec)	0.30–60
Inspiratory time (sec)	0.10–2.90
I:E ratio	1:01–1.99
Test	Verifies operation in the "vent" mode
Inspiratory phase light	Red LED illuminates during inspiratory phase in "vent" mode
Inverse I:E ratio light	Red LED indicates inverse I:E ratio

TABLE 21-84 **Classification of the Siemens-Elema Servo 900C**

Power source	Pressurized gas (35–100 psig)
Power source for control circuit	Electricity (115 volts AC at 60 Hz)
Control mechanism	Pressure, flow/volume
Triggering	Pressure, manual, time
Limiting	Pressure, volume, flow
Cycling	Time, pressure, flow

A small hood located beneath the "UPPER ALARM LIMIT" in the far left panel encloses push buttons for the following functions: inspiratory pause hold ("INSP PAUSE HOLD"), expiratory pause hold ("EXP PAUSE HOLD"), and "GAS EXCHANGE." Each function is activated for as long as the push button is depressed. The "INSP PAUSE HOLD" may be used to enhance alveolar gas mixing to provide an accurate mean expired carbon dioxide analysis. Stable end-expiratory pressure measurements may be affected by extending exhalation via "EXP PAUSE HOLD." To quickly change the patient's inspiratory gas mixture, the "GAS CHANGE" button is depressed, which rapidly "washes" the internal and external circuits with the "new" gas mixture.

□ CONTROL VARIABLES

The SERVO 900C can control either pressure or flow during inspiration. It controls flow in the volume control and volume control + sigh modes. It controls pressure in the pressure support and pressure control modes. In the SIMV mode, it switches between flow control for mandatory breaths and pressure control for spontaneous breaths or pressure support breaths (SIMV + pressure support).

Inspiratory Waveform

When functioning as a pressure controller (PSV and PCV), the ventilator provides a rectangular pressure waveform. As a flow controller, the operator can select either a rectangular (constant) or a simulated sine waveform (a waveform with ascending and descending ramps). A descending ramp flow waveform can be approximated by reducing the working pressure until it is at or slightly above peak inspiratory pressure (PIP) for the desired tidal volume with the waveform select switch on the rectangular pattern in volume-targeted modes and happens automatically in all pressure-targeted modes

□ PHASE VARIABLES

Triggering

Inspiration is pressure-triggered when the ventilator senses (based on sensitivity setting) a drop in baseline pressure. Sensitivity can be set from 0 to 20 cmH_2O below PEEP using the trigger sensitivity knob. The SERVO 900C is time-triggered based on the frequency

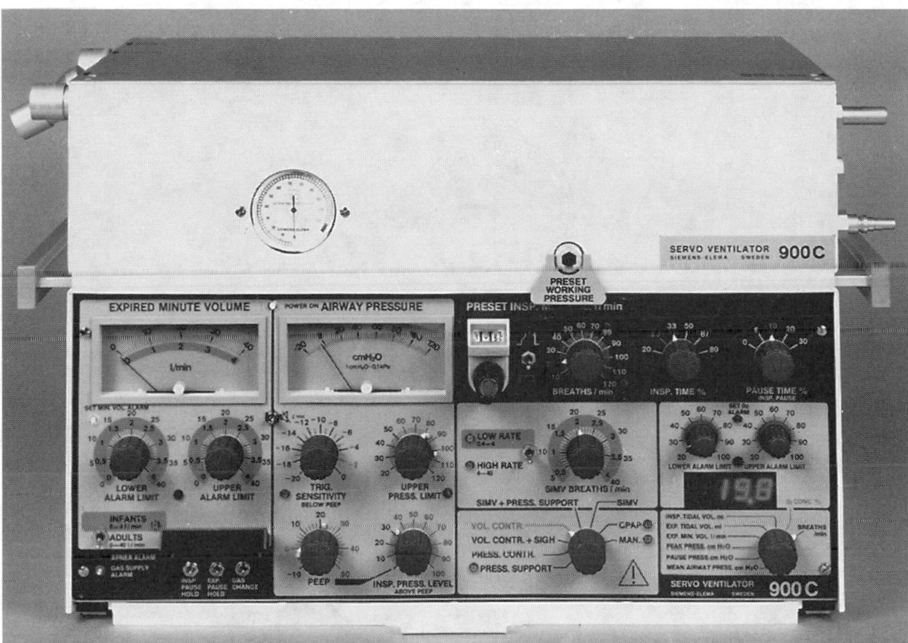

FIGURE 21-121. Siemens-Elema Servo 900C. (Courtesy of Siemens-Elema Corp., Danvers, MA)

setting. Frequency can be set with the breaths/min knob (5 to 120 breaths/min) or the SIMV breaths knob (0.4 to 4 breaths/min with the toggle switch on the low scale and 4 to 40 with the toggle switch on the high scale). When sigh is selected, the machine delivers a sigh breath once every 100 mandatory breaths.

Limiting

In the pressure control and pressure support modes, the ventilator is pressure-controlled. When PCV and PSV are not in use, a demand valve controls the inspiratory pressure by maintaining the set PEEP/CPAP level. When PCV and PSV are in use, the operator can select a pressure limit from 0 to 100 cmH_2O above PEEP/CPAP level using the inspiratory pressure level knob. This would allow peak pressure to go as high as 120 cmH_2O.

Inspiration is volume-limited when the pause time knob is above zero (range, 0% to 30%). Pause time increases I time and the I:E ratio. This can be calculated using the following equation:

$$\text{I:E} = [\text{I time }\% + \text{pause time }\%]/[100 - (\text{I time }\% + \text{pause time }\%)$$

For example, given an inspiration time set at 33% and a pause time set at 5%:

$$\text{I:E} = (33\% + 5\%)/[100 - (33\% + 5\%) = 38/62 = 1{:}1.6$$

Inspiration is flow-limited when the rectangular inspiratory waveform is selected. With this waveform, the peak and the mean values for flow are the same during inspiration. The mean (average) flow is controlled by the minute volume setting and the inspiratory time settings:

$$\text{Mean flow (L/min)} = \text{minute volume (L/min)}/\text{I time (as a fraction)}$$

For example, if the minute volume is 6 L/min and the I time is set at 20%, the mean flow will be 30 L/min.

Baseline Pressure

Baseline pressure can be adjusted in a range from −10 to +50 cmH_2O using the PEEP control knob. To achieve pressures below zero, a vacuum source needs to be connected to the expiratory side of the patient circuit to provide negative end-expiratory pressure (NEEP). The accessory to adapt for NEEP is no longer sold by the company and is not recommended for use.

TABLE 21-85 **Specifications for the Servo 900C**

Inspiration	
Rate (bpm)	SIMV, 0.4–40 High 5–120
Minute volume (L/min)	0.5–40
Pressure (cmH_2O)	0–100 above PEEP
Inspiratory time (%)	20, 25, 33, 50, 67, 80
Pause time (%)	0, 10, 20, 30
Effort (cmH_2O)	−20 to 0 (PEEP compensated)
Safety pressure (cmH_2O)	120
Pressure limit (cmH_2O)	16–120
Working pressure (cmH_2O)	0–120
Expiration	
PEEP/CPAP (cmH_2O)	0–50
Expiratory time	Not controlled
Retard	Not controlled
I/E ratio	1:4–4:1

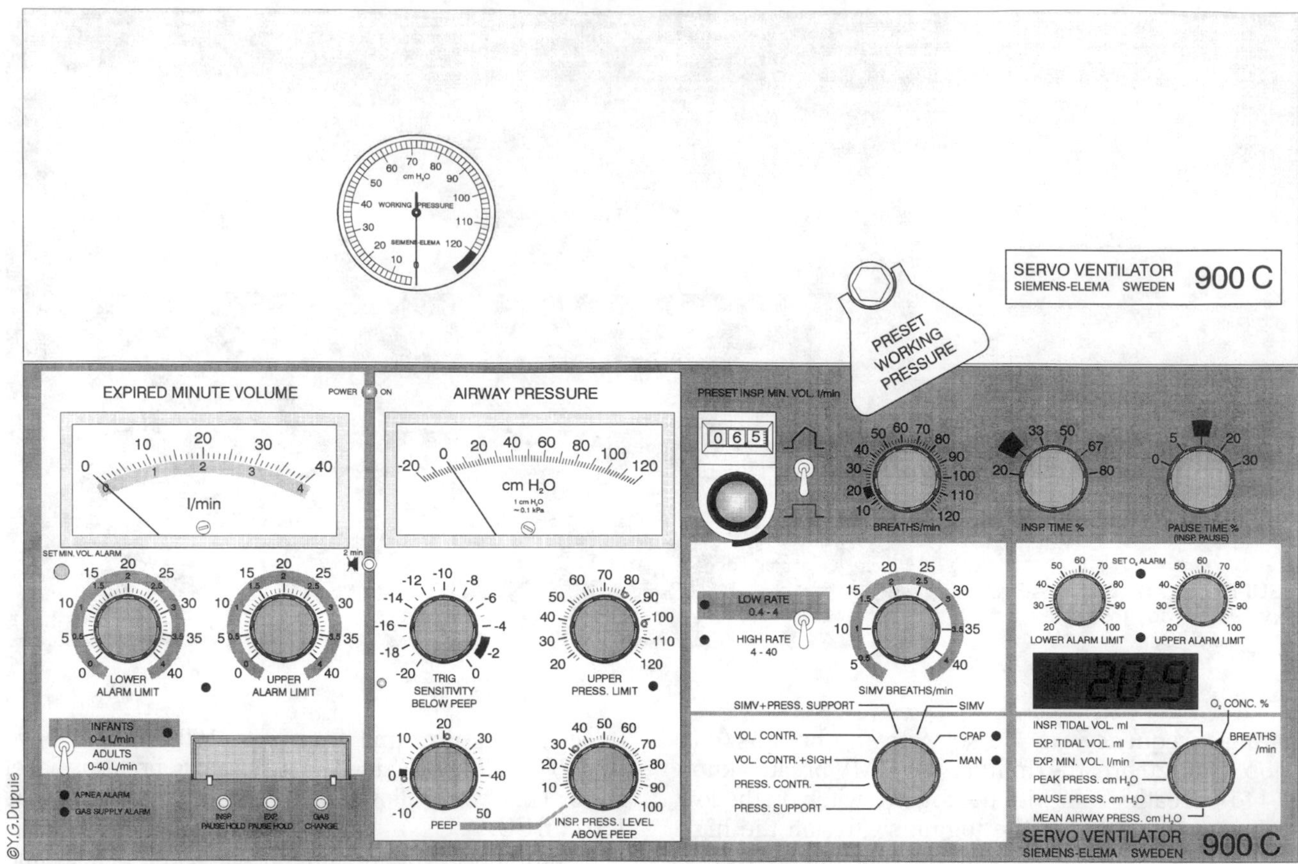

FIGURE 21-122. Control panel of the Servo 900C. (Courtesy of Yvon Dupuis, Ilderton, Ontario, Canada)

□ CONTROL SUBSYSTEMS

Control Circuit

The Servo 900C is electronically controlled but does not use a microprocessor. There are two pressure and two flow transducers, with a set of each for inspiratory and expiratory measurements. The pressures are measured inside the ventilator and not at the proximal airway. The inspiratory pressure transducer produces the reading on the airway pressure display. It is also used by the pressure alarm systems.

Information from the inspiratory and expiratory flow transducers is electrically integrated to measure volume. The volume signals are then used to display both inspiratory and expiratory tidal volumes.

Signals from both of the pressure and flow transducers on the inspiratory side control the inspiratory valve which determines the amount of pressure and the flow waveforms during inspiration. On the expiratory side, signals from the pressure transducer close the expiratory valve when the pressure reaches the preset PEEP/CPAP level.

Drive Mechanism

The Servo 900C has an internal plastic bellows that is under tension from an adjustable spring (Fig. 21-123). Air enters the bellows under pressure from the high-pressure gas source. The ventilator must have this external pressurized gas source to fill the bellows and compress the springs. The amount of working pressure is then established by the force exerted by the springs. The range of working pressure is from zero to 120 cmH_2O. Pressures in excess of this are vented to the atmosphere. The spring assembly moves the gas from the bellows into the patient circuit.

Output Control Valve

The output control valves are the two valves located in the inspiratory and expiratory sections inside the ventilator. When gas is being delivered to the patient from the inspiratory side, the inspiratory valve is open and its movement determines the amount of pressure and the shape of the flow waveform. At the same time the expiratory valve is closed. During exhalation, the inspiratory valve closes and the expiratory valve determines the expiratory baseline pressure above zero.

□ MODES OF OPERATION

The mode selection switch on the front panel of the Servo 900C has the following modes available (Table 21-86): pressure support, pressure control, volume control, volume control with periodic sigh, SIMV, SIMV with pressure support, CPAP, and manual.

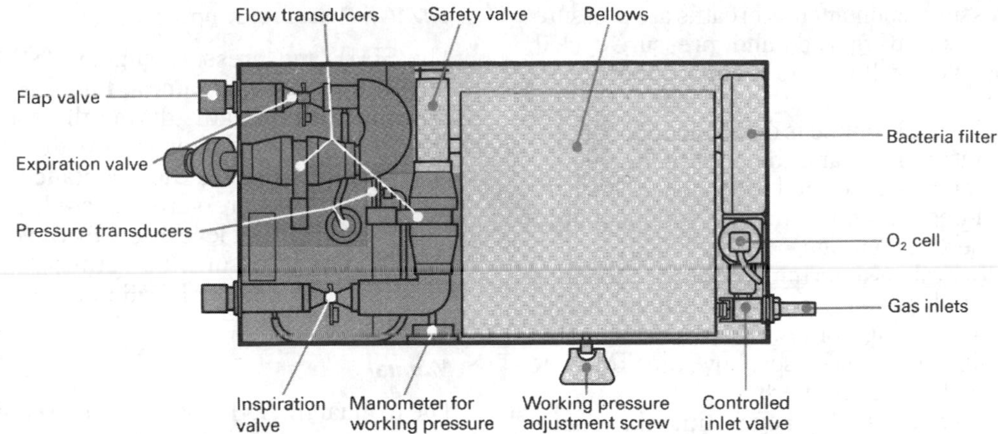

FIGURE 21-123. General view of the pneumatic unit of the Servo 900C. (Courtesy of Siemens-Elema Corp., Danvers, MA)

Pressure Support

PSV ("PRESS SUPPORT") provides an adjustable constant airway pressure during spontaneous breathing. These breaths are pressure controlled, pressure-triggered, pressure-limited, and flow-cycled. The operator sets the pressure using the inspiratory pressure level knob and must also set machine sensitivity. Inspiratory flow tends to characterize a decaying exponential flow waveform and varies depending on the set pressure and the patient's inspiratory demands and lung and circuit characteristics.

The inspiratory pressure support is normally terminated when the inspiratory flow, as measured by the inspiratory flow transducer, has decreased to approximately 25% of the peak flow. As a safety feature, pressure support will terminate if the expiratory pressure transducer senses an airway pressure of 3 cmH_2O preset inspiratory pressure level plus PEEP. If there is a leak in the circuit and flow does not drop, a safety backup system will end the breath when pressurized inspiration exceeds 80% of the breathing cycle, as determined by the existing control settings. In this circumstance the inspiratory valve closes, and the exhalation valve vents pressure to a preset end-expiratory pressure level. For this reason, the operator must be sure to check preset breaths/min when selecting this mode.

TABLE 21-86 **Modes of Ventilation for the Servo 900C Ventilator**

Volume control (assist, A/C, control)
Volume control + sigh
Pressure control
Pressure support (PS)
SIMV
SIMV + pressure support
CPAP (PEEP)
Manual (for anesthesia use)

Pressure Control

PCV ("PRESS CONTR") provides a constant airway pressure during a selected mechanical inspiratory time. The constant pressure is maintained by the inspiratory servo-feedback system (similar to "INSP PRESS SUPPORT" mode). In this mode, breaths are pressure controlled and can be time-triggered based on the set frequency or pressure-triggered with an appropriate sensitivity setting and a spontaneously breathing patient. Pressure-controlled breaths are normally time-cycled, but will also be terminated if the airway pressure exceeds the selected pressure level. Delivered mechanical V_T depends on inspiratory pressure, ventilatory rate, inspiratory time, patient and circuit characteristics, and patient effort. In this mode, the minute ventilation control is not active. Tidal volume can be checked on the digital display. The flow pattern forms a decaying exponential ramp.

Volume Control

The volume control ("VOL CONTR") mode provides tidal ventilation without a sigh. In this mode, inspiration is flow-controlled. It can be time-triggered based on the frequency set on the breaths per minute knob, or pressure-triggered if the patient is spontaneously breathing and the sensitivity is set correctly. Breaths are time-cycled out of inspiration under normal conditions in this mode.

With the Servo 900C, the operator sets a minute ventilation and a rate for the patient. There is no tidal volume control. Tidal volume is calculated by dividing the minute volume setting (L/min) by the frequency in breaths per minute.

Volume Control + Sigh

Volume control and sigh ("VOL CONTR + SIGH") mode provides consistent V_T delivery to the circuit, with every 100th breath being doubled in volume.

SIMV

In this mode, mandatory breaths are flow-controlled, time- or pressure-triggered, and time-cycled. Spontaneous ventilation occurs at baseline (ie, ambient or end-expiratory) pressure. Spontaneous breaths are pressure-controlled, pressure-triggered, and pressure-cycled. The inspiratory flow will vary to maintain the PEEP/CPAP settings.

The mandatory tidal volume is determined by the setting on the minute volume and the breaths per minute knob and calculated as described previously. The inspiratory flow will depend on the minute volume and inspiratory time percent settings.

The respiratory rate is determined by the rate setting on the SIMV rate knob and the toggle switch that selects a higher (4 to 40/min) or lower rate (0.4 to 4/min). The breaths/min knob must be set above the SIMV rate setting for rate to function properly.

Each SIMV breath has a total cycle time that equals 60 seconds divided by the SIMV rate. For example, with an SIMV rate of 2 breaths/min the total cycle time is 60 sec/2 or 30 seconds. This SIMV total cycle time is then divided into two portions, the SIMV period and the spontaneous period. The SIMV period is determined by the breaths/min knob and not the SIMV rate knob. The SIMV period will equal 60 seconds divided by the setting on the breaths/min knob. If the breaths/min knob is set at 10, the SIMV period will equal 60 sec/10 or 6 seconds. The spontaneous period is different between the SIMV total cycle time and the SIMV period. In the above examples, the spontaneous period would be (30 − 6 = 24 seconds) for the spontaneous period. The patient can breath spontaneously during the 24 seconds and not receive a mandatory (mechanical) breath.

The mandatory breath is normally pressure-triggered by patient effort when the sensitivity is set. The mandatory breath is then delivered at the beginning of the SIMV period. If no spontaneous effort is detected, then the mandatory breath is time-triggered at the end of the SIMV period. The patient can breathe freely without triggering a mandatory breath during the spontaneous period.

Continuing our example from above, if the patient initiated a mandatory breath during the SIMV period (6 seconds), following mandatory breath delivery the patient has 24 seconds to breathe spontaneously without triggering a mandatory breath. The cycle then repeats itself.

SIMV + Pressure Support

The SIMV and pressure support (SIMV + PRESS SUPPORT) mode is the same as the SIMV mode except that spontaneous breaths during the spontaneous period trigger pressure support breaths. The pressure support breaths during the spontaneous period are pressure-controlled, pressure-triggered, and flow-cycled. The pressure support level is set by the operator using the inspiratory pressure knob (inspiratory pressure above PEEP). Mandatory breaths are the same as in the SIMV mode.

Manual

The manual (MAN) mode is used in conjunction with an anesthesia bag and manual ventilation valve (accessory equipment) attached to the ventilator outflow port and connected to the inspiratory line of the breathing circuit (eg, anesthesia system). During manual inflation (bag compression), circuit pressure rises; when it reaches 4 cmH_2O the ventilator exhalation valve closes, diverting the compressed volume to the patient. During exhalation, as the circuit pressure decreases to less than 4 cmH_2O, the ventilator exhalation valve opens. When circuit pressure is $<cmH_2O$, demand flow from the ventilator refills the bag. Flow into the bag is regulated by the preset inspiratory minute volume control. The apnea alarm is deactivated while in the manual mode. Spontaneously breathing patients can breath from the bag. This requires a strong enough inspiratory effort to open the valve (-2.0 cmH_2O).

CPAP

In this mode, the spontaneous inspiratory breaths are pressure controlled. Inspiratory flow varies depending on the PEEP/CPAP level set and the patient's effort. It is pressure-triggered when a spontaneous breath is detected and flow-cycled.

Mechanism of Operation

The Servo 900C is electronically operated and pneumatically powered (see Fig. 21-123 and Fig. 21-124). An air–oxygen mixer (A) provides gas at the prescribed F_{IO_2}. Metered gas may be added by means of an auxiliary inlet (B). On demand, a valve (C) opens, allowing

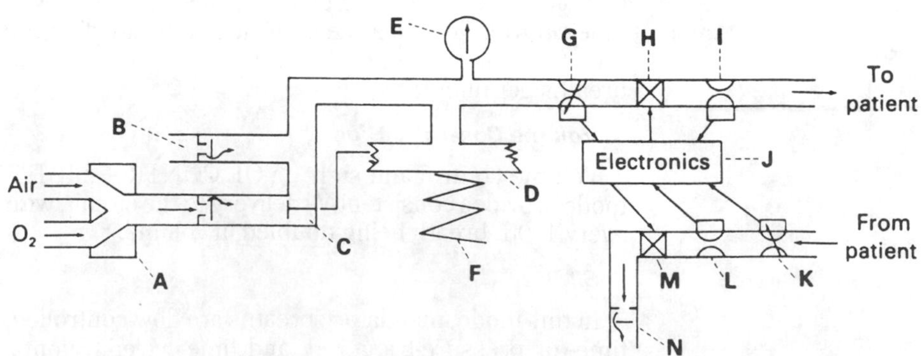

FIGURE 21-124. Schematic diagram of the 900C ventilator (see text).

mixed gas to flow by an oxygen sensor and through a bacterial filter (not illustrated) into a pressurized concertina bag (see Fig. 21-123). The pressure is indicated on manometer (E) (see Fig. 21-124) and is generated by adjustable spring tension (F). During mechanical inspiration, gas from the concertina bag is directed into the patient circuit by means of an inspiratory flow valve, controlled by a "closed feedback loop" or servo system. The servo system is composed of an inspiratory flow transducer, electronic comparator circuitry, and an inspiratory flow valve, which comprises a stepper motor that actuates a lever arm and a silicone rubber tube. The function of the lever is to open and close the rubber tubing by pinching it against a fixed part of the valve, thereby allowing or terminating flow through the silicone tube.

This pinching effect occurs in a series of 48 discrete steps. From the closed position, each additional step will increase the opening within the tube. Each step open will increase the flow through the silicone tubing by approximately 10%. The valve can be opened from the closed position in as little as 0.1 second, or at a rate of 480 steps per second. As inspiration begins, the inspiratory valve opens a predetermined number of steps, creating an appropriate aperture that permits the desired inspiratory flow as calculated by the front panel control settings. Flow passes the inspiratory flow transducer, where it is measured. If the measured and desired flows do not agree, the electronic comparator circuitry modulates the valve aperture to produce the specific flow required to guarantee volume delivery in the allotted inspiratory time.

In the pressure-support mode, the inspiratory pressure transducer signal is processed electronically and referenced to the set value. The inspiratory flow valve is subsequently modulated, allowing only sufficient flow to maintain the selected pressure.

The exhalation valve is also a lever arm and silicone tube assembly. The expiratory lever arm, however, is actuated by a two-position (opened/closed) electromagnetic solenoid or pull-magnet. During mechanical inspiration, the solenoid closes, pinching the silicone tube and permitting the delivery of the mechanical V_T. Termination of inspiration releases the lever arm and the patient exhales freely.

PEEP/CPAP is regulated by a second servoloop. Exhaled gas enters the expiratory servocircuit, comprising a flow transducer (K) (see Fig. 21-124), pressure transducer (L), and expiratory valve (M) interfaced in a feedback loop with the electronics. PEEP/CPAP is regulated as a function of flow resistance by altering the exhalation orifice. During exhalation, the pressure transducer signal to the electronics is compared with the selected PEEP level. The expiratory valve is then opened or closed by a process referred to as "pulse width modulation," which is various sequences of rapid open–close signals to the solenoid that will create a series of discrete apertures within the expiratory valve. The size of the exhalation orifice is thereby altered until the desired PEEP and the measured PEEP coincide. Exhaled gas is ultimately vented through a unidirectional valve (N).

□ OUTPUT DISPLAYS (MONITORS) AND ALARMS

The Siemens 900C provides extensive display, monitoring, and alarm capabilities (Table 21-87). Electronic signals are collected from two flow transducers and two pressure transducers, one of each being located in the inspiratory and expiratory limbs of the breathing circuit. After appropriate electronic conditioning, these signals provide information that is displayed or used to trigger alarm conditions. A digital display window located in the lower right panel is capable of presenting one measured variable at a time (see Fig. 21-122). It is controlled by an eight-position rotary knob. Selections include mean airway pressure ("MEAN AIRWAY PRESS"; cmH_2O), pause or inspiratory plateau pressure ("PAUSE PRESS"; cmH_2O), peak airway pressure ("PEAK PRESS"; cmH_2O), expired minute volume ("EXP MIN VOL"; L/min), inspired V_T ("INSP TIDAL VOL"; mL), expired V_T ("EXP TIDAL VOL"; mL), oxygen concentration ("O_2 CONC"; %), and breaths per minute ("BREATHS/min").

The primary patient monitors include expired minute volume and apnea. These controls are located in the far left panel (see Fig. 21-122). The lower and upper limit for exhaled minute volume is adjustable in two ranges: infants, 0 to 4 L/min and adults, 0 to 40 L/min. When either the lower or upper limit has been reached, an audible and visual alarm is activated. The exhaled minute volume is displayed on an analog meter in this same panel.

If the ventilator does not sense a trigger effect or a mandatory breath is not delivered within 15 seconds,

TABLE 21-87 **Monitors and Alarms for the Servo 900C Ventilator**

Digital Display Window
- Mean airway pressure (cmH_2O)
- Inspiratory plateau pressure (pause pressure) (cmH_2O)
- Peak (airway) pressure (cmH_2O)
- Expired minute volume (L/min)
- Inspired tidal volume (mL)
- Expired tidal volume (mL)
- Oxygen concentration (%)

Minute Volume Monitor
- Upper and lower limit for exhaled minute volume (L/min)
- Adjustable for infants (0–4 L/min) and adults (0–40 L/min)

Airway Pressure Monitor (cmH_2O)

Alarms and Indicators
- Upper pressure limit (cmH_2O)
- Apnea alarm (15-sec limit)
- Gas supply alarm
- Set oxygen alarm (%)—Lower and upper limit

the apnea alarm, in the lower left corner, provides both audible and visual alarms. Table 21-87 provides apnea alarm time, and a listing of digital displays, minute volume monitors, alarms, and indicators. A gas supply alarm in the same location will be activated if the gas supply fails to maintain adequate pressure in the concertina bag.

A visual and audible alarm for oxygen is located in the middle section of the far right panel (see Fig. 21-122). The lower and upper limits for oxygen are adjustable from 0.20 to 1.0. If either has been reached, an audible and visual alarm is activated.

Violation of the peak pressure threshold results in the ventilator immediately cycling to the exhalation phase and the initiation of audible and visual alarms. This indicator is located just below the upper pressure limit control.

□ TROUBLESHOOTING

Performance failures may be caused by internal system leaks in valve assemblies or in the concertina bag. Valve system leaks are correctable but may be difficult to detect. When the rubber valves are inserted, twisting must be avoided to prevent unnecessary flow resistance. If the meter reads erroneously elevated minute volume, the flow transducer screen may have accumulated moisture.

Despite its sophisticated electronics, the Siemens 900C has no electronic troubleshooting software and troubleshooting may be difficult, often requiring a trip to the factory for proper diagnosis and repair.

Siemens Servo 300*

□ CLASSIFICATION

The Siemens Servo 300 ventilator (Table 21-88) (Fig. 21-125) is an electronically and pneumatically powered, microprocessor controlled ventilator. It is pressure- or flow-controlled and pressure-, time-, flow-, or manually triggered into inspiration. The Servo SV 300 is pressure-, volume-, or flow-limited and pressure-, flow-, or time-cycled.

□ SPECIFICATIONS

Table 21-89 provides a list of the specifications for the Servo SV 300. The control panel can be selected for either adult, pediatric, or neonatal ranges.

□ INPUT VARIABLES

The Siemens Servo 300 uses external compressed gases (air and oxygen) at 29 to 94 psig, which provide the flow of gas to the patient. The control circuitry is powered by electricity (110 or 120 volts AC at 50 to 60 Hz).

* Thanks to Bruce Dammann with Siemens Medical Systems, Danvers, MA, for his technical assistance with the Siemens Servo ventilators.

TABLE 21-88 **Classification of the Siemens Servo SV 300 Ventilator**

Power source	Pressurized gas (29–100 psig)
Power source for control circuit	Electricity (110, 120 volts AC at 50 to 60 Hz)
Control mechanism	Pressure, flow/volume
Triggering	Pressure, manual, time, flow
Limiting	Pressure, volume, flow, time
Cycling	Time, pressure, flow

Operation

The front control panel contains eight panels providing controls or readout systems for the following: (1) patient range selection, (2) airway pressures, (3) mode selection, (4) respiratory pattern, (5) volumes, (6) oxygen concentration, (7) alarms and messages, and (8) pause hold. Figure 21-126 provides an overview of the operating panel for the SV 300.

1. Patient Range Selection (see Fig. 21-126A). The patient range selection knob permits the operator to select either adult, pediatric, or neonate ventilation. These settings affect the resolution of monitoring, continuous flow during expiration, maxi-

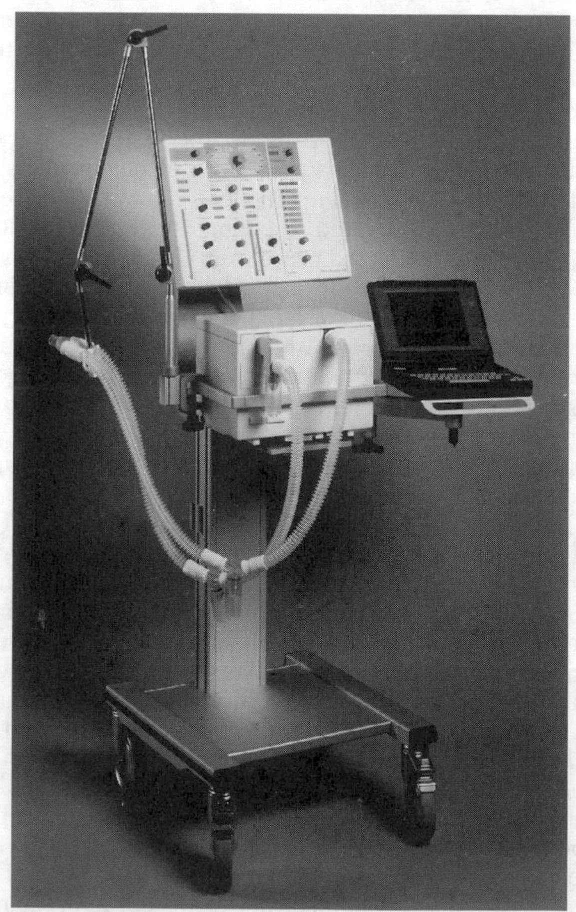

FIGURE 21-125. The Siemens Servo 300 ventilator. (Courtesy of Siemens Life Support Systems, Danvers, MA)

TABLE 21-89 **Specifications for the Servo SV 300 Ventilator**

Inspiration	
Rate (beats/min)	SIMV, 0.5–40
High 5–150	
Minute volume (L/min)	0.2–60
Tidal volume (mL)	2–4000
Flow of gas	Not controlled
Pressure control (cmH_2O)	0–100
Pressure support (cmH_2O)	0–100
Pressure monitored (cmH_2O)	0–120 above PEEP
Inspiratory time (%)	10–80 (continuous)
Pause time (%)	0–30
Trigger pressure (cmH_2O)	0–−17
Trigger flows (L/min)	Neonate 0.17–0.5
	Pediatric 0.3–1.0
	Adult 0.7–2.0
Pressure limit (cmH_2O)	15–120
Inspiratory rise time	0%–10% of cycle time
Expiration	
PEEP/CPAP (cmH_2O)	0 to 50
Expiratory time	Not controlled
Retard	Not controlled
Continuous expiratory flow (L/min)	
Neonates	0.5
Pediatric	1.0
Adult	2.0

mum peak flow during inspiration, maximum tidal volume settings, and apnea alarm time (Table 21-90).

2. Airway Pressure Settings (see Fig. 21-126A). The airway pressure settings include four controls. The upper pressure limit (range of 16 to 120 cmH_2O) will pressure-cycle breaths when the set limit is reached. The pressure control level above PEEP is used for pressure-controlled breaths. It is active in PCV and SIMV (pressure control) plus pressure support.

   The pressure support level above PEEP control sets the pressure level for pressure-support breaths (range 0 to 100 cmH_2O). It is active in the following modes: pressure support, SIMV (vol. control) + pressure support, SIMV (press. control) + pressure support. The PEEP knob sets the end expiratory pressure in all modes (range, 0 to 50 cmH_2O).

   The control marked "trig. sensitivity level below PEEP" establishes the sensitivity level for pressure-triggering or flow-triggering and is active in all modes. The pressure-triggering is activated when the patient has created a certain negative pressure below PEEP. Flow-triggering occurs when the patient has initiated a certain drop in flow through the expiratory flow transducer. The transducer sends information to the gas modules which then initiate inspiration. The flow-trigger level set by the operator is the amount by which expiratory flow must decrease to initiate a breath. Ranges for flow-trigger sensitivity are 0.7 to 2.0 L/min for adults, 0.3 to 1.0 L/min for pediatric patients, and 0.17 to 0.5 L/min for neonatal patients.

   Airway pressure displays include peak, mean, pause, and end expiratory pressure displays.
3. Mode selection (see Fig. 21-126B). The ventilator provides eight different modes of ventilation that can be selected with this control. They include the following (by manufacturer label) "pressure regulated volume control," "volume control," "pressure control," "volume support," "SIMV (vol contr.) + pressure support," "SIMV (press. contr.) + pressure support," and "Pressure support, CPAP."

   The modes themselves are described in greater detail later in this chapter. The mode selection switch also has positions for "ventilator off battery charging" (when the ventilator is not in use, it should be connected to an electrical wall outlet to allow the internal battery to charge), "standby" and "optional." In the standby mode, all the electrical circuits are receiving power for warming up and the ventilator is ready for use. Settings for a specific patient can be made in this position. In "standby" the inspiratory, expiratory, and safety valves are closed and a caution sound is heard. All displays are off except the "alarms and messages" display, which indicates the "standby" operation is active. The "optional" setting is intended for future upgrade.
4. Respiratory pattern (see Fig. 21-126C). The respiratory pattern panel contains controls for CMV frequency in breaths per minute (5 to 150 breaths/min); inspiratory percentage (10% to 80%); pause time (0% to 30%), which adds to inspiratory time; inspiratory rise time % (0% to 10%), which allows manipulation of the pressure and flow waveforms by altering the inspiratory gas flow; and SIMV frequency (0.5 to 40 breaths/min).
5. Volumes (see Fig. 21-126D). This panel permits selection and monitoring of volume-targeted breaths. The lower panel contains a bar graph for gas flows at high and low range. It also contains controls for upper and lower minute volume alarms.
6. Oxygen concentration (see Fig. 21-126E). A continuous readout of oxygen concentration is available in this panel. Desired oxygen delivery can also be selected by the knob provided in this section. An additional control provides access to the "start breath" and "oxygen breath."
7. Alarms and messages (see Fig. 21-126E).
8. Pause hold (see Fig. 21-126E).

The right-hand panel of the ventilator contains the alarm system indicators and the alarms and message window. These are discussed below. The inspiration pause control permits measurement of end inspiratory pressure (plateau pressure). The inspiratory pause is

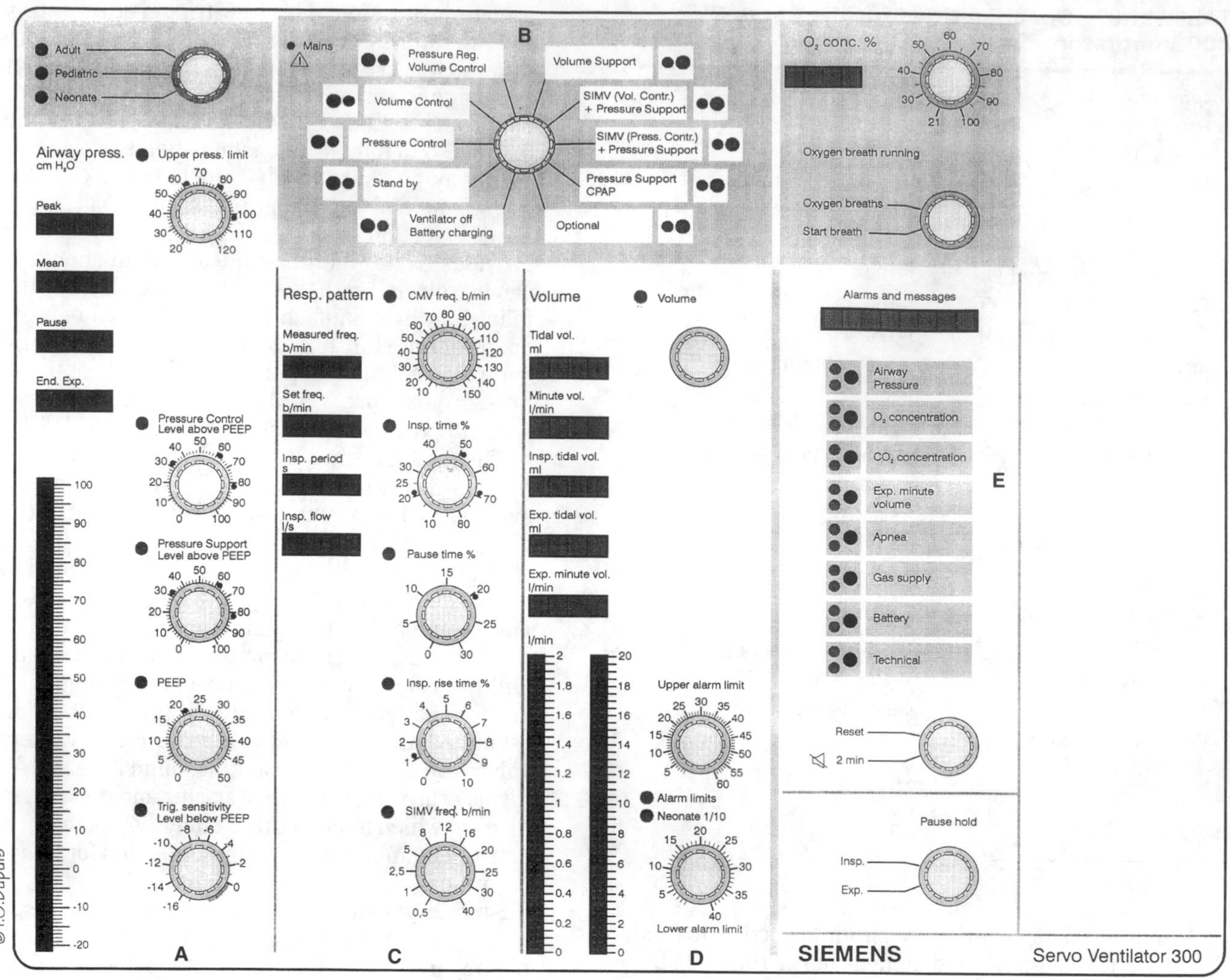

FIGURE 21-126. The control panel of the Servo SV 300. **(A)** The patient range selection panel and airway pressure settings. **(B)** The patient mode selection switch. **(C)** The panel for respiratory pattern. **(D)** The panel for volume control and monitoring. **(E)** Oxygen concentrations, start breath, alarms and messages, and pause hold controls and indicators are located in this panel. (Courtesy of Yvon Dupuis, Ilderton, Ontario, Canada)

held as long as the control is activated, but has a built in time limit of 5 seconds. The expiratory pause control measures end expiratory pressure for the estimation of auto-PEEP. The expiratory pause is held as long as the control is kept in position, but has a time limit of 30 seconds. A patient can take a breath during the expiratory pause hold.

TABLE 21-90 **Range for Continuous Flow, Inspiratory Flow, Maximum Tidal Volume and Apnea Alarm Time in the Servo SV 300 Ventilator**

Range	Continuous Flow	Max. Inspiratory Flow	Max. V_T	Apnea Alarm Time
Adult	2 L/min	200 L/min	3999 mL	20 sec
Child	1 L/min	33 L/min	399 mL	15 sec
Neonate	0.5 L/min	13 L/min	39 mL	10 sec

□ CONTROL VARIABLES

The Servo 300 controls either flow/volume or pressure. It controls flow/volume in the volume control mode and in SIMV (volume control) + pressure support for the mandatory volume breaths. The pressure support breaths in this case are pressure controlled. It controls pressure in PCV, PSV, SIMV (pressure control) + pressure support, pressure regulated volume control, and volume support modes and in CPAP. In the volume control modes, the ventilator will switch from flow-control to pressure-control if the patient's inspiratory demand exceeds the value of flow being provided, that is, the airway pressure drops below the baseline (PEEP) level. The flow to the patient is increased to maintain the set PEEP.

In the pressure-regulated volume control modes, the ventilator checks the set tidal volume with the delivered tidal volume and automatically resets the pressure control level between breaths in order to achieve the targeted volume.

Inspiratory Waveform

The flow pattern is rectangular (constant) in volume control. The pressure pattern is rectangular in pressure control. If the "INSPIRATORY RISE TIME (%)" is selected, this control allows the ventilator to trim the beginning edge of the pressure and flow waveforms to provide for patient comfort and avoid premature cycling of inspiration. The trim will last from 0% to 10% of the total cycle time. The pressure or flow, depending on which mode is selected, builds gradually at the beginning of the breath.

□ PHASE VARIABLES

Triggering

Breaths can be pressure-, time-, flow-, or manually triggered. Time-triggering is present with preset ventilator frequency. The frequency of mandatory breaths is determined either by the CMV "FREQUENCY" control or the "SIMV FREQUENCY" control. Pressure- or flow-triggering occurs when the patient makes an inspiratory effort and drops the system value below the preset sensitivity level. The operator uses the "TRI. SENSITIVITY LEVEL BELOW PEEP" control to select either pressure- or flow-triggering. Pressure-triggering occurs when the patient's inspiratory effort drops the pressure below a preset value (0 to -17 cmH_2O).

Flow-triggering occurs when the patient has started an inspiratory effort that drops the flow through the expiratory flow transducer below a certain level. Throughout exhalation a bias flow is constantly flowing through the ventilator circuit. When inspiration is triggered, the bias flow stops. The amount of bias flow is determined by the patient range selected by the operator. For adults it is 2.0 L/min, for pediatric patients 1.0 L/min, and for neonates 0.5 L/min. The total flow, bias flow plus patient exhaled gas, is measured by the expiratory transducer. When a spontaneously breathing patient begins inspiration, he or she takes gas from the bias flow. The flow measured by the expiratory transducer is lower than the preset value. When the inspiratory flow reaches the preset flow trigger level, the ventilator begins a new inspiration.

Normally, flow-triggering is used rather than pressure-triggering because it is easier for the patient to start a breath. It is set so that the ventilator is as sensitive as possible to the patient's effort without causing auto-triggering (self-triggering). If there is a known leak in the patient circuit, such as an uncuffed endotracheal tube, and the leak is higher than the bias flow, then pressure-triggering should be used. Flow- or pressure-triggering can be used in all modes.

Manual triggering can occur using the "START BREATH" switch. Triggering by any of the described methods can be overridden by using the inspiratory "PAUSE HOLD" control.

Limiting

Inspiration is pressure-limited in all modes except "VOLUME CONTROL" and "SIMV (VOLUME CONTROL)." The limit is set using the "PRESSURE CONTROL LEVEL ABOVE PEEP" or the "PRESSURE SUPPORT LEVEL ABOVE PEEP" control knobs.

Volume-limiting occurs with flow-controlled breaths when the pause time control is set above zero (available range is 0% to 30%).

Flow-limiting is available in the "VOLUME CONTROL" and "SIMV (VOLUME CONTROL)" settings. The rate of gas flow is dependent on the "CMV FREQUENCY" setting and the "INSPIRATORY TIME %" setting except in cases where the patient's inspiratory demand pulls pressure below PEEP. Gas flow can be estimated using the following equation:

$$\text{Mean inspiratory flow (L/min)} = \text{minute volume (L/min)} / \text{Insp. Time \%(as a decimal)}$$

For example, if minute volume is 12 L/min. and I% is 25%, the flow will be an average of 48 L/min.

Cycling

Ventilation can be pressure-, time-, or flow-cycled into exhalation. It is pressure-cycled when the preset upper pressure limit is achieved in volume-targeted (flow controlled) breaths. This helps avoid excessive airway pressures during volume ventilation. It will also pressure-cycle in the pressure support mode if the pressure in the system exceeds the preset upper pressure limit. This is also to avoid an excess pressure, but is not the normal cycling mechanism for pressure support.

This ventilator is normally flow-cycled for spontaneous breaths and for breaths in pressure support and volume support modes when inspiratory flow drops to 5% of peak flow. Time-cycling occurs in pressure control mode, volume control mode and SIMV mode. Inspiratory time is determined by the "INSPIRATORY TIME %" setting, and the "CMV FREQUENCY" setting in all modes except volume control and SIMV (volume control). Pause percent time will increase (add to) inspiratory time only in volume control and SIMV (volume control).

There is an emergency time-cycling system available in the pressure support mode. If inspiratory time exceeds 80% of the inspiratory time of the total cycle time as established by the "CMV FREQUENCY" settings, the ventilator will time-cycle.

Normal cycling can be overridden by using the inspiratory "PAUSE HOLD" switch to measure plateau (static) pressure during inspiration.

Baseline Pressure

The baseline pressure can be adjusted between 0 and 50 cmH_2O.

□ CONTROL SUBSYSTEMS

The Servo 300 consists of two separate units connected by a 3-meter cable. In general, the control unit contains the control panel and electrical circuits that actually control the pneumatic or patient unit. The separate pneumatic unit has a gas delivery system containing high-performance solenoid valves with a total response time of 6 milliseconds. Maximum flow delivery from these valves is 180 L/min.

Control Circiut and Drive Mechanism

The Servo 300 ventilator is microprocessor (electrically) controlled and powered by external compressed gas sources (drive mechanism). The gases must be pressurized in the range of 29 to 94 psig and connect into two flow control modules. These modules control the inspired oxygen concentration and the flow waveform of the inspired gas. Oxygen is measured before it enters the patient circuit.

Pressure is measured in two locations. Inspiratory pressure is measured just after the gas leaves the inspiratory side of the mix chamber. The expiratory pressure is measured just before the gas enters the exhalation valve. Flow is measured on the expiratory side just before the exhalation valve, also. These measured values are used to control the flow and pressure waveforms.

Output Control Valve

Figures 21-127 and 21-128 show the internal components of the pneumatic unit. Air and oxygen enter the unit at (1) and (2) (Fig. 21-127) under a pressure of 29 to 94 psig, pass through bacterial filters and enter the gas modules of the unit (3). The gases leave their individual modules to go to a mixing area (4). As gas exits the mixing area the pressure is measured by a pressure transducer (5). The gas then enters the inspiratory pipe (6). This pipe also contains a safety valve (120 cmH_2O limit), a holder for the oxygen analyzer (7) and the inspiratory outlet. Gas leaves the inspiratory pipe and passes into the patient circuit.

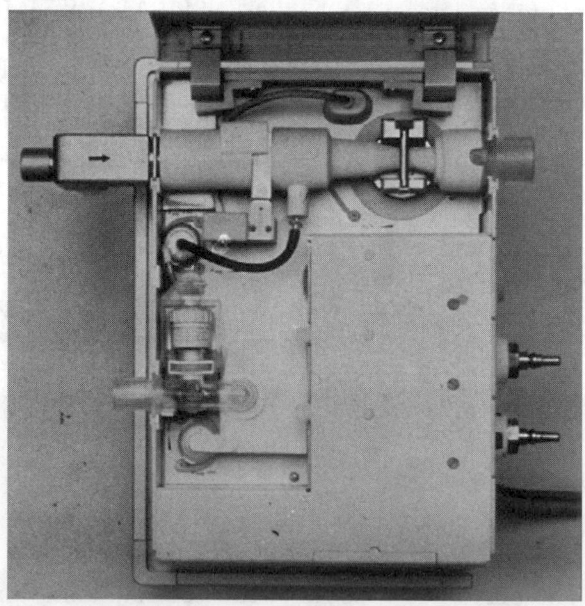

FIGURE 21-127. Photograph of the internal components of the Siemens Servo 300 ventilator. (Courtesy of Siemens Life Support Systems, Danvers, MA)

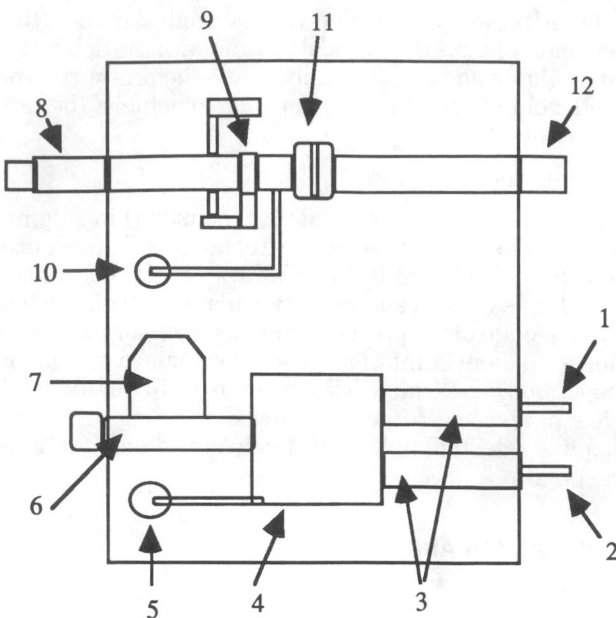

FIGURE 21-128. Internal components of the Siemens Servo 300 ventilator. See text for explanation.

Exhaled gas from the patient circuit passes through a moisture trap and into the expiratory inlet (8). The gas is then measured by the expiratory flow transducer (9), which also senses a drop in flow during patient inspiration and allows for flow-triggering. Gas then passes by the expiratory pressure transducer (10), which detects inspiratory pressure changes for pressure-triggering. PEEP levels are controlled by the expiratory pressure transducer and the expiratory valve (11). Gas exits the ventilator by the expiratory outlet (12).

□ MODES OF OPERATION

The modes that are named on the control panel will be described and are listed in Table 21-91.

Pressure Control

Pressure control mode is a pressure controlled, time-, flow-, or pressure-triggered, pressure-limited, and time-cycled mode of ventilation. The operator sets the patient

TABLE 21-91 **Modes of Ventilation as Named by the Manufacturer for the Siemens Servo SV 300 Ventilator**

Volume control (control, A/C)
Pressure regulated volume control (PRVC)
Volume support
Pressure control
Pressure support
SIMV (volume control) + pressure support
SIMV (pressure control) + pressure support
CPAP

range selector, the pressure control level above PEEP, the CMV frequency, the sensitivity setting, and the PEEP level. Time-cycling is established by the inspiratory time percentage setting and the CMV frequency. The pause time percentage is not active in this mode.

Volume Control

Volume control mode is a flow/volume controlled, time-, flow-, or pressure-triggered, flow-, volume-, and time-limited, and time- or pressure-cycled. Tidal volume delivery is based on the minute volume (L/min) and the CMV frequency (breaths/min): Tidal volume (L) = minute volume/frequency. Tidal volume remains constant from breath to breath

Inspiratory time is based on the inspiratory time percentage setting and the pause time percentage settings. Inspiratory time is limited to a maximum of 80% of the total cycle time of a set breath period. Flow is constant based on minute volume and inspiratory time percentage with two exceptions: (1) the use of the inspiratory rise time percentage, and (2) when patient's flow demand exceeds set flow.

First, when inspiratory rise time percentage is set, this tapers the start of the breath. Figure 21-129 shows the tapering effect with a flow/volume controlled breath (left) and pressure controlled breath (right). The curves on the left represent volume-targeted breaths. The top curve is pressure and the second curve is a normal flow pattern. The second set of curves on the left show the pressure and flow patterns using the "INSP. RISE TIME %." Notice how the flow curve at the bottom tapers during inspiration. The curves on the right represent pressure-targeted breaths. The top curve is pressure and the second curve is flow delivery with a normal pressure controlled breath pattern. The second set of curves on the right (bottom) use "INSP. RISE TIME %" to taper the beginning of the breath. Notice how the pressure curve is tapered (not squared) at the beginning of inspiration.

Second, if the patient's inspiratory flow demand exceeds the flow provided, the ventilator senses the pressure drop below the baseline (PEEP) level. It then switches to a pressure-controlled rather than a flow-controlled situation, giving enough flow to maintain the set PEEP level.

Pressure Regulated Volume Control (PRVC)

PRVC is a pressure-controlled, time-, flow-, or pressure-triggered, pressure-limited, time-cycled mode of ventilation. In this mode, the ventilator varies the inspiratory pressure level according to the patient's lung characteristics (lung/thorax/airway resistance) to achieve a preset tidal and minute volume. The first breath is delivered at 5 cmH_2O. The ventilator measures the volume achieved at this pressure. The next three breaths are delivered at a pressure that would achieve 75% of the preset volume as determined by the "CMV FREQUENCY" and the "VOLUME" settings and the calculated lung compliance. From that point on, the ventilator regulates the pressure for each breath based on the compliance calculated for the previous breath in order to achieve the preset volume. However, it will never vary the pressure from breath to breath by more the 3 cmH_2O. It will also limit the pressure so that it never goes below the baseline (PEEP) setting or above "UPPER PRESS LIMIT" minus 5 cmH_2O. For this reason, it is important that the operator set the maximum safety pressure for the patient. For each breath, pres-

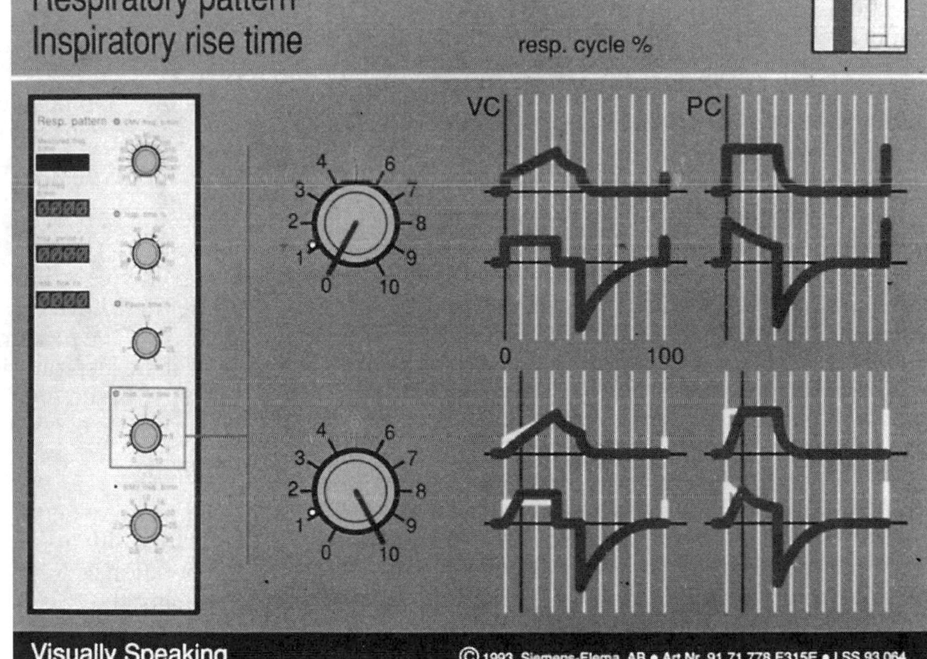

FIGURE 21-129. The top curves represent pressure during a volume-targeted breath (left) and a pressure-targeted breath (right) when the inspiratory rise time is zero. The second curves are the flow curves for these two breath types. The third set of curves represent pressure during the use of Inspiratory Rise Time set at 10 (pressure during a volume-targeted breath (left) and a pressure-targeted breath (right)). The fourth set of curves represents flow during these two breath types (Insp. Rise Time = 10). (Courtesy of Siemens Life Support Systems, Danvers, MA)

sure will be constant for the preset inspiratory time and breaths are given at the preset frequency.

Volume Support

In this mode, ventilation is pressure-controlled, pressure- or flow-triggered, pressure-limited, and flow-, time-, or volume-cycled. This is similar to pressure support ventilation in that a constant pressure is delivered when the patient triggers a breath. It also provides a descending waveform. The difference is that the operator can select a target volume using the "CMV FREQUENCY" (breaths/min) and "VOLUME" controls.

Pressure is regulated during a few breaths to ensure that the target volume is delivered at the lowest possible pressure. Each breath is at a constant pressure. As with PRVC, the pressure from one breath to the next does not change by more than 3 cmH_2O. Pressure will not go below the set baseline (PEEP) or more than 5 cmH_2O lower than the set "UPPER PRESS. LIMIT." The patient establishes the respiratory frequency and inspiratory time. If the patient fails to take a breath and the apnea alarm is triggered, the ventilator switches to controlled ventilation ("PRESSURE REGULATED VOLUME CONTROL" mode).

Inspiration normally ends when the flow is 5% of the measured peak flow. In addition, inspiratory time cannot exceed 80% of the total cycle time based on CMV FREQ.

In volume support, the operator sets the tidal volume and minute volume. The breath rate is generally set close to the expected spontaneous rate and the tidal volume is commonly set slightly below normal (10 to 15%). In the event that the patient's respiratory rate increases, the tidal volume remains constant and the minute ventilation increases. For this reason, it is important to set the upper alarm limit for minute volume to alert for an unacceptably high minute ventilation.

In the event that the patient's respiratory rate slows, the tidal volume will increase to guarantee the set minute volume. To avoid potential hyperventilation, the volume cannot exceed 150% of the preset tidal volume. For example, suppose the tidal volume is calculated at 500 mL and the minute volume at 5 L/min. and the rate at 10. If the patient's spontaneous rate drops to 8 breaths/min, the tidal volume of 500 mL will only give a minute volume of 4.0. The ventilator increases the pressure support level so that the tidal volume increases in order to maintain the preset minute ventilation value. In this example, the tidal volume could not exceed 750 mL, that is, 50% over the set tidal volume.

SIMV (Vol Contr) + Pressure Support

Triggering

In SIMV (vol contr) plus pressure support, mandatory breaths are flow/volume-controlled and are pressure- or flow-triggered (patient effort based on "TRIG. SENSITIVITY LEVEL BELOW PEEP" control setting). Breaths will time-trigger if the patient fails to take a breath during the mandatory time period. Spontaneous breaths between mandatory flow controlled breaths are pressure- or flow-triggered, again based on "TRIG. SENSITIVITY LEVEL BELOW PEEP" control setting. The spontaneous breaths are then pressure controlled based on the "PRESSURE SUPPORT LEVEL ABOVE PEEP" setting.

The SIMV cycle time is determined by dividing the SIMV FREQ B/min into 60. For example, if the SIMV FREQ is set at 2, the SIMV cycle time is 30 seconds. The SIMV cycle time is divided into two parts. The first is the "SIMV period" and the second is the "spontaneous period." The SIMV period is equal to the CMV FREQ. setting divided into 60. For example, if the CMV setting is 15 breaths/min, the SIMV period will be 60/15 or 4 seconds. The spontaneous period is equal to the SIMV cycle time minus the SIMV period. In the above example, this would be 30 seconds minus 4 seconds or 26 seconds.

Suppose the patient triggers a mandatory breath. Following that breath the SIMV cycle begins. The patient then has 26 seconds to breathe spontaneously and trigger pressure support breaths. At the end of the 26-second spontaneous period, the 4-second SIMV period begins. The ventilator waits for the patient to make an inspiratory effort. During this time frame, the breath will be flow- or pressure-triggered. If the patient fails to take a breath in this 4 seconds, the ventilator will automatically give a mandatory breath (time-triggered).

Limiting

Mandatory breaths are flow-/volume-limited. If the patient's inspiratory flow exceeds the flow value established by the "VOLUME" and "INSP TIME %" setting, the ventilator switches to pressure-control and flow matches patient demand. Spontaneous breaths are pressure-limited to either the "PEEP" or "PRESSURE SUPPORT LEVEL ABOVE PEEP" setting.

Cycling

Mandatory breaths are time-cycled depending on the "INSP TIME %," "PAUSE TIME %," and "CMV FREQ" settings. When pressure support is in use, spontaneous breaths are normally flow-cycled at 5% of the measured peak flow, or time-cycled (will not exceed 80% of the total cycle time based on the "CMV FREQ").

Pressure Support/CPAP

Pressure support/CPAP is a pressure control mode that can be pressure- or flow-triggered depending on the sensitivity setting. It is pressure-limited to the pressure setting above PEEP. Normally the mode is flow-cycled at 5% of the peak measured flow. It can also be time-cycled if the inspiratory time exceeds 80% of the set total cycle time based on CMV FREQ. It will pressure-cycle if the pressure exceeds the preset upper pressure limit.

Standby

The standby setting is not a mode. In standby, the ventilator's circuits are powered up, but the ventilator is not operational. All the parameters can be set for a patient using the "SET PARAMETER GUIDE" (SPG). A caution sound is heard in this setting.

Ventilator Off Battery Charging

In this setting, the ventilator is not operational. The ventilator is off and the internal battery is being charged. This is selected between patient use.

□ OUTPUT DISPLAYS (MONITORS) AND ALARMS

The front panel was described above (see Fig. 21-126). The output display for the monitoring system provides digital displays in both red and green. The red digital displays are measured values and the green are operator-set values. It also provides two vertical volume monitors or bar graphs. In the left panel is the vertical display (bar graph) for airway pressure monitoring. The two-column vertical display (bar graph) towards the center is for minute volume monitoring. The upper set limit on both is a nonflashing double bar, as is the lower set limit. The flashing diode on each is the actual value for pressure or minute volume.

Alarm Monitor/Display

The alarm monitor on the Servo 300 contains alpha numeric alarms and eight touchpad/light displays. A high-priority alarm exists when a red flashing light is present in an alarm display and an audible alarm is sounding. A text message in the alarm and message display will be present under these conditions.

A constant yellow light can indicate two conditions: (1) a manual reset action has been used to override certain alarms or, (2) a previous high-priority alarm situation has been corrected.

Input Power Alarms

Battery Alarm

When the main electrical power has failed, a battery alarm will alert the operator to the situation and the ventilator will operate off battery backup power. If the battery power should run low, an alarm message will indicate this condition. When no battery capacity is left, this alarm is activated and cannot be silenced.

Gas Pressure

If inlet gas pressure is outside the operating range of 29 to 94 psig, a gas supply alarm will activate and cannot be silenced.

Control Variable Alarms

Airway Pressure

The airway pressure alarm is activated under two conditions: (1) if the upper pressure limit (safety pressure) is exceeded or, (2) if the airway pressure is greater than PEEP + 15 cmH_2O for more than 15 seconds.

Oxygen Concentration

An oxygen concentration alarm will be activated if the oxygen concentration goes above or below 6% of the set alarm value, or if the oxygen fuel cell is not connected.

Expired Minute Volume

The expired minute volume alarm has a range of 0 to 60 L/min in adults and children and 0 to 6 L/min in neonates. The alarm will be activated when the measured exhaled minute volume is higher or lower than the set value. The set value for upper and lower minute volume are represented on the bar graph or vertical volume monitor by stationary double-bar diodes. The actual minute volume being measured is the flashing diode.

Apnea Alarm

The apnea alarm will be activated when the time between two patient-triggered spontaneous breaths or two mandatory breaths is more than the default value (20 seconds for adults; 15 seconds for children and 10 seconds for neonates).

Control Circuit Alarms

A ventilator control circuit alarm will be activated in several conditions. Below are a few examples:

1. In the event of loss of electrical power the "battery" alarm will activate. This indicates that the ventilator has switched to the internal battery for power. A fully charged battery has the capability to supply power for 30 minutes.
2. When the inlet gas pressure drops below 29 psig or rises above 94 psig for a certain time period, the ventilator will give a "gas supply" alarm. If one gas source fails, the ventilator automatically switches to the single available gas source and continues to operate at the previous settings with the exception that the FIO_2 will change (1.0 if air fails, 0.21 if oxygen fails).
3. When a microprocessor problem or mechanical problem is detected by the ventilator control system a "technical alarm" is activated.
4. If the exhalation valve becomes twisted or the check valve is reversed (not properly installed), the ventilator will give an upper-pressure limit alarm. If the problem is not resolved rapidly, the ventilator will give a continuous high-pressure alarm and, with pressure build-up, the internal safety pop-off device will activate.
5. Sometimes a technical alert will indicate a "leakage" alarm. This alarm may be too sensitive for practical usage. The manufacturer has now deleted this function from the ventilator.

Another technical message is the technical alert "check tubing." This message will appear in the message window if the ventilator measures a 25% difference between the inspiratory and expiratory pressure transducer measurements or if there is a 5 cmH_2O difference between the inspiratory and expiratory pressure transducers for a specific time frame set by the manufacturer. Examples of situations that will cause this alarm are the presence of water in the circuit or a kink in the circuit.

Other technical alerts require repair service and are not described in the operator's manual. When technical alerts occur, a service representative should be called.

Alarm Silence/Reset

Both an alarm silence and an alarm reset control are available. The alarm silence will silence the audible alarms under most circumstances for 2 minutes. The battery alarm is slightly different. It alarms, first, when the ventilator switches to battery power due to loss of electrical power. It will alarm again when voltage is getting low. It will alarm a third time and cannot be silenced when there is limited power left.

Several alarms cannot be reset. Examples of these are the power failure alarm and the internal microprocessor alarm.

□ TROUBLESHOOTING

Before disconnecting a patient, for example, during suctioning procedure, with the "Reset/2 min" control, turn the dial to "reset" and then immediately to "2 min." This silences the audible alarms for "minute volume," "overrange," and "check tubing."

Electromagnetic interference from such devices as cellular phones, walkie-talkies, and other types of handheld communication devices have the potential to interfere with ventilator operation if they are in close proximity of the ventilator. Their use should be prohibited around medical devices that use microprocessors.

BIBLIOGRAPHY

Barnhart SL, Czervinski P: Perinatal and Pediatric Respiratory Care. Philadelphia, WB Saunders, 1995

Branson RD, Chatburn RL: New generation of microprocessor ventilators. In Tobin MJ (ed): Principles and Practice of Mechanical Ventilation. New York, McGraw-Hill, 1994

Chatburn RL: Types of Ventilators. In Branson RD, Hess DR, Chatburn RL (eds): Respiratory Care Equipment. Philadelphia, JB Lippincott, 1995, pp 294–392

Desautels DA, Blanch P: Mechanical ventilators. In Koff PB, Eitzman D, Neu J (eds): Neonatal and Pediatric Respiratory Care, 2nd Ed. St. Louis, Mosby–Year Book, 1993, pp 345–373

Dupuis YG: Ventilators: Theory and Application. St. Louis, CV Mosby, 1986

McPherson SP: Respiratory Care Equipment, 5th ed. Chicago, Mosby-Year Book, 1995

Pilbeam SP: Mechanical Ventilation, Physiological and Clinical Applications, 2nd ed. Chicago, Mosby–Year Book, 1992

Sanborn WG: Microprocessor-based mechanical ventilation. Respir Care 38:72–109, 1991

Sorbello JG, Acevedo RA: Manual resuscitators, mechanical ventilators, and breathing circuits. In Eubanks DH, Bone RC (eds): Principles and Applications of Cardiorespiratory Care Equipment. St.Louis, Mosby–Year Book, 1994, pp 147–224

Whitaker KB: Comprehensive Perinatal and Pediatric Respiratory Care. Albany, NY, Delmar Publ., Inc, 1992

MANUFACTURERS INFORMATION

Bear Medical, 2085 Rustin Ave., Riverside, CA 92507

Bird Products Corp, 1100 Bird Center Drive, Palm Springs, CA 92262

Hamilton Medical Inc., P.O. Box 30008, Reno, NV 89520

Infrasonics, Inc., 3911 Sorrento Valley Blvd, CA 92121

Newport Medical Instruments, Inc., 300 N. Newport Blvd., Newport Beach, CA 92663

Nellcor Puritan Bennett Corp., 2200 Faraday Ave., Carlsbad, CA 92008

Sechrist Industries, Inc., Medical Products Div., Anaheim, CA

Siemens Medical Systems, Inc., 16 Electronics Ave., Danvers, MA 01923

22 Cardiopulmonary Resuscitation

Thomas A. Barnes
Karen M. Boudin

CLINICAL SKILLS

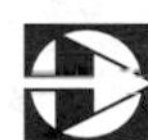

Upon completion of this chapter, the reader will be able to:

- Obtain, and interpret electrocardiograms (for dysrhythmias); electrolytes; fluid balance; vital signs (pulse, respiration, blood pressure); venous distension; capillary refill; auscultation of bilateral sound, stridor, rhonchi crackles, and wheeze; and position of endotracheal tube and tracheal cuff pressure
- Assemble and check for proper function of, and correct malfunctions of any equipment necessary for cardiopulmonary resuscitation, including mouth-to-valve mask resuscitators, manual resuscitators, and transport ventilators; oropharyngeal and nasopharyngeal airways; oral endotracheal tubes and intubation equipment; and automated, semiautomated, and manual defibrillators
- Evaluate and monitor patient's response to basic and advanced life support
- Initiate and interpret ECG monitoring
- Perform ventilation via mouth to mouth, mouth to valve, bag-valve-mask device, transport ventilation, or transtracheal catheter ventilation
- Perform airway management, including oropharyngeal and nasopharyngeal airways or tracheal intubation
- Perform external cardiac compressions
- Administer defibrillation, cardioversion, and oxygen
- Recommend administration of advanced cardiac life support (ACLS) drugs

KEY TERMS

Anaphylaxis
Cardiopulmonary resuscitation
Defibrillation
Dysrhythmia
Electrocardiogram
Heimlich maneuver
Hypovolemic shock
Pulmonary edema
Pulmonary embolus
Ventricular fibrillation
Xiphoid process

Resuscitation encompasses all the care required to treat acute and life-threatening events. There is a broad scope of patient problems affecting the cardiopulmonary system as well as settings for resuscitation. This chapter will focus on in-hospital care and interhospital transport. Since closed-chest cardiopulmonary resuscitation (CPR) was first described 34 years ago, it has become a commonly performed procedure in hospitals and has sparked the development of rapid response CPR "code teams."

Provision of emergency care within the hospital is a multifaceted team effort. Resuscitation includes identification of the patient, assessment of the problem, and implementation of an organized response. Respiratory care practitioners, physicians, and nurses compose the major components of that team. In addition to providing basic life support services, all three groups have expanded their abilities through the American Heart Association's advanced cardiac life support (ACLS) training. This includes (1) maintaining airways using adjunct equipment and advanced techniques, (2) monitoring electrocardiograms (ECG) and recognizing dysrhythmias, (3) using defibrillators, and (4) administration of supplemental oxygen and drugs via parenteral or endotracheal routes. The level of participation by the respiratory care practitioner (RCP) is defined by each medical institution. However, because of expertise in patient assessment and oxygen and airway management, an enhanced role is emerging.

INDICATIONS FOR CARDIOPULMONARY RESUSCITAION

Cardiac Arrest

Cardiovascular disease encompasses a variety of entities in which coronary heart disease (CHD) is a significant factor.[1] Sudden death related to CHD is the most prominent medical emergency in the United States today. Cardiac arrest may be the **first** sign of cardiovascular disease in up to 20% of patients. The highest priority of a rescuer suspecting a cardiac arrest is activation of the emergency medical system (EMS) or calling a code in the hospital setting. The primary survey includes **a**irway, **b**reathing, **c**irculation, and **d**efibrillation (ABCD). The hunt for ventricular fibrillation (VF) is paramount and, once diagnosed, its treatment supersedes all other interventions.[2]

In addition to treatment of acute events, the RCP also has a role in preventing CHD through awareness of risk factors that can be changed or modified (Table 22-1).

- **Heredity**. A family history of heart disease in siblings or parents suggests an increased risk.
- **Gender**. Women, before menopause, have a lower incidence of coronary atherosclerosis than men. However, the incidence increases significantly in postmenopausal women, who also have a worse clinical course (as compared with men).

TABLE 22-1 **Risk Factors for Coronary Disease**

Factors That Cannot Be Changed	Factors That Can Be Changed
Heredity	Cigarette smoke
Male gender	Hypertension
Increasing age	Lack of exercise
	Obesity
	Excessive stress
	Diabetes
	Blood cholesterol levels

- **Age**. The risk of death from heart disease increases with age, although nearly one-in-four deaths occur in persons under age 65.
- **Cigarette smoking**. The risk of death from heart attack is considerably higher in smokers than among people who do not smoke. Fortunately, if a smoker kicks the habit, the risk of death eventually declines almost to that of those who have never smoked. Unfortunately, passive smoking (environmental exposure to tobacco smoke) has been shown to be associated with an increased risk of smoking-related disease.[3]
- **Hypertension.** High blood pressure poses a major risk for stroke and heart attack but can be easily controlled by a program of weight reduction if overweight, salt restriction, or physician-prescribed medications.
- **Elevated blood cholesterol levels**. Narrowing of the arteries may result from a buildup of cholesterol on the walls of the arteries. A diet low in saturated fat and cholesterol helps reduce this risk factor; medications are also available to maintain cholesterol levels within the normal range.
- **Lack of exercise**. Physical inactivity has been clearly established as a risk factor for heart attack. When combined with overeating, it becomes difficult to maintain normal body weight. Physical activity becomes more difficult as people become more obese.
- **Diabetes**. Diabetes can greatly increase a person's risk of heart attack. Although the elevation in blood sugar level associated with diabetes can be controlled by proper eating habits and drugs, if necessary, the increased risk of heart disease cannot be eliminated. Control of other risk factors becomes even more important in this case.
- **Obesity**. Obesity places a great burden on the heart and other organs of the body. It is associated with coronary heart disease primarily because of its role in raising blood pressure, precipitating diabetes, and elevating cholesterol levels. Exercise combined with a low-fat, low-calorie diet may reduce this risk factor.
- **Excessive stress**. Although it is virtually impossible to define, measure, or totally eliminate a person's level of emotional and mental stress, most

doctors agree that reduction of stress benefits the health of the average person.

Prudent Heart Living

Risk factor reduction is an important part of any comprehensive approach to reducing cardiovascular disease, especially among children and young adults. A prudent heart lifestyle must begin at an early age. This lifestyle is really an attitude that includes weight control, physical fitness, smart eating habits, and avoidance of stress and cigarette smoking.

As respiratory care practitioners, we should feel an increased responsibility to promote smoking cessation. The CHD death rate is 70% greater for smokers than nonsmokers. Additionally, it acts together with other risk factors (most notably elevated cholesterol and hypertension) to increase the risk factor of CHD even more.[3] Because of the increased risk that smoking represents, cigarette smoking should be considered the most important modifiable risk factor. When combined with the awareness of the number of people in the population who smoke and who are affected by passive smoking, all efforts should be made to encourage the friends and relatives of patients to quit smoking.

Risk factor modification has clearly been shown to save lives. The knowledge held by respiratory care practitioners demands that they exercise their professional responsibility in educating patients and the public to actively participate in a healthier heart lifestyle.

Respiratory Arrest and Other Indications for CPR

There are a number of conditions other than CHD and life-threatening dysrhythmias that can lead to cardiopulmonary arrest. During hypovolemic shock or anaphylaxis, there is deterioration of vital signs. Respiratory problems that prevent adequate oxygenation and ventilation can occur due to an obstructed airway (partial or complete), interference with the respiratory drive mechanism (eg, spinal cord or head injury), or disorders of pulmonary gas transport (eg, pulmonary edema, and pulmonary embolus). Smoke inhalation can cause a toxic carboxyhemoglobinemia in addition to dysrhythmias, loss of consciousness, and airway burns. Newborns at high risk for respiratory or cardiac arrest during delivery pose a significant need for CPR. Box 22-1 summarizes indications for resuscitation, as listed in the AARC Clinical Practice Guidelines.

The Need for Medical Intervention

Since closed-chest CPR was first described in the early 1960s, it has become a commonly performed procedure (Protocol 22-1) and has evolved to an organized, rapid response by CPR "code teams."[5,6] Many studies of in-hospital survival following CPR, including one analysis of 75 such papers describing 19,190 patients, report that 35% of patients treated with CPR were resuscitated, with 15% of those treated surviving to hospital discharge.[5] The increased interest in the use of resources has lead

BOX 22-1

INDICATIONS FOR CARDIOPULMONARY RESUSCITATION[31]

- Airway obstruction—partial or incomplete
- Acute myocardial infarction with cardiodynamic instability
- Life-threatening dysrhythmias
- Hypovolemic shock
- Severe infections
- Spinal cord or head injury
- Drug overdose
- Pulmonary edema
- Anaphylaxis
- Pulmonary embolus
- Smoke inhalation
- High-risk delivery

Used with permission from American Association for Respiratory Care: Clinical Practice Guideline: Resuscitation in Acute Care Hospitals. Respir Care 38:1179, 1993.

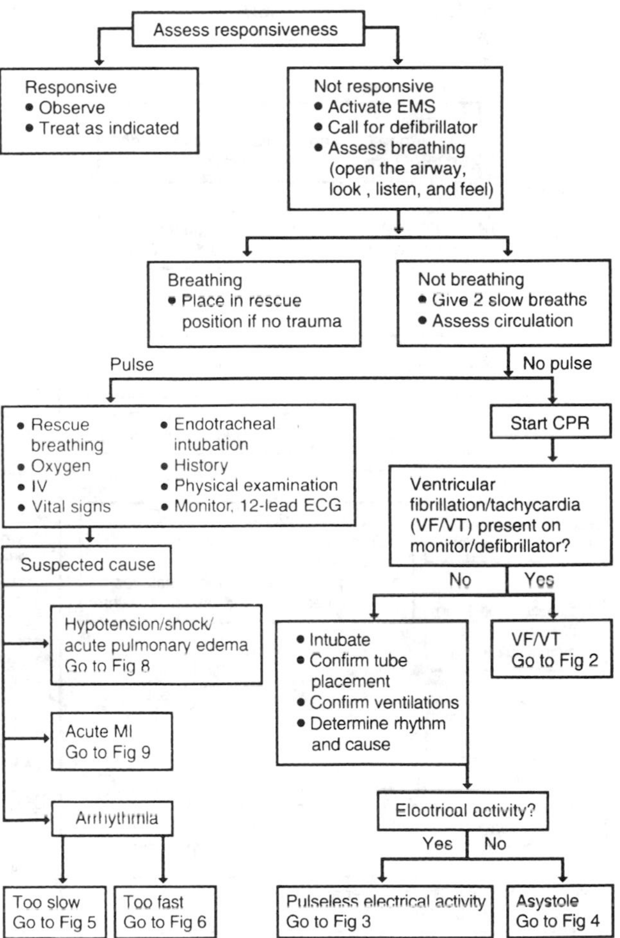

PROTOCOL 22-1. Universal algorithm for adult emergency cardiac care. (Emergency Cardiac Care Committee and Subcommittees. American Heart Association: Guidelines for cardiopulmonary resuscitation and emergency cardiac care, III: Adult advanced cardiac life support. JAMA 1992;268:2216. Reproduced with permission.)

to studies on long-term CPR outcomes. There has been a particular interest in tracking the long-term functional status after CPR, such as quality of life, ability to live independently on discharge from the hospital, and number of years of survival after CPR. Robinson and Hess[6] found 24 of 83 (29%) patients survived in-hospital CPR and were discharged. Follow-up of these 24 patients showed 13 (54%) of them were still alive a mean of 31 months after discharge, and 10 of those 13 (77%) were reported to be living independently. Robinson and Hess asked the continuing care physicians to characterize the patients' lives by choosing from four levels of functioning based on their subjective knowledge of resuscitated patients and not on objective findings. The 10 patients were described by primary physicians as "alive and well" and reported to be functioning "normally" without limitations. Two of these ten returned to their prehospitalization employment. Three patients were described as having health limitations that did not require institutionalization: angina in two patients and chronic renal failure in one patient.

Factors related to practitioner performance that are frequently reported to affect outcomes after CPR include initial rhythm, speed at which CPR is initiated, duration of CPR, and witnessed arrest. Practitioners should be keenly aware of the initial rhythm during resuscitation because ventricular fibrillation (VF) and tachyarrhythmias appear to be important determinants of CPR outcome.[7–11] Practitioners must be prepared to recognize VF and pulseless ventricular tachycardia (VT) and treat both with defibrillation quickly to increase the chances of restoring a spontaneous rhythm (Protocol 22-2; AARC Clinical Practice Guideline: Defibrillation During Resuscitation). The AHA lists a simple rationale for treatment of VF as early as possible:[12]

- The most frequent initial rhythm in sudden cardiac arrest is VF.
- The only effective treatment for VF is electrical defibrillation.
- The probability of successful defibrillation diminishes rapidly over time.
- Ventricular fibrillation tends to convert to asystole within a few minutes.

Survival rates from cardiac arrest can be unusually high if the event is witnessed and treated with defibrillation within minutes. In four studies of cardiac arrest in supervised cardiac rehabilitation programs, 90 of 101 victims (89%) were resuscitated.[7–10] The American Heart Association (AHA) has identified a sequence of

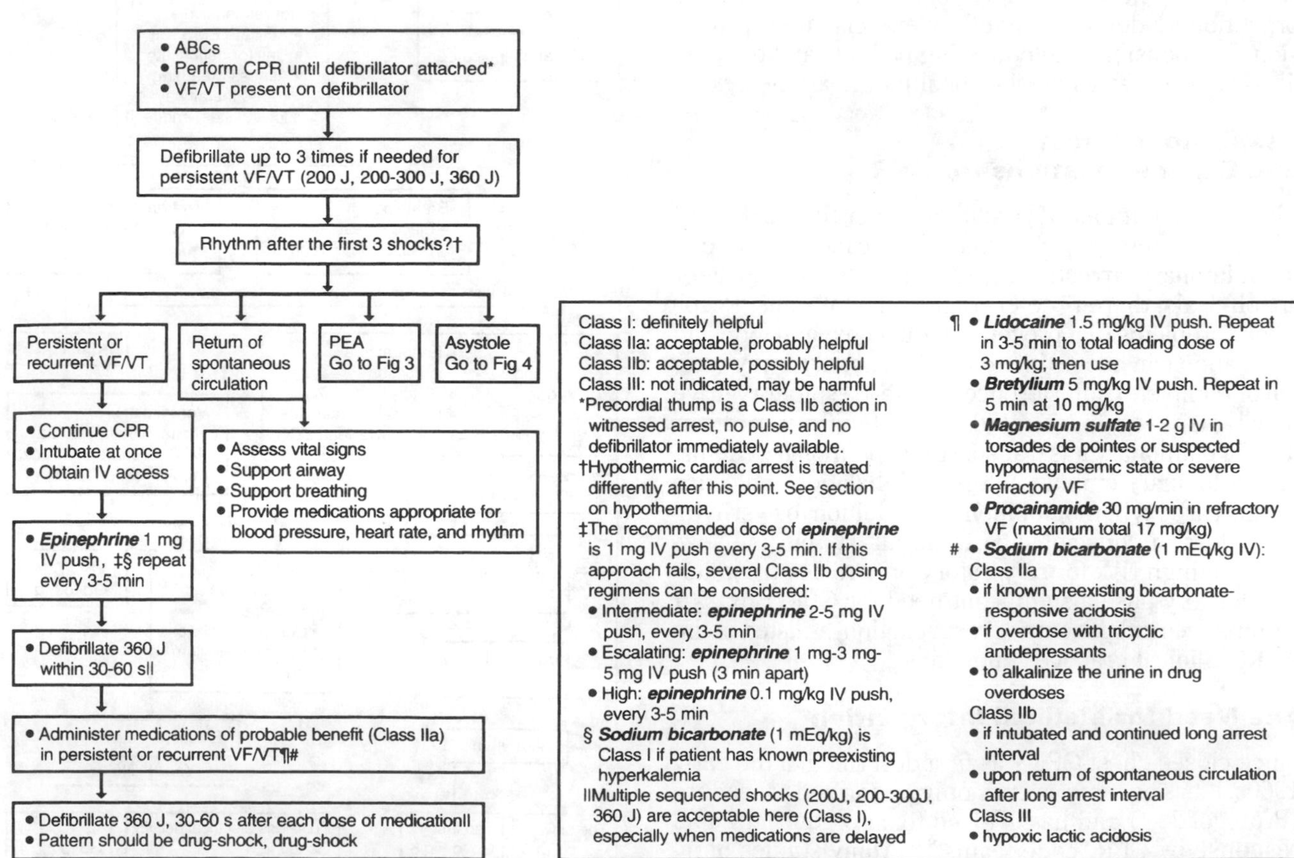
• ABCs
• Perform CPR until defibrillator attached*
• VF/VT present on defibrillator
Defibrillate up to 3 times if needed for persistent VF/VT (200 J, 200-300 J, 360 J)
Rhythm after the first 3 shocks?†
Persistent or recurrent VF/VT
Return of spontaneous circulation
PEA Go to Fig 3
Asystole Go to Fig 4
• Continue CPR
• Intubate at once
• Obtain IV access
• Assess vital signs
• Support airway
• Support breathing
• Provide medications appropriate for blood pressure, heart rate, and rhythm
• Epinephrine 1 mg IV push, ‡§ repeat every 3-5 min
• Defibrillate 360 J within 30-60 s||
• Administer medications of probable benefit (Class IIa) in persistent or recurrent VF/VT¶#
• Defibrillate 360 J, 30-60 s after each dose of medication||
• Pattern should be drug-shock, drug-shock
Class I: definitely helpful
Class IIa: acceptable, probably helpful
Class IIb: acceptable, possibly helpful
Class III: not indicated, may be harmful
*Precordial thump is a Class IIb action in witnessed arrest, no pulse, and no defibrillator immediately available.
†Hypothermic cardiac arrest is treated differently after this point. See section on hypothermia.
‡The recommended dose of epinephrine is 1 mg IV push every 3-5 min. If this approach fails, several Class IIb dosing regimens can be considered:
• Intermediate: epinephrine 2-5 mg IV push, every 3-5 min
• Escalating: epinephrine 1 mg-3 mg-5 mg IV push (3 min apart)
• High: epinephrine 0.1 mg/kg IV push, every 3-5 min
§ Sodium bicarbonate (1 mEq/kg) is Class I if patient has known preexisting hyperkalemia
||Multiple sequenced shocks (200J, 200-300J, 360 J) are acceptable here (Class I), especially when medications are delayed
¶ • Lidocaine 1.5 mg/kg IV push. Repeat in 3-5 min to total loading dose of 3 mg/kg; then use
• Bretylium 5 mg/kg IV push. Repeat in 5 min at 10 mg/kg
• Magnesium sulfate 1-2 g IV in torsades de pointes or suspected hypomagnesemic state or severe refractory VF
• Procainamide 30 mg/min in refractory VF (maximum total 17 mg/kg)
• Sodium bicarbonate (1 mEq/kg IV):
Class IIa
• if known preexisting bicarbonate-responsive acidosis
• if overdose with tricyclic antidepressants
• to alkalinize the urine in drug overdoses
Class IIb
• if intubated and continued long arrest interval
• upon return of spontaneous circulation after long arrest interval
Class III
• hypoxic lactic acidosis

PROTOCOL 22-2. Ventricular fibrillation/pulseless ventricular tachycardia algorithm. (Emergency Cardiac Care Committee and Subcommittees, American Heart Association: Guidelines for cardiopulmonary resuscitation and emergency cardiac care, III: Adult advanced cardiac life support. JAMA 1992;268:2217. Reproduced with permission.)

AARC Clinical Practice Guideline

DEFIBRILLATION DURING RESUSCITATION

Indications: Cardiac arrest with ventricular fibrillation or pulseless ventricular tachycardia.

Contraindications: Defibrillation is contraindicated when the patient's desire not to be resuscitated has been clearly expressed and documented in the patient's medical record or other legal document; continued resuscitation is determined to be futile by the treating physician; immediate danger to the rescuers is present due to the environment, patient's location, or patient's condition.

Assessment of Need: *Before arrival of defibrillator:* The patient should be assessed for lack of responsiveness, apnea, and pulselessness, and help should be summoned if needed. *After arrival of defibrillator:* The patient should be evaluated immediately for the presence of ventricular fibrillation or ventricular tachycardia by the operator (conventional device) or the defibrillator (automated or semiautomated device). Inappropriate defibrillation can cause harm.

Assessment of Process and Outcome: *Equipment management issues:* Use of standard checklists can improve defibrillator dependability. *Defibrillation process issues:* System access, response time, first-responder actions, adherence to established algorithms, patient selection and outcome, first-responder authorization to defibrillate.

Monitoring: *Resuscitation process:* Properly performed defibrillation has been shown to improve patient outcome. The most important determinant of survival in adult out-of-hospital ventricular fibrillation is defibrillation. Continuous monitoring of the process identifies components needing improvement. Among these components are response time, witnessed versus unwitnessed arrest, CPR performance, time-to-first defibrillation attempt, return of spontaneous circulation, complication rate, equipment function, equipment maintenance, and equipment availability. *Equipment:* All maintenance should be documented and records preserved. Included in documentation should be routine checks of energy output; condition of batteries; proper functioning of monitor and recorder; and presence of disposables needed for function of defibrillator, including electrodes and defibrillation pads. Defibrillators should be checked each shift for presence, condition, and function of cables and paddles; presence of defibrillating and monitoring electrodes, paper, and spare batteries (as applicable); and charging, message-light indicators, monitors, and ECG recorder (as applicable). *Training:* Records should be kept of initial training and continuing education of all personnel who perform defibrillation as part of their professional activities.

From AARC Clinical Practice Guideline; see Respir Care 40:744, 1995, for complete text.

critical actions that improve survival after cardiac arrest and has coined the phrase "chain of survival" to indicate their importance. The AHA concept of a linked chain applies to cardiac arrests in both the in-hospital and prehospital setting. The AHA chain of survival has four links (Fig. 22-1.)[13]

- Early access—a cardiac emergency must be recognized, and medical assistance must be called.
- Early CPR—some efforts at opening the airway, ventilation, and blood circulation must occur as soon as possible.
- Early defibrillation—identification and treatment of VF is the single most important intervention.
- Early ACLS—advanced airway control and rhythm-appropriate intravenous medications must be administered rapidly.

Research on ACLS training suggests that the AHA chain of survival should be modified for hospital use to emphasize the importance of early defibrillation (Fig. 22-2).[14] A study of 37 simulated cardiac arrests (SCAs) showed that respiratory care practitioners (RCPs) are among the first members of the resuscitation team to respond (mean response time was 3.2 min).[15] Thus, it appears that, along with registered nurses assigned to intensive care units, all RCPs carrying a code beeper should be trained as ACLS providers and retrained at frequent intervals. This level of training would allow respiratory care practitioners to defibrillate patients in VF and pulseless VT when they are the earliest, best-trained respondents to cardiac arrest calls.

Duration of the resuscitation effort impacts CPR outcome; that is, shorter codes have a better record of long-term survival.[8] Successful defibrillation depends on the metabolic state of the myocardium; that is, longer duration of VF leads to greater myocardial deterioration. Consequently, shocks are less likely to convert VF to a spontaneous rhythm (Fig. 22-3).[16–19] Also, early intubation of the trachea immediately following electrical therapy has been identified by the AHA as an important step in the VF treatment algorithm.[20] The study by RCPs at Duke Medical Center has shown that a specially trained group of respiratory therapists can perform emergency tracheal intubations with a 95% success rate.[21] The intubation success of RCPs in hospitals compares favorably with paramedics in the field.[22] The early placement of an endotracheal tube during CPR improves ventilation and oxygenation, and it provides a route for administering cardiac drugs when intravenous access can not be established quickly.

Contraindications to CPR

Initiating cardiopulmonary resuscitation is contraindicated when patients have clearly expressed and documented their desire that we "do not resuscitate" (DNR) them. The CPR approach presumes that the event precipitating the arrest can be corrected and the patient has the potential to be stabilized in the postarrest period. Therefore, resuscitation is not indicated if a patient has an underlying disease or condition that determines CPR to be futile.

Basic and Advanced Life Support Training

Respiratory therapy students are taught basic life support (BLS) and how to perform tracheal intubation before they are allowed to graduate, and many respiratory

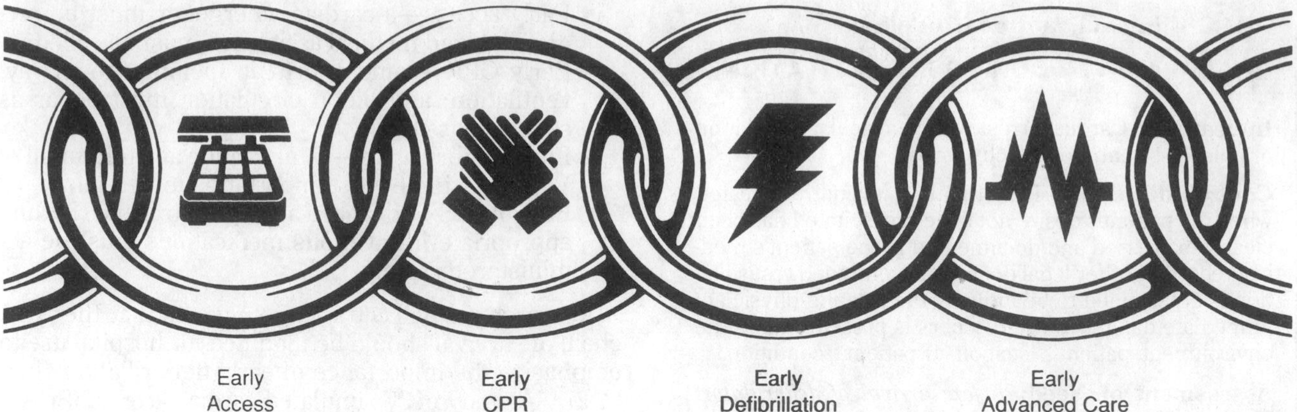

FIGURE 22-1. The emergency cardiac care systems concept is displayed schematically by the "chain of survival" metaphor. (Emergency Cardiac Care Committee and Subcommittees, American Heart Association: Guidelines for cardiopulmonary resuscitation and emergency cardiac care, IX: Ensuring effectiveness of community-wide emergency cardiac care. JAMA 268:2289–2295, 1992. Reproduced with permission.)

therapy schools require students to successfully complete an advanced cardiac life support (ACLS) provider course immediately before graduation. Everyone working in the hospital should be trained in basic life support. If a non–health professional in the hospital witnesses an arrest, it is critical that the person know how to initiate a code call and begin CPR. There must exist an integrated system that includes mechanisms for communication and rapid response by properly trained and equipped personnel. In many situations, unsuccessful outcome is the result of time delays. Early CPR and defibrillation after cardiac arrest substantially increases the long-term survival rate of victims and decreases the possibility of neurologic damage.[23,24] Accordingly, research on resuscitation within hospitals has shown that all personnel who have direct patient contact must be trained in CPR and early defibrillation as first responders.[14] The discussion here, however, focuses primarily on BLS provided by health care providers in acute care hospitals.

Automated external defibrillation is now considered by national authorities to be a basic life support skill and should be incorporated into all BLS training programs for health care providers expected to respond to a cardiac arrest (including physicians, respiratory therapists, nurses, and physician assistants), with rapid defibrillation taking priority over CPR.[14,25–27] The American Heart Association has provided a recommended curriculum and guidelines for an automated external defibrillation provider's course, and it encourages all emergency medical service agencies to adopt these materials and implement early defibrillation programs.

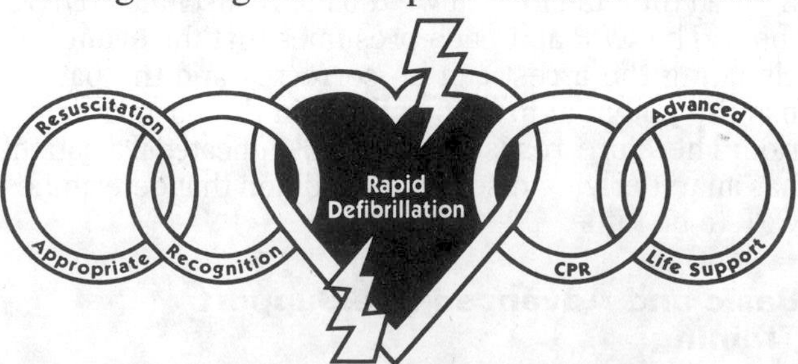

FIGURE 22-2. "Inhospital chain of survival" metaphor. (Kaye W, Mancini ME: Improving outcome from cardiac arrest in the hospital. Resuscitation 1996; In press. Reproduced with permission.)

Basic and advanced life support training and periodic retraining for hospital personnel are crucial. Resuscitation procedures must be reviewed and practiced periodically for maximum retention. Deliberate overtraining in the initial basic life support class has resulted in satisfactory skills retention for at least 1 year.[28] Maintaining skills requires opportunities for review and practice, even for those practitioners regularly involved with CPR.[21] However, motivating physicians, nurses, and respiratory care practitioners to attend review sessions is often a problem.[30] Including some advanced cardiac life support techniques and creativity in designing the training sessions may overcome this issue.[29] For example, simulated cardiac arrests can be used as a technique for identifying and correcting problems so that retraining can focus on areas where performance is inadequate.

The AARC Clinical Practice Guideline: Resuscitation in Acute Care Hospitals is a "profession-oriented" document that speaks directly to the responsibilities that RCPs on code teams should perform, given appropriate training.[31] There are some critical recommendations that should be implemented immediately and others that deserve serious consideration for development in the near future. Particularly important is the training, evaluation by performance, and retraining of Level I personnel in BLS and Level II personnel in emergency cardiac care (ECC) and ACLS, or pediatric advanced life support (PALS) and neonatal resuscitation program (NRP), as appropriate, at intervals that should not exceed 1 year.[31,32]

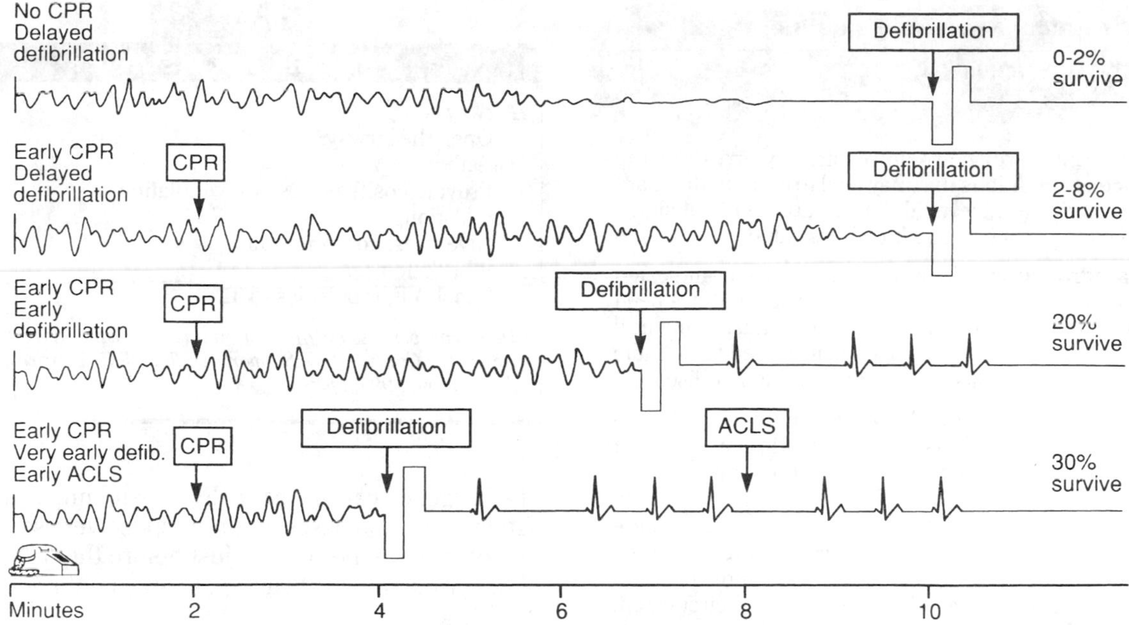

FIGURE 22-3. Survival rates are estimates of probability of survival to hospital discharge for patients with witnessed collapse and with ventricular fibrillation as initial rhythm. (Chandra NC, Hazinski MF (eds). Textbook of Basic Life Support for Healthcare Providers, p. 9–2. Dallas, American Heart Association, 1994. Reproduced with permission.)

Batenhorst et al[33] evaluated 516 CPR attempts and found no correlation between time of day and arrest incidence. Based on these data, many believe that 24-hour staffing for resuscitation teams is critical. Adequate staffing of resuscitation teams means that respiratory care departments should have a registered respiratory therapist continuously available (24 hours/day, 7 days/week) to respond to emergencies.[31] It is imperative for RCPs to assume five critical tasks when they are the best-trained responders at the scene:

- Emergency airway management: manual ventilation, oxygen administration, and tracheal intubation
- Defibrillation of ventricular fibrillation or pulseless ventricular tachycardia with manual, semiautomatic, or automated external defibrillators
- Chest compressions
- Tracheal instillation of cardiac drugs (ie, epinephrine, lidocaine, atropine) before an intravenous line is established
- Arterial blood gas and pH determinations

A resuscitation committee within the hospital can be designated for the purpose of reviewing and maintaining resuscitation records, assuring the continuing competence of the health care workers and making changes in CPR policies when appropriate. The committee should also assure that a postarrest conference be held after each CPR effort. Each resuscitation attempt is unique, and postarrest conferences can be useful in reinforcing good performance and identifying those tasks for which further team training is needed.

Maximal performance during CPR may also depend on the organization and maintenance of the "crash carts." Crash carts should be standardized throughout the facility, including the location of each item on the cart. They should include medications and supplies necessary for at least the first 10 minutes of resuscitation.[34] The cart should not include any unnecessary equipment or supplies. A method should be established for stocking and checking the cart. Sealing the cart assures that no one takes the supplies. A protocol should also be provided for nursing, respiratory therapy, and medical personnel to familiarize themselves with the organization of the cart. The respiratory care department should be responsible for assuring the presence and proper function of the equipment needed for an emergency intubation and a manual resuscitator capable of delivering 100% oxygen.

BASIC LIFE SUPPORT

The Primary ABCD Survey

Cardiopulmonary arrest needs to be treated quickly, starting with BLS and followed by early advanced cardiac life support (ACLS). The AHA recommends a primary–secondary approach during all major decision points in a difficult resuscitative effort, including not only cardiac and respiratory arrests but also prearrest and postarrest patients. The term "primary survey" calls attention to basic CPR and defibrillation and uses the acronym "ABCD" (Box 22-2).[12] Time drives all aspects

AARC Clinical Practice Guideline

RESUSCITATION IN ACUTE CARE HOSPITALS

Indications: Cardiac arrest, respiratory arrest, or the presence of conditions that may lead to cardiopulmonary arrest as indicated by rapid deterioration in vital signs, level of consciousness, and blood gas values.

Contraindications: Resuscitation is contraindicated when the patient's desire not to be resuscitated has been clearly expressed and documented in the patient's medical record, or resuscitation has been determined to be futile because of the patient's underlying condition or disease.

Assessment of Need: *Prearrest:* Identification of patients (including the fetus) in danger of imminent arrest and in whom consequent early intervention may prevent arrest and improve outcome. These are patients with conditions that may lead to cardiopulmonary arrest as indicated by rapid deterioration in vital signs, level of consciousness, blood gas values, or fetal monitoring data. *Arrest:* Absence of spontaneous breathing or circulation. *Postarrest:* Once a patient has sustained an arrest, the likelihood of additional life-threatening problems is high, and continued vigilance and aggressive action are indicated. Control of the airway and cardiac monitoring must be continued and optimal oxygenation and ventilation assured.

Assessment of Process and Outcome: Timely, high-quality resuscitation improves patient outcome in terms of survival and level of function. Despite optimal resuscitation performance, outcomes are affected by patient-specific factors. Patient condition postarrest should be evaluated from this perspective. Documentation and evaluation of the resuscitation process (eg, system activation, team member performance, functioning of equipment, and adherence to guidelines and algorithms) should occur.

Monitoring: *Patient clinical assessment:* Continuous observation of the patient and repeated clinical assessment by a trained observer provide optimal monitoring of the resuscitation process. Special consideration should be given to the following: level of consciousness, adequacy of airway, adequacy of ventilation, peripheral or apical pulse and character, evidence of chest and head trauma, pulmonary compliance and airway resistance, presence of seizure activity. *Assessment of physiologic parameters:* Repeat assessment of physiologic data by trained professionals supplements clinical assessment in managing patients throughout the resuscitation process. Monitoring devices should be available, accessible, functional, and periodically evaluated for function. These data include, but are not limited to, arterial blood gas studies (although investigators have suggested that such values may have a limited role in decision making during CPR); hemodynamic data; cardiac rhythm; ventilatory frequency, tidal volume, and airway pressure; exhaled CO_2; neurologic status. *Resuscitation process:* Properly performed resuscitation should improve patient outcome. Continuous monitoring of the process identifies areas needing improvement. Among these areas are response time, equipment function, equipment availability, team member performance, team performance, complication rate, and patient survival and functional status.

From AARC Clinical Practice Guideline; see Respir Care 38:1179, 1993, for complete text.

BOX 22-2

PRIMARY ABCD SURVEY

Airway
Open the airway.
Breathing
Provide positive-pressure ventilation.
Circulation
Give chest compressions.
Defibrillation
Shock VF or pulseless VT.

Used with permission from Cummins RO (editor): Textbook of Advanced Cardiac Life Support. Dallas, TX, American Heart Association, 1994, pp 1–4.

of emergency cardiac care (ECC), and important "first actions" such as assessing unresponsiveness and calling for help are performed just before the "A" (airway) of the primary ABCD survey.

☐ ASSESSING UNRESPONSIVENESS

Unresponsiveness (ie, clinically comatose) should be established by gently shaking the patient and shouting, "Are you OK?," at a level that would cause arousal if the patient was asleep or had a depressed sensorium. If trauma is likely, shaking the person can aggravate injuries, and "touch and talk" is a better approach.[2] There are many situations in which the unresponsiveness of the patient is obvious, and a call for help should be done simultaneously.

☐ ACTIVATION OF THE EMERGENCY MEDICAL SYSTEM

For cardiac arrest in adults, research has demonstrated the efficacy of early defibrillation.[26,27] The highest hospital discharge rate has been achieved in patients in whom CPR was initiated within 4 minutes of arrest and ACLS within 8 minutes.[35–37] Early CPR intervention and fast resuscitation team response are, therefore, essential in improving survival rates[36] and good neurologic recovery rates.[38] Some BLS instructors use the acronym "A^2" to teach rescuers to remember that assessment of unresponsiveness and activation of EMS should be done before starting the ABCs of adult CPR. For arrests in hospitals, health care professionals should call out loudly for someone to help, mentioning the room number; for example, "I need help at once in room 100." The person who responds should be told to activate the hospital's emergency response system. This approach brings advanced care in the form of a code team and crash cart to provide early defibrillation of VF and pulseless VT, advanced airway management, and intravenous medications.

☐ AIRWAY

Opening the airway is the first step in the primary "ABCD" survey; the mouth should be opened and the upper airway inspected for foreign objects, vomitus, or blood. AARC Clinical Practice Guideline: Management of Airway Emergencies outlines when and how to manage emergencies involving the airway. If present, these should be removed with a finger sweep, by suctioning, or by turning the patient on the side while paying attention to the possibility of a cervical spine injury. The posterior displacement of the tongue is the most common cause of airway obstruction in the unconscious person. The loss of tonicity of the submandibular muscles, which provide direct support to the tongue and indirect support to the epiglottis, allows the tongue to move posteriorly, obstructing the pharynx. Because the tongue is attached to the lower jaw, moving the jaw forward pulls the tongue away from the back of the pharynx and opens the airway. The rescuer should open the patient's airway using one of two maneuvers: head-tilt/chin-lift or jaw-thrust maneuver. The position that opens the airway must be maintained at all times. The *head-tilt/chin-lift* maneuver is accomplished by placing one hand on the victim's forehead and applying firm backward pressure with the palm to tilt the head back. The fingers of the other hand are placed under the bony part of the lower jaw near the chin and lifted to bring the chin forward and the teeth almost to occlusion (Fig. 22-4). Caution should be taken not to harm or increase an injury to the cervical spine. In the victim with a suspected neck injury, the initial step in opening the airway is the chin lift or jaw thrust without head tilt.

AARC Clinical Practice Guideline

MANAGEMENT OF AIRWAY EMERGENCIES

Indications: Conditions requiring management of the airway are impending or actual airway compromise, respiratory failure, and need to protect the airway.

Contraindications: Aggressive airway management (intubation or establishment of a surgical airway) may be contraindicated when the patient's desire not to be resuscitated has been clearly expressed and documented in the patient's medical record or other valid legal document.

Assessment of Need: The need for management of airway emergencies is dictated by the patient's clinical condition. Careful observation, the implementation of basic airway management techniques, and laboratory and clinical data should help determine the need for more aggressive measures. Specific conditions requiring intervention include inability to adequately protect airway; partially obstructed airway; complete airway obstruction; apnea; hypoxemia, hypercarbia, or acidemia seen on arterial blood gas analysis, oximetry, or exhaled gas analysis; respiratory distress.

Assessment of Outcome: Timely intervention to maintain the patient's airway can improve outcome in terms of survival and level of function. Under rare circumstances, maintenance of an airway by nonsurgical means may not be possible. Despite optimal maintenance of the airway, patient outcomes are affected by patient-specific factors. Lack of availability of appropriate equipment and personnel may adversely affect patient outcome. Monitoring and recording are important to the improvement of the process of emergency airway management. Some aspects (eg, frequency of complications of tracheal intubation or time to establishment of a definitive airway) are easy to quantitate and can lead to improvement in hospital-wide systems; patient condition following the emergency should be evaluated from this perspective.

Monitoring: Continuous observation of the patient and repeated clinical assessment by a trained observer provide optimal monitoring of the airway. Special consideration should be given to the following: level of consciousness; presence and character of breath sounds; ease of ventilation; symmetry and amount of chest movement; skin color and character (temperature and presence or absence of diaphoresis); presence of upper airway sounds (crowing, snoring, stridor); presence of excessive secretions, blood, vomitus, or foreign objects in the airway; presence of epigastric sounds; presence of retractions; presence of nasal flaring. Repeated assessment of physiologic data by trained professionals supplements clinical assessment in managing patients with airway difficulties. Monitoring devices should be available, accessible, functional, and periodically evaluated for function. These data include, but are not limited to, ventilatory frequency, tidal volume and airway pressure, presence of CO_2 in exhaled gas, heart rate and rhythm, pulse oximetry, arterial blood gas values, chest radiograph. Regardless of the method of ventilation used, the most important consideration is detection of esophageal intubation. Tracheal intubation is suggested, but may not be confirmed by, bilateral breath sounds over the chest, symmetrical chest movement, absence of ventilation sounds over the epigastrium, presence of condensate inside the tube corresponding with exhalation, visualization of the tip of the tube passing through the vocal cords. Esophageal detector devices may be useful in differentiating esophageal from tracheal intubation. Tracheal intubation is confirmed by detection of CO_2 in the exhaled gas, although cases of transient CO_2 excretion from the stomach have been reported. Tracheal intubation is confirmed by endoscopic visualization of the carina or tracheal rings through the tube. The position of the endotracheal tube (ie, depth of insertion) should be appropriate on chest radiograph.

From AARC Clinical Practice Guideline; see Respir Care 40:749, 1995, for complete text.

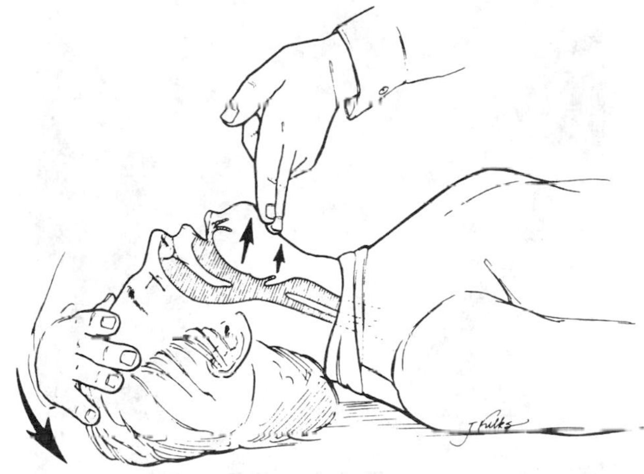

FIGURE 22-4. Opening the airway. (Barnes TA, Watson ME: Cardiopulmonary resuscitation and emergency cardiac care, In Barnes TA (ed), Core Textbook in Respiratory Care Practice, 2nd ed., p. 291. St. Louis, Mosby–Year Book, 1994. Reproduced with permission.)

If the airway remains obstructed, then the head tilt is added slowly and gently until the airway is opened.[39] If the head-tilt method of opening the airway is unsuccessful or contraindicated because of suspected cervical spine injury, the jaw thrust is accomplished by placing the fingers behind the angles of the jaw and displacing the mandible forward (Fig. 22-5).

□ BREATHING

Breathing, the second step in the primary survey, is confirmed by positioning the ear over the patient's nose and mouth while maintaining an open airway. In this position, the chest is observed for a rising and falling motion, and airflow is felt and heard during the expiratory phase: look, listen, and feel for breathing (Fig. 22-6). If breathing is observed, the patient should be placed in the recovery position, that is, a side-lying position (Fig. 22-7). Emergency ventilation should begin immediately for the patient who is apneic. If immediately available, an oropharyngeal airway should be inserted and ventilation started with a mouth-to-mask device or manual resuscitator. The airway is kept open by the head-tilt/chin-lift method. The rescuer gives two slow breaths, over 1.5 to 2 seconds per breath, while observing the chest rise. The recommended rate for ventilation during CPR in the adult is 10 to 12 breaths per minute, using a tidal volume of 800 to 1200 mL. Gastric distension occurs if the breath is delivered too fast because airway pressures exceed the esophageal opening pressures, allowing air to enter the stomach.

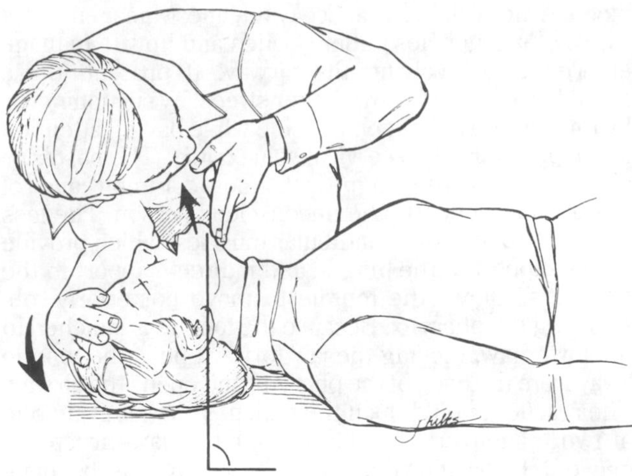

FIGURE 22-6. Confirming apnea. (Barnes TA, Watson ME: Cardiopulmonary resuscitation and emergency cardiac care, In Barnes TA (ed), Core Textbook in Respiratory Care Practice, 2nd ed., p. 292. St. Louis, Mosby–Year Book, 1994. Reproduced with permission.)

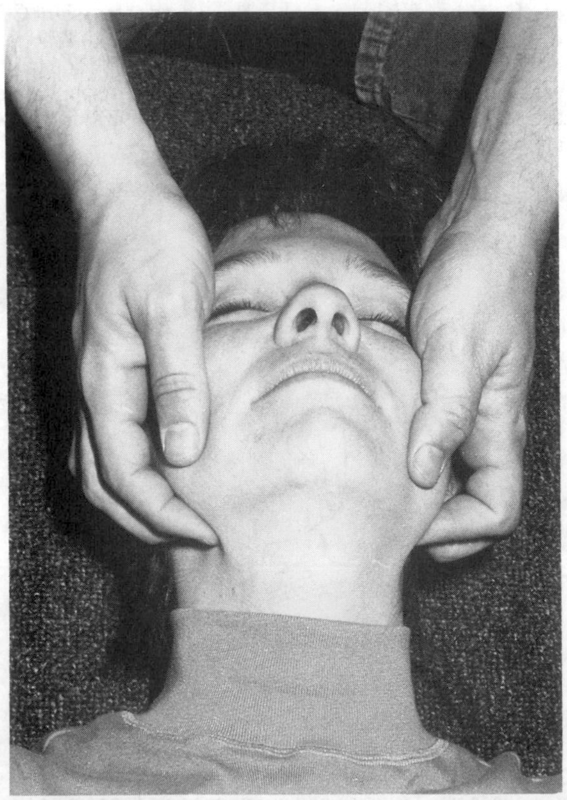

FIGURE 22-5. Jaw-thrust maneuver for use in cases of suspected cervical spine injury.

Masks with or without nonrebreathing valves are more effective than face shields (Fig. 22-8*A*) in delivering adequate ventilation (eg, 10 to 15 mL/kg per breath).[31] A manual resuscitator capable of delivering 100% oxygen may not be immediately available, but oxygen can be added to a mouth-to-mask device. Also, several studies have shown that mouth-to-mask breathing is more effective than bag-valve devices, especially when only one rescuer is available for rescue breathing.[40–45] Oxygen enrichment with some masks increases the delivered oxygen concentration to greater than 70%.[37] However, because of the larger tidal volume delivered, even a mask without oxygen enrichment capability should be used instead of barrier devices, or when the rescuer is unskilled in the use of a bag-valve device.

In addition to oxygen enrichers, other desirable characteristics of mouth-to-mask devices include a nonrebreathing valve to divert the exhaled gas away from the rescuer, an extension tube to separate the face-to-face proximity, transparency, easy application to the anatomy of the face, little resistance, and the capability to be easy for the rescuer to achieve a face seal.[43,46,47] In addition to the one-way valve, a bacterial filter should be placed proximal to the nonrebreathing valve.[43] The mask and the valve should not be affected by the presence of vomitus, and it should protect the rescuer from vomitus. The dead space volume should be as small as possible.

To effectively ventilate the victim, mouth-to-mask devices must be used correctly. The rescuer should be positioned at the head of the patient. The mask is placed over the patient's nose and mouth, and it is held in place with the rescuer's thumbs. The first fingers of each hand are placed under the patient's mandible, and the mandible is lifted as the head is tilted back. The mask is sealed using the rescuer's thumbs (Fig. 22-8*B*). Both of the rescuer's hands are used to hold the mask and open

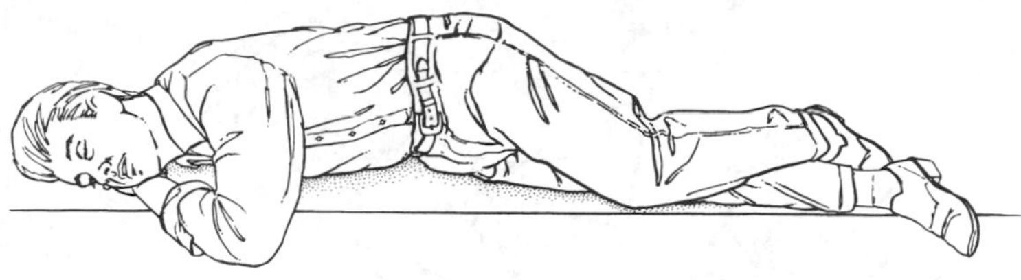

FIGURE 22-7. Placing the patient in the recovery position. (Emergency Cardiac Care Committee and Subcommittees, American Heart Association: Guidelines for cardiopulmonary resuscitation and emergency cardiac care, II: adult BLS. JAMA 268:2187, 1992. Reproduced with permission.)

the airway. In patients with cervical spine injury, the mandible should be lifted without tilting the head. Effective use of these devices requires instruction and supervised practice.[43,47]

□ CIRCULATION

Pulse Assessment

Circulatory inadequacy is determined by palpating the carotid artery in the adult patient; this should take no longer than 5 to 10 seconds. This artery is the most accessible for the respiratory care practitioner who is maintaining the airway. The area should be palpated gently to avoid compressing the artery. Simultaneous palpation of both carotid arteries should never be done because it can obstruct cerebral blood flow. The femoral artery is also a common alternative for establishing circulatory adequacy, but it is not as easily accessible in a clothed victim. If a pulse is absent, the patient is in cardiac arrest, and external cardiac compressions should be initiated immediately.

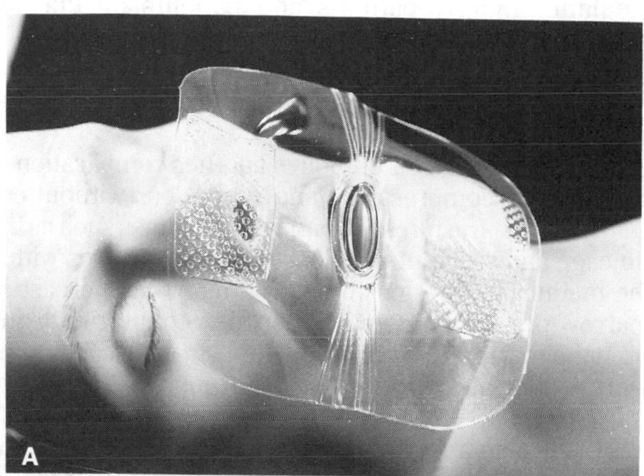

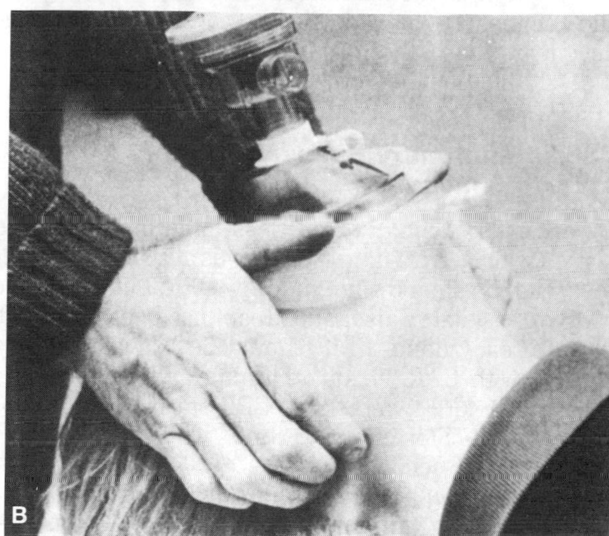

FIGURE 22-8. Mouth-to-mask ventilation devices **(A)** Microshield face shield with duckbill valve; **(B)** Mouth-to-mask ventilation in position using two-hand technique. (Hess D, Ness C, Oppel A, Rhoads K: Evaluation of mouth-to-mask ventilation devices. Respir Care 34:191, 1989. Reproduced with permission.)

Chest Compressions

The patient should be placed in the supine position to allow the maximum blood flow to the brain during cardiac compressions. Even when compressions are performed properly, cardiac output is reduced to approximately 25% to 30% of normal. If the head is elevated, blood flow to the brain may not be adequate. Elevation of the legs may also improve cardiac output by enhancing venous return.

For external chest compressions to be effective, the patient must be on a firm surface. If a patient is in bed, a board preferably the full width of the bed should be placed under the patient's back.[48] If a cardiac board is not readily available, the backs of some hospital beds are designed to be easily detached for this purpose. Chest compressions should not be delayed while waiting for this support.

External chest compressions are performed on the lower half of the adult sternum, above the notch where the ribs meet the lower sternum. The following technique is used to locate the safest hand position (Fig. 22-9):[48]

- Using your middle and index fingers, locate the lower margin of the patient's rib cage.
- Run your fingers along the rib cage to the notch where the ribs meet the sternum.
- Place your middle finger on this notch. The index finger is placed next to the middle finger and rests on the lower end of the sternum.
- The heel of the hand is placed on the lower half of the sternum close to the index finger, with the long axis of the hand perpendicular to the sternum.
- The first hand is then removed from the notch and placed on top of the hand on the sternum. The fingers are extended or interlaced to keep them off the chest.

Arms are kept straight with elbows locked, and the shoulders are directly over the sternum (Fig. 22-10). For an adult, pressure is exerted downward to depress the

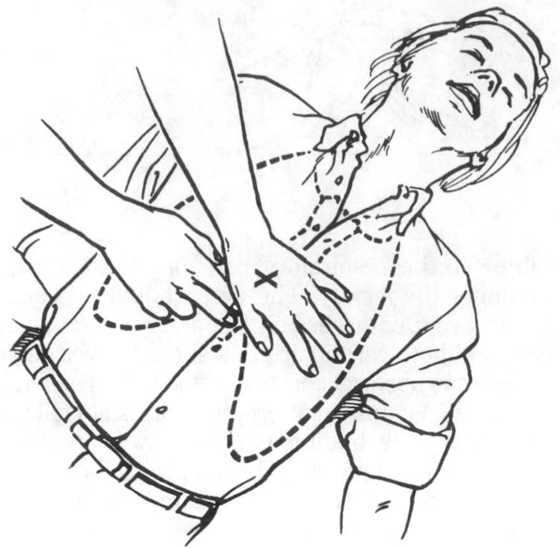

FIGURE 22-9. Hand position for cardiac compressions: Move the fingers up the rib cage to the notch where the ribs meet the lower sternum in the center of the lower part of the chest. (Cardiopulmonary Resuscitation. Washington, DC: American Red Cross; 1981:25. Reproduced with permission.)

sternum 1.5 to 2 inches (4 to 5 cm) at a rate of 80 to 100 times per minute. Hands must never be removed from the chest during relaxation. However, pressure must be completely released on the upward stroke of compressions to allow blood to flow into the chest and heart. Arterial blood pressure during chest compression is maximal when the duration of compression is 50% of the compression-release cycle.[48] Optimally, effectiveness of chest compressions are best evaluated by a second person who palpates the carotid or femoral pulse. Compressions are done in conjunction with artificial ventilation. The ratio of compressions to ventilation is 5:1, with a pause for ventilation for 1.5 to 2 seconds.

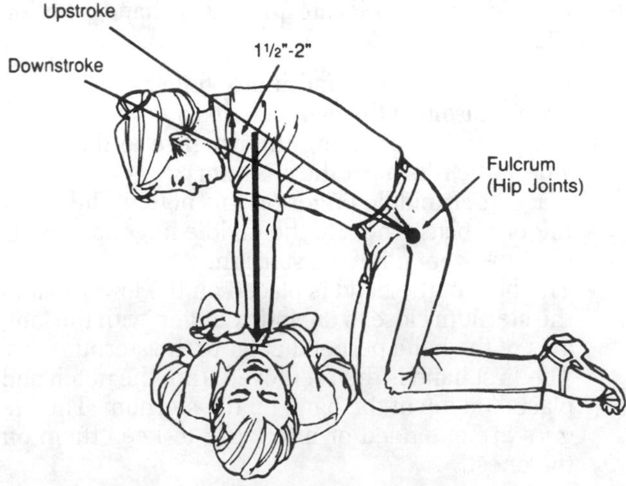

FIGURE 22-10. Arm position for chest compressions. (Cardiopulmonary Resuscitation. Washington, DC: American Red Cross; 1981:25. Reproduced with permission.)

Complications of Chest Compression

Compression of the xiphoid process can cause laceration of the liver that can lead to severe internal bleeding. The *xiphoid process* extends downward over the upper abdomen, and finding the correct position above it decreases the possibility of its lacerating the liver. This may be the most common complication of cardiac compressions in infants and children.

Rib fractures and costochondral separation can occur if the compressions deviate from midline or if pressure with the fingers is put on the rib cage. Interlocking the fingers helps to avoid this. Between compressions, the heel of the hand should remain on the chest. This helps prevent excessive compression of the rib cage or the costochondral cartilage. Even when compressions are being done correctly, there is still a possibility of causing fractured ribs or sternum. The broken ends of the ribs can in turn cause laceration of the lung. Elderly patients and patients on chronic steroids are the most susceptible. If cracking of the ribs is felt or heard, the compressor should check hand position and continue to compress (because the alternative is death of the patient).[49]

The formation of fat emboli is another complication of closed chest compressions and may occur without evidence of overt fractures.[49] Compressing bones such as the rib cage and sternum may lead to microfractures within the medulla of the ribs and sternum and an increase in marrow pressure. Fat may enter the venous circulation from the marrow. Cerebral fat emboli may be considered a cause of mental deterioration following CPR.

Improperly performed chest compressions may lead to less than optimal cardiac output, causing inadequate blood flow to the brain. Compressions that are smooth, regular, and uninterrupted provide the best cardiac output and reduce injury. Also, the correct amount of pressure to depress the sternum helps to optimize cardiac output.[49]

Cardiopulmonary Resuscitation by Two Rescuers

Two-rescuer techniques are less fatiguing. A second person with BLS training who arrives at a single-rescuer resuscitation should state, "I know CPR," and ask if the EMS or hospital resuscitation team has been activated. If not already done, EMS should be activated before helping with CPR. Next, breathing and pulse are reassessed before two-rescuer CPR starts. The second rescuer says, "Stop compressions," while assessing the pulse for 3 to 5 seconds.

When two people performing CPR want to switch, they must do so without interrupting the 5:1 compression-to-ventilation sequence. The person performing chest compressions initiates the switch by saying "switch" in place of "one" while counting with each compression, "switch, two, three, four, five," meaning that the change will take place at the end of the 5:1 sequence. After giving the breath, the person performing ventilation moves into position to give compressions. The person giving compressions moves to the head to ventilate and checks the pulse after giving the fifth compression. If there is no pulse, CPR is continued.

Adult Foreign Body Airway Obstruction

□ SUDDEN CHOKING

Most airway obstructions are foreign body obstructions (FBAOs) that occur while a person is eating. However, many cases of sudden choking are due to cardiac ischemia that simulates food obstructing the airway. Differentiating between these two emergencies can be important for successful management. In both situations, the person clasps his neck or upper chest because of pain, panic, and constriction of that area. In the case of complete foreign body obstruction, most patients do not lose consciousness immediately but are unable to speak, breathe, or cough. If the victim is becoming cyanotic, this means there is hypoxemia, which may indicate respiratory obstruction. A partial obstruction with poor air exchange should be treated as if it were a complete airway obstruction. This situation requires further attempts at dislodging the obstruction. Circulatory failure is indicated by pallor as opposed to frank cyanosis.[50]

Foreign bodies that cause partial obstruction result in some ability to ventilate. Varying degrees of retraction, agitation, respiratory noises, and activity of the accessory muscles are evident. If there is good air exchange, a strong cough may force the foreign body out of the airway. A normal cough is superior to any of the artificially induced coughs. Therefore, if a choking person can speak or breathe and is coughing with a moderately strong effort, intervention is unnecessary and potentially dangerous.[51]

Partial obstruction with poor air exchange or the presence of cyanosis requires immediate intervention. Poor air exchange is indicated by a weak, ineffective cough, high-pitched noises during inspiration, and use of accessory muscles. When these signs occur, the management protocol is the same as with a complete airway obstruction. Emergency maneuvers to relieve airway obstruction are designed to generate positive intrathoracic pressure to expel a foreign body from the trachea.

□ HEIMLICH MANEUVER

The maneuver recommended to relieve airway obstruction is the *Heimlich maneuver* (Fig. 22-11). This maneuver exerts upward, subxiphoid pressure with the fist. The rescuer stands behind the victim and puts both arms around the victim's waist. One fist is grasped with the other hand and placed thumb side against the victim's abdomen, in the midline slightly above the navel and well below the tip of the xiphoid process. Each quick thrust given should exert force inward and upward. Thrusts are repeated until the object is expelled from the airway or the patient becomes unconscious. If the victim becomes unconscious, the victim is eased to the floor and placed in a supine position. The emergency medical

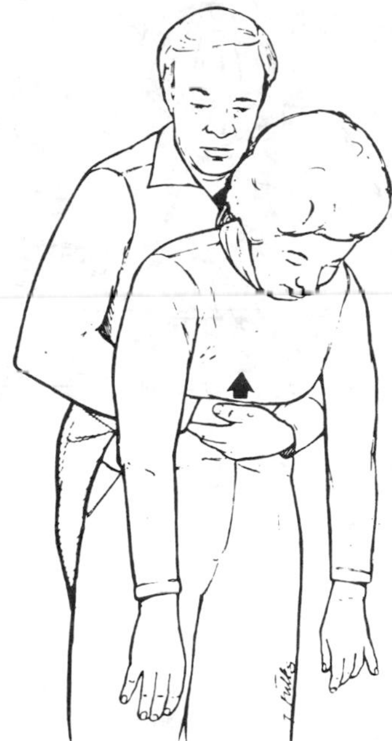

FIGURE 22-11. Performing the Heimlich maneuver. (Barnes TA, Watson ME: Cardiopulmonary resuscitation and emergency cardiac care, In Barnes TA (ed), Core Textbook in Respiratory Care Practice, 2nd ed., p. 300. St. Louis, Mosby–Year Book, 1994. Reproduced with permission.)

service (EMS) should be activated at this point, or a stat call for the hospital resuscitation team should be placed. If you witness an adult victim losing consciousness and suspect that a foreign body is present, perform the finger sweep.[48] The Heimlich maneuver is continued by placing one hand against the upper abdomen (same hand position as above) with the second hand on top applying force inward and upward. The abdominal thrusts are safer and most easily done by straddling the victim's legs (Fig. 22-12). If you are in the correct position, you are unlikely to misdirect the thrust right or left. The complications of abdominal thrusts are abdominal trauma including pneumoperitoneum, laceration or rupture of the stomach, fractured ribs, and regurgitation. Also, a possible danger in young children is that of liver laceration.[52] Therefore, abdominal thrusts should be limited to the older child and the adult.

□ CHEST THRUST

Another maneuver to relieve airway obstruction is a chest thrust. This maneuver is used in special situations, such as the late stages of pregnancy or extreme obesity. To perform a chest thrust, the rescuer's arms encircle the victim with arms directly under the armpits, and one fist is placed thumb side on the midsternum, taking care to avoid the xiphoid process and the margins of the rib cage. The other hand grasps the fist, and up to five backward thrusts are given. If the victim is unconscious, the hand position is the same as for applying closed-chest cardiac compressions.

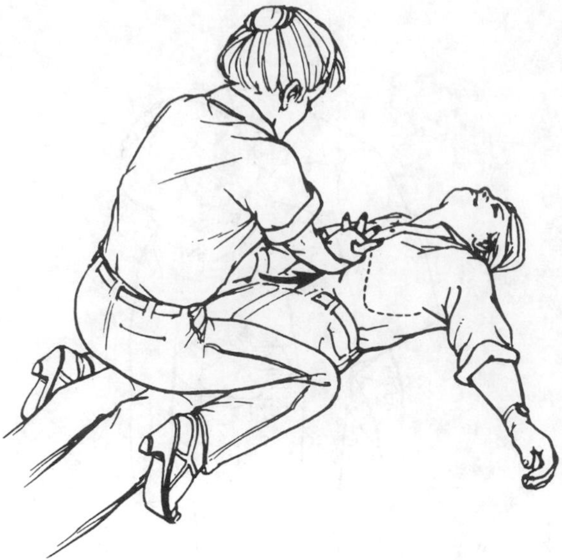

FIGURE 22-12. Abdominal thrusts administered to an unconscious victim of foreign-body airway obstruction who is lying down. (Emergency Cardiac Care Committee and Subcommittees, American Heart Association: Guidelines for cardiopulmonary resuscitation and emergency cardiac care, II: adult BLS. JAMA 268:2193, 1992. Reproduced with permission.)

□ FINGER SWEEP

Finger sweeps of the oropharynx should be avoided in infants and young children to prevent pushing the foreign body back and increasing the obstruction. Only if the foreign body is visualized should it be removed with the finger in a small child or infant. Finger sweeps may be effective in removing a foreign body in the older child or an adult. To perform this technique, the mouth is opened by grasping the lower jaw and tongue between the thumb and fingers and lifting the mandible (jaw lift). The index finger is inserted to the base of the tongue. A hooking action is used to dislodge the object. A Kelly clamp or Magill forceps may be useful if the object is visible. A laryngoscope may help to permit direct visualization.

□ RECOMMENDED SEQUENCE FOR THE ADULT

The Heimlich maneuver should be applied as soon as airway obstruction has been identified. This maneuver is continued until the airway is cleared or the victim becomes unconscious. When the victim becomes unconscious or unresponsive, he or she should be placed in a supine position; the EMS should be activated, or a stat call for the hospital resuscitation team should be placed (preferably by a second person at the scene). Next, the mouth should be opened using the tongue-jaw lift method, and a finger sweep done (Fig. 22-13). Two breaths are given with the airway repositioned between breaths, and if unable to ventilate, the abdominal thrusts should be performed up to five times. The sequence of abdominal thrusts, finger sweep, and attempt to ventilate should be repeated as long as necessary. In hospitals, the use (under direct visualization with laryngoscope or flashlight and tongue blade) of Kelly clamps, or Magill forceps, or suctioning the upper airway may facilitate the removal of an obstruction.

Breathing attempts between other efforts at removing the obstruction are important because they may help relieve the obstruction. Also, if the obstruction has been partially relieved, some air flow may be lifesaving. Advanced life support techniques used to open the airway are initiated as soon as skilled professionals are available.

Cardiopulmonary Resuscitation in Children and Infants

□ CAUSES OF PEDIATRIC AND NEONATAL CARDIOPULMONARY ARREST

The causes of pediatric and neonatal cardiopulmonary arrest are most often injury related. Attempts to prevent injury can reduce childhood death and disability, especially when prevention strategies are geared toward the six most common types of severe childhood injuries nationwide:[53,54]

- Motor vehicle passenger injuries
- Pedestrian injuries
- Bicycle injuries
- Submersion
- Fire- and burn-related injuries
- Firearm injuries

During infancy, the most common causes of cardiopulmonary arrest are respiratory emergencies, that is, respiratory diseases and airway obstruction including foreign body aspiration. Unlike adults, infants rarely suffer a sudden cardiac arrest. Instead, they experience a progressive deterioration in respiratory function that initiates the final cardiopulmonary arrest.[2] The following discussion focuses on the significant differences between BLS and FBAO treatment for children and infants as compared to adults (Tables 22-2 and 22-3).

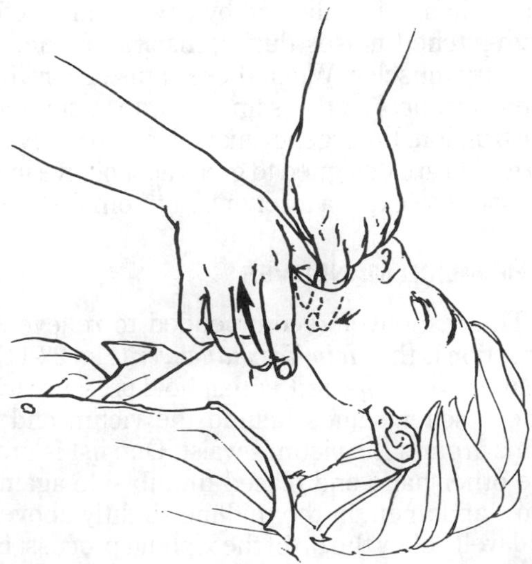

FIGURE 22-13. Finger sweep maneuver administered to an unconscious victim of foreign-body airway obstruction. (Chandra NC, Hazinski MF (eds). Textbook of Basic Life Support for Healthcare Providers, p. 4–19. Dallas, American Heart Association 1994. Reproduced with permission.)

TABLE 22-2 **Summary of BLS Maneuvers for Adults, Children, and Infants**

Maneuver	Infant (<1 y)	Child (1 to 8 y)	Adult
Assess responsiveness	Tapping and speaking loudly	Tapping and speaking loudly	Tapping, shaking, and speaking loudly
Activate EMS	After 1 min CPR, if alone	After 1 min CPR, if alone	Before opening the airway
Airway	Head tilt–chin lift (unless trauma present)	Head tilt–chin lift (unless trauma present)	Head tilt–chin lift (unless trauma present)
Breathing	Jaw thrust	Jaw thrust	Jaw thrust
Initial	2 breaths at 1 to 1.5 sec/breath	2 breaths at 1 to 1.5 sec/breath	2 breaths at 1.5 to 2 sec/breath
Subsequent	20 breaths/min	20 breaths/min	10–12 breaths/min
Circulation			
Pulse check	Brachial/femoral	Carotid	Carotid
Compression area	Lower half of sternum	Lower half of sternum	Lower half of sternum
Compression with	Two or three fingers	Heel of one hand	Heel of one hand on top of hand on sternum
Depth	0.5 to 1 in.	1 to 1.5 in.	1.5 to 2 in.
Rate	At least 100/min	100/min	80 to 100/min
Compression to ventilation	5:1 (pause for ventilation)*	5:1 (pause for ventilation)*	15:2 (pause for ventilation)[†]
Reassess	After 20 cycles*	After 20 cycles*	After 4 cycles[‡]

* One or two rescuers
[†] One rescuer 15:2, two rescuers 5:1
[‡] One rescuer after 4 cycles, two rescuers after 10 cycles

TABLE 22-3 **Summary of FBAO Maneuvers in Adults, Children, and Infants**

Conscious Adult	Conscious Child	Conscious Infant
1. Ask "Are you choking?"	1. Ask "Are you choking?"	1. Confirm complete or partial airway obstruction. Check for serious breathing difficulty, ineffective cough, **no** strong cry.
2. Give up to 5 abdominal thrusts (chest thrusts for pregnant or obese victim).	2. Give up to 5 abdominal thrusts (chest thrusts for obese victim).	2. Give up to 5 back blows and 5 chest thrusts.
3. Repeat thrusts until effective or victim becomes unconscious.	3. Repeat thrusts until effective or victim becomes unconscious.	3. Repeat step 2 until effective or victim becomes unconscious.
Adult Becomes Unconscious	**Child Becomes Unconscious**	**Infant Becomes Unconscious**
4. Activate EMS or code team.	4. If second rescuer is available, have him or her activate EMS or code team.	4. If second rescuer is available, have him or her activate EMS or code team.
5. Perform tongue-jaw lift followed by a blind finger sweep to remove the object.	5. Perform a tongue-jaw lift and, if you see the object, perform a finger sweep to remove it.	5. Perform a tongue-jaw lift and, if you see the object, perform a finger sweep to remove it.
6. Open airway and attempt to ventilate; if still obstructed, reposition and attempt to ventilate again.	6. Open airway and attempt to ventilate; if still obstructed, reposition and attempt to ventilate again.	6. Open airway and attempt to ventilate; if still obstructed, reposition and attempt to ventilate again.
7. Give up to 5 abdominal thrusts.	7 Give up to 5 abdominal thrusts.	7. Give up to 5 back blows and 5 chest thrusts
8. Repeat steps 5 through 7 until effective.*	8. Repeat steps 5 through 7 until effective.*	8. Repeat steps 5 through 7 until effective.*
	9. If alone and airway obstruction is not relieved after about 1 minute, activate the EMS system or code team.	9. If alone and airway obstruction is not relieved after about 1 minute, activate the EMS system or code team.

* Persist in these efforts as long as necessary; do not check pulse or attempt chest compressions until airway becomes unobstructed. If victim is breathing or resumes effective breathing, place in recovery (side-lying) position.

□ SEQUENCE OF PEDIATRIC AND NEONATAL BLS

The sequence of interventions used for treating children and infants in cardiorespiratory distress is very similar to that provided to adults, with the exception of when to activate EMS as a single rescuer. If a bystander or second rescuer is present during the initial assessment of a child or infant in respiratory or cardiac distress, that person should activate EMS immediately. However, the lone rescuer should shout for help, then provide approximately 1 minute of BLS, if necessary, before activating the EMS system. Shouting for help may alert a neighbor or someone in the vicinity of the accident. Waiting 1 minute before activating EMS is recommended for children and infants because the most common cause of distress is an obstructed airway or primary respiratory arrest. Consequently, assessment of the child or infant with intervention aimed at ventilation is more likely to be needed than defibrillation, which is more commonly needed in adults.

The short, fat neck of infants under 1 year of age makes palpation of the carotid artery difficult. Thus, the brachial artery or the femoral artery should be palpated.

The cardiac compression technique for children is similar to that of adults. The heel of only one hand is placed over the lower half of the sternum (between the nipple line and the notch), avoiding the xiphoid process. Compressions are delivered at the rate of 100 per minute by depressing the sternum 1 to 1.5 inches, depending on the size of the child. The other hand is used to maintain the child's head position so that it may be possible to ventilate without repositioning the head. A breath is delivered after every five compressions. With pauses for ventilation, the number of compressions are actually about 80 per minute.

Two or three fingers are used to compress the lower half of the sternum of an infant ½ to 1 inch. The compression rate should be at least 100 per minute, with a breath given every five compressions. A hand placed under the back can provide a firm surface, if necessary, for compressions with infants and small children (Fig. 22-14). Placing the infant on a hard surface frees the other hand to maintain head position for ventilation (Fig. 22-15). Table 22-2 compares the BLS maneuvers in adults, children, and infants.

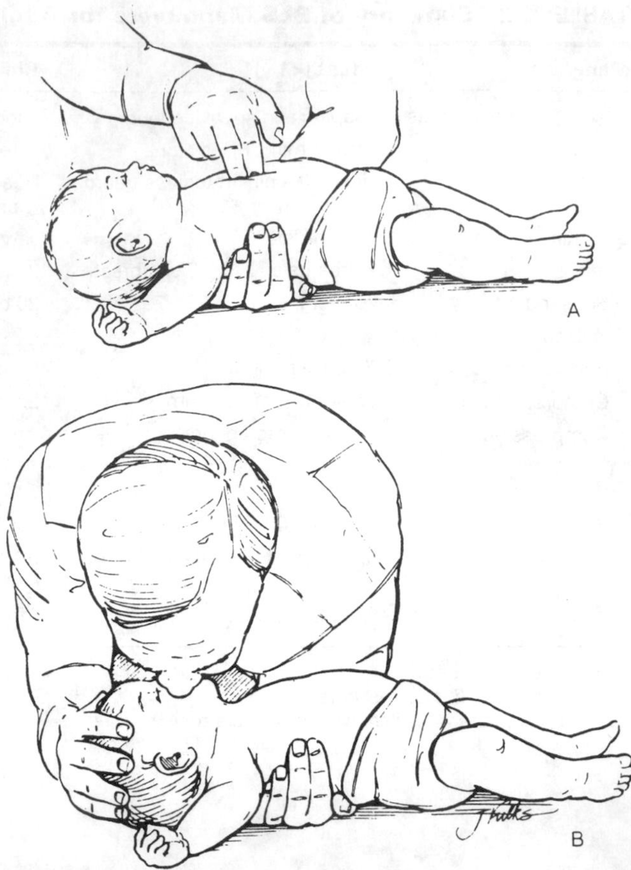

FIGURE 22-14. CPR for infants **(A)** External cardiac compression; **(B)** Mouth-to-mouth and nose ventilation. (Barnes TA, Watson ME: Cardiopulmonary resuscitation and emergency cardiac care, In Barnes TA (ed), Core Textbook in Respiratory Care Practice, 2nd ed., p. 299. St. Louis, Mosby–Year Book, 1994. Reproduced with permission.)

□ PEDIATRIC AND NEONATAL FOREIGN BODY AIRWAY OBSTRUCTION

Like adults, the Heimlich maneuver (subdiaphragmatic abdominal thrusts) is recommended for relief of airway obstruction in children. The sequence of interventions used for treating children with an obstructed airway is identical to that provided to adults; however **blind** finger sweeps should not be performed. A finger sweep may be used only when the foreign object is visible. When delivering abdominal thrusts to a child who is unconscious or who becomes unconscious, the heel of **one** hand is used rather than two as in the adult.

The sequence of interventions used for treating infants with an obstructed airway is very different from that provided to adults and children (see Table 22-3). In the infant, a combination of back blows and chest thrusts is recommended for relief of airway obstruction. The baby is sandwiched between the rescuer's forearms and hands, with the head lower than the trunk. With the infant face down, five forceful back blows should be delivered between the infant's shoulder blades with the heel of one hand. After turning the baby over to the supine position, with the head lower than the trunk, five quick downward chest thrusts should be delivered in the same location and manner as chest compressions. Rescue breathing is attempted when the infant loses consciousness.

Automatic External Defibrillation

The most important factors associated with neurologically intact survival following cardiac arrest include the presence of witnesses, ventricular fibrillation as the presenting rhythm, prompt initiation of bystander CPR, and the rapid provision of advanced life support.[55–57] A

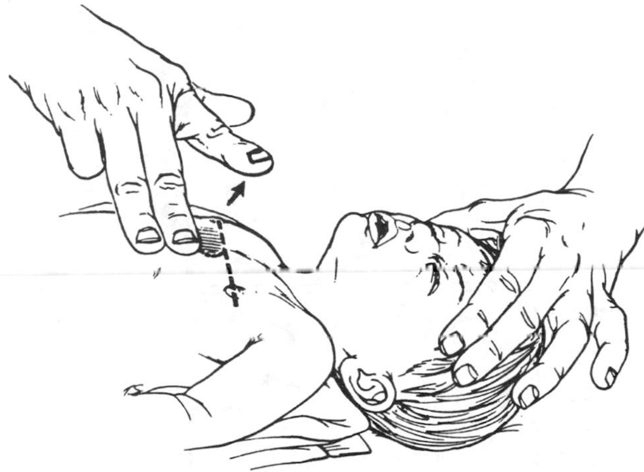

FIGURE 22-15. Locating the proper finger position for chest compression in the infant. The rescuer uses the other hand to maintain the head position for ventilation. (Emergency Cardiac Care Committee and Subcommittees, American Heart Association: Guidelines for cardiopulmonary resuscitation and emergency cardiac care, V: Pediatric BLS. JAMA 268:2256, 1992. Reproduced with permission.)

direct relationship has been established between neurologically intact survival and the speed with which defibrillation is administered (see Fig. 22-3).[58,59] The American Heart Association has deemphasized the sole benefit of CPR in recognition that a successful resuscitation requires the systematic linking of a number of elements, termed the chain of survival (see Fig. 22-1).[60–62] These linked elements include:

- Early access to the emergency system (call first and fast)
- Early initiation of CPR
- Early defibrillation
- Quick ACLS support

These four elements presuppose the ability to recognize cardiac arrest and the quick response times from emergency personnel. For early defibrillation to be possible, all BLS personnel must be trained, equipped, and permitted to operate a defibrillator if in their professional activities they are expected to respond to people in cardiac arrest.[63] The generic term *automated external defibrillators* (AEDs) refers to defibrillators that incorporate a rhythm analysis system. Some AEDs are fully automated, and others are semiautomated or shock-advisory defibrillators. All AEDs are attached to the patient by two adhesive pads and connecting cables,[54,55] as shown in Figure 22-16. All AEDs can be operated by the following four simple steps:[63,64]

- Turn on the power.
- Attach the device.
- Initiate the analysis.
- Deliver the shock, if necessary.

The American Heart Association AED treatment algorithm (Protocol 22-3) summarizes the sequence of assessment, CPR, defibrillation, pulse checks, and AED power settings. Health professionals with a duty to respond to patients in cardiac arrest should have a defibrillator immediately available or within 1- to 2-minute access.[63]

ADVANCED CARDIAC LIFE SUPPORT

Advanced cardiac life support (ACLS) demands a high level of training and retraining of the resuscitation team to maintain performance levels. Respiratory care practitioners, physicians, and nurses must understand the role of each member on a resuscitation team. The team must come together and function quickly and effectively to improve the patient's chances for long-term survival. The American Heart Association ACLS course is interdisciplinary and standardized to promote a common understanding of the algorithms used to manage respiratory or cardiac arrest (course participants are cross trained in all aspects of resuscitation). Health care professionals enrolled in ACLS courses are evaluated against the same performance criteria regardless of their professions or job titles. This leads to common ground and mutual respect among team members.

The tasks performed during an in-hospital resuscitation by respiratory care practitioners may vary depending on who is available at the resuscitation scene. Advanced cardiac life support training and retraining prepares therapists to deal with sudden life-threatening events affecting a patient's cardiopulmonary system. Most therapists with ACLS training are allowed to function as primary members of the hospital's resuscitation team. The AARC Clinical Practice Guideline: Resuscitation in Acute Care Hospitals on page 818 describes the respiratory care practitioner's responsibilities, which involve the identification, assessment, and treatment of patients in danger of or in frank arrest, including the high-risk delivery patient.

Core ACLS Educational Objectives

The "core" of the ACLS courses emphasizes the evaluation and management of the first 10 minutes of witnessed, adult ventricular fibrillation (VF) cardiac arrest.[2] This approach assumes that a single rescuer witnesses a VF collapse. The single rescuer must manage the patient alone for several minutes, performing basic CPR and automated defibrillation. When additional ACLS providers arrive, they must be directed in how to assist in the resuscitation attempt. If the patient responds, for example, he is defibrillated and reverts to other rhythms, then the patient has to be managed in the postarrest period. The *primary ABCD survey* (see the section on BLS) is always done first and involves the following performance skills: opening the airway, assessing apnea, ventilating the patient, confirming pulselessness, performing closed-chest compressions, and defibrillation of ventricular fibrillation and pulseless ventricular tachycardia.

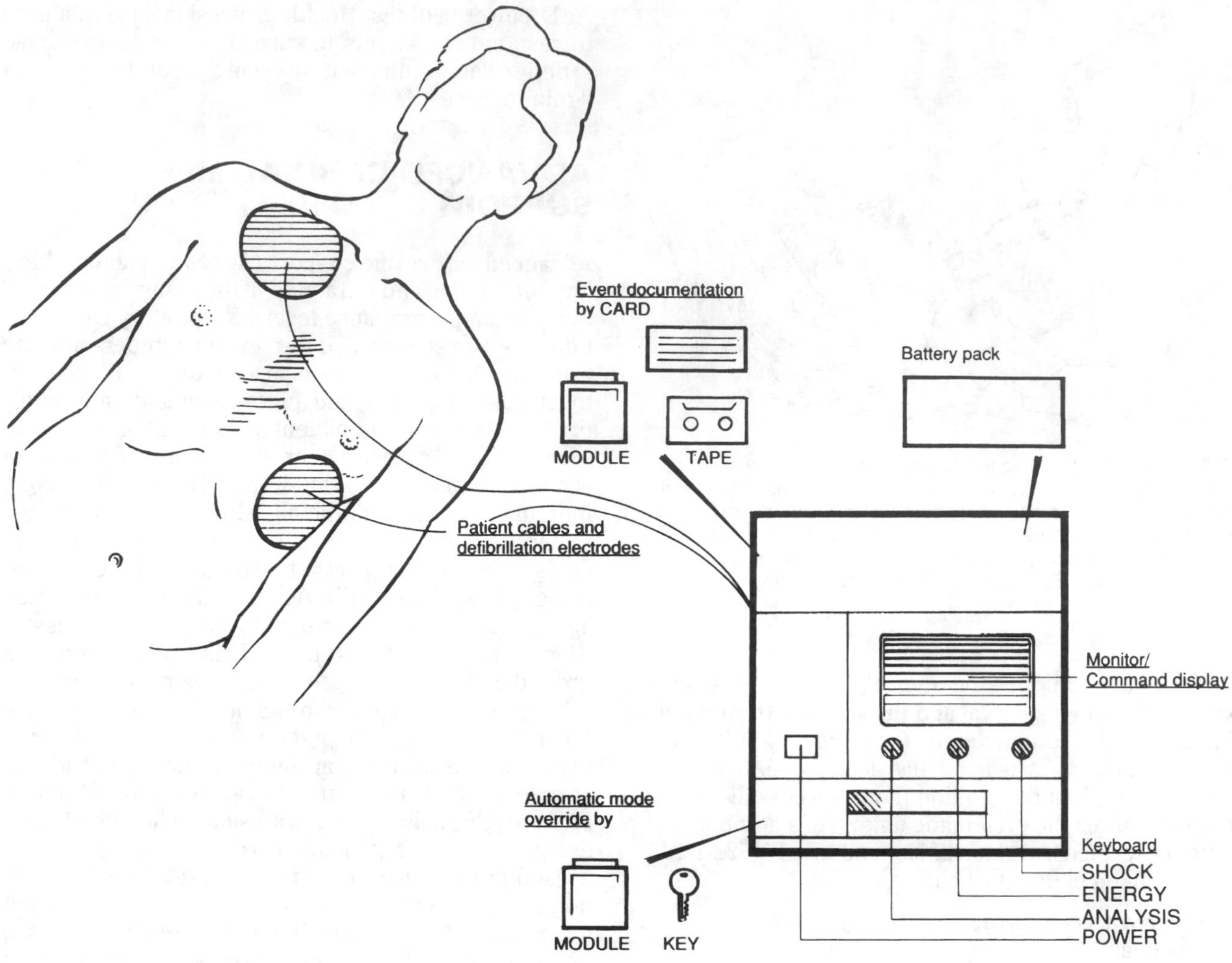

FIGURE 22-16. Schematic drawing of automated external defibrillator and its attachments to patient. (Chandra NC, Hazinski MF (eds). Textbook of Basic Life Support for Healthcare Providers, p. 9–4. Dallas, American Heart Association, 1994. Reproduced with permission.)

Secondary ABCD Survey

In the *secondary ABCD survey,* the resuscitation team returns to the ABCDs, but at a more advanced level (Box 22-3).[2] The assessments and actions of the secondary survey should be done simultaneously. However, the AHA recommends endotracheal intubation before gaining intravenous (IV) access.[2] It is acceptable to gain IV access before endotracheal intubation if ventilation, oxygenation, and airway protection appear satisfactory. A well-trained resuscitation team should delegate member responsibilities before the arrests occur. When all team members are not available, the team leader must be ready to step forward to perform the most essential next action.

Endotracheal Intubation

For airway management there is no equivalent substitute for *endotracheal intubation* (See Ch. 19). The team leader should make sure someone is preparing to perform endotracheal intubation. Typical steps include:

- Locating a tube of proper size with appropriate 15/22-mm connector
- Inflation and check of the cuff and pilot tube
- Checking the laryngoscope for proper blade and light function
- Preparing a suction method.

Endotracheal intubation can be delayed for other interventions if bag-valve-mask or mouth-to-mask ventilation appear to be temporarily adequate. A nasopharyngeal airway should be inserted for noninvasive ventilation techniques. Continuous cricoid pressure during intubation of adults may prevent regurgitation into the hypopharynx and aspiration of gastric contents.

There are some hospitals in which the primary responsibility for emergency intubation is shared between anesthesiologists and respiratory therapists.[65] In other hospitals, the respiratory therapists perform tracheal intubation during resuscitation only when they are the most experienced; for example, during the night shift when an anesthesiologist is not present. In hospitals where they do not actually perform the intubation,

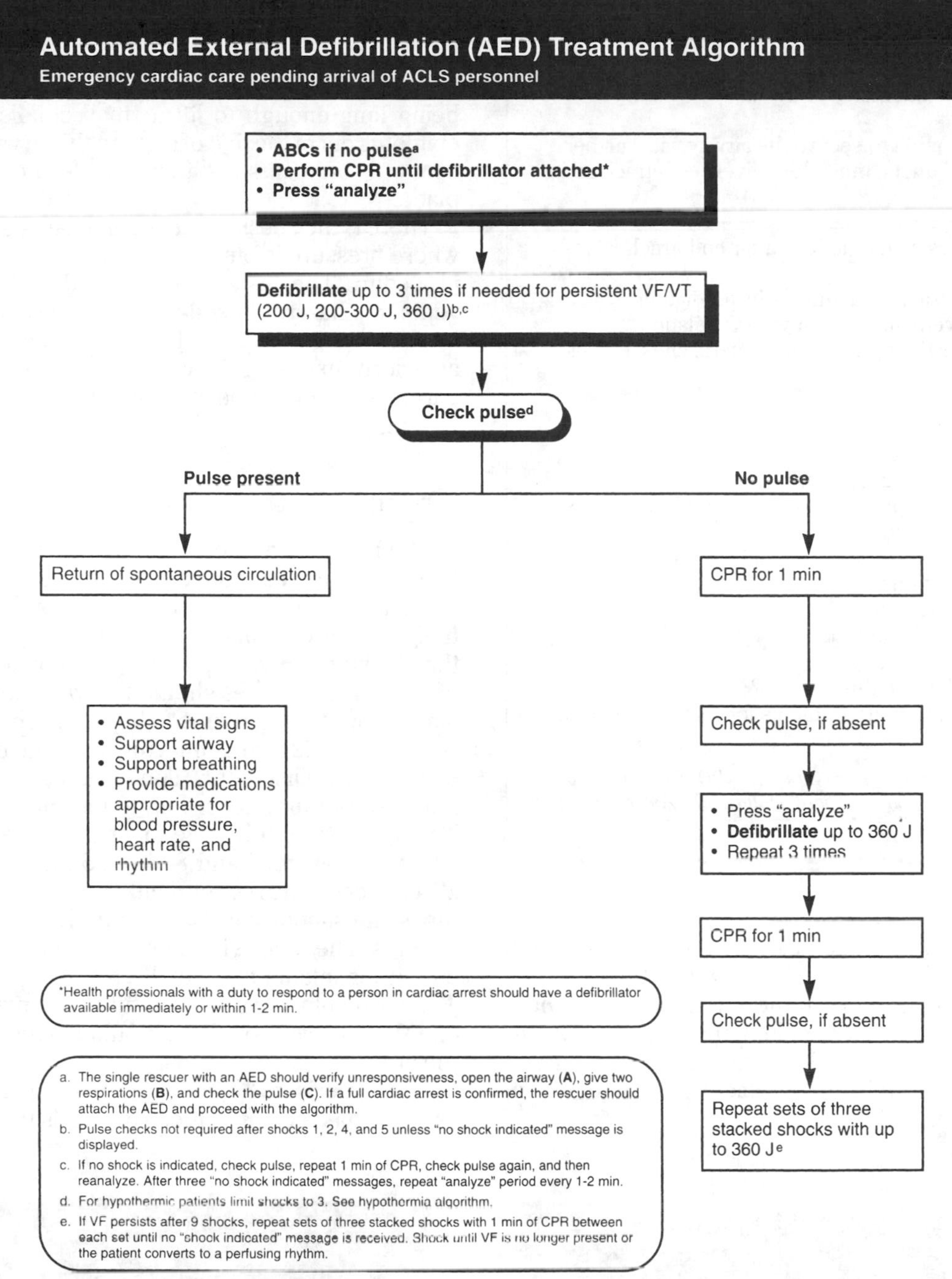
Automated External Defibrillation (AED) Treatment Algorithm
Emergency cardiac care pending arrival of ACLS personnel
• ABCs if no pulse[a]
• Perform CPR until defibrillator attached*
• Press "analyze"
Defibrillate up to 3 times if needed for persistent VF/VT (200 J, 200-300 J, 360 J)[b,c]
Check pulse[d]
Pulse present
No pulse
Return of spontaneous circulation
• Assess vital signs
• Support airway
• Support breathing
• Provide medications appropriate for blood pressure, heart rate, and rhythm
CPR for 1 min
Check pulse, if absent
• Press "analyze"
• Defibrillate up to 360 J
• Repeat 3 times
CPR for 1 min
Check pulse, if absent
Repeat sets of three stacked shocks with up to 360 J[e]
*Health professionals with a duty to respond to a person in cardiac arrest should have a defibrillator available immediately or within 1-2 min.
a. The single rescuer with an AED should verify unresponsiveness, open the airway (A), give two respirations (B), and check the pulse (C). If a full cardiac arrest is confirmed, the rescuer should attach the AED and proceed with the algorithm.
b. Pulse checks not required after shocks 1, 2, 4, and 5 unless "no shock indicated" message is displayed.
c. If no shock is indicated, check pulse, repeat 1 min of CPR, check pulse again, and then reanalyze. After three "no shock indicated" messages, repeat "analyze" period every 1-2 min.
d. For hypothermic patients limit shocks to 3. See hypothermia algorithm.
e. If VF persists after 9 shocks, repeat sets of three stacked shocks with 1 min of CPR between each set until no "shock indicated" message is received. Shock until VF is no longer present or the patient converts to a perfusing rhythm.

PROTOCOL 22-3. Automated external defibrillation (AED) treatment algorithm. (Chandra NC, Hazinski MF, editors. Textbook of Basic Life Support for Healthcare Providers, p. 9–8. Dallas American Heart Association 1994. Reproduced with permission.)

respiratory therapists are responsible for assisting the physician during the procedure. Therefore, the respiratory care practitioner must be familiar with the preparation, equipment, and procedure for intubation.

☐ LARYNGOSCOPES

Laryngoscopes are instruments designed to facilitate tracheal intubation. They consist of two parts; the handle and a detachable blade (Fig. 22-17). The handle contains batteries to light the bulb located near the end of the blade. The handle is designed to accommodate both adult- and pediatric-size blades. However, smaller handles for pediatric intubation are available for those who prefer a smaller grip. Straight (eg, Miller) and curved blades (eg, Macintosh) in several sizes are commonly available for intubation of both adults and children.

The curved blade conforms to the shape of the tongue, with the tip of the blade lying in the vallecula between the epiglottis and the base of the tongue (Fig.

BOX 22-3

SECONDARY ABCD SURVEY

Airway
- Reassess the adequacy of the airway-opening techniques.
- Direct personnel to secure the airway with further airway adjuncts, most definitively endotracheal intubation.

Breathing
- Assess status of ventilations after endotracheal intubation.
- Make necessary adjustments in ventilation.
- Assess movement of chest with ventilations.
- Examine for the presence of bilateral chest expansions.

Circulation
- Obtain IV access.
- Attach monitor leads.
- Identify rhythm and rates.
- Measure blood pressure (noninvasive blood pressure measurements).
- Provide rhythm-appropriate and vital-sign-appropriate medications.

Differential Diagnosis
- What caused the arrest?
- What is the rhythm?
- What could cause this rhythm?
- Look for underlying problems for refractory cardiac arrests.

Used with permission from Cummins RO (ed): Textbook of Advanced Cardiac Life Support. Dallas, TX, American Heart Association, 1994, Chap. 1.

22-18). The curved blade also has the advantage of a wider profile to help sweep the tongue to the side. Elevation in the direction of the laryngoscope handle should bring the vocal cords into full view (Fig. 22-19). Laryngospasm is potentially reduced with the curved blade because there is less contact with the highly innervated epiglottis.

The straight blade (Fig. 22-20) can be used to lift the epiglottis and expose the vocal cords. It allows a greater exposure of the glottic opening, which increases the chance that the tube can be seen passing through the cords. Also, the straight blade has the advantage of being long enough to lift a small child's large floppy epiglottis out of the line of sight to the larynx. The larger epiglottis of infants is difficult to elevate with a curved blade.

There is the possibility of dental damage in situations where pressure is put on the upper incisors during the procedure. The design of the curved blade partially prevents this hazard if used properly. The tongue is lifted by the laryngoscope blade and the epiglottis is pulled anteriorly, exposing the vocal cords (see Fig 22-20). Regardless of which type of blade is used, the teeth cannot be used as a fulcrum.

□ ENDOTRACHEAL TUBES

The respiratory therapist should take the responsibility to assure that both types of blades in various sizes are available on the emergency carts throughout the hospital. The equipment check should include assuring that the bulbs on the blades are functional. Several sizes of endotracheal tubes should be available to accommodate a variety of patients. The tubes should have the standard 15/22-mm connector that attaches to a mask or manual resuscitator. Tube sizes are designated in millimeters (mm) according to internal diameter (ID). The appropriate tube size for the average adult is 7 or 7.5 mm for women and 8.0 or 8.5 mm for men. Table 22-4 indicates the recommended sizes for endotracheal tubes and suction catheters for newborn through adult patients. The tubes should be cuffed for adults and uncuffed for infants and small children (<8 years old). The correct-fitting uncuffed tube for small children is one that allows a small leak on applying 20 cmH_2O to the airway.[66]

The American Society for Testing and Materials (ASTM) has recommended standards for endotracheal

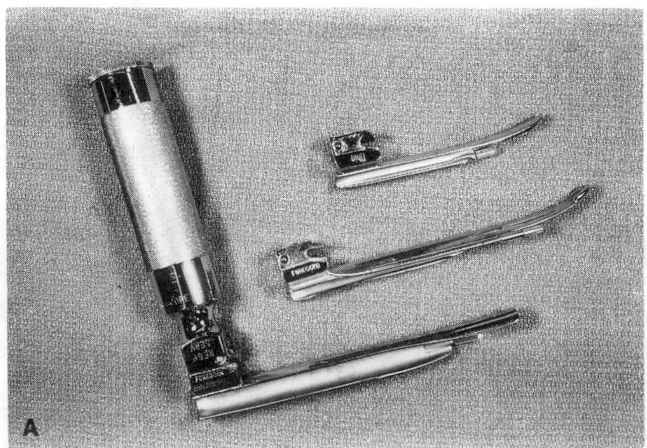

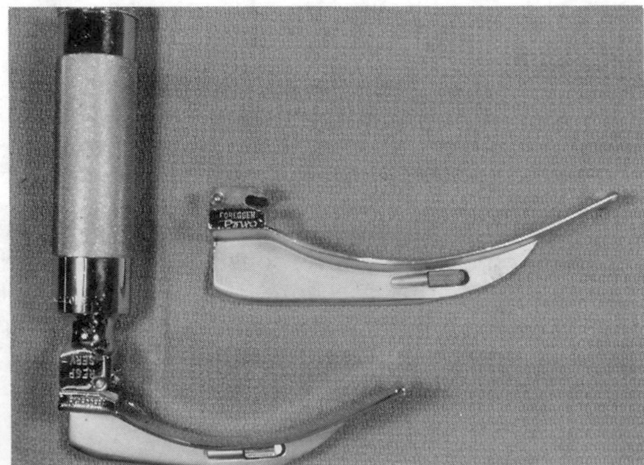

FIGURE 22-17. Laryngoscope handle and blades **(A)** straight; **(B)** curved (McIntosh) blades.

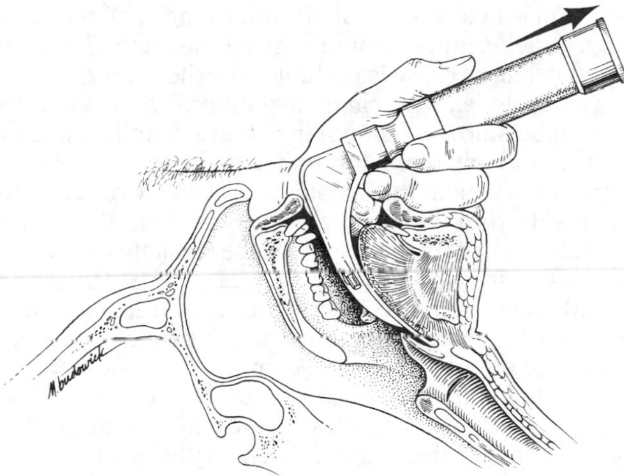

FIGURE 22-18. Adult laryngoscopy with curved blade. Note that the wrist is straight. (Finucane BT, Santora AH: Principles of Airway Management, p. 131. Philadelphia: FA Davis, 1988, Reproduced with permission.)

tubes and cuffs.[58] These standards do not prohibit the manufacture or use of tubes not conforming to the standards. However, ASTM standards are considered by the medical community to be important in delivering safe care to patients. The F29 stamped on tracheal tubes indicates the manufacturer has used an implantation or cell culture technique, according to ASTM testing specifications, to establish that the material used for the device is nontoxic. Implantation testing involves placing a small piece of the tube under the skin of a rabbit muscle to verify that the material does not trigger a tissue reaction.

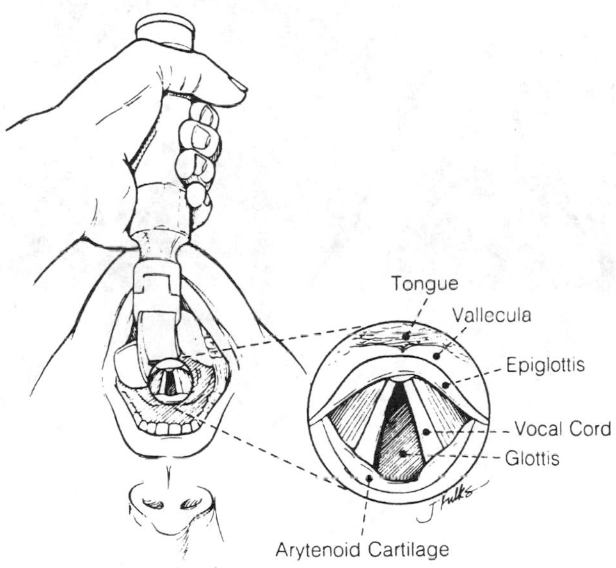

FIGURE 22-19. Visualization of vocal cords with laryngoscope. (Barnes TA, Watson ME: Cardiopulmonary resuscitation and emergency cardiac care, In Barnes TA (ed), Core Textbook in Respiratory Care Practice, 2nd ed., p. 308. St. Louis, Mosby–Year Book, 1994. Reproduced with permission.)

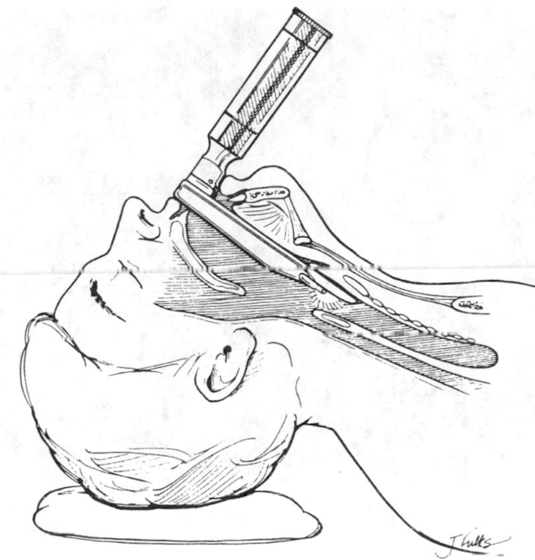

FIGURE 22-20. Adult laryngoscopy with straight blade. (Barnes TA, Watson ME: Cardiopulmonary resuscitation and emergency cardiac care, In Barnes TA (ed), Core Textbook in Respiratory Care Practice, 2nd ed., p. 308. St. Louis, Mosby–Year Book, 1994. Reproduced with permission.)

The tracheal tube package should have the ID, or internal diameter, size printed near the right corner and also on the side of the tube. The tube should also be marked oral or nasal. If it is smaller than 6.0 mm ID, the outside diameter in millimeters should also be shown.[67]

The most common material used for tracheal tubes is polyvinylchloride (PVC). The advantages of this mater-

TABLE 22-4 **Suggested Sizes for Endotracheal Tubes and Suction Catheters***

Age and Weight	Internal Diameter of Tube (mm)	Suction Catheters (Fr)
Newborn, <1 kg	2.5	5
Newborn, 1 to 2 kg	3.0	6
Newborn, 2 to 3 kg	3.5	8
6 months, >3 kg	3.5	8
18 months	4.0	8
3 years	4.5	8
5 years	5.0	10
6 years	5.5	10
8 years	6.0	10
12 years	6.5	10
16 years	7.0	10
Adult (female)	7.5 to 8.0	12
Adult (male)	8.0 to 8.5	14

* Endotracheal tube selection for a child should be based on the child's size, not age. One size larger and one size smaller should be allowed for individual variations.

Reproduced with permission from Emergency Cardiac Care Committee and Subcommittees, American Heart Association: Guidelines for cardiopulmonary resuscitation and emergency care, VI: Pediatric advanced life support. JAMA 268:2263, 1992.

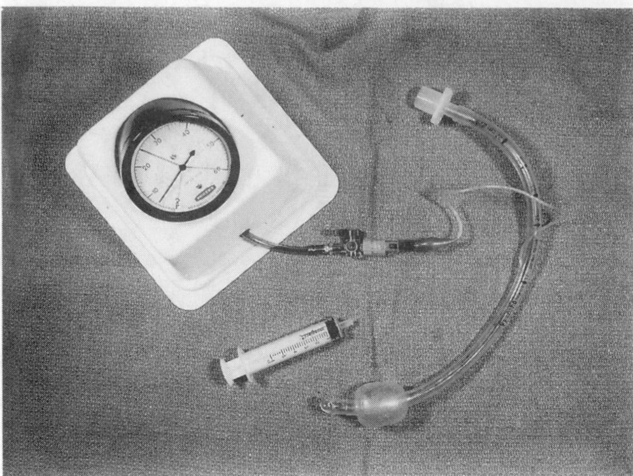

FIGURE 22-21. An aneroid pressure gauge and stopcock to monitor intracuff pressure.

ial are flexibility to mold at body temperature and nontoxicity so that no tissue reaction should occur. Sterilization of artificial airways made with PVC require the same precautions as other devices made with PVC. Tubes that are labeled "gamma-radiation sterilized" should not be resterilized because of the risk of toxic levels of ethylene chlorohydrin forming. The package of the tracheal tube should suggest the method of sterilization unless reuse is prohibited by the manufacturer; for example, as with single-use tubes. Tracheal tubes should be stored when not in use in a round container with a 14-inch diameter to maintain their required curved shape, and they should be relatively resistant to agents used in chemical cleansing and sterilization.[67] The slight curve of the tracheal tube facilitates easier introduction into the airway.

Although there are a variety of endotracheal tubes available for clinical use, those meeting the ASTM standards incorporate the same components. The bevel is the slanted end of the tracheal tube and faces left when viewed from the concave aspect. It is located at the distal end and is 45 degrees in relation to the long axis. The inflating tube provides a route for inflating the cuff and a place for monitoring cuff pressures (Fig. 22-21). The pilot balloon is fitted to the inflating tube and indicates cuff inflation. The cuff itself is the inflatable sleeve that is located at the distal end of the tube, and it provides a seal between the tube and the trachea. This allows ventilation, prevents aspiration, and positions the tube in the trachea. The cuff length and design varies by manufacturer. Cuffs may be circular or cylindrical, large or small in diameter, long or short, of thin- or thick-walled PVC, and air or foam filled (Fig. 22-22).[68] Emergency in-

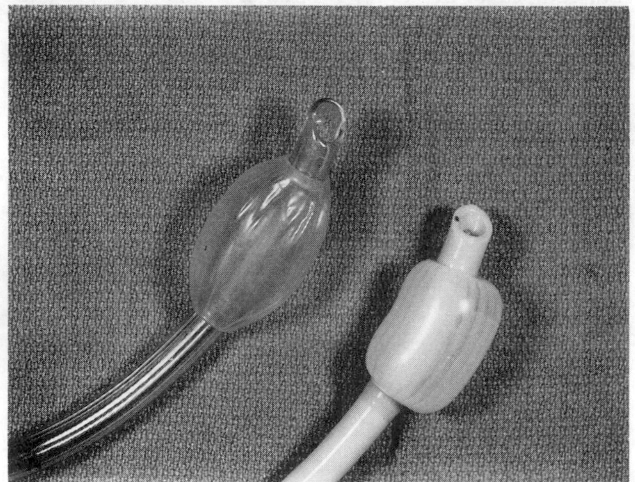

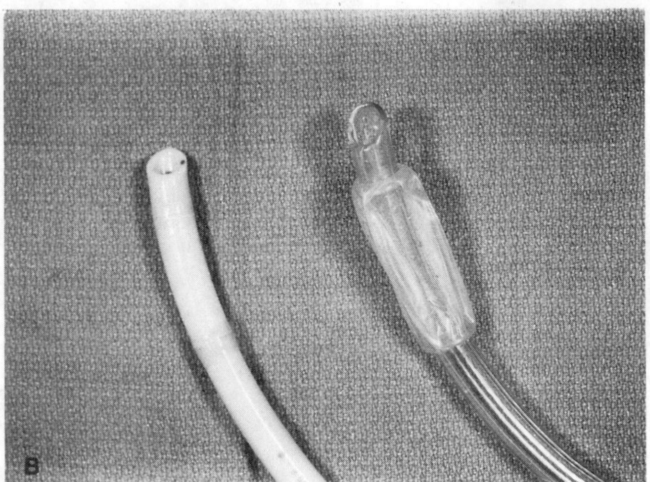

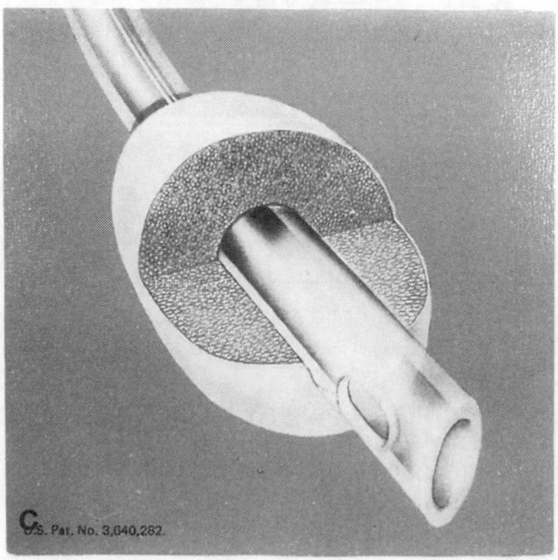

FIGURE 22-22. Endotracheal tube cuff designs demonstrating "trim" (*left*) and "bulky" (*right*) cuffs **(A)** Tubes with cuffs inflated to therapeutic levels; **(B)** The same tubes with cuffs completely evacuated of air; **(C)** Diagram of the Bivona Fome-Cuff endotracheal tube. (Courtesy Biovana, Inc., Gary, Indiana.)

tubations may be more difficult with a cuff that has a "bulky" profile when deflated (Fig. 22-22*B*).[69]

The most commonly used tracheal tubes incorporate a high-volume low-pressure cuff. Thin-walled, high-volume cuffs form thin folds against the tracheal mucosa. This design holds to a minimum the pressure needed to form a seal, and the folds provide redundancy to guard against aspiration. This type of tube decreases the risk of inhibiting capillary blood flow that may lead to tracheal necrosis and stenosis. High pressures on the tracheal wall are also associated with tracheoesophageal fistulas, which can be prevented with low-pressure cuffs. However, even cuffs designed for low pressure can exert high pressure on the trachea if too much air is inserted. Intracuff pressures must be monitored periodically to confirm that cuffs either contain a minimal occluding volume (MOV) or offer minimal leak as peak inspiratory pressure (MLT) is applied.

The proper-size tube for intubation must be chosen. If the tube is too large, pressure necrosis on the trachea is a hazard, even with small amounts of air in the cuff. If the tube is too small, more air is required to inflate the cuff. Also, suctioning may not be as effective because the suction catheter used for small tubes must also be smaller. The suction catheter should be less than one half the inside diameter of the tracheal tube.

□ INTUBATION PROCEDURE

The equipment necessary for orotracheal intubation should be on every emergency cart and checked frequently. The equipment should include a manual resuscitator capable of delivering 100% oxygen; masks in a variety of sizes; suction equipment including a large tonsil suction tip to clear the airway of mucus, blood, or vomitus; a variety of endotracheal tubes; laryngoscope with different sizes of straight and curved blades; a flexible metal stylet; and Magill forceps to aid insertion.

The endotracheal tube should be inspected before the intubation attempt to assure that the cuff inflates properly, and that a one-way valve is attached to the pilot tube with a syringe attached (the plunger of the syringe should be withdrawn to inject the appropriate amount of air into the cuff with one push). The tube should also be checked for appropriate size and to assure that a 15/22-mm connector is attached to the proximal end. While the equipment is being checked, the patient should be hyperventilated and hyperoxygenated with 100% oxygen for a minimum of 3 minutes with a bag-valve-mask device.

The head, neck, and shoulders of the patient should be positioned so a straight line is possible between the incisors and the glottis (Fig. 22-23). A small towel placed

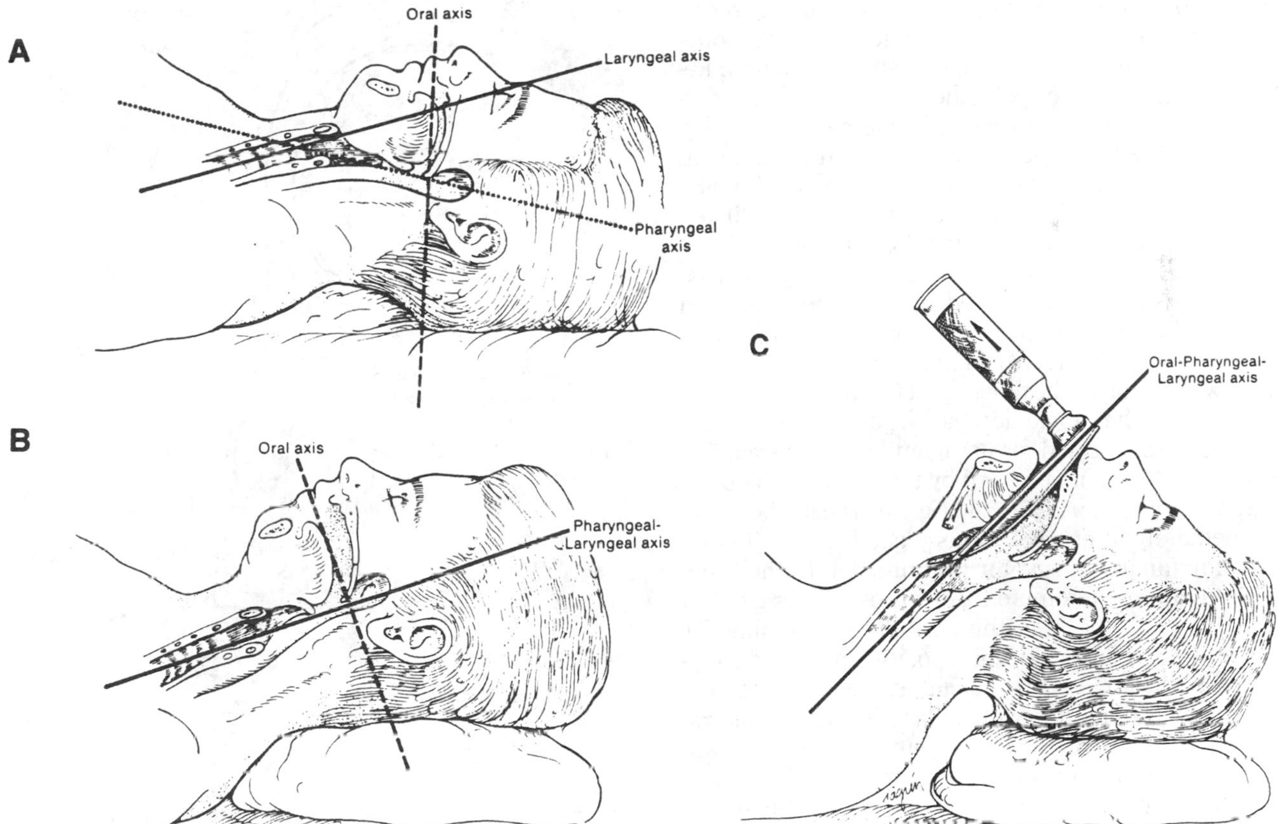

FIGURE 22-23. Proper head position is important for successful orotracheal intubation **(A)** The oral, pharyngeal, and laryngeal axes must be aligned for direct laryngoscopy; **(B)** Elevate the head 10 cm above the shoulders with a folded towel to align the pharyngeal and laryngeal axes; **(C)** Extend the atlanto-occipital joint to achieve the straightest possible line from the incisors to the glottis. (Cullen DJ: Endotracheal intubation, In Wilkins EW, ed; MGH Textbook of Emergency Medicine, p. 756–757. Baltimore, Williams & Wilkins, 1978. Reproduced with permission.)

under the head may facilitate the proper alignment (Fig. 22-23*B*), which is referred to as the "sniffing position." The blade is attached to the laryngoscope, which is held in the left hand. The blade is inserted on the right-hand side of the mouth, sweeping the tongue to the left as the blade is brought to the midline. The blade is advanced forward along the midline, pulling the mandible at a 45° angle in a straight line toward the ceiling. A slight lifting pressure is applied to the laryngoscope until the tip of the epiglottis is visualized. If a curved blade is used, the tip of the blade is then advanced into the vallecula (the epiglottis would be lifted if a straight blade was used). Contracting the forearm muscles as opposed to the upper arm muscles helps to assure the pressure is not exerted on the front teeth by the blade.

The primary landmarks of intubation are the epiglottis and the arytenoid cartilage. When these structures are recognized, the vocal cords and the opening of the glottis are known. The vocal cords should be continuously in view immediately before the endotracheal tube passes through the glottis. Direct visualization, at a minimum, should include observing the endotracheal tube pass by the arytenoid cartilage. The esophageal opening can also be seen so that incorrect placement of the tube is avoided.

With the blade in midline position, the endotracheal tube is inserted into the right side of the mouth, taking care not to obstruct the view down the laryngoscope blade. The endotracheal tube is advanced into the glottis and through the vocal cords in one smooth motion. Repeatedly trying to jab or poke the tube through the glottis must be avoided because glottic edema may develop and make subsequent intubation attempts more difficult, if not impossible. If the tube cannot be placed within 30 seconds, it should be taken out and the patient ventilated and reoxygenated before another attempt is made.

If the tube has lost its normal curve, a metal stylet can be used. This instrument is inserted into the tube but should not project beyond the tip of the tracheal tube or it could cause damage to the tracheal tissue. The stylet should be withdrawn as soon as the tube is past the vocal cords to reduce trauma to the subglottic area. The use of a stylet is absolutely contraindicated for nasal intubations because of the potential for trauma caused by the combination of an acute angle for tube passage and rigid tracheal tube.

Immediately after the tube is placed, the cuff is inflated, a manual resuscitator is connected to the tube, and ventilation is attempted. A stethoscope is used to verify that the tube is in the trachea by listening for breath sounds bilaterally while positive pressure is applied with the manual resuscitator. The stethoscope should be placed under each axilla to listen for bilateral breath sounds and on the epigastrium (to the left of the xiphoid process) to check for gurgling sounds created by air flow if the tube is in the esophagus. If the tube is in the esophagus, the cuff must be deflated, and the tube quickly removed. The patient is reoxygenated with a manual resuscitator and mask before reintubation is attempted. Experienced practitioners may prefer to leave the tube in the esophagus while a second attempt is made to intubate the trachea with another tube. This has the advantage of "plugging the wrong hole" and preventing aspiration of gastric fluids, but it must be done quickly because reoxygenation is not possible.

Placement of the tube in the right main stem bronchus is suspected if breath sounds are heard on the right side of the chest and are absent on the left side. If the 30-cm mark is at the incisor line following oral intubation, a right main stem intubation is likely. When this situation is present, the cuff is deflated and the tube pulled out 1 to 2 cm or until bilateral breath sounds are heard. The approximate orotracheal tube insertion distance at the incisor line is 21 to 23 cm. Approximately 2 to 4 cm need to be added for nasotracheal tubes (Fig. 22-24). The average distance from nose to midtrachea is approximately 25 cm in an adult.

When proper placement of the tube is determined, it must be secured in position. Marking the tube at the

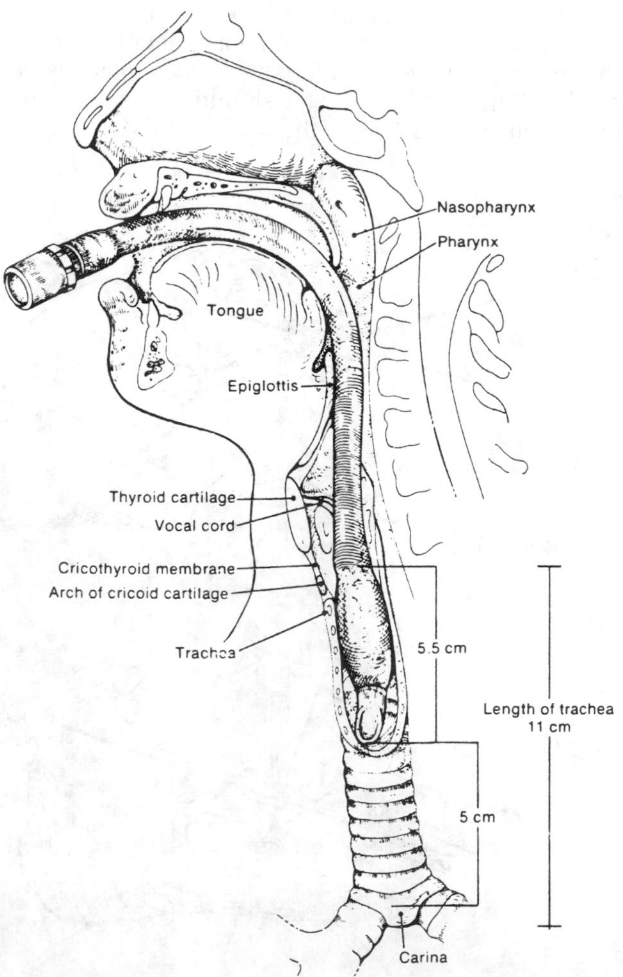

FIGURE 22-24. Malposition of the endotracheal tube can be suspected from the depth of insertion. In an average adult, the 18- to 24-cm mark will show at the incisors when the tip of the tube is midway between the vocal cords and the carina. (Cullen DJ: Endotracheal intubation, In Wilkins EW, (ed), MGH Textbook of Emergency Medicine, p. 758. Baltimore, Williams & Wilkins, 1978. Reproduced with permission.)

point where it meets the corner of the mouth assists in reevaluating the tube position. The tube is taped in place to prevent inadvertent extubation or problems with the tube going forward into the right main stem bronchus. There are a variety of acceptable techniques available for securing the tube. Adhesive tape secured to the face using benzoin so that the adhesive is not lost is a commonly used method (Fig. 22-25). In addition, there are a variety of commercially available endotracheal tube holders or harnesses available for securing tubes. Whichever method is used to secure the tube, correct positioning must be constantly monitored. A chest x-ray film confirms proper tube depth when the emergency situation has passed.[70] The tip of the tube lies in the middle portion of the trachea (near the level of the aortic knob).

☐ PEDIATRIC AND NEONATAL INTUBATION

Pediatric and neonatal patients should be positioned by placing a towel under the neck. The neck should be extended slightly for straight alignment of the airway. The patient should be oxygenated with a pediatric or neonatal manual resuscitator. The proper-size blade is attached to the laryngoscope, and it is placed in the left hand. Infants and small children have a relatively large epiglottis, which may require a straight blade to lift it out of the way. The blade is inserted into the center of the mouth and the tongue is moved to the left side. The blade is advanced into the base of the tongue, and the larynx is observed by lifting the laryngoscope and blade. Suctioning may be necessary, and then the tube is inserted along the right side of the blade and through the vocal cords. An uncuffed tube is used for infants because the cricoid cartilage forms the narrowest part of the airway and acts as a seal. Immediately, the lungs are auscultated to determine correct placement. Bilateral breath sounds should be heard under the axillae. If breath sounds are evident on the right but not the left, the tube should be pulled back slightly until bilateral breath sounds are auscultated. The tube is then secured using tape or a commercially available endotracheal tube holder. When the emergency situation is over, a chest x-ray film is taken to confirm tube position.

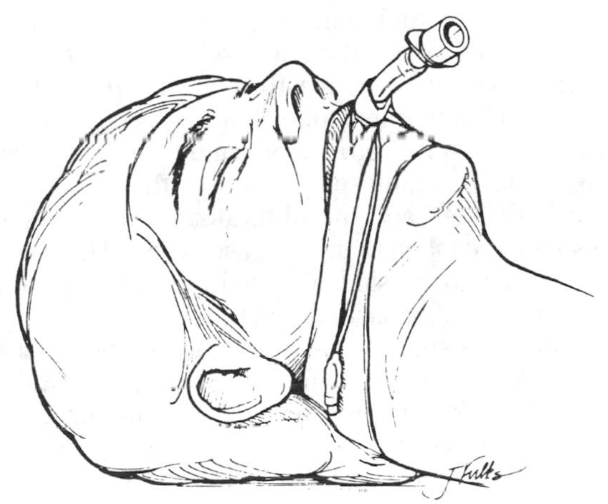

FIGURE 22-25. Securing the endotracheal tube. (Barnes TA, Watson ME: Cardiopulmonary resuscitation and emergency cardiac care, In Barnes TA (ed), Core Textbook in Respiratory Care Practice, ed 2, p. 312. St. Louis, Mosby–Year Book, 1994. Reproduced with permission.)

Airway Adjuncts

☐ OROPHARYNGEAL AND NASOPHARYNGEAL AIRWAYS

Oropharyngeal airways facilitate manual resuscitation by means of a face mask when an endotracheal tube is not in place. They are useful in preventing upper airway obstruction caused by the tongue falling back in the unconscious patient. Oropharyngeal airways are inappropriate for patients who are conscious because stimulation of the gag reflex could potentially cause vomiting and aspiration. Thus, the oropharyngeal airway should be removed immediately if the patient shows signs of returning consciousness. The insertion of the oropharyngeal airway is accomplished by opening the mouth, turning the airway upside down while placing it against the tongue. The airway is turned as it is introduced into the oropharynx alongside the tongue. This maneuver pulls the tongue forward, maintaining an open position of the upper airway. The two common types of oropharyngeal airways are the tubular Guedel and the Berman,[62] which has channels along its sides (Fig. 22-26*A,B*). Both types of oral airways allow a pathway for breathing and for pharyngeal suctioning. They are made with a rigid material at the point where the patient's teeth could clamp to prevent the patient from occluding the tube. The following sizes of oropharyngeal airways are recommended by the AHA:[39]

- Large adult: 100 mm (Guedel)
- Medium adult: 90 mm (Guedel)
- Small adult: 80 mm (Guedel)

Nasopharyngeal airways (Fig. 22-26*C*) are uncuffed tubes made of soft rubber or plastic. They are used in situations when insertion of an oropharyngeal airway is not possible, such as massive trauma around the mouth. They are also used with semiconscious or conscious patients who might not tolerate an oropharyngeal airway. However, a nasopharyngeal airway, although better tolerated than an oral airway, may precipitate laryngospasm and vomiting in these patients. If the tube is too long, it may enter the esophagus, causing gastric distension and hypoventilation during bag-valve-mask ventilation. The following sizes are recommended for nasopharyngeal airways by the AHA:[39]

- Large adult: 8.0 to 9.0 ID
- Medium adult: 7.0 to 8.0 ID
- Small adult: 6.0 to 7.0 ID

After lubrication with a water-soluble gel or anesthetic jelly, the nasopharyngeal airway may be gently inserted along the floor of the nostril into the posterior pharynx be-

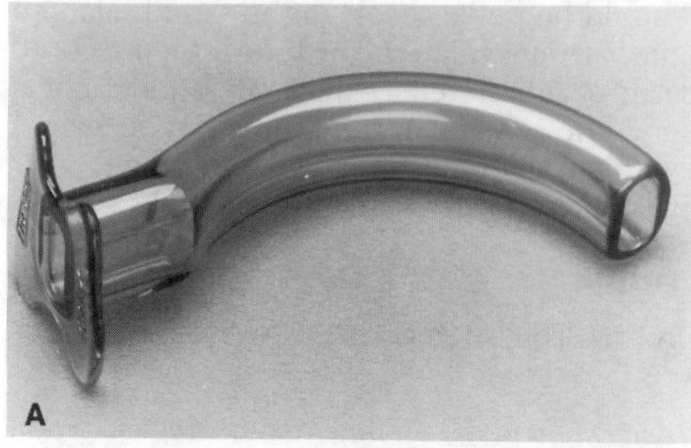

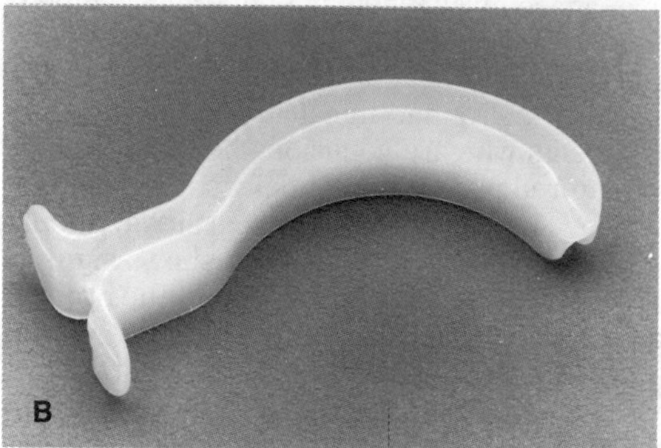

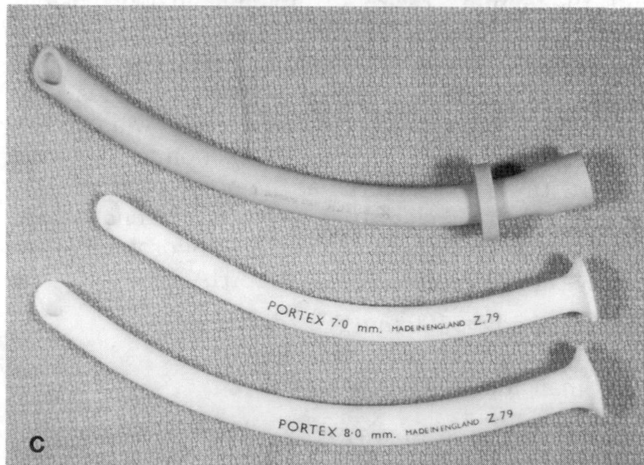

FIGURE 22-26. Various types of oro- and nasopharyngeal airways **(A)** Guedel oropharyngeal airway; **(B)** Berman oropharyngeal airway; and **(C)** Nasopharyngeal airways.

hind the tongue. The bevel on the tip of the airway should be kept close to the midline during insertion, and slight rotation may be necessary to ease insertion when the angle of the nasal passage and the nasopharynx is encountered. The insertion of a nasopharyngeal airway may injure the nasal mucosa with bleeding and possible aspiration of clots into the trachea. It is necessary to maintain head tilt with anterior displacement of the mandible by chin lift or jaw thrust when using this airway.[39]

□ ESOPHAGEAL OBTURATOR AIRWAY

A cardiac arrest victim may be admitted to the emergency room with an *esophageal obturator airway* (EOA) in place. The EOA consists of a mask attached to a cuffed tube (Fig. 22-27*A*). The mask is placed tightly around the nose and mouth to provide a seal (Fig. 22-28). This airway is inserted into the esophagus rather than the trachea and is designed so that the distal end is sealed. Air from a manual resuscitator is delivered to the laryngeal area through holes in the tube. The tube is cuffed to prevent gastric inflation and regurgitation.

The esophageal obturator presents problems that make it inferior to the endotracheal tube.[20,71,72] The endotracheal tube is the emergency airway of choice and can be successfully placed in patients without complications by trained health professionals.[20,73] The American Heart Association considers the EOA a Class IIb intervention (acceptable, possibly helpful) compared with the endotracheal tube, which is a Class I intervention (definitely helpful). The EOA is not appropriate for use in general hospitals because practitioners skilled in endotracheal intubation are readily available. The American Heart Association recommends that the EOA should not be used in victims younger than 16 years, conscious persons, those with spontaneous breathing, those with esophageal disease, or those who have swallowed caustic substances.[20]

Close monitoring of patients who arrive in the emergency room with an EOA is required to recognize the critical complications related to their use. Fatal complications have been reported to occur from esophageal rupture and inadvertent placement of the esophageal obturator into the trachea.[74,75] Esophageal rupture is suspected by the presence of subcutaneous emphysema, pneumomediastinum, pleural effusion, and chest pain. Placement of the tube into the trachea is recognized by absence of chest movement and breath sounds.[76] However, this may be difficult to observe in the obese patient, and sounds generated by air going into the stomach may be transmitted to the chest and misinterpreted.[77] The tube should be withdrawn immediately if signs indicate it has been placed in the trachea.

Another potential complication related to using the esophageal obturator is vomiting and aspiration when the tube is removed. When the unconscious patient is admitted to the emergency room with an esophageal obturator in place, an endotracheal tube should be inserted before the obturator is removed.[20] If the patient has become conscious and is breathing spontaneously, the cuff of the obturator is deflated and the obturator removed. Precautions should be taken to prevent aspiration. The patient's head is turned to the side and suction equipment should be available. Also, a nasogastric tube can be inserted to decompress the stomach before removing the obturator.

An EOA has been designed with a gastric tube in place to deal with the problem of vomiting during extubation. The esophageal gastric tube airway (EGTA) allows passage of a gastric tube through the esophageal tube into the esophagus and stomach (Fig. 22-27*B*). The EGTA allows the stomach to be decompressed and gastric contents suctioned while ventilation is continued. The extubation of the EGTA can then be accomplished with less risk of vomiting and aspiration of gastric contents into the lungs.

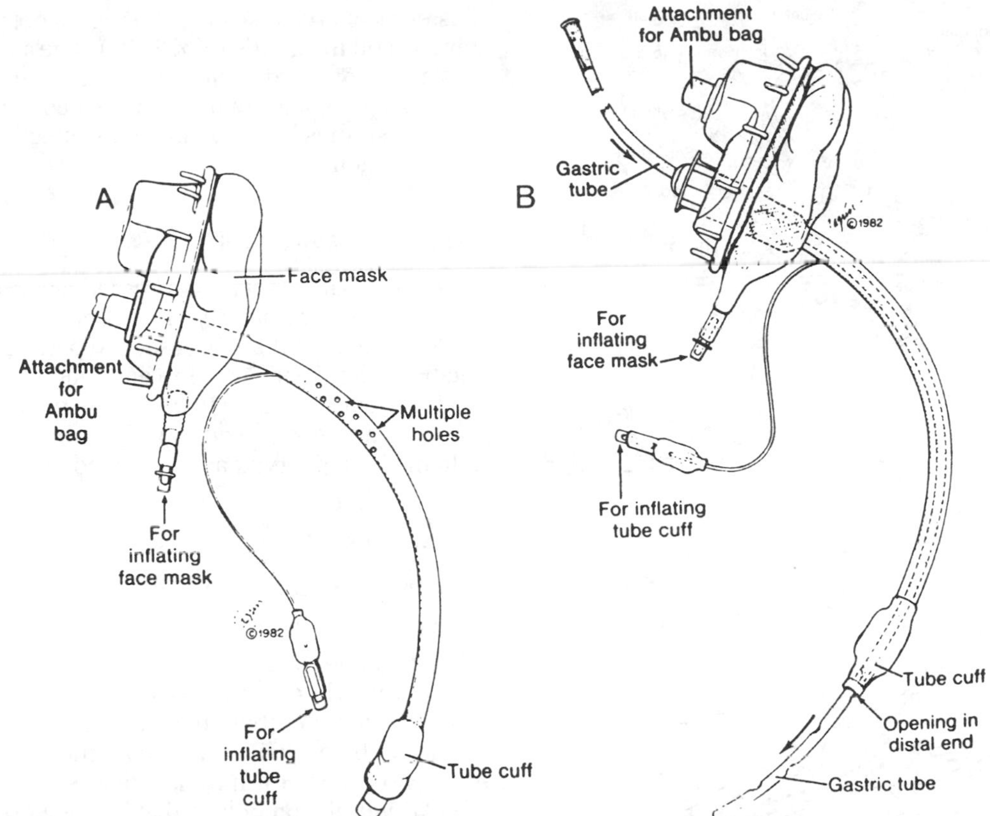

FIGURE 22-27. Esophageal obturator airways **(A)** Esophageal obturator airway (EOA); **(B)** Esophageogastric tube airway (ETGA). (McCabe BF: Prehospital medical care. In Wilkins EW (ed): MGH Textbook of Emergency Medicine, 3rd ed. Baltimore, Williams & Wilkins, 1989. Reproduced with permission.)

□ PHARYNGOTRACHEAL LUMEN AIRWAY

The *pharyngotracheal lumen airway* (PTL) is a double-lumen tube that is inserted into the oropharynx without the use of a laryngoscope (Fig. 22-29). One of the tubes is 31 cm in length and passes through the other, shorter lumen (21 cm). The longer tube of the PTL is placed in either the trachea or the esophagus without the practitioner knowing which structure the tube lies in until an assessment is made. After insertion, an airway seal is made by inflating a large proximal balloon that fills the oropharynx. A smaller cuff on the distal end of the tube is then inflated. If the long tube is in the trachea, ventilation can be accomplished in a way similar to using an endotracheal tube. If the long tube is in the esophagus, then the short tube is used to deliver air below the large proximal balloon inflated in the oropharynx. The smaller cuff on the long tube prevents air from traveling down the esophagus and air enters the trachea. The cuff on the long tube, similar to the EOA, prevents gastric contents from being aspirated into the lungs.

□ ESOPHAGEAL-TRACHEAL COMBITUBE

The *esophageal-tracheal combitube* (ETC) is similar to the PTL but has two tubes of the same length that are inserted blindly into the laryngopharynx. Depending on whether the trachea or esophagus is intubated, one of the lumina is used to ventilate the patient after the cuffs are inflated (Fig. 22-30). If the tubes are in the trachea, ventilation occurs through the lumen of one of the two tubes in a manner similar to that of an endotracheal tube. If the tubes sit in the esophagus, then the air enters the laryngopharynx through side holes from

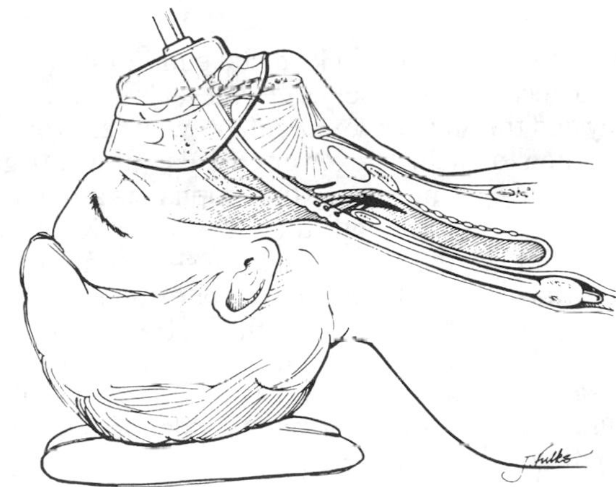

FIGURE 22-28. Esophageal obturator. The mask is placed tightly around the nose and mouth to provide a seal. (Barnes TA, Watson ME: Cardiopulmonary resuscitation and emergency cardiac care, In Barnes TA, (ed), Core Textbook in Respiratory Care Practice, 2nd ed., p. 315. St. Louis, Mosby–Year Book, 1994. Reproduced with permission.)

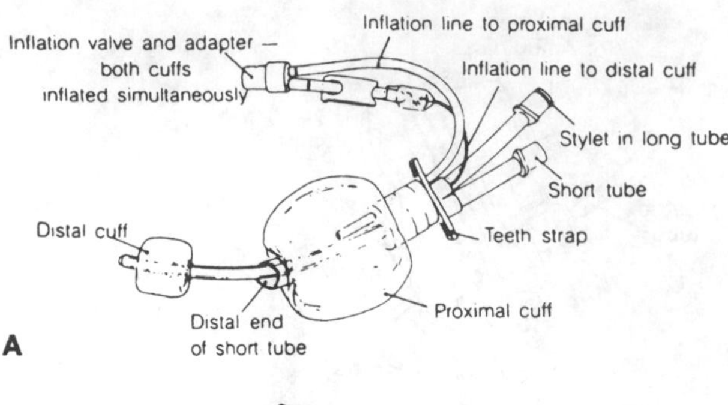

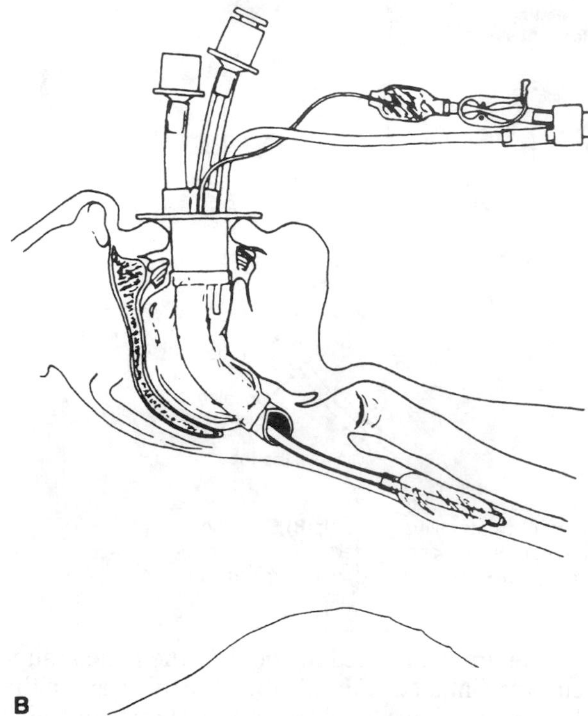

FIGURE 22-29. **(A)** Diagram of the pharyngotracheal lumen airway (PTL); **(B)** Representation of the PTL airway in position. (Niemann JT, Myers R, Scarberry EN: The pharyngotracheal lumen airway: Preliminary investigation of a new airway adjunct. Ann Emerg Med 13:591, 1984. Reproduced with permission.)

a lumen that has a plug in its distal end. Air enters the trachea because the upper large cuff seals off the upper airway and the smaller, lower cuff prevents air from entering the stomach. The lower cuff also prevents gastric material from moving up the esophagus around the tube. The use of the both the PTL and ETC has occurred clinically before objective assessment of their efficacy has been determined. Despite adequate training, serious complications with the PTL and ETC (similar to the EOA) have occurred. Accordingly, the endotracheal tube remains the airway of choice to achieve adequate airway protection and ventilation during resuscitation.[20]

□ LARYNGEAL MASK AIRWAY

The *laryngeal mask airway* consists of a tube similar to an endotracheal tube, with a small mask with a large inflatable circular cuff intended for placement in the posterior pharynx, sealing the region of the base of the tongue and the glottis (Fig. 22-31). The airway was used first in Europe under the controlled condition of the operating room, and its use requires considerable training. No studies have evaluated its effectiveness during resuscitation.[39]

□ SELLICK MANEUVER

In adult patients with depressed levels of consciousness, a *Sellick maneuver* should be performed during endotracheal intubation. A second person on the resuscitation team applies thumb and index finger pressure to the cricoid cartilage to compress the esophagus and prevent any gastric contents from being regurgitated into the hypopharynx and aspirated into the trachea.[78]

Emergency Ventilation

□ MANUAL RESUSCITATORS

Manual ventilations with bag-valve-mask devices often provide inadequate tidal volumes. This is especially true when the operator is untrained, and even trained team members need to practice at frequent intervals to be proficient. In recognition of this problem, many hospitals now have a two-person bag-valve-mask (BVM) ventilation policy; that is, one person holds the mask with two hands (to make a good seal with the patient's face and to extend the head), and the second person squeezes the bag of the resuscitator with two hands. Whenever possible, an exhaled volume respirometer should be connected to the exhalation port of the resuscitator to monitor ventilation on a breath-to-breath basis. If this is not possible, then chest excursion should be visually assessed for depth and bilateral symmetry. Checking breath sounds bilaterally over the midaxillary line is also recommended. An arterial blood gas and pH sample may be useful to assess the adequacy of ventilation and oxygenation. To assure that the tube is not in the esophagus, the epigastrium should also be auscultated. Tube placement should be confirmed with other techniques such as end-tidal CO_2 detectors, aspiration bulb devices, or direct visualization with a laryngoscope. If the location of the tube is in doubt, you should consider removing the tube and starting over. A stat chest x-ray film should be ordered after the intubation. This confirms the clinical assessment of tube depth and provides information on pulmonary conditions.

A variety of manual resuscitation units are currently available. These units are used to support the ventilation of patients who have a respiratory or cardiopulmonary arrest. Manual resuscitators (bag-valve devices) consist of a self-inflating bag, an air intake valve, a nonrebreathing valve, an oxygen inlet nipple, and oxygen reservoir. One end of the nonrebreathing valve connects to the bag, and the other end is connected to the patient's endotracheal tube or face mask. The self-inflating bag is compressed by the operator, and the nonrebreathing valve directs gas from the bag to the patient as the exhalation port closes. When the operator

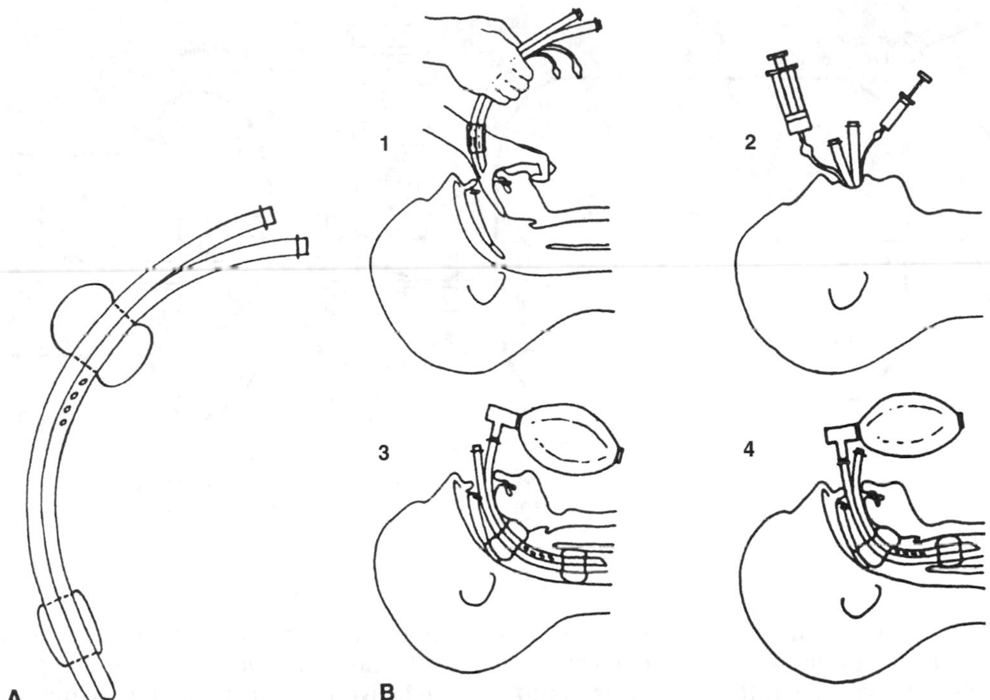

FIGURE 22-30. (A) Esophagotracheal combitube. (B) Insertion procedure: Intubation of either the esophagus or trachea will facilitate ventilation. (Frass M, Frenzer R, Rauscha F, Weber H, Pacher R, Leithner C: Evaluation of esophageal combitube in cardiopulmonary resuscitation. Crit Care Med 15:609, 1986, Williams & Wilkins. Reproduced with permission.)

releases the bag, the exhaled gas is directed through the exhalation port. The bag reinflates through a one-way air inlet valve opening directly into the bag. The gas inlet valve is part of the nonrebreathing valve in some units (Fig. 22-32) and part of the valve at the bottom of other units (Fig. 22-33).

During cardiac arrest, it is important to administer the highest oxygen concentration possible.[20] The American

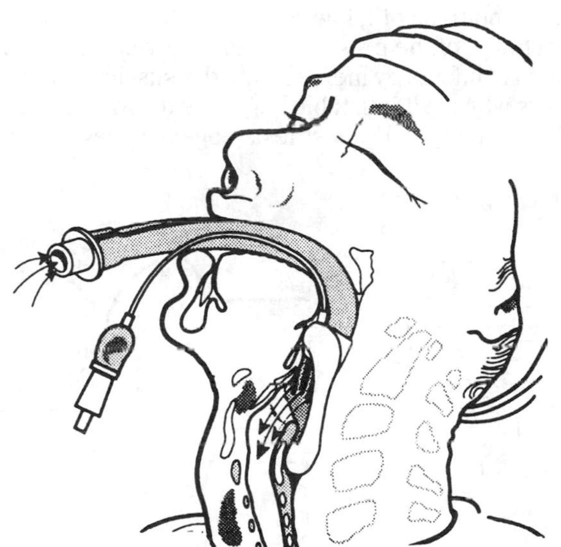

FIGURE 22-31. Laryngeal mask airway. (Donen M, Tweed WA, Dashfsky S, Guttormson B: The esophageal obturator: An appraisal. Can Anaesth Soc J 30:194, 1983. Reproduced with permission.)

Society for Testing and Materials (ASTM) and International Organization for Standardization (ISO) have recommended that manual resuscitators be capable of delivering at least 85% oxygen at a minute ventilation of 7.2 L/min (600 mL × 12 breaths/min) with an oxygen flow of 15 L/min.[79,80] However, 85% oxygen may not be optimal to treat a cardiopulmonary arrest, and most manual resuscitators available deliver greater than 95% oxygen. Some manual resuscitators, with poorly designed oxygen reservoirs, deliver less than 85% oxygen.[81]

Although all the criteria described below are important when choosing a manual resuscitator for emergency ventilation, the first consideration should be delivered oxygen capability. The respiratory care practitioner must know the capabilities and limitations of the manual resuscitators currently available to assure the delivery of adequate ventilation during a cardiopulmonary arrest.

When using a bag-valve device to ventilate a patient with an endotracheal tube in place, it is difficult to deliver a tidal volume of 0.8 to 1.2 L with one-hand compression of the bag. The following one-hand tidal volumes have been observed at a compliance of 0.02 L/cmH_2O and resistance of 20 to 28 cmH_2O/L/sec: ECRI, 660 mL;[82] Hess, 550 mL;[83] and Van Hooser, 546 mL.[84] At the same high lung impedance, a two-hand squeeze of the bag results in a tidal volume of 800 to 900 mL.[5,83] At normal lung impedance with a 7- to 8-mm endotracheal tube, a one-hand squeeze of the bag delivers only 600 mL, and a two-hand squeeze provides 900 to 1000 mL.[5,83,85] Practitioners with small hands tend to deliver 100 to 250 mL less with a one-hand squeeze of the bag than those

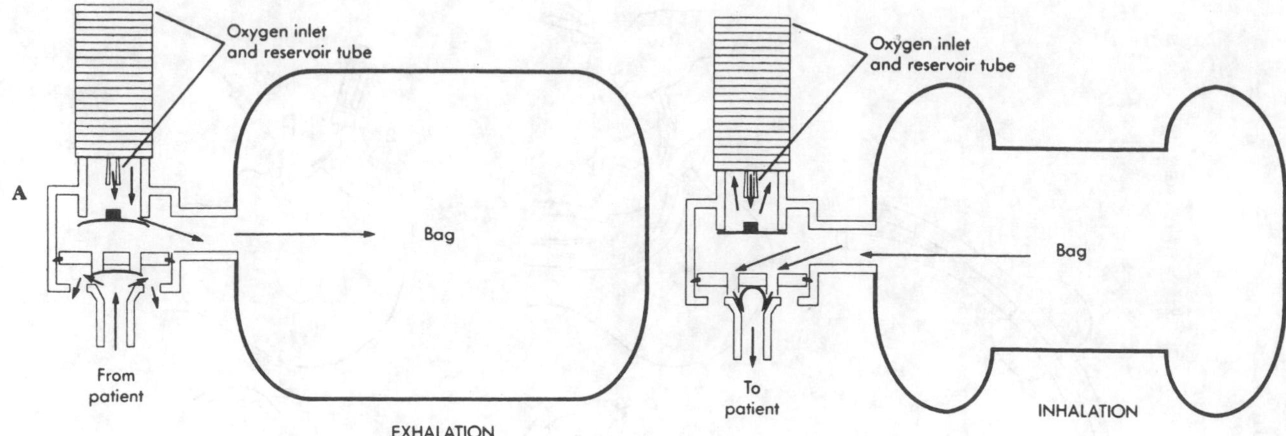

FIGURE 22-32. Manual resuscitator with gas intake valve located proximal to the patient valve. (McPherson SP: Respiratory Therapy Equipment, 4th ed., p. 134. St. Louis, Mosby–Year Book, 1990. Reproduced with permission.)

with large hands.[5,83] To adequately ventilate a patient during CPR with the tidal volume recommended by the AHA, most staff members need to use two hands to squeeze the bag. Teaching staff members how to best use bag-valve devices by using volumetric feedback has been shown to improve the tidal volume delivered.[86] This type of instruction should be given to all staff personnel involved in resuscitation.

Most practitioners cannot deliver adequate tidal volumes when holding the mask with one hand and squeezing the bag with the other hand.[83] With two-person bag-valve-mask ventilation and two-hand compression of the bag, Hess reported a tidal volume of 580 mL delivered to a Laerdal Recording Resusci-Anne.[87] Other investigators have reported higher tidal volumes for two-hand bag-valve-mask ventilation but used intubation models without lung impedance.[88,89] Thus, most hospitals now recommend two-person ventilation with bag-valve-mask devices. One person holds the mask in place with two hands and extends the head, opening the airway, and the other person uses two hands to squeeze the bag. Early tracheal intubation removes the need to assign two people to ventilating the patient and allows the second person to be reassigned to other CPR tasks.

In the presence of high airway resistance, Melker and Banner observed a dramatic improvement of volume delivered to an adult lung model when inspiratory time was lengthened from 0.5 to 2.0 sec.[90] The improvement created by lengthening inspiratory time was lost when the lung compliance fell below 0.04 L/cmH_2O.[90] The noteworthy study by Ornato reported that pulmonary edema during resuscitation causes a drop in compliance to 0.022 L/cmH_2O, and the peak inspiratory pressure required to deliver a tidal volume of 936 ± 322 mL is 43 ± 8 cmH_2O.[91]

The use of a mask with a soft, partially inflated balloon placed along the rim of the mask reduces leaks.[92] When the appropriate size and type of mask is used to ventilate an infant, the size of the bag (infant, child, or adult) does not affect the rate or volume delivered to the lung.[93] It takes an experienced neonatal practitioner to use a Mapleson type D anesthesia bag (Fig. 22-34) to ventilate an infant. The anesthesia bag tends to collapse due to poor mask fit, low source gas flow, and incorrect adjustment of the pressure release valve. The best ventilation of infants by inexperienced resuscitators usually occurs when self-inflatable bag-valve devices are used.[85] A Mapleson type D anesthesia bag-valve device can be

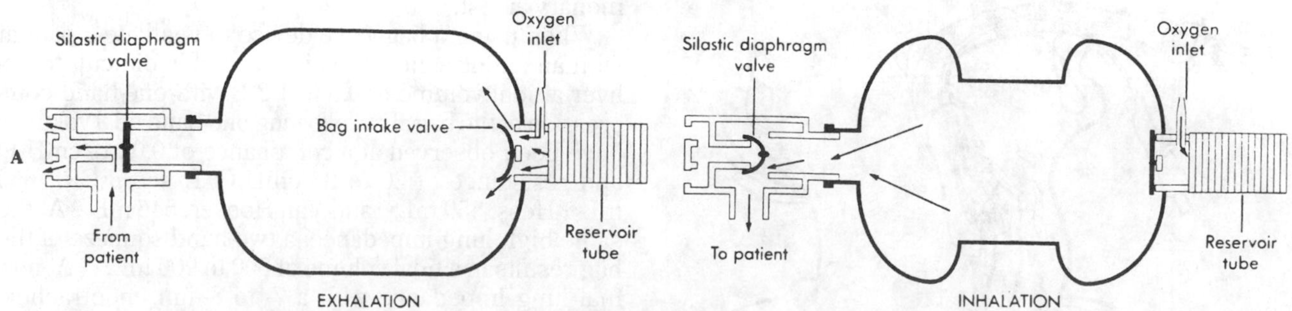

FIGURE 22-33. Manual resuscitator with gas intake valve located at the bottom of the bag. (McPherson SP: Respiratory Therapy Equipment, 4th ed., p. 135. St. Louis, Mosby–Year Book, 1990. Reproduced with permission.)

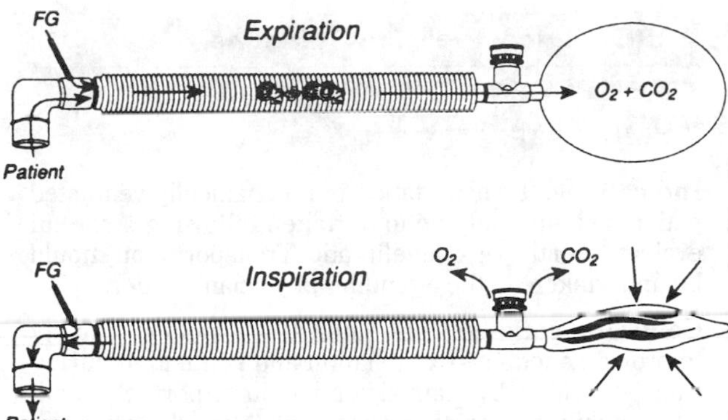

FIGURE 22-34. Mapleson D system. During expiration fresh gas (FG) flushes CO_2 and O_2 to the reservoir bag. During inspiration fresh gas is delivered to the patient and the contents of the reservoir bag exit through a pressure-relief valve. (Thompson JE, Farrel E, McManus M: Neonatal and pediatric airway emergencies. Respir Care 37:585, 1992. Reproduced with permission.)

used effectively during resuscitation by practitioners who use the bag routinely to ventilate neonatal patients.

Resuscitators for adult and pediatric patients should not have a pressure-limiting system. Some neonatal resuscitators have a pressure relief valve with an opening pressure of 40 cmH_2O. The 40 cmH_2O pressure limit should not be exceeded during normal ventilation conditions, but an override mechanism should be provided for times when lung impedance is high and the patient has a tracheal tube in place. The override mechanism must be designed so that its operating mode is readily apparent to the user.[94,95]

The ASTM and ISO standards for bag-valve devices used with infants require a release valve to limit peak inspiratory pressure (PIP).[79,80] This pop-off valve (POV) must provide an audible signal that gas is being vented, have a mechanism for overriding the POV, and visually indicate when the POV is on or off. The POV limit required by the ASTM standard is 40 ± 10 cmH_2O for children and 40 ± 5 cmH_2O for infants,[79] and the ISO standard specifies that the pressure should not exceed 45 cmH_2O for neonates and infants.[80] Some POV valves have been shown to vent gas at pressure varying from 38 to 106 cmH_2O.[96,97] The venting of gas through the POV reduces the FIO_2 significantly and lowers the tidal volume produced by one third to one half that produced when the POV is turned off.[97] Bag-valve ventilation by competent practitioners with an in-line manometer and without a POV (or with the POV turned off) may be safer for neonates, especially for delivery of the first breaths of a neonate's nonaerated lung, when higher pressures may be needed.[98] The PIP during ventilation with a Mapleson type D bag has been compared to PIP during mechanical ventilation. The PIP values delivered without a manometer were significantly higher than those delivered with a manometer.[99]

Practitioners using pressure manometers to monitor PIP during infant bag-valve ventilation need to ensure that the manometer is accurate at rates over 40 breaths per minute because some manometers underestimate the actual pressure.[100] As an alternative to solely pressure-monitored bag-valve ventilation, a neonatal volume-controlled resuscitator has been developed (Fig. 22-35). Studies report that the device is capable of providing adequate ventilation at lower mean airway pressure.[101–103] Lung rupture in the newborn infant has been reported at a relatively low PIP of 35 cmH_2O, suggesting that bag-valve ventilation cannot be regulated rationally by looking at airway pressure or delivered tidal volume, but must be monitored for adequacy of ventilation by observation of chest movement and by blood gas analysis.[104,105]

Resuscitation of newborns at birth often involves bag-valve-mask ventilation and, if correctly administered, spares the infant from the possible hazards associated with intubation.[104,106,107] The critical components for effective use include a self-expanding bag of suitable volume to compensate for face-mask leaks (450 to 750 mL),[108] properly functioning nonrebreathing and pressure-limiting valves, and a circular face mask.

A hard, molded mask (Rendall-Baker) should not be used to ventilate infants because it does not easily fit the contours of the baby's face, and leakage occurs.[109] Peak pressure was less than 80% of the opening pressure in 57% of the trials when a Rendall-Baker mask was used to ventilate a 1- to 2-day-old newborn, compared with a 4% failure rate for a soft circular mask.[109] Problems related to creating a seal with a mask may require tracheal intubation for resuscitation at birth. None of the initial three inflations delivered by bag-valve-mask device were adequate (4.4 mL/kg body weight was required) in a series of 200 resuscitations

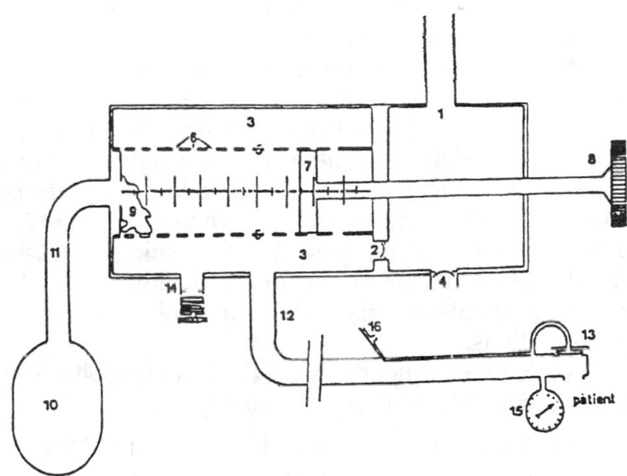

FIGURE 22-35. Schematic of the volume-controlled device for neonatal manual resuscitation. 1—Gas flow reservoir box, 2—one-way gas intake valve, 3—pressure chamber, 4—reservoir box gas outflow valve, 5—fixed graduated cylinder, 6—small holes that perforate graduated cylinder, 7—plunger-type platform for volume adjustment, 8—handle for volume adjustment plunger, 9—inflatable latex balloon, 10—squeeze bag, 11—tube connecting bag to latex balloon, 12—patient circuit, 13—patient valve with adjustable PEEP, 14—adjustable pressure-release valve, 15—pressure manometer, and 16—adjustable PEEP control. (Tiffin NH, Gallant JH, Pasquet EA, Kissoon N, Frewen TC: A neonatal volume controlled resuscitator. RRT 24(1):15, 1988. Reproduced with permission.)

at birth (no breathing after 1 minute), whereas 37% of the tidal volumes delivered to intubated infants met the criteria.[110] A prolonged and slow-rising inflation (3 to 5 seconds) in the resuscitation of the asphyxiated newborn has been reported to be more effective in producing a larger inflation volume than that seen during conventional 1-second square-wave inflation.[111,112] Healthy, full-term neonates at birth rarely show an inspiratory opening pressure of more than 10 cmH_2O.[113] However, some infants, particularly premature infants[114] and babies born by cesarean section,[115] may need ventilating pressures higher than 30 cmH_2O before they respond to resuscitation. Very low lung compliance of 0.3 mL/cmH_2O has been observed at birth with a premature infant, and it was still only 0.6 mL/cmH_2O after 1 minute.[114] To adequately ventilate infants with very low compliance, POV valves on self-inflatable bag-valve devices must be able to be turned off.

□ AUTOMATIC TRANSPORT VENTILATORS

Studies comparing the use of automatic transport ventilators (ATVs) with bag valve devices during intrahospital transport show that ATVs are better at maintaining adequate tidal and minute ventilation.[39] Manual resuscitators can also be effective if tidal and minute ventilation are monitored with a respirometer. However, some bag-valve devices do not have exhalation ports that allow respirometers to be easily attached. The use of ATVs provides a way to control inspiratory time, flow, tidal and minute volume, ventilatory frequency, and peak inspiratory pressure (AARC Clinical Practice Guideline: Transport of the Mechanically Ventilated Patient). In the United States, the ATVs are not used as often during resuscitation for cardiac arrest as in Europe, because Americans are concerned with coordinating ventilation with external chest compression. However, some ATVs allow for manual triggering of inspiration, which helps the rescuers synchronize ventilation with chest compressions. Once the patient is intubated, it is unnecessary to synchronize ventilation with chest compressions. Accordingly, ATVs should be used more often in the United States to ensure adequate ventilation and oxygenation during resuscitations.

The AHA recommends that ATVs have the following minimum functional characteristics:[39]

- A lightweight connector with a standard 15/22-mm connector coupling for a mask, endotracheal tube, or other airway adjunct
- A lightweight (2 to 5 kg), compact, rugged design
- Capability of operating under all common environmental conditions and extremes of temperature
- A peak inspiratory pressure limiting valve set at 60 cmH_2O, with an option of an 80 cmH_2O limit, that is easily accessible to the user
- An audible alarm that sounds when the peak inspiratory limiting pressure is generated to alert the rescuer that low compliance or high airway resistance is resulting in a diminished tidal volume delivery
- Minimal gas consumption (eg, at a tidal volume of 1 L and a rate of 10 breaths per minute, the device should run for a minimum of 45 minutes on an E cylinder)
- Minimal gas compression volume in the breathing circuit
- Ability to deliver an FIO_2 of 1.0
- An inspiratory time of 2 seconds in adults and 1 second in children, and maximal inspiratory flow rates of approximately 30 L/min in adults and 15 L/min in children (ATVs are unsuitable in children younger than 5 years of age)
- At least two rates, 10 breaths per minute for adults and 20 breaths per minute for children

AARC Clinical Practice Guideline

TRANSPORT OF THE MECHANICALLY VENTILATED PATIENT

Indications: Transportation of mechanically ventilated patients should only be undertaken following a careful evaluation of the risk-benefit ratio. Transportation should be undertaken on the attending physician's order.

Contraindications: Contraindications include inability to provide adequate oxygenation and ventilation during transport either by manual ventilation or portable ventilator, inability to maintain acceptable hemodynamic performance during transport, inability to adequately monitor patient's cardiopulmonary status during transport, inability to maintain airway control during transport. Transport should not be undertaken unless all the necessary members of the transport team are present.

Assessment of Need: The necessity for transport should be assessed by the attending physician. The risks of transport should be weighed against the potential benefits from the diagnostic or therapeutic procedure to be performed.

Assessment of Outcome: The safe arrival of the mechanically ventilated patient at the destination is the indicator of a favorable outcome.

Monitoring: Monitoring provided during transport should be similar to that during stationary care. Electrocardiograph should be continuously monitored for signs of dysrhythmias. Heart rate should be monitored continuously. Blood pressure should be monitored continuously if invasive lines are present. In the absence of invasive monitoring, blood pressure should be measured intermittently by means of sphygmomanometer. Respiratory rate should be monitored intermittently. Airway pressures should be monitored if a transport ventilator is used. Tidal volume should be monitored intermittently to assure appropriate ventilation. Continuous pulse oximetry may be useful in patients with borderline respiratory function. Breath sounds should be monitored intermittently.

From AARC Clinical Practice Guideline; see Respir Care 38: 1169, 1993, for complete text.

- If demand flow is incorporated into the ATV, it should deliver a peak inspiratory flow of 100 L/min at − 2 cmH_2O triggering pressure to minimize the work of breathing.

Problems that may occur with ATVs include gastric distension with unintubated patients, and a loss of the gas supply may make it inoperative. Accordingly, a manual resuscitator should always be available as a backup.

Three examples of ATVs are Life Support Products Autovent models 2000 and 3000 and Bio-Med Devices IC-2A. A brief description of each ATV summarizes the functional design of each device.

□ LIFE SUPPORT PRODUCTS AUTOVENT 2000 AND 3000

The LSP Autovent models 2000 and 3000 are time-cycled ventilators, both with a constant flow (rectangular) inspiratory waveform. The modes are controlled ventilation or intermittent mandatory ventilation (IMV), with the patient able to take spontaneous breaths (of ambient air) between the machine breaths by generation of −2 cmH_2O pressure. Ambient air augments the inspiratory flow if the patient's inspiratory flow exceeds the 48 L/min of gas supplied by the ventilator. The ventilators weigh 24 ounces and are compact in size (Fig. 22-36). They require gas supplied at 40 to 90 psig. The ventilators have an operating temperature range of −35° to +53°C. Controls include rate and tidal volume (LSP 2000) or ventilatory frequency, tidal volume, and inspiratory time (LSP 3000). The LSP 2000 is intended for patients weighing at least 40 kg; the LSP 3000, at least 20 kg. The patient valve assembly has a dead space of 8 mL. Table 22-5 lists the range for controls and other parameters.

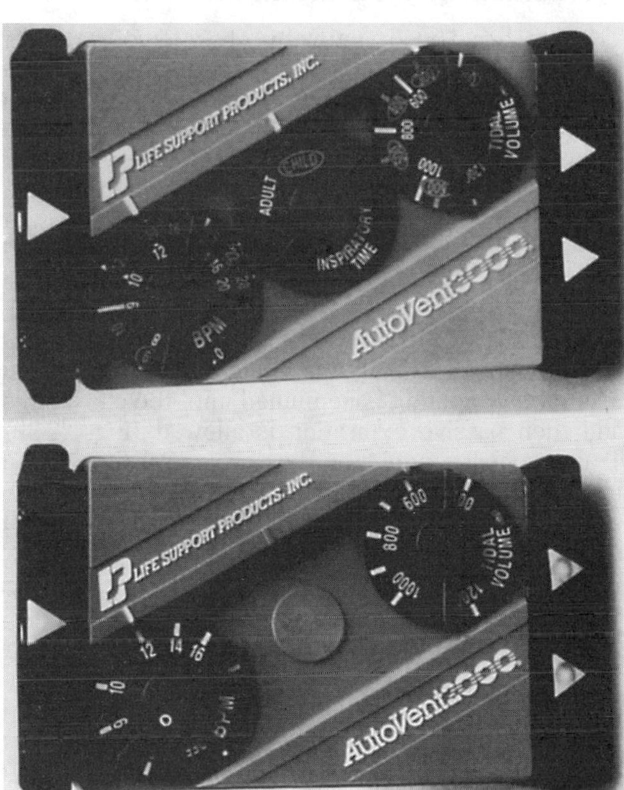

FIGURE 22-36. LSP Autovent 2000 and 3000 portable ventilators. (Courtesy of Life Support Products Inc., Irvine, Calif.)

□ BIO-MED DEVICES IC-2A

The IC-2A (Fig. 22-37) is a time-cycled, constant flow generator with SIMV, IPPV, CPAP, and manual modes; it has built-in PEEP. The IC-2A is about 10 inches high, 6 inches wide, and 3 inches deep and weighs about 9 pounds. It has controls for inspiratory time, expiratory time, flow rate, sensitivity, PEEP, manual breath, SIMV or IPPV, cycle or manual, CPAP, on or off, and maximum pressure (located on the rear panel). There are no integral alarms on the IC-2A; therefore, the respiratory care practitioner must always connect external alarms when the ventilator is operated without direct observation. The IC-2A operates from two sources of 50 ± 5 psig gas—one 100% oxygen for the logic control system, the other from a blender for patient gas. (Note that malfunction of the ventilator occurs if either gas supply is <35 or >80 psig.) Table 22-6 lists the ranges of the controls.[116]

Emergency Cricothyrotomy

An emergency *cricothyrotomy* is indicated when upper airway obstruction cannot be relieved and an endotracheal tube cannot be inserted.[117,118] The problem may result from aspiration of a foreign object or other causes of upper airway obstruction such as laryngeal edema, epiglottitis, or trauma. This situation is evident when mouth-to-mouth, mouth-to-nose, and ventilation with a manual resuscitator do not result in lung inflation. If repositioning of the airway and pushing the mandible

TABLE 22-5 **Range of Controls and Parameters for LSP 2000 and 3000**

	LSP 2000	LSP 3000
Respiratory rate (breaths/min)	8–20	8–28
Tidal volume (mL)	400–1200	200–1200
Inspiratory flow rate (L/min)	16–48	16–48
Inspiratory time (sec)	1.5	0.75 or 1.5
Expiratory time (sec)	1.5–6.0	1.5–6.0
I:E	1:1 to 1:4	1:1 to 1:4
Gas consumption (L/min)	≤0.5	≤0.5
Pressure limit (cmH_2O)	50 ± 5	50 ± 5

Reproduced with permission from Fluck RR: Intermittent Positive Pressure Breathing Devices and Transport Devices. In Barnes TA (ed): Core Textbook in Respiratory Care Practice, 2nd ed. St. Louis, Mosby–Year Book, 1994.

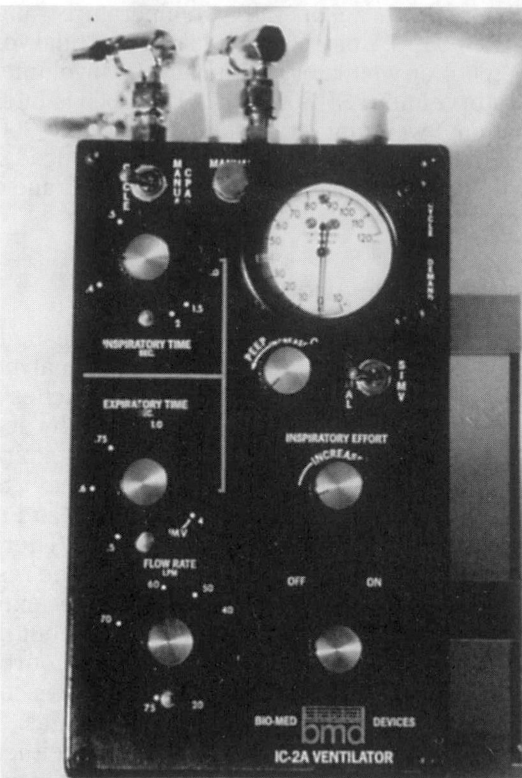

FIGURE 22-37. Bio-Med IC-2A portable ventilator. (Courtesy of BioMed Devices, Inc. Madison, Conn.)

TABLE 22-6 **Ranges of Controls for Bio-Med IC-2A**

Inspiratory time (sec)	0.4–2.0
Expiratory time (sec)	0.5–4.0 (may be set to more than 45 in SIMV)
Flow rate (L/min)	0–75
PEEP (cmH_2O)	0–25 ± 5
Maximum pressure (cmH_2O)	0–120 ± 20
Logic gas consumption (L/min)	12
Respiratory rate (breaths/min)	1.33–66
Tidal volume (mL)	0–3000
I:E	1:10 to 4:1
Sensitivity	Not specified

Reproduced with permission from Fluck RR: Intermittent Positive Pressure Breathing Devices and Transport Devices. In Barnes TA (ed): Core Textbook in Respiratory Care Practice, 2nd ed. St. Louis, Mosby–Year Book, 1994.

forward do not relieve obstruction and an endotracheal tube still cannot be placed, a cricothyrotomy is done. A cricothyrotomy is the procedure of choice in emergency situations, because the cricothyroid membrane is easily located, and it is the safest point of entry.[118] This portion of the airway is thin and relatively avascular, which limits the risk of hemorrhage. The chance of vocal cord damage is also minimal because the membrane is below the cords. The cricothyroid space is large enough to place at least a 6-mm endotracheal tube for ventilation.

The patient is positioned so the neck is fully extended and the larynx is prominent. The thyroid cartilage is located, and the finger is moved downward until the cricoid cartilage is palpated. The cricoid is a ridged structure just below the thyroid cartilage. A horizontal, midline incision is made between the two cartilages. The edges of the incision are separated and the membrane is cut horizontally just above the cricoid cartilage (Fig. 22-38). A tube is then inserted to maintain an open airway.[117] A cricothyrotomy should take less than a minute to complete, and the most experienced person available should perform this procedure. However, the respiratory therapist should thoroughly understand the emergency techniques so they may be performed safely and successfully in a life-threatening situation. An alternative to making an incision into the membrane is puncturing it with a large bore needle (14 to 16 gauge). The needle puncture procedure can be done easily by inexperienced therapists and may be lifesaving while waiting for a physician to arrive. Needle puncture allows easy access to the airway but has limited effectiveness for ventilation. Therefore, an incision is made and a tracheal tube inserted as soon as possible.

Transtracheal Jet Ventilation

Transtracheal jet ventilation may be a temporary alternative to a cricothyrotomy or tracheotomy for emergency ventilation.[20,117] This procedure requires the cricothyroid membrane be punctured with a needle catheter attached to a syringe. The needle is directed caudally at a 45° angle while negative pressure is maintained with the syringe. The return air indicates that the trachea has been entered. The catheter is then advanced, and its hub is attached to an oxygen delivery device. Intravenous tubing is extended from the catheter hub to a 50-psig oxygen outlet. A side hole cut near the distal end of the tubing is occluded by a finger during inspiration. Inflation is continued until the chest rises, and then passive expiration is allowed (Fig. 22-39). Transtracheal cannulation is quick and relatively atraumatic. Possible complications are local bleeding, subcutaneous or mediastinal emphysema, and esophageal injury from incorrect catheter placement.[117]

Circulation

The "C" in the secondary survey corresponds to circulation, which entails establishing IV access, attaching monitor leads, identifying rhythms and rates, measuring blood pressure, and providing rhythm-appropriate and vital-sign-appropriate medications. Respiratory care practitioners play a vital and increasing role in emergency cardiac care. As primary responders on hospital

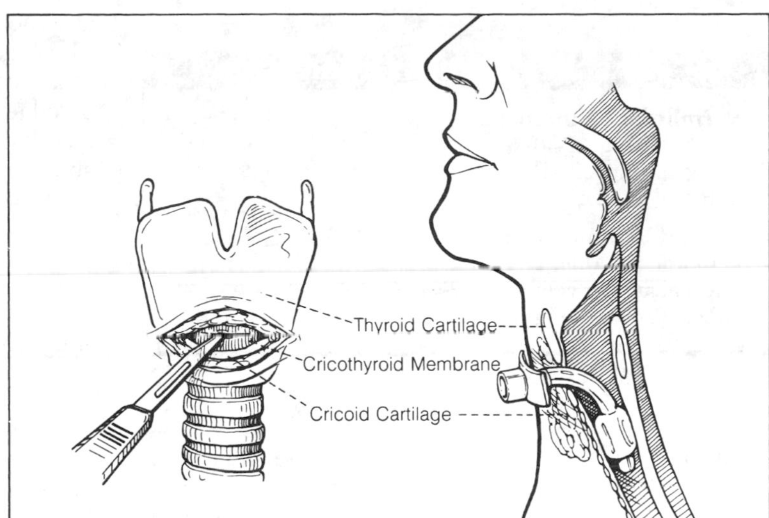

FIGURE 22-38. Emergency cricothyrotomy. (Barnes TA, Watson ME: Cardiopulmonary resuscitation and emergency cardiac care, In Barnes TA (ed), Core Textbook in Respiratory Care Practice, 2nd ed., p. 313. St. Louis, Mosby–Year Book, 1994. Reproduced with permission.)

code and trauma teams, they may make a significant difference in the survival of patients if the knowledge is mastered and effectively applied with the advanced skills that correspond to the "C" in circulation.

□ INTRAVENOUS ACCESS

Along with defibrillation and management of the airway, establishing intravenous (IV) access is one of the key priorities of cardiopulmonary resuscitation. Establishing IV access is essential during resuscitative attempts for several reasons: (1) to administer drugs and fluids, (2) to obtain venous blood for laboratory evaluations, and (3) to insert catheters into the central circulation for physiologic monitoring and electrical pacing.[119] This discussion is limited to a brief overview of selecting an IV access site and the alternative methods for medication administration when an IV site is not available.

□ SELECTION OF AN INTRAVENOUS SITE

If a central line is not in place, cannulation of a large, easily accessible peripheral vein is recommended because of the speed, ease, and safety with which it can usually be performed (Box 22-4). The site of choice is the antecubital fossa for the following three reasons: (1) the technique is easy to master, (2) antecubital vein cannulation does not interfere with continuing ventilation and chest compressions,[119] and (3) the largest of the su-

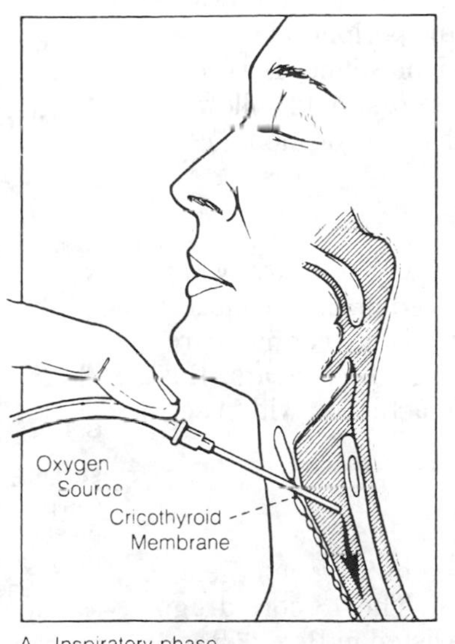

A Inspiratory phase

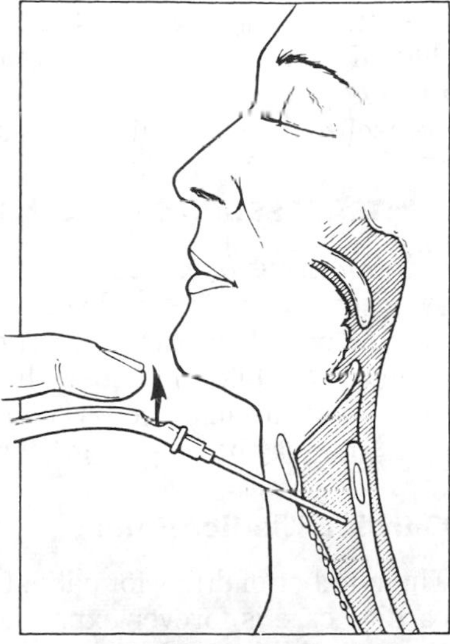

B Passive expiration

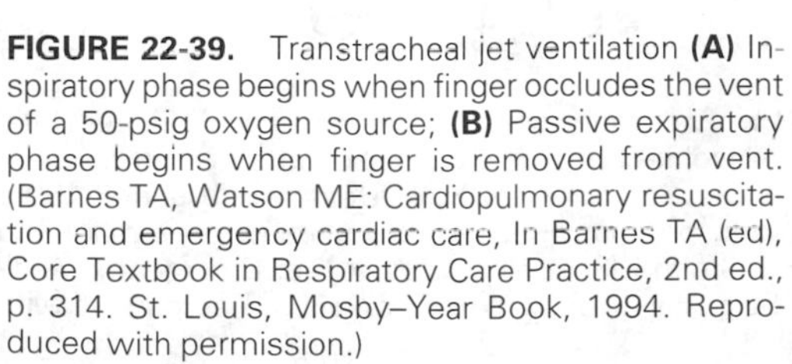

FIGURE 22-39. Transtracheal jet ventilation **(A)** Inspiratory phase begins when finger occludes the vent of a 50-psig oxygen source; **(B)** Passive expiratory phase begins when finger is removed from vent. (Barnes TA, Watson ME: Cardiopulmonary resuscitation and emergency cardiac care, In Barnes TA (ed), Core Textbook in Respiratory Care Practice, 2nd ed., p. 314. St. Louis, Mosby–Year Book, 1994. Reproduced with permission.)

BOX 22-4

VASCULAR ACCESS CHOICES

Peripheral Venipuncture
Arm vein (Fig. 22-40)
Leg vein (Fig. 22-41)
External jugular vein (Fig. 22-42)

Central Venipuncture
Femoral vein (Fig. 22-43)
Internal jugular vein (Fig. 22-44)
Subclavian vein (Fig. 22-45)

perficial veins of the arm are located in the antecubital fossa.[119] Although peripheral vessels may collapse during low-flow states making access difficult, once established they usually provide an effective route for drugs if the access site is elevated and flushed with a 20- to 30-mL bolus of IV fluid following drug administrations.

Central line cannulation offers some advantages over peripheral sites, but it is not without problems. The large size and greater flow of central vessels permits passage of large-bore catheters and infusion of solutions that would irritate peripheral vessels. Drugs delivered to a central vein reach the central circulation much faster than by peripheral site administration. The primary disadvantage of central venous cannulation is an increased complication rate, such as damage to adjacent structures, pneumothorax, air embolus, and hemorrhage from noncompressible sites.

□ ENDOTRACHEAL TUBE INSTILLATION

When IV access is not available, the endotracheal tube provides a route for administration of certain drugs. The mnemonic *ALE* can be used to remember the medications that can be administered via the ET tube: atropine, lidocaine, and epinephrine.[2] Although the optimal dosing strategy for endotracheal delivery is unknown, a dose that is at least 2 to 2.5 times the peripheral IV dose, diluted in 10 mL of sterile water or saline, is recommended. Several quick insufflations should follow to aerosolize the medication and hasten absorption.[120,121]

□ INTRAOSSEOUS INFUSION

Intraosseous infusion of drugs is an alternative when IV access cannot be readily achieved during resuscitation of pediatric patients. Primarily a technique reserved for children under the age of 6 years, this method of vascular access can be achieved within seconds and may be lifesaving.[2,121]

Cardiac Medications

The number of drugs for patients requiring emergency cardiac care is forever expanding. The 18 core drugs taught in AHA ACLS courses are listed in Box 22-5 and are each reviewed in Boxes 22-6 through Box 22-22. The American Heart Association has achieved an enormous educational success with their continually updated textbooks on basic life support and advanced cardiac life support. The reader requiring greater detail should refer to standard pharmacology textbooks or the

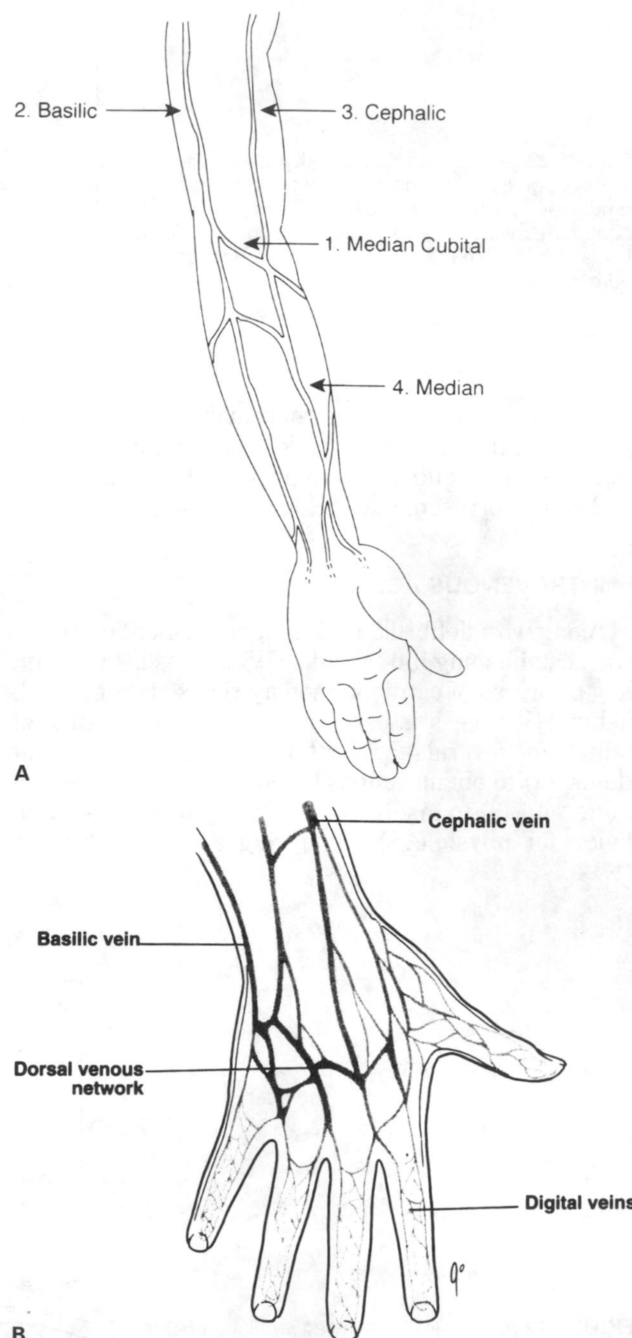

FIGURE 22-40. Vascular access via arm veins **(A)** Antecubital venipuncture. (Hoeltke LB: The Clinical Laboratory Manual Series: Phlebotomy, p. 54. Albany, New York, Delmar Publishers, 1995. Reproduced with permission); **(B)** Venipuncture of dorsal hand vein. (Snell RS, Smith MS: Clinical Anatomy for Emergency Medicine, p. 149. St. Louis, Mosby–Year Book 1993. Reproduced with permission.)

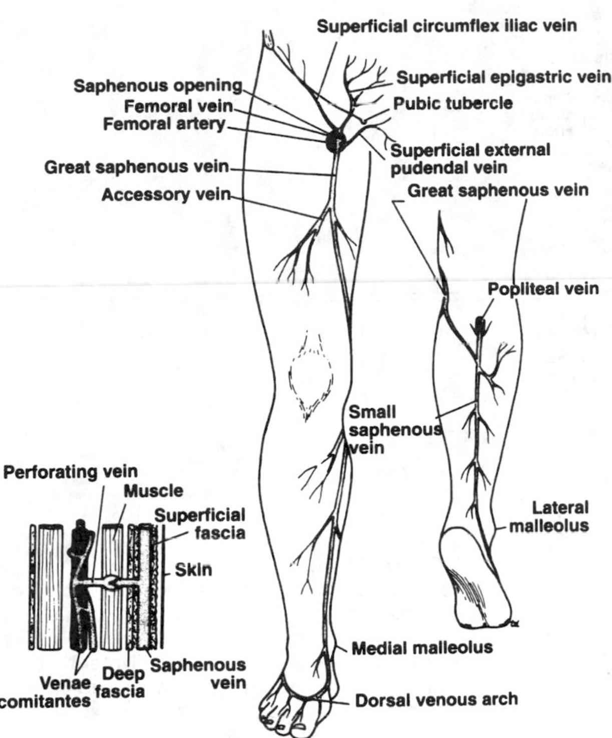

FIGURE 22-41. Superficial veins of the right lower limb. (Snell RS, Smith MS: Clinical Anatomy for Emergency Medicine, p. 557. St. Louis, Mosby–Year Book 1993. Reproduced with permission.)

AHA ACLS textbook for information beyond the basics of the overview presented in this chapter. This chapter's cardiac medications reference the AHA textbooks and are consistent with their approach, which lists the following four things to consider for each pharmacologic agent:

- *Why* an agent is used? (Actions)
- *When* to use an agent? (Indications)
- *How* to use an agent? (Dosing)
- What to *watch out* for? (Precautions)

To offer the simplest method for classifying and prioritizing the often complex therapeutic interventions in emergency cardiac care, the 1992 National Conference on CPR and ECC used a new classification system, based on the strength of the supporting scientific evidence. These classifications include:

- Class I: acceptable, definitely helpful
- Class IIa: acceptable, probably helpful
- Class IIb: acceptable, possibly effective
- Class III: not indicated, may be harmful

□ THROMBOLYTICS

Thrombolytic agents dissolve clots and are Class I agents in acute myocardial infarction when there is evidence of coronary thrombosis with no exclusionary cri-

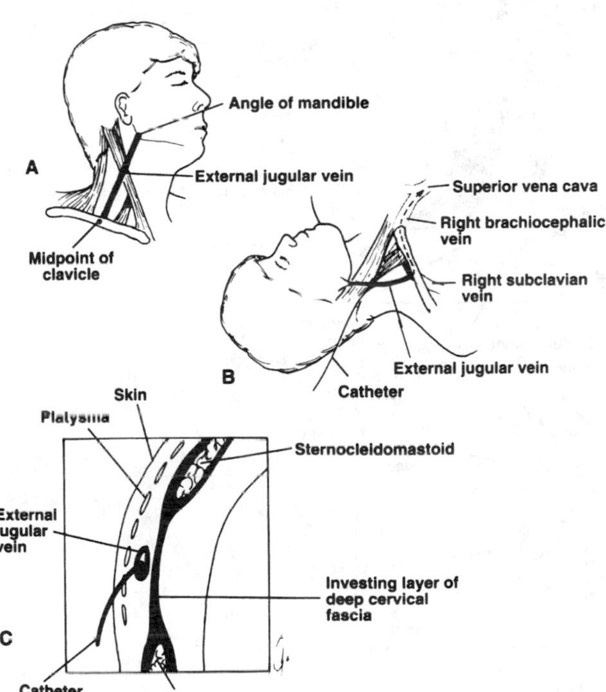

FIGURE 22-42. Catheterization of the right external jugular vein. **(A)** Surface marking of the vein. **(B)** Site of catheterization. **(C)** Cross section of neck showing relationships of external jugular vein as it crosses the posterior triangle of the neck. (Snell RS, Smith MS: Clinical Anatomy for Emergency Medicine, p. 195. St. Louis, Mosby–Year Book 1993. Reproduced with permission.)

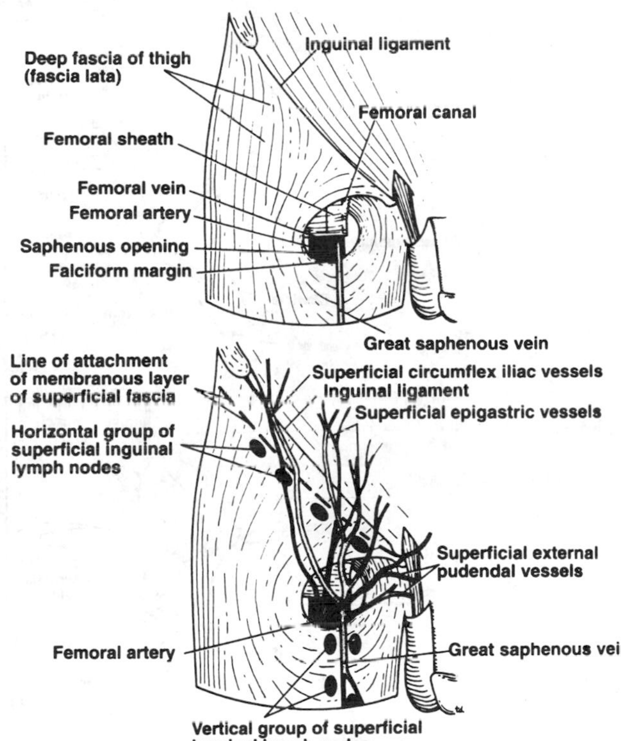

FIGURE 22-43. Superficial veins, arteries, and lymph nodes on the front of the right thigh. (Snell RS, Smith MS: Clinical Anatomy for Emergency Medicine, p. 558. St. Louis, Mosby–Year Book 1993. Reproduced with permission.)

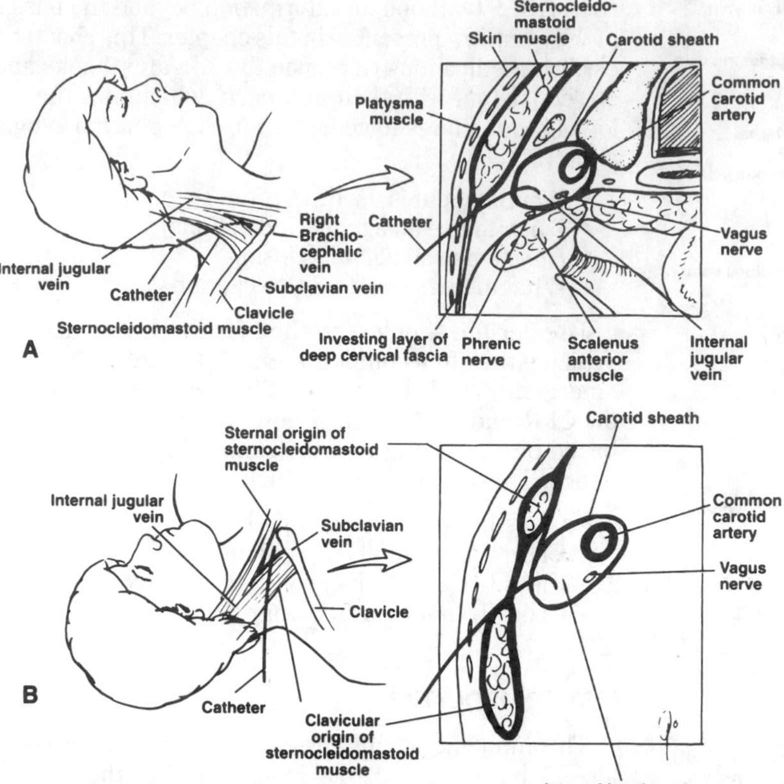

FIGURE 22-44. Catheterization of the right internal jugular vein. **(A)** Posterior approach. Note the position of the catheter relative to the sternocleidomastoid muscle and the common carotid artery. **(B)** Anterior approach. Note that the catheter is inserted into the vein close to the apex of the triangle formed by the sternal and clavicular heads of the sternocleidomastoid muscle and the clavicle. (Snell RS, Smith MS: Clinical Anatomy for Emergency Medicine, p. 198. St. Louis, Mosby–Year Book 1993. Reproduced with permission.)

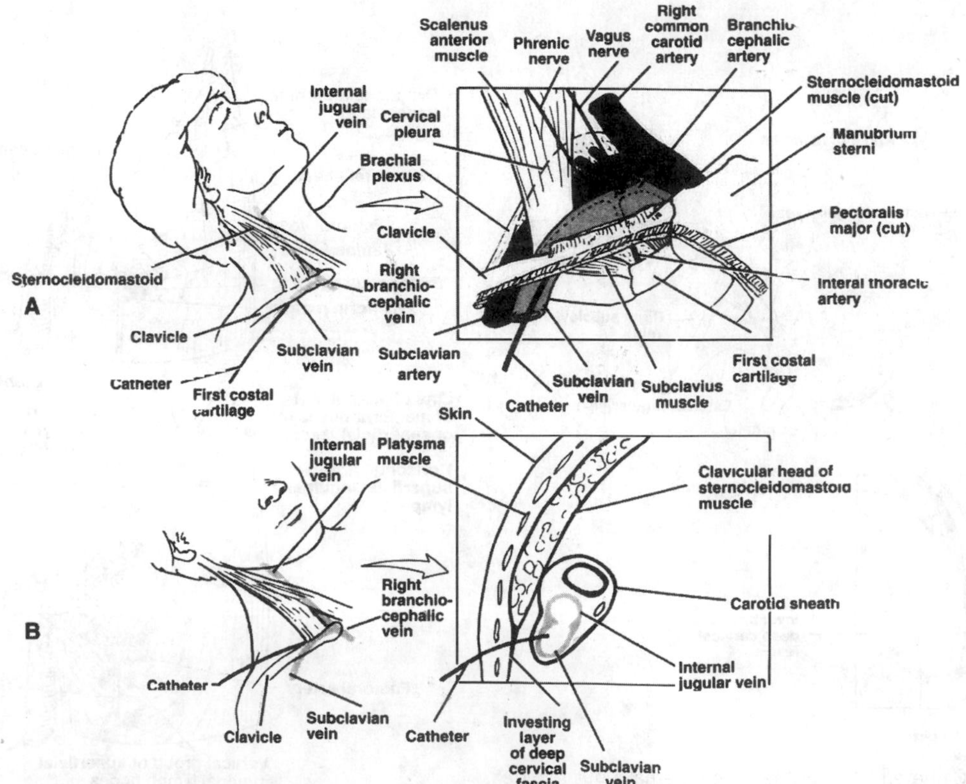

FIGURE 22-45. Subclavian vein catheterization. **(A)** Infraclavicular approach. Note the many important anatomical structures located in this region. **(B)** Superclavicular approach. The catheter enters the subclavian vein close to its junction with the internal vein to form the brachiocephalic vein. (Snell RS, Smith MS: Clinical Anatomy for Emergency Medicine, p. 161. St. Louis, Mosby–Year Book 1993. Reproduced with permission.)

teria. They should ideally be administered within the first 6 hours of the onset of symptoms. There is no absolute age limit for thrombolytic therapy. Thrombolytic therapy conveys the most benefit for patients older than 70 years of age; however, the risk of intracerebral bleeding also increases with age. The thrombolytic agents currently available in the United States include anistreplase, or anisoylated plasminogen streptokinase activator complex (APSAC); streptokinase; urokinase; and recombinant tissue-type plasminogen activator (t-PA, Alteplase).

ECG Monitoring

The initiation of ECG monitoring is a vital step in the treatment of patients who are in a state of cardiopulmonary compromise or are found unresponsive. As first responders, respiratory care practitioners must identify critical medical conditions that, if unrecognized or untreated, can lead to full cardiac arrest or death. After assessing the ABCs, the ECG monitor display leads the rescue team to the next step. No matter what setting, early defibrillation is the single most important intervention in adult resuscitation. If ECG monitoring is delayed for any reason, the initial tachyarrhythmia causing 80% to 90% of nontraumatic cardiac arrests in adults deteriorates to a nonviable rhythm.[122,123]

□ ATTACHING MONITORING LEADS

Electrical flow in the heart can be measured by externally applied electrodes that transmit the information to an electrocardiogram. Any two points on the body may be connected by electrical leads to register an ECG, but standardization is crucial, otherwise the

BOX 22-5

CORE ACLS DRUGS

Adenosine (Box 22-6)
Atropine (Box 22-7)
Beta-blockers (propranolol, metoprolol, atenolol, esmolol) (Box 22-8)
Bretylium (Box 22-9)
Calcium channel blockers (diltiazem, verapamil, nifedipine) (Box 22-10)
Dobutamine (Box 22-11)
Dopamine (Box 22-12)
Epinephrine (Box 22-13)
Furosemide (Box 22-14)
Isoproterenol (Box 22-15)
Lidocaine (Box 22-16)
Magnesium sulfate (Box 22-17)
Morphine sulfate (Box 22-18)
Nitroglycerin (Box 22-19)
Nitroprusside (Box 22-20)
Procainamide (Box 22-21)
Sodium bicarbonate (Box 22-22)
Thrombolytics (streptokinase, urokinase, anistreplase [APSAC], alteplase [t-PA])

BOX 22-6

ADENOSINE

Actions
Slows conduction through the AV node
Interrupts AV-nodal reentry pathways
Can restore normal sinus rhythm in patients with PSVT

Indications
Drug of choice (Class I) for hemodynamically stable PSVT
Second agent to use for wide-complex tachycardia of uncertain type, after two doses of lidocaine

Dosage (Stable Tachycardia)
First dose of 6-mg rapid IV bolus over 1–3 seconds, follow with saline flush
Second dose of 12-mg rapid IV bolus in 1–2 min, if necessary; 12-mg bolus may be repeated once after 1–2 minutes, if necessary

Precautions
A brief period of asystole (up to 15 seconds) is common after rapid administration
Flushing, dyspnea, and chest pain are transient but frequently observed
PSVT may recur
Cardiac transplant recipients are more sensitive to adenosine and may require only a small dose

BOX 22-7

ATROPINE

Actions
Parasympatholytic
Accelerates sinus node rate
Improves AV conduction
May restore rhythm in asystole

Indications
Initial drug of choice in symptomatic bradycardia
Asystolic cardiac arrest patients
PEA patients, but only when they have slow electrical activity

Dosage
Patients not in cardiac arrest: 0.5–1.0 mg IV repeated every 3–5 min, maximum of 0.03–0.04 mg/kg (about 2–3 mg)
Patients with cardiac arrest or PEA: 1.0 mg IV repeated every 3–5 minutes, 3.0 mg (0.04 mg/kg) is a fully vagolytic dose
Administration of atropine in doses < 0.5 mg can produce a paradoxical bradycardia
ET administration: 1.0–2.0 mg diluted to a total ≤ 10 mL with normal saline

Precautions
Atropine should not be given if bradycardia is not associated with symptoms (chest pain, dyspnea, lightheadedness, hypotension, or ventricular ectopy)
Increased myocardial oxygen demand
Ventricular tachycardia or fibrillation, although unlikely
Less effective in infranodal blocks
Unlikely to be effective in denervated hearts

BOX 22-8

BETA-BLOCKERS (PROPRANOLOL, METOPROLOL, ATENOLOL, ESMOLOL)

Actions

Attenuate the effects of circulating catecholamines by blocking their ability to bind to β-adrenergic receptors

Reduce heart rate, blood pressure, myocardial contractility, and myocardial oxygen consumption

Indications

For rate control in stable tachycardias such as atrial fibrillation or flutter

Acute MI with excess sympathetic activity (elevated heart rate and blood pressure)

Large MI treated early (less than 6 hours of pain)

Refractory chest pain or tachycardias due to excessive sympathetic tone

Dosage

Metoprolol: 5-mg IV infusion (slowly), every 5 min to a total of 15 mg

Atenolol: 5-mg IV infusion (over 5 min); wait 10 min, then give second dose of 5 mg IV (over 5 min)

Propranolol: 1-mg IV (slow) every 5 min to a total of 5 mg

Esmolol: 2.5 g in 250 mL of solution. Loading dose is 250–500 μg/kg for 1 min followed by a maintenance dose of 25–50 μg/kg per min for 4 min

Precautions

Congestive heart failure or pulmonary edema

Bronchospasm or history of asthma

Bradycardia (<50 to 60 beats/min)

Hypotension (systolic BP <100 mmHg)

BOX 22-9

BRETYLIUM

Actions

Antiarrhythmic

Suppresses ventricular ectopy

Elevates the VF threshold

Has transient sympathomimetic effects of elevated blood pressure, heart rate, and cardiac output

Indications

Refractory malignant ventricular arrhythmias

Third drug (after epinephrine and lidocaine) for VF and recurrent VF

Dosage

In VF, 5 mg/kg IV push, repeat in 5 min at 10 mg/kg, to a maximum of 30–35 mg/kg

In stable VT, 5–10 mg/kg over 8–10 min; if continuous drip, maintain at 1–2 mg/min

Precautions

Postural hypotension in the non–cardiac arrest patient

Nausea and vomiting with rapid IV injection in a conscious person, but for cardiac arrest it must be given by rapid bolus

BOX 22-10

CALCIUM CHANNEL BLOCKERS (DILTIAZEM, VERAPAMIL, NIFEDIPINE

Actions

Dilates coronary arteries

Dilates peripheral arteries

Depresses AV and SA node activity

Increases flow to ischemic areas

Slows heart rate

Reduces afterload

Overall, reduces ischemia and infarction

Indications

Diltiazem decreases sinoatrial and AV conduction and dilates coronary arteries. It is used for atrial fibrillation and angina.

Verapamil is a potent AV nodal depressor and thus is used for PSVT; however, because of its shorter duration of action, adenosine is preferable in PSVT.

Nifedipine is a powerful arterial dilator and thus is used for hypertensive emergencies; however, poor control of response makes it relatively contraindicated in acute MI.

Use of calcium channel blockers for unstable angina is a Class I recommendation.

Use of calcium channel blockers as a cardioprotective agent for non-Q-wave infarction is a Class IIa recommendation.

Use of calcium channel blockers for postinfarction angina is a Class IIb recommendation.

Overall, calcium channel blockers are not routine therapy for all acute MI patients, just for certain subsets.

Dosage

Diltiazem 30 to 60 mg by mouth 3 to 4 times daily

Diltiazem 0.25 mg/kg IV over 2 min; a second bolus of 0.35 mg/kg may be administered in 15 minutes (for PSVT, atrial fibrillation, or flutter conversion)

Verapamil, as a single dose, 2.5–5.0 mg IV, over 2 minutes; the repeat dose is 5–10 mg in 15 to 30 min after the first dose, to a maximum dose of 30 mg

Precautions

Hypotension

Bradycardia

Decreased left ventricular contractility

Signs of left ventricular failure or dysfunction

Giving verapamil to a patient with VT can be a lethal error, as it can accelerate the heart rate and decrease the blood pressure; do not give verapamil to patients with a wide-complex tachycardia unless the tachycardia is known with certainty to be supraventricular in origin.

rhythm strips would be confusing to anyone not familiar with that particular axis. An axis is simply the electrical flow in relation to a direct line between two poles. The locations of a set of electrodes (one negative pole, one positive pole, and one ground) is a lead. There are 12 established leads, each of which has a unique individual axis; some require a combination of electrodes. The four conventional locations for the placement of chest electrodes are illustrated in Figure 22-46*A–D*.

BOX 22-11

DOBUTAMINE

Actions
Synthetic sympathomimetic amine
Increases cardiac output by its direct β-adrenergic action
Directly increases myocardial contractility

Indications
Pulmonary congestion and low cardiac output
Hypotensive patients with pulmonary congestion and left ventricular dysfunction who cannot tolerate vasodilators
Improves left ventricular work in patients with septic shock

Dosage
2 to 20 μg/kg/min

Precautions
Higher doses may produce tachycardia
Dysrhythmias
Fluctuations in blood pressure
Myocardial ischemia, especially if tachycardia is induced
Headache
Nausea
Tremor
Hypokalemia

BOX 22-12

DOPAMINE

Actions
Catecholamine
Precursor of norepinephrine
Alpha- and beta-adrenergic effects
Low-dose dopamine dilates renal and mesenteric arterial beds (dopaminergic effect)

Indications
Dopamine is the first vasopressor recommended for moderate hypotension (systolic BP of 70–100 mmHg)
For hypotension that occurs with severe, symptomatic bradycardia, in the absence of hypovolemia

Dosage
Start at 2.5 μg/kg/min and titrate as needed to 20 μg/kg/min
Low dose (renal dose) 1–5 μg/kg/min
Moderate dose (cardiac dose) 5–10 μg/kg/min
High dose (vasopressor dose) 10–20 μg/kg/min

Precautions
Excessive vasoconstriction
Fall in blood pressure
Arrhythmias
Nausea and vomiting
Extravasation can cause tissue ischemia and sloughing
Effects are dramatically enhanced in conjunction with monoamine oxidase inhibitors or with pheochromocytoma
Taper dose slowly; rapid discontinuation can result in return of bradycardia and profound hypotension

Limb lead II and a modified chest lead I (MCL_1) are the two most commonly used monitoring leads. Lead II is the most traditional monitoring lead, where the positive electrode is below the left pectoral muscle and the negative electrode below the right clavicle (Fig. 22-46*B*). To connect MCL_1, the negative electrode is placed near the left shoulder, usually under the outer third of the left clavicle, and the positive is placed to the right of the sternum in the fourth intercostal space (Fig. 22-46*D*). The ground electrode in all four monitoring leads can usually be placed almost anywhere, but is commonly located below the right pectoral muscle or under the left clavicle. The negative lead is usually white, the positive lead is red, and the ground lead is black, green, or brown. The phrase "white-to-right, red-to-ribs, and black left over" can be used as an aid to remembering where the leads for lead II should be placed.[124]

It is important to remember that monitoring leads should be used for rhythm interpretation only. One should not try to read ST abnormalities or attempt more elaborate ECG interpretation without a 12-lead ECG. When monitoring patients, leads that show the P wave clearly should be used. Artifacts should be noted; a straight line or a bizarre, wavy baseline resembling ventricular fibrillation may appear if an electrode is loose or if the patient moves.[125] And of course, any ECG finding should be correlated with clinical observation and assessment (checking pulses, pressures, and mental status) of the patient.

□ THE NORMAL ELECTROCARDIOGRAM

To differentiate normal from abnormal readings, a basic understanding of the normal ECG rhythm is required. The key to dysrhythmia interpretation is the analysis of the form and interrelations of the P wave, the PR interval, and the QRS complex (Fig. 22-47).

The P wave represents depolarization of the atria, normally as a result of an impulse generated in the sinoatrial (SA) node. The P wave is typically small, rounded, and the first wave of the normal electrocardiographic cycle. It should always be upright in standard lead II with normal sinus rhythm. The PR interval is measured from the start of the P wave to the start of the QRS complex. It should not exceed 0.20 second as measured on ECG paper, where each small square represents 0.04 second. PR intervals less than 0.12 second are abbreviated, and values greater than 0.20 are prolonged. Depolarization of the ventricles produces the QRS complex: a series of waves (Q, R, and S waves) that occur so fast they are measured together. The Q wave is the first negative wave in the QRS complex that precedes the first positive wave. It is not unusual or abnormal for a QRS complex to have no Q wave. The R wave is the first positive wave. Occasionally, a QRS complex has two R waves; the second R wave is called the R-prime wave. The S wave is the first negative wave after

BOX 22-13

EPINEPHRINE

Actions
Sympathomimetic catecholamine with both α- and β-adrenergic agonist activity
Peripheral vasoconstriction
Produces favorable redistribution of blood flow from peripheral to central circulation during CPR

Indications
First drug to use for any pulseless rhythm: VF or VT, asystole, PEA

Dosage
1.0-mg IV push (10 mL of 1:10,000) repeated every 3–5 min
Class IIb dosing regimens may be considered
ET administration: 2.0–2.5 mg diluted in 10 mL of normal saline

Precautions
Increased myocardial oxygen demand
Don't mix with alkaline solution (sodium bicarbonate)
Delayed administration prolongs hypoxia

BOX 22-15

ISOPROTERENOL (ISUPREL)

Actions
Pure β-adrenergic stimulator (β_1 and β_2)
Potent inotropic and chronotropic effects and therefore increases cardiac output

Indications
Class IIa only for refractory torsades de pointes
Class IIa for immediate or temporary control of symptomatic bradycardia in denervated hearts of heart transplant patients
Class IIb only for symptomatic bradycardia while waiting for a pacer and only at low doses
Class III for full arrest and for hypotension

Dosage
Start with 2 μg/min with gradual titration upward, to a maximum of 10 μg/min

Precautions
Ability to induce serious dysrhythmias, including VT and VF
Increases myocardial oxygen consumption
Precipitates hypokalemia

the R wave. The complex is always called the QRS complex even if only one or two of the Q, R, or S waves are present. Normal values for the QRS interval vary, although a wide QRS (≥0.12 second) may imply that conduction arises from the ventricle or from supraventricular tissue, as prolonged conduction through the ventricle produces a widened QRS.

□ SYSTEMATIC APPROACH TO ECG ANALYSIS

The analysis of ECG strips is usually one of two types:[124] (1) sight reading, the technique used by many experienced ECG interpreters who regularly view rhythm strips, or (2) a systematic approach, in which questions are used to assist in the orderly evaluation of the ECG. One such method, recommended by the AHA, is tailored to the setting of cardiac arrest and asks three basic questions:

- Are there normal-looking QRS complexes?
- Are there normal-looking P waves? (or Is there a P wave?)
- What is the relationship between the P waves and QRS complexes?

Students as well as experienced practitioners must be able to immediately interpret the life-threatening dysrhythmias by sight. Other dysrhythmias can be identified by using a systematic approach. In the simplest sense, all rhythm diagnostics can be lumped into two classifications: cardiac arrest (lethal) rhythms and non–cardiac arrest (nonlethal) rhythms.[2]

BOX 22-14

FUROSEMIDE (LASIX)

Actions
Potent, rapidly acting diuretic

Indications
Emergency treatment of pulmonary congestion associated with left ventricular dysfunction

Dosage
20–40 mg IV, injected slowly over at least 1–2 min

Precautions
Dehydration and hypotension
Sodium, potassium, calcium, and magnesium depletion
Hyperosmolality and metabolic alkalosis
Allergic reaction in patients sensitive to sulfonamides

□ DYSRHYTHMIA RECOGNITION

To successfully manage a cardiac arrest, members of the code team should be able to rapidly and accurately diagnose cardiac dysrhythmias. The AHA uses the algorithm approach to emergency cardiac care, an illustrative method that summarizes the recommended interventions for a variety of patient conditions. Seven of the ten algorithms are titled according to the type of dysrhythmia seen on the ECG monitor. A clear understanding of the common dysrhythmias (Box 22-23) is essential for respiratory care practitioners, given their important role in ACLS. This section presents a brief overview of the four cardiac arrest (lethal) rhythms encountered in clinical practice that should be readily

BOX 22-16

LIDOCAINE

Actions

Antiarrhythmic
Suppresses ventricular ectopy
Decreases excitability in ischemic tissue
Elevates VF threshold
Prevents a patient from going into VF or VT

Indications

Class IIa in presence of PVCs, VF, VT
Routine prophylactic use to prevent VF and VT is no longer recommended before thrombolytic therapy or for acute MI patients

Dosage

In VF and VT, 1.5 mg/kg, followed by 1.5 mg/kg bolus in 3–5 min, to a total dose of 3 mg/kg
In stable VT, 1.0–1.5 mg/kg IV push, repeat every 5–10 min at 0.5–0.75 mg/kg IV push, to a total dose of 3 mg/kg; use infusion of 2–4 mg/min after termination of dysrhythmia
For ET administration, use 2 to 2.5 times the IV dose to obtain equivalent blood levels compared to IV administration

Precautions

Clinical indication of toxicity usually CNS related
Muscle twitching
Dizziness
Drowsiness
Slurred speech
Altered consciousness
Decreased hearing
Paresthesias
Seizures
Respiratory arrest
Move quickly to another Class IIa drug during VF or VT if lidocaine has no effect

recognized. Space constraints prevent an exhaustive analysis of all the common dysrhythmias, but several examples of electrocardiograms are provided for the dysrhythmias that are discussed in the ACLS case studies below.

□ CARDIAC ARREST (LETHAL) RHYTHMS

Imminently fatal, *ventricular fibrillation* is the single most important rhythm for the emergency care provider to recognize. If one could observe the heart, the myocardium would appear to be quivering. The ECG displays highly irregular waves of depolarization and repolarization that represent poorly defined QRS complexes. There is no organized ventricular depolarization; therefore, there is no cardiac output and no pulse. The terms coarse and fine are commonly used in reference to the amplitude of the waveforms (Fig. 22-48*A*,*B*). Coarse VF usually indicates the recent onset of VF, leading to fine VF and eventually asystole.

BOX 22-17

MAGNESIUM SULFATE

Actions

Antiarrhythmic
Magnesium affects energy transfer and electrical stability in the myocardium
Magnesium deficiency is associated with cardiac dysrhythmias, cardiac insufficiency, and sudden cardiac death
Magnesium possesses "cardioprotective" effect due to unknown mechanism

Indications

Drug of choice for torsades de pointes
Class I for cardiac arrest with suspected hypomagnesemia
For acute MI with known or suspected magnesium deficiency
Class IIa as a prophylactic antiarrhythmic in acute MI

Dosage

For cardiac arrest or VF, 1–2 g (2–4 mL 50% $MgSO_4$) IV push
For torsades de pointes, 1–2 g over 1–2 minutes
For acute MI prophylaxis, 1–2 g diluted in 100 mL of normal saline, over 5–60 min; follow with 0.5–1.0 g/h sufficient for control or as long as 24 h

Precautions

Too rapid administration may cause flushing, sweating, mild bradycardia, and hypotension
Hypermagnesemia may produce depressed reflexes, flaccid paralysis, circulatory collapse, respiratory paralysis, and diarrhea
Renal failure (adjust prolonged infusions)

Asystole essentially means without contractions or, more accurately, without electrical activity (Fig. 22-49). There are no waves; the rhythm is a flat line on the ECG. However, ventricular asystole, or ventricular standstill, may be present in which P waves may be seen with the complete absence of ventricular electrical activity. In ei-

BOX 22-18

MORPHINE SULFATE

Actions

Manifests both analgesic and hemodynamic effects
Increases venous capacitance and reduces systemic vascular resistance
Decreases myocardial oxygen requirements

Indications

Drug of choice for treatment of pain and anxiety associated with acute MI
Class IIb agent for acute cardiogenic pulmonary edema

Dosage

Small incremental doses of 1–3 mg slow IV (over 1–5 min)

Precautions

Like other narcotic analgesics, it is a respiratory depressant
Hypotension

BOX 22-19

NITROGLYCERIN

Actions

Decreases the pain of ischemia
Increases venous dilation
Decreases venous blood to the heart
Decreases preload and oxygen consumption
Dilates coronary arteries
Increases cardiac collateral flow

Indications

Suspected ischemic chest pain
Unstable angina (change in angina pattern)
Acute pulmonary edema (if systolic BP >100 mmHg)
Used routinely in acute MI (not just for continuing pain)
Elevated blood pressure in setting of acute MI (especially with signs of left ventricular failure)

Dosage

Sublingual, 0.3–0.4 mg, repeat every 5 min
Spray inhaler, repeat every 5 min
Paste, apply 1–2 in. with backing pad
IV infusion, 10–20 μg/min, increase 5–10 μg/min every 5–10 min

Precautions

Use nitroglycerin with extreme caution if systolic blood pressure is less than 90 mmHg
Limit blood pressure drop of 10% if patient is normotensive
Limit blood pressure drop of 30% if patient is hypertensive
Watch for headache, drop in blood pressure, syncope, and tachycardia
Instruct patient to sit or lie down

BOX 22-20

NITROPRUSSIDE

Actions

Direct peripheral vasodilator that decreases systemic vascular resistance (SVR) and increases cardiac output

Indications

Hypertensive emergencies and in congestive heart failure
Left ventricular heart failure

Dosage

0.5–8.0 μg/kg per min

Precautions

Ensure precise flow rate on infusion system
Nitroprusside-induced hypotension
Thiocyanate intoxication

ther case, patients with this rhythm do not have a pulse and are treated the same. If the patient does have a pulse with a "flat line," then the ECG is improperly connected, turned off, or improperly calibrated.

Ventricular tachycardia (Fig. 22-50) usually has a rate range of 100 to 220 beats per minute, although a run of three or more consecutive premature ventricular contractions (PVCs) is also considered ventricular tachycardia. More commonly, this dysrhythmia persists for an extended period of time and is life threatening when associated with hemodynamic compromise. The patient may have a pulse with this rhythm, or she may be pulseless if the fast rate of the tachycardia compromises ventricular filling time and reduces cardiac output. Surprisingly enough, VT can be well tolerated depending on the rate and the presence or absence of myocardial dysfunction. This is clearly a situation in which a rapid assessment is necessary to determine if the patient is stable or unstable. *Hemodynamically unstable* is defined by the following signs and symptoms: chest pain, shortness of breath, decreased level of consciousness, low blood pressure, shock, pulmonary congestion, congestive heart failure, and acute myocardial infarction.[125]

Ventricular tachycardia is differentiated from the supraventricular tachycardias based on the origin of the dysrhythmia; if the origin is above the ventricles (junctional or atrial), the dysrhythmia is supraventricular. Supraventricular tachydysrhythmias are not generally classified as life threatening, but they may lead to hemodynamic decompensation and progress to a lethal rhythm. Supraventricular tachydysrhythmias include sinus tachycardia, atrial tachycardia, atrial flutter, atrial fibrillation, and junctional tachycardia.

Simply said, *pulseless electrical activity* (PEA) is any ECG rhythm, other than VF or VT, in which a pulse cannot be palpated. Typically, the rhythms in this group include electromechanical dissociation (EMD), pseudo-

BOX 22-21

PROCAINAMIDE

Actions

Antiarrhythmic
Suppresses ventricular ectopy and elevates VF threshold

Indications

Class IIa for PVCs, recurrent VT, persistent VF, wide-complex tachycardias that cannot be distinguished from VT
Has prolonged time to reach adequate levels, which is a disadvantage for cardiac arrest

Dosage

20 mg/min, maximum total of 17 mg/kg, until dysrhythmia is suppressed
In urgent situations, as much as 30 mg/min may be given, up to same maximum; maintain at 1–4 mg/min for continuous IV infusion

Precautions

Hypotension and QRS widening, increased PR and QT interval, and AV block
Procainamide is slow to reach therapeutic doses

BOX 22-22

SODIUM BICARBONATE ($NaHCO_3$)

Actions
Buffering agent
May be beneficial in patients with preexisting metabolic acidosis, hyperkalemia, or aspirin overdose

Indications
Class I (definitely helpful) only for preexisting hyperkalemia
Class IIa (probably helpful)
For known preexisting bicarbonate-responsive acidosis
If overdose with tricyclic antidepressants
To alkalinize the urine in some drug overdoses
Class IIb (possibly helpful)
If intubated and long arrest interval
For return of spontaneous pulse after long arrest interval
Class III (may be harmful) in hypoxic lactic acidosis

Dosage
1 mEq/kg initially and repeat ½ dose every 10 min or when ABG indicates a need

Precautions
Increases mixed venous (intracellular) acidosis from CO_2 formation and retention
Enhances chances of hyperosmolality, hypernatremia, metabolic alkalosis, and acute hypokalemia

EMD, idioventricular rhythms, ventricular escape rhythms, and bradyasystolic rhythms.[2]

An *agonal rhythm* is marked by being extremely slow and irregularly becoming slower to the point of asystole. It usually occurs as a result of an escape ectopy, a compensatory mechanism for a slow rate, occurring in an underlying asystole. Surprisingly, this sporadic, usually ventricular, electrical activity may continue for minutes and sometimes hours. Clinically, it is similar to asystole and is managed the same.

Electromechanical dissociation is not really a dysrhythmia; rather, it is a condition. Literally, the heart is failing to mechanically respond to normal electrical depolarization and therefore has no associated pulse. Paradis has proposed the term "pseudo-EMD" in which electrical activity is associated with mechanical contractions, although these contractions do not produce a blood pressure detectable by the usual methods of palpation or blood pressure measurement.[126]

Any rhythm originating in the ventricles is technically considered *idioventricular*, although ventricular tachycardia or fibrillation have additional criteria that separate them from this category. Because the inherent automaticity of a ventricular pacemaker is 40 beats per minute or less, this rhythm is recognized as a fairly regular, wide-complex bradydysrhythmia. P waves are always absent. On occasion, a rhythm may have these characteristics but occur at a rate faster than 40 beats per minute. This is considered an accelerated idioventricular rhythm.

Differential Diagnosis

The last step, "D," in the ABCD secondary survey is an attempt to arrive at a differential diagnosis. The critical question that must be answered is "What caused the arrest?". Answering this question leads to identifying reversible causes that have a specific therapy. The same process is used in identifying the cause of refractory cardiac arrests that do not respond to the initial interventions. This process is also used before or after the arrest for any severe cardiorespiratory emergency.

In some instances, the only possibility of successfully resuscitating a person may lie in searching for, finding, and treating reversible causes (Table 22-7). Two algorithms, PEA (Protocol 22-4) and asystole (Protocol 22-5), emphasize the importance of considering the possible causes for the patient's condition. These algorithms include a list of common causes (see Table 22-7) and their interventions that must be learned and considered for every patient presenting with these two rhythms.

Precautions, Hazards, and Complications of Resuscitation

Both basic and advanced CPR interventions pose risks to those being resuscitated. Procedures or drugs may be provided inappropriately or incorrectly, or there may be

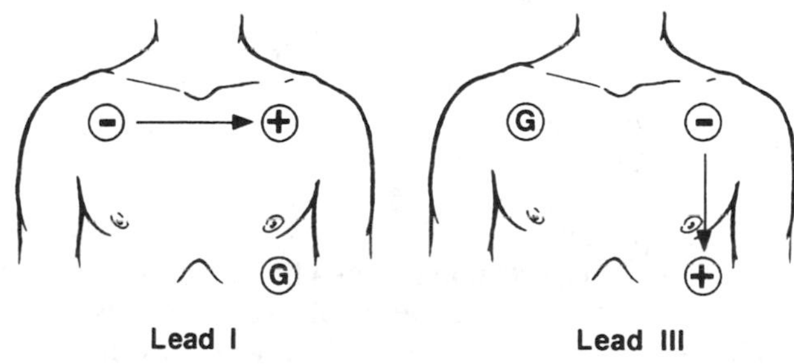

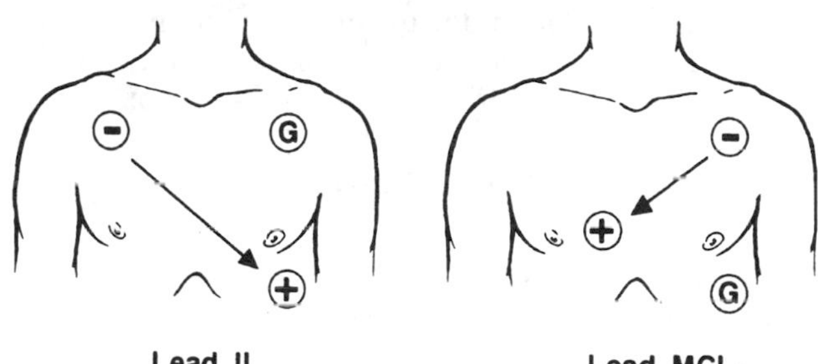

FIGURE 22-46. Location of chest leads. (Revised from Aehlert B: ACLS Quick Review Study Guide, pps. 118–119. St. Louis, Mosby–Year Book 1994. Reproduced with permission.)

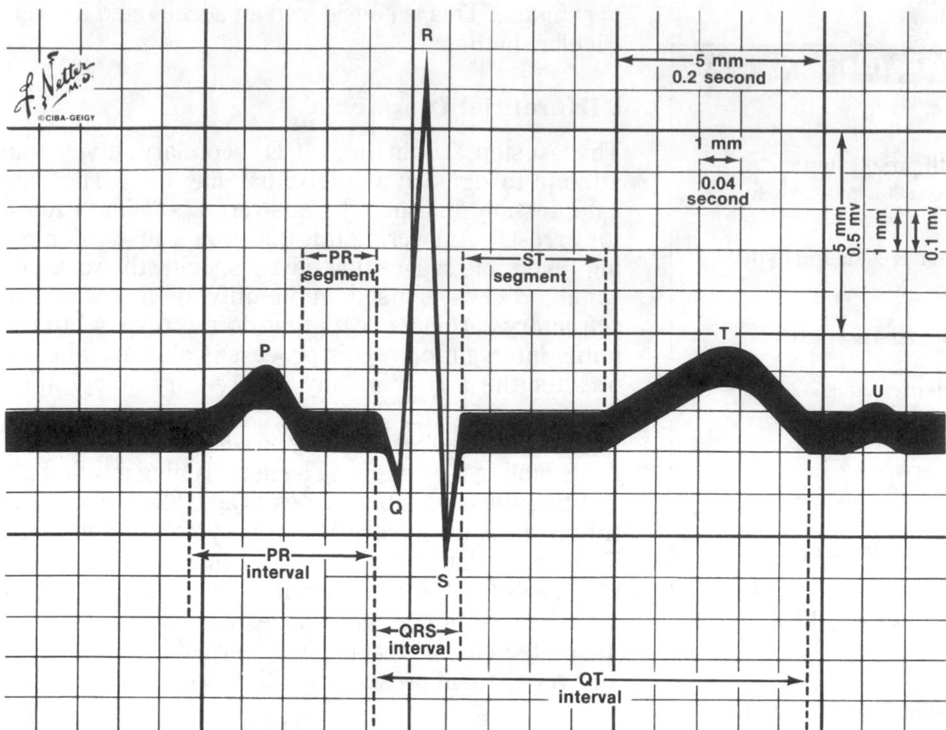

FIGURE 22-47. Electrocardiographic waves, intervals, and segments. (Scheidt S, Erlebacher JA: Basic Electrocardiography, p. 15. West Caldwell, NJ. 1986 Ciba-Geigy Corporation. Reproduced with permission.)

untoward responses from therapy. Box 22-24 lists possible problems within major facets of the resuscitative process according to AARC Clinical Practice Guidelines.[31]

The ACLS Cases

In support of the new case-based teaching philosophy recommended by the American Heart Association for ACLS courses taught after 1994, this section presents the nine core ACLS cases in a series of case-based clinical scenarios. This approach makes the cognitive knowledge and psychomotor skills more relevant as they are applied to clinical responsibilities that practitioners will face. Each case has a unique set of teaching points based on the scenario. Although the full ACLS course includes 18 separate cases, the essentials of ACLS are contained in the nine core cases. It is worth noting that there is an ACLS algorithm that goes with each core case. The deletion of the last nine cases is simply due to space constraints and is not intended to diminish their importance. All respiratory care practitioners are encouraged to become familar with all 18 of the ACLS cases (Box 22-25).

□ ACLS CASE 1—RESPIRATORY ARREST WITH A PULSE

Respiratory Arrest Scenario—COPD Patient Ordered for Stat Respiratory Treatment

An 82-year-old man with a long-standing history of COPD was transferred to the general medical floor from the ICU after being successfully extubated 2 days ago from a 4-day course on the ventilator. The patient

BOX 22-23

COMMON DYSRHYTHMIAS

- Sinus bradycardia
- Sinus tachycardia
- Premature atrial complex (contraction)
- Premature ventricular complexes (contractions, PVCs)
  - Unifocal
  - Multifocal (multiformed)
  - Couplets (pairs of PVCs)
  - Bigeminy
  - R-on-T phenomenon
- Atrial flutter
- Atrial fibrillation
- Paroxysmal supraventricular tachycardia (PSVT)
- Ventricular tachycardia
- Torsades de pointes
- Ventricular fibrillation
  - Coarse
  - Fine
- Atrioventricular (AV) blocks
  - First-degree AV block
  - Second-degree AV block, type I
  - Second-degree AV block, type II
  - Third-degree AV block
- Junctional escape rhythm
- Idioventricular rhythm
- Agonal rhythm
- Asystole (ventricular asystole and cardiac standstill)
- Paced rhythm (pacemaker spikes)
- Artifact
  - Detachment or movement
  - From electrical interference

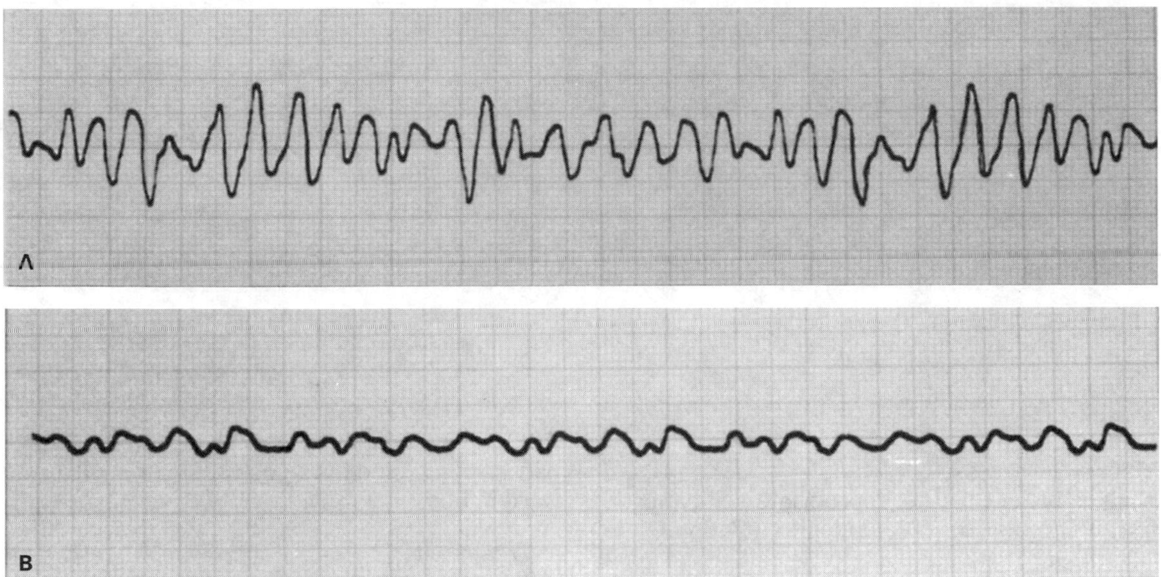

FIGURE 22-48. Ventricular fibrillation **(A)** Coarse ventricular fibrillation. Note high amplitude waveforms, which vary in size, shape, and rhythm, representing chaotic ventricular electrical activity. There are no normal-looking QRS complexes. **(B)** Fine ventricular fibrillation (coarse asystole). In comparison with (A), amplitude of electrical activity is much reduced. Note complete absence of QRS complexes. Slow undulations like this are virtually indistinguishable from asystole. (Laerdal Heartsim 2000 ECG Simulator Manual. Wappingers Falls, NY, 1996 Laerdal Medical Corporation. Reproduced with permission.)

receives respiratory treatments every 4 hours but was just evaluated by the physician for increasing shortness of breath over the last 2 hours. The respiratory therapist has been called to administer a stat treatment and finds the patient unresponsive.

Treatment

The respiratory care practitioner immediately calls for help and a defibrillator after determining unresponsiveness. Further assessment reveals the patient is not breathing but has a pulse. After opening the airway, the respiratory therapist provides bag-valve-mask ventilation with 100% oxygen. The code team members have arrived and preparations for IV access and intubation begin. The necessary history regarding intubation status is obtained from the nurse and confirmed in the medical chart. The patient's blood pressure is normal and an ECG monitor confirms normal sinus rhythm (Fig. 22-51). After intubation, the tube placement is assessed, and arrangements are made for a mechanical ventilator on transfer to the ICU.

Summary—Critical Actions

The following critical actions must be done to provide the best chance for recovery.

1. Perform initial steps of the primary ABCD assessment: Assess responsiveness, call the code team, determine breathing and pulse.
2. Initiate proper rescue breathing with 100% O_2 by means of a bag-valve-mask device.
3. Evaluate the patient for cause of respiratory arrest, and determine if intubation is appropriate.
4. Assess adequacy of ventilation before and after intubation.

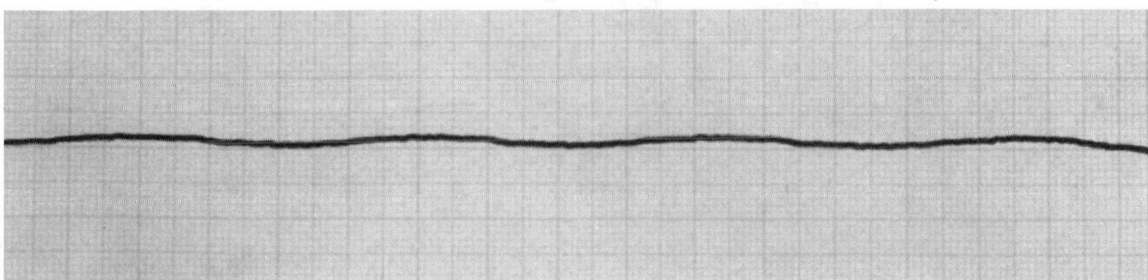

FIGURE 22-49. Asystole. (Laerdal Heartsim 2000 ECG Simulator Manual. Wappingers Falls, NY, 1996 Laerdal Medical Corporation. Reproduced with permission.)

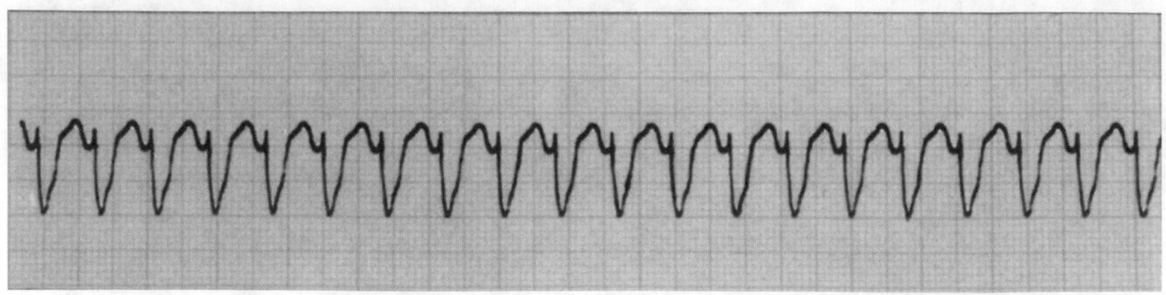

FIGURE 22-50. Ventricular tachycardia. (Laerdal Heartsim 2000 ECG Simulator Manual. Wappingers Falls, NY, 1996 Laerdal Medical Corporation. Reproduced with permission.)

5. Evaluate tube placement after intubation.
6. Establish IV access.
7. Transfer patient to the appropriate critical care unit, and arrange for mechanical ventilation.

☐ ACLS CASE 2—WITNESSED ADULT VF CARDIAC ARREST

Cardiac Arrest Scenario—Discussing the Risks and Benefits of AICDs

A 48-year-old man with a history of refractory ventricular dsyrhythmias partially suppressed by medical therapy has been admitted to the hospital for placement of an *automatic implantable cardioverter-defibrillator* (AICD). After discussing the risks and benefits of the procedure, the cardiologist instructs the patient to sign the surgery consent form. With a flourish of the pen, the patient completed his signature before collapsing backward in bed.

Treatment

The doctor at the bedside confirms unresponsiveness and presses the code button at the head of the bed. The bedside monitor displays coarse ventricular fibrillation (see Fig. 22-48*A*); the patient has no respirations or pulse. Seeing an automated external defibrillator (AED) at the bedside, the doctor turns the unit on and attaches the adhesive pads to the patient's chest. After pressing "analyze," the patient is defibrillated at 200 J, then 300 J, for persistent ventricular fibrillation. The rhythm converts to sinus bradycardia (Fig. 22-52) after the second shock, and a palpable pulse is detected. The

TABLE 22-7 **Conditions That Cause Pulseless Electrical Activity**

Asystole	PEA	Condition	Clues	Management
	+	Hypovolemia	History, flat neck veins	Volume infusion
	+	Cardiac tamponade	History (trauma, renal failure, thoracic malignancy), no pulse with CPR, vein distension; impending tamponade—tachycardia, hypotension, low pulse pressure—changing to sudden bradycardia as terminal event	Pericardiocentesis
	+	Tension pneumothorax	History (asthma, ventilator, COPD, trauma), no pulse with CPR, distended neck veins, tracheal deviation	Needle decompression
	+	Massive pulmonary edema	History, no pulse with CPR, distended neck veins	Thrombolytics, pulmonary arteriogram, embolectomy
	+	Acute, massive MI	History, ECG, enzymes	Pharmacologic data
+	+	Drug overdose (digoxin, tricyclics, β-blockers)	Bradycardia, history of ingestion, empty bottles at the scene, pupils, neurologic exam	Drug screens, intubation, lavage, activated charcoal
+	+	Preexisting acidosis		Sodium bicarbonate, hyperventilation
+	+	Hypothermia	History of exposure to cold, central body temperature	Passive or active rewarming
+	+	Hypoxia	Cyanosis, blood gases, airway problems	Oxygen, ventilations
+	+	Hyperkalemia	History of renal failure, diabetes, recent dialysis, dialysis fistulas, medications	Calcium chloride (immediate); then combination of insulin, glucose, sodium bicarbonate
+		Hypokalemia	History of diuresis, vomiting, diarrhea, malnutrition, trauma	Potassium, potassium with chloride

PEA includes
- Electromechanical dissociation (EMD)
- Pseudo-EMD
- Idioventricular rhythms
- Ventricular escape rhythms
- Bradyasystolic rhvthms
- Postdefibrillation idioventricular rhythms

- Continue CPR
- Intubate at once
- Obtain IV access
- Assess blood flow using Doppler ultrasound

↓

Consider possible causes
(Parentheses=possible therapies and treatments)
- Hypovolemia (volume infusion)
- Hypoxia (ventilation)
- Cardiac tamponade (pericardiocentesis)
- Tension pneumothorax (needle decompression)
- Hypothermia (see hypothermia algorithm, Section IV)
- Massive pulmonary embolism (surgery, ***thrombolytics***)
- Drug overdoses such as tricyclics, digitalis, β-blockers, calcium channel blockers
- Hyperkalemia*
- Acidosis†
- Massive acute myocardial infarction (go to Fig 9)

↓

- ***Epinephrine*** 1 mg IV push, *‡ repeat every 3-5 min

↓

- If absolute bradycardia (<60 beats/min) or relative bradycardia, give ***atropine*** 1 mg IV
- Repeat every 3-5 min up to a total of 0.04 mg/kg§

Class I: definitely helpful
Class IIa: acceptable, probably helpful
Class IIb: acceptable, possibly helpful
Class III: not indicated, may be harmful
****Sodium bicarbonate*** 1 mEq/kg is Class I if patient has known preexisting hyperkalemia.
†***Sodium bicarbonate*** 1 mEq/kg:
Class IIa
- if known preexisting bicarbonate-responsive acidosis
- if overdose with tricyclic antidepressants
- to alkalinize the urine in drug overdoses

Class IIb
- if intubated and long arrest interval
- upon return of spontaneous circulation after long arrest interval

Class III
- hypoxic lactic acidosis

‡The recommended dose of ***epinephrine*** is 1 mg IV push every 3-5 min.
If this approach fails, several Class IIb dosing regimens can be considered.
- Intermediate: ***epinephrine*** 2-5 mg IV push, every 3-5 min
- Escalating: ***epinephrine*** 1 mg-3 mg-5 mg IV push (3 min apart)
- High: ***epinephrine*** 0.1 mg/kg IV push, every 3-5 min

§ Shorter ***atropine*** dosing intervals are possibly helpful in cardiac arrest (Class IIb).

PROTOCOL 22-4. Pulseless electrical activity (PEA) algorithm. (Emergency Cardiac Care Committee and Subcommittees, American Heart Association: Guidelines for cardiopulmonary resuscitation and emergency cardiac care, III: Adult advanced cardiac life support. JAMA 1992;268:2219. Reproduced with permission.)

patient is assessed for spontaneous respirations and adequacy of blood pressure before transfer to the operating room for his surgery.

Summary—Critical Actions

The following critical actions must be done to provide the best chance for recovery.

1. Perform initial steps of the primary ABCD assessment: Assess responsiveness, call the code team, determine breathing and pulse.
2. Initiate defibrillation immediately.
3. Demonstrate proper defibrillation with an AED.
4. Recognize need to check pulse and need to support ventilation in the immediate postdefibrillation period.

□ ACLS CASE 3—ADULT REFRACTORY VF AND PULSELESS VT

Cardiac Arrest Scenario—A Collapsed Line Dancer

A 70-year-old man collapses while line dancing with his wife. His younger sister begins CPR as another witness activates EMS.

Treatment

Emergency medical technicians arrive within 2 minutes after the call and find the victim unresponsive with no respirations or pulse. A monitor indicates fine ventricular fibrillation is present (see Fig. 22-48*B*). Three successive countershocks are administered with no change in the rhythm; CPR is resumed after confirmation of pulselessness. Preparations begin for intubation and IV access. After establishing a peripheral IV line, 1 mg of epinephrine is administered followed by a 20-mL fluid bolus. Thirty seconds later, another countershock at 360 J is administered. Cardiopulmonary resuscitation resumes after the defibrillation attempt when the monitor confirms VF and no pulse is detected. At this point, several Class IIa medications are considered: (1) lidocaine at 1.0 to 1.5 mg/kg IV bolus every 3 to 5 minutes to a maximum of 3 mg/kg; (2) bretylium at 5 mg/kg IV bolus, repeated in 5 minutes at 10 mg/kg, to a maximum of 30 to 35 mg/kg; (3) procainamide at 20 to 30 mg/minute to a maximum of 17 mg/kg; and (4) magnesium sulfate 1 to 2 g IV bolus followed by 1 to 4 g/hour. The drugs are administered in a drug–shock, drug–shock sequence, with pulse and rhythm checks after each intervention. Cardiopulmonary resuscitation is continued whenever the patient is not receiving shocks at 360 J. Epinephrine is administered every 3 to 5 minutes between doses of the Class IIa medications. Sodium bicarbonate is considered early on if the patient has preexisting hyperkalemia or bicarbonate-responsive acidosis, otherwise not until return of spontaneous circulation after his long arrest interval.

Summary—Critical Actions

The following critical actions must be done to provide the best chance for recovery.

1. Perform initial steps of the primary ABCD assessment: Assess responsiveness, call the code team, determine breathing and pulse.
2. Provide ventilation and chest compressions until a monitor and defibrillator are available.
3. Attach the ECG monitor and recognize VF.
4. Deliver three stacked countershocks at 200 J, 300 J, and 360 J.

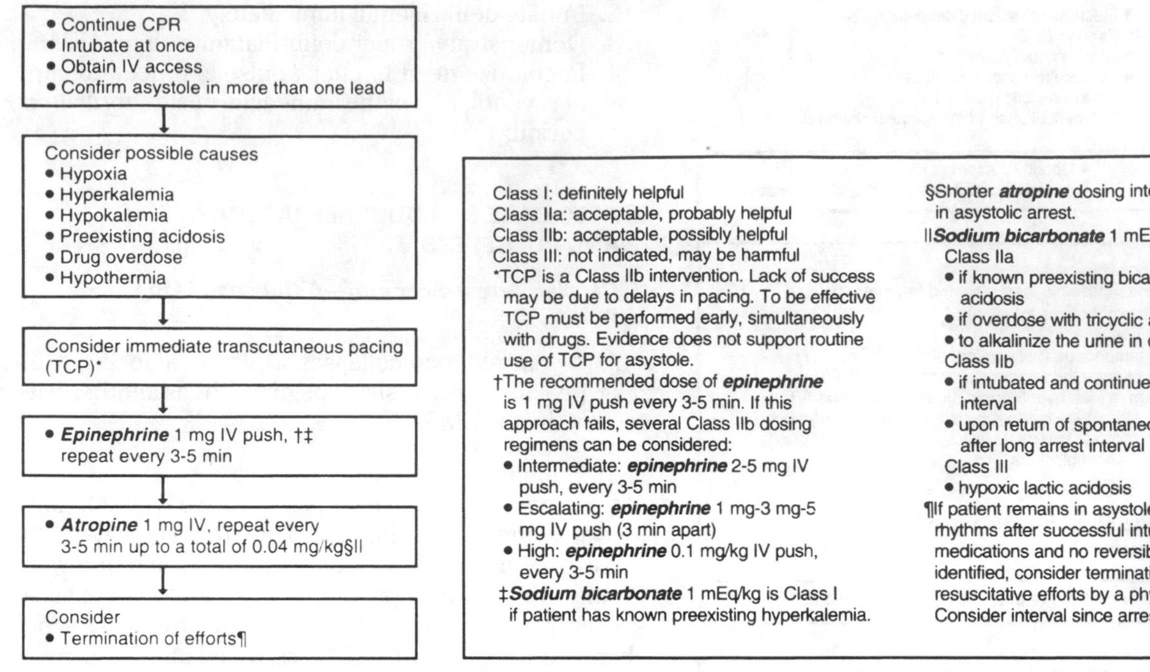
• Continue CPR
• Intubate at once
• Obtain IV access
• Confirm asystole in more than one lead
Consider possible causes
• Hypoxia
• Hyperkalemia
• Hypokalemia
• Preexisting acidosis
• Drug overdose
• Hypothermia
Consider immediate transcutaneous pacing (TCP)*
• Epinephrine 1 mg IV push, †‡ repeat every 3-5 min
• Atropine 1 mg IV, repeat every 3-5 min up to a total of 0.04 mg/kg§||
Consider
• Termination of efforts¶
Class I: definitely helpful
Class IIa: acceptable, probably helpful
Class IIb: acceptable, possibly helpful
Class III: not indicated, may be harmful
*TCP is a Class IIb intervention. Lack of success may be due to delays in pacing. To be effective TCP must be performed early, simultaneously with drugs. Evidence does not support routine use of TCP for asystole.
†The recommended dose of epinephrine is 1 mg IV push every 3-5 min. If this approach fails, several Class IIb dosing regimens can be considered:
• Intermediate: epinephrine 2-5 mg IV push, every 3-5 min
• Escalating: epinephrine 1 mg-3 mg-5 mg IV push (3 min apart)
• High: epinephrine 0.1 mg/kg IV push, every 3-5 min
‡Sodium bicarbonate 1 mEq/kg is Class I if patient has known preexisting hyperkalemia.
§Shorter atropine dosing intervals are Class IIb in asystolic arrest.
||Sodium bicarbonate 1 mEq/kg:
Class IIa
• if known preexisting bicarbonate-responsive acidosis
• if overdose with tricyclic antidepressants
• to alkalinize the urine in drug overdoses
Class IIb
• if intubated and continued long arrest interval
• upon return of spontaneous circulation after long arrest interval
Class III
• hypoxic lactic acidosis
¶If patient remains in asystole or other agonal rhythms after successful intubation and initial medications and no reversible causes are identified, consider termination of resuscitative efforts by a physician. Consider interval since arrest.

PROTOCOL 22-5. Asystole treatment algorithm. (Emergency Cardiac Care Committee and Subcommittees, American Heart Association: Guidelines for cardiopulmonary resuscitation and emergency cardiac care, III: Adult advanced cardiac life support. JAMA 1992;268:2220. Reproduced with permission.)

5. Recognize need to establish IV access and perform endotracheal intubation at the appropriate points in the resuscitation.
6. Administer the appropriate pharmacologic agents in the proper sequence.
7. Direct code team members so that interventions follow the drug-shock, drug-shock pattern, with the continuation of CPR after each countershock and confirmation of pulselessness.

□ ACLS CASE 4—PULSELESS ELECTRICAL ACTIVITY

PEA Scenario—Shark Bite Victim

Emergency medical service personnel were called to a beach where several lifeguards reported hearing screams from a surfer before he disappeared underwater while paddling near the shoreline. Found floating face down, the victim was brought to the shore where the lifeguards provided chest compressions and ventilation with a mouth-to-mask device. The victim was still unresponsive approximately 15 minutes later when EMS personnel arrived.

Treatment

A rapid assessment at the scene revealed a young, tanned, and muscular male lying in a large pool of blood with basic life support in progress. After confirmation of apnea and pulselessness, IV access preparations began immediately because of the obvious blood loss. The ECG monitor leads were attached, and the initial cardiac rhythm was identified as a slow idioventricular rhythm at a rate of 40 beats per minute (Fig. 22-53, see Protocol 22-4). A second pulse check confirmed the absence of pulse and therefore the presence of PEA. Because a shark bite was suspected, the probable cause for the surfer's condition was hypovolemia. As CPR continued, a volume infusion was begun while rescuers attempted to control the bleeding. Other potential causes for PEA were considered and treated: intubation for hypoxia, removal of wet clothing and application of blankets for hypothermia, and history of ingestion or abuse of drugs for possible drug overdose. After a 250-mL bolus of normal saline and no return of pulse or blood pressure, a 1-mg dose of epinephrine via IV push was administered. A second 250-mL bolus of normal saline followed by another dose of epinephrine and 1 mg of atropine resulted in a detectable pulse and systolic blood pressure of 70 mmHg. The patient was then taken to the nearest hospital.

Background Information

Pulseless electrical activity can be defined as the absence of a detectable pulse and the presence of some type of electrical activity. This group of rhythms, which includes electromechanical dissociation (EMD), pseudo-EMD, idioventricular rhythms, ventricular escape rhythms, postdefibrillation idioventricular rhythms, and bradyasystolic rhythms, represents an intermediate state before cardiac arrest. Success in treat-

BOX 22-24

PRECAUTIONS, HAZARDS, AND COMPLICATIONS[31]

- Airway management
  - Failure to establish a patent airway
  - Failure to intubate the trachea or recognize esophageal placement
  - Trauma to the upper airway or esophagus
  - Aspiration
  - Cervical spine trauma
  - Unrecognized bronchial intubation
  - Facial, dental, or ocular injuries
  - Bronchospasm or laryngospasm
  - Autonomic nervous system stimulation causing either hypotension and bradycardia or hypertension and tachycardia
- Ventilation (artificial)
  - Inadequate oxygen delivery
  - Hypo- or hyperventilation
  - Gastric insufflation or rupture
  - Pulmonary barotrauma or systemic hypotension induced by decreased venous return
  - Vomiting and aspiration
- Circulation (chest compression)
  - Ineffective chest compression
  - Fractured ribs or sternum
  - Hemo- or pneumothorax
  - Laceration of the spleen or liver
- Electrical therapy (defibrillation or cardioversion)
  - Failure of equipment
  - Inadvertent shock to CPR team
  - Induction of malignant dysrhythmias
  - Fire hazard
- Drug administration
  - Inappropriate drug or dose
  - Idiosyncratic or allergic response
  - Failure to establish parenteral route or ineffectiveness of endotracheal tube instillation

Used with permission from American Association for Respiratory Care: Clinical Practice Guideline: Resuscitation in Acute Care Hospitals. Respir Care 38:1179, 1993.

ing PEA depends on the rapid identification and treatment of the underlying causes. The American Heart Association lists 10 conditions that cause PEA, with clues for identification and management interventions (see differential diagnosis section above).

Summary—Critical Actions

The following critical actions must be done to provide the best chance for recovery.

1. Perform initial steps of the primary ABCD assessment: Assess responsiveness, call EMS, determine breathing and pulse.
2. Initiate proper CPR.
3. Reassess ABCDs, continue CPR, and properly attach monitor.
4. Recognize PEA.
5. Direct intubation.
6. Ensure IV access.
7. Assess associated injuries and symptoms, and consider the causes of PEA.
8. Determine appropriate management for the patient's condition.

□ ACLS CASE 5—ASYSTOLE

Asystole Scenario—Suctioning Episode Leads to Asystole

You are a nurse suctioning a patient on a mechanical ventilator. After inserting the catheter to its full length you notice the patient's oxygen saturation dropping rapidly. You remove the catheter and begin bagging with the resuscitation bag as you watch the cardiac monitor change from sinus rhythm to asystole.

Treatment

A quick check of all electrodes confirms they are securely attached, and a switch of the lead selector reveals asystole in leads I, II, and III (see Fig. 22-49). The patient appears cyanotic and is unresponsive, apneic, and pulseless. After pressing the code button at the head of the bed, you begin chest compressions and squeeze the resuscitation bag for ventilations at a ratio of 15:2 (see Protocol 22-5). Within 1 minute, a respiratory therapist and several other nurses enter the room. While describing the series of events leading to asystole, you notice the respiratory therapist attach the oxygen tubing from the resuscitation bag to the flow meter. As one of the nurses leaves to get a transcutaneous pacer (TCP), the respiratory therapist begins to hyperventilate the patient with the resuscitation bag, stating the patient may have suffered a hypoxic episode during suctioning as a result of

BOX 22-25

THE ACLS CASES RECOMMENDED BY AHA FOR CASE-BASED TEACHING

Case 1: Respiratory Arrest With a Pulse
Case 2: Witnessed Adult VF Cardiac Arrest
Case 3: Mega VF: Refractory VF and Pulseless VT
Case 4: Pulseless Electrical Activity
Case 5: Asystole
Case 6: Adult Acute Myocardial Infarction
Case 7: Bradycardia
Case 8: Unstable Tachycardia and Electrical Conversion
Case 9: Stable Tachycardia
Case 10: Hypotension, Shock, and Pulmonary Edema
Case 11: Cardiac Arrest Due to Drowning
Case 12: Hypothermia
Case 13: Cardiac Arrest Associated With Trauma
Case 14: Cardiac Arrest Due to Electrical Shock
Case 15: Acute Stroke
Case 16: ACLS Ethics
Case 17: Psychological Effects of CPR on the Rescuer
Case 18: Phased-Response Megacode

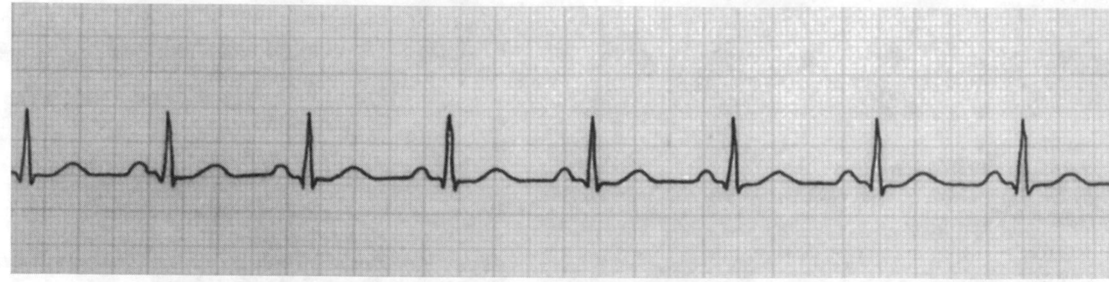

FIGURE 22-51. Normal sinus rhythm. (Laerdal Heartsim 2000 ECG Simulator Manual. Wappingers Falls, NY, 1996 Laerdal Medical Corporation. Reproduced with permission.)

the disconnected oxygen tubing. A 1-mg dose of epinephrine is administered via IV push followed by 1 mg of atropine, with return of a bradycardic rhythm on the monitor. Cardiopulmonary resuscitation is stopped for a pulse check, which confirms the patient has a spontaneous circulation with a heart rate of 45 beats per minute and blood pressure of 60/40. Despite return of spontaneous ventilations and improvement in the blood pressure, the arterial blood gas analysis revealed an acute respiratory acidosis. The suggestion to use sodium bicarbonate was rejected because the patient did not have a preexisting hyperkalemia or bicarbonate-responsive acidosis, and the ventilator rate was increased instead.

Background Information

Asystole, the absence of electrical activity in the heart, represents a grim prognosis without a rapid identification and treatment of the underlying causes. The American Heart Association lists six possible causes for asystole:

- Hypoxia
- Hyperkalemia
- Hypokalemia
- Hypothermia
- Preexisting acidosis
- Drug overdose

Although asystole often represents a confirmation of death rather that a "rhythm" to be treated, asystole occurring in a hospital may not be as bleak as in the prehospital setting. Asystole can occasionally result from a massive parasympathetic discharge and, consequently, may be quite responsive to atropine therapy and early institution of pacing. On the other hand, when the patient has received successful endotracheal intubation, IV access, basic CPR, and all rhythm-appropriate medications, persistent asystole necessitates cessation of efforts.

Summary—Critical Actions

The following critical actions must be done to provide the best chance for recovery.

1. Perform the initial steps of the primary ABCD survey, and call for help.
2. Initiate CPR.
3. Recognize asystole and confirm it in more than one lead.
4. Provide ventilatory support as hypoventilation and hypoxemia are frequent causes of asystole.
5. Establish IV access and administer epinephrine, atropine, and sodium bicarbonate in the proper dosages.
6. Consider the causes of asystole.
7. Articulate the indications for transcutaneous pacing.
8. Assess the presence of a pulse and the blood pressure, and identify changes in rhythm.
9. Articulate the indications for termination of resuscitation.

□ ACLS CASE 6—ADULT ACUTE MYOCARDIAL INFARCTION

Acute MI Scenario—The Proud Farmer

A 70-year-old farmer is brought to the hospital by his wife after their 50th wedding anniversary at the local Elks Club. Feeling fit as a fiddle and proud to have danced the

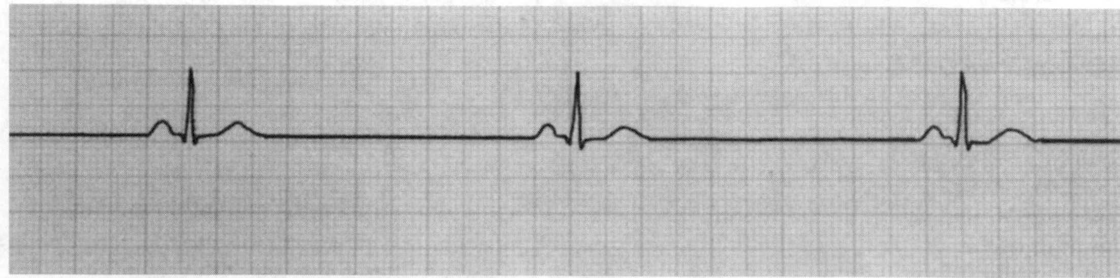

FIGURE 22-52. Sinus bradycardia. (Laerdal Heartsim 2000 ECG Simulator Manual. Wappingers Falls, NY, 1996 Laerdal Medical Corporation. Reproduced with permission.)

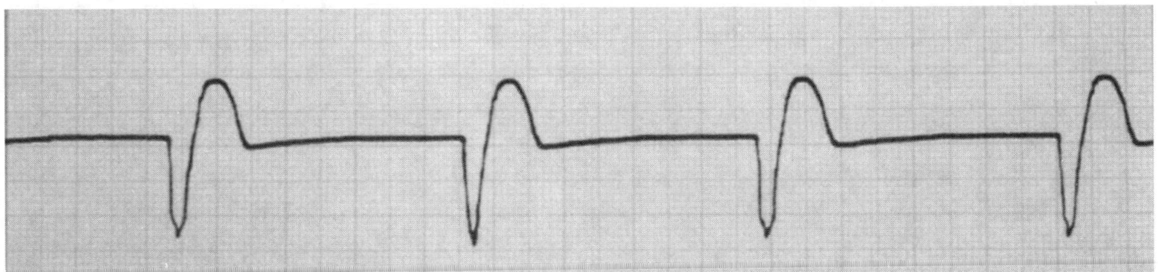

FIGURE 22-53. Slow idioventricular rhythm. (Laerdal Heartsim 2000 ECG Simulator Manual. Wappingers Falls, NY, 1996 Laerdal Medical Corporation. Reproduced with permission.)

night away, he refused his wife's insistent plea to call 911 after he complained of severe indigestion and shortness of breath on returning to their farm. Within minutes, he became pale and diaphoretic and stated he now had a bad cramp in his chest and left arm. He continued to refuse to let his wife call 911 until the pain became so bad he felt like an elephant was standing on his chest. When he finally gave in, his wife decided to drive him to the hospital in their truck, believing the ambulance would take too long and get lost trying to find their farm.

On arrival at the hospital, he is placed on a stretcher, and vital signs are taken. His blood pressure is 150/100, pulse is 118, respirations are 16, and oxygen saturation is 94%. A 12-lead ECG is ordered stat. He has never seen a doctor in his life, takes no medications, and reports no prior history of these symptoms. He remains diaphoretic and complains of severe chest pain. He is given oxygen at 6 L/min, monitor leads are attached, and an IV is started. A nurse asks him to chew an aspirin and swallow it, then sprays nitroglycerin into his mouth and on his tongue.

Treatment

It is essential to know the signals of a heart attack and respond appropriately and quickly. It is never acceptable to drive someone suspected of having a heart attack to the hospital when an EMS system is available. Continuous-recording ambulatory monitoring reveals that 85% of people with sudden cardiac death had VF or VT.[127] Therefore, a strong emphasis must be placed on early access to help at the first signs of chest pain and possible acute MI (Protocol 22-6).

Immediate assessment in the emergency department should include vital signs, placement on an ECG monitor, oxygen saturation, a brief history and physical examination, having a 12-lead ECG taken, and some decision made on the eligibility and appropriateness of thrombolytic therapy. The first things to be done can be remembered by the words **"oxygen, IV, monitor."** Oxygen is probably the most important and effective agent in the emergency setting. The AHA and the American College of Cardiology recommend that every patient suspected of having an acute MI should be given an aspirin to chew as soon as possible.[128] Patients who are suffering from an MI with severe pain can have an increased level of catecholamines that elevate blood pressure, heart rate, and oxygen demands. Both morphine and nitroglycerin are effective in relieving pain as well as altering hemodynamics in a positive manner. Beta-blockers are indicated for acute MI with elevated heart rate and blood pressure and for a large MI within 6 hours of pain onset. Because β-blockers can cause significant side effects, they should be given with caution

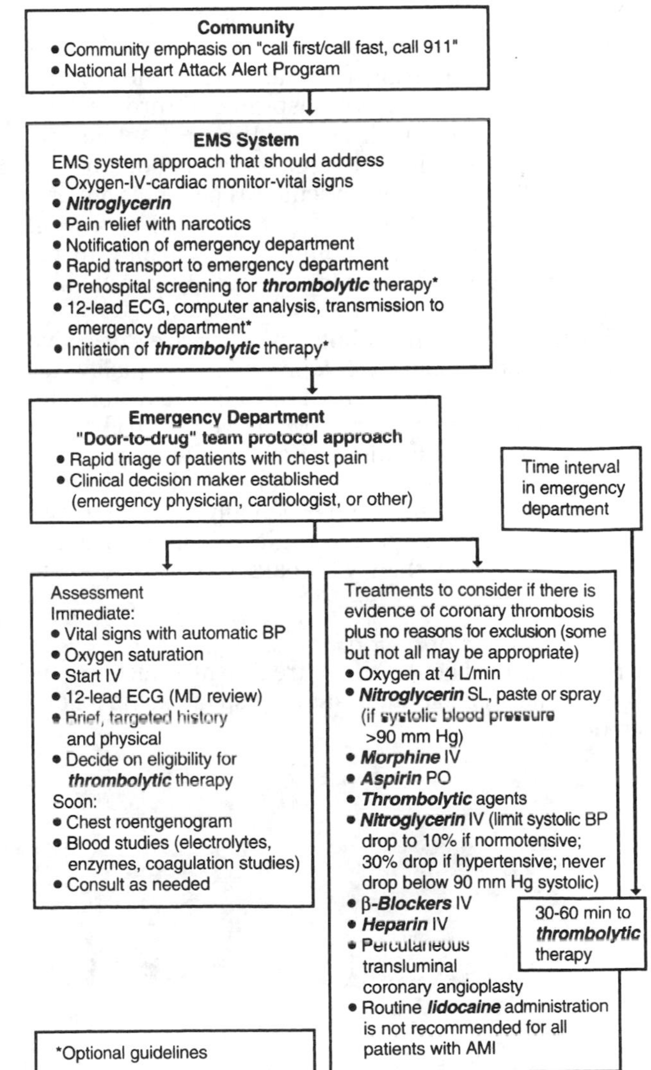

PROTOCOL 22-6. Acute myocardial infarction algorithm. (Emergency Cardiac Care Committee and Subcommittees, American Heart Association: Guidelines for cardiopulmonary resuscitation and emergency cardiac care, III: Adult advanced cardiac life support. JAMA 1992;268:2230. Reproduced with permission.)

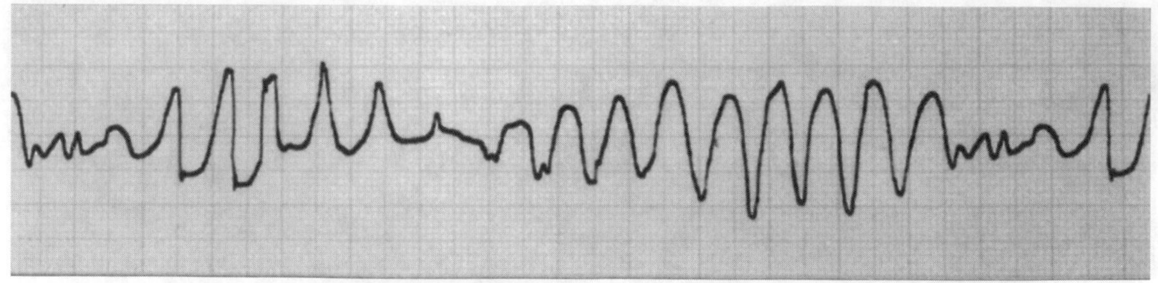

FIGURE 22-54. Torsades de pointes. (Laerdal Heartsim 2000 ECG Simulator Manual. Wappingers Falls, NY, 1996 Laerdal Medical Corporation. Reproduced with permission.)

and only when critical care monitoring is planned. Magnesium sulfate is a Class I agent in the following three conditions: (1) to suppress torsades de pointes (Fig. 22-54), (2) for cardiac arrest with known or suspected magnesium deficiency, and (3) for acute MI with known or suspected magnesium deficiency. Heparin is a Class IIa agent for the early management of MIs, but it has gained increasing favor as part of the "thrombolytic package," along with aspirin and thrombolytic agents, for patients with acute MI.[129,130] Routine prophylactic lidocaine is no longer recommended before thrombolytic therapy or for acute MI patients with premature ventricular contractions (Fig. 22-55) to prevent VF and VT. Lidocaine should be given only to patients with new onset of ventricular ectopy who are having an MI.

Treatment with thrombolytics is an area of active reasearch and rapid developments. To qualify for thrombolytic therapy, a patient must have a history and an ECG consistent with acute MI as well as no absolute or relative contraindications (Box 22-26).[122] Upper age limits for thrombolytic therapy were initially set at 70 to 75 years. More recent studies actually eliminated age restrictions on patients as significant clinical benefits for patients more than 75 years old were demonstrated.[131–133]

Background Information

For suspected acute MI, 10 treatments must be considered once the patient is at the hospital, in the following order:

- Oxygen at 4 L/min via mask or nasal cannula to start for $SaO_2 \geq 97\%$.
- Nitroglycerin, given sublingually or by spray inhaler, paste, or IV infusion, if systolic blood pressure > 90 mmHg.
- Morphine, 1 to 3 mg at frequent intervals, to eliminate pain.
- Aspirin, considered Class I, given as one chewable tablet, then another, by mouth.
- Beta-blockers given in the first 4 to 6 hours of acute MI via IV; consult with cardiology.
- Magnesium sulfate given via IV when hypomagnesemia is suspected or detected.
- Heparin, Class IIa, via IV bolus as part of the thrombolytic package
- Lidocaine is not for prophylaxis; must have symptomatic ventricular ectopy or VT
- Class I thrombolytic agent for those treated within 6 hours of symptoms
- Coronary angioplasty (PTCA) Class I for signs and symptoms of large acute MI for <6 hours and contraindications to thrombolytic therapy

Summary—Critical Actions

The following critical actions must be done to provide the best chance for recovery.

- Perform a rapid evaluation: ABCD assessment, physical examination and history, vital signs, and a 12-lead ECG.

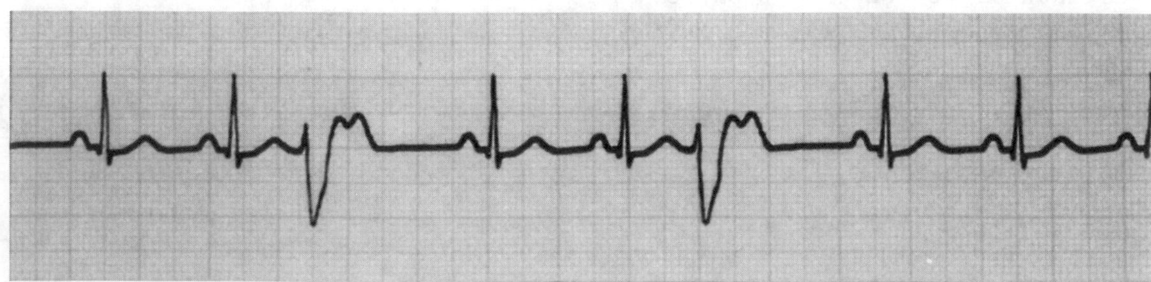

FIGURE 22-55. Premature ventricular contractions. (Laerdal Heartsim 2000 ECG Simulator Manual. Wappingers Falls, NY, 1996 Laerdal Medical Corporation. Reproduced with permission.)

BOX 22-26

CONTRAINDICATIONS FOR THROMBOLYTIC THERAPY

Absolute
Known traumatic CPR
Severe persistent hypertension despite pain relief and initial drugs
Recent head trauma or known intracranial neoplasm
History of stroke in past 6 months
Pregnancy

Relative
Recent trauma or major surgery in past 2 months
Initial systolic BP >180 mmHg or diastolic >110 mmHg controlled by medical treatment
Active peptic ulcer or guaiac-positive stools
Remote history of stroke, tumor, injury, or brain surgery
Known bleeding disorder or current use of warfarin
Significant liver dysfunction or renal failure
Exposure to streptokinase or anistreplase during the preceding 12 months
Known cancer or illness with possible thoracic, abdominal, or intracranial abnormalities
Prolonged CPR

- Articulate the indications, the exclusion criteria, and the ECG criteria for the use of thrombolytic therapy.
- Administer the proper medications in the acute MI algorithm, stating the major actions, indications, and contraindications for oxygen, nitroglycerin (SL and IV), morphine, aspirin, thrombolytic agents, β-blockers, heparin, lidocaine, and magnesium sulfate.
- Evaluate and treat the dysrhythmias associated with acute MI.

□ ACLS CASE 7—BRADYCARDIA

Bradycardia Scenario—The Card Dealer Overcome With Cigarette Smoke

A 42-year-old casino card dealer was seen by paramedics for loss of consciousness. En route to the hospital, she regained consciousness briefly and told the paramedic that it began with a feeling of nausea when all the players at her table began smoking cigarettes. Within minutes she became drowsy, pale, and sweaty and then slumped to the floor. She couldn't remember anything after that.

On arrival at the hospital, she was again unconscious with a palpable heart rate of 35 beats per minute and blood pressure of 74/50. She had a respiratory rate of 30 breaths per minute on a nonrebreather mask at 15 L/min. The ECG monitor revealed a second-degree type II AV block (Fig. 22-56). A 12-lead ECG was ordered stat, and the nurse began setting up a transcutaneous pacer (TCP) while the respiratory care practitioner established IV access. A trial dose of 0.5 mg atropine was given with a mild acceleration in the heart rate to 42 beats per minute, but no change in level of consciousness was seen. After 3 minutes, a second dose of 0.5 mg atropine was administered with a change in the ECG rhythm to third-degree AV block. The TCP was initiated at 80 beats per minute on a minimal energy setting and increased until mechanical capture was determined.

Treatment

Initial assessment should determine if the patient is responsive and breathing (Protocol 22-7). Evaluation of the pulse rate and strength is the next priority for an unstable patient. Initial preparation should include O_2, IV access, and monitoring. When the ECG rhythm is identified as bradycardia (see Fig. 22-56), with symptoms related to bradycardia (Box 22-27), preparation for TCP is the initial treatment because of the speed with which it can be instituted and because it is the least invasive pacing technique available. Atropine can be tried in all cases and should be used concurrently with setting up the TCP to give temporary stabilization only. Anticipatory pacing readiness is a Class I intervention in the setting of acute myocardial infarction (symptomatic sinus node dysfunction, see Fig. 22-52); second-degree type II AV block (see Fig. 22-56); third-degree AV block (Fig. 22-57); and newly acquired left, right, or alternating bundle branch block. Dopamine infusions may be helpful in patients who do not respond to atropine and when TCP is delayed or impossible due to noncapture, unavailability, or malfunction.

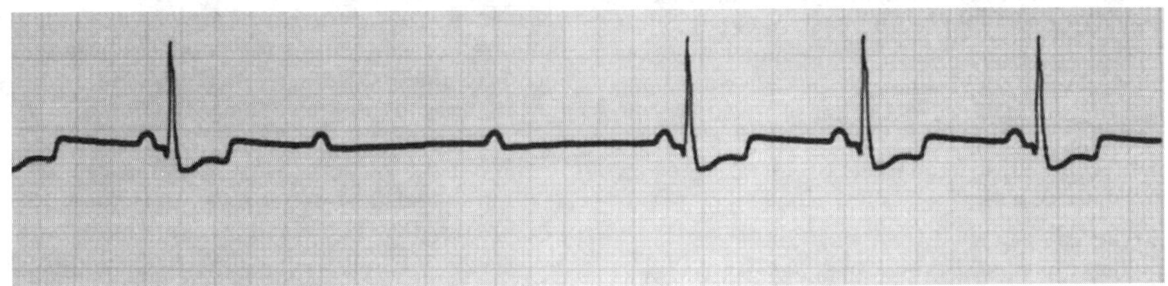

FIGURE 22-56. Second-degree type II AV block. (Laerdal Heartsim 2000 ECG Simulator Manual. Wappingers Falls, NY, 1996 Laerdal Medical Corporation. Reproduced with permission.)

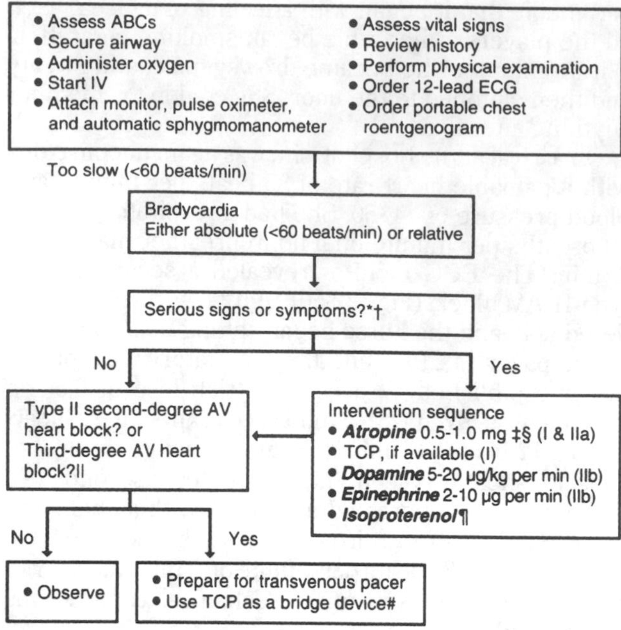

*Serious signs or symptoms must be related to the slow rate. Clinical manifestations include: *symptoms* (chest pain, shortness of breath, decreased level of consciousness) and *signs* (low BP, shock, pulmonary congestion, CHF, acute MI).
†Do not delay TCP while awaiting IV access or for ***atropine*** to take effect if patient is symptomatic.
‡Denervated transplanted hearts will not respond to ***atropine***. Go at once to pacing, ***catecholamine*** infusion, or both.
§***Atropine*** should be given in repeat doses in 3-5 min up to total of 0.04 mg/kg. Consider shorter dosing intervals in severe clinical conditions. It has been suggested that atropine should be used with caution in atrioventricular (AV) block at the His-Purkinje level (type II AV block and new third-degree block with wide QRS complexes) (Class IIb).
llNever treat third-degree heart block plus ventricular escape beats with ***lidocaine***.
¶***Isoproterenol*** should be used, if at all, with exteme caution. At low doses it is Class IIb (possibly helpful); at higher doses it is Class III (harmful).
#Verify patient tolerance and mechanical capture. Use analgesia and sedation as needed.

PROTOCOL 22-7. Bradycardia algorithm. (Emergency Cardiac Care Committee and Subcommittees, American Heart Association: Guidelines for cardiopulmonary resuscitation and emergency cardiac care, III: Adult advanced cardiac life support. JAMA 1992;268:2221. Reproduced with permission.)

Background Information

In patients with bradycardia, an appropriate history and physical exam cannot be emphasized enough. It is just as important to not treat a stable patient with a slow heart rate as it is to quickly manage a patient with symptomatic bradycardia to prevent primary arrest. Recognition of symptoms and primary use of atropine with rapid institution of transcutaneous pacing are the cornerstones of this case.

Summary—Critical Actions

The following critical actions must be done to provide the best chance for recovery.

- Recognize the signs and symptoms due to bradycardia by appropriately assessing a patient's history and performing a physical examination; differentiate the symptomatic patient from the asymptomatic patient with bradycardia.
- Provide oxygen and monitoring; order a 12-lead ECG.
- Ensure IV access, and prepare for intubation, if necessary.
- Administer the appropriate doses of atropine, and know the appropriate dose of a dopamine infusion, if necessary.
- Apply TCP while giving a trial of atropine, and recognize the need for transvenous pacing.
- Differentiate between second-degree type II and third-degree AV blocks.
- Know the importance of thrombolytics in the setting of an acute MI.

BOX 22-27

DEFINITIONS OF BRADYCARDIA

Absolute: (<60 beats per minute [bpm])

Symptomatic: important observations include blood pressure, shortness of breath, level of consciousness, signs of shock (cool, clammy), heart sounds, murmurs, rubs, signs of CHF (rales in the bases), chest pain, weakness, dizziness, syncope.

Asymptomatic: athletes and physically fit patients may have sinus rates below 40 bpm and still be completely asymptomatic. The history should be emphasized to help determine if this is a normal rate versus an acute event.

Relative: (≥60 beats per minute)

Symptoms are due to inability to accelerate an appropriate heart rate to maintain cardiac output. For example, a hypotensive patient that would normally exhibit a tachycardia but is unable to increase her heart rate due to sinus node disease or β-blockers.

☐ ACLS CASE 8—UNSTABLE TACHYCARDIA AND ELECTRICAL CONVERSION

Unstable Tachycardia Scenario—Woman With Family Crisis

A 38-year-old woman with history of depression and unstable angina is hospitalized in an unmonitored unit after a particularly stressful family crisis. The code alarm in her room is activated during visiting hours. On entering, the nurse finds the patient shouting at a visitor who immediately departs. The patient states she is having palpitations, chest pain, and shortness of breath and feels an impending sense of doom.

The patient has no IV access and is not on oxygen. The nurse feels a weak, thready pulse at a rate of approximately 180. The blood pressure is 78/48, and the skin is cool and moist. Auscultation of the lungs reveals bibasilar rales. The nurse calls for help and an ECG monitor stat. She places a nasal cannula at 6 L/min on the patient and attempts to calm her down. While waiting for help to arrive, the nurse listens for carotid bruits

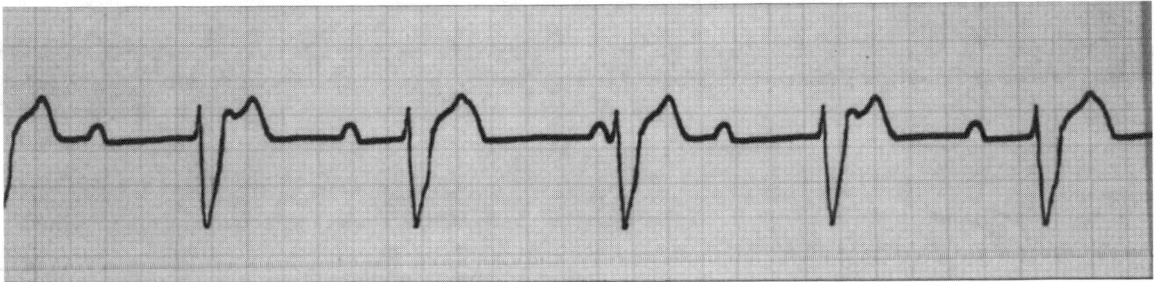

FIGURE 22-57. Third-degree AV block. (Laerdal Heartsim 2000 ECG Simulator Manual. Wappingers Falls, NY, 1996 Laerdal Medical Corporation. Reproduced with permission.)

and, when none are detected, turns the patient's head to the left and applies a firm massage to the right carotid sinus for about 5 seconds. When no change in the pulse rate is noted, the nurse turns the patient's head to the right and performs left carotid massage. When the monitor and defibrillator arrive, the patient is determined to be in paroxysmal supraventricular tachycardia (PSVT) (Fig. 22-58). As the physician attempts to insert an IV, the patient becomes hysterical and quickly loses consciousness. The nurse immediately charges the defibrillator and prepares for synchronized cardioversion.

Treatment

For stable dysrhythmias, vagal maneuvers or drugs, or both, should be attempted first before electrical cardioversion. Although this patient exhibited hemodynamic instability at the outset, the nurse was unable to perform synchronized cardioversion until the defibrillator arrived. Vagal maneuvers may serve both a diagnostic and therapeutic purpose as they increase parasympathetic tone and slow conduction through the AV node. A long list of vagal maneuvers have been described, ranging from the commonplace to the bizarre (Box 22-28).[2] Ideally, ECG monitoring, an IV line, atropine, and lidocaine should be readily available before vagal maneuvers are attempted.

The management of unstable narrow and wide-complex tachyarrhythmias requires synchronized cardioversion. Although a brief antiarrhythmic medication trial can be attempted while preparing for synchronized cardioversion, immediate electrical cardioversion is indicated and should not be delayed for any patient with serious signs and symptoms related to the tachycardia (Box 22-29). The use of sedatives for awake, hemodynamically unstable patients is recommended, but the potential for further deterioration should be considered. The procedure for cardioversion may vary between defibrillator models and from institution to institution; however, a representative procedure is provided in Box 22-30. The energy selection for PSVT begins with 50 J, followed by 100 J, 200 J, 300 J, and 360 J. Reassess the patient and the monitor between each shock. If the rhythm deteriorates to VF or pulseless ventricular tachycardia, proceed immediately to defibrillation at the energy level last used. Frequent monitoring of vital signs after cardioversion is essential until stabilization occurs. After resuscitation, antiarrhythmic medications such as lidocaine, procainamide, bretylium, or magnesium sulfate may be indicated.

Summary—Critical Actions

The following critical actions must be done to provide the best chance for recovery.

1. Perform the initial steps of the primary ABCD assessment, attachment of the monitor, and assessment of vital signs.
2. Evaluate the patient's condition for signs and symptoms of cardiovascular instability.
3. Recognize the rhythm.
4. Safely administer the appropriate energy levels while performing synchronized electrical cardioversion.

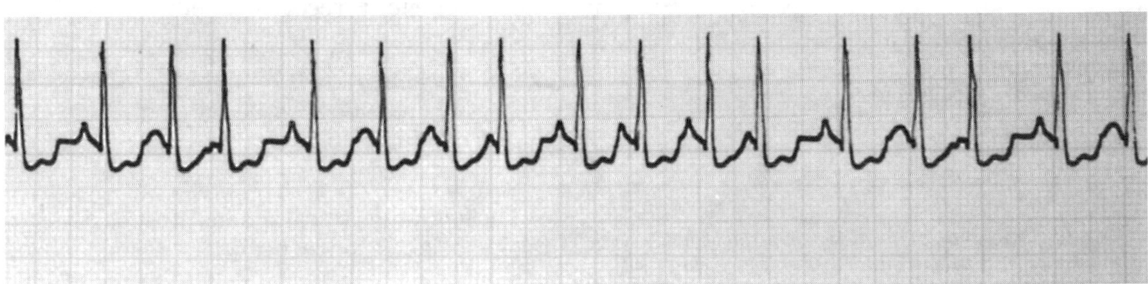

FIGURE 22-58. Paraoxymal supraventricular tachycardia (PSVT). (Laerdal Heartsim 2000 ECG Simulator Manual. Wappingers Falls, NY, 1996 Laerdal Medical Corporation. Reproduced with permission.)

BOX 22-28

VAGAL MANEUVERS

Carotid sinus massage
Breath holding
Facial immersion in ice water
Coughing
Nasogastric tube placement
Gag reflex stimulation by tongue blades, fingers, or oral ipecac
Eyeball pressure
Squatting
MAST garments
Trendelenburg position
Circumferential digital sweep of the anus

5. Reassess the ABCDs, rhythm, and blood pressure after synchronized shock.
6. Recognize the need to monitor vital signs and provide appropriate interventions, such as oxygen and IV access, and follow-up with antiarrhythmic therapy, if necessary.
7. Recognize the need to progress from synchronized to unsynchronized shock in a deteriorating patient.

□ ACLS CASE 9—STABLE TACHYCARDIA

Stable Tachycardia Scenario—Medical Student Observes "Funny" Rhythm on Monitor

A first-year medical student was observed entering a patient's room on the post–cardiovascular surgical step-down unit. Immediately, the student ran out of the room exclaiming to all at the nurses' station that there was a funny rhythm on the monitor and to bring a crash cart immediately. On entering the room, a middle-aged man was noted to be sitting upright in bed watching TV. The patient cheerily greeted the four nurses who had just run in and asked why there was so much commotion.

BOX 22-29

UNSTABLE CONDITIONS RELATED TO TACHYCARDIA*

Chest pain
Shortness of breath
Low blood pressure
Decreased level of consciousness
Shock
Pulmonary congestion
Congestive heart failure
Acute MI

** Most patients with a ventricular rate less than 150 bpm do not require and usually will not benefit from emergent synchronized cardioversion.*

BOX 22-30

SYNCHRONIZED CARDIOVERSION PROCEDURE

Attach monitor leads to the patient.
Apply conductive material to paddles if necessary.
Turn on the defibrillator.
Turn on the synchronization mode, or press the synch button.
Verify synchronization.
Select energy level.
Charge paddles.
Place paddles on the chest and apply pressure (if necessary).
Clear the area.
Press both buttons and hold pressure until discharge occurs.
Resynchronize the defibrillator after the initial synchronized shock.

One nurse proceeded to assess the patient's condition and determined the following: the ECG monitor displayed ventricular tachycardia at 160 beats per minute (see Fig. 22-50), the patient had no complaints of chest pain or shortness of breath, his blood pressure was 140/80, and his lungs were clear to auscultation. When asked how he felt, the patient replied that he was fine except for a pounding in his heart he had felt for the past 15 minutes or so.

Treatment

The patient was placed on a nasal cannula at 4 L/min of oxygen, and a 12-lead ECG was ordered. Assessment of the patient for serious signs and symptoms is the first priority. Recognition of the dysrhythmia follows. The drug treatment for VT is lidocaine, procainamide, then bretylium. Proceed to synchronized cardioversion if the drug therapy fails or the patient becomes unstable.

In summary, management of stable tachycardia can be simplified into three easy steps:

Step 1: Assess the patient for serious signs and symptoms.
Step 2: Identify the dysrhythmia.
Step 3: Treat the dysrhythmia.

For stable VT, the following general IV drug treatment sequence is recommended:

1. Lidocaine 1 to 1.5 mg/kg
2. Lidocaine 0.5 to 0.75 mg/kg
3. Procainamide 20 to 30 mg/min
4. Bretylium 5 to 10 mg/kg

Summary—Critical Actions

The following critical actions must be done to provide the best chance for recovery.

1. Perform the initial steps of the primary ABCD assessment.

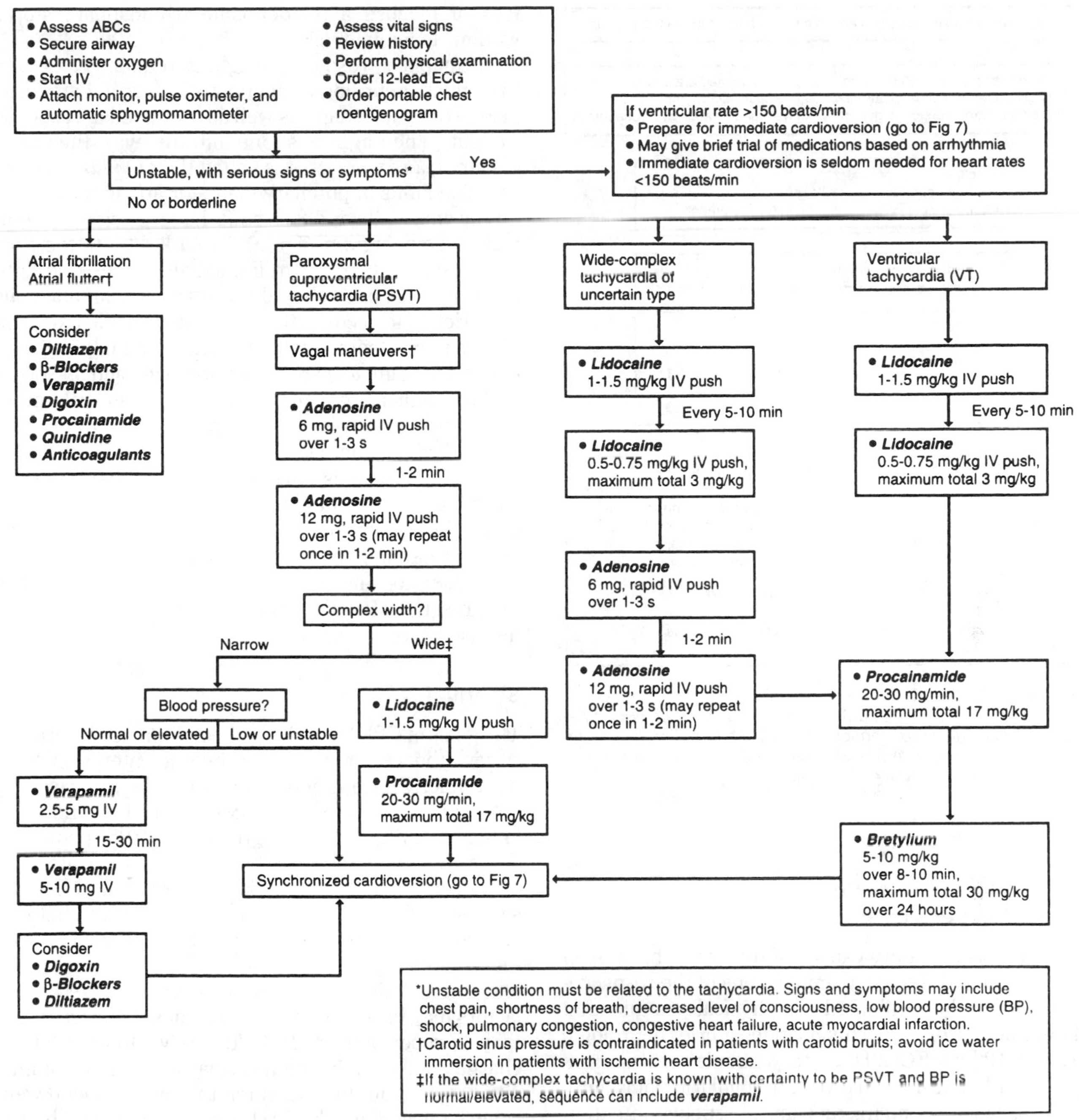

• Assess ABCs
• Secure airway
• Administer oxygen
• Start IV
• Attach monitor, pulse oximeter, and automatic sphygmomanometer
• Assess vital signs
• Review history
• Perform physical examination
• Order 12-lead ECG
• Order portable chest roentgenogram
Unstable, with serious signs or symptoms*
Yes
If ventricular rate >150 beats/min
• Prepare for immediate cardioversion (go to Fig 7)
• May give brief trial of medications based on arrhythmia
• Immediate cardioversion is seldom needed for heart rates <150 beats/min
No or borderline
Atrial fibrillation
Atrial flutter†
Consider
• Diltiazem
• β-Blockers
• Verapamil
• Digoxin
• Procainamide
• Quinidine
• Anticoagulants
Paroxysmal supraventricular tachycardia (PSVT)
Vagal maneuvers†
• Adenosine
6 mg, rapid IV push over 1-3 s
1-2 min
• Adenosine
12 mg, rapid IV push over 1-3 s (may repeat once in 1-2 min)
Complex width?
Narrow
Wide‡
Blood pressure?
Normal or elevated
Low or unstable
• Verapamil
2.5-5 mg IV
15-30 min
• Verapamil
5-10 mg IV
Consider
• Digoxin
• β-Blockers
• Diltiazem
• Lidocaine
1-1.5 mg/kg IV push
• Procainamide
20-30 mg/min, maximum total 17 mg/kg
Synchronized cardioversion (go to Fig 7)
Wide-complex tachycardia of uncertain type
• Lidocaine
1-1.5 mg/kg IV push
Every 5-10 min
• Lidocaine
0.5-0.75 mg/kg IV push, maximum total 3 mg/kg
• Adenosine
6 mg, rapid IV push over 1-3 s
1-2 min
• Adenosine
12 mg, rapid IV push over 1-3 s (may repeat once in 1-2 min)
Ventricular tachycardia (VT)
• Lidocaine
1-1.5 mg/kg IV push
Every 5-10 min
• Lidocaine
0.5-0.75 mg/kg IV push, maximum total 3 mg/kg
• Procainamide
20-30 mg/min, maximum total 17 mg/kg
• Bretylium
5-10 mg/kg over 8-10 min, maximum total 30 mg/kg over 24 hours
*Unstable condition must be related to the tachycardia. Signs and symptoms may include chest pain, shortness of breath, decreased level of consciousness, low blood pressure (BP), shock, pulmonary congestion, congestive heart failure, acute myocardial infarction.
†Carotid sinus pressure is contraindicated in patients with carotid bruits; avoid ice water immersion in patients with ischemic heart disease.
‡If the wide-complex tachycardia is known with certainty to be PSVT and BP is normal/elevated, sequence can include verapamil.

PROTOCOL 22-8. Tachycardia algorithm. (Emergency Cardiac Care Committee and Subcommittees, American Heart Association: Guidelines for cardiopulmonary resuscitation and emergency cardiac care, III: Adult advanced cardiac life support. JAMA 1992;268:2223. Reproduced with permission.)

2. Attach ECG monitor and categorize the rhythm. Emphasis should be placed on the management of stable PSVT, wide-complex tachycardia of uncertain type, and ventricular tachycardia.
3. Assess cardiovascular stability.
4. Safely administer therapeutic maneuvers in correct sequence, for example, vagal maneuvers, drugs, electrical cardioversion.
5. Reassess the ABCDs, rhythm, and blood pressure.
6. Recognize the need to monitor vital signs and provide appropriate interventions such as oxygen and IV access, and follow-up with antiarrhythmic therapy, if necessary.
7. Recognize the need to progress from synchronized to unsynchronized shock in a deteriorating patient.

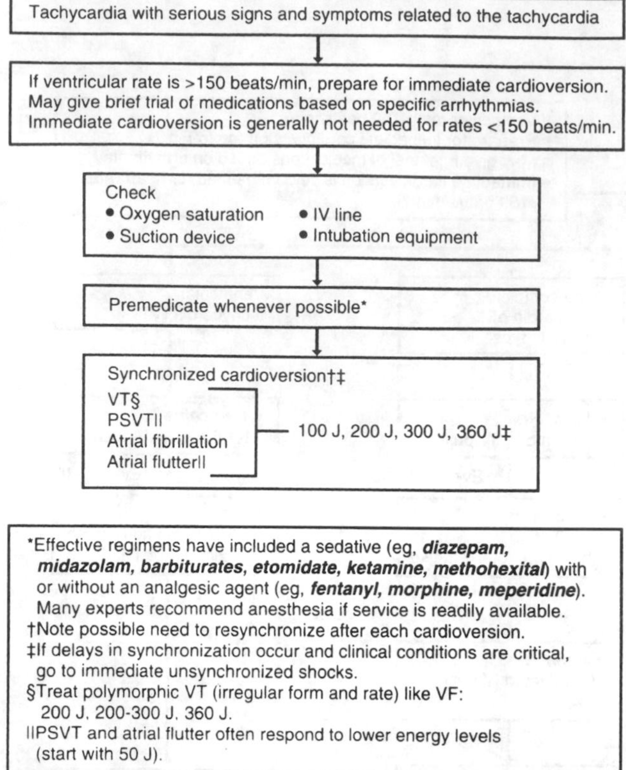

Tachycardia with serious signs and symptoms related to the tachycardia
If ventricular rate is >150 beats/min, prepare for immediate cardioversion. May give brief trial of medications based on specific arrhythmias. Immediate cardioversion is generally not needed for rates <150 beats/min.
Check
• Oxygen saturation
• Suction device
• IV line
• Intubation equipment
Premedicate whenever possible*
Synchronized cardioversion†‡
VT§
PSVT||
Atrial fibrillation
Atrial flutter||
100 J, 200 J, 300 J, 360 J‡
*Effective regimens have included a sedative (eg, **diazepam, midazolam, barbiturates, etomidate, ketamine, methohexital**) with or without an analgesic agent (eg, **fentanyl, morphine, meperidine**). Many experts recommend anesthesia if service is readily available.
†Note possible need to resynchronize after each cardioversion.
‡If delays in synchronization occur and clinical conditions are critical, go to immediate unsynchronized shocks.
§Treat polymorphic VT (irregular form and rate) like VF: 200 J, 200-300 J, 360 J.
||PSVT and atrial flutter often respond to lower energy levels (start with 50 J).

PROTOCOL 22-9. Electrical cardioversion algorithm. (Emergency Cardiac Care Committee and Subcommittees, American Heart Association: Guidelines for cardiopulmonary resuscitation and emergency cardiac care, III: Adult advanced cardiac life support. JAMA 1992;268:2224. Reproduced with permission.)

Cerebral Resuscitation After Cardiac Arrest

After the precipitating causes of the arrest have been considered and treated, complications of the resuscitation should be evaluated. A physical examination should be performed. This includes a brief neurologic exam, a 12-lead ECG, laboratory samples (cardiac enzymes and serum electrolytes, particularly potassium, sodium, calcium, and magnesium). Particular attention to pupil size and reactivity is provided at this point, as pupillary assessment can contribute to the diagnosis of many conditions. However, there is a potential for clinicians to place unwarranted emphasis on pupillary assessment, especially in the postresuscitation period. Physical examinations of neurologic status should not be used as a determining factor for considering the termination of resuscitative efforts.

With the onset of cardiac arrest, patients quickly lose consciousness, usually within 15 seconds. By the end of 1 minute, brain stem function ceases, respirations become agonal, and pupils are fixed or dilated. This clinical picture corresponds to the biochemical changes of oxygen depletion that occur over 15 seconds and the loss of glucose and adenosine triphosphate stores within 4 to 5 minutes.[134]

The pupillary response to light is frequently assessed to evaluate neurologic function, with careful attention paid to the pupil shape as well as the speed of response to light. When light is shone into the eyes, the pupils constrict, a reaction that is called the *pupillary light reflex.* The limits of pupillary diameter are about 1.5 mm on the small side and 8 mm on the large side, the normal range being 3 to 7 mm. Direct light into the eyes should cause the pupil to immediately constrict; light shone into one pupil should cause similar, simultaneous constriction to occur in the other pupil. While fixed and dilated pupils (completely unreactive, in midposition, 4 to 6 mm in diameter) are an ominous sign and one of the findings indicating brain death, they offer little information in the postresuscitative period. An absent pupillary reflex is nondiagnostic after administration of scopolamine, opiates, succinylcholine, other neuromuscular blocking agents, atropine, mydriatic eye drops, glutethimide, monoamine oxidase inhibitors, tricyclic antidepressants, high-dose catecholamines, bretylium overdose, cocaine, or high-dose magnesium and in the presence of ocular trauma or another relevant eye disease.[135]

Survival

The goals of CPR have always been reported in terms of survival, but recently there has been an interest in defining the long-term functional status. The increased interest in utilization of resources has lead to studies on long-term CPR outcomes. A review of 19,955 pooled patients, from 98 studies of in-hospital CPR survival to hospital discharge between 1960 and 1990, found that the success of CPR has not changed in 30 years (15% survival to hospital discharge).[136] This study also reported that community hospitals had higher CPR success than teaching hospitals (19% versus 14%). However, other factors may have influenced outcomes. Urbergand and Ways[137] report only a 11% CPR survival to hospital discharge after an in-hospital cardiac arrest in a community hospital, but they mention that patients who were living independently before hospitalization had a higher survival rate (19%) than homebound (3%) or nursing home (3%) patients. Another report from a 600-bed community hospital found that, of 272 patients receiving CPR in 1984, only 11% survived to hospital discharge.[138] This study also compared this data with 129 patients admitted to their critical care units in 1982 and 1983 in whom CPR was withheld based on their poor response to therapy. There was an 11% survival rate for patients who had received CPR compared to a 16% survival rate for the DNR group. Kyff suggested that the criteria for administering CPR to hospitalized patients should be improved.[138]

Respiratory care practitioners should be keenly aware of the initial rhythm during resuscitation because

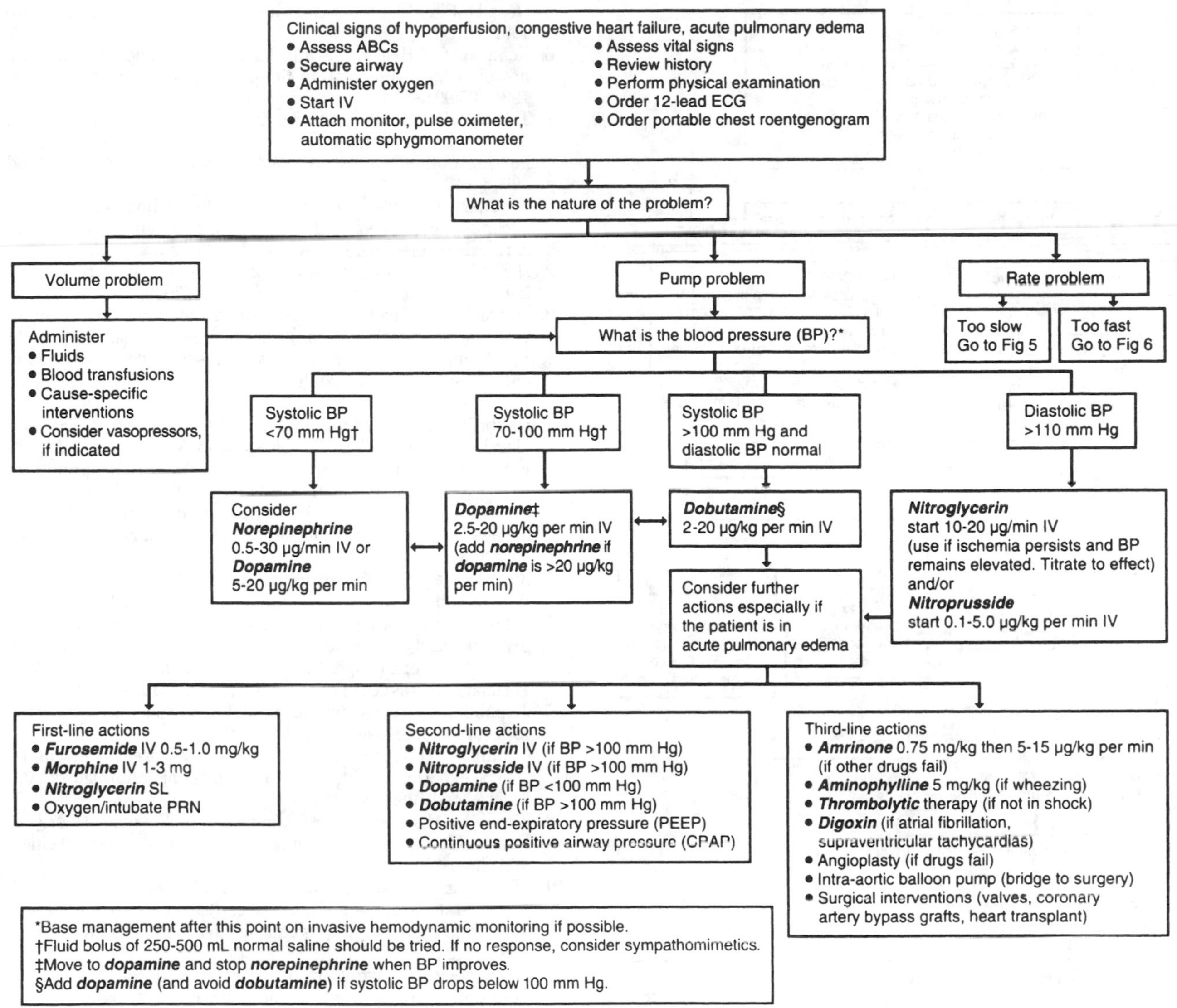
Clinical signs of hypoperfusion, congestive heart failure, acute pulmonary edema
• Assess ABCs
• Secure airway
• Administer oxygen
• Start IV
• Attach monitor, pulse oximeter, automatic sphygmomanometer
• Assess vital signs
• Review history
• Perform physical examination
• Order 12-lead ECG
• Order portable chest roentgenogram
What is the nature of the problem?
Volume problem
Pump problem
Rate problem
Administer
• Fluids
• Blood transfusions
• Cause-specific interventions
• Consider vasopressors, if indicated
What is the blood pressure (BP)?*
Too slow Go to Fig 5
Too fast Go to Fig 6
Systolic BP <70 mm Hg†
Systolic BP 70-100 mm Hg†
Systolic BP >100 mm Hg and diastolic BP normal
Diastolic BP >110 mm Hg
Consider Norepinephrine 0.5-30 μg/min IV or Dopamine 5-20 μg/kg per min
Dopamine‡ 2.5-20 μg/kg per min IV (add norepinephrine if dopamine is >20 μg/kg per min)
Dobutamine§ 2-20 μg/kg per min IV
Nitroglycerin start 10-20 μg/min IV (use if ischemia persists and BP remains elevated. Titrate to effect) and/or Nitroprusside start 0.1-5.0 μg/kg per min IV
Consider further actions especially if the patient is in acute pulmonary edema
First-line actions
• Furosemide IV 0.5-1.0 mg/kg
• Morphine IV 1-3 mg
• Nitroglycerin SL
• Oxygen/intubate PRN
Second-line actions
• Nitroglycerin IV (if BP >100 mm Hg)
• Nitroprusside IV (if BP >100 mm Hg)
• Dopamine (if BP <100 mm Hg)
• Dobutamine (if BP >100 mm Hg)
• Positive end-expiratory pressure (PEEP)
• Continuous positive airway pressure (CPAP)
Third-line actions
• Amrinone 0.75 mg/kg then 5-15 μg/kg per min (if other drugs fail)
• Aminophylline 5 mg/kg (if wheezing)
• Thrombolytic therapy (if not in shock)
• Digoxin (if atrial fibrillation, supraventricular tachycardias)
• Angioplasty (if drugs fail)
• Intra-aortic balloon pump (bridge to surgery)
• Surgical interventions (valves, coronary artery bypass grafts, heart transplant)
*Base management after this point on invasive hemodynamic monitoring if possible.
†Fluid bolus of 250-500 mL normal saline should be tried. If no response, consider sympathomimetics.
‡Move to dopamine and stop norepinephrine when BP improves.
§Add dopamine (and avoid dobutamine) if systolic BP drops below 100 mm Hg.

PROTOCOL 22-10. Acute pulmonary edema/hypotension/shock algorithm. (Emergency Cardiac Care Committee and Subcommittees, American Heart Association: Guidelines for cardiopulmonary resuscitation and emergency cardiac care, III: Adult advanced cardiac life support. JAMA 1992;268:2227. Reproduced with permission.)

ventricular fibrillation (VF) and tachyarrhythmias appear to be an important determinate of CPR outcome.[139–142] We must be prepared to recognize VF and pulseless ventricular tachycardia (VT) and treat both with defibrillation quickly to increase the chances of restoring a spontaneous rhythm.

Respiratory care practitioners and health care providers should define the goals of resuscitation in terms of long-term survival, quality of life, and years of useful life following CPR. The cost of paying inadequate attention to determining which patients should have DNR orders written is a drain on the entire health care system. Research on the impact of disease categories on CPR outcome should be used to educate physicians, nurses, and RCPs so they can help patients better understand the probability that they will return to the quality of life they experienced before CPR. Successful CPR outcome should be carefully defined using the patient disease category. Each patient should be individually evaluated for DNR orders. As suggested by Schwenzer,[143] "Patients' perception of their quality of life before and after CPR should guide their and our decisions." However, we must all accept the responsibility of defining the limitations of medical technology and try to determine when CPR is a futile effort.

ACLS Algorithms

Additional ACLS algorithms are shown in Protocols 22-8, 22-9, 22-10, and 22-11.

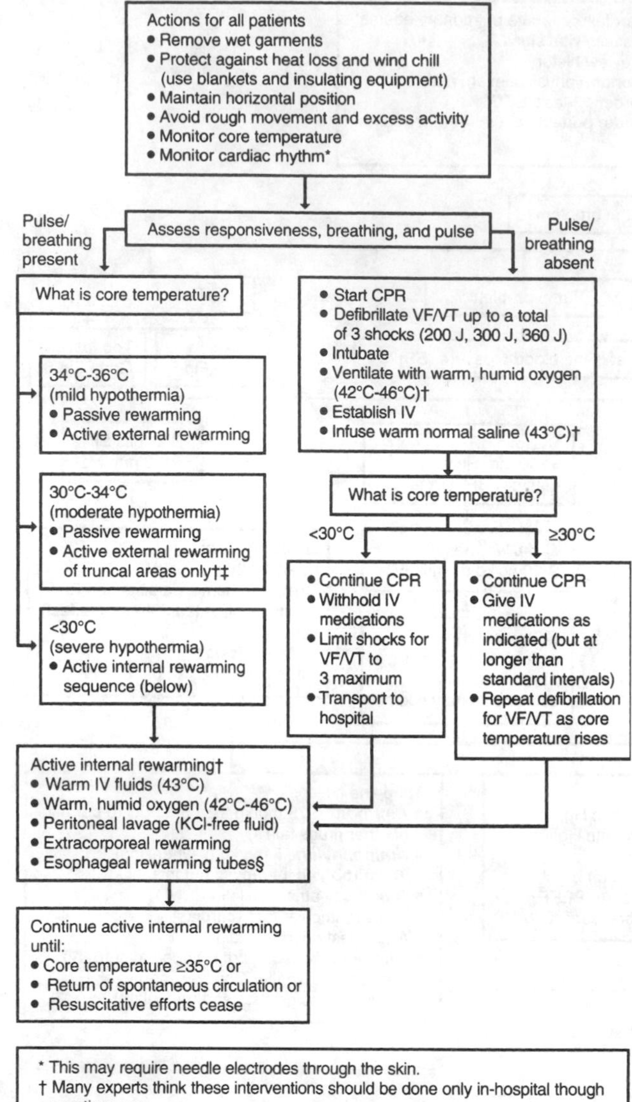

PROTOCOL 22-11. Algorithm for the treatment of hypothermia. (Emergency Cardiac Care Committee and Subcommittees, American Heart Association: Guidelines for cardiopulmonary resuscitation and emergency cardiac care, III: Adult advanced cardiac life support. JAMA 1992;268:2245. Reproduced with permission.)

REFERENCES

1. Emergency Cardiac Care Committee and Subcommittees, American Heart Association. Guidelines for cardiopulmonary resuscitation and emergency cardiac care, I: introduction. JAMA 1992;268:2172.
2. Essentials of ACLS. In: Cummins RO, ed. Textbook of advanced cardiac life support. Dallas: American Heart Association, 1994:1-1.
3. Risk Factors and Prudent Heart Living. In: Chandra NC, Hazinski MF, eds. Textbook of basic life support for healthcare providers. Dallas: American Heart Association, 1994:3-1.
4. Kouwenhoven WB, Jude JR, Knickerbocker GG. Closed chest cardiac massage. JAMA 1960;173:1064.
5. Hess D, Eitel D. Monitoring during resuscitation. Respir Care 1992;37:739.
6. Robinson GR, Hess D. Postdischarge survival and functional status following in-hospital cardiopulmonary resuscitation. Chest 1994;105:991.
7. Tresch DD, Neahring JM, Duthie EH, Mark DH, Kartes SK, Aufderheide TP. Outcomes of cardiopulmonary resuscitation in nursing homes: can we predict who will benefit? Am J Med 1993;95:123.
8. Fletcher GF, Cantwell JD. Ventricular fibrillation in a medically supervised cardiac exercise program: clinical, angiographic, and surgical correlations. JAMA 1977;238:2627.
9. Haskell Wl. Cardiovascular complications during exercise training of cardiac patients. Circulation 1978;57:920.
10. Hossack KF, Hartwig R. Cardiac arrest associated with supervised cardiac rehabilitation. J Cardiac Rehab 1982;2:402.
11. Van Camp SP, Peterson RA. Cardiovascular complications of out-patient cardiac rehabilitation programs. JAMA 1986;256: 1160.
12. Defibrillation. In: Cummins RO, ed. Textbook of advanced cardiac life support. Dallas: American Heart Association, 1994;4-1.
13. Emergency Cardiac Care Committee and Subcommittees, American Heart Association. Guidelines for cardiopulmonary resuscitation and emergency cardiac care, IX: Ensuring effectiveness of communitywide emergency cardiac care. JAMA 1992;268:2289.
14. Kaye W. Research on advanced cardiac life support training—Which methods improve retention? Respir Care 1995;40:538.
15. Palmisano JM, Akingbola OA, Moler FW, Custer JR. Simulated pediatric cardiopulmonary resuscitation: initial events and response times of a hospital arrest team. Respir Care 1994;39:725.
16. Tortalani AJ, Risucci DA, Rosati RJ, Dixon R. In-hospital cardiopulmonary resuscitation: patient arrest factors associated with survival. Resuscitation 1990;20:115.
17. Cummins RO. From concept to standard-of-care? Review of the clinical experience with automated electrical defibrillators. Ann Emerg Med 1989;18:1269.
18. Eisenberg MS, Horwood BT, Cummins RO, Reynolds-Haertie R, Heame TR. Cardiac arrest and resuscitation: a tale of 29 cities. Ann Emerg Med 1990;19:179.
19. Eisenberg MS, Cummins RO, Damon S, Larsen MP, Heame TR. Survival rates from out-of-hospital cardiac arrest: recommendations for uniform definitions and data to report. Ann Emerg Med 1990;19:1249.
20. Emergency Cardiac Care Committee and Subcommittees, American Heart Association. Guidelines for cardiopulmonary resuscitation and emergency cardiac care, III: Advanced cardiac life support. JAMA 1992;268:2199.
21. Thalman JJ, Rinaldo-Gallo S, MacIntyre NR. Analysis of an endotracheal intubation service provided by respiratory care practitioners. Respir Care 1993;38:469.
22. Stewart RD, Paris PM, Winter PM, Pelton GH, Cannon GM. Field intubation by paramedical personnel; success rates and complications. Chest 1984;85:341.
23. Murphy RJ. Citizen cardiopulmonary resuscitation training and use in a metropolitan area: the Minnesota Heart Survey. Am J Pub Health 1984;74:513.
24. Spaite DW, Hanlon T, Criss EA, Valenzuela TD, Wright AL, Keeley KT. Prehospital cardiac arrest: the impact of witnessed collapse and bystander CPR in a metropolitan EMS system with short response times. Ann Emerg Med 1990;19:1264.
25. Kaye W, Mancini JE, Giuliano KK, Richards N, Nagid DM, Marler CA, Sawyer-Silva S. Strengthening the inhospital chain of survival with rapid defibrillation by first responders using automated external defibrillators: training and retention issues. Ann Emerg Med 1995;25:163.
26. DeBono D. Resuscitation—Time for a rethink? Quarterly Journal of Medicine. 1991;81:959.
27. Brenner BE, Kaufman J. Reluctance of internists and medical residents to perform mouth-to-mouth resuscitation. Arch Intern Med 1993;153:1763.
28. Tweed WA, Wilson E, Isfeld B. Retention of cardiopulmonary resuscitation skills after initial overtraining. Crit Care Med 1980;8:651.

29. Kaye W, Mancini MF, Rallis S, Handel LP. Education Aspects: Resuscitation Training and Evaluation. In Kaye W, Bircher NG, eds: Cardiopulmonary resuscitation. New York: Churchill Livingstone, 1989.
30. Kaye W, Mancini ME. Use of the Mega Code to evaluate team leader performance during advanced cardiac life support. Crit Care Med 1986;14:99.
31. American Association For Respiratory Care. Clinical practice guideline: Resuscitation in acute care hospitals. Respir Care, 1993;38:1179.
32. Curry L, Gass D. Effects of training in cardiopulmonary resuscitation on competence and patient outcome. Can Med Assoc J 1987;137:491.
33. Batenhorst RL, Clifton GD, Booth DC, Hendrickson NM, Ryberg ML. Evaluation of 516 cardiopulmonary resuscitation attempts. Am J Hosp Pharm 1985;42:2478.
34. Schade J. An evaluation framework for code 99. Q Rev Bull 1983;9:306.
35. American College of Emergency Physicians. ACEP Policy Statement—Implementation of Early Defibrillation/Automated External Defibrillator Programs. Dallas: ACEP, 1992.
36. Eisenberg MS, Copass MK, Hallstrom AP, Blake B, Berger L, Short FA, Cobb LA. Treatment of out of hospital cardiac arrests with rapid defibrillation by emergency medical technicians. N Engl J Med 1980;302:1379.
37. Eisenberg MS, Bergener L, Hallstrom A. Cardiac resuscitation in the community: importance of rapid provision of and implications for program planning. JAMA 1979;241:1905.
38. Abramson NS, Safar P, Detre K, Kelsey S, Reinmuth O, Synder J. An international collaborative clinical study mechanism for resuscitation research. Resuscitation 1982;10:141.
39. Adjuncts for Airway Control. In: Cummins RO, ed. Textbook of advanced cardiac life support. Dallas: American Heart Association, 1994:2-1.
40. Barnes TA, Adams G. Ventilatory volumes using mouth-to-mouth, bag-valve-mask, and pocket face mask (abstract). Respir Care 1991;36:1292.
41. Cummins RO, Austin D, Graves JR, Litwin PE, Pierce J. Ventilation skills of emergency medical technicians: a teaching challenge for emergency medicine. Ann Emerg Med 1986;15:1187.
42. Hess D, Baran C. Ventilatory volumes using mouth-to-mouth, mouth-to-mask, and bag-valve-mask techniques. Am J Emer Med 1985;3:292.
43. Hess D, Ness C, Oppel A, Rhoads K. Evaluation of mouth-to-mask devices. Respir Care 1989;34:191.
44. Jesudian MC, Harrison RR, Keenan RL, Maull KI. Bag-valve-mask ventilation two rescuers are better than one: preliminary report. Crit Care Med 1985;13:122.
45. Johannigman JA, Branson RD, Davis K, Hurst JM. Techniques of emergency ventilation: a model to evaluate tidal volume, airway pressure, gastric insufflation. J Trauma 1991;31:93.
46. Johannigman JA, Branson RD. Oxygen enrichment of expired gas for mouth-to-mask resuscitation. Respir Care 1991;36:99.
47. ECRI. Evaluation: exhaled-air pulmonary resuscitators (EAPRs) and disposable manual resuscitators (DMPRs). Health Devices 1989;18:333.
48. Adult Basic Life Support. In: Chandra NC, Hazinski MF, eds. Textbook of basic life support for healthcare providers. Dallas: American Heart Association, 1994:4-1.
49. Emergency Cardiac Care Committee and Subcommittees, American Heart Association. Guidelines for cardiopulmonary resuscitation and emergency cardiac care, II: adult BLS. JAMA 1992;268:2184.
50. Howells TH. Disaster at the dining table. Br Med J 1984;289:510.
51. Greensher J, Mofenson HC. Aspiration accidents: choking and drowning. Pediatr Ann 1983;12:747.
52. Torrey SB. The choking child—a life threatening emergency. Clin Pediatr 1983;22:751.
53. CDC. Fatal injuries to children—US 1986. JAMA 1990;264:952.
54. Division of Injury Control, Center for Environmental Health and Injury Control, CDC. Childhood injuries in the U.S. Am J Dis Child 1990;144:627.
55. Aufderheide TP. Pacemakers and electrical therapy during advanced cardiac life support. Respir Care 1995;40:364.
56. Cobb LA, Werner JA, Trobaugh GB. Sudden cardiac death: a decade's experience with out of hospital resuscitation. Mod Concepts Cardiovasc Dis 1980;49:31.
57. Eisenberg M, Bergner L, Hallstrom A. Paramedic programs and out-of-hospital cardiac arrest: factors associated with successful resuscitation. Am J Public Health 1979;69:30.
58. Hargarten KM, Stueven HA, Waite EM, Olson DW, Mateer JR, Darin JC. Prehospital experience with defibrillation of coarse ventricular fibrillation: a ten-year review. Ann Emerg Med 1990;19:157.
59. Weaver WD, Cobb LA, Hallstrom AP, FahrenBruch C, Copass MK, Ray R. Factors influencing survival after out-of-hospital cardiac arrest. J Am Coll Cardiol 1986;7:752.
60. Newman M. Chain of survival concept takes hold. J Emerg Med Serv 1989;14:11.
61. Newman M. Early access, early CPR, and early defibrillation: cry of the 1988 Conference on Citizen CPR. J Emerg Med Serv 1988;13:30.
62. Cummins RO, Thies W. Encouraging early defibrillation: the American Heart Association and automated external defibrillators. Ann Emerg Med 1990;19:1245.
63. Automated External Defibrillation. In: Chandra NC, Hazinski MF, eds. Textbook of basic life support for healthcare providers. Dallas: American Heart Association, 1994:9-1.
64. Stultz KR, Brown DD, Cooley F, Kerber RE. Self-adhesive monitor defibrillation pads improve prehospital defibrillation success. Ann Emerg Med 1987;16:872.
65. Thalman JJ, Rinaldo-Gallo S, MacIntyre NR. Analysis of an endotracheal intubation service provided by respiratory care practitioners. Respir Care 1993;38:469.
66. Finucane BT, Santora AH. Principles of Airway Management. Philadelphia: FA Davis, 1988.
67. American Society for Testing and Materials: Standard Specification For Cuffed and Uncuffed Tracheal Tubes, Designation: F 1242-89. 1995 Annual Book of ASTM Standards, 1995;13.01:582.
68. Plevak DJ, Ward JJ. Airway Management. In: Burton GG, Hodgkin JE, Ward JJ, eds. Respiratory care—a guide to clinical practice, 3rd ed. Philadelphia: JB Lippincott, 1991:449.
69. Lindholm CE, Grenvik A. Tracheal tube and cuff problems. Int Anesthesiol Clin 1981;20:103.
70. Beamer WC, Prough DS. Technical and pharmacologic considerations in emergency translaryngeal intubation. Ear Nose Throat J 1983;62:11.
71. Lillenfield SM, Berman RA. Correspondence. Anesthesiology 1950;11:136.
72. Smith JP, Bodai BI, Palder S, Thomas V. The esophageal obturator. A review. JAMA 1983;250:1081.
73. Jacobs LM, Berrizbeitia LD, Bennett B, Madigan C. Endotracheal intubation in the pre-hospital phase of emergency medical care. JAMA 1984;250:2175.
74. Smith JP, Balazs IB, Aubourg R. A field evaluation of the esophageal obturator airway. J Trauma 1983;23:317.
75. Auerbach PS, Geehr EC. Inadequate oxygenation and ventilation using the esophageal gastric tube airway in the prehospital setting. JAMA 1983;250:3067.
76. Michael TA, Gordon AS. The oesophageal obturator airway: a new device in emergency cardiopulmonary resuscitation. Br Med J 1980;281:1531.
77. Yauncey W, Wears R, Kamajian G. Unrecognized tracheal intubation: A complication of the esophageal obturator airway. Ann Emerg Med 1980;9:18.
78. Selleck BA. Cricoid pressure to control regurgitation of the stomach contents during induction of anesthesia. Lancet 1962; 2:404.
79. American Society for Testing and Materials. Standard specification for performance and safety requirements for resuscitators intended for use with humans. Designation: F 920-93. 1995 Annual Book of ASTM Standards, 1995;13.01:266.
80. ISO Technical Committee ISO/TC 121, Anesthetic and Respiratory Equipment. International Standard ISO 8382: Resuscitators Intended For Use With Humans. Switzerland: International Organization for Standardization, 1988.
81. Barnes TA. Emergency ventilation techniques and related equipment. Respir Care 1992;37:673.

82. ECRI. Evaluation: exhaled-air pulmonary resuscitators (EAPRs) and disposable manual resuscitators (DMPRs). Health Devices 1989;18:333.
83. Hess D, Goff G. The effects of two-hand versus one-hand ventilation on volumes delivered during bag-valve ventilation at various resistances and compliances. Respir Care 1987;32:1025.
84. Van Hooser DT. Altitude and temperature effects on bag-valve resuscitator performance (abstract). Respir Care 1991;36:1293.
85. Augustine JA, Seidel DR, McCabe JB. Ventilation performance using a self-inflating anesthesia bag: effect of operator characteristics. Am J Emerg Med 1987;5:267.
86. Powers WE. Evaluation of a training method that uses volumetric feedback with bag-valve-mask ventilation techniques (abstract). Respir Care 1988;33:942.
87. Hess D, Goff G, Johnson K. The effect of hand size, resuscitator brand, and use of two hands on volumes delivered during adult bag-valve ventilation. Respir Care 1989;34:191.
88. Jesudian MC, Harrison RR, Keenan RL, Maull KI. Bag-valve-mask ventilation two rescuers are better than one: preliminary report. Crit Care Med 1985;13:122.
89. Seidelin PH, Stolarek IH, Littlewood DG. Comparison of six methods of emergency ventilation. Lancet 1986;2:1274.
90. Melker RJ, Banner MJ. Ventilation during CPR: two-rescuer standards reappraised. Ann Emerg Med 1985;14:397.
91. Ornato JP, Bryson BL, Donovan PJ, Farquharson RR, Jaeger C. Measurement of ventilation during cardiopulmonary resuscitation. Crit Care Med 1983;11:79.
92. Stewart RD. Influence of mask design on bag-mask ventilation. Ann Emerg Med 1985;14:403.
93. Terndrup TE, Kanter RK, Cherry RA. A comparison of infant ventilation methods performed by prehospital personnel. Ann Emerg Med 1989;18:607.
94. Kanter RK. Evaluation of mask-bag ventilation in resuscitation of infants. AJDC 1987;141:761.
95. Hirschman AM, Kaavath RE. Venting versus ventilating: a danger of manual resuscitation bags. Chest 1982;82:369.
96. Barnes T: Evaluation of four disposable pediatric manual resuscitators (abstract). Respir Care 1989;34:1059.
97. Finer NN, Barrington KJ, Al-Fadley F, Peters KL. Limitations of self-inflating resuscitators. Pediatrics 1986;77:417.
98. Kauffman GW, Hess DR. Modification of the infant Laerdal resuscitation bag to monitor airway pressure. Crit Care Med 1982;10:112.
99. Goldstein B, Catlin EA, Vetere JM, Arguin LJ. The role of in-line manometers in minimizing peak and mean airway pressure during the hand-regulated ventilation of newborn infants. Respir Care 1989;34:23.
100. Bizzle TL, Kotas RV. Positive pressure hand ventilation: potential errors in estimating inflation pressures. Pediatrics 1983; 72:122.
101. Pasquet EA, Frewen TC, Kissoon N, Gallant J, Tiffin N. Prototype volume-controlled neonatal/infant resuscitator. Crit Care Med 1988;16:55.
102. Terndrup TE, Cherry RA, McCabe JB. Comparison of ventilation performance: standard resuscitation bag and the resuscitation bag controller. JEM 1990;8:121.
103. Tiffin NH, Gallant JH, Pasquet EA, Kissoon N, Frewen TC. A neonatal volume controlled resuscitator. RRT 1988;24:15.
104. Chernick V. Lung rupture in the newborn infant. Respir Care 1986;31:628.
105. Palme C, Nystrom B, Tunell R. An evaluation of the efficiency of face masks in the resuscitation of newborn infants. Lancet 1985;1:207.
106. Cole AF, Rolbin SH, Hew EM, Pynn S. An improved ventilator system for delivery-room management of the newborn. Anesthesiology 1979;51:356.
107. Field D, Milner AD, Hopkin IE. Efficacy of manual resuscitators at birth. Arch Dis Childhood 1986;61:300.
108. Terndrup TE, Kanter RK, Cherry RA. A comparison of infant ventilation methods performed by prehospital personnel. Ann Emerg Med 1989;18:607.
109. Palme C, Nystrom B, Tunell R. An evaluation of the efficiency of face masks in the resuscitation of newborn infants. Lancet 1985;1:207.
110. Miller RD, Hamilton WK. Pneumothorax during infant resuscitation. JAMA 1969;210:1090.
111. Vyas H. Facemask resuscitation of the newborn. Indian J Pediatrics 1987;54:618.
112. Vyas H, Milner AD, Hopkin IE, Boon AW. Physiologic responses to prolonged and slow-rise inflation in the resuscitation of the asphyxiated newborn infant. J Pediatr 1981;99:635.
113. Milner AD, Saunders RA. Pressure and volume changes during the first breath of human neonates. Arch Dis Childhood 1977; 52:918.
114. Boon AW, Milner AD, Hopkin IE. Lung expansion, tidal volume, and formation of the functional residual capacity during resuscitation of asphyxiated neonates. J Pediatrics 1979;95:1031.
115. Hull D. Lung expansion and ventilation during resuscitation of asphyxiated newborn infants. J Pediatrics 1969;75:47.
116. Fluck RF Jr. Intermittent Positive Pressure Breathing Devices and Transport Ventilators. In: Barnes TA, ed. Core textbook in respiratory care practice. St. Louis, Mosby-Year Book, 1994:485.
117. Iserson K, Sanders AB, Kaback K. Difficult intubations: aids and alternatives. Am Fam Phys 1985;31:99.
118. Roven AN, Clapham MB. Cricothyrotomy. Ear Nose Throat 1983;62:68.
119. Intravenous Techniques. In: Cummins RO, ed. Textbook of advanced cardiac life support. Dallas: American Heart Association, 1994:6-1.
120. Aitkenhead AR. Drug administration during CPR: what route? Resuscitation 1991;22:191.
121. Hess D. Methods of emergency drug administration. Respir Care 1995;40:498.
122. Bayes de Luna A, Coumel P, Leclercg JF. Ambulatory sudden cardiac death: mechanism of production of fatal arrhythmia on the basis of data from 157 cases. Am Heart J 1989;117:151.
123. Greene HL. Sudden arrhythmic cardiac death: mechanisms, resuscitation and classification. Am J Cardiol 1990;65:4B.
124. Arrhythmias. In: Cummins RO, ed. Textbook of advanced cardiac life support. Dallas: American Heart Association, 1994:3-1.
125. Overview of Case-Based Teaching and Interactive Teaching. In: Billi JE, Cummins RO, eds. Instructor's manual for advanced cardiac life support. Dallas: American Heart Association, 1994:8-1.
126. Paradis NA, Martin GB, Goetting MG, Rivers EP, Feingold M, Nowak RM. Aortic pressure during human cardiac arrest: identification of pseudo-electromechanical dissociation. Chest 1992; 101;123.
127. ACLS Provider Training: Overview. Billi JE, Cummins RO, eds. Instructor's manual for advanced cardiac life support. Dallas: American Heart Association, 1994:2-1.
128. Gunnar RM, Bourdillon PO, Dixon DW, Fuster V, Korp RB, Kennedy JW, et al. ACC/AHA guidelines for the early management of patients with acute myocardial infarction. Circulation 1990;82:664.
129. Antman EM, Lau J, Kupelnick B, Mosteller F, Chalmers TC. A comparison of results of meta analyses of randomized control trials for myocardial infarction. JAMA 1992;268:240.
130. Lau J, Antman EM, Jimenez-Silva J, Kupelnick B, Mosteller F, Chalmers TC. Cumulative meta-analysis of therapeutic trials for myocardial infarction. N Engl J Med 1992;327:248.
131. Eisenberg MS, Aghababian RV, Bossaert L, Jaffe AS, Ornato JP, Weaver WD. Thrombolytic Therapy. Ann Emerg Med 1993; 22:417.
132. EMERAS (Estudio Multicentrico Estreptoquinasa Republicas de America del Sur) Collaborative Group. Late Assessment of Thrombolytic Efficacy (LATE) study with alteplase 6–24 hours after onset of acute myocardial infarction. Lancet 1993;342:759.
133. EMERAS (Estudio Multicentrico Estreptoquinasa Republicas de America del Sur) Collaborative Group. Randomised trial of late thrombolysis in patients with suspected acute myocardial infarction. Lancet 1993;342:767.
134. Cerebral Resuscitation: Treatment of the Brain After Cardiac Resuscitation. In: Cummins RO, ed. Textbook of advanced cardiac life support. Dallas: American Heart Association, 1994;14-1.
135. Grande CM, ed. Textbook of Trauma Anesthesia and Critical Care. St. Louis: Mosby-Year Book, 1993:999.
136. Schneider AP, Nelson DJ, Brown DD. Inhospital cardiopulmonary resuscitation: a 30 year review. J Am Board Fam Practice 1993;6:91.
137. Urberg M, Ways C. Survival after cardiopulmonary resuscitation for an inhospital arrest. J Fam Pract 1987;25:41.

138. Kyff J, Puri VK, Rheja, Ireland T. Cardiopulmonary resuscitation in hospitalized patients: continuing problems in decision-making. Crit Care Med 1987;15:41.
139. Fletcher GF, Cantwell JD. Ventricular fibrillation in a medically supervised cardiac exercise program: clinical, angiographic, and surgical correlations. JAMA 1977;238:2627.
140. Haskell Wl. Cardiovascular complications during exercise training of cardiac patients. Circulation 1978;57:920.
141. Hossack KF, Hartwig R. Cardiac arrest associated supervised cardiac rehabilitation. J Cardiac Rehab 1982;2:402.
142. Van Camp SP, Peterson RA. Cardiovascular complications of out-patient cardiac rehabilitation programs. JAMA 1986;256: 1160.
143. Schwenzer KJ, Smith WT, Durbin CG Jr. Selective application of cardiopulmonary resuscitation improves survival rates. Anesth Analg 1993;76:478.

23 Pulmonary Rehabilitation

John E. Hodgkin
Gerilynn L. Connors

PROFESSIONAL SKILLS

Upon completion of this chapter, the reader will:

- Define and state the goals of pulmonary rehabilitation
- Identify the essential components of a pulmonary rehabilitation program
- Use initial patient assessment information to tailor the pulmonary rehabilitation program to the individual needs of the patient
- Describe essential medical tests used to assess the pulmonary rehabilitation candidate
- Summarize the role of exercise testing in patient evaluation for pulmonary rehabilitation
- Address the nutritional needs of the pulmonary patient
- Recommend appropriate psychosocial interventions for the pulmonary patient
- Develop a typical exercise training program
- Formulate objective outcome measurements for tracking improvement of the pulmonary rehabilitation patient
- List potential benefits for the pulmonary rehabilitation patient
- Discuss various approaches to helping patients stop smoking

KEY TERMS

Activities of daily living
Assessment for lung disease
Exercise prescription
Exercise training
Nicotine addiction
Nicotine replacement therapy
Prevention of lung disease
Smoking cessation
Target heart rate
Treatment of lung disease

INTRODUCTION

The course and prognosis for many individuals with chronic pulmonary disease can be altered through a comprehensive process referred to as pulmonary rehabilitation (PR).[1,2] This process incorporates the concepts of preventive medicine into the patient's care plan.[3,4] The prescription of medications for the pulmonary patient is just one part of appropriate treatment that is addressed in a PR program. Pulmonary rehabilitation should be considered for patients at various ages with a variety of pulmonary diseases, including chronic obstructive pulmonary disease (COPD), asthma, cystic fibrosis, and restrictive disorders.[5–11] Pulmonary patients have specialized needs that often can best be met by members of a multidisciplinary health care team. The intent of this chapter is to provide an understanding of the process of assessment, patient training, psychosocial intervention, exercise, and follow-up known as pulmonary rehabilitation.

ECONOMIC IMPACT OF LUNG DISEASE

The cost of lung disease in terms of dollars spent and lives affected is immense, and it continues to grow each year. Lung disease is now the fourth leading cause of mortality in the United States, surpassed only by heart disease, cancer, and stroke.[12] The top 10 causes of death in the United States in 1994 are listed in Table 23-1.[12] Among the 32 industrialized countries studied in 1991, the United States ranked 14th in COPD mortality for males and 8th for females.[13]

Lung disease is the leading cause of disability in the United States and costs the economy in excess of $50 billion per year in direct and indirect expenditures.[14] In the United States in 1992, there were 91,400 deaths due to COPD and allied conditions, an age-adjusted death rate of 19.9 per 100,000 people. In 1994, there were 101,870 deaths due to COPD and allied conditions. The average mortality rate for COPD and allied conditions rose 14.2% per year between 1970 and 1993, while the average mortality rate for heart disease dropped 0.3% per year over the same period.[12]

TABLE 23-1 **Deaths from the Leading Causes, United States, 1994**

Rank	Cause of Death	Number
Total of all causes		2,286,000
1	Heart disease	734,090
2	Cancer	536,860
3	Stroke	154,350
4	COPD and allied conditions*	101,870
5	Accidents and adverse effects	90,140
6	Pneumonia and influenza	82,090
7	Diabetes mellitus	55,390
8	Human immunodeficiency virus (HIV) infection	41,930
9	Suicide	32,410
10	Chronic liver disease and cirrhosis	25,730
All other causes		431,140

* Includes COPD, chronic and unspecified bronchitis, emphysema, and asthma.

Men and women have similar COPD mortality rates before the age of 55, but the rate for men rises thereafter: at age 70, the rate for men is more than double that for women; and at 85 and older, the COPD death rate for males is more than 3.5 times that for females.[15,16]

In the United States in 1993, there were an estimated 13.07 million people with asthma, including 4.8 million children, 13.82 million people with chronic bronchitis, and 1.93 million people with emphysema.[17,18] There are an estimated 14.2 million Americans with COPD.[19] The 1991 economic cost estimates for COPD from the National Heart, Lung and Blood Institute were $18.1 billion, which included $9.6 billion in direct health care expenditures, $4.3 billion in indirect morbidity costs, and $4.2 billion in indirect mortality costs.[17]

In 1991, asthma cost the U.S. economy an estimated $9.5 billion, of which $6.9 billion was for direct medical expenditures and $2.6 billion for indirect costs.[14,16] The age-adjusted death rate from asthma was 1.4 per 100,000 people in 1992. This is low, but it has risen over 40% since 1980. In asthmatic children ages 5 to 17, asthma accounts for the loss of over 10 million school days per year.[16] In individuals 18 years of age or older, more than 3 million work days per year are lost. Asthma causes a serious economic burden on the U.S. economy through the loss of productivity and because of increasing health care costs due to morbidity.

There are currently about 46.3 million smokers (25.7% of the adult population) in the United States and an estimated 419,00 deaths caused by smoking-related diseases every year.[14] Smoking costs approximately $68 billion each year in assessment, health care, and lost productivity.[19] Occupational lung disease is the leading cause of work-related illness in the United States.

Tuberculosis has been on a resurgence, but during the last 2 years it has stabilized, with reported cases of 10.5 per 100,000 in the United States in 1992.[14]

DEFINITION

The concept of rehabilitation is not new. In 1942 the Council on Rehabilitation defined rehabilitation as "the restoration of the individual to the fullest medical, mental, emotional, social and vocational potential of which he/she is capable." Pulmonary rehabilitation is concerned not only with the control of symptoms and disease but also with the promotion and maintenance of health. Rehabilitation is a process whereby a patient moves toward better health and an increased level of wellness.

Patients must understand their rehabilitative potential so that they have the information needed for decision making. Rehabilitation helps the person to identify his or her "assets and liabilities," as well as the available avenues for change.

In 1974, the American College of Chest Physicians adopted the following definition of pulmonary rehabilitation:[20]

> *An art of medical practice wherein an individually tailored multidisciplinary program is formulated, which, through accurate diagnosis, therapy, emotional support and education, stabilizes or reverses both the physio- and psychopathology of pulmonary disease and attempts to return the individual to the highest possible functional capacity allowed by his pulmonary handicap and overall life situation.*

As pointed out in the official American Thoracic Society Statement on Pulmonary Rehabilitation in 1981,[21] "in the broadest sense, pulmonary rehabilitation means providing good, comprehensive respiratory care for patients with pulmonary disease."

In 1994, the National Institutes of Health Consensus Conference on Pulmonary Rehabilitation developed the following definition to describe the process:[22]

> *A multi-dimensional continuum of services directed to persons with pulmonary disease and their families, usually by an interdisciplinary team of specialists, with a goal of achieving and maintaining the individual's maximum level of independence and functioning in the community.*

ESSENTIAL COMPONENTS OF PULMONARY REHABILITATION

A PR program must be individualized to meet the needs of each patient. The essential components of PR are depicted in Figure 23-1 and Figure 23-2. They include team assessment, patient training, psychosocial intervention, exercise, and follow-up.[2]

PATIENT SELECTION AND SEQUENCE

Pulmonary rehabilitation is not just an exercise or education program, but a carefully integrated comprehensive program that follows a logical sequence. Conditions which are appropriate for pulmonary rehabilitation are listed in Box 23-1. The sequence of PR begins with patient selection and assessing the patient's needs. Factors to be evaluated when selecting a patient for PR are listed in Box 23-2. Any patient with symptoms and abnormal lung function should be considered for PR.

Conditions that may be considered contraindications to PR include psychiatric disturbances, such as dementia and organic brain syndrome; acute congestive heart failure; recent myocardial infarction; acute cor pulmonale; substance abuse; significant liver dysfunction; metastatic cancer; and disabling stroke. The next step is to develop reasonable goals with the patient and the family that allow the PR team members to individualize the patient's treatment program. Throughout the program, the team members need to assess the patient's progress, making any changes warranted in the treatment program. Before the completion of the program, the PR team determines the patient's home program and arranges for follow-up.

ASSESSMENT

The initial patient assessment lays the foundation for the entire PR program.[23] An evaluation by the team's director or coordinator and the team physician helps to determine what other team member assessments would be useful, such as a physical therapist, occupational therapist, and so forth. The initial evaluation of the patient includes a thorough history and physical examination and appropriate medical testing to determine or confirm the pulmonary diagnosis. It is important to determine if there are problems with other systems, such as nasal or sinus, gastrointestinal, cardiovascular, neurologic, or musculoskeletal, that need to be considered when outlining a comprehensive treatment plan.[24]

The assessment should include a review of symptoms such as dyspnea, cough, sputum production, wheezing, hemoptysis, edema, and chest pain. Smoking history, occupational and environmental exposure, hobby or recreational exposure to pulmonary irritants, alcohol history, medications used and how prescribed, childhood pulmonary problems, and family history of pulmonary disease should all be determined.

In addition to basic vital signs, the physical examination should assess the heart, lungs, use of accessory muscles on quiet breathing, neck veins, and legs (for edema). Tests to be considered as part of the initial evaluation are listed in Box 23-3.

Comparison of previous test results with current tests can help determine the impact and progression of the patient's disease. Additional tests that may be ordered as a result of the initial assessment are listed in Box 23-4.

The exercise assessment helps to determine an appropriate exercise training program and detects if hypoxemia occurs with activity or exercise, if supplemental oxygen during training is needed, if there are any orthopedic problems that may impede the patient's exercise program, and if there is any cardiac dysfunction. The type of exercise testing may vary from a simple 6-minute walk to a pulmonary exercise stress test with gas exchange measurements.[25]

The psychological assessment can be done using standardized questionnaires.[26] This evaluation should assess for depression, anxiety, anger management, effectiveness of the patient's rehabilitation-related behaviors, family support and dependency issues, perception of stress, coping styles, general neuropsychological status, overall adaptation to disease, drug usage, compliance with the medical regimens, and the impact of role change due to disease.[27] The assessment focuses on the

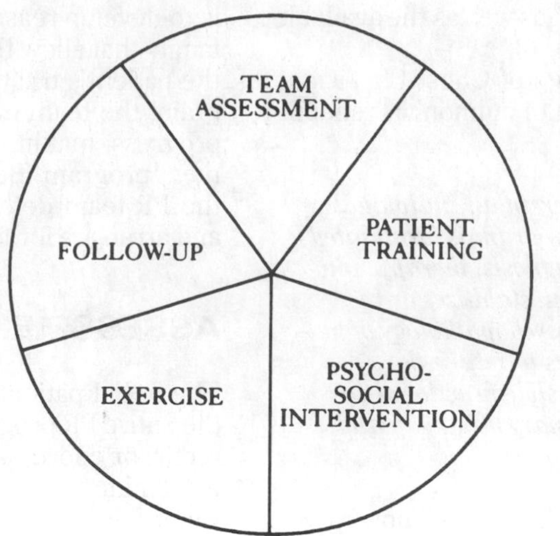

*Team Assessment**
PR team medical director
Respiratory care practitioner
Nurse
Occupational therapist
Physical therapist
Exercise physiologist
Psychologist
Vocational counselor
Recreational therapist
Social worker
Nutritionist

Exercise
Exercise conditioning
Respiratory muscle strength
Upper extremity strength
Home program plan

Follow-up
Patient outcomes
Maintenance exercise group
Group meetings
Reevaluation as necessary

Patient Training
Breathing retraining
Bronchial hygiene
Medications
Proper nutrition
ADL training
Panic control/relaxation
Energy conservation
Warning signs of infection
Sexuality for COPD patient and others

Psychosocial Intervention
Support system and dependency issues
Anger management
Treatment of depression
Counseling
Self-efficacy for rehabilitation-related behaviors
Impact of role change
Coping styles

* An individualized pulmonary rehabilitation program will meet the specific needs of the patient. Not every member of the pulmonary rehabilitation program team may be involved with the patient.

FIGURE 23-1 Essential components of a pulmonary rehabilitation program. NOTE. Patient training or exercise alone does not constitute a pulmonary rehabilitation program. (From Beytas L, Connors GL: Organization and management of a pulmonary rehabilitation program. In Hodgkin JE, Connors GL, Bell CW [eds], Pulmonary Rehabilitation: Guidelines to Success [2nd ed]. Philadelphia, JB Lippincott, 1993. Reprinted with permission)

patient's reaction to his or her disease, how to handle the illness, and its effects on daily life. It deals with the patient's work, social, recreational, interpersonal, and family relationships and sexual functioning. Psychotherapy and psychopharmacologic agents may be necessary for some patients. Counseling and support therapy are essential for many patients.

Assessment of basic life management skills, including activities of daily living (ADL), vocational issues, and leisure function, is essential. Nutritional assessment should include an evaluation of body weight, dietary history, fluid intake, and sodium intake.[28]

PATIENT TRAINING

To achieve success with a rehabilitation program, the patient and significant other must have a thorough understanding of the patient's lung disease and the principles of management, treatment, and prevention. The patient must make behavioral changes to optimize his or her health and become an active participant in the treatment program. The process by which a patient learns best varies from patient to patient and may be auditory, visual, or kinesthetic (by doing). Determining the patient's learning style allows the educator to en-

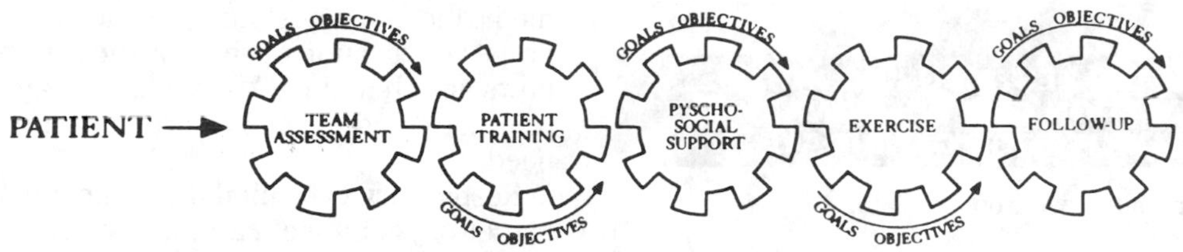

PATIENT → TEAM ASSESSMENT — PATIENT TRAINING — PYSCHO-SOCIAL SUPPORT — EXERCISE — FOLLOW-UP

GOALS OBJECTIVES

The essential components of pulmonary rehabilitation are very specific. Once the initial assessment is completed, the foundation of the patient's individualized program is developed from the goals and objectives established. It is essential for each component to be incorporated into a comprehensive pulmonary rehabilitation program.

FIGURE 23-2 Essential components of pulmonary rehabilitation. NOTE: Reprinted with permission from Connors GL, Hilling LR, Morris KV. "Assessment of the Pulmonary Rehabilitation Candidate." In Pulmonary Rehabilitation: Guidelines to Success (2nd Ed.) by Hodgkin JE, Connors GL and Bell CW, (eds). Philadelphia: J.B. Lippincott, 1993.

hance the patient's learning. The information covered in the education and training program should be contained in a patient education manual. The development of the patient's training program is based on the patient's needs as determined by the initial assessment and ongoing assessments.

Areas of training include self-assessment, bronchial hygiene, activities of daily living, medication use, respiratory care modalities, psychosocial intervention, and exercise.[2] The self-assessment training may include the following: (1) anatomy and physiology of the respiratory system and disease process; (2) an understanding of the medical tests performed on the patient; (3) importance of avoiding environmental and occupational irritants; (4) principles of exercise and physical fitness; (5) nutritional needs; (6) management of symptoms;[29] (7) knowledge of trigger signals for the asthmatic; (8) warning signals of an infection; (9) appropriate use of pneumococcal and influenza vaccines; (10) other areas of self-assessment training depending upon the patient's needs, such as pedal edema, sugar level, and so forth; and (11) avoidance of active and passive smoking.

Bronchial hygiene training should teach the patient proper breathing, including pursed lip and diaphragmatic breathing, cough techniques, and postural drainage therapy including positioning and percussion

BOX 23-1

CONDITIONS APPROPRIATE FOR PULMONARY REHABILITATION

Obstructive Pulmonary Disease
Chronic obstructive pulmonary disease (COPD)
Asthma
Asthmatic bronchitis
Chronic bronchitis
Emphysema
Bronchiectasis
Cystic fibrosis

Restrictive Pulmonary Disease
Interstitial fibrosis
Rheumatoid pulmonary disease
Collagen vascular lung disorders
Pneumoconiosis
Sarcoidosis
Kyphoscoliosis
Rheumatoid spondylitis
Severe obesity
Poliomyelitis

Other Conditions
Pulmonary vascular diseases
Lung resection
Lung transplantation
Occupational or environmental lung diseases

Note: Reprinted with permission from Beytas L, Connors GL: Organization and Management of a Pulmonary Rehabilitation Program. In Hodgkin JE, Connors GL, Bell CW (eds), Pulmonary Rehabilitation: Guidelines to Success (2nd ed). Philadelphia, JB Lippincott, 1993.

BOX 23-2

CRITERIA TO BE EVALUATED IN SELECTING A PATIENT FOR PULMONARY REHABILITATION*

Disease effect on patient's quality of life
Reduction in physical activity
Changes in occupational performance
Dependence vs. independence in activities of daily living
Disease effect on the patient's psychosocial status (ie, anxiety, depression, etc.)
Use of medical resources (ie, hospitalizations, emergency room visits, etc.)
Presence of other medical problems
Pulmonary function assessment
Smoking history
Patient motivation
Patient commitment to time and active program participation
Patient transportation needs
Financial resources
Patient's background

* *Any patient with impairment because of lung disease and who is motivated should be a candidate for pulmonary rehabilitation.*

Note: Reprinted with permission from Beytas L, Connors GL: Organization and Management of a Pulmonary Rehabilitation Program. In Hodgkin JE, Connors GL, Bell CW (eds), Pulmonary Rehabilitation: Guidelines to Success (2nd ed). Philadelphia, JB Lippincott, 1993.

BOX 23-3

SUGGESTED TESTS DURING INITIAL EVALUATION OF A PULMONARY REHABILITATION CANDIDATE

Spirometry pre- and post-bronchodilator
Lung volumes
Diffusing capacity
Chest radiograph
Resting electrocardiogram
Exercise test with cutaneous oximetry or arterial blood gas or both (simple or modified test such as 6- or 12-minute walk, calibrated cycle ergometer, or motorized treadmill)
Complete blood count
Basic blood chemistry panel

Note: It is acceptable to not repeat these tests if done within the 3 months prior to entering the pulmonary rehabilitation program or as determined by the pulmonary rehabilitation medical director.

Note: Reprinted with permission from Selection and Team Assessment of the Pulmonary Rehabilitation Candidate. In AACVPR, Guidelines for Pulmonary Rehabilitation Programs. Champaign, IL, Human Kenetic Publishers, 1993.

if appropriate. Positive expiratory pressure and autogenic drainage are techniques that have been recommended for patients with excessive mucus due to bronchiectasis and cystic fibrosis.

Activities of daily living training covers time and energy conservation techniques, leisure time activities, panic control and relaxation, sexuality, travel recommendations for the pulmonary patient, community resources, and vocational retraining.

Medication training in the proper use, side effects, and role of medication in the treatment and prevention of lung impairment is crucial. Areas to include in this training are proper use of aerosolized medications, medication changes during an acute exacerbation, and proper medication dosing for the asthmatic when peak flows are changing. Many patients are either on inappropriate medications or are not on medications they need.

Respiratory care modalities include the appropriate use of oxygen; use, care, and cleaning of aerosol devices; suctioning in the home; ventilator management in the home; sleep disturbances; and home care issues.

Psychosocial training may cover coping with lung disease, stress management techniques, support system and dependency issues, anger management, and depression.

The components of patient training are different for each patient depending on the individual's needs. The goal of PR is to help the patient achieve the best quality of life through improving compliance with the treatment program and optimizing prevention.

BOX 23-4

OTHER TESTS TO CONSIDER FOR SELECTED PATIENTS

Maximal voluntary ventilation
Maximal inspiratory and expiratory pressures
Theophylline level
Pulmonary exercise stress test (metabolic study) with continuous ECG monitoring
Postexercise spirometry
Bronchial challenge (eg, methacholine)
Cardiovascular test (eg, holter monitor, echocardiogram, radionuclide exercise stress test)
Polysomnography
Sinus radiography
Upper gastrointestinal series
Skin tests

Note: Reprinted with permission from Selection and Team Assessment of the Pulmonary Rehabilitation Candidate. In AACVPR, Guidelines for Pulmonary Rehabilitation Programs. Champaign, IL, Human Kinetics Publishers; 1993.

PSYCHOSOCIAL INTERVENTION

Once the psychosocial assessment is complete, the treatment intervention can be outlined for each individual patient. It is important to teach patients how to restore their self-esteem, learn adaptive coping skills, and control or manage their symptoms.

Knowing the patient's personal strengths, weaknesses, and available resources helps determine the extent of intervention required. The psychosocial issues are addressed throughout the program by PR team members. In some cases, a psychologist or psychiatrist is required. Determining the patient's needs helps to define the type of intervention needed: individual counseling, group support, family therapy, biofeedback, stress management, panic control, anger management, traditional psychotherapy, or use of psychotropic medications (eg, antidepressants, relaxants). When anxiety and depression coexist, the symptoms of anxiety often mask the depression. If the anxiety alone is treated, the depression may worsen significantly.

Other areas to be addressed include community resources, patient advocacy, durable power of attorney for health care, living will, CPR, outpatient home care, follow-up, and vocational counseling.

EXERCISE

The patient with pulmonary impairment often decreases his or her activity level because of dyspnea or fatigue, resulting in reduced exercise endurance. This results in a worsening condition and leads to a cycle of increasing deconditioning. The benefits of exercise training in patients with lung impairment include improved appetite, better sleep, enhanced tolerance of dyspnea, and ability to achieve a higher level of work.

The *exercise prescription* consists of four parts: (1) the mode of exercise, (2) the intensity of exercise, (3) the duration of exercise, and (4) the frequency of exercise.[30] The modes of exercise that could be selected include walking, swimming, riding a stationary bicycle, circuit training, or weight training. The mode selected for the patient should be the one that the patient will be compliant with, is feasible in relation to economic status, and is easy to perform on a routine basis at home. Walking is the most commonly selected exercise.

There has been considerable controversy over how to determine the appropriate intensity level of exercise for the COPD patient.[31–33] A *target heart rate* (THR) can be used by most patients with lung disease. Karvonen's formula, using 0.6 as the factor in the equation, is a reasonable way to select a THR that works well for most patients initiating a home exercise program.

$$THR = [0.6 \times (PHR - RHR)] + RHR$$

where PHR is the peak heart rate during a maximal exercise stress test or 6-minute walk, and the RHR is the resting heart rate. Karvonen's formula is particularly helpful in that it takes both the PHR and the RHR into account when determining a THR. In patients who undergo a pulmonary exercise stress test (including gas exchange measurements), if an anaerobic threshold is identified, it would be appropriate to select the heart rate at the anaerobic threshold as the THR.

In patients with very severe impairment, for whom a THR may be a less reliable indicator of the level of work, and in those who have difficulty monitoring their heart rate, an acceptable alternative for determining the intensity of exercise is to teach the patient the level of dyspnea or "perceived exertion" that would be safe to achieve during exercise. On a Borg scale of 0 to 10, aiming for a value of 4 to 8 would be reasonable.[34]

It is important to increase the intensity of exercise gradually to achieve improved conditioning. Patients who exercise at a higher intensity will achieve a higher level of fitness than those who exercise at a lower level. The duration of exercise should be at least 20 to 30 minutes, with the patient exercising at least three to four times a week.

Interval exercise (breaking up the exercise session into shorter segments) may be necessary for the limited patient. If the patient's O_2 saturation decreases to 88% or below during exercise training, supplemental oxygen should be used to achieve an O_2 saturation of 90% or above.

FOLLOW-UP

Follow-up varies from program to program, but to track outcomes and to improve patient compliance a follow-up program is critical. A goal of PR is for the patient to maintain the long-term benefits started during the program.[35–39] Follow-up activities are listed in Table 23-2.

A listing of the tools used in evaluating patient outcomes are described in Table 23-3. It is important to be able to demonstrate an improved status to justify the existence of the pulmonary rehabilitation program.

TABLE 23-2 **Follow-up Options for Pulmonary Rehabilitation Programs**

Regular physician visits
Maintenance exercise group
Program graduate group outings and trips
Program graduate group meetings
Referral to community groups (eg, American Lung Association's "Better Breathers Clubs")
Phone follow-up by program staff
Newsletters
Postprogram questionnaires
Re-evaluation as indicated
Home-health referral
Home visits
National Pulmonary Rehabilitation Week (observed during the first week of spring)

Note: Reprinted with permission from Beytas L, Connors GL: Organization and Management of a Pulmonary Rehabilitation Program. In Hodgkin JE, Connors GL, Bell CW (eds), Pulmonary Rehabilitation: Guidelines to Success (2nd ed). Philadelphia, JB Lippincott, 1993.

BENEFITS OF PULMONARY REHABILITATION

The benefits of pulmonary rehabilitation include reduced respiratory symptoms, reversal of anxiety and depression and an improved ego strength, an enhanced ability to carry out activities of daily living, improved exercise ability, better quality of life, the ability to continue or return to gainful employment for some patients, and a reduction in the number of days of hospitalization required for patients with COPD.[40–45] Improved survival as a result of participating in a pulmonary rehabilitation program has been reported by some groups.[41] It is hoped that by implementing the components of PR described in this chapter in patients with relatively mild obstructive airway disease, the course of the disease may be altered favorably.[46–49] See Protocol 23-1 for an overview of the pulmonary rehabilitation protocol.

SMOKING INTERVENTION

Dr. C. Everett Koop, one of the recent surgeons general of the United States, stated that smoking was the single largest preventable cause of premature death and disability in our society.[50] There are more than 22 surgeon general reports on the health consequences of tobacco dependence. Almost 50 million Americans continue to smoke. Smoking has a variety of effects, including acting as a stimulant, a sedative, and an euphoriant. Many people are unsuccessful in attempts to stop smoking because they are addicted to nicotine. Nicotine is a psychoactive drug. The major addictive components of nicotine are habit, pleasure seeking, and self-medication.[51] A description of the addictive components

TABLE 23-3 **Evaluating Patient Outcomes**

Changes in Exercise Tolerance
Before and after 6- or 12-minute walk
Before and after pulmonary exercise stress test
Review of patient home exercise training logs
Strength measurement
Flexibility and posture
Performance on specific training modalities (eg, ventilatory muscle, upper extremity)
Changes in Symptoms
Dyspnea measurements comparison
Frequency of cough, sputum production, or wheezing
Weight gain or loss
Psychological test instruments
Other Changes
Activities of Daily Living changes
Postprogram follow-up questionnaires
Before and after program knowledge test
Compliance improvement with pulmonary rehabilitation medical regimen
Frequency and duration of respiratory exacerbations
Frequency and duration of hospitalizations
Frequency of emergency room visits
Return to productive employment

Note: Reprinted with permission from Beytas L, Connors GL: Organization and Management of a Pulmonary Rehabilitation Program. In Hodgkin JE, Connors GL, and Bell CW (eds), Pulmonary Rehabilitation: Guidelines to Success (2nd ed). Philadelphia, JB Lippincott, 1993.

of nicotine, the clinical relevance, and treatment approaches are described in Table 23-4.

The burning cigarette produces more than 4,000 different chemicals caused by heat and fire, gases (especially carbon monoxide), and particulates such as tars and nicotine. It is the gases and tars that negatively impact the lungs of susceptible people. The smoker can achieve satisfaction quickly from nicotine because it takes less than 8 seconds for nicotine to travel from the lungs to the brain. If one assumes that a person takes 10 puffs per cigarette and smokes about one pack (20 cigarettes) per day, this would result in 73,000 immediate "fixes," or nicotine highs, per year!

The withdrawal symptoms reported from nicotine include sweats, tremor, nausea, depression, anxiety, inadequate sleep, irritability, impatience, difficulty concentrating, restlessness, craving tobacco, hunger, gastrointestinal problems, headaches, and drowsiness. The withdrawal symptoms peak during the first 72 hours and are persistent for the first 1 to 2 weeks after discontinuing tobacco. Patients may also notice changes in cognitive ability and decreases in psychomotor performance, heart rate, and blood pressure. A concern for many smokers is that a person gains an average of about 6 pounds after smoking cessation. Part of the reason for this gain in weight is that the metabolic rate decreases when nicotine is withdrawn. Stopping smoking decreases the rate of caffeine metabolism, so if caffeine consumption remains the same, there is a 250% increase in caffeine concentration. Patients on theophylline medications may need their dosage reduced by ¼ to ⅓ after quitting cigarettes.

Smoking intervention early in adult life can prevent serious, disabling lung disease and slows down the decline in lung function in patients with obstructive airways disease.[52,53]

The benefits of quitting smoking are numerous.[54] The carbon monoxide level returns to normal in 8 to 20 hours (increasing availability of oxygen to tissues); cough and phlegm subside within a few days to weeks; increased immunity occurs rapidly; heart attack rate and risk of stroke begin to drop immediately, reaching the risk of a nonsmoker in approximately 5 years; total cholesterol decreases and HDL increases; survival in patients with COPD improves with a reduction in respiratory infections; lung cancer risk decreases gradually, taking 15 years or more to reach the risk of a nonsmoker; risk for a multitude of cancers decreases; sense

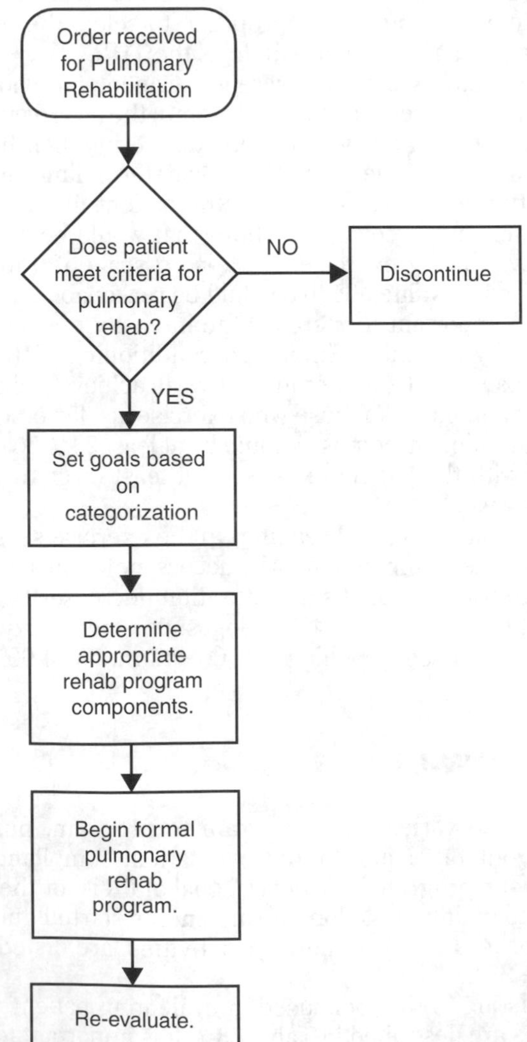

Protocol 23-1 Pulmonary rehabilitation protocol.

TABLE 23-4 **Multiple Components of Tobacco Dependence with Corresponding Clinical Implications and Interventions**

Addictive Components	Clinical Relevance	Treatment Approaches
Habit (smoking cued by daily activities)	▪ Smoking-associated activities and stimuli produce urges. ▪ Smokers may relapse without awareness when performing smoking-associated activities (eg, talking on the phone, driving in a car).	1. Training to anticipate, modify, or avoid smoking-related activities. 2. Training in cognitive and behavioral strategies to reduce urges and craving. 3. Adoption of a substitute habit (eg, chewing gum or toothpicks, drinking water).
Pleasure (smoking to increase pleasure)	▪ Experiencing pleasure (eg, after a meal, at a party) may "prime" urges to heighten pleasure through smoking. ▪ About 25% of relapses occur when smokers are happy.	1. Identification and encouragement of alternative routes to enjoyment (eg, exercise, hobbies). 2. Anticipation of and preparation for high-risk pleasure situations (eg, parties, taverns).
Self-medication (smoking to reduce negative affect and physical symptoms)	▪ Negative moods arising from stress or tobacco withdrawal produces powerful urges to smoke. ▪ Craving may arise from withdrawal or stressors and is decreased rapidly by smoking. ▪ Weight gain is a key withdrawal sign and causes many smokers to relapse. ▪ About 65% of relapses occur when smokers are sad, angry, or anxious.	1. Pharmacologic nicotine replacement to reduce withdrawal symptoms and stress reactions. 2. Training to anticipate and cope with stressors. 3. Healthy eating and exercise habits may reduce negative physical feelings and weight gain. 4. Cognitive and behavioral strategies for coping with negative moods (eg, relaxation, using social support).

Note: Reprinted with permission from Fiore MC, Jorenby DE, Baker TB, Kenford SL: Tobacco dependence and nicotine patch, clinical guidelines for effective use. JAMA 268:2687, 1992.

of smell improves; money is saved; and sense of control over oneself improves.

Factors affecting smoking cessation include:[54,55] age, with smokers over 55 years of age more likely to quit; gender, with men having better success in quitting; cigarette consumption, with lighter smokers more successful; marital status, with persons in stable marriages more successful; health, with those with chronic disease more likely to quit; education, with more educated people more likely to quit; occupation, with smokers in higher-level occupations and in the upper socioeconomic status more successful; and the presence of other smokers in the home worsening the chance for success with quitting.

There are numerous smoking-cessation techniques. Education techniques emphasize that all one needs to do is to teach the smoker about the dangers and hazards of cigarette smoking and they will quit. The reported 1-year success rate is 10% to 15%. Special cigarette filters have been tried but have not been shown to be of any significant value in helping people to quit.

Group-counseling programs, which include lectures, films, group interaction, and recommendations on diet and exercise, have reported a success rate of 15% to 25% at 1 year. The Seventh-Day Adventist Five-Day Plan, the American Lung Association Freedom from Smoking for You and Your Family, and the American Cancer Society I Quit Kit are just a few examples of group-counseling programs.

Hypnosis is another technique used in smoking cessation, with no good studies to support efficacy and with reported success rates of 1% to 100%.

Acupuncture has been variously reported in the literature as to its success rate, without convincing data for efficacy, and with a success rate of 12% reported at 6 months.[56]

Aversive conditioning, based on the premise to create a strong association between smoking and an unpleasant sensation, has included electrically shocking the smoker; breath holding; inhaling hot, smoky air; giving nausea-inducing drugs; and rapid smoking. Currently there is no conclusive evidence to justify the use of adversive-conditioning techniques.

Switching to low-nicotine cigarettes causes most smokers to regulate the nicotine dosage, so that when they switch from a high-nicotine to a low-nicotine cigarette, they inhale the smoke more rapidly and more deeply, smoking more cigarettes.[57] One advantage is that smokers of low-nicotine cigarettes are exposed to less tar, and smokers of low-tar cigarettes are a little less likely to develop lung cancer.[58]

The effects of monetary gain or loss may help some people to quit smoking. Tapering cigarette use fails for most people at a level of about 5 to 15 cigarettes per day. Setting a firm quit date and stopping "cold turkey" is a key element to success.[59] Physician advice is better than nonintervention, but the 1-year success rate is only about 5%.[60] Studies have shown that half or more of smokers have **never** been advised by a physician to stop smoking.[61,62]

Self-help manuals, when used alone, have a 1-year success rate of only about 5%. These manuals may serve as an adjunct to a smoking cessation program.

Chemical approaches have used a variety of drugs, including meprobamate, lobeline sulfate, doxepin hydrochloride, corticotropin, anticholinergics, amphetamines, quinine sulfate, garlic, and various tranquilizers. These have not shown any significant benefit.[63] Clonidine hydrochloride (Catapres) is available as a tablet or patch and has been reported to decrease tobacco withdrawal symptoms and enhance smoking cessation rates. Clonidine has not been approved for use as a smoking cessation agent. Because it is an antihypertensive agent, a patient may become hypotensive with its use. Its role in smoking cessation is yet to be determined.

Nicotine replacement therapy is based on the fact that nicotine addiction can be as difficult a habit to break as other forms of drug dependence. Relapse rates for heroin, alcohol, and smoking were virtually identical in one report, with two thirds of those treated resuming the habit within 3 months.[64] To help with the loss of the pleasurable effects of cigarette smoking and to cope with the withdrawal symptoms, nicotine polacrilex (nicotine gum) and transdermal nicotine patches have been developed. These are designed to achieve a blood nicotine level that prevents major withdrawal symptoms but avoids the pleasure-inducing levels. Nicotine replacement should be considered for people who are highly addicted to nicotine according to the Fagerstrom scale, for those who stopped smoking but relapsed, or for those who feel they have to start smoking again. Nicotine replacement therapy increases the initial and permanent smoking abstinence by two- to three-fold.

The majority of patients who use the nicotine gum chew the gum incorrectly. The nicotine patch helps avoid these problems. The 24-hour patch has the potential to lessen early morning craving and may lessen the potential for early morning relapses.[65] Prescribing the nicotine gum or patches alone, without any concomitant counseling or advice, produces very low rates of cessation.[66] There seems to be little reason to use nicotine patches beyond 6 to 8 weeks duration. The largest dosage in the patch may be skipped in those smoking less than 10 cigarettes a day or weighing less than 45 kg. The nicotine patch has been reported to be safe in individuals with stable coronary artery disease.[67] However, these people should be cautioned against smoking during patch therapy. Nicotine gum has a potential advantage in acute, high-stress situations, because it allows the user to make an active coping response that delivers a dose of nicotine. Nicotine nasal spray has been reported in research to be an aid to smoking cessation.[68]

The reason people smoke, the addiction each individual experiences, and the type of smoking cessation technique used vary greatly from person to person. It is important to individualize the smoking cessation program just as has been discussed with a pulmonary rehabilitation program. The PR team is responsible for addressing behavior modification techniques, teaching strategies for coping with symptoms from nicotine withdrawal, and determining who should use nicotine replacement treatment.[69]

It has been reported that the greatest barrier to smoking cessation is inadequate motivation and commitment. Exercise should be an integral component to a smoking cessation program because of its own positive benefits and to help prevent weight gain. Patients with alcohol addiction should get treatment for the alcoholism first, because continuing to drink alcohol makes it very difficult to stop smoking. One can confirm a nonsmoking status in patients by using measures of saliva, plasma, or urinary cotinine, a metabolite of nicotine. Cotinine can be detected in the urine, blood, or saliva for up to 7 days.

The National Cancer Institute's program suggests a four-stage intervention for medical professionals:[70] *ask* patients about their smoking status at each visit; *advise* them in a clear, direct manner to quit smoking; *assist* the interested smoker in quitting by setting a quit date, and consider prescribing nicotine replacement therapy; and *arrange* follow-up visits.

It has been reported that the highest rates of successful smoking cessation occur when patients are hospitalized for a smoking-related illness.[71] Don't ever pass up the opportunity to recommend smoking cessation to patients during their acute hospitalization.

REFERENCES

1. Ries AL: Position paper of the American Association of Cardiovascular and Pulmonary Rehabilitation: Scientific basis of pulmonary rehabilitation. J Cardiopulm Rehab 10:418, 1990
2. AACVPR Guidelines for Pulmonary Rehabilitation Programs: Connors GL, Hilling L, (eds.) Champaign, IL, Human Kinetics Publishers, 1993
3. Peter, JA: Preventive care in pulmonary rehabilitation. In JE Hodgkin, GL Connors, CW Bell (eds), Pulmonary Rehabilitation Guidelines to Success (2nd ed). Philadelphia, JB Lippincott, 1993, pp. 102–118
4. Connors GL: A primary role in secondary prevention. RT Feb–Mar:31, 1994
5. Kyes K: Pulmonary rehabilitation for children, a conversation with Mark Spaingard, M.D. RT, Feb–Mar:19, 1994
6. Detwiler DA, Boston LM, Verhulst SJ: Evaluation of an educational program for asthmatic children ages 4–8 and their parents. Respir Care 39(3):204, 1994
7. Make B: COPD: Management and rehabilitation. Am Fam Physician 43:1315, 1991
8. Foster S, Thomas HM: Pulmonary rehabilitation in lung disease other than COPD. Am Rev Respir Dis 141:601, 1990
9. Hodgkin JE: United States audit of asthma therapy. Chest 90(suppl):625, 1986
10. Orensteim DM: Cystic fibrosis. Respir Care 36(7):746, 1991
11. Mason RJ, Katz JL, Bethel RA: Time out for asthma: Rationale for a comprehensive evaluation. Semin Respir Crit Care Med 15(2):97, 1994
12. U.S. Department of Commerce: Deaths and death rates, by selected causes: 1970–1993. In Statistical Abstract of the United States, 1995 (115th ed), the National Data Book (Publication no. 125). Washington, DC, Dept. of Commerce, Issued Sept, 1995
13. World Health Organization: Unpublished death rates for chronic obstructive pulmonary diseases and allied conditions by country for each year from 1980 to 1991. Geneva: World Health Organization, 1990 and 1993

14. California Thoracic Society: California Lung Health: A selection of Lung Health Statistics for California. American Lung Association of CA, 1995
15. ATS Statement: Standards for the diagnosis and care of patients with chronic obstructive pulmonary disease. Am J Respir Crit Care Med 152:S77, 1995
16. Weiss DB, Gergen PJ, Hodgson TA: An economic evaluation of asthma in the United States. N Engl J Med 326:862, 1992
17. Current Estimates from the National Health Interview Survey, 1982–93. Series 10: Data from National Health Survey. National Center for Health Statistics
18. American Lung Association: Asthma research initiative. New York, American Lung Association 1995
19. Other Drivers of Change Deserve Consideration. AARC Times Dec:36, 1995
20. Petty TL: Pulmonary rehabilitation. In Basics of RD (vol 4). New York, American Thoracic Society, 1975, p. 1
21. Hodgkin JE, Farrell MJ, Gibson SR, et al: Pulmonary rehabilitation: Official ATS statement. Am Rev Respir Dis 124:663, 1981
22. Fishman AP: Pulmonary rehabilitation research: NIH workshop summary. Am J Resp Crit Care Med 149:825, 1994
23. Connors GL, Hodgkin JE, Asmus RM: A careful assessment is crucial to successful pulmonary rehabilitation. J Cardiopul Rehab 8(11):435, 1988
24. Branscomb BV: Aggravating factors and coexisting disorders. In JE Hodgkin, TL Petty (eds), Chronic Obstructive Pulmonary Disease: Current Concepts. Philadelphia, WB Saunders, 1987, p. 183.
25. Ries AL: The importance of exercise in pulmonary rehabilitation. Clin Chest Med 15(2):327, 1994
26. Guyatt G, Feeny D, Patrick D: Measuring health related quality of life. Ann Intern Med 118:622, 1993
27. Weaver T, Narsavage G: Physiological and psychological variables related to functional status in chronic obstructive pulmonary disease. Nurs Res 41:286, 1992
28. Donahoe M, Rogers RM: Nutritional assessment and support in chronic obstructive pulmonary disease. Clin Chest Med 11(3):487, 1990
29. Stulbarg MS:A contemporary approach to dyspnea management. RT Oct–Nov:75, 1994
30. Hodgkin JE: Exercise testing and training. In JE Hodgkin, TL Petty (eds), Chronic Obstructive Pulmonary Disease: Current Concepts. Philadelphia, WB Saunders, 1987, p. 120
31. Punzal PA, Ries AL, Kaplan RM, Prewitt LP: Maximum intensity exercise training in patients with chronic obstructive pulmonary disease. Chest 100:618, 1991
32. Hodgkin JE, Litzau KL: Exercise training target heart rates in chronic obstructive pulmonary disease. Chest 94:305, 1988
33. Belman MJ: Exercise in patients with chronic obstructive pulmonary disease. Thorax 48:936, 1993
34. Borg GAV: Psychophysical bases of perceived exertion. Med Sci Sports Exerc 14:377, 1982
35. Ries AL, Kaplan RM, Limberg TM, Prewitt LM: Effects of pulmonary rehabilitation on physiologic and phychosocial outcomes in patients with chronic obstructive pulmonary disease. Ann Intern Med 122:823, 1995
36. McSweeney A, Labuhn J, Labuhn KT: Chronic obstructive pulmonary disease. In B Spilker (ed), Quality of life assessment in Clinical Trials. New York, Raven Press Ltd, 1990, pp. 391–417
37. Peske GW: The power of outcomes research. RT 8(2):18, 1995
38. Kretz SE, Meyer LC: Improving patient outcomes for severe asthma through comprehensive, specialized treatment: A report of the prototype project to develop a center of excellence model for the treatment of severe asthma. John Hancock Managed Care Group, National Jewish Center for Immunology and Respiratory Medicine, 1993
39. Make BJ: Pulmonary rehabilitation: What are the outcomes? Respir Care 35(4):329, 1990 (Editorial)
40. Sneider R, O'Malley JA, Kahn M: Trends in pulmonary rehabilitation at Eisenhower Medical Center: Our 11 years experience (1976–1987). J Cardiopul Rehab 11:453, 1988
41. Hodgkin JE: Prognosis in chronic obstructive pulmonary disease. Clin Chest Med 11(3):555, 1990
42. Bebout DE, Hodgkin JE, Zorn EG, et al: Clinical and physiological outcomes of a university-hospital pulmonary rehabilitation program. Respir Care 28:1468, 1983
43. Mall RW, Medeiros M: Objective evaluation of results of a pulmonary rehabilitation program in a community hospital. Chest 94:1156, 1988
44. Holden DA, Stelmach KD, Curtis PS, et al: The impact of a rehabilitation program on functional status of patients with chronic lung disease. Respir Care 35(4):332, 1990
45. Radovich JL, Hodgkin JE, Burton GG, et al: Cost effectiveness of pulmonary rehabilitation programs. In JE Hodgkin, GL Connors, CW Bell (eds), Pulmonary Rehabilitation: Guidelines to Success (2nd ed). Philadelphia, JB Lippincott Co, 1993, pp. 548–561
46. Canter R, Nicrota B, Blevins W, et al: Altered exercise, gas exchange and cardiac function in patients with mild chronic obstructive pulmonary disease. Chest 103:745, 1993
47. Petty TL: Pulmonary rehabilitation for early COPD: COPD as a systemic disease. Chest 105:1636, 1994
48. Connett JE, Kusek JW, Bailey W, et al: Design of the Lung Health study: A randomized clinical trial of early intervention for chronic obstructive pulmonary disease. Controlled Clin Trials 14:35, 1993
49. Petty TL: Pulmonary rehabilitation in perspective: Historical roots, present status, and future projections. Thorax 48:855, 1993
50. U.S. Department of Health and Human Services: The health consequences of involuntary smoking, a report of the surgeon general. Rockville, MD, Public Health Service, Centers for Disease Control, Center for Health Promotion and Education, Office on Smoking and Health, 1986
51. Fiore MC, Jorenby DE, Baker TB, Kenford SL: Tobacco dependence and the nicotine patch: Clinical guidelines for effective use. JAMA 268:2687, 1992
52. Anthonisen NR, Connett JE, Kiley JP, et al: Effects of smoking intervention and the use of an inhaled anticholinergic bronchodilator on the rate of decline of FEV1. JAMA 272(19): 1497, 1994
53. Huber FL, Byrne B, Pandina RJ (Guest Editors): Economic, health and social implications of tobacco use and smoking cessation. Semin Respir Crit Care Med 16(2):69, 1995
54. Flay BR, Phil D, OcKene JD, et al: Smoking: Epidemiology, cessation, and prevention. Chest 102:277S, 1992
55. Daughton D, Fix AJ: Smoking intervention techniques: Historical and practical applications. In JE Hodgkin, GL Connors, CW Bell (eds), Pulmonary Rehabilitation: Guidelines to Success (2nd ed). Philadelphia, JB Lippincott, 1993
56. Lamontage Y, Annable L, Gagnon MA: Acupuncture for smokers: Lack of longterm therapeutic effect in a controlled study. Can Med Assoc J 122:787, 1980
57. U.S. Public Health Service Smoking and Health: Report of the advisory committee to the Surgeon General of the Public Health Service (PHS Publication No. 1103). Bethesda, MD; U.S. Dept. of Health, Education, and Welfare, Public Health Service: Centers for Disease Control; 1964
58. Hammond EC, Garfinkel C, Seidman H, Lee EA. Tar and nicotine content of cigarette smoke in relation to death rates. Environ Res 12:263, 1976
59. Flaxman J: Quitting smoking now or later: Gradual, abrupt, immediate or delayed quitting. Behav Ther 9:260, 1978
60. A round-table discussion: Cigarette smoking. J Cardiopul Rehab 12:385, 1992
61. Dawley HH, Wingfield CW: Assessing the attitude of veterans toward a smoking cessation program in a hospital setting. Percept Mot Skills 40:448, 1975
62. The American Cancer Society. A survey concerning: Cigarette smoking, health check-ups, cancer detection tests: A summary of the findings. Conducted by the Gallup Organization, 1977
63. Ornish SA, et al: Effects of transdermal clonidine treatment on withdrawal symptoms associated with smoking cessation. Arch Intern Med 148:2027, 1988
64. Hunt WA, Barnett LW, Branch LG: Relapse rates in addiction programs. J Clin Psychol 27:455, 1971
65. Fagerstrom KO, Lunell E, Molander L, et al: Continuous and intermittent transdermal delivery of nicotine and blockade of withdrawal symptoms. In The Global War: Proceedings of the Seventh World Conference on Tobacco and Health; Arpil 1–5, 1990. Perth, Australia; Health Dept. of Western Australia; 1990; pp. 687–689
66. Sachs DL: Nicotine polacrilex: Practical use requirement. Curr Pulmonol 10:141, 1989

67. Rennard S, Daughton D, Fortmann S, et al: Transdermal nicotine enhances smoking cessation in coronary artery disease patients. Chest 100:5S, 1991
68. Silagy C, Mant D, Fowler G, Lodge M. Meta-analysis on efficacy of nicotine replacement therapies in smoking cessation. Lancet 343:139, 1994
69. Daughton DM, Fix AJ, Kass I, Patil KD. Smoking cessation among patients with chronic obstructive pulmonary disease (COPD). Addict Behav 5:125, 1980
70. Glynn TJ, Manley MW. How to help your patients stop smoking: A national cancer institute manual for physicians (Publication NIH 90-3064). Washington, DC; US Dept of Health and Human Services (Public Health Service), National Institutes of Health; 1990
71. Schwartz JL: Review and evaluation of smoking cessation methods: The United States and Canada, 1978–1985. Washington, DC; US Dept of Health and Human Services, Public Health Service; 1987

24 Respiratory Care in the Home and Alternate Sites

Susan L. McInturff
Walter J. O'Donohue, Jr.

PROFESSIONAL SKILLS

Upon completion of this chapter, the reader will:

- Denote reasons for the shift in health care from the acute setting to the home setting
- Delineate the roles of the medical professionals involved in the care of patients in the home setting
- Discuss the importance of the discharge plan
- Select appropriate equipment for oxygen delivery in the home care setting
- Use Medicare's criteria for reimbursement for home oxygen therapy
- Describe the various types of respiratory and nonrespiratory medical equipment the clinician may be responsible for setting up in the home
- Explain the complexities of home mechanical ventilation, including patient selection, discharge planning, education and training, and follow-up care
- Describe the clinician's role in providing respiratory care in other alternate sites

KEY TERMS

Bilevel positive airway pressure
Compressor nebulizer
Continuous positive airway pressure
Cool or heated aerosol
Environmental assessment
Gaseous systems
Intermittent positive pressure breathing
IV pumps
Liquid oxygen
Long-term mechanical ventilation
Long-term oxygen therapy
Oxygen conserving devices
Oxygen concentrator
Patient education
Peak flow meters
Physical assessment
Plan of treatment
Portable gas system
Pulse oximetry

INTRODUCTION

Home care has been viewed in the past as an addendum to the care patients receive in the hospital rather than an integral part of their overall care. Home care has also been viewed as a location of care rather than a specialty field of practice for Respiratory Care Practitioners (RCPs). The last several years have brought a change in the focus of health care from hospitalizing patients for treatment of acute illnesses to practicing preventive medicine and cost containment. This has brought about a like change in the perception of home care; instead of aftercare as an afterthought, home care has become a major focus in the health care continuum.

The goal of home care is to allow patients to maintain their independence and to manage their medical care at home. This chapter highlights many of the therapies that are used in the management of patients in the home and identifies how a patient is provided with this type of care, including assessment of the patient and his or her environment, patient education, and setting up a plan of treatment. We will also review the various types of medical equipment used in the home, from oxygen therapy to the management of a home ventilator.

Current Shift in the Health Care Setting

Since the inception of our government-funded health care programs, Medicare and Medicaid, health care costs have been growing at an exponential rate. Health care expenditures in this country consumed 14% of the gross national product (GNP) at the end of 1993, and it is estimated that this figure will increase to 17% by the year 2000.[1,2] Costs for hospital care have been reported to account for two-thirds of the Medicare dollars spent![3] These burgeoning expenses have resulted in changes in reimbursement to hospitals in an effort to control costs and reduce expenditures. Hospitals, in an effort to come into line with these changes, look for ways to reduce their costs. Discharging patients earlier in their course of treatment is an obvious solution.

Patients who are discharged "quicker and sicker," as the saying goes, often require continued medical treatment at home. This treatment frequently requires some type of medical device, as well as the personnel to monitor the patient and the equipment. This need has propelled great advances in the technology of home medical equipment (HME), making it possible to treat a patient at home with anything from oxygen therapy to intravenous (IV) therapy, enterostomal care, and even continuous mechanical ventilation.

In the past, visiting nurses were the only health care professionals following patients at home. The change in the health care focus from hospital to home has brought many other health care professionals out of the hospital; RCPs, physical therapists, social workers, and speech therapists are now integral components of the patient's home care team. The availability of technology and personnel has allowed the health care industry to provide care in a less costly and more amenable environment and can encompass nearly every therapy found in the acute care setting.

The Benefits of Home Care

It would seem that the primary benefit of home care is its cost-effectiveness. Indeed, studies looking at hospital versus home care have shown that home care can reduce the total health care dollars spent by third-party payers, such as Medicare.[4–7]

There are many other benefits to home care. Patients being treated at home have a reduced risk of nosocomial infection.[8] Cancer patients have shown statistically significant improvement in their mental health and social dependency when receiving home care services.[9] Rehospitalization and emergency room visits can often be averted in patients with acute problems when they are being monitored by health care professionals.[5]

These are only a few of the benefits of home care. A more complete listing of the benefits can be found in Table 24-1.

Candidates for Home Care Services

The American Medical Association's Department of Geriatric Health has stated that "44% of all patients discharged from the hospital by primary care physicians require posthospital medical or nursing care that cannot be provided by family or friends alone."[10] They go further to state that an estimated 20% of patients over age 65 have functional impairments with related home care needs. This would seem to identify a very large population of patients that are candidates for home care.

Generally speaking, patients with functional or physical impairments that require continuing medical treatment would benefit from receiving home care. One group of patients we commonly see are those with pulmonary diseases necessitating some type of respiratory therapy at home. These patients are usually at greater risk for relapses, infections, frequent emergency room visits, and rehospitalizations and are often so physically debilitated that they or their family members are unable to manage their care alone. There are a variety of functional and physical impairments that may identify a patient as being a candidate for home care (Table 24-2).

The Role of the Physician

According to the AMA's Home Care Advisory Panel, "it is the role of the physician to prescribe, in consultation with members of the home care team, a home care plan of treatment."[10] It is the physician that leads the team of

TABLE 24-1 **The Benefits of Home Care**

- Improves quality of life
- Is cost-effective
- Encourages self-management and independence
- Allows for ongoing monitoring of patient response to treatment
- Reduces the need for clinic visits, emergency room visits, and hospital readmissions
- Reduces risk of nosocomial infections
- Improves mental health and social independence

TABLE 24-2 **Candidates for Home Care**

- Patients with the desire to be treated at home
- Patients with adequate family, care givers, and financial resources
- Patients with physical limitations
  - -dyspnea that limits activities of daily living (ADLs)
  - -ambulatory difficulties
  - -difficulties with vision, speech, or hearing
- Patients with functional impairments
  - -cognitive disabilities
  - -inability to perform ADLs
  - -inability to monitor and administer medications and other treatments
- Patients requiring medical devices that necessitate monitoring and maintenance

nurses, RCPs, and other professionals, along with the patient and family, as they strive to manage the patient's medical problems. The physician reviews the short- and long-term goals that the team has established and provides the support necessary to assist the patient in achieving those goals. With the information provided by the home health professionals during their visits, the physician evaluates and treats the patient for emergent problems that might otherwise require hospitalization. The physician truly is the link to continuity of care from hospital to home.

The Role of the RCP

The primary function of the RCP in home care is to provide patient education.[11] Instructing patients and their care givers in the safe and proper use of the medical equipment they require is a very important aspect of patient education, but it is certainly only a part of it.

The RCP also educates patients and their care givers in symptom recognition and management, when it is appropriate to call the RCP or the HME provider, and when it is appropriate to call the physician. The patient should be able to understand the intent of the physician's prescription and the consequences of noncompliance. The patient must be educated about infection control, energy-conservation techniques, and how to take medications properly. The RCP frequently instructs patients and care givers in specific care procedures such as suctioning and tracheostomy care.

Another very important function of the RCP is to provide clinical assessment. Physical assessment is an integral part of the overall assessment performed by the RCP. The RCP also performs an assessment of the patient's environment, however, to insure that it is an optimum site for care and offers no impediments or safety hazards. Assessment of the patient and care givers for their ability to learn, understand procedures, and retain information is also important, as well as determining that the procedures can be performed satisfactorily. The RCP must have good assessment skills to troubleshoot physical, psychosocial, and mechanical problems.

Communicating with the patient's physician and the rest of the home care team is part of the RCP's role. The physician relies on the observations of the team members to assist in decision making essential in the care of the patient. The RCP is responsible for communicating with the physician and other members of the team in both oral and written form. The RCP must also communicate with the patient and the care givers and present information in a manner that is easy for them to understand.

TRANSITION FROM HOSPITAL TO HOME

As stated previously, there is a large population of patients who would benefit from home care because they have functional and physical limitations that require continuing care once they leave the hospital or physician's office. The physician may identify the need for home care before discharging the patient, or the hospital's discharge planner may be the one who identifies this need and communicates it to the physician. Once the need has been established the process begins to provide the patient with both the therapy and the health care professionals necessary to administer therapy and monitor the patient.

The Discharge Plan

An essential component of the home care process is the discharge plan (see AARC Clinical Practice Guideline: Discharge Planning for the Respiratory Care Patient). This plan is the vehicle that coordinates the services needed to carry out the physician's plan of treatment. The discharge planner is the hospital representative who coordinates these services; some hospitals use the RCP as a discharge planner when oxygen or other respiratory therapy modalities are going to be used at home.

The discharge plan should establish and dispatch several key components: (1) the physicians's plan of treatment; (2) the professional services needed to administer the plan of treatment; (3) the equipment needed to administer the plan of treatment; (4) reimbursement issues; (5) care giver issues; and (6) advanced directives, when indicated. Careful attention to these components goes a long way to insure a safe and positive home care experience for the patient and the family.

The physician's *plan of treatment* is a prescription for the medical interventions needed by the patient. For example, a patient who has been hospitalized for an exacerbation of chronic obstructive pulmonary disease (COPD) may be quite debilitated and still require oxygen therapy and aerosolized bronchodilators when discharged. The physician writes orders for the patient to be discharged with oxygen and a compressor nebulizer. The discharge plan should include the physician's specific order for oxygen therapy, for example, O_2 at 2 liters per minute continuous, and for the nebulizer therapy, for example, compressor nebulizer with unit dose albuterol four times daily. The discharge planner must then consider the professional services the patient may

AARC Clinical Practice Guideline

DISCHARGE PLANNING FOR THE RESPIRATORY CARE PATIENT

Indications: Discharge planning is indicated for all respiratory care patients who are being considered for discharge or transfer to alternate sites including the home. The alternate site may provide a higher or lesser level of care (depending on the patient's condition). The discharge plan should always be developed and implemented as early as possible before transfer.

Contraindications: There are no contraindications to the development of a discharge plan.

Assessment of Need: All patients with a primary respiratory diagnosis should be assessed for the need for a discharge plan.

Assessment of Outcome: The desired outcome of the discharge plan is determined by no readmission to an alternate care site due to discharge plan failure; satisfactory performance of all treatments and modalities by care givers as instructed; care givers' ability to assess the patient, troubleshoot, and solve problems as they arise; the treatments' meeting the patient's needs and goals; the equipment's meeting the patient's needs; the site's providing the necessary services; the patient and family's satisfaction.

Monitoring: The discharge plan coordinator and the physician should monitor the progress of the discharge plan. Each team member should participate in regularly scheduled team conferences to assess the progress of the discharge plan. Modifications may be made according to the individual patient's goals and needs.

From AARC Clinical Practice Guideline; see Respir Care 40:1308, 1995, for complete text.

require. In this case, the patient might benefit from intermittent visits by a nurse from the hospital's home health agency, as well as by a nurse's aide to assist with personal care, and a physical therapist to assist with increasing the patient's physical strength and activities of daily living. Home visits by a RCP would also be helpful to the patient. The services of the RCP are usually provided in conjunction with the home medical equipment ordered.

The equipment needed to administer the physician's plan of treatment must be determined and supplied. In this case home oxygen equipment must be ordered, and a portable oxygen system must be set up for the trip home from the hospital. A compressor nebulizer, as well as the proper medications, also must be ordered.

Establishing reimbursement for these services and equipment, before discharge, is useful. Medicare and Medicaid have very strict reimbursement guidelines for home oxygen and nebulizer therapy, so it should never be assumed that these services will be reimbursed. Private insurance companies and managed care organizations also have specific guidelines and will most likely need to be contacted before the services are delivered to establish coverage. Identifying whether the patient has a mechanism for copayment for these services is also important. There are times when the copayment is so high that the patient may be unable to meet it, especially when there are large amounts of equipment and supplies ordered. Home health agencies and medical equipment providers will bill patients for services that are not covered or are denied by their insurance, and the discharge planner should appreciate the impact this can have on patients' finances. In fact, it is common for patients to refuse the service if it is not reimbursed by insurance, even if the doctor feels it is medically necessary.

Identifying care-giver issues before discharge is very important. For example, an oxygen-dependent patient who is very debilitated may have a spouse whose health is also poor and who may be physically unable to care for the patient; or no care giver may be available. Persons identified as care givers must be evaluated for their willingness to learn, ability to be responsible for the things required of them, competence, physical capacity, and other commitments.[10] These care givers may need training in some of the care procedures (suctioning, stoma care, bladder care, and so on) before discharge and must be able to dedicate the time required for learning these processes as well as performing them satisfactorily.

Advanced directives should be established before going home. It is certainly preferable to understand and document the patient's wishes regarding withholding or withdrawing life support before the patient's medical condition worsens to the point where such measures would be necessary to keep the patient alive. The patient's physician can assist the patient in making this decision and should discuss this with the patient before discharge. In fact, the Patient Self-Determination Act of 1991 requires that patients be advised of their right to accept or refuse treatment and that they are asked if they have decided on advanced directives on admission to the hospital. Patients who haven't already made such decisions are supposed to be provided with written information that helps explain the impact of these decisions.[12] Home nursing agencies and home medical equipment providers can also provide this information to the patient once he or she goes home, if this is still necessary.

The Initial Home Visit

Once all the elements of the discharge plan have been dispatched, the medical equipment has been delivered, and the patient leaves the hospital for home, the home care RCP makes an initial home visit. The initial visit should contain several key elements: an environmental assessment; an initial physical assessment including a patient interview and history taking; assessment of care givers; and patient and care giver education.

An *environmental assessment* should be performed to determine the suitability of the patient's home in concert with the medical interventions ordered by the physician.[10]

The home must be inspected for any hazards that may be present. The electrical outlets should be checked for proper grounding to reduce risk of shock. Electrical circuit capability may need to be evaluated when patients are using multiple pieces of medical equipment, particularly when that equipment is placed on the same circuit as home appliances patients may already be using. It may be necessary to choose alternate types of equipment, remove appliances, or even have some rewiring done to accommodate the equipment.

Other hazards or impediments could be stairways, narrow passageways, objects on the floor, and inadequate lighting.[13] Electrical power cords may need to be taped down, scatter rugs may need to be removed, and oxygen tubing may need to be secured in such a fashion as to avoid an ambulation problem for the patient. Poor housekeeping habits can create health and fire hazards, particularly when papers, trash, and food have been left about the home.

The home should have adequate storage space for the medical equipment and supplies the patient needs, as well as adequate working space for the care givers. Access to telephone, emergency services, and an alternate source of electrical power if life-support equipment is being used are all necessary. An emergency evacuation plan should be devised taking into consideration any assistive devices necessary to remove the patient, such as a Stryker frame or other device if the patient is unable to walk.

A history and physical examination are done during the first visit. This should include a thorough interview with the patient to obtain a complete medical history.[14,15] This history taking helps identify the patient's symptom profile, current illness and previous health history, cognitive ability, and any cultural and socioeconomic factors that may play a role in the patient's care. A number of areas that should be covered when taking the patient's medical history are shown in Table 24-3.

A complete physical assessment should also be done. This evaluation usually includes standard assessment techniques such as blood pressure, temperature, and pulse rate as well as inspection and auscultation of the chest. Expansion of the chest and respiratory rate should be evaluated, the fingers should be inspected for clubbing, and the patients should be checked for any evidence of cyanosis. The patient's feet and ankles should be examined for edema, and the patient can be weighed and questioned about change in weight. Oximetry should also be performed during this initial assessment.

TABLE 24-3 **Information to Obtain During the Initial Interview**

- Demographic information
- Current condition, chief complaint
- Symptom profile
- Medical history, past, present, and familial
- Environmental factors
- Psychosocial factors—family, social, environmental, and cultural factors
- Medication profile
- Nutritional profile
- Ability to self-manage medical problems

The RCP also does an assessment of care givers, although this may already have been done by the hospital's discharge planner. It is difficult to know if patients and their family members or other care givers can manage equipment such as oxygen devices and the like until they are actually at home and the equipment is in place. The care givers need to be assessed for willingness, competency, and availability. It is important to identify any functional or physical impairments the care givers may have that could negatively impact the patient's care, such as a spouse who is arthritic and cannot turn on an oxygen tank, or one whose eyesight is so poor as to impair his or her ability to read medication labels or measure them properly.

As stated earlier, *patient education* is the primary function of the home care RCP. The therapist instructs the patient and care givers not only on how to use the medical devices ordered but also on how to properly use any medications. The RCP also educates the patient and care givers on the health consequences of noncompliance; this is particularly important for home oxygen patients who tend to take their oxygen off at night and when they leave home. Energy-conservation techniques, breathing retraining, and symptom recognition may also be reviewed by the RCP. The patient should always receive instructions regarding cleaning, infection control, and safety issues during this home visit.

Instruction must be customized to meet the demands of each patient. Cognitive ability, cultural background, and primary language all impact how a patient receives information. Teaching tools such as written instructions, videotapes, and repeated demonstrations can be used to help the patient and care givers learn to perform the required techniques. Patience and the use of simple terminology go a long way to insure that what is being taught is actually being heard and understood.

The purpose of the initial evaluation is to identify areas of concern that could hinder the care of the patient or that need modification. The RCP may find that the patient's hands shake so much that measurement or mixture of medications is impossible. The patient or the care giver may be so forgetful that he or she cannot remember the instructions given on how to use the equipment. These physical and functional limitations, once identified, are what the plan of care is based on.

The plan of treatment is the vehicle that identifies the physician's orders for the medical interventions that are necessary for the patient, as well as the types of assessments that should be performed. For a patient receiving home oxygen, the plan of treatment might be written as follows: "Oxygen at 2 L/min at rest, and 3 L/min with activity, via oxygen concentrator and portable gaseous system. Clinical assessments are to be done monthly and should include measurements of blood pressure, pulse, respiratory rate, and auscultation of the chest. Pulse oximetry with prescribed oxygen flows should be monitored when there is a clinical change."

The next step in this formula is to develop the *plan of care*. This plan is a statement that identifies individual needs, treatment goals, and the resulting plan of action for patients receiving home care services.[16] The home care RCP uses the physician's orders for treatment and assessments as well as the information gathered during the initial evaluation to determine an action plan for the patient. The plan of care encompasses a "triad" approach of identifying a problem or need, establishing a goal based on that problem or need, and then outlining the services that will be provided to meet that goal.[17]

Using the patient receiving home oxygen as an example, there are several potential problems. We can identify hypoxemia as problem number one. The goal for this patient might be to maintain oxygen saturations at or above 90%, per physician order. The services that would be provided to reach this goal would be to (1) set up and instruct patient and care givers in the use of an oxygen concentrator; (2) instruct in cleaning, infection control, and safety issues; (3) maintain and service concentrator according to manufacturer's specifications; (4) measure oxygen saturations monthly per physician order.

Problem number two might be that the patient's spouse is too ill to care for the equipment, and the goal would be that the equipment is used and maintained properly. The service necessary to meet this goal would be to identify another care giver besides the spouse, to instruct that care giver on use, oxygen safety, and cleaning techniques, and to monitor the patient and care givers.

The environmental assessment also likely identifies problems that should be addressed in the plan of care, such as lack of grounded outlets, hazardous walkways, or poor heating. Thorough examination of the patient and a complete medical history also identify problems or needs.

The plan of treatment and plan of care help the physician and RCP determine an appropriate follow-up schedule for the patient. Patients with complicated medical needs or who have have a large number of problems identified require more frequent follow-up than stable patients with few needs. A follow-up schedule may be as frequent as daily or as infrequent as every 6 months, but it should be based on the clinical evaluation of the patient.

Follow-up visits include many of the same elements as the initial visit. The environmental, physical, and care giver assessments should all be done to identify changes and emergent problems, and the plan of care should be updated any time a new problem or need is identified. The patient may need to be reeducated in some aspects of care, and the follow-up schedule may need to be altered based on what has been found. Communication with the physician is essential so that it can be determined if there is a need to change the patient's plan of treatment. This can be done either in written form or by telephone if there is a problem that requires immediate attention.

Assessment of Outcomes

An important part of the home care follow-up program is the assessment of outcomes. A lot of effort is put into establishing goals for the patient and in providing services to help the patient achieve those goals; however, without looking at the outcomes of those services, we would be unable to determine when or if those goals are met.

One of the most positive roles of RCPs in providing home care services is their ability to assess patient outcomes, determine response to therapy, and affect the decision to continue or discontinue treatment. It was common in the past for patients to receive such services as oxygen therapy for indefinite periods without anyone determining whether they still use or need it. This is particularly true when the patient is only being followed by the physician on an annual basis.

Part of every follow-up visit should be devoted to the evaluation of the clinical goals and the determination of progress toward those goals. Some patients may require oxygen or compressor nebulizer therapy only during the immediate convalescent phase of their posthospital course. For patients requiring long-term therapy, the goal might be for total self-management of their care. Periodic assessment of the outcomes of therapy and services provided helps identify the continued need for therapy or the achievement of treatment goals, which might signify that services or treatment can be discontinued.

LONG-TERM OXYGEN THERAPY

There is a great deal of information in the literature supporting the benefits of *long-term oxygen therapy* (LTOT). The Nocturnal Oxygen Therapy Trial (NOTT) showed that patients who received nearly continuous oxygen therapy had a reduced mortality rate. Other benefits to LTOT include an improved quality of life, reduced hospitalizations, increased exercise tolerance, and decreased pulmonary vascular resistance (see AARC Clinical Practice Guideline: Oxygen Therapy in the Home or Extended Care Facility).[18,19,20]

Oxygen Delivery Equipment

Oxygen delivery equipment is one of the most common types of HME placed in the home. It has been reported that there are more than 600,000 patients currently receiving home oxygen therapy in this country.[19] It is recommended that home oxygen equipment be categorized as stationary, portable, or ambulatory.[21] *Stationary systems* are considered to be such by virtue of their size and weight; they are usually large and heavy and are not intended to be moved about. The stationary system is the primary source of oxygen for the patient. *Portable oxygen systems* are small enough in size and weight to allow the patient to move them about, usually on a wheeled cart. *Ambulatory systems* are smaller and lighter still and allow the patient to carry the system on

AARC Clinical Practice Guideline

OXYGEN THERAPY IN THE HOME OR EXTENDED CARE FACILITY

Indications: In adults, children and infants older than 28 days: $PaO_2 \leq 55$ mmHg (or $SaO_2 \leq 88\%$ in subjects breathing room air) or PaO_2 of 56 to 59 torr (or SaO_2 or $SpO_2 \leq 89\%$) in association with specific clinical conditions (eg, cor pulmonale, congestive heart failure, or erythrocythemia with hematocrit > 56). Some patients may not qualify for oxygen therapy at rest but qualify for oxygen during ambulation, sleep, or exercise. Oxygen therapy is indicated during these specific activities when SaO_2 is demonstrated to fall to ≤ 88%.

Contraindications: No absolute contraindications to oxygen therapy exist when indications are present.

Assessment of Need: Initial assessment: Need is determined by the presence of clinical indicators as previously described and the presence of inadequate oxygen tension or saturation, or both, as demonstrated by the analysis of arterial blood. Concurrent pulse oximetry values must be documented and reconciled with the results of the baseline blood gas analysis if future assessment is to involve pulse oximetry. **Ongoing evaluation or reassessment:** Additional arterial blood gas analysis is indicated whenever there is a major change in clinical status that may be cardiopulmonary related. Arterial blood gas measurements should be repeated in 1 to 3 months when oxygen therapy is begun in the hospital in a clinically unstable patient to determine the need for long-term oxygen therapy. Once the need for long-term oxygen therapy has been documented, repeated arterial blood gas analysis or oxygen saturation measurements are unnecessary other than to follow the course of the disease, to assess changes in clinical status, or to facilitate changes in the oxygen prescription.

Assessment of Outcome: Outcome is determined by clinical and physiologic assessment to establish adequacy of patient response to therapy.

Monitoring: Clinical assessment should routinely be performed by the patient or the care giver to determine changes in clinical status. Patients should be visited and monitored at least once a month by credentialed personnel unless conditions warrant more frequent visits. Measurement of baseline oxygen tension and saturation is essential before oxygen therapy is begun. These measurements should be repeated when clinically indicated or to follow the course of the disease. Measurements of SaO_2 also may be made to determine appropriate oxygen flow for ambulation, exercise, or sleep. **Equipment maintenance and supervision:** All oxygen delivery equipment should be checked at least once daily by the patient or care giver. Facets to be assessed include proper function of the equipment, prescribed flow rates, F_DO_2, remaining liquid or compressed gas content, and backup supply. A respiratory care practitioner or equivalent should, during monthly visits, reinforce appropriate practices and performance by the patient and care givers and assure that the oxygen equipment is being maintained in accordance with manufacturers' recommendations. Liquid systems need to be checked to assure adequate delivery. Oxygen concentrators should be checked regularly to assure that they are delivering ≥ 85% O_2 at 4 L/min.

From AARC Clinical Practice Guideline; see Respir Care 37:918, 1992, for complete text.

their person. A stationary system is combined with a portable or ambulatory system to allow continuous oxygen administration inside and outside the home.

There are three types of delivery systems for home oxygen therapy: gaseous oxygen, liquid oxygen, and oxygen concentrators. *Gaseous systems* are the steel and aluminum cylinders that are familiar to all RCPs. Figure 24-1 illustrates a *portable gas system* as it is used in the home. These cylinders are filled with oxygen gas usually to a pressure of 2000 psi. Common sizes used in the home are the larger H or K tanks (244 cu ft), E tanks (22 cu ft), and D tanks (13 cu ft).

Due to their limited volume, H or K tanks are not commonly used as a stationary oxygen system for patients requiring continuous oxygen. These tanks last only about 3 days with a continuous flow of 2 L/min, necessitating the placement of several of these bulky tanks in the home or very frequent oxygen deliveries by the home oxygen provider. H or K tanks are most often used as a backup to other stationary systems. Size E and D cylinders are commonly used as portable systems when the patient needs to be away from the stationary source. Aluminum portable tanks are preferred over steel because they are much lighter in weight. Some patients find the steel cylinders too heavy to move, even when in a wheeled cart. Patients who are highly mobile and require frequent deliveries of portable gas cylinders may encounter difficulties in receiving the tanks at the time that they want them and need to plan ahead as much as possible.

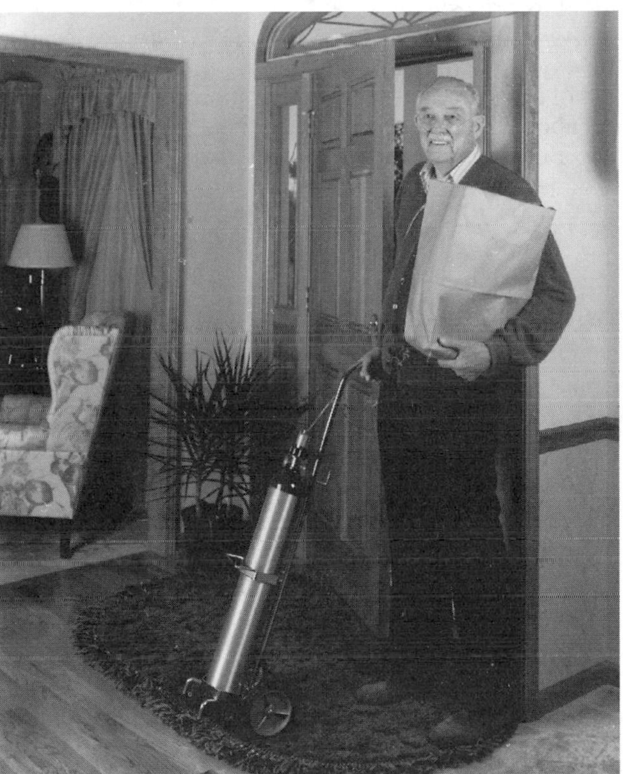

FIGURE 24-1. Gaseous portable oxygen tank used in the home. (Photo courtesy of Puritan Bennett, Lenexa, KS).

The regulators used on gaseous oxygen tanks can pose a problem for some patients. Those with arthritis or a loss of hand strength may be unable to open the valve on the tank. Other patients forget to turn off the tank resulting in the inadvertent loss of contents. Assessing the patient's ability to use the equipment is essential, and employing adaptive techniques or alternative equipment may be necessary to insure compliance.

Liquid oxygen (LOX) systems provide an excellent method of oxygen administration for patients who are active. The oxygen is kept in a special steel container called a "dewar" where it is held in its liquid state at −273°F. The dewar has a withdrawal tube and warming coils that allow the liquid to convert to a gas that is then delivered to the patient. An average dewar that is placed in the home holds about 100 pounds of liquid oxygen. At a flow rate of 2 L/min, 100 pounds of oxygen lasts about a week, reducing the number of visits necessary by the home oxygen provider to refill the stationary tank.

The prime advantage of the liquid system is that it allows the patient to have a greater degree of mobility. The patient uses a small tank that holds about 3 pounds of liquid oxygen, and the patient is able to transfill this portable unit from the stationary unit ad lib. These portable tanks weigh from 5 to 12 pounds when full and provide the patient with up to 8 hours of oxygen at a flow of 2 L/min. Lighter weight units and longer periods of oxygen delivery are possible when oxygen conserving devices are used. The lighter weight, increased running time, and patient transfill capability make the LOX system very useful for patients who leave the home frequently. Figure 24-2 illustrates stationary and portable liquid oxygen systems.

There are drawbacks to the LOX system. Because the oxygen is held in a liquid state, there is a continual loss of contents caused by evaporation and venting, usually about 1 pound per day when the equipment is not in use. Between patient usage and evaporative loss, the stationary tank has to be refilled with some frequency, usually once per week. Some patients have difficulty filling the portable unit. The noise created during the transfill can be quite loud and frightening, and some patients overfill the unit, causing the connections to freeze up. The portable unit must also be kept upright or it can vent rather loudly, which can frighten the patient; this poses a particular problem if the unit tips over in a moving vehicle while the patient is driving. The patient may need to have repeated demonstrations on how to transfill the portable tank, and he or she may need assistance in devising a method to secure the tank when it is taken in the car. Another drawback to the LOX system is that it is a more expensive method of home oxygen therapy when compared with the oxygen concentrator.

The *oxygen concentrator* is the third method of oxygen delivery used at home. This is an electrically powered device that draws in room air and separates the oxygen molecules from the nitrogen by means of a molecular sieve. The resultant gas that is delivered to the patient is usually at a concentration of 90% to 97% oxygen. Most concentrators can deliver flow rates from 0 to 5 L/min. Refer to Figure 24-3 to see an example of an oxygen concentrator.

There are several advantages to the oxygen concentrator. Because it is electrically powered, the concentrator provides a continuous source of oxygen to the patient as long as there is electricity available and no mechanical failure of the equipment. This eliminates the need for repeated deliveries by the home oxygen provider, and herein lies its cost-effectiveness. The patient does need to have an oxygen tank in the home as a backup in case of power outages; this is usually an H or K tank. There is an alarm built into the unit to alert the patient when the concentrator stops running, as occurs with a power outage or compressor malfunction. Some machines have an oxygen concentration indicator (OCI) built in to alert the patient of a drop in oxygen

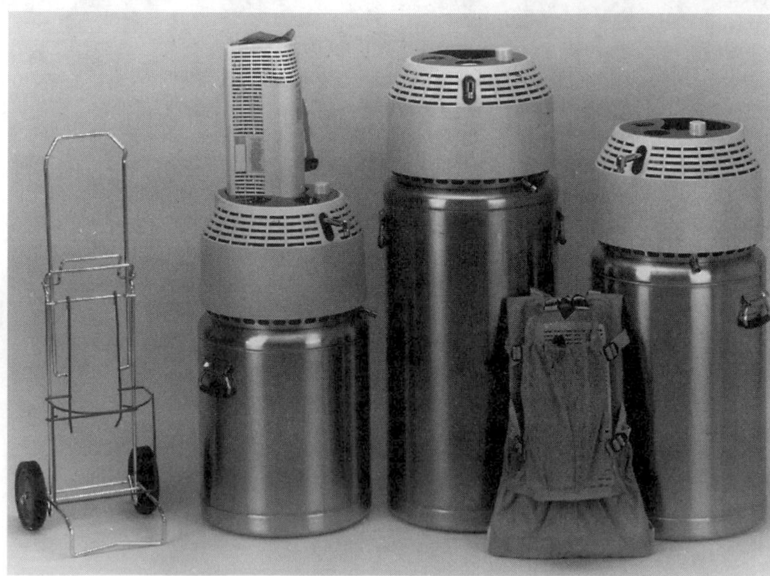

FIGURE 24-2. Stationary and portable liquid oxygen systems. (Photo courtesy of Puritan-Bennett, Lenexa, KS)

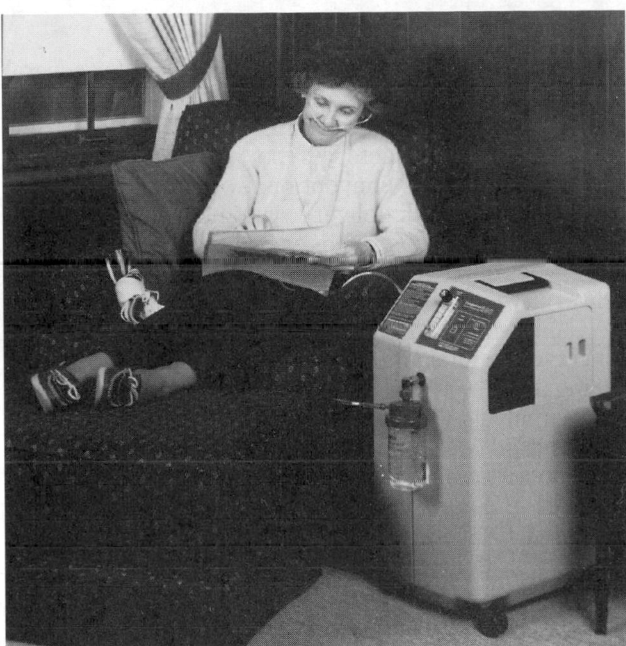

FIGURE 24-3. Oxygen concentrator. (Photo courtesy of Puritan-Bennett, Lenexa, KS)

concentration below acceptable levels. Patients using machines without an OCI (and that number composes the vast majority) have no indication of an inadequate oxygen concentration except by how they feel and by regular checks by the oxygen supplier. Concentrators can be retrofitted with OCIs, which many people feel should be required. Oxygen concentrators are very easy for the patient to use and maintain, usually requiring only that a filter be washed by the patient weekly.

There are disadvantages to using oxygen concentrators. Being a machine, the oxygen concentrator is eventually going to break down, and it does require maintenance. These machines do produce some noise, particularly when they are older, and the patient can find this bothersome. Placing the unit in a room away from the patient can alleviate this to some degree. Concentrators also produce some heat from the compressor; and because concentrators use electricity, patients see an increase in their utility bill. Patients on a fixed income may find this increase intolerable because it can be as much as $20 to $50 per month. It must also be remembered that oxygen concentrators provide a stationary source of oxygen only and must be supplemented by a portable or ambulatory system if the patient is active and mobile.

Oxygen concentrators, as well as liquid oxygen systems, do require periodic inspection and maintenance by the provider. LOX systems should have their liter flows checked routinely for accuracy, and they periodically need to have seals and gaskets replaced. Concentrators have filters that must be cleaned by the patient and internal filters that must be changed on a periodic basis by the provider. Each machine must be temporarily replaced after a manufacturer's specified number of hours for preventive maintenance or overhaul, and they should also have an electrical safety check. Liter flow accuracy and oxygen concentration should be checked by the provider; this should be done every 6 weeks to 6 months, depending on the manufacturer. If the equipment is being rented to the patient, these services should be provided at no additional charge.

Selecting the Appropriate Equipment

Patients should receive the oxygen equipment that best suits their needs, but sometimes this may not be possible. This decision requires evaluation of the patient and how the equipment is to be used. If the physician does not specify what type of equipment the patient should have, the home oxygen provider makes that decision.[19] Reputable providers give the patient the most appropriate equipment, but when Medicare pays the provider the same amount regardless of the type of system placed, there is a financial incentive to provide the patient with the system that costs the supplier the least.

It is essential that patients be evaluated individually for how they will be using the oxygen system. Factors to consider are whether the patient is ambulatory and, if so, to what degree; whether the patient can manage the equipment; the electrical capability of the home; and others. The criteria used to select the most appropriate system for the patient are listed in Table 24-4.

Medicare Guidelines

As stated before, it is very important to determine whether the equipment that is ordered will be reimbursed by the patient's insurance company. Medicare is the third-party payer that HME providers bill most fre-

TABLE 24-4 **Criteria for Selecting the Appropriate Oxygen System**

- Stationary oxygen delivery system, alone
  - -patient is bed bound or unable to ambulate beyond the limits of a 50-ft length of tubing
  - -patient requires nocturnal oxygen only
  - -patient requires oxygen source for ventilator, CPAP, and so on
- Stationary and portable oxygen delivery system (eg, concentrator with E tank or liquid O_2 system)
  - -continuous oxygen therapy is needed for a patient who only occasionally travels beyond the limits of a 50-ft length of tubing (eg, occasional visits to the physician)
- Stationary and ambulatory oxygen delivery system (eg, concentrator with lightweight cylinders $<$10 lb)
  - -continuous oxygen therapy is needed for a patient who frequently travels beyond the limits of a 50-ft length of tubing (eg, frequent visits outside the home)
- Oxygen conserving device
  - -continuous oxygen therapy is needed
    - a. with portable or ambulatory system to reduce weight, extend functional time, and reduce need for refills
    - b. with refractory hypoxemia and increased O_2 requirement
  - -nasal cannula or transtracheal oxygen catheter requires the decision of physician and patient

TABLE 24-5 **Indication and Requirements for Home Oxygen Therapy for Medicare Patients**

A. Continuous long-term oxygen therapy when:
   1. $PaO_2 \leq 55$ mmHg or $SaO_2 \leq 88\%$, or
   2. PaO_2 56–59 mmHg or SaO_2 of 89%, with
      a. edema due to heart failure, or
      b. evidence of cor pulmonale, or
      c. elevated hematocrit ≥ 56
   3. ABGs or arterial oxygen saturation by pulse oximetry obtained following optimum medical management
   4. Repeat ABGs or pulse oximetry 3 months after initial certification when
      a. initial $PO_2 \geq 56$ mmHg or $SaO_2 \geq 89\%$, or
      b. the physician's initial estimated length of need was 1–3 months
   5. Certification of medical necessity and a prescription for therapy completed by the physician
   6. Revised certification when there is a change in O_2 prescription

B. Oxygen with exercise when:
   1. $SaO_2 \leq 88\%$ or $PaO_2 \leq 55$ mmHg during exercise, while resting $PaO_2 \geq 56$ mmHg or $SaO_2 \geq 89\%$ and
   2. Demonstration of improvement in hypoxemia that was evidenced when the patient exercised breathing room air

C. Nocturnal oxygen when:
   1. $SaO_2 \leq 88\%$ or $PaO_2 \leq 55$ mmHg evidenced during sleep, with $PaO_2 \geq 56$ mmHg or $SaO_2 \geq 89\%$ during day, or
   2. A decrease in arterial PO_2 more than 10 mmHg or saturation more than 5% associated with nocturnal restlessness, insomnia, or other physical or mental impairment attributable to nocturnal hypoxemia

quently because of the predominately older patients that they serve. Medicare's guidelines are fairly rigid, and it should never be assumed that, just because the physician orders oxygen, Medicare will pay for it.

Current Medicare guidelines allow for the payment of home oxygen therapy when the patient's PaO_2 is less than or equal to 55 mmHg on room air (or SaO_2 less than or equal to 88%). They will also pay for oxygen when the PaO_2 is 56 to 59 mmHg (or SaO_2 is 89%) in the presence of cor pulmonale or erythrocytosis. The indications and requirements for home oxygen therapy in the United States that have been approved for Medicare patients are summarized in Table 24-5.

Oxygen Conserving Devices

Oxygen conserving devices (OCDs) are used for several reasons: they allow for lighter, longer-lasting ambulatory systems for patients requiring portability; they allow for patients with refractory hypoxemia requiring high-flow oxygen to use conventional equipment at lower flows instead of bulk delivery systems; and they can reduce the overall cost of oxygen contents. There are three types of OCDs available: the transtracheal oxygen delivery system; the reservoir cannula; and the electromechanical demand, or pulsed-oxygen, system. All three conserve the total amount of oxygen used either by reducing the flow necessary to maintain an adequate PaO_2 or by supplying the oxygen flow only during inspiration (as opposed to continuously). OCDs have slowly become an accepted component of home oxygen therapy, although their use varies regionally and may be discouraged because Medicare does not reimburse the provider for their cost. Most OCDs can reduce the total amount of oxygen required to correct hypoxemia by 50% or more.[22] The use of OCDs should be encouraged, and they should be prescribed by the physician whenever they are appropriate to enhance patient care. They can be combined with light-weight ambulatory units for increased patient mobility and physical activity.

□ TRANSTRACHEAL OXYGEN

Transtracheal oxygen is a total system for oxygen delivery rather than simply an OCD. Oxygen is delivered through a small catheter that is inserted percutaneously into the trachea (Figure 24-4). Because the oxygen is delivered directly into the trachea, the total flow required to oxygenate the patient is reduced. Careful patient selection is necessary when considering transtracheal oxygen therapy because of its invasive nature and the care and maintenance the catheter requires.

□ RESERVOIR DEVICES

These cannulas use a reservoir from which the patient breathes oxygen. The reservoir is either directly

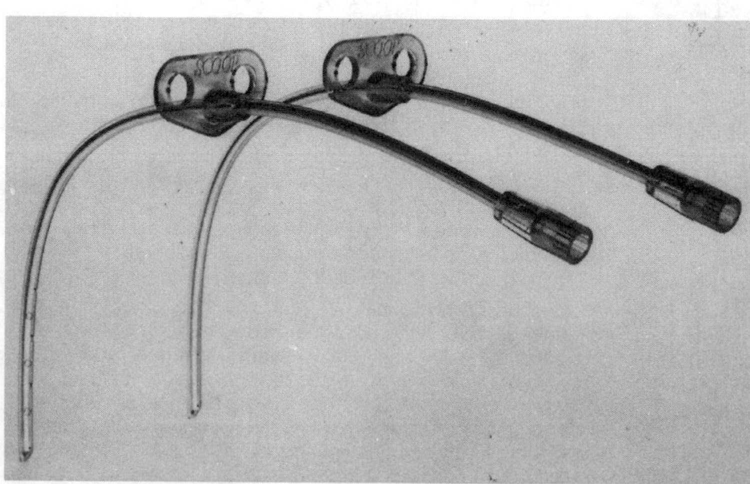

FIGURE 24-4. Transtracheal Oxygen Catheter. (Photo courtesy of Transtracheal Systems, Englewood, CO).

attached to the nasal prongs, forming a "mustache" (Figure 24-5), or is designed as a "pendant" hanging at the patient's chest (Figure 24-6). Many patients feel that these devices are unsightly and may use them only in the privacy of their home.

□ PULSED-OXYGEN SYSTEMS

Electromechanical OCDs work by pulsing small volumes of oxygen to the patient as they inspire. The oxygen savings occur by delivering oxygen only during the first part of inspiration rather than continuously. These units can be attached to either liquid or gaseous systems (Figure 24-7), or they may be built into ambulatory LOX units. As stated earlier, use of these devices not only reduces the flow rates needed but also increases the length of time an oxygen tank lasts, enabling patient activity.

Traveling With Oxygen

Patients are encouraged to maintain an activity level as high as possible, and ambulatory oxygen allows for that. Patients who wish to travel encounter some additional challenges, however. Although traveling with oxygen is fairly common, there are several details that must be considered and worked out before the patient's journey.[23]

The mode of travel may influence the type of oxygen system patients might use, both during travel and once they are at their destination. Airlines, railways, and bus and cruise lines should be contacted well in advance of the patient's departure date to determine their requirements. It is necessary also to contact oxygen suppliers along the travel route and at the final destination to arrange for oxygen to be available on arrival.

The physician should evaluate the patient before airline travel or if the patient is traveling to a destination at a higher elevation. There may be a need to change the oxygen prescription to compensate for the desaturation that occurs during flight and at higher altitudes.[23]

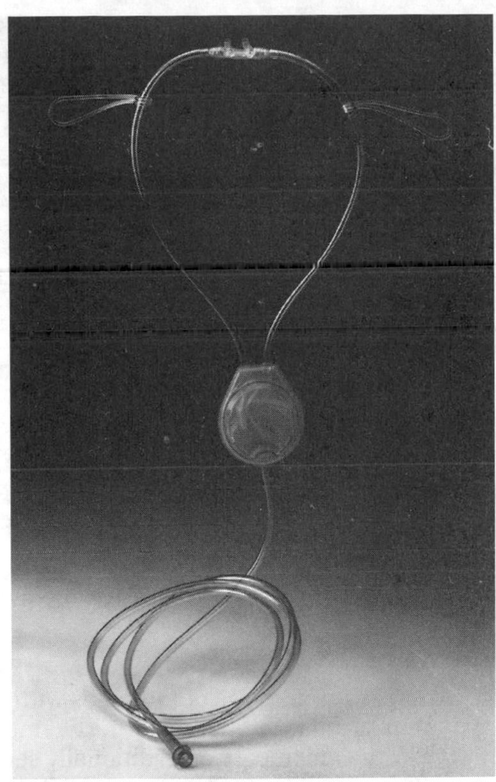

FIGURE 24-6. Pendant-type reservoir cannula. (Photo courtesy of Chad Therapeutics, Chatsworth, CA).

OTHER HOME CARE EQUIPMENT

The physician has the ability to order a wide array of medical devices to be used by the pulmonary patient at home, and the home care RCP can expect to set up and instruct the patient in the use of many of these devices. Many patients receive oxygen delivery equipment and may also receive aerosol therapy, positive pressure breathing therapy, and many monitoring and diagnos-

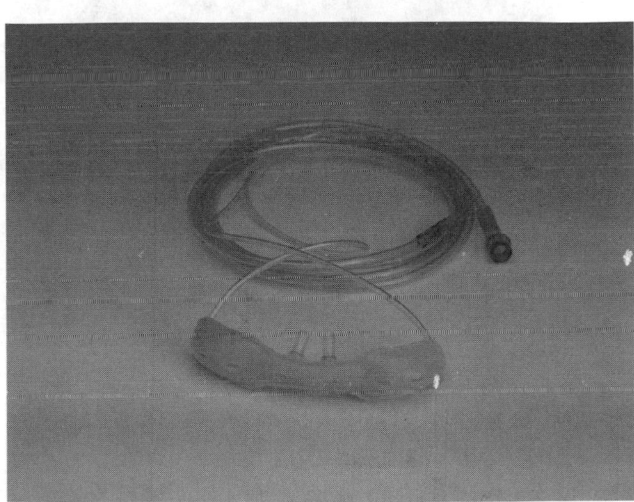

FIGURE 24-5. Reservoir Cannula, mustache type. (Photo courtesy of Chad Therapeutics, Chatsworth, CA).

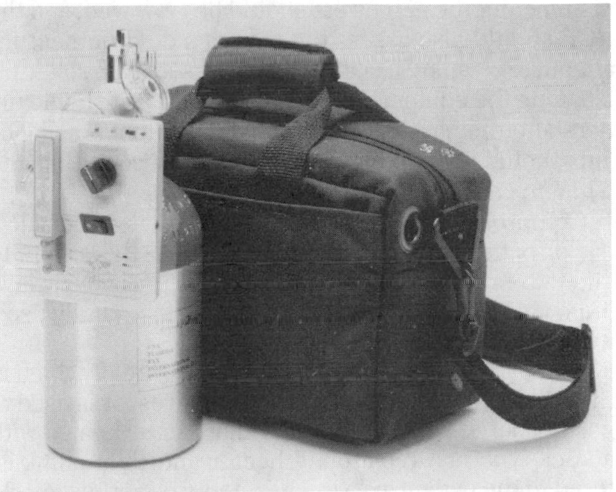

FIGURE 24-7. Oxygen conserving device, pulsed-oxygen type. (Photo courtesy of DeVilbiss Health Care, Somerset, PA).

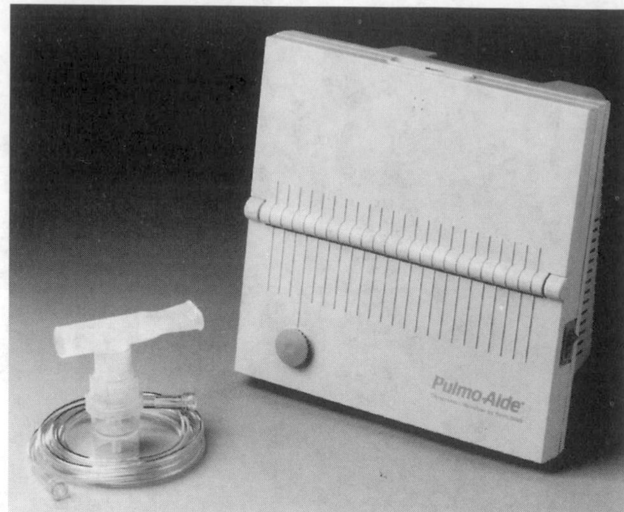

FIGURE 24-8. Compressor nebulizer. (Photo courtesy of DeVilbiss Health Care, Somerset, PA).

tic devices. These are all types of therapies with which the RCP is familiar, but the home care RCP may also have to work with equipment not traditionally set up by respiratory therapists. Home phototherapy, IV therapy equipment, and enteral therapy devices may all be used by the home care RCP.

Aerosol Therapy

The most common type of aerosol therapy used in the home is by means of a *compressor nebulizer* for bronchodilator administration. A small compressor with an output of 7 to 10 L/min is used with either a disposable or permanent hand-held nebulizer (Figure 24-8). The RCP instructs the patient in how to operate the compressor and how to use the nebulizers, as well as how to draw up or mix the medications and take a proper treatment according to the physician's order. Cleaning and disinfecting the nebulizers should be reviewed, and the RCP should also assess the patient's environment for adequate cleaning facilities (a bucket set aside solely for cleaning the equipment is ideal). The patient should understand the possible consequences of noncompliance and should also understand symptom recognition and when to call the physician.

Compressor nebulizers are available as either electric or battery-operated devices, allowing the patient to take a treatment virtually anywhere. This is especially important for the patient who cannot successfully use a metered-dose inhaler.

Cool or heated aerosol therapy can also be provided in the home. A high-output (50 psi) compressor is used to power a large-volume nebulizer that can be heated with a stick-type or wrap-around heater and then administered to the patient via a tracheostomy or aerosol mask. Wick-type, temperature-controlled aerosol delivery systems are also used when strict temperature control is desired, such as with the pediatric patient or the patient with a tracheostomy.

The RCP should instruct the patient regarding the physician's intent for this therapy (whether it is continuous or intermittent) and about infection control in conjunction with a tracheostomy. The tracheostomy patient may also need to be instructed in the use of a home suction machine (Figure 24-9) as well as home suctioning procedures.[24] Teaching patients to use clean or sterile technique and the proper cleaning of equipment, as well as frequent hand washing, is an essential element of the training program.

Positive Pressure Devices

Although not used frequently, ***intermittent positive pressure breathing*** (IPPB) therapy does have its place in the home. Electrically powered IPPB machines (Figure 24-10) are being used for patients with respiratory insufficiency secondary to neuromuscular disorders, such as muscular dystrophy, as a component of noninvasive ventilation. It may also be used for bronchodilator administration in patients unable to take a deep enough breath on their own due to neuromuscular weakness.[25]

One of the most rapidly growing areas of home care has been in the treatment of sleep-disordered breathing. Once the diagnosis of obstructive sleep apnea is made by polysomnography, the physician frequently orders the patient to be set up with a *continuous positive airway pressure* (CPAP) machine. The CPAP is a small blower that delivers a continuous flow through a special mask that fits over the patient's nose (Figure 24-11). This flow creates a pressure of 3 to 20 cmH_2O, preventing closure of the upper airway and acting as a "pneumatic splint" to eliminate the patient's airway obstruc-

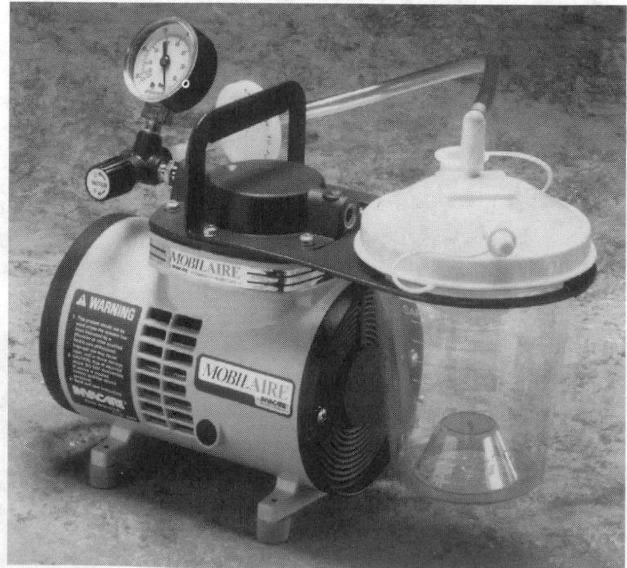

FIGURE 24-9. Home suction machine. (Photo courtesy of Invacare, Inc., DeVilbiss Health Care, Somerset, PA).

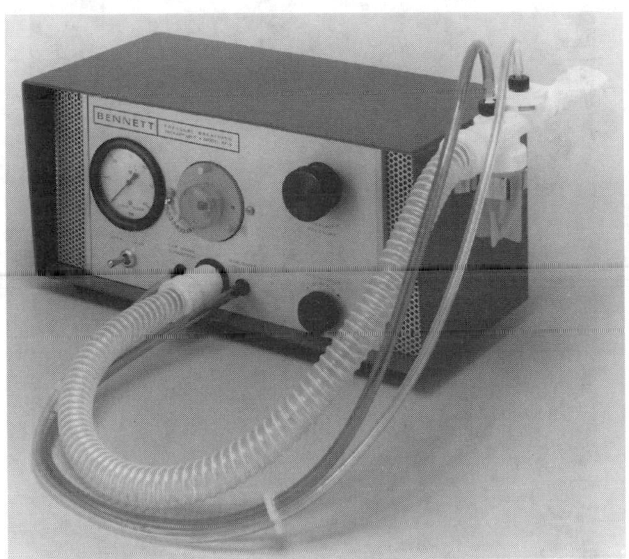

FIGURE 24-10. Home-type IPPB machine. (Photo courtesy of Puritan-Bennett, Lenexa, KS)

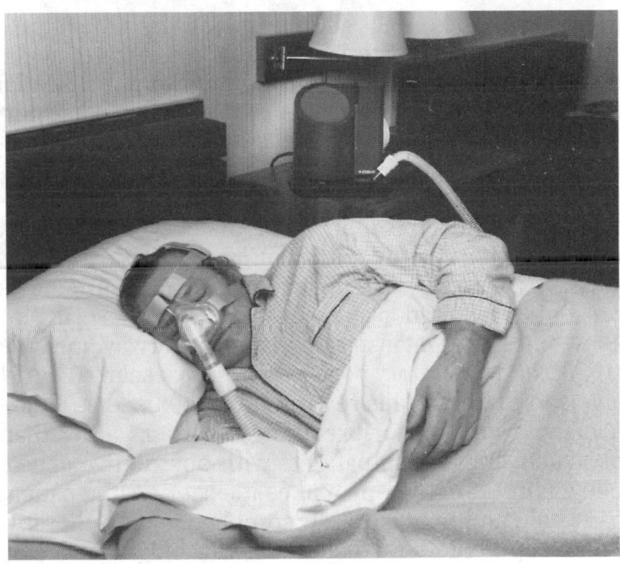

FIGURE 24-12. Nasal CPAP mask. (Photo courtesy of Respironics, Inc., Murrysville, PA)

tion.[26] There are many types of nasal masks currently on the market, as well as "nasal pillows," which are small silicone seals that fit in the nares (Figures 24-12, 24-13). Nasal pillows are useful for patients who are unable to tolerate a nasal mask.

Patients receiving CPAP therapy require a good deal of follow-up and support when therapy is first begun. It is often difficult for the patient to tolerate the nasal mask, necessitating refit or trials with other types of masks or the nasal pillows to achieve the greatest level of comfort for the patient. The CPAP patient may be unable to tolerate the high flows necessary to achieve the pressure ordered by the physician and may benefit from a "ramp" feature on the machine; the ramp feature starts out at a very low pressure and gradually increases that pressure over a preset number of minutes until the prescribed pressure is reached. The benefit of the ramp feature is that it can make it easier for patients to fall asleep with the CPAP on, and they are usually unaware when the pressure has reached its therapeutic level.

Patients on CPAP therapy need to be instructed about compliance when they receive a CPAP machine. Many patients have very negative feelings about the therapy and often feel they don't need the therapy at all. Some may feel that they have been forced into the therapy because of complaints from their sleeping partner. These patients may have difficulties with compliance and should understand how noncompliance affects

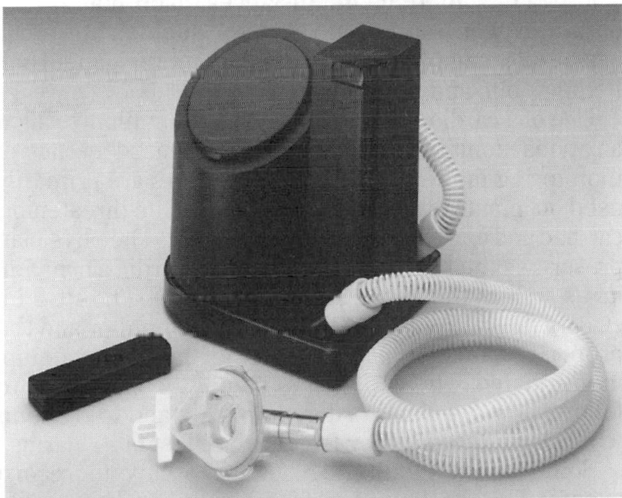

FIGURE 24-11. CPAP device for home therapy. (Photo courtesy of Respironics, Inc., Murrysville, PA)

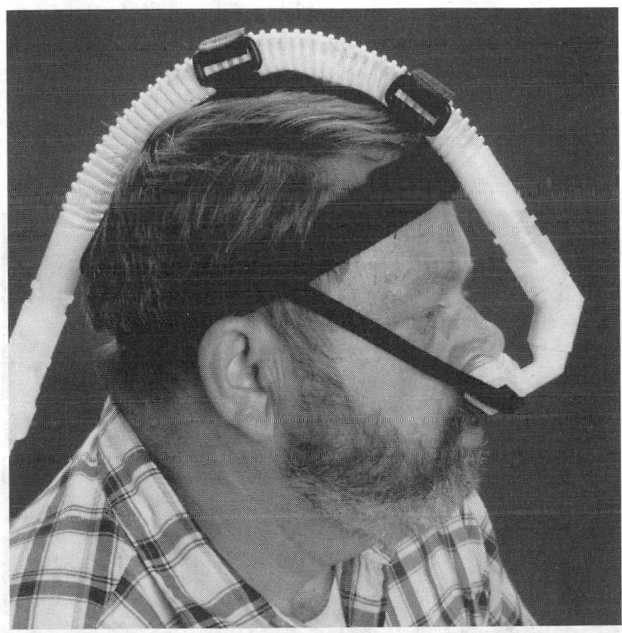

FIGURE 24-13. Nasal pillows for CPAP. (Photo courtesy of Puritan-Bennett, Lenexa, KS)

their health. The RCP should use all the educational tools and support material available to educate the patient. Careful interviewing during follow-up is essential to help determine if there are problems, such as snoring, chin drop, or nasal or sinus irritation, and to identify compliance issues.

For patients who feel that CPAP is unbearable because they find it too difficult to exhale against the back pressure, there is the option of *bilevel positive airway pressure* (Figure 24-14). Instead of a set pressure that is present on inspiration and expiration, the bilevel device allows independent inspiratory positive airway pressure (IPAP) and expiratory positive airway pressure (EPAP) levels to be set. In this regard, it can be used as a noninvasive ventilator for breathing disorders other than obstructive apnea. In patients with obstructive apnea, bilevel pressure therapy makes it easier for the patient to exhale and may increase compliance with therapy. Follow-up is the key to success with either device so that the patient isn't suffering with problems that can be solved, becoming so discouraged as to give up on the therapy altogether. Transtracheal oxygen has been reported to help in patients with obstructive sleep apnea, and it should be considered when the patient is unwilling to use nasal CPAP.[27]

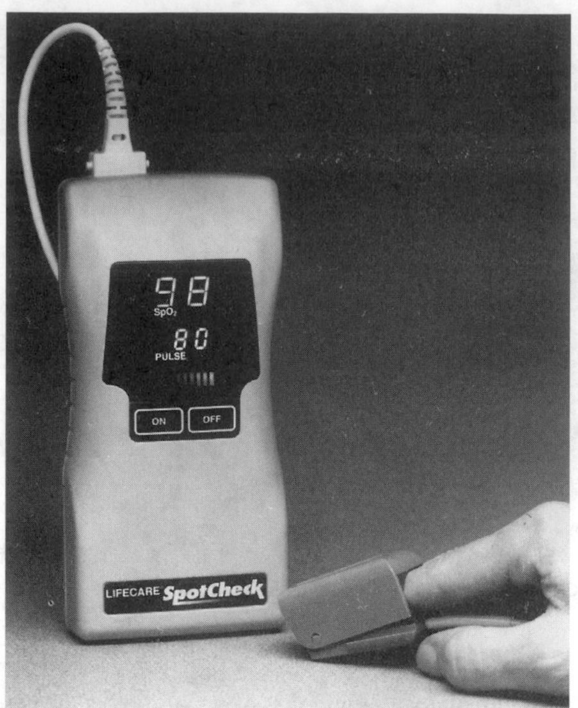

FIGURE 24-15. Pulse oximeter. (Photo courtesy of Lifecare, Intl., Inc., Westminster, CO)

Monitoring and Diagnostic Devices

Some of the most positive aspects of home care are the ability to monitor patients without sending them to the doctor's office or hospital and the ability to perform certain diagnostic tests at home. Venous and arterial blood sampling are commonly done at home now, as well as mobile electrocardiograms (ECGs) and x-ray films.

Home care RCPs may be called on to monitor oxygen saturation levels by *pulse oximetry* in the form of "spot checks," overnight studies, or even continuous monitoring (Figure 24-15). Physicians often order continuous oximetry for pediatric patients due to their instability; most other patients should not require ongoing oxygen saturation monitoring. Reimbursement for oxygen saturation studies may be provided by private insurance, usually on a case-by-case basis. Medicare does not pay for this type of monitoring in the home. In any event, home care should not be an attempt to create an intensive care facility in the home, but should use the simplest means possible to manage the patient's problems.

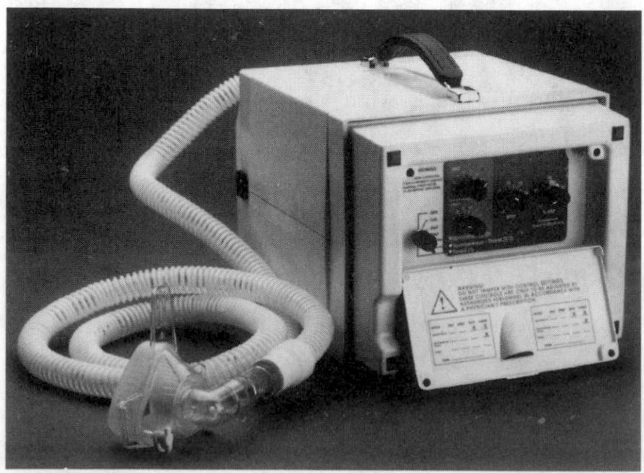

FIGURE 24-14. BiPAP (R) machine for bilevel pressure therapy. (Photo courtesy of Respironics, Inc., Murrysville, PA)

Patients and care givers must be carefully instructed on the usefulness of oximetry readings when continuous monitoring is done. They should understand that the oximetry readings should be used in conjunction with other aspects of the patient's status and that oximetry alone should not be used to make decisions regarding changing oxygen flows. They should also be made aware of the different circumstances that produce inaccurate oxygen saturation readings, such as improper sensor placement or poor perfusion, motion, abnormal hemoglobin, and fingernail polish.[28]

Use of a cardiorespiratory monitor (commonly called an apnea monitor) is another frequently used method of monitoring in the home. Apnea monitors are primarily used on infants to alert the care givers of life-threatening cardiac and apneic events (Figure 24-16). The physician prescribes the brachycardia and tachycardia alarm limits as well as the apnea alarm time delay. The RCP instructs the care givers in the use of the monitor and the proper response to alarms, whether human or equipment related. The care givers should be instructed to follow the physician's orders implicitly and to respond to all alarms even if they feel they are just false alarms.

Some apnea monitors have the ability to record events. This documented monitoring can help verify compliance because such units record not only alarm situations but also every time the monitor is turned on and off. They can also help identify truly life-threatening

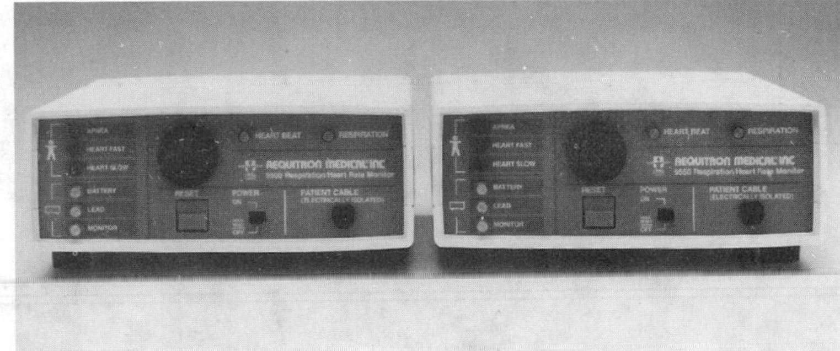

FIGURE 24-16. Infant Apnea Monitor. (Photo courtesy of Aequitron Medical, Inc., Minneapolis, MN)

events and can help the physician with treatment decisions. Care givers should always be instructed in how to perform cardiopulmonary resuscitation (CPR) in the event of a life-threatening event, and they should be cautioned that the monitor does not prevent an event but warns them of one.

Diagnostic monitoring in the form of sleep recording is being performed with more frequency in the home. Sleep recording devices are most often used to screen patients for sleep-disordered breathing (Figure 24-17); a positive home screening would indicate the need for a comprehensive polysomnography test in a sleep lab. The home care RCP applies the recording electrodes and instructs the patient how to turn the unit on at bedtime and off again in the morning. The RCP retrieves the equipment, downloads the information, and sends the study printout to the physician for interpretation. The patient with abnormal findings may then be studied in a sleep lab; however, it is becoming increasingly more common for CPAP to be initiated solely on the results of the home sleep study. This requires the home care RCP to evaluate the patient and titrate the therapeutic CPAP level based on subjective data from the patient.

Peak flow meters (Figure 24-18) are used by patients at home to detect reductions in air flow and to monitor the effectiveness of their bronchodilator therapy. The physician should define the parameters on the peak flow meter from which the patient can make adjustments in medication or seek medical attention.

The home care RCP may instruct the patient on the proper use of the peak flow meter and review the parameters ordered by the physician. Patients should be encouraged to use their own peak flow meter when having these measurements assessed in the doctor's office or pulmonary function lab because of the inherent and significant differences between brands and between peak flow meters within the same brand.[29]

Other Equipment

Home care therapists are occasionally called on to set up equipment not usually considered respiratory therapy equipment. Phototherapy lights for the treatment of hyperbilirubinemia (Figure 24-19) and for the treatment of sleep-related disorders, such as as seasonal affective disorder and delayed sleep phase syndrome (Figure 24-20), are frequently set up by the RCP. It is essential that the RCP receive thorough training and have a good understanding of the disorders being treated before setting up these types of equipment.

There are times when the RCP is called on to set up equipment such as enteral therapy pumps and *IV pumps*, although these are traditionally considered nursing procedures. This occurs because most home medical equipment providers do not employ both a nurse and an RCP, thus leaving the RCP as the only licensed professional available. It is certainly preferable that a nurse from a home health agency be involved in the set up of

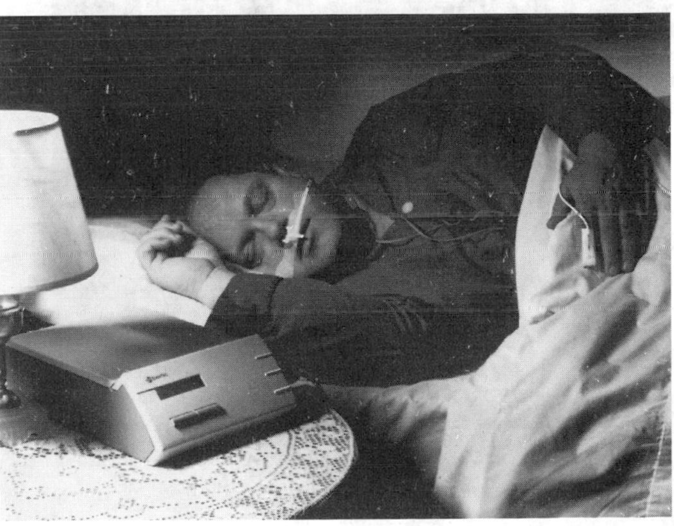

FIGURE 24-17. Home sleep recording system. (Photo courtesy of EdenTec, Eden Prairie, MN)

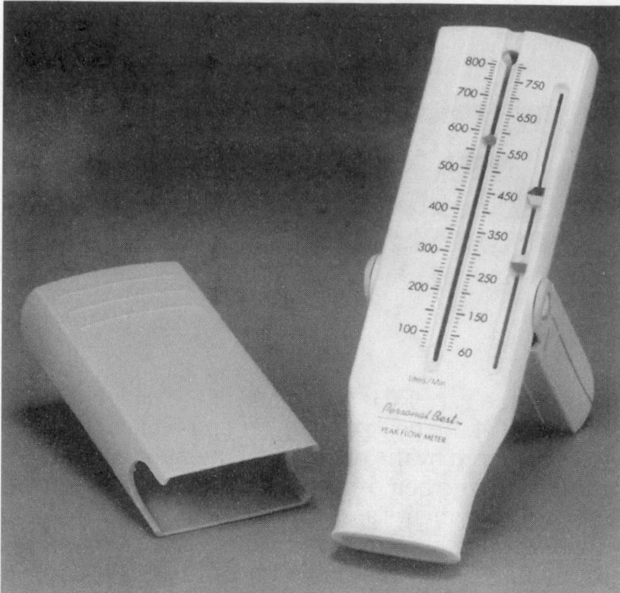

FIGURE 24-18. Peak flow meter. (Photo courtesy of Healthscan Products, Inc., Cedar Grove, NJ)

these types of equipment, and the physician is encouraged to order home health nursing visits for the patient. The RCP can instruct the care givers in the use of the pump and delivery device, such as the enteral pump, but should not instruct in the care of feeding tubes or IV lines unless specially trained to do so.

HOME MECHANICAL VENTILATION

As stated at the beginning of this chapter, patients are able to receive virtually any type of treatment they need at home, including *long-term mechanical ventilation*

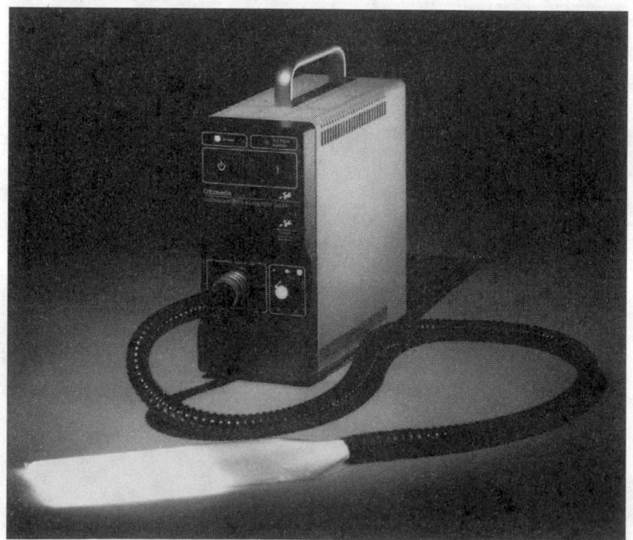

FIGURE 24-19. Phototherapy lights for treatment of hyperbilirubinemia. (Photo courtesy of Ohmeda, Inc., Columbia, MD).

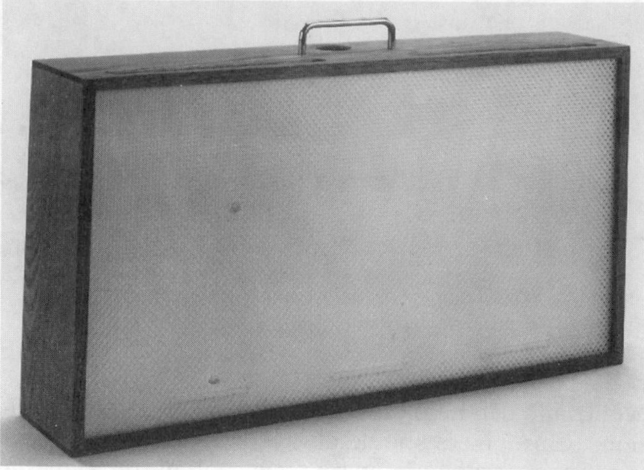

FIGURE 24-20. Phototherapy lights for treatment of sleep-related disorders. (Photo courtesy of Apollo Lights, Inc., Orem, UT).

(LTMV) (see AARC Clinical Practice Guideline: Long-Term Invasive Mechanical Ventilation in the Home). Although the process of getting the patient home is very complex, once the patient is home, it can be a very positive and rewarding experience for all concerned.

Patients are placed on mechanical ventilation in the acute care setting for any number of reasons, and in most cases, the ventilator is required for only a short duration. There are patients, however, who are unable to be weaned from the ventilator or who have chosen mechanical ventilation knowing that they may require it for the rest of their lives. If these patients are kept in the hospital (and many times they are) on a long-term basis, the cost of their care is exorbitant. Many hospitals begin looking for alternate sites of care as soon as it appears that weaning is going to be prolonged. Ventilator weaning facilities and subacute or skilled nursing facilities are potential sites for discharge, and home is another.

Candidates for Home Mechanical Ventilation

Patients requiring LTMV are not always good candidates for ventilator care at home. There are many factors to evaluate when considering home mechanical ventilation (HMV) as a discharge option, such as medical stability, whether the patient has adequate care givers, and reimbursement issues.[30] The factors shown in Table 24-6 should be considered when determining if a patient would be a good candidate for a home ventilator program.

The patient's family members are usually the primary care givers, and it is essential that they be counseled on the realities of home ventilator management. Quality of life issues should be discussed, and the patient and family should be aware of what daily life will be like. They should also understand that they will be performing many of the procedures the nurses and RCPs are doing in the hospital. They should be informed of the psychosocial and financial burdens that HMV places on the

AARC Clinical Practice Guideline

LONG-TERM INVASIVE MECHANICAL VENTILATION IN THE HOME

Indications: Patients requiring long-term invasive ventilatory support are those who have demonstrated an inability to be completely weaned from invasive ventilatory support or a progression of disease etiology that requires increasing ventilatory support. Conditions that meet these criteria may include, but are not limited to, ventilatory muscle disorders, alveolar hypoventilation syndrome, primary respiratory disorders, obstructive diseases, restrictive diseases, and cardiac disorders including congenital anomalies.

Contraindications: Long-term invasive mechanical ventilation is contraindicated in the presence of a physiologically unstable medical condition requiring a higher level of care or resources than available in the home. Indicators of a medical condition too unstable for the home and long-term care setting are FIO_2 requirement > 0.40, PEEP > 10 cmH_2O; need for continuous invasive monitoring in adult patients; lack of mature tracheostomy; patient's choice not to receive home mechanical ventilation; lack of an appropriate discharge plan; unsafe physical environment as determined by the patient's discharge planning team; presence of fire, health, or safety hazards including unsanitary conditions; inadequate basic utilities (such as heat, air conditioning, electricity); inadequate resources for care in the home; inability of ventilator-assisted individual to care for self if no care giver is available; inadequate respite care for care givers; inadequate numbers of competent care givers.

Assessment of Need: Need is determined when indications are present and contraindications are absent, when continued need exists for higher level of services, and when frequent changes in the plan of care are not needed.

Assessment of Outcome: At least the following aspects of patient management and condition should be evaluated periodically: implementation and adherence to the plan of care, quality of life, patient satisfaction, resource usage, growth and development in the pediatric patient, and unanticipated morbidity or mortality.

Monitoring: The frequency of monitoring should be determined by the ongoing individualized care plan and based on the patient's current medical condition. The ventilator settings, proper function of equipment, and the patient's physical condition should be monitored and verified with each initiation of invasive ventilation to the patient, including altering the source of ventilation, as from one ventilator or resuscitation bag to another ventilator; with each ventilator setting change; on a regular basis as specified by individualized plan of care. All appropriately trained care givers should follow the care plan and implement the monitoring that has been prescribed. These care givers may operate, maintain, and monitor all equipment and perform all aspects of care after having been trained and evaluated on their level of knowledge for that equipment and the clinical response to each of the interventions. Lay care givers should monitor the following regularly: patient's physical condition (respiratory rate, heart rate, color changes, chest excursion, diaphoresis, lethargy, blood pressure, body temperature), ventilator settings (the frequency at which alarms and settings are to be checked should be specified in the plan of care), peak pressures, preset tidal volume, frequency of ventilator breaths, verification of oxygen concentration setting, PEEP level, appropriate humidification of inspired gases, temperature of inspired gases, heat and moisture exchanger function, equipment function (appropriate configuration of ventilator circuit, alarm function, cleanliness of filters according to manufacturer's recommendation, battery power levels, overall condition of equipment), self-inflating manual resuscitator cleanliness and function. A practitioner should perform a thorough, comprehensive assessment of the patient and the patient-ventilator system on a regular basis as prescribed by the plan of care. The practitioner should implement, monitor, and assess results of other interventions as indicated by the clinical situation and anticipated in the care plan; pulse oximetry should be used in patients requiring a change in prescribed oxygen levels or in patients with a suspected change in condition; specimen collection (and analysis, as applicable) as prescribed by physician, including but not limited to sputum and blood work; cardiorespiratory monitoring (electrocardiogram, heart-rate trending), pulmonary function testing, ventilator settings, exhaled tidal volume, analysis of fraction of inspired oxygen. Personnel are also responsible for maintaining interdisciplinary communication concerning the plan of care. Personnel should integrate respiratory plan of care into the patient's total care plan. Plan of care should include all aspects of patient's respiratory care and ongoing assessment and education of the care givers involved.

From AARC Clinical Practice Guideline; see Respir Care 40:1313, 1995, for complete text.

family before making the decision to go home with a ventilator.

The Discharge Plan

Planning for the discharge of the HMV patient uses the same components of the discharge plan discussed earlier in this chapter. The major difference in planning the discharge of the HMV patient is that every aspect of the evaluation, assessment, and teaching must be done before the patient leaves the hospital. Potential problems need to be anticipated and solutions planned. The patient and care givers must know who and where their

TABLE 24-6 Factors to Consider for Candidacy Into a Home Ventilator Program

- Medical stability
- Patient and family are desirous of going home with a ventilator
- A physician familiar with home ventilator care is willing to follow the patient after discharge
- Adequate numbers of trainable care givers can be assured
- The home environment is acceptable
- Adequate financial resources (eg, insurance coverage, and so forth) are available
- Necessary community services (eg, medical equipment provider, nursing agency, social services) are available

resources are, because the goal of discharging the HMV patient from the hospital is to avoid complications and readmissions.

The *environmental assessment* is critical when considering HMV and should be done very early in the discharge process to allow sufficient time for any electrical, structural, or other modifications to be made. Patients going home with a ventilator usually go home with several additional pieces of medical equipment, such as oxygen concentrators, hospital beds, and suction machines. Careful evaluation of the home's electrical capabilities is necessary. Again, patients are going to want to continue to use lamps, televisions, heaters, and so forth, which may overtax a circuit when used in conjunction with medical equipment. Electrical rewiring and other modifications are the financial responsibility of the patient, and it must be determined whether the patient can afford to pay for them.

Geographic location also may be a factor in the patient's HMV discharge. Those living in remote areas may not have access to an HME provider that is capable of managing home ventilator care. Patients living in areas that might prove to be unreachable during severe weather also may not be ideal candidates. Alternate sites may need to be considered for these patients.

Care giver evaluation is crucial to the safe discharge of the HMV patient. Taking care of a single piece of equipment like an oxygen concentrator may not be difficult for a care giver; but when highly technical equipment such as a ventilator is added and the care giver is expected to learn how to suction, clean a tracheostomy, and perform bladder and bowel care, it may prove to be too overwhelming. Parents of pediatric patients have been shown to accept care responsibilities most readily, and female spouses are often willing care givers. Elderly men have more difficulty with the role reversal and may be less willing to accept the burdens of care as easily.

Because ventilator care is usually an around-the-clock job, more than one care giver should be designated, and at least three trained care givers are preferable. This can prove to be very difficult when family members work and have their own families to care for in addition to the HMV patient. Some insurance companies will pay for home nursing care for up to 16 and occasionally 24 hours per day; this is not a benefit for the Medicare patient, however. Insurance benefits often terminate after a period of time, and this must be taken into account. Nurses are not used in many home ventilator cases, and properly trained paid attendants are used successfully in many instances.

Home Ventilators

There are several brands of mechanical ventilators used at home; they are generally piston driven, volume cycled, and pressure limited, with the ability to be powered by electricity, an internal battery, or a 12-volt external battery (Figures 24-21 and 24-22). They are small enough in size to allow them to be mounted beneath the seat of a wheelchair (Figure 24-23) and light enough in weight

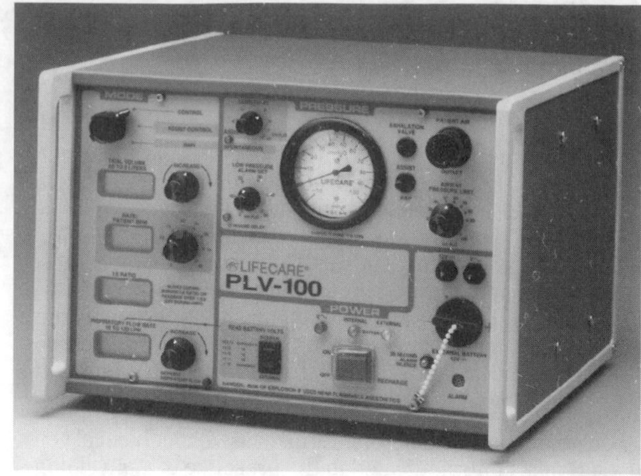

FIGURE 24-21. One brand of home ventilator. (Photo courtesy of Lifecare, Intl., Inc., Westminster, CO)

to hand carry. They are capable of performing in control, assist-control, and sometimes synchronized intermittent mandatory ventilation (SIMV) modes. Home ventilators cannot yet supply pressure support or CPAP modes, but continuous flow by means of a CPAP blower can be added in line to the ventilator circuit. Although this is commonly used with pediatric patients, the intent is to maintain simplicity in the home ventilator and not to try to introduce a critical care ventilator in the home.

All home ventilators can have oxygen added to the patient's inspired gas either through a reservoir attached to the air intake or by bleeding it into the air outlet. When supplemental oxygen is added at the air outlet, the ventilator's tidal volume needs to be reduced to compensate for the volume the oxygen adds to the minute ventilation.

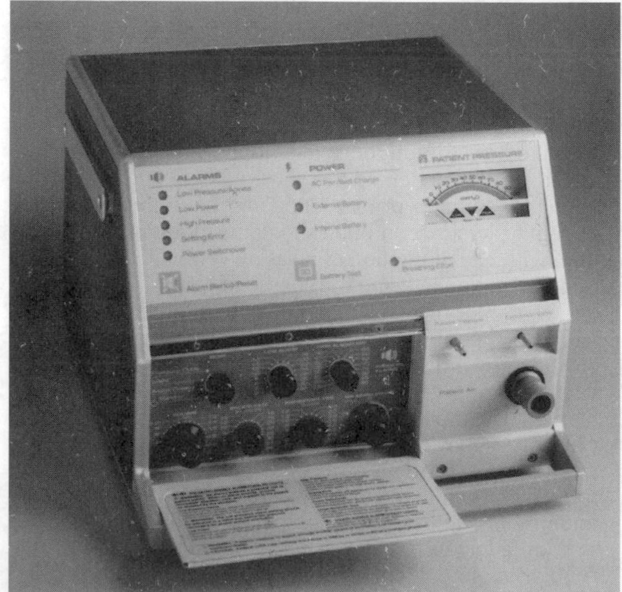

FIGURE 24-22. Another common home ventilator. (Photo courtesy of Aequitron Medical, Inc., Minneapolis, MN)

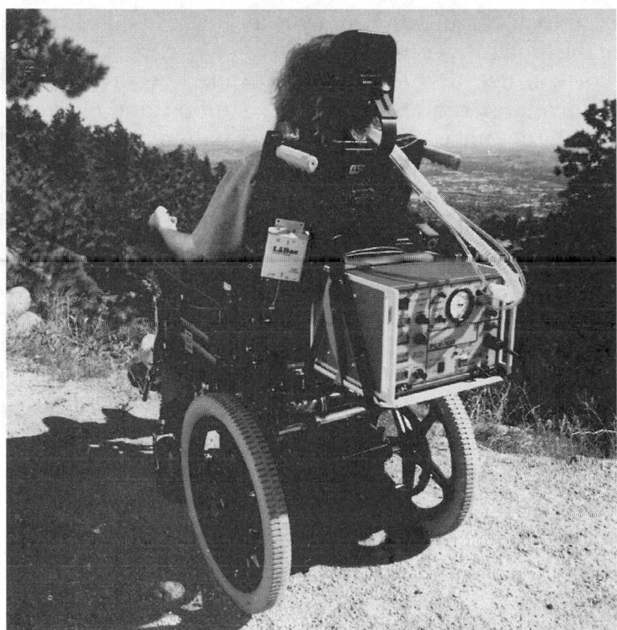

FIGURE 24-23. Ventilator mounted to a wheelchair. (Photo courtesy of Lifecare, Intl., Inc., Westminster, CO)

As stated before, home ventilators can be operated from a battery. An internal battery powers the ventilator for 1 to 2 hours, depending on the tidal volume and respiratory rate. Due to this limited battery time, the internal battery should be used only for transport or to move the ventilator from room to room. An external battery should always be included with the home ventilator setup. A 12-volt, deep-cycle, marine-type battery can provide 10 to 20 hours of power, enough time to allow the user to go to school, work, or attend many other activities outside the home. Home ventilators automatically switch to battery power in the event of an electrical power failure, so it is important to have an external battery hooked up to the ventilator at all times in anticipation of this.

Home ventilators are machines that have the potential to malfunction; and, although malfunctions occur infrequently, an alternate ventilator is recommended for patients using HMV for life support (20 or more hours per day).[31] Placing an alternate ventilator in the home allows the care givers to use the backup ventilator in the event of a mechanical problem, requiring the patient to endure only a brief interruption in mechanical ventilation. Not having an alternate ventilator in the home would necessitate ventilating the patient using a mask-valve-bag device until another ventilator is brought to the home, which could take several hours or longer. This alternate ventilator is also commonly used as the "wheelchair ventilator" for patients who are mobile.

All home ventilators require maintenance to be performed by the provider. Intake filters need to be changed routinely (usually every 30 days), and ventilator setting accuracy and battery function should also be verified. Home ventilators need to be replaced periodically (after several thousand hours) for more extensive servicing; this is done according to the manufacturer's specifications.

Patient Education

Education as the home care RCP's primary function is very apparent in HMV. Consider that the care givers are being expected to perform as therapists and nurses and being taught to do so in a very short period of time. The RCP's skills in patient education are put to the test to bring care givers up to speed in performing some very complex tasks.

Patient and care giver education and training compose most of the discharge process. Each care giver must be thoroughly trained on not only the respiratory therapy techniques and ventilator management, but also on the nursing care procedures. The patient should be instructed in self-management, to the degree possible, whenever this is appropriate.

The teaching process is best done using a team approach and using hospital staff as well as the home care personnel who will follow the patient after discharge. Specialists, such as physical and speech therapists, stoma care nurses, and social workers, should be called on to work with the patient and care givers on the areas of patient care in which they specialize.

The RCP plays an important role in the educational process. The types of things the RCP must teach the patient and care givers before discharge are presented in Table 24-7. All care givers, including nurses, must be able to manage the care of the ventilator patient satisfactorily before the patient is allowed to go home.

The ventilator that the patient will have at home should be used while the patient is still in the hospital. This accomplishes several different things, including but not limited to the following: (1) it allows the patient to adjust to the sensations of a different ventilator; (2) it

TABLE 24-7 **Aspects of Respiratory Care the HMV Patient and Family Must Learn Before Discharge**

- Use of the ventilator
  - -settings
  - -troubleshooting
  - -responding to alarms
  - -circuit maintenance
  - -use of supplemental oxygen, if needed
  - -portability of the ventilator, battery maintenance
- Tracheostomy tube management
  - -suctioning procedures
  - -stoma care
  - -tracheostomy tube care
  - -troubleshooting problems with the cuff
  - -speech (communication)
  - -elective and emergency tube changes
- Infection control and cleaning procedures
- Signs and symptoms
  - -when to call the physician
  - -when to call the medical equipment provider
  - -symptom management
- Ventilator-free time, when appropriate

allows the hospital staff to fine tune the patient's ventilator settings in relation to this new ventilator (this is particularly true when the patient has to be taken off of pressure support and placed on a conventional mode of ventilation); and (3) it allows the patient and care givers to hear and learn to respond to the ventilator alarms. The hospital staff can assist in reinforcing the education process by reviewing alarm sounds and the proper response to them when care givers are there to witness an alarm.

Follow-up Care

HMV patients can require a great deal of follow-up during the initial postdischarge phase, sometimes as frequently as daily for a while. The care givers should be able to call the home health nurse or HME provider at any hour for advice, answers to questions, or just for reassurance. The HME provider should have an RCP immediately available 24 hours a day 7 days a week, and only HME providers that can guarantee this level of service should be used.

Ventilator patients have a plan of care similar to the one developed for other types of respiratory home care patients. Follow-up visits should be based on patient need as outlined in the plan of care; frequent visits are often necessary in the beginning and are gradually reduced as the patient and home situation stabilize (eg, daily for 1 week, twice weekly for 2 weeks, then monthly or PRN for problems).

Follow-up visits should include not only ventilator maintenance but a thorough patient assessment as well. This may include oximetry, vital signs, and measurement of spontaneous tidal volume and vital capacity when ordered by the physician. The RCP should also evaluate the care givers for problems with patient care, troubleshooting alarms, or cleaning procedures and for any problems related to the other respiratory therapy equipment. The RCP is in an ideal position to identify many types of problems that may require reeducation or contacting the physician for assistance.

The Physician's Role

The physician plays a key role in the success of the home ventilator experience for the patient. The physician assists the patient in making the decision to go home with a ventilator and then is a part of the team that counsels the patient and family members on life with a home ventilator.

It is helpful to have the physician attend discharge planning conferences whenever possible. During these conferences, the physician can get the input of all the health care specialists involved in the patient's discharge and make decisions for patient care accordingly. The physician is the patient's continuous link in the hospital-to-home process and so should take an active role in the discharge planning process.

Once the patient is home, the physician supervises the program of care given by the various members of the home health care team. The physician relies on this team to act as his or her "eyes and ears" and to report all information pertinent to the patient's care. The physician can use this information to change orders, add medications, request laboratory studies, and even add treatments necessary to keep the patient at home and avoid a clinic or hospital visit. (Even for stable ventilator patients, a trip to the doctor's office or outpatient lab can be difficult at best, and if the patient is transported by ambulance, it can be very costly.)

Careful patient selection and discharge planning, thorough education of all care givers, and consistent follow-up can allow many patients to have a safe and positive home ventilator experience. The RCP is a key member of the team that can achieve this outcome.

RESPIRATORY CARE IN ALTERNATE SITES

There are patients who for any number of reasons are not good candidates for home care but still require treatment of their medical problems. Keeping them in the hospital is an extremely expensive option, and hospitals are becoming increasingly creative with alternative placement.

Subacute, skilled nursing, and acute rehabilitation hospitals are common options for alternate sites of care; in fact, a patient may go to one of these facilities before being discharged home. Patients may in some instances enter these facilities directly from home rather than being admitted to an acute facility.

RCPs are playing an ever-expanding role in the care of patients in these alternate facilities. They are a standard part of the staff of ventilator "weaning" hospitals (such as Vencor); these types of facilities are reimbursed for care at a per diem rate rather than on a Diagnosis Related Groups (DRG) basis. RCPs may also work on subacute or special weaning units that are part of the hospital where they are employed. These units are sometimes placed in another wing or ward of the hospital.

RCPs are also finding themselves caring for patients in skilled nursing facilities or nursing homes. The role of RCPs in such long-term care facilities is more that of a consultant, where RCPs evaluate the patient and determine the need for respiratory therapy modalities that they and the nursing staff administer.

These RCPs are very often employees of a hospital that has a transfer agreement with the skilled nursing facility. This is caused by the fact that Medicare currently reimburses for services provided for Medicare patients in these facilities as long as the RCPs are employees of a hospital with a transfer agreement. Non-Medicare patients may not receive these services.

RCPs in these alternate sites perform similar functions to those in the acute facility, using many of the same therapies, particularly in ventilator weaning facilities. They may assist with the teaching and discharge plan for patients being sent home. They do not have the independence of the RCP working in the home care setting, however. Probably the most striking difference is that in most instances the home care RCP's services are not currently reimbursed, whereas the services provided in the alternate sites are.

SUMMARY

Whatever the venue, RCPs are playing a major part in the treatment of patients outside the hospital setting, and their role in the home continues to gain in importance. RCPs are seeking to practice in this arena with greater frequency and are becoming increasingly recognized as a beneficial part of the pulmonary patient's plan of treatment. RCPs do not function as equipment technicians but rather as clinicians providing a full range of services.

Although their services are frequently not reimbursed by third-party payers, home care therapists are assisting physicians and case managers in determining the best and most cost-effective methods of treatment in the home, administering that therapy, and assessing the outcome. They use many of the same types of equipment found in the hospital and often assist patients in the use of equipment not commonly set up by RCPs. They educate patients and their families in the use of the most simple of therapies or the most complex. It is hoped that in the near future third-party payers such as Medicare will acknowledge the important role the RCP plays in assisting the patient at home and in keeping that patient out of the hospital and will begin to reimburse for these services.

REFERENCES

1. Dunne PJ: Demographics and financial impact of home respiratory care. Respir Care 39(4):309, 1994
2. Zabludoff J: A capital plan for reform. Home Health Care Dealer 4(2):31, 1992
3. Balinsky W and Starkman J: The impact of DRGs on the health care industry. Health Care Manage Rev 12(3):61, 1987
4. Rosell S and D'Amico FJ: The effect of home respiratory therapy on hospital readmission rates of patients with chronic obstructive pulmonary disease. Respir Care 27(10):1194, 1982
5. Haggerty MD, Stockdale-Woolley R, and Nair S: Respi-Care: An innovative home care program for the patient with chronic obstructive pulmonary disease. Chest 100(3):607, 1991
6. McAleese KA, Knapp MA, and Rhodes TT: Financial and emotional cost of bronchopulmonary dysplasia. Clin Pediatr (Phila) 32(7):393, 1993
7. Bach JR, Intintola R, Alba AS, et al: The ventilator-assisted individual: Cost analysis of institutionalized vs rehabilitation and inhome management. Chest 101(1):26, 1992
8. Bradley JS: Pediatric considerations (discussion 63). Hosp Pract (Off Ed) Suppl 1:28, 1993
9. McCorkle R, Jepson C, Malone D, et al: The impact of posthospital home care on patients with cancer. Res Nurs Health 17(4):243, 1994
10. Home Care Advisory Panel: Guidelines for the Medical Management of the Home Care Patient. Chicago, IL, AMA, 1992
11. Dunne PJ: The role of the respiratory care practitioner in home care. NBRC Horizons 18(4):2, 1992
12. Massong JI: Legal Issues. In J Turner, G McDonald, and N Larter (eds): Handbook of Adult and Pediatric Respiratory Home Care. St. Louis, Mosby-Year Book, 1994, pp. 394–405
13. Safety for Older Consumers: Home Safety Checklist. Washington DC, U. S. Consumer Product Safety Commission, June 1986
14. Krider SJ: Interviewing and the Respiratory History. In RL Wilkins, RL Sheldon, and SJ Krider (eds): Clinical Assessment in Respiratory Care (2nd ed). St. Louis, CV Mosby, 1990
15. ATS: Standards of Nursing Care for Adult Patients with Pulmonary Dysfunction. Am Rev Resp Dis 144(1):231, 1991
16. The Joint Commission on Accreditation of Health Care Organizations: Accreditation Manual for Home Care, Vol. 1: Standards. Oakbrook Terrace, IL, JCAHO, 1995
17. McInturff SL: A model plan of care. Home Health Care Dealer May–June, 5(3):35, 1992
18. Nocturnal Oxygen Therapy Trial Group: Continuous or Nocturnal Oxygen Therapy in Hypoxemic Chronic Obstructive Lung Disease. Ann Intern Med 93(3):391, 1980
19. O'Donohue WJ Jr, Plummer AL: The magnitude of use and cost of home oxygen therapy in the United States. Chest 107:301, 1995
20. Tiep BL: Long term oxygen therapy. Clin Chest Med 11(3):505, 1990
21. Petty TL and O'Donohue WJ Jr: Further recommendations for prescribing, reimbursement, technology development, and research in long-term oxygen therapy. Am J Respir Crit Care Med 150:875, 1994
22. Hoffman LA: Novel strategies for delivering oxygen: Reservoir cannula, demand flow, and transtracheal oxygen administration. Respir Care 39(4):363, 1994
23. Stoller JK: Travel for the technology-dependent individual. Respir Care 39(4):347, 1994
24. Shiley Tracheostomy Products: Tracheostomy Tube Adult Home Care Guide. Irvine, CA, Sorin Biomedical, 1992
25. Aerosol Therapy Guidelines Committee: AARC Clinical Practice Guideline: Intermittent Positive Pressure Breathing. Respir Care 38(11):1189, 1993
26. Sullivan CE and Grunstein RR: Continuous Positive Airway Pressure in Sleep Disordered Breathing. In MH Kruger, T Roth, and WC Dement (eds): Principles and Practice of Sleep Medicine. Philadelphia, WB Saunders, 1989, pp. 559–570
27. Farney RJ, Walker JM, Elmer JC, et al: Transtracheal oxygen, nasal CPAP and nasal oxygen in five patients with obstructive sleep apnea. Chest 101:1228, 1992
28. Craig KC: Clinical Application of Pulse Oximetry. In GH Hicks (ed): Problems in Respiratory Care: Applied Noninvasive Respiratory Monitoring. Philadelphia, JB Lippincott, 1989, pp. 255–290
29. Simmons M, Wynegar T, and Hess D: Evaluation of the agreement between portable peak flow meters and a calibrated pneumotachometer. Respir Care 38(8):916, 1993
30. O'Donohue WJ, Giovanonni RM, Goldberg AJ, et al: Long-term mechanical ventilation: Guidelines for management in the home and at alternative community sites. Chest 90(1):1s, 1986
31. Plummer AL, O'Donohue WJ, and Petty TL: Consensus conference on problems in home mechanical ventilation. Am Rev Respir Dis 140:555, 1989

SECTION

5

APPLICATION OF RESPIRATORY CARE TECHNIQUES

25 Neonatal Lung Disease and Respiratory Care

John M. Fiascone and Patricia N. Vreeland

CLINICAL SKILLS

Upon completion of this chapter, the reader will be able to:

- Describe development of the fetal lung and fetal circulation
- Explain the pulmonary and circulatory adaptations necessary for a neonate to sustain extrauterine life
- Administer resuscitative procedures to neonates at birth based on rapid patient assessment
- Describe the prevention, pathophysiology, testing, and treatment of infant respiratory distress syndrome
- Select a method to deliver infant CPAP with consideration of the indications, pulmonary effects, and potential hazards
- Select appropriate settings for infant mechanical ventilation while minimizing potential hazards
- Explain the basic principles that are responsible for the effectiveness of high-frequency ventilation
- Discuss indications, patient monitoring, and weaning techniques associated with high-frequency oscillatory ventilation
- Identify the clinical features and treatment options for common pulmonary disorders of the newborn
- Describe the clinical presentation of neonates with congenital heart disease
- Discuss various approaches to the treatment of central, obstructive, and mixed apnea of the infant
- Identify the clinical presentation, treatment, and prognosis of chronic lung disease of infancy

- Summarize methods of oxygen delivery for infants
- Describe characteristics of infant mechanical ventilators
- Select the appropriate mode and ventilator settings for infants requiring mechanical ventilation
- Adapt bronchial hygiene therapies to the needs of the neonate
- Monitor the arterial oxygenation and carbon dioxide levels of the sick neonate

KEY TERMS

Alveolar period
Apgar scoring system
Bronchopulmonary dysplasia
Bulk convection
Canalicular period
Capnography
Cardiogenic mixing
Chronic lung disease of infancy
Congenital diaphragmatic hernia
Designated neonatal resuscitators
Embryonic period
Fetal hemoglobin
High-frequency jet ventilation
High-frequency oscillatory ventilation
High-frequency positive pressure ventilation
Hypoxic pulmonary vasoconstriction
Infant mortality rate
Lamellar bodies
Lecithin to sphingomyelin ratio
Lung maturity
Meconium aspiration
Meconium staining of amniotic fluid
Minute ventilation
Molecular diffusion
Neonatal mortality rate
Nitric oxide therapy
Pendelluft
Persistent fetal circulation
Pneumomediastinum
Pneumopericardium
Pseudoglandular period
Pulmonary interstitial emphysema
Pulmonary surfactant
Pulse oximetry
Reid's first law of lung development
Reid's second law of lung development
Rescue therapy
Saccular period
Surface tension
Surfactant deficiency disease
Surfactant inhibitor
Taylor dispersion
Transient tachypnea of the newborn

Since early in this century, the *infant mortality rate,* defined as the number of deaths in the first year of life per 1000 live births, has been falling steadily. Initially this decline was caused by a reduction in deaths from infection, malnutrition, and diarrheal disease. More recently, however, the decline in infant mortality has been caused by a reduction in *neonatal mortality rate,* the number of deaths in the first 28 days of life per 1000 live births. Currently, in developed countries, neonatal mortality is the major determinant of infant mortality. Most deaths in the first year of life happen in the first 28 days of life. Fatal disease in newborns most often involves the respiratory system. These facts underscore the importance of fetal lung development and neonatal pulmonary disease within the field of respiratory care.

FETAL LUNG DEVELOPMENT

Structural Development

Development of the human lung[1–3] can be conveniently divided into five phases, each with distinct morphologic alterations that mark its beginning and end. The *embryonic period* begins between the fourth and fifth week of gestation. Its most prominent feature is the formation of the proximal conducting airways. This period begins when the embryonic foregut, an endodermal derivative, gives rise to a single lung bud as an outpouching structure at the caudal end of the laryngotracheal groove (Fig. 25-1). Shortly after its appearance, the single lung bud divides to give rise to two bronchial buds. Subsequent divisions and growth form the segmental bronchi. Formation of the segmental bronchi establishes the future bronchopulmonary segments, occurs by the end of the sixth postconceptional week, and marks the end of the embryonic period.

The *pseudoglandular period* of lung development extends from the 7th through the 16th week. During this time, all of the conducting airways are formed. Study of this period gives rise to *Reid's first law of lung development:* the entire bronchial tree is developed by the 16th week of intrauterine life, and this development with its subsequent deposition of cartilage proceeds from lung hilum to periphery (centrifugal development). *Reid's second law of lung development* also applies to the pseudoglandular period and states that preacinar blood vessels (ie, arteries and arterioles leading to alveoli or to structures that will be alveoli) develop in parallel with the conducting airways (Box 25-1). However, the intraacinar arteries and veins (ie, those vessels closest to the future gas-exchanging units) develop in parallel with alveoli and, thus, will make their appearance and begin to develop in the next period of lung development. The pseudoglandular stage takes its name from the microscopic appearance of the lung (Fig. 25-2), which resembles that of an exocrine gland, with columnar epithelial cells surrounding lumina that are approximately circular.

The *canalicular period* is characterized by the beginning of formation of the pulmonary gas-exchanging unit—the acinus. This period lasts from the 17th through the 28th week of gestation. The acinus may be thought of as the functional gas-exchanging unit of the mature lung and, ultimately, consists of a respiratory

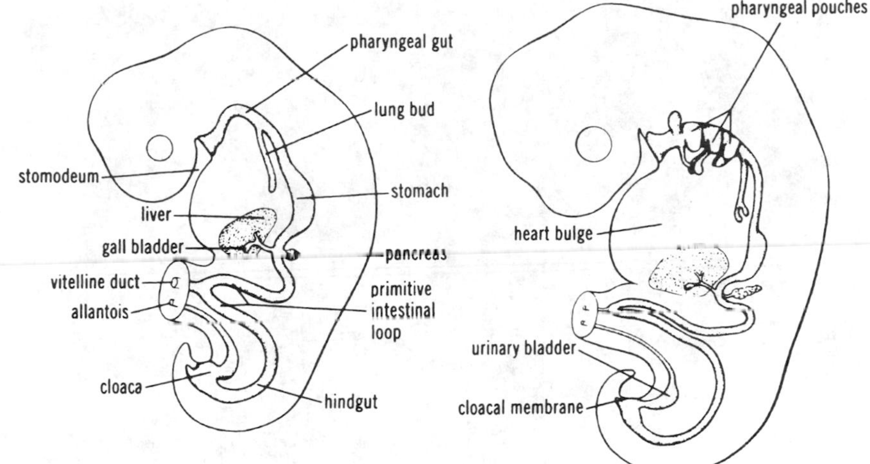

FIGURE 25-1. Diagrammatic embryos at different stages of development between 4 and 8 weeks illustrating the endodermal origin of the lungs. The single lung bud shown in the figure on the *left* is a derivative of the gastrointestinal tract. The figure on the *right* illustrates the subsequent appearance of the bronchial buds. (Reproduced with permission from Langman J: Medical Embryology [3rd ed.] 1975, Williams & Wilkins Co, Baltimore)

bronchiole, with its subsequent 6 to 10 additional generations of airways, and their blood supply. During the canalicular period, the basic structure of the acinus is formed, and the vascularization process is begun as intraacinar vessels develop within the mesenchyme adjacent to the forming acini (Reid's second law). Histologically, the fetal lung shows potential airspaces that are lined with cuboidal epithelium; a thick, cellular interstitium is present; and the lung as a whole contains more tissue space than potential airspace (Fig. 25-3).

During the *saccular period,* 29 through 36 weeks after conception, formation of the gas-exchanging units continues in association with a dramatic change in the microscopic appearance of the lung (Fig. 25-4). There is reversal of the tissue-airspace relationship that was present in the previous period, and the lung comes to contain much more potential airspace than tissue space. The interstitium is thin, and the walls between airspaces become very compact. Capillary networks are present and are easily visible within the lung interstitium.

BOX 25-1

REID'S LAWS OF LUNG DEVELOPMENT

1. All the conducting airways of the tracheobronchial tree are formed by the end of the 16th week of gestation. Deposition of cartilage proceeds from hilum to periphery.
2. The preacinar blood vessels follow the development of the conducting airways, and the intraacinar vessels develop along with the alveoli. The cannalicular phase is characterized by capillary invasion of the acini.
3. Alveolar development takes place predominantly during postnatal life. Alveoli increase in number during the first 8 years and in size until adulthood. Alveolar development proceeds from the periphery to the hilum; alveoli first appear on saccules and later in life on terminal bronchioles.

Used with permission from Reid LM: Structural Development of the Lung and Pulmonary Circulation. In P Ballard (ed): Respiratory Distress Syndrome, London, Academic Press, 1984

The final period of lung development is the *alveolar period,* which begins at 37 weeks after conception but continues into postnatal life to the 8th year. However, primitive alveoli can first be seen at 29 weeks, and by full term the infant lung should be extensively alveolarized (Fig. 25-5). The absolute number of alveoli varies linearly with body weight. There is an average of 150 million alveoli present at term, although the range of normal appears to be quite wide. At term there are 50% as many alveoli present as in the adult lung, but the infant lung weighs only 5% as much as the adult lung. New alveoli continue to form until 8 years of age and increase in size until adulthood (Table 25-1).

Cytodifferentiation

The human lung contains more than 40 cell types.[1,2] The two cell types of greatest interest are the type I alveolar epithelial cells, which line alveoli and across which gas exchange occurs, and the type II alveolar epithelial cells, which synthesize, store, and secrete pulmonary surfactant. Neither of these two cell types is recognizable before the canalicular stage of development. After 20-weeks gestational age, the respiratory epithelial cells accumulate large quantities of glycogen, probably in preparation for differentiation and surfactant synthesis. Distinct type II cells appear between 22 and 26 weeks of gestation, but they become more prominent after 34 weeks. These cells are distinguished by easily identified subcellular organelles involved in surfactant metabolism: polyribosomes, endoplasmic reticulum, Golgi apparatus, multivesicular bodies, and lamellar bodies.

The lamellar bodies contain surfactant and are eventually excreted by the type II cell. Type II cells constitute less than 15% of the lung parenchyma but have great functional importance. At the same time that type II cells are first identified, other alveolar cells are differentiating into type I cells. These cells are flat, with long extensions of thin cytoplasm, a large surface area, and few subcellular organelles. Most gas exchange takes place across these cells because they cover the major portion of the alveolar surface. Junctions between

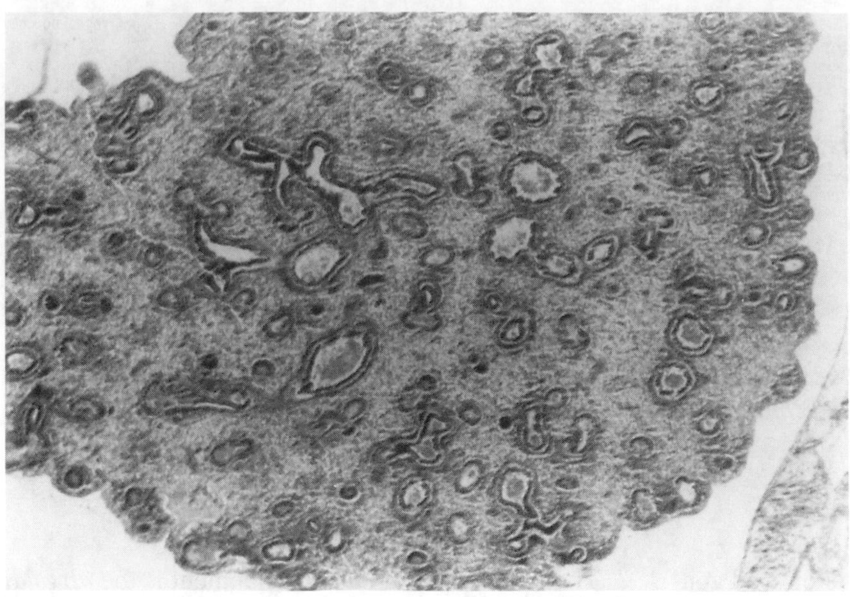

FIGURE 25-2. Microscopic appearance of the lung during the pseudoglandular stage. This stage is named for the resemblance of the lung to an exocrine gland.

type I cells constitute the alveolar epithelial barrier to fluids and molecules. This barrier, in the normal lung, is virtually impermeable to protein.

Connective Tissue Development

Relatively little is known about the developmental aspects of lung connective tissue. Pulmonary fibroblasts, located in the interstitium, synthesize and secrete both collagen and elastin. Collagen synthesis is required for branching of airways and, as such, has a major influence on airway development. Elastin, in contrast, is more intimately involved with the structure of the lung parenchyma distal to the conducting airways. Whereas collagen is present in lung primordia from very early in gestation, elastin does not appear earlier than 20 weeks. Elastin, subsequent to its appearance, is closely involved in the structure of the acinus. Elastin has both immature and mature forms. In human development, immature forms appear first and then are replaced with more mature elastin as gestation progresses.

The human fetal lung parenchyma contains only small quantities of collagen and elastin. Postnatally there is a rapid deposition of these proteins and, at approximately 6 months of age, adult levels (12% of dry lung weight) are reached.

Biochemical Development and Surface Tension in the Lung

Surface tension[4] can conveniently be thought of as the attractive force between molecules in a liquid at an air–liquid interface. The alveolar surface is lined by a thin liquid layer; hence, any expansion of alveoli, as dur-

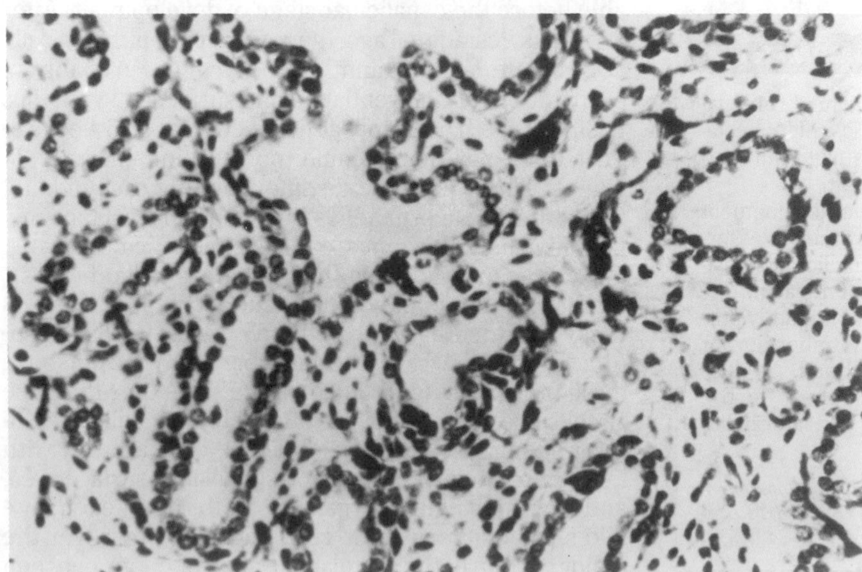

FIGURE 25-3. Microscopic appearance of the lung during the canalicular stage. Potential air spaces are present but are lined with cuboidal epithelium, the interstitial tissue is thick, and there is more tissue space than air space. (DW Thibeault, GA Gregory (eds): Neonatal Pulmonary Care [2nd ed.] Norwalk, Conn, Appleton & Lange, 1987, with permission)

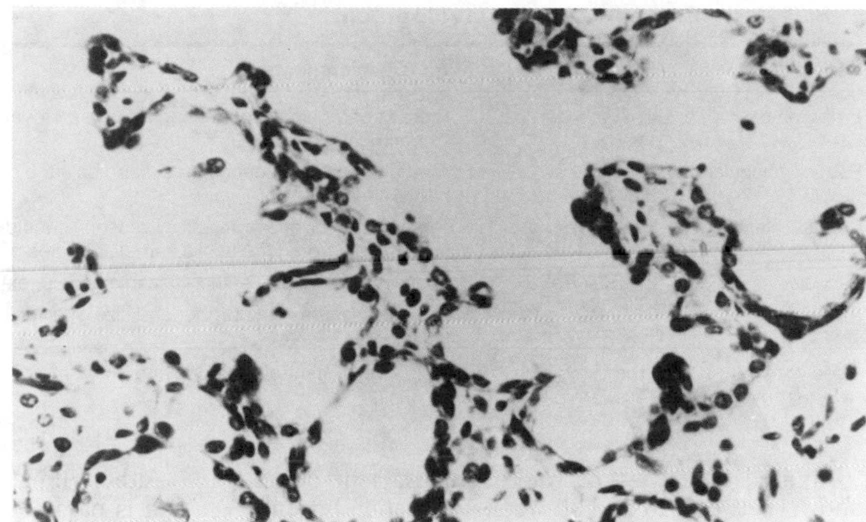

FIGURE 25-4. Saccular stage microscopic appearance of the lung: Potential airspace now exceeds tissue space, the interstitial area is much thinner, and epithelial lining cells are flatter than in previous stages. (DW Thibeault, GA Gregory (eds): Neonatal Pulmonary Care [2nd ed.] Norwalk, Conn, Appleton & Lange, 1987, with permission)

ing inspiration, requires not only the force necessary to expand the lung tissue itself (referred to as frictional resistance) but also that force necessary to overcome surface tension.

Pulmonary surfactant is a complex phospholipid and protein mixture secreted into the alveolus by type II cells (Table 25-2). The function of pulmonary surfactant is to reduce surface tension within the alveolus at the air–liquid interface and thereby greatly decrease the force or pressure required for alveolar expansion. In the absence of adequate quantities of surfactant as a result of surface tension, the alveolus has a force directed toward collapse that becomes strongest at end-expiration when the alveoli are smallest. The presence of adequate quantities of surfactant reduces surface tension at end-expiration to nearly zero and, in this manner, stabilizes alveoli. An inadequate quantity of surfactant, leading to end-expiratory alveolar collapse and to a requirement for greater pressure to produce lung expansion (ie, decreased lung compliance), is the central feature of the infant respiratory distress syndrome (RDS), or hyaline membrane disease (HMD). Recognition of the critical role of surfactant in RDS has led to the term *surfactant deficiency disease* to replace both of the preceding names, as this new term is more specific in its description.

The term *lung maturity* is generally used to describe the fetal or newborn lung when it comes to contain adequate quantities of surfactant in the airspaces to support alveolar stability and gas exchange. In uncomplicated pregnancies, type II cells are first discernible shortly after 20 weeks of gestation, during the canalicular period. As these cells increase in number, the subcellular synthetic organelles involved in surfactant synthesis become more prominent, and surfactant synthesis increases. *Lamellar bodies,* the intracellular storage sites of surfactant, can first be found between 20 and 24 weeks.

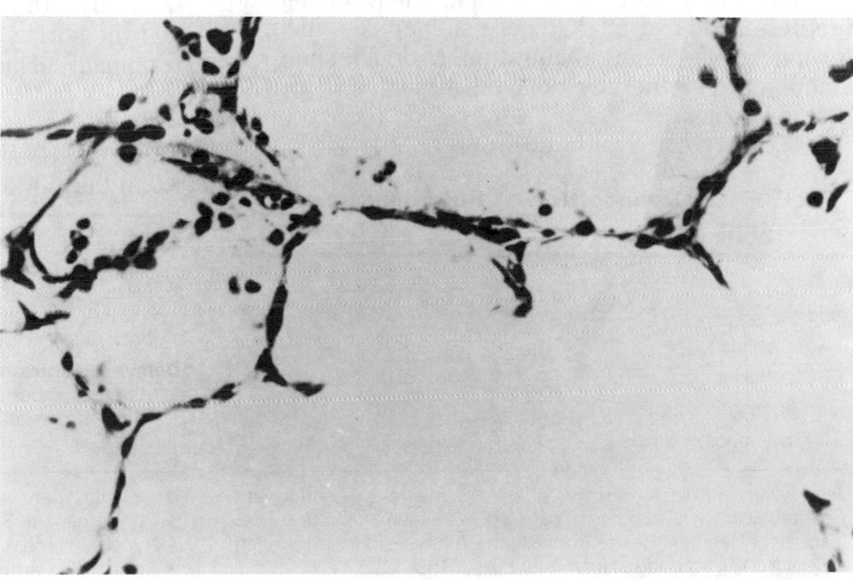

FIGURE 25-5. Early, histologic structure of the alveolar period lung: Microscopic appearance is now very similar to that of a mature lung. (DW Thibeault, GA Gregory (eds): Neonatal Pulmonary Care [2nd ed.] Norwalk, Conn, Appleton & Lange, 1987, with permission)

TABLE 25-1. **Stages of Lung Development**

Period	Time	Major Developments
Embryonic	4–6 weeks	Formation of proximal conducting airways to level of segmental bronchi; establishment of bronchopulmonary segments
Pseudoglandular	7–16 weeks	Formation of all conducting airways, preacinar blood vessels; columnar epithelial cells surround future airspaces
Cannalicular	17–28 weeks	Formation of acini and intra-acinar vessels; cuboidal cells line future airspaces; type II cells distinguishable from type I cells; lamellar bodies present in type II cells
Saccular	29–36 weeks	Decrease in tissue space, increase in airspace, extensive capillary network
Alveolar	37 weeks on	Progressive increase in number and size of alveoli

Used with permission from Reid LM: Structural Development of the Lung and Pulmonary Circulation. In P Ballard (ed): Respiratory Distress Syndrome. London, Academic Press, 1984.

Limited quantities of released surfactant can be shown between 25 and 30 weeks; secretion becomes more extensive after 35 weeks. There is wide variation in the timing of normal development relative to the quantity of surfactant synthesized, stored, and available for secretion should birth occur earlier than 37 weeks (full term). There is an approximate 10-week window, from 25 to 35 weeks, when early lung maturity may be present. Several conditions of pregnancy, and specific pharmacologic interventions, are capable of accelerating or delaying fetal lung maturity (Tables 25-3 and 25-4).

Large amounts of information from both laboratory and clinical studies indicate that corticosteroid exposure results in increased synthesis of surfactant and in precocious maturation of the fetal lung. Similar, although not as extensive, data indicate that the thyroid hormones triiodothyronine (T_3), thyroxine (T_4), and thyrotropin-releasing hormone (TRH), as well as aminophylline, have similar effects. Corticosteroids do not act on type II cells directly. Rather, they induce the production of small polypeptides such as fibroblast pneumonocyte factor in surrounding lung fibroblasts. This peptide, in turn, accelerates surfactant production by alveolar type II cells. On the other hand, chronic hyperglycemia, as found in infants of diabetic mothers, leads to fetal hyperinsulinemia, which, in turn, delays fetal lung maturation. Male fetal lung development is generally delayed in comparison with that of females.

TABLE 25-2. **Composition of Pulmonary Surfactant**

Protein	7%
Lipid	93%
Neutral lipid	9%
Phospholipid	91%
Phosphatidylcholine	92%
Other phospholipids	8%

Used with permission from Jobe A: Surfactant Function and Metabolism. In BR Boynton, WA Carlo, AH Jobe (eds): New Therapies for Neonatal Respiratory Failure: A Physiological Approach. New York, Cambridge University Press, 1994

Although maturity of the pulmonary surfactant system is paramount in determining lung function after birth, there are other biochemical systems within the lung, the development of which is important to the neonate. The system of enzymes that function to prevent lung tissue damage by oxygen radicals is one example. Molecular oxygen in tissue is capable of undergoing several reactions that may lead to the formation of unstable molecular species such as hydrogen peroxide (H_2O_2), the hydroxyl radical (OH^-), and the superoxide anion (O_2^-). These species may interact with membrane lipids in a reaction called *peroxidation,* which results in cellular and tissue damage. Iron may accelerate and exacerbate this process. The enzymes of the pulmonary antioxidant system are catalase, glutathione peroxidase, and superoxide dismutase. Their activity in fetal lung tissue, as gestation progresses, parallels the increasing activity of the pulmonary surfactant system. In addition to the antioxidant enzymes, there are nonenzymatic antioxidant compounds, such as vitamin E and ascorbic acid, that can interfere with lipid peroxidation. Tissue stores of these compounds also accumulate as pregnancy progresses. Exposure of the fetus to corticosteroids accelerates the development of at least the enzymatic portion of the antioxidant system.

At birth, the degree of maturation of lung structure and the surfactant system are the most important determinants of lung function. When oxygen therapy is re-

TABLE 25-3. **Maternal Conditions Influencing Fetal Lung Maturation**

Accelerated Maturation
- Chronic hypertension
- Placental insufficiency
- Prolonged rupture of the membranes
- Black race

Delayed Maturation
- Maternal diabetes
- Rh isoimmunization with fetal hydrops
- Male sex

Used with permission from Jobe A: Surfactant Function and Metabolism. In BR Boynton, WA Carlo, AH Jobe (eds): New Therapies for Neonatal Respiratory Failure: A Physiological Approach. New York, Cambridge University Press, 1994

TABLE 25-4. **Drugs Accelerating Fetal Lung Maturation**

Corticosteroids
Thyroid hormones
Methylxanthines: theophylline, caffeine
Estrogens

Used with permission from Jobe A: Surfactant Function and Metabolism. In BR Boynton, WA Carlo, AH Jobe (eds): New Therapies for Neonatal Respiratory Failure: A Physiological Approach. New York, Cambridge University Press, 1994

quired in high concentrations and for prolonged periods of time, there can be formation within the newborn lung of oxygen radicals, and the potential for lung damage from these species exists. Additionally, during severe neonatal lung diseases, polymorphonuclear leukocytes migrate into the lung and release toxic products that can lead to lipid peroxidation reactions. The degree of maturity of the antioxidant system and the ability of the lung to control an inflammatory response may determine, in part, if and how much secondary lung damage will occur when oxygen therapy is required for treatment of severe neonatal lung disease.

FETAL PULMONARY FLUID

In fetal life, the pulmonary epithelial cells secrete fluid into the alveoli.[5] This fluid fills the potential airspaces during development, is very rich in chloride, has almost no protein, and exhibits a net flux up the conducting airways and outward into the amniotic fluid. As term approaches, mammalian lungs contain a volume of fetal pulmonary fluid that exceeds their functional residual capacity (approximately 20 to 30 mL/kg body weight of fluid). This pulmonary fluid is essential for normal lung development. In animal experiments in which this fluid is removed, abnormal lung growth and pulmonary hypoplasia develop.

Although fetal pulmonary fluid is essential for normal lung development, this liquid must be removed from the airspaces before or very soon after birth for gas exchange to occur. Evidence indicates that the process of removal of lung fluid begins before delivery. As part of preparation for the onset of labor, the pulmonary epithelium decreases its secretion of fluid. When labor commences, further reductions in lung fluid are initiated. The processes that determine fetal lung fluid content are incompletely understood, but regulation by several hormones is involved. The stress of labor for the fetus and the accompanying high levels of circulating epinephrine and perhaps arginine vasopressin (AVP) seem to be responsible, in large part, for the reduction in fluid content. There is some evidence that prostaglandin E_2 (PGE_2) may also be involved.

Animal and human infants delivered by cesarean section without prior labor have increased volumes of pulmonary fluid in comparison with the amount found after vaginal delivery following labor. Premature birth is associated with a higher lung fluid content than is found after term birth, regardless of the manner of delivery.

Removal of fluid from airspaces continues in the several hours that follow birth. The onset of respiration creates a transpulmonary pressure gradient. Conducting airways pressure is equal to atmospheric pressure, whereas intrapleural pressure is -5 to -8 cmH_2O. This transpulmonary pressure gradient favors shifting of the remaining fluid in the airspaces into the perivascular spaces around large blood vessels and conducting airways (the pulmonary interstitium), where lymphatic vessels and small blood vessels take the fluid up and remove it. In addition to this fluid shift, caused by a pressure gradient, there is reason to believe that active transport of sodium and fluid across the pulmonary epithelium contributes to removal of fluid from the airspaces. At present, the site of this active transport seems to be the type II cell. Following its displacement from airspaces to perivascular and peribronchial spaces, most fluid is removed by small vessels in the lung microcirculation, with a small amount (11% in lambs) being removed through the lymphatics. On the basis of animal experiments, the final clearance of this pulmonary fluid occurs within 6 hours after delivery.

FETAL CIRCULATION

Most of the information on fetal circulation[6] has been obtained from the study of fetal lambs; it is generally believed that the human fetal circulation is similar. Recent studies of the fetal circulation in humans, which used pulsed Doppler ultrasonography and Doppler color-flow mapping technology, indicate that this is true. Several features of the circulation that are present before birth are very different from the circulation that exists shortly after birth (Fig. 25-6). These prenatal features are (1) the presence of the placenta, which functions as the organ of gas exchange and as a very low resistance circuit for blood flow; (2) a very high pulmonary vascular resistance owing to constriction of the pulmonary arterioles, resulting in very little flow of blood through the fetal lungs; and (3) two channels for shunting of blood from the pulmonary system to the systemic circulation, the patent ductus arteriosus and the foramen ovale.

Blood returning from the placenta is carried in the umbilical vein, which has a PaO_2 close to 35 mmHg and an SaO_2 in the range of 85% to 90%. Some 50% of umbilical venous blood is shunted through the liver by the ductus venosus to the inferior vena cava, with no change in oxygen content. The remainder is divided between the hepatic venous system, supplying the major circulation to the left lobe of the liver, and the portal venous system, supplying blood to the right lobe of the liver. Blood distributed through the liver in this manner delivers oxygen to those tissues; as a consequence, there is a decrease in blood oxygen content.

The distal vena cava, the ductus venosus, and the right and left hepatic veins all contribute blood flow to the thoracic inferior vena cava (IVC). Blood entering the thoracic IVC from each of these sources has a dif-

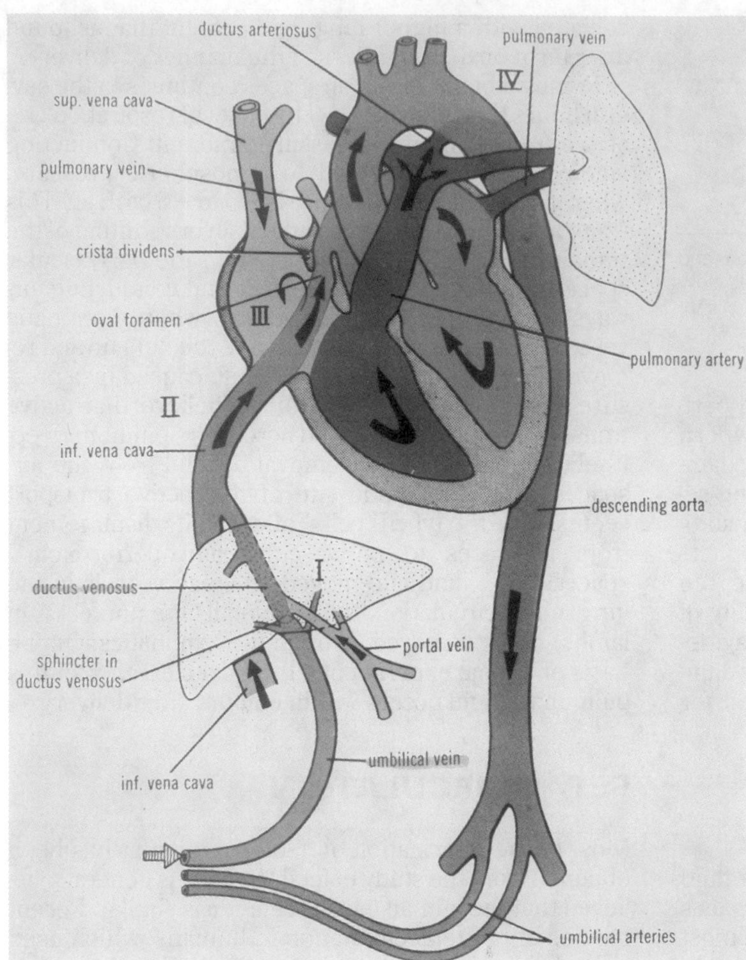

FIGURE 25-6. The fetal circulation. Note selective streaming of blood returning form the placenta, with the highest PO_2 across the foramen ovale. This blood supplies the coronary arteries and brain selectively, as these vessels leave the aorta proximal to the entry of the ductus arteriosus. (Reproduced with permission from Langman J: Medical Embryology [3rd ed.] Baltimore, Williams & Wilkins, 1975)

ferent oxygen content. Blood from the ductus venosus has the highest oxygen content because it has not participated in tissue oxygen delivery.

Recent information indicates that within the thoracic IVC there is selective streaming of blood. Blood from the ductus venosus is directed into the right atrium and across the patent foramen ovale (in the atrial septum) into the left atrium. From the left atrium, this blood, with its relatively high oxygen content, is pumped into the left ventricle and then out into the proximal aorta from which the coronary arteries and the cerebral vessels arise. In this manner, the heart and brain tissues are selectively supplied with the fetal blood that has the highest oxygen content.

In contrast, blood in the thoracic IVC returning to the heart from the liver or lower body, on reaching the heart, is selectively directed to the right atrium where atrial contractions then force it, along with blood returning to the right atrium from the superior vena cava, into the right ventricle, with subsequent ventricular contractions ejecting this more desaturated blood into the main pulmonary artery. Once in the main pulmonary artery, approximately 90% of blood crosses the patent ductus arteriosus, with only 10% entering the pulmonary circulation because of the high pulmonary vascular resistance.

Blood that crosses the patent ductus arteriosus enters the descending thoracic aorta, where it mixes with blood ejected from the left ventricle, which has a higher oxygen content. The fetal arrangement places the ventricles in parallel rather than in series, as they will be in extrauterine life. Of the combined ventricular output into the aorta, approximately 60% enters the placenta, and 35% is distributed to supply other organs.

FETAL HEMOGLOBIN

The hemoglobin molecule synthesized by fetal red blood cells is structurally different from that synthesized after several months of age. All hemoglobin molecules consist of four peptide chains. Both fetal and adult hemoglobin contain two α chains, but these hemoglobins differ in that adult hemoglobin also contains two β chains, whereas *fetal hemoglobin* instead has two δ chains. The β and δ chains differ in their amino acid sequence, and this structural difference confers functional differences that are of consequence for the fetus. The β chains of adult hemoglobin bind small phosphate-containing compounds involved in energy metabolism, and such binding results in a diminished binding affinity for oxygen. The most important of these compounds is 2,3-diphosphoglycerate (2,3-DPG) because it is present in significant amounts in red blood cells. Binding of 2,3-DPG results in a rightward shift of the oxyhemoglobin dissociation curve; adult hemoglobin binds less oxygen at any given PO_2 within the physiologic range (Fig. 25-7). In contrast, the δ chains of fetal hemoglobin do not bind 2,3-DPG and, as a result, have an oxyhemoglobin dissociation curve that lies to the left of that for adult hemoglobin.

Thus, at any given PO_2 fetal hemoglobin has a greater affinity for oxygen and a higher percentage saturation than adult hemoglobin. The increased binding of oxygen by fetal hemoglobin, in comparison with adult hemoglobin, is responsible for the transplacental passage of oxygen from mother to fetus. However, the high affinity of fetal hemoglobin for oxygen may be a disadvantage in the setting of neonatal anemia, during which the total oxygen content of blood is reduced because of a reduced amount of hemoglobin, and the high affinity of fetal hemoglobin for oxygen results in less release of oxygen to tissues.

ADAPTATION TO EXTRAUTERINE LIFE

The first few minutes after delivery of an infant are a critical time when marked pulmonary and cardiovascular changes in function must occur smoothly if the newborn is to survive.[6,7] At the moment of delivery, the infant has no functional residual capacity (FRC) and, hence, is unable to perform gas exchange. As a result of stimulation from touch and the abrupt change in temperature, newborns in good condition initiate a series of deep inspiratory efforts. These initial inspirations or cries are very forceful and can generate pressures in excess of 60 cmH_2O. Their purpose is to rapidly establish the newborn's FRC, which forms the basis for effective gas exchange. At the end of several minutes of crying, a normal infant has a well-established FRC.

This initial inflation of the lungs leads to the secretion of large amounts of surfactant from type II cells into the airways, which in turn assists in stabilizing the neonate's FRC and leads to normal lung mechanics. Premature infants who have severe surfactant deficiency, the basis for RDS, often have difficulty initiating effective respirations because of their inability to expand the lungs repeatedly and achieve a stable FRC.

Sustained inflation of the lungs, along with removal of the placenta from the circulation, are critical for the transition from the fetal to the neonatal pattern of circulation. As a direct consequence of lung expansion and an increase in alveolar PO_2, the pulmonary arteriolar vasoconstriction, which maintained a high pulmonary vascular resistance in fetal life, remits, and pulmonary vascular resistance falls. Removal of the placenta from the circulation causes a marked increase in systemic vascular resistance. With the expansion of the lungs, arterial PO_2 rises, and the ductus arteriosus constricts. As a result of these changes, blood in the right ventricle is pumped into the main pulmonary artery and flows into the lungs, with their newly decreased resistance to blood flow. Blood that has perfused the lungs returns to the left atrium, where a high left atrial pressure, the result of increased blood flow and increased systemic vascular resistance, results in functional closure of the foramen ovale.

With functional closure of the foramen ovale and ductus arteriosus and with a reversal of the relationship between pulmonary and systemic vascular resistances, the transition to the normal neonatal circulation is complete. It is, however, important to realize that early on in neonatal life the transition is tenuous. Hypoxia, acidosis, cold stress, hypoglycemia, and unstable pulmonary function may be associated with a partial return of the fetal pattern of circulation. In the absence of a placenta, this leads to shunting of blood from the right side of the circulation (pulmonary) to the left side of the circulation (systemic), resulting in arterial desaturation.

The molecular basis for the transition from the fetal to the neonatal circulation has only recently begun to be understood. Vascular endothelial cells are active participants in the control of blood vessel constriction and dilation. They accomplish this by the synthesis and local release of short-lived vasoactive molecules. At the time of birth, in response to ventilation, a high FiO_2 (compared to that in utero), and the sheer stress associated with increased pulmonary blood flow, the endothelial cells of the pulmonary vascular bed elaborate and release *endothelium-derived relaxing factor (EDRF)*. Endothelium-derived relaxing factor diffuses a very short distance into smooth muscle cells, where it stimulates the activity of guanylate cyclase, resulting in the production of increased intracellular levels of cyclic guanosine monophosphate (cGMP) in smooth muscle. The

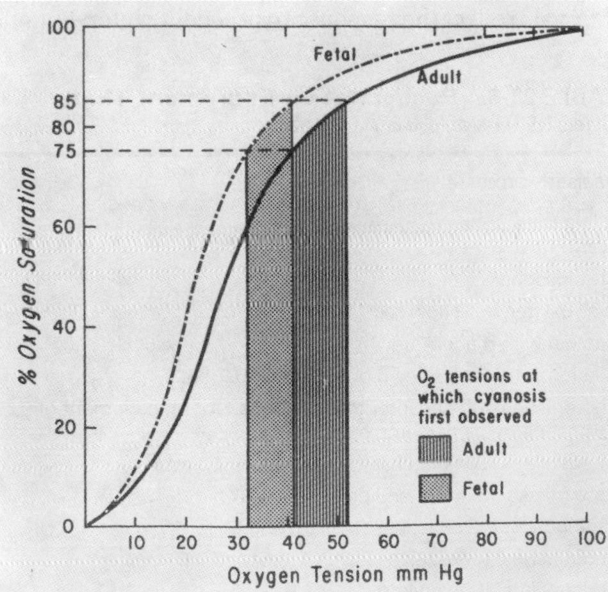

FIGURE 25-7. Fetal and adult oxyhemoglobin dissociation curves. Note that the neonate, with a high proportion of fetal hemoglobin, will have a low PaO_2 (33 to 42 mmHg) before cyanosis will be observed. (Reproduced by permission from Lee MH, King DH: Cyanosis in the newborn. Pediatr Review 9:36–42, 1987)

presence of increased amounts of cGMP leads to reduced amounts of intracellular calcium, and this, in turn, leads to relaxation of smooth muscle.[7]

Endothelium-derived relaxing factor has recently been identified as *nitric oxide (NO)*, which the endothelial cells synthesize from arginine by the action of nitric oxide synthetase. Ongoing synthesis of NO is responsible for the sustained dilation of the pulmonary circulation that begins at birth. The vasodilatory action of NO is confined to cells very close to the site of its synthesis and release because hemoglobin has a very high affinity for NO; NO that reaches the blood stream rapidly combines with hemoglobin, leading to the formation of methemoglobin and to inactivation of NO.[7]

NEONATAL RESUSCITATION AND STABILIZATION

Anticipation and Planning

As previously stated, the first moments of life are critical because of the need for rapid establishment of a new system for gas exchange and a new pattern of circulation. Approximately 80% of full-term neonates have a smooth transition and require no help beyond avoidance of cold stress, suctioning of the airway, and gentle tactile stimulation. Approximately 6% of all newborns require more extensive resuscitative care in the delivery room. However, among those infants whose birth weight is less than 1500 g, nearly 80% require resuscitation. Some infants require supplemental oxygen; others require positive-pressure ventilation with bag and mask for a time; and a small number require a combination of endotracheal intubation, chest compressions, and therapy with drugs.[8]

An important aspect of stabilization of those neonates who require more than minimal help at delivery is anticipation. Although it is not possible to foresee all situations in which resuscitation is required, there are warning signs that should alert the responsible personnel to the increased risk of need for resuscitation at birth (Table 25-5).

TABLE 25-5. **Conditions With Increased Risk of Need for Neonatal Resuscitation**

Prematurity (less than 37 weeks of gestation)
Intrauterine growth retardation
Fetal heart rate pattern indicating fetal distress
Acidosis in fetal scalp pH assessment
Birth by emergency cesarean section
Umbilical cord prolapse
Abnormal presentation with difficult extraction
Meconium staining of the amniotic fluid
Multiple gestation
Maternal drug therapy General anesthesia Magnesium sulfate Narcotics
Placental abruption
Maternal cardiorespiratory compromise

Used with permission from American Heart Association, American Academy of Pediatrics: Neonatal Resuscitation. In L Chameides (ed): Textbook of Pediatric Advanced Life Support. American Heart Association, 1988

The preparation for resuscitation of a newborn involves having both the appropriate people (in some centers termed *designated neonatal resuscitators*) and the proper equipment in place in advance of the actual delivery. At least two people are required, and a third is highly desirable. Tables 25-6 and 25-7 list the equipment required. Two types of resuscitation bags are available: self-inflating bags and anesthesia bags. Self-inflating bags are easier to use and, hence, require less training and experience, whereas anesthesia bags provide more control over pressure delivery. Self-inflating bags are preferred, unless the operators are experienced in the use of anesthesia bags.

In addition to having the appropriate number of people and equipment available for deliveries when the need for resuscitation is anticipated, each person on the team should have a clear understanding of his or her role and tasks before the infant is delivered. In general, it is wise to have one person assigned to manage the airway; a second person for the task of assessing the heart rate, respiratory effort, and breath sounds; and a third person available to perform other tasks.

One way of assessing newborns that is currently in widespread use is the *Apgar scoring system.* In this method, an infant is assessed by hands-on examination and scored on the basis of specific findings at age 1 minute and again at age 5 minutes. For distressed infants, scoring is repeated at 10 minutes of age and again every 5 minutes until stabilization. On the basis of the score given at 1 minute of age, the type of intervention required is determined. Subsequent scores at 5-minute intervals reflect the response to preceding interventions

TABLE 25-6. **Resuscitation Equipment That Should Always Be Available**

Radiant warmer
Bulb syringe
Warm towels
Stethoscope
Wall oxygen with flow meter
Suction with manometer
Suction catheters, sizes 5 or 6, 8, and 10 French
Endotracheal tube adaptor to wall suction for management of meconium stained amniotic fluid
Neonatal resuscitation bag (volume 250–500 mL)
Face masks (full-term and preterm sizes)
Laryngoscope with blades, Miller 0 and Miller 1
Endotracheal tubes, sizes 2.5, 3.0, 3.5, and 4.0
Endotracheal tube stylets

Used with permission from American Heart Association, American Academy of Pediatrics: Neonatal Resuscitation. In L Chameides (ed): Textbook of Pediatric Advanced Life Support. American Heart Association, 1988

TABLE 25-7. **Equipment That Should Be Readily Available For Neonatal Resuscitation**

ECG with oscilloscope
Umbilical catheters, 3.5 and 5.0
Three-way stopcocks
Sterile umbilical artery catheterization tray
Needles, syringes
Drugs in these forms:
- Epinephrine, 1:10,000 dilution
- Albumin, 5%
- Sodium bicarbonate, 0.5 mEq/mL
- Neonatal naloxone (Narcan), 0.02 mg/mL

10% dextrose in water IV solution
IV therapy equipment

Used with permission from American Heart Association, American Academy of Pediatrics: Neonatal Resuscitation. In L Chameides (ed): Textbook of Pediatric Advanced Life Support. American Heart Association, 1988

and again determine what further interventions are necessary. Box 25-2 summarizes the Apgar scoring system.

When the infant is delivered, he or she should be placed under the radiant warmer and dried off with warm towels. The head should be placed in the slightly extended "sniffing" position while the mouth and hypopharynx are gently suctioned with a bulb syringe by the person assigned the responsibility of airway management. During this same time, the person responsible for heart rate and breath sounds should be assessing these findings. As this is being done, other characteristics of the infant that should also be noted are muscle tone and whether the child is crying and turning pink or making less than desirable respiratory effort and remaining cyanotic. Very rapid and accurate assessment of the condition of a newborn at delivery is possible by determining the heart rate, respiratory effort, and rapidity of color change.

Infants whose score is 7 or higher at 1 minute require only protection from hypothermia by warming and drying and continued maintenance of an airway free of secretions. Continuous observation is also required. *Newborns whose Apgar score at 1 minute is between 4 and 6* are those babies who at delivery have a heart rate of approximately 100 beats per minute or faster and have some muscle tone; however, they may have inadequate respiratory effort or apnea. In general, they require blow-by oxygen, continued tactile stimulation and warming with repositioning of the head, and bulb suctioning to ensure airway patency. Those infants with scores in this range who exhibit no or ineffective respirations require a brief period of positive-pressure ventilation with the resuscitation bag and face mask. Infants in this group generally do not require extended positive-pressure ventilation.

Newborns whose Apgar scores are 3 or less as 1 minute approaches are in definite need of intervention. Although continued warming is important, continued tactile stimulation of babies exhibiting this degree of depression is unlikely to be productive and generally wastes time. These infants should have their airway repositioned, and positive-pressure ventilation with bag and mask should commence without delay. For ventilation to be effective, the infant's chest must be seen to rise and fall, and breath sounds must be audible. Often, surprisingly high amounts of pressure (40 cmH_2O) are required for the first few breaths for this to occur. This relates to the need to expand atelactatic alveoli, remove lung liquid, and establish an FRC. Infants in this group sometimes require extended periods of positive-pressure ventilation. Effectively performed bag-and-mask ventilation with 100% oxygen results in a rapid increase in heart rate to values faster than 100 beats per minute (bpm) in less than 1 minute in almost all children. Failure to obtain this response rapidly or the need for extended positive-pressure ventilation is an indication for endotracheal intubation.

Once effective ventilation is established, either by bag and mask or bag and endotracheal tube, 15 to 30 seconds should be allowed to ascertain the response of the heart rate to ventilation. Ventilation is the foundation of good neonatal resuscitation, and as stated, almost all babies respond to ventilation with a prompt increase in heart rate and change in color to pink. The most frequent cause of failure to respond to ventilation is failure of the resuscitator to ventilate the infant appropriately. Reasons for inadequate ventilation include inadequate seal between infant and mask, improper positioning of the head, obstructed airway, equipment failure, use of inadequate pressure to expand the lungs, and malpositioning of the endotracheal tube. If at the

BOX 25-2

APGAR SCORING

Sign	0	1	2
Heart rate	None	Below 100	Above 100
Respirations	Absent	Slow, gasps	Good, crying
Muscle tone	Limp	Some flexion	Active motion
Irritability	None	Grimace	Cough, sneeze
Color	Blue	Pink body, dusky extremities	Completely pink

Used with permission from American Heart Association, American Academy of Pediatrics: Neonatal Resuscitation. In L Chameides (ed): Textbook of Pediatric Advanced Life Support. American Heart Association, 1988

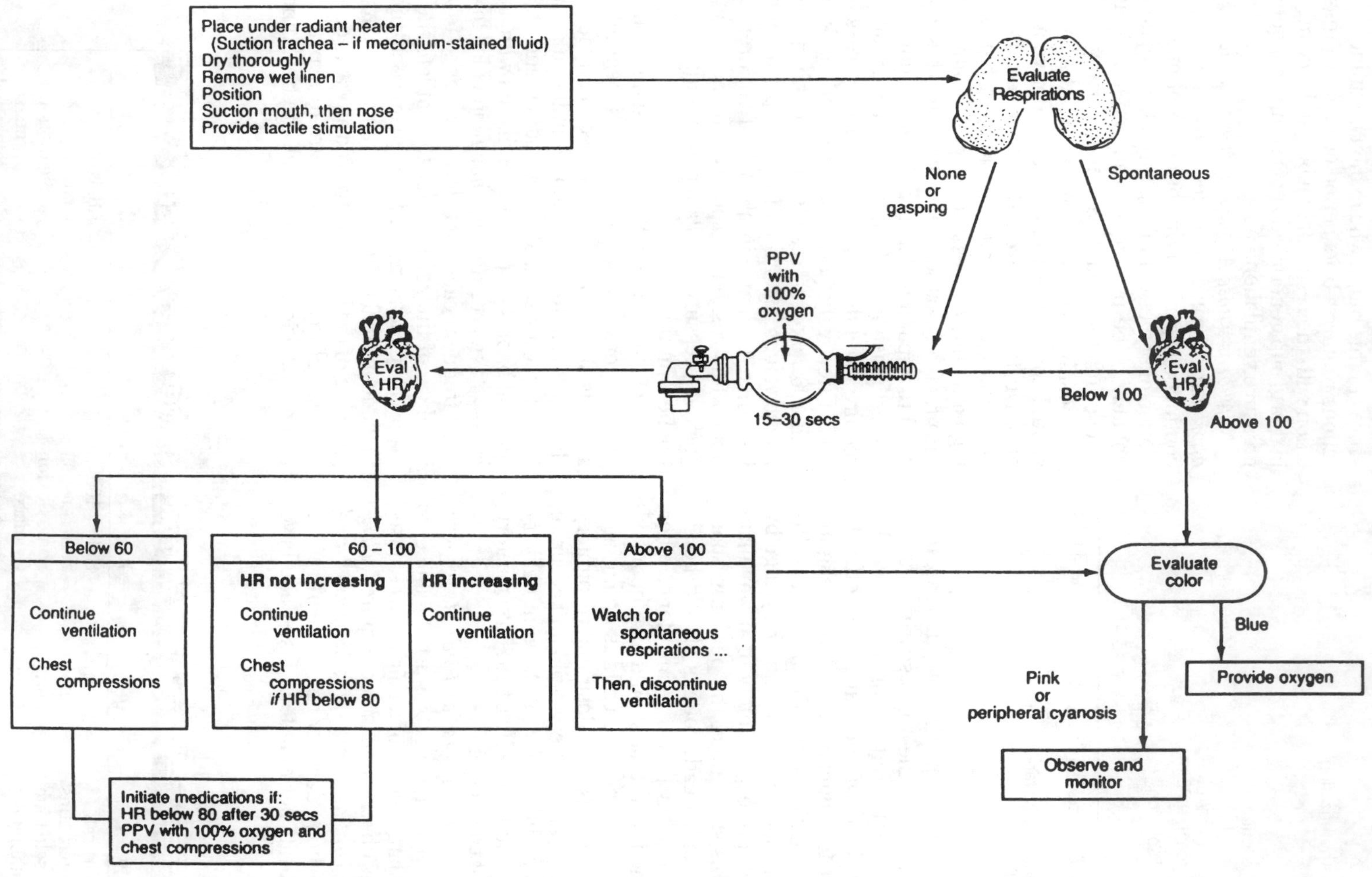

FIGURE 25-8. Overview of resuscitation of the newborn in the delivery room. Note that babies are assessed based on spontaneous respirations, a heart rate above or below 100 bpm and color. Ventilation forms the cornerstone of successful resuscitation. (Reproduced with permission from the American Heart Association.)

end of 15–30 sec of effective ventilation the heart rate is below 60 bpm or is 60–80 bpm but not increasing rapidly, external cardiac compressions are indicated. This infrequent circumstance is also the one in which placement of an umbilical venous catheter, vascular volume expansion, and cardiotonic drugs may be indicated if the infant does not respond to the combination of chest compressions with continued, effective positive-pressure ventilation after 30 sec (Fig. 25-8).

A course of instruction and standards for neonatal resuscitation have been developed and adopted under the combined auspices of the AHA and the American Academy of Pediatrics. It is highly recommended that individuals with responsibilities for newborns participate in this course and become certified.

Delivery of an infant with *meconium staining of the amniotic fluid* requires modification of the foregoing principles. Infants with meconium-stained amniotic fluid are at risk for aspiration of this highly irritating material and for the subsequent development of the meconium aspiration syndrome. This is a severe disease with a significant mortality rate; the prevention of this disease deserves high priority. Before the delivery of an infant with meconium-stained amniotic fluid, the oropharynx and hypopharynx should be thoroughly suctioned while the infant's head is still on the mother's perineum. Following delivery of the baby, no attempt should be made to stimulate the infant to initiate respiration. Instead, the baby should be rapidly given to the resuscitation team. Many infants cry spontaneously at delivery, and this imposes an unavoidable risk of meconium aspiration that can be minimized by predelivery suctioning as described. However, under no circumstances should positive-pressure ventilation be administered until the trachea has been suctioned.

The person responsible for airway management should clear the newborn's hypopharynx of secretions and meconium; perform direct laryngoscopy and endotracheal intubation; and suction the trachea with wall suction at approximately 80 mmHg while slowly withdrawing the endotracheal tube. This procedure should be repeated until the tracheal secretions seen in the tube are free of meconium, and it may require two or three intubations, although most commonly one is sufficient. At the time of laryngoscopy, endotracheal intubation should be performed even if no meconium is seen "on the cords," because it is still possible that there are substantial quantities of meconium in the trachea below the level of the vocal cords. When the pharynx and trachea are free of meconium, the management of the infant should proceed as described previously, and Apgar scores should be assigned.

CLINICAL ASSESSMENT OF RESPIRATORY STATUS

In the immediate hours that follow delivery, there are ongoing adaptations to extrauterine life.[5,6,8] Fluid continues to be removed from alveoli; recruitment of new lung units is ongoing; central control of respiratory effort stabilizes; and the infant, for the first time, participates in her own thermoregulation. The usual signs of respiratory difficulty in newborns are an elevated respiratory rate (the normal range being 40 to 60 breaths per minute), intercostal or sternal retractions, grunting, nasal flaring, and central cyanosis or a requirement for supplemental oxygen to avoid cyanosis.

Although these are signs of respiratory difficulty, it is not unusual for normal infants to have these findings in a mild form for the first 4 to 6 hours of life as part of transition to extrauterine life. Arterial blood gas values obtained during this period may show mild hypercarbia and the need for small amounts of supplemental oxygen in babies who, at 6 or 8 hours of age, are completely well and no longer have an oxygen requirement. It is often difficult to distinguish the infant who will be well after a several-hour transition period from the infant who is in the initial stages of RDS, transient tachypnea of the newborn, pneumonia, or meconium aspiration syndrome. The exact point at which diagnostic and therapeutic interventions are indicated in infants such as these is a matter of judgment that is based on the constellation of various risk factors present in the maternal history, the exact findings on physical examinations, and the clinical sense of whether the child is improving or worsening during a period of observation.

MANAGEMENT OF NEONATAL RESPIRATORY PROBLEMS

Respiratory Distress Syndrome

□ GENERAL CONSIDERATIONS

Respiratory distress syndrome (RDS),[9] or hyaline membrane disease (HMD), remains a major cause of illness and death for newborns. It is involved in 30% of all neonatal deaths and 70% of deaths among preterm newborns. The greatest risk factor for RDS is preterm birth, and the more premature the baby, the greater the risk. Other factors that increase the risk at any gestational age are maternal diabetes, maternal bleeding, perinatal asphyxia, and birth by cesarean section. The size and maturity of infants with RDS have been decreasing progressively for the past several years, a finding that is consistent with an increasing birth weight–specific survival rate during the same period.

□ PREVENTION OF RDS BY ANTENATAL CORTICOSTEROID ADMINISTRATION

The most effective way to prevent RDS would be to prevent premature delivery. Despite extensive efforts in this direction, 7% to 10% of all births in the United States occur before full term. A large amount of experimental data indicate that endogenous corticosteroids are involved in the final steps of fetal maturation in a variety of organs. The lung is the best studied of these organs. In animals and in humans, there is a late-gestation surge in the production and secretion of hydrocortisone, which is followed by the appearance of surfactant in the amniotic fluid and pulmonary maturity. In various animal models, giving corticosteroids to mothers before premature delivery of fetuses results in acceleration of surfactant synthesis, the presence of greater amounts of surfactant in the lung, and greatly improved survival with marked improvement in lung function.

Studies in humans conducted during the 1970s demonstrated that both betamethasone (two 12-mg doses given 24 hours apart) and dexamethasone (four 6-mg doses every 12 hours) given to mothers at high risk of delivering early resulted in a significant decrease in the occurrence and severity of RDS and a decrease in mortality caused by RDS. For patients to achieve maximal benefit, a complete course had to be given and 24 hours had to pass before delivery occurred. The benefit of the steroids was apparent for 1 week following administration. Partial benefit was demonstrated when the treatment course was interrupted by delivery. No significant side effects were observed. Debate has been ongoing about whether this therapy should be used in the setting of premature, prolonged rupture of fetal membranes (P, PROM) and at very young gestational ages. For reasons that remain in large part unclear, the great risk reduction for death and RDS demonstrated in human studies has not been widely translated into clinical obstetrical practice.[10]

Recently, the National Institutes of Health convened a consensus conference[10] motivated in large part to address the issue of underutilization of antenatal corticosteroids. This conference concluded the following:

1. Compelling data exist to demonstrate a 50% reduction in mortality when antenatal corticosteroids are used.
2. In 12-year follow-up studies of the babies, no adverse effects of this therapy have been found.
3. No long-term maternal adverse effects have been demonstrated.
4. All fetuses between 24- and 34-weeks' gestational age with threatened premature delivery are candidates for treatment.
5. There is no convincing evidence that gender or race affects the response to corticosteroid treatment.
6. There is controversy regarding the use of corticosteroids in P, PROM, but their use is appropriate when gestational age is less than or equal to 30 to 32 weeks of gestation in the absence of overt chorioamnionitis.
7. The decision to use antenatal corticosteroids should not be altered by the availability of surfactant replacement therapy.
8. There is significant evidence that antenatal corticosteroids can also reduce the likelihood of intracranial hemorrhage in premature infants.

□ PATHOPHYSIOLOGY

In recent years, the understanding of the functional abnormalities of RDS has expanded and may be conveniently described as consisting of four basic elements: (1) a quantitative deficiency of pulmonary surfactant, (2) immaturity of the lung structure, (3) pulmonary capillary leak, and (4) patency of the ductus arteriosus. These elements in varying combinations lead to progressive alveolar atelectasis, pulmonary edema, right-to-left shunting of blood through atelectatic alveoli, poor lung compliance, and a markedly increased work of breathing. The result is hypoxemia, hypercarbia, and metabolic acidosis. The abnormalities of lung mechanics and gas exchange bring about the clinical picture that is associated with RDS.[9]

Pulmonary surfactant has been recognized for several decades as a complex of phospholipids (90%) and proteins (10%) that is synthesized, stored, and secreted by alveolar type II cells. It is widely believed that the essential action of surfactant is to lower surface tension at an air–liquid interface, such as occurs within aveoli. Such lowering of surface tension is believed to result in stable lung volumes at end-expiration and to be required for normal lung compliance. As noted previously, there is a window of time during gestation within which the pulmonary surfactant system matures; this window is between 25 and 35 weeks.

In addition to a deficiency of surfactant, premature babies have lungs whose structure corresponds to their gestational age. Accordingly, a 25-week-old infant has lungs in the canalicular stage, with a paucity of alveoli. In the absence of surfactant and with the presence of an immature lung structure, there is a leak of serum proteins into the alveolar space from the vascular space. Several of these serum proteins have the unique ability to inhibit the function of surfactant in lowering surface tension and, thus, have the potential to further aggravate the alveolar deficiency of surfactant. One protein in particular with a molecular weight of 110 kDa is very potent at inhibiting surfactant. This protein is known as the *surfactant inhibitor.*

Although in full-term, healthy infants, functional closure of the ductus arteriosus occurs within several hours of birth, this is not necessarily true for premature infants with RDS. In these newborns, a patent ductus arteriosus (PDA) is common. The smaller and less mature the baby, the more common is a PDA. In the presence of a PDA, there is shunting of blood from the aorta to the main pulmonary artery and subsequent overcirculation through the pulmonary vascular bed. This leads to pulmonary edema. Pulmonary edema in turn worsens lung compliance and thereby exacerbates the consequences of surfactant deficiency.

□ FETAL LUNG MATURITY TESTING

In pregnancies complicated by maternal or fetal illness, and when labor begins before 37 weeks of gestation, it may be desirable to know whether or not the fetal lungs contain an adequate quantity of surfactant to prevent RDS.[4,9] Several laboratory studies currently in use are able to accurately predict fetal lung maturity by quantifying the amount of surfactant present in the amniotic fluid.

One such test is the *lecithin to sphingomyelin (L:S) ratio*, which has been in use for several years. Lecithin is phosphatidylcholine, and its concentration in amniotic fluid increases with increasing duration of gestation, as the components of lung surfactant move from within the type II cell to the alveoli to amniotic fluid as part of the outward flux of fetal pulmonary fluid. Sphingomyelin is a phospholipid derived primarily from nonsurfactant sources, and its concentration in amniotic fluid is relatively constant as gestation progresses. The L:S ratio that predicts fetal lung maturity varies somewhat among laboratories, depending on the exact methodology used, but it is usually close to a value of 2:1. In pregnancies that are not complicated by diabetes, an L:S ratio indicating maturity correctly predicts the absence of RDS in 98% of fetuses. The L:S ratio is a less reliable indicator in pregnancies complicated by diabetes, and it cannot be measured in amniotic fluid samples contaminated by meconium or blood. Another shortcoming of the L:S ratio test is its technical difficulty, which creates the need for great attention to detail and leads to a 3- to 4-hour time required to perform the test. A further limitation of the test is its inability to accurately predict lung immaturity. Approximately 50% of fetuses with an L:S ratio indicating immature lungs, if delivered, do not develop RDS. An L:S ratio indicating immature lungs at term, a time in gestation when RDS is very rare, is not uncommon.

Phosphatidylglycerol (PG) is a surfactant phospholipid, the appearance of which in amniotic fluid is coincident with lung maturity. The presence of detectable PG in the amniotic fluid correctly predicts lung maturity virtually 100% of the time. However, the absence of PG does not predict lung immaturity with any degree of accuracy. Approximately 50% of full-term pregnancies with L:S ratios indicating mature lungs still do not have detectable quantities of PG present in the amniotic fluid. Determination of PG is most helpful in diabetic pregnancies, for which the L:S ratio may falsely indicate mature lungs, and on occasions when the amniotic fluid is contaminated with blood or meconium. This test is now commercially available as a slide agglutination test (AmnioStat-FLM).

Several other tests for fetal lung maturity exist and are used by specific medical center laboratories with experience in using their own results to predict fetal lung maturity in their population. Examples include saturated phosphatidylcholine concentration, fluorescence polarimetry, and the delta optical density 650 test. Each of these methods has specific advantages and disadvantages. None has found acceptance beyond that of the L:S ratio and the presence or absence of PG.

□ CLINICAL FEATURES

The delivery of an infant at risk for RDS can be anticipated on the basis of gestational age and the presence or absence of risk factors in the pregnancy history.[9] At the time of delivery, larger, more mature infants who later develop RDS may initially be vigorous and have good Apgar scores. It may be only later in the newborn nursery that the typical symptoms of tachypnea, grunting, flaring, retracting, and cyanosis in room air, or a requirement for supplemental oxygen to avoid cyanosis, become manifest. The chest radiograph in RDS shows hypoinflation and a unique pattern of reticulogranularity and air bronchograms that are diagnostic of RDS (Fig. 25-9).

Infants such as these are usually symptomatic by several hours of age at the latest. In contrast, smaller, less mature infants (under 30 weeks of gestation or under

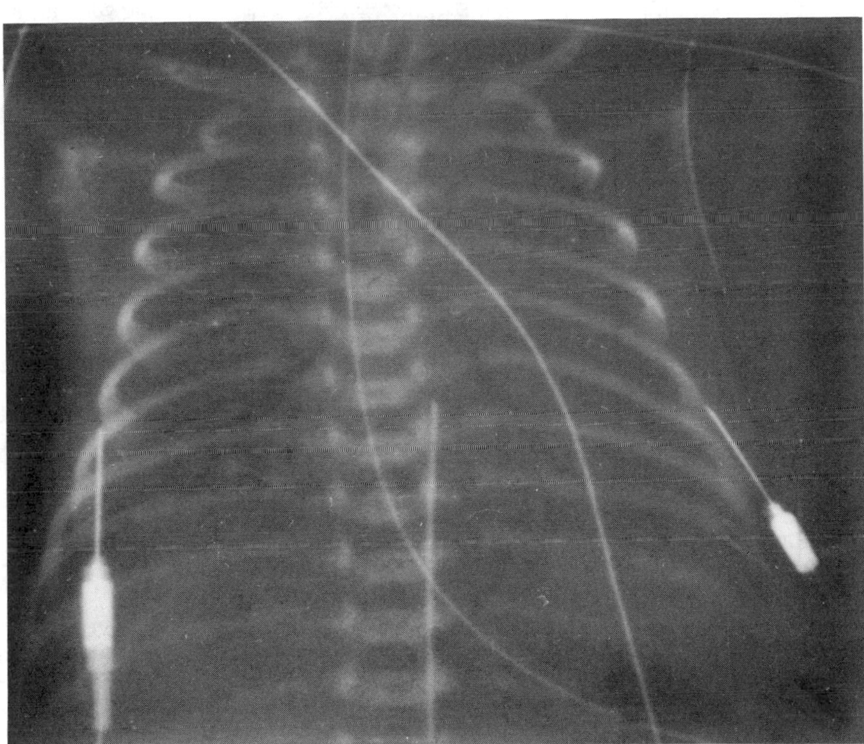

FIGURE 25-9. Chest radiograph of an infant with respiratory distress syndrome. Note the reticulogranularity and gray background with superimposed air bronchograms.

1500 g) destined to develop RDS may not be strong enough to initiate respirations and establish an FRC at the time of delivery. They may be apneic or have only ineffective gasping. Such infants require resuscitation and positive-pressure ventilation in the delivery room if they are to survive.

Newborns with RDS typically exhibit an increasing degree of illness for some 3 to 5 days after birth. The smaller and more immature the infant, the greater the duration of illness. Many infants with RDS exhibit respiratory failure, despite supplemental oxygen, and require mechanical ventilation. The smaller the infant, the greater the duration of mechanical ventilation that can be anticipated. Ultimate survival from RDS is birth weight– and gestational age–specific, with the larger, more mature infants having distinctly better survival. Most neonatal units report a greater than 90% survival in infants with birth weight heavier than 1250 g, in contrast to the less than 10% survival seen when birth weight is between 500 and 600 g. An unintended consequence of successful mechanical ventilation of smaller infants with lung disease has been a chronic pulmonary illness, referred to as *bronchopulmonary dysplasia (BPD)* or *chronic lung disease of infancy.*

Although successful mechanical ventilation of the newborn has been the single largest contributor to the increased survival of preterm infants, there are other aspects of their care that deserve mention. Obstetric management in relation to the avoidance of perinatal asphyxia and the readiness to provide respiratory support in the delivery room have produced babies in better condition to undergo the mechanical ventilation that supports them during RDS. Cautious administration of glucose, fluids, and electrolytes, with frequent monitoring of body weights, has been helpful, in that overhydration exacerbates a PDA and increases the risk of bronchopulmonary dysplasia, whereas underhydration leads to metabolic acidosis. Availability of total parenteral nutrition has improved the survival and the developmental outcome of the smallest infants whose duration of lung disease precludes adequate caloric intake by the gastrointestinal tract.

□ SURFACTANT REPLACEMENT THERAPY

In the past 5 years, correction of the surfactant deficiency state, which is the central feature of RDS, by exogenous surfactant has become possible and widespread.[11–18] This therapy has dramatically shortened the course of RDS and improved the prognosis for premature babies. In fact, this therapy has proven so effective at reducing mortality that U.S. vital statistics record a drop in infant mortality associated with and caused by the availability of surfactant replacement therapy. Here we will consider the preparations available for surfactant replacement therapy, strategies for use, a summary of clinical trials done to date, and the newer uses of surfactant preparations that may come in the next few years. (See AARC Clinical Practice Guideline: Surfactant Replacement Therapy for indications, contraindications, assessments of need and outcome, and monitoring.)

AARC Clinical Practice Guideline

SURFACTANT REPLACEMENT THERAPY

Indications: Prophylactic administration of natural or artificial surfactant may be indicated in infants at high risk of developing RDS because of short gestation (<32 weeks) or low birth weight (<1300 g), which strongly suggests lung immaturity; infants in whom there is laboratory evidence of surfactant deficiency such as lecithin–sphingomyelin ratio less than 2:1, bubble stability test indicating lung immaturity, or the absence of phosphatidylglycerol; rescue or therapeutic administration is indicated in preterm or full-term infants who require endotracheal intubation and mechanical ventilation because of increased work of breathing as indicated by an increase in respiratory rate, substernal and suprasternal retractions, grunting, and nasal flaring; increasing oxygen requirements as indicated by pale or cyanotic skin color, agitation, and decreases in PaO_2, SaO_2, or SpO_2 mandating an increase in FIO_2 above 0.40 and by clinical evidence of RDS, including chest radiograph characteristic of RDS, mean airway pressure greater than 7 cmH_2O to maintain an adequate PaO_2, SaO_2, or SpO_2.

Contraindications: Relative contraindications to surfactant administration are the presence of congenital anomalies incompatible with life beyond the neonatal period, respiratory distress in infants with laboratory evidence of lung maturity.

Assessment of Need: Determine that valid indications are present. Assess lung immaturity prior to prophylactic administration of surfactant by gestational age and birth weight or by laboratory evaluation of tracheal or gastric aspirate. Establish the diagnosis of RDS by chest radiographic criteria and the requirement for mechanical ventilation in the presence of short gestation or low birth weight.

Assessment of Outcome: Reduction in FIO_2 requirement, reduction in work of breathing, improvement in lung volumes and lung fields as indicated by chest radiograph, improvement in pulmonary mechanics (eg, compliance, airways resistance, V_T, $\dot{V}_E$, transpulmonary pressure) and lung volume (ie, FRC), reduction in ventilator requirements (PIP, PEEP, $\bar{P}aw$), improvement in ratio of arterial to alveolar PO_2 or $[P(A - a)O_2]$.

Monitoring: *Variables to be monitored during surfactant administration:* proper placement and position of delivery device, FIO_2 and ventilator settings, reflux of surfactant into endotracheal tube, position of patient (ie, head direction), chest-wall movement, oxygen saturation by pulse oximetry, heart rate, respirations, chest expansion, skin color, and vigor. *Variables to be monitored after surfactant administration:* invasive and noninvasive measurements of arterial blood gases, chest radiograph, ventilator settings (PIP, PEEP, $\bar{P}aw$) and FIO_2, pulmonary mechanics and volumes, heart rate, respirations, chest expansion, skin color and vigor, breath sounds, blood pressure.

From AARC Clinical Practice Guideline; see Respir Care 39:824,

Preparations Available for Use

Two general types of surfactants are available for replacement therapy. The *modified natural surfactants* are produced by adaptation of bovine or porcine surfactant. Surfactant is first obtained from lungs either by saline lavage of intact lungs or by rinsing minced lung tissue with saline. The natural surfactant is then isolated from the saline suspension by centrifugation, extra phospholipids are added, and the protein content is reduced.

The final phospholipid composition of these surfactants is similar to that of natural mammalian surfactants: 60% disaturated phosphatidylcholine, 24% unsaturated phosphatidylcholine, and 15% phosphatidylglycerol and other phospholipids. These preparations differ from natural surfactant in the amount and composition of the surfactant-associated proteins. The surfactant proteins described to date, A, B, C, and D, are glycoproteins of differing molecular weights and solubilities and are involved in the regulation of surfactant secretion and reuptake by type II cells, enhancement of intraalveolar spreading and adsorption, maintenance of surface tension lowering capabilities, and defense of the lung against pathogens.

The surfactant-associated proteins constitute approximately 6% by weight of unmodified natural surfactant. However, the process by which surfactant is prepared for clinical use eliminates essentially all SP-A, and the final product contains about 2% SP-B and SP-C by weight. Beractant (Survanta) is of bovine origin and is FDA approved for use in the United States. A similar product (Infasurf), also of bovine origin, is not yet FDA approved, and a surfactant that is of porcine origin (Curosurf) is widely used in Europe.

The other type of surfactant that is currently available is referred to as *synthetic surfactant.* Exosurf is the only artificial surfactant that is available at present in the United States. This surfactant is a mixture of dipalmitoylphosphatidylcholine, hexadecanol and tyloxapol. The latter two compounds are used to enhance the spreading and absorption of the surfactant at the air–liquid interface within the alveoli. A similar preparation, artificial lung-expanding compound (ALEC), has undergone extensive testing in Europe.

Strategies for the Use of Surfactant

There are two fundamental approaches to the use of surfactant replacement therapy. *Rescue therapy* is the use of surfactant to treat established RDS. *Prophylactic or at birth therapy* refers to the administration of surfactant shortly after (ie, within minutes) the birth of an infant known to be at high risk for RDS, without any effort to ascertain whether the child actually develops RDS. Prophylactic therapy is usually given in the delivery room. Studies using animal models of RDS indicate that, while rescue therapy is highly effective, the administration of surfactant at birth is associated with a more even distribution of surfactant throughout the lungs, a greater magnitude and duration of effect, and less histologic evidence of lung damage when compared to rescue therapy.

Summary of Clinical Trials

Several types of clinical trials of surfactant replacement therapy have been done.[11,13,16–18] The first generation of studies were single-dose studies, wherein infants with established RDS were given one dose of surfactant, and the physiologic endpoints of oxygenation, ventilation, and ventilatory requirements were monitored. Safety of the preparations, the route of delivery (which involves the endotracheal administration of large fluid volumes), and formation of air leaks were also studied.

As a group, these studies showed that there was a dramatic, beneficial physiologic response to surfactant and a reduction in air leak events, and the administration procedure and drug were not associated with any untoward effects. Many of these studies were not large enough to determine differences in the important endpoints of mortality and the incidence of chronic lung disease.

The second generation of surfactant replacement therapy trials involved multiple doses of surfactant and were designed to determine whether surfactant replacement therapy would alter overall mortality, mortality caused by RDS, or the occurrence of chronic lung disease, and to further study the issues of safety and air leak events. Babies of lower birth weights and gestational ages have long been known to have the highest rates of mortality and chronic lung disease, so this population was chosen for these studies. Some studies employed rescue therapy, whereas others attempted to prevent RDS with prophylactic therapy; all studies employed placebo (air) controls and were double blind in design.

Table 25-8 summarizes the results of four representative trials,[11,13,16,17] two of beractant (Survanta) and two of synthetic surfactant (Exosurf). The important endpoints of overall mortality within 28 days of birth, mortality caused by RDS, and the occurrence of pneumothorax have all been shown to be significantly reduced in these and other studies. The incidence of chronic lung disease (bronchopulmonary dysplasia, BPD) was not reduced in the studies shown or in several other studies. This may be because the use of surfactant prevents death in babies who are subsequently left with residual chronic lung disease. Direct comparison of the results of these studies is not appropriate because of differing enrollment criteria and because the children were cared for according to different protocols in different neonatal ICUs. The very large magnitude of the difference in mortality caused by RDS between control and surfactant-treated infants is particularly striking. This is most true in the study that used beractant prophylactically, where there was nearly a 10-fold decrease in mortality caused by RDS, from 15.6% in controls to 1.9% in beractant recipients.[13]

Comparative Trials of Surfactant Replacement Therapy

There are two issues beyond efficacy that have been studied regarding the use of surfactant replacement therapy:[12,14,15,18] rescue therapy versus prophylaxis[12,15] and synthetic surfactant (Exosurf) versus beractant (Survanta).[14] Several small trials have compared administration of surfactant at birth with rescue therapy. All of these trials have involved modified natural surfactants, probably because the original efficacy trials did

TABLE 25-8. **Clinical Trials of Surfactant Replacement Therapy**

Study Population	Drug and Dosage	Design	Mortality Due to RDS:			Overall Mortality:			Pneumothorax:			Chronic Lung Disease:		
			C	*T*	*p*	*C*	*T*	*p*	*C*	*T*	*p*	*C*	*T*	*p*
BW* 600 to 1750 g, n = 798	Beractant, up to four doses in 48 hours	Rescue after RDS established	20.3%	9.0%	$p < 0.001$	27.3%	18.4%	$p = 0.002$	25.9%	11.5%	$p < 0.001$	62.7%	57.9%	$p = 0.318$
BW 600 to 1250 g, n = 430	Beractant, up to four doses in 48 hours	At birth treatment of at risk infants	15.6%	1.9%	$p < 0.001$	18.8%	11.4%	$p = 0.031$	20.8%	9.6%	$p = 0.002$	52.0%	55.4%	$p = 0.600$
BW 700 to 1350 g, n = 419	Synthetic surfactant, two doses 12 hours apart	Rescue after RDS established	9.9%	3.4%	$p = 0.007$	23.4%	11.2%	$p = 0.001$	29.1%	19.4%	$p = 0.022$	14.0%	11.7%	$p = 0.107$
BW 700 to 1100 g, n = 446	Synthetic surfactant, one dose at birth	Single dose prophylaxis	10.3%	4.5%	$p = 0.011$	22.0%	13.0%	$p = 0.22$	19.3%	10.7%	$p = 0.011$	17.0%	20.0%	$p = 0.671$

* BW is birth weight; C is control; T is treatment; p is probability value.

not show that synthetic surfactants could decrease the occurrence of RDS. One trial[12] involved 182 infants of less than 30-weeks gestational age and compared treatment in the delivery room with treatment after RDS was diagnosed up to 6 hours later; the mean age at treatment in the latter group was 2.9 hours. The mortality rate was not different between the two groups, and there was some increase in chronic lung disease in the group treated in the delivery room. Overall, there was no clear advantage to either treatment strategy.

Another study involving a larger group of 479 infants with gestational age less than 30 weeks had a multicenter design.[15] This study also compared delivery room treatment with rescue therapy, but the rescue occurred at a mean age of 5.6 hours. This study demonstrated a higher proportion of infants surviving to discharge home in the prophylaxis group; an even greater advantage to prophylaxis was shown in infants with gestational age at or below 26 weeks at birth. There was also a lower risk of pneumothorax in infants at or less than 26 weeks' gestational age who were randomized to prophylactic treatment.

Finally, a third study[18] involved infants with gestational ages of 29 to 32 weeks and compared surfactant given immediately following delivery with "early treatment" that was given at a mean age of 1.5 hours. This trial analyzed data from 1248 babies. Prophylaxis was associated with less severe RDS and reduced need for mechanical ventilation and supplemental oxygen over the first 4 days of life. Prophylaxis was also associated with a reduction in the occurrence of the combined outcome of death and chronic lung disease. The benefits to prophylactic treatment were more striking in babies less than 30-weeks gestational age.

Overall, there is a consensus that early treatment is better than delayed treatment, but the exact definitions of early and late vary. The data indicate that there is likely to be a population of very immature infants who have decreased mortality when surfactant is given immediately following birth. However, the safe administration of surfactant, which involves endotracheal instillation of large volumes of liquid during positioning maneuvers for the child, requires an experienced team. Experience is necessary both in management of the neonatal airway and in the actual delivery of surfactant. Such expertise may not be available at all hospitals. The Boston Perinatal Center's recommendations for the use of surfactant are summarized in Table 25-9.

TABLE 25-9. **Boston Perinatal Center Guidelines for Use of Surfactant**

Administer surfactant within 15 minutes of delivery when gestational age is less than 27 weeks.
When gestational age is 27 to 30 weeks, administer surfactant in the delivery room if endotracheal intubation is required for respiratory difficulty or apnea.
When gestational age is greater than 30 weeks, administer surfactant when presence of RDS is established.

Another question that has arisen regarding surfactant replacement therapy is whether there is an advantage to one type of surfactant over another, that is, is modified natural surfactant superior to synthetic surfactant, or vice versa? One multicenter randomized trial that involved 617 infants with birth weights between 501 and 1500 g compared beractant (Survanta) to synthetic (Exosurf) for the treatment of RDS. Infants given beractant had a superior initial physiologic response with a greater reduction in the need for supplemental oxygen and ventilatory pressure than the response seen in infants given synthetic. The combined endpoint of death or chronic lung disease at 28 days of age was not significantly different between treatments with the two preparations. Of some note, in the smallest weight group, there may have been a trend toward increased survival in recipients of beractant (birth weight 501 to 750 g, 51% mortality with synthetic vs 36% with beractant). However, the study was not designed to detect differences between treatment preparations by weight group, and so no firm conclusion can be drawn.[14]

Safety and Outcome Data

The surfactant preparations that have been in use for the past 5 years have shown remarkably few untoward effects. The administration procedure can lead to transient arterial desaturation and agitation, but in skilled hands this is minimal and brief. These effects essentially always can be managed by a pause in the administration procedure and continuation of mechanical ventilation, sometimes with slightly higher rates and pressures.[11 18]

Pulmonary hemorrhage has been reported to occur in infants who have received surfactant. However, the frequency of this event is very low, and its relationship to surfactant administration is not entirely clear. Some increase in the occurrence of apnea has also been associated with the receipt of surfactant.[11–18]

The available neurodevelopmental follow-up data demonstrates that recipients of surfactant fare equally well or better than comparable infants who did not receive surfactant. In other words, despite a large increase in survival of very small babies, there has not been an increase in the rate of neurodevelopmental handicap. Pulmonary function has also been studied at 2 years after birth in recipients of surfactant during the original efficacy trials. Pulmonary function in children treated with surfactant as babies did not differ in any detrimental way from that in surviving control-group infants.[19]

Newer Use of Surfactant Replacement Therapy

Currently, beractant and colfosceril are approved by the U.S. FDA only for the prevention and treatment of RDS in infants.[20 24] However, inactivation of endogenous surfactant in infants born with a mature and sufficient surfactant system may play a role in several common neonatal lung diseases. Under laboratory conditions, meconium, even in dilute amounts, is able to interfere with the surface tension lowering properties of pulmonary surfactant. Pneumonia in full-term infants can also be associated with inactivation of surfactant. There are currently two reports in the literature, each involving a small number of full-term infants with meconium aspiration syndrome or pneumonia, who had a substantial improvement in their clinical status following a dose of a modified natural surfactant. Future investigations will be needed to determine what additional lung diseases, if any, consistently respond to surfactant replacement therapy.[20–22]

A particularly interesting possibility for surfactant replacement therapy involves its use in countries where mechanical ventilation of newborns is scarce or not routinely available. In a study done at the Kuwait Maternity Hospital,[23] 14 premature infants with an average gestational age of 32 weeks with severe RDS were treated with endotracheal intubation and administration of a modified natural surfactant, ventilated by hand for several minutes to disperse the surfactant, and then extubated and placed into hood oxygen. Twelve of the fourteen infants ultimately survived; this was a much better survival rate than would have been anticipated based on historical controls in that nursery. A recently published multicenter Scandinavian study[24] tested the hypothesis that the combination of surfactant replacement therapy and nasal CPAP would reduce the need for mechanical ventilation in preterm infants with RDS. Results of this study, which involved 68 infants with moderately severe RDS, supported the author's hypothesis, with 83% of surfactant-only treated babies, but only 43% of surfactant- and CPAP-treated babies, requiring mechanical ventilation.

VENTILATION OF THE NEWBORN

Continuous Positive Airway Pressure

The application of continuous positive airway pressure (CPAP)[25] to the airways of newborns with respiratory difficulty has been thought to be beneficial in a number of circumstances. The pulmonary effects of CPAP are (1) to prevent end-expiratory collapse of alveoli in the setting of surfactant deficiency, and thereby help to increase and stabilize an infant's FRC, and (2) to cause a redistribution of alveolar fluid into the lung interstitium, which results in improved lung function without alteration in total lung water content. These effects result in an increase in PaO_2 after the application of CPAP that can be very dramatic and occurs in two stages. The early increase is related to an improvement in FRC, which leads to superior gas exchange; the later increase is related to the redistribution of pulmonary water.

Consistent with its mode of action, the use of CPAP seems to be most effective in the setting of RDS and in diseases, such as transient tachypnea of the newborn (TTNB), in which the alveoli are filled with retained fetal lung fluid. Continuous positive airway pressure has also been used to treat infants with apnea of prematurity when the basis for the apnea is hypotonia and incoordination of the muscles of the upper airway. In these infants, the increased airway pressure is believed to maintain patency of the upper airway and prevent obstruction. Infants with lung disease respond to the application of CPAP with a decrease in respiratory rate, a decrease in retractions, and an increase in PaO_2 values, usually with no change in the $PaCO_2$ value. The decrease in respiratory rate in the setting of a stable $PaCO_2$ implies an improvement in matching of ventilation to perfusion within the lung.

The use of CPAP may actually result in a decrease in dynamic lung compliance, whereas it increases static lung compliance. The effect of CPAP on airways resistance is inconsistent. The application of excessive levels of CPAP results in a worsening of arterial blood gas values. During CPAP therapy for RDS, there is a very rapid loss of FRC when CPAP is interrupted, as for suctioning or with inadvertent disconnection. In infants and experimental animals with normal lungs, application of CPAP results in prompt transmission of approximately 60% of applied pressure to the thoracic vasculature. This has the potential to decrease venous return to the heart and thereby compromise cardiac output. However, in the setting of lung disease, reduced transmission of airway pressures to thoracic vessels occurs, perhaps as little as 25% of airway pressure is transmitted, and cardiac output is usually unimpaired. As an infant's lung condition improves, transmission of pressures increases, and compromise of cardiac output may supervene during the recovery phase of an illness such as RDS.

There are several methods for application of CPAP. Nasal prongs are perhaps the most frequently used at present (Fig. 25-10). A major difficulty with this approach is frequent inadvertent dislodgment with subsequent rapid loss of FRC and clinical deterioration. Also, secretions may plug the prongs and result in failure to deliver pressure and supplemental oxygen. This is easily determined when the sounds of gas flow are no longer audible over the infant's lung fields. Gastric distension may occur with this technique, and decompression with a nasogastric tube should be accomplished during the application of nasal CPAP. Prongs may also cause local irritation and ischemia, and infants must be examined for these inadvertent effects.

An endotracheal tube may also be used to apply CPAP. Appropriately sized endotracheal tubes must be used. Advantages are the increased stability of the delivery system compared with nasal prongs, and the ability to deliver a more constant FIO_2 and CPAP level. The disadvantage of this delivery method relates to the increased resistance to airflow through the endotracheal tube, which is narrower and longer than the trachea. This increased resistance increases the newborn's work of breathing and may result in carbon dioxide retention or frank respiratory failure.

Therapy with CPAP should be considered for any newborn who exhibits clinical signs of respiratory difficulty, such as tachypnea, grunting, flaring, and retracting, and who requires substantial amounts of supplemental oxygen. It is especially easy to begin nasal CPAP in this circumstance, and 5 cmH_2O is a reasonable starting point. Opinions differ on how high CPAP should be raised if the response to lower levels is not satisfactory. Levels as low as 7 cmH_2O and as high as 15 cmH_2O have

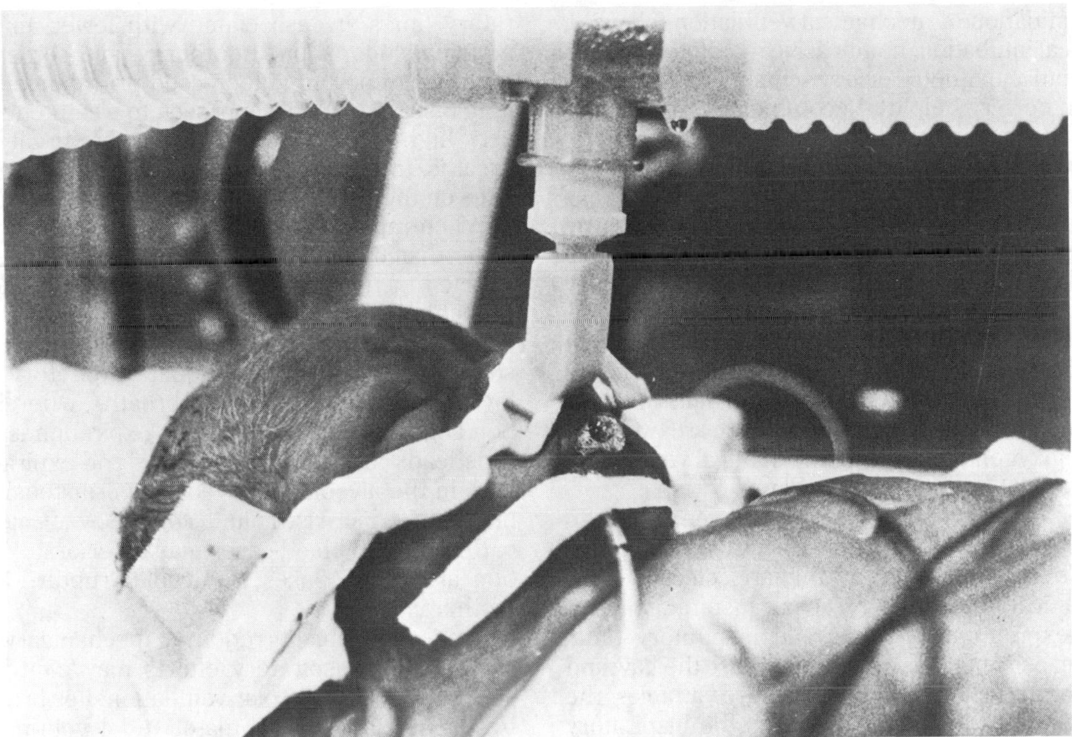

FIGURE 25-10. Use of the nasal CPAP cannula with prongs (see text). (Reproduced by permission of Sherwood Medical Industries)

been recommended by various authors. In general, if the required F_{IO_2} exceeds 0.8, the CPAP is 10 cmH_2O, and if the PaO_2 is not consistently greater than 50 mmHg, then mechanical ventilation is required.

Mechanical Ventilation

Indications for mechanical ventilation[26,27] in neonates are (1) respiratory failure, which is defined by arterial blood gas criteria; (2) apnea, which is common in neonates; (3) impending cardiovascular collapse, as in severe sepsis or shock; and (4) clinical evidence of respiratory difficulty in premature infants with birth weight less than 1500 g, such as tachypnea, inspiratory retractions, and poor air entry on auscultation of the chest. Arterial blood gas criteria for respiratory failure vary somewhat from one author to another. A PaO_2 of less than 50 mmHg with an F_{IO_2} in excess of 0.60, or a $PaCO_2$ more than 50 mmHg, is in the range constituting respiratory failure given by most authors.

Ventilators for use on newborns generally function in a time-cycled, pressure-limited manner. A high flow of fresh gas is circulated by the endotracheal tube at a rate rapid enough to preclude rebreathing of exhaled carbon dioxide; flow rates are usually 5 to 15 L/min. This permits the infant to breathe spontaneously at whatever respiratory rate is desired. Mechanical inspiration occurs by periodic partial obstruction of the expiratory limb of the gas flow, which results in an increase in pressure proximal to the endotracheal tube. This pressure is conducted down the tube and applied to the infant's lungs. When a preset pressure limit is reached, the expiratory obstruction is modified to maintain the set pressure limit for the duration of the prescribed inspiratory time.

The frequency of these ventilator breaths, the duration of expiratory limb obstruction, and the preset pressure limit are chosen by the operator of the ventilator. The frequency of periodic obstructions is the ventilator rate or intermittent mandatory ventilation (IMV) rate, the duration of obstruction of the expiratory limb is the inspiratory time, and the pressure limit chosen becomes the peak inspiratory pressure. By manipulating the degree of resistance in the expiratory circuit, the positive end-expiratory pressure (PEEP) can also be chosen by the operator of the ventilator.

Choosing the initial ventilator settings can be done well by careful observation of the child during ventilation with a resuscitation bag and in-line manometer, immediately following endotracheal intubation and stabilization of heart rate and color. Chest excursions with inflation should be approximately 0.25 to 0.50 cm in the anteroposterior plane. On auscultation of the chest, air entry should be clearly audible. If the infant has RDS, then faint end-inspiratory crackles, corresponding to opening of the terminal air sacs, should be audible. The peak inspiratory pressure that produces these findings is the one with which ventilation should be initiated. Ventilation at a rate of between 30 and 50 breaths per minute is a common starting point. The F_{IO_2} chosen should be that which produces a pink infant and generally is similar to that required before beginning mechanical ventilation.

During initiation of mechanical ventilation following endotracheal intubation, noninvasive monitoring of oxygenation (pulse oximetry or transcutaneous PO_2 monitoring) can be very helpful. Recommended inspiratory times during mechanical ventilation differ greatly among authors and depend on the type of ventilatory strategy to be employed.

The concept of mean airway pressure, Paw, is one that is of considerable importance in newborn ventilation. The Paw can be thought of as the average airway pressure over the course of a respiratory cycle, and its importance lies in the linear relationship between Paw and PaO_2 in infants with RDS (Fig. 25-11). That is, for any given FIO_2, an infant's PaO_2 rises or falls in direct proportion to the Paw applied. Thus, there are two ways to improve oxygenation during mechanical ventilation: increase the FIO_2 or increase the Paw.

However, standard infant mechanical ventilators do not allow the operator to directly select the Paw to be applied. The determinants of Paw that are selectable during mechanical ventilation are peak inspiratory pressure, end-expiratory pressure, and inspiratory time. Increases in any of these variables increase the Paw and result in improved oxygenation. Of these variables, the most powerful in determining Paw is the inspiratory time; hence, this variable is particularly important.

Longer inspiratory times (equal to or more than 0.6 sec) are associated with an ability to use lower peak inspiratory pressures and low end-expiratory pressures, because of the impact of inspiratory time on Paw (which is the principal determinant of PaO_2 at any given FIO_2). However, this ventilatory strategy is associated with a higher frequency of pneumothorax. Conversely, use of a shorter inspiratory time (between 0.3 and 0.6 sec) requires the use of a higher peak inspiratory pressure, a faster rate, and higher end-expiratory pressure to achieve comparable oxygenation. These shorter inspiratory times are associated with fewer air leak phenomena, such as pneumothorax, and some investigators have reported a decreased prevalence of chronic lung disease with this approach to treatment. Except at very high ventilator rates (eg, a rate greater than 60 breaths/min), the rate chosen has only a small influence on the Paw.

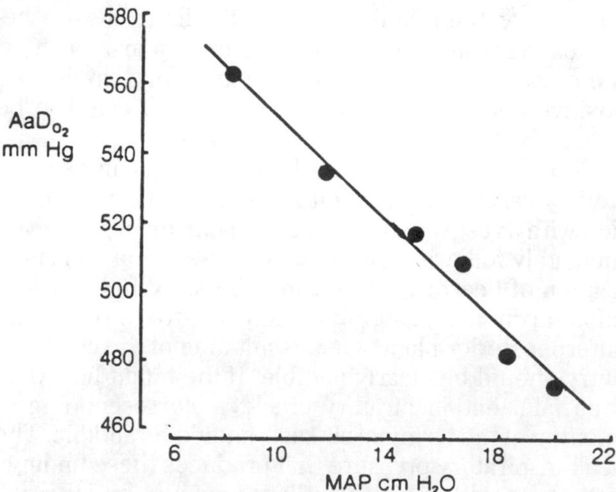

FIGURE 25-11. A linear relationship exists between the alveolar–arterial O_2 gradient and mean airway pressure (MAP) in infants with surfactant deficiency disease undergoing mechanical ventilation. (Herman S, Reynolds ER: Methods for improving oxygenation in infants mechanically ventilated for hyaline membrane disease. Arch Dis Child 48:612–617, 1973, with permission)

When rapid ventilator rates are used, as with rates faster than 60 breaths per minute, there may not be adequate time for complete exhalation. This is especially probable if the ventilator rate is increased by a large amount, without a compensatory shortening of the inspiratory time. When inadequate expiratory time is allowed, there is "stacking" of breaths, wherein inspiration begins before the previous expiration is complete. This leads to increasing positive end-expiratory pressure in the alveoli and alveolar overdistension, with a progressive increase in lung volume over time. Because of this, arterial blood gases may deteriorate. This situation also predisposes to alveolar rupture and pneumothorax.

Even among infants requiring mechanical ventilation, spontaneous respiratory efforts may contribute substantially to total alveolar ventilation. For breaths given by the mechanical ventilator, tidal volume is determined by the difference between the peak inspiratory pressure and the end-expiratory pressure. Therefore, the determinants of minute ventilation that involve the mechanical ventilator are the rate and the difference between peak inspiratory pressure and end-expiratory pressure. The influence of mechanical ventilation on arterial pH is mainly through changes in arterial carbon dioxide levels. Table 25-10 is helpful in assessing the most likely effects of various parameter changes in ventilator management.

Alterations in flow rate through the mechanical ventilator alter the inspiratory waveform delivered to the baby, which may increase the Paw. The physiologic effects of altering the waveform are complicated, and only rarely is manipulation of this variable required. Delivered flows should always be twice a baby's minute ventilation; rates of 5 to 15 L/min are usually chosen.

High-Frequency Ventilation

Although standard mechanical ventilation has been very successful at achieving adequate gas exchange and preventing mortality in newborns, there have been undesirable consequences to this therapy. Pulmonary air leak syndromes, especially pneumothorax and pulmonary interstitial emphysema, and chronic lung disease, also known as bronchopulmonary dysplasia, occur with excessive frequency. Additionally, some infants do not achieve adequate gas exchange with conventional mechanical ventilation. For these reasons, alternate forms of mechanical ventilation have been developed and tested; high-frequency ventilation (HFV) is one such approach to ventilation.[28,29]

There are several types of HFV and several types of ventilators to deliver each type of HFV. This has resulted in considerable confusion within this field. What

TABLE 25-10. **Ventilatory Management Considerations**

Variable	Physiologic and Clinical Effects
F_IO_2	P_AO_2 and PaO_2 will change in the same direction as F_IO_2 administered.
PIP	Increases and decreases in PIP produce changes that are in the same direction for both Paw and in tidal volume. PaO_2 varies directly with Paw, and $PaCO_2$ changes in the opposite direction in which tidal volume (and thus minute ventilation) is changed.
PEEP	Changes in PEEP produce changes in Paw that are in the same direction. Paw and PaO_2 change in the same direction. Application of PEEP reduces ventilation-perfusion mismatch, leading to an increase in PaO_2.
Rate	Changes in ventilator rate change minute ventilation and P_ACO_2 in the opposite direction, leading to alteration of $PaCO_2$.
T_I	Lengthening T_I (inspiratory time) increases Paw, leading to an increase in PaO_2; shortening T_I has the opposite effect.
Flow rate	Changes in flow rate alter the respiratory waveform and may change Paw. Effects of manipulating flow rate may be complicated.

all types of HFV have in common is the use of respiratory rates that are faster than conventional rates and the use of tidal volumes that are smaller than those usually found during conventional mechanical ventilation.

□ TYPES OF HIGH-FREQUENCY VENTILATION AND MECHANISMS OF GAS EXCHANGE

High-Frequency Positive Pressure Ventilation (HFPPV) is the use of conventional ventilators at unconventional rates. Many conventional infant ventilators can now cycle at rates of up to 150 breaths per minute. During this type of ventilation, tidal volume is larger than anatomic dead space, and gas exchange takes place in the usual manner, by bulk convection. It is important to understand that each brand of ventilator has a rate, specific to that brand of ventilator, above which the tidal volume delivered to the patient begins to decrease. If this is not taken into account, minute ventilation (the product of rate and tidal volume) may paradoxically fall as the ventilator rate is increased.

High-Frequency Jet Ventilation (HFJV) requires a unique endotracheal tube with two small side lumina for "jet" ventilation and monitoring of tracheal pressure. Jet ventilation occurs when a pinch valve delivers rapid pulses of gas at very high speeds into a side port that leads into the endotracheal tube lumen. High-frequency jet ventilation frequencies range from 4 to 11 hertz (Hz; one Hz is one cycle per second). The "jet" of gas through the side port leads to the entrainment of a large volume of gas through the standard endotracheal tube lumen; exhalation is passive and occurs through the regular endotracheal tube lumen. As a result of entrainment, the tidal volume delivered to the infant is probably larger than anatomic dead space, and gas exchange probably occurs in large part through bulk convection. Inspiratory times are extraordinarily short, on the order of 20 to 30 msec. The tracheal pressure is servo-controlled, and mean airway pressure can range between 8 and 50 cmH_2O. Aspects of such ventilators that are under operator control include peak pressure, inspiratory time, and frequency. Positive end-expiratory pressure is provided by a conventional ventilator attached in tandem at the endotracheal tube. High-frequency jet ventilation has had some success in the management of air leaks such as bronchopleural fistula and pneumothorax.

High-Frequency Oscillatory Ventilation (HFOV) is created when an oscillatory waveform is superimposed on a bias flow of gas. The height of the wave is referred to as the amplitude. Different ventilators create the oscillation by different mechanisms. The Infant Star HFOV uses pulses of gas from metered pneumatic valves controlled by a microprocessor, whereas the Sensor Medics 3100A uses a diaphragm attached to a piston that is made to oscillate in a magnetic field. The mean airway pressure is created by imposing a resistance on the bias flow and adjusted by changing the resistance; mean airway pressure can range from 3 to 45 cmH_2O. Frequency ranges from 3 to 15 Hz, and the percent of inspiratory time can be adjusted on the Sensor Medics but not on the Infant Star.

High-frequency oscillatory ventilation is unique for two reasons. First, the expiratory phase is active. The negative motion of the diaphragm on the Sensor Medics ventilator and a Venturi system on the Infant Star promote lung emptying. Second, the delivered tidal volume during HFOV is less than the anatomic dead space. For alveolar ventilation to occur with tidal volumes smaller than anatomic dead space, gas exchange must occur by mechanisms other than bulk convection.

Mechanisms of Gas Exchange in HFV are at least in part novel. In spontaneous ventilation and conventional mechanical ventilation, alveolar ventilation is the product of ($V_T - V_D$) and rate. Tidal volume (V_T) must be larger than anatomic dead space (V_D) for any alveolar ventilation to occur. With HFOV, V_T is smaller than V_D. Proposed mechanisms for gas exchange during HFOV in are listed in Table 25-11 and represented schematically in Figure 25-12.

Bulk convection (also called direct alveolar ventilation) probably does occur to an unknown extent during HFV. Certain gas exchanging units within the lung that are in close proximity to the large conducting airways can be ventilated with small tidal volumes. *Pendelluft* refers to circulating currents of gas that occur between different regions of the lung because of differences in filling and emptying times (inspiratory and

TABLE 25-11. **Proposed Mechanisms of Gas Exchange During HFOV**

- Bulk convection
- Pendelluft
- Asymmetrical velocity profiles
- Taylor dispersion
- Cardiogenic mixing
- Molecular diffusion

expiratory time constants) between those regions. Pendelluft can be thought of as ventilation by cross currents between units.

Asymmetric velocity profiles may enhance gas exchange at airway branch points; it has been demonstrated that bulk gas transport can occur when the velocity profile in one direction is parabolic and alternates with an opposite velocity profile that is flat; this situation occurs at airway branch points during HFV.

Taylor dispersion, which is also known as augmented diffusion, occurs when bulk flow of gas is superimposed on diffusion; the contribution of this mechanism to gas exchange during HFV is unclear. *Cardiogenic mixing* may participate in gas exchange if cardiac motion is enough to generate airflow. *Molecular diffusion,* the final step in gas exchange in conventional ventilation or HFV, is diffusion of gas through the alveolar region. Although all of the above mechanisms may participate in gas exchange during HFV, the relative contribution of each of these mechanisms and the conditions that influence their relative contributions remain unknown.

☐ USE OF HFV IN NEWBORNS

High-frequency ventilation, mainly in the forms of HFOV and to a lesser extent HFJV, currently has an important role in neonatal intensive care. It is generally accepted that infants with intractable pneumothoracies or pulmonary interstitial emphysema have an improved recovery rate when managed with HFOV or HFJV. Several extracorporeal membrane oxygenation (ECMO) centers have reported that critically ill full-term or near-term newborns with respiratory failure from any of several causes who were close to meeting, or met, criteria for ECMO were successfully treated with HFOV using the Sensor Medics 3100 approximately 50% of the time. Finally, HFV is often considered for infants requiring conventional mechanical ventilation with rates and inspiratory pressures that portend the development of either air leaks or severe chronic lung disease (Table 25-12).

Several basic principles direct the use of a high-frequency oscillatory ventilator. First, *minute ventilation* is more dependent on tidal volume than on frequency, as shown in the equation

$$\dot{V}CO_2 = (f)\ (V_T^2)$$

where f is the frequency in hertz, V_T is tidal volume, and $\dot{V}CO_2$ is alveolar ventilation. Generally, the starting frequency chosen is 10 to 15 Hz, and this is not changed during operation of the ventilator. The pressure-time waveform produced during HFOV is very different from that seen during conventional ventilation, as shown in Figure 25-13. The Infant Star HFOV refers to the peak-to-trough waveform height simply as "amplitude," whereas the Sensor Medics 3100 and 3100A refer to this property as "oscillatory pressure amplitude." V_T is controlled by adjusting the amplitude of the oscillations. Initially, the ventilator is set up with an amplitude that produces gentle but easily visible oscillations of the baby's chest wall. Subsequent blood gas analysis is used to determine whether increased alveolar ventilation is required. Increasing the amplitude leads to an increased tidal volume, which in turn leads to a lower $PaCO_2$; decreasing amplitude has the opposite effect.

In a very few babies, amplitude adjustment may not allow for adequate ventilation. Careful reduction in frequency may allow the ventilator to generate higher tidal volumes and improve minute ventilation. Also, the Sensor Medics ventilator allows the operator to vary the percentage of the respiratory cycle that is inspiratory

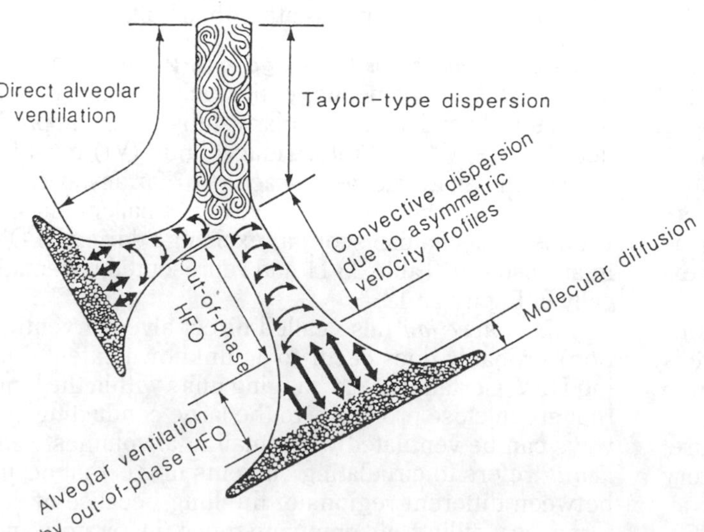

FIGURE 25-12. Potential mechanisms of gas exchange during HFV. All modes are probably active with the predominant mechanism being different at different areas within the lung. (Reproduced with permission of the American Physiological Society from HK Chang, J Appl Physiol 56:553–563, 1984)

TABLE 25-12. **Potential Indications for HFV**

I. Pneumothorax or pulmonary interstitial emphysema
II. Severe respiratory failure unresponsive to conventional ventilation
III. Requirement for very high inspiratory pressures and rates conventional ventilation

time; increasing the percent inspiratory time from 33% toward 50% increases VT.

The second principle of HFOV is that *mean airway pressure* is adjusted directly, with the goal of producing the lung volume that minimizes ventilation-perfusion mismatch and thus maximizes oxygenation. When an infant is switched from a conventional ventilator to HFOV, it is necessary to use a mean airway pressure that is 1 to 2 cmH_2O greater. Conceptually, HFOV allows the use of high end-expiratory pressure for oxygenation without requiring the use of high peak inspiratory pressure to maintain ventilation.

During HFOV, as during conventional ventilation, oxygenation is determined by FIO_2 and mean airway pressure. However, during HFOV, not only is the mean airway pressure important, but how the baby is brought to that mean airway pressure also influences oxygenation. It is important to remember that the lung pressure-volume curve shows hysteresis, with distinct inspiratory and expiratory limbs. At any given pressure, lung volume is higher on the expiratory limb than on the inspiratory limb. This is shown in Figure 25-14.

The best results in oxygenation of patients during HFOV are obtained when patients are maintained on the expiratory limb of their pressure-volume curve. Practically, this means that the mean airway pressure should be reached by inflating the child very well, as with an anesthesia bag and manual breaths, and then attaching him to the HFOV machine at the chosen mean airway pressure. To maintain lung volume, it may be necessary to periodically remove the patient from HFOV and give him a series of manual inflations followed by reattachment to HFOV. Alternatively, the Infant Star, but not the Sensor Medics 3100A, HFOV allows the addition of conventional "sigh" breaths. These types of approaches are often referred to as volume recruitment maneuvers.

Monitoring during HFOV is directed at detecting the two most common untoward effects of HFOV: diminished cardiac output and lung overdistension. The use of high mean airway pressures, as is common during HFOV, has the ability to compromise cardiovascular function. High intrathoracic pressures can impair the return of venous blood to the heart with the result that cardiac output may diminish. The manifestations of this may be overt or subtle and include decreased blood pressure, increased heart rate, diminished capillary refill, metabolic acidosis, and diminished urine output. During HFOV, the patient should be monitored for signs of diminished cardiac output and, if seen, treated with intravascular volume expansion. Over time, the presence of a high mean airway pressure can lead to a progressive increase in lung volume. Lung hyperinflation, if not detected and reversed, can lead to deterioration of arterial blood gases and impairment of cardiac performance. Frequent chest radiographs and a constant awareness of this possibility can prevent severe problems.

Weaning from HFOV involves a gradual reduction in mean airway pressure, as arterial oxygenation and FIO_2

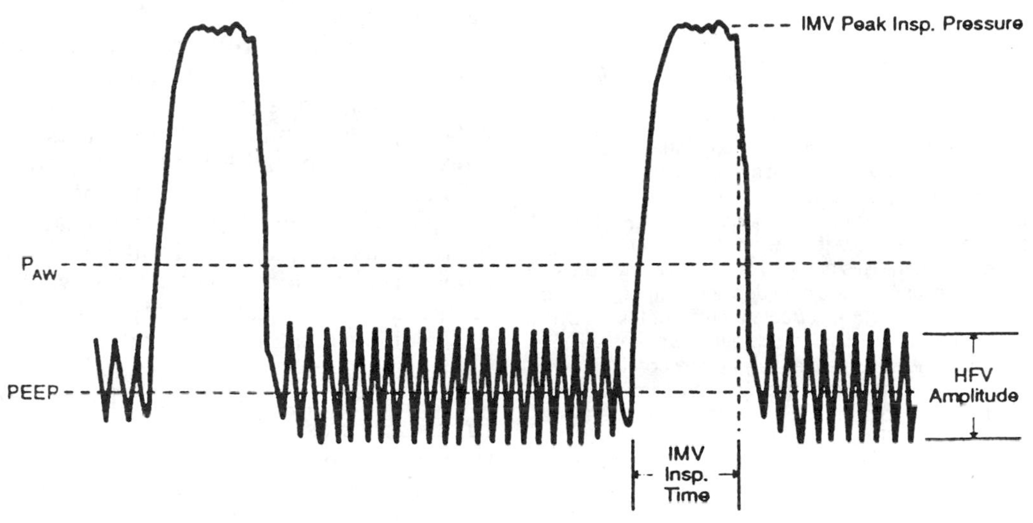

FIGURE 25-13. Pressure waveforms of HFOV compared to conventional ventilation. Note that the HFOV amplitude is the peak-to-trough magnitude of the waveform and that there is a negative component to the pressure swing. This "active expiration" may be in part responsible for the efficacy of this type of ventilation in lowering $PaCO_2$.

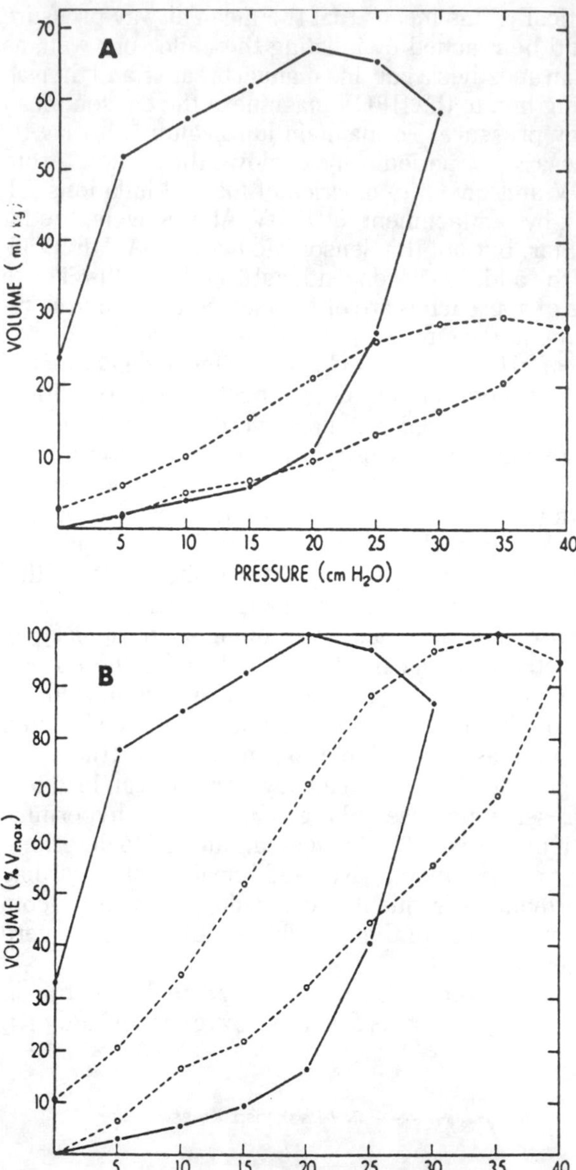

FIGURE 25-14. Pressure-volume curves of lung inflation and deflation. The solid line is a mature, surfactant sufficient lung while the dashed line is an immature, surfactant deficient lung. For each curve, the inflation limb is lower than the deflation limb so that at any transpulmonary pressure there is a greater lung volume during deflation than during inflation. This property is known as hysteresis and is present even if the lung is surfactant deficient, although there is greater hysteresis in the mature, surfactant-sufficient lung. During HFOV, at any given mean airway pressure lung volume will be greater if that mean airway pressure was reached by coming down from a higher pressure rather than by inflating the lung from a lower pressure. This illustrates the importance of volume recruitment and maintenance during HFOV. (Reproduced with permission of the Johns Hopkins University Press from Scarpelli, Surfactant and the lining of the lung, 1988.)

requirement permit, and gradual reduction in amplitude, as permitted by arterial carbon dioxide tension. Patients can either be weaned to continuous positive airway pressure or back to conventional ventilation. There is no level of support (Paw, amplitude, FIO_2) during HFOV at which it is generally agreed that it is safe to return a baby to conventional mechanical ventilation. An example of reasonable criteria to be met before changing a baby back to conventional ventilation would be resolution of any pneumothorax or pulmonary interstitial emphysema, mean airway pressure requirement less than 10 to 12 cmH_2O, and amplitude less than 30 cmH_2O.

TRANSIENT TACHYPNEA OF THE NEWBORN

Transient tachypnea of the newborn (TTNB)[29–31] is a common entity, which has several names in common use: wet lung syndrome, retained fetal lung fluid, and RDS type II. Incidence data are not widely available, but TTNB is a quite common illness and is probably the most common reason for respiratory symptoms in larger babies who are nearly full term or full term. Among unselected deliveries, this disorder may be as common as 2 per 100 births; among infants admitted to a neonatal intensive care nursery with symptoms of respiratory difficulty, the final diagnosis is TTNB as often as 40% of the time.

The functional disorder of TTNB is a delay in removing fetal pulmonary fluid from the alveoli. Retention of this fluid results in partial airway obstruction, which has two effects. First, there is obstruction to air entry, which results in lung units with low ventilation to perfusion ratios. Lung units that function with low ventilation-perfusion ratios result in arterial hypoxemia. Second, there is inadequate emptying of these units during expiration, resulting in air trapping and lung hyperinflation. As a result of hyperinflation, the lung compliance is lower than normal; the infant's work of breathing increases, and excessive respiratory effort is required to maintain normal gas exchange.

There is evidence from echocardiographic studies of children with TTNB that sometimes the high pulmonary artery pressure that characterizes fetal life does not completely remit.[31,32] These infants seem to have a more severe form of the disease. The cause for the high pulmonary artery pressures may be hyperinflation of groups of alveoli, leading to mechanical compression of the pulmonary capillary bed and, thereby, resistance to blood flow. Resistance to blood flow would then lead to an increased pulmonary artery pressure. In babies with this additional feature to their illness, the persistently high pulmonary artery pressure may lead to shunting of blood from the pulmonary circulation to the systemic circulation across fetal channels, with subsequent arterial desaturation.

Another recent development in the understanding of TTNB relates to the role of pulmonary surfactant. Several authors have offered preliminary data that indicate that some babies with TTNB may have a mild deficiency, in quantity or function, of pulmonary surfactant. Whether this deficiency is quantitative or qualitative, or whether it really exists at all, is not completely clear at present.

Risk factors for TTNB are considered to be borderline prematurity with gestational age 34 to 37 weeks, delivery by cesarean section without preceding labor, absent phosphatidylglycerol from the amniotic fluid, and low Apgar scores. Clinically, these infants usually come to attention because of persistent tachypnea, retractions, nasal flaring, grunting, and a requirement for supplemental oxygen to prevent cyanosis. The chest radiograph shows hyperinflation to varying degrees, fluid in one or both lung fissures, perihilar haziness, and a normal to slightly large heart size (Fig. 25-15).

The course of this illness is usually uncomplicated, with infants remaining tachypneic in the range of 80 to 90 breaths per minute for 2 to 5 days, with gradual improvement noted toward the end of this time. Some infants may require an FIO_2 of 0.30 to 0.40, although some authors believe that infants with TTNB have no requirement for supplemental oxygen. It is important to note, however, that there are a few infants who have a much more severe illness. These infants are discernible by their extreme elevation in respiratory rate, to faster than 90 to 100 breaths per minute, and their need for high FIO_2 in the 0.60 to 0.80 range. Some of these infants benefit from a constant distending pressure (such as with nasal CPAP), whereas others experience frank respiratory failure and require mechanical ventilation. Echocardiographic data indicate that these latter infants are those with persistence of a high pulmonary artery pressure.

The diagnosis of TTNB is best thought of as one of exclusion. Other diagnoses that must be considered are sepsis, pneumonia, RDS, and aspiration syndromes. The prognosis for infants with TTNB is quite good, with most recovering rapidly and completely.

PNEUMONIA AND SEPSIS IN THE NEONATAL PERIOD

Infections in newborn infants (sepsis) often take the form of pneumonia and, generally, have a bacterial origin.[33,34] The most common etiologic agents are group B streptococci, *Escherichia coli, Klebsiella pneumoniae,* and *Listeria monocytogenes,* although other bacteria can produce illness as well. Less typically, a newborn may be infected by cytomegalovirus or herpesvirus, and the infection may manifest as pneumonia. In the last few years, it has become clear that approximately two-thirds of cases of neonatal sepsis and pneumonia are acquired during labor. Thus, affected children are most often ill at the time of birth or within several hours immediately following birth. These children have acquired infection with an organism that ascended from the maternal vagina and cervix into the amniotic space during labor. Less commonly, babies develop pneumonia and sepsis some 24 to 48 hours after birth. These infants were well at delivery, but were colonized with a pathogenic organism during the birth process. Following birth, bacteria multiply for a time locally, as in the nasopharynx, and then disseminate to create systemic illness.

There are many reports that describe various constellations of perinatal events thought to increase the risk of pneumonia. Often these reports are not in agreement with one another. Important risk factors for newborn sepsis or pneumonia include maternal cervical or rectal colonization with group B streptococci; premature labor or a low-birth-weight infant; prolonged rupture of the membranes longer than 18 hours; and evidence of maternal chorioamnionitis during labor, such as fever, high white blood cell count, or abdominal ten-

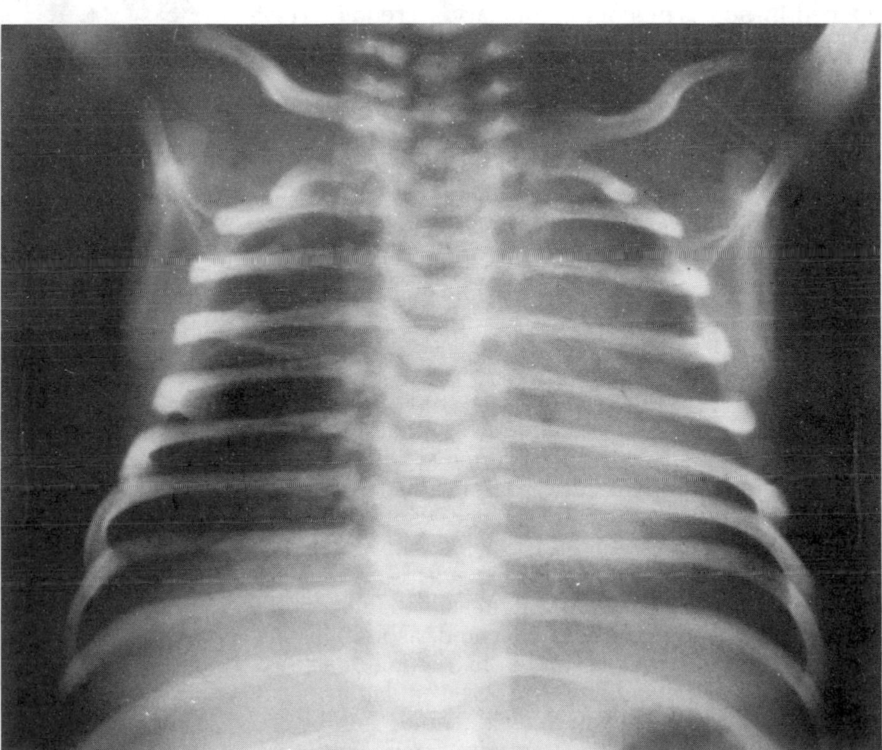

FIGURE 25-15. Chest radiograph typical of transient tachypnea of the newborn. Note the presence of adequate to increased lung volumes, perihilar congestion, and fluid in the minor fissure of the right lung.

derness. Maternal urinary tract infection is also an important risk factor. Premature birth not only is a powerful risk factor for pneumonia but also for a fatal outcome with pneumonia.

The clinical findings in pneumonia are virtually the same as those for RDS or TTNB. When faced with an infant displaying the typical signs of respiratory difficulty, it is not possible to differentiate with certainty among RDS, TTNB, and pneumonia. The chest radiograph in infants with pneumonia may show only a diffuse haze, resemble RDS in all respects, or show a typical localized infiltrate. It is not possible to definitively distinguish pneumonia from RDS or TTNB on a single chest radiograph; this is especially true when the study is obtained in the first few hours after birth. As a result of the similarity in clinical and radiographic appearance of pneumonia and RDS, these two entities must always be considered when either of them is being considered. The inability to distinguish between these diseases with confidence is why virtually all children with respiratory symptoms that are not a mere reflection of transition to extrauterine life are appropriately treated with antibiotics.

The treatment of neonatal pneumonia consists of antibiotic therapy as well as support of respiratory function. Treatment decisions are made on the basis of both arterial blood gas determinations and serial examinations with assessment of interval improvement or worsening. Among babies with pneumonia who require mechanical ventilation, there are two clues that favor the diagnosis of pneumonia over that of RDS. First, infants with pneumonia generally have a higher pulmonary compliance and so require less pressure from the ventilator. Second, copious, purulent secretions in the endotracheal tube favor the diagnosis of pneumonia, as opposed to RDS. In contrast, RDS is generally accompanied by scant, mucoid pulmonary secretions. However, it is important to remember that RDS and pneumonia may coexist.

The prognosis for pneumonia in full-term infants is good unless the disorder is accompanied by septic shock or is so overwhelming as to make adequate oxygenation impossible. Preterm infants have a higher mortality, which varies with the degree of prematurity.

PERINATAL ASPIRATION SYNDROMES

Before the onset of labor, fetuses intermittently make breathing movements, which are essential for normal lung development. During these movements, the net flux of material remains outward from lungs to amniotic fluid. However, certain conditions or events that occur during labor can result in deep gasping movements by the fetus. If at the time of such a gasp the fetal hypopharynx is filled with meconium-stained fluid, blood, infected secretions, or amniotic fluid, aspiration may occur. Aspiration may result in obstruction of airways and lead to sections of lung with low ventilation–perfusion ratios and filling of alveoli with liquid, thereby creating an intrapulmonary shunt with arterial desaturation. Moreover, there is a later inflammatory reaction to inhalation of any of these substances that results in an additional component of impaired lung function several hours after the initial event.[33,34]

Risk factors for aspiration include fetal distress, a postdate gestational age, meconium staining of the amniotic fluid, and placental abruption. Initiation of positive-pressure ventilation of a meconium-stained infant before proper tracheal suctioning can cause meconium aspiration syndrome. Infants who aspirate exhibit respiratory difficulty that creates a clinical picture identical with that seen with other neonatal respiratory disorders. The chest radiograph may only show diffuse haziness or, in severe cases, bilateral "white out." The fluffy, diffuse densities of meconium aspiration syndrome are rather specific for that disorder (Fig. 25-16).

Treatment of these syndromes is supportive. More severely affected children exhibit respiratory failure and require mechanical ventilation. The prognosis depends on the severity of the aspiration and is generally worse if the inhaled substance is meconium.

PERSISTENT PULMONARY HYPERTENSION OF THE NEWBORN

The fetal circulation is characterized by pulmonary arteriolar vasoconstriction, which occurs as a consequence of the low P_{AO_2} values seen in utero. This reflex

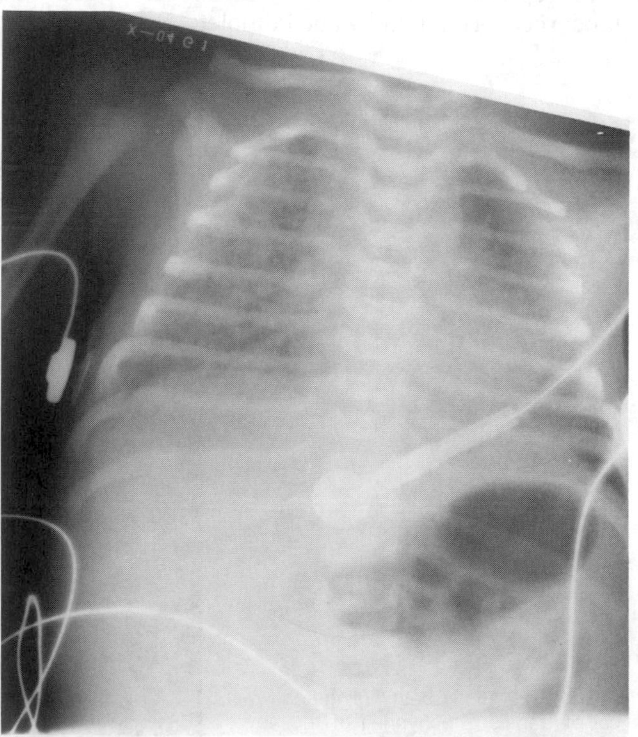

FIGURE 25-16. Chest radiograph of an infant with meconium aspiration syndrome. Note the diffuse, fluffy densities extending out to the periphery of the lung.

is often referred to as *hypoxic pulmonary vasoconstriction,* and it is retained after birth and into adult life.[35] The fetal circulation is also characterized by the shunting of blood from right to left across a patent foramen ovale and an open ductus arteriosus (see Fig. 25-6). Although this circulatory pattern is appropriate for a fetus, it is very detrimental for a newborn because it results in intracardiac shunting of desaturated blood into the systemic arterial circulation. If the shunt is large enough, it precludes adequate tissue oxygenation, and a metabolic acidosis results from tissue hypoxia. The situation wherein there is failure of the fetal circulation to make an appropriate transition to the neonatal circulation is referred to as *persistent fetal circulation* (PFC), or *persistent pulmonary hypertension of the newborn* (PPHN).

Persistent pulmonary hypertension of the newborn can occur alone without any pulmonary disease in its so-called idiopathic form. However, PPHN most often occurs in the setting of, and complicates the management of, other lung diseases. Common settings in which PPHN may supervene are RDS in infants of advanced gestational age; pneumonia, especially when the cause is group B streptococci; and meconium aspiration syndrome. Congenital diaphragmatic hernia is also associated with PPHN. Rarely, an infant who initially is thought to have TTNB has a course complicated by the development of PPHN.

Infants with PPHN in the setting of lung disease initially show the signs of their primary pulmonary illness; PPHN becomes apparent when they fail to respond to the usual therapy or when their course is particularly severe. Babies with the idiopathic form of PPHN have a clear chest radiograph and resemble those with cyanotic congenital heart disease. The diagnosis may be suggested by the history, physical examination, and clinical course. Certain diagnosis requires echocardiographic study, to exclude structural heart disease, and a demonstration of a right-to-left shunt by contrast saline injection or color flow mapping, along with other characteristic findings of pulmonary artery hypertension.

Treatment of this disorder virtually always requires mechanical ventilation with an FIO_2 of 1.0. Support of the systemic circulation with fluid therapy and the use of vasoactive drugs is often required. Administration of sodium bicarbonate to treat a metabolic acidosis may be necessary, and the use of sodium bicarbonate to create a metabolic alkalosis has been advocated by some.

The specifics of ventilatory management of these children are controversial. There are some data to suggest that hyperventilation to produce $PaCO_2$ values in the range of 20 to 25 mmHg and arterial pH values greater than 7.55 reverses pulmonary artery vasoconstriction; this approach to management has been called hyperoxic hyperventilation. Others have pointed out the high mortality that has existed in the past with this approach (most reports describe an approximate 50% mortality rate before the availability of extracorporeal membrane oxygenation) and the lung damage that this type of management engenders.

Other authors have advised a minimal intervention that avoids deliberate hyperventilation. This approach involves managing the mechanical ventilator in a more conventional manner, while using an FIO_2 of 1.0, supporting the systemic circulation, and maintaining a normal arterial pH and accepting lower than usual values for PAO_2. No direct comparisons of results with these differing approaches have been made.

In the past 5 years, substantial advances in the treatment of PPHN have been seen. It is now known that the normal transition from the high pulmonary vascular resistance of fetal life to the low pulmonary vascular resistance of extrauterine life is mediated by *nitric oxide* (NO). Pulmonary arteriolar endothelial cells synthesize NO, which in turn diffuses to the smooth muscle layer and produces vasodilatation. A large body of experimental data demonstrates that the administration of exogenous, inhaled NO lowers pulmonary vascular resistance and raises arterial PO_2 in several animal models of PPHN. Several groups have investigated the use of inhaled NO for the treatment of human infants with PPHN. Doses used to date have ranged from 6 to 80 ppm of inhaled NO. The observed response has very often been favorable, with significant rises in PaO_2 and avoidance of ECMO in children who would otherwise have required ECMO.

Ongoing studies in this area are focused on determining the dose necessary; whether any toxicities exist and how frequent they might be; how often a response can be anticipated; the duration of responses; whether unique conditions such as congenital diaphragmatic hernia respond in a predictable manner; and whether there is benefit from combined therapies such as HFOV, exogenous surfactant, and inhaled NO. Although the use of inhaled NO for the treatment of PPHN remains investigational at present (NO is not currently FDA approved for any medical use), it seems very likely that this modality will soon be accepted as a management option for PPHN.

Another relatively new approach to the management of PPHN has been the use of HFOV. Several ECMO centers have reported that approximately 50% of patients referred because of failure of conventional ventilation in anticipation that ECMO is required can be managed without ECMO by using HFOV.

Extracorporeal Membrane Oxygenation

Extracorporeal membrane oxygenation (ECMO)[36,37] is an established treatment modality in PPHN as well as in other forms of severe neonatal respiratory failure. Extracorporeal membrane oxygenation has been reserved for those infants who, by criteria that vary among institutions, are failing conventional management and are perceived as having potentially fatal disease. The use of ECMO involves the creation of a temporary cardiopulmonary bypass (Fig. 25-17). In venoarterial ECMO (VA ECMO, Fig. 25-17*A*) catheters are placed in the right carotid artery and right atrium. Venous blood is drained from the right atrium to a reservoir and subsequently pumped across a membrane oxygenator, where gas exchange occurs. Oxygenated blood is rewarmed and then returned to the aortic arch by way of the right

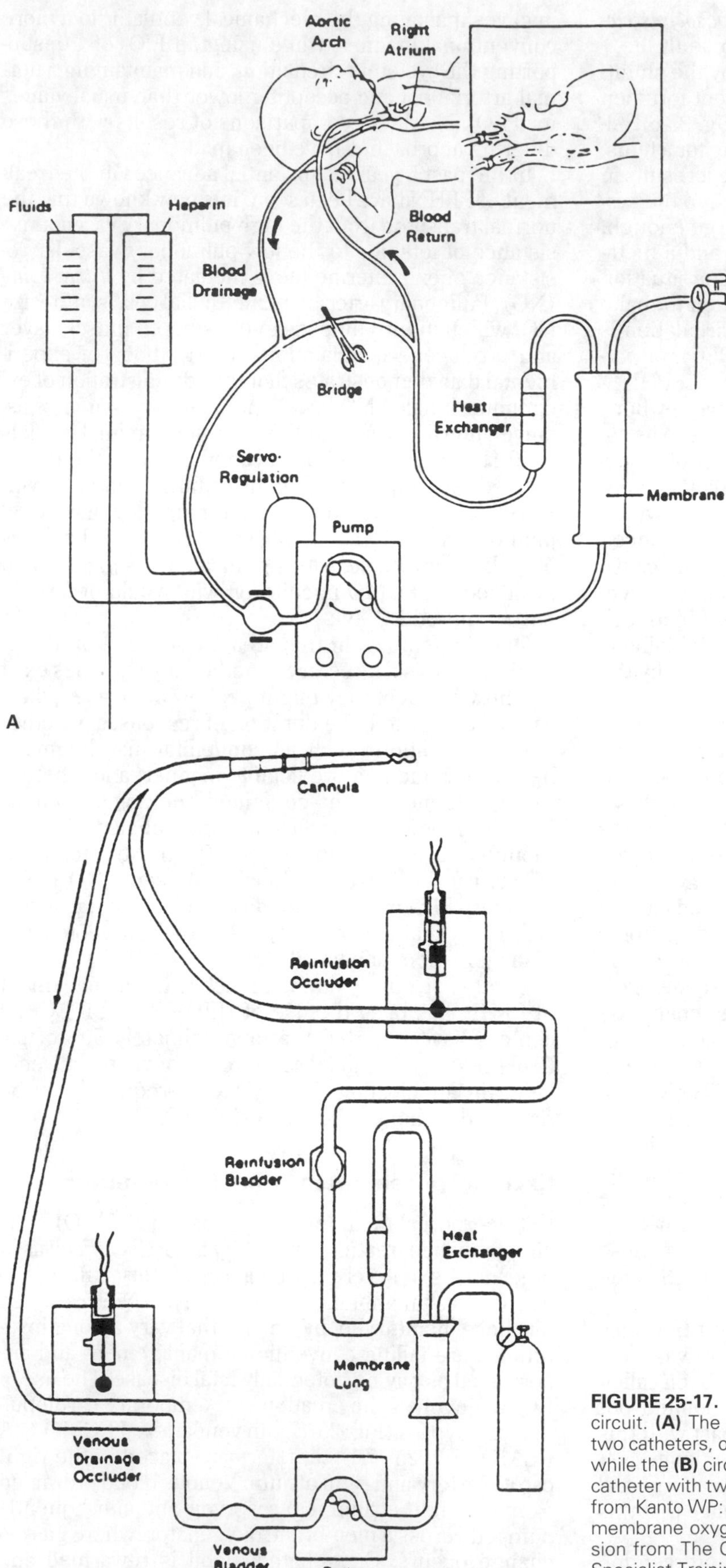

FIGURE 25-17. The extracorporeal membrane oxygenation (ECMO) circuit. **(A)** The circuit for venoarterial ECMO (VA ECMO) involves two catheters, one in the right atrium and the other in the aortic arch while the **(B)** circuit for venovenous ECMO (VV ECMO) uses a single catheter with two separate lumena. See text for details. (Reproduced from Kanto WP: A decade of experience with neonatal extracorporeal membrane oxygenation, J Pediatr 124:335–347, 1994 with permission from The CV Mosby Company and from the Neonatal ECMO Specialist Training Manual, with permission from the Extracorporeal Life Support Organization.)

carotid artery catheter. This technique sometimes involves permanent ligation of the right carotid artery when the baby is removed from ECMO; some ECMO centers have been reconstructing the carotid artery at the time of decannulation. With this system, arterial PO_2 can be raised into the physiologic range, and the lungs can be "put to rest" to heal for several days. Reporting institutions generally state that 2 to 5 days of therapy are required before it is possible to return the patients to the mechanical ventilator and more conventional management.

Another technique of cardiopulmonary bypass is venovenous ECMO (VV ECMO, Fig. 25-17*B*). In this method, a single, large, double-lumen catheter is placed in the right atrium; blood is removed via one lumen and treated as described for VA ECMO, but it is then returned to the right atrium via the other catheter lumen. The child's own cardiac output then circulates the blood without further assistance. As a result of mixing of oxygenated blood and deoxygenated blood, VV ECMO raises the final arterial PO_2 to a lesser degree than seen in VA ECMO, but the final value is one that supports the infant, provided that the hematocrit and cardiac output are adequate. Additionally, for VV ECMO to succeed, the infant's cardiac output must be good. The advantage of VV over VA ECMO is that the carotid artery is left undisturbed.

Long-Term Outcome After PPHN

Children who recover from PPHN generally do well in terms of their development, although hearing loss has been reported to occur with a higher than expected frequency.[34] However, children treated for PPHN sometimes have residual chronic lung disease. This is a consequence of the therapy for PPHN. In general, children treated with ECMO have neurodevelopmental outcomes that are similar to those who survive without ECMO when the degree of illness of the patients is taken into account. Long-term outcome after VA ECMO is of special concern because of the permanent loss of the right carotid artery (unless it has been reconstructed), which this therapy involves.

PULMONARY AIR LEAK SYNDROMES

The pulmonary air leak syndromes[38] include pneumothorax, pulmonary interstitial emphysema, pneumomediastinum, and pneumopericardium. Pulmonary air leaks begin with the rupture of an overdistended alveolus or terminal airway. This rupture gives rise to air within the pulmonary interstitium, which is able to traverse along the tissue planes that accompany vessel and lymphatics until it reaches the mediastinum. If the air remains within the mediastinum, the result is a *pneumomediastinum.* Rarely, in infants, the air dissects into the pericardial space and creates a *pneumopericardium* (Fig. 25-18). Most commonly, the air breaks through the mediastinum, and a *pneumothorax* results (Fig. 25-19).

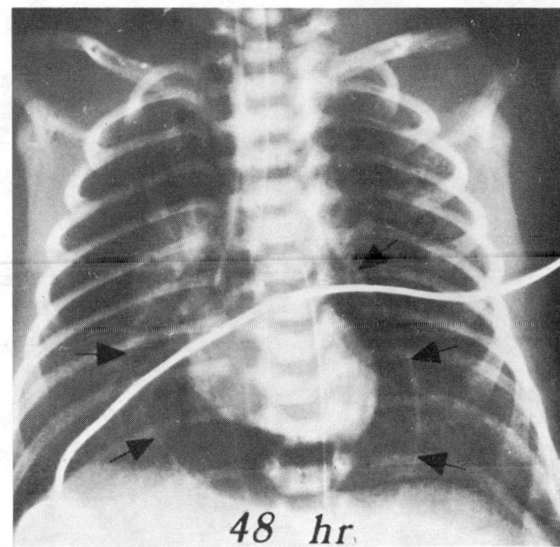

FIGURE 25-18. Pneumopericardium. Air completely encircles the heart and may cause tamponade. Even though the endotracheal tube was down the right mainstem bronchus, no perforation of the tracheobronchial tree was present at postmortem examination.

In babies who are free of pulmonary disease, pneumothorax may occur as a consequence of the high airway pressures, often close to 60 cmH_2O, that accompany the onset of respirations immediately following birth. In fact, an incidence of spontaneous pneumothorax of 1% has been found in this setting. These are most often asymptomatic and of no significance. Treatment is required only rarely, as when there is a mediastinal shift indicating the presence of tension.

The use of positive-pressure ventilation at birth, meconium aspiration syndrome, RDS, and pneumonia all increase the frequency of pneumothorax. Incidences of pneumothorax as high as 20% to 50% have been found in children with meconium aspiration syndrome. Other aspiration syndromes are also associated with an increased risk of pneumothorax. Transient tachypnea of the newborn also predisposes babies to pneumothorax and represents one of the major morbidities of this disease.

A common theme in all of these conditions is the presence of abnormal pulmonary mechanics that require the infant to generate high intrathoracic pressures to effect gas exchange. The increased pressures predispose newborns to alveolar rupture. In meconium aspiration syndrome, there is also increased resistance to expiratory (and inspiratory) flow because of the partial obstruction of airways by meconium. The resulting incomplete expiratory flow leads to progressive alveolar distension, which further increases the risk of alveolar rupture. The incidence of pneumothorax is increased whenever mechanical ventilation is used. In preterm infants undergoing mechanical ventilation for RDS, an incidence as high as 40% has been reported in the era before surfactant replacement therapy. The availability of surfactant has reduced the occurrence of pneumothorax by approximately 50%.

In contrast with the pneumothoraces that occur spontaneously, those that occur in the setting of lung disease

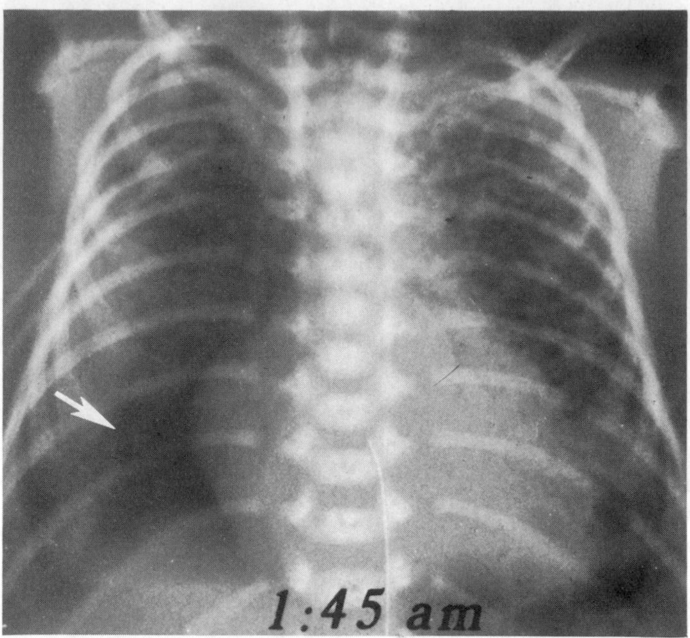

FIGURE 25-19. Pneumothorax and interstitial emphysema: Pneumothorax is seen on the right, with a chest tube in place. Note the accumulation of air anteriorly and medially (*arrow*) because of noncompliance of the lungs and their inability to collapse concentrically. Interstitial pulmonary emphysema involves the left lung; a left pneumothorax occurred shortly after this film was taken.

generally do result in compromise of arterial blood gas levels and cardiac output; consequently, drainage with tube thoracotomy is often required. This is especially true in patients undergoing mechanical ventilation, in whom pneumothorax is often a catastrophic event owing to the presence of tension in the thorax, with a consequent mediastinal shift. Arterial blood gas levels deteriorate with pneumothorax because of right-to-left intrapulmonary shunting of blood through the atelectatic lung. Cardiac output is compromised with tension pneumothorax because the high intrathoracic positive pressure and shifting of the mediastinum lead to compression of the great veins. Compression of the great veins diminishes cardiac return, and subsequently, cardiac output falls.

Most often, a *pneumomediastinum* is a silent abnormality and usually is not a cause of respiratory or cardiac dysfunction. Its pathogenesis is analogous to that of a spontaneous pneumothorax. It does have the potential to decompress to form a pneumothorax and, accordingly, deserves careful observation. Generally, it is unwise to attempt to drain a pneumomediastinum. *Pneumopericardium* is rare and is essentially always seen in children who are undergoing mechanical ventilation. It may be asymptomatic, or it may cause the picture of cardiac tamponade. Drainage may be lifesaving in the latter event.

Pulmonary interstitial emphysema (PIE) begins when air dissects out of the alveolar bases or ducts and remains as cysts of air within the perivascular tissues of the lung, rather than following tissue planes to the hilum and leading to pneumothorax. These cysts range in size from 0.1 to 1.0 cm and extend radially from the hilar regions outward (see Fig. 25-19). This type of air leak is strongly associated with use of mechanical ventilation. Two types of PIE are recognized: diffuse and localized. Early onset of diffuse and bilateral PIE in infants undergoing mechanical ventilation for RDS is a poor prognostic sign. Localized PIE does not have the same significance for outcome. Beyond reducing the amount of pressure used for ventilation to that which is absolutely essential, no specific management is usually required. On occasion, PIE is asymmetric, with one side markedly more affected and hyperinflated, whereas the contralateral side is atelectatic. In such cases, positioning the severely affected side down may be of benefit as the weight of the mediastinum and atelectatic lung may prevent progression or lead to reversal of the air leak. Selective intubation of the main stem bronchus leading to the atelectatic side has been reported to be of benefit in specific cases.

In the past several years, the treatment of PIE has improved with the addition of HFPPV, HFJV, and especially HFOV being successfully used to manage patients with this form of air leak. The very short inspiratory time common to each of these types of ventilation allows for adequate ventilation of normal airspaces while avoiding filling of the abnormal intraparenchymal spaces, which in turn leads to the gradual resolution of the PIE.

CONGENITAL HEART DISEASE

There are three basic modes of presentation by which newborns with *congenital heart disease* (CHD) can come to attention: (1) cyanosis, (2) congestive heart failure, and (3) low cardiac output states. When cyanosis is the mode of presentation, the infant is noted to be dusky in room air but generally does not have the grunting, flaring, and retracting characteristic of infants with lung disease. If an arterial blood gas analysis is obtained, the PaO_2 is typically in the 30- to 60-mmHg range. The presence of cyanotic CHD is made more likely by demonstrating that the PaO_2 does not rise significantly in 100% oxygen. A rise in PaO_2 to greater than 200 mmHg in response to an FIO_2 of 1.0 would greatly favor the diagnosis of lung disease. Also, lung disease should be accompanied by abnormal lung parenchyma on a chest radiograph, and this is not seen in infants with CHD.

As a second type of presentation, infants may come to attention because of congestive heart failure. Infants presenting with congestive heart failure exhibit the typical signs of respiratory difficulty in a newborn, but also have an enlarged liver on examination and cardiomegaly with pulmonary edema on a chest x-ray film. Some of these infants may also exhibit cyanosis, and the two presentations of cyanosis and congestive heart failure are not mutually exclusive.

Congenital heart disease may also appear as a low cardiac output state, as when there is obstruction to left ventricular outflow. In its extreme form, this represents cardiogenic shock. Respiratory signs occur later in this type of presentation. Lethargy, poor feeding, poor systemic perfusion, and metabolic acidosis are the early indications of disease.

The immediate newborn history, physical examination, chest radiograph, and a comparison of arterial blood gas levels obtained while the baby is breathing room air or 100% oxygen should differentiate between CHD and lung disease in the majority of cases. Table 25-13 lists the specific lesions categorized by their typical mode of presentation. Some diseases may have more than one possible presentation; only the more common diseases are listed. The specific issues of diagnosis and therapy are beyond the scope of this discussion.

APNEA

Apnea[39,40] is the cessation of effective airflow for longer than 20 seconds or for long enough to produce arterial desaturation, or bradycardia, or both. Apneic episodes are very common in preterm infants, occurring in approximately 50% of infants whose birth weights are less than 1500 g. The apneic episodes may be secondary to environmental circumstances or to another disease process, or they may occur as a reflection of an immature respiratory control system. These latter episodes are referred to as idiopathic apnea of prematurity. Table 25-14 lists the specific causes of apnea. Idiopathic apnea of prematurity is the most common cause of apneic events in preterm infants, but it remains a diagnosis of exclusion. Specific causes must be sought in infants who develop new apnea.

The immaturity of respiratory control that gives rise to apnea of prematurity may take several forms. *Central apnea* results when, because of insensitivity of peripheral chemoreceptors or poor central integration of information from these receptors, there is cessation of central respiratory drive. *Obstructive apnea* results when immaturity of upper airway reflex events allows collapse of the airway, leading to absence of airflow, despite continued respiratory effort. However, the predominant type of apnea in infants is *mixed apnea,* wherein elements of both impaired central control and obstruction from poor reflex activity are operative.

Although *idiopathic apnea of prematurity* is common (present in approximately 50% of babies less than 1500 g), it is not necessarily benign. Doppler flow studies of the anterior cerebral artery have demonstrated reverse diastolic flow when apneic episodes have led to heart rates slower than 100 beats per minute. Some reports have associated recurrent episodes of apnea accompanied by cyanosis with a less favorable developmental outcome.

Several approaches to treatment are available. Removal of any underlying precipitant is the first step. A

TABLE 25-13. **Presentations of Congenital Heart Disease**

Cyanosis
- Pulmonary atresia
- Tricuspid atresia
- Ebstein's anomaly
- Transposition of the great vessels
- Total anomalous pulmonary venous return
- Pulmonary stenosis
- Tetralogy of Fallot

Congestive Heart Failure
- Common atrioventricular canal
- Truncus arteriosus
- Atrial septal defect with patent ductus arteriosus
- Ventricular septal defect

Low Cardiac Output States
- Hypoplastic left heart syndrome
- Aortic coarctation
- Aortic stenosis
- Interrupted aortic arch

TABLE 25-14. **Specific Causes of Apnea**

Infection
- Sepsis
- Meningitis
- Necrotizing enterocolitis

Decreased oxygen delivery
- Hypoxemia
- Anemia
- Shock
- Left-to-right shunting (as through a PDA)

CNS disease
- Asphyxia and cerebral edema
- Hemorrhage
- Seizures
- Malformations

Drugs
- Maternal narcotics
- Fetal narcotics

Metabolic diseases
- Hypoglycemia
- Hypocalcemia
- Hyponatremia
- Hypernatremia-dehydration
- Hyperammonemia

Thermal instability

Idiopathic apnea of prematurity

common example of this would be the finding of a borderline low PaO_2 in a child with apnea. Often, correction of this situation with small amounts of supplemental oxygen greatly reduces the frequency of apneic episodes. Treatment with nasal CPAP has been advocated. It is possible that this is effective either because it improves oxygenation or because it "stents" open the soft tissues of the upper airways and improves the course of children with obstructive apnea.

The methylxanthines theophylline and caffeine have both been used to treat apnea in preterm infants. It is widely believed that these agents act to stimulate central respiratory drive, although definitive proof of their mechanism of action is lacking. Methylxanthines increase the mean inspiratory flow rate, increase respiratory flow rate output, and also lead to an approximate 20% increase in metabolic rate. This latter finding is a disadvantage of therapy with these agents. Theophylline levels of 5 to 10 μg/mL and caffeine levels of 8 to 20 μg/mL are recommended. Generally, apnea of prematurity remits when the children are approximately 34 weeks' gestational age, and it is possible to discontinue drug therapy, although continued cardiorespiratory monitoring for a period during and after discontinuance is prudent.

CONGENITAL DIAPHRAGMATIC HERNIA

Congenital diaphragmatic hernia (CDH)[41–44] is an infrequent but life-threatening neonatal disorder. These newborns come to attention either because of the typical signs of respiratory distress or because of profound cyanosis that does not remit with oxygen therapy. The chest radiograph usually shows loops of bowel in the thorax, although films obtained before significant amounts of air have been swallowed may show a unilateral "white out" with a mediastinal shift. In this latter case, repeat films show the typical appearance of bowel in the thorax (Fig. 25-20). Approximately 80% of diaphragmatic hernias are left sided. In several reported series, 20% to 25% of children with CDH have associated major congenital abnormalities. These anomalies have included trisomies, several types of congenital heart disease, tracheoesophageal fistula, and genitourinary malformations.

Although definitive repair of this lesion involves surgery, the preoperative management is important. A nasogastric tube attached to suction is used for gastric decompression. In symptomatic infants, elective endotracheal intubation is required and should be followed by muscle relaxation and sedation. This approach provides minimal inflation of the gastrointestinal tract and aims to minimize lung and heart compression by preventing the gastrointestinal tract from filling with air. These patients should be mechanically ventilated with an a FIO_2 of 1.0 and with great care given to minimize inspiratory pressures, as pneumothorax is common in this setting and is associated with a less favorable prognosis.

Surgical repair of this lesion is important, but survival is dictated by the degree of pulmonary hypoplasia that is present.[42–44] In CDH, both lungs are hypoplastic, although the ipsilateral lung is more hypoplastic than the contralateral lung. The earlier in gestation the diaphragmatic hernia appears, the greater the degree of pulmonary hypoplasia, and the less the chances for survival. Arterial blood gas abnormalities in CDH are caused, in part, by decreased lung surface area, but a more important determinant is right-to-left shunting of blood across fetal channels. This shunting of blood is a

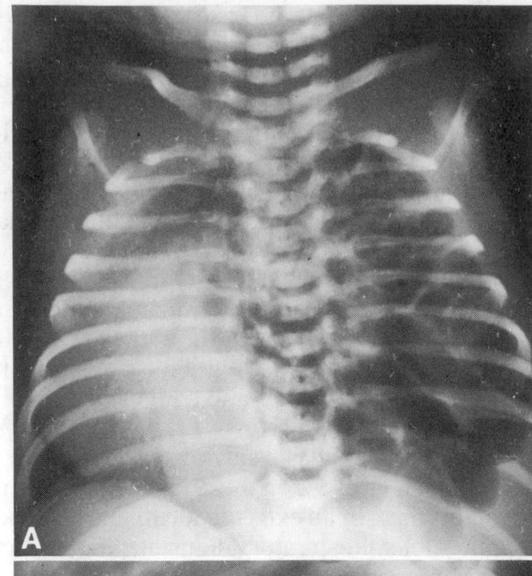

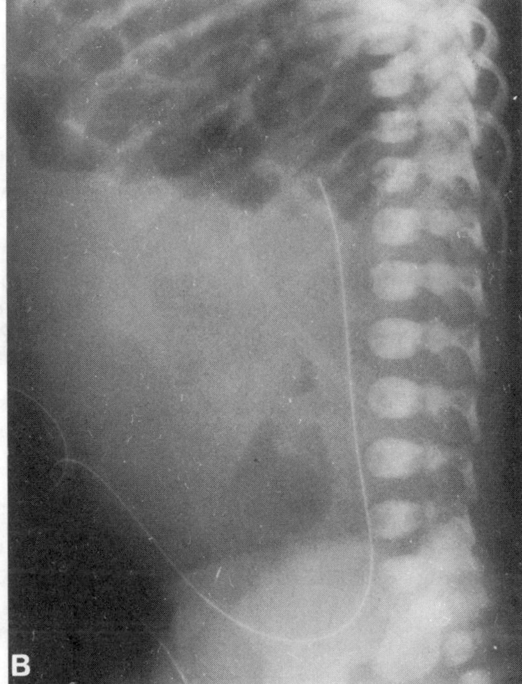

FIGURE 25-20. **(A)** Anteriposterior view of a diaphragmatic hernia. This full-term newborn had respiratory distress from birth. Heart tones were heard on the right. Note the multiple loops of bowel in the left pleural space, with herniation of the heart and mediastinum toward the right. **(B)** Lateral view of the same diaphragmatic hernia. Physical examination of the abdomen revealed a scaphoid configuration. The only air below the level of the diaphragm is in the stomach. Note the multiple loops of small bowel in the chest.

consequence of both the anatomic hypoplasia itself and the pulmonary vasoconstriction that frequently precedes or follows surgical repair of these infants.

After surgical repair, infants can be separated into three groups. The first group consists of those children who do well and have an uncomplicated course. The second group of children have a degree of pulmonary hypoplasia that is fatal, and their arterial blood gas levels are incompatible with life, despite extensive efforts to support them. The third group of infants do well for several hours after surgery (the so-called "honeymoon period") and then experience extensive right-to-left shunting of blood across fetal channels caused by an elevation in pulmonary vascular resistance. The management of this third group of children is similar to that for PPHN.

Before the availability of ECMO, the mortality rate for diaphragmatic hernia remained unchanged at approximately 50% for many years.[41] It was widely believed that the availability of ECMO would significantly reduce this mortality rate. However, it is unclear whether this promise has been achieved, as some ECMO centers continue to report mortality rates that are not significantly different from those seen before the use of ECMO. Currently, this issue is a matter of debate and ongoing investigation.

The occurrence of pulmonary hypoplasia is not limited to the setting of CDH. It is also seen in the oligohydramnios malformation sequence, with Potter's syndrome, and with several other chromosomal or malformation syndromes.

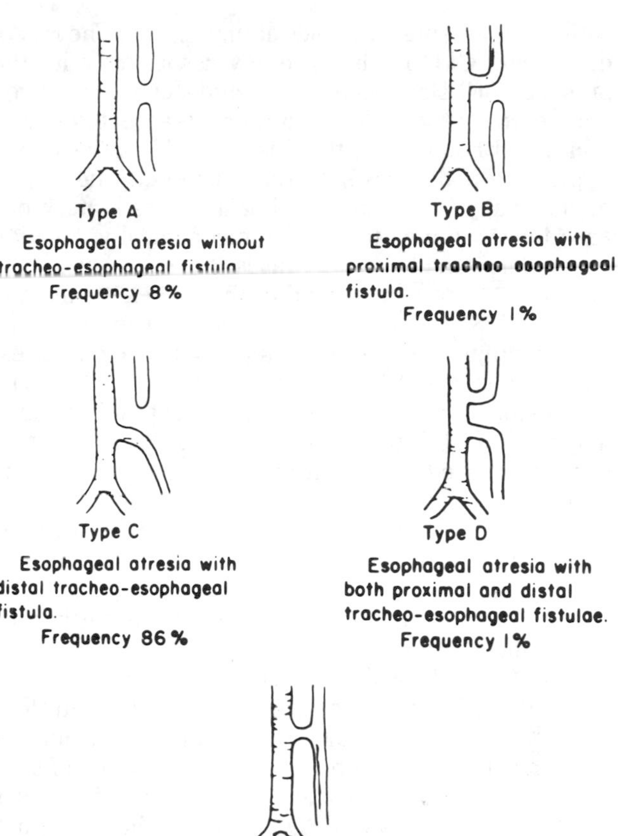

FIGURE 25-21. Tracheoesophageal anomalies: type and incidence. (Reproduced by permission from Sunshine P et al: Gastrointestinal disorders. In MB Fanaroff, RJ Martin [eds]: Berman's Textbook of Neonatal–Perinatal Medicine: Diseases of the Fetus and Infant [3rd ed.] St Louis, The CV Mosby Company, 1983)

ESOPHAGEAL ATRESIA WITH TRACHEOESOPHAGEAL FISTULA

An abnormality of separation between the trachea and esophagus during the fourth to sixth week of intrauterine life leads to this anomaly, the incidence of which is approximately 1 per 3,000 live births. Several anatomic arrangements are possible, as shown in Figure 25-21. Data indicate that 35% of children with tracheoesophageal fistula (TEF) also have a preterm delivery. Approximately 50% of infants with TEF have a recognizable constellation of anomalies that include vertebral abnormalities, imperforate anus, abnormalities of the radius, and congenital heart disease. This constellation of anomalies is referred to as the VATER or VACTERL complex.

Polyhydramnios, caused by the inability of the fetus to swallow amniotic fluid, is a clue to the presence of this defect. The combination of polyhydramnios and prematurity further suggests this condition. Although these infants are generally well at the time of delivery, they rapidly come to attention because of an inability to handle oral secretions or as a result of choking and coughing during feedings. Over time, lung damage occurs because of reflux of gastric secretions directly into the lungs. Diagnosis is usually made when a nasogastric tube is seen (on a chest radiograph) to coil in the esophageal pouch rather than enter the stomach.

Immediate management of this condition includes placing the infant in the reverse Trendelenburg position to minimize reflux of gastric contents into the lungs, and placing a catheter with constant suction in the proximal esophageal pouch to eliminate upper airway compromise. Adequate temperature control, ventilatory stability, and hydration should be assured. Surgical treatment is definitive and is always required; the procedure of choice depends on the exact characteristics of the defect. The prognosis is generally good except when premature birth or associated congenital anomalies add their own morbidities and mortality risk.

CHRONIC LUNG DISEASE OF INFANCY

Chronic lung disease of infancy (CLD),[45,46] or *bronchopulmonary dysplasia* (BPD), is a pulmonary disorder that has emerged in parallel with the increasing survival of prematurely born infants with respiratory disease. Its occurrence is closely linked to gestational age at birth, with younger, smaller babies at higher risk. The risk of developing CLD is also strongly associated with the presence of RDS. Attempts to study CLD have been hampered by the lack of a uniformly accepted definition. Most commonly, the onset of CLD is insidious. Typically, the diagnosis is first considered when a premature baby who is recovering from respiratory disease but continues to require mechanical ventilation and supplemental oxygen ceases to improve or begins to worsen during the second or third week of life. If, at an age of 28 days, an infant recovering from lung disease continues to require supplemental oxygen, exhibits tachypnea and retractions with crackles heard by auscultation, and has an abnormal chest radiograph, a diagnosis of CLD may be made (Fig. 25-22). A more recently proposed definition would require these same findings to be present at a corrected gestational age of 36 weeks. There are data to suggest that this latter definition may be the more useful one, and its acceptance is increasing.

The incidence of CLD varies among reporting authors. This variation in reported occurrence ranges between 6% and 62%, with an average of approximately 30% in infants with birth weights less than 1500 g and RDS. Most of the variation in incidence is due not to actual differences in outcome of patients but, rather, to differing populations being studied and to different definitions of CLD. The frequency of CLD is strongly linked to birth weight, as is shown in Table 25-15. These data were obtained before the availability of surfactant replacement therapy.

Although there is no generally agreed on, single cause for CLD, it is generally agreed that the high concentrations of inspired oxygen and positive-pressure ventilation interact with an immature lung such as to lead to the alterations that constitute CLD. The mechanism by which these factors interact to produce CLD involves uncontrolled inflammation within the lung that alters the morphology and physiologic properties of the developing tissue. Pathologically, CLD is characterized by several findings. The alveolar structure is abnormal, with fibrosis of alveolar septae and with areas of alveolar overdistension immediately adjacent to areas of atelectasis. Some acini are destroyed.

Pulmonary edema is universally present. The small conducting airways exhibit increased thickness of the submucosal muscular layer and abnormal extension of the muscular layer down the bronchial tree. Additionally, there is excessive production of mucus and alteration in function of the mucociliary escalator. A newly emerging feature of this disease is the frequent involvement of the large airways, manifested as tracheomalacia, bronchomalacia, inspissation of secretions, and occlusion of airways by growth of granulation tissue. The microscopic examination of the pulmonary vascular bed shows abnormal muscular thickening and abnormal extension of the muscular layer down through succeeding generations of vessels. Pulmonary artery hypertension is commonly present. Cor pulmonale may occur in children who are severely affected.

These anatomic abnormalities have pathophysiologic consequences. The presence of atelectatic alveoli leads to venous admixture and hypoxemia, whereas the result of emphysematous overdistension in other lung units with high ventilation–perfusion ratios is carbon dioxide retention. Pulmonary fibrosis and pulmonary edema both decrease lung compliance. As a result of the small-airways abnormalities, there is increased resistance to airflow caused by anatomic narrowing of the lumen and the presence of excessive quantities of

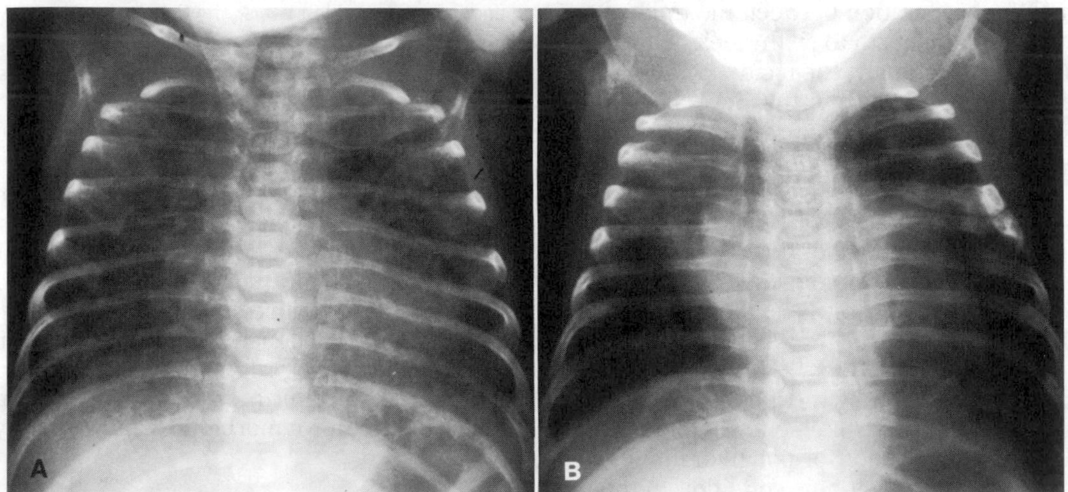

FIGURE 25-22. (A) Bronchopulmonary dysplasia in a 2-month-old child with severe hyaline membrane disease and prolonged oxygen and ventilatory therapy. Bilateral diffuse interstitial fibrosis and cystic change are present, consistent with stage IV bronchopulmonary dysplasia of Northway (see text). **(B)** Bronchopulmonary dysplasia in a 2½-month-old patient who had severe hyaline membrane disease, prolonged ventilator and oxygen therapy, and ligation for persistent patient ductus arteriosus. There is now advanced bronchopulmonary dysplasia, with areas of cystic overexpansion of the lower lobes and considerable interstitial fibrosis, not well seen because of the marked cystic changes. The heart is enlarged by cor pulmonale.

TABLE 25-15. **Frequency of Bronchopulmonary Dysplasia as a Function of Birth Weight**

Birth Weight (g)	Infants With BPD (%)
701–800	76.1
801–900	68.8
901–1000	46.4
1001–1250	26.0
1251–1500	12.9

Adapted from Avery ME, Tooley WH, Keller JB et al: Is chronic lung disease in low birth weight infants preventable? Pediatrics 79:26, 30, 1987

mucus. Abnormalities of the large conducting airways may lead to persistent wheezing or stridor. Persistent elevation of pulmonary artery pressures has the potential to lead to cor pulmonale, with heart failure as the ultimate consequence.

As a result of these abnormalities, children with CLD have hypoxemia and hypercarbia, and elevated respiratory rate, retractions, and crackles on examination. They generally have an increased work of breathing. The increased work of breathing often leads to growth failure, despite a caloric intake that would be adequate for normal children. Patients with CLD may have acute worsening of their respiratory condition if their fluid intake leads to a worsening of their pulmonary edema. Another cause of acute deterioration is reactive airways disease.

Treatment of these children is difficult and complicated. Most aspects of therapy have not undergone rigorous trials to establish proof of benefit. Babies with CLD generally require prolonged administration of supplemental oxygen and, often, prolonged mechanical ventilation. Diuretic agents that ameliorate the abnormalities of pulmonary mechanics related to pulmonary edema are frequently used, but they have not been shown to improve the ultimate outcome. Abnormalities in electrolyte balance are common among children treated with diuretics. Fluid restriction may be helpful, but the associated caloric restriction can be a problem because of the frequent requirement for a supranormal caloric intake to achieve growth. Often the feeding of formulas with increased caloric density is helpful in producing weight gain.

Therapy with bronchodilators, such as theophylline or various inhaled β-adrenergic agents, has produced beneficial changes in pulmonary mechanics, but whether this corresponds to improvement in long-term outcome is not known with certainty. Treatment with corticosteroids has been shown to hasten weaning from mechanical ventilation and improve pulmonary mechanics; one study has also shown improved neurodevelopmental outcome. However, complications of corticosteroids are not uncommon when they are used for the amelioration of CLD.

Chronic lung disease has a significant mortality rate; before the availability of surfactant replacement therapy the mortality rate was approximately 30%. Most deaths occur before discharge from the hospital. Children with CLD often require home oxygen therapy, diuretic therapy, bronchodilator therapy, and special formulas, but they have a prognosis for recovery that is good. Hospital readmissions during the first year of life are common and generally occur in association with viral respiratory tract infections. Growth failure is common in babies with CLD, and generally, growth improves simultaneously with improvement in lung function as indicated by clinical assessment.

Pulmonary function testing is able to detect abnormalities for many years in children who have recovered from CLD. The children generally do not have exercise intolerance and are able to keep up with their peers. Respiratory symptom questionnaires have, in some studies, detected a higher incidence of symptoms, such as cough and wheezing, in children who have recovered from CLD. Provocation with methacholine inhalation in the pulmonary function testing laboratory and assessment of response to inhaled bronchodilators have supplied evidence that there is a higher than anticipated incidence of reactive airways in children with CLD. Physician-diagnosed reactive airways disease (asthma) is not uncommon in these children. Despite these findings, the great majority of children discharged with BPD gradually recover, wean from oxygen and medications, and have pulmonary function that permits participation in normal childhood activities.

The majority of information available regarding CLD was obtained before the availability of surfactant replacement therapy. The impact of surfactant replacement on CLD is not yet entirely clear. The early, randomized, controlled surfactant trials did not show a reduction in the incidence of CLD. However, CLD was defined merely by the requirement for supplemental oxygen at 28 days of life; no physical or radiographic findings were considered. Additionally, no attempt was made to determine whether the severity of CLD was altered by surfactant therapy. Data that have emerged since the early studies and involve more mature babies do indicate a reduction in both the incidence and severity of CLD with surfactant therapy. This area is one that will receive continued study in the future.

PRACTICAL ASPECTS OF NEONATAL RESPIRATORY THERAPY

Oxygen Administration

Oxygen is a drug critical for the survival of newborns with respiratory problems. As with other drugs, it must be administered in the proper dosage to avoid unintended effects. Therapy with oxygen is complicated in that the appropriate "dosage" varies widely from one patient to another and even from one time to another for the same patient. Whatever the mode of delivery, oxygen therapy requires continuous monitoring of the FIO_2, continuous monitoring of the temperature of the delivered gas, and ongoing assessment of the adequacy of therapy.

□ OXYGEN TOXICITY

Two organs seem to be at risk for adverse effects during oxygen therapy—the retina and the lungs. The toxic effects of oxygen on the retina are related to the PaO_2 that is achieved. The effect of oxygen on the retina depends on the stage of development of the retinal vessels and the duration of exposure to excessive levels of oxygen. Preterm infants are most at risk, and the more premature a baby is, the greater the risk. Currently, most infants with significant retinopathy of prematurity are born with birth weight less than 1000 g. The exact values for PaO_2 that are dangerous are not known with certainty. However, current recommendations are to maintain the PaO_2 below the 100-mmHg level.

The toxic effects of high concentrations of inspired oxygen on the lungs are well described in animals, in which a specific sequence of pathologic changes can be observed. Infants who require therapy with high concentrations of inspired oxygen are at greater risk for the development of BPD.

□ METHODS OF OXYGEN DELIVERY

Hood Oxygen Therapy

For infants who are breathing without the need for positive airway pressure, hood oxygen delivery systems provide the most precise control of FIO_2, temperature, and humidification of gases. Hood oxygen delivery requires flow rates of fresh gas that are adequate to expel carbon dioxide and maintain the intended FIO_2. The minimum flow rate that ensures that an infant will not rebreathe expired gases is 8 L/min. The hood chosen should fit comfortably around the infant's neck, but have only a minor leak. The use of a blender system with hood oxygen delivery is preferred because it offers easier control of FIO_2 and reduces the level of noise within the hood. Blender systems also permit quicker and more precise alterations in the delivered FIO_2. The FIO_2 and temperature should be continuously monitored as close to the baby's face as possible. It is important to recognize that radiant warmers and phototherapy lights can alter the temperature within the hood.

Newborns are not able to precisely control their body temperatures, in part because of their large surface area to body mass ratio. As a result, they are best cared for in a thermoneutral environment—that is, the environment that allows the lowest possible oxygen consumption. The range of temperatures that leads to a thermoneutral environment for a newborn varies with age after birth and with weight. This means that each newborn has an ideal ambient temperature that avoids cold stress, the need to burn calories, and the need to increase oxygen consumption to maintain body temperature. Failure to maintain a thermoneutral environment is the most common cause of hypothermia and can substantially worsen an infant's condition. Circulation of cold gas across the face and head of an infant can disrupt a thermoneutral environment and lead to hypothermia.

Nasal Cannula and Face Mask

Oxygen may be delivered by nasal cannula to larger infants who are in the convalescent stage of a respiratory illness or who have BPD. The use of this delivery system during an acute illness is not appropriate. For successful use, the FIO_2 that is required by the infant should be 0.35 or less. In general, nasal cannula flow rates should be no greater than 1.0 L/min, because excessive drying of the nasal mucosa and gastric distension can occur at higher flow rates. The most important use of nasal cannula oxygen therapy is a part of a home oxygen therapy program, allowing early discharge of infants with CLD.

Face masks for oxygen delivery are available in sizes that are appropriate for newborns. These are only occasionally useful, as for short-term administration of oxygen during transport or special procedures. It is important to realize that the flow rate chosen must be sufficient to prevent the rebreathing of exhaled gases. Delivery of oxygen at any chosen liter per minute flow rate gives no information about the alveolar PO_2. Therefore, when infants are transferred from one delivery system to another (oxygen hood, mask, or nasal cannula), the adequacy of therapy must be assured by pulse oximetry or blood gas determination.

Continuous Positive Airway Pressure Delivery

Continuous positive airway pressure (CPAP) can be delivered in several ways, no one of which is clearly superior to the others for all circumstances. Most commonly, CPAP is delivered by nasal prongs (Hudson prongs), but it can also be delivered by a single nasopharyngeal tube or by an endotracheal tube. Nasal prongs are subject to displacement but do not become obstructed very frequently and do not increase expiratory resistance. A disadvantage to this delivery system is the loss of CPAP and FIO_2 that may occur during mouth breathing or crying. Nasopharyngeal tubes are more secure in their placement but can become plugged with secretions, resulting in loss of pressure and FIO_2. An endotracheal tube has the advantages of security of placement and very constant pressure and FIO_2 delivery, but it has the disadvantages of requiring endotracheal intubation, creating increased resistance to airflow, with the possibility of inducing respiratory fatigue and the need for repeated tracheal suctioning. The use of face masks and head chambers are of historical interest only.

The most efficient way to create CPAP is by using a mechanical ventilator in the CPAP mode. This has the additional advantage of in-line monitoring of FIO_2 and alarm systems. It is possible, however, to construct a CPAP system using a gas flow system, water column with the pressure exhaust tubing submerged to a depth (in cm) equal to the desired level of CPAP and a screw valve attached to an anesthesia bag, as shown in Figure 25-23. A major disadvantage of such a system is the need for additional equipment to continuously monitor FIO_2 and to alarm for unwanted pressure changes.

Mechanical Ventilators for Infants

This section is concerned with mechanical ventilator itself; refer to the previous section concerning mechanical ventilation of the newborn for issues concerning patient management.

Since the 1970s, when mechanical ventilation of very low birth weight infants became widespread, major ad-

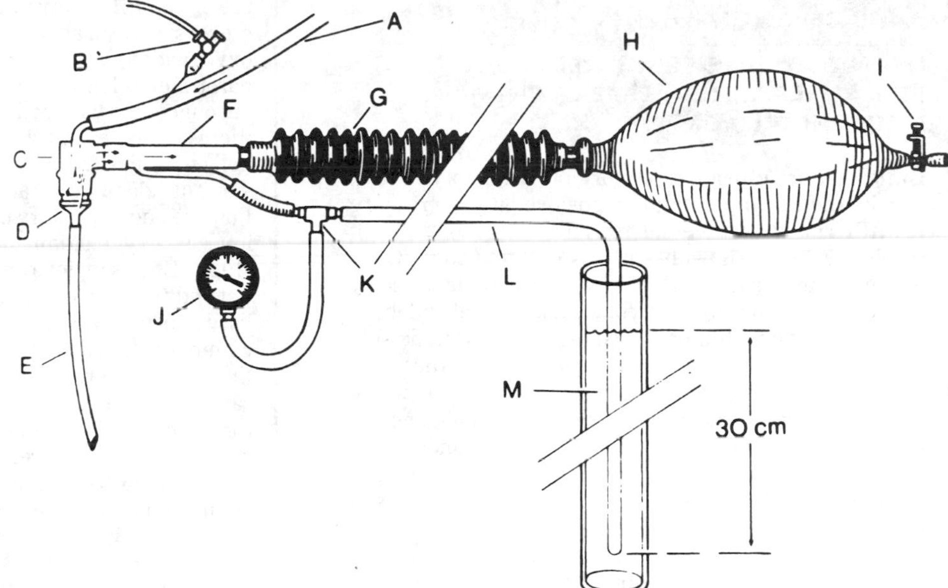

FIGURE 25-23. System for applying CDP by endotracheal tube: *A*, gas inflow; *B*, oxygen monitor; *C*, Norman elbow; *D*, endotracheal tube connectors; *E*, endotracheal tube; *F*, Sommers T-piece; *G*, corrugated tubing; *H*, anesthesia bag; *I*, screw clamp; *J*, pressure manometer; *K*, T-connector; *L*, pressure exhaust tube; *M*, underwater seal. (DW Thibeault, GA Gregory (eds): Neonatal Pulmonary Care [2nd ed.] Norwalk, Conn, Appleton & Lange, 1987, with permission)

vances have been made in ventilator technology. Ventilators are classified by a combination of pressure, volume, flow, or time control. When using a volume ventilator, a predetermined volume is delivered to the patient circuit, and there is no control over the pressure generated. Volume ventilation is infrequently seen in the neonatal intensive care unit, and this discussion will be limited to time-cycled, pressure-limited ventilators. There have been several advances in ventilator design in recent years. We will first discuss the basic workings of a time-cycled, pressure-limited ventilator before discussing the many modes of ventilation now available.

□ PRESSURE-LIMITED, TIME-CYCLED VENTILATION

When using a pressure-limited, time-cycled ventilator, a preset pressure limit is reached during inspiration and terminated by an operator-chosen inspiratory time (see AARC Clinical Practice Guideline: Neonatal Time-Triggered, Pressure-Limited, Time-Cycled Mechanical Ventilation). The flow rate is chosen by the operator and is usually between 4 and 10 L/min. A sufficient flow rate is necessary to reach the desired peak pressure and maintain the chosen I:E ratio. Unlike some adult ventilators, there is not a control on most neonatal ventilators to choose the waveform; instead, adjustment of flow rate determines the waveform. The two waveforms usually used in neonatal ventilation are the sine wave and the square wave (Fig. 25-24). A sine wave is shaped more like the wave of a spontaneous breath and is seen with low flow rates. This waveform produces a lower mean airway pressure and causes less barotrauma, but hypercapnia may occur, and delivery of the assigned peak inspiratory pressure may not be possible. The most common waveform used in neonatal ventilation is the square wave. Square wave ventilation produces a higher mean airway pressure for equivalent peak airway pressures and a longer time at the chosen peak inspiratory pressure. This ventilatory strategy opens up atelectatic areas of the lung and improves distribution of ventilation.

The volume of gas delivered to the baby by a pressure-limited, time-cycled ventilator is unknown unless devices to measure it are specifically placed in line. This volume is dependent on the gas flow rate, inspiratory time, pressure limit, the baby's lung compliance, airway resistance, and compliance of the ventilator circuit. This is especially important: if the baby's endotracheal tube is kinked or plugged, the preset pressure can still be reached, but no tidal volume is delivered to the lungs.

□ CONTINUOUS FLOW VERSUS DEMAND FLOW

Most pressure-limited, time-cycled ventilators used today have a constant flow of gas during both inspiration and expiration, thus allowing the baby to draw on this flow during spontaneous breathing without rebreathing exhaled gas. In the recently designed demand-flow systems, the basic flow rate for mechanical breaths is chosen by the operator to be the constant backup flow, but if the patient's spontaneous flow requirements increase, as with an increase in respiratory rate or tidal volume, the ventilator delivers added flow. (These systems are different than the older systems used in adult ventilation, which had zero flow until a spontaneous breath was initiated; in this sense they are not true demand-flow systems.) Demand-flow systems for infants work by sensing a drop in airway pressure and opening a flow valve without relying on patient triggering. Demand-flow systems may be useful because the ventilator circuit, humidifier, and endotracheal tube all add resistance to the delivery system and may intensify the work of breathing required of the baby; demand systems may decrease this work and facilitate weaning from the ventilator. The Babylog 8000, Infant Star, and

AARC Clinical Practice Guideline

NEONATAL TIME-TRIGGERED, PRESSURE-LIMITED, TIME-CYCLED MECHANICAL VENTILATION

Indications: Apnea; respiratory or ventilatory failure, despite the use of continuous positive airway pressure (CPAP) and supplemental oxygen (ie, $F_{IO_2} \geq 0.60$); respiratory acidosis with a pH $<$ 7.20 to 7.25; $PaO_2 >$ 50 mmHg; increased work of breathing demonstrated by grunting, nasal flaring, tachypnea, and sternal and intercostal retractions; the presence of pale or cyanotic skin and agitation; alterations in neurologic status that compromise the central drive to breathe such as apnea of prematurity, intracranial hemorrhage, congenital neuromuscular disorders; impaired respiratory function resulting in a compromised functional residual capacity (FRC) due to decreased lung compliance or increased airways resistance, including but not limited to respiratory distress syndrome (RDS), meconium aspiration syndrome, pneumonia, bronchopulmonary dysplasia, bronchiolitis, congenital diaphragmatic hernia, sepsis; radiographic evidence of decreased lung volume; impaired cardiovascular function; persistent pulmonary hypertension of the newborn (PPHN); post resuscitation; congenital heart disease; shock; postoperative state characterized by impaired ventilatory function.

Contraindications: No specific contraindications for neonatal ventilation exist when indications are judged to be present.

Assessment of Need: Determination that valid indications are present by physical, radiographic, and laboratory assessment.

Assessment of Outcome: Establishment of neonatal assisted ventilation should result in improvement in patient condition or reversal of indications; reduction in work of breathing as evidenced by decreases in respiratory rate, severity of retractions, nasal flaring, and grunting; radiographic evidence of improved lung volume; subjective improvement in lung volume as indicated by increased chest excursion and aeration by chest auscultation; improved gas exchange; ability to maintain a PaO_2 $\geq$50 torr with F_{IO_2} $<$0.60; ability to reverse respiratory acidosis and maintain a pH $>$7.25; subjective improvement as indicated by a decrease in grunting, nasal flaring, sternal and intercostal retraction, and respiratory rate.

Monitoring: Patient-ventilator system checks should be performed every 2 to 4 hours and should include documentation of ventilator settings and patient assessments; O_2 and CO_2 monitoring; periodic sampling of blood gas values by arterial, capillary, or venous route. PaO_2 should be kept below 80 mmHg in preterm infants to minimize the risk of retinopathy of prematurity. The unstable infant should be monitored continuously by transcutaneous O_2 monitor or pulse oximeter. The unstable infant should be monitored continuously by transcutaneous or end-tidal CO_2 monitoring. Fractional concentration of oxygen delivered by the ventilator should be monitored continuously. Continuous monitoring of cardiac activity (by means of electrocardiograph) and respiratory rate. Monitoring of blood pressure by indwelling arterial line or by periodic cuff measurements. Continuous monitoring of proximal airway pressures including peak inspiratory pressure (PIP), PEEP, and mean airway pressure. Increases in mean airway pressure may result in improved oxygenation, but $>$12 cmH_2O has been associated with barotrauma. The difference between PIP and PEEP (ΔP) in conjunction with patient mechanics determines V_T. As the ΔP changes, V_T varies. PIP should be adjusted initially to achieve adequate V_T as reflected by chest excursion and adequate breath sounds or by V_T measurement. Positive end-expiratory pressure increases FRC and may improve oxygenation and ventilation-perfusion relationship (PEEP is typically adjusted at 4 to 7 cmH_2O—levels beyond this range may result in hyperinflation, particularly in patients with obstructive airways disease). Many commercially available neonatal ventilators provide continuous monitoring of ventilator frequency, T_I, and I:E ratio. If only two of these variables are directly monitored, the third should be calculated (eg, the proportion of the T_I for a given frequency determines the I:E ratio). Lengthening T_I increases mean airway pressure and should improve oxygenation. An I:E ratio in excess of 1:1 may lead to the development of auto-PEEP and hyperinflation. Frequencies of 30 to 60 breaths per minute with shorter T_I (eg, I:E of 1:2) are commonly used in patients with RDS. Depending on the internal diameter of the ventilator circuit, excessive flow rates can result in expiratory resistance that leads to increased work of breathing and automatic increases in PEEP. Some ventilators are equipped with demand-flow systems that permit the use of lower baseline flow rates but provide the patient with additional flow as needed. Because of the possibility of complete obstruction or kinking of the endotracheal tube and the inadequacy of ventilator alarms in these situations, continuous tidal volume monitoring by means of an appropriately designed (minimum dead space) proximal airway flow sensor is recommended. Periodic physical assessment should be performed of chest excursion and breath sounds and for signs of increased work of breathing and cyanosis. Periodic evaluation of chest radiographs to follow the progress of the disease, identify possible complications, and verify endotracheal tube placement.

From AARC Clinical Practice Guideline; see Respir Care 39:808, 1994, for complete text.

Bird VIP all have demand systems that can be selected for use by the operator.

□ T_I, T_E, AND I:E RATIO

Independent control of the inspiratory time is essential when ventilating infants. The time necessary for the lungs to inflate and deflate is dependent on both resistance and compliance. The product of resistance and compliance is called the time constant of the lung. The time constant is also the time necessary for the alveolar pressure to reach 63% of a change in airway pressure. The effects of changing the T_I and T_E on gas exchange are dependent on the time constant of the lung. Both too short and too long an inspiratory time can adversely affect gas exchange. An inspiratory time that is too short leads to an "incomplete" inspiration and may lead to a decreased tidal volume and mean airway pressure resulting in hypercapnia and hypoxemia. An incomplete

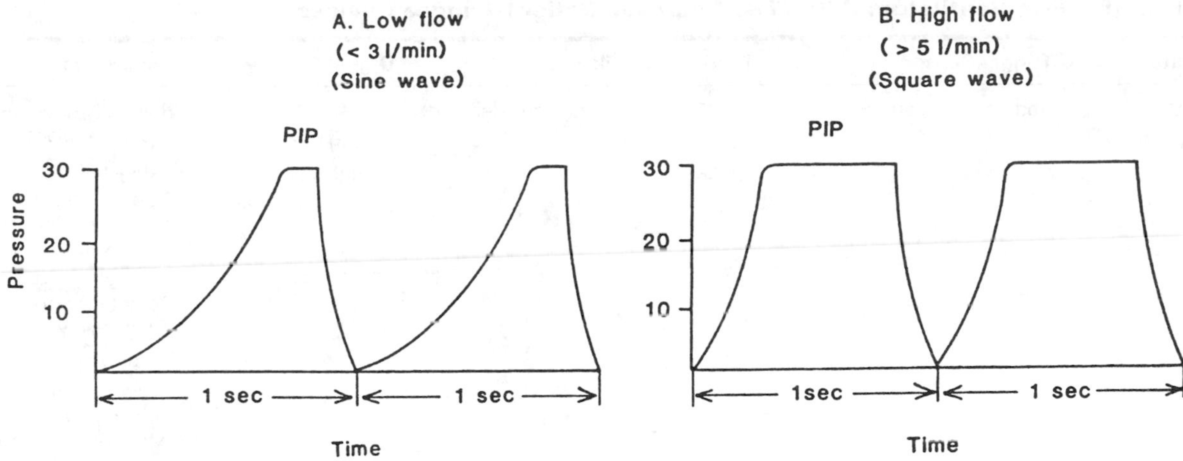

FIGURE 25-24. Comparison of sine wave ventilation with square wave ventilation. The difference between sine and square wave ventilation can be created by changing the flow rate through the patient circuit. Note that the area under the sine wave curve is less than that under the square wave, thus the mean airway pressure will be less for the sine wave. (Reproduced with permission from W.B. Saunders Company, Assisted Ventilation of the Neonate [2nd ed.], JP Goldsmith and EH Karotkin [eds], 1988, p. 148)

expiration, from an excessively long inspiratory time, can lead to hyperinflation of the lung, a decrease in compliance, and increased mean airway pressure. These may result in hypercapnia without hypoxemia.

Incomplete expiration can also result in air trapping, decreased venous return, and subsequent decreased cardiac output. Pulmonary air leaks may also occur. It is also important to be conscious of the I:E ratio when ventilating the infant, and it is both convenient and somewhat safer to have the ventilator display all these variables. However, if any two of the four variables (T_I, T_E, rate, and I:E ratio) are known, then the other two can be calculated. The ideal I:E ratio, like the optimal inspiratory time, varies depending on the disease. Generally, the inspiratory time is less than or equal to one-half of the total respiratory cycle. It is important when changing ventilatory rate to avoid an unintentional inversion of the I:E ratio. In general, an inverse I:E ratio is not recommended because of the high rate of occurrence of air leaks and chronic lung disease seen with this ventilatory strategy. However, occasionally, an inverse ratio such as 2:1 is used in certain disease states.

□ OTHER CONSIDERATIONS

Other desirable features to consider when comparing ventilators from different manufacturers are (1) a comprehensive alarm package that indicates which alarm was triggered even if the condition corrects spontaneously, (2) an oxygen blender capable of giving 21% to 100% O_2 and which displays the FIO_2, and (3) direct control of PEEP with the ability to deliver 0 to 24 cmH_2O. The circuit (lower compliance and smaller dead space volume) and humidifier to be used are also important considerations. It is important to remember that the gas must be humidified and heated. Inadequate humidification of the respiratory gas may result in increased viscosity of mucus leading to obstruction of airways and distal atelectasis. Heating the gas is not only important to the infant's temperature but, if the temperature varies, then the compressible volume of the gas will change, which could cause a change in the tidal volume delivered to the infant. Under most circumstances, the change in tidal volume caused by changes in gas temperature is small, but some particularly ill children may be adversely affected by such a change.

The information displayed by the ventilator has improved, and many ventilators now have a separate monitor that can be used to calculate and display flow-volume loops and other breath-to-breath measurements (Table 25-16). One important display is a mean airway pressure display. Mean airway pressure is the average airway pressure during one respiratory cycle. The mean airway pressure is determined by the PIP, waveform, inspiratory time, and PEEP. Figure 25-25 shows the mean airway pressure and four ways it can be increased. In neonates with RDS, an increase in oxygenation is directly related to an increase in mean airway pressure. Thus, it is important to be able to directly monitor Paw during various manipulations of the ventilator.

□ MODES OF VENTILATION

The most common modes of ventilation currently found on neonatal ventilators include (1) continuous positive airway pressure (CPAP), also called spontaneous ventilation (SV) on some ventilators; (2) intermittent mandatory ventilation (IMV); (3) assist-control (A-C), sometimes seen as patient-triggered ventilation (PTV) or synchronized assisted ventilation of infants (SAVI); (4)

TABLE 25-16. **Five Ventilators With FDA-Approved Patient-Trigger Devices**

Ventilator	Trigger Sensor	Modes+	Flow	Digital Display	Comments
Infant Star Star Sync*	Abdominal capsule	A-C* IMV CPAP SIMV*	Continuous demand	T_I (spont)* Paw I:E ratio Breaths per minute	Reliability depends on capsule placement Apnea backup Able to avoid inadvertent PEEP by exhalation-value assist venturi Do not have to adjust sensitivity Sensitive detector of spontaneous breaths Does not have a problem with autocycling
Bear Cub NVM1 volume monitor* CEM for A-C & SIMV*	Flow hot-wired anemometer	CMV, IMV A-C SIMV CPAP	Continuous	Continuous MV* % Leak*	Needs NVM1 to trigger CEM Apnea backup Addition of NVM1 has been found to cause CO_2 retention because dead space is same as other vents; thought to be because of wire-mesh screen filters In-lab study of the three flow-triggering systems had highest rate of auto cycling
Babylog 8000	Flow hot-wired anemometer	A-C SIMV	Continuous demand	T_I I:E tv Pressure-flow wave Minute ventilation % Leak	Flow sensor at the "Y" provides bidirectional measurements of patient flow Variable insp. and variable exp. flow allows you to adjust to infants' expiratory needs and the delivery needs of the ventilator for inspiration Able to avoid inadvertent PEEP by exhalation-value assist venturi
Bird VIP Partner*	Flow variable orifice pneumotachometer	IMV CPAP SIMV*	Continuous demand	T_I $\overline{P}aw$ I:E ratio Breath rate Minute ventilation Pressure-flow wave Leak LPM	Low rate of autocycling Breath termination at % of peak inspiratory flow
Sechrist IV-100B IV-200 Hewlett Packard cardio-resp monitor*	Chest leads	CPAP VENT SAVI*		I:E ratio T_I T_E Rate	Reliability depends on chest lead placement Breath termination on active expiration Triggers on every breath so, SAVI and A-C mode not SIMV

* Separate module.
\+ Modes for time cycled mode; for example, Bird also has volume-cycled modes.
T_I: Inspiratory time
T_E: Expiratory time

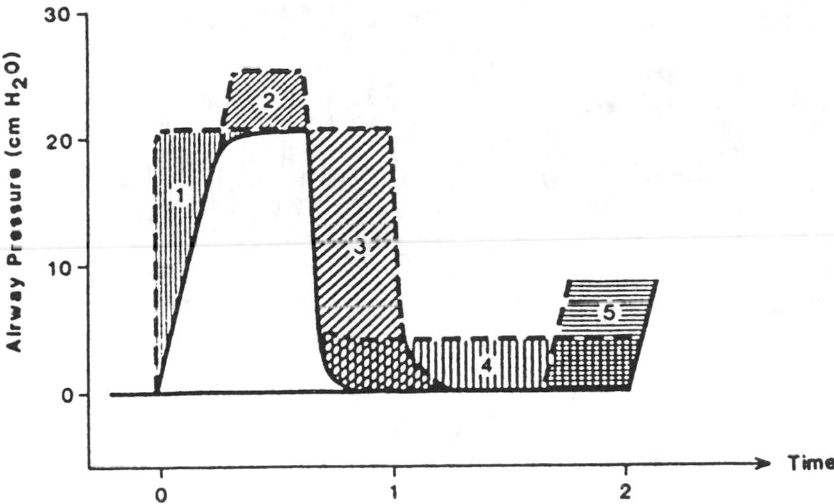

FIGURE 25-25. Mean airway pressure during conventional ventilation may change with any of several changes in ventilator settings. Changes illustrated result in increased mean airway pressure; changes made in the opposite direction would result in decreased mean airway pressure. (1) Increase flow through ventilator circuit, (2) increased peak inspiratory pressure, (3) prolongation of the inspiratory time, (4) application of greater positive end expiratory pressure. (Reproduced with permission. Int Anesthesiol Clinics 12: 259, 1974)

synchronous IMV (SIMV); and (5) the newest mode, proportional assisted ventilation (PAV).[47–49]

Continuous Positive Airway Pressure (CPAP). This has been discussed in a previous section.

Intermittent Mandatory Ventilation (IMV). This is the traditional manner in which infants have been ventilated. In the IMV mode of ventilation, the patient is allowed to breathe spontaneously from the ventilator's continuous flow or demand system. Ventilator breaths are delivered at preset intervals and may occur between spontaneous breaths, or spontaneous breaths may be interrupted by machine breaths. In this mode, ventilator breaths **cannot** be triggered by the patient on demand.

Assist Control, Patient-Triggered Ventilation, and Synchronized Assisted Ventilation of Infants. Almost all of the newly designed ventilators have at least one of these three modes. The goal of PTV is to allow the infant to trigger the ventilator breath early enough during inspiration to preclude active exhalation by the infant against a ventilator breath. These systems produce a ventilator breath for **every** spontaneous breath. The infant determines her own ventilator rate and therefore her own minute ventilation.

A new mode of ventilation used for synchronization in conjunction with the Sechrist IV-100B ventilator uses an impedance-based system and is referred to as synchronized assisted ventilation of infants (SAVI). The developers of this system believed that the pressure-based systems were not sensitive enough for very low birth weight infants, and that electrical measurements of the respiratory cycle would be more sensitive. Pneumography signals from a standard cardiorespiratory monitor with electrodes placed on the right and left sides of the chest trigger the exhalation solenoid valve of the ventilator. Figure 25-26 contrasts flow-volume loops from a baby on SAVI and then conventional IMV. Adjustment of a sensitivity control during SAVI allows the trigger point to be anywhere on the inhalation curve and termination anywhere on the exhalation curve. This mode, similar to assist-control and PTV modes, triggers the ventilator with every infant breath. These modes are useful for higher respiratory rates, but in infants with less lung disease, triggering every breath can cause hyperventilation and apnea. This mode may prove to be useful in the future in weaning infants from mechanical ventilation. One study with infants whose birth weight was <850 g showed infants on SAVI had a significantly shorter time on the ventilator than the infants on conventional ventilation.

Synchronous Intermittent Mandatory Ventilation (SIMV). During synchronized IMV, the prescribed ventilator rate is used by the ventilator to divide each minute into epochs of time. When the infant breathes his first breath within an epoch, the ventilator cycles in synchrony with the infant; subsequent spontaneous infant breaths within that same epoch of time do not trigger a ventilator breath. If the infant is apneic within any given time epoch, the ventilator cycles at the end of that epoch. The advantage of SIMV is the ability to synchronize the baby to a selected ventilator rate. Infants ventilated with SIMV have more consistent tidal volumes and flow-volume loops for both machine and spontaneous breaths than infants receiving IMV. Figure 25-27 contrasts these loops from a baby ventilated on IMV and then SIMV with the Infant Star ventilator.

It is widely accepted that asynchrony of spontaneous breaths and ventilator breaths can cause serious problems in infants. Especially in very-low–birth-weight babies, asynchrony of breaths can lead to increased airway pressure, exhaustion of the baby, and pneumothorax. Such asynchrony may also contribute to the development of chronic lung disease and intraventricular hemorrhage (IVH). The response time (the time between the onset of the baby's inspiration and the cycling of the ventilator) of these trigger systems is important. Although the maximum acceptable response time for triggering is not known, based on research on the tim-

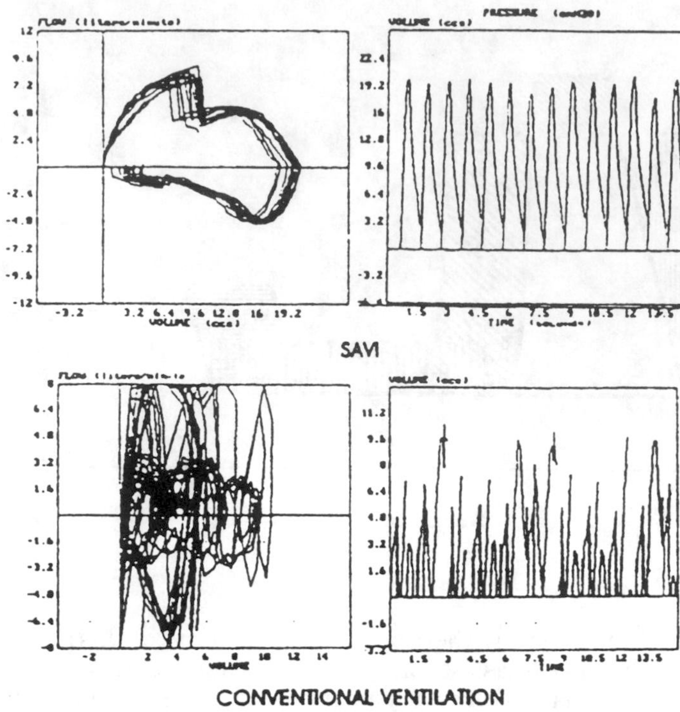

FIGURE 25-26. The effects of synchronized assisted ventilation of infants (SAVI, *top*) versus intermittent mandatory ventilation (*bottom*). Airway flow is more reproducible and tidal volumes are more consistent during SAVI. (Reproduced with permission from Stoutenborough T: Synchronized assisted ventilation of infants [SAVI]: A thoracic impedance-based method description and case histories. Neonatal Intensive Care: The Journal of Perinatology-Neonatology 7: 20–26, 1993.)

ing of spontaneously breathing infants, a response time of <100 msec is thought to be adequate. Table 25-16 shows data for five ventilators now on the market with FDA-approved triggering devices. All five of these ventilators now have response times of <100 msec.

The Star Sync (Infrasonics) promotes patient triggering by a connection between an abdominal respiration sensor (Graseby MR10) and the Infant Star ventilator. Because infants are primarily abdominal breathers and diaphragmatic movement is the first indication of a spontaneous breath, developers at Infrasonics believe

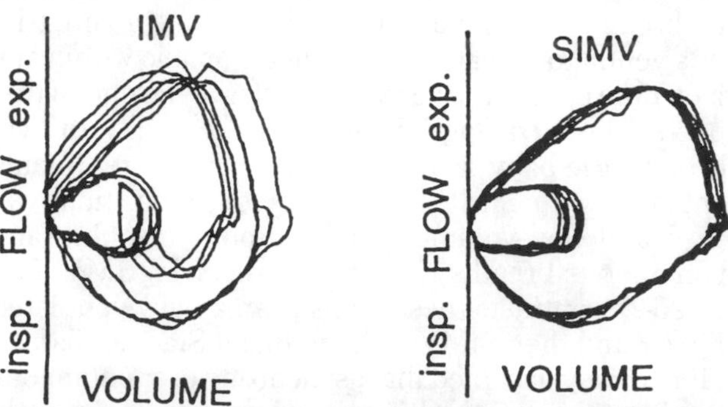

FIGURE 25-27. A comparison of sequential flow-volume loops for a single premature infant with RDS during conventional intermittent mandatory ventilation (*left*) and synchronized mandatory ventilation (*right*). The left figure demonstrates that during conventional IMV tidal volume is very variable and that ventilatory breaths may be initiated during the late inspiratory and early expiratory phases of spontaneous infant breaths. In comparison, the right figure shows no interference between spontaneous breaths and ventilator breaths and more consistent tidal volumes during SIMV. (Reproduced with permission from Boynton BR, Carlo WA, Jobe AH, [eds] New Therapies for Neonatal Respiratory Failure: A Physiological Approach, p 162. New York, Cambridge University Press, 1994.)

this is a more efficient way of triggering a breath than waiting until a pressure change occurs. In a small, randomized, crossover-designed study using the Infant Star ventilator for IMV and Star Sync for SIMV, very low birth weight infants were found to have significantly higher PaO_2 values and lower $PaCO_2$ values with SIMV versus IMV. A multicenter, prospective, controlled trial of SIMV is currently underway.

The Babylog 8000 (Draeger), Bear Cub (Bear Medical Systems), and the Bird VIP (Bird Products) all use airway flow sensors to detect the initiation of a spontaneous inspiration. The Babylog and the Bear Cub use a hot-wired anemometer flow sensor, while the Bird VIP uses a variable-orifice pneumotachometer flow sensor. All three provide data on the infant's tidal volume and minute ventilation; the Infant Star does not provide this information. The Babylog and Bird VIP both display the leak flow rate. This is helpful in setting the sensitivity above the leak to prevent autocycling. Autocycling of the ventilator can occur if the leak around the endotracheal tube is large enough to create a large pressure drop or changes in flow that trigger the ventilator. The Infant Star, Babylog 8000, and Bird VIP all have demand as well as continuous flow, which may decrease the work of breathing. Comparisons of triggering systems using the same ventilator and electronic equipment have favored these airway pressure systems over the Graseby capsule. However, adding a flow sensor to the circuit may increase resistance that might have to be compensated for by an increase in peak inspiratory pressure or ventilator rate.

When using any of the triggering modes, the infant must be carefully observed clinically to determine that the system is not missing breaths. All ventilators listed in Table 25-16 have a display to indicate whether a breath is machine-delivered or spontaneous, assisted or controlled. Any of the sensors may fail or become insensitive for a variety of reasons. For example, low spontanous flow rates, large air leaks, thick secretions in the flow systems, improper placement of capsule or leads, infant position, and autocycling (inappropriate triggering) can lead to failure in any system. The most common cause of autocycling is vibration of water in the tube (the to-and-fro motion of the water can create a pressure drop or change in flow large enough to trigger the ventilator).

Other causes are leaks in the flow systems and fluctuations in the flow of the ventilator itself. Ventilators can not distinguish between patient or artifact triggering, and artifacts can result in a falsely rapid rate readout. A study of the Sechrist, Infant Star, Bear Cub, and SLE2000 showed all four triggering systems were significantly more reliable in infants at >27 weeks of gestation; this difference was even more significant in infants with chronic lung disease.

Patient-Assisted Ventilation is the newest mode of ventilation. Instead of a set airway pressure waveform being given with each breath, the amount of support is continuously proportional to the patient's respiratory effort throughout the cycle. This mode can be found on the Stephan ventilator, but it does not yet have FDA approval. Experience in newborns to date is limited.

Aerosol Administration

Administration of β-adrenergic agonists improves pulmonary function measurements in children with CLD, at least as assessed over the course of several hours. Spontaneously breathing infants may receive these drugs through a nebulizer after dilution with normal saline. Racemic epinephrine may also be given in this manner to extubated infants who are having difficulty with upper airway swelling. Intubated infants can be removed from the mechanical ventilator, a nebulizer can be placed in line between an anesthesia circuit and the baby, and the medication may be administered by manual inflations. When using this technique, care must be taken not to increase the FIO_2 or the inflating pressures beyond those with which the infant is being ventilated. It is important to note that the delivery of aerosolized medications to intubated infants is both extremely inefficient and highly variable from treatment to treatment and between babies as well. There is no uniformly agreed on manner in which to optimally deliver aerosolized medications. The use of spacing devices for metered-dose inhalers in intubated and spontaneously breathing newborns is an area of very active research.

Chest Physical Therapy

Chest physical therapy (CPT), or bronchopulmonary segmental drainage, uses three techniques—percussion, vibration, and postural drainage—to loosen secretions and move them into a larger airway for removal. In the absence of a therapist-driven protocol, it is helpful for a prescribing physician to specify the frequency, mode, and area of concentration of this therapy. The duration of therapy is chosen by the amount of secretions and on how well the baby tolerates the procedure.

For maximal effectiveness, the lobe or segment of the lung at which therapy is directed should be known to the person performing the CPT. It is also important for the therapist to know the anatomic location of each bronchus and the position that drains each bronchus. Therapy should emphasize the area most involved, and that area should be in the most vertical (superior) position to facilitate movement of secretions from smaller to larger airways. Drainage from one area usually means drainage into another area, and consequently, the opposite lobe or segment should also be treated if all positions are not being done.

Percussion uses mechanical energy applied to the chest wall to detach secretions from airway walls and allow drainage. A common way to do this is with an infant resuscitation mask with the 15-mm adapter occluded to make a cushion of air. Speed and force of percussion need not be excessive; a relaxed rhythmic rate achieves adequate segmental drainage. Each area should be percussed for 3 to 5 minutes.

Chest physical therapy given to adults includes vibration during expiration. The high respiratory rate typical of newborns precludes exclusive expiratory-phase vibration. Commonly, a mechanical vibrator is used; a padded electric toothbrush functions very well for this purpose also. Two minutes of vibration to each area is recommended.

Sometimes CPT constitutes a significant stress for ill infants. This is often manifested as arterial desaturation during therapy, which may continue after therapy is completed. For this reason CPT should not be given within one-half hour of feedings. Percussion is not recommended for infants weighing less than 1500 g because of the possibility of bruising and rib fracture. Most infants generally do well with vibration only, although a few may tolerate changes in position as the sole form of CPT.

Respiratory Monitoring

Management of newborns receiving oxygen therapy requires accurate and continuous monitoring to ensure both the adequacy and safety of therapy. Both hyperoxia and hypoxia must be avoided. Arterial blood gas levels are the gold standard for patient management, but even when an indwelling arterial line is present, this information is available only intermittently. It has been demonstrated that the use of transcutaneous PO_2 monitors and pulse oximeters has the potential to reduce the amount of time that the infant spends with undesirable oxygenation.

□ TRANSCUTANEOUS GAS MONITORS

Transcutaneous monitors measure the partial pressure of oxygen and sometimes carbon dioxide that diffuses through the skin. This is accomplished by heating the skin to produce local vasodilatation and to facilitate diffusion. The transcutaneous PO_2 ($tcPO_2$) approximates the PaO_2 closely, and for a given infant, the differences between these two values should be constant over several hours time. For safety considerations, as well as for concerns about accuracy, these devices should be used in strict compliance with the manufacturer's guidelines. This is of particular concern for skin temperature and the interval between changing of sites with recalibration. During the warm-up time, readings are unreliable. It is especially important that the membrane be in good contact with the skin and that bony areas be avoided. Several conditions, including hypothermia, poor peripheral perfusion, hypovolemia, and subcutaneous edema, as well as the drug tolazoline, make $tcPO_2$ values less reliable.

□ PULSE OXIMETRY

Pulse oximetry is widely used in the monitoring of oxygenation. A color difference between oxygenated and deoxygenated hemoglobin makes this method of monitoring possible. Extinction is a measure of how dark or absorptive a given material, in this case, hemoglobin, is at a specified wavelength of light. Oximetry is based on an empirically derived extinction curve for hemoglobin in human subjects. The extinction at 660 nm is compared with the extinction at 940 nm, and this ratio is translated into a percentage saturation of hemoglobin by comparison with an internal calibration curve. The value given on the digital display is oxygen saturation, or SpO_2.

The pulse oximeter is extremely accurate. When the ECG-determined heart rate agrees with the pulse oximeter heart rate, and the oximeter waveform is regular and of good amplitude, the accuracy of a pulse oximeter is $\pm 2\%$. The response time of the oximeter is very short, measured in seconds. This high degree of accuracy and the short response time are advantages of oximetry over $tcPO_2$ monitoring.

Despite the usefulness of this technique, there are several limitations to pulse oximetry. The oximeter is unable to give accurate data if it cannot detect an adequate waveform. This sometimes represents a problem in location of the oximeter lead. This problem can be minimized by using the oximeter in exact accordance with the manufacturer's recommendations. When an infant has significant compromise of cardiac output, as during cardiogenic or hypovolemic shock, the oximeter may be unable to detect arterial pulsations and, thus, unable to determine saturation values.

Another limitation of pulse oximetry relates to the shape of the oxyhemoglobin dissociation curve. Adult hemoglobin becomes essentially 100% saturated at a PaO_2 of 75 mmHg, and fetal hemoglobin at the significantly lower value of 55 mmHg. Thus, a pulse oximeter is unable to discriminate between the newborn with a PaO_2 of 60 mmHg and the newborn with a PaO_2 of 250 mmHg. Hyperoxia can be avoided when it is important to do so, as with preterm infants, by administering oxygen to obtain an oxygen saturation of 93% to 95%. This allows the oxygen content of the blood to be nearly maximal while ensuring that the PaO_2 is not dangerously high.

□ CAPNOGRAPHY

Capnography, or end-tidal carbon dioxide determination, is currently undergoing evaluation to determine its role in neonatal respiratory management. End-tidal carbon dioxide is the carbon dioxide in the last portion of an expired breath; these terminal gases have their origins in the alveolar space. When the lung consists of multiple homogeneous units, end-tidal carbon dioxide reflects alveolar PCO_2 accurately. Under most circumstances, alveolar PCO_2 equals arterial PCO_2. Expired gas is analyzed for absorption of infrared light, and the carbon dioxide content is read at a specific wavelength. Thus, these devices have the potential to continuously determine and display arterial PCO_2. However, the assumption that the lung is made of homogeneously emptying smaller units is often untrue when lung disease, which tends to be heterogeneous, is present. The relation between end-tidal carbon dioxide and alveolar carbon dioxide concentrations then becomes uncertain. Other assumptions made in the use of end-tidal carbon dioxide monitoring include a constant rate of carbon dioxide production by the baby and constant pulmonary capillary blood flow. In certain disease states, either of these assumptions may be untrue as well. These considerations have to date limited the use of this type of monitoring to intraoperative monitoring of infants with healthy lungs and confirmation of tracheal positioning of the endotracheal tube. Whether further refinements in this technique will lead to greater applicability remains to be seen.

REFERENCES

1. Boyden EA: Growth and Development of the Airways. In WA Hodson (ed): Development of the Lung. New York, Marcel Dekker, 1977, pp 3–35
2. Gross I: Regulation of Fetal Lung Maturation. In P Ballard (ed): Respiratory Distress Syndrome. London, Academic Press, 1984, pp 51–64
3. Reid LM: Structural Development of the Lung and Pulmonary Circulation. In P Ballard (ed): Respiratory Distress Syndrome. London, Academic Press, 1984, pp 3–18
4. Jobe A: Surfactant Function and Metabolism. In BR Boynton, WA Carlo, AH Jobe (eds): New Therapies for Neonatal Respiratory Failure: A Physiological Approach. New York, Cambridge University Press, 1994, pp 16–35
5. Bland RD: Pathogenesis of pulmonary edema after premature birth. Adv Pediatr 34:175, 1987
6. Teitel D, Rudolph AM: Perinatal oxygen delivery and cardiac function. Adv Pediatr 32:321, 1985
7. Roberts JD, Abman SH: Physiology of Nitric Oxide in the Perinatal Lung. In BR Boynton, WA Carlo, AH Jobe (eds): New Therapies for Neonatal Respiratory Failure: A Physiological Approach. New York, Cambridge University Press, 1994, pp 339–348
8. American Heart Association, American Academy of Pediatrics: Neonatal Resuscitation. In L Chameides (ed): Textbook of Pediatric Advanced Life Support. American Heart Association, 1988, pp 69–76
9. Mannino FL, Merritt TA: The Management of Respiratory Distress Syndrome. In DW Thibeault, GA Gregory (eds): Neonatal Pulmonary Care, 2nd ed. Norwalk, CT, Appleton-Century-Crofts, 1986, pp 349–366

10. National Institutes of Health Consensus Conference: Effect of corticosteroids for fetal maturation on perinatal outcomes. JAMA 273:413, 1995
11. Corbet A, Bucciarelli R, Goldman S, et al: Decreased mortality rate among small premature infants treated at birth with a single dose of synthetic surfactant: A multicenter controlled trial. J Pediatr 118:277, 1991
12. Dunn MS, Shennan A, Zayack D, and Possmayer F: Bovine surfactant replacement therapy in neonates of less than 30 weeks gestation: A randomized, controlled trial of prophylaxis versus treatment. Pediatrics 87:377, 1991
13. Hoekstra RE, Jackson JC, Myers TF, et al: Improved neonatal survival following multiple doses of bovine surfactant in very premature neonates at risk for respiratory distress syndrome. Pediatrics 88:10, 1991
14. Horbar JD, Wright LL, Soll RF, et al: A multicenter randomixed trial comparing two surfactants for the treatment of neonatal respiratory distress syndrome. J Pediatr 123:757, 1993
15. Kendig JW, Notter RH, Cox C, et al: A comparison of surfactant as immediate prophylaxis and as rescue therapy in newborns of less than 30 weeks' gestation. N Engl J Med 324:865, 1991
16. Liechty EA, Donovan E, Purohit D, et al: Reduction of neonatal mortality after multiple doses of bovine surfactant in low birth weight neonates with respiratory distress syndrome. Pediatrics 88:19, 1991
17. Long W, Thompson T, Sundell H, et al: Effects of two doses of a synthetic surfactant on mortality rate and survival without bronchopulmonary dysplasia in 750–1350 gram infants with respiratory distress syndrome. J Pediatr 118:595, 1991
18. Kattwinkel J, Bloom BT, Delmore P, et al: Prophylactic administration of calf lung surfactant extract is more effective than early treatment of respiratory distress syndrome in neonates of 29 through 32 weeks gestation. Pediatrics 92:90, 1993
19. Soll RF, Merritt TA, Hallman W: Surfactant in the Prevention and Treatment of Respiratory Distress Syndrome. In BR Boynton, WA Carlo, AH Jobe (eds): New Therapies for Neonatal Respiratory Failure: A Physiological Approach. New York, Cambridge University Press, 1994, pp 74–75.
20. Auten RL, Notter RH, Kendig JW, et al: Surfactant treatment of full term newborns with respiratory failure. Pediatrics 87:101, 1991
21. Khammash H, Perlman M, Wojtulewicz J, et al: Surfactant therapy in full-term neonates with severe respiratory failure. Pediatrics 92:135, 1993
22. Davis JM, Notter RH: Lung Surfactant Replacement for Neonatal Abnormalities Other than Primary Respiratory Distress Syndrome. In BR Boynton, WA Carlo, AH Jobe (eds): New Therapies for Neonatal Respiratory Failure: A Physiological Approach. New York, Cambridge University Press, 1994, pp 81–92
23. Victorin LH, Deveragan LV, Curstedt T, et al: Surfactant replacement is spontaneously breathing babies with hyaline membrane disease: A pilot study. Biol Neonate 58:121, 1990
24. Verder H, Robertson B, Greisein G, et al: Surfactant therapy and nasal continuous positive airway pressure for newborns with respiratory distress syndrome. N Engl J Med 331:1051, 1994.
25. Gregory GA: Continuous Positive Airway Pressure. In DW Thibeault, GA Gregory (eds): Neonatal Pulmonary Care, 2nd ed. Norwalk, CT, Appleton-Century-Crofts, 1986, pp 349–366
26. Boynton BR, Hammond MD: Pulmonary Gas Exchange: Basic Principles and the Effects of Mechanical Ventilation. In BR Boynton, WA Carlo, AH Jobe (eds): New Therapies for Neonatal Respiratory Failure: A Physiological Approach. New York, Cambridge University Press, 1994, pp 115–129
27. Carlo WA, Greenough A, Chatburn RL: Advances in Conventional Mechanical Ventilation. In BR Boynton, WA Carlo, AH Jobe (eds): New Therapies for Neonatal Respiratory Failure: A Physiological Approach. New York, Cambridge University Press, 1994, pp 131–151
28. Clark RH: High frequency ventilation. J Pediatr 124:661, 1994
29. Cronin JH: High frequency ventilator therapy for newborns. J Intensive Care Med 9:71, 1994
30. Fox WW, Murray JP, Martin RJ: Transient Tachypnea. In AA Fanaroff, RJ Martin (eds): Behrman's Neonatal-Perinatal Medicine: Diseases of the Fetus and Infant. St Louis, CV Mosby, 1983, pp 447–448
31. Bucciarelli RL, Egan EA, Gessner IH, Eitzman DV: Persistence of fetal cardiopulmonary circulation: One manifestation of transient tachypnea of the newborn. Pediatrics 58:192, 1976
32. Halliday HL, McClure G, Reid MAC: Transient tachypnea of the newborn: Two distinct clinical entities? Arch Dis Child 56:322, 1981
33. Givner LB, Baker CJ: The prevention and treatment of neonatal group B streptococcal infections. Adv Pediatr Infect Dis 3:65, 1988
34. Fox WW, Gewitz MH, Dinwiddie R, et al: Pulmonary hypertension in the perinatal aspiration syndromes. Pediatrics 59:205, 1977
35. Fox WW, Duara S: Persistent pulmonary hypertension in the neonate: Diagnosis and management. J Pediatr 103:505, 1983
36. Bartlett RH, Roloff DW, Cornell RG, et al: Extracorporeal circulation in neonatal respiratory failure: A prospective randomized study. Pediatrics 76:479, 1985
37. Kanto WP: A decade of experience with neonatal extracorporeal membrane oxygenation. J Pediatr 124:335, 1994
38. Madansky DL, Lawson EE, Chernick V, Taeusch HW: Pneumothorax and other forms of pulmonary air leak in newborns. Am Rev Respir Dis 120:729, 1979
39. Martin MJ, Miller RJ, Carlo WA: Pathogenesis of apnea in preterm infants. J Pediatr 109:733, 1986
40. Perlman JM, Volpe JJ: Episodes of apnea and bradycardia in the preterm newborn: Impact on cerebral circulation. Pediatrics 76:333, 1985
41. Harrison MR, Adzick S, Estes JM, et al: A prospective study of the outcome for fetuses with diaphragmatic hernia. JAMA 271:382, 1994
42. Bohn D, Tamura M, Perrin D, et al: Ventilatory predictors of pulmonary hypoplasia in congenital diaphragmatic hernia, confirmed by morphologic assessment. J Pediatr 111:423, 1987
43. Reynolds M, Luck SR, Lappen R: The "critical" neonate with diaphragmatic hernia: A 21 year perspective. J Pediatr Surg 19:385, 1984
44. Hansen J, James S, Burrington J, Whitfield J: The decreasing incidence of pneumothorax and improving survival of infants with congenital diaphragmatic hernia. J Pediatr Surg 19:385, 1984
45. Fiascone JM, Rhodes TT, Grandgeorge SR, Knapp MA: Bronchopulmonary dysplasia: A review for the pediatrician. Curr Probl Pediatr 19:169, 1989
46. O'Brodovich HM, Mellins RB: Bronchopulmonary dysplasia: Unresolved neonatal lung injury. Am Rev Respir Dis 132:694, 1985
47. Heldt GP, Bernstein G: Patient-initiated mechanical ventilation. In BR Boynton, WA Carlo, AH Jobe (eds): New Therapies for Neonatal Respiratory Failure: A Physiological Approach. New York, Cambridge University Press, 1994, pp 152–170
48. Chan V, Greenough A: Randomized controlled trial of weaning by patient triggered mechanical ventilation or conventional ventilation. Europ J Pediatr 152:51, 1993
49. Cleary JP, Bernstein G, Heldt GP, et al: Improved oxygenation during synchronized versus intermittent mandatory ventilation in VLBW infants with respiratory distress: A randomized cross over design. Pediatr Res 33:207A, 1993

26 Respiratory Care for the Infant and Child

Jackie L. Long-Goding

CLINICAL SKILLS

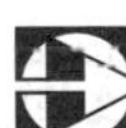

Upon completion of this chapter, the reader will be able to:

- Identify how a family adapts to having a sick child
- Explain how the anatomy of a child makes the physical examination different
- Conduct a patient interview with the patient and family
- Assess a patient through inspection, palpation, percussion, and auscultation
- Explain the methods of oxygen therapy to patient and family
- List situations in which chest physiotherapy may be necessary
- Determine when age, size, and physical condition of a child permits use of incentive spirometry
- Correctly administer aerosol and humidity therapy to a pediatric patient
- Determine whether intubation is necessary, and intubate a pediatric patient
- Suction a patient's airway by means of orotracheal or nasotracheal suctioning
- Select a ventilator for mechanical ventilation of a pediatric patient, set it up, and successfully monitor and then wean a pediatric patient
- Recognize the major respiratory disorders in infants and children, and provide the necessary therapies

KEY TERMS

Auscultation
Autogenic drainage (AD)
Croup tents
Forced expiration technique (FET)
Functionalism
Heat and moisture exchanger (HME)
High-frequency compression
Inspection
Near drowning
Palpation
Percussion
Pneumonia
Positive expiratory pressure (PEP) therapy
Postural drainage
Prodrome
Tuberculosis
Vibration

Health care professionals who provide care to pediatric patients must recognize that they are not only interacting with the child as the patient, but also with all members of the child's family. Consequently, clinicians should have a basic understanding of human growth and development as well as family dynamics. Theories of child development are well documented in works by Sigmund Freud, Lawrence Kohlberg, Jean Piaget, Erik Erikson (Boxes 26-1 and 26-2), and B. F. Skinner, as well as others in the fields of psychology and sociology.[1–4] A complete discussion of these theories is beyond the scope of this chapter; however, the reader is referred to almost any introductory psychology text for an overall discussion of the theoretical frameworks. The tools provided by psychoanalytic theory can be extremely helpful when caring for children, because the clinician can use those tools to objectively evaluate the behavior of both the patient and the family. Motives, emotions, and fantasies influence human behavior,[4] and the health care provider needs to be able to recognize how each of these can influence patient and family compliance with the care plan.

Each member of a family, as well as each member of the health care team, is expected to play certain *roles* within his or her environment. Although role definition is changing to reflect contemporary life-styles, conflict and misunderstandings between health care providers and families often arise when the health care providers apply their expectations to the behavior of the parents (both mother and father). The sociologic paradigm of *functionalism*, as described by Talcott Parsons,[5] is useful in allowing the clinician to evaluate and understand what may appear, at first glance, to be unusual behaviors by various family members. Parsons used the concept of *systems* as his theoretical framework. Consequently, a family can be viewed as a system, and the Parsonian theory of functionalism can be used to analyze and describe how a family functions when a child is ill enough to require hospitalization.

The familial structure grounds the family as a primary social system. Because the family has shared values (returning the family member to his or her baseline health status), it also functions as a cultural system. Stability and control of the family as a functional unit are maintained through the tenets of the cultural system. Parsons assumed that all systems would want to remain in equilibrium, or a state of balance. Clearly, the stresses associated with having a sick child are disruptive to the equilibrium of the family unit. Parson's theory of functionalism assumes that the family returns to equilibrium through four functions: Adaptation, Goal attainment, Integration, and Latent pattern maintenance—tension management (AGIL).

The family is the primary source of psychosocial support during an illness.[6] A health care provider can use Parsonian theory to identify elements of disequilibrium and develop strategies to assist the family with returning to a "normal state," or equilibrium. According to Parsonian theory, the family maintains itself as a unit through adaptive functions, which may be observed as mechanisms for coping; goal attainment functions, such as returning the sick child to health; and integrative functions and latent pattern maintenance–tension management, both of which allow the family to adjust to the new structure and its concomitant tensions and conflicts. The integrative function, or integration, allows family members to adjust to systematic change to keep the family intact. Latent pattern maintenance means that family members are motivated to assume their roles in the family, and tension management means that there is some mechanism for managing tension within the family.

Health care providers can play an important role in the integration of the family by empowering family members through communication and education. A review of nursing care plans frequently identifies alter-

BOX 26-1

INFANCY

Erik Erikson describes infancy as a period of conflict between trust and mistrust. The infant develops trust when his or her needs are met by the parents or other primary care givers. When an infant is hospitalized he or she may have difficulty determining whether the clinician who is approaching the crib represents safety, or whether another painful incident is about to occur. The infant's mistrust of the clinician is illustrated when the infant begins to cry before the treatment begins.

Respiratory care practitioners may find that an infant responds better during an aerosolized bronchodilator treatment when the parent is allowed to hold the infant. A parent could also be encouraged to touch or caress the infant on a limb during positioning for chest physical therapy.

BOX 26-2

ADOLESCENCE

Adolescence is generally defined as those years that span the period between the onset of puberty and maturity. During adolescence, one is trying to establish a sense of identity. To establish that identity, the adolescent uses cultural and familial norms, or expectations. Teenagers are, by and large, healthy individuals who are growing and rapidly becoming young men and women. Even healthy adolescents, or teenagers, experience episodes of identity conflict that manifest as confusion, frustration, and isolation. When a teenager is confronted with an illness that is serious enough to require hospitalization, there is conflict between the role the teenaged patient is forced to assume and the role that is perceived as normal. This conflict is sometimes displayed as anger, preoccupation, withdrawal, or rude behavior. When an adolescent is faced with a chronic illness, it may be difficult to establish a sense of identity. Erik Erikson characterized the psychosocial crises experienced by adolescents as "identity versus identity confusion." Practitioners can use Erikson's theoretical framework to assist them in developing a therapeutic relationship with adolescent patients.

ations in the family process as a nursing diagnosis,[7] which describes mechanisms wherein the nurse, and by extension other health care providers, can work with family members to enable them to adapt to the illness of the child.

The benefits of empowering the family and involving them in the care of a child were identified by Harrison and Mitchell.[8] Children of empowered families are much less likely to be abandoned by the family, especially when the family is involved in the care of the patient from the beginning of the illness. Many laypeople feel inadequate when interacting with highly educated physicians and other allied health professionals. These feelings of inadequacy can translate into issues surrounding communication and empowerment. The health care provider, therefore, has a responsibility to explain the therapeutic goals in language that can be understood by the patient's family. Care-giving tasks must be divided into multiple components. Education and training programs for the primary care giver must begin with simple information and progress through more complex aspects of each task. The health care provider also has a responsibility to evaluate how well the family understands the therapeutic goals. This can easily be accomplished by asking members of the family to repeat what has been said to them, or by asking them to perform a procedure that has been explained and demonstrated to them.

As the health care system in this country continues to respond to cost-saving strategies, families will assume more of the responsibility for providing care for chronically ill children. The concept of family-centered care requires the participation of all family members in the care of the sick child. Family involvement must begin at diagnosis and continue through recovery or, in the case of a terminal illness, the death of the child.[9] To function effectively within the family-centered care model, respiratory care practitioners, as well as all members of the health care team, need to understand the basis of child-family interactions, concepts of family dynamics, strategies for stress management and stress reduction, and case management designs in both the acute care and long-term care environments.

ASSESSMENT OF THE CHILD WITH RESPIRATORY DISEASE

Characteristics of the Pediatric Airway

The first, and perhaps most important, thing to remember when assessing an infant or child in respiratory distress is that the pediatric airway is **not** just a smaller version of the adult airway. As a result of the anatomic and physiologic differences, children may confront the respiratory care practitioner with a higher sense of urgency than an adult with a similar illness. In the newborn, the trachea is shorter and narrower than the larynx, which is approximately one third the size of an adult's. The cricoid cartilage, which is the only complete cartilage ring in the upper airway, forms the narrowest part of the upper airway. The epiglottis is narrower and more vertically positioned than in an adult. For approximately the first 18 months of life, the epiglottis makes frequent contact with the infant's soft palate, thus transforming the infant's larynx into two channels. The anterior channel serves as the passageway for air into the trachea, while the posterior channel allows suckled liquids to pass into the esophagus. The characteristic ability of an infant to "lock" the soft palate and larynx led to the use of the term "obligatory nasal breather" to describe human infants.[10] We now know, however, that all infants can breathe through the oral passageway if the nasal route becomes obstructed; therefore, a more accurate term to describe an infant's respiratory maneuvers is "preferential, or predominant, nasal breathing."[11]

The epiglottis in an infant or young child is softer and more bulky than in an adult. The arytenoid mounds are also more prominent. These anatomical differences are largely responsible for stridor being a more frequent finding in an infant than in an adult. The epithelial cells in the larynx and trachea of an infant differ from the adult only in the distribution and the size of the area that contains cilia. The airway mucosa in an infant becomes edematous quite readily when it is exposed to irritate.[10] These anatomic and physiologic differences in the infant and child make upper airway diseases such as epiglottitis, croup, and subglottic laryngitis more dangerous in this patient population.

At birth, the larynx is located relatively high in the newborn's neck. The larynx descends as the infant grows into a child, primarily because of changes in the shape of the skull related to growth and the movement of the tongue downward toward the pharynx. By age six, children have an upper airway that closely resembles that of an adult, with the lower border of the cricoid cartilage anatomically located at the level of the sixth cervical vertebra.[10] The pharynx has become a common passageway for both food and inspired gases. Though this anatomical configuration has advantages related to speech, it presents several hazards associated with aspiration of food and other foreign bodies.

Obtaining a History Through Interviewing

Respiratory care practitioners, as well as all other health care providers, should recognize the value of an interview when attempting to assess a patient. The patient or, in the case of a young child, the parent or primary caretaker can provide valuable insight into symptoms that can be used to establish a diagnosis. Each patient brings a unique presentation of the illness, because each individual personalizes signs and symptoms.

Talking with a patient during an interview serves three purposes: (1) the clinician learns about the patient's illness as the patient or family member perceives it, (2) important clinical data are gathered, and (3) the therapeutic relationship is established when the patient, or family members, feel that they have been heard and understood.[12] The respiratory care practitioner does not usually take a multisystem, comprehensive history; however, the history section of the medical record should be reviewed before seeing the patient. The components of a complete medical history are illustrated in Box 26-3. The practitioner can identify relevant areas of the history that should be expanded when the practitioner completes a focused interview as part of the initial respiratory therapy session.

Establishing a therapeutic relationship with the child and his or her family requires the practitioner's full attention. Having first reviewed the chart, the practitioner approaches the patient's room with not only a sense of who the patient is, but also a mental picture of the diagnosis and how respiratory care can play a role in the resolution of this episode or illness. Immediately on entering the patient's room, the practitioner should begin the process of patient evaluation. The first component of a physical examination, *inspection,* actually begins during the interview process. If the patient is an infant or very young child, the practitioner should address questions to the parent or primary caretaker. Although it is acceptable to use a first name when addressing a child, questions to the parent should be prefaced with the surname, for example, Mr. Jones or Mrs. Smith. Children who are school aged can answer questions themselves and, in so doing, provide an opportunity for the practitioner to assess the child's perceptions of his or her own illness.

Interviewing an adolescent patient often presents a source of frustration for both the practitioner and the patient. Much of the frustration may be linked to the adolescent's self-perception, while another source is frequently the manner in which the practitioner approaches the patient. It must be remembered that, although an adolescent may physically resemble an adult, the adolescent responds to stresses and crises very differently than an adult. Consequently, the practitioner needs to focus on the adolescent patient as a person, rather than focusing on the illness or its manifestations.

During the interview, the practitioner should observe factors that indicate the work of breathing. Is there alar flaring in an infant or young child? If the child's chest is visible, is there evidence of chest wall retractions? Is there observable use of the accessory muscles of inspiration? During expiration, does the abdomen appear to rise? Does the child or adolescent speak in full sentences, or is it necessary for the patient to stop after every two or three words to take a breath? Skin color can also be observed during the interview. Is there evidence of cyanosis? Is the child pale? If the patient was admitted with acute asthma, is there evidence of allergic shiners (the skin below the eyes appears discolored or bruised)?

Physical Examination

The respiratory care practitioner can obtain valuable information concerning the patient's respiratory status through the four components of patient assessment: inspection, palpation, percussion, and auscultation.

BOX 26-3

COMPONENTS OF A COMPREHENSIVE HISTORY FOR A PEDIATRIC PATIENT

Date of History
This establishes the historical reference for the history. The time is sometimes included.

Identifying Data
The date and place of birth is included. The child's nickname, if one is used, should be included. Parental information, such as first and last names and their occupations, may be found here.

Chief Complaints
The person who offers the complaint must be clearly identified in this section. For example, is the complaint offered by the parent, the child, or another relevant party?

Present Illness
This section expands the chief complaints. The symptoms should be described in full detail and in chronological order. The events that led to the development of each symptom should be included. Also found in this section is information concerning how both the child and the family respond to the illness.

Past History
This section includes information about the birth history, relevant prenatal and neonatal incidents, the feeding history and eating habits, and growth and development history. The growth and development history contains information related to physical growth, attainment of developmental milestones, and a review of social development. Previous hospitalizations and illnesses, as well as recent exposures to other childhood illnesses, appear in this section.

Current Health Status
Important information concerning allergies, immunization status, and the dates and results of screening tests is found in this section.

Family History
Information contained in this section assists the health care provider in determining the degree of risk for certain illnesses with familial associations. The psychosocial history, also frequently found in this section, assists the practitioner in evaluating how the patient and family respond to illness and hospitalization. This is also an important source of information that allows the practitioner to take the initial steps in developing a therapeutic relationship with the patient and his family.

Review of Systems
During the review of systems, focused questioning can help the practitioner determine if problems, other than the chief complaints, exist.

Adapted with permission from Bates B, Hoekelman RA: Interviewing and the Health History. In B Bates: A Guide to Physical Examination and History Taking, 6th ed. Philadelphia, JB Lippincott, 1995

□ INSPECTION

Inspection, or simple observation, allows the practitioner to evaluate the patient's growth and development. The size (height and weight) of the child should be compared to the normal ranges for the age of the child. The frequency and pattern of respirations should be noted. Normal vital sign measurements for various age groups of patients can be found in Table 26-1. The respiratory rate and heart rate increases more significantly in children than in adults in response to activity, emotional stress, and illness. Consequently, the respiratory rate should be measured while the child is either at rest or sleeping. Abdominal movement during respiration is more pronounced than thoracic expansion in an infant and young child; therefore, it is easier to monitor the respiratory rate by counting the abdominal movements.[13] The respiratory rate should be determined by counting the number of respirations in 1 full minute (60 seconds).

□ PALPATION

Palpation can be used to determine the heart rate when the practitioner palpates either the brachial or femoral arteries in an infant or small child. The radial artery can be successfully palpated in cooperative small children and in adolescents. Tactile fremitus, or vibrations of the chest wall caused by vibrations that originate in the vocal cords and travel down the tracheobronchial tree, can be assessed using palpation. When the patient is an infant, tactile fremitus can be assessed by the examiner's placing a hand, palm side down, over the child's chest while the child is crying. The hand should be moved in a systematic manner to cover all areas of the chest, including anterior, lateral, and posterior areas of the thorax. Just as in the adult patient, fremitus is increased when there is an increase in the density of the lung tissue, such as may occur when consolidation is present. Fremitus is decreased when there is an abnormal accumulation of either air or fluid in the chest.

Palpation of the chest can also be used to confirm the presence of mucus in the airways. As the child breathes, air travels through the mucous-laden airways and produces vibrations that can be felt through the chest wall. In this instance, the practitioner can almost always hear rhonchi during auscultation of the chest.

Finally, palpation can be used to determine the position of the trachea. The finding of a trachea that is displaced from midline carries the same implications in the pediatric patient as in the adult. In the case of atelectasis, the trachea is shifted toward the atelectatic lung. When the patient has a pneumothorax, the trachea is shifted toward the unaffected side, or away from the pneumothorax, during exhalation. During inhalation, the trachea moves toward the side on which the pneumothorax has occurred.[14]

□ PERCUSSION

Percussion is not particularly useful when assessing a small child. Because of the small amount of soft tissue on the chest and the relatively high compliance of the chest wall, the percussion note sounds much like that heard in a hyperinflated adult chest. Perceived changes in percussion note may be instructive, for example, when compared with previous examination or from left to right in the chest. In an older child or an adolescent patient, the principles of assessing percussion notes in the adult are applicable.

□ AUSCULTATION

A systematic approach is essential when auscultating the chest of all patients, including children. It may be helpful in establishing a trust relationship with a small child if the practitioner allows the parent to hold the child during auscultation. The examiner may gain even more rapport with the patient by letting him or her listen through the stethoscope first. Before beginning an auscultatory examination, the practitioner should warm the chest piece on the stethoscope by holding it in the palms of his hand. The practitioner should locate the anatomic position of the lobes and segments by linking them to surface landmarks and ensure that each segment is auscultated during the examination.

Auscultation should begin at the posterior bases and move toward the apical segments, with a comparison of the sounds heard on the right and left sides. Finally, auscultation of the anterior and lateral chest should be performed. If the child is lying in the supine position, it may be preferable to auscultate the anterior chest first, then reposition the child and auscultate the posterior chest. The same terms used to describe normal and adventitious breath sounds in the adult are used in pediatrics (vesicular, bronchovesicular, crackles, rhonchi, wheezes, and pleural friction rubs).

TABLE 26-1. **Vital Signs for the Pediatric Patient**

	Body Temperature		Heart Rate (in bpm)		Respiratory Rate (per minute)	Blood Pressure (in mmHg)
Age	***°F***	***°C***	***Range***	***Average***	***Average***	***Systolic/Diastolic***
Infant	99.7	37.7	80–180	125	40	74–100/50–70
Toddler	99.0	37.2	80–140	110	25	80–112/50–80
Preschooler	98.6	37.0	80–120	100	23	82–110/50–78
School-age child	98.3	36.8	70–115	100	20	84–120/54–80
Adolescent	97.8	36.6	50–110	80	16–18	94–140/62–88

The practitioner should first evaluate the degree of air movement. In an infant, the chest wall is thinner than in an adult. Consequently, normal breath sounds seem more harsh than vesicular sounds in the older child and adult. The presence of abnormal bronchial breath sounds, crackles, rhonchi, and wheezes carries the same implications in pediatrics as in adult care. For example, crackles may be indicative of congestive heart failure, atelectasis, pneumonia, or asthma. Wheezes can be either diffuse, in which case they likely indicate bronchoconstriction, or localized, in which case they are indicative of an airway obstruction such as might be encountered when the child aspirates a foreign body. Rhonchi are indicative of airway secretions. Stridor is another important auscultatory finding; however, a stethoscope is not required to hear it. Stridor indicates airflow through an obstructed larynx or trachea.

RESPIRATORY CARE PROCEDURES APPLIED TO THE PEDIATRIC PATIENT

Most, if not all, of the therapeutic procedures used to treat adults can be applied to the pediatric patient. The practitioner needs to consider the age and size of the patient, as well as the ability of the patient to understand and follow instructions, when preparing to administer respiratory care in the pediatric setting.

Oxygen Therapy

The indications for oxygen administration and the treatment goals for pediatric patients are the same as for an adult. Oxygen is a drug; therefore, the physician must prescribe either an FIO_2 or a delivery flow. When selecting an appropriate oxygen delivery device for children, the practitioner should consider the indications for oxygen administration, the prescribed FIO_2, and the age of the child. Delivery devices are provided in a variety of sizes to accommodate patients of various ages and sizes. Children receiving oxygen therapy should be routinely monitored, using either pulse oximetry (continuous or intermittent spot-checks) or periodic arterial blood gas analysis.

Nasal cannulae are frequently used to provide oxygen to infants and children.[15] Though relatively easy to use, nasal cannulae present problems related to controlling the oxygen concentration received by the patient. The oxygen concentration (FIO_2) delivered by the device is 1.0; however, the oxygen concentration received by the patient varies according to the oxygen flow, the patient's minute volume, the patient's peak inspiratory flow, whether the patient is breathing through the mouth or nose, and the manner in which the prongs are positioned within the nares.[15–17] A nasal cannula is usually considered a low-flow device that delivers low to medium oxygen concentrations; however, nasal cannulae can actually deliver medium to high oxygen concentrations in a small child or infant. The relationship between the delivered oxygen concentration, oxygen flow, and the size of the child can be understood by (1) converting oxygen flow from liters per minute to liters per second, (2) approximating an inspiratory time by determining the respiratory rate and I:E ratio, and (3) calculating an estimated FIO_2 (Equation Box 26-1).[18] If any of these variables change, the resulting change in FIO_2 can cause the patient's oxygenation to increase or decrease significantly.

EQUATION BOX 26–1

ESTIMATING FIO_2 BASED ON OXYGEN FLOW TO NASAL CANNULA AND PATIENT SIZE

Assume that two patients with respiratory rates of 30 breaths/min are each receiving oxygen via nasal cannula at 1 L/min. The first patient is a 5 kg infant with a tidal volume of 30 mL. First, convert 1 L/min oxygen to mL/sec:

1 L/min = 1000 mL/min = 16.7 mL oxygen/sec coming through the nasal cannula

Next, assume that observation of the infant's respiratory pattern indicates that the I:E ratio is 1:3. Inspiratory time can then be approximated as follows:

Total cycle time can be determined by dividing 60 seconds by the respiratory rate: 60/30 = 2 seconds. Next, add the parts of the I:E ratio (1 + 3 = 4), and divide the total cycle time by the total parts (2/4) to obtain the portion of the total cycle time that is allotted to inspiration (0.5 seconds). The remainder of the total cycle time is then allotted to the expiratory cycle.

16.5 mL/second × 0.5 second = 8.3 mL × FIO_2 1.0 = 8.3 mL oxygen coming through the the nasal cannula

The remainder of the patient's tidal volume, 21.7 mL, is entrained room air with an FIO_2 of .21 (21.7 × .21) Therefore, 4.6 mL of oxygen is being added.

To estimate the FIO_2, the following calculation can be performed:

8.3 + 4.6 = 12.9/30 = .43

The second patient is a 50 kg adolescent with a tidal volume of 325 mL. For consistency, let's assume that this patient's I:E ratio is also observed to be 1:3. The FIO_2 can be calculated following the same steps used for the first patient. The amount of oxygen coming through the nasal cannula is the same, 16.7 mL/second. This patient's inspiratory time is also 0.5 second; therefore, 8.3 mL oxygen comes through the cannula. This patient's tital volume, however, is significantly larger at 325 mL. Therefore, 316.7 mL of the tidal volume represents entrained room air, and 66.50 mL of oxygen are being added.

8.3 + 66.50 = 74.8/325 = 0.23

This is only a rough estimation of FIO_2; remember, it will change as the respiratory rate, inspiratory time (which is being used as an approximation of inspiratory flow) and tidal volume change. It does illustrate, however, the need for practitioners to consider the oxygen concentration that will ultimately be delivered when a nasal cannula is used to administer oxygen to an infant or small child.

Adapted from Aoki BY and McCloskey K.[18] Evaluation, Stabilization, and Transport of the Critically Ill Child. St. Louis (MO): Mosby Year Book, Inc., 1992:14

Low-flow flow meters (calibrated to 1 L/min in 1 mL increments, and calibrated to 3 L/min in 1/8 L increments) are available and should be used when administering oxygen to infants and small children. These flow meters allow the practitioner to control more precisely the amount of oxygen being delivered to the patient. Pediatric patients may be quite active and tend to remove extraneous (to them) items, such as oxygen cannulae. Consequently, it is often necessary to secure the device in place. Commercial fasteners and tape used to secure intravenous lines (Tegaderm, 3M Medical Surgical Division, St. Paul, MN) can be used to minimize dislodging of the cannulae. The use of adhesive tape should be avoided because it may cause breakdown of the skin.

Oxygen hoods are most suited for use with neonates and quiet infants. Oxygen hoods can be either disposable or nondisposable, and they are composed of clear plastic or Plexiglass. Oxygen hoods provide a chamber that encloses the head of the infant while allowing easy access to the infant's body for nursing care. A relatively stable oxygen concentration can be provided in a variety of clinical environments. Oxygen hoods can be used on radiant warmers, in cribs, and in isolettes.

Oxygen is delivered to an inlet port, which is usually located in the rear of the chamber, using wide-bore or aerosol tubing. The delivered oxygen concentration is controlled either by using an oxygen blender that is set at the prescribed FIO_2 or by using a large-volume nebulizer. When a nebulizer is used, it is recommended that the air entrainment be set at 100% and powered using compressed air, while bleeding oxygen from a flow meter into the aerosol tubing using a T-piece adapter. The noise levels generated when the air-entrainment port on a nebulizer is used to control the delivered FIO_2,[19] as well as the potential for the particulate water carrying airborne bacteria, both create unacceptable hazards for the newborn. The respiratory care practitioner can use air-oxygen entrainment ratios to efficiently establish the flows of compressed air and oxygen necessary to deliver the desired FIO_2.

The delivered FIO_2 should be continuously monitored using an oxygen analyzer sensor placed as close to the infant's face as possible. The temperature inside the oxygen hood should also be monitored continuously and maintained between 34° and 36°C, because delivery of gas that is either too hot or too cold increases the infant's oxygen consumption. Finally, it should be remembered that oxygen hoods can accumulate exhaled carbon dioxide. As a result, flows of at least 7 L/min should be provided to prevent the infant's rebreathing carbon dioxide. Oxygen hoods are provided in a variety of sizes and can generally be used on infants who weigh up to 5.4 kg. When infants exceed the size limits for an oxygen hood, a flexible, plastic tent that covers the infant's head and thorax, called a Tenthouse (Nova Health Systems Inc. Blackwood, NJ), can be used to provide oxygen therapy.

Oxygen tents, also known as croup tents, have limited use as an oxygen delivery device. This is related to the difficulty in delivering and maintaining a desired FIO_2. Oxygen is delivered into the canopy, or tent, through a nebulizer. The nebulizer also produces the aerosol particles that are circulated into the tent. Tents are prone to leaks from tears in the canopy itself, as well as from loose seals around the crib or bed mattress. As a result, the delivered oxygen concentration varies considerably, and it is usually not possible to deliver greater than 50% oxygen. Children tend to object strenuously to being placed inside an oxygen tent, partly because they find the enclosure confining, and also because of separation from the parents and other care givers. When a croup tent is in use, parents and other care givers must be warned against allowing the patient to use any toy capable of generating a spark. The use of these toys presents a fire hazard in the oxygen-enriched environment.

Oxygen masks are also provided in pediatric sizes. Pediatric masks function similarly to adult masks with respect to the delivered oxygen concentrations and oxygen delivery flows. However, it must be remembered that masks are not well tolerated by children, and in fact, it is difficult to persuade a sick child to wear an oxygen mask at all. Masks are usually used only for short-term oxygen delivery in situations such as emergency transport and stabilization and in the postanesthesia care unit (PACU).

Chest Physical Therapy

Gaining the confidence of a child before beginning a chest physical therapy (CPT) treatment is critical to being able to deliver effective therapy. The patient, as well as the parent or primary care givers, may believe CPT to be painful. This perception may be related to the sound of effective percussion, or because they have witnessed other children crying during therapy. A young child may respond to attempts to deliver therapy by exhibiting signs of emotional stress such as crying, whining, becoming rigid, or kicking and biting. An older child, or adolescent, may respond by trying to negotiate a delay in the treatment and complaints of pain. By initially establishing a therapeutic relationship, which includes truthful communication and trust building, the respiratory care practitioner can provide effective CPT with a minimum of emotional and physical discomfort for the patient.

Chest physical therapy has traditionally included four elements: (1) postural drainage, (2) percussion, (3) vibration, and (4) coughing. Although the utility of CPT is debated in the literature, it may be considered in the therapeutic plan for patients who have undergone thoracic or abdominal surgery, or who have bronchiectasis, cystic fibrosis, atelectasis, and neuromuscular conditions that impair the cough reflex.[20–28] Table 26-2 illustrates the indications, hazards or contraindications, and therapeutic considerations for CPT. *Postural drainage* is performed by positioning the patient to allow gravity to aid in the drainage of secretions from specific areas of the lung. Postural drainage employs the anatomy of the bronchial tree; therefore, the respiratory care practitioner must have a thorough understanding of segmental anatomy of the lung. Specific drainage po-

TABLE 26-2. **Indications, Hazards or Contraindications, and Therapeutic Goals for Chest Physiotherapy**

Component of CPT	Indications	Hazards or Contraindications*	Therapeutic Goal(s)
Postural drainage	Atelectasis; respiratory distress syndrome (after the acute phase); diseases that result in an increase in secretion production, such as pneumonia, cystic fibrosis, chronic bronchitis, asthma; diseases that result in limited ability to inspire deeply and cough, such as neuromuscular diseases or thoracic cage injuries	May produce increased work of breathing in patients with advanced obstructive disease May cause transient hypoxemia due to ventilation-perfusion mismatching May produce postural hypotension in some patients Should not be used in patients with an untreated pneumothorax, status asthmaticus or in the immediate postoperative period	To reverse alveolar collapse in atelectasis To promote maintenance of a patent airway by using gravity to assist the patient in mobilizing and removing secretions Determine the effectiveness by evaluating breath sounds and X-ray
Percussion	Atelectasis; diseases that result in excessive secretion production such as cystic fibrosis and chronic bronchitis; and diseases or conditions that limit thoracic expansion	May produce bronchospasm in patients with hyperreactive airways Airway obstruction may result in patients who are unable to cough and expectorate when excessive secretions become mobile Should not be used in patients with an untreated pneumothorax or unstable cardiac status Should not be used in patients with status asthmaticus or in the immediate postoperative period	To reverse alveolar collapse in atelectasis To promote maintenance of a patent airway by using the energy created by the vibrations on the bronchi to assist the patient in mobilizing and removing secretions Determine the effectiveness by evaluating breath sounds and X-ray
Vibration	Atelectasis; respiratory distress syndrome (after the acute phase); diseases that result in an increase in secretion production, such as pneumonia, cystic fibrosis, chronic bronchitis, asthma; diseases that result in limited ability to inspire deeply and cough, such as neuromuscular diseases or thoracic cage injuries	May produce bronchospasm in patients with hyperreactive airways Airway obstruction may result in patients who are unable to cough and expectorate when excessive secretions become mobile Should not be used in patients with status asthmaticus, in the immediate postoperative period for patients undergoing neurosurgical procedures, or patients with active pulmonary bleeding	To reverse alveolar collapse in atelectasis To promote maintenance of a patent airway by using the energy created by the vibrations on the bronchi to assist the patient in mobilizing and removing secretions

*All modalities should be used with caution if increased work of breathing occurs.

sitions used for adults can easily be modified for use with children (Figures 26-1 to 26-11). It is difficult to place small children and infants in specific positions for an extended period of time; however, specific positioning can be used during the application of percussion and vibration.

Percussion, or clapping, of the chest wall is thought to work by sending a pressure wave through the chest wall to the lung, thereby loosening secretions. Percussion is performed by lightly striking the patient's chest wall with a slightly cupped hand. It is difficult to perform percussion using an adult hand when the patient is a small child or infant; consequently, either the hand position is modified to use "tented" fingers or a commercial device that resembles a cup can be used. Percussion is administered using a rhythmic pattern. The patient's skin should be covered with a light covering such as a gown, sheet, or thin towel. The treatment should last between 1 and 5 minutes per segment. Percussion must not be applied below the posterior ribs because of the potential for injury to the kidneys, and below the anterior ribs because of risk of injury to the liver, spleen, and stomach.

Vibration is also thought to assist in moving secretions from small to large airways. The efficacy of vibration is debatable;[29,30] however, it does appear to benefit patients who have large amounts of secretions.[31] The respiratory care practitioner performs vibrations by placing her hands, with her arms held straight, on the patient's chest wall. An isometric contraction of the arm muscles causes a fine tremor that is transmitted to the patient's chest wall. Vibration is performed only during expiration. Not only does the size of the adult hand make it difficult to administer vibrations to the chest of an infant or small child, it is also difficult to coordinate the timing of vibrations with exhalation. For these reasons, it may be helpful to use a commercially available vibrator to administer vibrations.

Coughing is the fourth component of chest physiotherapy. Most patients cough spontaneously when secretions have been moved into the large airways where irritant receptors can be stimulated. The effectiveness

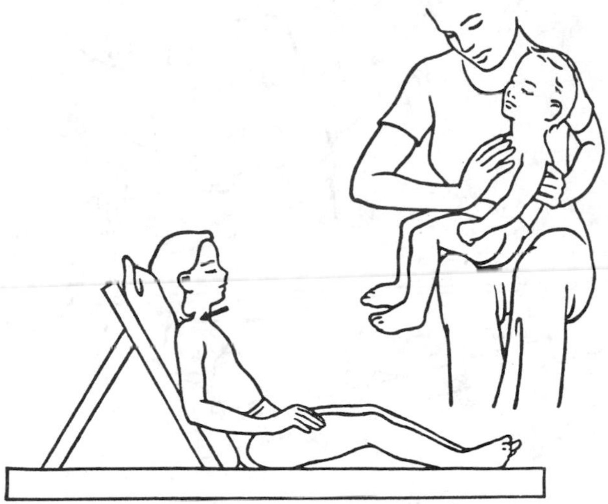

FIGURE 26-1. Postural drainage positions: *apical segments, right and left upper lobes.* Position patient in semi-Fowler's position, leaning forward at a 30° angle. Percuss and vibrate between the clavicle and scapula. (From Blodgett D: Manual of Pediatric Respiratory Care Procedures. Philadelphia. JB Lippincott, 1982.)

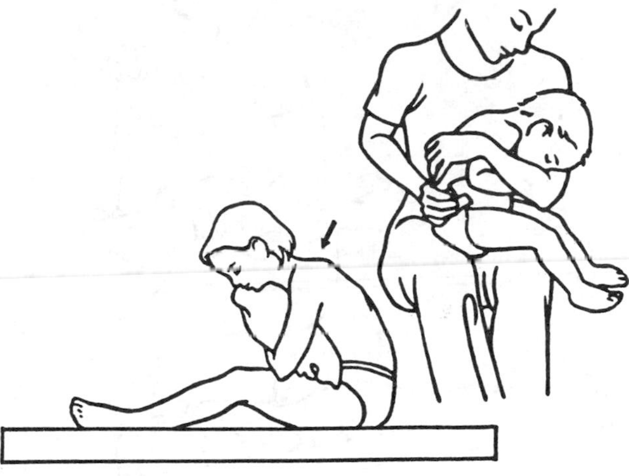

FIGURE 26-3. Postural drainage positions: *posterior segments, upper lobes.* Position patient sitting up, leaning forward at a 30° angle. A pillow can be used to provide support. Percuss and vibrate the upper posterior thorax, above the scapula. (From Blodgett D: Manual of Pediatric Respiratory Care Procedures. Philadelphia. JB Lippincott, 1982.)

of coached coughing depends on the age of the child and his ability, or desire, to follow instructions. During coached coughing, the patient should be instructed to inhale deeply through the nose, hold his breath briefly while simultaneously contracting the abdominal muscles, and, finally, exhale forcefully while coughing. If a patient either cannot or will not cough, it may be necessary to perform nasotracheal suctioning to remove secretions and clear the airway.

□ NEW MODALITIES IN CPT

Four new modalities have been incorporated into the therapeutic application of chest physiotherapy: (1) positive expiratory pressure therapy, (2) forced expiration technique, (3) autogenic drainage, and (4) high-frequency chest compression. *Positive expiratory pressure therapy* (PEP therapy) uses expiratory resistance to prevent dynamic airway collapse and promote secretion removal.[32]

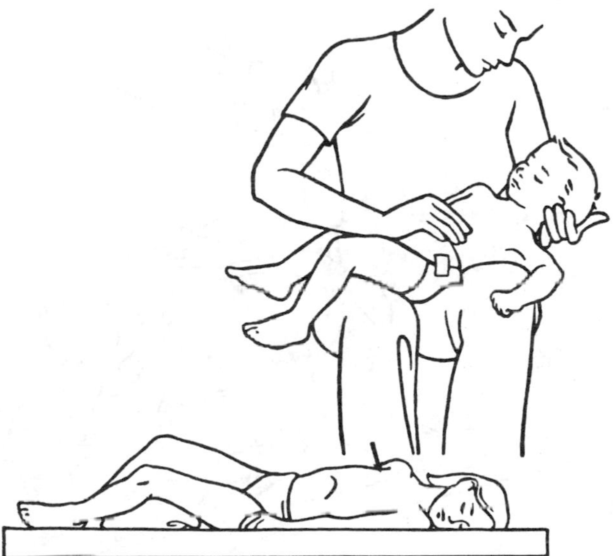

FIGURE 26-2. Postural drainage positions: anterior segment, upper lobes. Position patient lying flat on back (supine). Place a pillow or towel roll under the knees to reduce strain on the abdominal muscles. Percuss and vibrate over the anterior chest just below the clavicles to slightly above the nipple area (the levels of the 2nd to 4th ribs), taking care to avoid the sternum. (From Blodgett D: Manual of Pediatric Respiratory Care Procedures. Philadelphia. JB Lippincott, 1982.)

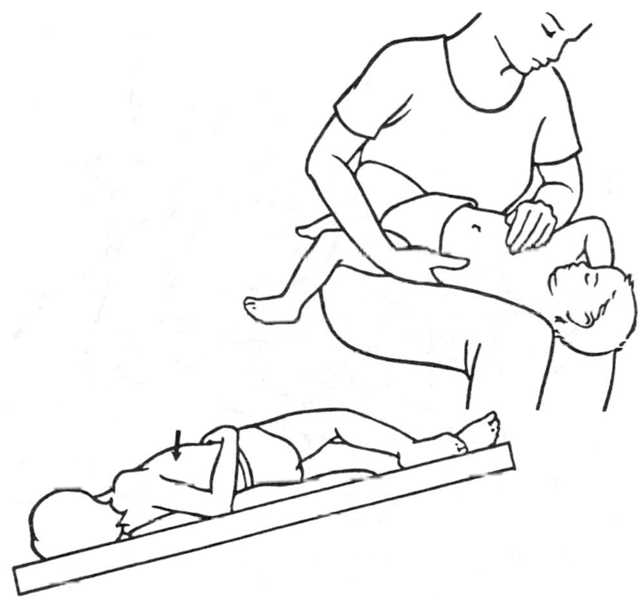

FIGURE 26-4. Postural drainage positions: right medial lobe (lateral medial). Place the patient in Trendelenburg's position at a 15° angle. Percuss and vibrate over the right anterolateral portion of the right breast, from the 3rd to the 6th rib. (From Blodgett D: Manual of Pediatric Respiratory Care Procedures. Philadelphia. JB Lippincott, 1982.)

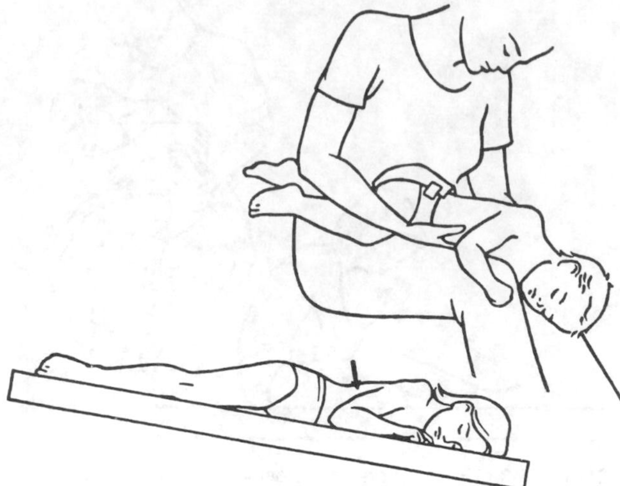

FIGURE 26-5. Postural drainage positions: right lower lobe (medial basal). Position the patient prone with the foot of the bed elevated about 20″ (30°) and the right side turned up slightly. Percuss and vibrate over the lower portion of the right anterolateral rib cage. (From Blodgett D: Manual of Pediatric Respiratory Care Procedures. Philadelphia. JB Lippincott, 1982.)

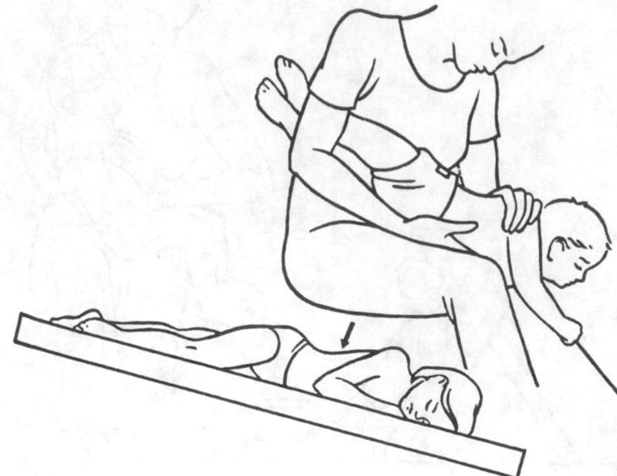

FIGURE 26-7. Postural drainage positions: lower lobes (lateral basal). Place patient in Trendelenburg's position, with the patient lying on the abdomen and rotated 1/4 turn to position the appropriate side. The foot of the bed is raised about 20″ (30°). Percuss and vibrate on the lateral thorax at the level of the 8th rib (From Blodgett D: Manual of Pediatric Respiratory Care Procedures. Philadelphia. JB Lippincott, 1982.)

Positive expiratory pressure therapy can be self-administered, and this may be the major advantage of the therapy. The use of PEP therapy for patients with cystic fibrosis has been evaluated;[23,33–42] however, it has not been found to be more beneficial than autogenic drainage, postural drainage, and physical exercise.

Forced expiration technique (FET) is a form of huff coughing in which the patient forcefully exhales while keeping the glottis open. The term "active cycle of breathing" also refers to FET. After the patient has performed several repetitions of FET, a normal cough is performed to remove secretions. This technique also reduces dynamic airway collapse, so it is useful in those conditions in which the structural integrity of the airways is compromised. The benefit of FET, much like that of PEP, appears to be in the simplicity of the ther-

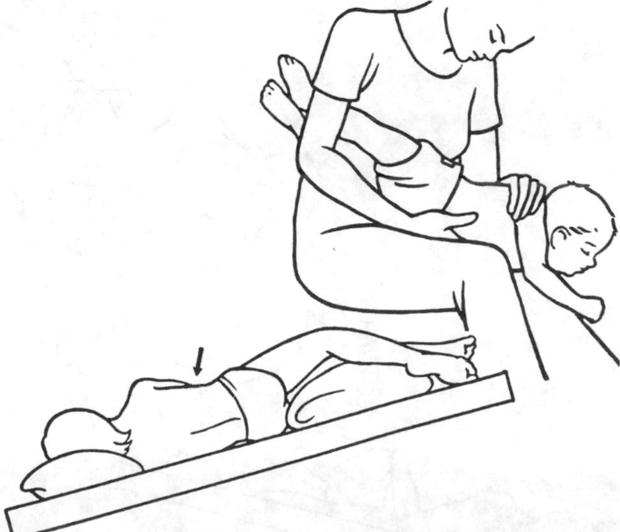

FIGURE 26-6. Postural drainage positions: lower lobes (anterior basal). For the RLL, position the patient on the left side with the foot of the bed elevated about 20″ (30°). A pillow should be placed under the knees and the head for support. Percuss and vibrate slightly above the lower ribs, on the anterolateral aspect of the chest. If the LLL is to be drained, position the patient on the right side with the foot of the bed elevated about 20″ (30°). (From Blodgett D: Manual of Pediatric Respiratory Care Procedures. Philadelphia. JB Lippincott, 1982.)

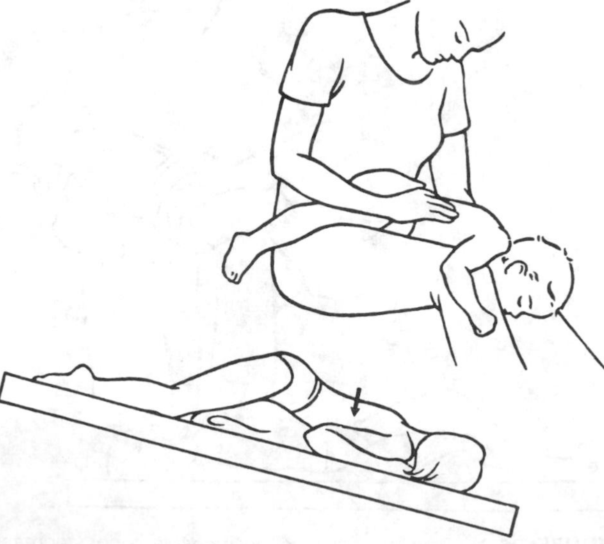

FIGURE 26-8. Postural drainage positions: lower lobes (posterior basal). Position the patient in Trendelenburg's position, lying on the abdomen (prone) with the foot of the bed elevated about 20″ (30°). A pillow should be placed under the hips. Percuss and vibrate just above the 11th and 12th ribs. (From Blodgett D: Manual of Pediatric Respiratory Care Procedures. Philadelphia. JB Lippincott, 1982.)

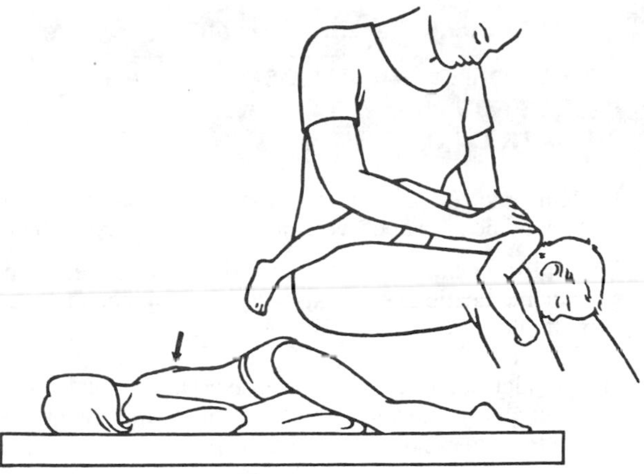

FIGURE 26-9. Postural drainage positions: lower lobes (superior segment). Position the patient on the abdomen (prone), with the bed flat. Two pillows placed under the patient's hips will produce a 15° elevation. Percuss and vibrate just below the scapula. (From Blodgett D: Manual of Pediatric Respiratory Care Procedures. Philadelphia. JB Lippincott, 1982.)

apy and the ease of self-administration. Studies have failed to document a clinical advantage of its use over other forms of CPT.[23,33,38–42]

The goal of *autogenic drainage* (AD) is to enhance secretion removal by using controlled breathing maneuvers and delaying the cough as long as possible. It is useful in patients who have cystic fibrosis and bronchiectasis.[43,44] Autogenic drainage can be self-administered; however, the manner in which breathing is performed and controlled during treatment is fairly sophisticated, and some patients may find it difficult to master. The primary benefit of AD, as with FET, may be the ability for self-administration. Clinical research has not demonstrated an increase in efficacy when AD is used to facilitate secretion removal.[23,39,40]

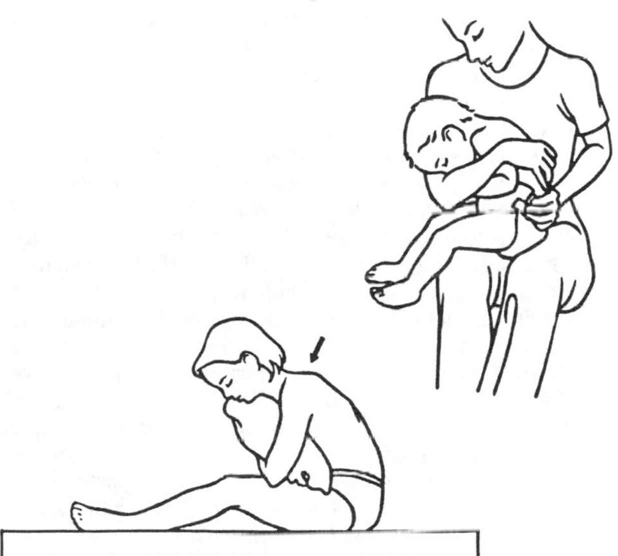

FIGURE 26-10. Postural drainage positions: left upper lobe (apical posterior segment). Position the patient in a sitting position, leaning forward over a pillow at a 30° angle. Percuss between the clavicle and scapula. (From Blodgett D: Manual of Pediatric Respiratory Care Procedures. Philadelphia. JB Lippincott, 1982.)

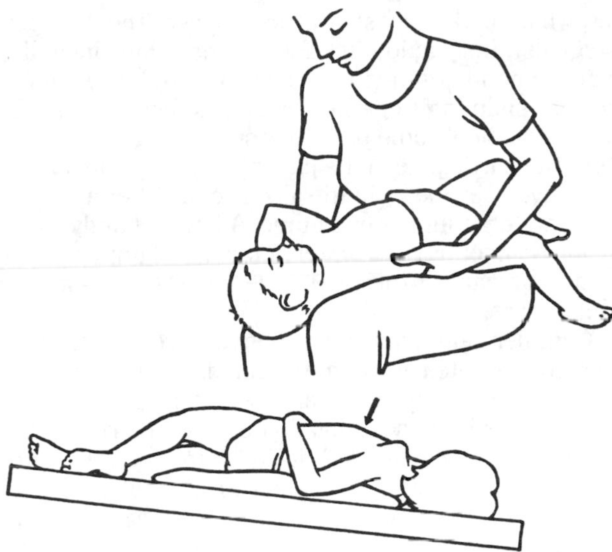

FIGURE 26-11. Postural drainage positions: left upper lobe (lingula, superior and inferior segments). Position the patient in Trendelenberg's position, lying on the right side with a ¼ turn backwards. A pillow should be placed behind the patient for support. The foot of the bed is elevated about 15°, or 12″. Percuss and vibrate over the left chest, in line with the nipple. (From Blodgett D: Manual of Pediatric Respiratory Care Procedures. Philadelphia. JB Lippincott, 1982.)

High-frequency chest compression is administered using a commercially available device (ThAIRpy Bronchial Drainage System, American Biosystems Inc., St. Paul, MN). The patient wears an inflatable vest that fits snugly around the chest. The chest wall is intermittently compressed. The alternating compression and relaxation produces episodic intervals during which expiratory airflow is increased. As a result, mucus becomes loosened and more easily removed from the walls of the airways.[44–46]

Lung Hyperinflation Procedures

Lung hyperinflation procedures include incentive spirometry and intermittent positive-pressure breathing (IPPB) therapy. Intermittent positive-pressure breathing therapy has limited use in the pediatric population; therefore, the discussion of lung hyperinflation therapy will be directed to incentive spirometry.

The use of incentive spirometry is limited to children who are cooperative and able to understand and follow directions. Incentive spirometry can be effective only in those children who do not have preexisting conditions that limit the ability to inhale deeply. When a child is to receive postoperative incentive spirometry, the therapy should be taught preoperatively. Family members should also be included in the teaching sessions. Information given to the patient and family during the teaching session should include a description of the therapy and device, why it has been ordered for the patient, clear instructions for the use of the incentive spirometer, what the therapy should accomplish (the therapeutic goals), instruction in effective coughing (including an explanation of the importance of coughing), and incisional splinting (together with an explanation that the patient will feel some pain after surgery). Family members can participate in the patient's care by supervising incentive spirometry in the absence of either a respiratory care practitioner or a nurse. Allowing family supervision of incentive spirometry enhances family empowerment and allows them to be active participants in their child's care.

Commercially available incentive spirometers are either flow oriented or volume oriented. If the device is volume oriented, a volume goal is set for the patient. Flow-oriented devices use a flotation device that rises when negative flow is generated during inspiration. Pediatric versions of incentive spirometers are available; however, adult versions of incentive spirometers can easily be used in the pediatric setting. If a volume-oriented device is being used, the respiratory care practitioner must remember to set a realistic volume goal for the patient.

Aerosol and Humidity Therapy

Pediatric patients require increased humidity when breathing dry gases, such as oxygen. Breathing dry gases produces the same complications in a pediatric patient as in an adult. These complications include (1) increased viscosity of the mucous blanket and a reduction in ciliary action, both of which may contribute to increased airway resistance; (2) mucosal crusting; (3) destruction of the ciliated pulmonary epithelium; (4) atelectasis; and (5) pneumonia.[46–48] The same equipment used in the adult patient population to deliver aerosol and humidity therapy can be used for pediatric patients (AARC Clinical Practice Guideline: Selection of an Aerosol Delivery Device for Neonatal and Pediatric Patients).

Nonheated bubble humidifiers are frequently used with nasal cannulae and masks. These devices are capable of providing approximately 30% to 40% relative humidity at body temperature.[49] Inspired gas that bypasses the upper airway, for example, through an endotracheal or tracheostomy tube, should provide approximately 100% relative humidity at 32° to 34° C.[50]

The water vapor content of a volume of gas can be significantly increased by adding heat to the device. Heated pass-over humidifiers can be used on ventilators and in other circuits in which there is high gas flow. These devices produce the least amount of humidity of the heated humidifiers. Heated wick humidifiers are capable, under most circumstances, of delivering 100% relative humidity at body temperature.

When heat has been added to a humidity device, it becomes necessary to monitor the temperature of the delivered gas. This can be done by placing an in-line thermometer in the circuit. If the patient is intubated, the thermometer should be placed near the Y, in the inspiratory limb of the circuit. If the heated vapor is being delivered to an oxygen hood, the thermometer should be placed inside the hood, near the patient's head. When

AARC Clinical Practice Guideline

SELECTION OF AN AEROSOL DELIVERY DEVICE FOR NEONATAL AND PEDIATRIC PATIENTS

Indications: An aerosol delivery system is indicated when a medication approved for inhalation is prescribed.

Contraindications: Contraindications associated with specific medications may exist. Pharmaceutical information should be consulted for relative contraindications. An MDI or DPI should not be used for patients with known allergies to medication preservatives, or for patients unable to perform the respiratory maneuver required to disperse or deliver the drug.

Assessment of Need: Small-volume nebulizers are indicated when there is a need to deliver aerosolized medications that are approved in solution form to the lower airway of spontaneously breathing patients with or without an instrumented airway; to provide supplemental gas flow in conjunction with aerosol treatment; to modify drug concentration; to deliver a particular aerosolized medication that is only available in solution form; to deliver aerosolized medications to patients in acute distress or with reduced inspiratory flow; to deliver aerosolized medications to patients who are unable to coordinate or perform the necessary inspiratory maneuvers required with an MDI or DPI. Small-volume nebulizers with mouthpiece and extension reservoir are indicated when there is a need to deliver aerosolized medications approved in solution form to the lower airways of spontaneously breathing patients without an instrumented airway who are able to utilize a mouthpiece (patients <3 years). Small-volume nebulizers with face mask are indicated for the need to deliver aerosolized medications that are approved in solution form to the lower airways of spontaneously breathing patients without an instrumented airway who are unable to negotiate a mouthpiece (usually <3 years); the need to deliver aerosolized medications to the upper airway. Small-volume nebulizers with T connector (15-mm and 22-mm openings) are indicated for the need to deliver aerosolized medications approved in solution form in line with a mechanical ventilator circuit or manual resuscitation bag; the need to deliver aerosolized medications approved in solution form to patients with instrumented airways who are spontaneously breathing. Metered-dose inhalers are indicated for the need to deliver aerosolized medications that are approved in MDI form; the need to deliver a particular medication that is only available in MDI form; the need to reduce the length of time for the aerosol treatment; the need for maximum portability. Metered-dose inhalers with spacer device with one-way valve and face mask are appropriate for small children (usually <3 years) and others unable to use a mouthpiece; for the need to eliminate actuation and inspiratory maneuver coordination; for the need to reduce oropharyngeal impaction, particularly with the delivery of corticosteroids by inhalation. The valved-spacer device with mouthpiece is the method of choice if patient is able to use a mouthpiece. A specially designed spacer device is used for MDI delivery during mechanical ventilation or with manual resuscitators. Metered-dose inhalers with a non-valved spacer device are indicated for the need to use a MDI when a patient can coordinate inspiration and actuation; the need to reduce oropharyngeal impaction, particularly with the delivery of corticosteroids by inhalation. Dry-powder inhalers are indicated for the need to deliver aerosolized medications approved in DPI form; the need to deliver a particular medication that is only available in DPI form; the need to eliminate chlorofluorocarbon propellants. Large-volume nebulizers are indicated for the need to deliver continuously aerosolized medication, approved in solution form, to the lower airway of spontaneously breathing patients without an instrumented airway.

Assessment of Outcome: Desired medication effect is observed as indicated by an improvement in subjective (physical examination) and objective (pulmonary function measurements) assessments. Health care providers demonstrate competency with proper technique and patient instruction of aerosol delivery systems. Patients and patients' family members demonstrate proper technique and compliance with the application of aerosol delivery systems.

Monitoring: Observe delivery technique of spontaneously breathing patients who are able to self-administer aerosolized medications. A slow, deep inhalation with an inspiratory pause or hold is performed during SVN treatments. A flow of 6 to 8 L/min and fill volume of 4 mL (dependent upon the brand of SVN used) provide a maximum volume of delivered drug. The sides of the SVN are periodically tapped to minimize the dead volume (ie, volume of solution not nebulized) and maximize the volume nebulized. Metered-dose inhaler actuation occurs at end-exhalation followed by a slow inspiration and breath hold for 10 seconds. Patient is able to produce a rapid inhalation to fully activate and discharge DPI. Observe patient or patient's family member following instruction and demonstration. Proper understanding and return demonstration of delivery device and accompanying equipment is observed. Proper understanding and preparation of medication is observed. Observe response to medication by performing subjective (eg, physical examination) and objective (eg, pulmonary function measurements) assessments and other diagnostic techniques that are appropriate for the specific medication being delivered. Ensure that medication volume is nebulized over desired amount of time when using LVN. Continuous monitoring of ECG is recommended when delivering a bronchodilator by LVN. Monitor ventilator function for inadvertent increases in tidal volume or airway pressures, changes in FIO_2, difficulty with patient triggering and patient-ventilator synchrony, or other system problems.

From AARC Clinical Practice Guideline; see Respir Care 40:1325, 1995, for complete text.

an infant is either in an isolette or on a radiant warmer, the thermometer should be placed in the circuit just before the point where the circuit enters the heated environment. Most humidification devices designed recently incorporate a servo-controlled heating system, as well as audible and visual alarm systems for high and low temperature. The temperature-sensing probe, or thermistor, in a servo-controlled heating device should be placed in similar positions to the thermometer in non–servo-controlled devices.

A *heat and moisture exchanger (HME)* may be used to provide humidity for an intubated child. When deciding to use an HME, the following factors must be considered: (1) compliance of the device, (2) amount of mechanical dead space contributed by the device, (3) the weight of the device, (4) resistance to flow through the device, (5) the patient's body temperature, and (6) the patient's size and tidal volume.[50,51] Although use of an HME is limited in neonates and small infants, it provides an effective alternative to conventional humidifiers for short-term use. Heat and moisture exchanger use should not be initiated when the patient has thick or copious secretions, and it should be terminated if the character of mucoid secretions changes in consistency (becomes thickened, for example) or if the amount of secretions produced increases or decreases significantly.

Aerosol therapy may be used to increase ambient humidity, to deliver medications, and in conjunction with chest physiotherapy. A large-volume nebulizer may be used to deliver bland aerosol therapy to patients who are not intubated, as well as to those patients who have an endotracheal or tracheostomy tube. Therapy can be administered either continuously or intermittently when using a large-volume nebulizer. These devices commonly have an air-entrainment port that allows the FIO_2 to be varied from approximately 0.30 to 1.0. Heat can be added to the device using a heating rod or a collar device.

Small-volume nebulizers are typically used for the administration of medications such as bronchodilators and antibiotics. The procedure should be explained to children in clear and age-appropriate terms. Children as young as 3 or 4 years old can often be convinced to breathe through a mouthpiece; older children readily do so, therefore facilitating the administration of medication using a small-volume nebulizer. Particle deposition can be maximized by having the patient inhale deeply through the mouth, followed by an end-inspiratory pause (breath holding). If the child either cannot or will not hold the mouthpiece in her mouth, a face mask (aerosol mask) can be attached to the nebulizer and the treatment administered in this manner.

When delivering medication to an adult patient using a small-volume nebulizer, the flow to power the nebulizer is usually set at 6 to 8 L/min. This flow, however, is excessive for children and infants. The respiratory care practitioner should titrate the flow to the patient's inspiratory demand.

Metered-dose inhalers (MDI) are frequently employed to deliver medications used in the treatment of asthma. Currently, β_2-agonist bronchodilators, anticholinergics, and steroids are commonly administered using an MDI. Metered-dose inhalers offer the advantages of delivering precise doses of medication and convenience because of their portability.[52,53] The difficulty in using MDIs to treat children can be related to the difficulty in coordinating the actuation of the device with an inspiratory effort. Consequently, several inhalation aids (also known as spacers or holding chambers) have been developed and can be used with children. Lee and Evans evaluated the use of three inhalation aids (InspirEase, Aerochamber, and Aerosol Bag) and found that children who demonstrate the appropriate technique for inhalation do not benefit from the use of a spacer; however, children who do not demonstrate correct technique show a significant increase in their FEV_1 when a spacer is used.[54] Children as young as 2 to 3 years of age can be taught to use an MDI when a spacer is employed.[55,56]

Increased compliance with therapy can be found in some children who use a dry-powder inhaler (DPI) instead of an MDI. This may be related to the operation of a DPI, which is breath activated. Cromolyn sodium (Intal) is administered using the Spinhaler, while albuterol (Ventolin) is administered using the Rotahaler.[52,56] The problems encountered when using a DPI may be related to the high inspiratory flow needed to activate the device and the difficulty some patients may experience when trying to load the drug capsule into the device. Though the problem of coordinating inspiration and actuation is eliminated when using a DPI, patients still need to be taught how to use the device. The main factor related to inappropriate use of both MDIs and DPIs is absent or incomplete instruction, with repeated return demonstrations required to document patient competency in using the device. Though the devices are supplied with written instructions and diagrams, these materials cannot replace patient education by health professionals who are themselves competent in the use of the equipment.

ESTABLISHMENT AND CARE OF ARTIFICIAL AIRWAYS

Endotracheal Tubes

The ability to rapidly and effectively establish an artificial airway in infants and children requires expert knowledge of the anatomy of the upper airway, including the anatomic differences between infants and young children and older pediatric patients. In addition, the respiratory care practitioner must be competent in the use of intubation equipment that is functionally the same as that used in adult care, but with different technical and performance characteristics. The sizes and styles of endotracheal tubes vary, not only with the size of the patient, but also with the laryngeal anatomy.

Endotracheal tube sizes typically used for infants and children of various ages are shown in Table 26-3. When preparing for an intubation, it is usually wise to obtain tubes that are one-half size smaller and one-half size larger than the size expected to be used. Endotracheal tubes used with children who are less than 7 to 8 years old are generally uncuffed. The airway is sealed because the cricoid cartilage is the smallest part of the airway in this age group. Should a cuffed endotracheal tube be used in an infant or young child, the tube itself may exert sufficient pressure on the tracheal mucosa to produce many of the same problems seen in adults when the intracuff pressure is excessive (eg, submucosal edema, mucosal necrosis, and potentially stenosis).

Intubation

Indications for endotracheal intubation in children are the same as in adults: (1) to facilitate mechanical ventilation, (2) to protect or maintain the airway, (3) and to provide a route for suctioning. Equipment that must be selected and checked for proper functioning once the decision to intubate has been made is listed in Table 26-4.

Pharmacotherapy (sedatives and neuromuscular blocking agents) may be used to facilitate intubation, particularly if the child is awake. Morphine sulfate is a good first choice because it has both analgesic and sedative qualities. Benzodiazepines, for example, diazepam (Valium), lorazepam (Ativan), and midazolam (Versed), can be used in conjunction with morphine for their sedative effects.[18] Neuromuscular blocking agents such as succinylcholine (Anectine) can be used for short-term muscle relaxation (<8 minutes); longer-acting agents such as pancuronium bromide (Pavulon)

TABLE 26-3. **Pediatric Endotracheal Tube and Suction Catheter Sizes**

Patient Age*	Internal Diameter (mm)	Distance to Lips (cm)	Suction Catheter (in Fr)
Newborn	3.0 uncuffed	9	6
1 to 6 months	3.5 uncuffed	10	8
6 to 18 months	4.0 uncuffed	11	8
18 months to 2 years	4.5 uncuffed	12	8
3 to 4 years	5.0 uncuffed	14	10
5 to 6 years	5.5 uncuffed	16	10
7 to 8 years	6.0 uncuffed	18	10
9 years	6.0 cuffed	18	10
10 to 11 years	6.5 cuffed	20	10
12+ years	7.0 cuffed	22	10

* Assumes normal growth and development

From Aoki BY, McCloskey K: Evaluation, Stabilization, and Transport of the Critically Ill Child. St Louis, Mosby–Year Book, 1992, 25, with permission.

TABLE 26-4. **Equipment and Supplies for Airway Intubation**

Equipment	Comments
Oxygen	100% oxygen source must be available
Suction	Check vacuum pressure and ensure that both rigid (Yankauer) and flexible catheters are available
Manual resuscitator	Check for leaks and refilling when using a self-inflating unit; check for leaks when using a flow-dependent bag
Face masks	Various sizes should be available
Laryngoscope with proper handle and blades	Check for bulb tightness and illumination; have extra bulbs and batteries available
Endotracheal tubes	Have several sizes available; if a cuffed endotracheal tube is being used, the cuff should be inflated and checked for symmetry and leaks
10-cc syringe	If a cuffed endotracheal tube is being used
McGill forceps	For nasal intubation
Tape and benzoin	Prepare tape according to institutional policy for securing endotracheal tubes; have long-handled cotton-tipped swabs available for applying benzoin
Teflon-coated stylet*	May be used to "stiffen" endotracheal tube during oral intubation

* Stylets are used to facilitate insertion of the endotracheal tube. When placing the stylet inside the tube, care must be taken to ensure that the tip of the stylet does not protrude beyond the distal end of the endotracheal tube. A protruding stylet can perforate the larynx.

and vecuronium bromide (Norcuron) can exert their effects for approximately half an hour.[57] Neuromuscular blocking agents produce apnea; therefore, it is essential that a person who is capable of providing ventilation using a bag-valve-mask unit be present whenever these agents are administered.

Both the necessity of placing the endotracheal tube and the procedure should be explained to the family. Age-appropriate explanations should be given to the child. The route of tracheal intubation in the pediatric patient includes oral and nasal intubation. Personal preference, institutional policy, and the condition that produced the need for intubation are all factors in the decision to place the tube either orally or nasally. When preparing to orally intubate an adult, the practitioner usually facilitates alignment of the mouth, pharynx, and larynx by hyperextending the patient's head. When intubating an infant or young child, however, this positioning actually decreases the practitioner's ability to visualize the larynx. The head position that maximizes the ability to visualize the larynx in a child is referred to as the "sniffing" position.[58–60]

During the intubation procedure, the child's vital signs should be carefully monitored. Monitoring the child's color, along with pulse oximetry, provides valuable information concerning oxygenation status. If oxygen saturation (SpO_2), heart rate, or color deteriorates during attempts to place the endotracheal tube, the procedure should be interrupted and effective ventilation established using a bag-valve-mask unit and 100% oxygen. All vital signs, including SpO_2, must return to an acceptable baseline before further attempts to place the endotracheal tube.

Pediatric laryngoscope handles and Miller (straight) and Macintosh (curved) blades are available. The practitioner holds the laryngoscope in his or her left hand, and the blade is inserted in the right side of the patient's mouth. The blade is used to sweep the tongue to the left, then it is centered and advanced in a midline position. Some practitioners find the Macintosh blade easier to position at the base of the tongue than the Miller, probably because it is broader.[61] The Macintosh blade is positioned in the vallecula, then the laryngoscope is lifted up and forward. This movement lifts the epiglottis. The Miller blade is placed under the tip of the epiglottis and lifts it directly. The upward and forward movement of the laryngoscope occurs when using either the Miller or the Macintosh blade. An easy way to produce this movement is to imagine bringing the laryngoscope toward the line where the wall behind the patient's head meets the ceiling. This movement minimizes the likelihood of using the blade as a lever, a motion that produces much of the oral trauma (lacerations of the gum or broken teeth) associated with intubation. The endotracheal tube is held in the practitioner's right hand and passed into the larynx. The practitioner should visualize the glottic opening and observe the tube as it passes through the glottis. If the tube is uncuffed, the practitioner should note the black ring near the distal tip of the tube and ensure that the line is slightly distal to the glottic opening. If the tube is cuffed, the cuff must be placed distal to the glottic opening.

Immediately following placement of the tube, the practitioner must assess the airway to determine the position of the tube within the trachea. Initially, the patient should be ventilated using a manual resuscitation bag and the chest auscultated to determine if bilateral, equal breath sounds are present. If the practitioner determines the breath sounds are more distinct on the right, for example, it is likely that right main stem intubation has occurred. Bilateral thoracic expansion should be observed during the positive pressure breath. The stomach should also be auscultated during a positive-pressure breath to make sure that esophageal intubation has not occurred. A disposable end-tidal carbon dioxide (ET_{CO2}) monitor can also be placed in line between the endotracheal tube and the manual resuscitation bag to verify the presence of carbon dioxide in the exhaled gas.[62] Finally, the practitioner can observe the tube for the presence of condensate from exhaled gases. Although these measures support the presence of the endotracheal tube within the trachea, they cannot provide information about the position of the tube. For this reason, a chest radiograph must be obtained.

The tip of a properly positioned endotracheal tube should lie approximately 2 cm above the carina. A chest radiograph is required to document that the endotracheal tube is in the proper position.

Suctioning the Airway

Suctioning is the procedure by which secretions are removed from the airway of a patient who cannot, or will not, cough and expectorate either spontaneously or on command. Patients who are intubated require assistance to effectively remove secretions from the airway. Failure to remove secretions causes a reduction in the lumen of the airway and a concomitant increase in airway resistance. There is a direct relationship between increased airway resistance and the patient's work of breathing; for example, as the airway resistance increases, the patient must expend more energy and effort during breathing. Retained secretions also increase the possibility of aspiration.

Suctioning should not be routinely performed on a regularly scheduled basis such as every 2 hours. Instead, suctioning should only be done when it is indicated, or on an as-needed basis. Indications for suctioning include the visible presence of secretions in the endotracheal tube, the presence of rhonchi or decreased breath sounds during auscultation of the chest, an acute onset of dyspnea, an increase in the amount of positive pressure required to deliver the tidal volume during mechanical ventilation, and a decrease in oxygen saturation. Decreases in oxygen saturation can be noted by monitoring the SpO_2 display on a pulse oximeter. Finally, endotracheal suctioning may be indicated when a sputum specimen is required for diagnostic testing.[63]

Suctioning the airway of a newborn or very young infant is usually performed manually by using a bulb syringe. Secretions are suctioned from the mouth and pharynx first, and then the nares. When using a bulb syringe, the practitioner must remember to squeeze the bulb **before** the tip is placed in the mouth or nares. If the bulb is squeezed after the tip is placed in the infant's mouth or nares, it can stimulate gasping that enhances the possibility of the infant aspirating upper airway secretions.

Orotracheal and nasotracheal suctioning can be performed on pediatric patients; however, it is very difficult to enter the trachea using these methods. As a result, orotracheal and nasotracheal suctioning are generally used only to stimulate a cough or to clear the upper airway. The procedure must be carefully explained to the child, using terms he or she can understand.

Infants are not able to understand an explanation of the procedure before beginning the suctioning; however, as soon as the procedure is completed, the infant should be comforted using both physical and verbal measures. Toddlers may verbalize protests and anger; the practitioner should recognize this as an expression of the child's psychological defenses. Preschoolers may express their fears and anger more definitively than toddlers. The practitioner should respond to the preschooler's verbal communication and physical actions clearly and firmly. When the procedure is completed the child should be praised and rewarded in concrete ways, such as giving the child "smiley face" stickers. School-aged children and adolescents often fear more the loss of control over their situations than they fear pain. As a result, these age groups are more cooperative when the procedure is fully explained to them.

Suctioning the endotracheal tube of a pediatric patient follows the same basic procedure as with an adult patient, with appropriate modifications in the size of the catheter (based on the size of the endotracheal or tracheostomy tube) and vacuum pressure. The catheter selected to perform orotracheal and nasotracheal suctioning depends on the size of the patient. In general, a small infant requires a size 6 to 8 French (FR) catheter. An older infant or young preschooler requires an 8 FR catheter. A 10 FR catheter is usually required for older children. The equipment (which includes a sterile suction catheter, sterile gloves, sterile normal saline, and a supplemental oxygen source) must be collected and prepared before beginning the suctioning procedure. The procedure should be completed quickly and efficiently.

Table 26-5 describes the suctioning procedure for a pediatric patient. It is preferable to have two people working together when suctioning is to be performed. One person manipulates the suction catheter while the other provides manual ventilation between passes of the suction catheter and monitors the patient's vital signs.

The suctioning procedure has several associated hazards, or side effects. In infants and young children, the most often encountered hazard, or side effect, is bradycardia. Bradycardia is most likely the result of either stimulation of the vagus nerve or hypoxia as a result of the suctioning procedure. The onset of bradycardia can be minimized by limiting the amount of time the catheter is inserted into the airway to 10 seconds or less, with suction being applied for no more than 5 seconds, and by ensuring that the patient is hyperoxygenated before beginning the procedure. The incidence of suctioning-related atelectasis can be lessened by providing manual ventilation (using a manual resuscitator bag connected to an oxygen source) before, during, and after suctioning.

Damage to the tracheal mucosa can be minimized by using a shallow suctioning technique, during which the tip of the suction catheter is not allowed to extend more than slightly beyond the end of the endotracheal tube. When deep tracheal suctioning is avoided, the tip of the suction catheter does not impact the carina or the tracheal walls. Lower-airway contamination can be minimized or avoided by ensuring that sterile technique is followed throughout the suctioning procedure. The risk of accidental extubation can be decreased by

TABLE 26-5. **Suctioning the Artificial Airway**

Task or Procedure	Comments
1. Gather all equipment before beginning the suctioning procedure.	Sterile suction catheters, sterile gloves, sterile normal saline or water and container to be used for moistening and clearing the catheter, sterile normal saline for lavage, stethoscope, oxygen source, manual resuscitation bag-valve-mask unit, and a suction source must be available before beginning the procedure.
2. Obtain baseline readings of SpO_2, heart rate and rhythm, and blood pressure.	Oxygen saturation, heart rate and rhythm, and blood pressure can all be adversely affected by suctioning. They must be carefully monitored throughout the procedure.
3. Wash hands.	Prepare all equipment for use. Sterility of sterile materials must be maintained during preparation.
4. Put on gloves.	Identify one hand (usually your dominant hand) as the "sterile" hand. Do not touch anything other than the sterile suction catheter with this hand. The other hand is your "dirty" hand and is used to perform all manual requirements of the suctioning procedure.
5. Attach catheter to suction system.	The size of the catheter depends on the size of the endotracheal or tracheostomy tube. The catheter size can be determined by the following formula: French size = tube ID (in mm) multiplied by 3, then divided by 2.
6. Moisten the suction catheter by dipping it into sterile water or sterile normal saline. Test the vacuum pressure by occluding the suction port and noting the vacuum pressure on the suction regulator.	The vacuum pressure should not exceed 60 to 80 mmHg in an infant or 80 to 100 mmHg in a child.
7. Administer an increased FIO_2 and increase ventilation to the patient.	Hypoxemia and atelectasis are two of the hazards of endotracheal suctioning. Both can be minimized by ventilating the patient using a manual resuscitator bag (at the same PIP and PEEP as being used on the mechanical ventilator) with an FIO_2 set approximately 0.10 higher when suctioning an infant, and set up to 100% when the patient is 6 months of age or older.
8. Instill normal saline, if necessary.	Normal saline may be used to help loosen and thin secretions. In infants, 0.3 to 0.5 mL is instilled, in older patients up to 3.0 mL may be instilled. Following each instillation, the patient should be given several manual breaths by means of a manual resuscitation bag.
9. Insert the suction catheter.	Suction is not applied during insertion. The length to which the suction catheter is to be inserted should be predetermined by measuring the length of the endotracheal or tracheostomy tube (including the 15-mm male adapter) and noting the corresponding length markings (in cm) on the suction catheter. The suction catheter should extend just past the tip of the endotracheal tube, but should not be allowed to make contact with the carina.
10. Apply intermittent suction while the catheter is withdrawn from the airway.	The catheter should be rotated during withdrawal. The time during which the catheter remains in the airway should be 10 seconds or less; the time during which suction is actually applied should not exceed 5 seconds.
11. Manually ventilate the patient.	During manual breaths the patient is oxygenated and ventilated. The practitioner should observe all monitors to determine how much deviation from the baseline has occurred.
12. Determine the need for additional suctioning.	Auscultation of the chest allows the practitioner to evaluate the quality of breath sounds and the need for additional suctioning.
13. Dispose of the gloves and catheter and return the remaining equipment to its proper storage place.	When the suctioning procedure has been completed, the catheter can be "wrapped" around the practitioner's hand and the glove removed and turned inside out and over the catheter prior to disposal. All other equipment should be properly stored.
14. Wash hands.	The practitioner should always wash his or her hands on completion of any therapeutic procedure. This action minimizes the possibility of cross contamination.
15. Document the suctioning procedure.	Documentation should include notes regarding how well the child tolerated the procedure and the amount and character of secretions obtained. If diagnostic samples were obtained, the samples must be labeled and sent for analysis.

having two people available to perform the suctioning procedure.

MECHANICAL VENTILATION OF THE PEDIATRIC PATIENT

Mechanical ventilation of the pediatric patient uses basic principles from both the neonatal and adult patient populations. Infants weighing up to 10 kg are usually ventilated using time-cycled, pressure-limited ventilation (AARC Clinical Practice Guideline: Application of Continuous Positive Airway Pressure to Neonates via Nasal Prongs or Nasopharyngeal Tube). Larger infants and children are generally ventilated using volume-cycled ventilation. The indications for mechanical ventilation in infants and children are similar to those for adults, and they are illustrated in Box 26-4. Ventilator classification systems and modes of operation are fully described by Pilbeam and Payne in Chapter 21 of this text; therefore, this section will address the clinical application of mechanical ventilation in the pediatric patient.

Selection of Ventilator Settings

When using a time-cycled, pressure-limited, continuous-flow IMV system to ventilate an infant, the practitioner must establish the peak inspiratory pressure (PIP), the positive end-expiratory pressure (PEEP), the frequency (respiratory rate), the inspiratory-expiratory (I:E) ratio, the flow, and an FIO_2. If the infant is receiving assisted ventilation using a manual resuscitation unit, the practitioner can establish initial ventilator settings for PIP, PEEP, frequency, and FIO_2 consistent with those being delivered with the manual resuscitator. Suggestions for initial ventilator settings for an infant with normal lungs and one with pulmonary pathology are shown in Table 26-6. The practitioner must modify the initial settings based on the disease state or condition for which mechanical ventilation was initiated.

Adequacy of the set peak inspiratory pressure (PIP) can be assessed by evaluating the degree of chest expansion, presence of bilateral air movement during auscultation of the lungs, and oxygenation. Oxygenation can be assessed using the PaO_2 on an arterial blood gas analysis or by monitoring the SpO_2. Levels of positive end-expiratory pressure (PEEP) are evaluated by monitoring oxygenation. Positive end-expiratory pressure is used to restore or maintain the functional residual capacity (FRC). The FIO_2 is set at a level to ensure adequate oxygenation. Adequacy of the frequency is determined by evaluating the degree of ventilation, which is reflected by the $PaCO_2$ on an arterial blood gas analysis.

Although ventilator gas flow should be set at twice, at least, the patient's minute volume, an initial setting is usually between 6 and 8 L/min. By observing the patient and the pressure manometer, the practitioner can determine whether the flow setting needs to be increased or decreased. Turbulence and an associated increase in airway resistance occur if the flow is set too

AARC Clinical Practice Guideline

APPLICATION OF CONTINUOUS POSITIVE AIRWAY PRESSURE TO NEONATES VIA NASAL PRONGS OR NASOPHARYNGEAL TUBE

Indications: Abnormalities on physical examination include the presence of increased work of breathing as indicated by a 30% to 40% increase above normal in respiratory rate, substernal and suprasternal retractions, grunting, and nasal flaring; the presence of pale or cyanotic skin color and agitation. Inadequate arterial blood gas values indicate CPAP when there is an inability to maintain a PaO_2 >50 mmHg with $FIO_2 \geq 0.60$, provided $\dot{V}E$ is adequate as indicated by a $PaCO_2 \leq 50$ mmHg and a pH ≥ 7.25. The presence of a condition thought to be responsive to CPAP shows the following clinical presentations: presence of poorly expanded and/or infiltrated lung fields on chest radiograph, respiratory distress syndrome, pulmonary edema, atelectasis, apnea of prematurity, recent extubation, tracheal malacia or other similar abnormality of the lower airways, transient tachypnea of the newborn.

Contraindications: Although CPAP has been used in bronchiolitis, this application may be contraindicated; other contraindications include the need for intubation and mechanical ventilation, upper airway abnormalities that make CPAP ineffective or potentially dangerous (eg, choanal atresia, cleft palate, tracheoesophageal fistula), severe cardiovascular instability and impending arrest, unstable respiratory drive with frequent apneic episodes resulting in desaturation or bradycardia, ventilatory failure as indicated by the inability to maintain $PaCO_2 \geq 60$ mmHg and pH ≤ 7.25. Application of CPAP in patients with untreated congenital diaphragmatic hernia may lead to gastric distension and further compromise of thoracic organs.

Assessment of Need: Determine that valid indications are present by physical, radiographic, and laboratory assessments.

Assessment of Outcome: Initiate CPAP at levels of 4 to 5 cmH_2O, and gradually increase to 10 cmH_2O to provide the following: stabilization of FIO_2 requirement ≤ 0.60 with PaO_2 levels ≥ 50 mmHg or the presence of clinically acceptable noninvasive monitoring of oxygen ($PtcO_2$), while maintaining an adequate $\dot{V}E$ as indicated by $PaCO_2$ ≤ 50 to 60 mmHg and pH ≥ 7.25; reduction in the work of breathing as indicated by a decrease in respiratory rate and a decrease in the severity of retractions, grunting, and nasal flaring; improvement in lung volumes and appearance of lung as indicated by chest radiograph; improvement in patient comfort as assessed by bedside care giver.

Monitoring: Patient-ventilator system checks should be performed at least every 2 to 4 hours and should include documentation of ventilator settings and patient assessments. Oxygen and carbon dioxide levels should be monitored, including periodic sampling of blood gas values by arterial, capillary, or venous route; continuous noninvasive blood gas monitoring by transcutaneous O_2 and CO_2 monitors; continuous noninvasive monitoring of oxygen saturation by pulse oximetry; continuous monitoring of electrocardiogram and respiratory rate. Continuously monitor proximal airway pressure, PEEP, and mean airway pressure. Continuously monitor FIO_2; periodically assess breath sounds and signs of increased work of breathing; periodically evaluate chest radiographs.

From AARC Clinical Practice Guideline; see Respir Care 39(8):817, 1994, for complete text.

BOX 26-4

INDICATIONS FOR MECHANICAL VENTILATION IN INFANTS AND CHILDREN

Neonates and Infants	Children
Apnea from any cause that results in bradycardia and decreases in oxygen saturation.	**Acute respiratory failure** from any cause, when the $PaCO_2$ is >50 mmHg and results in a pH <7.25, and the PaO_2 is <70 mmHg on supplemental oxygen.
Respiratory failure from any cause, when the $PaCO_2$ is > 55 mmHg and results in a pH <7.25, and the PaO_2 is <50 mmHg on supplemental oxygen.	**Chronic respiratory failure** that is primarily associated with diseases involving the lungs (chronic lung disease), neurologic or neuromuscular dysfunction, and congenital defects.
Pulmonary diseases that result in an increased work of breathing and impending respiratory failure.	Following **cardiopulmonary resuscitation** and **surgery**.
In neonates only, to treat **persistent pulmonary hypertension of the newborn** (PPHN).	Following **trauma**, particularly when the trauma results in an elevated intracranial pressure.

high. On the other hand, if the flow is set too low, the infant's work of breathing increases when the inspiratory demand is not met and air hunger occurs. The practitioner can determine inadequate flow by observing the ascent of the needle on the pressure manometer. If there are needle fluctuations instead of a smooth rise to the preset PIP, or if the inspiratory phase is terminated by the inspiratory time setting before reaching the PIP, the flow likely needs to be increased.

Inspiratory time should be set by considering the pathologic condition that required initiation of mechanical ventilation. The effect of inspiratory time on the I:E ratio should always be considered, and the I:E ratio usually should not be allowed to go below 1:1. When the infant's compliance is low, longer inspiratory times may enhance alveolar ventilation. Patients with obstructive diseases, in which there is significant air trapping, generally require smaller I:E ratios (long expiratory times and low frequency) to maximize alveolar emptying.

When using a time-cycled, pressure-limited ventilator, tidal volume is a function of the pressure gradient (PIP − PEEP) interacting with the patient's lung compliance and airway resistance. Tidal volume can be considered to vary directly with the pressure gradient between PIP and PEEP. This is true, however, only if there is sufficient time during which the alveolar pressure and proximal airway pressure can equalize.[64–67] The equilibration time, or time constant, applies to both inspiration and expiration.

A time constant is determined by multiplying compliance (in L/cmH_2O) by resistance. It takes one time constant for approximately 63% of the airway pressure to equilibrate with alveolar pressure, and approximately 95% of airway pressure equilibrates with alveolar pressure in three time constants. Within five time constants, approximately 99% of airway pressure equilibrates with alveolar pressure.[64,68–69] We usually think of time constants in terms of exhalation; therefore, under normal conditions, approximately 63% of the tidal volume is emptied in one time constant. It takes three time constants to allow 95% of the tidal volume to be exhaled.[65] Though calculating time constants may seem laborious, doing so has practical value when attempting to maximize ventilation while minimizing adverse effects such as air trapping and barotrauma. Equation Box 26-2 illustrates how a time constant can be calculated and used to establish inspiratory and expiratory times and an I:E ratio.

Although it is not a ventilator parameter set by the respiratory care practitioner, mean airway pressure should be monitored while the patient is receiving mechanical ventilation. Mean airway pressure can be measured directly by using airway pressure monitors that are commercially available,[70] or calculated using the formula:

$$Paw = (PIP)(T_I/T_{TOT}) + (PEEP)(T_E/T_{TOT})$$

T_I is inspiratory time (in seconds), T_E is expiratory time (in seconds), and T_{TOT} is the total cycle time (in

TABLE 26-6. **Initial Ventilator Settings for Time-Cycled, Pressure-Limited, Mechanical Ventilators**

	Infants With Respiratory Distress Syndrome	Infants With Normal Lungs
Peak inspiratory pressure (PIP)	20 to 25 cmH_2O	12 to 18 cmH_2O
Positive end-expiratory pressure (PEEP)	4 to 5 cmH_2O	2 to 3 cmH_2O
Frequency	20 to 40 cycles/min	10 to 20 cycles/min
Inspiratory/Expiratory (I:E) ratio	1:1 to 1:2	1:4 to 1:8

Reproduced with permission from Chatburn RL: Assisted Ventilation. In Blumer JL: A Practical Guide to Pediatric Intensive Care (3rd ed.) St Louis, 1990, Mosby–Year Book

EQUATION BOX 26–2

CALCULATION OF TIME CONSTANTS AND THE I:E RATIO

The formula for calculating a **time constant** (K_t) is

$$K_t = \text{compliance } (L/cmH_2O) \times \text{resistance}$$

Compliance can be calculated by obtaining a measurement of exhaled tidal volume and dividing by (PIP-PEEP). If we assume normal compliance of 0.005 L/cmH_2O in a newborn and normal resistance of 50 $cmH_2O/L/sec$, we can calculate the K_t as follows:

$$K_t = 0.005 \times 50$$
$$= 0.25 \text{ sec}$$

Therefore, to allow emptying of 95% of the tidal volume, an expiratory time of 0.75 seconds would be required.

To calculate an **I:E ratio**, first determine the time allotted to each respiratory cycle:

60 seconds/ventilator rate = time allotted to each respiratory cycle

Next, determine the appropriate I:E ratio for the disease state, and add the parts of the ratio (for an I:E ratio of 1:2, for example, 1 + 2 = 3). Assuming a ventilator rate of 30,

60 sec/30 cycles = 2 sec per respiratory cycle

Divide the time per respiratory cycle by the sum of the parts of the ratio (sum of parts of the ratio = 3)

2 sec/3 = 0.66 sec

The time allotted to inspiration is 0.66 second. The expiratory time can then be determined by subtracting the inspiratory time from the total cycle time.

2.0 sec − 0.66 sec = 1.44 sec

If compliance were to decrease, however, such as might be expected in an infant with pneumonia or RDS, the time required for pressure equilibration (time constant) would increase. Inspiratory time would need to be increased to deliver an adequate tidal volume; consequently, either the I:E ratio would be altered, or the expiratory time would need to be decreased to maintain an I:E ratio of 1:2. If resistance were to increase, for example, in an infant with meconium aspiration or a child with asthma, the expiratory time would need to be increased to allow complete emptying of the lungs and avoid air trapping.

seconds). This formula is applicable only when the ventilator is delivering a square wave flow form and is pressure limited. By examining the formula, the practitioner can determine that mean airway pressure is influenced by PEEP, PIP, inspiratory time, and frequency (which is a function of expiratory time). In addition, the inspiratory flow and pressure waveforms also influence mean airway pressure.

When using a volume-cycled ventilator to mechanically ventilate older infants and children, the following ventilatory parameters must be established: tidal volume, inspiratory and expiratory time, ventilator frequency, and PEEP.

☐ TIDAL VOLUME

The guideline for establishing the tidal volume to be delivered via the ventilator to a child is the same as is used for the adult patient, that is, 10 to 15 mL/kg. The smallest tidal volume that can achieve effective ventilation, as determined by the $PaCO_2$ on an arterial blood gas analysis, should be used to minimize airway pressures and barotrauma.

The delivered tidal volume may vary significantly from the preset tidal volume as a result of the ventilator circuit compliance. During mechanical ventilation using standard ventilator circuits, a variable portion of the preset volume is compressed in the circuitry and, therefore, is not delivered to the patient. Consequently, the preset tidal volume does not indicate the tidal volume that is received by the patient. The portion of tidal volume lost in the ventilator circuit, which is referred to as the compressible volume, can be minimized by using ventilator circuits that are noncompliant. When a standard ventilator circuit is used, it is necessary to determine the compressible volume and adjust the preset tidal volume to compensate for that loss.

The first step in determining compressible volume is to determine the compliance of the ventilator circuit. This can be done by having the ventilator deliver a known volume into the ventilator circuit (with the patient connection at the Y occluded) while observing the pressure generated (with no PEEP applied). The volume is then divided by the observed pressure, yielding compliance for the circuit. Once the compliance of the ventilator circuit is known, the amount of volume that is compressed in the ventilator circuit can be calculated. Equation Box 26-3 illustrates how ventilator circuit compliance can be used to adjust the preset tidal volume so that the desired tidal volume and the compressible volume are included.

☐ VENTILATOR FREQUENCY, INSPIRATORY AND EXPIRATORY TIMES

The ventilator frequency should be established in concert with the tidal volume so that a normal minute volume is delivered to the patient. Ventilator frequencies for children are generally set between 20 and 40 cycles per minute.[64] As children enter adolescence and approach adulthood, optimum ventilator frequencies begin to approximate those commonly used in the adult patient. Inspiratory and expiratory times are not set directly on most volume ventilators. Expiratory time is a function of the preset ventilator frequency. Inspiratory time can be increased by decreasing the inspiratory flow; conversely, inspiratory time is decreased when the inspiratory flow is increased. The concept of time constants, discussed previously, is also applicable to the pediatric patient.

☐ POSITIVE END-EXPIRATORY PRESSURE

Similar to its use in infants, positive end-expiratory pressure (PEEP) is used in children to increase the patient's arterial oxygenation and to maintain the FRC.

EQUATION BOX 26–3

CALCULATING A CORRECTED TIDAL VOLUME

Step 1
To determine the tubing compliance, set the tidal volume to deliver 300 mL into the ventilator circuit. Occlude the patient Y with a cap or with your hand, using a sterile gauze pad placed between your hand and the patient outlet. Attach a volume-measuring device to the exhalation valve to verify the delivered volume. Manually cycle the ventilator, and observe the pressure generated on the pressure manometer.

Assume that the volume-measuring device indicates a volume of 300 mL and the manometer indicates a peak pressure of 100 cmH_2O. To determine the ventilator circuit compliance, divide

$$300 \text{ mL}/100 \text{ cmH}_2\text{O} = 3 \text{ mL}/\text{cmH}_2\text{O}$$

Step 2
Determine the desired tidal volume using the patient's weight. Start by using a tidal volume of 10 mL/kg and a patient weight of 40 kg.

$$40 \text{ kg} \times 10 \text{ mL/kg} = 400 \text{ mL}$$

Step 3
Set the tidal volume control to deliver 400 mL, and attach the patient Y to the patient's endotracheal tube. Allow the ventilator to cycle several times, and observe the peak inspiratory pressure being generated while the tidal volume is delivered.

Step 4
To determine the amount of volume sequestered in the ventilator circuit, multiply the tubing compliance by the peak inspiratory pressure observed during delivery of a tidal volume to the patient. Assume the PIP is 32 cmH_2O.

$$32 \text{ cmH}_2\text{O} \times 3 \text{ mL}/\text{cmH}_2\text{O} = 64 \text{ mL}$$

This exercise assumes that PEEP is not being used. If PEEP were applied, compressible volume would be determined by using the **change in pressure** (PIP − PEEP), not the observed PIP. The amount of volume retained in the ventilator circuit as a result of PEEP is constant.

Step 5
Determine the effective tidal volume by subtracting the compressible volume from the preset tidal volume.

$$400 \text{ mL} - 64 \text{ mL} = 335 \text{ mL}$$

As can be seen, the effective tidal volume is considerably less than 10 mL/kg. The compressible volume can then be added to the desired tidal volume, resulting in a preset tidal volume of approximately 465 mL.

Some microprocessor-controlled ventilators display a corrected tidal volume. The practitioner must understand technical aspects of the mechanical ventilators being used to maximize the effectiveness of mechanical ventilatory support.

Positive end-expiratory pressure is titrated to maintain an acceptable PaO_2 with the lowest FIO_2.[71] Positive end-expiratory pressure is generally initiated at 3 to 5 cmH_2O, and adjusted in increments of 1 to 2 cmH_2O. Adjustments in the level of PEEP are usually made based on the PaO_2 on an arterial blood gas analysis. Positive end-expiratory pressure can also be adjusted by monitoring static compliance.[72]

Monitoring During Mechanical Ventilation

Safe and effective performance of the mechanical ventilator must be documented during the entire time the patient is receiving mechanical ventilatory support. Many ventilators have built-in alarm systems to monitor the patient–ventilator interface and to alert care givers to events that compromise patient safety. At a minimum, alarm systems should alert care givers to interruptions in the ventilator circuit (failure to meet a preset pressure, failure to meet a low volume threshold, loss of PEEP/CPAP), obstructions in the ventilator circuit (high pressure alarms), and loss of power supply (electrical or pneumatic). In addition, alarm systems can signal care givers when the patient's respiratory rate changes significantly (either an increase or a decrease) and when minute volume varies from preset parameters (high and low).

Complete monitoring also must include an ongoing evaluation of the patient. The patient's breath sounds should be evaluated at the beginning of each shift so the practitioner has a basis from which to evaluate changes that may occur over time. The quality of breath sounds can be used to alert the practitioner to the presence of bronchospasm, atelectasis, or secretions. The degree and symmetry of chest expansion should be noted. Cardiac status can be evaluated by monitoring heart rate and rhythm. Blood pressure, color, and perfusion are also important indicators of the adequacy of ventilation. Pulmonary function can be evaluated by determining compliance and resistance and looking for trends. Oxygenation status can be continuously evaluated by using a pulse oximeter to monitor SpO_2. The adequacy of ventilation can be assessed using end-tidal carbon dioxide monitoring. Intermittent arterial blood gas analysis should be performed to verify oxygenation and ventilation status.

Weaning From Mechanical Ventilation

Weaning from mechanical ventilation, or the process of decreasing and ultimately removing mechanical support for breathing, can vary from rapid and uncomplicated to slow and complex. Basically, weaning can begin (1) as soon as the condition that necessitated intubation and the initiation of mechanical ventilation has resolved, (2) when cardiovascular status is stable, (3) when arterial blood gas values return to normal for the child, and (4) when muscle strength has returned to a level that supports spontaneous respirations and the ability to cough and maintain a patent airway. Methods used for weaning include (1) decreasing the rate on IMV, (2) CPAP, (3) T-piece trials, and (4) pressure support. The decision process for determining the weaning methods includes consideration of the child's condition and the underlying pathology.

Both the patient and the primary care givers require psychosocial support during the weaning process. Parents and other care givers should be encouraged to ask questions and participate in the care of the child. When patients are older children or adolescents, they should be fully informed throughout the weaning process. They should be made to feel that they have some element of control over what is happening. Patients should be able to indicate when they perceive the need to rest, and that request should be honored by the health care team.

Removal of the Artificial Airway

The procedure for extubating a pediatric patient is the same as for an adult. Before removing the endotracheal tube, equipment required for reintubation should be prepared and available in the event that an emergency reintubation is required. Before extubation, the patient is hyperoxygenated and the endotracheal tube suctioned. The patient is reoxygenated, usually by giving several breaths using a manual resuscitation bag unit. The tape securing the endotracheal tube is loosened. If the patient is intubated with a cuffed endotracheal tube, the cuff is deflated. The patient is given a final manual breath from the manual resuscitation bag, and the tube is quickly and smoothly removed at peak inspiration.

Following extubation, the child is given humidified oxygen at an FIO_2 sufficient to maintain an acceptable level of oxygenation. The child is carefully monitored for signs of respiratory distress, including inspiratory stridor, and symptoms of an increased work of breathing, including accessory muscle use. Mild postextubation inspiratory stridor usually responds to aerosolized racemic epinephrine.

BOX 26–5

CAUSES OF UPPER AIRWAY OBSTRUCTION AND STRIDOR IN CHILDREN

Acute

With the exception of foreign body aspiration, acute stridor is usually associated with an infectious process.

Viral croup (laryngotracheobronchitis)*
Epiglottitis
Bacterial tracheitis (membranous croup)
Retropharyngeal abscess
Foreign body

Chronic

The presence of chronic stridor is usually attributed to abnormal anatomic structure.

Laryngomalacia*
Laryngeal papillomas
Soft tissue bleeding
Vocal cord paralysis
Scarring or stenosis from artificial airway
Burns
Compression by mediastinal masses
Vascular compression syndrome (vascular rings)
Foreign body

** Most frequently occurring in each category*

Adapted with permission from Aoki BY and McCloskey K: Evaluation, Stabilization, and Transport of the Critically Ill Child. St Louis, Mosby–Year Book, 1992; and Schidlow DV, Smith DS. Stridor and Upper Airway Obstruction. In *DV Schidlow and DS Smith (eds): A Practical Guide to Pediatric Respiratory Diseases. Philadelphia, Hanley & Belfus, 1994*

MAJOR RESPIRATORY DISORDERS IN INFANTS AND CHILDREN

Stridor is the breath sound most frequently associated with an obstruction of the upper airway, whether the obstruction is caused by a pathologic process or from aspiration of a foreign body. Though there are a number of diseases capable of producing stridor (Box 26-5), this section will cover only the three most commonly seen in clinical practice. Foreign body aspiration will also be discussed later in this chapter because children, particularly toddlers, are likely to put objects into their mouth; consequently, the risk for either swallowing or aspirating the object is high.

Laryngotracheobronchitis

Commonly referred to as simply "croup," laryngotracheobronchitis usually occurs in children between 3 months and 3 years of age. The etiologic organisms are most frequently viral, and they include the parainfluenza viruses (types 1, 2, and 3) and influenza virus A. Laryngotracheobronchitis may be caused by bacterial agents, including *Mycoplasma pneumoniae* and *Corynebacterium diphtheriae;* however, a bacterial basis is rarely seen.[73] The incidence of laryngotracheobronchitis is increased during the fall and winter months.

Children with laryngotracheobronchitis typically present following several days of symptoms consistent with a viral upper respiratory infection: coryza, sore throat, cough, hoarseness, and low-grade temperature. A typical "croupy" cough and stridor develop as a result of swelling of the airway (glottic and subglottic edema). Very young infants appear more acutely ill and are frequently in more respiratory distress than older infants and children because their airways have a smaller diameter; as a result, a modest amount of edema produces a greater degree of airway obstruction.

A child who presents with a croupy cough, stridor, and respiratory distress must be carefully evaluated. The degree to which the airway is obstructed can be assessed by determining the presence and severity of inspiratory stridor, retractions, and tachypnea and by evaluating the quality of air movement during auscultation of the chest. An anteroposterior neck radiograph usually depicts subglottic narrowing (referred to as the "steeple sign.")[73–75]

Treatment for laryngotracheobronchitis is usually symptomatic. Children who are appropriately active and moving air with minimal distress can generally be managed at home. The efficacy of cool mist therapy has not been demonstrated;[73] however, many physicians still recommend its use.[73–75] In the home environment, mist therapy can be provided using a room humidifier. If respiratory distress increases, activity decreases, or the child is unable to take oral feedings, hospitalization is indicated. Children who are hospitalized are usually treated with cool humidity and supplemental oxygen, delivered by means of a croup tent. Continuous monitoring of oxygenation status can easily be accomplished using pulse oximetry. Anxiety and its associated increase in the work of breathing can be minimized by decreasing the number of times the patient is approached by hospital staff. The use of visual observations and noninvasive monitoring can allow safe, effective care for most patients with laryngotracheobronchitis.

Aerosolized racemic epinephrine, delivered using a small-volume nebulizer, can provide transient reductions in stridor. A recurrence of airway obstruction, manifested by rebound stridor, frequently occurs approximately 30 minutes to 1 hour after treatment with racemic epinephrine; therefore, a decision to initiate this therapy mandates a hospital admission. The use of steroids remains controversial. However, the administration of a single dose of dexamethasone has been incorporated as part of the care plan for most cases of moderate to severe disease.[73,74] Endotracheal intubation and mechanical ventilation are rarely required during the treatment of laryngotracheobronchitis.

Bacterial Tracheitis

Bacterial tracheitis is thought to be a complication of croup. Bacterial tracheitis can produce a complete airway obstruction as a result of copious, mucopurulent secretions.[18] Although bacterial tracheitis is diagnosed in only a very small number of children who present with stridor and crouplike symptoms, it is a life-threatening condition, and the respiratory care practitioner should be familiar with its presentation and treatment.[18,76]

The child may actually appear to be improving following an episode of viral croup, when suddenly there is a new onset of stridor. Typically, the child develops a fever and appears quite ill. A lateral neck film shows subglottic swelling. The etiologic agent for bacterial tracheitis is most frequently *Staphylococcus aureus*. The diagnosis is established by obtaining cultures of the purulent material. The child usually requires anesthesia to obtain the cultures.

Treatment includes appropriate antibiotic coverage. Approximately 50% of infected children require intubation to secure the airway. A superimposed bacterial pneumonia may exist, and this is likely to cause the child to require mechanical ventilation.[18,73]

Epiglottitis

The incidence of epiglottitis is declining since the implementation of vaccination against the primary causative agent, *Haemophilus influenzae* type B;[73,74,77,78] however, all respiratory care practitioners must be aware of this disease entity because it can result in an acute, total airway obstruction. Epiglottitis is an acute bacterial infection of the epiglottis and surrounding structures. As a result, it causes a supraglottic obstruction.

Epiglottitis occurs most frequently in children between 3 and 6 years of age. It can, however, occur in infants and, on occasion, in adults. Unlike laryngotracheobronchitis, which has a prodrome of several days, epiglottitis presents abruptly. The child is typically asymptomatic, then has a sudden onset of a severe sore throat and difficulty swallowing. Additional presenting symptoms include fever, drooling (because of the severe sore throat), irritability, restlessness, and anxiety. Unlike other causes of airway obstruction, in which the patient is coughing spontaneously, patients with epiglottitis usually are not coughing.[7,79] Often the child assumes a characteristic sitting posture, in which he or she is leaning forward with the mouth open and the jaw thrust forward. This is referred to as the "tripod position." The child does not usually have tachypnea, although respiratory distress is apparent.

Because of the danger of an acute airway obstruction, it is imperative to establish the diagnosis and implement initial treatment immediately. The presumptive diagnosis of epiglottitis can be made on the basis of history and presenting symptoms. If the child is in little distress, a lateral neck radiograph can be used to visualize the swollen epiglottis (Figure 26-12). The child should not be stressed during attempts to complete any medical procedures, including taking the radiograph. Some institutions allow the parent to continue holding the child during all diagnostic procedures. This approach minimizes emotional distress for both the patient and the family.

Direct visualization of the throat should not be attempted until the child is in a controlled environment, such as an operating room, and a person skilled in intubation and tracheostomy is available to establish an artificial airway in the event that examination induces laryngospasm and an acute airway obstruction. When an artificial airway has been established and secured, the physician may wish to visualize the airway using direct laryngoscopy. The epiglottis is enlarged and has a characteristically bright, cherry-red color. Cultures from the epiglottis can be obtained to verify the causative organism.

The primary treatment for epiglottitis is to establish a patent airway by intubating the child. When preparing to assist with intubation, the practitioner should select a variety of different-sized endotracheal tubes. The intubation protocol may differ between institutions; however, it is usually preferable to initially intubate the child using an orotracheal tube. The orotracheal tube may be changed to a nasotracheal tube once the child has been stabilized. Usually, intubation is accomplished with a tube that is one-half to one size smaller than would normally be used for the child. Once the airway has been established, intravenous lines can be inserted and blood cultures drawn. Because the source of infection is bacterial, intravenous antibiotic coverage is implemented. Table 26-7 illustrates categories of antibiotics used in the treatment of *Haemophilus influenzae* type B.

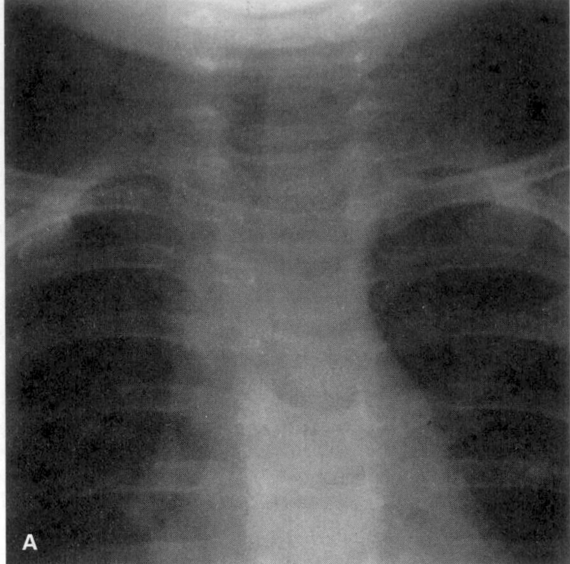

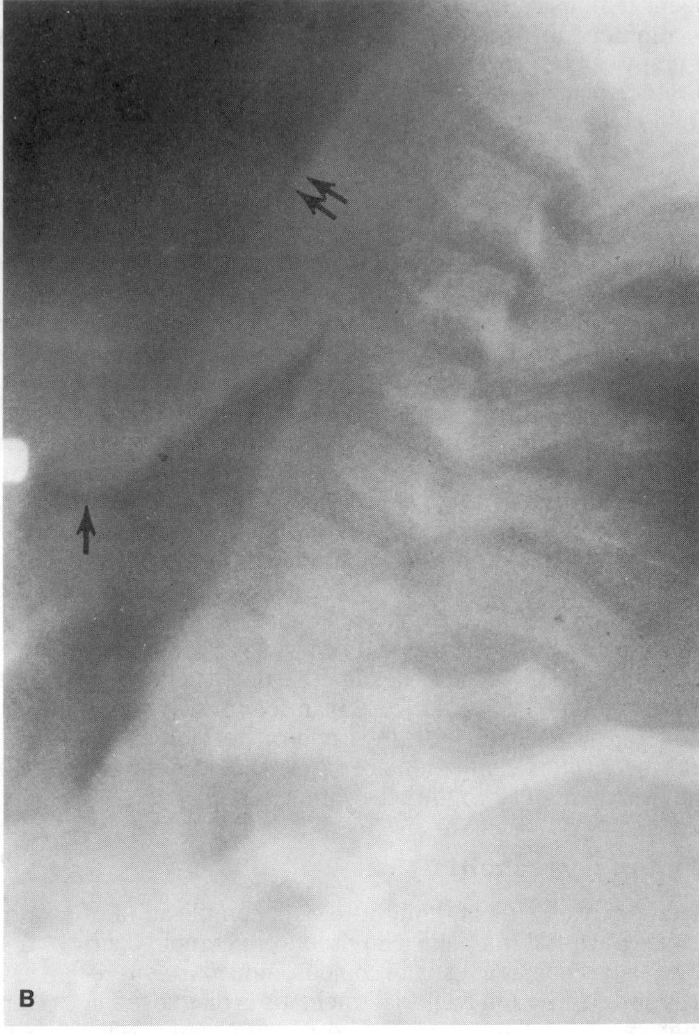

FIGURE 26-12. Radiographs of the neck can be used to differentiate laryngotracheobronchitis **(A)** from epiglottitis **(B)**.

Care must be taken to protect the patency of the airway and to prevent accidental extubation. Supplemental humidity must be provided. Some institutions supply humidity using a nebulizer and T piece, whereas others use a mechanical ventilator and provide low levels of pressure support ventilation (PSV) to minimize airway resistance caused by breathing through the endotracheal tube. Finally, some institutions place the intubated child in a high-humidity croup tent. Suctioning should be performed only when clinically indicated. To minimize the likelihood of accidental self-extubation, the child is usually restrained and sedated with agents that do not depress respirations. Mechanical ventilation is usually required only for those children who require heavy sedation or pharmacologic paralysis to protect the airway.

Antibiotic therapy usually leads to resolution of the inflammation in the epiglottic area within 24 to 36 hours; therefore, extubation usually takes place within 1 to 3 days. Direct laryngoscopy can be used to verify resolution of epiglottic inflammation. Other clinical signs that can be used to evaluate the readiness for extubation include return to a normal temperature, a general improvement in the child's appearance, and auscultation of a leak around the endotracheal tube.

Asthma

Asthma has been recognized for at least 300 years as a complex disease that causes an obstructive defect in the airways. The contributions of the inflammatory process and the autonomic nervous system were described by Sir Thomas Willis in 1685. In 1870, Austin Flint described the clinical features of asthma. During the early 20th century, Freud introduced an erroneous theory of a psychogenic basis for the disease. These early medical writings about asthma are included by Reed[80] in a historical review of airway obstruction. According to Reed, "it should not come as a surprise that our understanding of asthma as airway inflammation associated with hyperresponsive airway has progressed by rediscovering old ideas." Despite the length of time during which the medical community has researched and treated asthma, the disease continues to present diagnostic and management challenges in the contemporary practice of respiratory care.

TABLE 26-7. **Pharmacotherapy for the Treatment of *Haemophilus influenzae* type B**

Penicillins	
Ampicillin and sulbactam sodium (Unasyn)	Parenteral
Cephalosporins and Other β-Lactam* Drugs	
Cefuroxime (Ceftin, Kefurox, Zinacef), second-generation cephalosporin	Oral, parenteral
Cefotaxime (Claforan), third-generation cephalosporin	Parenteral
Ceftazidime (Fortaz, Tazidime), third-generation cephalosporin	Parenteral
Ceftriaxone (Rocephin), third-generation cephalosporin	Parenteral
General-Purpose Sulfonamides	
Trimethoprim and sulfamethoxazole (generic, Bactrim, Septra, and others)	Oral, parenteral

* More than 30% of the *Haemophilus influenzae* population is not responsive to penicillin therapy because it is capable of producing β-lactamase.

From Katzung BG: Basic and Clinical Pharmacology (6th ed.) Norwalk, CT, Appleton & Lange, 1995

In 1991, an expert panel convened by the National Heart, Lung, and Blood Institute (NHLBI) of the National Institutes of Health defined asthma as follows:

Asthma is a lung disease with the following characteristics: (1) AIRWAY OBSTRUCTION (or airway narrowing) that is reversible (but not completely so in some patients) either spontaneously or with treatment, (2) AIRWAY INFLAMMATION, and (3) AIRWAY HYPERRESPONSIVENESS to a variety of stimuli.[81]

The NHLBI definition focuses attention on two components of the disease that were not emphasized in earlier definitions. First, it is now clearly recognized that not all asthma is completely reversible, and secondly, there is renewed emphasis on the role of inflammation in the disease.[82] Inflammation appears to be the primary pathophysiologic basis for the airway hyperresponsiveness. Close scrutiny of the pathophysiologic events of an asthma attack clearly reveals that the disease can be controlled if the airway inflammation is controlled.[83] The NHLBI definition also provides a descriptive cue that enables the practitioner to create a visual image of the pathophysiology of an asthmatic episode. When participating in the development of a respiratory care plan, the practitioner can use the NHLBI definition of asthma to provide a logical framework from which to recommend diagnostic and therapeutic procedures, as well as to create an educational program for the patient and family.

The pathogenesis of asthma that occurs in the pediatric patient does not differ from that in the adult. Li provides a thorough discussion of the pathology of asthma in Ch. 27. Therefore, this section will primarily focus on the specific presentation, diagnosis, and treatment of the pediatric patient.

It is estimated that more than 4 million children in the United States suffer from asthma.[84] Though asthma is often considered by the public, as well as some medical professionals, as a fairly benign disease, every year children die as a result of asthma and its complications.[85] The rate of pediatric deaths during an asthma attack is well documented in the literature.[86–88] The highest incidence of asthma is noted in urban settings; among blacks in all geographic locations; and among children who were born to mothers who smoke cigarettes, children who reside in poverty, children who had low birth weight, and children who were born to mothers who were less than 20 years old.[85] A recent study suggests that maternal smoking is the only risk factor associated with children who were found to have transient early childhood wheezing (defined as those children who wheezed during the first 3 years of life, but who did not have a definitive diagnosis of asthma), as well as with children who had persistent wheezing (defined as children who continued to wheeze for the first 6 years of life and who had a significant decrease in their lung function at that age).[86] The economic impact of asthma is felt by both the patient (or family unit) and by society as a whole.[86,87] In a cost estimate for 1990, it was found that the direct cost of caring for children under the age of 18 with asthma exceeded $1.6 billion.[82] This figure does not include the costs of medications or the wages that were lost by parents who needed to stay home with their sick child.

The social and opportunity costs of asthma are also evident. More school days are missed because of asthma than any other childhood disease. Parents of children with asthma report missing work; exacerbations of asthma are a major cause of work absenteeism.

□ EVALUATION OF KNOWN OR SUSPECTED ASTHMA

The diagnosis of asthma in a young child is usually made on the basis of the history and findings from the physical examination. The physician usually compiles a complete history (see Box 26-3), performs a physical examination with emphasis on an assessment of the upper and lower airways and the extremities, and orders diagnostic tests. The final component in the diagnosis of asthma is an evaluation of the patient's response to bronchodilator administration.

The history may provide valuable insight into precipitating events, such as the presence of a common cold or upper respiratory infection, exposure to a known or suspected allergen, changes in environmental conditions, or an event that is associated with emotional distress. Examination of the upper airways allows the physician to determine whether an infection of the ears, sinuses, or throat contributed to the onset of symptoms that are consistent with a diagnosis of asthma. The physician and the respiratory care practitioner should observe the patient's respiratory rate and pattern. The presence of accessory muscle use should be noted. The quality of air movement during both the inspiratory and expiratory phases should be evaluated, and the I:E ratio should be assessed. Air movement in all lung segments should be determined. The examiner should listen carefully to determine the presence of wheezing and any other adventitious sounds. If wheezing is heard, the practitioner must determine whether it is generalized throughout the lung fields or unilaterally located, and if it is associated with either inspiration or expiration, or both. Wheezing during inspiration is usually associated with severe obstruction. A combination of decreased air movement and the absence of wheezes may indicate that the patient has severely obstructed airways and that airflow is so diminished that sounds are not being produced. Finally, the configuration of the chest should be observed.[12]

□ LABORATORY STUDIES

Pulmonary Function Testing. It is essential that an objective assessment of airway patency be obtained, because neither the patient nor the health care providers, including the physician, can accurately determine the degree of airway obstruction on the basis of symptoms and the physical examination.[89–92] The use of an objective measurement of airflow has been incorporated into the NHLBI Guidelines for the Diagnosis and Management of Asthma,[81] and Tinkelman argues "the single most important laboratory study in evaluating the child who has or is suspected of having asthma is spirometry."[83] The NHLBI recommends that spirometry be performed during the initial assessment of a patient who is being evaluated for asthma and periodically thereafter. The NHLBI also recommends that patients be followed with either spirometry or measurements of peak expiratory flow rate (PEFR) using a peak flow meter. Peak flow meter assessments of PEFR can be accomplished quite easily in the hospital, either in the emergency room or on a general patient floor; in the physician's office or clinic; and in the patient's home. The ease with which they can be used and the cost efficiency of peak flow meters allow rapid and repeated gross assessments of airway patency.

The use of peak flow meters may also empower the patient and family by allowing them to participate more fully in the therapeutic plan. When used in conjunction with a well-planned and well-understood care plan, PEFR measurements can allow the patient to exercise more control over his or her disease. The issue of self-control may be especially important when working with an adolescent patient. The concept of allowing control to originate from within a sense of self was explained by Cooley in 1902.[4,93] The adolescent is capable of understanding complex systems and making linkages between behaviors and outcomes. When the adolescent is allowed to exercise control over observable outcomes, such as improved activity levels and an ability to be more like friends who do not have asthma, he or she is more likely to comply with the prescribed therapeutic regimen.

Peak flow meters typically provide a nomogram so the patient can determine a normal value for an individual of the same sex, age, and height. By using this typical normal value, a patient can evaluate the degree to which his or her lung function approximates normal function. There are two problems related to using standard nomograms to follow PEFR. First, according to the British Thoracic Society, PEFR "values expressed as percentages of the predicted normal are not useful in patients with chronically impaired lung function."[94] Second, normal PEFR values vary widely among normal people, so the "normal values" may or may not accurately predict a person's PEFR.[92] Consequently, the physician and the patient should determine the patient's "personal best" PEFR. Then, routine PEFR measurements should be compared to the patient's "personal best" instead of using the prepared nomogram.

Technical performance standards for peak flow meters are described in a report published by the NHLBI in 1991.[95] The performance of peak flow meters has been researched and documented in the literature.[96–101] The respiratory care practitioner should remember that, from a practical perspective, repeated test results are constant when a patient uses a peak flow meter from a single manufacturer. If it becomes necessary to change to a peak flow meter manufactured by a different company, the patient should notify his primary health care provider so that potential differences in the absolute value can be evaluated. A single value that is inconsistent with other clinical findings should be evaluated for the possibility of peak flow meter malfunction. There is evidence that peak flow meter performance and accuracy may deteriorate as the unit ages;[98] as a result, the patient and health care providers need to evaluate declining trends within the context of other clinical findings.

Chest Radiograph. When a person suffers an acute asthma attack, his or her chest radiograph usually shows hyperinflation. The chest film may show areas of segmental or subsegmental atelectasis in the presence of mucous plugs. There may be some mild interstitial thickening.[102]

Arterial Blood Gas Analysis. An assessment of arterial blood gases provides information regarding both the acid–base balance and oxygenation status of the patient. Arterial blood gas analysis should be performed when the child's peak flow is less than 25% of that predicted, in younger children who demonstrate use of accessory muscles,[82] and in infants with an $SpO_2 < 90\%$.[81] During the initial asthma attack, a mild respiratory alkalosis is likely to occur as a result of hyperventilation. The PaO_2 may be slightly low or normal. Changes in the $PaCO_2$ and pH should be evaluated within the context of the clinical situation. Many patients with mild hypercarbia, in whom oxygenation is adequate, respond to conservative therapy, and intubation can be avoided.

Capillary blood gas studies are frequently used in the pediatric setting; however, during an asthma attack, the utility of capillary blood gas assessments is limited. Treatment with β agonists may produce peripheral resistance sufficient to prevent obtaining an adequately arterialized sample for analysis.[82]

Other Laboratory Tests. If the patient is being treated with oral theophylline on a maintenance basis, it is necessary to obtain a serum theophylline level. Complete blood counts may be useful. The presence of eosinophilia is consistent with a diagnosis of asthma. The presence of leukocytosis is often indicative of a bacterial infection that may be a predisposing factor for exacerbation of the asthma. In general, laboratory tests should be ordered on an individual basis and within the context of the clinical situation.

Response to Bronchodilator Administration. During spirometric testing, it is common to obtain tracings of expiratory air flow before and after the administration of a β_2 agonist. In the pediatric patient, reversibility of bronchospasm has been demonstrated when the FEV_1 increases by at least 10%.[103]

□ TREATMENT

The goals of therapy, as described by the NHLBI, are as follows:

(1) Maintain (near) "normal" pulmonary function rates; (2) maintain normal activity levels (including exercise); (3) prevent chronic and troublesome symptoms (eg, coughing or breathlessness in the night, in the early morning, or after exertion); (4) prevent recurrent exacerbations of asthma; and (5) avoid adverse effects from asthma medications.[81]

The goals of treatment in the pediatric patient do not differ from the goals of treatment in the adult; therefore, the reader is once again referred to Chapter 27 for a thorough discussion of pharmacotherapy in the treatment of asthma. This section will focus on the treatments or delivery methods that are specific to the pediatric patient, and on considerations regarding therapies that are pertinent only to a pediatric patient. Tables 26-8 and 26-9 provide the NHLBI treatment protocols for the child who is experiencing an acute asthma attack.[81] Table 26-10 provides a summary of the clinical signs and symptoms, level of activities of daily living (ADL) disturbance, diagnostic evaluations, and treatment goals for asthma.

Bronchiolitis

One of the most common illnesses in infancy and early childhood, *bronchiolitis* typically causes the child to present with tachypnea, dyspnea, and wheezing. The etiologic agent is viral, most frequently the respiratory syncytial virus (RSV). Parainfluenza viruses (types 1 and 3), adenovirus, influenza viruses, rhinovirus, and enterovirus are also capable of causing the disease. The diagnosis of bronchiolitis is based on symptoms and presentation, and it is confirmed by the presence of RSV in nasal washings. Respiratory syncytial virus is identi-

TABLE 26-8. **NHLBI Treatment Protocols: Mild and Moderate Asthma**

Chronic Mild Asthma	Chronic Moderate Asthma
Clinical Characteristics	Clinical Characteristics
Intermittent symptoms (wheeze, cough, dyspnea, tightness) no more than twice weekly; nocturnal symptoms less than twice monthly	Symptoms occur more than 1 or 2 times weekly
Asymptomatic between exacerbations	Exacerbations last several days
Symptoms last less than 1/2 hour following activity	Requires occasional emergency care
Assessment of Lung Function (FEV_1 or PEFR)	Assessment of Lung Function (FEV_1 or PEFR)
Equal to or >80% baseline when asymptomatic	Less than 60% of baseline
Varies more than 20% from baseline when symptomatic	Highly variable: changes 20% to 30% with medication
Therapy	Therapy
PRN pretreatment with β agonists or cromolyn before exposure to exercise, allergen, or other stimuli when asymptomatic	Inhaled β agonist PRN 3 to 4 times daily and
When symptomatic and <5 years old, use PRN aerosolized β agonist at age-appropriate dose	Cromolyn or other antiinflammatory agent twice daily, or sustained-release theophylline or oral β agonist
When symptomatic and >5 years old, use β agonist delivered via MDI every 4–6 hours PRN	If symptoms persist, may eliminate cromolyn and theophylline and add inhaled corticosteroids
Outcome	Outcome
Prevent and control symptoms	Improve pulmonary function
Promote normal activity	Reduce PEFR variability
Eliminate nocturnal cough or wheeze	Promote almost normal activity
Reduce PEFR variability	Reduce frequency of awakening at night
Promote normal lung function	Reduce frequency of exacerbations
	Reduce frequency of PRN inhaled β agonists

TABLE 26-9. **NHLBI Treatment Protocols: Severe Asthma**

Clinical Characteristics
- Continuous symptoms
- Limited activity level
- Frequent exacerbations
- Frequent nocturnal symptoms
- Occasional hospitalization and emergency treatment

Assessment of Lung Function (FEV_1 or PEFR)
- Less than 60% of baseline
- Highly variable: changes 20 to 30% with routine medications

Therapy
- Inhaled β agonists PRN TID or QID
  - With patient <5 years old, use nebulizer
  - With patient >5 years old, use MDI with spacer
- Following β agonist therapy, use antiinflammatory agent, such as inhaled corticosteroid BID to QID
- If nocturnal symptoms are present, use oral sustained-release theophylline or oral β agonist, or both

Outcome
- Improved pulmonary function
- Reduced peak flow variability
- Almost normal activity
- Infrequent awakening at night
- Reduced frequency of exacerbations
- Reduced frequency of PRN inhaled β agonists
- Reduced need for corticosteroid burst
- Reduced need for emergency treatment

fied using an enzyme-linked immunosorbent assay (ELISA).[104] Bronchiolitis occurs most frequently during the winter months and primarily among infants between 1 and 6 months of age. It can also be seen in toddlers. In most children, bronchiolitis is a self-limiting disease; it generally improves within 7 to 10 days.[105] Children under 6 months of age are most likely to experience episodes of cyanosis and are more likely to require hospitalization. This is probably related to the degree of edema and airway obstruction relative to the size of the airway.

In addition to tachypnea, dyspnea, and wheezing, the physical examination may reveal an elevated temperature and mild dehydration. Mild hypoxemia, which responds readily to oxygen therapy, may be present. The airway becomes obstructed from the inflammatory process that accompanies the disease. Airway narrowing and a concomitant increase in airway resistance can occur as a result of bronchoconstriction. Aerosolized bronchodilator therapy may produce significant clinical improvement, for example, a decrease in wheezing and tachypnea. Because it is difficult to know which patients benefit from aerosolized bronchodilator therapy, it is useful to administer a trial of nebulized β agonists and evaluate each patient's response to the therapy. If no clinical improvement is noted, the treatments should be discontinued.[105]

Most children with mild symptoms can usually be cared for at home. Treatment consists of humidity therapy, saline nose drops, bulb suctioning of the nose and oropharynx, and increased fluids. Children with congenital heart disease and those with preexisting cardiopulmonary illness frequently require hospitalization and more intensive treatment. Children who have a respiratory rate >45 breaths/minute, marked retractions, decreased breath sounds, and an SpO_2 of <95% on room air require hospitalization. Children who are listless and unable to take adequate fluids also require admission.[7,105,106]

Treatment for hospitalized children is based on the symptoms. Humidity and oxygen therapy can be provided using an oxygen hood, a Tot Tent, or a croup tent. The FIO_2 is titrated to maintain an acceptable SpO_2. Intravenous fluids may be necessary if the child cannot tolerate oral feedings. Antibiotics are not indicated unless there is a superimposed bacterial infection. Aerosolized bronchodilators should only be used when there is clinical evidence of their effectiveness.[7,106]

Children who are severely ill from bronchiolitis, and those with underlying cardiopulmonary disease, may benefit from the administration of ribavirin (Virazole). Ribavirin is the only drug developed and approved specifically for the treatment of RSV. The mechanism of action is not clearly understood; however, it is known that ribavirin disrupts viral RNA and DNA.[105,107] It appears that early treatment with ribavirin may decrease the length of time mechanical ventilation is required, the length of time and the amount of supplemental oxygen required, and the length of stay in the hospital.[108,109]

Ribavirin is administered for 12 to 18 hours each day. It is nebulized, using a small particle aerosol generator (SPAG-2 nebulizer, ICN Pharmaceuticals, Costa Mesa, CA), and delivered to the patient using large-bore (aerosol) tubing connected to a mask, hood, or croup tent. Initially, it was recommended by the manufacturer that ribavirin not be administered to mechanically ventilated patients. When it was recognized that the patient group requiring mechanical ventilation was also the patient group for whom ribavirin would most likely be indicated, a method by which to administer ribavirin to patients requiring mechanical ventilation was sought.

Ribavirin can be administered to patients who are being mechanically ventilated by means of either a pressure-cycled or volume-cycled ventilator. The ventilator circuit is modified to receive the input of aerosolized ribavirin from the SPAG-2. With a pressure-cycled ventilator, the respiratory care practitioner must monitor peak inspiratory pressure and PEEP levels carefully throughout the ribavirin run. Inspiratory flow and PEEP may require adjustments after the SPAG-2 is connected to the ventilator circuit to ensure that the prescribed parameters are maintained. With a volume-cycled ventilator, the respiratory care practitioner must remember that exhaled volume monitors are erroneously high because of the added flow from the SPAG-2 unit. Ventilator alarm systems, such as low exhaled tidal volume, cannot be used to detect small disruptions in the integrity of the ventilator circuit. External monitors for high and low pressure, including PEEP, must be used to monitor the patient-ventilator interface and to ensure patient safety.

Ribavirin precipitates in the ventilator circuit and on the exhalation valve. Clogging of the exhalation valve causes inadvertent increases in PEEP as well as pro-

TABLE 26-10. **Asthma**

Severity of Asthma	ADL Disturbance	Clinical Signs	Lab & PFT Findings	Therapeutic Plan
Mild	Minimal; child engages in age-appropriate play activities Sleep not usually disturbed as a result of asthma Acute episode: child may modify play activities by selecting quiet games, watching television, reading or drawing instead of games that require physical activity such as running or jumping; feeding difficulty may be noticed in younger children or infants	Mild cough or wheezing up to twice a week Acute episode: respiratory rate increases during activity, pulsus paradoxus <10 mmHg, end-expiratory wheezes, good color, no change in alertness, mild retractions may be present	Lung volumes and expiratory flows obtained by spirometry WNL (>80%) PEFR is stable on a day-to-day basis Acute episode: PEFR varies 10% to 30% below baseline, SpO_2 >95%	Patient and family asthma education, monitor PEFR, oral or inhaled β agonists on a PRN basis for symptoms, may use cromolyn before exercise or potential allergen exposure Goals of therapy: prevent or control symptoms, enable child to participate in age appropriate activities, prevent sleep disturbances, promote normal lung function
Moderate	Mild; exercise and play limited by coughing and wheezing Sleep disturbed at least one time each week by asthma symptoms such as coughing and wheezing Acute episode: all activities, including sleeping, playing, and feeding, are negatively impacted by coughing and wheezing; parents and other primary care givers may notice that the child begins to look anxious	Frequent episodes of coughing and wheezing (>2 days each week) Acute episode: respiratory rate is increased during rest; I&E wheezing; work of breathing is increased, but the child does not appear in distress while at rest; pulsus paradoxus 10 to 20 mmHg; moderate retractions with accessory muscle use; no change in alertness; color good	Obstructive defect on expiratory flows (60% to 80%) PEFR shows day-to-day variation Acute episode: PEFR varies 30% to 50% below baseline, SpO_2 90% to 95%	Patient and family asthma education, monitor PEFR, daily treatment with anti-inflammatory agents via MDI (cromolyn, nedocromil; low-dose corticosteroids may be used), inhaled β agonists used on a PRN basis (up to QID) Goals of therapy: control symptoms, optimize lung function, enable child to participate in age appropriate activities, minimize sleep disturbances, decrease frequency of β_2-agonist requirement, minimize need for emergency care
Severe	Severely limited; unable to engage in age-appropriate play activities Sleep disturbed; child awakens with "tight chest" nearly every day Acute episode: all activities, including talking and eating, require increased effort; child is obviously anxious	Wheezing on an almost continual basis Coughing with minimal activity Acute episode: wheezing is usually audible to care givers; however, the absence of wheezing must be considered with all other findings because it may be indicative of severe airway obstruction with concomitant severely decreased airflow; severe retractions are observable in young children; alar flaring	Chronic reduction in expiratory flows (60%) PEFR shows day-to-day variation Acute episode: PEFR <50% of baseline	Patient and family asthma education, PEFR monitoring, daily treatment with β agonists (inhaled or oral), daily treatment with antiinflammatory agents (Cromolyn may not be controlling inflammation; therefore, it may be discontinued; if already on low-dose corticosteroids, dosage may be increased; oral corticosteroids may be used during an exacerbation of symptoms, or low-dose daily therapy may be initiated); daily treatment with inhaled anticholinergics (MDI) Goals of therapy: improve lung function, promote ability to engage in age-appropriate activities, minimize sleep disturbances, decrease need for corticosteroid burst, minimize need for emergency care, minimize exacerbations of disease

longation of inspiratory time. Precipitation within the ventilator circuit can be minimized by using a heated wire circuit. Precipitation of ribavirin on the exhalation valve can be minimized by using a series of two bacteria filters, placed in the ventilator circuit immediately proximal to the exhalation valve. The filters should be changed every 2 to 4 hours, and the ventilator circuit itself should be changed every shift.

Respiratory syncytial virus is highly contagious; therefore, all care givers must be diligent in washing their hands after caring for patients admitted with bronchiolitis. In addition, care givers should avoid touching their own faces with hands that are possibly contaminated with RSV. Ribavirin has been shown to have carcinogenic, mutagenic, and teratogenic properties in laboratory animals (prescription insert, ICN Pharmaceuticals, Costa Mesa, CA). Care givers should exercise caution when administering ribavirin and follow institutional policies and procedures that minimize the likelihood that the drug is inadvertently inhaled.

Cystic Fibrosis

Cystic fibrosis (CF) is the most common fatal genetic disease in the United States, occurring approximately 1 in 2,000 births. While CF can occur in African Americans and Asian Americans, it is primarily a disease of whites who descended from European ancestry. Cystic fibrosis is transmitted as an autosomal recessive disorder, which means both parents must carry the genetic mutation for the disease to be transmitted to their children. In 1989, the gene responsible for CF was identified and cloned.[110–112] The CF gene, cystic fibrosis transmembrane conductance regulator (CFTR), is located on chromosome 7. *Cystic fibrosis transmembrane conductance regulator* is a protein that regulates the normal movement of electrolytes through epithelial cell membranes.[113] In organs lined with epithelial cells, including the lungs and intestinal system, dehydration and an increase in the viscosity of sections results from the abnormal movement of sodium and chloride. In the United States, approximately 5% of the population, or 1 in 20, carry the gene. When both parents are carriers, each of their children have a 25% chance of developing the disease, a 50% chance of carrying the gene but not having the disease, and a 25% chance of neither carrying the gene nor developing CF. Male and female offspring appear to be equally effected.

While advances in pharmacotherapy and therapeutic modalities have extended the life expectancy of a patient with CF to the mid-to-late 20s,[113–115] as of this writing there is no cure for the disease. As a result, emotional support for the patient and family is essential from diagnosis throughout the course of the disease. Parents and extended family members frequently need to learn to deal with feelings of guilt and self-recrimination. Because CF is a chronic disease, the family must modify many, if not all, of its activities. Parental employment options may be limited due to concerns about insurance and access to medical care. Because CF is ultimately fatal, all family members must learn coping strategies that enable them to live with the almost certain knowledge that the child will die. All members of the health care team, including respiratory care practitioners, should be well versed in the psychology of chronic illness and dying to provide maximal support to the patient and family.

Cystic fibrosis typically affects the exocrine glands; therefore, abnormalities occur in bronchiolar, pancreatic, and biliary secretions as well as in sweat.[116] Table 26-11 summarizes the major organ systems impacted by CF, along with the clinical manifestations. Clearly, CF is a disease with multisystemic consequences for the body. The overwhelming majority of patients, however,

TABLE 26-11. **Cystic Fibrosis**

Organ System or Structure	Abnormality	Clinical Effect
Upper airways	Nasal polyps and chronic sinusitis	Airway obstruction and increased airway resistance
Lower airways	Hypertrophy of mucous-secreting glands	Increased production of thick secretions
	Decreased ciliary motility and secretion retention	Airway obstruction and increased airway resistance
	Airway hyperreactivity	Increased airway resistance
	Bronchiectasis	Colonization and chronic infections with multiple organisms, including *Pseudomonas aeruginosa, Pseudomonas cepacia, Hemophilus influenzae,* and *Staphylococcus aureus*
Lungs	Cystic areas	Increased incidence of pneumothorax
	Atelectasis	Hypoxemia and hypercapnia related to V/Q mismatching
Respiratory musculature	Decreased muscle strength	Increased work of breathing, increased oxygen consumption, carbon dioxide retention (late stages), difficulty clearing secretions
Pancreas	Thickening of pancreatic enzymes Obstruction of secretory ducts	Difficulty in digesting and using dietary fats and proteins leading to chronic, large, foul-smelling stools; chronic diarrhea; and malnutrition
Intestines	Intestinal obstruction	Abdominal pain

experience pulmonary morbidity and mortality.[114] Lower respiratory tract infections are frequently seen in infants, and this finding, along with **failure to thrive,** often prompts the physician to consider CF as a differential diagnosis. Children and adolescents usually have begun to demonstrate characteristic clinical findings such as generalized plugging of the airways and atelectasis, both of which can be attributed to thickened and retained secretions.

□ EVALUATION

Physical examination of a patient with CF usually reveals rhonchi during auscultation of the chest. Wheezes are likely to be present during an acute infection. The patient is usually tachypneic and may have a prolonged expiratory phase; the child may, however, deny dyspnea because of having become accustomed to the breathing pattern. Inspection of the chest may reveal a widened anteroposterior diameter. In late disease, percussion may reveal a hyperresonant note because of chronic air trapping and an increased in the FRC.

Though not a component of a medically oriented physical examination, a significant physical finding that frequently prompts parents and other primary care givers to seek a medical consultation is the presence of a salty taste when an infant or child is kissed.

□ LABORATORY STUDIES

Diagnostic Testing. The definitive diagnostic test for CF is the sweat test. During a sweat test, the levels of sodium and chloride are determined using pilocarpine electrophoresis. Because the sweat glands are exocrine glands, abnormally high levels of sodium chloride are found in the sweat of patients with CF. The diagnosis of CF is established when the levels of sodium and chloride in the sweat are greater than 60 mEq/L.

Genetic Testing. The gene for CF can now be detected as early as the 10th week of gestation, using chorionic villus sampling and DNA analysis. Genetic testing is generally reserved for those families in which there is a history of CF; routine screening as part of prenatal care is not recommended.[113]

Pulmonary Function Testing. Results of spirometric testing typically reveal an obstructive defect. Tests of expiratory air flow typically show a decrease, while the FRC and TLC may be increased, particularly in the advanced disease state.

Sputum Cultures. The sputum is generally colonized with bacterial growth. During an acute exacerbation, however, a sputum culture is very beneficial in identifying the specific pathogen causing the infection.

Arterial Blood Gas Analysis. During periods of relative stability of the disease, the arterial blood gas analysis results may be nearly normal or reveal mild hypoxemia. As the disease progresses, chronic hypoxemia and hypercarbia appear.

Chest Radiograph. Radiographs can be used to monitor the degree of hyperinflation and other pulmonary changes, as well as to monitor the size of the heart (cardiomegaly occurs as a result of chronic hypoxemia). In an acute exacerbation, radiographs are used to identify and localize areas of consolidation. If a patient experiences a sudden onset of chest pain associated with dyspnea, a chest x-ray film can confirm the presence and size of a pneumothorax.

□ TREATMENT

Treatment programs vary for each child according to the severity of the disease and the existing symptoms. As a result, primary care givers for infants and young children, and the patients themselves in cases of school-aged children and adolescents, must be knowledgeable about the disease state and be able to respond appropriately to changes from baseline. Because most patients with CF experience pulmonary disease, respiratory care modalities play an important role in the treatment plan.

Most patients benefit from a bronchial hygiene program including chest physiotherapy and postural drainage. Chest physiotherapy and postural drainage should be performed before meals. If the patient is receiving bronchodilator therapy, using either a small-volume nebulizer or MDI, the bronchodilator should be administered before chest physiotherapy and postural drainage. This treatment schedule maximizes the effectiveness of the therapy. Newer methods of chest physiotherapy, including PEP mask therapy and autogenic drainage (AD), have been shown to be at least as effective as the traditional treatment of percussion, vibration or shaking, and postural drainage.[23–27] Positive expiratory pressure mask therapy and AD can be more cost-effective because they are typically self-administered. Finally, the use of PEP mask therapy and AD may be more accepted by older children and adolescents when they are allowed to be more in control of their disease and its treatment.

Aerosolized bronchodilators may be used in those patients for whom airway hyperreactivity has been demonstrated, or during an acute exacerbation when wheezing is present. Intravenous antibiotic therapy is usually required during an acute infection. Some patients require hospitalization for intravenous antibiotic therapy administration; other patients can be treated successfully at home when the primary care givers have demonstrated the ability to care for an indwelling intravenous catheter. Aerosolized antibiotics (tobramycin, gentamicin, and penicillin) have been shown to enhance the treatment of gram-negative bacterial infections.[113,115] Aerosolized antibiotics are likely to induce bronchospasm; therefore, they should always be administered in conjunction with an aerosolized bronchodilator. The bronchodilator can be administered immediately before administering the aerosolized antibiotic, or if the drugs are chemically compatible, they can be mixed and administered in a single treatment. Albuterol and tobramycin, for example, have been found to be stable for up to 7 days when mixed and stored in a refrigerator.[117]

In the past few years, a number of new and innovative drug therapies have been developed for the treatment of CF. When the gene responsible for causing CF was identified, researchers were hopeful that normal genetic material could be introduced into the body using an adenovirus as the carrier and could thus correct the genetic defect. Unfortunately, the adenovirus has been found to be ineffective as a carrier.[118] Research is continuing in the area of gene therapy. Aerosolized amiloride (Midamor), a potassium-sparing diuretic, has been shown to block the absorption of sodium from respiratory secretions. Recombinant human deoxyribonuclease I (rhDNase I), a medication that breaks the DNA bond in sputum and thus reduces viscosity, is used to increase sputum removal and therefore maintain airway patency.[113] Recently, the effectiveness of daily, high-dose ibuprofen in slowing the progression of the disease has been documented.[119,120]

Normal growth and development is supported by nutritional therapy. Although respiratory care practitioners are not usually directly involved in nutritional support, the entire health care team must be aware of the importance of appropriate nutrition intake. The diet for a patient with CF provides a high daily calorie content and additional protein. Fats are usually limited because of their negative impact on the absorption of other nutrients. Supplemental vitamins, including vitamins A, D, and E, are provided. Supplemental pancreatic enzymes are required with all meals.[113] Familial and cultural norms surrounding diet must be taken into consideration when caring for a child with CF. The family can usually maintain its normal dietary habits, as long as the dietary needs of the child or children with CF are known and incorporated into the daily meals.

Surgical treatment for patients with CF has had good success. Lung resection may be used when there is recurrent segmental or lobar collapse. Transplantation of one or both lungs has been used to treat patients with advanced CF. Although the mortality remains high with these procedures, refinements in patient selection and the surgical technique, combined with improvements in postoperative management, hold promise for these therapeutic interventions.[115,121]

Infectious Diseases

□ PNEUMONIA

Pneumonia is defined as an inflammation of the pulmonary parenchyma. Pneumonia occurs frequently in children, and the etiology may range from an infectious process (bacteria, viruses, chlamydia, mycoplasma) to aspiration of food or upper airway secretions into the lung to the inhalation of noxious substances such as chemicals. Most infectious pneumonias occur when organisms are inhaled and lodge in the nasopharyngeal secretions and are subsequently carried into the lungs as aerosol particles. Pneumonia in the pediatric patient is identified anatomically, the same as in adults. Lobar pneumonia refers to an infiltrate that occupies most or all of one of the lobes in the lung. Bronchopneumonia refers to an infiltrate that originates in the terminal bronchiole and extends into nearby lobules. Interstitial pneumonia refers to an inflammatory process of the interstitium.

The clinical presentation in infants and children is similar to that in adults and depends on a number of variables, including the age and immune system status of the child and the causative organism. Most children with pneumonia present with tachypnea, fever, and cough. Auscultation of the chest may reveal fine crackles or decreased breath sounds, depending on the degree of lung involvement. Though the etiologic agent for approximately one half of all pneumonias is not identified, the physician uses a variety of assessment tools (physical examination, history of the onset of illness, laboratory and radiographic findings) to determine the treatment plan. The ability to obtain and examine a sputum sample is limited in infants and children because of the high likelihood of specimen contamination by upper airway secretions. Older children can usually produce an adequate sputum sample.[7,122]

Treatment protocols in pediatric patients are similar to those for adults. Hypoxia is treated or prevented by the administration of oxygen. Oxygenation can be monitored using pulse oximetry. Children with an elevated temperature and a high minute volume are at risk for dehydration; therefore, adequate fluid administration is essential. The respiratory care practitioner should monitor the consistency of airway secretions and report any changes. Chest physiotherapy and aerosolized bronchodilator therapy may be ordered. The respiratory care practitioner should evaluate the response to these therapies (an improvement in breath sounds, for example, or a decrease in respiratory distress) and make appropriate recommendations for either continuing or modifying the respiratory care treatments. When there is no documentable change in the patient's breath sounds or respiratory rate, there may be little, if any, indication for continued therapy. Most children recover from pneumonia without incident; however, children with compromised immune systems or those with chronic pulmonary conditions are at increased risk of morbidity and mortality.

Aspiration pneumonia results when a patient aspirates a foreign substance into the lung and there is a resulting inflammatory reaction. Aspiration pneumonia is seen when the patient aspirates gastric contents, suffers from smoke inhalation, or aspirates hydrocarbon-based products such as household cleaners. When a patient aspirates a foreign substance into the airway, there is irritation to the airway mucosa and lung parenchyma. This results in mucosal edema and impairment of the mucociliary escalator. The pathophysiologic events are the same as in the adult, where aspiration pneumonia may lead to atelectasis and V/Q mismatching with resulting hypoxemia. Alveolar-capillary leaking may occur when the alveolar epithelium is disrupted. Treatment is directed at supporting gas exchange and maintaining a patent airway. This may require simple therapies such as aerosolized bronchodilators or, in some cases, intubation and mechanical ventilation.

☐ TUBERCULOSIS

The etiologic agent for *tuberculosis* is *Mycobacterium tuberculosis.* Until recently, the incidence of tuberculosis in the United States was declining; however, there has been an increase in the number of reported cases over the past few years. This increase is attributed, in part, to an increase in immigration of tuberculosis-infected people from third-world countries, and to the increase in the incidence of acquired immunodeficiency syndrome (AIDS).[123] Children develop tuberculosis when they are exposed to a source, which is usually an adult who has active disease. The route of transmission is direct contact with contaminated respiratory secretions from a person who has the disease.[7,123]

Children with tuberculosis exhibit similar signs and symptoms as an adult: fever, loss of appetite, weight loss, night sweats, and cough. The diagnosis of tuberculosis is established by skin testing and confirmed by isolation of the bacillus in sputum. Pharmacotherapy for tuberculosis consists of multiple drug treatment, usually using isoniazid (INH) and rifampin. Children should be placed in respiratory isolation until therapy has been in place for at least 24 hours. Parents and older children should be taught about the disease and the importance of complying fully with all prescribed treatments, including testing of other family members and any known contacts. Respiratory care practitioners play an important role in the diagnosis and treatment of tuberculosis.

☐ INCIDENCE AND PATHOPHYSIOLOGY

Drowning is the fourth leading cause of death in the pediatric population (defined as ages 0 to 19 years old) in the United States, following only motor vehicle accidents as a cause of accidental death.[124,128,129] Children under 4 years of age, who were being supervised by one or both parents, and adolescent males (between 15 and 19 years old) are most commonly involved in submersion injuries. When an adolescent male is involved in a submersion accident, alcohol is involved in up to 50% of the cases.[124,126] Children under 6 years of age are most frequently involved in submersion injuries; however, the fatality rate is highest in the adolescent patient population.[124] Although there is some variation across states and patient age groups regarding the environments (swimming pools, rivers, lakes, bathtubs, open containers of water, and so forth) for submersion injuries, residential swimming pools are involved in approximately 90% of pediatric drownings and near drownings.[124,126,129] More fatalities occur, however, among patients who were submerged in rivers and lakes. This may be related to the length of submersion, which is impacted by the depth and the clarity of the water, both of which hinder rescue efforts.[124]

The sequence of events during a submersion injury were described by Noble and Sharpe in 1963.[130] Generally, there is an initial episode of panic. The victim then begins struggling and making swimming efforts. The victim usually holds her breath for a period of time, following which there is gasping and swallowing of large amounts of water. Vomiting and aspiration of both vomitus and water occur next. Laryngospasm, which is mediated by the vagus nerve, occurs as a result of aspiration. The victim looses consciousness as a result of hypoxia; in approximately 85% to 90% of submersion injuries, the larynx then relaxes, and the protective mechanisms for the airway are absent. As a result, a large amount of water is allowed to enter the lungs. In the remaining 10% to 15% of victims, laryngospasm persists and death occurs without significant aspiration of water. In either case, the victim experiences cardiac arrest as a result of prolonged hypoxia.[124,126,130]

Much of the literature focuses on the differences in pathophysiology that occur secondary to freshwater drowning when compared with saltwater drowning. These differences, while significant in animal studies in which large amounts of water were aspirated into the lungs, do not appear to be clinically important in human victims of submersion injury. Serum electrolytes do not usually require correction, and the hypervolemia that was thought to occur with freshwater submersion has rarely been found clinically important.[124,127] The most important result of submersion injury, whether in saltwater or freshwater, is the onset of hypoxemia and its effect on other organ systems, most notably the brain.[124,125,129] Hypoxemia initially develops during the apneic episode that occurs during the process of drowning. It is compounded when water that has been aspirated causes a disruption of the pulmonary surfactant, which leads to atelectasis and intrapulmonary shunting.

Pulmonary edema often develops in both saltwater and freshwater submersion injuries; however, experimental studies indicate the process by which pulmonary edema develops differs according to the water type.[124] Pediatric patients, especially young children, are more likely to survive the hypoxic-ischemic injuries associated with submersion injuries. This appears to be related to two factors. First, small children become hypothermic more quickly than adults. This appears to be related to the relative body surface area, proportional amount of subcutaneous body fat, and the amount of activity engaged in during the submersion.[124,127,128] Second, children appear to be more impacted by the diving reflex. The reflex, which occurs when an apneic child's face is submerged in cold water (<20°C), results in bradycardia and a shunting of blood flow to the heart and brain. This results in an increased ability of the body to withstand long periods of hypoxia.[124,128]

☐ TREATMENT

The initial treatment for submersion injury is cardiopulmonary resuscitation (CPR). Kyriacou et al demonstrated that patients who receive immediate CPR (administered by family members or other laypeople before the arrival of emergency medical personnel) survived with a significantly better neurologic outcome than those patients who do not receive immediate CPR.[129] Clearing of the airway, using a finger sweep, and mouth-to-mouth breathing can be started before the victim has been removed from the water. Neck injuries are frequently seen in submersion injuries, especially if the victim was diving or engaged in play activities. Therefore, while establishing the airway and in subsequent rescue breathing, the neck must be protected by immobilizing the cervical spine. The risk of aspiration is high during resuscitation efforts. To minimize the likelihood of vomiting and aspiration, the rescuer can apply cricoid pressure during all rescue breaths. Once the patient has been moved to a solid area (to a boat, the shore, or pool decking, for example), cardiac massage should be initiated.

Oxygen therapy with an FIO_2 of 1.0 should be initiated as soon as possible.[131] A patient who has responded to CPR and begun to breathe spontaneously can be given oxygen using a nonrebreathing mask. If the patient has ineffective respiratory efforts or is apneic, an artificial airway should be established, and a manual resuscitation bag with supplemental oxygen should be used. Serial arterial blood gas analyses provide valuable information about the patient's oxygenation and acid–base balance and are used to guide the treatment of hypoxia and acidosis.

Aspiration of water produces pathophysiologic changes in the alveoli that are consistent with acute respiratory distress syndrome (ARDS). These changes include alteration or inactivation of pulmonary surfactant, destruction of the cells that line the alveoli as well as those of the capillary endothelial cells, loss of alveolar volume, decreased compliance, intrapulmonary shunting, and ventilation-perfusion abnormalities. As a result, mechanical ventilation and early application of PEEP can help restore the patient's FRC, minimize intrapulmonary shunting, and maximize oxygen delivery to the tissues while using the lowest FIO_2 possible. Tidal volume, respiratory rate, FIO_2, and PEEP can be titrated to provide adequate oxygenation and ventilation.[124,127]

The initial chest radiograph may show little, if any, abnormality. However, chest radiographs should be monitored to evaluate the progression of ARDS. In patients with significant pulmonary involvement, the chest radiograph is likely to show evidence of pulmonary edema and atelectasis. If new infiltrates appear, or the chest radiograph fails to improve within several days, the presence of a pulmonary infection should be considered.[127]

Sputum for Gram's stain and cultures should be obtained to determine whether a secondary pulmonary infection, which may result from aspiration of either gastric contents or contaminated water, exists. Appropriate antibiotic therapy should be started when there is evidence of an infection; there is no evidence that prophylactic antibiotic therapy is beneficial.[124,127]

Additional pharmacotherapy for the pulmonary injuries may include aerosolized β agonists, especially in those patients with known reactive airways disease. If the patient requires mechanical ventilation, appropriate sedation and pharmacologic paralysis may be needed to facilitate effective ventilation. There is no evidence that the use of corticosteroids is beneficial in controlling the inflammatory component of ARDS.[124,126,127,132]

Cardiovascular status usually stabilizes once the patient is oxygenated and the acidosis is corrected. Fluid status must be monitored carefully. Excessive fluid administration may worsen any existing pulmonary edema. If intravascular volume is low, however, cardiac function may be compromised during positive-pressure ventilation. Measurements of hemodynamic function, using a flow-directed pulmonary artery catheter, may be required to allow the physician to monitor fluid status and cardiac function.[124,127,132]

The outcome of a submersion injury is primarily dependent on the extent of the hypoxic-ischemic injury to the brain.[124,125,127–129,133] As a result, much of the treatment is directed toward preventing expansion of the initial neurologic injury. The respiratory care components of treatment, including effective ventilation and oxygenation, minimize poor outcomes related to hypoxia and hypercapnia. When intracranial pressure (ICP) is increased, therapeutic measures may include mild hyperventilation (maintaining the $PaCO_2$ between 25 and 35 torr),[127] elevating the head of the bed, suctioning and stimulating coughing only when clinically indicated (ie, using breath sounds and increasing inspiratory pressures as guidelines), appropriate sedation, and carefully monitoring and maintaining fluid balance.[124,127,132]

The psychosocial impact on the family of a victim of either a drowning or a near-drowning accident is substantial. Because most submersion accidents occur in a home environment, often with multiple members of the immediate family in the vicinity, feelings of guilt and anger are frequently experienced by the family. If the patient survives and is admitted to either the pediatric floor or the pediatric intensive care unit (PICU), the family is likely to have some interactions with the respiratory care practitioner. The respiratory care practitioner, as an integral member of the health care team, must be aware of not only the pathophysiologic events, but also the psychosocial trauma inflicted on both the patient and the patient's family as a consequence of submersion injury.

PEDIATRIC EMERGENCIES

Trauma

When a child presents to the emergency department with an acute injury or illness, the medical team must immediately implement a comprehensive, multisystem assessment to establish and implement a treatment plan. Resuscitation efforts follow the same basic protocols as in adults: establishing and maintaining a patent airway, insuring effective ventilation (breathing), and maintaining adequate circulation. In addition to the physiologic challenges encountered when providing emergency care to a pediatric patient, members of the health care team are likely to be faced with a number of behavioral responses by both the patient and his family.

Pediatric patients respond to pain and the environmental stimuli from the emergency department in various ways, primarily dependent on the age of the child. For example, an infant or toddler is not able to assist the health care team in the assessment by communicating verbally. Therefore, during the physical observation, hospital personnel must take into consideration the age-appropriate response of fear and use calming strategies, such as allowing the parents or other primary care givers access to the patient or by remembering to soothe the infant by the use of comforting touches. School-age children have reasonably well-developed language skills and can participate by verbalizing an account of the injury and identifying the origin of pain. However, this age group also exhibits fear related to pain, disfigurement, and, in some cases, death. Adolescents are able to participate more fully in giving a history of the injury and by using descriptive language to identify sources of pain. Adolescent patients are usually more cooperative in participating in the therapeutic plan if they are involved in making some decisions about their own care.[134]

Although trauma is relatively rare when one considers the pediatric population as a whole, it accounts for the death of more than 8,000 children each year.[135,136] Most of the injuries to children occur as the result of motor vehicle accidents; however, in pediatric patients, the injuries most frequently occur as the consequence of a child–motor vehicle collision (pedestrian accident) rather than two motor vehicles colliding and causing injury. Widespread injury, in which chest trauma may be only one of the systems involved, is likely to be present.

Because of their lower absolute blood volume, children are at greater risk for hypovolemia than adults when a relatively small amount of blood is lost. Also, children are frequently able to initially maintain a relatively normal blood pressure because of arteriolar constriction. As a result, children tend to maintain a normal blood pressure for a period of time and then rapidly decompensate by developing significant hypotension. This is in contrast to adults, whose blood pressure tends to drop over a longer period of time. When the patient is hemodynamically unstable, it is essential to establish intravenous access to assure a route for adequate fluid administration. If a peripheral line can not be established, the intraosseous route is recommended.[134,137] In the prehospital setting, an intraosseus line may be placed in children who are less than 5 years old. Within the hospital, intraosseus placement is usually used in children who are 3 years old or less.[134] Fluid administration may consist of blood products when the hemoglobin is low. When hemoglobin is adequate, either crystalloids or colloids can be administered.[134,138]

Pulmonary contusions are encountered in pedestrian–motor vehicle collisions, in falls from significant height, and as a result of child abuse.[136,137] A high-speed impact is necessary to produce pulmonary contusion; therefore, the presence of other injuries should be evaluated. Tachypnea and abnormal breath sounds may or may not be present. The pathophysiologic process in pulmonary contusion includes alveolar-capillary disruption; V/Q imbalances; and, in extreme cases, respiratory failure. Treatment of the pulmonary contusion includes oxygen therapy and monitoring of oxygenation status, as well as coughing and deep-breathing exercises to minimize the onset of atelectasis. Fluids may be restricted to minimize leaking of intravascular fluid into the alveoli and the development of pulmonary edema.[135–137]

Because the ribs of young children are more compliant than in older children and adults, it is relatively rare to encounter rib fractures in young children. The trauma required to produce a rib fracture is a severe blow or crushing impact; therefore, the presence of rib fractures should lead the clinician to suspect other organ system involvement.[136] Treatment for rib fractures includes pain control to enhance effective ventilation (splinting is minimized and ventilation improved), deep-breathing exercises, and using a pillow or other external support when the child coughs. Pneumothorax and hemothorax can be seen in children who have sustained significant chest injury. When hemothorax is involved, venous access must be established to provide fluid resuscitation. Chest tubes and closed thoracic drainage are used in the treatment of pneumothorax and hemothorax.

Traumatic brain injuries are relatively common in children, accounting for most of the accidental deaths in children older than 1 year of age.[134] Regardless of the origin of injury, the goal of treatment is to maintain normal cardiopulmonary function. Intracranial pressure (ICP) is usually monitored, and the therapeutic plan is directed toward preventing intracranial hypertension. The respiratory care plan generally includes intubation and mechanical ventilation to maintain a mild respiratory alkalosis (the $PaCO_2$ is usually kept between 30 and 35 torr). The patient is usually sedated or pharmacologically paralyzed. Other therapeutic measures include diuretic therapy, often using osmotic agents such as mannitol (Osmitrol).

Smoke Inhalation

Smoke inhalation and burn injuries account for only a small percentage of annual pediatric deaths;[139] however, the respiratory care practitioner should have a working knowledge of the pathophysiologic events because of their deleterious effect on the airway and on oxygenation. Chemical by-products, some of which are toxic in and of themselves, are produced during combustion. Carbon monoxide (CO) is readily produced during combustion. The CO molecule readily combines with the hemoglobin molecule, forming COHb, thus severely limiting effectiveness of the oxygen-transport system and producing significant levels of hypoxia. Other chemicals produced during combustion (aldehydes, crolein, ammonia, anhydrides, carbon dioxide, cyanide, hydrogen chloride, hydrogen fluoride, and nitrogen dioxide) are capable of producing significant airway and lung injuries, including irritation, inflammation, and pulmonary edema.[139,140]

Early administration of 100% oxygen is recommended to minimize the effects of CO inhalation. This can be accomplished by using a nonrebreathing mask with a tight fit on a spontaneously breathing patient, or by either manual resuscitator bag or mechanical ventilator for a patient who requires ventilatory support. Delivery of 100% oxygen should be maintained until the COHb level drops below 10%.[140] Oxygenation status must be monitored using a co-oximeter to measure COHb levels, rather than relying on either the SpO_2 obtained by means of pulse oximetry or the PaO_2/SaO_2 on an arterial blood gas analysis.

The upper airway and potentially the lower airway are exposed to superheated gases during a fire. The patient is at risk for airway obstruction as a result of mucosal swelling that results from heat injury. In addition, chemical by-products of combustion are capable of producing an inflammatory response that includes swelling and fluid shifting. When these factors are considered together with the smaller diameter of the pediatric airway, it is easy to understand why a primary, and initial, goal in treating the patient is to assess the airway and take measures to maintain airway patency.

The initial airway injury is related to mucosal edema. Within a few hours to days following exposure to smoke, the patient is at risk for severe pulmonary edema as a result of injuries to the pulmonary capillary membranes. As capillary membrane permeability increases, fluid leaks from the intravascular space into the interstitium and alveoli. Within 2 or 3 days, the patient frequently develops pneumonia. Pneumonia may be the result of atelectasis that develops as a result of a decreases in pulmonary compliance, secretions retained distal to obstructions in the airway, and a decreased ability to cough and sigh as a result of pain or sedation. The etiologic agents in pneumonia that occurs secondary to pulmonary burns are usually gram-negative organisms, including *Staphylococcus aureus* and *Pseudomonas aeruginosa*.[139] A sputum culture and sensitivity are used to identify the etiologic agent and establish specific antibiotic therapy.

In addition to oxygen therapy, establishing and maintaining an airway, and providing ventilatory support, the respiratory care plan may include aerosolized bronchodilators (β agonists and anticholinergics), bronchial hygiene procedures, and hyperbaric oxygen therapy.

Gun-Shot Injuries

A relatively new phenomenon in pediatric trauma has emerged over the past few years: gun-shot injuries. While all other forms of traumatic death have decreased during the last decade in the United States, firearm fatalities have increased.[141] Firearm deaths result from homicide, suicide, and unintentional injury. The majority of firearm injuries occur within the familial residence (either the home of the victim or that of a relative). The highest incidence of firearm fatalities occurs among black males.[142] Gun shots produce a penetrating injury, and the mechanism of injury in children is not unlike that in adults. Though the degree of injury varies according to the characteristics of the bullet and the distance the bullet travels before striking the victim, the initial injury produces crushing of the affected tissue and the production of an associated cavity.

Primary assessment of the patient with a gun-shot wound revolves around the principles of basic life support: establishing an airway, assuring effective ventilation, and maintaining adequate circulation. Children are at risk for hypovolemia because a penetrating injury can produce significant bleeding. Penetrating wounds to the head are associated with intracranial hypertension and seizures. Penetrating wounds in the area of the neck frequently cause an airway obstruction. Penetrating wounds to the thorax disrupt the integrity of the thoracic wall and can cause severe gas exchange deficiencies. Specific treatment is governed by the organ systems involved in the traumatic event.

The psychosocial effects of trauma can be significant. Parents, or the family members who were responsible for caring for the child at the time of the accident, may experience feelings of guilt. Other family members may direct anger toward the injured person, and this accentuates disruption of the family system. The injured child may be overwhelmed by having been removed from her home and other familiar environments because of hospitalization. Siblings may experience uncertainty and fear that the child will die. Family-centered care recognizes the impact of an injury to a child on the family as a whole, and thus allows the child and the family to begin to participate in care-giving activities as soon as it is feasible.[142]

Near Drowning

Respiratory care practitioners in all geographic areas should be aware of the pathophysiology and treatment of submersion injuries, which include both drowning and near drowning. The term *drowning* indicates death from injuries related to submersion within 24 hours of the event. *Near drowning* indicates patient survival for at least 24 hours following the submersion event, even though the patient may ultimately die from related injuries.[124–128] Injuries to the pulmonary, cardiovascular, and central nervous systems are most frequently associated with the morbidity and mortality of victims of submersion events.

RESPIRATORY CARE OF THE IMMUNOCOMPROMISED CHILD

Immunocompromised children are found in two primary patient populations: (1) children with cancer, where immunosuppression results either from the malignancy itself or from the treatment of the malignancy, and (2) children with acquired immunodeficiency syndrome (AIDS). Respiratory symptoms in children who have compromised immune systems require immediate attention because of the rapidity with which the child can develop significant respiratory compromise.[143–145]

The incidence of pediatric AIDS is increasing.[145] The etiologic agent for AIDS is the human immunodeficiency virus (HIV). When a patient is infected with HIV, the immune system looses its ability to mount an effective response when the body is invaded by an organism capable of producing disease. As a result, all patients infected with HIV are susceptible to bacterial and viral infections, as well as opportunistic infections. The most frequent infectious agent in the adult with AIDS is opportunistic; however, in children, bacterial infections occur more frequently.[143,144]

The primary source of AIDS infection in young children is exposure to an AIDS-infected mother; the disease may be transmitted across the placenta or acquired during delivery and, potentially, through breast feeding. In adolescents, AIDS is related to the same high-risk behaviors responsible for transmissions of the disease in adults. A small number of children have acquired AIDS by receiving an HIV-infected blood product.[145] The clinical manifestations in children with AIDS differ from those of adults. The immune systems in children are more profoundly compromised, and symptoms appear more quickly after exposure. In infants, symptoms are often seen as early as 2 months after birth, and usually always appear by 2 years of age.[146] Pulmonary complications in children infected with HIV are similar to those in adults, with pneumonia occurring frequently. Lymphocytic interstitial pneumonitis and *Pneumocystis carinii* pneumonia are the most commonly seen pneumonias in children with AIDS. While Kaposi's sarcoma is frequently seen an adults infected with HIV, it is not commonly seen in pediatric patients.[145]

Chemotherapy suppresses the immune system and places the child at risk for infection with many of the same organisms seen in the child with AIDS. Respiratory care for the immunocompromised child is primarily supportive. Oxygen therapy is titrated to maintain acceptable levels of oxygenation. The respiratory care practitioner may be asked to collect sputum samples for Gram's stain and culture and sensitivity studies. Bronchoscopy and bronchial lavage may also be used to identify the etiologic agent of pneumonia. The practitioner may be asked to assist the physician during a thoracentesis procedure when a pleural effusion exists. Aerosolized pentamidine may be used to prevent and treat *P. carinii* pneumonia.

Health care providers are potentially exposed to HIV whenever therapeutic procedures cause exposure to blood or body fluids of a child infected with HIV. Consequently, universal precautions should be employed at all times.

SUMMARY

Pediatric respiratory care requires all members of the health care team to recognize the importance of actively involving the family in the decision-making process and in care-giving procedures. A solid understanding of pathology and therapeutic procedures is not enough to ensure that a respiratory care practitioner does well in the pediatric environment. The needs of patients and their families are a primary feature of today's health care paradigm. Consequently, respiratory care practitioners need to have a functional understanding of some of the basic theories from the social sciences, most notably, sociology, medical sociology, and psychology. Respiratory care practitioners can enhance the medical management of a pediatric patient, but only if they are able to work with the family and members of the health care team to identify and resolve issues related to medical, psychological, and social barriers.

REFERENCES

1. Piaget J: The Language and Thought of the Child. New York, Harcourt, Brace, 1926
2. Piaget J: The Origins of Intelligence in Children. New York, International Universities Press, 1952
3. Kolhberg L: Stages in the Development of Moral Thought and Action. New York, Holt, Rinehart & Winston, 1969
4. Newman BM, Newman PR: Adolescent Development. Columbus, OH, Merrill, 1986
5. Wallace RA, Wolf A: Contemporary Sociologic Theory. Englewood Cliffs, NJ, Prentice Hall, 1991
6. Kazak A: Families of chronically ill children: A systems and social-ecological model of adaptation and challenge. J Consult Clin Psychol 57:25, 1989
7. Whaley L, Wong D: Essestials of Pediatric Nursing, 4th ed. St. Louis, Mosby, 1993
8. Harrison GM, Mitchell MB: The medical and social outcome of 200 respiratory and former respiratory patients on home care. Arch Phys Med Rehabil 4:590, 1961
9. Mosely KW, Perdue JD, Casillas CS, Brady DK: Family-Centered Health Care. In SL Barnhart, MP Czevinske: Perinatal and Pediatric Respiratory Care. Philadelphia, WB Saunders, 1995
10. O'Connor DM: Developmental Anatomy of the Larynx and Trachea. In CM Myer, RT Cotton, SR Shott: The Pediatric Airway: An Interdisciplinary Approach. Philadelphia, JB Lippincott, 1995
11. Rodenstein DO, Perlmutter N, Stanescu DC: Infants are not obligatory breathers. Am Rev Respir Dis 131:343, 1985
12. Bates B, Hoekelman RA: Interviewing and the Health History. In B Bates: A Guide to Physical Examination and History Taking, 5th ed. Philadelphia, JB Lippincott, 1991
13. Hoekelman RA: The Physical Examination of Infants and Children. In B Bates: A Guide to Physical Examination and History Taking, 5th ed. Philadelphia, JB Lippincott, 1991
14. Cloutier MM: History and Physical Examination. In DV Schidow, DS Smith (eds): A Practical Guide to Pediatric Respiratory Diseases. Philadelphia, Hanley & Belfus, 1994
15. Vain NE, et al: Regulation of oxygen concentration delivery to infants via nasal cannulas. Am J Dis Child 143:1458, 1989
16. Fan LL, Voyles JB: Determination of inspired oxygen delivered by nasal cannula in infants with chronic lung disease. J Pediatr 103:923, 1983
17. Poulton TJ, Comer PB, Gibson RL: Tracheal oxygen concentration with a nasal cannula during oral and nasal breathing. Respir Care 25:739, 1980
18. Aoki BY, McCloskey K: Evaluation, Stabilization, and Transport of the Critically Ill Child. St. Louis, Mosby–Year Book, 1992
19. Beckham RW, Mishoe SC: Sound levels inside incubators and oxygen hoods used with nebulizers and humidifiers. Respir Care 27:33, 1982
20. Telfar H, Willis S: Nursing perspectives in the management of infants and children requiring thoracic surgery. Prog Pediatr Surg 17:30, 1991
21. Scott AA, Koff PB: Airway Care and Chest Physiotherapy. In PB Koff, D Eitzman, J Neu (eds): Neonatal and Pediatric Respiratory Care. St. Louis, Mosby–Year Book, 1993
22. Blodgett D: Manual of Pediatric Respiratory Care Procedures. Philadelphia, JB Lippincott, 1982
23. Miller S, Hall DO, Clayton CB, Nelson R: Chest physiotherapy in cystic fibrosis: A comparative study of autogenic drainage and the active cycle of breathing teachniques with postural drainage. Thorax 2:165, 1995

24. Pryor JA, Webber Ba, Hodson ME, Warner JO: The Flutter VRP1 as an adjunct to chest physiotherapy in cystic fibrosis. Respir Med 88(9);677, 1994
25. Williams MT: Chest physiotherapy and cystic fibrosis: Why is the most effective form of treatment still unclear? Chest 106(6);1872, 1994
26. Baldwin DR, Hill AL, Peckcham DG, Knox AJ: Effect of addition of exercise to chest physiotherapy on sputum expectoration and lung function in adults with cystic fibrosis. Respir Med 88(1):49, 1994
27. Natale JE, Pfeifle J, Homnick DN: Comparison of intrapulmonary percussive ventilation and chest physiotherapy: A pilot study in patients with cystic fibrosis. Chest 105(6);1789, 1994
28. Stiller K, Montarello J, Wallace M, et al: Efficacy of breathing and coughing exercises in the prevention of pulmonary complications after coronary artery surgery. Chest 105(3);741, 1994
29. Anderson JB, Faml M: Chest physiotherapy in the pediatric age group. Respir Care 36;546, 1991
30. Sutton PP: Chest physiotherapy: Time for reappraisal. Br J Dis Chest 82;127, 1988
31. Gallon A: Evaluation of chest percussion in the treatment of patients with copious sputum production. Respir Med 85;45, 1991
32. Mahlmeister MJ, Fink JB, Hoffman GL, et al: Positive-expiratory-pressure mask therapy: Theoretical and practical considerations and a review of the literature. Respir Care 36;1218, 1191
33. Lannefors L, Wollmer P: Mucus clearance with three chest physiotherapy regimes in cystic fibrosis: A comparison between postural drainage, PEP and physical exercise. Eur Respir J 5(6);748, 1992
34. Groth S, Stafanger G, Dirksen H, et al: Positive expiratory pressure (PEP-mask) physiotherapy improves ventilation and reduces volume of trapped gas in cystic fibrosis. Bull Eur Physiopathol Respir 21(4);339, 1985
35. Tyrrell JC, Hiller EJ, Martin J: Face mask physiotherapy in cystic fibrosis. Arch Dis Child 61(6);598, 1986
36. Van Asperen PP, Jackson L, Hennessy P, Brown J: Comparison of a positive expiratory pressure (PEP) mask with postural drainage in patients with cystic disease. Aust Paediatr J 23(5);283, 1987
37. Oberwaldner B, Evans JC, Zach MS: Forced expirations against a variable resistance: A new chest physiotherapy method in cystic fibrosis. Pediatr Pulmonol 2(6);358, 1986
38. Braggion C, Cappelletti LM, Cornacchia M, et al: Short-term effects of three chest physiotherapy regimens in patients hospitalized for pulmonary exacerbations of cystic fibrosis: A crossover randomized study. Pediatr Pulmonol 19(1);16, 1995
39. Thomas Y, Cook DJ, Brooks D: Chest physical therapy management of patients with cystic fibrosis: A meta-analysis. Am J Respir Crit Care Med 151(3 Pt 1);846, 1995
40. Pfleger A, Therissl B, Oberwaldner B, Zach MS: Self-administered chest physiotherapy in cystic fibrosis: A comparative study of high-pressure PEP and autogenic drainage. Lung 170(6);323, 1992
41. Mortensen J, Falk M, Groth S, Jensen C: The effects of postural drainage and positive expiratory pressure physiotherapy on tracheobronchial clearance in cystic fibrosis. Chest 100(5);1350, 1991
42. Steen HJ, Redmond AO, O'Neill D, Beattie F: Evaluation of the PEP mask in cystic fibrosis. Acta Paediatr Scand 90(1);51, 1991
43. Schoni MH: Autogenic Drainage: A modern approach to physiotherapy in cystic fibrosis. J Soc Med 82(16, Suppl);32, 1989
44. Rosen HK: Lung Volume Expansion Therapy. In SL Barnhart, MP Czervinske: Perinatal and Pediatric Respiratory Care. Philadelphia, WB Saunders, 1995
45. Warwick WJ, Hanson LG: The long-term efficacy of high-frequency chest compression on pulmonary complications of cystic fibrosis. Pediatr Pulmonol 11;26, 1991
46. Kacmarek RM: Humidity and Aerosol Therapy. In DJ Pierson, RM Kacmarek: Foundations of Respiratory Care. New York, Churchill Livingstone, 1992
47. Shapiro BA, Kacmarek RM, Cane RD, et al: Clinical Application of Respiratory Care, 4th Ed. St. Louis, Mosby–Year Book, 1991
48. Benson DM: Systemic and pulmonary changes with inhaled humid atmospheres. Anesthesiology 30;199, 1969
49. Chatburn RL, Primiano FP: A rational basis for humidity therapy. Respir Care 32(4);249, 1987
50. Fink JB, Jue PK: Humidity and Aerosol Therapy for Pediatrics. In SL Barnhart, MP Czervinske: Perinatal and Pediatric Respiratory Care. Philadelphia, WB Saunders, 1995
51. Scanlon CL: In Egan: Fundamentals of Respiratory Care, 5th Ed. St. Louis, CV Mosby, 1990
52. Hess DR, Branson RD: Humidification: Humidifiers and Nebulizers. In RD Branson, DR Hess, RL Chatburn RL: Respiratory Care Equipment. Philadelphia, JB Lippincott, 1995
53. Cottrell GP, Surkin HB: Pharmacology for Respiratory Care Practitioners. Philadelphia, JB Lippincott, 1995
54. Lee H, Evans HE: Evaluation of inhalation aids of metered dose inhalers in asthmatic children. Chest 91(3);366, 1987
55. Sly RM, Barbera JM, Middleton HB, Eby DM: Delivery of albuterol aerosol by Aerochamber to young children. Ann Allergy 60(5);403, 1988
56. Oldaeus G, Kubista J, Stahl E: Comparison of Bricanyl Turbohaler and Ventolin Rotahaler in children with asthma. Ann Allergy Asthma Immunol 74(1);34, 1995
57. Miller RD: Skeletal Muscle Relaxants. In BG Katzung: Basic and Clinical Pharmacology, 6th ed. Norwalk, CT, Appleton & Lange, 1995
58. Pettignano MM, Pettignano R: Airway Management. In SL Barnhart, MP Czervinske: Perinatal and Pediatric Respiratory Care. Philadelphia, WB Saunders, 1995
59. Westhorpe RN: The position of the larynx in children and its relationship to the east of intubation. Anaesth Intensive Care 15;384, 1987
60. Gregory GA: Respiratory care of the child. Crit Care Med 8;852, 1980
61. Arnold J, Casto C: Endotracheal Intubation. In JL Blumer: A Practical Guide to Pediatric Intensive Care, 3rd ed. St. Louis, Mosby–Year Book, 1990
62. Tochen ML: Orotracheal intubation in the newborn infant: A method for determining depth of tube insertion. J Pediatr 95;1050, 1979
63. American Association for Respiratory Care: Clinical practice guideline: Endotracheal suctioning of mechanically ventilated adults and children with artificial airways. Respir Care 38:501, 1993
64. Chatburn RL: Assisted Ventilation. In JL Blumer: A Practical Guide to Pediatric Intensive Care, 3rd ed. St. Louis, Mosby–Year Book, 1990
65. Goldsmith JP, Karotkin EH: Assisted Ventilation of the Neonate, 2nd ed. Philadelphia, WB Saunders, 1988
66. Hargett KD: Mechanical Ventilation of the Neonate. In SL Barnhart, MP Czervinske: Perinatal and Pediatric Respiratory Care. Philadelphia, WB Saunders, 1995
67. Whitaker K: Comprehensive Perinatal and Pediatric Respiratory Care. Albany, NY, Delmar Publishers, 1992
68. Betit P, Thompson JE, Benjamin PK: Mechanical Ventilation. In PB Koff, D Eitzman, J Neu (eds): Neonatal and Pediatric Respiratory Care. St. Louis, Mosby–Year Book, 1993
69. Carlo W, Chatburn RL: Assisted Ventilation of the Newborn. In RL Chatburn, W Carlo (eds): Neonatal Respiratory Care, 2nd ed. Chicago, Mosby–Yearbook, 1988
70. Branson RD: Airway Pressure Monitoring Devices. In RD Branson, DR Hess, RL Chatburn: Respiratory Care Equipment. Philadelphia, JB Lippincott, 1995
71. Witte MK, Galli SA, Chatburn RL, Blumer JL: Optimal positive end-expiratory pressure therapy in infants and children with acute respiratory failure. Pediatr Res 24;217, 1988
72. Suter PM, Fairley HB, Isenberg MD: Optimum end-expiratory pressure in patients with acute pulmonary failure. N Engl J Med 292;284, 1975
73. Schidlow DV, Smith DS: Stridor and Upper Airway Obstruction. In DV Schidlow, DS Smith (eds): A Practical Guide to Pediatric Respiratory Diseases. Philadelphia, Hanley & Belfus, 1994
74. Saladino McManus: Manual of Pediatric Therapeutics.
75. Allen ED, McCoy KS: Airway Disorders. In K Whitaker: Comprehensive Perinatal and Pediatric Respiratory Care. Albany, NY, Delmar Publishers, 1992
76. Sofer S, Daoan R, Tal A: The need for intubation in serious upper respiratory tract infection in pediatric patients. Infection 19;131, 1991

77. Progress toward elimination of *Haemophilus influenzae* type B disease among infants and children: United States, 1993–1994. MMWR Morb Mortal Wkly Rep 44(29);545, 1995
78. Vetter RT, Johnson GM: Vaccination update: Hib, hepatitis, polio, varicella, influenza, pneumococcal and meningococal disease. Postgrad Med 98(5), 1995
79. Mauro RD, Poole SR, Lockhart CH: Differentiation of epiglottitis from laryngotracheitis in the child with stridor. Am J Dis Child 142;679, 1988
80. Reed CE: Mechanisms of airway obstruction in the asthmatic patient: From past to present. Ann Allergy 69:245, 1992
81. National Asthma Education Program, National Heart, Lung, and Blood Institute: Guidelines for the Diagnosis and Management of Asthma. Publication No. 91-3042. Washington, DC, National Institutes of Health, 1991
82. Cloutier MM: Quick: What's first-line therapy for acute asthma? Contemporary Pediatrics (March) 1993
83. Tinkelman DG: Asthma. In DV Schidlow, DS Smith (eds): A Practical Guide to Pediatric Respiratory Diseases. Philadelphia, Hanley & Belfus, 1994, p 61
84. Mrazek DA: Psychiatric complications of pediatric asthma. Ann Allergy 69:285, 1992
85. Sly MR: Asthma mortality, East and West. Ann Allergy 69:81, 1992
86. Martinez FD, et al: Asthma and wheezing in the first six years of life. N Engl J Med 332:133, 1995
87. Spitzer WO, et al: The use of β agonists and the risk of death and near death from asthma. N Engl J Med 326:501, 1992
88. Ryan-Wenger NM, Walsh M: Children's perspectives on coping with asthma. Pediatr Nurs 20(3):224, 1994
89. Shim CS, Williams MH: Evaluation of severity of asthma: Patients versus physicians. Am J Med 68:11, 1980
90. Shim CS, Williams MH: Relationship of wheezing to the severity of obstruction in asthma. Arch Intern Med 143:890, 1983
91. Burdon JGW, et al: The perception of breathlessness in asthma. Am Rev Respir Dis 126:825, 1982
92. Li JTC: Home peak expiratory flow rate monitoring in patients with asthma. Mayo Clin Proc 70:649, 1995
93. Cooley CH: Human Nature and the Social Order. New York: Scribner's, 1902
94. Woodhead M (ed): Guidelines on the management of asthma. Thorax 48(Suppl):S1, 1993
95. Cherniak RM, Chatburn R, Gardner RM, et al: Statement on Technical Standards for Peak Flow Meters. Publication No. NIH 92-2113a. Bethesda, MD, National Institutes of Health, 1992
96. Gardner RM, Crapo RO, Jackson BR, Jensen RL: Evaluation of accuracy and reproducibility of peak flowmeters at 1,400 m. Chest 101:948, 1992
97. van Schayck CP, Dompeling E, van Weel C, et al: Accuracy and reproducibility of the Assess peak flow meter. Eur Respir J 3:338, 1990
98. Shapiro SM, Hendler JM, Ogirala RG, et al: An evaluation of the accuracy of Assess and MiniWright peak flowmeters. Chest 99:358, 1991
99. Pistelli R, Fuso L, Muzzolon R, et al: Comparison of the performance of two mini peak flow meters. Respiration 56:103, 1989
100. Miller MR, Dickinson SA, Hitchings DJ: The accuracy of portable peak flow meters. Thorax 47:904, 1992
101. Eichenhorn MS, Beauchamp RK, Harper PA, Ward JC: An assessment of three portable peak flow meters. Chest 82:306, 1982
102. Williams JL: Radiographic Evaluation. In PB Koff, D Eitzman, Neu J: Neonatal and Pediatric Respiratory Care, 2nd ed. St. Louis, Mosby–Year Book, 1993, p 73
103. Allen JL: Office Pulmonary Function Testing. In DV Schidlow, DS Smith (eds): A Practical Guide to Pediatric Respiratory Diseases. Philadelphia, Hanley & Belfus, 1994, p 281
104. Wren CG, Bate BJ, Masters HB, Lauer BA: Detection of respiratory syncytial virus antigen in nasal washings by Abbott Testpac Enzyme Immunoassay. J Clin Microbiol 28(6);1395, 1990
105. Panitch HB: Wheezing and Lower Airway Obstruction. In DV Schidlow, DS Smith (eds): A Practical Guide to Pediatric Respiratory Diseases. Philadelphia, Hanley & Belfus, 1994, p 39
106. Kurth CD, Goodwin SR: Obstructive Airway Diseases in Infants and Children. In PB Koff, D Eitzman, J Neu (ed): Neonatal and Pediatric Respiratory Care. St. Louis, Mosby–Year Book, 1993
107. Jawetz E: Antiviral Chemotherapy and Prophylaxis. In BG Katzung: Basic and Clinical Pharmacology. Norwalk, CT, Appleton & Lange, 1995
108. Smith DW, Frankel LR, Mather LH, et al: A controlled trial of aerosolized ribavirin in infants receiving mechanical ventilation for severe respiratory syncytial virus infection. N Engl J Med 325;24, 1991
109. Hall CB, McBride JT, Gala CL, et al: Ribavirin treatment of respiratory cyncytial viral infection in infants with underlying cardiopulmonary disease. JAMA 254;3047, 1985
110. Riordan JR, Rommens JM, Kerem B, et al: Identification of the cystic fibrosis gene: Cloning and characterization of complementary DNA. Science 245:1006, 1989
111. Rommens JM, Iannuzzi MC, Karem B, et al: Identification of the cystic fibrosis gene: Chromosome walking and jumping. Science 245:1059, 1989
112. Karem B, Rommens JM, Buchanan JA, et al: Identification of the cystic fibrosis gene: Genetic analysis. Science 245:1073, 1989
113. Schidlow DV: Cystic Fibrosis. In DV Schidlow, DS Smith (eds): A Practical Guide to Pediatric Respiratory Diseases. Philadelphia, Hanley & Belfus, 1994
114. Fick RB, Stillwell PC: Controversies in the management of pulmonary disease due to cystic fibrosis. Chest 95:1319, 1989
115. McCoy K: Parenchymal Dieases. In PB Koff, DV Eitzman, J Neu (ed): Neonatal and Pediatric Respiratory Care. St. Louis, Mosby–Year Book, 1993
116. Snyder JD: Gastroenterology. In JW Graef (ed): Manual of Pediatric Therapeutics, 5th ed. Boston, Little, Brown, 1994
117. Gooch MD: Stability of albuterol and tobramycin when mixed for aerosol administration. Respir Care 36:1387, 1991
118. Knowles MR, Hohneker KW, Zhaoqing Z, et al: A controlled study of adenoviral-vector-mediated gene transfer in the nasal epithelium of patients with cystic fibrosis. N Engl J Med 333:823, 1995
119. Raloff J: Ibuprofen stalls advance of cystic fibrosis. Science News 147(13):197, 1995
120. Konstan MW, Byard PJ, Hoppel CL, Davis PB: Effect of high-dose ibuprofen in patients with cystic fibrosis. N Engl J Med 332:848, 1995
121. Theodore J, Lewiston N: Lung transplantation comes of age. N Engl J Med 322:772, 1990
122. Long SS: Pneumonia in Older Infants, Children, and Adolescents. In DV Schidlow, DS Smith (eds): A Practical Guide to Pediatric Respiratory Diseases. Philadelphia, Hanley & Belfus, 1994
123. Callahan CW: Tuberculosis. In DV Schidlow, DS Smith (eds): A Practical Guide to Pediatric Respiratory Diseases. Philadelphia, Hanley & Belfus, 1994
124. Fields AI: Near-drowning in the pediatric population. Crit Care Clin 8:113, 1992
125. Abrams RA, Mubarak S: Musculoskeletal consequences of near-drowning in children. J Pediatr Orthop 11(2):168, 1991
126. Walsh EA, Ioli JG: Childhood near-drowning: Nursing care and primary prevention. Pediatr Nurs 20(3):265, 1994
127. Witte MK: Near-Drowning. In JL Blumer: A Practical Guide to Pediatric Intensive Care, 3rd ed. St. Louis, Mosby–Year Book, 1990, p 313
128. Biggart MJ, Bohn DJ: Effect of hypothermia and cardiac arrest on outcome of near-drowning accidents in children. J Pediatr 117:179, 1990
129. Kyriacou DN, Arcinue EL, Peek C, Kraus JF: Effect of immediate resuscitation on children with submersion injury. Pediatrics 94(2):137, 1994
130. Noble CS, Sharpe N: Drowning: Its mechanism and treatment. Can Med Assoc J 89:402, 1963
131. Joffe M: Near-Drowning. In DV Schidlow, DS Smith (eds): A Practical Guide to Pediatric Respiratory Diseases. Philadelphia, Hanley & Belfus, 1994
132. Saladino R, McManus M: Acute Care. In JW Graef (ed): Manual of Pediatric Therapeutics, 5th ed. Boston, Little, Brown, 1994, p 48
133. Kemp AM, Sibert JR: Outcome in children who nearly drown: A British Isles study. BMJ 302(6789):1404, 1991
134. Vernon-Levett P: Pediatric emergencies. Crit Care Nurs Clin North Am 7(3):457, 1995
135. Eichelberger MR, Anderson KD: Sequelae of Thoracic Injuries in Children. In MR Eichelberger, Pratsch G (eds): Pediatric Trauma Care. Rockville, MD, Aspen, 1988

136. Loiselle J: Chest Trauma. In DV Schidlow, DS Smith (eds): A Practical Guide to Pediatric Respiratory Diseases. Philadelphia, Hanley & Belfus, 1994
137. Peclet MH, Eichelberger MR: Approach to the Child with Multiple Trauma. In JL Blumer: A Practical Guide to Pediatric Intensive Care, 3rd ed. St. Louis, Mosby–Year Book, 1990
138. Kaufman B: Fluid resuscitation of the critically ill: Consensus and controversies (Editorial). Anesthesiol Rev 17:2, 1990
139. Ruddy RM: Smoke inhalation injury. Pediatr Clin North Am 41(2):317, 1994
140. O'Sullivan BP: Respiratory Complications of Burns and Smoke Inhalation. In DV Schidow, DS Smith (eds): A Practical Guide to Pediatric Respiratory Diseases. Philadelphia, Hanley & Belfus, 1994
141. Moloney-Harmon PA, Czerwinski SJ: Caught in the crossfire: Children, guns, and trauma. Crit Care Nurs Clin North Am 6(3):525, 1994
142. Titler MG, Bombei C, Schutte DL: Developing family-focused care. Crit Care Nurs Clin North Am 7(2):375, 1995
143. Bye MR: Respiratory Disease in the Immunocompromised Child. In DV Schidow, DS Smith (eds): A Practical Guide to Pediatric Respiratory Diseases. Philadelphia, Hanley & Belfus, 1994
144. Albano EA, Pizzo PA: The evolving population of immunocompromised children. Pediatr Infect Dis J 7:S79, 1988
145. Dowe DA, Heitzman ER, Larkin JJ: Human immunodeficiency virus infection in children. Clin Imaging 16:145, 1992
146. Berry RK: Home care of the child with AIDS. Pediatr Nurs 14:314, 1988

27 Bronchial Asthma

James T. C. Li
and Charles E. Reed

PROFESSIONAL SKILLS

Upon completion of this chapter, the reader will:

- Describe the inflammatory and bronchospastic components of asthma
- Assess the asthmatic patient by means of medical history and physical examination
- Use laboratory studies to determine the presence and severity of asthma
- Provide a differential diagnosis for acute and chronic asthma
- Administer bronchodilators by wet nebulization or metered-dose inhaler to patients with acute asthma
- Adjust ventilator settings to minimize barotrauma in mechanically ventilated asthmatic patients
- Identify risk factors for fatal asthma
- Instruct patients on metered-dose inhaler use
- Instruct patients on peak expiratory flow meter use
- Instruct patients on the pathophysiology of asthma, indications and risks of asthma medications, home peak flow monitoring, and early recognition and treatment of asthma exacerbation
- Develop a written plan for asthma patients discharged from the hospital or emergency room

KEY TERMS

Allergen
Allergy
Anti-inflammatory
Arachidonic acid
Asthma
β_2-adrenergic
Bronchial hyperresponsiveness
Bronchitis
Bronchodilator
Corticoid (corticosteroid)
Cromolyn
Cytokines
Eosinophil
Immunotherapy
Interleukin-4 and -5
Leukotrienes
Metered-dose inhaler
Methacholine
Nedocromil
Prostaglandins

INTRODUCTION

Asthma is a common disorder affecting approximately 5% of the people in the United States (roughly, 13 million).[1] Although precise figures are not available, asthma exacerbations account for about 1.5 to 3 million emergency room visits and 500,000 hospitalizations annually.[2–4]

Of particular significance is the increasing mortality, hospitalization rate, and prevalence of asthma over the past two decades. The prevalence of asthma in school-age children has increased from 48 per 1,000 in the early 1970s to 76 per 1,000 in 1980,[5] but it has decreased by 3% from 1982 through 1992.[1] From 1982 to 1992, the prevalence of asthma has increased by 42%, from 34.7 per 1,000 people to 49.4 per 1,000.[1] Hospitalization rates in the United States have increased fourfold from 1965 to 1983.[6] The prevalence of asthma for persons aged 5 to 34 years increased by 52% (from 35 per 1,000 to 53 per 1,000) from 1982 to 1992.[1] From 1982 through 1991, the death rate for asthma in the United States rose 40%, from 13.4 per one million (3,154 deaths) to 18.8 per one million (5,106 deaths).[1] The cause of this increase in asthma is unknown at the present time. However, asthma experts agree that morbidity and mortality from asthma can be significantly reduced through effective application of the appropriate asthma management principles.

The total cost of illness related to asthma in 1990 was estimated at $6.2 billion.[7] Forty-three percent of this cost was associated with emergency room use, hospitalization, and asthma deaths. The economic cost of loss of school days alone approached $1 billion in 1990.

Nevertheless, asthma can be well controlled in the vast majority of patients, and the human and economic costs can be reduced. Current management strategy rests on three major principles:[8]

1. Objective measurement of pulmonary function for the diagnosis and management of asthma.
2. Anti-inflammatory therapy for stable asthma and acute asthma.
3. Self-care of asthma through education and the use of written plans.

DEFINITION

Asthma is a condition characterized by variable or intermittent obstruction of the lower airways that results in shortness of breath, wheezing, chest tightness, and cough. The American Thoracic Society and American College of Chest Physicians have offered the following definition of asthma:[9] "A disease characterized by an increased responsiveness of the airways to various stimuli and manifested by slowing of forced expiration which changes in severity either spontaneously or as a result of therapy." The Expert Panel Report of the National Education Program agreed on this working definition: "Asthma is a lung disease with the following characteristics: 1) Airway obstruction that is reversible (but not completely so in some patients) either spontaneously or with treatment; 2) Airway inflammation; and 3) Increased airway responsiveness to a variety of stimuli."[8] These definitions address the bronchial hyperresponsiveness and reversible obstruction of the airways in asthma.

A specific kind of airway inflammation is the underlying cause of airway obstruction in asthma. This airway inflammation is characterized by bronchial infiltration with inflammatory cells (in particular, eosinophils) and epithelial injury. This eosinophilic inflammation of the airways is the target of anti-inflammatory treatment of asthma. Hence, an alternative definition of asthma is "chronic eosinophilic desquamating bronchitis," which is a concise summary of the histology in asthma.[10]

PATHOPHYSIOLOGY

Pathology

Over the past decades, pathologic study of persons with fatal asthma clearly demonstrated the inflammatory nature of this disease.[11–16] Typically, the lungs of such patients are overdistended, with mucus exudate and plugging that obstructs the airway lumen of segmental airways. The thick and tenacious mucus plugs contain fibrin and inflammatory cells such as eosinophils, macrophages, and plasma cells. Furthermore, epithelial injury leads to disruption of the airway epithelium with epithelial cells present in airway mucus.

Histologic examination of the airway in fatal asthma shows an inflammatory cell infiltration, primarily with eosinophils. Mast cells, lymphocytes, macrophages, and plasma cells are also present in the cellular infiltrate. The epithelial injury often progresses to complete denudation of ciliated cells from the epithelium.

The entire bronchial wall may be thickened because of tissue edema, smooth muscle hypertrophy or hyperplasia, and vascular congestion. There may be hyperplasia of the submucosal mucous glands, as is seen in patients with chronic bronchitis. The basement membrane zone appears thickened because of collagen deposition beneath the basement membrane itself. This basement membrane zone thickening may be an important cause of fixed airway obstruction that can occur in long-standing asthma.

Study of bronchial biopsy specimens from patients with mild asthma clearly shows that eosinophilic desquamating bronchitis is present even in these patients.[17–26] Patients with untreated, newly diagnosed asthma show increased numbers of eosinophils, mast cells, lymphocytes, and macrophages in the epithelium and lamina propria. Likewise, the deposition of collagen beneath the basement membrane found in bronchial biopsy specimens obtained from patients with mild asthma is similar to such changes found in fatal asthma.[23] At least one study suggested that neutrophils are not increased in the mucosa of patients with mild asthma, although neutrophils are present in sputum.[22] On the other hand, there is an increase in the number of T lymphocytes in the airway of asthmatics.[27–29] These T lymphocytes may be a source of cytokines relevant to the airway inflammation in asthma.

Mechanisms of Airway Inflammation

☐ CYTOKINES

Study of bronchial mucosal biopsies and bronchoalveolar lavage fluid obtained from patients with mild or moderate asthma strongly suggests that cell-derived *cytokines* are integrally involved in the airway inflammation of asthma.[30–35] Cytokines and interleukins are cell-derived soluble factors that have specific actions on other cells. Interleukin-5, interleukin-3, and granulocyte-macrophage colony-stimulating factor are important eosinophil active cytokines that stimulate eosinophil differentiation, maturation, activation, and degranulation.[36–38] These three cytokines are found in bronchoalveolar lavage fluid obtained from asthmatics, and the mRNA for these cytokines are found in cells obtained by bronchial biopsy or bronchoalveolar lavage from patients with asthma. Although a variety of cell types can synthesize interleukin-5 (IL-5), interleukin-3 (IL-3), and granulocyte-macrophage colony-stimulating factor, the predominant source of *interleukin-4* (IL-4) and *interleukin-5* in asthma may be the TH2 type of lymphocyte.[31,39,40]

In mice, helper T cells can be classified as TH1 and TH2 derived from precursor TH0 cells. The TH2 lymphocyte produces IL-4 and IL-5, while the TH1 lymphocyte preferentially produces interleukin 2 (IL-2) and interferon-γ.[31,39,40] Similar division of T-helper function occurs in humans, although the distinction into cell lines is not so precise. Our current model of airway inflammation in asthma involves an important role for the TH2-like lymphocyte with the production of eosinophil active cytokines. Moreover, because interleukin-4 induces IgE antibody production, whereas interferon-γ inhibits IgE production, preferential activation of TH2 lymphocytes would lead to both eosinophil activation and IgE production.

☐ HYPERSENSITIVITY

Mast cells and basophils express high affinity IgE Fcε receptors on the cell's surface. In patients with allergic asthma, specific IgE antibodies bind to these high affinity Fc receptors. In the presence of specific antigen, the Fcε receptors are cross-linked, and the mast cell or basophil is degranulated, which results in the release of preformed mediators such as histamine and the production of cytokines, *arachidonic acid* metabolites, *leukotrienes*, and *prostaglandins*. Macrophages, platelets, and some lymphocytes express low affinity receptors for IgE and may contribute to the immediate allergic response to antigen. This sequence of events is responsible for the immediate bronchial response to antigen challenge. The predominant airway response to antigen 15 minutes after aerosol challenge is contraction of smooth muscle, or bronchospasm.

Airway caliber returns toward normal 1 or 2 hours following aerosol allergen challenge. However, 4 to 6 hours after challenge, there is a subsequent or late response characterized by a cellular inflammation of the airway dominated by the eosinophil. Hence, the dual response of the asthmatic airway to antigen challenge parallels the bronchospasm and airway inflammation found in chronic asthma.

Bronchial Hyperresponsiveness

As described above, patients with allergic asthma respond to exposure to allergen with an immediate response characterized by smooth muscle contraction (bronchospasm) and a late phase response characterized by inflammation with eosinophils. A hallmark of all patients with asthma, whether allergic or nonallergic, is the increased responsiveness of the airways to nonantigen-specific stimuli. When compared with nonasthmatic individuals, patients with asthma develop greater bronchoconstriction to inhaled *methacholine*, histamine, cold air, and exercise. The level of airway hyperresponsiveness roughly correlates with the clinical severity of asthma. The degree of airway hyperresponsiveness can be quantitated by standard inhalation testing with methacholine or histamine. Typically, airway hyperresponsiveness to histamine or methacholine is expressed as the concentration of challenge agent required to produce a 20% fall in FEV_1 (PD_{20}).

Closely related to airway hyperresponsiveness is the exaggerated fluctuation of airway caliber in asthma. Individuals without asthma generally show a small daily fluctuation in peak expiratory flow rate of about 5% (airway caliber typically is lowest in the morning). Individuals with asthma, particularly poorly controlled asthma, may exhibit fluctuations in peak expiratory flow rate of 20% to 50%, with airway obstruction also greatest in the morning. Clinically, patients with asthma often describe worsening symptoms in the morning, and asthma deaths and respiratory arrests occur more frequently between midnight and 6 A.M.[41–43]

Management of asthma includes measures that can improve airway hyperresponsiveness. Therapy with inhaled corticosteroids as well as inhaled nedocromil and cromolyn can reduce airway hyperresponsiveness in asthma.[44–50] In the allergic individual, allergen avoidance and specific immunotherapy also can reduce airway hyperresponsiveness.[51]

Physiologic Abnormalities

The primary physiologic abnormality in asthma is widespread airway obstruction that varies spontaneously or with treatment. Patients with very mild asthma may show normal pulmonary physiology, whereas those with severe asthma may demonstrate severe airway obstruction, decreased expiratory flow rates, increased lung volumes from air trapping, and severe hypoxemia and carbon dioxide retention.

Typically, a patient with asthma shows an obstructive pattern on pulmonary function such as a reduced FEV_1,

FEV_1 to FVC ratio, and flow rate. There may be an increased residual volume, functional residual capacity, total lung capacity, and RV to TLC ratio. These changes occur because airways in asthma close at higher than normal lung volumes resulting in air trapping and increased lung volumes.

Expiratory flow rates are commonly reduced in asthma. In more severe asthma, disordered gas exchange results from ventilation-perfusion inequality. In this situation, pulmonary blood flow does not match the uneven ventilation caused by severe asthma. The resultant hypoxemia is commonly associated with hyperventilation and a decreased $PaCO_2$. On the other hand, the $PaCO_2$ rises in very severe asthma when the airway obstruction and respiratory muscle fatigue become so great that hypoventilation and hypercapnia ensue.

MEDICAL HISTORY

The medical history is directed toward establishing the diagnosis of asthma and assessing its severity. The typical symptoms of asthma are episodes of shortness of breath, wheezing, cough, and chest tightness. Common provoking factors or asthma triggers include exercise, cold air, respiratory irritants, upper and lower respiratory infections, and allergen exposure. Exercise tolerance and routine daily activity are important components of the medical history because some patients with asthma significantly curtail their activities when asthma is troublesome. Frequency of symptoms is especially important because patients with mild asthma experience symptoms only once or twice a week, patients with moderate asthma may experience asthma symptoms several times a week, and patients with severe asthma may experience continuous symptoms.

Respiratory infections are a common cause of asthma exacerbations, especially in children. Typically, a symptomatic viral infection (common cold) can lead to asthma exacerbation. Common cold viruses such as rhinovirus are common asthma triggers, although *Mycoplasma* and *Chlamydia* may also trigger acute asthma.[52,53]

A detailed allergy history is important for all patients with asthma. Specific questions should be directed toward the seasonal variation in symptoms; aggravation of asthma following exposure to pets or other animals; and the possibility of allergy to dust mites, cockroaches, and other indoor allergens. Dust mites produce highly sensitizing allergens and are found in microenvironments where humidity is high. Such environments include damp, musty basements; homes in humid climates with carpet laid over concrete slabs; bedding and upholstered furniture; and where tight, energy efficient construction results in high indoor humidity. Allergens from cockroaches and rodents may be present in warmer climates or in unsanitary urban housing.

An open-ended inquiry into hobbies and recreation can provide useful information about clinically important allergen exposure. Of course, active and passive smoking are both important triggers of asthma.

It is particularly important that all patients with asthma give a thorough occupational history. Occupational asthma is the cause of 2% to 15% of asthma in the United States.[54] Furthermore, the number of work (or school) days lost due to asthma is helpful in assessing asthma severity. Attention to alleviating factors is helpful in establishing the diagnosis of asthma by history and is helpful in assessing asthma severity. Patients with asthma generally report improvement in symptoms following inhaled bronchodilators or systemic steroids. Lack of response to these therapies by history may cast doubt about the diagnosis of asthma (or, alternatively, may indicate severe asthma).

The medical history must include current and past medication use. The frequency of inhaled bronchodilator use, response to inhaled corticosteroids, and requirements for systemic corticosteroids all help the clinician judge the severity of asthma. Moreover, medications such as β-adrenergic blocking agents often aggravate asthma, and aspirin or other nonsteroidal anti-inflammatory drugs can trigger severe asthmatic reactions in sensitive individuals.

Assessment of severity of asthma must include a detailed past medical history of asthma such as emergency room use, hospitalizations, corticosteroid use, and intensive care unit admission. Recent hospitalization for asthma, repeated emergency room treatment for asthma attacks, and previous life-threatening asthma are all very important indicators of high risk for another severe, even fatal, episode.[55]

The medical history should include inquiry into associated conditions such as allergic rhinitis, sinusitis, and gastroesophageal reflux as well as comorbid conditions such as coronary artery disease, hypertension, congestive heart failure, and emphysema. The family history is useful not only for evaluating familial tendency for asthma or atopy, but also for the diagnosis of hereditary diseases such as α_1-antitrypsin deficiency and cystic fibrosis.

PHYSICAL EXAMINATION

Wheezing in asthma is caused by the vibration of at least one severely obstructed airway during expiration or inspiration. It is important to note that, while wheezing usually indicates airway obstruction, the presence or absence of wheezing does not by itself indicate mild or severe asthma. Other physical findings of asthma include prolonged forced expiratory time, chest hyperinflation, and cough. In severe acute asthma, there may be the use of accessory muscles of respiration and pulsus paradoxus of more than 10 mmHg (Table 27-1).[56] During an asthma attack, the patient may generate high negative inspiratory pleural pressures at higher than normal lung volumes. There is an increased afterload on the right ventricle during inspiration that may cause a transient inspiratory decline in systolic blood pressure. An inspiratory decline in systolic blood pressure of greater than 10 mmHg (pulsus paradoxus) can be found in severe acute asthma. Finally, the physical examination is helpful in

TABLE 27-1 **How to Measure Pulsus Paradoxus**

1. Inflate the cuff to a level higher than the systolic blood pressure.
2. Lower the cuff pressure slowly as the patient breathes (normally or quietly, if possible).
3. Note the pressure level at which the first sounds (Korotkoff sounds) can be heard during the respiratory cycle (ie, at expiration).
4. Continue to lower the cuff pressure slowly.
5. Note the pressure level at which sounds can be heard throughout the respiratory cycle (ie, at inspiration and expiration).
6. The difference between these two levels (ie, step 3 and step 5) is the pulsus paradoxus.

Note: A paradoxical pulse of 10 mmHg or more is abnormal. When pronounced, the pulsus paradoxus can be detected as a palpable decrease in pulse amplitude.

the differential diagnosis of asthma and in establishing comorbid medical conditions.

LABORATORY STUDIES

Pulmonary function studies are essential to document the severity of airflow obstruction and to establish reversibility or variability in airflow obstruction with treatment or spontaneously over time. Although the medical history and physical examination are also essential for diagnosis and severity assessment, several clinical studies have shown that health care providers and even patients themselves are not able to accurately estimate airflow obstruction by history and physical examination alone.[57–60]

Patients with mild or well-controlled asthma may show normal pulmonary function. Others with more severe asthma may demonstrate airway obstruction on spirometry with improvement in pulmonary function following inhaled bronchodilator. Generally, an increase in FEV_1 of 15% or 200 mL or more is considered significant and supports the diagnosis of asthma. Patients with airway obstruction that does not improve following bronchodilator administration may have another obstructive lung disease characterized by "fixed" airway obstruction (eg, chronic obstructive pulmonary disease or emphysema), or they may have airway obstruction that is temporarily irreversible from asthma caused predominately by airway inflammation. In the latter case, treatment with corticosteroids or other anti-inflammatory drugs may reveal significant improvement in pulmonary function after several days of therapy.

The peak expiratory flow (PEF) as measured by a peak flow meter is a simple test that can be performed at home, in the office, or at the bedside. Measurement of peak expiratory flow is especially well suited to home or ambulatory monitoring. Wide variation in peak expiratory flow rate aids in the diagnosis and severity assessment of asthma. Decreased morning expiratory flows and wide swings in flows during the course of a day support the diagnosis of nocturnal asthma. The peak expiratory flow is measured at high lung volume and is very effort dependent, whereas the FEV_1 measures flow at both high and intermediate lung volumes. The FEV_1 is the preferred study for the diagnosis of asthma.

The chest radiograph in asthma is often normal, but it may show hyperinflation; infiltrates caused by atelectasis; and, in rare situations, mucus plugs that appear as linear infiltrates. The chest radiograph is most useful in the evaluation of other cardiopulmonary conditions or for complications such as pneumothorax or pneumonia. The complete blood cell count with differential count can reveal a peripheral eosinophilia in some asthmatic patients. There is a rough correlation between the level of peripheral blood eosinophilia and the severity of asthma.[61] In the acute setting, a leukocytosis with a predominance of neutrophils may indicate a pulmonary or systemic bacterial infection. The sputum from an asthmatic patient may contain increased numbers of eosinophils, desquamated epithelial cells, and inflammatory mucus plugs. Although sputum examination is uncommonly used for the diagnosis of asthma, it may be useful in the evaluation of possible respiratory infection (eg, pneumonia or tuberculosis).

All patients with asthma should give a detailed history regarding the role of respiratory allergy as an important asthma trigger. Patients with suspected inhalant allergy are candidates for allergy skin testing or in vitro testing. Allergy testing should be strongly considered for patients with uncontrolled asthma, asthma beginning before the age of 40, severe asthma, or recurrent asthma exacerbations, or for patients who are developing adverse effects to asthma pharmacotherapy. Skin testing is the preferred method of allergy evaluation because it is more sensitive and less expensive than in vitro testing. In vitro tests of IgE antibody may be preferred for patients with severe skin disease, for those who are taking antihistamines, or for those few patients for whom skin testing is considered hazardous.

DIFFERENTIAL DIAGNOSIS

A differential diagnosis should be considered when patients present with acute symptoms of shortness of breath or wheezing. The differential diagnosis for patients presenting with chronic or stable symptoms of asthma is similar but not identical (Box 27-1).

MANAGEMENT OF ASTHMA

Overview

As a chronic medical condition, asthma is managed primarily by the patient in an outpatient setting. The patient and the patient's family assume the major responsibility for avoidance of asthma triggers, monitoring of pulmonary function, and administration of medication. The patient with asthma must have the knowledge and skill to appropriately manage asthma exacerbations when they occur.

BOX 27-1

MAJOR DIFFERENTIAL DIAGNOSES OF ASTHMA

Chronic Asthma
Fixed airway obstruction
Laryngeal dysfunction
Chronic obstructive lung disease
Congestive heart failure
Sarcoidosis
Hypersensitivity pneumonitis
Hyperventilation syndrome
Habit cough

Acute Asthma
Common cold
Sinusitis
Pneumonia
Pulmonary embolus
Congestive heart failure
Coronary artery disease
Fixed airway obstruction
Hyperventilation syndrome
Panic attack

The role of the physician or health care provider is to provide the expertise in identifying important asthma triggers, designing a medical regimen suitable for the individual patient, and to insure that the patient and the patient's family develop the necessary knowledge and skills for proper asthma management. Thus, successful management of asthma revolves around a constructive physician-patient partnership.

Virtually all patients with moderate and severe asthma can expect episodes of asthma exacerbation. Prompt recognition and treatment of these asthma flare-ups usually result in successful resolution of the attack in the outpatient setting. Management of acute asthma in the emergency room often (but not always) indicates a failure of outpatient management. Therefore, an important goal of managing acute asthma in the emergency room or hospital setting is the review and modification of the outpatient therapeutic regimen.

In addition to recognition of asthma triggers, the clinician should judge asthma severity using the results of pulmonary function tests. Because stepcare of chronic stable asthma and management of acute asthma both rely on the clinician's assessment of asthma severity, pulmonary function tests play a crucial role in the management of asthma.

The pharmacologic treatment of asthma is directed toward both eosinophilic inflammation of the airway and smooth muscle contraction. Hence, anti-inflammatory therapy and bronchodilators are useful in the management of asthma. In moderate stable asthma, the patient's condition may be well controlled by the regular use of an inhaled corticosteroid combined with the as-needed use of a β-adrenergic bronchodilator. Likewise, patients with severe acute asthma or status asthmaticus should be treated with intravenous corticosteroids combined with the regular administration of a β-adrenergic aerosol by nebulization. For reasons that are unclear, the anti-inflammatory component of asthma therapy is often neglected by clinicians. Most asthma experts agree that patients with moderate or severe stable asthma should be treated with the routine use of anti-inflammatory aerosol therapy, and that acute asthma exacerbations should be treated early in the course of development with systemic corticosteroids.

Management of Acute Asthma

Exacerbations of asthma are characterized by worsening symptoms of shortness of breath, wheezing, chest tightness, or cough. Asthma exacerbations may develop over the course of days or weeks, or they may rapidly progress over a few hours. In the ideal setting, prompt recognition of worsening asthma accompanied by appropriate intensification of asthma treatment at home results in rapid and complete resolution of the asthma exacerbation in the outpatient setting. However, patients on a less than optimal outpatient regimen, patients with severe asthma, patients with unavoidable asthma triggers, and patients with highly labile airways present to the emergency department with acute exacerbations of asthma.

The primary goals of the immediate treatment of acute asthma are (1) reversal of airway obstruction and (2) adequate oxygenation (Box 27-2).

Emergency Room Management of Acute Asthma

☐ INITIAL ASSESSMENT

The strategy and methods in managing acute asthma in the emergency room are summarized by the algorithm in Protocol 27-1. The clinician's first task is the initial and rapid assessment of the severity of the asthma

BOX 27-2

ROLES AND RESPONSIBILITIES OF RESPIRATORY CARE PRACTITIONERS IN THE MANAGEMENT OF ACUTE ASTHMA*

- Assess severity of asthma
- Administer bronchodilator treatment and supplemental oxygen
- Measure pulmonary function by spirometry or handheld peak expiratory flow meter (PEF)
- Assess patient response to bronchodilators
- Obtain and interpret arterial blood gas analyses
- Intubate patients in respiratory failure or impending respiratory failure
- Monitor mechanically ventilated patients to minimize barotrauma
- Provide patient education before discharge

**Intensity of evaluation and treatment should be individualized. All patients do not require all steps summarized in this table.*

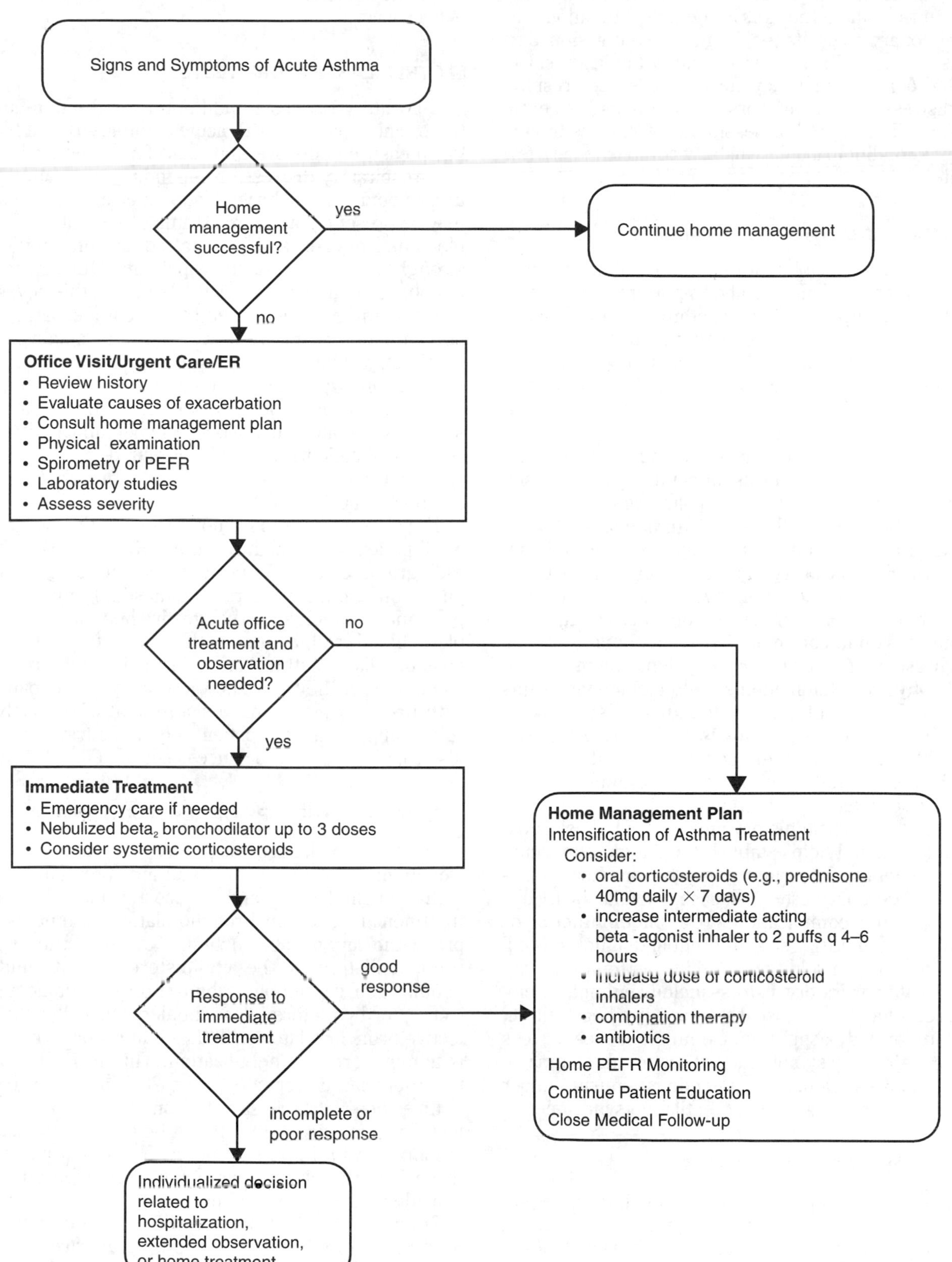

PROTOCOL 27-1. Management of acute asthma in adults. (From Institute for Clinical Systems Integration: Guidelines for Diagnosis and Management of Asthma, 1994, with permission)

attack and the general medical condition of the patient. This essential triage function should determine whether the patient requires immediate intubation, cardiopulmonary resuscitation, immediate admission to an intensive care unit, or other life support measures. Depressed consciousness, cyanosis, and severe respiratory distress are all indicators of a severe asthma exacerbation. This initial assessment of the asthmatic patient's condition usually can be accomplished in a few minutes.

☐ HISTORY AND PHYSICAL EXAMINATION

A focused medical history should be obtained from the patient and patient's family. Important components of the focused history in acute asthma include severity of symptoms, duration of asthma attack, possible causes of the asthma attack, previous hospitalizations and emergency room visits for asthma, previous or current use of corticosteroids, and complete medication history including inhaler use.

Viral respiratory tract infections and allergen exposure are two common causes for acute asthma. Sensitization to indoor and outdoor inhalants is an important risk factor for acute asthma or asthma death.[62–64] Outbreaks of acute asthma can be caused by episodic increases in airborne allergen (such as soybean dust)[65] or by increases in air pollution.[66] Although exercise is a common trigger of asthma symptoms in the outpatient setting, it is an uncommon cause of asthma exacerbations presenting to the emergency department.

The physical examination should include vital signs and examination of the heart and lungs. Use of accessory muscles, pulsus paradoxus, tachycardia (greater than 120 beats per minute), tachypnea (greater than 30 breaths per minute), diaphoresis, and cyanosis all suggest severe airways obstruction.

The initial medical history and focused physical examination should help establish the diagnosis of acute asthma, identify important comorbid medical conditions (eg, coronary artery disease, valvular heart disease), identify complications (eg, pneumothorax or pneumonia), and trigger a differential diagnosis. Medical conditions in addition to acute asthma that can cause acute respiratory distress include pulmonary embolus, coronary artery disease, congestive heart failure, and foreign body aspiration. Common causes for less severe respiratory symptoms that can mimic asthma include upper respiratory tract infections, sinusitis, upper airway obstruction, and hyperventilation syndrome.

☐ PULMONARY FUNCTION TESTS

Measurement of pulmonary function is very helpful for narrowing the differential diagnosis of the patient presenting with symptoms of acute asthma and for determining the severity of the attack. Virtually all but the most critically ill patients should have spirometry or peak expiratory flows measured in the emergency department. Furthermore, if airway obstruction is demonstrated by pulmonary function tests, improvement in lung function is an important factor that helps the clinician decide whether hospital admission is necessary.

☐ OTHER LABORATORY TESTS

Laboratory studies should not delay the immediate treatment of patients with acute asthma. Arterial blood gas measurements are important for patients with severe respiratory distress or impending respiratory failure. Hypoxia caused by ventilation/perfusion inequality may be present in a severe asthma exacerbation.[67] Supplemental oxygen and hospital admission should be strongly considered for these patients. During the initial phases of an asthma exacerbation of this severity, the PCO_2 may be decreased from a compensatory hyperventilation resulting in a respiratory alkalosis. As respiratory failure develops, there is worsening airway obstruction, worsening hypoxemia, and hypoventilation. The arterial blood gas pattern in these patients shows a respiratory acidosis with hypercapnia. All these severely ill patients should be admitted to an intensive care unit, and many such patients require intubation and mechanical ventilation.

The chest radiograph is not needed in the evaluation of all patients with acute asthma. However, the chest radiograph can be important for the diagnosis of pneumonia, pneumothorax, mediastinal emphysema, pulmonary embolus, and congestive heart failure. Complete blood cell counts with differential can show eosinophilia in asthma or other eosinophilic medical conditions, or they may show a leukocytosis in patients with bacterial infection. Measurement of electrolytes can be important if the patient requires intravenous fluids or if electrolyte imbalance is suspected.

☐ PHARMACOTHERAPY OF ACUTE ASTHMA

Treatment of the acute asthma exacerbation involves treatment of bronchospasm and airway inflammation with bronchodilators and corticosteroids. The initial treatment focuses on bronchodilators to quickly improve the airway obstruction of acute asthma. The bronchodilators can be administered by intermittent nebulization, continuous nebulization, subcutaneous injection, or by metered-dose inhaler. Typically, a β_2 selective bronchodilator such as albuterol or terbutaline is administered by nebulization. This bronchodilator treatment can be repeated every 20 minutes for a total of three doses if necessary. Spirometry or peak expiratory flow measurements should be repeated to assess response to therapy. Patients who respond poorly to three bronchodilator treatments should be strongly considered for hospital admission.[68,69]

Continuous rather than episodic administration of bronchodilators by nebulization is an alternative delivery method advocated by some asthma investigators.[70,71] Continuous nebulization may be particularly suitable for patients with severe obstruction. Subcutaneous injection of epinephrine or terbutaline is effective in achieving bronchodilation in many patients with acute asthma.[72,73] There is concern that patients with very severe airway obstruction may not achieve sufficient ventilation for aerosol therapy to be effective. For these patients, subcutaneous administration of bronchodilators offers some theoretical advantage over aerosol therapy. However, most asthma experts recommend episodic administration of bronchodilators by nebulization as a first-choice therapy of acute asthma.[8]

There is evidence that the repeated administration of bronchodilators by metered-dose inhaler is as effective as jet nebulization in acute asthma.[74–76] In clinical trials, bronchodilators delivered by metered-dose inhalers and spacers were equivalent to that achieved by jet nebulizers.[74–76] Further experience is needed before bronchodilator administration by metered-dose inhaler can be considered the treatment of choice in acute asthma.

Intravenous aminophylline is not necessary in the treatment of acute asthma in the emergency room and often adds unwanted toxicity.[77,78] Aerosol anticholinergic agents are not routinely used in the emergency setting, although they may be helpful in unusual circumstances.[79,80] Routine antibiotic treatment of acute asthma is not necessary and should be avoided. However, patients with suspected bacterial infection such as pneumonia or sinusitis should be treated with antibiotics.

Some patients with acute asthma may show a good and complete response after treatment with bronchodilators. This response should be assessed not only by symptoms and physical examination but especially by pulmonary function tests. Many of these patients should receive a course of oral corticosteroids for continuation of asthma treatment initiated in the emergency room. Because acute asthma exacerbations are usually caused by increased airway inflammation in addition to bronchospasm, anti-inflammatory therapy is necessary to achieve full recovery and to prevent relapse.[81] A single dose of oral or intravenous corticosteroids administered in the emergency department does not substitute for a 7- to 10-day course of oral corticosteroids. A full response requires several days. Some patients with acute asthma who recover fully following bronchodilators and who generally describe a brief duration of illness can be discharged without corticosteroids.

Patients with respiratory distress following treatment with bronchodilators should be admitted to a hospital room or an intensive care unit, whereas patients with a good or complete response can be discharged home. Those patients with a partial or incomplete response following 1 or 2 hours of bronchodilator therapy must have an individualized decision regarding hospitalization. When corticosteroids are administered in the emergency room, it usually takes 4 to 6 hours before clinical improvement becomes evident and several days for a full response. In general, patients with acute asthma should not be treated in the emergency room for longer than 4 hours. Factors that favor hospitalization include peak expiratory flow or FEV_1 less than 50% of the predicted value, previous life-threatening asthma, hospitalizations or emergency room use, prolonged duration of asthma exacerbation, and prior systemic corticosteroid use. The clinician may favor discharge home if good home care and medical follow-up is available.

HOSPITAL MANAGEMENT OF ASTHMA

The patient hospitalized for an acute asthma exacerbation should receive systemic corticosteroids[81] and aerosol bronchodilators. In addition to pharmacotherapy, the major benefit for hospital treatment is close observation with rapid intervention if the patient's condition deteriorates. Careful discharge planning and patient education is crucial for continued recovery following discharge from the hospital and prevention of asthma relapse.

Hospital treatment should include the continued administration of a bronchodilator aerosol such as albuterol or terbutaline delivered by nebulization. If the patient is in acute respiratory distress, bronchodilator nebulization treatments can be continued every 1 to 2 hours, usually in an intensive care setting. Those patients not as acutely ill can receive aerosol β agonists every 3 to 4 hours or as symptoms and pulmonary function indicate. As in the emergency room setting, bronchodilator delivery with a metered-dose inhaler or continuous nebulization of a wet aerosol may be an appropriate alternative in treating selected patients. Repeated systemic administration of sympathomimetics (eg, epinephrine or terbutaline) and continuous intravenous sympathomimetics (eg, isoproterenol) are potentially hazardous practices and generally should be avoided.

On the other hand, there may be a role for intravenous aminophylline in the adult patient hospitalized with asthma.[82] Whereas the routine use of aminophylline in the emergency room setting is discouraged, therapy with intravenous theophylline in adult hospitalized patients may be beneficial. The decision to include aminophylline in the hospital treatment of asthma must be individualized. Risks are increased in patients with coronary artery disease, and the dosage should be carefully monitored by blood levels. On the other hand, intravenous aminophylline may not be effective in children hospitalized with severe asthma.[83,84]

Virtually all patients hospitalized with asthma should receive systemic corticosteroids. Traditionally, corticosteroids are administered intravenously four times daily (eg, methylprednisolone 40 mg QID). Because oral corticosteroids are well absorbed from the gastrointestinal tract, the route of administration can be changed from intravenous to oral as the patient recovers. Some clinical studies suggest that intravenous corticosteroids can be omitted altogether in the treatment of acute asthma (ie, administered entirely by the oral route).[85] However, most asthma experts recommend that corticosteroids be given intravenously during the initial phases of hospital treatment.[8]

Supplemental oxygen should be included for most patients hospitalized for asthma. Generally, low-dose supplemental oxygen (eg, 2 to 3 L/min by nasal cannula) is sufficient to reverse the hypoxemia associated with acute asthma. Oxygen therapy can be guided by arterial blood gas measurements or oximetry. In acutely ill patients, it should be noted that oximetry does not include the measurement of $PaCO_2$ or pH, both of which are useful in treating patients with impending respiratory failure.

Replacement of water and electrolytes must be individualized for each patient. Dehydration and hypovolemia are common, especially if the duration of respiratory distress is longer than a few hours. Close attention to the blood potassium level is important. Both β agonists and glucocorticoids lower potassium, and many patients with coexisting cardiovascular disease may be taking diuretics. Antibiotic therapy should be included when bacterial infections such as sinusitis or pneumonia are suspected. Routine use of antibiotics for hospitalized patients with asthma is not necessary.

Patients hospitalized with acute asthma are at risk for respiratory arrest and should be monitored closely. Because respiratory arrests and asthma deaths occur more often between midnight and 6 A.M.,[41–43] medical supervision must be especially vigilant during these early morning hours.

The patient's progress should be assessed by symptoms, physical examination, and peak expiratory flow. Bedside spirometry can be useful, especially in those patients in whom accurate measurement of pulmonary function is important.

Mechanical Ventilation

Some patients with extreme respiratory distress or impending respiratory failure, and all patients with frank respiratory insufficiency, should be intubated and mechanical ventilatory support begun. The decision to proceed with endotracheal intubation and mechanical ventilatory support is based on the clinical evaluation of the patient (eg, fatigue, exhaustion), pulmonary function tests (FEV_1 or PEF less than 25% of the predicted value), and arterial blood gas measurements ($PaCO_2$ greater than 40 mmHg). Frequent administration of nebulized bronchodilators and intravenous corticosteroid therapy are continued when the asthmatic patient is mechanically ventilated. Inhalational anesthetic agents such as halothane, enflurane, and isoflurane have bronchodilator properties and may be helpful in the treatment of severe asthma unresponsive to standard therapy. Fortunately, intubated asthma patients usually recover rapidly with treatment, and most intubated asthma patients can be extubated within 72 hours. Clinical reports show that about 2% to 8% of all asthma patients who are hospitalized require endotracheal intubation and mechanical ventilation.[86,87]

The management goal of the intubated asthma patient is to insure adequate oxygenation as the corticosteroids and bronchodilators reverse the airways obstruction. Complications from the use of mechanical ventilation in patients with severe asthma are associated with barotrauma.[88] The use of low pressure, controlled mechanical ventilation carries the lowest risk of barotrauma complication.[89] The peak airway pressure should be less than or equal to 35 cmH_2O. Relative hypoventilation with an elevated $PaCO_2$ and mild acidemia is generally well tolerated.

Many patients with severe asthma develop dynamic hyperinflation because of reduced expiratory ability. In mechanically ventilated patients, this pulmonary hyperinflation can lead to hypotension and barotrauma. Generally, low tidal volumes (5 to 7 mL/kg) and greater inspiratory flow rates (> 80 mL/min) help reduce pulmonary hyperinflation.

Mechanically ventilated asthma patients can receive aerosol β agonists by nebulization or by metered-dose inhaler. Delivery of bronchodilator by jet nebulization is most effective at low flow rates (eg, 40 mL/min) and tidal volumes of 700 to 1,000 mL at 20 respirations per minute.[90,91] Assessing the response to aerosol bronchodilator treatment can be difficult in the intubated patient because direct measurement of expiratory resistance is not available. Generally, an increase in heart rate of 10% to 15% indicates that an adequate dose of bronchodilator has been delivered.

Recovery

Continued treatment with corticosteroids and bronchodilators leads to decreased airway obstruction and improvement in symptoms, physical findings, and pulmonary function. As the patient improves, administration of corticosteroids (and theophylline, if administered) can be changed from the intravenous to the oral route, and inhaled bronchodilators can be changed from wet nebulization to metered-dose inhaler. Remember that the presence or absence of wheezing is not a reliable indicator of airway obstruction. Thus, the asthma exacerbation is rarely completely resolved at the time the patient is discharged from the hospital (or the emergency department). Careful discharge planning and medical follow-up should result in full recovery without relapses and in the prevention of future exacerbations.

Risk Factors for Asthma Deaths

Patients with the most severe asthma are at greatest risk for asthma death. Life-threatening asthma attacks, recent hospitalizations or emergency room visits for asthma, and increased diurnal variation in peak flow rates are all important indicators of severity and high risk asthma (Box 27-3).[55,92] Most asthma experts believe that underestimating asthma severity, undertreatment with corticosteroids, and delays in seeking medical care contribute significantly to asthma mortality.

Psychiatric illness complicates asthma management and increases the risk of a fatal asthma attack.[55] Reduced chemosensitivity and perception of asthma can lead to poor patient perception of airway obstruction and delays in seeking medical care.[93] Other asthma patients may have inadequate access to medical care because of economic or social obstacles.

BOX 27-3

RISK FACTORS FOR ASTHMA DEATH

Hospital admission for asthma in past year
Previous life-threatening asthma
Emergency room visit for asthma in past year
African American race
Psychosocial problems
Decreased perception of asthma
Asthma severity underestimated
Poor access to medical care

Some patients with fatal or near-fatal asthma experience rapidly progressive asthma attacks that develop within 1 to 3 hours.[94] Histologic study of airway mucosa from such patients reveals a predominance of neutrophils, rather than eosinophils.[95] Whether or not asthmatics who experience sudden asphyctic episodes represent a distinct subset of the asthma population remains uncertain.

DISCHARGE PLANNING FROM THE HOSPITAL AND EMERGENCY DEPARTMENT

The clinical study of fatal and near-fatal asthma indicates that recent hospitalization or an emergency room visit for asthma are important risk factors for asthma deaths.[55] Hence, all hospitalized patients and many emergency room patients with asthma should be considered high risk. Discharge planning from the hospital or emergency department should include continued anti-inflammatory and bronchodilator treatment, home peak flow monitoring for many patients, and close medical follow-up. Patients should have sufficient knowledge to avoid asthma triggers, adhere to the medical regimen, and manage exacerbations promptly. Patients should have the proper skill to use the metered-dose inhaler effectively and to keep a peak expiratory flow diary, if so instructed. Finally, effort should be made for each patient to establish continuing care with a clinician for the ongoing management of this chronic condition. Education of the asthmatic patient is effective in reducing asthma exacerbations and hospitalizations.[96,97]

Patient Education

Whereas patient education should be an integral part of the ongoing care of the patient with stable asthma,[98] preparation for discharge from the hospital is an opportune time for the patient to learn about self-care of asthma (Table 27-2). Key points include knowledge of the inflammatory and bronchospasm components of asthma, the actions of bronchodilator and anti-inflammatory medications, and the potential adverse effects of these drugs. Patients should understand that aerosol corticosteroids do not have a bronchodilator effect, nor do these agents cause clinically important adverse effects usually associated with systemic corticosteroid therapy. Patients should receive careful written instructions of their discharge treatments, including how to continue and taper oral corticosteroids.

TABLE 27-2 **Patient Education for Asthma**

Knowledge

Roles of inflammation and bronchospasm in asthma
Asthma triggers and how to avoid or control them (eg, allergens, smoke, respiratory infections, exercise)
How asthma medications work
Adverse effects of medications

Skills

Proper use of metered-dose inhalers
Peak expiratory flow rate measurement
Self-care based on written guidelines

Attitude

Continuing relationship with health care provider
Early recognition and prompt treatment of asthma exacerbations

Metered-Dose Inhaler Use

Virtually all patients discharged from the hospital should be using inhaled corticosteroid therapy along with a continued course of oral prednisone or equivalent. The respiratory care practitioner is an effective teacher of metered-dose inhaler technique (Table 27-3).[99] A comparative study of physicians, nurses, and respiratory care practitioners showed that respiratory care practitioners demonstrated and taught metered-dose inhaler technique more effectively than the other health care providers.[100] Breath-activated devices and the use of spacer devices are helpful for patients who have difficulty coordinating hand motion and lung inflation.

Management of Allergic Triggers

If an important allergy or allergen exposure was identified during the hospital evaluation, patients should be instructed on effective avoidance measures. Pollens and molds are important triggers of asthma exacerbations in allergic patients.[62–65] Occupational asthma or asthma triggered by allergens related to pets or hobbies often is unrecognized for many years. If these are important

TABLE 27-3 **How to Use a Metered-Dose Inhaler***

1. Remove cap.
2. Shake inhaler.
3. Exhale normally.
4. Position inhaler 2 inches from open mouth.
5. Start to inhale slowly, then squeeze cartridge to release spray.
6. Inhale slowly, over 5 seconds, if possible.
7. Hold breath for 10 seconds, if possible.

*Breath-actuated inhalers and metered-dose inhalers used with a spacer device require a different technique.

asthma triggers for an individual patient, avoidance measures should be instituted. Dust mite allergy is also often unrecognized, in part, because the dust mite–sensitive patient may not report seasonal variation in symptoms. Dust mite avoidance measures can be very effective in sensitive patients and should be reviewed in detail with those selected individuals.

Written Action Plan

Because all patients recovering after hospital treatment of acute asthma are at increased risk of relapse, respiratory arrest, and asthma death, all or most of these patients should receive a written contingency plan for managing future exacerbations. Frequently referred to as an "action plan" or "crisis plan," this written plan usually includes home peak expiratory flow monitoring. The respiratory care practitioner is well suited to review the proper use of the home peak flow meter and the recommended actions based on peak flow measurements and symptoms (Table 27-4). Ambulatory peak expiratory flow rate monitoring warns of impending asthma attacks, allows the patient to assume more responsibility for self-care, and tracks the effectiveness of therapy. The action plan should include clear instructions on when the patient should increase bronchodilator treatment, increase aerosol anti-inflammatory treatment, begin oral prednisone, and call the physician. Telephone numbers, medication dosage, and timing of treatment should be part of the written plan.

Medical Follow-up

A follow-up visit with the patient's physician should be arranged at the time of hospital or emergency room discharge. Pulmonary function tests with spirometry should be part of this follow-up visit. The medical regimen of oral corticosteroids, inhaled anti-inflammatory therapy, and bronchodilator therapy is reviewed and modified during this visit. As the patient recovers from the asthma exacerbation, he or she can resume therapy for chronic stable asthma.

TABLE 27-4 **How to Measure the Peak Expiratory Flow Rate**

1. Place the indicator at the base of the numbered scale.
2. Stand or sit up.
3. Take a deep breath.
4. Place the meter in the mouth and close lips around the mouthpiece.
5. Blow out as hard and fast as possible.
6. Write down the achieved measurement.
7. Repeat the process once or twice.
8. Record the highest measurement achieved.

(Modified from National Asthma Education Program: Expert Panel Report: Guidelines for the Diagnosis and Management of Asthma. U.S. Department of Health and Human Services, Public Health Service, National Institutes of Health, Publication No. 91-3042, August 1991)

MANAGEMENT OF CHRONIC STABLE ASTHMA

Overview

The principles of anti-inflammatory therapy, bronchodilator therapy, and avoidance of asthma triggers apply to the management of chronic stable asthma just as they do to acute asthma. Whereas an important goal of treating acute exacerbations of asthma is the prompt reversal of airway obstruction using bronchodilators, an important goal of managing chronic stable asthma is control of airway inflammation using inhaled anti-inflammatory drugs, namely aerosol corticosteroids, nedocromil or cromolyn. The overall goals of stable asthma, then, are prevention of exacerbations, achieving normal or near-normal pulmonary function, and reaching normal or near-normal activity levels. These goals should be achieved while minimizing adverse effects from asthma medications.

As described earlier, patient and family education, environmental control, and objective monitoring of pulmonary function with spirometry or peak expiratory flow measurements are important components of asthma therapy. Allergy testing is appropriate for those patients for whom respiratory allergy is an important asthma trigger. Allergy test results help guide environmental control and avoidance measures. Immunotherapy, or allergy shots, can be effective in desensitizing allergic patients.[51]

Guidelines for the management of stable asthma often are presented as "stepcare," where recommended therapy is described for mild, moderate, or severe disease (Protocol 27-2).[8] Of course, individual patients with asthma may defy categorization as mild, moderate, or severe, and the management plan for these and other patients must be individualized.

Mild Asthma

The typical patient with mild asthma experiences symptoms of asthma at most two times weekly and is asymptomatic between exacerbations. Generally, patients with mild asthma show pulmonary function that is normal or near normal (greater or equal to 80% of predicted values).

Most patients with mild asthma can be successfully managed with an intermediate-acting β agonist metered-dose inhaler (eg, albuterol, terbutaline, or pirbuterol) as needed. Some patients with mild asthma experience exercise-induced asthma or allergen-induced asthma, and these patients can use their bronchodilator inhaler before exercise or exposure. Patients with allergic asthma may benefit from aerosol cromolyn or nedocromil before allergen exposure.

Moderate Asthma

Typically, the patient with moderate asthma experiences symptoms of asthma more than two times per week and may experience occasional symptoms of asthma at night or during early morning hours. These patients may experience more severe asthma exacer-

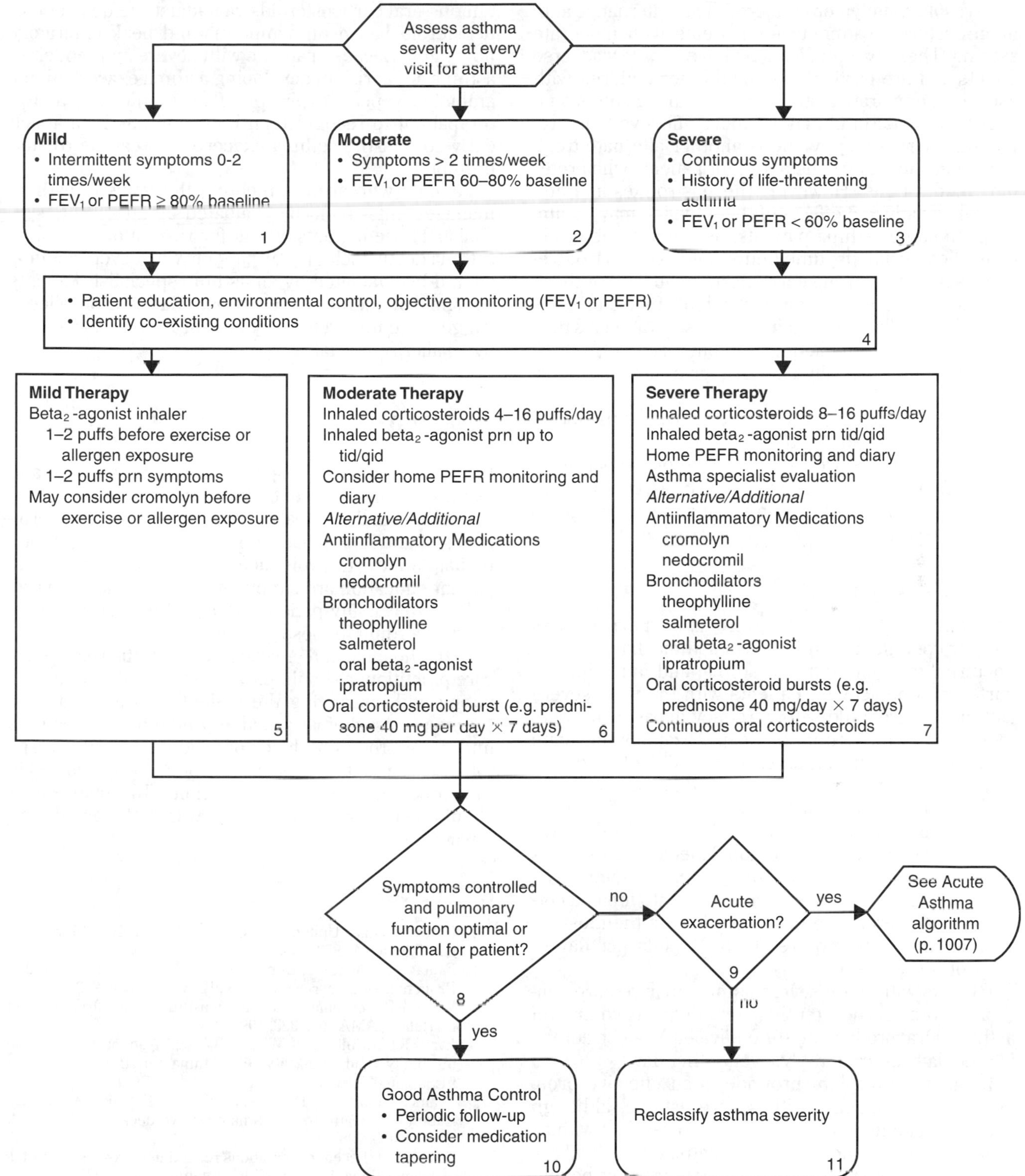

PROTOCOL 27-2. Stepcare management of chronic asthma in adults (ages 18 and older). (Modified from: Institute for Clinical Systems Integration: Guidelines for Diagnosis and Management of Asthma. 1994; with permission.)

bations and require occasional treatment of acute asthma on an urgent basis. Baseline pulmonary function in patients with moderate asthma is in the range of 60% to 80% of normal predicted values.

All patients with moderate asthma should take asthma medications, usually aerosol corticosteroids, on a regular and continuous basis. Patients in this category with milder disease may be controlled with as little as 4 puffs daily of an inhaled corticosteroid. Patients with more severe disease may require up to 16 puffs daily (or more) of inhaled corticosteroid medication to successfully reach all treatment goals.

Aerosol cromolyn or nedocromil are alternative anti-inflammatory treatments for patients with moderate asthma. These two medications have very few adverse effects and are particularly suitable for children with asthma. Comparative studies in asthmatic adults suggest that nedocromil may be more effective than cromolyn.[101] Oral theophylline is another alternate treatment and should be considered for patients who prefer oral medications. However, the gastrointestinal and neurologic adverse effects of theophylline may be limiting. In some asthma patients, asthma can be easily controlled during daytime hours but becomes troublesome at night or during early morning hours. For these patients, the evening administration of sustained release theophylline or sustained release β_2 agonists may be helpful. The long-acting β agonist aerosol, salmeterol, may be especially effective for treatment of nocturnal asthma.[102]

Another possible approach in managing moderate asthma is combination therapy (eg, aerosol corticosteroids combined with theophylline or nedocromil). Although not well studied in clinical trials, combination therapy may be successful in some patients with moderate or severe asthma.

Severe Asthma

Typically, the patient with severe asthma experiences daily or continuous symptoms of asthma, has frequent nocturnal awakening from asthma, and must limit or curtail routine activity. Patients with the most severe asthma require multiple emergency department treatments for acute asthma or hospitalizations for acute asthma. Pulmonary function may be 60% of predicted values or less, with large swings in pulmonary function.

Generally, patients with severe asthma should administer inhaled corticosteroids 8 to 16 puffs daily (or more) and often require additional medications such as cromolyn, nedocromil, theophylline, or salmeterol. There is a dose response relationship with inhaled corticosteroid therapy, so that patients with the most severe asthma may require 20 to 24 puffs per day of aerosol corticosteroid.

Patients with more severe asthma may require continuous oral corticosteroids for adequate control of asthma. Oral prednisone (or equivalent) can be administered daily or, preferably, every other day.

Inhaled ipratropium bromide is an effective bronchodilator in patients with severe asthma, although peak bronchodilatation is generally lower than with albuterol.[103] Nevertheless, some patients, particularly those with moderate or severe asthma, may benefit from a trial of anticholinergic bronchodilator therapy. The International Consensus Report on the Diagnosis and Management of Asthma suggests that ipratropium bromide should "be considered as an alternative for patients who experience such adverse effects as tachycardia or tremor from β agonists."[104]

All patients with severe asthma and most patients with moderate asthma should measure peak expiratory flow rates at home. For example, patients requiring continuous oral corticosteroids can adjust the dose of corticosteroid based on symptoms and peak expiratory flow rates. Because patients with severe and moderate asthma are at risk of developing asthma exacerbations, ambulatory peak expiratory flow monitoring allows the patient to recognize an impending asthma attack early so that the asthma exacerbation can be treated promptly.

Patients who are not meeting the goals of asthma management should be evaluated by an asthma specialist. Those patients at risk for respiratory arrest or asthma death, including all patients with severe asthma, should be evaluated by an asthma specialist. Patients with mild, moderate, or severe asthma for whom allergy triggers are important may benefit from an evaluation by an allergy specialist.

SUMMARY

In many respects, hospitalizations for asthma and asthma deaths represent a failure to successfully manage asthma in the outpatient setting. Although the principles of anti-inflammatory therapy, monitoring of pulmonary function, avoidance of asthma triggers, and patient education are simple in concept, many experts believe that many patients with asthma are not managed according to these guidelines.

In the hospital and emergency room, the respiratory care practitioner should play an important role in evaluating and instructing the patient with asthma. Furthermore, as clinical practice guidelines for asthma underscore the importance of patient education, respiratory care practitioners may become more involved in the outpatient care of this condition. This involvement should be welcomed by patients with asthma and their physicians.

REFERENCES

1. CDC: Asthma—United States, 1982–1992. MMWR Morb Mortal Wkly Rep 43:953, 1995
2. Fanta CH: Acute Asthma. In EB Weiss, M Stein, (eds): Bronchial Asthma. Boston, Little, Brown, 1993, p. 972
3. Weiss KB: Seasonal trends in US asthma hospitalizations and mortality. JAMA 263:2323, 1990
4. Evans R III, Mullally DI, Wilson RW, et al: National trends in the morbidity and mortality of asthma in the U.S. Chest 91:Suppl6:65S, 1987
5. Evans R III, Mullally DI, Wilson RW, et al: Prevalence, hospitalization and death from asthma over two decades: 1965–1984. Chest 91:65, 1987
6. Evans R III: Recent observations reflecting increases in mortality from asthma. J Allergy Clin Immunol 80:337, 1987
7. Weiss KB, Gergen PJ, Hodgson TA: An economic evaluation of asthma in the United States. N Engl J Med 326:862, 1992
8. National Asthma Education Program: Expert Panel Report: Guidelines for the Diagnosis and Management of Asthma. U.S. Department of Health and Human Services, Public Health Service, National Institutes of Health, Publication No. 91-3042; August 1991
9. American College of Chest Physicians, American Thoracic Society: Pulmonary terms and symbols. Chest 67:583, 1975
10. Reed CE: New therapeutic approaches in asthma. J Allergy Clin Immunol 77:537, 1986

11. Hogg JL: Pathology of Asthma. In E Middleton Jr, CE Reed, EF Ellis (eds): Asthma: Principles and Practice. St. Louis, Mosby, 1993, p. 1215
12. Reid LM: The presence or absence of bronchial mucus in fatal asthma. J Allergy Clin Immunol 80:415, 1987
13. Ellis AG: The pathological anatomy of bronchial asthma. Am J Med Sci 136:407, 1980
14. Huber HL, Koessler KK: The pathology of bronchial asthma. Arch Int Med 30:689, 1992
15. Dunnill MS: The pathology of asthma with special reference to changes in the bronchial mucosa. J Clin Path 13:27, 1960
16. Naylor B: The shedding of the mucosa of the bronchial tree in asthma. Thorax 8:207, 1962
17. Laitinen LA, Heino M, Laitinen A, et al: Damage of the airway epithelium and bronchial reactivity in patients with asthma. Am Rev Respir Dis 131:599, 1985
18. Lozewicz S, Gomez E, Ferguson H, Davies RJ: Inflammatory cells in the airways of mild asthma. Br Med J 297:1515, 1988
19. Beasley R, Roche WR, Roberts JA, Holgate ST: Cellular events in the bronchi of mild asthma and after bronchial provocation. Am Rev Respir Dis 139:806, 1989
20. Bousquet J, Chanez P, Lacoste JY, et al: Eosinophilic inflammation in asthma. N Engl J Med 323:1033, 1990
21. Ohashi Y, Motojima S, Fukuda T, Makino S: Airway hyperresponsiveness, increased intracellular spaces of bronchial epithelium and increased eosinophils and lymphocytes in bronchial mucus in asthma. Am Rev Respir Dis 145:1469, 1992
22. Poston RN, Chanez P, Lacoste JY, et al: Immunohistochemical characterization of the cellular infiltration in asthmatic bronchi. Am Rev Respir Dis 145:918, 1992
23. Ollerenshaw SL, Woolcock AJ: Characteristics of the inflammation in biopsies from large airways of subjects with asthma and subjects with chronic airflow limitation. Am Rev Respir Dis 145:922, 1992
24. Pesci A, Foresi A, Bertorelli G, et al: Histochemical characteristics and degranluation of mast cells in epithelium and lamina propria of bronchial biopsies from asthmatic and normal subjects. Am Rev Respir Dis 147:684, 1993
25. Laitinen LA, Laitinen A, Haahtela T: Airway mucosal inflammation even in patients with newly diagnosed asthma. Am Rev Respir Dis 147:697, 1993
26. Montefort S, Gratziou C, Goulding D, et al: Bronchial biopsy evidence for leukocyte infiltration and upregulation of leukocyte-endothelial cell adhesion molecules 6 hours after local allergen challenge of sensitized asthmatic airways. J Clin Invest 93:1411, 1994
27. Corrigan CJ, Hartnell A, Kay AB: T-lymphocyte activation in acute severe asthma. Lancet 1:1129, 1988
28. Azzawi M, Bradley B, Jeffery PK, et al: Identification of activated T lymphocytes and eosinophils in bronchial biopsies in stable atopic asthma. Am Rev Respir Dis 142:1410, 1990
29. Walker C, Kaegi MK, Braun P, Blaser K: Activated T cells and eosinophilia in bronchoalveolar lavages from subjects with asthma correlated with disease severity. J Allergy Clin Immunol 88:935, 1991
30. Walker C, Virchow J-C, Bruijnzeel PLB, Blaser K: T cell subsets and their soluble products regulate eosinophilia in allergic and nonallergic asthma. J Immunol 146:1829, 1991
31. Robinson DS, Hamid Q, Ying S, et al: Predominant Th2-like bronchoalveolar T lymphocyte population in atopic asthma. N Engl J Med 326:298, 1992
32. Ying S, Robinson DS, Varney V, et al: TNF-α mRNA expression in allergic inflammation. Clin Exp Allergy 21:745, 1991
33. Hamid Q, Azzawi M, Ying S, et al: Expression of mRNA for interleukin-5 in mucosal bronchial biopsies from asthma. J Clin Invest 87:1541, 1991
34. Broide DH, Lotz D, Cuomo AJ, et al: Cytokines in symptomatic asthma airways. J Allergy Clin Immunol 89:958, 1992
35. Robinson DS, Ying S, Bentley AM, et al: Relationships among numbers of bronchoalveolar lavage cells expressing messenger ribonucleic acid for cytokines, asthma symptoms, and airway methacholine responsiveness in atopic asthma. J Allergy Clin Immunol 92:397, 1993
36. Lopez AF, Sanderson CJ, Ganble JR, et al: Recombinant human interleukin-5 is a selective activator of human eosinophil function. J Exp Med 167:219, 1988
37. Yamaguchi Y, Hayashi Y, Sugama Y, et al: Highly purified murine interleukin-5 (IL-5) stimulates eosinophil function and prolongs in vitro survival. J Exp Med 167:1737, 1988
38. Rothenberg ME, Owen WF Jr, Silberstein DS, et al: Human eosinophils have prolonged survival, enhanced functional properties, and become hypodense when exposed to human interleukin-3. J Clin Invest 81:1986, 1988
39. Robinson D, Hamid Q, Bentley A, et al: Activation of $CD4^+$ T cells, increased Th2-type cytokine mRNA expression, and eosinophil recruitment in bronchoalveolar lavage after allergen inhalation challenge in patients with atopic asthma. J Allergy Clin Immunol 92:313, 1993
40. Walker C, Bode E, Boer L, et al: Allergic and nonallergic asthmatics have distinct patterns of T-cell activation and cytokine production in peripheral blood and bronchoalveolar lavage. Am Rev Respir Dis 146:109, 1992
41. Hetzel MR, Clark TJH, Branthwaite MA: Asthma: Analysis of sudden deaths and ventilatory arrest in hospital. Br Med J 1:80, 1977
42. Cochrane GM, Clark TJM: A survey of asthma mortality in patients between ages 35 and 64 in the Greater London hospitals in 1971. Thorax 30:300, 1975
43. Bateman JRM, Clark SW: Sudden death in asthma. Thorax 34:40, 1979
44. Ryan G, Latimer KM, Juniper EF, et al: Effect of beclomethasone dipropionate on bronchial responsiveness to histamine in controlled nonsteroid-dependent asthma. J Allergy Clin Immunol 75:25, 1985
45. Mattoli S, Rosati G, Mormile F, Ciappi G: The immediate and short-term effects of corticosteroids on cholinergic hyperreactivity and pulmonary function in subjects with well-controlled asthma. J Allergy Clin Immunol 76:214, 1985
46. Svendsen VG, Frolund L, Madsen F, et al: A comparison of the effects of sodium cromoglycate and beclomethasone dipropionate on pulmonary function and bronchial hyperreactivity in subjects with asthma. J Allergy Clin Immunol 80:68, 1987
47. Lowhagen O, Rak S: Modification of bronchial hyperreactivity after treatment with sodium cromoglycate during pollen season. J Allergy Clin Immunol 75:460, 1985
48. Aalbers R, Kauffman HF, Groen H, et al: The effect of nedocromil sodium on the early and late reaction and allergen-induced bronchial hyperresponsiveness. J Allergy Clin Immunol 87:993, 1991
49. Rodwell LT, Anderson SD, DuToit J, Seale JP: Nedocromil sodium inhibits the airway response to hyperosmolar challenge in patients with asthma. Am Rev Respir Dis 146:1149, 1992
50. Sont JK, Bel EH, Dijkman JH, Sterk PJ: The long-term effect of nedocromil sodium on the maximal degree of airway narrowing to methacholine in atopic asthmatic subjects. Clin Exp Allergy 22:554, 1992
51. Bousquet J, Michel F-B: Specific immunotherapy in asthma: Is it effective? J Allergy Clin Immunol 94:1, 1994
52. Hudgel DW, Langston L Jr, Selner JC, McIntosh K: Viral and bacterial infections in adults with chronic asthma. Am Rev Respir Dis 120:393, 1979
53. Minor TE, Dick EC, DeMeo AN, et al: Viruses as precipitants of asthmatic attacks in children. JAMA 227:292, 1974
54. Blanc P: Occupational asthma in a national disability survey. Chest 92:613, 1987
55. Sly RM: Mortality from asthma. J Allergy Clin Immunol 84:421, 1989
56. Jardin F, Farcot J-C, Biosante L, et al: Mechanism of paradoxic pulse in bronchial asthma. Circulation 66:887, 1982
57. Shim CS, Williams MH: Evaluation of severity of asthma: Patients versus physicians. Am J Med 68:11, 1980
58. Shim CS, Williams H: Relationship of wheezing to the severity of obstruction in asthma. Arch Intern Med 143:890, 1983
59. Burdon JGW, Killian KJ, Hargreave FE, Campbell EJM: The perception of breathlessness in asthma. Am Rev Respir Dis 126:825, 1982

60. McFadden ER, Kiser R, DeGroot WJ: Acute bronchial asthma: Relationships between clinical and physiological manifestations. N Engl J Med 288:221, 1973
61. Gleich GJ, Motojima S, Frigas E, et al: The eosinophilic leukocyte and the pathology of fatal bronchial asthma: Evidence for pathologic heterogeneity. J Allergy Clin Immunol 80:412, 1987
62. Gelber LE, Seltzer LH, Bouzoukis JK, et al: Sensitization and exposure to indoor allergens as risk factors for asthma among patients presenting to hospital. Am Rev Respir Dis 147:573, 1993
63. Pollart SM, Chapman MD, Fiocco GP, et al: Epidemiology of acute asthma: IgE antibodies to common inhalant allergens as a risk factor for emergency room visits. J Allergy Clin Immunol 83:875, 1989
64. O'Hollaren MT, Yunginger JW, Offord KP, et al: Exposure to an aeroallergen as a possible precipitating factor in respiratory arrest in young patients with asthma. N Engl J Med 324:359, 1991
65. Anto JM, Sunyer J, Rodriguez-Roisin R, et al: Community outbreaks of asthma associated with inhalation of soybean dust. N Engl J Med 320:1097, 1989
66. Schwartz J, Slater D, Larson TV, et al: Particulate air pollution and hospital emergency room visits for asthma in Seattle. Am Rev Respir Dis 147:826, 1993
67. Ferrer A, Roca J, Wagner PD, et al: Airway obstruction and ventilation-perfusion relationships in acute severe asthma. Am Rev Respir Dis 147:579, 1993
68. Fanta CH, Rossing TH, McFadden ER Jr: Emergency room treatment of asthma: Relationships among therapeutic combinations, severity of obstruction and time course of response. Am J Med 72:416, 1982
69. Kelsen SG, Kelsen DP, Fleegler BF, et al: Emergency room assessment and treatment of patients with acute asthma: Adequacy of the conventional approach. Am J Med 64:622, 1978
70. Lin RY, Sauter D, Newman T, et al: Continuous versus intermittent albuterol nebulization in the treatment of acute asthma. Ann Emerg Med 22:1842, 1993
71. Rudnitsky GS, Eberlein RS, Schoffstall JM, et al: Comparison of intermittent and continuously nebulized albuterol for treatment of asthma in an urban emergency department. Ann Emerg Med 22:1847, 1993
72. Brenner BE: Bronchial asthma in adults: Presentation to the emergency department. Part II: Sympathomimetics, respiratory failure, recommendations for initial treatment, indications for admission, and summary. Am J Emerg Med 1:306, 1983
73. McFadden ER Jr: Therapy of acute asthma. J Allergy Clin Immunol 84:151, 1989
74. Kerem E, Levison H, Schuh S, et al: Efficacy of albuterol administered by nebulizer versus spacer device in children with acute asthma. J Pediatr 123:313, 1993
75. Morgan MDL, Singh BV, Frame MH, Williams SJ: Terbutaline aerosol given through pear spacer in acute severe asthma. BMJ 285:849, 1982
76. Idris AH, McDermott MF, Raucci JC, et al: Emergency department treatment of severe asthma: Metered dose inhaler plus holding chamber is equivalent in effectiveness to nebulizer. Chest 103:665, 1993
77. Siegel D, Sheppard D, Gelb A, Weinberg PF: Aminophylline increases the toxicity but not the efficacy of an inhaled β agonist in the treatment of acute exacerbations of asthma. Am Rev Respir Dis 132:283, 1985
78. Rossing TH, Fanta CH, Goldstein DH, et al: Emergency therapy of asthma: Comparison of the acute effects of parenteral and inhaled sympathomimetics and infused aminophylline. Am Rev Respir Dis 122:365, 1980
79. Patrick DM, Dales RE, Stark RM, et al: Severe exacerbations of COPD and asthma: Incremental benefit of adding ipratropium to usual therapy. Chest 98:295, 1990
80. Higgins RM, Stradling JR, Lane DJ: Should ipratropium bromide be added to β_2 agonists in treatment of acute severe asthma? Chest 94:718, 1988
81. Fanta CH, Rossing TH, McFadden ER Jr: Glucocorticoids in acute asthma: A critical controlled trial. Am J Med 74:845, 1983
82. Huang D, O'Brien RG, Harman E, et al: Does aminophylline benefit adults admitted to the hospital for an acute exacerbation of asthma? Ann Intern Med 119:1155, 1993
83. Carter E, Cruz M, Chesrown S, et al: Efficacy of intravenously administered theophylline in children hospitalized with severe asthma. J Pediatr 122:470, 1993
84. DiGiulio GA, Kercsmar CM, Krug SE, et al: Hospital treatment of asthma: Lack of benefit from theophylline given in addition to nebulized albuterol and intravenously administered corticosteroid. J Pediatr 122:464, 1993
85. Ratto D, Alfaro C, Sipsey J, et al: Are intravenous corticosteroids required in status asthmaticus? JAMA 260:527, 1988
86. Santiago SM Jr, Klaustermeyer WB: Mortality in status asthmaticus: A nine-year experience in a respiratory intensive care unit. J Asthma Res 17:75, 1980
87. Scoggin CH, Sahn SA, Petty TL: Status asthmaticus: A nine-year experience. JAMA 238:1158, 1977
88. Mansel JK, Stogner SW, Petrini MF, Norman JR: Mechanical ventilation in patients with acute severe asthma. Am J Med 89:42, 1990
89. Dworkin G, Kattan M: Mechanical ventilation for status asthmaticus in children. J Pediatr 114:545, 1989
90. O'Riordan TG, Palmer LB, Smaldone GC: Aerosol deposition in mechanically ventilated patients: Optimizing nebulizer delivery. Am J Respir Crit Care Med 149:214, 1994
91. O'Riordan TG, Greco MJ, Perry RJ, Smaldone GC: Nebulizer function during mechanical ventilation. Am Rev Respir Dis 145:1117, 1992
92. Boulet L-P, Deschesnes F, Turcotte H, Gignac F: Near-fatal asthma: Clinical and physiologic features, perception of bronchoconstriction, and psychologic profile. J Allergy Clin Immunol 88:838, 1991
93. Kikuchi Y, Okabe S, Tamura G, et al: Chemosensitivity and perception of dyspnea in patients with a history of near-fatal asthma. N Engl J Med 330:1329, 1994
94. Wasserfallen J-B, Schaller M-D, Feihl F, Perret CH: Sudden asphyxic asthma: A distinct entity? Am Rev Respir Dis 142:108, 1990
95. Sur S, Crotty TB, Kephart GM, et al: Sudden-onset fatal asthma: A distinct entity with few eosinophils and relatively more neutrophils in the airway submucosa? Am Rev Respir Dis 148:713, 1993
96. Wilson SR, Scamagas P, German DF, et al: A controlled trial of two forms of self-management education for adults with asthma. Am J Med 94:564, 1993
97. Osman LM, Abdalla MI, Beattie JA, et al: Reducing hospital admission through computer supported education for asthma patients. BMJ 308:568, 1994
98. Bone RC: The bottom line in asthma management is patient education. Am J Med 94:561, 1993
99. Interiano B, Guntupalli KK: Metered-dose inhalers: Do health care providers know what to teach? Arch Intern Med 153:81, 1993
100. Guidry GG, Brown WD, Stogner SW, George RB: Incorrect use of metered dose inhalers by medical personnel. Chest 101:31, 1992
101. Lal S, Dorow PD, Venho KK, Chatterjee SS: Nedocromil sodium is more effective than cromolyn sodium is the treatment of chronic reversible obstructive airway disease. Chest 101:438, 1993
102. Fitzpatrick MF, Mackay T, Driver H, Douglas NJ: Salmeterol in nocturnal asthma: A double blind, placebo controlled trial of a long acting inhaled β2 agonist. BMJ 301:1365, 1990
103. Gross NJ: Ipratropium bromide. N Engl J Med 319:486, 1988
104. International Consensus Report on Diagnosis and Treatment of Asthma. U.S. Department of Health and Human Services, Public Health Services, National Institutes of Health, Publication No. 92-3091; June 1992

ANNOTATED BIBLIOGRAPHY

Barnes PJ, Pedersen S: Efficacy and safety of inhaled corticosteroids in asthma. Am Rev Respir Dis 148:S1, 1993. This rather lengthy review includes mechanisms of action, pharmacokinetics, adverse effects, and efficacy of inhaled corticosteroids. Clinicians caring for patients should be knowledgeable about inhaled corticosteroids because this therapy is safe and effective for most patients with chronic stable asthma.

Beasley R, Burgess, Crane J, Pearce N, Roche W: Pathology of asthma and its clinical implications. J Allergy Clin Immunol 92:148, 1993. The histopathologic studies of fatal asthma and of endobronchial biopsy specimens from mild asthma patients are reviewed in this paper. These studies clearly indicate that eosinophilic inflammatory changes are present in the airways of patients with mild and severe asthma. The authors suggest that anti-inflammatory drugs should be used in patients with both mild and severe asthma.

Bousquet J, Michel F-B: Specific immunotherapy in asthma: Is it effective? J Allergy Clin Immunol 94:1, 1994. The authors review most of the clinical studies evaluating the effectiveness of immunotherapy in asthma. Guidelines for patient selection and referral to allergy specialists are presented. Allergy immunotherapy can be effective for selected patients with asthma.

Kavura MS: β agonists for acute asthma: Which way to deliver? J Respir Dis 15:312, 1994. This review practically addresses the alternative methods of administering β-adrenergic agonists for acute asthma. The relative merits and limitations of intermittent jet nebulization, continuous nebulization, metered-dose inhaler delivery, and subcutaneous injection are discussed.

Mayo PH, Richman J, Harris HW: Results of a program to reduce admissions for adult asthma. Ann Intern Med 112:864, 1990. Asthma patients who had previously required multiple hospitalizations for asthma attacks were able to successfully decrease hospital use as a result of an intensive educational program. This is one of several studies that suggest that asthma education results in improved outcomes.

National Asthma Education Program, Expert Panel Report: Guidelines for the Diagnosis and Management of Asthma. U.S. Department of Health and Human Services, Public Health Service, National Institutes of Health, Publication No. 91-3042; August 1991. This 130-page monograph details the diagnosis and management of asthma. A multidisciplinary team, the expert panel, developed these consensus guidelines. The report is thorough, practical, and well referenced to 1990. A must read for those interested in learning about asthma.

Sly RM: Mortality from asthma. J Allergy Clin Immunol 4:421, 1989. Epidemiologic studies showing the increases in morbidity and mortality from asthma are summarized in this review. Risk factors for asthma deaths are discussed in detail, and strategies to manage the high-risk asthma patient are clearly presented.

Weiss KB, Gergen PJ, Hodgson TA: An economic evaluation of asthma in the United States. N Engl J Med 326:862, 1992. In this unique report, the direct and indirect costs related to asthma in 1990 in the United States are estimated. The high overall costs ($6.2 billion) and the high cost of managing asthma exacerbations emphasize the importance of effective ambulatory care.

28 Chronic Obstructive Pulmonary Disease

Yancy Y. Phillips
Oleh W. Hnatiuk
Kenneth Torrington

CLINICAL SKILLS

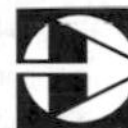

Upon completion of this chapter, the reader will:

- Describe the interrelationship between chronic bronchitis, emphysema, and asthma
- Categorize chronic pulmonary disease into stages of severity
- List risk factors for acquiring chronic obstructive pulmonary disease
- Assess the chronic obstructive pulmonary diseased patient via history and physical examination
- Use appropriate laboratory studies to determine the presence and/or the severity of chronic obstructive pulmonary disease
- Guide pulmonary patients toward measures that prevent complications and worsening of their disease
- Discuss pharmacologic, surgical, and rehabilitative therapy options for patients with chronic obstructive pulmonary disease
- Describe common complications that may accompany and help determine the course of chronic obstructive pulmonary disease
- Advise pulmonary patients to take appropriate measures to reduce the possibility of hypoxemia while traveling by airplane
- Summarize the effects of chronic obstructive pulmonary disease on sleep-related disorders
- Predict increased surgical risks for patients with chronic obstructive pulmonary disease

KEY TERMS

Acute respiratory failure
Air Travel
Alpha-1 antitrypsin inhibitor deficiency
Bullectomy
Chronic bronchitis
COPD
Cor pulmonale
Dyspnea
Emphysema
Lung transplantation
Pharmacotherapy
Pulmonary rehabilitation
Reduction pneumoplasty
Smoking cessation

DEFINITION OF CHRONIC OBSTRUCTIVE PULMONARY DISEASE

Chronic obstructive pulmonary disease (COPD) is a distinct clinical entity and one of the most common problems seen by pulmonologists and respiratory care practitioners in both the inpatient and ambulatory care settings. The American Thoracic Society (ATS) defines COPD "as a disease state characterized by the presence of airflow obstruction due to chronic bronchitis or emphysema; the airflow obstruction is generally progressive, may be accompanied by airways hyper-reactivity and may be partially reversible."[1]

After decades of increasing use by clinicians and patients, the acronym COPD has supplanted "emphysema" and "bronchitis" as the common clinical diagnosis for most American adults with chronic airways disease associated with cigarette smoking. Those two entities—emphysema and bronchitis—are actually pathologic diagnoses (see below), and their presence in a patient is almost always inferred from clinical history and physiology. One rarely has a tissue specimen on which to base such labels. The terms "pink puffer" and "blue bloater" have often been applied to patients with classic clinical syndromes associated with ***emphysema*** and ***chronic bronchitis***, respectively. Using the inclusive term COPD obviates the need to split hairs, since most patients have some overlap of the two pathologic and syndromic entities. Putting the spectrum of disease under one name is attractive because our diagnostic and therapeutic approaches to emphysema and bronchitis are identical. Lumping them together to make one broad disorder—COPD—makes sense.

Historically, a number of other terms have been proposed for the spectrum of adult obstructive airways disease. Chronic airflow obstruction (CAO), chronic airflow limitation, chronic obstructive airways disease (COAD), and chronic obstructive lung disease (COLD) have been used by some authors, but COPD has won the battle of acronyms. Importantly, the ATS definition of COPD differs from the other category definitions by specifically excluding patients with an unambiguous diagnosis of a specific disorder such as asthma. There is clearly overlap between asthma and COPD in some individuals, for example, a heavy smoker with allergies who has a pronounced bronchodilator response. However, a patient with asthma, as defined by substantial airflow reversibility, has a more benign clinical course and prognosis than one with COPD with a similar degree of airways obstruction measured prebronchodilator.[2,3] Here it is useful to be specific—differentiating asthma from COPD.

Figure 28-1 illustrates the overall interrelationships among the various adult airways disorders. To make a diagnosis of COPD, one should exclude asthma and other diseases of known cause, such as bronchiectasis, bronchiolitis obliterans, or tracheal abnormalities. This differentiation of COPD from everything else is typically made on the basis of history, radiographic appearance, and the results of pulmonary function testing (see below). Occasionally, a tissue diagnosis of a specific airway disorder can be made. This is often the case when airway obstruction is associated with interstitial lung disease, and an open lung biopsy is necessary to make a diagnosis of the parenchymal process (see Chapter 31).

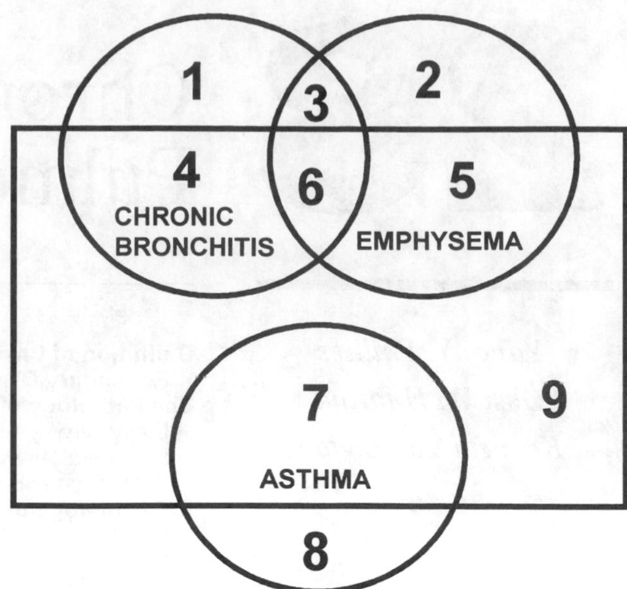

FIGURE 28-1. Nonproportional Venn diagram depicting the interrelationships between adult obstructive lung diseases and COPD (Reproduced with permission from Snider GL. Chronic bronchitis and emphysema. In *Textbook of Respiratory Medicine*, Murray JF and Nadel JA. (Eds) Philadelphia, WB Saunders Company, 1994, and modified in accordance with the 1995 ATS Statement on COPD). The presence of airway obstruction, as indicated by the rectangle, is defined as an FEV_1, which is significantly less than predicted even when measured after the administration of a bronchodilator. Subset 1 is the patient with a history of excessive mucus production but with a normal FEV_1. Subset 2 is a patient with anatomic evidence of emphysema but with a normal FEV_1. Subset 3 has elements of both emphysema and chronic bronchitis but no airflow obstruction. Subset 4 has chronic phlegm production and post-bronchodilator airflow obstruction. Subset 5 has emphysema and obstruction. Subset 6 has features of both chronic bronchitis and emphysema. COPD is comprised of subsets 4, 5, and 6. Subset 7 is asthma with persistent obstruction. Subset 8 is asthma in which airflow can be normalized with a bronchodilator. Subset 9 is the large number of disorders with airflow obstruction which are not COPD or asthma, eg, bronchiectasis, bronchiolitis obliterans, sarcoidosis, or hypersensitivity pneumonitis. This schema shows no overlap between asthma and COPD. In reality it may be difficult to determine the etiology of airflow obstruction in a patient who both smokes and has allergies.

Distinguishing asthma from COPD can be difficult. It may be impossible to determine whether a smoking, atopic patient with persistent airflow obstruction has COPD, asthma, or some overlapping syndrome. The ATS definition even allows for a degree of airway hyperresponsiveness—the ***sine qua non*** of asthma—in patients with COPD. For simplicity's sake, overlapping syndromes of bronchitis, emphysema, and asthma are not depicted in Figure 28-1 but would include patients historically labeled as having asthmatic bronchitis. From a therapeutic standpoint it does not really matter because the prescription of smoking cessation, bronchodilators, and antiinflammatory medications will be identical. Basically, a patient with a long smoking history who has symptoms associated with airflow obstruction but who normalizes his or her forced expired volume in 1 second (FEV_1) with a bronchodilator is labeled as an asthmatic. A similar individual whose FEV_1 does not come back to the normal range is labeled as having COPD.

An important aspect of the ATS definition of COPD is the requirement that a decrease in airflow be present after the administration of a bronchodilator.[1] This is defined as FEV_1, which is below standard deviations two the expected value.[4] That means that patients with normal airflow who are believed to be at risk for obstructive airways disease because of their smoking (subsets 1, 2, and 3 of Fig. 28-1) are not considered to have COPD. That is, they are not obstructed. However, they may already have significant pathologic changes in their lungs[5] and are an important target for smoking cessation efforts.

Patients who are diagnosed with COPD will have a history of exposure to an inhalational irritant (almost always cigarette smoke in the United States) and abnormal spirometry. The clinical diagnosis of chronic bronchitis is made by history alone with the patient reporting expectoration of excessive mucus on most days out of 3 months of the year for at least 2 years in a row.[6] It is important to remember that a patient may have chronic bronchitis but not COPD (subset 1 of Fig. 28-1). One would only make a diagnosis of COPD if the patient with such excessive phlegm production also had significantly decreased airflow.

THE PATHOLOGY OF COPD

COPD is a syndromic, clinical entity but it is associated with distinct pathologic changes in the lungs. These changes are found in the major airways, the conducting bronchioles, and the lung parenchyma. These pathologic abnormalities may be present in a wide spectrum of severity. They are united in their common origin—tobacco smoke—and in their contribution to airflow obstruction and respiratory symptoms.

Major Airway Abnormalities

The most important abnormality in the major airways is mucous gland hyperplasia and hypersecretion (Fig. 28-2). Most anatomic studies in patients with the clinical diagnosis of chronic bronchitis have shown an increase in the aggregate size of the submucosal mucous glands. This is commonly expressed as the Reid index or gland-to-bronchial-wall–thickness ratio. Surprisingly, the degree of mucous gland hypertrophy does not correlate with the degree of airflow obstruction.[7] Some degree of smooth muscle hyperplasia or inflammation of bronchial wall may also be found in smokers, but their relationship to airflow obstruction is unclear.

Peripheral Airway Involvement

Inflammation and its sequelae in the small or peripheral airways have been increasingly recognized as common and important lesions in the lungs of smokers.[8,9] In the small airways of smokers there is often evidence of an active inflammatory process with infiltration of neutrophils and macrophages. This is presumably the result of chronic irritation from tobacco smoke. As a consequence of these activated cellular components and the cytotoxic mediators that they release, the small airways ultimately develop mucous gland metaplasia and hypertrophy, muscular hypertrophy, fibrosis and distortion or tortuosity of the airway channel, and loss of alveolar attachments to the airway external wall (Fig. 28-2). All of these factors contribute to airflow obstruction in the peripheral airways to some degree. However, bronchiolitis in its most severe form is generally associated with an increasing severity of emphysematous

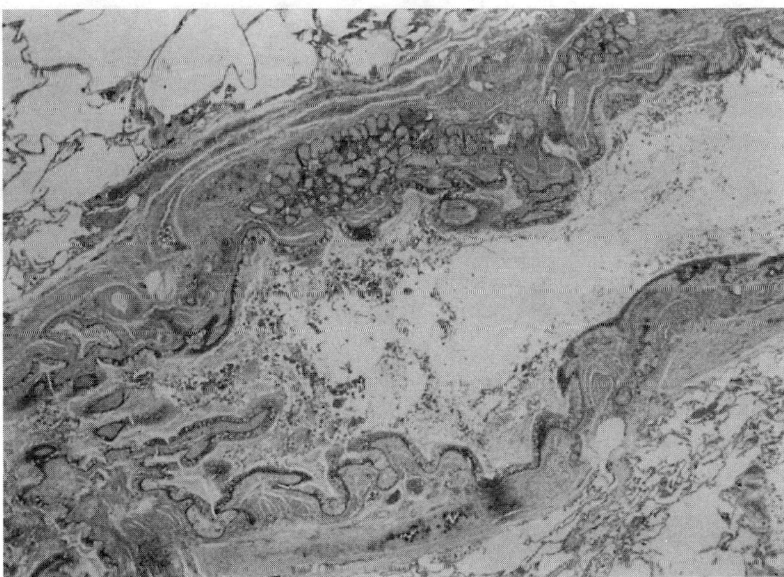

FIGURE 28-2. Low-power (100×) photomicrograph of a small bronchus with cartilage showing changes consistent with chronic bronchitis. There is a thickened muscular layer and goblet cell hyperplasia. There is mucus in the airway lumen. The surrounding alveolar walls show some loss of attachment to the airway and emphysematous change.

change, which is the cause of the greatest degree of airflow obstruction.[10]

Parenchymal Emphysema

Emphysema is defined as "an anatomic alteration of the lung characterized by abnormal, permanent enlargement of the airspaces distal to the terminal bronchiole, accompanied by destruction of their walls and without obvious fibrosis."[11] Emphysematous and normal lung are compared in Figure 28-3.

Emphysema is the most important pathologic lesion in patients with severe airflow obstruction.[9] However, even significant degrees of emphysema may not be clinically recognized during life and are only discovered at autopsy. Loss of alveolar walls results in a decrease in airflow through a loss in elastic recoil of the lung (the driving pressure for expiration) and a loss of supporting tissue "tethering" the airways open.[12]

The destructive process evident in emphysema is clearly associated with tobacco smoke. We know that smoking causes an influx of inflammatory cells such as neutrophils and macrophages into the alveoli and the delicate interstitium of the lung. These activated cells can release inflammatory mediators including proteases, which have the capacity to digest the substrate of the alveolar walls. Cigarette smoke has also been shown to inhibit the naturally occurring antiproteases in the lung.

Antiprotease *(alpha-1 antitrypsin) inhibitor deficiency* is a natural model for severe emphysema in smokers.[13] This is an autosomally recessive genetic disorder in which an individual inherits a gene coding for the enzyme from each parent. The homozygous deficiency state is characterized by the onset of severe emphysema at an early age with a predilection for bullous changes at the bases. It is estimated that antiprotease deficiency accounts for about 1% of emphysema patients in the United States. It should be suspected and screened for in patients with the onset of severe COPD before the age of 50 years.

Pathologists often subdivide airspace enlargement and emphysema into several categories. Table 28-1 illustrates a general schema adapted from that of Thurlbeck.[9] The emphysema found in smokers is most often centrilobular and is predominantly located in the upper lung zones. Patients with antiprotease deficiency have panacinar emphysema, which may be worse in the lung bases. However, from a practical, clinical viewpoint there is little to be gained by making such differentiations. The degree of airflow obstruction is more a function of the extent and severity of emphysema than its precise anatomic form.

EPIDEMIOLOGY OF COPD

It is difficult to quantitate the extent of disability and lost productivity in the workplace, that occur secondary to COPD. Data regarding COPD deaths are more readily available but suffer from potential errors occurring when physicians fill out death certificates. Statistical information collected by the National Heart Lung and Blood Institute reveals that COPD (including asthma) was the 4th leading cause of death in the United States in 1992, with approximately 87,000 deaths.[14] Between 1972 and 1992, the COPD death rate increased by 48%, whereas death rates from all other causes decreased by 12%. This alarming increase in overall mortality affected both men and women, with the greatest percent of increase in COPD deaths among women. The importance of COPD mortality as a significant international problem is readily apparent, when one considers that US mortality from COPD ranked 15th among men and 7th among women from 32 industrialized countries.[14]

The increasing COPD incidence and mortality have paralleled the increasing incidence of tobacco smoking. In the United States, smoking-related health care ex-

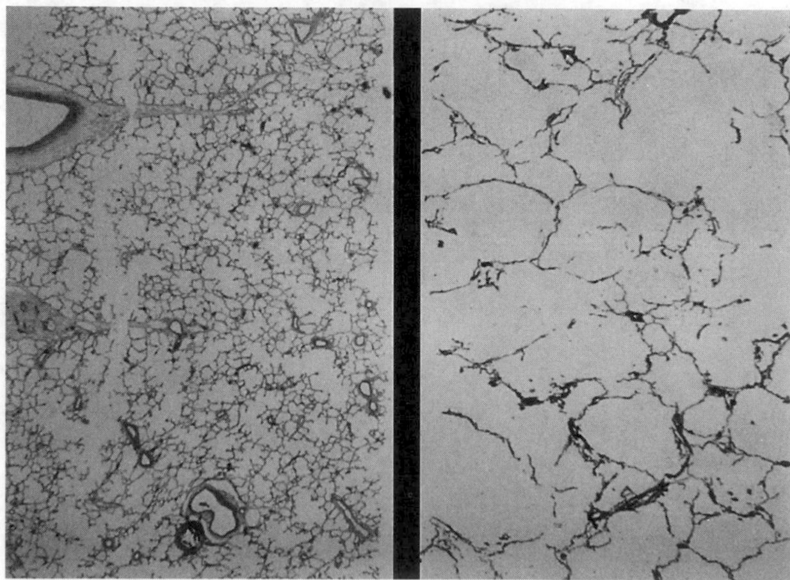

FIGURE 28-3. Low-power (100×) photomicrographs of normal and emphysematous lung. The similar size of blood vessels confirms that the magnification is similar. The normal lung shows small, fairly regular alveolar spaces. The emphysematous lung shows distention of the airspaces and a loss of septal walls. Overall there is a loss of alveolar area in the emphysematous specimen.

TABLE 28-1. **A Schema for Classifying Enlargement of the Alveoli and Airspaces of the Lung**

Simple airspace enlargement
- Congenital
- Compensatory for volume loss
- Senescent

Emphysema
- Proximal acinar emphysema
  - Centrilobular
  - Simple pneumoconiosis
- Panacinar emphysema
- Distal emphysema
- Bullae

Airspace enlargement with fibrosis
- Irregular or paracicatricial
- Honeycomb lung

Modified from Thurlbeck WM: Pathophysiology of chronic obstructive pulmonary disease. Clin Chest Med 11:389–403, 1990; reproduced with permission.

penditures were approximately $50 billion in 1993.[15] Based on the total number of cigarettes smoked, the health costs of smoking were calculated at $2.06 per pack, of which $0.89 was paid from public sources. Smoking-attributable mortality accounted for 20% of all U.S. deaths.[16]

Risk Factors for COPD

COPD risk factors can be divided into those extrinsic and intrinsic to the host and are described in Box 28-1. They can be further subdivided as known causes or possible/probable causes. Tobacco smoking clearly represents the predominant COPD risk factor in the industrialized world.[17] It is not known why certain smokers are unusually susceptible to the adverse effects of tobacco smoke while others are relatively resistant. Other probable, extrinsic risk factors include occupational exposure to dusts, fumes, or gases (eg, in industries such as underground mining, grain storage, and textiles), passive exposure to cigarette smoke, and childhood respiratory diseases.[18] Severe air pollution, such as existed in London in the 1950s, was epidemiologically correlated with COPD. It is more difficult to prove adverse effects from low levels of air pollution.

Antiprotease inhibitor deficiency is the intrinsic risk factor known to cause COPD.[13] The lungs of individuals suffering from this uncommon, hereditary condition are attacked by enzymes released from leukocytes. The patients are susceptible to lung injury because they lack the proteins that should prevent white blood cell enzymes from damaging the lung. Antiprotease inhibitor deficiency affects only about 1% of COPD patients, as opposed to cigarette smoking, which is the major cause of COPD in approximately 95% of patients. Additional hereditary causes of COPD may eventually be identified to explain familial clustering of cases and increased susceptibility of certain individuals to the deleterious effects of cigarette smoke or other pollutants.

BOX 28–1

RISK FACTORS FOR THE DEVELOPMENT OF COPD

Known	Possible/Probable
Inciting Agent	
Cigarette smoke	Air pollution Occupational dusts, fumes, gases Passive smoking Childhood respiratory disease Socioeconomic factors Alcohol
Host Factors	
Antiprotease deficiency	Age Gender Familial Airway hyperresponsiveness

Prognosis in COPD

Table 28-2 lists the factors that influence the survival of COPD patients.[19] Most important are the FEV_1 at the time of the patient's diagnosis, age, and whether the patient continues smoking. Figure 28-4 illustrates the dominant effect of airflow limitation on mortality in COPD.[2] The natural history of COPD is described visually by the Fletcher Diagram (Fig. 28-5).[17] The figure illustrates that smokers can be divided into two groups, one susceptible to the adverse effects of smoking and the other resistant. Susceptible smokers have an accel-

TABLE 28-2. **Factors Related to Morbidity and Early Mortality in Chronic Obstructive Pulmonary Disease**

- Continued smoking
- Decreased FEV_1
- Increased age
- Poor bronchodilator response
- Decreased exercise capacity
- Decreased diffusing capacity
- Decreased vital capacity
- Loss of FEV_1 on serial testing
- Resting tachycardia
- Increased $PaCO_2$
- Increased pulmonary artery pressure
- Cor pulmonale
- Increased total lung capacity
- Perceived physical disability/dyspnea
- Malnutrition/weight loss
- Antiprotease deficiency

Adapted from Hodgkin JE: Prognosis in chronic obstructive pulmonary disease. Clin Chest Med 11:555–569, 1990; reproduced with permission.

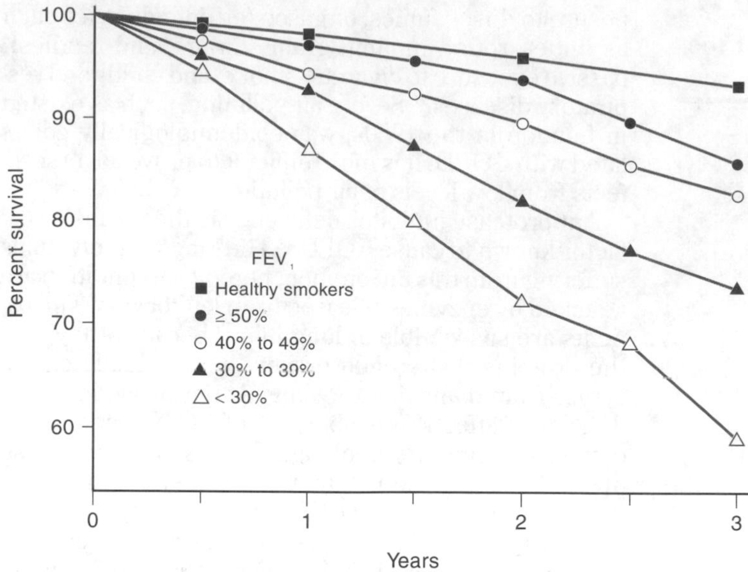

FIGURE 28-4. Survival curves for smokers with varying degrees of obstruction based upon postbronchodilator FEV_1. (Reproduced with permission from Anthonisen NR, Wright EC, Hodgkin JE, et al: Prognosis in chronic obstructive pulmonary disease. Am Rev Resp Dis 1986; 133:14–20.)

erated decline in lung function, which is two and a half to three times that occurring as the result of the normal aging process. Several large population studies have shown that the typical patient develops significant COPD symptoms around age 60 years when the FEV_1 drops to approximately 1 L. In patients who are able to stop smoking before lung function has deteriorated to that level, the accelerated loss of function can be averted and the onset of symptomatic COPD can be postponed or prevented. This concept emphasizes the enormous importance of smoking cessation among susceptible individuals.

The other prognostic factors listed in Table 28-2 are easily understood when considered as surrogates of the FEV_1. For example, patients with a significant reversible (asthmatic) component or history of atopy (allergy) are more likely to be treatable than patients with primarily emphysematous changes (eg, antiprotease deficiency). Patients with better preserved pulmonary function (ie, greater vital capacity, better diffusing capacity, and better exercise capacity) have improved survival. Finally, the absence of extrapulmonary signs of COPD such as weight loss or tachycardia also portends an improved prognosis.

SEVERITY STAGING OF COPD

There is presently no widely accepted schema for staging the patient with COPD. A clinical staging system would allow categorization of the heterogeneous population of patients with COPD for epidemiologic studies, health resource planning, and prognostic implications. Such a stratification would greatly facilitate the application of clinical practice guidelines and improve communication between professionals. At present we are limited to describing COPD patients as pink puffers or blue bloaters and to grading their disease based on some objective physiologic measure of pulmonary function, usually the spirometric measure of FEV_1.

Although FEV_1 and age are the most powerful predictors of prognosis,[2,19] the impact of COPD on a patient and his or her ability to perform the normal activities of a vocation or of daily living are incompletely described by the spirometric variables.[20,21] The severity of dyspnea

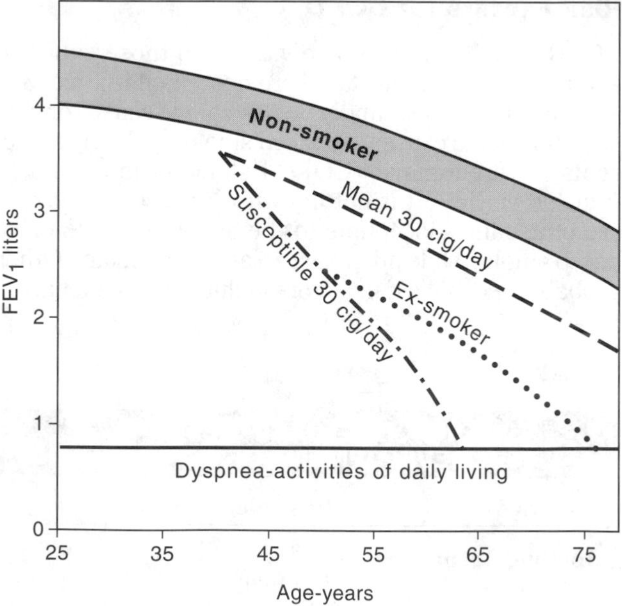

FIGURE 28-5. Visual model showing the loss of lung function over time for normals and smokers (a modified Fletcher Diagram). Nonsmokers lose about 30 mL/year. Smokers average a slightly greater loss over time. However, a subset of susceptible individuals (about 10%–15%) will show substantially greater losses with smoking such that the FEV_1 falls to a level which interferes even with the activities of daily living sometime in the 6th or 7th decade of life. If a susceptible smoker stops smoking, he or she will not regain much function but will revert to a more gradual loss of FEV_1. The later was proven in the NIH sponsored Lung Health Study. (Reproduced with permission from Snider GL: Chronic bronchitis and emphysema. In *Textbook of Respiratory Medicine,* Murray JF and Nadel JA (eds.). Philadelphia: WB Saunders, 1994.)

that a patient perceives plays a major role in how COPD affects his or her life.

The presence of hypoxemia and hypercapnia also affects mortality and the complexity of care that a patient requires.

COPD is a chronic disorder that may affect the life of a patient for decades, limiting his or her ability to work and even impairing the normal activities of daily living. An ideal staging system would provide a composite picture of disease severity based on the inter-relationships between the sensation of breathlessness (dyspnea), the impairment in airflow (FEV_1), and the derangement in gas exchange (arterial blood gases). Within each factor, there can be a progressive increase in severity. The impact of these factors and their magnitude on disease severity and disability is clearly interactive but not necessarily additive. Unfortunately, there is no comprehensive database that reveals how these factors can be integrated into a single, clinical whole.

The ATS has taken an interim step by breaking COPD into three stages of severity.[1] The stages were first defined on the basis of the overall impact of the disease and the complexity of care required.

Stage 1 (mild to moderate) COPD comprises the majority of patients. In these patients, COPD has only minimal impact on health-related quality of life and results in only a modest per capita health care expenditure. Stage 1 patients will usually be cared for on a continuing basis by a generalist. The presence of severe dyspnea, hypoxemia, or hypercarbia in a patient with stage 1 COPD warrants evaluation by a respiratory specialist.

Stage 2 (severe) COPD includes a minority of patients with COPD. In these patients, COPD has a significant impact on health-related quality of life and results in a large per capita health care expenditure. Stage 2 patients will usually require an evaluation by a respiratory specialist and may receive continuing care by such a specialist.

Stage 3 (very severe) COPD includes a small minority of patients. In these patients, COPD has a profound impact on health-related quality of life and results in a large per capita health care expenditure. Stage 3 patients will usually be under the care of a respiratory specialist.

In this interim system, patients are assigned to a stage based on the severity of airflow limitation based on the severity grading system espoused by the ATS[4]:

Stage 1 COPD—mild or moderate COPD
$FEV_1 \geq 50\%$ predicted (after bronchodilator)

Stage 2 COPD—severe COPD
$FEV_1 <50\%$ and $\geq 34\%$ predicted (after bronchodilator)

Stage 3 COPD—very severe COPD
$FEV_1 <34\%$ predicted (after bronchodilator)

Ideally, the staging system should provide practitioners a means for categorizing disease which takes into account the interactions between physiology and symptoms. There is a generally expected increase in symptoms and blood gas abnormalities as the FEV_1 falls. This is depicted in Box 28-2. In general, patients with relatively well preserved airflow (stage 1) should not have disabling dyspnea, hypoxemia, or hypercapnia. The presence of any one of these factors in a stage 1 COPD patient should prompt an evaluation for complicating conditions such as congestive heart failure, interstitial lung disease, and pulmonary vascular disease. This will usually warrant referral to a pulmonary specialist.

Future refinements of this staging system may incorporate information on dyspnea, hypoxemia, and hypercarbia directly. Until that is the case, the provider should annotate the FEV_1-based stage with comments on the severity of dyspnea and the results of blood gas analysis. For example, a classic pink puffer might be described as a stage 3 COPD patient with very severe dyspnea without hypoxia or hypercapnia and a classic blue bloater as having stage 1 COPD with hypoxemia and hypercapnia.

DIAGNOSIS AND EVALUATION OF COPD

The Medical History

As is true of most diseases, the key to diagnosing COPD is the history, which can be strongly suggestive. Table 28-3 lists important historic features, many of which correspond to the COPD risk factors discussed earlier in this chapter. It is critical for the health care practitioner

BOX 28–2

USUAL CLINICAL CHARACTERISTICS OF PATIENTS WITH COPD

COPD Stage	I	II	III
FEV_1 predicted (postbronchodilator)	≥50%	<50% and ≥34%	<34%
Dyspnea	Mild	Moderate	Severe
Hypoxemia	Very rare	Infrequent	Common
Hypercarbia	Very rare	Very rare	May be present

From American Thoracic Society: Statement on the evaluation and management of patients with chronic obstructive pulmonary disease. 1995; reproduced with permission.

TABLE 28-3. **Key Points in the History for Patients With COPD**

General
- History of cardiopulmonary diseases
- Smoking history—duration, intensity, current?
- Family history—COPD, heart disease, asthma
- Occupation—industrial dusts and fumes
- Overall health
- History of respiratory infections—frequency and severity
- Pulmonary medications

Pulmonary Symptoms
- Cough—frequency, phlegm production
- Sputum production—quantity, quality, duration, hemoptysis
- Wheezing
- Dyspnea—quantitate severity

to elicit a detailed history. For example, smoking history should include an estimate of the number of pack-years (number of packages of cigarettes smoked per day multiplied by the number of years of smoking), the number of cigars smoked per day, or the number of bowls of pipe tobacco smoked together with information about inhalation. A family history of lung diseases may suggest asthma, cystic fibrosis, or antiprotease deficiency. The occupational history may contain vital information, which can only be discovered by inquiring about every job the patient has ever performed.

Specific pulmonary symptoms (cough, sputum production, wheeze, and dyspnea) must also be individually evaluated and quantitated as accurately as possible. No symptom is specific for COPD. For example, chronic undiagnosed cough is much more likely to be caused by postnasal drip syndrome, asthma, or gastroesophageal reflux disease. When patients confirm that they are producing sputum, the volume should be estimated and the color and characteristics described. The presence of hemoptysis should be sought. Wheezing may accompany or be exacerbated by coughing, cold air exposure, exercise, allergen exposure, or lower respiratory tract infections. Wheezing may also occur in patients with upper airway obstruction or cardiac disease and thus cannot be considered a specific symptom of pulmonary disease.

Dyspnea, the patient's subjective sensation of breathlessness, should be quantitated. One may use the Borg Category Scale[22] or the Magnitude of Task component of the Baseline Dyspnea Index[21] shown in Table 28-4. Like wheezing, dyspnea can occur in patients with normal lungs who are suffering from nonpulmonary conditions such as heart disease, anemia, or neuromuscular weakness. Accurate assessment of the patient's symptoms will provide a rapid, noninvasive method for sequential patient evaluations.

Physical Examination

General evaluation and assessment skills for the respiratory care practitioner are described in Chapter 6; skills specific to COPD are listed in Box 28-3. The physical examination may be essentially normal in patients with mild COPD but reveals a variety of extrathoracic and thoracic abnormalities in those with advanced disease (Box 28-4). Accurate recording of the vital signs may reveal several potential abnormalities. A paradoxic

TABLE 28-4. **Quantification of Dyspnea Based On the Magnitude of Task Component of the Baseline Dyspnea Index**

Mild dyspnea—Becomes short of breath only with major activities such as walking up a steep hill, climbing more than three flights of stairs, or carrying a moderate load on the level

Moderate dyspnea—Becomes short of breath with moderate or average tasks such as walking up a gradual hill, climbing less than three flights of stairs, or carrying a light load on the level

Severe dyspnea—Becomes short of breath with light activities such as walking on the level, washing, or standing

Very severe dyspnea—becomes short of breath at rest, while sitting, or lying down

Adapted from Mahler DA, Weinburg DH, Wells CK, Feinstein AR: The measurement of dyspnea: contents, inter-observer agreement, and physiologic correlates of two new clinical indexes. Chest 85:751–758, 1984; reproduced with permission.

BOX 28-3

ASSESSMENT, THERAPY, AND EDUCATION OF THE PATIENT WITH COPD

RCPs have three major areas of responsibility in their interactions with COPD patients. These roles can be performed in acute, subacute, or chronic care facilities as well as in patients' homes.

1. Patient assessment
   - Perform and evaluate peak flow testing or pulmonary function tests.
   - Draw and interpret results of ABGs.
   - Perform patient assessment (eg, on hospitalized patients, who develop respiratory problems when the physician is not available in house).
   - Assess chest x-rays (eg, during the night, when the therapist may have more knowledge of radiographic abnormalities than the nurses).
2. Therapeutic maneuvers
   - Administer oxygen (appropriate flow and delivery system).
   - Administer medication via nebulizer or MDIs (including beta agonists, anticholinergics, steroids, antibiotics such as pentamidine).
   - Set up, monitor, and adjust ventilators.
   - Assist with mobilizing secretions (CPT, suctioning).
3. Education
   - Oxygen therapy
   - Aerosols and MDIs
   - Mucolytics/expectorants
   - Secretion mobilization (CPT, suctioning)
   - Breathing retraining
   - Perioperative care
   - CPAP, ventilator management (inpatient and outpatient)
   - Smoking cessation
   - Rehabilitation programs

BOX 28–4

IMPORTANT PHYSICAL FINDINGS IN PATIENTS WITH COPD

Extrathoracic
- Tachycardia
- Paradoxic pulse
- Accessory muscle use
- Jugular venous distention
- Peripheral edema
- Clubbing
- Cyanosis

Thoracic
- Tachypnea
- Barrel chest
- Low, flat diaphragms
- Hyperresonant percussion
- Reduced breath sounds
- Prolonged expiration
- Adventitious sounds

pulse, defined as >10-mm reduction in systolic blood pressure during inspiration, is thought to result from the accentuated fluctuation in intrathoracic pressure that occurs in COPD patients. Jugular venous distention and peripheral edema are manifestations of right sided congestive heart failure (cor pulmonale). Clubbing is rarely encountered in COPD patients unless bronchogenic carcinoma or chronic suppurative lung disease such as bronchiectasis or lung abcess is also present. Cyanosis, usually noted in chronic bronchitic patients, indicates advanced disease when it develops in emphysematous patients. It is not a sensitive sign of hypoxemia.

Thoracic findings in advanced COPD may include a barrel chest deformity, in which the anteroposterior dimension of the chest is increased. Inspiratory expansion of the thorax is minimal, and respiration is primarily accomplished by the diaphragm and the accessory respiratory muscles. The percussion note may be hyperresonant in patients whose lungs are hyperinflated, and the diaphragms may be low and fixed. Auscultation reveals reduced or occasionally absent breath sounds; crackles, rhonchi, or wheezes may be present. COPD patients typically have prolonged expiration and expiratory wheezing during forced expiratory maneuvers.

Radiographic Evaluation

The chest roentgenograph of the COPD patient may be normal or may manifest the changes listed in Box 28-5. Abnormalities can be grouped into two patterns, one resulting from pulmonary hyperinflation and the other from right heart failure. Typical radiographs are illustrated in Chapter 7. The radiographic abnormalities are neither sensitive nor specific, in that patients with severe emphysema may have normal chest radiographs and patients with asthma may have marked hyperinflation. Furthermore, chronic bronchitis is a historical diagnosis and cannot be diagnosed radiographically. Routine chest radiographs are of minimal value in the stable COPD patients. Their real importance is their ability to diagnose complications (eg, pneumothorax, pneumonia) or associated conditions (eg, bronchogenic carcinoma).

BOX 28–5

COMMON CHEST RADIOGRAPHIC FINDINGS IN PATIENTS WITH COPD

Evidence of Hyperinflation
- Hyperlucent lung fields
- Bullae
- Vascular pruning
- Flattened diaphragms
- Increased anteroposterior diameter on lateral view
- Increased retrosternal airspace

Evidence of Cor Pulmonale
- Right ventricular enlargement
- Enlarged proximal pulmonary arteries
- Prominent interstitial markings

Computed tomography (CT) of the chest greatly enhances the health care practitioner's ability to visualize emphysematous changes, interstitial abnormalities, and airways disease, especially when the images are reconstructed using high-resolution algorithms. Thoracic magnetic resonance imaging (MRI) adds little to the information gained by chest CT and is extremely expensive. In the future, technologic advancements such as the development and widespread availability of spiral CT will facilitate image reconstruction in the sagittal and coronal planes and may further enhance the value of chest CT scanning.

Evaluation of Blood and Sputum

Laboratory testing is of limited value in stable patients with COPD. Potentially useful tests are listed in Box 28-6. In chronically hypoxemic patients, the complete blood count (CBC) may reveal polycythemia, an elevated hemoglobin. The white blood cell differential count may show eosinophilia in patients with an allergic component of their COPD. Serum electrolytes usually demonstrate increased total CO_2 (TCO_2) in COPD patients with chronic CO_2 retention, because of renal

BOX 28–6

USEFUL LABORATORY TESTS IN PATIENTS WITH COPD

Hematology
- Complete blood count
  - Polycythemia
  - Eosinophilia
  - Neutrophil count
- Serum electrolytes
  - Increased TCO_2
  - Sodium and potassium

Arterial Blood Gases

Sputum
- Wet prep for eosinophils
- Gram stain
- Culture
- Cytology

compensation for the patient's chronic respiratory acidosis. Reduced sodium and potassium values sometimes occur and are usually noted in patients being treated with diuretic therapy for symptoms of right heart failure.

Arterial blood gas analysis and interpretation were discussed in detail in Chapter 9. Typical changes in COPD patients include the frequent finding of hypoxemia, usually in patients with more severely reduced FEV_1. Carbon dioxide retention may develop late in the course of the disease and indicates a poorer prognosis.

Expectorated sputum can be examined with several techniques. The sputum wet prep is a simple, rapid, inexpensive, and underused test that can effectively distinguish infectious or inflammatory bronchitis from asthma (eosinophilic bronchitis). This assessment helps guide therapy, as patients with sputum eosinophilia usually respond to steroid therapy. Sputum gram stains are useful for identifying the type of pathogenic bacteria causing an infectious exacerbation of COPD. Only good quality gram stains will provide reliable information.

Sputum culture is overused and often provides misleading results. Sputum cultures will occasionally reveal a pathogen that will affect therapy and suggest a clinical diagnosis (eg, the isolation of *Pseudomonas aeruginosa* suggests bronchiectasis or cystic fibrosis). Sputum can be cultured for nonbacterial pathogens such as viruses, mycobacteria, and fungi. Respiratory care practitioners should be constantly aware of the possibility of tuberculosis, a disease many clinicians fail to consider. Expectorated sputum can also be evaluated for malignant cells, an assessment requiring the analysis by a skilled cytopathologist. Even if malignant cells are identified, the cancer may be located anywhere between the lips and the lower respiratory tract.

Pulmonary Function Testing

An obstructive ventilatory defect is defined by the ATS as "a disproportionate reduction of maximal airflow from the lung with respect to the maximal volume (VC) that can be displaced from the lung."[4] Chapter 8 covers the performance standards for pulmonary function testing.

By definition, COPD patients have a reduction in FEV_1.[1] They also typically have a reduction in the FEV_1/FVC ratio. In more severe stages of COPD, the FEV_1/FVC ratio becomes a less useful index of severity, because the decreases in FVC may result in plateauing or increasing values for FEV_1/FVC. Quantification of the severity of airflow obstruction should be based on FEV_1 rather than FEV_1/FVC.

In contrast to asthma, the obstruction to expiratory airflow obstruction in COPD does not reverse completely with bronchodilator therapy. In most cases, the FEV_1 does not improve significantly at all. It is important to remember that the week-to-week (>20% change) and year-to-year (>15% change) variabilities in FEV_1 and FVC are greater than in normal individuals, and this level of change must be exceeded before considering a change as significant. The importance of the magnitude of the common partial response to bronchodilator on morbidity and mortality in COPD is not known.

Increases in total lung capacity (hyperinflation) along with increases in residual volume and functional residual capacity (air trapping) are commonly seen in patients with COPD, but are not useful in distinguishing between COPD and asthma clinically. Correlation between these variables and underlying pathology has also shown mixed results. However, the diffusing capacity for carbon monoxide (DL_{CO}) has been shown to correlate significantly with pathologic assessments of underlying emphysema and can be used to differentiate between emphysema and asthma. The DL_{CO} is usually normal or increased in patients with asthma and decreased in patients with emphysema.

The PaO_2 and the $PaCO_2$, although important in the management of a patient's acute exacerbations and prescribing long-term oxygen therapy, are not useful in separating COPD patients with emphysema from those with predominantly chronic bronchitis or from patients with asthma. The arterial blood gases of the classic pink puffer (normal PaO_2 and $PaCO_2$) and the blue bloater (reduced PaO_2 and increased $PaCO_2$ with cor pulmonale) have *not* proven to reliably predict presence of emphysema or chronic bronchitis, respectively. Other tests of lung function such as frequency dependence of lung compliance, closing volume, and helium–oxygen flow curves are not very useful in separating patients into diagnostic categories and are seldom used outside of the research setting.[23]

MANAGEMENT OF THE PATIENT WITH COPD

General Considerations

The majority of patients with COPD are of an age when other significant health problems arise. They are older and predominantly male and are therefore at risk for the common diseases of aging men. Their chronic cigarette abuse puts them at particular risk of cardiovascular problems and malignancies of the aerodigestive tract. They, like most patients, are best served by a health care delivery system that is oriented to preventive measures and to providing health maintenance services. The respiratory therapist can play an important role as a patient advocate in assuring that the patient with COPD receives appropriate routine preventive care.

Respiratory symptoms and complaints often dominate the health care concerns of patients with COPD. However, it is important that the individual and his or her physician not overlook the other elements of good, general preventive care. This includes periodic physical examinations, blood pressure checks, mammograms, and other studies as appropriate to age and gender.[24] Table 28-5 summarizes some of the recommendations of the U.S. Preventive Services Task Force.

Prevention of upper respiratory tract infections is important in patients with COPD. Infections are common causes of exacerbation, which often leads to significant

TABLE 28-5. **U.S. Preventive Services Task Force Selected Recommendations for Physical Examinations and Selected Screening Tests for Routine Health Maintenance in Adults**

Test	Age (years) or Other Criteria
Oral cavity examination	>18 if using tobacco or alcohol
Breast examination	>40
Blood pressure	Every visit or every 1–2 years
Eyesight	>65 with visual symptoms
Hearing	>65, earlier if exposed to loud noises
Urinalysis	>60 or diabetic
Fasting glucose	Family history diabetes, extreme obesity
Electrocardiogram	>40 and risk factors for heart disease
Intraocular pressure	>65
Tuberculosis skin testing	If exposed; if taking high-dose steroids
Mammography	>50 annually; >35 if family history of breast cancer
Cervical cytology	Age 20–65, every 1–3 years
Stool for blood	>40 if history of inflammatory bowel disease or colon cancer

From Sox HC: Preventive health services in adults. N Engl J Med 330:1589–1595, 1994; reproduced with permission.

morbidity. Patients may help themselves in preventing common viral infections by avoiding contact with people who are obviously ill and by regularly washing hands after shaking hands with or touching individuals with colds.

All patients with COPD should receive influenza vaccine annually.[25] This not only prevents infection but has been shown to decrease total health care costs by reducing hospitalization.[26]

Pneumococcal vaccine should be administered to all patients with COPD.[25] Immunization has been shown to decrease the incidence of infection with covered serotypes in patients with chronic illnesses including COPD. Because of reports of severe local reactions, the original guidance on pneumococcal vaccination was that it was to be given only once in a lifetime. More recent evidence suggests that immunity wanes but can be safely boosted with revaccination at 6 years.[27] This is even more important as drug-resistant pneumococci emerge.

The Health Benefits of Smoking Cessation

Cigarette smoking is the most important cause of COPD and its continuation has major adverse consequences for health and longevity. Most patients acknowledge that smoking is bad for them but typically underestimate the risks of continued smoking. They often believe that "the damage is done" and are unaware of the benefits to be derived from quitting. Smoking cessation is the cornerstone of preventive care for an active smoker. The respiratory care practitioner can play a key role in the multidisciplinary team approach to smoking cessation.

In a prospective survey of 1.2 million American adults conducted during the period between 1982 and 1986, the mortality rate for current smokers was more than twice that of nonsmokers for both men and women.[28] This excess mortality was reduced by smoking cessation, although it took more than a decade to approach that of individuals who had never smoked (Table 28-6). Figure 28-6 summarizes similar outcomes from a registry of Dutch patients.[29] Clearly, smokers who continue to smoke have higher mortality from all causes compared with smokers who quit.

Mortality from lung cancer is decreased by smoking cessation. About 90% of lung cancers are attributable to cigarette smoking. The incidence of lung cancer in current smokers is more than 15 times that of people who have never smoked. With smoking cessation, the rate changes little for the first 4 years, falls to approximately 5 times from 5 to 14 years after quitting, and levels out to twice the baseline risk after 15 years.[30] Part of this phenomenon is attributable to a survivor effect wherein those destined to get lung cancer do so within a decade of quitting smoking, and we are left with a cohort of relatively healthy survivors.

Smoking is strongly implicated in coronary artery disease, peripheral arteriosclerotic vascular disease, and stroke. All other factors being equal, smokers have an estimated risk of myocardial infarction three times that of nonsmokers. With smoking cessation, the rate of infarction falls nearly to baseline within 2 years.[31] Unfortunately, many smokers wait until they have a catastrophic event, like a heart attack, before they actually quit smoking. Even then, quitting has benefits. Patients who stopped smoking after their first myocardial infarction had a 40% reduction in 5-year mortality compared with smokers who did not quit.[32] The former smokers had similar cardiac morbidity to people who never smoked.

Mortality is not the only outcome that is improved by smoking cessation. Worker absenteeism is a global

TABLE 28-6. **Mortality Ratios for Smokers and Former Smokers Who Were Well at Time of Smoking Cessation**

	Current Smokers	Years of Abstinence				
		1–2	*3–5*	*6–10*	*11–15*	*≥16*
Males						
1–20 cig/d	2.34	2.05	1.89	1.48	1.29	1.01
≥20 cig/d	2.73	2.15	1.90	1.77	1.65	1.19
Females						
1–20 cig/d	1.82	1.26	1.42	1.01	1.09	1.00
≥20 cig/d	2.46	2.15	1.44	1.46	1.18	0.95

cig = cigarette.
Comparison is to age-matched individuals who had never smoked. From U.S. Department of Health and Human Services: The Health Benefits of Smoking Cessation: A report of the Surgeon General, US GPO 1990; reproduced with permission.

index of health status and perception. Workers who quit smoking have a 10% to 20% reduction in work-days lost to illness from all causes.[33]

Smoking cessation can alter the rate of loss of lung function in a COPD patient. The NIH Lung Health Study was a multicenter survey of almost 6000 middle-aged smokers who were observed for up to 5 years.[34] It showed convincingly that individuals who quit smoking lose function at a different rate (an average of 34 mL/y) than those who continued to smoke (63 mL/y). Figure 28-7 illustrates this disparity over the 5 years of the study.

COPD patients who continue to smoke should be advised that there are considerable health benefits to smoking cessation no matter how long they have smoked. It is never too late to quit. The only exception to an unwavering policy advocating smoking cessation may be in a patient with incurable lung cancer who has a short expected life span where the denial of a pleasurable habit is more punitive than therapeutic.

Multiple factors such as nicotine addiction and social reinforcers act together to maintain a smoking habit. Few patients respond to advice alone, and a successful smoking cessation program often involves multiple ap-

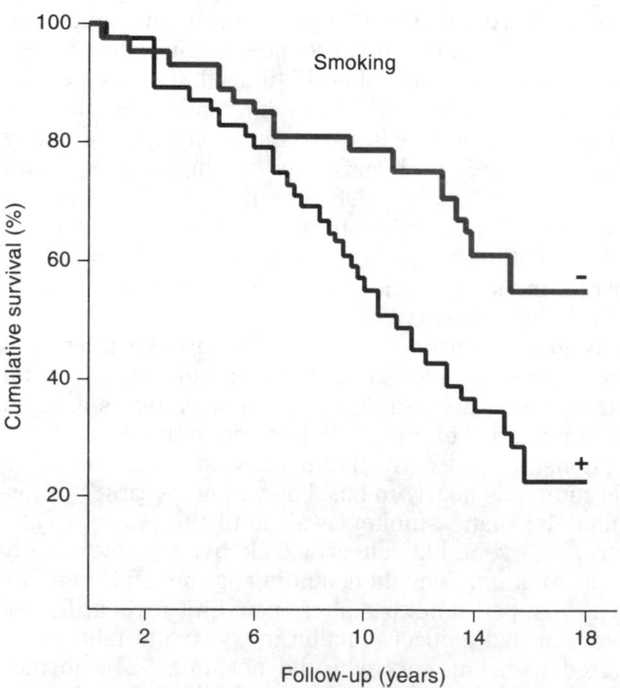

FIGURE 28-6. Survival curves for Dutch adults who quit smoking (−) or continue smoking (+). (From Postma DS, Sluiter HJ: Prognosis in chronic obstructive pulmonary disease: the Dutch experience. Am Rev Resp Dis 1989; 140:S100-S104 with permission.)

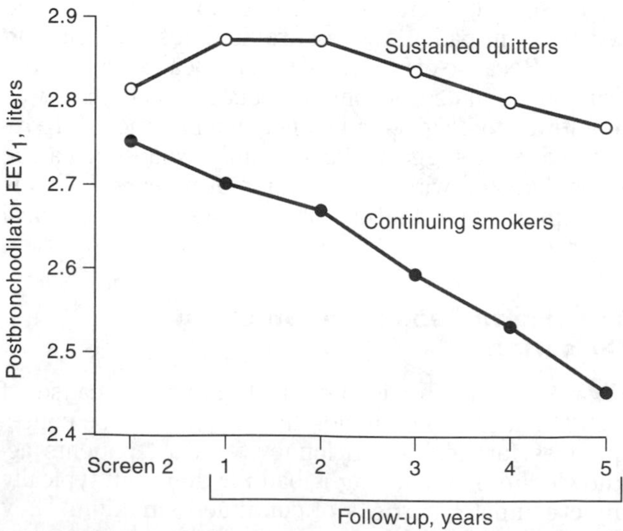

FIGURE 28-7. Changes in postbronchodilator FEV_1 for sustained quitters and continuing smokers from the NIH Lung Health Study. Quitters had both an initial improvement in airflow and a slower rate of decline in FEV_1 (34 mL/yr versus 64 mL/yr for continuing smokers). (Reproduced with permission from Anthonisen NR, Connett JE, Kiley JP, Altose MD, et al: Effects of smoking intervention and the use of an inhaled anticholinergic bronchodilator on the rate of decline of FEV_1: the Lung Health Study. JAMA 1994; 272: 1497–1505.)

proaches and many disciplines. The therapist can play an important role in smoking cessation efforts at all stages, from patient identification through education and into maintenance. Chapter 23 reviews approaches to smoking cessation.

An intensive, multidisciplinary approach can work. The Lung Health Study reported a 35% 1-year quit rate, with 22% sustained for 5 years.[34] Abstinence was validated by carbon monoxide analysis. This was obtained with an intensive 12-class education and behavior modification program, nicotine replacement, and an active follow-up during maintenance. There was only a 5% sustained quit rate in the usual care group.

Pharmacologic Therapy of COPD

All symptomatic COPD patients are candidates for therapeutic interventions. The individuals most likely to benefit are those with cough or wheeze, evidence of reversibility on postbronchodilator pulmonary function testing, or eosinophilia of the sputum or the peripheral blood. Before *pharmacotherapy* is considered, environmental factors contributing to COPD should be minimized, even if this necessitates early retirement or job dislocation, changing the home's internal environment by installing new heating or air conditioning systems, or moving to a less polluted location. Exposure to cigarette smoke must be curtailed. This includes passive smoke exposure in the workplace and at home.

The medications most commonly used for COPD pharmacotherapy are summarized in Tables 28-7 and 28-8. They have been divided into respiratory and nonrespiratory agents. More detailed descriptions of the specific respiratory drugs is provided in Chapter 16. The three types of bronchodilator medications (anticholinergic, beta agonist, and methylxanthine) are the most widely used drugs for treating COPD patients.[35] They are often used concurrently and, either singly or in combination, may result in improvement of objective measures of lung function or more subjective measures of quality of life. Some investigators consider anticholinergics the bronchodilators of choice for COPD, although many patients seem to prefer the more rapid onset of bronchodilation seen with inhaled beta agonists. The beneficial effects of theophylline may result from improved diaphragmatic contractility in addition to its mild bronchodilation.

Anti-inflammatory medications include corticosteroids, cromolyn, and nedocromil. At some point in their disease, all COPD patients should be treated with representative anti-inflammatory drugs. Many physicians administer a 2-week trial of high-dose oral corticosteroids and look for an objective improvement measured by pre- and post-steroid spirometry.[35] Unless an objective response is documented (>15% improvement in FEV_1), the patient cannot be judged a steroid responder. Systemic steroid therapy should be stopped to avoid the multiple severe side effects associated with long-term use. Measurement of an objective improvement is especially important, because most patients experience improved appetite, energy, and an overall sense of well-being from systemic steroids. Individuals who do respond should be tapered to the lowest dose of daily or alternate day steroids and/or inhaled steroids that sustains the clinical improvement. The addition of cromolyn or nedocromil to a therapeutic regimen may provide benefit to some patients with partially reversible COPD. In general, these drugs are less likely to benefit COPD patients than asthmatics. Individuals with viscid, tenacious secretions may benefit from the addition of mucolytic or expectorant medications.

Oxygen as a respiratory gas is described in Chapter 13. The pioneering work on long-term oxygen therapy was performed on COPD patients and confirmed its multiple benefits, such as reduced hospitalizations, improved patient function and quality of life, improved cognitive function, and delayed development of cor pulmonale and polycythemia.[36] A series of consensus conferences has further refined medical and reimbursement issues regarding this expensive therapeutic modality. Recent technologic advances including reservoir devices, flow demand valves, and lightweight aluminum cylinders have improved the portability and duration of oxygen systems. Transtracheal oxygen provides an additional oxygen delivery system, which is particularly useful in patients requiring high-flow oxygen.

Of the nonrespiratory medications used to treat COPD patients, antibiotics are the most frequently pre-

TABLE 28-7. **Respiratory Medications Commonly Used to Treat Patients With COPD**

Class of Medication	Indication	Route(s)
Anticholinergics	Reduce bronchomotor tone	Inhaled
$Beta_2$ agonists	Bronchospasm	PO, SQ, inhaled (MDI or Neb)
Methylxanthines	Bronchodilation Diaphragm weakness	PO, IV
Corticosteroids	Anti-inflammatory	PO, IM, IV, inhaled
Cromolyn/nedocromil	Anti-inflammatory	Inhaled
Mucolytics	Tenacious secretions	Inhaled
Expectorants	Thick secretions	PO
Oxygen	Hypoxemia	Inhaled

TABLE 28-8. **Nonrespiratory Medications Commonly Used for Patients With COPD**

Class of Medication	Indication	Route(s)
Antibiotics	Infection	PO, IV, IM
Digitalis	Congestive heart failure	PO, IV
Diuretics	Congestive heart failure	PO, IV, IM
Psychopharmacologic	Depression	PO

scribed. Lower respiratory tract infections are the most frequent causes for COPD exacerbations. Although viruses initiate most such infections, bacterial superinfection often supervenes. Most broad-spectrum antibiotics are useful for shortening the duration of the bronchial infection and lessening the risk of pneumonia. The choice of antibiotic is empiric but should be influenced by the patient's history of allergy, medication cost, results of current sputum gram stain testing or prior sputum culture results, and type and severity of underlying disease. Antiviral therapy with amantadine or rimantadine may be considered for unvaccinated COPD patients during community outbreaks of influenza A.

Diuretics and digitalis are used to treat right-sided congestive heart failure. Because digitalis glycoside toxicity is more likely in COPD patients and is exacerbated by diuretic-induced hypokalemia, clinical and laboratory evidence of drug toxicity must be monitored carefully.

Depression occurs frequently in patients with chronic, debilitating diseases such as COPD. Recently developed antidepressant medications may be superior to older tricyclic antidepressants, because they lack anticholinergic side effects, possess minimal respiratory depressant activity, and are less dangerous if taken in overdose. The patient's quality of life may improve substantially in response to appropriate antidepressant treatment.

Surgical Treatment of COPD: Bullectomy and Transplantation

Surgical treatment of patients with COPD falls into two general categories: treatment of bullous emphysema and *lung transplantation*. Surgical resection of bullous emphysema *(bullectomy)* has been proposed as a useful modality in those individuals with predominantly upper lobe, nondiffuse disease. In symptomatic patients, removal of bullae theoretically should improve pulmonary function because the bullae can reduce lung compliance, increase dead space ventilation, reduce cardiac output by increasing intrathoracic pressure, decrease diaphragmatic excursion, and compress normal lung causing a reduction in pulmonary function. Although changes on chest radiograph and spirometry and large differences between measurement of (functional residual capacity) FRC by helium dilution and body plethysmography can be seen in these individuals, computed tomography remains the best way to evaluate the volume of hemithorax involved. Pulmonary angiography or whole lung tomography have been advocated to provide confirming evidence of compression of normal tissue.[37] Recent evidence suggests that surgery improves lung function in individuals with bullous involvement of more than one third of their hemithorax.[38] Successful bilateral *reduction pneumoplasty* has also been attempted in small numbers of these patients.[39] Other indications for surgery in patients with bullous emphysema include patients with a history of spontaneous pneumothorax, those with infected bullae that do not respond to antibiotics, and patients with massive hemoptysis.[40]

Criteria for single lung transplantation (SLT) have recently been extended to include end-stage nonsuppurative COPD. The first successful SLT for treatment of emphysema was performed in France in 1988, followed closely by the first SLT in the United States in 1989. Double lung transplant (DLT) is usually performed on patients with obstruction and suppuration, such as patients with cystic fibrosis or bronchiectasis, but can also used for nonsuppurative COPD. Heart–lung transplantation (HLT) is performed in individuals with pulmonary disease and unrelated cardiac disease. In the past it was thought that, compared with the transplanted lung, the compliant parenchyma of the native lung would receive the majority of the ventilation while the newly transplanted lung would receive the majority of blood flow. This would create large ventilation perfusion mismatching and compression of the transplanted lung by the overdistended native lung.[41] Although ventilation–perfusion mismatching and distention of the native lung do occur postoperatively, the changes are not prohibitive.

Recipient selection is currently based on a number of factors, which vary from center to center (Table 28-9). The use of systemic steroids is controversial because of the theoretic risk of increased wound complications. However, more centers are performing transplants for patients who cannot be weaned from steroids. Patients with a history of systemic disease or prior malignancy, as well as patients with renal or hepatic dysfunction (due to possible adverse effects of immunosuppressives) are generally not considered candidates for transplantation. Notably, psychosocial selection criteria are just as important as the medical criteria in the transplantation decision. Individuals must have normal psychiatric evaluations, good compliance, a strong support network, and

TABLE 28-9. **General Selection Criteria for Recipients of Single Lung Transplantation**

Expected survival less than 12–18 months
Age less than 60 years
Appropriate psychological status
Good nutritional status
No recent steroid use (controversial)
No concomitant systemic illness
Discontinued smoking
Strong family or social support

Each transplant center has its own specific guidelines, including some criteria not listed here.

be well motivated. Usually, smoking must be discontinued for at least 1 year before transplantation.

Evaluation of transplant candidates is extensive and includes a wide variety of tests depending on the institution. Patients may be on waiting lists for long periods of time. Participation in an outpatient respiratory rehabilitation program during this waiting period may potentially improve these patients' quality of life.

Donor criteria are less stringent, but great care is taken to rule out infection. Size matching of donors and recipients is done using chest radiography or predicted lung volumes. The choice of side in SLT is traditionally the left side because it is technically easier to perform the surgery. However, some transplant surgeons prefer transplanting the right side because the native left lung can then expand inferiorly (no liver to limit it) and not as much across the midline.[42]

Since 1989 more than 250 SLTs for end-stage obstructive lung disease have been performed worldwide. More than 50% of referrals to large transplant centers are related to obstructive pulmonary disease. To date, results have been very promising, with significant improvements in symptoms, oxygenation, vital capacity, FEV_1, and 6-minute walk distances. Actuarial survival at 3 years is 76% for SLT compared with 80% for DLT. Some studies have shown that patients who have undergone DLT have higher postoperative FEV_1s; however, they were not able to show a difference in exercise capacities.

Postoperative immunosuppression regimens are variable and can include cyclosporin, Minnesota antilymphocyte globulin (MAG), azathioprine, prednisone, and OKT3. However, transplant rejection still occurs. Fever, leukocytosis, hypoxemia, and parenchymal infiltrates herald the onset of this complication, although the most reliable indicator of rejection is transbronchial lung biopsy. Transplant rejection is usually treated with intravenous pulse steroids.

Pulmonary Rehabilitation

Pulmonary rehabilitation for the COPD patient constitutes a spectrum of interventions ranging from basic office-based instruction to comprehensive residential programs. Rehabilitation should not be viewed as a last-ditch effort to help a patient but as a continuum of services designed to improve quality of life. It starts with the physician encouraging exercise, smoking cessation, weight control, and other healthy living habits. It often involves the respiratory care practitioner as an educator in one-on-one instructions for breathing exercises, coping techniques, and medication use. The goal of rehabilitation is to minimize airflow limitation, to decrease respiratory symptoms, and to prevent or treat complications such as hypoxemia. Chapter 23 provides an in-depth coverage of pulmonary rehabilitation.

Considerations in Late-Stage COPD

Because of the stringent selection criteria used in identifying lung transplant recipients, as well as the large disparity between the number of lung transplant candidates and donors, the majority of patients with late stage COPD will not undergo transplantation. Of these patients, there will be a subgroup who might benefit from long-term mechanical ventilation. Intermittent positive-pressure ventilation via nasal mask has been shown to improve gas exchange and rest the respiratory muscles. Criteria for initiation of this type of therapy do not exist, although it has been suggested that individuals with hypercapnia, nocturnal symptoms, and frequent hospitalizations may benefit. Continuous home mechanical ventilation is infrequently used for late-stage patients because of associated complicated medical illnesses and clinical instability. There have been no large, controlled clinical trials to evaluate the benefits and risks of such management, although there have been anecdotal reports published revealing successes with long-term home mechanical ventilation.

Consideration of home mechanical ventilation (see Chapter 24) is usually given to COPD patients who are unable to wean from total ventilator support over a period of weeks. The patients' health status should be stable, their PaO_2 >60 mmHg on FIO_2 <40% without wide fluctuations in PaO_2 or $PaCO_2$; they should have an active gag and cough reflex, be free of active infection, have stable comorbid disease, not require frequent suctioning, and have an adequate support network and caregiver support at home. A tracheostomy tube should be in place.[43] Transfer of the patient to the home environment takes great planning and coordination on the part of every member of the health care team to assure that the transition to home care is smooth. A key role during this transfer should be played by the respiratory therapists involved in the patient's inpatient and outpatient care.

In late-stage COPD patients, one of the most important things that can be done is to assure that decisions regarding quality of life issues and the use of life-sustaining treatments have been made. Compassionate communication with patients and their families regarding wishes for withholding and withdrawing of life support are paramount. Information should be provided to allow individuals to make informed decisions regarding their preferences for dealing with cardiopulmonary arrest, while assuring that the individuals are competent to make these decisions. Published guidelines should be adhered to when dealing with issues of initiation, continuation, and withdrawal of intensive care.[44,45]

Table 28-10 lists the respiratory therapy modalities commonly used in the treatment of COPD. This table lists the currently accepted signs to clinically justify administration of such therapy (part 1), indications (part 2), sample treatment plans, including frequencies for such therapy (part 3), indications that more or less intense application of individual therapies is indicated (part 4), and suggested boundaries when additional physician input is present (part 5).

COMPLICATIONS OF COPD

Cor Pulmonale

Cor pulmonale is defined as an alteration of right ventricular structure or function resulting from diseases affecting the lungs. It is a term that is often misused to de-

TABLE 28-10. **Specific Respiratory Care Modalities for COPD**

Part 1 **Treatment**	**Assessment (What is Seen Clinically to Justify Treatment)**
O_2 therapy	Hypoxemia <60 mmHg PaO_2 SaO_2 <90% for patients who chronically retain CO_2, maintain the SaO_2 at 88%–90% Signs and symptoms include Confusion/disorientation Somnolence Cyanosis
Bronchodilator therapy	Wheezing Increased sputum Impending respiratory failure (accessory muscle use, pursed lip breathing)
Directed cough with incentive spirometry (DB&C w/IS)	Done on all patients receiving bronchodilator therapy that have secretions present, specifically those patients with: Inability to mobilize secretions History of color/consistency change in sputum Increased respiratory rate with low volumes
Postural drainage	Patients generally unable to tolerate this procedure in the acute care setting; however, it may be tried if unable to mobilize secretions after bronchodilator therapy and DB&C.
IPPB	Not indicated

Part 2 **Treatment**	**Indications for Therapy**
O_2 therapy	Hypoxemia <60 mmHg PaO_2 SaO_2 <90% while breathing room air for patients who chronically retain CO_2, maintain SaO_2 at 88% Cyanosis
Bronchodilator therapy	Diffuse wheezing Documented airway obstruction (FEV_1/FVC <70) Sputum acute or chronic Home use
Directed cough w/ incentive spirometry (DB&C w/IS)	Always include with bronchodilator therapy given to mobilize secretions
Postural drainage	Patient unable to mobilize secretions after bronchodilator therapy and coughing A trial of postural drainage could be tried and discontinued if procedure does not appear to be clinically efficacious
IPPB	Not indicated

Part 3 **Treatment**	**Initial Treatment Plan With Frequencies**
O_2 therapy	Continuous Check O_2 sats Q/AM and PRN according to patient's condition Long-term therapy If indicated (SaO_2 <88%–89% on RA) at discharge, O_2 must be given 15–18 hours/day, not PRN, as a therapy to slow pulmonary artery hypertension
Bronchodilator therapy	If neb used, 0.5 mL albuterol w/2.5 mL Ipratropium (no saline added) Q/4–6 hours upon admission Reduce to Q/6 hours Change to MDI with chamber if appropriate after 24 hours MDI Dosage: Albuterol 2–4 puffs Q/2–4 hours* Ipratropium 4–12 puffs Q/2–4 hours* * Q/2–4 hours PRN according to patient's condition and patient request

(continued)

TABLE 28-10. **Specific Respiratory Care Modalities for COPD** (Continued)

Part 3 (continued) **Treatment**	**Initial Treatment Plan With Frequencies**	
Directed cough with incentive spirometry (DB&C w/IS)	Include with bronchodilator procedure if sputum present	
Postural drainage	Usually not indicated; however, 24-hour trial if unable to mobilize secretions after above attempted Most patients unable to tolerate flat position Evaluate hydration and ambulatory status of patient	
IPPB	Not indicated	
Part 4 **Treatment**	**Outcome**	
	When to Increase	***When to Decrease***
O_2 therapy	PRN to keep sat between 88%–90% (if high liter flow needed, check O_2 sats Q/shift) with blood gases done Q/day (For patients who chronically retain CO_2, maintain sat @88%–89%. When blood gases are drawn, do O_2 sats simultaneously to correlate with ABG sat)	PRN to keep sat 88%–90% Sat at 90% (For patients who chronically retain CO_2, maintain sat @88%–89%. When blood gases are drawn, do O_2 sats simultaneously to correlate with ABG sat)
Bronchodilator therapy	Worsening airway obstruction Inability to mobilize secretions	Signs of bronchodilator toxicity: Pulse rate >180/min Atrial fibrillation or developed tachyarrhythmia Documented clinical improvement
Directed cough w/incentive spirometry (DB&C w/IS)	As per bronchodilator therapy protocol	As per bronchodilator therapy protocol
Postural drainage	Not applicable	If patient unable to tolerate
IPPB	Not applicable	Not applicable
Part 5 **Treatment**	**Boundaries (when to call MD)**	
O_2 therapy	If O_2 needs required to be >2 lpm to maintain sats Confused, restless Unarousable Cyanotic despite appropriate sats All other signs of impending respiratory failure	
Bronchodilator therapy	We would call when: Pulse increase >180/min Patient has tachyarrhythmias Unable to decrease wheeze after consecutive treatments within a 2-hour period Patient is unable or unwilling to take bronchodilator therapy Evidence of difficulty clearing secretions	
Directed cough w/incentive spirometry (DB&C w/IS)	Not applicable	
Postural drainage	Not applicable	
IPPB	Not applicable	

scribe the presence of pulmonary arterial hypertension or edema in a patient with COPD. Development of cor pulmonale in patients with COPD is classically described as following a natural progression from chronic pulmonary hypertension to increased right ventricular work finally resulting in right ventricular hypertrophy and dilation. However, the exact mechanisms causing cor pulmonale have not yet been worked out.

It is postulated that hypoxic vasoconstriction, elevation in $PaCO_2$, destruction of alveolar vessels, reduction in caliber of blood vessels from increased alveolar pressures, increased blood volume, and increased blood viscosity lead to pulmonary hypertension. These factors, along with smooth muscle proliferation within small pulmonary arteries and intimal thickening and medial hypertrophy in the muscular pulmonary arteries then lead to the development of cor pulmonale. The relative contribution of each of these factors to the overall level of pulmonary hypertension is difficult to quantitate.

Cor pulmonale is found at autopsy in 9% to 40% of COPD patients. Its prevalence increases with increasing hypoxemia, polycythemia, hypercapnia, and decreasing FEV_1. The presence of pulmonary artery hypertension in patients with COPD is a poor prognostic sign.

Assessment of cardiac function in these patients can be difficult. Clinical signs that are normally used to identify pulmonary hypertension such as elevated jugular venous pressure, peripheral edema, systolic right-sided parasternal heave, and accentuation of the pulmonary component of the second heart sound may be obscured by lung hyperinflation and tend to occur late in the disease process. Noninvasive techniques such as chest radiography, M-mode and two-dimensional echocardiography, radionuclide ventriculography, and MRI have all been reported to be useful in identifying pulmonary hypertension in patients with COPD to varying degrees.[46,47]

Treatment of pulmonary hypertension in patients with COPD has focused in two areas: pulmonary vasodilators and long-term oxygen therapy. Alpha blockers, beta agonists, calcium channel blockers, hydralazine, theophylline, angiotensin-converting enzyme inhibitors, prostaglandin, and atrial natriuretic peptide (ANP) have all been tried to reduce pulmonary artery pressures in patients with COPD. However, to date, no study has been able to show a long-term survival benefit using any of these drugs. Only long-term oxygen therapy has been shown to improve survival in patients with COPD. Interestingly, this improvement in survival is not always associated with an improvement in pulmonary hemodynamics.[48]

Lung Cancer

In the United States, lung cancer is the most common type of malignancy causing death in both men and women. The 5-year survival rate in Americans has improved only slightly from 12% to 13% from 1974 through 1987. About 95% of lung cancers in men and 80% to 85% of lung cancers in women result from cigarette smoking.[49] There is a dose-dependent relationship between the degree of cigarette abuse and relative risk of death from lung cancer. Several studies have shown that the presence of COPD is an independent risk factor for the development of lung cancer and that the risk of lung cancer increases in proportion to the degree of airways obstruction.[50,51] It is postulated that impaired mucociliary clearance allows pooling of carcinogens within the airways, and that increased exposure time to the carcinogen or the combination of lung tissue damage and exposure to carcinogen may be responsible.

Pneumothorax

COPD is the disease most commonly associated with secondary spontaneous pneumothorax. In the Veterans Administration cooperative study of 185 patients with spontaneous pneumothorax, 70% of participants had an FEV_1/FVC ratio below 0.7.[52] Clinical symptoms such as dyspnea are usually more severe in COPD patients because of reduced pulmonary reserve. Signs such as diminished breath sounds and resonance on percussion are unreliable owing to underlying pulmonary disease. Radiographic assessment with posteroanterior, lateral, and end-expiratory films is essential. Small pneumothoraces may be very difficult to locate, especially with the hyperlucent parenchyma found in the apices of many patients with COPD. Larger pneumothoraces are easier to spot especially when causing tracheal and mediastinal shift or depression of the diaphragm.

The recommended treatment for secondary spontaneous pneumothorax is tube thoracostomy. In the patient with severe COPD and initial spontaneous pneumothorax, pleurodesis should be considered because of documented reductions in recurrence rates. Although tetracycline has been used effectively for this purpose in the past, it is currently not available in the injectable form, and alternative tetracycline derivatives, as well as talc, are now commonly used.[53] Video-assisted thoracoscopy has recently been introduced as a potentially cost-effective alternative to tube-thoracostomy and pleurodesis.

Consideration must be given to the possible effect of pleurodesis on potential lung transplantation. Depending on the transplant center involved, patients may be excluded from transplantation if pleurodesis has been done on the side of the transplant. This is because of the potential for increased bleeding and technical difficulty in performing the transplant surgery.

Pulmonary Infections

Infection may contribute to the course of COPD in many ways. Recurrent acute infectious exacerbations or chronic bacterial colonization may accelerate the natural loss of lung function with age. Unfortunately there is little hard data to support this. However, epidemiologic studies have shown that acute lower respiratory tract infections (usually viral) in childhood are a significant risk factor for the development of adult COPD.[54]

Viral and mycoplasma infections cause approximately one third of COPD exacerbations. *Streptococcus pneumoniae, Haemophilus influenzae*, and recently *Branhamella catarrhalis* are the most common bacterial pathogens associated with exacerbations. Over the past several decades little has changed in the management of infections in COPD patients, with the exception of the increased use of the influenza and pneumococcal vaccines.

There is considerable controversy regarding the role of antibiotics in managing COPD exacerbations. The reasons for the controversy center around the fact that the usual pathogenic organisms make up part of the normal oropharyngeal flora of many patients with COPD. Their presence in the sputum of patients experiencing exacerbations does not always imply that they are responsible for symptoms, making the decision to treat with antibiotics more difficult.

The goals of antibiotic therapy are to shorten the duration of exacerbation and to prevent further acute deterioration in airflow or gas exchange. More symptomatic patients and those with more severe exacerbations tend to benefit most from antibiotic therapy. Studies evaluating efficacy of antibiotics during exacerbations have been favorable, showing either trends toward improvement or statistically significant acceleration of recovery. The choice of antibiotic is guided by the most likely pathogen. Morphology of the predominant organism on an adequate gram stain is helpful in guiding therapy if something other than normal pathogens are found. Sputum cultures can also be helpful especially when first-line therapy fails, exacerbations are frequent, or drug allergies exist but are not usually used for routine exacerbations. Azithromycin, clarithromycin, trimethoprim-sulfamethoxazole, tetracycline, amoxicillin/clavulanate, second- or third-generation cephalosporins, and certain quinolones have all been used effectively in this setting. It should be noted that resistance to trimethoprim-sulfamethoxazole, tetracycline, and amoxicillin is increasing. Antibiotics may also be useful in preventing exacerbations in patients with four or more exacerbations per year.

Pneumonia is increasingly common among the elderly and those with comorbid disease such as chronic lung disease. COPD is considered a risk factor for mortality. It is predictive of a complicated course in community-acquired pneumonia and is a justifiable reason for admitting a patient to the hospital.[55] When the choice of antibiotic is empiric in the hospitalized COPD patient with community-acquired pneumonia, activity against beta-lactamase–producing strains of *Branhamella catarrhalis* and *Haemophilus influenzae* is essential. Recommendations are for a second- or third-generation cephalosporin or beta-lactam/betalactamase inhibitor with or without a macrolide. In hospitalized COPD patients with severe community-acquired pneumonia, a macrolide and a third-generation cephalosporin with anti-pseudomonas activity is recommended.

Acute Respiratory Failure in COPD

Acute respiratory failure is one of the most common reasons for admission to the intensive care unit in patients with COPD. Small insults to the respiratory or other organ systems can rapidly lead to respiratory failure in these individuals. Acute respiratory failure is usually defined using arterial blood gases because FEV_1 and PaO_2 correlate poorly in patients with COPD.[56] A PaO_2 less than 55 mmHg and a $PaCO_2$ greater than 50 mmHg in the setting of respiratory distress is usually considered acute respiratory failure. Common signs and symptoms of respiratory distress in patients with COPD include worsening dyspnea, decreased exercise tolerance, altered mental status, tachypnea, accessory muscle use, cyanosis, and right-sided heart failure. Respiratory muscle fatigue is believed to be the primary determinant of ventilatory failure in patients with COPD. A visual model depicting the balance between respiratory muscle strength and endurance and imposed respiratory mechanical load is shown in Figure 28-8.[57] It has been used to conceptualize the pathophysiology of acute respiratory failure. In this model, inspiratory muscle contraction generating negative intrathoracic pressure to drive inspiratory gas flow must be sufficient to overcome both airway resistance and elastic recoil of the lung and chest wall. When it is inadequate, the model helps to identify the factors contributing to ventilatory failure. Increases in load include increased airways resistance or decreased lung/chest wall compliance, gas exchange abnormalities, and increased metabolic requirements. Decreases in respiratory muscle output arise from depressed ventilatory drive or muscle weakness. The most common precipitants of respiratory failure in COPD are listed in Box 28-7. These factors are important because they are potentially reversible, and a diligent search for them must always be undertaken in the patient with COPD and acute respiratory failure.

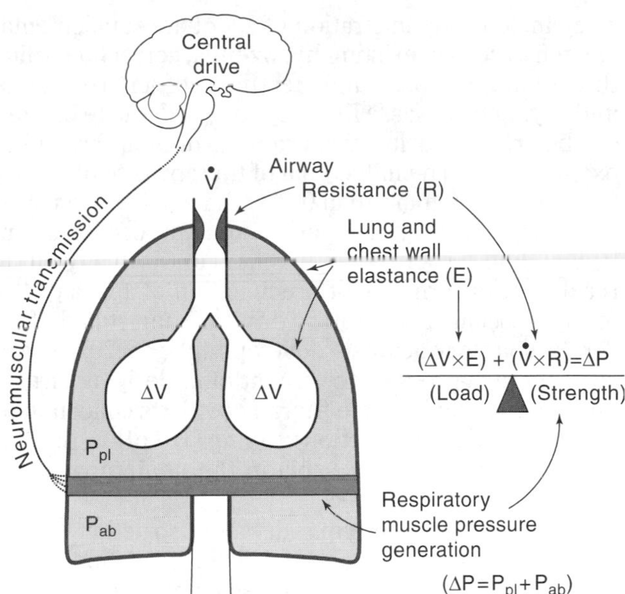

FIGURE 28-8. Depiction of the balance between the mechanical load on the respiratory muscles (airway resistance times the inspiratory flow and chest wall elastance times the tidal volume) and the force of contraction of the muscles (determined by neural input and muscle strength). Each part of the mathematical relationship on the right is related to it's pictorial counterpart by an arrow. When load outweighs strength then respiratory failure occurs with decreased ventilation and elevated $PaCO_2$. (Reproduced with permission from Schmidt GA, Hall JB: Acute or chronic respiratory failure; Assessment and management of patients with COPD in the emergent setting. JAMA 1989;261:3444–53.)

The principles of management of acute respiratory failure in COPD patients are detailed in Chapter 33.

BOX 28–7

COMMON, REVERSIBLE CONDITIONS THAT MAY PRECIPITATE ACUTE RESPIRATORY FAILURE IN PATIENTS WITH COPD

Noncompliance with medications
Pulmonary infection
Congestive heart failure
Pneumothorax
Pulmonary embolism

They include administration of adequate supplemental oxygen to correct existing hypoxemia, correction of life-threatening acidosis, and treatment of any reversible underlying diseases.[58] In many cases adequate oxygen can be provided using nasal cannula or nonrebreathing oxygen mask. The initial goal of therapy is to obtain an O_2 saturation of more than 90% with PaO_2 between 55 to 65 mmHg. Delivery of oxygen should proceed in a controlled and progressive manner until this goal is reached. Concerns about precipitation of apnea owing to suppression of respiratory drive are unjustified. If severe respiratory acidosis develops (pH <7.20), it may respond to aggressive treatment of underlying airflow obstruction. Bicarbonate therapy (with its concomitant increase in CO_2 production) to improve pH in the setting of profound hypercarbia in the nonintubated patient is not recommended.

Treatment of underlying airway obstruction can be accomplished by using aerosolized bronchodilators, administered either by nebulizer or metered-dose inhaler (MDI) with spacer, as long as the patient can cooperate and use the MDI correctly. Parenteral beta agonists are rarely necessary. The choice of drug—beta agonist or ipratropium bromide—does not seem to matter in the acutely worsening COPD patient when only one or the other is used.[59] However, the addition of ipratropium to beta-agonist therapy has been shown to shorten duration of treatment in emergency room stays compared with monotherapy with either agent.[60] Despite this improved outcome, pulmonary function was not different in any treatment group. Certainly, if one drug is used and fails to produce the desired results, the other agent should be added. Administration of corticosteroids is recommended in this setting since it has been shown to significantly improve FEV_1 at 12 hours.[61] The role of theophylline in this setting is controversial. Most studies have found no beneficial effect to initiating theophylline. If the patient is already on theophylline on admission, it is usually continued and a level is checked.

A new modality that has recently been reported to be effective in the treatment of respiratory failure in patients with COPD is noninvasive positive pressure ventilation (NIPPV) by face mask. This modality is thought to reduce the work of breathing by overcoming intrinsic positive end-expiratory pressure (PEEP). If this fails, intubation and mechanical ventilation is the next step. The immediate purpose of mechanical ventilation is to halt progression to apnea and death. The long-range goal is to rest the respiratory muscles and allow improvement in muscle function. Although different authors propose different thresholds of values for PaO_2, $PaCO_2$, and pH as indications for intubation, the decision should be individually based on the patient's response to therapy, baseline status, and reversibility of the initiating event. A rapid respiratory rate (>40 breaths per minute), accessory muscle use, inability to speak in full sentences, and thoracoabdominal paradox can all suggest deterioration, but by themselves are not definite indications for mechanical ventilation. In many instances the patient's mental status is the primary determinant regarding the decision to intubate. Somnolence and inability to cooperate with treatment are usually indications for mechanical ventilation.

The in-hospital mortality in patients with COPD and respiratory failure varies from 6% to 40%, with studies after 1975 reporting mortalities of less than 20%. Long-term prognosis in these patients is not influenced once a patient survives an episode. Because of this, mechanical ventilation should not be withheld from these patients solely on the basis of presumed poor outcome. The fear of prolonged ventilator dependence should be tempered with the knowledge that withholding and withdrawing life support are considered the same by most ethicists today. Thus, the decision to intubate is not a sentence to ventilator dependency for the rest of one's life.

Patients with very severe COPD (stage 3) and their health care providers can anticipate that at some time the patient will suffer an episode of respiratory failure. Together they can determine the circumstances under which mechanical ventilation should be withheld or withdrawn. Advanced directives and living wills do not usually include enough specifics regarding these issues and make the decision more difficult than it should be for family members and health care providers.

SPECIAL CIRCUMSTANCES IN COPD

Air Travel for Patients With COPD

The number of passengers using supplemental oxygen while flying commercial airlines is unknown, but it is estimated to be several thousand each year. Ascent to high altitudes resulting in a reduction in the inspired partial pressure of oxygen is the primary hazard of *air travel* to patients with chronic obstructive pulmonary disease. Commercial aircraft usually operate between 22,000 feet and 44,000 feet above sea level. Cabin pressurization usually results in a cabin altitude of 5000 feet to 8000 feet. Cabin altitudes above 10,000 feet are prohibited because of the requirement for supplemental oxygen for all flight crew members and passengers. During flights at less than 22,500 feet, sea-level cabin pressure can be maintained, attempting to preserve aircraft structural integrity by avoiding multiple pressurization-depressurization cycles. However, this is rarely done. Newer aircraft appear to fly at higher mean cabin altitudes than older models. In doing so they expose COPD patients to greater degrees of hypoxemia.

Physiologic responses to high altitude in normal individuals include hyperventilation, pulmonary vasoconstriction, and an initial increase in cardiac output. This results in a PaO_2 of 50 to 60 mmHg with O_2 saturations of 80% to 90% at 8000 to 10,000 feet in normal individuals. In patients with COPD, the PaO_2 can fall to 40 mmHg or lower during commercial air travel. This decrease in oxygenation at altitude in patients with COPD depends on several factors including rate of ascent, duration at altitude, and the underlying mechanism for hypoxemia. Despite all of this, the incidence of exacerbations of pulmonary disorders and respiratory-related deaths during air travel is extremely low.[63]

Owing to the difficulties of measuring PaO_2 in flight, investigations have focused on methods for predicting oxygenation at altitude (PaO_2-alt) from measurements made at ground level (PaO_2-ground). A multiple regression equation describing this relationship for patients with COPD has recently been published[63]:

$$PaO2\text{ alt (mmHg)} = 0.453(PaO2\text{-ground}) + 0.386(FEV_1\ \%\text{predicted}) + 2.440$$

Supplemental oxygen is generally recommended if the predicted arterial blood oxygen tension at altitude (PaO_2-alt) is expected to be below 50 mmHg. The necessary oxygen flow rate in liters per minute can be estimated as (55-PaO_2-alt)/5.

Airlines usually require written medical clearance and recommendations for oxygen from the individual's physician more than 48 hours before scheduled departure. If the individual's condition meets the individual airline's policy regarding medical clearance, there is usually little difficulty in providing oxygen during transit on the major carriers. If possible, humidification of oxygen is helpful to counteract the dry air found inside of an aircraft. The charge for this service varies from $40 to $150, and this cost may be reimbursed by the patient's insurance company or Medicare. In-flight use of personal oxygen systems is prohibited by FAA regulations. Oxygen equipment on board airplanes usually consists of a rebreather mask or nasal cannula. Compressed oxygen is the most frequently available form of O_2 and may have a fixed flow rate.

Because each airline establishes their own policies regarding in-flight oxygen, it is imperative for COPD patients to be familiar with the regulations of the airline on which they are traveling. Also important is planning a trip with a reputable vendor who may be able to provide oxygen during layovers, at the airport, and during transit to and from the airport. Other alternative methods to improve oxygenation during air travel include avoidance of in-flight alcohol, sedatives, and overeating carbohydrate-rich meals before departure.

Sleep-Related Breathing Disorders

During sleep, worsening of hypoxemia and mild carbon dioxide retention are common in patients with COPD. The episodes of hypoxemia can be severe and occur predominantly during REM sleep. The extent of this nocturnal hypoxemia is related to daytime oxygenation and prediction equations exist that estimate the level of nocturnal hypoxemia and saturation from daytime values.[64] The cause of nocturnal hypoxemia in COPD patients is predominantly hypoventilation during rapid eye movement (REM) sleep, although reductions in FRC and ventilation/perfusion mismatching also contribute. There is also a small subset of people with COPD who have obstructive sleep apnea.

The consequences of nocturnal hypoxemia in COPD patients are largely unknown. It has been theorized that nocturnal desaturation may lead to pulmonary hypertension, but this has not been definitively proven. Mean nocturnal SaO_2 and lowest nocturnal SaO_2 are both related to survival, with lower values associated with worse prognoses. Neither factor improves the prediction of survival compared with daytime SaO_2 measurements or vital capacity. COPD patients with obstructive sleep apnea are more likely to develop pulmonary hypertension and right heart failure. Routine clinical sleep studies as described in Chapter 11 are indicated only in COPD patients who are suspected of having obstruction. This may be suspected when either symptoms compatible with obstructive sleep apnea such as heroic snoring or excessive daytime somnolence are present or when cor pulmonale or polycythemia occur despite adequate daytime oxygenation.

Treatment of patients with COPD who only have hypoxemia at night includes avoidance of bedtime hypnotics and alcohol, both of which may worsen nocturnal hypoxemia and hypercapnia. Although nasal intermittent positive pressure ventilation and various drugs such as almitrene bismesylate, medroxyprogesterone acetate, acetazolamide, and theophylline have been tried during sleep, oxygen therapy remains the only proven treatment for COPD patients with nocturnal hypoxemia. Improvement in pulmonary artery pressures has been reported by using nocturnal supplemental oxygen for COPD patients with desaturation during sleep and daytime PaO_2 greater than 60 mmHg.[65] However, further long-term studies evaluating the effect on mortality are needed before mass screening with nocturnal polysomnography and initiation of oxygen therapy can be recommended in this group of individuals.

Surgery in the Patient With COPD

Patients with COPD have been identified as a group that is at increased risk of perioperative pulmonary complications during and after surgery, particularly upper abdominal procedures. Box 28-8 lists some of the many different pulmonary function criteria that have been proposed as suggesting an increased risk of postoperative pulmonary complications after abdominal surgery.[66,67] Hypoxemia and hypercapnia also have been touted as markers of increased risk of perioperative pulmonary complications. However, the data are

BOX 28–8

SELECTED PREOPERATIVE PULMONARY FUNCTION CRITERIA THAT SUGGEST AN INCREASED RISK OF POSTOPERATIVE COMPLICATIONS FOLLOWING ABDOMINAL SURGERY

FVC	<70% predicted
FEV_1	<70% predicted
FEV_1/FVC	<65% predicted
MVV	<50% predicted
$PaCO_2$	>45 mmHg

From Gass GD, Olsen GN: Preoperative pulmonary function testing to predict postoperative morbidity and mortality. Chest 89:127–135, 1986; reproduced with permission.

anecdotal, and there has been no large prospective study to support this hypothesis. Some investigators have found that in patients with severe COPD, spirometry does not independently predict postoperative complications.[68] To date, there is no consensus regarding the magnitude of perioperative risk for patients with COPD and no precise correlation with underlying lung function. With the exception of lung resection, no study has clearly defined a lower limit of FEV_1 or FVC below which a patient should not be subjected to anesthesia and surgery. Noncardiac surgery in patients with severe COPD has been shown to have a low operative risk (29% complications, 1.3% mortality) leading to the conclusion that "with present day supportive techniques, operations can be safely performed in the majority of patients with severe pulmonary disease."[69]

In individuals undergoing lung resection, the American College of Physicians notes that "severe chronic obstructive pulmonary disease increases the risk associated with lung resection, and persistent elevations in $PaCO_2$ greater than 45 mmHg suggests a very high risk relative to the benefit of the procedure."[70] They recommend preoperative spirometry in all patients undergoing lung resection to identify high-risk and inoperable patients (Table 28-11).[71]

Although the magnitude of risk remains unknown, once an individual is identified as having COPD, it is reasonable to attempt to decrease this risk. Interventions such as deep-breathing maneuvers, chest physiotherapy, bronchodilators, antibiotics (for clinical infection), and smoking cessation have been shown to decrease the incidence of postoperative complications in patients with COPD undergoing surgery. They are described in some detail in Chapters 17 and 18. It seems reasonable to initiate some combination of these modalities in every patient with significant COPD (stages 2 and 3) who are undergoing major surgery. Comprehensive programs such as the perioperative respiratory therapy (PORT) program may help to further identify even higher risk patients, allowing more aggressive intervention in these individuals.[72]

TABLE 28-11. **Selected Pulmonary Function Criteria Suggesting Increased Risk of Postoperative Pulmonary Complications in Patients Undergoing Resectional Lung Surgery**

Increased Risk of Complications
Preoperative FEV_1 <2 L
Preoperative FVC <50% predicted
Preoperative MVV <50% predicted
Preoperative DL_{CO} <50% predicted
Preoperative $VO_{2\,max}$ <15 mL/kg/min
Predicted postoperative (PPO) FEV_1 <40% predicted
Probably Inoperable
Predicted postoperative FEV_1 <0.8 L
PaO_2 <45 mmHg with exercise and balloon occlusion of pulmonary artery to area to be resected
Mean PA pressure >35 mmHg with exercise and balloon occlusion of pulmonary artery to resected area

From Olsen GN, Block AJ, Swenson EW, Castle JR, Wynne JW: Pulmonary function evaluation of the lung resection candidate: A prospective study. Am Rev Respir Dis 111:379–387, 1975; and Markos J, Mullan BP, Hillman DR, Musk AW, et al: Preoperative assessment as a predictor of mortality and morbidity after lung resection. Am Rev Respir Dis 139:902–910, 1989; reproduced with permission.

REFERENCES

1. American Thoracic Society: Statement on the evaluation and management of patients with chronic obstructive pulmonary disease. 1995
2. Anthonisen NR, Wright EC, Hodgkin JE, et al: Prognosis in chronic obstructive pulmonary disease. Am Rev Respir Dis 133: 14–20, 1986
3. Traver GA, Cline MG, Burrows B: Predictors of mortality in chronic obstructive pulmonary disease. Am Rev Respir Dis 119: 895–902, 1979
4. American Thoracic Society: Lung function testing: Selection of reference values and interpretative strategies. Am Rev Respir Dis 144:1202–1218, 1991
5. US Department of Health and Human Services: Reducing the Health Consequences of Smoking: 25 (DHHS publication No. (CDC) 89-8411). Atlanta, US Department of Health and Human Services, Centers for Disease Control, Center for Chronic Disease Prevention and Health Promotion, Office on Smoking and Health, 1989
6. Ciba Foundation Guest Symposium: Terminology, definition and classifications of chronic pulmonary emphysema and related conditions. Thorax 14:286–299, 1959
7. Nagai S, West WW, Thurlbeck WM: The National Institute of Health Intermittent Positive Pressure Breathing Trial: Pathologic studies II. Correlation between morphologic findings, clinical findings, and evidence of expiratory air-flow obstruction. Am Rev Respir Dis 132:946–953, 1985
8. Hogg JC: Bronchiolitis in asthma and chronic obstructive pulmonary disease. Clin Chest Med 14:733–740, 1993
9. Thurlbeck WM: Pathophysiology of chronic obstructive pulmonary disease. Clin Chest Med 11:389–403, 1990
10. Snider GL: Chronic obstructive pulmonary disease: A definition and implications of structural determinants of airflow obstruction for epidemiology. Am Rev Respir Dis 140(S):S3–S8, 1989
11. American Thoracic Society: Chronic bronchitis, asthma and pulmonary emphysema. Am Rev Respir Dis 85:762–768, 1962
12. Hogg JC, Wright JL, Wiggs BR, Coxson HO, et al: Lung structure and function in cigarette smokers. Thorax 49:473–478, 1994
13. Snider GL: Pulmonary disease in alpha-1 antitrypsin deficiency. Ann Intern Med 111:957–959, 1989
14. National Heart Lung and Blood Institute FY 1993 Fact Book, pp 34–45
15. Medical care expenditures attributable to cigarette smoking—United States, 1993. MMWR Morb Mortal Wkly Rep 43: 469–472, 1994
16. Cigarette smoking-attributable mortality and years of potential life lost—United States, 1990. MMWR Morb Mortal Wkly Rep 42:645–649, 1993
17. Snider GL: Chronic bronchitis and emphysema. In Murray JF, Nadel JA (eds): Textbook of Respiratory Medicine. Philadelphia, WB Saunders, 1988, pp 1069–1106
18. Sherrill DL, Lebowitz MD, Burrows B: Epidemiology of chronic obstructive pulmonary disease. Clin Chest Med 11:375–387, 1990
19. Hodgkin JE: Prognosis in chronic obstructive pulmonary disease. Clin Chest Med 11: 555–569, 1990
20. Sweer L, Zwillich CW: Dyspnea in the patient with chronic obstructive pulmonary disease. Clin Chest Med 11(3):417–445, 1990
21. Mahler DA, Weinburg DH, Wells CK, Feinstein AR: The measurement of dyspnea: Contents, inter-observer agreement, and physiologic correlates of two new clinical indexes. Chest 85: 751–758, 1984
22. Borg G: Psychophysical basis of perceived exertion. Med Sci Sports Exerc 14:377–381, 1982
23. Clausen JL: The diagnosis of emphysema, chronic bronchitis, and asthma. Clin Chest Med 11:405–416, 1990
24. Sox HC: Preventive health services in adults. N Engl J Med 330:1589–1595, 1994
25. American College of Physicians Task Force on Adult Immunization, Infectious Disease Society of America: Guide for Adult Im-

munization, 3rd ed. Philadelphia, American College of Physicians, 1994
26. Nichol KL, Margolis KL, Wuorenma J, Von Sternberg T: The efficacy and cost effectiveness of vaccination against influenza among elderly persons living in the community. N Engl J Med 331:778–784, 1994
27. Davidson M, Bulkow LR, Grabman J, Parkinson AJ, et al: Immunogenicity of pneumococcal revaccination in patients with chronic disease. Arch Intern Med 154:2209–2214, 1994
28. US Department of Health and Human Services: The Health Benefits of Smoking Cessation (DHHS publication No. (CDC) 90-8416. Atlanta, US Department of Health and Human Services, Centers for Disease Control, Center for Chronic Disease Prevention and Health Promotion, Office on Smoking and Health, 1990
29. Postma DS, Sluiter HJ: Prognosis in chronic obstructive pulmonary disease: The Dutch experience. Am Rev Respir Dis 140:S100–S104, 1989
30. Doll R, Peto R: Mortality in relation to smoking: 20 years observations on male British doctors. BMJ 2:1525, 1976
31. Rosenburg L, Kaufman DW, Helmrich SP, et al: The risk of myocardial infarction after quitting smoking in men under 55 years of age. N Engl J Med 313:1511, 1985
32. Vliestra RE, Kronmal RA, Oberman A, et al: Effect of cigarette smoking on survival of patients with angiographically documented coronary artery disease: Report from the CASS Registry. JAMA 255:1023, 1986
33. US Department of Health and Human Services: The health consequences of smoking: Cancer and chronic lung disease in the workplace: A Report of the Surgeon General (DHHS Publication No. PHS 85-50207). Washington, DC, US Government Printing Office, 1985
34. Anthonisen NR, Connett JE, Kiley JP, Altose MD, et al: Effects of smoking intervention and the use of an inhaled anticholinergic bronchodilator on the rate of decline of FEV_1: The Lung Health Study. JAMA 272:1497–1505, 1994
35. Ferguson GT, Cherniack RM: Management of chronic obstructive pulmonary disease. N Engl J Med 328: 1017–1022, 1993
36. Walters MI, Edwards PR, Waterhouse JC, Howard P: Long term domiciliary oxygen therapy in chronic obstructive pulmonary disease. Thorax 48:1170–1177, 1993
37. Connolly JE, Wilson A: The current status of surgery for bullous emphysema. J Thorac Cardiovasc Surg 97:351–361, 1989
38. Nickoladze GD: Functional results of surgery for bullous emphysema. Chest 101:119–122, 1992
39. Trulock EP, Cooper JD: Reduction pneumoplasty for COPD. Chest 106:52S, 1994
40. Harpole DH, Sugarbaker DJ: Surgical procedures in bullous emphysema. Pulmonary & Critical Care Updates 9:1–6, 1994
41. Patterson GA: Lung transplantation for chronic obstructive pulmonary disease. Clin Chest Med 11:547–554, 1990
42. Levine SM, Bryan CL, Jenkinson SG: Transplantation for obstructive lung disease. Pulmonary & Critical Care Update 8:1–9, 1993
43. American Thoracic Society: Standards for the diagnosis and care of patients with chronic obstructive pulmonary disease (COPD) and asthma. Am Rev Respir Dis 136:225–244, 1987
44. ACCP/SCCM Consensus Panel: Ethical and moral guidelines for the initiation, continuation, and withdrawal of intensive care. Chest 97:949–958, 1990
45. Position Paper: American College of Physicians Ethics Manual, 3rd ed. Ann Intern Med 117:947–960, 1992
46. Klinger JR, Hill NS: Right ventricular dysfunction in chronic obstructive pulmonary disease: Evaluation and management. Chest 99:715–723, 1991
47. Salvaterri CG, Rubin LJ: Investigation and management of pulmonary hypertension in chronic obstructive pulmonary disease. Am Rev Respir Dis 148:1414–1417, 1993
48. MacNee W: State of the Art: Pathophysiology of cor pulmonale in chronic obstructive pulmonary disease, Parts 1 & 2. Am J Respir Crit Care Med 150:833–52 and 1158–1168, 1994
49. Lin AY, Ihde DC: Recent development in the treatment of lung cancer. JAMA 267:1661–1664, 1992
50. Tockman MS, Anthonisen NR, Wright E, Donithan MG: Airways obstruction and the risk for lung cancer. Ann Intern Med 106: 512–518, 1987
51. Skillrud DM, Offord KP, Miller D: Higher risk of lung cancer in chronic obstructive pulmonary disease; A prospective, matched, controlled study. Ann Intern Med 105:503–507, 1986
52. Light RW, O'Hara VS, Moritz TE, McElhiney J, et al: Intrapleural tetracycline for the prevention of recurrent spontaneous pneumothorax: Results of a Department of Veteran's Affairs cooperative study. JAMA 264:2224–2230, 1990
53. Light RW: Management of spontaneous pneumothorax. Am Rev Respir Dis 148:245–248, 1993
54. Murphy TF, Sanjay S: Bacterial Infection in chronic obstructive pulmonary disease. Am Rev Respir Dis 146:1067–1083, 1992
55. American Thoracic Society: Guidelines for the initial management of adults with community-acquired pneumonia: Diagnosis, assessment of severity, and initial antimicrobial therapy. Am Rev Respir Dis 148:1418–1426, 1993
56. Emerman CL, Connors AF, Lukens TW, et al: Relationship between arterial blood gases and spirometry in acute exacerbations of chronic obstructive pulmonary disease. Ann Emerg Med 18:523–527, 1989
57. Schmidt GA, Hall JB: Acute or chronic respiratory failure: Assessment and management of patients with COPD in the emergent setting. JAMA 261:3444–3453, 1989
58. Curtis JR, Hudson LD: Emergent assessment and management of acute respiratory failure in COPD. Clin Chest Med 15:481–500, 1994
59. Karpel JP, Pesin J, Greenberg D, Gentry E: A comparison of the effects of ipratropium bromide and metaproterenol sulfate in acute exacerbations of COPD. Chest 98:835–839, 1990
60. Shrestha M, O'Brien T, Haddox R, Gourlay HS, Reed G: Decreased duration of emergency department treatment of chronic obstructive pulmonary disease exacerbations with the addition of ipratropium bromide to beta-agonist therapy. Ann Emerg Med 20:1206–1209, 1991
61. Albert RK, Martin TR, Lewis SW: Controlled clinical trial of methylprednisolone in patients with chronic bronhitis and acute respiratory insufficiency. Ann Intern Med 92:753–761, 1980
62. Gong H: Air travel and oxygen therapy in cardiopulmonary patients. Chest 101:1104–1113, 1992
63. Dillard TA, Berg BW, Rajagopal KR, Dooley JW, Mehm WJ: Hypoxemia during air travel in patients with chronic obstructive pulmonary disease. Ann Intern Med 111:362–367, 1989
64. Douglas NJ, Flenley DC: State of the Art: Breathing during sleep in patients with obstructive lung disease. Am Rev Respir Dis 141:1059, 1990
65. Fletcher EC, Luckett RA, Goodnight-White S, Miller CG, et al: A double blind trial of nocturnal supplemental oxygen for sleep desaturation in patients with chronic obstructive pulmonary disease and a daytime PaO_2 above 60 mm Hg. Am Rev Respir Dis 145:1070–1076, 1992
66. Gass GD, Olsen GN: Preoperative pulmonary function testing to predict postoperative morbidity and mortality. Chest 89:127–135, 1986
67. Olsen GN, Block AJ, Swenson EW, Castle JR, Wynne JW: Pulmonary function evaluation of the lung resection candidate: A prospective study. Am Rev Respir Dis 111:379–387, 1975
68. Kroenke K, Lawrence VA, Theroux JF, Tuley MR, Hilsenbeck S: Postoperative complications after thoracic and major abdominal surgery in patients with and without obstructive lung disease. Chest 104:1445–1451, 1993
69. Kroenke K, Lawrence VA, Theroux JF, Tuley MR: Operative risk in patients with obstructive pulmonary disease. Arch Intern Med 152:967–971, 1992
70. American College of Physicians Position Statement: Preoperative pulmonary function testing. Ann Intern Med 112:793–794, 1990
71. Markos J, Mullan BP, Hillman DR, Musk AW, et al: Preoperative assessment as a predictor of mortality and morbidity after lung resection. Am Rev Respir Dis 139:902–910, 1989
72. Torrington KG, Henderson CJ: Perioperative respiratory therapy (PORT): A program of perioperative risk assessment and individualized postoperative care. Chest 93:946–951, 1988

The opinions or assertions contained herein are the private views of the authors and are not to be construed as official or as reflecting the views of the Department of the Army or the Department of Defense.

29 Neuromuscular Disease

Douglas R. Gracey

CLINICAL SKILLS

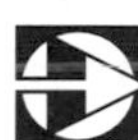

Upon completion of this chapter, the reader will:

- Describe the neuromuscular control of ventilation
- Correlate cerebral blood flow with changes in arterial carbon dioxide tension
- Evaluate abnormal breathing patterns seen in neurogenic disorders
- Determine the extent of respiratory muscle paralysis in spinal cord trauma
- Identify the causes, epidemiology, and clinical features of diseases causing diaphragmatic paralysis
- Predict the progression and need for supportive care for the patient with Guillain-Barré syndrome
- Identify the causes, pathology, and treatment of disorders of neuromuscular transmission
- Predict the progression and need for supportive care for the patient with muscular dystrophy
- Assess diaphragmatic function via physical examination and pulmonary function measurements
- Recommend noninvasive mechanical ventilation for the maintenance of neuromuscular diseased patients in the home setting

KEY TERMS

Acute intermittent porphyria
Amyotrophic lateral sclerosis
Autoregulation of cerebral blood flow
Botulism
Central (medullary) chemoreceptors
Cheyne-Stokes breathing
Duchenne's muscular dystrophy
Guillain-Barré syndrome
Lambert-Eaton myasthenic syndrome
Medullary respiratory center
Muscular dystrophy
Myopathy
Neurogenic pulmonary edema
Organophosphate insecticide poisoning
Peripheral chemoreceptors
Poliomyelitis
Post-polio syndrome
Spinal cord trauma
Tensilon test

The neuromuscular system is clearly the most complex system of the human body. The relation of the neuromuscular system to the respiratory system is also complex. Commands from the central nervous system activate the muscles of the respiratory system, producing the cyclic activity that we recognize as the process of breathing. A host of defects or problems can arise in the central nervous system, in the respiratory muscles, or in the process that transmits the signals from the nervous system to the respiratory muscles. In this chapter specific neuromuscular disorders are reviewed with a discussion of pathologic site(s), etiology, and pathophysiology. Emphasis is on the respiratory manifestations, treatment, and supportive care. The objective of this chapter is to provide a background for clinicians and to discuss guidelines for respiratory care in patients with neurologic disorders. Box 29-1 summarizes the application of this information as clinical skills needed in the respiratory care of such patients.

NEUROMUSCULAR COMPONENTS OF THE RESPIRATORY SYSTEM

The signal that drives the periodic activation of the muscles that ventilate the lungs originates mainly in the pons and medulla. Rhythmic contraction and relaxation of the muscles of respiration is produced from signals generated in the medullary respiratory center, the apneustic center of the lower pons, and the pneumotaxic center of the upper pons. *The medullary respiratory center* is the primary source of the inspiratory signal to the respiratory muscles. However, the cortex of the brain can voluntarily control respiration as well.

Ventilation control is complex, with the respiratory center output modified by a number of sensors that supply input signals. These sensors, which provide feedback to the respiratory center, include the central chemoreceptors, the peripheral chemoreceptors, pulmonary stretch receptors, J receptors, irritant receptors, upper airway receptors, joint and muscle receptors, and arterial baroreceptors.

The *central chemoreceptors* are located near the surface of the medulla where the hydrogen ion concentration of the extracellular fluid is monitored. Increases in hydrogen ion concentration stimulate ventilation, and decreases have the opposite effect. The hydrogen ion concentration of the extracellular fluid of the medulla is related to that of the cerebrospinal fluid and local blood flow. The metabolic activity of the brain and brain stem is also important in determining hydrogen ion concentration.

The *peripheral chemoreceptors* are located in the carotid and aortic bodies. The peripheral chemoreceptors respond to a fall in arterial pH and oxygen tension (PaO_2) and an increase in arterial carbon dioxide tension ($PaCO_2$) by increasing input to the respiratory center and increasing ventilatory drive. Other receptors are important for airway protective mechanisms, cough, stimulation of respiration with exercise, and other situations that require increased ventilation, production of the sensation of dyspnea, and so on.

BOX 29-1

CLINICAL SKILLS NEEDED IN THE CARE OF PATIENTS WITH NEUROMUSCULAR DISORDERS

Select, review, obtain, and interpret data relative to neuromuscular diseases, syndromes, or complications

- Review patient records
  - Physician notes on pathologic findings with special reference to:
    - Family history and hereditary background
    - Previous results of neurologic tests including:
      - Muscle biopsy, EMG, EEG
      - Sleep studies
    - Description of damage/trauma to neurologic structures as seen by lab test or imaging
    - Microbial culture of blood, sputum or CSF
    - Toxologic screens
    - Arterial blood gases or pulse oximetry
  - Pulmonary function tests with special reference to VC, P_{Imax} and P_{Emax}
- Assess patient status
  - Physical examination with special reference to:
    - Ability/deficit of neuromuscular function, muscle strength, muscle wasting, evidence of diaphragmatic movement, accessory muscle activity, breathing pattern
    - Chest auscultation
    - Inspect chest radiograph
- Perform and/or interpret bedside procedures to determine
  - Pathophysiological state:
    - eg, VC, VT, MEP and MIP
    - arterial blood gases
  - Sleep studies
- Participate in the development of respiratory care plan(s)

Select, assemble, and check equipment for proper function, operation, and cleanliness

- Equipment for oxygenation
- Equipment for airway management
- Equipment for mechanical ventilation (acute and chronic care devices)

Initiate, conduct, and modify therapeutic procedures

- Evaluate, monitor, and record patient's response to respiratory care
- Conduct therapeutic procedures to maintain airway, assure/maintain ventilation, and achieve removal of bronchopulmonary secretions
- Establish a respiratory care plan based on the needs of the patient
- Make modifications in therapeutic procedures based on patient tolerance and response to therapy

Modified from: Matrices and Detailed Content Outlines for the Entry Level CRTT and Written Registry (RRT) Examinations given by the National Board for Respiratory Care, Inc., Lenexa, KS, 1993; reproduced with permission.

The efferent or output signal from the respiratory center passes to the anterior horn cells of the spinal cord via three groups of neurons. One group carries the signal for involuntary rhythmic breathing. A second group is responsible for the voluntary control of breathing such as is necessary for speech. A third group controls nonrhythmic functions such as cough.

Two types of efferent motor neurons pass from the anterior horn cells to the muscles of respiration. Thick (alpha) efferent neurons go to the neuromuscular junction of the main skeletal muscle fiber, whereas thin (gamma) efferent neurons supply the intrafusal muscle spindle fibers. The muscles of respiration innervated by the thick and thin efferent neurons include the diaphragm, intercostal muscles, abdominal muscles, and the accessory muscles of respiration.

Clinical respiratory compromise can occur with disease at any level of the central or peripheral nervous system, the neuromuscular junction, or with primary muscle disease.

DISEASES OF THE BRAIN

Disease of the brain and especially the brain stem can affect the respiratory system. Alterations in the brain may produce abnormal respiratory patterns, respiratory failure, inability to protect the airway, inability to clear the airway by coughing, and other respiratory complications.

Cerebral Blood Flow–Intracerebral Pressure

Cerebral blood flow is *autoregulated* by the arterial CO_2 tension. Rising arterial CO_2 tensions increase cerebral blood flow, whereas lowering the $PaCO_2$ has the opposite effect. This is the reason that patients with acute cerebral trauma and associated increased *intracranial pressure* (ICP) are frequently hyperventilated with mechanical ventilation acutely (eg, for 1 or 2 days) after the traumatic event. Hyperventilating the patient to reduce the $PaCO_2$ causes temporary cerebral vasoconstriction, reduces cerebral blood flow, and decreases ICP. A substantial increase in ICP can reduce cerebral perfusion pressure to critically low levels, and frequently, patients with head injuries are monitored by continuously measuring ICP.

In patients with very high ICPs, the brain is forced inferiorly with compression of the brain stem, especially the medulla into the foramen magnum. This herniation of the brain stem can compromise the blood supply to the brain stem and cause acute inactivation of the respiratory center and death. As noted previously, attempts may be made to reduce cerebral blood flow, and thereby ICP, by hyperventilating the patient with a mechanical ventilator to reduce the arterial CO_2 tension ($PaCO_2$) below 30 mmHg.[1,2] In addition, corticosteroids and hypertonic solutions such as mannitol may be administered intravenously to reduce cerebral edema and ICP. Significant elevation of ICP is a contraindication to lumbar puncture because the rapid decompression of cerebral spinal fluid pressure may precipitate herniation of the brain stem into the foramen magnum.

Neurogenic Pulmonary Edema

Another complication of acute brain injury is *neurogenic pulmonary edema*. The exact mechanisms of neurogenic pulmonary edema have been debated for some time.[3] One theory is that massive sympathetic discharge produces transient systemic vasoconstriction and a shift of blood volume to the pulmonary vascular bed with resulting high pulmonary vascular pressures and secondary pulmonary edema. Some authors have suggested sudden pulmonary venous constriction with transient high pulmonary vascular pressures and secondary pulmonary edema as the cause. Elevation of both systemic and pulmonary arterial pressures occurs within seconds of the injury to the central nervous system and probably results from massive alpha-adrenergic sympathetic discharge caused by stimulation of the hypothalamic centers; this has also been suggested as the cause of neurogenic pulmonary edema. Whatever the mechanisms, acute noncardiogenic pulmonary edema can result from acute brain injury and may require mechanical ventilation with positive end-expiratory pressure and high inspired oxygen fractions (FIO_2).

Central Neurogenic Breathing Disorders

Abnormal patterns of breathing commonly result from intracranial disorders and indicate bilateral hemispheric or brain stem injury. Head trauma, intracranial tumors, and vascular events can all lead to neurogenic breathing disorders. The abnormal breathing patterns associated with damage at different levels of the brain and brain stem include the following (Fig. 29-1):

□ CHEYNE-STOKES BREATHING

This disordered breathing pattern is characterized by alternating patterns of hyperventilation followed by either apnea or marked hypoventilation. Some authors state that the variation is in tidal volume alone and that true apnea is not part of the periodic breathing pattern. The cause of *Cheyne-Stokes breathing* is not well understood, although a number of factors including enhanced ventilatory response to CO_2 and disordered cerebral blood flow have been suggested. Severe heart failure is probably the major cause of Cheyne-Stokes respiration. Although the pattern of breathing in Cheyne-Stokes respiration is striking, arterial blood gas abnormalities are not necessarily present. Respiratory alkalosis in this condition is, however, a poor prognostic sign.

□ APNEUSTIC BREATHING

This pattern of breathing is characterized by a prolonged cessation of breathing in an inspiratory position. Apneustic breathing indicates damage to the pons.

□ CENTRAL NEUROGENIC HYPERVENTILATION

This marked hyperventilation persists despite arterial O_2 tensions well in excess of 75 mmHg. Persistent hyperventilation produces minute ventilations in excess of four times normal and is related to damage to the midbrain and upper pontine tegmentum from infarction, trauma, or severe anoxia. As with Cheyne-Stokes breathing, central neurogenic hyperventilation has a high mortality rate if accompanied by respiratory alka-

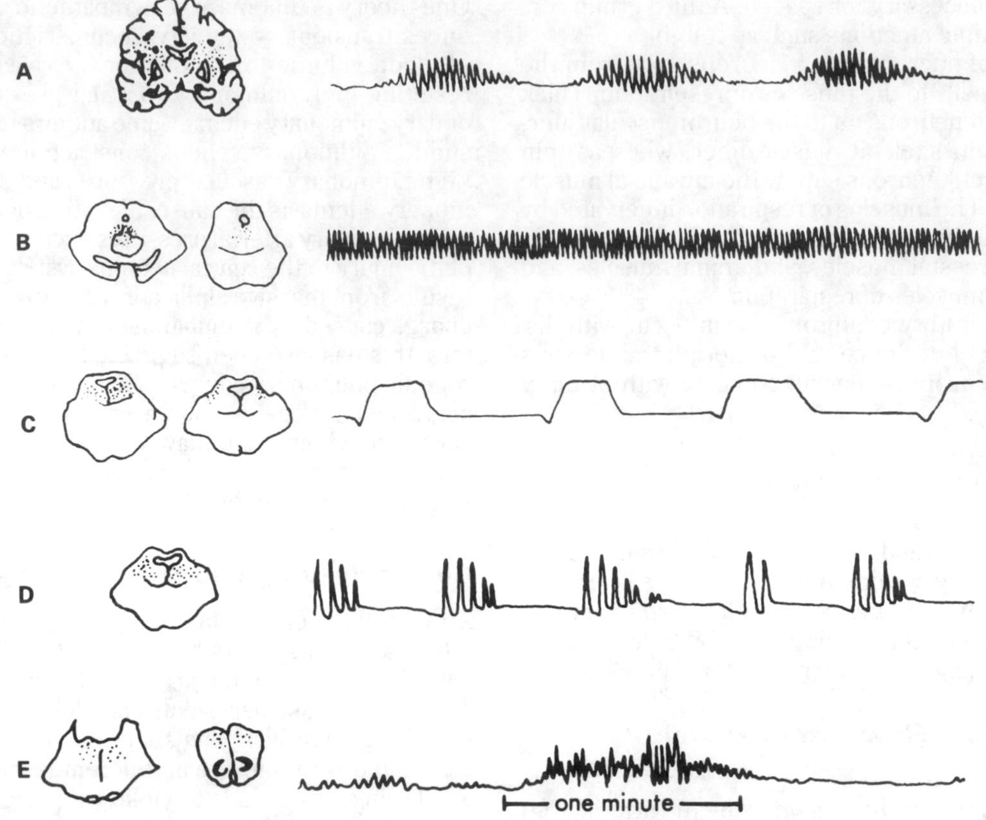

FIGURE 29-1. Abnormal respiratory patterns associated with pathologic lesions (shaded areas) at various levels of the brain. The dotted areas in the brain and brain stem represent the postulated sites of lesions producing the various rhythm abnormalities. Tracings are by chest–abdomen pneumograph: inspiration leads up. (**A**) Cheyne-Stokes respiration. (**B**) Central neurogenic hyperventilation. (**C**) Apneusis. (**D**) Cluster breathing. (**E**) Ataxic breathing. (Plum F, Postner JB: *The Diagnosis of Stupor and Coma,* ed 2. Philadelphia: FA Davis, 1972.)

losis. Central neurogenic hyperventilation is very rare, and stimulatory drugs such as acetylsalicylic acid must be excluded as the cause.

□ CENTRAL NEUROGENIC HYPOVENTILATION

This breathing disorder is associated with narcotic suppression of the respiratory center, head trauma, vascular accidents, and central nervous system infections and is characterized by CO_2 retention. Chronic obstructive pulmonary disease must be ruled out as the cause of alveolar hypoventilation in these patients.

□ CENTRAL SLEEP APNEA

This condition has also been called Ondine's Curse. When these patients sleep, apneic spells occur with secondary hypoxemia and respiratory acidosis. Obstructive sleep apnea may accompany central sleep apnea. Whether this condition is congenital or is due to prior infection of the central nervous system, such as encephalitis, is not clear. Central sleep apnea and idiopathic central neurogenic hypoventilation can be treated with the implantation of phrenic nerve pacemakers.[4] The assessment and treatment of obstructive sleep apnea is reviewed in Chapter 11. Progesterone administration may produce an improvement in idiopathic central neurogenic hypoventilation.

□ CLUSTER BREATHING

Damage to the low pons or high medulla can produce an abnormal pattern of breathing characterized by normal breaths separated by irregular pauses.

□ ATAXIC BREATHING

This pattern of breathing is seen in narcotic poisoning, hypercarbic stupor, brain stem infarcts, meningitis, and with brain tumors. It is characterized by a totally chaotic pattern of breathing with periodic hyperventilation, inspiratory gasps, and apneustic-like inspiratory pauses. This pattern of breathing indicates low pontine and medullary damage.

Movement Disorders

There are a number of diseases of the extrapyramidal system that can cause respiratory complications. Parkinson's disease can cause respiratory muscle rigidity just as it does with other muscle groups, and this can compromise respiration. Irregular breathing patterns and incoordination of swallowing make patients with severe Parkinson's disease prone to aspiration with resulting respiratory embarrassment. Tardive dyskinesia is another movement disorder associated with respiratory difficulties.

It is clear from this brief discussion of the brain and neurogenic breathing disorders that a large number of conditions can cause malfunction of the signal from the respiratory center to the neuromuscular respiratory apparatus below the brain stem. These include the following: vascular events such as thrombosis and embolism; suppression by drugs such as narcotics and anesthetics; trauma; tumors; metabolic abnormalities such as alkalosis and myxedema; movement disorders; and idiopathic problems such as sleep apnea and central hypoventilation.

DISEASES OF THE SPINAL CORD, ANTERIOR HORN CELLS, AND PERIPHERAL NEURONS

Trauma is the most common cause of death in young people in their teens and early twenties. Motor vehicle and sports accidents are the most frequent causes of trauma. One of the most devastating sequelae of trauma is spinal cord injury.

The extent of paralysis following *spinal cord trauma* is related to the degree of injury and the location of the injury. Traumatic transection of the cord above the level of the third cervical segment leads to complete respiratory muscle paralysis and death unless mechanical ventilation is instituted. If the lesion of the cord is below the level of the third cervical segment, diaphragmatic function is spared. However, in quadriplegia with spared diaphragm function, the work of breathing is totally maintained with the diaphragm, which must greatly increase its level of work. In addition, respiratory function is not normal and the potential for respiratory complications is great.

These patients, even with intact diaphragm function, have compromise of their ability to cough. Paralysis of the abdominal muscles is one reason for this ineffective cough because an important part of the cough mechanism requires tensing the abdominal muscles to be effective. Although the inspiratory capacity of these quadriplegic patients may be good, the actual act of coughing causes paradoxical motion of the abdominal wall, and effective cough pressures are difficult to generate unless the abdomen is supported or assisted with inward pressure by the hands of an attendant.

Such patients need to be treated with a chest physical therapy protocol that includes the following: frequent assessment, frequent turning, and assistance in maintaining adequate clearance of airway secretions.[5] (Refer to Chapter 17 for a complete discussion of bronchial hygiene therapy.) With time, spasticity of the intercostal and abdominal muscles helps to improve the patient's spontaneous cough.

Diaphragmatic Paralysis

Unilateral diaphragm paralysis is not uncommon following cardiovascular surgery due to trauma to the phrenic nerve. This paralysis may be temporary or permanent. In patients with normal pulmonary function, unilateral diaphragm paralysis is usually asymptomatic. However, patients with significant obstructive lung disease or restrictive disease may be extremely symptomatic if they sustain unilateral diaphragm paralysis, and this is one of the causes of inability to wean patients from mechanical ventilation postoperatively following cardiac and thoracic surgery. In addition to trauma, there are a number of other causes of diaphragm paralysis, including progressive motor neuron disease (amyotrophic lateral sclerosis), poliomyelitis, tetanus, diphtheria, acute porphyria, Guillain-Barré syndrome, malignancy, and cervical cord trauma. The diaphragmatic paralysis can be unilateral or bilateral, depending on the cause. In many patients, the cause of unilateral paralysis of the diaphragm is never found and termed idiopathic.[6]

Multiple Sclerosis

Although respiratory complications occur with multiple sclerosis, they are rare. This demyelinating disease can affect the cervical spinal cord pyramidal tracts and possibly anterior horn cells. Bulbar involvement with multiple sclerosis can affect the respiratory center and airway protective reflex mechanisms and produce respiratory failure.[7]

Poliomyelitis

Poliomyelitis is the disease that launched the field of respiratory care. Although polio rarely is seen in the developed world today, it is still a problem in developing countries without large-scale vaccination programs to eradicate the disease. Mechanical ventilation of large numbers of these patients in the polio epidemics of the 1950s provided a great deal of experience in acute short-term and chronic mechanical ventilation. Negative pressure tank ventilators (iron lung), cuirass ventilators, and positive pressure ventilators were all developed in response to the needs of polio patients. Interestingly, serologic studies done during polio virus epidemics have shown that less than 1% of individuals with serologic evidence of acute infection with the virus develop symptoms. The incidence of paralytic illness in those individuals with symptoms is thought to have been 30% to 60%. The risk of paralysis increases with age, and adults are 10 times as likely to have paralysis.

The first sign of poliomyelitis infection is usually a brief febrile illness, usually a gastroenteritis, followed in 1 to 2 weeks with the onset of acute paralysis. The poliomyelitis virus attacks the anterior horn cells and may lead to paralysis of the limbs and trunk associated with recurrence of fever, headache, and frequently, stiff neck. If high cervical segments supplying the respiratory muscles are involved, varying degrees of respiratory compromise result. If the brain stem is involved (bulbar poliomyelitis), hypoventilation or apnea may result.

Today it is apparent that some patients who had poliomyelitis in the 1950s and survived with minimal and, at times, inapparent respiratory muscle and bulbar compromise are presenting with clinical compromise of their respiratory system function as they grow older.[8] This is termed the *post-polio syndrome*. Frequently these patients required some type of respiratory support at the time of their acute poliomyelitis infection, and, as they age, may do so again.

Amyotrophic Lateral Sclerosis

Amyotrophic lateral sclerosis (ALS) (Lou Gehrig disease) is a progressive motor neuron disease involving the anterior horn cells and is of unknown cause. The disease causes anterior horn cell neuronal degeneration and loss. It is the most common motor neuron disease, with a rate of occurrence of 2/100,000 per year. The occurrence of the disease is more common in men than in women. Symptomatic limb weakness is the presenting complaint in most patients. These patients can develop involvement of the respiratory muscles, especially the diaphragm, early or late in the course of disease and develop progressive respiratory failure. Involvement of the brain stem by this disease produces bulbar dysfunction with hoarseness, slurring of speech, and difficulty swallowing. Aspiration is common. Some of these patients elect to undergo elective tracheostomy for airway care and prolonged mechanical ventilation to prolong their life.[9] There is no known effective treatment for ALS. Some of the patients with predominantly lower motor involvement may have a prolonged course with late onset of respiratory muscle and/or bulbar involvement.

Guillain-Barré Syndrome

Acute inflammatory demyelinating polyradiculopathy is an acute and sometimes slowly evolving paralytic disease frequently called *Guillain-Barré syndrome*. First described by Landry in 1859 and later by Guillain, Barré, and Strohl, the etiology of this disease process is unknown. This disease is caused by a lymphocytic and macrophagic infiltration of the peripheral nerves with destruction of myelin. In severe cases, there may even be axonal degeneration. The incidence has been found to range from 0.6 to 2.4 cases per 100,000 population per year. Although the syndrome can occur at any age, there appear to be two peaks in incidence, in early adult life and between the fifth and eighth decades, the latter being the larger group.

There are several antecedent acute illnesses of infectious cause that appear to be related to the development of Guillain-Barré syndrome. Two thirds of these patients relate a history of an acute illness frequently described as influenza-like, with fever and upper respiratory symptoms from 1 to 3 weeks before the onset of neurologic symptoms. Approximately 10% of the patients with Guillain-Barré syndrome relate a history of a preceding gastrointestinal illness. *Campylobacter jejuni* enteritis has been implicated in this latter group of patients. Most commonly related to the former group has been cytomegalovirus (CMV), Epstein-Barr virus (EBV), human immunodeficiency virus (HIV), respiratory syncytial virus (RSV), and *Mycoplasma pneumoniae. Mycoplasma pneumoniae* is the second most common nonviral pathogen that has been linked to the development of Guillain-Barré syndrome. There are a number of other events, including surgery, which have been linked to the syndrome. Probably the best known is the swine flu vaccine, which was given in the fall of 1976. Much controversy still exists about the relationship of this vaccine to the Guillain-Barré syndrome. No other lot of influenza vaccine has been implicated in this syndrome before or since 1976.

Typically these patients first note paresthesias in the distal lower extremities followed by ascending paralysis. The degree of muscle paralysis may be mild or severe. In severe cases, complete paralysis of the voluntary muscles may occur, and severe respiratory muscle involvement results in death unless support with mechanical ventilation is undertaken. Examination of the spinal fluid reveals increased levels of protein without an increased number of leukocytes. This finding is classic for Guillain-Barré syndrome. Experience at the Mayo Clinic with 79 acute Guillain-Barré patients showed that 25% of them were admitted to a respiratory intensive care unit, and 17% of the patients required mechanical ventilation.[10] Three of the 79 patients died of complications of the disease or its treatment. The usual complications include aspiration, nosocomial infections, pulmonary embolism, and labile autonomic function. Careful attention to airway care, nutritional support, prevention of venous thrombosis and pulmonary embolism, and a physical medicine program are key to the successful treatment of these patients. On the whole, if the Guillain-Barré patient requires mechanical ventilation, tracheostomy should be performed early, as the mean number of days on the ventilator in the Mayo Clinic study was 37 ± 29 days.

Once the symptoms of Guillain-Barré syndrome begin to evolve, the neurologic defects are complete in 2 weeks in 50% of patients and, at 4 weeks, in 90% of patients. After a variable plateau phase, recovery commences. Recovery is usually, but not always, complete. Fifteen percent of patients have permanent residual motor defects, and in some series, 5% have been permanently disabled. The main complaint, weakness, usually begins in the legs but can begin in the arms and rarely presents as a facial diplegia. Proximal weakness is more frequent than distal, and loss of deep tendon reflexes in the affected areas is characteristic.

Significant neuropathic or muscular pain is seen in up to 30% of patients and may be severe and refractory to drug intervention. Autonomic dysfunction may occur leading to sinus tachycardia, bradycardia, hypotension, and hypertension.

The prevention of complications is key to the successful supportive care of Guillain-Barré syndrome and respiratory failure in other neuromuscular disorders. The major complications are respiratory failure, vascular collapse, pulmonary embolism, aspiration, and pressure neuropathy. Careful monitoring for respiratory failure and endotracheal intubation when appropriate is key. Table 29-1 summarizes the general indications for that intervention. Appropriate treatment of autonomic lability and the prevention of deep venous thrombosis is crucial. Appropriate use of feeding tubes when indicated can usually prevent aspiration. Frequently these patients are immobile, and excellent nursing care and physical therapy are key to preventing complications. Physical therapy can help to avoid contractures. Foot boards or foot splints help to prevent foot drop or contraction of the Achilles tendons. Wrist splints may also be indicated. Padding the peroneal and ulnar nerves can prevent pressure neuropathy. The newer special beds such as the rescue bed are helpful in preventing decubitus ulcers and skin breakdown. Frequent turning of the patient is also important. The key to preventing pneumonia and atelectasis is good airway care and chest physical therapy.

The treatment of Guillain-Barré syndrome, with other than supportive care, has been controversial. Studies have failed to show any benefit to giving corticosteroids, and in fact, they may lead to further complications. A consensus appears to have been reached that plasma exchange is beneficial, but the clinical trials published thus far are not very convincing. In 1992 van der Meché reported on a randomized trial comparing intravenous immune globulin and plasma exchange in Guillain-Barré syndrome; the study was carried out by the Dutch Guillain-Barré Study Group. The results indicate no apparent difference in the response of acute Guillain-Barré syndrome to immune globulin as opposed to plasma exchange. It also suggested that neither of these modalities had any true advantage over just good supportive treatment.[11] Furthermore, clinically significant relapses may occur in patients more often following use of humane immune globulin therapy than after either plasma exchange or no therapy.[12,13]

Critical Illness Polyneuropathy

Recently, both polyneuropathy and myopathy have been described in association with critical illness and may be linked with respiratory muscle weakness and may lead to ventilatory dependence. There is a great deal of controversy about critical illness polyneuropathy and myopathy and their cause. Some investigators feel that the use of high-dose corticosteroids and muscle-relaxing drugs in critically ill patients leads to the development of myopathy, which can adversely affect the respiratory muscles, and they feel that critical illness polyneuropathy is a distinct entity. The diagnosis is confirmed by electromyography, which shows a polyneuropathy and, at times, polyradiculopathy.[14] Critical illness polyradiculopathy may be so severe that it causes quadriplegia in some patients. Some investigators have suggested that moderate to severe malnutrition during critical illness is associated with critical illness polyneuropathy. Studies using diaphragmatic electromyograms have suggested that respiratory muscle weakness due to critical illness polyneuropathy is a major cause of failure to wean from mechanical ventilation.

TABLE 29-1. Possible Indications for Endotracheal Intubation

- Decreased respiratory muscle strength
  - $P_{Imax} \leq 30$ cmH_2O
  - $P_{Emax} \leq 30$ cmH_2O
  - Vital capacity $\leq$10–15 mL/kg
- Hypoventilation
  - $PaCO_2 \geq 50$ mmHg (acutely)
- Hypoxemia
  - $PaO_2 < 60$ mmHg when on supplemental oxygen with $FIO_2 \geq 0.7$
- Acidemia
  - pH < 7.35
- Tachypnea
  - Respiratory frequency > 30 breaths/min

Acute Intermittent Porphyria

Porphyrins are side products of the synthesis of heme. *Acute intermittent porphyria* is the most important of the group of porphyria cutanea tarda, congenital porphyria, and acute intermittent porphyria. (Acute intermittent porphyria is always listed as a cause of respiratory failure, but it is an exceedingly rare cause.) Patients with acute intermittent porphyria have a hereditary partial deficiency of porphobilinogen (PBG) deaminase and excrete excessive amounts of d-aminolevulinic acid and PBG in the urine.

Attacks of acute intermittent porphyria occur in susceptible individuals when precipitated by the administration of certain drugs including barbiturates, menstruation and pregnancy, infection, and excessive alcohol use. Neurologic features of acute intermittent porphyria can include motor paralysis or paresis varying from mild limb weakness to quadriplegia. Upper and lower motor neuron lesions have been described. The respiratory muscles can be involved and acute respiratory failure can occur.[15]

DISORDERS OF NEUROMUSCULAR TRANSMISSION

Myasthenia Gravis

Myasthenia gravis (MG) is caused by a defect in neuromuscular transmission and is characterized by muscle weakness, which worsens with repetitive effort. The defect is confirmed by electromyography. Repeat compound nerve stimulation causes a decremental response in the amplitude of the evoked muscle action potential. In addition, approximately 90% of patients with myasthenia gravis exhibit acetylcholine receptor antibodies in their serum. Those without radioimmunoassay detected antibodies have antibodies that can be demonstrated in cultured muscle cell assay systems. There is a significant association between the thymus gland and myasthenia gravis. Approximately 75% of patients with MG have thymic abnormalities; 85% have thymic hyperplasia; and 15% have thymomas.

Regardless of the underlying pathology, thymectomy can produce significant improvement of myasthenic weakness; 35% undergo complete remission and another 50% improve after surgery. The pharmacologic treatment consists of the administration of anticholinesterase drugs such as pyridostigmine. One test for myasthenia gravis, the *Tensilon test,* consists of giving edrophonium chloride (Tensilon), a very short-acting anticholinesterase drug and noting its effects on muscle strength. In "myasthenic crisis" or undermedication, muscle strength should improve following Tensilon administration. If the patient exhibits respiratory muscle weakness, the vital capacity and maximum inspiratory and expiratory airway pressures can be measured before and after Tensilon. In addition to anticholinesterase drugs, patients with myasthenia gravis are frequently treated with long-term, alternate day corticosteroids and with a short course of plasma exchange to reduce the level of antibody to the acetylcholine receptor sites.

Myasthenia gravis produces compromise of the respiratory system in a number of ways. First there is frequently weakness of the respiratory muscles with impairment of cough and vital capacity. Bulbar weakness may be significant and lead to aspiration and pneumonia. Anticholinesterase drugs increase airway secretions, and this may be a problem in patients with impaired ability to cough. Too much anticholinesterase medication may produce a "cholinergic crisis" and aggravate muscle weakness. These patients can be very difficult to manage, and respiratory failure can be precipitated by any number of events.[16] Meticulous respiratory care, including chest physical therapy and monitoring of respiratory muscle strength, is the key to the treatment of these patients.

Patients with myasthenia gravis are extremely sensitive to nondepolarizing myoneural blocking drugs and certain other drugs such as aminoglycosides. At times, unsuspected cases of myasthenia gravis are precipitated into acute respiratory failure by these medications when patients are in the hospital for treatment of other medical problems.

Some patients who are in prolonged respiratory failure and ventilator dependent with myasthenia gravis may be weaned from ventilator support after multiple plasma exchanges.[17] Subsequent control of acetylcholine receptor antibody production frequently requires high-dose alternate day corticosteroids and even immunosuppression with azathioprin.

Lambert-Eaton Myasthenic Syndrome

Lambert-Eaton myasthenic syndrome (LEMS) is a disease of the myoneural junction usually associated with bronchogenic small cell carcinoma. It is associated with proximal muscle weakness, easy fatigability, dry mouth, and impotence in men. The electromyogram in LEMS characteristically shows a progressive increase in amplitude of compound muscle action potentials with rates of nerve stimulation above 10 per second. On clinical examination these patients may exhibit this progressive increase in muscle strength with repeated stimulation of a deep tendon reflex or repeated testing of a weak muscle group. Clinical and electromyographic evidence of LEMS can be transferred via serum from human to laboratory animal, but the specific antibody has not been isolated and plasma exchange has little effect on the syndrome. Respiratory failure may occur in LEMS.[18]

Tetanus

Tetanus is a disease caused by infection by *Clostridium tetani*, a gram-positive bacillus that has a spore form. The spores, when introduced into a wound, can multiply in anaerobic conditions and produce a toxin. Penicillin kills the organism, and persons who have received a previous series of tetanus toxoid injections with periodic booster shots are not susceptible to tetanus. However, nonimmunized individuals who become infected with *Clostridium tetani* develop tetanus. The organisms liberate a toxin that eventually fixes to the presynaptic terminals of spinal inhibitory interneurons and interferes with the release of inhibitory transmitter substance. This produces the classic picture of tetanic muscle spasm and rigidity. Trismus may occur with inability to open the mouth and rigidity of the facial muscles produces an expression called "risus sardonicus." Opisthotonus, dysphagia, aspiration, and respiratory muscle spasm occurs in severe cases and respiratory failure may ensue.

Treatment consists of antibiotics, usually penicillin, surgical debridement of the infected wound, intravenous human tetanus immune globulin, active immunization with tetanus toxoid, fluids, and nutritional support. In severe tetanus, control of the airway and muscle spasms requires that the patient be paralyzed, sedated with diazepam or narcotics, and mechanically ventilated. Autonomic nervous system dysfunction causing arrhythmias and labile blood pressure can occur and require treatment. Usually after treatment as outlined, a trial of weaning the patient from muscle relaxants can be attempted after 1 to several weeks.

Botulism

Botulism is a severe paralytic disease caused by toxin produced by *Clostridium botulinum.* The most common source of botulism is from food poisoning, but it can occur from wound infection with the organism. Botulism from food poisoning involves the ingestion of preformed toxin in infected food. The toxin binds to the presynaptic neuromuscular junction and prevents acetylcholine release. This results in hypotonia and symmetrical paralysis. Ingestion of the toxin first produces gastrointestinal symptoms followed by symptoms of dry mouth, diplopia, and then descending motor paralysis including the muscles of respiration.

Treatment consists of ventilatory support, elimination of residual toxin in the gastrointestinal tract, and antitoxin. If the toxin type, designated A through G, has been determined from examination of the patient's serum or stool, specific antitoxin is given.

PHARMACOLOGIC NEUROMUSCULAR TRANSMISSION DEFECTS

Depolarizing and nondepolarizing muscle relaxant drugs are frequently used in surgery and the respiratory care unit. Meticulous attention to detail and ventilatory support is required if problems are to be avoided. In addition, a large number of substances such as antibiotics (ie, aminoglycosides), anticholinesterases (ie, parathione), phenothiazine intoxication, methyl alcohol, magnesium, and clinical hypokalemia can produce neuromuscular transmission defects and respiratory failure.

Organophosphate insecticide poisoning can occur by ingestion, inhalation, or absorption through mucous membranes. Two forms of organophosphate poisoning affect the respiratory system: acute organophosphate toxicity and an intermediate toxicity syndrome that occurs 1 to 4 days after exposure.

Organophosphate insecticides are potent lipid-soluble anticholinesterases. The anticholinesterase inhibits hydrolysis of acetylcholine. This leads to decreased respiratory muscle strength and may lead to "cholinergic crisis" with respiratory failure requiring mechanical ventilation.

Treatment consists of the cholinesterase reactivator pralidoxime and atropine, the latter to counter parasympathetic overactivity resulting from pralidoxime. Mechanical ventilation may be required for up to 2 weeks, depending on the severity of the poisoning.

DISEASES OF THE MUSCLES

Muscular Dystrophies

There are a number of hereditary diseases that lead to degeneration of skeletal muscles, the progressive muscular dystrophies. These diseases are distinguished from one another based on their mode of inheritance, distribution of muscle involvement, age at onset of symptoms, and rate of progression of symptoms. Characteristically, the involved muscles are symmetrically involved, and muscle fibers as they degenerate are replaced by fat and fibrous tissue.

The most common form of muscular dystrophy is the Duchenne form, which is sex-linked and carried on the x chromosome. Because the gene is recessive, it does not produce disease in the mother, but male offspring who inherit this defective x chromosome will develop the disease, which begins in utero. Females who carry this genetically defective x chromosome can be detected by measuring serum creatine kinase, which is elevated in two thirds of carriers and by performing an electromyogram. This carrier screening in families with the history of *Duchenne's muscular dystrophy* is key to preventing the disease. The incidence of the disease is estimated to be around 1 per 3000 live male births.

Duchenne's muscular dystrophy is the most important form in respiratory medicine because of its universal fatal outcome of respiratory failure. The disease is usually manifested around the age of 3 to 6 years with symptoms of difficulty walking or running and enlarged calf muscles. Initially the involved muscles appear hypertrophied but eventually they atrophy. The muscles of the lumbosacral spine, pelvis, and shoulder girdle become wasted. Eventual wasting of the muscles providing support to the spine leads to scoliosis, and most patients are no longer able to walk by the age of 12 years.

Involvement of the muscles of respiration eventually leads to restrictive pulmonary disease, hypoxemia, and then eventual hypercarbia. Before medical intervention with noninvasive mechanical ventilation, tracheostomy and mechanical ventilation, chest physical therapy, and airway care, survival beyond the age of 20 years was infrequent. With such intervention, survival well beyond 20 years of age is common.

Another form of pseudohypertrophic x-linked muscular dystrophy is the Becker type. For unknown reasons, the clinical onset of disease is much later in life; patients may live well into their 6th decade; and respiratory failure is less severe and scoliosis much less common. It is said the Duchenne form is twice as common as the Becker form. A rare form of benign x-linked muscular dystrophy has been reported to be associated with contractures but apparently not with respiratory failure.

Myotonic dystrophy is of dominant autosomal inheritance. The defective gene is believed to be on chromosome 19. Onset of symptoms is usually in the second decade of life. The disease has a slowly progressive course, but myotonic dystrophy and progressive muscular dystrophy can lead to progressive respiratory failure.[19] As noted previously, patients with Duchenne's muscular dystrophy almost invariably die of respiratory infections complicating chronic progressive respiratory failure.[20] Limb-girdle type of muscular dystrophy patients appear to have early involvement of the diaphragm associated with respiratory insufficiency.[21] Fasciocapulohumeral dystrophy does not appear to be associated with serious respiratory dysfunction.

Myopathies

A number of myopathies can lead to respiratory failure. These rather rare diseases include centronuclear myopathy, progressive congenital myopathy, Isaac's syndrome, and acid maltase deficiency.

Acid maltase deficiency is a hereditary defect of recessive autosomal inheritance and was originally recognized as a fatal disease of infancy in which glycogen accumulates in tissues, including the muscles, leading to generalized weakness. In infants, glycogen storage in the liver, heart, and tongue leads to organ enlargement. In adults, however, organomegaly is typically absent and the disease is slowly progressive. In adult patients, the respiratory muscles can be selectively affected, and these patients may present with clinically unexplained ventilatory failure. The diagnosis is made by biopsy of the muscle and chemical assay for acid maltase and histopathologic studies.[22]

Polymyositis and Dermatomyositis

Polymyositis is an inflammatory disease of the skeletal muscle. Characteristically in polymyositis, the muscles of the neck, pharynx, and limb girdle are involved. Weakness is the primary complaint. Dysphagia caused by weakness of the posterior pharyngeal muscles can lead to aspiration with pneumonia and also respiratory failure.[23] Similar problems occur in dermatomyositis where inflammation of both skin and muscle occur. In both diseases, associated malignancy must be ruled out as the cause of the disease, especially in adults. The incidence of associated malignancy is rare but increases with aging.

RESPIRATORY CARE OF NEUROMUSCULAR PATIENTS

Assessment of the Patient

The status of the respiratory muscles can be assessed in a number of ways. Because the most important respiratory muscle is the diaphragm, assessment of this muscle is of most interest.

The physical examination of the patient may suggest that the patient has a paralyzed diaphragm in that paradoxical (inward) movement of the abdomen may be observed during inspiration. This paradox of the abdomen may be subtle or absent in unilateral diaphragm paralysis. Normally the abdomen moves out on inspiration as the descending diaphragm pushes down on the abdominal contents. In addition, the patient with diaphragm paralysis may be observed to have dyspnea when supine or may complain of being unable to lie supine.

The function of the diaphragm may be checked with fluoroscopy. Because unilateral diaphragm paralysis may be missed on fluoroscopy with quiet breathing, it is common practice to ask the patient to sniff while being fluoroscoped. Sniffing causes sudden contraction of the diaphragm and if one side is paralyzed it will be observed to move paradoxically, that is, cephalad instead of caudad. In addition, each side of the diaphragm can be paced transcutaneously in the neck while being observed fluoroscopically, and its action potential with esophageal or surface electrodes can be recorded.

The transdiaphragmatic pressure (P_{di}) can be measured by using pressure transducers to measure intrathoracic (esophageal) and intra-abdominal (gastric) pressures during a maximum inspiration. The P_{di} in normal individuals is greater than 60 cmH_2O. There is a grey zone of normal individuals who have P_{di} measurements of 40 to 60 cmH_2O. Patients with weak or paralyzed diaphragms will exhibit gradations of pressure less than 40 cmH_2O.

The most simple means of measuring diaphragmatic function is to measure the vital capacity (VC) and maximum static inspiratory pressure (P_{Imax}). Both of these measurements are greatly dependent on diaphragm function and strength.[24] The maximum static expiratory pressure (P_{Emax}) is less useful in measuring diaphragm function but is helpful for evaluating the ability to produce adequate cough pressures. In Guillain-Barré syndrome with ascending paralysis, patients may have an excellent VC and P_{Imax} but exhibit a drop in P_{Emax}. This is usually a sign that the abdominal muscles have become paralyzed. Since the ability to hold the abdominal muscles rigid is key to producing an adequate P_{Emax} and also cough, this measurement is of great value in patients with neuromuscular disease. In Guillain-Barré syndrome, a fall in P_{Emax}, certainly to ≤ -30 cmH_2O, frequently heralds impending secretion retention and acute respiratory failure. In such patients, waiting for the development of hypoxemia or a low vital capacity may lead to the need for emergency endotracheal intubation or a cardiopulmonary arrest.

Arterial blood gases are essential to the evaluation of patients with neuromuscular disease. Abnormalities of the arterial blood gases will vary from hypoxemia, perhaps only when supine with diaphragm paralysis, to varying degrees of CO_2 retention owing to alveolar hypoventilation. As a general rule, the progression of hypoxemia and CO_2 retention in neuromuscular disease is gradual, and the CO_2 retention is metabolically compensated. Because of this, many chronic neuromuscular disease patients may develop serious pulmonary artery hypertension and cor pulmonale before their hypoxemia and CO_2 retention are discovered.

□ HEAD TRAUMA

Patients with trauma to the skull are frequently unconscious or severely obtunded. Therefore, as a rule, they require endotracheal intubation for protection of the airway and secretion management. If respiratory function is compromised, assisted or controlled mechanical ventilation is required. Since significant hypoxemia or hypercapnia causes an increase in cerebral blood flow and, therefore, increased ICP, avoidance of both of these situations is desirable. As noted earlier, the production of hypocapnia with controlled mechanical ventilation may be desirable in some head trauma patients to reduce cerebral blood flow, ICP, and cerebral edema.[1] It is also desirable to avoid high intrathoracic pressures because the resulting compromise of venous return elevates systemic venous pressure, which is transmitted to the central nervous system and has an adverse effect on cerebral spinal fluid drainage. If positive end-expiratory pressure (PEEP) must be used in these patients, it should be used carefully. Monitoring of ICP is very helpful in the management of these patients.

□ SPINAL CORD INJURY

As stated earlier, the degree of respiratory compromise with spinal cord trauma depends on the level of the trauma. Cord lesions above the level of C-3 cause the loss of diaphragm function, and to maintain life, chronic mechanical ventilation is required. Although lesions below C-3 will leave the patient with diaphragm function, special attention will usually be required to maintain adequate tracheobronchial toilet. The management of the patient with a high spinal cord injury is best done with a protocol, and the one used in one neurosurgical ICU is shown in Table 29-2.

□ CHRONIC MECHANICAL VENTILATION

The most common reason for long-term mechanical ventilation is neuromuscular disease. In addition, appreciation of the fact that respiratory muscles fatigue when overworked and function much more efficiently when rested has led to the use of nocturnal intermittent positive and negative pressure assisted mechanical ventilation in patients such as those with chronic obstructive lung disease.[25–27]

Extensive experience with home negative pressure ventilation has shown this mode of therapy to be useful in a number of neuromuscular diseases.[28,29] Home positive pressure assisted ventilation is now commonly used for patients with amyotrophic lateral sclerosis[9] and muscular dystrophy.[30] Both negative and positive pressure home mechanical ventilators have been modernized and made more convenient to use. It is now possible to maintain many patients with neuromuscular disease on nocturnal positive pressure ventilation using a nasal mask or full face mask.[31,32] This noninvasive method of positive pressure ventilation avoids the need for tracheostomy in patients whose only problem is alveolar hypoventilation. This noninvasive ventilation is used as either a bridge to tracheostomy or a final attempt to prolong life, depending on the wishes of the patient.

TABLE 29-2. **Respiratory Care After Spinal Cord Injury**

In the Emergency Room

1. Assess respiratory function
   Vital capacity, MIP, MEP
   Arterial blood gases
   Chest x-ray
2. Supply O_2, humidification, mechanical ventilatory support as necessary to maintain PaO_2 above 70 mmHg
3. Pass a nasogastric tube for gastric decompression and prevention of aspiration
4. Be aware of the possibility of pulmonary edema following overtransfusion. (In the absence of other injuries, a systolic blood pressure of 90 mmHg may provide adequate perfusion as monitored by a urine output greater than 30 mL/h. When other injuries have resulted in hypovolemia, a central venous catheter may be needed to monitor fluid balance.)

In the ICU

1. Once the cervical spine is stabilized with Crutchfield tongs or other device and on a turning frame, turn the patient prone for 2 h at 4-h intervals, eg, 1, 5, 9 AM, 1, 5, 9 PM, with approval of the neurosurgeon.
2. Order chest physical therapy to be done immediately before and after pronation
   Breathing exercises
   Assisted coughing
   Incentive spirometry
3. In the presence of secretion retention
   Order IPPB with a nebulized bronchodilator to be given before pronation
   Consider bronchoscopy if lobar collapse is present on chest radiograph
   Sputum for Gram stain culture and sensitivities
4. Obtain chest radiograph and arterial blood gases the day after admission.
5. Obtain vital capacity MIP and MEP the day after admission and then twice weekly while in the intensive care unit.

After Leaving the ICU

1. Order side-to-side turning every 2 h
2. Order chest physical therapy (breathing exercises and assisted coughing) and incentive spirometry every 2 h except between 10 PM and 6 AM
3. Obtain vital capacity, MIP and MEP once a week

SUMMARY

As can be seen from the preceding discussion, the neuromuscular and respiratory systems are related in complex and important ways. Disease of either one can have complex and often devastating effects on the other. No chapter on this subject in a text on respiratory care can possibly be complete. The reader is referred to comprehensive texts on neurologic disease for a more complete review of specific diseases.

REFERENCES

1. Bozza Marrubini ML, Rossanda M, Tretola L: The role of artificial hyperventilation in the control of brain tension during neurosurgical operations. Br J Anaesth 36:415, 1964
2. James HE, Langfitt TW, Kumar VS, Ghostine SY: Treatment of intracranial hypertension: Analysis of 105 consecutive recordings of intracranial pressure. Acta Neurochir 36:189, 1977
3. Theodore J, Robin ED: Speculations on neurogenic pulmonary edema (NPE). Am Rev Respir Dis 113:405, 1976
4. McMichan JC, Piepgras DG, Gracey DR, et al: Electrophrenic Respiration. Report of six cases. Mayo Clin Proc 54:662, 1979
5. McMichan JC, Michel L, Westbrook PR: Pulmonary dysfunction following traumatic quadriplegia. JAMA 243:528, 1980
6. Piehler JM, Pairolero PC, Gracey DR, et al: Unexplained diaphragmatic paralysis: A harbinger of malignant disease? J Thorac Cardiovasc Surg 84:861, 1982
7. Boor JW, Johnson RJ, Carnales L, et al: Reversible paralysis of automatic respiration in multiple sclerosis. Arch Neurol 34:686, 1977
8. Lane DJ, Hazleman B, Nichols PVR: Late onset respiratory failure in patients with previous poliomyelitis. Q J Med 172:551, 1974
9. Sivak ED, Gipson WT, Hanson MR: Long-term management of respiratory failure in amyotrophic lateral sclerosis. Ann Neurol 12:18, 1981
10. Gracey DR, McMichan JC, Divertie MB, et al: Respiratory failure in Guillain-Barré Syndrome: A 6-year experience. Mayo Clin Proc 57:742, 1982
11. van der Meché FGA, Schmitz PIM, and the Dutch Guillain-Barré Study Group: A randomized trial comparing intravenous immune globulin and plasma exchange in Guillain-Barré syndrome. N Engl J Med 326:1123, 1992

12. Irani DN, Cornblath DR, Chaudhry V, Borel C, Hanley DF: Relapse in Guillain-Barré syndrome after treatment with human immune globulin. Neurology 43:872, 1993
13. Castro LHM, Ropper AH: Human immune globulin infusion in Guillain-Barré syndrome: Worsening during and after treatment. Neurology 43:1034, 1993
14. Wijdicks EFM, Lichty WJ, Harrison BA, Gracey DR: The clinical spectrum of critical illness polyneuropathy. Mayo Clin Proc 69: 955, 1994
15. Goldberg A: Acute intermittent porphyria: A study of 50 cases. Q J Med 110:183, 1959
16. Gracey DR, Divertie MB, Howard FM Jr: Mechanical ventilation for respiratory failure in myasthenia gravis: Two-year experience with 22 patients. Mayo Clin Proc 58:597, 1983
17. Gracey DR, Howard FM Jr, Divertie MB: Plasmapheresis in the treatment of ventilator-dependent myasthenia gravis patients: Report of four cases. Chest 85:739, 1984
18. Gracey DR, Southorn PA: Respiratory failure in Lambert-Eaton Myasthenic Syndrome. Chest 91:716, 1987
19. McCormack WM, Spalter HF: Muscular dystrophy, alveolar hypoventilation and papilledema. JAMA 197:957, 1966
20. Inkley SR, Oldenburg FC, Vigno PJ Jr: Pulmonary function in Duchenne muscular dystrophy related to stage of disease. Am J Med 56:297, 1974
21. Newsom DJ: The respiratory system in muscular dystrophy. Br Med Bull 36:135, 1980
22. Rosenow EC III, Engel AG: Acid maltase deficiency in adults presenting as respiratory failure. Am J Med 64:485, 1978
23. James JL, Park HWJ: Respiratory failure due to polymyositis treated by intermittent positive-pressure respiration. Lancet 2: 1281, 1961
24. Black LF, Hyatt RE: Maximal static respiratory pressures in generalized neuromuscular disease. Am Rev Respir Dis 103:641–650, 1971
25. Sharp JT: Respiratory muscles: A review of old and newer concepts. Lung 157:185–199, 1980
26. Cohen CA, Zagelbaum G, Gross D, et al: Clinical manifestations of inspiratory muscle fatigue. Am J Med 73:308, 1982
27. Rochester DF, Braun NMT: The respiratory muscles. New York, American Thoracic Society: Basics of RD, 1978, p 6
28. Splaingard ML, Frates RC, Jefferson LS, et al: Home negative pressure ventilation: Report of twenty years' experience in patients with neuromuscular disease. Arch Phys Med Rehabil 66:239, 1985
29. Holtackers TR, Loosbrock LM, Gracey DR: The use of the chest cuirass in respiratory failure of neurologic origin. Respir Care 27:271, 1982
30. Alexander MA, Johnson EW, Petty J, et al: Mechanical ventilation of patients with late stage Duchenne muscular dystrophy: Management in the home. Arch Phys Med Rehabil 60:289, 1979
31. Carrey Z, Gottfried SB, Levy RD: Ventilatory muscle support in respiratory failure with nasal positive pressure ventilation. Chest 97:150, 1990
32. Gay PC, Patel AM, Viggiano RW, Hubmayr RD: Nocturnal nasal ventilation for the treatment of patients with hypercapnic respiratory failure. Mayo Clin Proc 68:427, 1993

30 Infectious Disease Aspects of Respiratory Therapy

John A. Washington

CLINICAL SKILLS

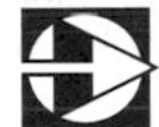

Upon completions of this chapter, the reader will:

- Classify microorganisms according to structure, parasitic domain, and survival capabilities
- Distinguish between saprophytic and parasitic microorganisms
- Recognize indigenous microflora in normal hosts
- Describe factors that may alter the normal indigenous microflora
- Discuss common microbial pathogenic mechanisms
- Identify the major host-defense mechanisms used by the host to avoid pulmonary infection
- List the normal anatomic barriers that are unimportant in host defense against pneumonia
- Describe alterations in oropharyngeal flora that may occur in seriously ill patients
- Identify the potential risks for the development of pneumonia posed by intubation and mechanical ventilation
- Discuss the etiology of community-acquired and hospital-acquired pneumonia
- Identify the major limitations of sputum culture
- Use invasive techniques for processing bronchoalveolar lavages and protected specimen brushes to allow interpretation of bacterial culture
- Avoid the spread of infectious diseases by using handwashing, universal precautions, and isolation procedures and list the essential features of each method
- Distinguish between universal precautions and body substance precautions
- Use physical and chemical means to sterilize, disinfect, and maintain respiratory equipment
- Take precautions to prevent the development of infusion-related sepsis

KEY TERMS

Adhesions
Bronchoalveolar lavage
Bronchoscopy
Disinfection
Eukaryotes
Neutralization
Open-lung biopsy
Opsonization
Prokaryotes
Protected catheter brush
Sterilization
Surfactant
Viruses

Pulmonary infections may be caused by a variety of microorganisms acquired either in the community or in the hospital, including bacteria, mycobacteria, chlamydiae, mycoplasmas, fungi, parasites, and viruses. Initial management of the patient with pulmonary infection therefore requires an understanding of various host factors, including age, sex, and occupation; underlying diseases or conditions; medications; sexual practices and preferences; place of acquisition of the infection (ie, community, hospital, or nursing home); circumstances surrounding onset of infection, such as the season of the year, recent travel or environmental exposures; and the type of presentation, including the mode of onset of illness and its rate of progression.

MICROBIAL CLASSIFICATION AND PATHOGENICITY

There are many approaches to the classification of microorganisms. First, they may be classified according to their structural characteristics as (1) viruses, which are the smallest infectious agents, have the simplest structure, and are obligate intracellular parasites; (2) prokaryotes, which lack a nuclear membrane enclosing chromosomal material, do not reproduce by mitosis, and include bacteria, chlamydiae, mycoplasmas, rickettsiae, and spirochetes; and (3) eukaryotes, which have chromosomes enclosed within a membrane, reproduce by mitosis, and include fungi and protozoa.

Bacteria have a rigid, relatively thick cell wall external to a cytoplasmic membrane that encloses their nuclear bodies, ribosomes, and a variety of small molecular structures, inorganic ions, and enzymes. The thickness of the bacterial cell wall is a major determinant of the Gram stain reaction in that the crystal violet–iodine complex is retained by the relatively thick cell wall of gram-positive (purple) bacteria but not by the thin cell wall of gram-negative (red) bacteria. Bacteria are further categorized morphologically as bacilli or cocci, and as aerobic, facultatively anaerobic, or anaerobic, according to their requirements for growth in air (aerobic), in the absence of oxygen (anaerobic), or their ability to grow under either condition (facultatively anaerobic). Chlamydiae and rickettsiae are obligate intracellular bacteria.

Fungi include yeast and filamentous (mold) forms and differ structurally from bacteria not only in having a nuclear membrane and in their mode of reproduction, but also by the presence of sterols in their cytoplasmic membranes and chitin in their cell walls. The protozoa, by contrast, share many structural properties with human cells.

Viruses contain a central core of DNA or RNA that is surrounded by a protein coat (capsid), which protects the viral nucleic acid from physical or chemical inactivation and facilitates attachment of the virus to the host cell. Other than their simple organization, viruses differ from prokaryotes or eukaryotes in their mode of reproduction in that, after their invasion of the host cell, viruses use the cell's machinery to synthesize their separate components and then assemble them into complete viral particles.

A second approach to classification of disease-producing microorganisms is according to whether they are extracellular parasites that produce infection by multiplying outside cells and are usually killed when ingested by phagocytes; facultative intracellular parasites that can be ingested, although not killed, by phagocytes; or obligate intracellular parasites that can multiply only within cells. Examples of the first category are *Streptococcus pneumoniae, Staphylococcus aureus, Escherichia coli, Pseudomonas aeruginosa,* and *Haemophilus influenzae.* Examples of the second category are mycobacteria (other than *Mycobacterium leprae*), *Legionella, Nocardia,* and fungi, such as *Candida, Cryptococcus,* and *Coccidioides.* Obligate intracellular parasites include chlamydiae, rickettsiae, and viruses.

Microorganisms are sometimes classified as *saprophytic* (ie, they can exist independently of a living host) or *parasitic* (ie, their survival depends on other living cells or tissue). Parasitic microorganisms may be commensals that coexist harmlessly with host cells or pathogens that damage host cells. The separation between commensals and pathogens has now become quite blurred in this era of immunocompromised patients, in that microorganisms previously thought to be harmless commensals (eg, coagulase-negative staphylococci) have been found to be pathogenic in patients with impaired host defenses or with implanted prosthetic devices or intravascular lines.

INDIGENOUS MICROBIAL FLORA

Many microorganisms are normally present on the skin and mucous membranes and therefore represent indigenous or commensal flora (Table 30-1). The oropharynx, for example, normally harbors more than 200 bacterial species in quantities of up to 10^8 bacteria per milliliter of saliva. Certain components of the indigenous flora vary because of occupational exposure. For example, *Staphylococcus aureus* is found in the nares of approximately 30% of the normal, healthy population; however, it may be found in the nares of up to 70% of hospitalized patients and health care personnel. Carriage of *S. aureus* on the hands is also significantly higher in health care personnel. Although not normally present on the skin, gram-negative bacilli, such as *Pseudomonas aeruginosa* and *Klebsiella pneumoniae,* may be transiently present on the skin. The transient carriage of such pathogenic microorganisms on the skin of health care personnel constitutes an important mechanism for nosocomial spread of infection within hospitals and underscores the importance of handwashing between treatment of each patient to limit the transmission of infectious agents.

The composition of indigenous flora can also be influenced by disease, environment, and antimicrobial agents. For example, enteric bacilli seldom constitute the indigenous flora of the oropharynx; however, they

TABLE 30-1. **Microorganisms Encountered on Healthy Human Body Surfaces***

Organism	**Skin**	**Conjunctiva**	**Upper Respiratory Tract**	**Mouth**	**Terminal Ileum, Cecum, Large Intestine**	**Genitourinary Tract**		
						External Genitalia	*Anterior Urethra*	*Vagina*
Bacteria								
Actinomyces			+	+	±			
Bacteroides					++	+	+	+
Bifidobacteria				+	++			
Clostridia	±			±	++		±	±
Corynebacteria	++	+	+	+	+	+	+	+
Enterobacteriaceae	±		±	±	++	+	+	±
Enterococcal			±	+	+	+	+	+
Eubacteria	±		±	+	++			±
Fusobacteria			+	++	+	+	+	±
Haemophili		±	++	+				+†
Lactobacilli				+	+		±	++
Neisseriae		±	++	+			±	±
Potphyromonae			++	++		++		++
Prevotelis				+		++	+	+
Propionibacteria	++	+	+	±	±			+
Staphylococci	++	+	+	+	±	++	+	+
Streptococci								
Pyogenic			±	±				± to ++‡
Viridans	±	±	±	++	+	+	+	+
Cocci, anaerobic								
Gram-positive	+	±	+	++	++	+	±	+
Gram-negative			+	++	+		±	+
Chlamydiae							±	±
Mycoplasmas			+	+			+	+
Spirochetes		+		±	+			
Fungi								
Aspergillus	±	±		+				
Candida	±	±	+	++	+			+
Cryptococcus	±			±				
Fusarium	±	±		±				
Penicillium	+	+		+				
Rhodotorula	±	±		+				

(Washington JA: Laboratory Procedures in Clinical Microbiology, 2nd ed, pp 2–3, Springer-Verlag, Mayo Foundation, 1985)

* ±, irregular or infrequent; +, common; ++, prominent.

† *Gardnerella vaginalis.*

‡ Group B.

are frequently found in this site in chronic alcoholics and in seriously ill and debilitated intensive care unit patients, regardless of whether such patients are receiving ventilatory assistance or antimicrobial therapy. Antimicrobial therapy may suppress the susceptible indigenous flora and allow colonization by pathogenic antibiotic-resistant microorganisms. Experimental data derived from animals have shown that a reduction in the normal gut flora facilitates colonization by pathogenic bacteria, such as *Salmonella, Pseudomonas,* or *Enterobacter.* Although the mechanism by which the indigenous flora of the gut plays a role in colonization resistance is unclear, selective decontamination regimens with antibiotics that spare the anaerobic bacterial flora of the gut have shown some success in some studies in preventing gram-negative infections in seriously ill intensive care unit patients, as well as during maximal immunosuppression of patients undergoing bone marrow transplantation. The most common lower respiratory pathogens are listed in Table 30-2.

MICROBIAL PATHOGENICITY

The first requirement for microbial pathogenicity is the microorganism's ability to adhere to epithelial surfaces. This process occurs through rather specific surface interactions involving *adhesins,* which are microbial surface molecules or organelles that bind to a receptor with complementary substrate molecules. Many bacteria, for example, possess fimbriae, which are filamentous structures that serve as adhesins that may be host-specific or specific for certain epithelial surfaces. For example, the meningococcus adheres by means of its fimbriae to nasopharyngeal cells more than to buccal or urethral cells. Pneumococci that are associated with oti-

TABLE 30-2. **Common Lower Respiratory Pathogens**

Class	Pathogens
Viruses	Influenza A Influenza B Adenoviruses Repiratory syncytial virus Parainfluenza viruses
Bacteria	*Streptococcus pneumoniae* *Staphylococcus aureus* *Haemophilus influenzae* *Enterobacteriaceae* *Klebsiella pneumoniae* *Pseudomonas aeruginosa* *Legionella* sp *Mycoplasma pneumoniae* *Chlamydia* sp
Fungi	*Coccidioides immitis* *Histoplasma capsulatum* *Blastomyces dermatitidis* *Aspergillus* sp *Cryptococcus neoformans* *Candida* sp
Protozoa	*Pneumocystis carinii**

* Taxonomy uncertain.

tis media adhere firmly to pharyngeal cells, whereas *P. aeruginosa* adheres more to nasal and tracheal cells than to buccal cells.

Once attached to an epithelial cell surface, the microorganism may multiply on the surface without invading the cell and produce disease by elaborating a soluble toxin that is absorbed by the cell to produce local or distant damage. Examples of such pathogens include *Corynebacterium diphtheriae*, which causes diphtheria, and *Bordetella pertussis,* which causes whooping cough.

Alternatively, microorganisms can multiply and cause disease by penetrating and damaging the cell, passing through the cell to the submucosa, and perhaps, spreading to other parts of the body, or, as with viruses, using the cell's machinery to reproduce themselves before damaging the cell.

HOST-DEFENSE MECHANISMS

The first line of host defense against microorganisms is the skin, which provides a mechanical barrier, except where its continuity is broken. An intact mucosal epithelial surface, including that of the conducting airways of the lung, is also important to host defense, but constitutes an appreciably less efficient barrier than does the skin. No bacteria are known to penetrate the intact skin. In fact, the acidic pH of normal skin, along with long-chain fatty acids that are located in sebaceous glands and have antibacterial activity, prevent the survival of pathogenic bacteria on the skin for any length of time. Moreover, many of the bacteria that make up the indigenous flora of the skin and mucous membranes produce bacteriocins, which are toxins directed at other bacteria. Nonetheless, because pathogenic microorganisms may survive transiently on the skin, the skin does serve as an important vehicle for transmission of infection, and careful handwashing, especially by health care workers, is an important control measure to prevent the transmission of infection.

An important internal defense mechanism is the inflammatory response. Once microorganisms penetrate the mechanical barrier of the skin or mucous membrane, they stimulate an inflammatory response, which consists of a variety of phagocytic cells, including neutrophils, monocytes, lymphocytes, and tissue macrophages. The functions of these cells is to ingest and destroy invading microorganisms, as well as to remove microbial and host debris and dispose of inflammation-producing toxins. Macrophages are normally present in the alveoli, in the interalveolar and peribronchial tissue, and near the surfaces of airways in the lungs. Pulmonary macrophages, therefore, are uniquely situated to interact with microorganisms and other particulate matter that have penetrated the normal mechanical barriers.

Many microorganisms resist phagocytosis by means of surface components, such as a capsule or a specific cell wall antigen. In such cases, plasma proteins may contain specific antibody that interacts with a plasma component (complement) that promotes phagocytosis.

Antibodies or immunoglobulins (Ig) are normally present in the body and bind to numerous foreign substances (antigens) that the host may encounter over a lifetime. Antibodies mediate humoral immunity and are intended to eliminate or destroy an antigen. Antibody is formed after a latent period of several days when the host is first exposed to an antigen (primary response). Antibody, predominantly IgM, increases exponentially, peaks in 1 or 2 weeks, and then decreases; however, reexposure to the same antigen provokes a secondary response in which the amount of antibody produced is substantially greater than that in the primary response and is predominantly of the IgG class.

Antibodies promote opsonization, whereby microorganisms become coated with antibody and complement and are prepared for ingestion by phagocytic cells; activation of the complement system that causes lysis of cells; neutralization of toxins; prevention of bacterial adherence to epithelial cells; and neutralization of viral infectivity, whereby viruses are prevented from attaching to cells.

Lymphocytes play a major role in the immune response in several ways. Lymphocytes are divided into two classes, B and T cells, according to their tissue of differentiation (bone marrow and thymus). The B lymphocytes synthesize immunoglobulins following exposure to specific antigens and are precursors of plasma cells, which are the major cells involved in antibody production. T lymphocytes have a number of functions in immunity. Some T lymphocytes enhance the immune response, whereas others suppress it. In general, however, cell-mediated immunity (CMI) is effected by T lymphocytes and contributes to host defenses against a variety of intracellular parasites, such as *Legionella, Mycobacterium, Chlamydia, Histoplasma,* and cytomegalovirus (CMV). Immunity to such infections cannot be transferred from immunized to nonimmunized hosts by serum-containing antibodies directed against the microorganisms causing these infections; rather, it may be transferred by lymphocytes from an immunized host to a nonimmunized host.

In brief, an antigen interacting with a macrophage is taken up by the macrophage, processed, and presented to B lymphocytes that are activated to synthesize antibody and to T lymphocytes that are stimulated to produce other factors responsible for CMI. At the same time, however, T lymphocytes may generate inhibitory or suppressor factors for cells, so that ultimately immunity represents a highly complex and as yet little understood process representing a balance between activation and regulation.

PATHOGENESIS OF PNEUMONIA

Host defenses that are specific to the respiratory tract include not only humoral-mediated immunity and CMI but also the ciliated and squamous epithelium in the nasopharynx, anatomic barriers such as the epiglottis and larynx, mucociliary clearance, coughing, bronchoconstriction, and secretory IgA.

The nasal ciliated epithelium overlies a submucosa with abundant plasma cells and secretes fluid containing predominantly IgA immunoglobulins, which may diminish bacterial attachment. IgA is also present in high concentrations in the large airways. At the alveolar level neither mucous-secreting cells nor ciliated epithelium is present, and microbial clearance depends on humoral and cellular factors. In addition, surfactant, which is excreted by pneumocytes in the alveoli, may inactivate certain bacteria. IgA and complement opsonize bacteria and prepare them for ingestion by alveolar macrophages. CMI is of particular importance for control of intracellular microorganisms, including mycobacteria, *Legionella, Listeria monocytogenes, Pneumocystis carinii,* and cytomegalovirus.

From the foregoing, it should be obvious that alteration of mechanical barriers, depressed cough reflex, immunoglobulin defects, complement deficiencies, and immunosuppression can predispose to pulmonary infection. Many factors contribute to the development of pneumonia, including those that are host specific, such as smoking, alcoholism, obesity, underlying disease (eg, diabetes, chronic obstructive pulmonary disease, prior viral illness, acidosis, trauma, altered consciousness), and immunosuppression (eg, hematologic malignancy, AIDS); invasive procedures, such as surgery, nasogastric and endotracheal intubation, and tracheostomy; and medications, such as antimicrobial agents, corticosteroids, cytotoxic agents, antacids or histamine type 2 receptor antagonists, and central nervous system depressants.

Microorganisms usually reach the lung by inhalation or, far less frequently, through the bloodstream from another infected site. Inhaled or aspirated microorganisms may originate from the oropharynx (endogenous) or from aerosols created exogenously, either from the environment or from other persons who are coughing or sneezing nearby.

As previously discussed, the oropharynx harbors a wide variety of bacterial species and a multitude of bacteria overall. This microbial flora is acquired shortly after birth and varies slightly in its composition from person to person. It may also vary because of interpersonal transmission from other family members or in other settings of close interpersonal contact, such as day care centers and nursing homes. Certain bacterial species have a predisposition for adherence to specific sites such as tooth surfaces, the tongue, or the buccal mucosa. Thus, potentially pathogenic bacteria must not only effectively compete with the indigenous flora of the oropharynx but also overcome local physical, chemical, and immunologic factors.

In seriously ill hospitalized patients, the oropharynx often becomes colonized with gram-negative bacilli, such as *E. coli, K. pneumoniae,* or *P. aeruginosa.* The mechanisms by which such colonization occurs are complex and not completely understood. One interesting observation is that colonization of the stomach may precede oropharyngeal colonization, as the result of enteral feedings or the administration of antacids or histamine type 2 receptor antagonists that increase gastric pH and allow bacterial overgrowth to occur.[1] Disruption of the esophagogastric junction by the presence of the nasogastric tube allows retrograde flow of gastric secretions containing bacteria into the oropharynx. Another observation is that antimicrobial therapy eradicates the largely susceptible indigenous flora of the oropharynx and allows it to be replaced by antibiotic-resistant "opportunistic" bacteria. Other potential mechanisms include transmission of pathogenic microorganisms from contaminated sources, such as respiratory equipment, hands of health care workers, and uncooked vegetables and fruits.

Whatever the mechanisms, oropharyngeal colonization with potentially pathogenic bacteria constitutes a major risk factor for the development of pneumonia. It should be emphasized, however, that because we normally aspirate small amounts of oropharyngeal secretions during sleep, factors such as the number of microorganisms aspirated, their pathogenicity, and the integrity of multiple host-defense mechanisms are important determinants of whether infection results.

Intubation poses a number of unique risk factors for the development of pneumonia: (1) The tube[1] reduces the natural warming and humidification of inspired air and bypasses the normal mechanical host defense barriers; (2) acts as a foreign body that causes local inflammation and alters bacterial colonization and causes obstruction and secondary infection of the paranasal sinuses; (3) traumatizes the tracheal epithelium, causing decreased bacterial clearance; (4) reduces the cough reflex and increases the need for suctioning to clear secretions; (5) allows bacterial access to the trachea; and (6) alters swallowing, oral hygiene, and nutritional status. The nasogastric tube also causes local trauma to and inflammation in surrounding tissues; acts as a foreign body, serving as a conduit for bacteria from the stomach to the pharynx; and prevents closure of the lower esophageal sphincter, which increases the reflux of gastric bacteria. For all of these reasons, the incidence of nosocomial pneumonia is about four times greater in the intubated patient than in the nonintubated patient.

The intubated patient is often connected to a mechanical ventilator with nebulization equipment that may become contaminated with bacteria and, thereby, poses risks for the development of pneumonia, depending on the size of the aerosol particles, the concentration of bacteria, and whether the aerosol is delivered directly through an endotracheal or tracheostomy tube. Only particles smaller than 4 μm in size will reach the terminal bronchioles and alveoli. Large-volume nebulizers with large (>500 mL) reservoirs and ultrasonic nebulizers pose the greatest risk of contamination and, therefore, of colonizing the patient with gram-negative bacilli. Although in-line nebulizers have small-volume reservoirs, contamination occurs frequently within 24 hours of use. Craven and Driks[1] have listed the possible sources of contamination of nebulizers as follows: (1) oxygen, (2) room air, (3) hands of hospital personnel, (4) use of contaminated water to fill the reservoir, (5) reflux of contaminated material into the reservoir, and (6) inadequate sterilization or disinfection of the equipment. In contrast with equipment for nebulizers, cascade humidifiers used in volume ventilators do not generate microaerosols and therefore substantially reduce the risk of colonization of the patient.

ETIOLOGIC AGENTS OF PULMONARY INFECTION

Although the microbial etiologies of pneumonias are quite diverse, age, underlying disease or condition, and place of acquisition of the infection are helpful in assessing therapeutic approaches to the patient. For example, respiratory syncytial virus, *Chlamydia trachomatis, Streptococcus pneumoniae,* and *Haemophilus influenzae* are the most frequent causes of pneumonia in 2-week-old to 6-month-old infants, whereas *S. pneumoniae, H. influenzae,* and adenoviruses are the most frequent causes of pneumonia in 7-month-old to 5-year-old children, and *S. pneumoniae,* adenoviruses, *Chlamydia pneumoniae,* and *Mycoplasma pneumoniae* are the most frequent causes of pneumonia in children over 5 years of age.[2]

For patients older than 15 years of age, *S. pneumoniae* remains the most frequent cause of community-acquired pneumonia; however, its incidence appears to have declined from 60% to 70% in the 1960s and 1970s to as low as 15% in more recent studies.(3) *Staphylococcus aureus, H. influenzae*, enteric gram-negative bacilli, *P. aeruginosa, Legionella,* and *Chlamydia pneumoniae,* have become more frequently associated with community-acquired pneumonias in adults, either because they were missed in earlier studies because methods were not available for their recovery (e.g., *Legionella* and *C. pneumoniae*) or because the populations that constitute the "community" changed(4). An aging population, changing life styles, increasing outpatient management of patients with serious underlying diseases and conditions, and evolving antibiotic resistance patterns have all contributed to a changing spectrum of the microorganisms that cause community-acquired pneumonia.

The place of acquisition of pneumonia is another important variable in determining its etiology. In some settings, for example, *Mycobacterium tuberculosis* may be a frequent cause of community-acquired pneumonia. The spectrum of microorganisms causing hospital-acquired (nosocomial) pneumonias differs from that causing community-acquired pneumonia and is predominantly gram-negative bacillary, including especially *P. aeruginosa, E. coli, K. pneumoniae,* and *Enterobacter* species.

Legionellosis may result from inhalation of dust from excavation sites or from aerosols from contaminated cooling towers, shower heads, and respiratory therapy humidification reservoirs.

Blastomyces dermatitidis, Coccidioides immitis, and *Histoplasma capsulatum* are found in soil in the mold (mycelial) form and produce spores that may be inhaled and cause, in most instances, asymptomatic infection in individuals present in endemic areas. Individuals who have not previously encountered the fungus (such as upper Midwesterners) and who encounter unusually large concentrations of the fungus may develop clinically apparent infection (in this example, coccidioidomycosis). Thus, travel history is an important component of a careful history.

DIAGNOSTIC TECHNIQUES FOR LOWER RESPIRATORY INFECTIONS

Diagnosis is suggested by the patient's age, clinical presentation, underlying disease, environmental and historical factors, and radiographic and laboratory tests. Definitive diagnosis depends on the detection or isolation of an etiologic agent from lower respiratory secretions or on the detection of antibodies specific for a particular etiologic agent. A variety of diagnostic techniques are available and are recommended by the American Thoracic Society[4] for community-acquired pneumonia and by the American College of Chest Physicians for ventilator-associated pneumonia.[5,6]

Because of the number and variety of microorganisms that are normally present in the oropharynx, culture of specimens collected through the oropharynx are more difficult to interpret than are those obtained by bypassing this site. Normally, the tracheobronchial tree below the level of the larynx is sterile or only minimally colonized with bacteria so that specimens taken directly from lung tissue or by methods designed to minimize contamination by oropharyngeal flora facilitate diagnosis. Exceptions to these rules are microorganisms that usually represent pathogens, regardless of their source and whether that source is contaminated by other microorganisms. Among the usually pathogenic microorganisms are *M. tuberculosis, B. dermatitidis, C. immitis, H. capsulatum, M. pneumoniae,* respiratory viruses, and *Legionella.*

The procedure selected for obtaining specimens for the diagnosis of lower respiratory infection depends on the suspected diagnosis or disease, underlying diseases or conditions, prior antimicrobial therapy, and the availability of technical expertise for performing invasive procedures.[5] Communication between the clinician and the pathologist or microbiologist is important, especially when unusual pathogens are being considered and when special laboratory procedures are required. In certain instances, such as with bronchoalveolar lavage (BAL) and open-lung biopsy, it is desirable for the clinician and the pathologist or microbiologist to establish protocols to ensure that specimens are routinely examined carefully for the most likely pathogen.

SPECIMEN TYPES AND COLLECTION

Noninvasive Procedures

Expectorated sputum is the specimen most frequently collected for diagnosis of pneumonia; however, its value remains highly controversial because of the difficulties involved in obtaining lower respiratory secretions that are uncontaminated by upper respiratory flora and, therefore, in interpreting results of cultures. Sputum for Gram stain and culture generally should be obtained from patients who have pneumonia or acute airways infection; however, it is important to instruct the patient to remove any dentures and to rinse or gargle the mouth with water before attempting to expectorate, into a specimen container, a specimen resulting from a deep cough. When asked simply to spit into a jar, most patients will usually oblige by providing a sample of saliva, the bacteriology of which is well established in the literature and culture of which provides no clinically useful information.

The expectoration of sputum requires, among other things, an alert, cooperative patient who may have to try several times to produce a satisfactory specimen. One method used in many laboratories today to assess the suitability of sputum for bacterial culture is to examine the specimen microscopically for the presence of squamous epithelial cells. Squamous epithelial cells are normally present in the oropharynx so that their presence in large numbers in sputum means that the specimen is substantially contaminated with oropharyngeal secretions (spit) and, therefore, is not suitable for bacterial culture. The absence of alveolar macrophages or bronchial epithelial cells microscopically indicates the absence of any lower respiratory secretions whatsoever in the specimen. Under these circumstances, the laboratory should reject the specimen as being unacceptable for culture and request that another specimen be collected. Because the recovery of mycobacteria (eg, *M. tuberculosis*) and certain fungi (eg, *H. capsulatum*) is clinically significant, regardless of the quality of the specimen, rejection of specimens for mycobacterial and fungal cultures on the basis of microscopic examination is inappropriate; however, there is no disputing the fact that mycobacteria and fungi are far more likely to be recovered from specimens consisting predominantly of lower respiratory secretions than from those consisting predominantly of saliva.

Given all of the problems associated with collection of a valid sputum specimen, it should not be surprising that in some hospitals the responsibility for patient instruction and collection of specimens lies with the respiratory therapist.

For the diagnosis of bacterial pneumonia, it is generally sufficient to obtain a single sputum specimen; however, for the diagnosis of mycobacterial or deep fungal infections, it is recommended that specimens be obtained on three to five successive mornings. Formerly, it was routine practice to collect and pool specimens over a 24-hour period for mycobacterial culture; however, this practice has been abandoned because overgrowth by normal oropharyngeal flora interfered with the recovery of mycobacteria from cultures.

In some instances, patients with pneumonia do not have a productive cough, and a productive cough is induced by having these patients inhale an aerosol or hypertonic salt solution. Such *sputum induction* is helpful in the diagnosis of mycobacterial, deep fungal, and, in acquired immune compromised patients, *Pneumocystis carinii* pneumonias.

Invasive Procedures

There is a wide variety of invasive techniques, ranging from nasotracheal suctioning to open-lung biopsy, that are considered for use in patients who are not able to produce sputum (spontaneous or induced), whose sputum examination provides equivocal or inconclusive results, or whose condition either fails to improve or worsens following the initiation of antimicrobial therapy. When performed skillfully, nasotracheal suction can be used to obtain sputum; however, when repeated attempts must be made to get the catheter into the trachea, oropharyngeal secretions are greatly stimulated, and it becomes nearly impossible not to contaminate the specimen.

In some instances *transtracheal aspiration* was considered to be useful for the detection of bacterial pathogens and, especially, for anaerobic bacteria because this method bypasses the oropharynx, which is heavily colonized with such bacteria. The procedure has been largely replaced by bronchoscopy procedures.

In the intubated patient, lower respiratory secretions often are contaminated by oral flora from upper respiratory secretions that pool around and leak past the cuff of the tube; therefore, the distinction between bacterial colonization and infection becomes difficult.

Bronchoscopy is often used in patients with acute severe infections, in chronic or refractory infections, and in immunocompromised patients for whom a diagnosis cannot be made from an expectorated or induced sputum specimen. There are two special procedures that warrant discussion. The first is bronchoscopy with a *protected catheter brush* consisting of a double-lumen, distally occluded brush catheter. The catheter is inserted through the bronchoscope channel to an area of infection, and the inner protected brush catheter is then advanced through the outer cannula; the distally occluding propylene glycol tip is jettisoned, and the brush is extended beyond the catheter tip into the area of the infection. Once the specimen has been obtained, the brush is retracted into the inner catheter and the entire catheter is withdrawn from the bronchoscope. The brush is then transected with a sterile scissors and placed into 1 mL of sterile lactated Ringer's solution (without preservative) for transport to the laboratory. The protected brush catheter is intended to minimize contamination of the lower respiratory tract by upper respiratory flora that is carried into the lower respiratory tract by the bronchoscope.

When quantitative culture of the brush is performed, it is often possible to distinguish between contamination and infection.[6] Once again, because the recovery of mycobacteria and deep fungi in any quantity is significant and because selective techniques are used for the recovery of mycobacteria and fungi in cultures, use of the protected brush catheter is most useful in the diagnosis of bacterial infection.

A second, special bronchoscopy procedure is BAL, whereby the tip of the bronchoscope is wedged into an infected bronchus and isotonic saline is instilled into the bronchus, aspirated, and collected in a suction trap. Several instillations are usually collected to obtain 40 to 70 mL of lavage fluid. The fluid is then concentrated by centrifugation and the concentrate used for microscopic examination and culture.[6] Although quantitative culture of BAL fluid is helpful in distinguishing between bacterial colonization and infection, the procedure of BAL is usually performed to diagnose opportunistic infections caused by microorganisms other than bacteria, such as mycobacteria, fungi, *P. carinii,* and viruses. Either the protected brush catheter or BAL may be helpful in the diagnosis of ventilator-associated pneumonia. Histopathologic examination of a transbronchial lung biopsy taken during the course of bronchoscopy may yield additional diagnostic information, especially in cases with chronic fungal infections or noninfectious causes of pulmonary infiltrates.

In a few instances, the aforementioned invasive procedures will still be nondiagnostic and an open-lung biopsy is performed for definitive diagnosis. Obviously, this procedure involves general anesthesia, a chest incision, and the risk of postoperative complications, such as pneumothorax, hemorrhage, or infection. Use of the open-lung biopsy appears to be declining as a result of the increasing use and diagnostic yield of BAL. Also, obtaining a lung biopsy through a thoracoscope that has been passed into the pleural space avoids a large thoracotomy incision and is becoming increasingly popular as a method for obtaining a sample of lung tissue.

Once a protected specimen brush, BAL, or lung biopsy specimen has been collected, it is imperative that the specimen be transported to the laboratory as soon as possible so that microbial viability is not lost. It is also essential that the microbiology laboratory has protocols in place to ensure that these specimens are processed for microscopic examination for bacteria (including *Legionella*), mycobacteria, fungi, viruses, and *Pneumocystis carinii.* In addition, a protocol should be in place for culture of such specimens for bacteria (including *Legionella*), mycobacteria, fungi, and viruses.

PREVENTION OF INFECTION

Because of the high morbidity, and especially in the case of nosocomial pneumonia, prevention represents the major component of any program for control of pneumonia. Prevention may focus on three areas: host defenses, colonization, and aspiration. Immunization (eg, pneumococcal and influenza vaccines), therapy and control of underlying diseases or conditions, and nutritional support contribute to or enhance host defenses. A variety of experimental approaches to stimulate CMI are under investigation and may be helpful in preventing pneumonia in the immunocompromised patient in the future.

Measures to prevent colonization by potentially pathogenic microorganisms take many forms. One form is environmental control, including handwashing, isolation procedures, control of contamination of equipment; maintenance of an acidic gastric pH; and, perhaps in the future, measures that prevent microbial adhesion to mucous membranes and foreign objects.

Measures to prevent aspiration include the avoidance of central nervous system depressants and, perhaps in the future, novel intubation devices that would minimize aspiration of pharyngeal flora into the lung.

Of the three areas just described for prevention of pneumonia, those of colonization and environmental control are most germane to respiratory therapy. An ongoing assessment of the effectiveness of environmental and colonization control falls within the purview of a nosocomial infection control program, the essential components of which are an effective surveillance program designed to establish and maintain a data base that describes the endemic infection rates of nosocomial infection and therefore allows recognition of epidemic occurrences; the establishment of a series of regulations and policies to reduce the risk of nosocomial infection; and the maintenance of a continuing education program.[7] Ordinarily, these functions are the responsibility of an infection-control practitioner who works with a hospital epidemiologist, both of whom are responsible to the hospital's infection-control committee, which develops guidelines, regulations, or policies that ideally are designed to foster habits and attitudes that lead to reduced nosocomial infections.

Handwashing

The fact that disease-producing microorganisms are frequently present on the hands of health care personnel has been recognized for more than a century. Transfer of microorganisms between the patient and the hands of health care personnel is well documented, and personnel hands have been shown to be a major vector of transmission of bacterial, fungal, and viral infections in burn units, intensive care units, and a variety of other hospital settings. The risk of skin and postoperative wound infections has also been related to general handwashing practices. Although plain soap appears to be sufficient to reduce fecal–oral transmission, antiseptic products may have added benefits in reducing nosocomial infections.[8] Evidence of the benefits of handwashing notwithstanding, the major difficulty is compliance with handwashing policies on busy wards or intensive care units without a conveniently located sink.

Handwashing should be carried out before and after contact with patients or their body fluids or secretions, even though gloves are worn. Gloves should not be washed because washing may cause the rubber to deteriorate, and washing gloves does not remove microorganisms from gloves. Gloves must therefore be removed and the hands washed immediately and before regloving to examine or treat another patient.

Universal Precautions

Whereas isolation procedures that are either disease- or category-specific have been in use in hospitals for decades, the advent of the epidemic of infections caused by the human immunodeficiency virus (HIV) resulted in a major change in isolation procedures, to include universal precautions for blood-borne pathogens in which all patients are regarded as being potentially infectious for HIV or hepatitis B virus (HBV). The key element in universal precautions is that of protective barriers to be used by health care workers (ie, gloves, gowns, masks, and eyewear). The major difference between universal precautions and the established isolation procedures is that the latter are applied when infection has been established or is suspected, whereas with universal precautions all patients are considered to be potentially infectious for HIV or HBV.[9] Because the focus of universal precautions is on blood-borne pathogens, there remain instances in which category- or disease-specific isolation is still required. Under universal precautions, gloves should be worn when touching blood and other specified body fluids in which blood-borne pathogens might be present (ie, pleural, pericardial, peritoneal, and synovial fluids; semen and vaginal secretions; and any body fluid visibly contaminated with blood). Masks and protective eyewear should be worn to protect the mucous membranes of the nose and mouth and the eyes when procedures are performed that are likely to produce droplets of blood or other body fluids, and gowns are to be worn during procedures when blood or other body fluids are likely to be splashed or sprayed.

Isolation Procedures

Isolation procedures for patients with non–blood-borne infections may be approached by the traditional methods recommended by the Centers for Disease Control and Prevention (CDC) or by an alternative method described as body substance isolation.[9] Gloves should be worn for any contact with mucous membranes, skin, secretions, wound drainages, and other body fluids, such as urine or feces. Handwashing should be performed whenever the gloves become visibly soiled and when the gloves are changed between patients. Although body substance isolation is a comprehensive approach, it does not totally replace the CDC's isolation guidelines.[9]

Under existing CDC isolation precautions or body substance isolation, specific measures must be taken with patients with known or suspected tuberculosis. These measures are aimed at reducing airborne tubercle bacilli by removing and diluting the air in the patient's room and by the use of protective respirators. Air in the patient's room must be under negative pressure with respect to the anteroom or hallway. The room air must be exchanged at least 6 times per hour and must be discharged to the outdoors, where it is diluted, or if this is not possible, the air must be subjected to high-efficiency particulate air (HEPA) filtration before its recirculation. A private room is recommended. The type of respirator that should be used is the object of considerable debate at this time. In 1990 the CDC recommended the use of a disposable particulate respirator for health care workers who enter an isolation room with a patient with known or suspected tuberculosis. In October, 1994 the CDC issued guidelines recommending use of the HEPA respirators on the basis that these represented the only class of respirators that were known to consistently meet or exceed the performance criteria previously specified by the CDC and because such respirators were certified by the National Institute for Occupational Safety and Health (NIOSH) as required by the Occupational Safety and Health Administration (OSHA). Since that time NIOSH has announced its intention to change its certification process so that users should be able to select from a broader range of certified respirators for use in the hospital. Further information on these changes is being awaited.

Confusion over body substance isolation and category-specific isolation precautions that have been published and updated over the years by the CDC has led to new recommendations for isolation precautions in hospitals that have been presented in a draft outline in the Federal Register.[9] The document reviews the history of isolation precautions developed by the CDC and proposes revisions of these guidelines based on modes of transmission of pathogens. These include contact transmission, direct and indirect; droplet transmission; airborne transmission; and common vehicle transmission. These proposed guidelines are subject to public comment and revision before publication in final form.

Although HIV has been isolated from blood, vaginal secretions, semen, saliva, tears, urine, cerebrospinal fluid, breast milk, and amniotic fluid, transmission of HIV has been linked only to blood and blood products, semen, vaginal secretions, and possibly breast milk. It occurs through sexual contact; parenteral (intravenous) exposure, including transfusion of blood or blood products, sharing of needles and syringes with illicit drug use, occupational needlestick injuries, and contact of blood with mucous membranes or skin lesions; and perinatal exposure.

Occupational exposure to HIV among health care workers has been under surveillance by the CDC since

1981. Between 1981 and 1992 the CDC identified 32 documented and 69 possible occupationally acquired HIV infections in health care workers.[10] Of those with documented occupationally acquired infection, 84% had percutaneous exposure and the remainder had mucocutaneous or mucocutaneous *and* percutaneous exposure. Only one of the documented occupationally acquired cases was in a respiratory therapist; the majority of cases were in clinical laboratory workers and in nurses. Studies conducted by the CDC and at several major medical centers, for example, indicate the risk of HIV infection following injury with a needle contaminated with the blood of an HIV-infected patient is less than 0.5%, compared with a 6% to 30% risk of HBV infection following an injury from a needle contaminated with the blood of a patient with HBV infection. The reason is that HIV is present at concentrations of only about 100 tissue culture infectious doses (TCID)/mL of blood, whereas HBV is present at concentrations of 10^8 to 10^9 TCID/mL of blood.

Persons who become infected with HIV usually develop antibodies within 6 to 12 weeks after infection. These antibodies, which are not protective but, rather, indicate infection with HIV, can be detected by an enzyme immunoassay (EIA). Although EIAs are highly sensitive and highly specific, false-negative results may occur during the first several weeks of infection before detectable antibody appears. Conversely, the presence of nonspecific and cross-reactive antibodies may cause a false-positive EIA result. Consequently, positive results of EIA must be regarded with caution and require confirmation with a more specific antibody test, such as the Western blot. As with any test, the sensitivity, specificity, false-negative, and false-positive rates of the HIV EIA will vary according to the population tested and the incidence and prevalence of HIV in such populations. Thus, it is customary to retest any serum sample that yields a positive EIA result for HIV antibody and, then, to perform a confirmatory test on any sample that has been repeatedly positive by the EIA method.

Although there is now a commercially available rapid EIA test for HIV antibodies, the test is quite expensive and therefore not suitable for routine purposes. Moreover, because of universal precautions and body substance isolation, there should be no need for a stat test for detecting HIV antibodies. Even if a rapid test is found to be positive, the result would still require confirmation with a Western blot, which is not a rapid test. For the diagnosis of HIV infection in patients in the early stages of HIV infection before the formation of detectable antibodies with the EIA test, there is now available the polymerase chain reaction (PCR), which is used to detect the virus by means of a gene amplification technique; however, this also is not a rapid test and is very expensive to perform.

More specific guidelines for the care of patients are as follows[10]:

1. Gloves should be worn for direct contact with blood, body fluids and secretions, wounds, and for handling all items or surfaces that are contaminated with blood, body fluids, or secretions. Gloves should be worn for venipuncture and for handling vascular access lines or intravascular monitoring devices.
2. Gloves should be changed between patients, when they are torn, or whenever a perforation occurs, as with a needlestick injury. Hands should be washed whenever gloves are removed.
3. Hands should be washed immediately whenever contamination with blood or body fluids or secretions occurs.
4. Masks and protective eyewear or face shields should be worn during procedures in which splattering, splashing, or generation of droplets of blood, body fluids, or secretions is likely to occur.
5. Gowns or aprons should be worn under conditions described in item 4.
6. Precautions should be taken when handling needles and sharp instruments. Used disposable needles and syringes, scalpels, and other sharp items should be placed into puncture-resistant containers for disposal. Used needles should not be bent, broken, recapped, or cut.
7. Mouthpieces, resuscitation bags, and other ventilatory devices should be available to minimize the need for mouth-to-mouth resuscitation.
8. All blood and body fluid specimens should be placed into a sturdy, leakproof container (eg, ziplock bag) for transport to the laboratory. The laboratory requisition form should be placed outside this container to minimize contamination.
9. Health care workers with exudative skin lesions should refrain from patient care activities.

DISINFECTION AND STERILIZATION

Disinfection means the removal of microorganisms capable of causing infection; sterilization means the elimination of all viable microorganisms. The principal difference between the two is, for all practical purposes, the elimination of bacterial spores by sterilization, but not by disinfection. In either case, the elimination of microorganisms does not take place instantaneously, but, rather, occurs over time in the form of a straight-line killing curve. The number of microorganisms killed is proportional to the number that is initially present. Thus, a particular process may be disinfecting or sterilizing, depending on the exposure time.

There are many physical and chemical methods available for disinfection and sterilization. Moist heat under pressure (autoclaving) and ethylene oxide gas are the principal sterilization methods in use today. In the autoclave, killing of organisms is achieved at high temperatures (121°C), using steam at 2 atm of pressure. Ethylene oxide (ETO) is a gas that is widely used to sterilize many heat-sensitive products. This technique is particularly useful in respiratory therapy, with its wide use of plastic products. Under specified conditions and use, chemical germicides that are ordinarily used as disinfectants may be used for sterilization purposes.

Disinfectants have been classified in three levels: high, intermediate, and low. A high-level disinfectant is effective against bacterial spores (sporicidal), vegetative bacteria, tubercle bacilli (tuberculocidal), fungi, and viruses. Intermediate-level disinfectants may, but do not necessarily, exert some sporicidal activity. They do exert tuberculocidal, bactericidal, fungicidal, and limited virucidal activity. HBV and HIV are inactivated by several intermediate- to high-level disinfectants, including aqueous glutaraldehyde, stabilized hydrogen peroxide, peracetic acid, aqueous formaldehyde, iodophors, and chlorine compounds.

In all instances, proper physical cleaning of any item is an absolute prerequisite for disinfection because blood, mucus, feces, or soil may shield microorganisms from the disinfectant or sterilant or may actually inactivate the disinfectant or sterilant. Moreover, it is essential to carefully follow the manufacturer's instructions for use of the disinfectant and for its suitability for the purposes intended. The selection and final concentration of disinfectant will depend on the surface to be disinfected.

Household bleach in a 1:10 to 1:100 dilution (made up fresh on a daily basis) may be used for surface decontamination; however, bleach may be corrosive to metallic surfaces and, as with other disinfectants, is less effective if serum, blood, or other proteinaceous materials are not first removed by cleaning with detergent. Low-level quaternary ammonium compounds should not be used for disinfection purposes, and phenolics should not be used on HIV- or HBV-contaminated medical devices. For blood spills, the blood should be absorbed with disposable towels; the spill site is then cleaned of all visible blood with a detergent, and finally wiped down with disposable towels soaked with an intermediate- to high-level disinfectant. All disposable materials used in the decontamination process should be placed into a biohazard container.

DECONTAMINATION AND MAINTENANCE OF VENTILATORY EQUIPMENT

There are many measures to be taken in the prevention of nosocomial pneumonia that have been recommended by the CDC in a document published in draft form in the Federal Register[11] and in final form in the *The American Journal of Infection Control.*[12] Among these recommendations are those specific to sterilization, disinfection, and maintenance of mechanical equipment and devices. Guidelines are categorized according to scientific evidence, theoretical applicability, and economic impact. Category IA contains guidelines that are strongly recommended for all hospitals and that are strongly supported by either experimental or clinical evidence. Category IB guidelines are also recommended for all hospitals and are viewed as effective by experts and a consensus process based on strong rationale and suggestive evidence. Category II guidelines are strongly suggested for many hospitals; recommendations in this category may be supported by suggestive clinical or epidemiologic studies, a strong theoretical rationale, or definitive studies applicable to some but not all hospitals. In addition, in the document there are a number of unresolved issues for which no recommendations could be made because no data were available as to efficacy of some specific measures.

Specific measures that were recommended in the section on sterilization, disinfection, and maintenance of mechanical equipment are summarized in Table 30-3.

INFUSION THERAPY

Although not directly related to lower respiratory infection, infusion therapy[13] for blood or blood products, drugs, fluids, or nutrition is used in many seriously ill patients. Approximately one half of all epidemics of nosocomial bloodstream infections (bacteremias and candidemias) are related to intravascular catheters. The sources of the infection are infected cannulas (ie, devices used for temporary vascular access, including plastic catheters used for hyperalimentation, hemodynamic monitoring, and hemodialysis) and, less frequently, contaminated infusates. Infection of cannulas is generally caused by introduction of microorganisms either along the external surface or within the lumen of the catheter, with organisms present on the skin of the patient or from the hands of the person inserting or manipulating the cannula. Bacteria adhere to irregularities in the surface of the cannula and form a biofilm consisting of proteins and polysaccharides. Within this biofilm, bacteria multiply that are resistant to high concentrations of antibiotics and phagocytosis.

The frequency of cannula-associated infection varies widely and is often related to the care exercised during insertion and the length of time the cannula is left in place. Contaminated infusate may result from the introduction of microorganisms during preparation and administration in the hospital.

Prevention of infusion-related sepsis depends on careful handwashing before cannula insertion, the use of sterile gloves, and aseptic technique when inserting cannulas into high-risk patients; or when inserting high-risk cannulas, the daily surveillance of all intravascular lines, limiting the use of lines for hemodynamic monitoring to 4 days, exercising care when compounding parenteral admixtures, and routinely replacing the entire delivery system including infusion sets every 72 hours.[13]

The laboratory diagnosis of intravascular device-associated bacteremia has been the subject of much study and controversy. A variety of approaches have been used, including the following: (1) microscopic examination of the catheter surface for the presence of bacteria; (2) semiquantitative culture of the skin surrounding the catheter insertion site; (3) culture of the catheter hub; (4) semiquantitative culture of solution flushed through a catheter segment; (5) semiquantitative culture of the external surface of the catheter by rolling it across the surface of an agar plate; (6) semiquantitative culture of the external and internal surfaces

TABLE 30-3. **Recommendations for the Sterilization, Disinfection, and Maintenance of Mechanical Equipment**

Recommendation	Category
General Measures	
Thoroughly clean all equipment and devices to be sterilized or disinfected.	Category 1A
Sterilize or use high-level disinfection for all semicritical equipment or devices (ie, items that come in contact with the mucous membranes of the lower respiratory tract). Follow disinfection with appropriate rinsing, drying, and packaging, taking care not to contaminate the item in the process.	Category 1B
Use sterile (not distilled, nonsterile water) for rinsing reusable semicritical equipment or devices used in the respiratory tract after they have been chemically disinfected.	Category 1B
No recommendation for using tap water as an alternative to sterile water for rinsing reusable, semicritical equipment or devices used in the respiratory tract following high-level disinfection, whether or not rinsing is followed by drying with or without alcohol.	Unresolved issue
Do not reprocess any equipment or device that is manufactured for single use only, unless data show that reprocessing the equipment or device poses no threat to the patient, is cost-effective, and does not change the structural integrity or function of the equipment or device.	Category 1B
Mechanical Ventilators, Breathing Circuits, Humidifiers, and Nebulizers for Respiratory Therapy	
Mechanical Ventilators	
Do not routinely sterilize or disinfect the internal machinery of mechanical ventilators.	Category 1A
Ventilator Circuits With Humidifiers	
Do not routinely change the breathing circuit more frequently than every 48 hours, including tubing and exhalation valve, and the attached bubbling or wick humidifier of a ventilator that is in use on an individual patient.	Category IA
No recommendation on the maximum length of time after which the breathing circuit and the attached bubbling or wick humidifier of a ventilator in use on a patient should be changed.	Unresolved issue
Sterilize reusable breathing circuits and bubbling or wick humidifiers or subject them to high-level disinfection between their uses on different patients.	Category IB
Periodically drain and discard any condensate that collects in the tubing of a mechanical ventilator, taking precautions not to allow condensate to drain towards the patient. Wash hands after performing procedure or handling the fluid.	Category IB
No recommendation for placing a filter or trap at the distal end of the expiratory-phase tubing of the breathing circuit to collect condensate.	Unresolved issue
Do not place bacterial filters between the humidifier reservoir and the inspiratory-phase tubing of the breathing circuit of a mechanical ventilator.	Category IB
Humidifier Fluids	
Use sterile water to fill bubbling humidifiers.	Category II
Use sterile, distilled, or tap water to fill wick humidifiers.	Category II
No recommendation for the preferential use of a closed, continuous-feed humidification system.	Unresolved issue
Ventilator Breathing Circuit With Hygroscopic Condenser-Humidifiers or Heat-Moisture Exchangers	
No recommendation for the preferential use of any hygroscopic condenser-humidifier or heat-moisture exchanger rather than a heater humidifier to prevent nosocomial pneumonia.	Unresolved issue
Change the hygroscopic condenser-humidifier or heat-moisture exchanger according to manufacturer's recommendations and/or when evidence of gross contamination or mechanical dysfunction of the device is present.	Category IB
Do not routinely change a breathing circuit attached to a hygroscopic condenser-humidifier or heat-moisture exchanger while it is in use on a patient.	Category IB
Wall Humidifiers	
Follow manufacturer's instructions for use and maintenance on wall oxygen humidifiers unless data show that modification of their use or maintenance poses no threat to the patient and is effective.	Category IB
Between patients, change the tubing, including any nasal prongs or mask used to deliver oxygen from any wall outlet.	Category 1B
Large-Volume Nebulizers and Mist Tents	
Do not use large-volume room-air humidifiers that create aerosols and thus are really nebulizers, unless they can be sterilized or subjected to high-level disinfection at least daily and filled only with sterile water.	Category IA
Sterilize large-volume nebulizers that are used for inhalation therapy (eg, for tracheostomized patients) or subject them to high-level disinfection between patients and after every 24 hours of use on the same patient.	Category IB
Use sterile nebulizers and reservoirs that have undergone sterilization or high-level disinfection and replace between patients.	Category IB
No recommendations regarding the frequency of changing mist-tent nebulizers and reservoirs while in use on one patient.	Unresolved issue

(continued)

TABLE 30-3. **Recommendations for the Sterilization, Disinfection, and Maintenance of Mechanical Equipment** (Continued)

Other Devices Used for Respiratory Therapy	
Between patients, sterilize or use high-level disinfection respirometers, oxygen sensors, and other respiratory devices used on multiple patients.	Category 1B
Between patients, sterilize or use high-level disinfection reusable hand-powered resuscitation bags.	Category 1A
No recommendation regarding the frequency of changing hydrophobic filters placed on the connection port of resuscitation bags.	Unresolved issue

* See text for category definitions.
Data from Tablan OC, Arden NH, Breiman RF, et al: Guidelines for prevention of nosocomial pneumonia. Am J Infect Control 22:247–292, 1994.

of the catheter by sonicating it in a solution and culturing a specified volume of the solution quantitatively on agar; and (7) differential blood cultures in which quantitative cultures are performed of blood drawn concurrently from a peripheral vein and from the catheter. All but the last technique require removal of the catheter. Controversial issues surrounding all of these methods include, first and foremost, what should be the "gold standard" for defining intravascular catheter-related bacteremia (ie, clinical signs and symptoms versus positive culture).

The first problem regarding the use of a positive culture is the criterion used to define a positive culture; that is, the number of colonies per plate (in the case of the roll method) or the number of colonies per milliliter (in the case of the sonication method). Published breakpoints for each method are designed primarily to distinguish between contamination and infection caused by *Staphylococcus epidermidis*, which is the most frequent isolate from such cultures. Using clinical criteria as the gold standard for identifying intravascular catheter-related sepsis, neither catheter tip culture method is particularly sensitive nor specific, and adjusting the breakpoints in either direction to increase sensitivity, for example, results in a loss of specificity. An added complication has been the introduction of molecular epidemiologic techniques, which now permit one to establish with a high level of certainty that any two isolates of *S. epidermidis* are or are not genetically related, whereas previously they might have been assumed to have been so on the basis of species identity and antibiotic susceptibility pattern identity. Now we know that isolation of *S. epidermidis* from both the blood and a catheter tip may or may not represent the same organism and that this fact can only be established by molecular epidemiologic techniques. Such techniques further diminish the sensitivity and specificity of catheter cultures. The same problem also applies to differential blood cultures in that the isolation of *S. epidermidis* from both peripheral and catheter-drawn blood cultures does not guarantee their genetic relatedness. In summary, the value of intravascular catheter cultures is limited and has led some to conclude that the practice should be discontinued altogether except when there is obvious purulence at the catheter insertion site.

REFERENCES

1. Craven DE, Driks MR: Nosocomial pneumonia in the intubated patient. Semin Respir Infect 2:20–33, 1987
2. Klein JO: Emerging perspectives in management and prevention of infections of the respiratory tract in infants and children. Am J Med 78 (Suppl 6B):38–44, 1985
3. Fang G-D, Fine M, Orloff J, et al: New and emerging etiologies for community-acquired pneumonia with implications for therapy. Medicine 69:309–316, 1990
4. Niederman MS, Bass JB Jr, Campbell GD, et al: Guidelines for the initial management of adults with community-acquired pneumonia: Diagnosis, assessment of severity, and initial antimicrobial therapy. Am Rev Respir Dis 148:1418–1426, 1993
5. Meduri U: Standardization of bronchoscopic techniques for ventilator-associated pneumonia, Chest 102:557S–564S, 1992
6. Baselski VS, El-Torky M, Coalson J, et al: The standardization of criteria for processing and interpreting laboratory specimens in patients with suspected ventilator-associated pneumonia. Chest 102:571S–579S, 1992
7. Ponce de Leon RS: Organizing for infection control. In Wenzel RP (ed): Prevention and Control of Nosocomial Infections, Baltimore, Williams & Wilkins, 1987, pp 56–69
8. Larson E: A causative link between handwashing and risk of infection? Examination of the evidence. Infect Control Hosp Epidemiol 9:28–36, 1988
9. Centers for Disease Control and Prevention. Draft Guideline for Isolation Precautions in Hospitals: Part 1. Evolution of Isolation Precautions and Part 2. Recommendations for Isolation Precautions in Hospitals: Notice of Comment. Fed Reg 59:5552–5570, 1994
10. CDC: Surveillance for occupationally acquired HIV infection-United States, 1981–1992. MMWR 41:923–825, 1992
11. Centers for Disease Control and Prevention: Draft guideline for the prevention of nosocomial pneumonia: Notice of comment period.59 Fed Reg 4980, 1994
12. Tablan OC, Arden NH, Breiman RF, et al: Guidelines for prevention of nosocomial pneumonia. Am J Infect Control 22:247–292, 1994
13. Maki DG: Infections due to infusion therapy. In Bennett JV, Brachman PS, Sanford JP (eds): Hospital Infections, 3rd ed. Boston, Little, Brown & Company, 1992, pp 849–898

BIBLIOGRAPHY

Townsend TR Jr: Infection in the ICU: How to protect yourself and others. J Crit Illness 2:29–37, 1987

Washington JA: Techniques for noninvasive diagnosis of lower respiratory tract infections. J Crit Illness 3:97–103,

31 Interstitial Lung Disease

Udaya B. S. Prakash

CLINICAL SKILLS

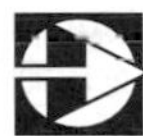

Upon completion of this chapter, the reader will:

- Recognize the general concepts of interstitial lung diseases and their classification based on varied etiologies.
- Understand the common physiologic abnormalities encountered in interstitial lung diseases and the pathologic basis for these changes.
- Recognize the role and limitation of various diagnostic methods that include imaging studies, serologic tests, and biopsy techniques.
- Understand clinical aspects of common interstitial disorders such as idiopathic pulmonary fibrosis, sarcoidosis, hypersensitivity pneumonitis, and rheumatologic diseases.
- Recognize that several uncommon disorders such as Langerhan's cell granuloma, pulmonary alveolar proteinosis, and lymphangioleiomyomatosis can cause significant interstitial pulmonary disorders.
- Identify several commonly used drugs that can contribute to the development of lung disease.
- Understand the role and limitation of various therapies used to treat interstitial lung disease.

KEY TERMS

Ankylosing spondylitis
Bronchoalveolar lavage
Eosinophilic granuloma
Histiocytosis X
Hypersensitivity pneumonitis
Idiopathic pulmonary fibrosis
Interstitial lung disease
Lymphangioleiomyomatosis
Lymphocytic interstitial pneumonitis
Neurofibromatosis
Polymyositis
Pulmonary alveolar phospholipoproteinosis
Sarcoidosis
Scleroderma
Sjögren's syndrome
Systemic lupus erythematosus

DESCRIPTION OF INTERSTITIAL LUNG DISEASE

Definition

The term *interstitial lung disease* (ILD) refers to disorders that result from injury to the pulmonary interstitium. Simply defined, the lung interstitium represents the major portion of the pulmonary parenchyma and consists of structures situated in between the alveoli. These structures include epithelial cells that constitute the walls of alveoli, reticular and elastic fibers (connective tissue), capillary network, and lymphatics. The term *alveolar disease* (sometimes referred to as air-space disease) is used when a pathologic process primarily affects the alveoli. In alveolar diseases, the intra-alveolar space is filled with fluid, pus, blood, cells, or other materials. In clinical practice, however, the derivation of these terms is based on chest radiographic findings.

It is often difficult to clearly separate interstitial lung diseases from alveolar diseases. It is important to recognize that many interstitial lung diseases begin as alveolar processes, and lung diseases that begin as interstitial processes may develop an alveolar appearance as a result of complications. Indeed, many lung diseases demonstrate an alveolar-interstitial pattern on chest radiography. Because of this overlap in radiographic and pathologic findings, the term *diffuse lung disease* is frequently employed. In this chapter, both terms, namely interstitial lung disease and diffuse lung disease, are used interchangeably. When the term *interstitial lung disease* is used by clinicians, it generally refers to diffuse involvement of the lungs; at least several segments of the lung are involved, often bilaterally. The majority of these disorders are subacute or chronic. Infectious processes are usually not included in this group, although they should be included in the differential diagnosis.

The term ILD encompasses a large number of heterogeneous disorders. Nevertheless, the common features of ILD include a relatively subacute to chronic course (usually longer than 6 months), progressive dyspnea on exertion, bilateral interstitial-alveolar infiltrates, restrictive pulmonary dysfunction, diminished diffusing capacity for carbon monoxide, exercise-induced hypoxemia, hypocarbia in the initial stages, nonspecific histologic findings (occasionally includes noncaseous granulomas), and absence of infection.

Etiology

Clinically, the starting point to consider the possibility of ILD is the abnormal chest radiograph (Figure 31-1). In the early stages of many types of ILD, an incidental chest radiograph may be the first indicator of ILD because many patients are asymptomatic. Interstitial lung diseases are caused by an unusually large number of heterogeneous etiologies. Causes and clinical situations associated with ILD number more than 160, and the number continues to grow. In the majority of patients, however, a specific cause is not identified. Often, the etiologic diagnosis is one of exclusion; when an etiology cannot be identified, the terms *cryptogenic alveolar fibrosis* and *usual interstitial pneumonitis* (UIP) are applied. For clinical purposes, the various etiologies can be grouped as shown in Table 31-1. Such broad classification helps the clinician to consider almost all causes of interstitial lung diseases. Some confusion has resulted because of the large number of disease entities under the broad categorization of ILD and various abbreviations used to describe them (Box 31-1).[1] The end stage of many forms of ILD is represented by nonspecific fibrosis. The terms *usual interstitial pneumonitis* (UIP), *fibrosing alveolitis,* and *cryptogenic fibrosing alveolitis* are frequently used interchangeably to describe this process. Indeed, approximately two thirds of disorders under the broad title of ILD have no known etiology.[2,3]

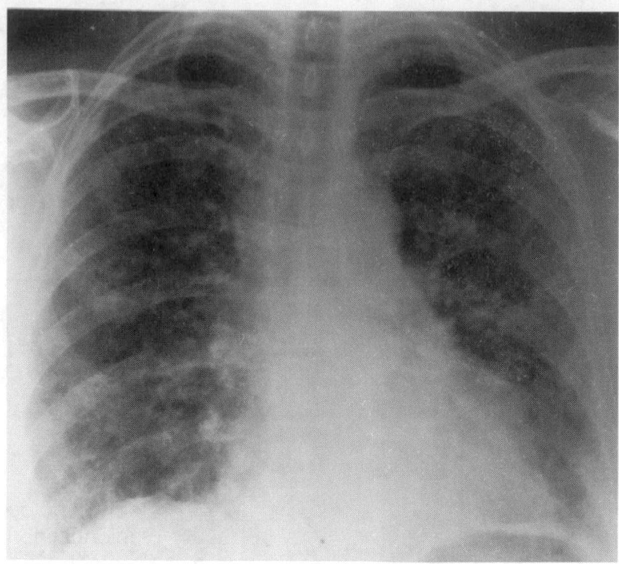

FIGURE 31-1. Chest roentgenograph of a patient who presented with progressive dyspnea of 8 months' duration. Diffuse interstitial process with predominant lower lung involvement is evident in this patient who was found to have moderately severe idiopathic pulmonary fibrosis.

Idiopathic pulmonary fibrosis is the prototype of ILDs. Despite extensive investigations, the etiology of idiopathic pulmonary fibrosis remains unknown. Infectious etiology (viral), genetic predisposition, individual susceptibility, environmental exposure, and other etiologies have been suggested as the basis for idiopathic pulmonary fibrosis.[4–7] Individual susceptibility seems to play a major role in certain types of ILD. For example, radiation-induced ILD occurs in only 5% to 15% of patients exposed to thoracic radiation.[8] A similar percentage of patients exposed to inhaled organic antigens develop hypersensitivity pneumonitis.[9,10] Less than 15% of subjects exposed to chemotherapeutic agents, such as bleomycin, methotrexate, and so on, develop cytotoxic ILD.[11]

Pathology

As indicated above, ILD as a group of diseases has innumerable etiologies, and thus the histologic findings vary from one disease entity to another. Often, the end

TABLE 31-1. **Clinical Classification of Diffuse Lung Diseases***

Collagen Diseases	***Malignant Diseases***
Scleroderma	Lymphangitic metastasis
Rheumatoid arthritis	Diffuse alveolar cell carcinoma
Polymyositis-dermatomyositis	***Idiopathic Diseases (Common)***
Others	Diffuse alveolar damage from ARDS
Occupational Diseases	Idiopathic pulmonary fibrosis
Asbestosis	Sarcoidosis
Silicosis	Eosinophilic lung diseases
Coal workers' pneumoconiosis	Bronchiolitis obliterans with organizing pneumonia (BOOP)
Hypersensitivity pneumonitis	Lymphocytic interstitial pneumonitis
Others	***Idiopathic Diseases (Uncommon)***
Drug-Induced Lung Diseases	Eosinophilic granuloma (histiocytosis X)
Radiation pneumonitis	Alveolar proteinosis
Chemotherapeutic agents	Lymphangiomyomatosis
Oxygen toxicity	Alveolar microlithiasis
Others	Others
Infectious Diseases	
Chronic mycobacterioses	
Chronic mycoses	

* The diffuse lung diseases include both interstitial and alveolar lung diseases; ARDS is adult respiratory distress syndrome.

BOX 31-1

ABBREVIATIONS USED TO DESCRIBE DIFFUSE LUNG DISEASES

HRS	Hamman-Rich syndrome (acute IPF)
UIP	Usual interstitial pneumonitis (an earlier terminology for IPF)
IAF	Idiopathic alveolar fibrosis (same as IPF)
GIP	Giant cell interstitial pneumonitis (very rare)
BIP	Bronchiolitis with interstitial pneumonitis (a form of BOOP)
BOOP*	Bronchiolitis obliterans with organizing pneumonia
COP	Cryptogenic organizing pneumonitis (same as BOOP)
PIP	Plasma cell interstitial pneumonitis (uncommon)
CIPF	Classic interstitial pneumonitis with fibrosis (IPF)
DIP	Desquamative interstitial pneumonitis (may predispose to IPF)
LIP*	Lymphocytic interstitial pneumonitis (many etiologies)
IPF*	Idiopathic pulmonary fibrosis
DAD*	Diffuse alveolar damage (as in ARDS)
RAD	Regional alveolar damage (nonspecific)

* *For clinical purposes, these entities are important because they constitute more than 90% of the diseases listed above. Table reproduced with permission from Prakash UBS: Pulmonary Diseases. In Mayo Internal Medicine Board Review 1996–97. Rochester, MN; Mayo Foundation for Education and Research; 1995; pp 673–770.*

stage of many diseases that are considered under the broad title of ILD exhibit nonspecific pulmonary fibrosis without providing clues as to the precise etiology. In a simplified scheme of the pathogenesis of ILD, injury to the alveoli or the interstitium is the initial event. The injury can be extrinsic (inhaled) or intrinsic as a result of another pathologic process within the body. An example of the extrinsic etiology is the hypersensitivity pneumonitis that results from the inhalation of certain antigens. Another example of the extrinsic cause is the ILD caused by administration of chemotherapeutic agents. Scleroderma, rheumatoid arthritis, and other nonpulmonary diseases can be considered as examples of the intrinsic etiologies for the development of ILD in these disorders.

The initial injury is often followed by altered permeability of the alveolar-capillary interphase and resultant alveolar exudation, followed by invasion of various cell types into the alveolar and interstitial spaces. Infiltration of interstitial spaces by mononuclear cells, neutrophils, and other cells (interstitial inflammation) increases the thickness of the pulmonary interstitium. Capillary damage causes increased permeability and edema formation within interstitial spaces or alveolar spaces, or both. As the disease process progresses, fibroblasts are recruited to the interstitium where the process of interstitial fibrosis begins. The terminal event in the pathology of most forms of ILD is the development of diffuse interstitial fibrosis. The degree of fibrosis, however, is variable and not always uniform or homogeneous. Depending on whether the predominant pathologic feature is alveolar or interstitial, the chest radiograph exhibits the corresponding abnormality. In chronic cases, deposition of fibrous tissue in the interstitium (interstitial fibrosis) contributes to the typical interstitial infiltrate seen on the chest radiograph.

Continuing research has shed light on the major role played by many cell-derived factors in the pathogenesis of ILD. Among these are cytokines, cell-derived proteins whose primary physiologic role is the regulation of cell function. A typical cytokine is a glycoprotein that is transiently secreted by an appropriately stimulated effector cell.[12] The cytokine group of chemical mediators include several interleukins, tumor necrosis factor, insulin-like growth factors, transforming growth factor-β, platelet-derived growth factor, and several other cytokines. Virtually all cells are capable of producing cytokines under appropriate circumstances. Fibroblasts are primarily responsible for the production of fibrotic matrix in areas of inflammation. Cytokines are important controllers of fibroblast function. A large number of ILDs, many discussed below, have strong association with cytokine-mediated pathogenetic mechanisms.[12]

Clinically, only a subset of persons exposed to extrinsic factors or those with intrinsic nonpulmonary diseases develop ILD. Individual susceptibility and the integrity of the immune system are likely to be the major reasons for this variability. Several types of ILD, such as familial interstitial pulmonary fibrosis, familial sarcoidosis, familial pulmonary hemosiderosis, tuberous sclerosis, neurofibromatosis, and pulmonary alveolar microlithiasis, demonstrate genetic predisposition. Racial differences also seem to affect the behavior of certain types of ILD. For instance, sarcoidosis, a relatively benign disease among whites, exhibits more severe pathology and clinical course in blacks. Even in a distinct type of ILD (for example, idiopathic pulmonary fibrosis), the course and severity of the disease show great variations.

Physiology

Pulmonary function tests in diffuse ILD typically show a restrictive type of pulmonary dysfunction manifested by reduced lung volumes, diminished diffusing capacity for carbon monoxide, and exercise-induced hypoxemia.[13] The degree of the abnormalities depend on the severity of the underlying pulmonary disorder. With progression of the ILD, the lung volumes may diminish significantly and suggest the "shrinking lung" phenomenon. Total lung capacity (TLC), vital capacity (VC), and residual volume (RV) continue to decrease with progression of disease. The loss of lung volumes is best correlated with interstitial fibrosis, although it can be marked in some alveolar diseases. Early in the disease, lung volumes may be normal. The diffusing capacity for carbon monoxide is perhaps the most important test in patients with ILD. The airflow rates and FEV_1/FVC ratio are usually normal or only minimally diminished unless an associated obstructive disease is also present. However, it should be recognized that cigarette smoking has been identified as a risk factor for idiopathic pulmonary fibrosis.[14] The static compliance is decreased, but airway resistance is normal in the absence of associated airway obstruction.[15]

The "stiff lung" resulting from the progressive deposition of fibrous tissue in the interstitium increases the work of breathing. As a result, patients with significantly fibrotic lungs are unable to maintain deep breathing maneuvers on a continual basis as is the case in normal subjects. To counteract this physiologic disadvantage, patients with ILD typically exhibit rapid, shallow breathing, a type of hyperventilation. This in turn leads to hypocarbia (diminished arterial carbon dioxide). Retention of carbon dioxide, occurring in the later stages of ILD, is caused by "respiratory exhaustion." Indeed, carbon dioxide retention in patients with ILD is a sign of impending respiratory failure.

Gas exchange is impaired because of the increased thickness of the alveolar-capillary interphase as well as the presence of ventilation/perfusion inequality. This leads to exercise-induced hypoxemia and decreased diffusing capacity for carbon monoxide (D_{LCO}). The latter physiologic abnormalities are among the earliest abnormalities to occur in ILD. Hypoxemia induced by exercise is a well-recognized phenomenon in ILD.[16–18] In patients with idiopathic pulmonary fibrosis and occupationally induced ILD, an exercise-associated increase in $P(A-a)$ has been shown to correlate best with morphologic changes.[16] However, the gas exchange abnormalities do not seem to provide prognostic information.[19]

Roentgenology

The routine chest roentgenogram is often the first indicator of ILD in a significant proportion of patients. The chest radiographic findings in ILD are determined by the etiology, pathology, severity, duration, and associated complications of the disease.[20] In certain forms of ILD, the chest roentgenogram may demonstrate abnormalities predominantly in the upper lung zones (Figure 31-2; Table 31-2), whereas lower lung involvement is more common in most forms of ILD (Figure 31-3). The radiologic abnormalities in ILD can be broadly classified into alveolar (air space) and interstitial patterns. It is important to recognize that many disease entities exhibit both radiologic forms. Furthermore, the interstitial or alveolar forms of infiltrates can be associated with other radiologic abnormalities such as nodular, cavitating, and honeycomb infiltrates.

The abnormalities observed on a routine chest roentgenogram do not establish definitive pathologic diagnoses, but provide hints as to the possibility of certain disease entities. For instance, the alveolar pattern is limited to a smaller number of diseases, that is, pulmonary edema (cardiogenic and noncardiogenic), alveolar sarcoidosis, uremic lung, intraalveolar hemorrhage, aspiration pneumonia, pulmonary alveolar phospholipoproteinosis, certain bacterial pneumonias, desquamative pneumonia, certain viral and protozoal

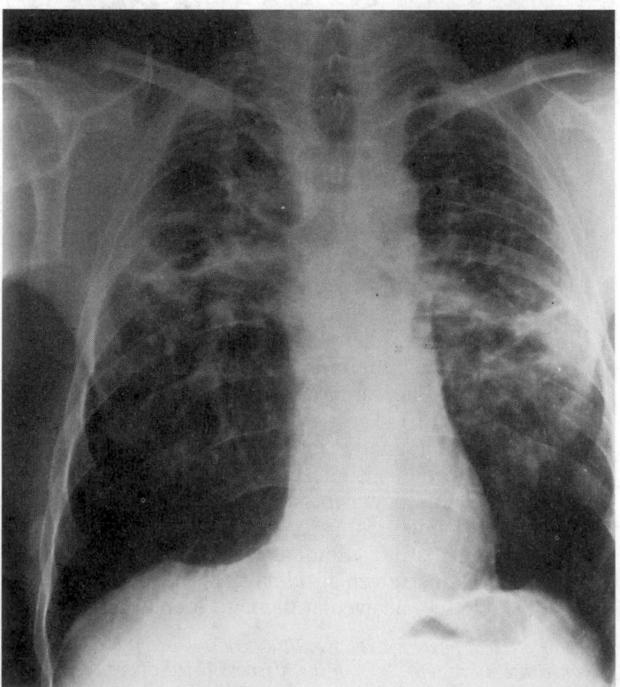

FIGURE 32-2. Predominantly upper lung involvement with interstitial and nodular changes noted in this chest roentgenograph in a patient who had chronic ankylosing spondylitis.

TABLE 31-2. **Types of Interstitial Lung Disease That Predominantly Affect the Upper Lungs**

Silicosis
Coal workers' pneumoconiosis
Sarcoidosis
Mycoses (histoplasmosis, coccidioidomycosis)
Mycobacterioses
Cystic fibrosis
Pulmonary eosinophilic granuloma (histiocytosis X)
Pulmonary lymphangiomyomatosis
Acute silo filler's lung disease
Certain gaseous exposures
Pneumocystis carinii infection in those on aerosolized pentamidine

pneumonias, diffuse alveolar cell carcinoma, and diffuse pulmonary lymphoma. Pulmonary edema, whether cardiogenic or noncardiogenic, is the commonest cause of alveolar pattern seen on chest roentgenogram.

On the other hand, the interstitial pattern of chest radiographic abnormality includes many diseases. Therefore, it is convenient to group them into the following broad categories as follows (also see Table 33-1): idiopathic pulmonary fibrosis, systemic diseases (eg, rheumatologic diseases), occupational lung diseases (including pneumoconioses and toxic exposures), drug-induced lung diseases (including radiation pneumonitis), granulomatous lung diseases (sarcoid, and so on), lymphangitic pulmonary metastasis, chronic mycotic and mycobacterial infections, unusual diseases (histiocytosis X, lymphangioleiomyomatosis, tuberous sclerosis), and others (chronic bronchiectasis, cystic fibrosis, and so on). As noted above, the anatomical distribution of the infiltrates is an important clinical consideration. Certain diseases, for instance, predominantly affect upper lung zones (see Table 31-2).

Currently, the high-resolution computed tomography (CT) of the chest has become an almost indispensable technique in the diagnosis of various types of ILD. The anatomic details provided by this technique permit identification of lobular units of the lung and highly dependable definition of interstitial and parenchymal processes. As a result, many types of ILD can be diagnosed with a great degree of confidence on the basis of high-resolution computed tomography. In the presence of appropriate clinical features, a high-resolution computed tomogram can establish the diagnosis of idiopathic pulmonary fibrosis, pulmonary eosinophilic granuloma (histiocytosis X), lymphangioleiomyomatosis (Figure 31-4), lymphangitic pulmonary metastasis, pulmonary veno-occlusive disease, and certain granulomatous diseases such as sarcoidosis. It appears that the increasing importance of this technique may obviate the need for lung biopsy in some of these diseases.

Magnetic resonance imaging (MRI) has a minimal role in the diagnosis of ILD. Magnetic resonance imaging may be useful in patients with renal failure or contrast allergy when CT is likely to require contrast administration. Magnetic resonance imaging may be superior to CT in evaluating pulmonary sequestration, arteriovenous malformation, and tumor recurrence in patients with total pneumonectomy. It is also useful in imaging the vascular structures within the thorax.

Radionuclide Imaging

Lung scan using gallium-67 was initially thought to help in assessing the activity of certain forms of ILD. This conclusion was based on the observation that the radionuclide selectively accumulated in the leukocytes, which are found in areas of active inflammation. This phenomenon was thought to localize areas of active process in patients with disease. Further studies have

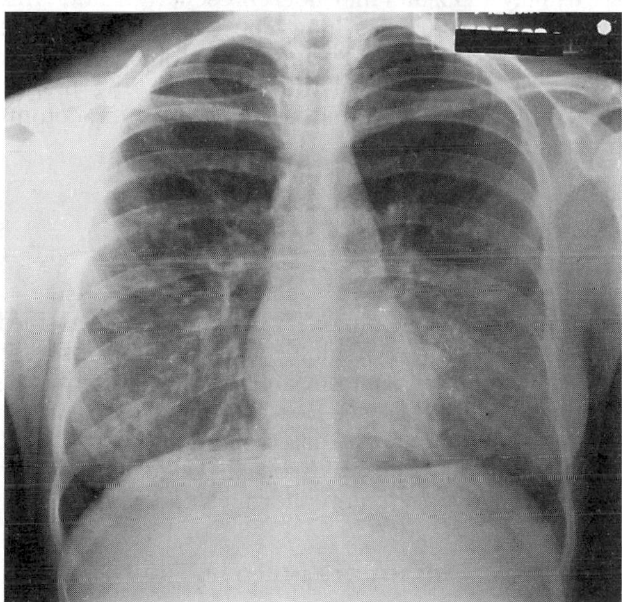

FIGURE 31-3. Chest roentgenograph demonstrates lower lung involvement caused by noncardiogenic pulmonary edema in this patient. The etiology of noncardiogenic edema was fluid overload during and following urologic surgery.

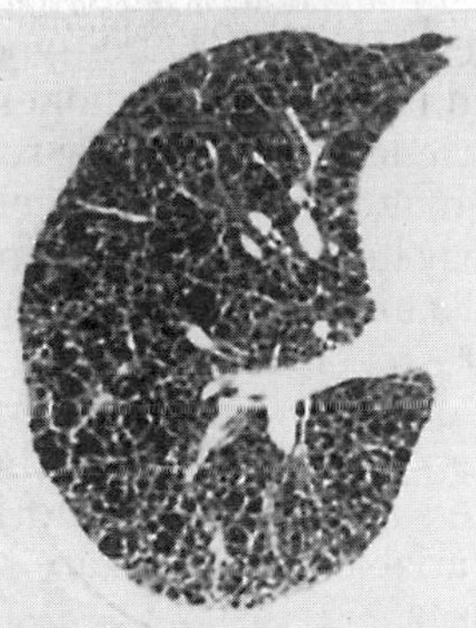

FIGURE 31-4. A section of the right lung depicted by high-resolution computed tomographic scan in a patient with lymphangioleiomyomatosis; the diffuse well-defined cystic changes are considered characteristic of the disease.

shown that this technique is nonspecific and the interpretation of results is subjective because there are no standardized indexes to evaluate the disease process.[21] The reported sensitivity of gallium scan in the diagnosis of sarcoidosis varies from 60% to 90%.[22] Presently, there is no clinical role for gallium scan in the diagnosis of ILD.

Serologic Tests

Routine blood tests are generally unhelpful in the diagnosis of most forms of ILD. Complete blood counts and a chemistry workup do not aid in the diagnosis. If abnormal, they may indicate complications of the disease or treatment. Serologic tests, on the other hand, are often helpful in supporting the clinical diagnosis in certain forms of ILD. For example, the presence of hypersensitivity pneumonitis may be indicated by the presence of specific antibodies in the serum. Serum angiotensin converting enzyme levels have been used in the diagnosis and follow-up of sarcoidosis, as discussed below. Certain abnormal tests, such as antinuclear antigen, rheumatoid factor, and immunoglobulins, may aid in pointing toward specific diagnosis. All these serologic tests, however, are nonspecific, and therefore caution should be exercised in using these tests in establishing specific diagnoses.

Bronchoscopy and Other Biopsy Techniques

Bronchoscopy with diagnostic bronchoalveolar lavage (BAL) or lung biopsy, or both, is extremely valuable in the diagnosis of several types of ILD.[23] BAL is performed by wedging a flexible bronchoscope into a segmental bronchus and instilling 100 to 150 mL of normal saline into the distal (abnormal) segments of the lung. The instilled saline is aspirated back by means of the bronchoscope and can be analyzed for cell counts, morphology, and typing. Protein and other constituents can be measured in the lavage fluid. The cells obtained represent the cell populations in the alveoli.

Bronchoalveolar lavage effluent in normal subjects shows pulmonary alveolar macrophages (93% ± 3%) and lymphocytes (7% ± 1%). Other types of leukocytes are rarely found in normal nonsmokers. Because several of the diffuse lung diseases are reported to result from the inflammatory and immune cells, the presence of these cells may help in understanding the pathogenesis. Increased numbers of neutrophils with normal lymphocytes are reported in idiopathic pulmonary fibrosis, familial pulmonary fibrosis, and asbestosis. Increased numbers of lymphocytes without neutrophilia have been noted in sarcoidosis and hypersensitivity pneumonitis. Variable cell counts are seen in other diffuse lung diseases.

Bronchoalveolar lavage should be considered a research tool to study the pathogenesis of lung diseases. Bronchoalveolar lavage currently has no value in the diagnosis of sarcoid or idiopathic pulmonary fibrosis. However, it may be helpful in diagnosing alveolar proteinosis, some infections, histiocytosis X, and lymphangitic pulmonary metastasis. The CD4:CD8 ratio is reversed in BAL obtained from patients with AIDS complicated by lymphocytic interstitial pneumonitis and many patients with hypersensitivity pneumonitis.[24,25] Bronchoalveolar lavage is extremely helpful in the diagnosis of *Pneumocystis carinii*, tuberculosis, mycoses, and other infections. It is necessary to stress that BAL has a limited role in the diagnosis of sarcoid, idiopathic pulmonary fibrosis, nonorganic pneumoconioses, and other forms of ILD.

Lung biopsy can be obtained by means of bronchoscopy, thoracoscopy, or thoracotomy. The indications for lung biopsy in diffuse lung disease should be based on the clinical features, treatment planned, and risks from biopsy and from treatment without a pathologic diagnosis. Bronchoscopic lung biopsy provides a higher diagnostic yield in sarcoidosis, pulmonary eosinophilic granuloma (histiocytosis X), eosinophilic pneumonitis, lymphangioleiomyomatosis, infections, pulmonary alveolar proteinosis, lymphangitic carcinomatosis, drug-induced lung disease, rejection process in transplanted lungs, and hypersensitivity pneumonitis.[26]

The major advantages of bronchoscopic techniques include the ease with which they can be performed and the relatively low risk of complications. The procedure can be performed in the outpatient setting under topical anesthesia. Complications from bronchoscopy and BAL are minimal in patients with ILD. The two major risks associated with bronchoscopic lung biopsy include bleeding and pneumothorax. The incidence of these complications is approximately 2%. The risk of bleeding is increased in patients with renal failure, thrombocytopenia, and other bleeding diatheses.

Specimens obtained by bronchoscopic lung biopsy are usually small and may not represent the underlying disease process. Larger lung biopsy specimens can be obtained by performing thoracotomy and open lung biopsy or video-assisted thoracoscopic lung biopsy. General anesthesia is required for the thoracotomy procedure.

CLASSIFICATION OF INTERSTITIAL LUNG DISEASE

Many of the diffuse pulmonary processes are classified on the basis of morphologic features. As observed above, the number of abbreviations used to describe the various forms of ILD (see Box 31-1) has resulted in significant confusion for the practicing physician. The following paragraphs describe the clinical features of several commonly encountered forms of ILD.

Idiopathic Pulmonary Fibrosis

In Western countries, idiopathic pulmonary fibrosis, sometimes referred to as usual interstitial pneumonitis, or UIP, is the commonest cause of chronic diffuse interstitial lung disease. Idiopathic pulmonary fibrosis is estimated to occur in approximately 3–5/100,000 people.[27] This is perhaps an underestimation because many patients have subclinical disease and may not seek medical assistance until they reach a symptomatic stage. To firmly establish the diagnosis of idiopathic pulmonary fibrosis, it is important that other causes of pulmonary fibrosis are excluded. Despite a careful analysis of clinical and environmental exposure, an etiologic diagnosis remains unknown in an overwhelming majority of patients with idiopathic pulmonary fibrosis. This is because many forms of ILD (see Table 31-1) demonstrate clinical and radiographic features akin to those in idiopathic pulmonary fibrosis. Therefore, the diagnosis of idiopathic pulmonary fibrosis is one of exclusion. The disorder is more commonly diagnosed in the fifth to seventh decades of life.[14,19] Familial incidence has been observed.[28] Males are slightly more likely to develop the disorder.

The diagnosis of idiopathic pulmonary fibrosis is generally based on clinical features, which include gradually progressive dyspnea, cough, and clubbing in more than 70% of patients. Weight loss, fatigue, and arthralgia can occur. Even though the presence of Velcro-type crepitant crackles during late inspiration is characteristic of diffuse ILDs, they are best heard in patients with idiopathic pulmonary fibrosis. In late stages, signs and symptoms of secondary pulmonary hypertension and cor pulmonale may be present. Laboratory tests reveal positive rheumatoid factor in 30%, presence of antinuclear antibody in 35%, or polyclonal gammopathy in more than 50%. Tachypnea is a common clinical finding, as is the cough associated with attempts at deep inspiration.

Pulmonary function tests show restrictive pulmonary dysfunction, low diffusing capacity, hypoxemia worsened by exercise, and hypocapnia. Chest radiography usually exhibits asymmetric interstitial process beginning in the peripheral zones of lower lungs, with gradual progression upward as the disease advances. In late stages of the disease, honeycombing may occur (Figures 31-5, 31-6). Chest radiographic findings in idiopathic pulmonary fibrosis are nonspecific because many other forms of ILD also demonstrate similar findings. High-resolution computed tomography of the lungs typically reveal subpleural honeycombing and interstitial process in the basal areas (Figure 31-7). Indeed, many clinicians currently accept the diagnosis of idiopathic pulmonary fibrosis based on clinical features and typical findings of high-resolution computed tomography. However, it is worthwhile to note that several forms of ILD such as scleroderma lung and rheumatoid lung may demonstrate clinical and computed tomographic features observed in idiopathic pulmonary fibrosis.

Lung biopsy in idiopathic pulmonary fibrosis reveals nonspecific fibrosis without granulomatosis. Many disease entities can produce nonspecific lung fibrosis; therefore, it is difficult to differentiate idiopathic pulmonary fibrosis from these diseases, which include rheumatoid lung, scleroderma lung, late stages of sarcoidosis, certain drug-induced lung diseases (eg, nitrofurantoin), radiation pneumonitis, end-stage hypersensitivity pneumonitis, certain pneumoconioses (asbestos), noxious gases,

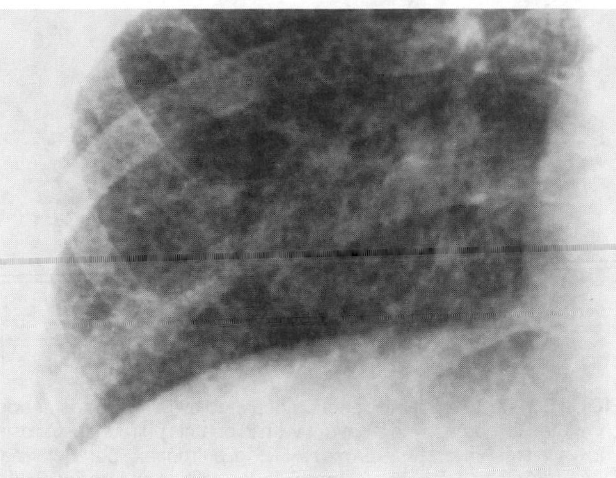

FIGURE 31-5. A roentgenologic view of the right lower lung zone in a patient with idiopathic pulmonary fibrosis; diffuse interstitial infiltrates with honeycomb changes can be seen. This type of abnormality is not limited to idiopathic pulmonary fibrosis; it can be seen in the end-stage of many fibrotic lung diseases.

paraquat, recurrent pulmonary edema, end-stage histiocytosis X, end-stage cystic fibrosis and bronchiectasis, chronic aspiration pneumonia, and recurrent intra-alveolar hemorrhage (eg, mitral stenosis, pulmonary hemosiderosis, and Goodpasture's syndrome). The limited role of bronchoalveolar lavage in idiopathic pulmonary fibrosis is discussed above.

Treatment of idiopathic pulmonary fibrosis has been disappointing. Standard therapy has consisted of corticosteroids (prednisone, 1 to 2 mg/kg/d) for 9 to 12 months. Less than 20% of patients thus treated show measurable improvement. Various immunosuppressive drugs (cyclophosphamide, azathioprine, cyclosporine), and anti-inflammatory agents (colchicine, plaquenil,

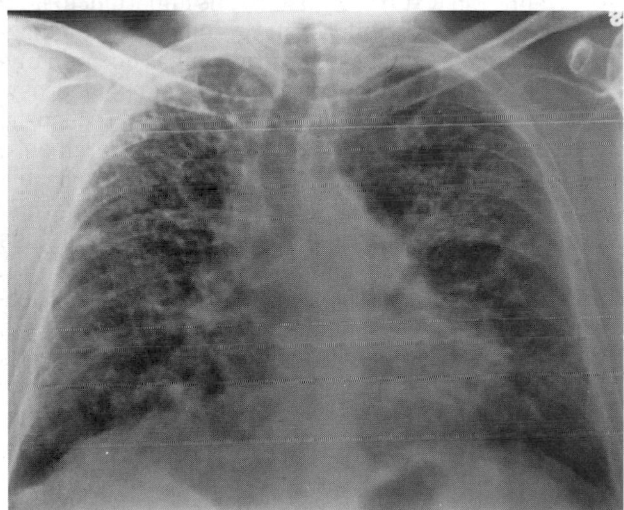

FIGURE 31-6. Diffuse advanced interstitial changes in a patient with progressive idiopathic pulmonary fibrosis; mild cardiomegaly caused by secondary pulmonary hypertension and cor pulmonale was also present.

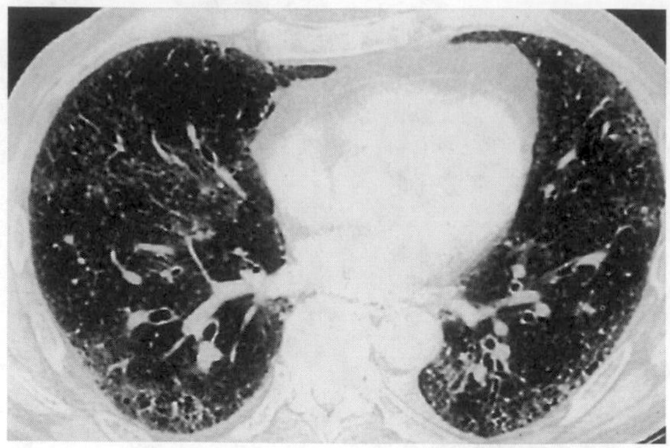

FIGURE 31-7. A mid-lung section depicted by this high-resolution computed tomography in a patient with idiopathic pulmonary fibrosis shows typical interstitial process in the pulmonary parenchymal periphery along with honeycomb abnormalities (posteriorly). Increased diameter of the bronchi is caused by "traction" bronchiectasis.

chloroquine) have been tried with varying success.[27] As the disease advances, the majority of patients develop disabling dyspnea, hypoxemia, and cor pulmonale. The mainstay of therapy for this group of patients is supplemental oxygen. Selected patients have undergone lung transplant. The overall prognosis in patients with idiopathic pulmonary fibrosis is poor, with 5-year survival of less than 30%.

Sarcoidosis

Sarcoidosis is a multisystemic granulomatous disease of unknown etiology. It is usually encountered in persons in the 25- to 45-year age group. It is a common form of ILD in Western countries. The disorder is characterized by development of noncaseous epithelioid cell granulomas in various organs; depression of delayed type hypersensitivity (as a result of decreased number of T lymphocytes); hyperglobulinemia (as a result of proliferation of B lymphocytes); and, frequently, positive Kveim skin test (rarely used). It is important to note that the presence of noncaseous granuloma is not diagnostic of sarcoid. Noncaseous granulomas occur in mycobacterioses (noncaseous in early stages), leprosy, mycoses, syphilis, mononucleosis, carcinoma, silicosis, hypersensitivity pneumonitis, zirconium, berylliosis, talcosis, Bakelite exposure, Crohn's ileitis, primary biliary cirrhosis, cat-scratch disease, foreign-body granulomas, hypogammaglobulinemia, and granulomatous arteritis.

Sarcoidosis commonly presents with pulmonary features, although any organ in the body may be affected. Traditionally, the clinical staging of sarcoidosis has been based on chest radiographic abnormalities rather than clinical severity, even though the chest radiographic changes roughly parallel the clinical course of the disease. The radiologic classification includes five types (formerly known as stages) of disease: (1) type 0: normal chest roentgenogram, with demonstration of noncaseous granulomas in other sites such as conjunctiva, liver, lymphoid tissue, skin, and so on; (2) type I: bilateral hilar and paratracheal lymphadenopathy (40% to 50% of all cases);[29,30] (3) type II: bilateral hilar and paratracheal lymphadenopathy with pulmonary parenchymal involvement; approximately 25% of patients present this way;[29,31] (4) type III: diffuse pulmonary parenchymal disease without lymphadenopathy (14% to 16% of all cases)[30] (Figure 31-8); and (5) type IV: end-stage pulmonary fibrosis with bullous changes (< 5% of all cases). Computed tomography is excellent for the evaluation of hilar lymphadenopathy. High-resolution computed tomography is more helpful in the assessment of the pulmonary parenchymal changes.[32–34] The role of computed tomography in the staging and management of sarcoidosis remains unclear.[22]

Intrathoracic disease is present in more than 90% of patients, even though almost all organ systems can be involved. Generalized lymphadenopathy occurs in 25% of patients, skin (lupus pernio, nodules) excluding nodosum in 25%, eyes (lacrimal enlargement, corneal band opacities, iridocyclitis, glaucoma, and choroidoretinitis) in 25%, hepatic disease in 25%, splenomegaly in 14%, endobronchial involvement in 11%, central nervous system involvement (paralysis of seventh cranial nerve, chronic meningitis, hypopituitarism) in 7%, bone cysts in 6%, and kidney involvement in 5%. Other manifestations include salivary gland involvement (uveoparotid fever, or Heerfordt's syndrome) in 6%, nasal mucosal lesions, keloid in areas of surgical scars, diffuse arthralgias of small joints, heart (arrhythmias) in 5%, persistent violaceous skin plaques, transient vesicular eruptions on fingers, and persistent scars of old trauma on the knees. Clinically, patients may present with the following initial complaints: lymphadenopathy (8% to 20%), cough (30%), dyspnea (28%), weight loss (20% to 28%), fatigue (20% to 27%), skin lesions (14% to 25%), visual complaints (10% to 21%), and fever (10% to 15%). Asymptomatic disease is seen in 12% to 34% of the patients.

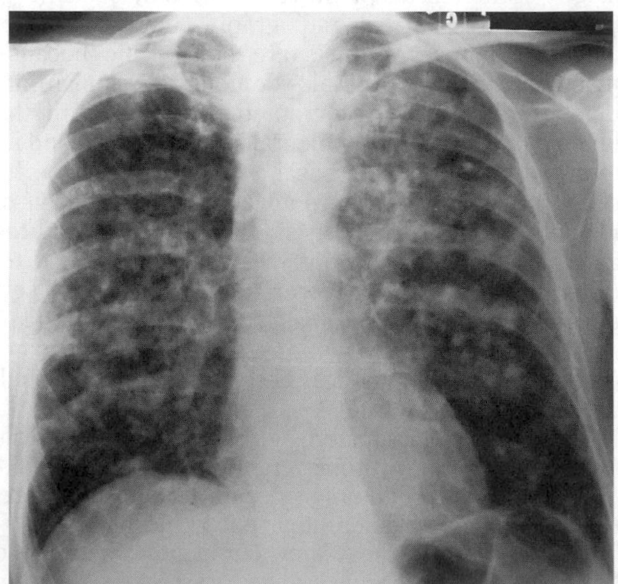

FIGURE 31-8. Diffuse nodular–interstitial pulmonary parenchymal process in a patient with type III sarcoidosis. The abnormalities are more pronounced in the upper two thirds of both lungs.

Complete or partial anergy to skin tests (PPD and others) is seen in 60% of patients. Other abnormalities in laboratory testing include increased CD4:CD8 ratio, high serum antibodies to mycoplasma viruses (Epstein-Barr virus, rubella, parainfluenza, herpes simplex), autoantibodies to rheumatoid factor, and positive antinuclear antibody. Hypercalcemia results from increased sensitivity to vitamin D and increased gastrointestinal absorption of calcium; hypercalciuria; increased levels of IgG, IgA, and IgM; and elevated serum alkaline phosphatase.

Serum angiotensin converting enzyme (SACE) levels have been used in the diagnosis and follow-up of patients with sarcoidosis. The diagnostic SACE levels are applicable only to adults (> 20 years), because children and teenagers have high and widely variable levels. Nearly 80% of patients with active sarcoidosis have increased levels of SACE, 70% with type I disease, 80% with type II, and 90% with type III. Serum angiotensin converting enzyme levels are increased in 5% of normal subjects. Changes in levels may correspond to the activity of sarcoid. Some physicians use SACE levels to monitor disease activity, but the clinical usefulness of this practice is limited. Elevated SACE levels are not diagnostic of sarcoidosis. Increased SACE level occurs in many granulomatous diseases including primary biliary cirrhosis, Gaucher's disease, leprosy, atypical mycobacteriosis, miliary tuberculosis, acute histoplasmosis, silicosis, hyperparathyroidism, and histiocytic lymphoma.

Pulmonary function tests are normal in most patients with type I disease. As the disease progresses to involve lung parenchyma, progressive restrictive lung dysfunction with diminished diffusing carbon monoxide capacity results.[35,36] Significant pulmonary dysfunction and hypoxemia do not result unless the disease has progressed to type IV. Because up to 10% of patients with sarcoidosis develop endobronchial sarcoidosis, pulmonary function testing may reveal mild obstructive phenomena in this group of patients.[37,38]

Histologic diagnosis of sarcoidosis is easy to accomplish. Biopsy of involved organs provides a high-diagnostic rate. Commonly, mediastinal nodes, lung, or tracheobronchial mucosa are biopsied. Noncaseous granulomas can be identified in nearly 100% of biopsies from epitrochlear nodes, mediastinal nodes, lung, nasal mucosal lesions, and subcutaneous nodules. Bronchoscopic lung biopsy provides the diagnosis in 76% of patients, irrespective of the stage of the disease.[39] Diagnostic rates of 80% to 90% can be obtained from biopsies of skin lesions, palpable scalene nodes, bronchial lesions, conjunctival lesions, and liver. Diagnostic accuracy falls to less than 65% with biopsies of bone marrow, scalene fat pad, and normal-appearing bronchial mucosa.

Not all patients with sarcoidosis require therapy. Approximately 80% of patients with type I disease exhibit resolution or regression of chest radiographic abnormalities within 5 years.[40] The prognosis is even better for those with either erythema nodosum or iridocyclitis.[41] Approximately 50% of patients with type II disease show spontaneous resolution.[40] Systemic corticosteroids (prednisone, 1 to 2 mg/kg/d) for prolonged periods (6 to 12 months) may be required in progressive or symptomatic type II and type III disease, ocular sarcoid, persistent hypercalcemia or calciuria, progressive or disfiguring skin lesions, neurosarcoid, myocardial sarcoid, and progressive systemic disease. Phenylbutazone and antimalarial drugs have been tried when sarcoidosis has failed to respond to corticosteroid therapy. Periodic follow-up evaluation of patients by means of clinical examination, chest roentgenogram, and pulmonary function tests is important.

Lymphocytic Interstitial Pneumonitis

Lymphocytic interstitial pneumonitis is a form of ILD with many etiologies.[42] The diagnosis is almost always dependent on lung biopsy. The main histologic feature is the diffuse lymphocytic infiltration of the lung parenchyma and interstitium. This type of pulmonary pathology can be caused by almost all types of lymphoproliferative disorders. Lymphocytic interstitial pneumonitis may result from Hodgkin's lymphoma, non-Hodgkin's lymphoma, early lymphomatoid granulomatosis, chronic lymphocytic leukemia, Waldenström's macroglobulinemia, angioimmunoblastic lymphadenopathy, Sézary syndrome, pseudolymphoma, acquired immune deficiency syndrome (AIDS), graft-versus-host disease, and congenital agammaglobulinemia.

Currently, almost all cases of lymphocytic interstitial pneumonitis are thought to represent low-grade B-cell lymphoma. Therefore, it is usual to conduct special lymphocyte studies on the lung biopsy specimens in all patients with lymphocytic interstitial pneumonitis so that the type of lymphoma can be determined. Idiopathic lymphocytic interstitial pneumonitis is a diagnosis of exclusion. Treatment is aimed at the underlying lymphoproliferative disorder. If the diagnosis of idiopathic lymphocytic interstitial pneumonitis is firmly established, by excluding other causes of lymphocytic interstitial infiltrates, a trial of systemic corticosteroid therapy is warranted.

Hypersensitivity Pneumonitis

Hypersensitivity pneumonitis, also known as extrinsic allergic alveolitis, is a form of organic pneumoconiosis.[43] The disorders under this entity are caused by immune-mediated mechanisms. There are many etiologic factors responsible for causing hypersensitivity pneumonitis. Many fungal precipitins (*Mycopolyspora faeni, Thermoactinomyces vulgaris, Thermoactinomyces viridis, Aspergillus* species) and several avian proteins (pigeon breeder's lung), animal proteins, chemicals (isocyanates), and metals (trimellitic anhydride, phthalic anhydride) are among the many precipitating factors known to cause this condition. The time required for sensitization to antigens may take months or years after exposure.

Clinically, three forms of hypersensitivity pneumonitis are encountered: acute (classic), subacute, and chronic.[44,45] The acute form of the disease is usually the result of intense or intermittent exposure to environmental antigen or antigens. Acute farmer's lung is the prototype of the acute form of the disease. Symptoms appear 4 to 6 hours after exposure and include fever, chills, sweats, tightness in the chest, dry cough, and dyspnea. Headaches and arthralgias are common. Sputum production is scanty. Patients may exhibit tachypnea and basal crackles without wheezing. Blood tests, if performed during the acute illness, usually reveal leukocytosis, hyperglobulinemia, and serum precipitating antibody (particularly after repeated exposure to the same antigenic material). Chest roentgenogram may show increased bronchovascular markings and fine reticular and nodular defects (Figure 31-9). Significant hypoxemia may be observed. Lung biopsy is rarely indicated in acute cases; histologic analysis of lung tissue may show bronchiolitis obliterans with organizing pneumonia. Symptoms usually resolve within 18 to 24 hours, and the entire clinical complex recurs on reexposure. In the acute stage, patients require observation, supplemental oxygen, and high-dose corticosteroid therapy (prednisone, 1 to 2 mg/kg/d) for several days. The most important aspect of managing hypersensitivity pneumonitis involves a thorough education of the patient in avoiding future exposures to known antigens so that the chronic form of the disease can be prevented. Unfortunately, many cases of acute hypersensitivity pneumonitis are wrongly diagnosed as community-acquired pneumonia. This inadvertent step may lead to subacute and chronic forms of the disease because of repeated exposure to offending antigens.

A subacute form of the disease is caused by continuous exposure to antigens. However, the degree of exposure in the subacute form of the disorder is not as intense as it is in the acute variety. Bird fancier's lung disease or pigeon breeder's lung disease are excellent examples of the subacute disease where the subject is exposed to small doses of avian protein on a continual basis. Clinical features include gradual onset of exertional dyspnea, cough with production of smaller amounts of mucoid sputum, anorexia, low-grade fever, malaise, and weight loss. Chest radiography may reveal subtle interstitial infiltrates, and the radiologic features may suggest granulomatous lung diseases such as sarcoidosis, chronic mycoses, or other ILDs. Serum precipitins are more likely to be positive than in the acute disease. A lung biopsy is also more likely to disclose an interstitial granulomatous process.

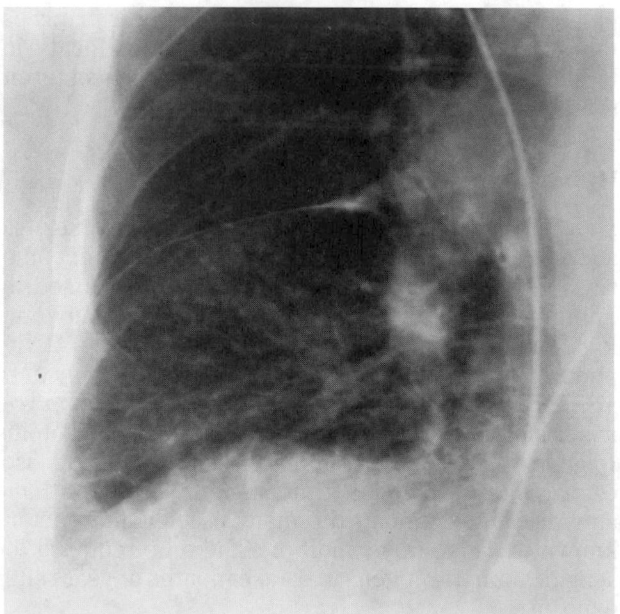

FIGURE 31-9. Chest roentgenographic depiction of the right lower lung in a farmer with chronic hypersensitivity pneumonitis caused by extrinsic allergens; diffuse fine interstitial infiltrates are seen.

Chronic farmer's lung results from repeated or chronic exposure to precipitins. The disease is insidious and may remain undiagnosed for months to years. Obtaining a detailed occupational history of various exposures is important in arriving at the diagnosis. In many patients with the chronic form, a history of recurrent episodes of acute disease, as described above, may not be present. Repeated and small exposures to offending antigens are often the mechanism for the insidious onset of symptoms and gradual progression of the disease, eventually resulting in progressive fibrosis. Clinically and radiologically, the chronic form of hypersensitivity pneumonitis may resemble chronic interstitial pulmonary fibrosis. Significant weight loss may be observed. Tachypnea, diffuse crackles, and clubbing (in more than 50% of patients)[46] are among the common findings. Wheezing is not typical. A chest roentgenogram may show honeycomb changes in the late stages of the disease. Pulmonary function tests typically demonstrate decreased lung volumes, compliance, and diffusing capacity and exercise-induced hypoxemia.

In pigeon breeder's lung disease, an avian-protein-derived hypersensitivity pneumonitis, the histologic features consist of foamy macrophages along with interstitial granulomas. Serologic testing is available to corroborate the diagnosis of various forms of hypersensitivity pneumonitis. It should be noted, however, that positive serology is not diagnostic of the disease because 20% of asymptomatic farmers and 40% of asymptomatic pigeon breeders have positive precipitins, and 10% of symptomatic farmers have negative precipitins.[47,48] A positive serologic finding supports the clinical diagnosis in the appropriate clinical setting. Lung biopsy usually reveals a granulomatous reaction with round cell infiltrates, epithelioid cells, and septal swelling with lymphocytes and plasma cells. Therapy includes avoidance of causative precipitins and use of corticosteroids on a long-term basis. Unfortunately, many patients do not seek medical attention until late and thus develop irreversible fibrosis. Even though a trial of high-dose corticosteroid (prednisone, 1 to 2 mg/kg/d) is recommended for most patients, supplemental oxygen becomes the mainstay of therapy for those with irreversible disease with significant hypoxemia.

INTERSTITIAL LUNG DISEASE CAUSED BY NONPULMONARY DISORDERS

A sizable number of disorders that are nonpulmonary in origin (they primarily arise in nonpulmonary organ systems) can be complicated by pulmonary involvement. In many such entities, respiratory manifestation may be the initial or presenting feature of the nonpulmonary disease. Rheumatologic disorders are the prototypes of nonpulmonary disorders with major respiratory manifestations.[49,50] Interstitial lung disease is an important and well-known manifestation of these diseases. The following are some examples of ILD associated with nonpulmonary diseases.

Rheumatoid Lung

Among the several pulmonary complications that occur in patients with rheumatoid arthritis, diffuse interstitial lung disease is perhaps the most serious.[51] Respiratory manifestations are more common in those with active rheumatoid arthritis, and indeed, the pulmonary features may precede the arthritic manifestations in some patients. The incidence of ILD, as judged by the chest radiographic abnormalities, is 1% to 5%.[52,53] Restrictive pulmonary dysfunction can be demonstrated in more than one-third of patients with rheumatoid lung disease.[51,54] The diffusing capacity for carbon monoxide is diminished in 40% of patients with rheumatoid arthritis.[55]

Clinically, physiologically, and histologically, the pulmonary involvement is identical to that in idiopathic pulmonary fibrosis.[56] Cough and dyspnea are common symptoms. Clubbing of finger and toe nails has been noted in up to 70%.[54] Chest roentgenograms in patients with ILD usually reveal a bibasilar interstitial process or micronodules (Figure 31-10). Honeycombing occurs in late stages of the disease. Lung biopsy usually demonstrates nonspecific inflammatory changes and fibrosis, and therefore many clinicians do not proceed with lung biopsy in patients with rheumatoid lung disease. However, the histologic findings in diffuse rheumatoid lung disease may consist of several abnormalities including rheumatoid nodules, nonspecific interstitial pneumonitis, bronchiolitis obliterans with patchy organizing pneumonia, lymphoid hyperplasia, and cellular interstitial infiltrates.[57]

A favorable response to high-dose corticosteroid therapy can be expected in the early stages of the disease. It is important to recognize that several drugs used to treat rheumatoid arthritis, such as gold salts, penicillamine, and methotrexate, are known to cause pulmonary complications.

Systemic Lupus Erythematosus

Even though pleurisy, pleural effusion, and diffuse alveolar hemorrhage are common in *systemic lupus erythematosus*, diffuse ILD is distinctly uncommon. The prevalence of diffuse interstitial process has been estimated to be about 3%.[58] Instead of diffuse lung infiltrates, patchy, asymmetric, and irregular areas of interstitial pneumonitis and fibrosis develop in 15% to 45% of patients with active systemic lupus erythematosus (Figure 31-11). In one study of 18 patients with systemic lupus erythematosus–induced ILD, the average age was 45.7 years and the mean duration of the disease was 10.3 years; pulmonary symptoms were present for a mean of 6 years.[59]

Pulmonary function tests in patients with diffuse lung disease demonstrate a restrictive pattern and diminished diffusing capacity for carbon monoxide. Plate-like

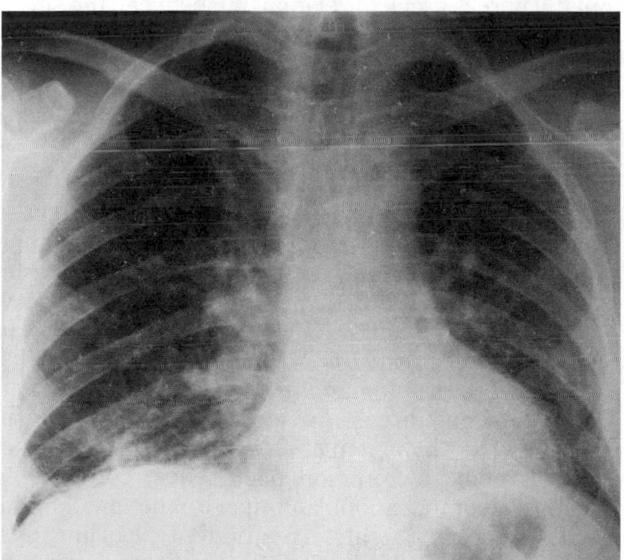

FIGURE 31-10. Chest roentgenograph discloses patchy, bilateral, interstitial process in a patient with active rheumatoid arthritis.

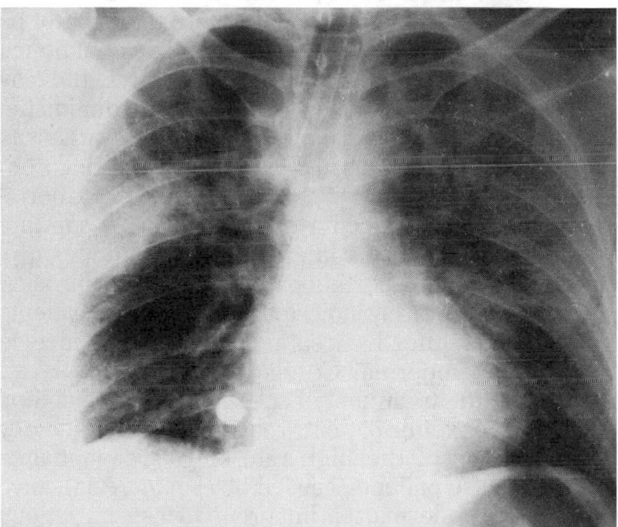

FIGURE 31-11. Patchy, bilateral, interstitial/alveolar infiltrates demonstrated by chest roentgenograph in a patient with systemic lupus erythematosus; the alveolar infiltrates were thought to be caused by intra-alveolar hemorrhage, occasionally encountered in these patients.

or discoid atelectasis is much more common and occurs in the lower two thirds of the lung fields.[59] Biopsy and immunofluorescent staining of lung in patients who develop ILD show patchy and lumpy or bumpy staining of alveolar wall. Clinical manifestations of a diffuse interstitial process are similar to those of rheumatoid arthritis and scleroderma. Infectious processes, particularly in patients receiving immunosuppressive therapy for systemic lupus erythematosus, are the commonest cause of pulmonary parenchymal infiltrates.[60] The mainstay of treatment of pulmonary complications in systemic lupus erythematosus is high-dose corticosteroids.

Scleroderma

Scleroderma, or progressive systemic sclerosis, is a systemic connective tissue disease characterized by a vascular disorder and excessive deposition of collagen and other matrix proteins in the skin and internal organs. Of all the nonpulmonary disorders, scleroderma is perhaps more often associated with diffuse ILD. Indeed, autopsy studies have shown diffuse interstitial pulmonary fibrosis in up to 80% of patients, even though many patients are minimally symptomatic during life.[61,62] The frequency of radiographically identified ILD is increased in patients with serum anti-Scl-70 antibody and decreased in those with anticentromere antibody.[63] Pulmonary involvement is more severe in the CREST (*c*alcinosis, *R*aynaud's phenomenon, *e*sophageal involvement, *s*clerodactyly, and *t*elangiectasia) variant of scleroderma. Chronic progressive interstitial pulmonary fibrosis is seen in two thirds of patients and is the commonest respiratory complication of scleroderma.

Clinical and histologic features mimic those of idiopathic pulmonary fibrosis.[64] At times, it is difficult to separate idiopathic pulmonary fibrosis from scleroderma lung. Other (nonpulmonary) manifestations may point to the correct etiology for the lung process. Although only one third of patients exhibit an abnormal chest radiograph (Figure 31-12), more than 50% of patients complain of exertional dyspnea. The commonest abnormality on pulmonary function testing is the slow but progressive restrictive dysfunction with diminished diffusing capacity for carbon monoxide. The earliest abnormality is the decreased diffusing capacity for carbon monoxide, and it is an important predictor of mortality.[65–67] Exercise-induced hypoxemia is also a common feature of scleroderma lung. The pathologic features are identical to those of idiopathic pulmonary fibrosis.[64] A lung biopsy is rarely indicated in this group of patients.

There is no effective treatment for the lung involvement in scleroderma. Corticosteroid therapy is not effective in the treatment of scleroderma or its complications. Hypoxemic patients require supplemental oxygen. Because of the high rate of gastroesophageal reflux in these patients, caused by esophageal involvement by scleroderma, it is important to instruct patients in measures to prevent reflux and aspiration. As in some cases of idiopathic pulmonary fibrosis,[68] chronic lung fibrosis secondary to scleroderma has been reported to predispose patients to lung cancer (so called "scar-cancer").[69]

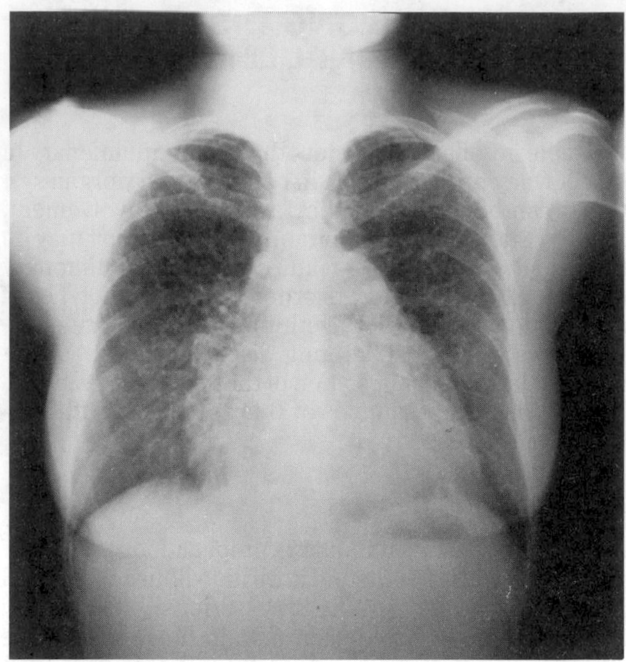

FIGURE 31-12. Chest roentgenographic appearance of chronic scleroderma-induced diffuse interstitial lung disease complicated by severe pulmonary hypertension and cor pulmonale.

Polymyositis-Dermatomyositis

Polymyositis and *dermatomyositis* caused by immunologic mechanisms should be differentiated from the polymyositis-dermatomyositis that occurs as a paraneoplastic syndrome in patients with lung cancer.[70] In the immunologic variety of the disease, diffuse ILD involving the basal regions of the lungs is the most common pulmonary abnormality encountered in 5% to 10% of patients.[51,70,71] The disease is more common in women. In one-third of the patients, the respiratory manifestations may precede the musculocutaneous signs and symptoms.[7] There is a lack of relationship between the severity and progression of the myositis and the severity of respiratory disease.[58] Lung disease associated with polymyositis-dermatomyositis may present as acute pneumonitis with alveolar or mixed alveolar-interstitial infiltrates.

There is no correlation between the severity and progression of the polymyositis-dermatomyositis and the severity of pulmonary disease.[58] However, more than 50% of patients with a disease-specific antibody (anti-Jo-1 antibody) exhibit diffuse interstitial lung disease, although not all patients demonstrate this antibody in their serum.[72–74] In one third of patients, respiratory disease precedes the skin and myopathic features by 1 to 24 months. Lung disease presents as progressive dyspnea, cough, and hypoxemia. The presence of gastroesophageal reflux, a common occurrence, complicates pulmonary complications and may be the initial manifestation in some patients. A restrictive type of lung dysfunction is present in nearly 50% of patients. Response to corticosteroids and other immunologic drugs is varied.

Patients with combined clinical features of systemic lupus erythematosus, scleroderma, and polymyositis-dermatomyositis and high titers of a specific circulating antibody to an extractable nuclear ribonucleoprotein antigen are considered to have mixed connective tissue disease. The majority of patients are women, and the average age at time of diagnosis is 37 years. Lung involvement is observed in 20% to 80% of patients. The clinical and pathophysiologic respiratory manifestations are similar to those in systemic lupus erythematosus, scleroderma, and polymyositis-dermatomyositis. More than two thirds of patients exhibit a restrictive pattern on pulmonary function tests and chest radiographs.[75,76]

Ankylosing Spondylitis

Ankylosing spondylitis, also referred to as rheumatoid spondylitis or Marie-Strümpell disease, is a chronic disorder of unknown cause characterized by progressive inflammatory disease involving the axial spine and adjacent soft tissues. It is distinctly a disease of males, with a male to female ratio of 10:1. Extraskeletal manifestations include incompetence of the aortic valve, varying degrees of heart block, acute anterior uveitis, fever, anemia, fatigue, and weight loss. Pulmonary involvement is reported in 2% to 70% of the patients.[77] In a review of more than 2,000 patients with ankylosing spondylitis, pleuropulmonary manifestations were noted in 1.3% of patients.[78] The commonest abnormality is the fibrobullous apical lesion, which is noted in 14% to 30% of cases.[79,80] The process begins as linear strands in the upper lobes, beginning medially and radiating laterally (see Figure 31-2). Computed tomography may reveal bullous changes, mycetomas, parenchymal fibrosis, pleural thickening, and bronchiectasis.[81] Diffuse ILD is an uncommon finding.[82] Costovertebral ankylosis seldom produces pulmonary symptoms, even though pulmonary function testing shows diminished total lung capacity, vital capacity, and diffusing capacity. Increased residual volume and functional residual capacity are common findings.

Sjögren's Syndrome

Sjögren's syndrome is a chronic inflammatory and autoimmune disorder characterized by diminished lacrimal and salivary gland secretion (sicca complex) resulting in keratoconjunctivitis sicca and xerostomia. Initial description of the syndrome consisted of a triad of dry eyes, dry mouth, and rheumatoid arthritis. However, only about 50% of patients with suspected Sjögren's syndrome have an autoimmune disease. Pulmonary complications are seen in both the primary and secondary forms of Sjögren's syndrome and occur in 1.5% to 75% of patients. In a large study of 343 patients with Sjögren's syndrome, 9% were found to have respiratory involvement.[83] Diffuse ILD, however, has been observed in 15% to 37% of patients.[84,85] The pulmonary process may represent nonspecific interstitial pneumonia and fibrosis or lymphocytic interstitial pneumonitis.

Studies using bronchoalveolar lavage have shown an increase in the percentages of lymphocytes and neutrophils, indicating a high frequency of subclinical alveolitis in this disease.[86] Chest roentgenograms in lymphocytic interstitial pneumonitis usually show a diffuse interstitial process, predominantly basal in distribution.[87] Lymphocytic interstitial pneumonitis may indeed represent low-grade lymphomas.[88] The physiologic dysfunction is usually mild in patients with ILD. It should be noted, however, that pulmonary function tests may demonstrate obstructive phenomenon caused by airway disease in some patients with Sjögren's syndrome.

Langerhan's Cell Granuloma of Lung

Langerhan's cell granuloma of the lung, also known as *pulmonary eosinophilic granuloma* or *histiocytosis X*, is an uncommon disorder that belongs to the reticuloendothelioses, a group of diseases of unknown cause in which an abnormal proliferation of Langerhan's cells occurs.[89] Pathologic features consist of proliferation of histiocytes in sheet-like masses with numerous eosinophils interspersed. More than 90% of patients are smokers. The disease is more frequent in whites and rare in blacks. Approximately one-third of the patients have nonspecific symptoms, namely fatigue, fever, and weight loss. Exertional dyspnea, observed in 40% of patients, is more likely caused by a spontaneous pneumothorax or an osteolytic rib lesion (both of which are well-known complications of the disease) than the pulmonary parenchymal involvement by the disease.

Pulmonary function tests show a restrictive type of defect, with decreased lung volumes, normal flow rates, and slightly reduced diffusing capacity for carbon monoxide. It is usual to see good pulmonary function even when the chest radiograph reveals extensive abnormalities. As the disease progresses, fibrosis replaces the granulomatous process, with formation of characteristic honeycomb cysts. Typically, the involvement is diffuse, bilateral, and most pronounced in the upper two thirds of the lung fields (Figure 31-13).

Spontaneous resolution is seen in a significant number of patients. In progressive disease, corticosteroids and *Vinca* alkaloid derivatives have been used.

Pulmonary Alveolar Proteinosis

Pulmonary alveolar proteinosis, a rare disease of unknown cause, affects mostly young adults.[90] It is more common in smokers, and the male to female ratio is 3:1. The pathogenesis is likely related to excessive production of surfactant or diminished clearance of surfactant by alveolar macrophages. The alveolar material contains large amounts of dipalmitoyl lecithin (surfactant). Similar pathologic features are found in patients with silica exposure, mycobacterial infections, fungal infections, tuberculosis, leukemia, and pneumocystis. An initial febrile episode is followed (after an interval of weeks to months) by progressive dyspnea with productive cough, low-grade fever, chest pain, and weight loss.

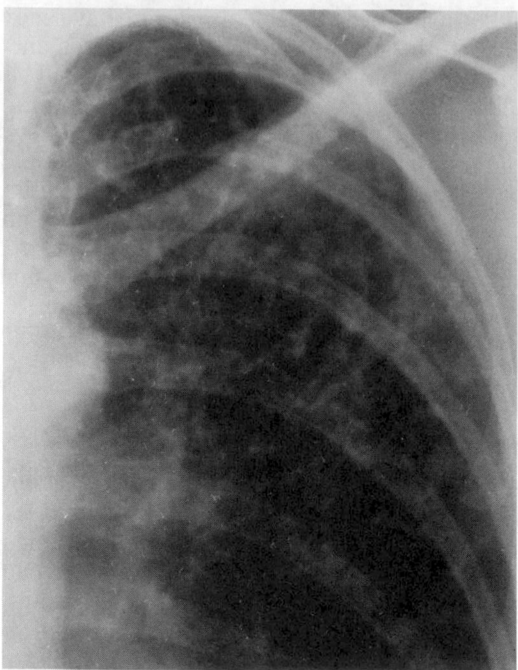

FIGURE 31-13. Roentgenograph of upper half of left lung showing nodular/interstitial infiltrates with cystic spaces in a patient with Langerhan's granuloma of lung (pulmonary eosinophilic granuloma or histiocytosis-x).

A restrictive pattern is typically seen on pulmonary function testing in combination with a decreased diffusing capacity. Lung biopsy may be needed to make the diagnosis. Chest radiographic features resemble those of pulmonary edema (alveolar infiltrates), but costophrenic angles are spared. Infections by *Nocardia* occur with a higher frequency.

Spontaneous resolution is seen in one third of patients. Symptomatic patients require whole lung lavage to remove the excessive collection of phospholipids from the alveolar spaces.

Lymphangioleiomyomatosis

Lymphangioleiomyomatosis is an uncommon progressive disorder of women of childbearing age. It is characterized by nodular and diffuse interstitial proliferation of the smooth muscle in lungs, lymph nodes, and thoracic duct. Dyspnea, hemoptysis, and spontaneous pneumothorax are common. Two thirds of the patients have chylous pleural effusion, and many of these develop chylous ascites, a result of obstruction of the thoracic duct. Chest radiograph may show diffuse nodular-interstitial infiltrates with multiple small cystic areas. High-resolution computed tomography of chest demonstrates characteristically diffuse, small, and well-defined cystic lesions in the pulmonary parenchyma (see Figure 31-4). Pulmonary function tests show obstructive features and decreased diffusing capacity. Rapidly progressive airway disease occurs in a significant number of patients. This condition is thought to be a forme fruste of tuberous sclerosis (see below). Treatment includes hormonal therapy, oophorectomy, and lung transplantation.

Tuberous Sclerosis

An inherited autosomal dominant disease of mesodermal development, tuberous sclerosis is characterized by epilepsy; mental retardation; congenital tumors; and malformations of the brain, skin, and viscera. Interstitial lung disease occurs in a small number (0.1% to 1%) of patients, most of whom are women.[91,92] The average age at the onset of symptoms caused by ILD is 34 years. Pulmonary function tests and chest radiographs reveal abnormalities similar to those in lymphangioleiomyomatosis. High-resolution computed tomography of the chest discloses typical diffuse cystic changes in the lung parenchyma often indistinguishable from lymphangioleiomyomatosis.[93] Spontaneous pneumothorax is common. Pulmonary tuberous sclerosis is usually accompanied by involvement of other organs.

An interesting note of clinical significance is that several of the ILDs discussed above demonstrate an unusual combination of diffuse interstitial, alveolar, and nodular changes on chest radiography that suggests restrictive lung disease, but pulmonary function testing shows an obstructive instead of a restrictive pattern. Examples of this unusual combination include pulmonary lymphangioleiomyomatosis, Langerhan's cell granuloma (histiocytosis X), tuberous sclerosis, cystic fibrosis, bronchiectasis, sarcoidosis with endobronchial involvement, and rheumatoid lung.

Neurofibromatosis of von Recklinghausen

Neurofibromatosis is a relatively common disease of dominant inheritance. The incidence of the disease is 1 in 3,000 births. It is manifested clinically by café-au-lait spots, freckling, Lisch nodules, hamartomas of the iris, and neurofibromas of skin and internal organs. ILD occurs in less than 10% of patients.[94] The onset of symptomatic lung disease is usually encountered between 35 and 60 years of age. The interstitial fibrosis is usually seen in the basal areas of the lungs and is radiologically and histologically indistinguishable from idiopathic pulmonary fibrosis.[95,96] Clinical manifestations are usually mild, consisting of exertional dyspnea. A restrictive pattern on pulmonary function testing and decreased diffusing capacity may be observed. Intrathoracic neurofibromas and meningoceles may occur.

Drug-Induced Lung Diseases

Lung damage from drugs is also considered under the heading of ILD. Mechanisms of drug-induced pulmonary disease include hypersensitivity, direct damage from toxic metabolites and oxygen radicals, alkylation of pulmonary tissue macromolecules, antigen-antibody reaction (type III), and type-I immune reactions. A large number of drugs are known to cause respiratory disease. Among these, the agents known to cause ILD are listed in Table 31-3. Many of the drugs initially produce acute pleuropulmonary manifestations and, with continued use, may result in ILD. Nitrofurantoin-induced lung disease is an excellent example of this.

Drug-induced lupus erythematosus is more common in older whites. Clinical manifestations include arthralgias, arthritis, fever, and malaise. Serologic abnormalities include antinuclear antibody, lupus erythematosus cell clot, rheumatoid factor, and hypocomplementemia. It is caused by cardiac drugs (procainamide, quinidine, and practolol), antibiotics (nitrofurantoin, penicillin, griseofulvin, sulfa, tetracycline), anticonvulsant agents (phenytoin, mephenytoin, carbamazepine), antihypertensive drugs (hydralazine, methyldopa, L-dopa), antituberculous drugs (isoniazid, streptomycin, para-aminosalicylic acid), phenothiazines (chlorpromazine, promethazine), and miscellaneous agents (D-penicillamine, methysergide, oral contraceptives, phenylbutazone, propylthiouracil, tolazamide, and so on). Pulmonary infiltrative disease is noted in one third of patients.

Nitrofurantoin, a commonly used urinary antibiotic, is the drug most commonly reported to produce pulmonary abnormalities. Acute reaction following ingestion of the drug may occur within a few hours to 8 weeks. The clinical features include dyspnea, cough, fever, crackles, wheezes, eosinophilia, patchy process, and pleural effusions. Chronic pulmonary reaction has occurred from 6 months to 7 years after drug therapy began. The chronic cases are uncommon but show similar features, although diffuse process is more common.[97]

Chemotherapeutic agents are among the more significant group of drugs associated with ILD. However, the mechanism of pulmonary reaction to chemotherapeutic agents remains unclear. Many chemotherapeutic drugs produce cytotoxic changes characterized by "bizarre-appearing" type II pneumocytes. Nonspecific changes are common. Symptoms include cough, dyspnea, and fever. Fever is present in most patients and may precede the onset of dyspnea or chest radiographic abnormalities (Figure 31-14).

TABLE 31-3. **Drug-Induced Interstitial Lung Disease**

Chemotherapeutic agents
Nitrofurantoin (chronic toxicity)
Drug-induced lupus erythematosus
Gold salts
Talc (intravenous use)
Aspirated oil
D-Penicillamine
Pituitary snuff
Radiation pneumonitis and/or fibrosis
Oxygen toxicity
Sulfasalazine
Cromolyn sodium
Methysergide
Hexamethonium, pentolinium, mecamylamine

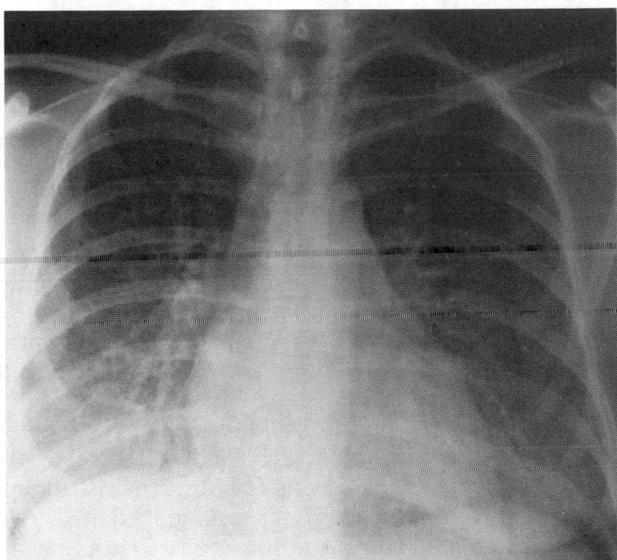

FIGURE 31-14. Chest roentgenograph demonstrates bleomycin-induced pulmonary parenchymal damage characterized by predominantly basal alveolar infiltrates in a patient who developed this "cytotoxic pneumopathy" following chemotherapy that included bleomycin for treatment of leukemia.

Pulmonary function tests reveal a restrictive pattern. Arterial oxygen desaturation is common. Busulfan (Myleran) causes "busulfan lung" in about 8% of patients. Findings on pulmonary function tests may be abnormal without clinical or radiologic evidence of disease. Pulmonary reaction is usually seen after 6 months of therapy. Chest radiograph shows diffuse interstitial and alveolar infiltrates. Death may occur despite stopping the use of the drug and using steroids. Cyclophosphamide (Cytoxan) produces (but less commonly) similar reactions. However, changes are seen earlier than with busulfan. Bleomycin has a 10% incidence of pulmonary toxicity, which increases with increasing age (> 70 years) and increasing dosage (> 450 units). Simultaneous use of a high concentration of the inhaled form increases the risk of pulmonary toxicity.

Acute hypersensitivity reaction with eosinophilia has been reported in some patients. Chlorambucil (uncommonly) produces complications similar to those caused by busulfan, cyclophosphamide, and bleomycin. Carmustine produces pulmonary reactions in 1% of patients within 8 months, similar to those seen with other chemotherapeutic agents. A higher incidence of pneumothorax has been noted. Methotrexate is the only antimetabolite known to produce pulmonary disease that is self-limiting and is frequently associated with peripheral eosinophilia. Most pulmonary reactions reported have been in children treated for acute lymphatic leukemia, and symptoms begin within a few days to several weeks after initiation of therapy. Chest radiograph shows diffuse fine interstitial infiltrates, hilar adenopathy, or pleural effusion in 10% of patients.

Radiation pneumonitis is a well-recognized cause of iatrogenic ILD. Type II pneumocytes and pulmonary capillary endothelial cells are initially affected by radiation. Radiation effects may be cumulative; the rate at which it is given is most important. A second or third course of radiation to the lung is more likely to result in a pneumonitis that can occur earlier and be devastating. During the acute phase, type II pneumocyte changes and an inflammatory process can be seen. In the chronic stage, nonspecific fibrosis is common. Symptoms of radiation pneumonitis begin insidiously 1 to 3 months after completion of radiation. Cough, fever, and dyspnea may precede the onset of chest radiographic changes (Figure 31-15). The late phase begins 6 months after radiation therapy. Dyspnea is usually out of proportion to the chest radiographic changes. Steroid therapy has varying response.

Oxygen toxicity can be avoided if the FIO_2 is kept below 0.5. If the duration of FIO_2 of 1.0 exceeds 24 hours, or if FIO_2 of 0.6 exceeds 72 hours, the risk of pulmonary damage increases. Oxygen-induced adult respiratory distress syndrome is not amenable to any treatment, and the patients usually succumb to lung failure. Histologic features include an early exudative phase followed by an irreversible proliferative and fibrotic phase.

With aspiration of oil, abnormalities range from solitary nodules to various types of infiltrates, especially in the dependent lower lung fields. Mineral oil for softening stools, oily nose drops, ophthalmic drops, and other oily preparations are used frequently.

Interstitial Lung Disease in HIV-Infected Patients

Nonspecific interstitial pneumonitis is a common occurrence in patients with chronic AIDS and represents 30% to 40% of all episodes of lung infiltrates in these patients. More than 25% of patients with this problem have either concurrent Kaposi's sarcoma, previous experimental therapies, or a history of *P. carinii* pneumonia or drug abuse. The clinical features are similar to those of patients with *P. carinii* pneumonia. Chest roentgenograms reveal patchy, diffuse interstitial infiltrates bilaterally (Figure 31-16). Histopathologic features of the lung in interstitial pneumonitis associated with AIDS may include varying degrees of edema, fibrin deposition, and interstitial inflammation with lymphocytes and plasma cells. There is no known therapy.

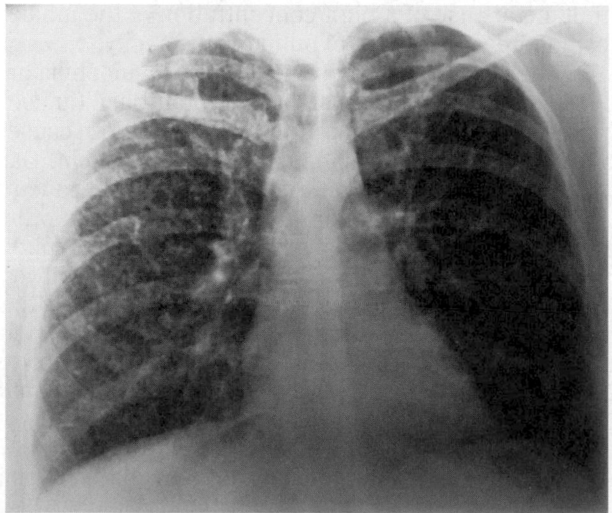

FIGURE 31-15. Radiation-induced interstitial lung disease seen in this chest roentgenograph of a patient who received high-dose radiotherapy for treatment of inoperable carcinoma of the esophagus.

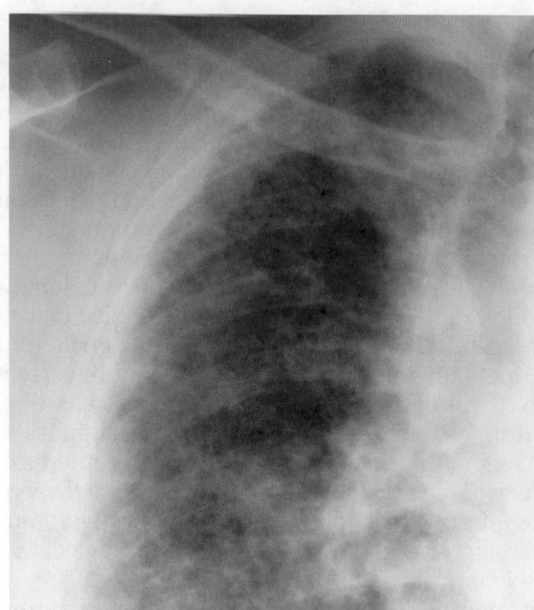

FIGURE 31-16. Upper half of the right lung depicted in this chest roentgenograph of a patient with acquired immunodeficiency syndrome; the diffuse interstitial infiltrates evaluated by lung biopsy revealed nonspecific interstitial infiltrates.

Lymphocytic interstitial pneumonitis is caused by pulmonary infiltration with mature polyclonal B lymphocytes and plasma cells. It occurs in children of mothers in groups at high risk for AIDS, Haitians, and patients with AIDS. Systemic corticosteroid therapy may produce significant improvement. Lymphocytic interstitial pneumonitis is a nonspecific entity in adults with AIDS.

Cystic lung disease is more common in patients with *P. carinii* infections and in those receiving aerosolized pentamidine therapy. Cystic lesions are more common in the upper- and mid-lung zones. Chest CT identifies these small- to medium-sized cystic lesions. Pneumothorax occurs with increasing frequency in patients with *P. carinii* pneumonia and in those receiving pentamidine aerosol therapy. Other causes of pneumothorax include Kaposi sarcoma, tuberculosis, and other infections. Pneumothorax in patients with AIDS carries a poor prognosis.

FUTURE APPROACHES TO INTERSTITIAL LUNG DISEASES

Newer insights into the pathogenesis of interstitial lung disease may help us understand the precise etiologic and pathologic mechanisms that lead to life-threatening pulmonary disease. Increasing numbers of etiologic factors have been identified in recent years. Endogenous chemical mediators and genetic factors responsible for interstitial lung disease have been identified.[98] A simplified diagnostic approach, aided by the more sophisticated imaging techniques, may obviate the need for invasive diagnostic procedures.[99]

In most cases of idiopathic interstitial lung diseases, the mainstay of therapy has included systemic corticosteroids. Other drugs have consisted of cytotoxic agents such as cyclophosphamide, azathioprine, chlorambucil, methotrexate, colchicine, penicillamine, or cyclosporine. Unfortunately, the response to these treatments is dismal, with less than 20% of patients thus treated demonstrating response. Newer modalities may include cytokine inhibitors, growth factor inhibitors, antifibrotic agents, antiproteases, antioxidants, surfactant, regulation of white cell traffic within the alveolar regions, gene therapy, and newer anti-inflammatory agents.[100–102]

Considering that idiopathic pulmonary fibrosis is a highly lethal disease in most patients, with a prognosis similar to that of lung cancer,[100] it is imperative that future research address the role of various etiologic factors and appropriate therapies.

REFERENCES

1. Prakash UBS: Pulmonary Diseases. In UBS Prakash (ed): Mayo Internal Medicine Board Review 1994–95. Rochester, Minnesota; Mayo Foundation; 1994; p 697
2. Crystal RG, Bitterman PB, Rennard SI, et al: Interstitial lung diseases of unknown cause. Disorders characterized by chronic inflammation of the lower respiratory tract. N Eng J Med 310:154 and 235, 1984
3. Crystal RG, Gadek JE, Ferrans VJ, et al: Interstitial lung disease: Current concepts of pathogenesis, staging, and therapy. Am J Med 70:542, 1981
4. King TE Jr: Idiopathic Pulmonary Fibrosis. In MI Schwratz, TE King Jr (eds): Interstitial Lung Disease. Philadelphia, BC Decker, 1988, p 139
5. Vergnon JM, Vincent M, DeThe G, et al: Cryptogenic fibrosing alveolitis and Epstein-Barr virus: An association? Lancet 2:768, 1984
6. Takashi U, Suzuki N, Yamaguchi M, et al: Idiopathic pulmonary fibrosis and high prevalence of serum antibodies to hepatitis C virus. Am Rev Respir Dis 146:266, 1992
7. Crystal RG, Fulmer JD, Roberts WC, et al: Idiopathic pulmonary fibrosis: Clinical, histologic, radiographic, physiologic, scintigraphic, cytologic, and biochemical aspects. Ann Intern Med 85:769, 1976
8. Gross N: Pulmonary effects of radiation therapy. Ann Intern Med 86:81, 1977
9. Christensen LT, Schmidt CD, Robbins L: Pigeon breeder's disease: A prevalence study and review. Clin Allergy 5:417, 1975
10. Roberts RC, Moore VL: State of the art: Immunopathogenesis of hypersensitivity pneumonitis. Am Rev Respir Dis 116:1975, 1977
11. Cooper JAO, White DA, Matthay RA: Drug-induced pulmonary disease: Parts I and II. Am Rev Respir Dis 133:321 and 488, 1986
12. Rochester CL, Elias JA: Cytokines and cytokine networking in the pathogenesis of interstitial and fibrotic lung disorders. Semin Respir Med 14:389, 1993
13. Robertson HT: Clinical application of pulmonary function and exercise tests in the management of patients with interstitial lung disease. Semin Respir Med 15:1, 1994
14. Turner-Warwick M, Burrows B, Johnson A: Cryptogenic fibrosing alveolitis: Clinical features and their influence on survival. Thorax 35:171, 1980
15. Gibson GJ, Pride NB: Pulmonary mechanics in fibrosing alveolitis. Am Rev Respir Dis 116:637, 1977
16. Gaensler EA, Carrington CB, Coutu RE, et al: Radiographic-physiologic-pathologic correlations in interstitial pneumonias. Prog Respir Res 8:223, 1975
17. Austrian R, McClement JH, Renzetti AD, et al: Clinical and physiologic features of some types of pulmonary diseases with impairment of alveolar-capillary diffusion. Am J Med 11:667, 1951
18. Fulmer JD, Roberts WC, von Gal ER, et al: Morphologic-physiologic correlates of the severity of fibrosis and degree of cellularity in idiopathic pulmonary fibrosis. J Clin Invest 63.65, 1979
19. Carrington CB, Gaensler EA, Coutu RE, et al: Natural history and treated course of usual and desquamative interstitial pneumonia. N Eng J Med 298:801, 1978
20. Godwin JD, Holt RM: Imaging of interstitial lung disease. Semin Respir Crit Care Med 15:10, 1994
21. Kirtland SH, Winterbauer RH: Pulmonary sarcoidosis. Semin Respir Med 14:344, 1993
22. Kirtland AH, Winterbauer RH: Pulmonary sarcoidosis. Semin Respir Med 14:344, 1993
23. Utz JP, Prakash UBS: Indications for and Contraindications to Bronchoscopy. In UBS Prakash (ed): Bronchoscopy. New York, Raven Press, 1994, p 81
24. Costabel U, Bross KJ, Marxen J, et al: T-lymphocytosis in bronchoalveolar lavage fluid of hypersensitivity pneumonitis. Chest 85:514, 1984
25. Semenzato G, Agostini C, Zambello R, et al: Lung T cells in hypersensitivity pneumonitis: Phenotypic and functional analyses. J Immunol 137:1164, 1986
26. Prakash UBS, Utz JP: Bronchoscopic lung biopsy. In KP Wang, AC Mehta (eds): Flexible Bronchoscopy. Cambridge, Massachusetts; Blackwell Scientific; 1995; p 119
27. Meier-Sydow J, Weiss SM, Buhl R, et al: Idiopathic pulmonary fibrosis: Current clinical concepts and challenges in management. Semin Respir Crit Care Med 15:77, 1994
28. Hughes EW: Familial interstitial pulmonary fibrosis. Thorax 19:515, 1964
29. Sharma OP: Sarcoidosis. Dis Mon 36:471, 1990
30. Kirks DR, McCormick VD, Greenspan RH: Pulmonary sarcoidosis: Roentgenologic analysis of 150 patients. AJR Am J Roentgenol 177:777, 1973
31. Thrasher DR, Briggs DD: Pulmonary sarcoidosis. Clin Chest Med 3:537, 1986
32. Dawson WB, Muller NL: High-resolution computed tomography in pulmonary sarcoidosis: Am Rev Respir Dis 107:609, 1973
33. Muller NL, Kullnig P, Miller RR: The CT findings of pulmonary sarcoidosis: Analysis of 25 patients. AJR Am J Roentgenol 152: 1179, 1989
34. Sider LS, Horton ES: Hilar and mediastinal adenopathy in sarcoidosis as detected by computed tomography. J Thoracic Imaging 5:77, 1990
35. Winterbauer RH, Hutchinson JF: Clinical significance of pulmonary function tests. Chest 78:640, 1980
36. Bradvik I, Wollmer P, Blom-Bulow B, et al: Lung mechanics and gas exchange during exercise in pulmonary sarcoidosis. Chest 99:572, 1991
37. Harrison BDW, Shaylor JM, Stokes TC: Airflow limitation in sarcoidosis: A study of pulmonary function in 107 patients with newly diagnosed disease. Respir Med 85:95, 1991
38. Sharma OP, Johnson RJ: Airway obstruction in sarcoidosis. Chest 94:343, 1988
39. Roethe RA, Fuller PB, Byrd RB, et al: Transbronchoscopic lung biopsy in sarcoidosis. Chest 77:400, 1980
40. Hillerdahl G, Osterman NR, Schmekel B: Sarcoidosis: Epidemiology and diagnosis: A 15-year European study. Am Rev Respir Dis 130:29, 1984
41. Neville E, Walker AN, Gerant-James D: Prognostic factors predicting the outcome of sarcoidosis: An analysis of 818 patients. Q J Med 208:525, 1983
42. Schwarz MI: Interstitial lung disease associated with bronchiolitis, eosinophilic granuloma, and other unique entities. Semin Respir Med 14:375, 1993
43. Selman M, Chapela R, Raghu G: Hypersensitivity pneumonitis: Clinical manifestations, pathogenesis, diagnosis, and therapeutic strategies. Semin Respir Med 14:353, 1993

44. Sharma OP: Clinical Features. In OP Sharma (ed): Hypersensitivity Pneumonitis: A Clinical Approach. Progress in Respiration Research, vol 23. Basel, S Karger, 1989, p 41
45. Richerson HB, Bernstein IL, Fink JN, et al: Guidelines for the clinical evaluation of hypersensitivity pneumonitis. J Allergy Clin Immunol 84:839, 1989
46. Sansores R, Salas J, Chapela R, et al: Clubbing in hypersensitivity pneumonitis: Its prevalence and possible prognostic role. Arch Intern Med 150:1849, 1990
47. Cormier Y, Belnager J, Durand P: Factors including the development of serum precipitins to farmer's lung antigen in Quebec dairy farmers. Thorax 40:138, 1985
48. McSharry C, Banham SW, Lynch PP, et al: Antibody measurement in extrinsic allergic alveolitis. Eur J Respir Dis 65:259, 1984
49. Prakash UBS: Rheumatological Diseases. In JF Murray (ed): Pulmonary Manifestations in Systemic Diseases, vol 59: Lung Biology in Health and Disease. New York, Marcel Dekker, 1992, p 1385
50. Prakash UBS: Pulmonary Manifestations in Rheumatologic Diseases. In Baum and Wolinsky (eds): Textbook of Pulmonary Diseases (5th ed). Boston; Little, Brown; 1994; p 1471
51. Hunninghake GW, Fauci AS: Pulmonary involvement in the collagen vascular diseases. Am Rev Respir Dis 119:471, 1979
52. Jurik AG, Davidsen D, Graudal H: Prevalence of pulmonary involvement in rheumatoid arthritis and its relationship to some characteristics of the patients. Scand J Rheum 11:217, 1982
53. Hyland RH, Gordon DA, Broder I, et al: A systematic controlled study of pulmonary abnormalities in rheumatoid arthritis. J Rheumatol 10:395, 1983
54. Roschmann RA, Rothenberg RJ: Pulmonary fibrosis in rheumatoid arthritis: A review of clinical features and therapy. Semin Arthritis Rheum 16:174, 1987
55. Roschmann RA, Rothenberg RJ: Pulmonary fibrosis in rheumatoid arthritis: A review of clinical features and therapy. Semin Arthrits Rheum 16:174, 1987
56. Keogh BA, Crystal RG: Chronic Interstitial Lung Disease. In DH Simmons (ed): Current Pulmonology. Chichester, Wiley, 1981, pp 237–240
57. Yousem SA, Colby TV, Carrington CB: Follicular bronchitis/bronchiolitis. Hum Pathol 16:700, 1985
58. Wiedemann HP, Matthay RA: Pulmonary manifestations of the collagen vascular diseases. Clin Chest Med 10:677, 1989
59. Eisenberg, H, Dubois EL, Sherwin RP, et al: Diffuse interstitial lung disease in systemic lupus erythematosus. Ann Intern Med 79:37, 1973
60. Haupt HM, Moore GW, Hutchins GM: The lung in systemic lupus erythematosus: Analysis of the pathologic changes in 120 patients. Am J Med 71:791, 1981
61. D'Angelo WA, Fries JF, Masi AT, et al: Pathologic observations in systemic sclerosis(scleroderma): A study of fifty-eight autopsy cases and fifty-eight matched controls. Am J Med 46:428, 1969
62. Weaver AL, Diverite MB, Titus JL: Pulmonary scleroderma. Dis Chest 54:490, 1968
63. Schumacher HR (ed): Primer on Rheumatic Diseases (9th ed). Atlanta, Georgia; Arthritis Foundation; 1988
64. Harrison NK, McAnulty RJ, Haslam PL, et al: Evidence for protein oedema, neutrophil influx, and enhanced collagen production in lungs of patients with systemic sclerosis. Thorax 45:606, 1990
65. Bagg LR, Hughes TD: Serial pulmonary function tests in progressive systemic sclerosis. Thorax 34:224, 1979
66. Owens GR, Fino GJ, Herbert DL, et al: Pulmonary function in progressive systemic sclerosis: Comparison of CREST syndrome variant with diffuse scleroderma. Chest 84:546, 1983
67. Wells AU, Hansell DM, du Bois RM: Interstitial lung disease in the collagen vascular diseases. Semin Respir Med 14:333, 1993
68. Mizushima Y, Kobayashi M: Clinical characteristics of synchronous multiple lung cancer associated with idiopathic pulmonary fibrosis: A review of Japanese cases. Chest 108:1272, 1995
69. Peters-Golden M, Wise RA, Hochberg M, et al: Incidence of lung cancer in systemic sclerosis. J. Rheumatol 12:1136, 1985
70. Bohan A, Peter JB: Polymyositis and dermatomyositis. N Engl J Med 292:344, 1975
71. Frazier AR, Miller RD: Interstitial pneumonitis in association with polymyositis and dermatomyositis. Chest 65:403, 1974
72. Arnett FC, Hirsch TJ, Bias WB, et al: The Jo-1 antibody system in myositis: Relationships to clinical features and HLA. J Rheumatol 8:925, 1981
73. Hochberg MC, Feldman D, Stevens MB, et al: Antibody to Jo-1 in polymyositis/dermatomyositis: Association with interstitial pulmonary disease. J Rheumatol 11:663, 1984
74. Wasicek CA, Reichlin M, Montes M, et al: Polymyositis and interstitial lung disease in a patient with anti-Jo-1 prototype. Am J Med 76:538, 1984
75. Prakash UBS, Luthra HS, Divertie MB: Intrathoracic manifestations in mixed connective tissue disease. Mayo Clin Proc 60:813, 1985
76. Prakash UBS: Lungs in mixed connective tissue disease. J Thorac Imaging 7:1, 1992
77. Prakash UBS: Pulmonary Manifestations in Skeletal Diseases. In G Baum and E Wolinsky (eds): Textbook of Pulmonary Diseases (5th ed). Boston; Little, Brown; 1994: p 1691
78. Rosenow EC III, Strimlan CV, Muhm JR, et al: Pleuropulmonary manifestations of ankylosing spondylitis. Mayo Clin Proc 52:641, 1977
79. Chakera TM, Howarth FH, Kendall MJ, et al: The chest radiograph in ankylosing spondylitis. Clin Radiol 26:455, 1975
80. Cruickshank B: Pathology of ankylosing spondylitis. Bull Rheum Dis 10:211, 1960
81. Rumancik WM, Firooznia H, Davis MS Jr, et al: Fibrobullous disease of the upper lobes: An extraskeletal manifestation of ankylosing spondylitis. J Comput Tomogr 8:225, 1984
82. Cohen AA, Natelson EA, Fechner RE: Fibrosing interstitial pneumonitis in ankylosing spondylitis. Chest 59:369, 1971
83. Strimaln CV, Rosenow EC III, Divertie MB, et al: Pulmonary manifestations of Sjögren's syndrome. Chest 70:354, 1976
84. Segal IE, Fink G, Machtey I, Gura V, et al: Pulmonary function abnormalities in Sjögren's syndrome and the sicca complex. Thorax 36:286, 1981
85. Papathanasiou M, Constantopoulos SH, Tsampoulas C, et al: Reappraisal of respiratory abnormalities in primary and secondary Sjögren's syndrome: A controlled study. Chest 90:370, 1986
86. Hatron P, Wallaert B, Gosset D, et al: Subclinical lung inflammation in primary Sjögren's syndrome. Arthritis Rheum 30:1226, 1987
87. Adamson T, Fox RI, Frisman D, Howell FV: Immunohistologic analysis of lymphoid infiltrates in primary Sjögren's syndrome monoclonal antibodies. J Immunol 130:203, 1983
88. Hansen LA, Prakash UBS, Colby TV: Pulmonary lymphoma in Sjögren's syndrome. Mayo Clin Proceed 64:920, 1989
89. Prakash UBS: Pulmonary Eosinophilic Granuloma. In JP Lynch III, RA DeRemee (eds): Immunologic Pulmonary Diseases. Philadelphia, JB Lippincott, 1991, p 432
90. Prakash UBS, Barham SS, Carpenter HA, et al: Pulmonary alveolar phospholipoproteinosis: Experience with 34 cases and a review. Mayo Clin Proc 62:499, 1987
91. Medley BE, McLeod RA, Houser OW: Tuberous sclerosis. Semin Roentgenol 11:35, 1976
92. Dwyer JM, Hickie JB, Garvan J: Pulmonary tuberous sclerosis: Report of three patients and a review of the literature. Q J Med 40:115, 1971
93. Rapport DC, Weisbrod GL, Herman SJ, et al: Pulmonary lymphangiomyomatosis: High resolution CT findings in four cases. J Roentgenol 152:961, 1989
94. Prakash UBS: Pulmonary Manifestations in Dermatologic Diseases. In G Baum and E Wolinsky (eds): Textbook of Pulmonary Diseases (5th ed). Boston; Little, Brown; 1994; p 1707
95. Webb WR, Goodman PC: Fibrosing alveolitis in patients with neurofibromatosis. Radiology 122:289, 1966
96. Massaro D, Katz S: Fibrosing alveolitis: Its occurrence, roentgenographic and pathologic features in von Recklinghausen's neurofibromatosis. Am Rev Respir Dis 93:934, 1966
97. Prakash UBS: Pulmonary reaction to nitrofurantoin. Semin Respir Med 2:70, 1980
98. Jimenez SA: New insights into the pathogenesis of interstitial pulmonary fibrosis. Thorax 49:193, 1994
99. Raghu G: Interstitial lung disease: A diagnostic approach. Am J Respir Crit Care Med 151:909, 1995
100. Hunninghake GW, Kalica AR: Approaches to the treatment of pulmonary fibrosis. Am J Respir Crit Care Med 151:915, 1995
101. Phan SH: New strategies for treatment of pulmonary fibrosis. Thorax 50:415, 1995
102. Goldstein RH, Fine A: Potential therapeutic initiatives for fibrogenic lung diseases. Chest 108:848, 1995

32 Work-Related, Environmentally Caused, and Self-Induced Pulmonary Diseases

George G. Burton

CLINICAL SKILLS

Upon completion of this chapter, the reader will:

- Understand the role of the respiratory care practitioner (RCP) in the diagnosis and treatment of work-related pulmonary disorders.
- Understand the clinical presentation and treatment of the reactive airways dysfunction syndrome (RADS).
- Be able to recognize the respiratory hazards that may be present in the health-care industry workplace, including tuberculosis, hepatitis, and HIV infection.
- Recognize the health effects of urban air pollution including those of carbon monoxide, ozone, sulfur oxides, and particulates.
- Understand the respiratory care of patients with pulmonary burns and smoke inhalation.
- Describe the health effects of tobacco smoking and strategies available for effective smoking cessation behavior.
- Understand the respiratory manifestations associated with alcoholism and illicit drug use.

KEY TERMS

Addiction
Air quality advisories ("smog alerts")
Alcoholism
Americans With Disabilities Act
Amphetamines
Asbestosis
Asphyxiants
Auto-PEEP
Behavioral modifications
B-readers
Bronchial provocation testing
Burn team
Carbon monoxide poisoning
Carboxyhemoglobinemia
"Cold turkey" method of smoking cessation
Co-oximetry
"Crack" cocaine
Cyanide intoxication
Disability
"Eggshell" calcifications
Fasciotomy
Heroin
ILO classification
Impairment
Marijuana
Material Safety Data Sheets (MSDS)
Mesothelioma
Negative pressure room ventilation
Nicotine dependency
Nicotine polacrilex gum
Nicotine withdrawal
NIOSH
OSHA
Ozone
Pleural plaques
Pneumoconiosis
RADS (Reactive Airways Dysfunction Syndrome)
Silicosis
"Slow taper" (nicotine fading) technique

Smoking cessation
Substance abuse
"Tight building" syndrome
Transdermal nicotine patches
Worker's compensation

The role of the respiratory care practitioner (RCP) expands as his or her capability as a diagnostician and educator matures. This chapter describes those nontraditional activities in the areas of the patient's respiratory compromise secondary to often unintentional exposure in the workplace and the environment, and to intentional exposures to tobacco smoke and abused controlled substances. Treatment of these disorders is described only briefly, as these topics have been covered in other sections of this book. The newer practice domains of prevention and diagnostic evaluation are discussed in more detail.

ASSESSMENT AND EVALUATION

Occupational and environmental exposures to a large variety of allergens, gases, fumes, dusts and other particulates, noxious gases, bacteriologic agents, and physical risk factors contribute to significant morbidity and mortality each year.[1,2] To a large extent, the symptoms caused by such exposures, for example, bronchospasm, cough, mucosal irritation, and dyspnea, are nonspecific, and their treatment does not differ significantly from symptoms caused by other, more widely recognized causes.

Only by a careful exposure history will the work factor- or environmental factor-relatedness of these symptoms become apparent, as will their relationship to long-term outcome and disability.[3] Bresnitz[4] recently observed that few physicians are trained in evaluating an occupational history to assess the cause of pulmonary disease. Himmelstein and Frumkin[5] reached the same conclusion with respect to physician awareness of the less dramatic environmental causative factors. Review of 2- and even 4-year respiratory care curricula reveal the basis for a similar lack of preparedness among RCPs. It is not unthinkable that in the future, RCPs may find themselves evaluating the nature and degree of exposure(s), assessing causation, performing physiologic tests to determine levels of impairment (see Chapter 8), assessing reversibility of impairment, preparing job evaluations to assist the physician in recommending work restrictions and modifications, as suggested in the *Americans with Disabilities Act* in suggesting preventive measures, and in helping to develop recommendations for disability payments in the form of *Workers Compensation.*

A detailed occupational/environmental exposure history outline is shown in Table 32-1[4] and is essential to estimating the possibility or probability of clinically significant exposure. With training, an RCP could be expected to elicit such a careful history from an exposed individual. Exposure to agents at concentrations in excess of *Occupational Safety and Health Administration (OSHA)* permissible levels, or *National Institute for Occupational Safety and Health (NIOSH)* recommended exposure limits would be appropriately investigated. In cases of suspected toxic exposure, all *material safety data sheets (MSDS)* regarding materials in use by the worker should be obtained, and the potential respiratory effects of the suspected agents should be evaluated.

Resting pulmonary function testing in all, and exercise testing in selected cases, both determined in a standardized manner, are the cornerstones for assessing work or environmentally caused impairment.[6,7] Table 32-2[4] lists the American Thoracic Society classification[7] for respiratory impairment in such cases. Serial worsening in pulmonary function is especially important. The role of the RCP in performing such measures has been discussed in Chapter 8.

Physical Examination and Radiographic Studies

With the exception of high-level, high-toxicity gaseous, liquid, and fume exposure (eg, H_2SO_4 mist, N_2O exposure, and CO intoxication), the physical examination is seldom helpful in determining the work-relatedness

TABLE 32-1. **Components of an Occupational History**

Current work history
- Specifics of the job
  - Employer's name
  - Duration of employment
  - Process description
  - Job description
  - Adjacent processes

Hazardous exposures

Health effects
- Suspicious health problems
- Temporality of symptoms
- Affected coworkers
- Medical surveillance records
- Biologic monitoring

Control measures
- Environmental sampling and monitoring
- Engineering controls
- Work practice protocols
- Administrative controls
- Personal protective equipment
- Worker education and training
- Medical monitoring

Work history

Nonoccupational exposures
- Hobbies
- Outdoor activities
- Residential exposures
- Community contamination

From Bresnitz EA, Rubenstein H, Rast KM: Recognition and follow-up of workplace poisonings. *In* Goldfrank LR, Flomenbaum NE, Lewin NA, et al (eds): Goldfrank's Toxicologic Emergencies. Norwalk, CT, Appleton & Lange, 1994, 1154–1157; with permission.

TABLE 32-2. **American Thoracic Society Classification Scheme for Respiratory Impairment***

American Thoracic Society*	Normal	Mildly Impaired	Moderately Impaired	Severely Impaired
FVC	≥80% predicted	60%–79% predicted	51%–59% predicted	≤50% predicted
	AND	**OR**	**OR**	**OR**
FEV_1	≥80% predicted	60%–79% predicted	41%–59% predicted	≤40% predicted
	AND	**OR**	**OR**	**OR**
$FEV_1/FVC \times 100$	≥75%	60%–74%	41%–59%	≤40%
	AND	**OR**	**OR**	**OR**
DLCOsb	≥80% predicted	60%–79% predicted	41%–59% predicted	≤40% predicted
Estimation of impairment based on VO_2 max; assumes comfortable performance of job at 40% VO_2 max	≥25 mL/(kg min); capable of all but the most exerting jobs	15–25 mL/(kg min) **AND** 40% of VO_2 max observed ≥ average metabolic work of job: able to perform the job comfortably		≤15 mL/(kg min); unable to perform most jobs because of discomfort traveling to and from work

From American Thoracic Society: Evaluation of impairment/disability secondary to respiratory disorders. Am Rev Respir Dis 133:1205–1209, 1996; with permission.

*Predicted values based on height, age, and sex of white Americans. These prediction values should be used when applying the American Thoracic Society criteria for respiratory impairment.

FVC = forced vital capacity; FEV_1 = forced expiratory volume in the first second; DLCOsb = single-breath carbon monoxide diffusing capacity of the lungs; VO_2 max = maximal oxygen consumption.

of the patient's condition. Such subtle findings as fine end-inspiratory crackles (*pneumoconiosis*) or transient pleural friction rubs (*asbestosis*) may be difficult to pick up, unless the examiner has a high degree of suspicion.

The RCP can assist the physician by assembling any and all chest radiographs that are available. "Old films" may allow serial assessment of subtle roentgenographic findings. In the dust and particulate diseases (coal worker's pneumoconiosis, *silicosis*, asbestosis), films should be interpreted by specially qualified radiologists, called "*B-readers*," using the International Labor Organization (ILB) classification of pneumoconiosis standards.

Table 32-3 lists common sense criteria used in assessing a causal relationship between workplace exposure and occupation-related pulmonary disease, impairment, and disability.[4] The Social Security Administration defines the *impaired individual* as having "medically demonstrable anatomical, physiological or psychological abnormalities" that *disable* the worker as defined by "the inability to engage in any substantial activity by reason of . . . impairment which can be expected to result in death or which has lasted or can be expected to last for a continuous period of not less than 12 months."[8] It is during this protracted period that the more traditional (treatment) skills of the RCP will come into play.

TABLE 32-3. **Criteria for Establishing the Work-Relatedness of Occupational Disease**

Known and documented occupational exposure to a suspected causative agent
Symptoms compatible with the suspected workplace exposure
Suggestive or diagnostic physical signs
Similar problems in fellow workers or workers in related occupations
Periodicity of complaints related to work
Confirmatory industrial hygiene or other environmental monitoring data
Scientific biologic plausibility
Biologic (tissue or fluid) confirmation in the patient
Lack of an obvious nonoccupational cause

OCCUPATIONAL PULMONARY DISORDERS

Asbestosis

Most cases of asbestosis develop from exposure to asbestosis fibers decades ago, when the material was widely used in ship insulation, heating and air conditioning, and building construction. Literally thousands of cases are currently in litigation, and at least one large manufacturer, Johns-Mansville Corporation, was forced into bankruptcy because of the litigation costs.

Today, workers are exposed to asbestos in the handling of brake shoe linings, ceiling acoustical tile, electrical equipment, and boiler insulation. Construction workers engaged in removing asbestos insulation from schools and other public buildings may also be heavily exposed, if they lack appropriate protective equipment or fail to use it. High-level exposure is required to produce parenchymal asbestosis. High- *or* low-level exposure may result in lung cancer or *mesothelioma*, both of which are usually fatal.

Dyspnea, dry cough, tachypnea, and mid- to late-inspiratory crackles characterize asbestosis. Calcified *pleural plaques* may be seen on CT scans of the chest and are virtually pathognomic of the condition. Small irregular opacities are seen in x-ray examination of the lung parenchyma and are nonspecific. A "shaggy heart" image is sometimes seen on chest radiograph and is highly suggestive of the disorder (see Chapter 7).

No specific treatment for asbestosis is available. Thus, treatment is symptomatic.[10]

Silicosis

Silicosis occurs in workers in the sandblasting, quarrying, brickmaking, cement, and pottery industries. The primary symptoms are dry cough and dyspnea. Discrete random nodules may be seen in the midzone of the chest radiograph, and highly characteristic *"eggshell" calcifications* of the hilar lymph nodes may be observed. A restrictive disorder appears on pulmonary function testing, but only after years of exposure. Patients with silicosis are at extremely high risk for later developing pulmonary tuberculosis.[10]

Tuberculosis: Another Workplace Hazard

Tuberculosis is an occupational disease for health care workers, and those who deliver care in high-incidence urban settings should feel especially vulnerable.[11] OSHA has mandated that hospitals and certain other facilities provide training, skin tests, and respiratory protective equipment for personnel, and isolation rooms and *negative pressure ventilation rooms* for patients. These rooms are arranged so that the ambient pressure is always negative, a strategy which is thought to keep harmful bacteria from escaping into adjoining hallways and rooms.

The risk of tuberculous infection is heightened by its airborne person-to-person transmission, especially among health care workers who come in contact with HIV-infected patients, homeless persons, drug users, and prison inmates. In some instances, individual tuberculosis patients have accounted for tuberculin skin test conversions among more than 30% of hospital personnel exposed, even when the employees were exposed for only a few hours.

The drug-resistant nature of certain strains of tuberculosis organisms affecting nearly 20% or more of all patients in some urban settings is also cause for concern. A recent nationwide survey found that nearly 10% of tuberculosis infections were resistant to isoniazid and/or rifampin.[12]

Workplaces outside the health care system may also pose a hazard for tuberculosis development. A single unsuspected worker has the ability to infect many others. Several tuberculosis carriers have infected scores of their co-workers, and one shipyard employee transmitted *Mycobacterium tuberculosis* to more than 400 coworkers. Ten persons have died of health occupation-acquired tuberculosis in the past 2 years in this country.

Specialists suggest that a patient believed to have tuberculosis—with cough, weight loss, and fever—should be placed in an isolation room and possibly provided with a mask with a no room-venting exhalation valve. Abnormal chest films help to confirm the diagnosis. Several sputum smears should be obtained because some negative smears are followed by positive findings. Sputum cultures are also appropriate.

Therapy typically includes isoniazid and rifampin. Most authors recommend, however, that a four-drug regimen be used in geographic areas where drug resistance is elevated. They suggest use of either isoniazid, rifampin, pyrazinamide, and ethambutol HCl (Myambutol), or the first three combined with streptomycin sulfate instead of ethambutol. Prompt and vigorous treatment is essential because pharmacotherapy is hampered by noncompliance as well as drug resistance.

ENVIRONMENTALLY CAUSED PULMONARY DISORDERS

Occupational Asthma

Work-induced asthma resembles conventional extrinsic asthma in symptoms and physical findings. However, it can be distinguished by a history of on-the-job exposure to any one of a variety of provocative substances. There is a general perception that the condition is underdiagnosed, though it is treatable and may become more severe if neglected.

Table 32-4 lists common causes of occupational asthma.[13] Substances that commonly induce asthma include isocyanates, wood dust, baking flour, organic dusts, hexavalent chromate compounds, and printing inks. Animal danders, enzymes, anhydrides, and pharmacologic agents may also cause asthma, as well as insect larvae and plant extracts.

The history will reveal occupational asthma's work-relatedness: onset of symptoms on starting a new job or job process; occurrence of symptoms within minutes or hours of starting work; offset on weekends while the patient is on vacation, and reoccurrence when he or she returns to work. Information in MSDS often warn of untoward health effects in susceptible individuals.

Simple pre- and post-exposure spirometry is often diagnostic, although clinically useful data can also be obtained from the use of a peak flow meter and symptom diary. A methacholine challenge test is usually positive for bronchial hygiene hyperreactivity in patients with occupational asthma.[14]

Reactive Airways Dysfunction Syndrome

Work-aggravated or caused asthma without a significant post-exposure latency period is illustrated by the *reactive airways dysfunction syndrome (RADS)*, which has been related to exposure to numerous irritants and inhalants. RADS is described in Table 32-5.[15]

When the multiple inhalant allergy syndrome occurs in the settings of new, often poorly ventilated construction environments, it has been termed the *"Tight Building Syndrome."* The existence of this latter entity is currently a topic of intense debate.

Medical therapy to permit a patient to "better tolerate" a noxious workplace environment is not generally recommended.[15] It would be preferable for the worker to be completely removed from such a setting. At the very least, work-site modification (eg, removal of offending inhalants, better ventilation, and the use of respiratory protective devices) should be considered.

TABLE 32-4. **Causes of Occupational Asthma**

Agents	Industries/Occupations	Agents	Industries/Occupations
High-Molecular-Weight Compounds			
Animals, animal products		**Insects**	
Birds		Bee moth	Fish bait breeders
Budgerigar	Bird fanciers	Cockroach	Laboratory workers
Chicken	Poultry workers	Cricket	Field workers
Pigoon	Pigeon breeders	Grain mite	Grain workers
Crab	Crab processing	Larva of silkworm	Sericulture
Prawn	Shrimp processing	Locust	Laboratory workers
Rabbit, rodent	Laboratory workers, veterinarians, animal handlers	Moth, butterfly	Entomologists
		River fly	Power plants along rivers
		Screwworm fly	Flight crews
Enzymes		**Plants**	
Bromelain, pancreatin, and pepsin	Pharmaceutical manufacturing	Buckwheat	Bakers
Fungal amylase	Manufacturing, baking	Castor bean	Oil industry workers
Papain	Laboratory workers, packaging industry	Coffee bean	Food processors
Subtilisin	Detergent industry	Grain dust	Grain handlers
Trypsin	Plastic and pharmaceutical manufacturing	Gum acacia	Printing
		Gum tragacanth	Gum manufacturing
		Hops	Brewery chemists
		Tea	Tea workers
		Tobacco leaf	Tobacco workers
		Wheat/rye flour	Bakers, millers
Low-Molecular-Weight Compounds			
Anhydrides		**Metals**	
Phthalic, tetrachlorophthalic, or trimellitic anhydrides	Epoxy resins, plastics	Chromium	Tanning
		Cobalt, tungsten carbide, vanadium	Hard metal industry
		Nickel	Metal plating
		Platinum	Platinum refining
Diisocyanates		**Other chemicals**	
Diphenylmenthan diisocyanate	Foundries	Azodicarbonamide	Plastics and rubber processing
Hexamethylene diisocyanate	Automobile spray painting	Diazonium salt	Photocopying and dyeing
Toluene diisocyanate	Plastics, varnish	Dimethylethanolamine	Spray painting
Drugs		Ethylenediamine	Photography
Albuterol, cephalosporins, methyldopa, penicillin, phenylglycine acid chloride, spiramycin, tetracycline	Pharmaceutical manufacturing	Formalin, hexachlorophene	Hospital staff
		Freon	Refrigeration
		Furfuryl alcohol	Foundry mold making
Amprolium HCl	Poultry feed mixing	Paraphenylenediamine	Fur dyeing
Piperazine HCl	Chemical processing	Persulfate salts, henna	Hairdressing
Psyllium	Laxative manufacturing	Urea formaldehyde	Insulation, resin
Sulfone chloramide	Manufacturing, brewing		
Fluxes		**Wood dust**	
Aminoethyl ethanolamine	Aluminum soldering	African maple, cedar, oak, mahogany, redwood, walnut, and zebra wood	Carpentry, construction, cabinetmaking, sawmills
Rosin	Electronics industry		

Adapted from Chan-Young M, Lam S: Occupational asthma. Am Rev Respir Dis 33:689–690, 1986; with permission.

Ambient Air Pollution Health Effects

It is beyond the scope of this book to describe in detail the numerous reported health effects of polluting dusts, fumes, smokes, mists, and gases. It is sufficient to say that such effects do certainly exist, usually in a dose-related manner, and that respiratory function usually suffers as a result. The extent of the health effects depends on the population at risk (eg, the very young and the aged are generally thought to be at greatest risk, as are those with known cardiorespiratory diseases such as coronary artery disease or asthma), the exertion level at the time of exposure, and the conditions at the time of exposure (eg, pollutant concentration, duration, pattern, presence of co-irritants).

TABLE 32-5. **The Reactive Airways Dysfunction Syndrome (RADS): A Definition**

1. No preceding respiratory complaints.
2. Onset of symptoms after a single exposure incident or accident.
3. Exposure to a gas, smoke, fume, or vapor with irritant properties in very high concentrations.
4. Onset of symptoms occurs within 24 hours after exposure, which persists for at least 3 months.
5. Symptoms simulate asthma with cough, wheeze, and dyspnea.
6. Airflow obstruction is demonstrated on pulmonary function tests.
7. There is evidence of subsequent nonspecific bronchial hyperresponsiveness ("Multiple Inhalant Allergy Syndrome").
8. Other pulmonary diseases have been ruled out.

Most large cities, and many small ones, now report daily air quality condition reports for *ozone*, nitrogen oxides, carbon monoxide, particulates, and aeroallergens (pollens). These reports form the basis for *"air pollution advisories"* or *"smog alerts,"* during which time susceptible individuals are advised to curtail their activities and to stay indoors. Cold and dampness may exacerbate the health effects of atmospheric pollutants.

Air quality indices vary from location to location, and many have diurnal and seasonal fluctuations as well. Accordingly, each blood gas laboratory must have its own "normal" values for carboxyhemoglobin (COHb) levels based on ambient (atmospheric) carbon monoxide concentrations. In no urban setting does the normal COHb level exceed 2.5 volumes %.

Air pollution associated with exposure to sulfur dioxide (SO_2), nitrogen dioxide (NO_2), and ozone (O_3) can and does trigger asthma exacerbations.

Burns and Smoke Inhalation

In more than 70,000 patients admitted with burn injuries to intensive care units in the United States each year, the most common causes of death are severe infection and/or cardiopulmonary failure.[16] The respiratory effects and complications of flame and smoke inhalation are many, and include upper airway obstruction, pulmonary edema, carbon monoxide poisoning, bronchitis and pneumonia, pulmonary embolism (secondary to burn-induced thrombophlebitis and immobility), and ARDS.[17] These effects are exacerbated by the effects of inhalation of gases, toxins, and particulate substances from the fire itself.

Irritant toxins that may be inhaled in fires include nitrogen and sulfur dioxide, isocyanates, hydrogen chloride, phosgene, and halogen gases such as chlorine, ammonia, and acrolein esters. *Asphyxiants* that complicate the effects of smoke and flame inhalation include cyanides and carbon monoxide.

□ PATIENTS AT RISK

Clinical predictors of thermal and irritant injuries in burned patients are important to recognize. They include facial, neck and oropharyngeal burns; expectoration of dark, carbonaceous sputum; irritating cough; stridor; and the presence of cough, dyspnea and chest pain. Auscultation will reveal wheezes, crackles, and rhonchi. Tachypnea and cyanosis may indicate the severity of the pulmonary injury.

□ AIRWAY MANAGEMENT

Ritz[16] has recently reviewed this subject and points out the importance of presumptive treatment in the presence of the signs and symptoms listed above. Airway edema usually occurs instantly or within 24 hours of injury. Prophylactic intubation may be indicated before edema and inflammation of the oropharyngeal airway and larynx makes it difficult or impossible, particularly if there is evidence of mucosal burns in the oral cavity, if there are singed nasal hairs, or if there is carbonaceous material in the airway itself. Intubation may also be indicated if the cutaneous burn injury exceeds 30% to 40% of the total body surface area, if there is loss of consciousness and attendant poor voluntary cough and secretion expectoration, and/or if there is hemodynamic instability (often as a result of volume depletion).

Although early tracheotomy should be avoided if possible because of the high risks of secondary infection, a later procedure may be required if long-term mechanical ventilation is necessary. Initial endotracheal intubation should be accomplished with as large-diameter an endotracheal tube as possible, as secretion control is better facilitated in this manner, including therapeutic suctioning and repeated bronchoscopic aspirations of eschar. The endotracheal tube should be long enough to allow for possible swelling of the facial tissues, and tube stabilization should be achieved in the best manner to prevent or at least minimize trauma to the surrounding skin and soft tissues.

Weaning from ventilator support and extubation in such patients must be approached with extreme caution, as muscle weakness, stenosis or webbing of the vocal cords, and tightness of the thoracic skin often make adequate alveolar ventilation difficult for the patient to achieve.

□ TREATMENT OF TOXIC AND ASPHYXIANT INHALATION

The treatment of *carbon monoxide intoxication* with hyperbaric oxygen (HBO) therapy is discussed in Chapter 14. *Carboxyhemoglobinemia* can be suspected by the presence of a "cherry red" appearance of the mucous membranes and lips[18] and confirmed by determination of carboxyhemoglobin (COHb) levels on either venous or arterial blood samples with *co-oximetry* (differential spectrophotometry). When carbon monoxide intoxication is suspected, initial treatment should be started with 100% oxygen. The general belief is that COHb levels of 40% or greater should be treated with HBO therapy[19].

The treatment of *cyanide intoxication* is pharmacologic, with current treatment consisting of intravenous sodium thiosulfate and methylene blue dye.

☐ TREATMENT OF HYPOVOLEMIA, ELECTROLYTE AND NUTRITIONAL ABNORMALITIES, AND INFECTIOUS DISEASE COMPLICATIONS

Although these topics go beyond the therapeutic purview of RCPs, understanding that skillful management in each of these domains often spells the difference between survival and death does not. *Burn teams* in large medical centers are accordingly complete with experts in these disciplines as well as surgeons who have special training in burns and wound care.[19]

The RCP will recognize that fluid volume mismanagement in burn patients may be related to the development of pulmonary edema, particularly in the 3rd to 5th day following injury, though iatrogenic fluid overloading may occur at any time.

Ventilator Management

Factors unique to mechanical ventilation in the burn patient are listed in Table 32-6. The increased metabolic rate seen in many burn patients may require extremely high minute ventilation on the mechanical ventilator. Not all ventilators have such capability (see Chapter 21), either in their inability to deliver high inspiratory pressures, flows, or both. Laryngeal spasm often occurs immediately following inhalation and burn injuries, and is treated in the standard manner, with inhaled vasoconstrictor bronchodilators such as racemic epinephrine. Exfoliation of burned mucosa may also cause airway obstruction. Many of these patients develop bronchorrhea as well, and the need for frequent suctioning and its attendant spasmodic coughing may present a real challenge to the RCP. The use of bland aerosols, and, as a last resort, aerosolized topical anesthetics should be considered.

When patients have burns that extend completely around the chest wall, skin tightness may limit chest wall expansion. Atelectasis may subsequently develop unless the problem is promptly recognized. Incisions in the chest wall (*fasciotomies*) may be necessary to allow adequate alveolar ventilation.

As discussed earlier, both hypovolemia and hypervolumia occur in burn patients. Careful monitoring of fluid intake and output records, allowing for losses from the burned skin surfaces, may be helpful. More accurate estimates of fluid homeostasis may be obtained with consideration of daily body weights, central venous pressure determinations, and pulmonary capillary "wedge" pressure measurements.

A common complication of high minute ventilation is the development of *auto-PEEP* (positive end-expiratory pressure). Patients should be monitored for this very real complication of ventilatory care, and techniques such as intermittent mandatory ventilation (IMV), low I:E ratio ventilation, and permissive hypercapnia may all be helpful. Once auto-PEEP is controlled, applied PEEP may be indicated, both to treat atelectasis and to reduce the work of breathing. Despite these adjustments, many of these patients will remain difficult to ventilate. The RCP may need to accept PaO_2s on the ventilator in the 60 to 70 mmHg range, and the $PaCO_2$ may need to be as high as 80 mmHg, as long as the pH does not drop below 7.35.[16]

TABLE 32-6. **Factors to Consider in the Mechanical Ventilation of Patients With Extensive Burn Injuries**

- High metabolic rate (from pain, anxiety, fever, secondary injection, demands of healing process)
- Laryngeal spasm
- Bronchospasm and spasmodic coughing
- Chest wall tightness from burn eschar
- Hypovolemia
- Auto-PEEP secondary to high minute ventilation on ventilator

SELF-INDUCED PULMONARY DISORDERS

In a novel approach to systematic patient evaluation, a group at the Mayo Clinic Foundation recently reported the effect of a mandated smoking history on subsequent caregiver attempts at intervention (smoking cessation).[9] The study points up the reluctance of many health workers to rely on anything as simple as history-taking to diagnose illness with anything short of "high-tech" (and high cost!) instrumentation.

In the evaluation of several diverse pulmonary disorders, self-induction of respiratory damage emerges as a real possibility (Table 32-7).

Tobacco Addiction and Smoking Cessation

Despite years of effort, a large portion of the American public still remains unconvinced that tobacco smoking is the chief avoidable cause of mortality and morbidity in our society. Epidemiologic studies show that 1 in 6 U.S. deaths are related to tobacco consumption as a result of cancer, and cardiovascular and obstructive pulmonary diseases. Although convinced of the magnitude of the problem, few physicians, and fewer allied health personnel, actively advise and assist their patients to quit smoking. The Centers for Disease Control and Prevention recently reported that less than 60% of U.S. smokers have ever been advised by their physicians to stop smoking.[20]

TABLE 32-7. **Self-Induced Pulmonary Disorders**

Lung cancer secondary to tobacco smoking
Chronic obstructive pulmonary disease secondary to tobacco smoking
Interstitial lung disease secondary to tobacco smoking
Poor control of asthma secondary to tobacco smoking
Aspiration pneumonitis secondary to bulimia, alcoholism
Acute bronchitis from marijuana and crack cocaine smoking

Entirely on their own, about 800,000 Americans stop smoking each year. Public information programs of the American Heart Association, American Cancer Society, and American Lung Association are credited with much of this success. Currently, about 65% of smokers say they want to stop smoking and have made at least one attempt to do so.[21] RCPs must join their physician colleagues in an aggressive effort to effect this important behavioral change in their patients, if a more significant effect on this nationwide health problem is to be achieved.[22]

Smoking Cessation Strategies

Various strategies have been implemented to achieve successful *smoking cessation* outcomes (see Box 32-1). In addition to various self-help methods, an intelligent comprehensive smoking cessation program must have the basic elements outlined in Table 32-8.[22]

□ INDIVIDUAL PATIENT EVALUATION

Each patient seeks, or is told he or she must seek, help in smoking cessation in a different manner. He or she may have been "data loaded" in the public media, or by his or her friends and family, or by his or her personal physician. Undiagnosed cardiorespiratory symptoms or specifically diagnosed medical conditions may have prompted his or her referral. His or her cardiorespiratory functional improvement may or may not have been specifically characterized by laboratory studies; for example, pulmonary function tests, cardiopulmonary exercise studies, chest radiographs, arterial blood gas studies, carboxyhemoglobin levels, or urinary continene levels. If these tests have not already been performed, they should be at the time of intake into the smoking cessation program.

BOX 32-1

SMOKING CESSATION STRATEGIES

Self-help individualized programs
- Slow taper method
- "Cold turkey" method
- Smoke-free environments

Formal stop-smoking programs
- American Lung Association
- American Cancer Association
- American Heart Association
- Smoke-enders
- 5-Day Plan to Stop Smoking
- Hospital-sponsored programs

Personal physician intervention (outpatient)
- Problem analysis
- Education
- Pharmacologic assistance
- Relapse prevention

Inpatient hospital intervention
- Case finding
- NHLBI/AARC programs[26]

TABLE 32-8. **Basic Elements Common to Successful Smoking Cessation Programs**

Individual patient evaluation
Patient-specific education
Addiction therapy
Nonpharmacologic
Pharmacologic
Follow-up and relapse prevention

The patient's history of previous attempts at smoking cessation must be carefully reviewed: What has "worked" (at least for a short time) before? What hasn't? As has recently been pointed out, *nicotine dependence* and *nicotine withdrawal* are mental disorders[23] associated with *addiction* and at least four of six cardinal withdrawal symptoms during attempts at smoking cessation (see Box 32-2).[22]

Other patients may claim a brief period of paradoxical worsening of pulmonary function in the few weeks or months following smoking cessation. Specific treatments for each of these withdrawal symptoms is available, and should be applied by the health care team as necessary (see below).

□ EDUCATION

The informed patient is more successful in any attempt at behavior modification than one who is not. In addition to videotapes and printed materials available from the national organizations listed in Box 32-1, RCPs and other health practitioners must discuss both the short- and long-term benefits of smoking cessation with their patients. Help in this respect is available in an excellent resource jointly prepared by the American Association for Respiratory Care and the National Heart, Lung and Blood Institute.[24]

□ THERAPY

Smoking cessation may be achieved by behavioral (nonpharmacologic) and pharmacologic means. Oral gratification by use of such nontoxic items as chewing gum, toothpicks, candy, and objects to handle (pencils, paper clips, rubber bands) have been initially used by patients attempting to stop smoking. Daily recording of withdrawal symptoms is helpful as both diagnostic (what and when do symptoms occur?) and therapeutic (as symptoms are seen to reduce in frequency and severity) tools.

BOX 32-2

NICOTINE WITHDRAWAL SYMPTOMS

- Craving for tobacco
- Irritability, frustration, or anger
- Anxiety or restlessness
- Reduced concentration/mental alertness
- Cardiac irritability/bradycardia
- Increased appetite or weight gain

Although most self-help patients have tried to stop smoking suddenly and completely by the *"cold-turkey method"*[25] others will have tried a *"slow taper"* or *nicotine-fading technique*. This latter approach is the basis for the nicotine replacement techniques described below.

The availability of premeasured doses of nicotine in the form of *nicotine polacrilex* ("Nicorette") chewing gum in 1991 and *transdermal nicotine patches* in 1994 has added a new dimension (and enhanced success) to smoking cessation efforts.[26–28] Patients should be placed on a physician-monitored program of nicotine replacement therapy, in which the daily dose of nicotine, which is the addicting substance in tobacco smoke, is slowly reduced to zero over a period of several weeks. This therapy provides nicotine blood levels adequate to modulate the withdrawal symptoms described in Box 32-2. Breakthrough anxiety and depression do occur and should be treated with psychotropic medications if they compromise the smoking cessation program's effectiveness. The common mistake made by health care practitioners who use these pharmacologic aids is to forget that support and counseling is necessary in all the comprehensive programs. Just recently, nicotine polacrilex chewing gum has become available over-the-counter, that is, without physician order. Time will tell whether or not this is in the public interest or not, but RCPs should be aware of this situation.

☐ FOLLOW-UP AND RELAPSE PREVENTION

Patients with smoking-induced cardiorespiratory symptoms, smokers who have failed in their own attempts to stop smoking, heavy smokers, and women, in particular, may seek medical assistance in formal smoking cessation programs. Relapse occurrence in all is, unfortunately, a fact of life in even the best of programs, and follow-up and skillful use of relapse prevention techniques must be built into every successful smoking cessation effort. Continual improvement of the lessons learned must be provided by every member of the health care team. Only with each aggressive problem identification will long-term intervention attempts be successful. Patients will appreciate and benefit from support, rather than criticism, during a process that requires both commitment and persistence.

Substance Abuse

Recent years have seen accumulating evidence that abusive behaviors other than tobacco addiction are on the rise, particularly among young and economically disadvantaged people. The RCP must enhance his or her background knowledge with an awareness of alcohol addiction (*alcoholism*) as it affects pulmonary function, as well as an appreciation of the respiratory health effects of the so-called "recreational drugs," for example, amphetamines, *marijuana*, *heroin*, and "crack" cocaine.

The pulmonary complications and conditions associated with acute and chronic alcohol consumption are listed in Table 32-9.

TABLE 32-9. **Pulmonary Complications of Alcoholism**

Tuberculosis
Recurrent pulmonary infections, eg, bronchitis, pneumonia
Aspiration pneumonia
Obesity and recurrent atelectasis
Hemoptysis (decreased coagulation parameters)
Poor compliance with medication and therapy regimens
High association with tobacco consumption
Delirium tremens—associated apneic spells
Susceptibility to trauma
Malnutrition

Use of *amphetamines*, once thought to be diminishing, is again being seen as a major public health problem, particularly in association with the current public fascination with a thin, trim body image. Activation of the sympathetic nervous system occurs with this substance, as it does with use of heroin and cocaine, producing tachycardia, hypertension, vasoconstriction, dilated pupils, hyperthermia, and predisposition to cardiac arrythmias.

The health effects of marijuana smoking have been carefully studied in recent years in several centers, identifying effects not unlike the amphetamine results discussed above and with bronchitis developing from the smoke itself.

Since *"crack" cocaine* was developed in 1980, it has become the most frequently abused controlled substance in the United States. Six percent of high school seniors have been estimated to use cocaine, and inhalation of the vapors from heated "crack" cocaine has been found in 27% of these individuals.[29] The pulmonary complications of "crack" cocaine inhalation are listed in Table 32-10.

TABLE 32-10. **Pulmonary Complications of Smoked "Crack" Cocaine[29]**

- Acute respiratory symptoms (cough productive of blackish sputum, dyspnea, chest pain, hemoptysis)
- Exacerbations of asthma
- Airway burns
- Worsening pulmonary function—questionable effect on diffusion capacity
- Pneumothorax/pneumomediastinum
- Bronchiolitis obliterans with organizing pneumonia
- Intrapulmonary hemorrhage
- Noncardiogenic pulmonary edema
- Pulmonary infiltrates with eosinophilia
- Pulmonary vascular occlusive disease/pulmonary infarction
- Increased incidence of HIV-related infections, multiple drug–resistant tuberculosis

REFERENCES

1. Landrigan PJ, Baker DB: The recognition and control of occupational disease. JAMA 266:676, 1991
2. Bureau of Labor Statistics: Occupational injuries and illnesses in the United States by industry, 1991. Washington, DC, U.S. Department of Labor, U.S. Government Printing Office Bulletin #2424, 1993
3. Bresnitz EA: Occupational history as the key to the recognition and prevention of workplace-related lung disease. Curr Opin Pulm Med 1:76, 1995
4. Bresnitz EA: The pulmonologist as expert: medicolegal aspects of occupational lung disease. Clin Pulm Med 3:142, 1996
5. Himmelstein JA, Frumkin H: The right to know about toxic exposures: Implications for physicians. N Engl J Med 312:687, 1985
6. American Medical Association: Guide to the evaluation of permanent impairment, 4th ed. Chicago, American Medical Association, 1993
7. American Thoracic Society: Evaluation of impairment/disability secondary to respiratory disorders. Am Rev Respir Dis 133:1205, 1986
8. Social Security Administration: Disability evaluation under Social Security. Washington, DC, U.S. Department of Health and Human Services, Social Security Administration Publication #64-039, 1994
9. Fiore MC, Jorenby DE, Schensky AE, et al: Smoking status as a new vital sign: Effect on assessment and intervention in patients who smoke. Mayo Clin Proc 70:209, 1995
10. Epler GR: Clinical overview of occupational lung disease. Radiol Clin North Am 30:1121, 1992
11. Sepkowitz KA: Tuberculosis and the health care worker: A historical perspective. Ann Intern Med 120:7, 1994
12. Bloch AB, Cauthen GM, Onorato IM, et al: Nationwide survey of drug-resistant tuberculosis in the United States. JAMA 271:665, 1994
13. Chan-Yeung M, Lam S: Occupational asthma. Am Rev Respir Dis 133:689, 1986
14. Chan-Yeung M: ACCP consensus statement—assessment of asthma in the workplace. Chest 108:1084, 1995
15. Brooks SM, Weiss MA, Bernstein IL: Reactive airways dysfunction (RADS). Chest, 88:376, 1985
16. Ritz RH: Respiratory care of the patient with burns or smoke inhalation. In Pierson DJ, Kacmarek RM (eds): Foundations of Respiratory Care. New York, Churchill Livingtone, 1992
17. Haponik EF, Summer WR: respiratory complications in burn patients: Diagnosis and management of inhalation injury. J Crit Care 2:121, 1987
18. Smith TS, Brandon S: Acute carbon monoxide poisoning: 3-year experience in a defined population. Postgrad Med J 46:65, 1990
19. Deitch EA: The management of burns. N Engl J Med 323:1249, 1990
20. Centers for Disease Control and Prevention: Physician and other health-care professional counseling of smokers to quit—United States 1991. MMWR Morb Mortal Wkly Rep 42:854, 1993
21. Fiore M, Novotny T, Lynn W, et al: Smoking cessation: Data from the 1986 adult use of tobacco survey. Excerpta Medica International Congress Series, #780, 1987, p 189
22. Nett LM, Pierson DJ: Smoking cessation. In Pierson DJ, Kacmarek RM (eds): Foundations of Respiratory Care. Churchill Livingstone, New York, 1992
23. American Psychiatric Association: Diagnostic and statistical manual of mental disorders, 3rd ed, revised. American Psychiatric Association, Washington, DC, 1987
24. U.S. Department of Health and Human Services: How You Can Help Patients Stop Smoking—Opportunities for Respiratory Care Practitioners. NIH Publications #89-2961. Public Health Service, National Institute of Health (National Heart, Lung, and Blood Institute), Bethesda, MD, 1989
25. Fiore M, Novotny TE, Pierce JP, et al: Methods used to quit smoking in the United States. JAMA 263:2760, 1990
26. Hjalmarson AI: Effect of nicotine chewing gum in smoking cessation. JAMA 252:2835, 1984
27. Tonnesen P, Fyrd V, Hansen M, et al: Two and four mg nicotine chewing gum and group counseling in smoking cessation: An open randomized controlled trial with a 22-month follow-up. Addict Behav 13:17, 1988
28. Transdermal Nicotine Study Group: Transdermal nicotine for smoking cessation: Six-month results from two multicenter controlled clinical trials. JAMA 266:3133, 1991
29. Haim D, Lippman ML, Goldberg SK, Wackenstein MD: The pulmonary complications of crack cocaine. Chest 107:233, 1995

33 Acute/Adult Respiratory Distress Syndrome

Neil R. MacIntyre and William J. Fulkerson

PROFESSIONAL SKILLS

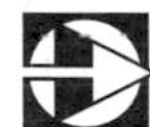

Upon completion of this chapter, the reader will be able to:

- Define ARDS, trace its pathophysiology, and identify its manifestations
- Identify the mediators of lung injury and explain how they contribute to the pathologic process of ARDS
- Define lung specific injury and systemic vascular injury, and explain how each contributes to ARDS
- Explain the goals of supportive therapy and give examples
- Understand the various experimental therapies available and determine a patient's possible need for them
- Recognize any underlying disease or development of ICU complications that may cause multiple organ failure or hemodynamic collapse in an ARDS patient

KEY TERMS

Acute/Adult respiratory distress syndrome
Complement cytokines
Extracorporeal membrane oxygenation
High-frequency ventilation
Neutrophil-related cytokines
Nitric oxide
Platelet-activating factor
Reactive oxygen species

In 1967, Ashbaugh and colleagues described a syndrome of acute respiratory failure associated with sepsis, trauma, and selected drug overdoses.[1] This syndrome was characterized by severe hypoxemia, diffuse pulmonary infiltrates, poor lung compliance, and absence of left heart failure. The term *acute/adult respiratory distress syndrome* (ARDS) was subsequently proposed as a label to characterize these patients because the syndrome was rapid in onset and there were physiologic and pathologic similarities to the neonatal respiratory distress syndrome.[2]

Specific definitions of ARDS vary in different reports. For our purposes, ARDS is defined as an acute clinical illness characterized by the development of bilateral pulmonary infiltrates on chest radiographs and severe hypoxemia (PaO_2/FIO_2 <200) in the absence of congestive heart failure. This is compatible with the position of the Joint European–American Consensus Conference on ARDS.[3]

PATHOPHYSIOLOGY

The pathophysiology of ARDS begins with an inflammatory "trigger" that initiates a host of cellular and biochemical mediators resulting in an alveolar–capillary injury (Fig. 33-1). Pathologically, the process is often divided into three phases, the exudative, the proliferative, and the fibrotic (Table 33-1), that evolve over days or weeks.[4–9]

The manifestations of the syndrome are a result of these pathologic changes coupled with surfactant dysfunction (both abnormal components as well as inactivation by exudative material[10]), and the effects of supervening complications. The alveoli in ARDS collapse due to the inflammatory infiltrate, blood, edema fluid, surfactant dysfunctioning, and small airways narrowing secondary to interstitial infiltration and bronchial obstruction. Resulting right-to-left shunting of blood through nonventilated lungs and ventilation-perfusion mismatching lead to severe hypoxemia. As the lung reacts to injury with increased proliferation of inflammatory cells and fibroblasts, pulmonary vascular obstruction produces increased physiologic dead space.[11] Capillary endothelial integrity is disrupted in ARDS, leading to edema formation. If the capillary injury is systemic, distribution defects in tissue oxygen delivery and impaired oxygen utilization by mitochondria result in diffuse hypoxic cellular injury and multiple organ failures. Pulmonary vascular injury may also interfere with the lungs' role in modulating inflammatory mediators.

Decreased thoracic compliance is characteristic of ARDS. This is the result of abnormal surfactant function coupled with alveolar edema, inflammation, and fibrosis affecting elastance of lung tissue. Given the heterogeneity of lung injury demonstrated by CT scans in ARDS, however, the decreased overall compliance may also be caused, at least in part, by decreased lung volume available for ventilation.[12]

Pulmonary hypertension occurs commonly in ARDS secondary to vasoconstriction, thrombosis, perivascular edema and inflammation, and eventual interstitial fibrosis.[12] Overt right ventricular failure may develop if pulmonary hypertension is severe.[13] Ventricular function may also be compromised by impaired myocardial oxygen delivery, suboptimal fluid management, dysrhythmias, malnutrition, and myocardial depressant factors associated with systemic capillary injury (eg, sepsis).[14]

Other respiratory system abnormalities associated with ARDS include respiratory muscle overload and fatigue (often potentiated by poor nutrition; reduced muscle oxygen delivery; systemic capillary injury; and the

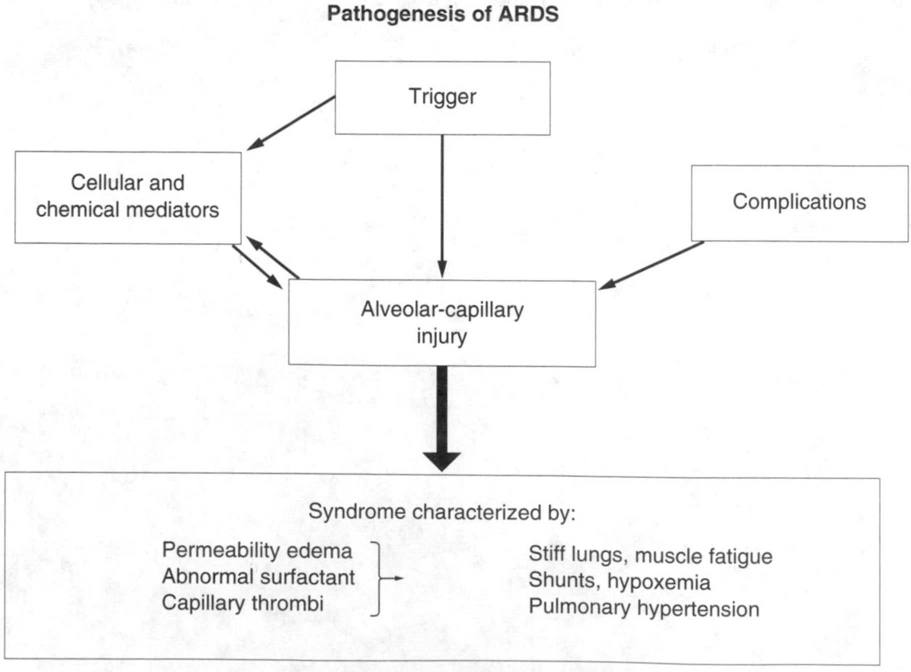

FIGURE 33-1. Pathogenesis of ARDS

TABLE 33-1. **Stages of ARDS**

	Exudative	Proliferative	Fibrotic
Timing	Edema early (<1 wk)	Organization (repair) intermediate	Fibrosis late (3 wks)
Macroscopic			
consistency	Rigid, heavy	Firm, consolidated	Spongy, cystic
appearance	Hemorrhagic	Pale gray	Pale
Microscopic			
Vasculature	Endothelial injury (mild),* congestion, neutrophil aggregates, minimal thrombi	Endothelial injury, intimal fibroproliferation, medial hypertrophy, thrombi	Endolthelial injury, distortion, compressed, proliferation
Alveoli	Type I pneumocytes necrosis, inflammatory exudate, hyaline membranes,‡ partial collapse	Type 2 pneumocyte proliferation,† myofibroblast invasion, increased fibronectin, collagen deposition	Fibrosis microcysts
Basement membrane	Denuded	Gaps with myofibroblast invasion	Disruption
Alveolar wall	Edema	Myofibroblast proliferation	Thick collagen
Alveolar duct	Dilated	Myofibroblast proliferation	Fibrosis
Interstitium	Volume ↑ edema	Volume ↑↑ myofibroblast proliferation	Volume ↑↑↑ fibrosis
Pleura	Subpleural ischemic changes	Subpleural necrosis	Subpleural necrosis

↑, increased.
* The endothelial cell layer is usually continuous with intact cell junctions. Endothelial gaps are rarely observed.
† Stem cell function for the entire epithelium.
‡ Hyaline membranes are composed of condensed plasma proteins casting the alveolar septum wherever the epithelium lining is destroyed.
Reprinted with permission from Meduri GU: Late adult respiratory distress syndrome. New Horizons 1:563, 1993

use of drugs such as steroids, paralytics, and aminoglycosides) and a deranged respiratory drive (secondary to CNS involvement in a systemic process, abnormal mechanoreceptors in the lung, sleep disturbance, and the use of sedatives or paralytics).[14]

MEDIATORS OF LUNG INJURY

A number of biochemical and cellular mediators are thought to contribute to the pathologic responses of ARDS.

Complement- and neutrophil-related cytokines appear to be major factors in injury to the lung and other organ systems.[6,15–17] In ARDS, complement-activated neutrophils release cytokines such as tumor necrosis factor (TNF) and interleukins that participate in the inflammatory response. These processes lead to coagulopathy, platelet-activating factor (PAF) and prostanoid release, platelet aggregation, induction of nitric oxide synthase, and enhanced cellular oxidant production.[15–17] Expression of adhesion molecules for leukocytes, for example ICAM-1, is increased, and enhanced neutrophil migration and activation in tissues leads to secretory product release and oxidant generation, which damages cell structural components.[14–17]

Cyclooxygenase products of arachidonic acid are present in increased amounts in animal models and human studies of sepsis and ARDS.[18–20] Thromboxane A_2 and prostacyclin have potent, opposing vascular effects that may play significant roles in pulmonary vascular autoregulation (hypoxic vasoconstriction) and systemic vasodilation. Thromboxane A_2 may interact with neutrophils to accentuate cell aggregation.[19] Lipoxygenase products are also released in large quantities in acute lung injury models and may contribute to pulmonary vascular changes, permeability characteristics, and airway dysfunction in this syndrome.[20]

Platelet-activating factor (PAF) is a phospholipid metabolite released by a number of cells including neutrophils, platelets, monocytes, basophils, eosinophils, and endothelial cells.[21] The response to platelet-activating factor at the endothelial surface results in enhanced superoxide production by circulating neutrophils.[22] In addition, PAF release enhances platelet aggregation and production of cyclooxygenase and lipoxygenase products, alters pulmonary vascular reactivity, and increases endothelial permeability.[22]

Reactive oxygen species develop as part of the initial inflammatory response as well as during reperfusion of previously ischemic tissues ("reperfusion injury").[14] These substances cause direct cell damage by oxidation of the lipids of cell membranes.[23] By-products of lipid peroxidation have been found in lavage fluid in animal models of ARDS.[24] The lung interstitial matrix and basement membrane is also damaged by oxygen-derived radicals, which leads to increased edema formation. Oxygen-derived radicals generate potent chemotaxins and stimulate the release of other mediators. Activated neutrophils and other phagocytic cells respond by increased oxygen radical production. Oxidative reactions involving free radicals and subsequent tissue damage are normally limited by endogenous antioxidant defenses. These defenses consist of both enzymatic and nonenzymatic antioxidant pathways. Oxidant tissue injury proceeds when these defenses are overwhelmed by oxidant production or when antioxidant defenses are depleted. In the lung, reduced glutathione (GSH) is a major antioxidant in the epithelial lining fluid. Patients with ARDS have been shown to have decreased levels of GSH in bronchoalveolar lavage fluid.[25] N-Acetylcysteine (NAC) is an antioxidant that repletes reduced glutathione and reduces pulmonary edema formation in endotoxin-induced lung injury in sheep.[26]

Nitric oxide (NO) is a powerful endogenous vasodilator and inflammatory mediator,[27] and enhanced NO production may contribute to the pathophysiology and vasodilation of septic shock. Nitric oxide (NO) is synthesized by a diverse cell population including endothelial cells, macrophages, platelets, neutrophils, smooth muscle cells, and neurons.[27] The enzymes responsible for NO synthesis are NO synthases (NOS). Many of the effects of NO are mediated by stimulation of guanylyl cyclase. The increases in intracellular cGMP concentration translate the NO signal into a remarkable array of functional responses.[27,28]

The reactions of NO with oxygen and superoxide can form nitrogen dioxide and peroxynitrite, respectively, which are highly reactive oxidants mediating significant cytotoxic actions of nitric oxide in biological systems.[27,28] The regulation of nitric oxide in biological systems in general, and in the lung in particular, is very poorly understood. Thus, the potential toxicity of nitric oxide in the oxygen-rich environment of the lung must be reconciled with growing evidence for its role as a beneficial biological mediator. Biochemical pathways must exist to stabilize NO in a bioactive form (ie, one that retains smooth muscle relaxant and antimicrobial activity) and also limits its toxicity. The reactions of nitrogen oxides with thiols may be very important in this regard.[28]

CLINICAL RISK FACTORS

The annual incidence of ARDS in the United States is difficult to calculate because of the nonuniformity of reporting data. Nevertheless, estimates range up to 150,000 cases per year.[3,29]

Clinical risk factors for the development of ARDS fall into two general categories: lung-specific injuries (direct) and systemic vascular injuries (indirect) (Box 33-1).[3,30] These two categories are important to distinguish because of the markedly different outcome (patients with ARDS from lung-specific injuries are often reported to have markedly better survival than those with ARDS from systemic injuries; see below), and because of the different impact of these categories on patient management strategies and clinical study design.[31]

Lung-specific injuries associated with the development of ARDS initiate the inflammatory cascade in the lung through either inhalation injuries (eg, toxic gas, aspiration) or vascular "emboli" (eg, amniotic fluid and IV drug use). All of these insults directly injure the alveolar–capillary interface. Whether the patient develops clinical ARDS appears to depend on the magnitude of the initial injury, the underlying host defense capabilities, and the development of iatrogenic injuries (eg, barotrauma, oxygen toxicity) or lung-related complications of ICU care (eg, gastric aspiration).[14,30]

BOX 33-1

TRIGGERS OF ARDS

Direct	Indirect
Aspiration of gastric contents	Bacterial sepsis
Infectious pneumonia	Trauma, nonthoracic
Inhalation of toxic gas or aerosol	Multiple blood transfusions
Lung contusion	Pancreatitis
Near drowning	Opiate and other drug overdose
	Disseminated intravascular coagulation
	Other infectious causes

Systemic vascular injuries involve all of the capillary beds of the body, and thus lung inflammation can be considered just one of many organ injuries by a systemic inflammatory response syndrome (SIRS).[32] Once initiated, SIRS can be self-perpetuating as one organ dysfunction leads to further metabolic derangements in others. The gut may play a particularly important role in SIRS because an injured intestinal epithelial barrier may permit continuous bacterial product entry into the blood stream to perpetuate the inflammatory response.

Sepsis is the most common example of SIRS, and other organ dysfunctions associated with sepsis include kidney, liver, marrow, brain, coagulation system, and heart. The risk of developing ARDS from sepsis depends on the severity of the septic episode and overall host defenses. Common sources of sepsis include GI tract, GU tract, pneumonia, and various intravascular appliances. Estimates of the risk of developing ARDS with sepsis range from 10% to 50%.[3,14,30,33,34] Note that sepsis developing in the ICU can convert an ARDS that resulted from lung-specific injury to an ARDS associated with SIRS.

Because risk factors for ARDS are recognized, there has been interest in "prophylactic" strategies to prevent ARDS. These include early administration of expiratory airway pressure,[35] aggressive early nutritional support,[36] corticosteroids,[14] gut sterilization,[37] and aggressive fluid restriction.[38] Although there appears to be some benefit to gas exchange with early positive end-expiratory pressure (PEEP) and some reduction in nosocomial pneumonia with gut sterilization, none of these strategies has clearly been shown to alter the development of ARDS.[14]

THERAPY OF ARDS

Conventional Therapy

Conventional therapy of ARDS (Fig. 33-2) consists of both *treating* the initiating injury and *supporting* the deranged metabolic functions. Unfortunately, the only initiating injury that has specific therapy available is infection, for which surgical drainage or antibiotics, or both, can be effective.

Supportive therapy has two goals: maintain metabolic function and minimize iatrogenic complications. Effec-

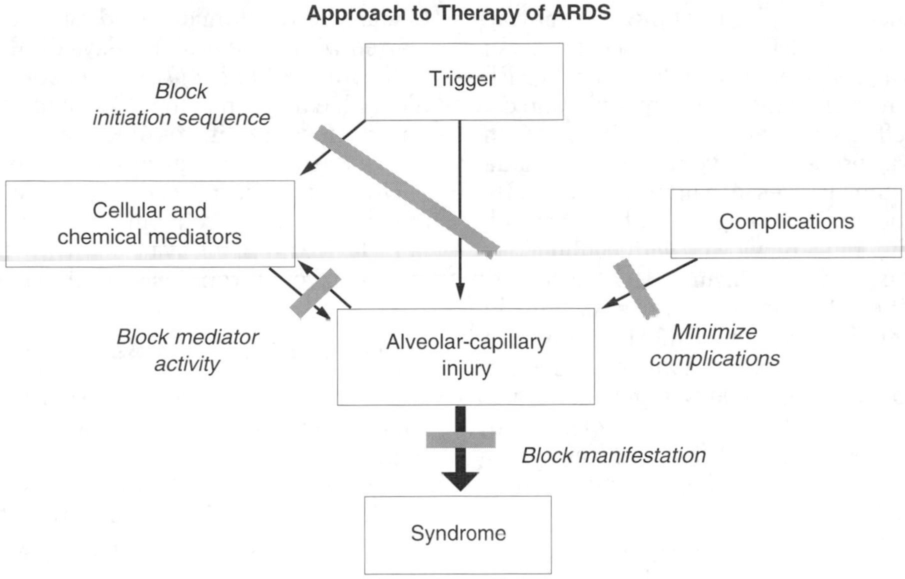

Approach to Therapy of ARDS

Trigger
Block initiation sequence
Cellular and chemical mediators
Complications
Block mediator activity
Alveolar-capillary injury
Minimize complications
Block manifestation
Syndrome

FIGURE 33-2. Approach to therapy of ARDS

tive supportive therapy exists for the respiratory system, cardiovascular system, kidney, coagulation system, and GI and nutrition systems.

Respiratory support consists of positive-pressure ventilation and supplemental oxygen. Generally, high levels of mechanical support (ie, volume- or pressure-targeted assist control) are provided initially.[39] The goal is to have the patient contribution to ventilatory work virtually abolished. Ventilatory muscles can thus be rested while the ventilator provides all of the needed ventilation. Unnatural breathing patterns (eg, long inspiratory time strategies) or uncomfortably high airway pressures usually need total mechanical support in conjunction with heavy sedation or paralysis.[40,41] If the lung injury is less severe or if the patient is in the recovery phase, lower levels of ventilatory support (ie, partial support such as intermittent mandatory ventilation, airway pressure release ventilation, or pressure-support ventilation) can be used to permit the patient to contribute some portion to the work of ventilation. With partial support, delivered pressures to the lung are generally less, and sedation requirements are usually lower. To date, no one mode of either total or partial support has proven superior to any other in terms of ultimate outcome of ARDS.

As noted above, alveolar collapse and consequent reduction in functional residual capacity are characteristic of ARDS. Moreover, collapse is more likely to occur during expiration when transalveolar pressures are lowest. The application of positive end-expiratory pressure (PEEP) may thus prevent collapse, thereby recruiting functional alveoli and increasing functional residual capacity (FRC).[35] This appears to improve ventilation-perfusion ($\dot{V}/\dot{Q}$) matching, reduce shunting, and thus lower the need for potentially toxic levels of inspired oxygen. Lung compliance may also improve with appropriate levels of PEEP because alveoli that do not collapse have improved mechanical properties. Excessive PEEP, however, can overdistend alveoli and thus worsen the compliance.[40] Selecting the appropriate level of PEEP requires appreciation of the balance between gas exchange improvement and the potential for harm. Generally, a minimal level of 5–7 cmH_2O is almost always applied to prevent alveolar collapse. Higher levels can be titrated according to criteria such as compliance or oxygen delivery. Levels above 15–20 cmH_2O, however, are usually avoided because of the risk of overdistending healthier lung regions. In patients who do not require concomitant ventilatory support, expiratory pressure can be provided as continuous positive airway pressure (CPAP).

Positive-pressure respiratory support also has the potential to injure the lung, primarily through overdistension of more compliant lung units.[42,43] The most serious form of lung injury is pneumothorax. The most important, clinically relevant risk factors for pneumothorax appear to be maximal transalveolar distending pressure and length of time receiving mechanical support. In recent years, more subtle lung abnormalities have been demonstrated in animal models using transalveolar pressures as low as 30 cmH_2O.[42] Because of this, a recent consensus conference has recommended maintaining maximal alveolar pressures (estimated by the "plateau pressure" during an inspiratory hold with no flow) below 35 cmH_2O.[39] This may require limiting both PEEP (to less than 15 to 20 cmH_2O) and tidal volume (to less than 8 mL/kg) and tolerating lower arterial saturations (eg, 85% to 89%) and higher levels of $PaCO_2$ (permissive hypercapnia).[43] Prolonging inspiratory time (without air trapping) can increase mean alveolar pressures without increasing maximal alveolar pressures. This may help recruit slower-filling alveoli and increase gas mixing time to improve $\dot{V}/\dot{Q}$ matching and arterial PaO_2.[39,41] Effects on other potential mechanisms of iatrogenic lung injury (ie, shearing), however, are not known. Moreover, whether this strategy affects outcome is not known.

If long inspiratory time strategies are being employed, one must also be alert to the development of air trapping from inadequate expiratory times.[39,41] Air trapping produces "intrinsic" PEEP that can have similar effects on collapsed alveoli to applied or "extrinsic" PEEP. Intrinsic PEEP, however, is difficult to monitor and can have significant effects on ventilator settings (eg, increases peak airway pressures in volume-cycled mode, decreases tidal volume in pressure-limited modes). Because of these concerns, strategies that deliberately produce air trapping must be viewed with caution.

Supplemental oxygen, by raising P_{AO_2}, can raise PaO_2, although the effect becomes less as lung injury and $\dot{V}/\dot{Q}$ matching worsen. Unfortunately, prolonged exposure to high concentrations of supplemental oxygen can produce pathologic changes identical to ARDS.[44] The safe level of F_{IO_2} that can be tolerated by patients with ARDS is unclear. Most clinicians, however, are usually comfortable with an $F_{IO_2} < 0.4$, and become concerned when $F_{IO_2} > 0.6$.

Other aspects of respiratory support include good pulmonary toilet, aspiration protection, patient turning, and endotracheal tube care. Proper endotracheal tube care involves the use of low pressure cuffs, clearance of secretions above the cuff, and consideration for tracheostomy if prolonged support (eg, >2 to 3 weeks) is needed.[14]

Cardiovascular support consists of proper fluid management, vasoactive drugs, and inotropes.[45] The optimal fluid and hemodynamic management of patients with ARDS, however, is not clear.[38,46] Some have shown improved outcome in euvolemic ARDS patients with fluid restriction and pulmonary artery occlusion pressure reduction. The rationale for this approach is that reductions in lung edema fluid should improve oxygenation and promote lung healing. Others, however, argue for aggressive volume support and inotropic management to achieve supranormal physiologic values for oxygen delivery.[14] The rationale for this approach is that systemic oxygen delivery is the critical goal in treating SIRS. Although data in otherwise healthy trauma patients would support this latter approach, the older medical ICU patient may, in fact, be harmed by excessive cardiovascular stimulation.[47] In this population, a normal wedge pressure and oxygen delivery goal would thus seem preferable.

Diagnosing and treating dysrhythmias is an additional management goal. Indeed, cardiac output may be substantially improved with maneuvers to control heart rate or restore atrial "kick" in patients with atrial fibrillation or flutter.

Renal management consists of maintaining renal perfusion and avoidance of renal toxic medications (eg, aminoglycosides, dyes, and so forth). Maintaining urine flow with a diuretic helps management of fluid balance but does not affect renal recovery. Dialysis may be needed for fluid and electrolyte management.

Nutritional support is aimed at preventing further organ dysfunction and immune suppression from inadequate intake of essential nutrients such as amino acids and vitamins.[14,36] Enteral nutrition is generally preferable as it is less invasive and may serve to maintain gut mucosal function.[36] Aspiration, however, is a risk, particularly with stomach feeding. Nutrition should be started within the first few days of ARDS.

Gastrointestinal support consists of control of stress ulcer bleeding,[48] maintenance of mucosal function with enteral feeding (if possible), and prevention of pulmonary aspiration of gastric contents.

Other support methodologies include replacing coagulation factors, frequent assessment of invasive support devices (eg, intravascular catheters) for infection, and deep vein thrombosis prophylaxis.[49,50]

Experimental Therapies

Novel therapies that remain experimental include both support and therapeutic modalities, such as the following.

High-frequency ventilation (HFV) uses very rapid breathing frequencies (up to 300 breaths/min in adults) with small tidal volumes (approaching anatomic dead space).[51] The rationale behind HFV is that this form of support would provide adequate gas exchange with smaller pressure changes in the lungs, thereby reducing injury associated with alveolar distension. There is concern, however, about shearing injury, standing waves, and air trapping with HFV. In infants at risk for barotrauma, HFV appears to improve outcome.[51] No such data exist, however, in adults, and thus this form of support for them remains experimental.

Extracorporeal membrane oxygenation (ECMO) for patients with severe hypoxemic respiratory failure was studied in a controlled, prospective, multicenter study.[52] Overall mortality in this study was not improved by ECMO, but mortality was exceedingly high in both ECMO and conventionally treated groups. Extracorporeal membrane oxygenation–treated patients continued to receive high inspired oxygen concentrations and conventional high-pressure mechanical ventilation in this protocol, which may have affected the results. Subsequent trials with a strategy combining venovenous bypass, extracorporeal CO_2 removal, partial oxygenation across the artificial membrane, and apneic oxygenation with nontoxic oxygen concentrations resulted in improved survival in patients with ARDS compared with historical controls.[53] A trial of this strategy in patients who failed pressure preset, inverse-ratio ventilation compared to patients who received tightly controlled routine support, however, showed lower mortality in both groups compared with historical data, but no survival advantage with the extracorporeal technique.[54]

Other experimental respiratory support strategies include liquid ventilation (using a fluorocarbon to either maintain FRC or to provide actual gas delivery into the lung) and apneic oxygenation and diffusive respiration. These approaches are still in early developmental stages.

Surfactant replacement therapy has been successful in improving morbidity and mortality in premature newborns with respiratory distress syndrome.[55] Because surfactant is deficient or denatured in animal models and patients with acute lung injury,[10] exogenously administered surfactant could potentially maintain alveolar stability during expiration, improve recruitment of alveoli on inspiration, and decrease the driving force for edema formation in this condition. Surfactant is also an important mediator of immune cell function, although this is a less well understood function than its surface tension–lowering effect.[14] Initial reports from a clinical trial of synthetic surfactant in ARDS were promising, demonstrating evidence of improved lung compliance and oxygenation in the treatment group. Unfortunately, recent analyses of patients recruited in a multicenter, randomized, placebo-controlled trial showed no significant survival benefit for patients who received aerosolized artificial surfactant.[56] The multifactorial nature of the lung injury in ARDS and the heterogeneity of the patient population may explain the disappointing results compared with newborn treatment. Drug delivery is also more complicated in intubated adults, and there is inadequate information regarding the optimal route or interval of drug dosing, amount required, and the critical timing for surfactant administration.

Pulmonary vasoactive therapies could improve V/Q matching and reduce right ventricular afterload. Indeed, pulmonary hypertension can be severe and progressive in ARDS and cause right ventricular dysfunction, limit cardiac output, and enhance edema formation.[11,13,45] Nonspecific vasodilators have been used in clinical trials of ARDS, but they have led to systemic hypotension and increased venous admixture due to worsening ventilation-perfusion relationships. A randomized, double-blind, placebo-controlled trial of prostaglandin E_1 (PGE_1) in ARDS showed no survival benefit.[57]

The vasodilating property of inhaled NO has been investigated in animal models and human subjects with pulmonary hypertension. Because of the presumed preferential distribution of inhaled NO to better-ventilated lung units, ventilation-perfusion matching may be improved in injured lungs.[58] Rapid and tight binding of NO to hemoglobin in the pulmonary circulation and subsequent biological inactivation likely prevent inhaled NO from acting on the systemic vasculature.

Clinical studies of inhaled NO in seriously ill infants with persistent pulmonary hypertension showed an improved arterial oxygenation without systemic hypotension.[59] A multicenter, randomized, placebo-controlled trial of NO in persistent pulmonary hypertension of the newborn is in progress. Children with pulmonary hypertension due to congenital heart disease have also responded to inhaled NO with decreased pulmonary artery pressures and improved pulmonary vascular resistance, without changes in systemic arterial pressure, while receiving the inhaled drug.[60]

Inhaled NO in adults with chronic pulmonary hypertension from a variety of causes has resulted in decreased pulmonary vascular resistance without changes in systemic hemodynamic values.[61] Inhaled NO in adults undergoing cardiac surgery and cardiopulmonary bypass had similar hemodynamic effects. A recent study compared the effects of inhaled NO with intravenous prostacyclin in nine adult patients with ARDS.[62] Inhaled NO resulted in decreased pulmonary artery pressure and improved oxygenation caused by decreased venous admixture.

To date, NO has not been studied in a prospective, randomized manner in ARDS, and no information exists about potential impact on survival. There should be concerns over potential toxicity of this therapy in this condition. Acute lung injury is likely associated with overproduction of endogenous nitric oxide rather than a deficit. Accordingly, it is possible that NO may contribute to lung injury in these clinical settings. One might argue, for example, that the elevated pressures and platelet activation seen in ARDS derive from endothelial dysfunction mediated by NO, and that the reduction in oxygen requirement seen with inhaled NO may merely be the substitution of one toxic gas with another. Concomitant administration of effective antioxidants may theoretically limit the toxic potential of nitric oxide and its by-products.

Corticosteroids can inhibit complement-induced neutrophil aggregation and the production of TNF by macrophages. Randomized, placebo-controlled, multicenter trials of high-dose corticosteroids failed to show improved survival in patients with ARDS, however.[63,64] There was also no evidence for a protective role in patients with predisposing conditions. Anecdotal reports describe improved gas exchange after corticosteroid treatment in patients with "late stage" ARDS and no ongoing, demonstrable infectious problems.[65] These observations have not been confirmed in prospective randomized studies.

Monoclonal antibodies directed against the lipid A component of endotoxin showed improved survival in certain subsets of patients with gram-negative infections.[66] Improvement in end-organ dysfunction including hypoxemic respiratory failure in patients who received antiendotoxin was also reported. A subsequent unpublished trial of the antiendotoxin HA1A was prematurely halted because of excess deaths in patients without gram-negative infections, and additional trials of the murine antiendotoxin E5 have failed, so far, to show survival benefits in patients with gram-negative infections.[67]

Proinflammatory cytokine neutralization could be used to modulate the intense inflammatory response of ARDS. Indeed, the presence and degree of cytokinemia has been associated with the occurrence of organ system failure and death.[68] Experimental data has established that blocking the effects of TNF or IL-1 with antibodies, receptor antagonists, or soluble receptors prevents lethal shock in animal sepsis models. Studies utilizing monoclonal antibodies and soluble receptors for TNF are underway. Report of a recent randomized, double-blind trial of interleukin-1 receptor antagonist (IL 1ra) in patients with sepsis syndrome showed no overall survival benefit.[69] A retrospective analysis of patients with more severe disease, however, did show a significant reduction in mortality in patients treated with IL-1ra. Therefore, cytokine blocking or inhibition may offer hope for patients with severe sepsis, but additional data and analysis are necessary.

Cyclooxygenase inhibitors have been shown to improve survival in animal models of sepsis.[70,71] Other studies have defined the role of excess prostanoid production in lung dysfunction. Pretreatment of endotoxin-challenged sheep with meclofenamate blocked early pulmonary hypertension and improved dynamic compliance.[72] Ibuprofen treatment in a similar model improved lung mechanics and pulmonary hemodynamics. A pilot study of ibuprofen in human sepsis showed decreased heart rate, temperature, peak airway pressure, and minute ventilation in the ibuprofen-treated group.[20] There were also trends toward increased blood pressure in hypotensive patients and improved oxygenation. Leukotrienes are also elevated in patients with sepsis and ARDS. Pretreatment of sheep with experimental lung injury with a 5-lipoxygenase inhibitor decreased pulmonary hypertension, improved lung mechanics, and decreased pulmonary edema.[73] The effects of intravenous ibuprofen in sepsis syndrome is currently being investigated in a multicenter, randomized, double-blind trial. No large-scale clinical studies of leukotriene inhibitors have been reported.

Antioxidant therapy has potential impact in patients with severe infections, ARDS, and SIRS. Treatment with vitamin E, superoxide dismutase (SOD), SOD and catalase, and SOD and the xanthine oxidase inhibitor allopurinol improve survival in some animal models of sepsis,[74,75] but the effect has been inconsistent. N-Acetylcysteine (NAC) is an antioxidant that repletes reduced glutathione and reduces the severity of pulmonary edema formation in endotoxin-induced lung injury in sheep.[26] N-Acetylcysteine infusion in patients with ARDS has resulted in increased plasma and erythrocyte glutathione levels, a trend toward improvement in oxygenation and chest radiograph scores, and increased cardiac output in the treatment group.[76]

Xanthine derivatives (eg, pentoxifylline) appear to inhibit oxygen radical release, phagocytosis, and response to PAF in human neutrophils.[14] These products may also affect other cytokine releases (eg, TNF) as well. In addition, xanthines have also been reported to improve diaphragm function in patients with ventilatory failure.

OUTCOME

Because of effective respiratory support systems, initial gas exchange severity is not a good predictor of outcome, and true respiratory failure is rarely the cause of death in patients with ARDS.[30,77] Rather, either the underlying disease or the development of ICU complications (especially sepsis)[78] is the usual cause of death through the development of multiple organ failures and hemodynamic collapse. Indeed, the best predictors of increased mortality risk are the presence of sepsis syndrome, evidence of tissue hypoxia or acidosis, and advanced age.[14] It should not be surprising, therefore, that young, relatively healthy patients with only lung-specific injury have generally twice the survival rate than older, severely immunocompromised patients with sepsis or SIRS as their cause for ARDS (Table 33-2). Estimating prognosis and designing clinical trials must take these factors into account.[31] Similarly, evaluating new respiratory support technologies must recognize that inadequate respiratory support capabilities is not a major cause of mortality.

TABLE 33-2. **ARDS Mortality**

	n	Mortality (%)
Ashbaugh (1967)	12	66
Fowler (1985)	88	65
Montgomery (1985)	47	68
Gillespie (1986)		
Lung injury alone	20	40
Lung injury plus multiorgan failure	60	82
Peters (1989)	166	71

The overall mortality from ARDS has been reported to be unchanged over the last 20 years (see Table 33-2).[30] This may reflect the fact that specific therapies for ARDS remain few, primarily consisting of only antibiotics and infection draining, which is similar to 20 years ago. On the other hand, the population getting ARDS in the 1990s has poorer host defenses than the population 20 years ago because patients with AIDS, patients surviving aggressive chemotherapy, and an older population are being treated. The fact that the mortality rate has not worsened under these circumstances may thus be reflecting beneficial effects of better management.

If a patient survives the initial episode of ARDS, long-term prognosis appears reasonably good.[79] One-year mortality after hospital discharge for ARDS is estimated at 10% to 20% (primarily from underlying disease), and pulmonary function tests in ARDS survivors 6 months later show remarkably good return of function (Table 33-3).

TABLE 33-3. **Lung Function In Survivors of ARDS**

	Follow-up <3 mo (*n* = 34)	Follow-up 3–6 mo (*n* = 23)	Follow-up >6 mo (*n* = 105)
Restrictive pattern	32%	26%	20%
Obstructive pattern	12%	17%	16%
Reduced DL	44%	30%	21%
Normal	44%	57%	65%

Used with permission from Ingbar DH, Matthaw RA: Lung function in survivors. Crit Care Clin 2:377, 1986

REFERENCES

1. Ashbaugh DG, Bigelow DB, Petty TL, Levine BE: Acute respiratory distress in adults. Lancet 2:319, 1967
2. Petty TL, Ashbaugh DG: The adult respiratory distress syndrome: Clinical features, factors influencing prognosis, and principles of management. Chest 60:233, 1971
3. Bernard GR, Artigas A, Brigham KL, et al, and the Consensus Committee: American-European consensus conference on ARDS. Am J Resp Crit Care Med 149:818, 1994
4. Meduri GU: Late adult respiratory distress syndrome. New Horizons 1:563, 1993

5. Lamy M, Fallat R, Koeniger E, et al: Pathologic features and mechanisms of hypoxemia in adult respiratory distress syndrome. Am Rev Respir Dis 114:267, 1976
6. Ratliff N, Wilson J, Mikat F, et al: The lung in hemorrhagic shock, IV: The role of the polymorphonuclear leukocyte. Am J Pathol 65:325, 1971
7. Pratt PC: Pathology of the Adult Respiratory Distress Syndrome. In WM Thurlbeck, MR Abel (eds): The Lung: Structure, Function and Disease. Baltimore, Williams and Wilkins, 1978, pp 43–57.
8. Pratt P, Vollmer R, Shelburne J, Crapo J: Pulmonary morphology in a multihospital collaborative extracorporeal membrane oxygenation project, I: Light microscopy. Am J Pathol 95:191, 1979
9. Zapol WM, Trelstad RL, Coffey W, et al: Pulmonary fibrosis in severe acute respiratory failure. Am Rev Respir Dis 119:547, 1979
10. Pison U, Seeger W, Buchhorn R, et al: Surfactant abnormalities in patients with respiratory failure after multiple trauma. Am Rev Respir Dis 140:1033, 1989
11. Zapol WM, Snider MT: Pulmonary hypertension in severe acute respiratory failure. N Eng J Med 296:476, 1977
12. Gattinoni L, Pesenti A, Bombino M: Relationships between lung computed tomographic density, gas exchange, and PEEP in acute respiratory failure. Anesthesiology 69:824, 1988
13. Brunet F, Dhainaut J, Devaux J, et al: Right ventricular performance in patients with acute respiratory failure. Intensive Care Med 14:474, 1988
14. National Heart, Lung, and Blood Institute: Report of the task force on research in cardiopulmonary dysfunction in critical care medicine. October, 1994, Bethesda, MD, National Institutes of Health, pp 1–119
15. Till GO, Johnson KL, Kunkel R, et al: Intravascular activation of complement and acute lung injury: Dependence on neutrophils and toxic oxygen radicals. J Clin Invest 69:1126, 1982
16. Henson P, Larsen G, Webster R, et al: Pulmonary microvascular alterations and injury induced by complement fragments: Synergistic effect of complement activation, neutrophil sequestration, and prostaglandin. Ann N Y Acad Sci 384:287, 1982
17. Tate R, Repine J: Neutrophils and the adult respiratory distress syndrome. Am Rev Respir Dis 128:552, 1983
18. Demling RH, Smith M, Gunther R, et al: Pulmonary injury and prostaglandin production during endotoxemia in conscious sheep. Am J Physiol 240:348, 1981
19. Henderson W: Eicosanoids and lung inflammation. Am Rev Respir Dis 135:1176, 1987
20. Bernard GR, Reines HD, Halushka P, et al: Prostacyclin and thromboxane A_2 formation is increased in human sepsis syndrome. Am Rev Respir Dis 144:1095, 1991
21. Braquet P, Touqui L, Shen T, Vargaftig B: Perspectives in platelet activating factor research. Pharmacol Rev 39:97, 1987
22. Koltai M, Hosford D, Grienot P, et al: Platelet-activating factor (PAF): A review of its effects, antagonists, and possible future clinical applications. Drugs 42:9, 1991
23. Freeman BA, Crapo JD: Biology of disease: Free radicals and tissue injury. Lab Invest 47:412, 1982
24. Cochrane G, Spragg R, Revak S: Studies on the pathogenesis of the adult respiratory distress syndrome: Evidence of oxidant activity in bronchoalveolar lavage fluid. J Clin Invest 71:754, 1983
25. Pacht E, Timerman A, Lykens M, et al: Deficiency of alveolar fluid glutathione in patients with sepsis and the adult respiratory distress syndrome. Chest 100:1397, 1991
26. Bernard G, Lucht W, Niedermeyer M, et al: Effect of N-acetylcysteine on the pulmonary response to endotoxin in the awake sheep and upon in vitro granulocyte function. J Clin Invest 73: 1772, 1984
27. Moncada S, Palmer R, Higgs E: Nitric oxide: Physiology, pathophysiology and pharmacology. Pharmacol Rev 43:109, 1991
28. Stamler JS, Singel DJ, Loscalzo J: Biochemistry of nitric oxide and its redox-activated forms. Science 258:1898, 1992
29. Villar J, Slutsky AS: The incidence of the adult respiratory distress syndrome. Am Rev Respir Dis 140:814, 1989
30. Hyers TM: Prediction of survival and mortality in patients with adult respiratory distress syndrome. New Horizons 1:466, 1993
31. Dellinger RP: Clinical trials in adult respiratory distress syndrome. New Horizons 1:584, 1993
32. Bone RC, Sibbald WJ, Sprunz CL: The ACCP-SCCM consensus conference on sepsis and organ failure. Chest 101:1481, 1992
33. Pepe PE, Potkin RT, Reus D, et al: Clinical predictors of the adult respiratory distress syndrome. Am J Surg 144:124, 1982
34. Fowler A, Hamman R, Good J, et al: Adult respiratory distress syndrome: Risk with common predispositions. Ann Intern Med 98:593, 1983
35. Kacmarek RM, Pierson DJ (ed): Positive end expiratory pressure. Respir Care 33:419, 1988
36. Anderson JD, Moore FA, Moore EE: Enteral feeding in the critically injured patient. Nutrition in Clinical Practice 7:117, 1992
37. SDD Collaborative Group: Meta analysis of randomized controlled trials of selective decontamination of the digestive tract. Br Med J 307:525, 1993
38. Schuster DP: The case for and against fluid restriction and occlusion pressure reduction in adult respiratory distress syndrome. New Horizons 1:478, 1993
39. Slutsky AS and the ACCP Mechanical Ventilation Consensus Group: Mechanical ventilation. Chest 104:1833, 1993
40. Marini JJ: New options for the ventilatory management of acute lung injury. New Horizons 1:489, 1993
41. MacIntyre NR: Clinically available new strategies for mechanical ventilatory support. Chest 104:560, 1993
42. Tsuno K, Prato P, Kolobow T: Acute lung injury from mechanical ventilation at moderately high airway pressures. J Appl Physiol 73:123, 1990
43. Hickling K, Henderson S, Jackson R: Low mortality associated with permissive hypercapnia in severe adult respiratory distress. Intensive Care Med 16:372, 1990
44. Jenkinson SG: Oxygen toxicity. New Horizons 1:504, 1993
45. Foex P: Right ventricular function during ARDS. Acta Anaesthesiol Scand 35:72, 1991
46. Dartzker DR: Oxygen transport and utilization in ARDS. European Respir J 11:485s–489s, 1990
47. Hayes MA, Timmins AC, Yan EH, et al: Elevation of systemic oxygen delivery in the treatment of critically ill patients. N Engl J Med 330:1717, 1994
48. Smythe MA, Zarowitz BJ: Changing perspectives of stress gastritis prophylaxis. Ann Pharmacother 28:1073, 1994
49. Wheeler AP: Sedation, analgesia and paralysis in the intensive care unit. Chest 104:566, 1993
50. Clagett, GP: Prevention of venous thromboembolism. Chest 102:391s, 1992
51. Villar J, Winston B, Slutsky AS: Non-conventional techniques of ventilatory support. Crit Care Clin 6:579, 1990
52. Zapol W, Snider M, Hill J, et al: Extracorporeal membrane oxygenation in severe acute respiratory failure: A randomized prospective study. JAMA 242:2193, 1979
53. Gattinoni L, Pesenti A, Mascheroni D, et al: Low frequency positive-pressure ventilation with extracorporeal CO_2 removal in severe acute respiratory failure. JAMA 256:881, 1986
54. Morris AH, Wallace CJ, Clemmer T, et al: Extracorporeal CO_2 removal therapy for adult respiratory distress syndrome patients: A computerized protocol controlled trial. Reanimation Soins Intensits Medicine d'Urgence 6:485, 1990
55. Hoekstra R, Jackson J, Myers T, et al: Improved neonatal survival following multiple doses of bovine surfactant in very premature neonates at risk for respiratory distress syndrome. Pediatrics 88:10, 1991
56. Anzueto A, Baughman R, Guntupalli K, et al: Aerosolized surfactant in adults with sepsis induced ARDS. New Engl J Med 334: 1417–1421, 1996
57. Bone RC, Slotan G, Maunder R, et al: Randomized double-blind, multicenter study of prostaglandin E_1 in patients with the adult respiratory distress syndrome. Chest 96:114, 1989
58. Pison U, Lopez F, Heidelmeyer C, et al: Inhaled nitric oxide reverses hypoxic pulmonary vasoconstriction without impairing gas exchange. J Appl Physiol 74:1287, 1993
59. Roberts J, Polaner D, Lang P, et al: Inhaled nitric oxide in persistent pulmonary hypertension of the newborn. Lancet 340:818, 1992
60. Roberts J, Long P, Bigatello L, et al: Inhaled nitric oxide in congenital heart disease. Circulation 87:447, 1993
61. Zapol WM, Hurford WE: Inhaled nitric oxide in the adult respiratory distress syndrome and other lung diseases. New Horizons 1:638, 1993

62. Rossaint R, Falke K, Lopez F, et al: Inhaled nitric oxide for the adult respiratory distress syndrome. N Engl J Med 328:399, 1993
63. Bone RC, Fischer CJ, Clemmer TP, et al: A controlled clinical trial of high-dose methylprednisolone int he treatment of severe sepsis and septic shock. N Engl J Med 317:653, 1987
64. Bernard GR, Luce JM, Sprung CL, et al: High-dose corticosteroids in patients with the adult respiratory distress syndrome. N Engl J Med 317:1565, 1987
65. Meduri GU, Belendria JM, Estes RJ, et al: Fibroproliferative phase of ARDS: Clinical findings and effects of corticosteroids. Chest 100:943, 1991
66. Ziegler E, Fisher C, Sprung C, et al: Treatment of Gram negative bacteremia and septic shock with HA-1A human monoclonal antibody against endotoxin: A randomized, double-blind, placebo-controlled trial. N Engl J Med 324:429, 1991
67. Wenzel R, Bone R, Fain A, et al: Results of a second double-blind, randomized, controlled trial of antiendotoxin antibody E_5 in gram-negative sepsis (Abstract 1170). In Program and Abstracts of the 31st Interscience Conference on Antimicrobial Agents and Chemotherapy. Washington, DC, American Society for Microbiology, 1991, p 294
68. Casey LC, Balk R, Bone R: Plasma cytokine endotoxin levels correlate with survival in patients and with the sepsis syndrome. Ann Intern Med 119:771, 1993
69. Fisher C, Dhalnaut J-F, Pribble J, Knaus W, and the IL-1 Receptor Antagonist Study Group: A study evaluating the safety and efficacy of human recombinant interleukin-1 receptor antagonist in the treatment of patients with sepsis syndrome. Presented at the 13th International Symposium on Intensive Care and Emergency Medicine; Brussels, Belgium; March 23, 1993
70. Fletcher J, Ramwell P: Indomethacin improves survival after endotoxin in baboons. Adv Prostaglandin Thromboxane Leukotriene Res 7:821, 1980
71. Beck R, Abel F: Effect of ibuprofen on the course of canine endotoxin shock. Circ Shock 23:59, 1987
72. Snapper JR, Hutchison AA, Ogletree ML, et al: Effects of cyclooxygenase inhibitors on the alteration of lung mechanics caused by endotoxemia in the unanesthetized sheep. J Clin Invest 72:63, 1983
73. Coggeshall J, Christmas B, Lefferts P, et al: Effect of inhibition of 5-lipoxygenase metabolism of arachidonic acid on response to endotoxemia in sheep. J Appl Physiol 65:1351, 1988
74. Powell R, Machiedo G, Rush B, et al: Effect of oxygen free radical scavengers on survival in sepsis. Am Surg 57:86, 1991
75. Kunimoto F, Morita T, Ogawa R, et al: Inhibition of lipid peroxidation improves survival rate of endotoxemic rats. Circ Shock 21:15, 1987
76. Bernard G: N-Acetylcysteine in experimental and clinical acute lung injury. Am J Med 91(Suppl 3c):54, 1991
77. Montgomery AB, Stager MA, Carrica CJ, Hudson LD: Causes of mortality in patients with ARDS. Am Rev Respir Dis 132:148, 1985
78. Pingleton S: Complications of respiratory failure. Am Rev Respir Dis 137:1463, 1988
79. Ingbar DH, Matthaw RA: Lung function in survivors. Crit Care Clin 2:377, 1986

34 Acute Respiratory Failure

Brent Van Hoozen
Timothy E. Albertson

PROFESSIONAL SKILLS

Upon completion of this chapter, the reader will:

- Denote the criteria that suggest the presence of acute respiratory failure
- Distinguish acute hypoxemic respiratory failure and acute hypercapnic respiratory failure
- Identify clinical manifestations suggestive of acute respiratory failure
- Formulate a differential diagnosis for acute respiratory failure based on clinical assessment
- Understand the basic pathophysiology of common causes of acute respiratory failure
- Recommend appropriate diagnostic and therapeutic intervention based on clinical assessment, radiographic features, and arterial blood gas findings
- Describe the staging of adult respiratory distress syndrome
- Outline general therapeutic approaches for reversing hypercapnea and respiratory acidosis in the patient with acute respiratory failure
- Calculate the alveolar-arterial PO_2 difference and PaO_2/FIO_2 ratio
- Use techniques to minimize complications of mechanical ventilation
- Outline diagnostic steps and treatment for acute distress associated with mechanical ventilation

KEY TERMS

Acute hypoxemic (Type I) respiratory failure
Acute hypercapnic (Type II) respiratory failure
Alveolar overdistension
APACHE scoring
Controlled hypoventilation
Dynamic hyperinflation
Multiple organ dysfunction syndrome (MODS)
Permissive hypercapnia
Volutrauma
Wasserman number

Despite the many technical advances in diagnosis, monitoring, and therapeutic intervention that have occurred over the past four decades, acute respiratory failure continues to be a major cause of morbidity and mortality in the intensive care unit setting. Acute respiratory failure is commonly considered synonymous with chronic obstructive pulmonary disease exacerbations. However, acute respiratory failure is a diagnosis that spares no age group and can be induced by many disease processes. Because some causes of respiratory failure can be readily reversible and often require rapid diagnosis and intervention, it is important for all members of the health care team to have a firm grasp on the assessment, differential diagnosis, and treatment of various causes of respiratory failure.

The precise incidence of acute respiratory failure is difficult to estimate due to the variability in disease classification and definition. However, one can generalize that it may be responsible for as many as 10% to 15% of admissions to medical intensive care units. Moreover, acute respiratory failure may become a complication for as many as 50% to 75% of those patients who require intensive care unit stays longer than 7 days. The mortality rate associated with acute respiratory failure is reported to range from 6% to 40%.[1–4] This wide range is caused by multiple factors including the heterogeneity of the various populations studied. This variability of causes of respiratory failure is discussed in more detail later in this chapter.

HISTORICAL PERSPECTIVE

Before the development of arterial blood gas analysis in the 1950s, acute respiratory failure was diagnosed predominantly on clinical grounds. At that time, barbiturate overdoses and poliomyelitis were the most common causes of respiratory failure.[5] Shortly thereafter, the introduction of the Salk vaccine virtually eliminated polio. With refinements in detection of impaired gas exchange, it became apparent that many other disease processes could also cause acute respiratory failure. Advancements in the 1960s brought about refinements in regulating oxygen delivery, routine measuring of arterial blood gases, renewed interest in positive pressure ventilation, and the birth of the modern-day intensive care unit (ICU). These advancements ushered in a new era, allowing for aggressive diagnosis and support of a host of conditions associated with respiratory failure such as shock, sepsis, burns, and trauma.

Improvements of the past two decades have brought about enhanced monitoring techniques such as continuous pulse oximetry, which is now an accepted monitoring standard for all ICUs, operating rooms, and procedure labs. Most recently, techniques for continuous capnic monitoring and intraarterial blood gas monitoring have been developed that promise to further our ability to manage critically unstable patients. The past decade has also seen proliferation of microprocessor-controlled mechanical ventilation, which has led to a bewildering array of ventilatory support modes and approaches.

The goal of these advancements has been to improve survival associated with respiratory failure. Unfortunately, the harsh reality may be that we are merely delaying mortality in some settings. The aggressive treatment required to sustain someone through respiratory failure may leave one vulnerable to multiple complications including barotrauma, sepsis, stress ulceration, acute renal failure, nosocomial pneumonia, and opportunistic infections.[5–7] Therefore, although hypoxemia is now treatable, complications of this therapy may promote mortality secondary to multiple organ system failure.

Moreover, the heightened complexity associated with technical advancements may lead to an increased risk for iatrogenic complications that may further negate any survival advantage conferred by these enhancements. Given that intensive care unit service constitutes a large percentage of total health care expenditures, this strategy may be evaluated with closer scrutiny due to the managed care movement currently sweeping the country.

DEFINITION

Acute respiratory failure can be thought of as a dysfunction in the respiratory system that leads to the buildup of carbon dioxide or a critical shortage of oxygen delivery to the tissues. Although respiratory failure usually implies a disorder involving the lungs, it is useful to recall that other organ systems are also involved in the process of respiration. Therefore, severe impairment of other involved systems such as the musculoskeletal, circulatory, or central nervous systems may also lead to acute respiratory failure. Figure 34-1 shows the many subsystems involved in the process of respiration as well as respective disease processes that may result in respiratory failure.[5]

Commonly cited criteria for the establishment of acute respiratory failure in a patient include any two of the following four factors:[5]

1. Presence of acute dyspnea
2. PaO_2 less than 50 mmHg while breathing room air
3. $PaCO_2$ greater than 50 mmHg
4. An arterial blood pH compatible with significant respiratory acidosis

Although these criteria serve mainly as guidelines and are not "set in stone," a fifth criteria is common and could be included as well:

5. Presence of altered mental status plus one or more of the above criteria

This fifth criterion is included because acute respiratory failure remains primarily a clinical diagnosis that should be confirmed by laboratory studies, rather than based solely on the results of arterial blood gas criteria. For example, in chronic obstructive pulmonary disease, patients may present with PaO_2s as low as 50 mmHg and $PaCO_2$s higher than 50 mmHg with few or no clinical symptoms to suggest acute respiratory failure. When these respiratory changes occur slowly

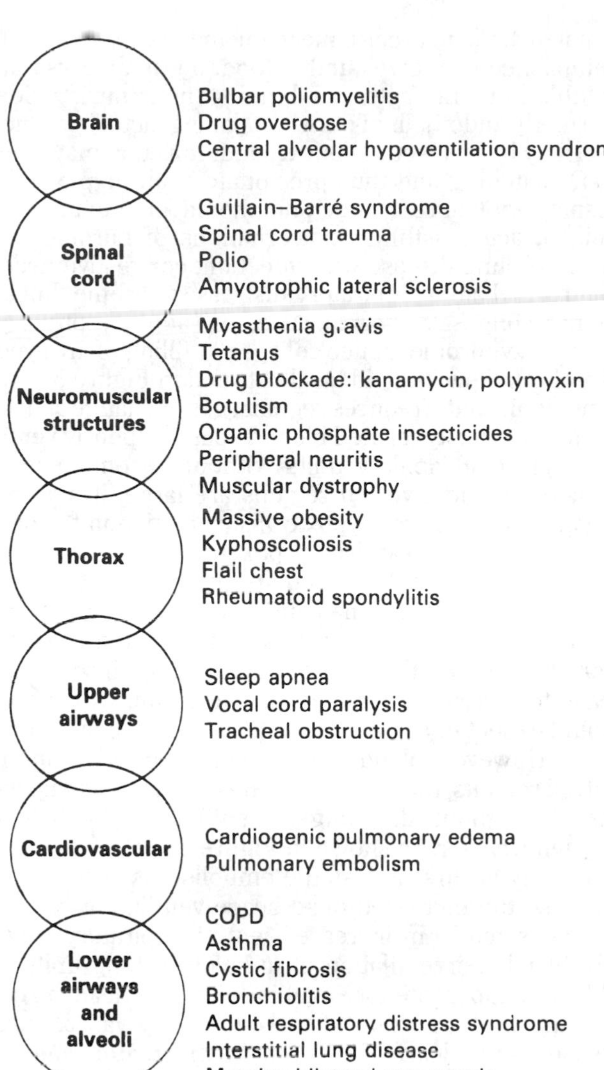

FIGURE 34-1. The causes of acute respiratory failure by organ system. (Reprinted with permission from Bone RC: Acute respiratory failure. In Burton GG, Hodgkin JE, Ward JJ [eds]: Respiratory Care: A Guide to Clinical Practice, 3rd ed. Philadelphia, JB Lippincott, 1991, p. 847.

over several months, increases in red cell mass and red blood cell 2,3-diphosphoglycerate levels augment tissue delivery of oxygen despite a reduced PaO_2. Likewise, if CO_2 retention occurs slowly over time, CO_2-induced central nervous system narcosis is blunted, and renal compensation with increased bicarbonate reabsorption results in near normalization of arterial pH. In this circumstance, modest supplemental oxygen is often indicated to correct the hypoxemia, but intubation and mechanical ventilation are usually not required.

Another example of the clinical diagnostic nature of respiratory failure is the unresponsive person who presents to the emergency department with obvious rapid and labored respirations. Aggressive therapeutic interventions including intubation and mechanical ventilation may be required immediately. Waiting the precious few minutes required to obtain a blood gas sample in this situation may result in cardiac arrest or anoxic brain damage before the results are known. A common error of physicians, respiratory therapists, and nurses is the feeling that the problem of respiratory failure is solved once mechanical ventilation is instituted. Clinical and laboratory documentation of improved status after initiating mechanical ventilation is needed.

Acute respiratory failure is actually a syndrome that may be precipitated by a multitude of underlying conditions. Most of these may require additional specific intervention such as diuretics, anticoagulants, antibiotics, or bronchodilators. As a respiratory practitioner, knowledge of the underlying diagnosis is required to formulate a comprehensive care plan including prioritization of care and frequency of follow-up assessments.

Classification

Acute respiratory failure can be classified as *acute hypoxemic respiratory failure* or *acute hypercapnic respiratory failure.* Acute hypoxemic respiratory failure, or Type I failure, refers to a primary defect in oxygenation; whereas acute hypercapnic respiratory failure, or Type II failure, refers to a primary defect in ventilation. Unfortunately, in clinical practice, the distinction is less than clear, and many patients present with features of combined Type I and Type II respiratory failure.

☐ ACUTE HYPOXEMIC RESPIRATORY FAILURE

This type of failure occurs when the predominant gas exchange defect is the result of failure to oxygenate. Typically, patients with Type I failure demonstrate a $PaO_2 \leq 50$ mmHg. The $PaCO_2$ is typically ≤ 40 mmHg unless there is also a cause for hypercapnic respiratory failure. There are at least six types of conditions that can result in Type I failure.[8] These types include an abnormally low inspired partial pressure of oxygen, (low PIO_2); oxygen diffusion impairment; ventilation/perfusion ($\dot{V}/\dot{Q}$) mismatch; right-to-left shunt; alveolar hypoventilation; and high tissue oxygen consumption. Of these, oxygen diffusion impairment and low PIO_2 are rarely seen, whereas $\dot{V}/\dot{Q}$ mismatch, right-to-left shunt, and alveolar hypoventilation are the most clinically significant causes. Because alveolar hypoventilation induces predominantly acute hypercapnic respiratory failure, it is discussed in the section under that heading. The major clinical causes of Type I respiratory failure are listed in Box 34-1.

Ventilation/Perfusion ($\dot{V}/\dot{Q}$) Mismatch. The effect of gravity on an upright human causes an unequal distribution of blood flow to the lungs; the lungs can therefore be divided into three basic zones, as in Figure 34-2. Zone 1, at the apexes, receives the smallest proportion of blood flow, while zone 3, located at the bases, receives the most generous supply. During tidal volume respirations in the normal person, a greater proportion of each breath is provided to the bases where perfusion

BOX 34-1

CAUSES OF HYPOXEMIC RESPIRATORY FAILURE

Diffuse parenchymal involvement
Cardiogenic pulmonary edema
- Congestive heart failure, mitral stenosis, fluid overload

Noncardiogenic pulmonary edema
- Adult respiratory distress syndrome, fat embolism syndrome
- Near drowning, neurogenic pulmonary edema

Bilateral pneumonia
- Bacterial: *S. aureus, P. aeruginosa, Legionella, H. influenzae, Mycoplasma*
- Viral: influenza, CMV, varicella, adenovirus, RSV, parainfluenza
- Parasitic: *Pneumocystis carinii*

Infiltrative
- Pulmonary fibrosis, tumor infiltration, cytotoxic drug reactions

Other
- Transfusion reactions, gastric contents aspiration, inhalation injury
- Toxic: salicylate and cyanide poisoning

Focal Parenchymal Involvement
Atelectasis, pleural effusion
Pneumonia, pulmonary contusion

No Parenchymal Involvement
Pneumothorax, pulmonary embolism, intracardiac shunt
Obstructive lung disease
- Asthma, chronic obstructive pulmonary disease

Increased metabolic demands
- Sepsis, shock, excessive feeding

Categorized by Radiographic Findings

is also the greatest. Therefore, ventilation and perfusion are closely matched. The lungs also regulate $\dot{V}/\dot{Q}$ matching through hypoxic vasoconstriction, which allows for the redistribution of pulmonary blood flow away from areas that are not well ventilated with oxygenated air. The precise mechanism for how this is accomplished is not well understood, but it appears that soluble humoral factors and endogenous nitric oxide (formerly endothelium-derived relaxing factor) production may be involved.[9] Clinical conditions that may alter $\dot{V}/\dot{Q}$ matching and thus precipitate acute hypoxemic respiratory failure include pneumonia, pulmonary embolism, acute asthma, exacerbations of chronic obstructive lung disease with infection, congestive heart failure, and adult respiratory distress syndrome. Pneumonia, congestive heart failure, and adult respiratory distress syndrome induce collapse or filling of involved alveolar units with fluid, as illustrated in Figure 34-3*A*. This significantly reduces regional gas exchange and allows some deoxygenated blood to pass by poorly ventilated alveolar-capillary units without becoming oxygenated. If the involved regions are large, it may be beyond the ability of hypoxic vasoconstriction to compensate, leading to arterial hypoxemia.

Pulmonary embolism produces hypoxemia through a slightly different mechanism. When a pulmonary embolus lodges in a pulmonary artery, afflicted alveolar units become ventilated but not perfused. This initially leads to increased dead space ventilation, which one would expect to cause hypercapnia rather than hypoxemia. However, blood flow is then diverted to uninvolved regions, thereby disrupting optimal $\dot{V}/\dot{Q}$ matching throughout the lungs, resulting in inefficient oxygen transfer, as shown in Figure 34-3*B*. Hypercapnia rarely occurs (unless the embolism is very large) because the increased dead space ventilation can be compensated for by increased central respiratory drive. Alveolar hyperventilation of uninvolved lung units is able to compensate for small increases in dead space. Occlusion of a portion of the pulmonary vasculature also leads to release of inflammatory mediators and vasoactive substances such as thromboxane A_2 and serotonin.[10,11] This regional inflammatory response also contributes to alteration in local blood flow and may also promote regional bronchoconstriction, accounting for reports of wheezing that may accompany pulmonary embolism.[12,13]

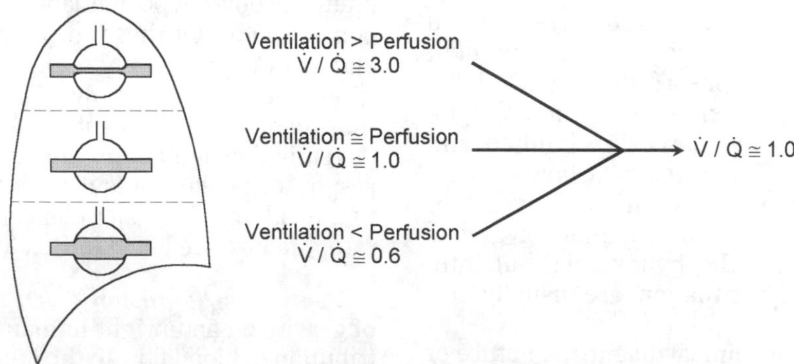

FIGURE 34-2. Normal ventilation/perfusion ($\dot{V}/\dot{Q}$) relationships within the lung. In an upright, normal host, a perfusion gradient exists such that perfusion is highest at the base (zone 3) and least at the apex (zone 1). When averaged for the entire lung, the ventilation and perfusion are essentially matched ($\dot{V}/\dot{Q} \approx 1.0$). (Data from Wagner PD, Laravuso RB, Uhl RR, et al: Continuous distributions of ventilation-perfusion ratios in normal subjects breathing air and 100% O_2. J Clin Invest 54:54–68, 1974.)

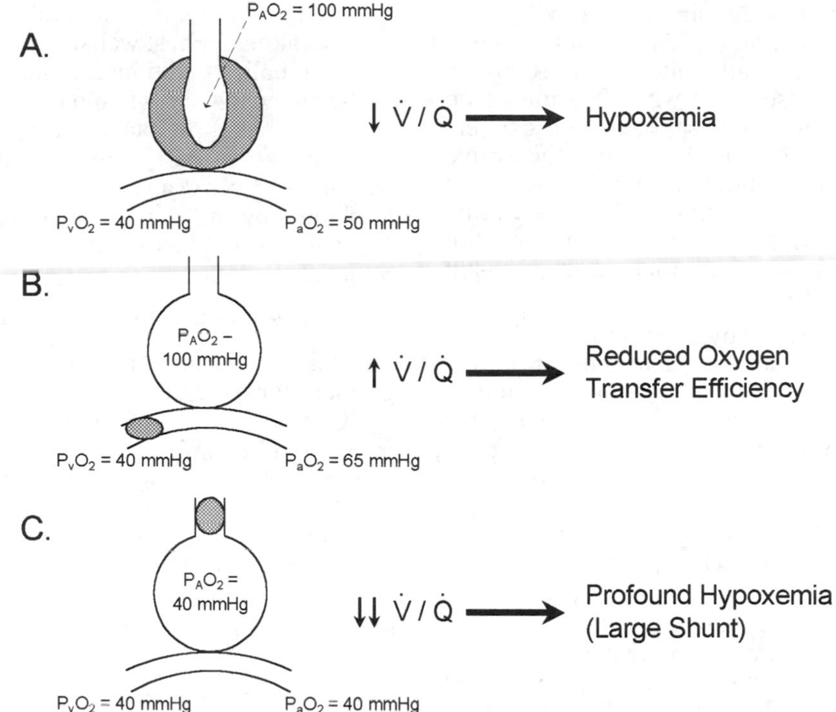

FIGURE 34-3. Abnormalities in ventilation/perfusion ($\dot{V}/\dot{Q}$) relationships. **(A)** In situations such as pulmonary edema and pneumonia, alveolar filling with fluid or cellular debris reduces the surface area available for gas exchange and results in a reduced $\dot{V}/\dot{Q}$ ratio and hypoxemia. **(B)** Pulmonary emboli disrupt normal $\dot{V}/\dot{Q}$ matching within the lung through two mechanisms. The blood clot itself blocks blood flow to ventilated alveoli resulting in increased dead space ventilation (elevated $\dot{V}/\dot{Q}$). Blood flow is then redistributed to other regions, decreasing their relative $\dot{V}/\dot{Q}$ ratio. The net effect is a reduced oxygen transfer efficiency which may lead to widening of the alveolar–arterial PO_2 difference and hypoxemia. Hypercapnia is usually not observed due to compensation by increased minute ventilation, however this cannot correct the reduced oxygen transfer efficiency. **(C)** Airway obstruction from mucus plugging, endobronchial tumors or aspirated foreign bodies can produce right-to-left shunt which may result in profund hypoxemia. In this situation, deoxygenated pulmonary artery blood continues to flow past nonventilated alveoli and fails to become oxygenated. If the shunt is sufficiently large (≥30%), administration of supplemental oxygen even at high flow rates, cannot compensate for this.

Right-to-Left Shunt. Shunting represents an extreme example of $\dot{V}/\dot{Q}$ mismatch whereby an involved region of the lung receives perfusion but no ventilation. This is usually termed right-to-left shunt as blood is able to pass through the pulmonary circulation and enter the systemic circulation without becoming oxygenated. In the normal person, there is a small amount of shunt present. Some of the bronchial blood flow is drained by the pulmonary venous system after it has been partially depleted of oxygen. Likewise, some of the coronary artery perfusion is drained into the left ventricle via the thebesian veins. This accounts for the nominal 2% to 3% shunt observed in the normal person.[8] Pathologic right-to-left shunting can be at the level of the heart (intracardiac shunt) or pulmonary vasculature (intrapulmonary shunt). Intracardiac shunts include atrial or ventricular septal defects and patent foramen ovale, which allow deoxygenated blood to mix with the left-sided, oxygenated blood. In adult clinical practice, acquired intrapulmonary shunts are more common than either congenital intracardiac or congenital intrapulmonary shunts such as pulmonary arteriovenous malformations.

Conditions normally associated with altered $\dot{V}/\dot{Q}$ matching such as pneumonia, congestive heart failure, and adult respiratory distress syndrome can produce right-to-left shunt in severe cases. Also, atelectasis of a lung or lung segment caused by mucus plugging or endobronchial obstruction with tumor can lead to right-to-left shunt, as depicted in Figure 34-3*C*. Atelectasis is important to recognize as a cause for shunt in that it is readily treatable through vigorous suctioning, percussion and postural drainage, or fiberoptic bronchoscopy. Although atelectasis is usually diagnosed by observing focal collapse of a lung segment on chest radiograph, abrupt onset hypoxemia may precede focal collapse, and the initial chest radiograph may be unremarkable. In this circumstance, atelectasis may be clinically confused with an acute pulmonary embolism.

Distinguishing right-to-left shunt from $\dot{V}/\dot{Q}$ mismatch can be determined on clinical grounds by comparing the PaO_2 response to administration of 100% oxygen. The hypoxemia associated with $\dot{V}/\dot{Q}$ mismatch can usually be corrected with supplemental oxygen, whereas even 100% oxygen does not correct the hypoxemia associated with right-to-left shunt $\geq$ 30%. The equation for calculating the shunt percentage can be found in Appendix A. Hypercapnia rarely occurs with shunt and, if present, suggests that the right-to-left shunt is greater than 50%.[8]

Diffusion Impairment. Any process that thickens the lining separating the alveolus and capillary lumen can produce hypoxemia by slowing the diffusion of oxygen across the alveolar-capillary membrane. This is rarely clinically significant as the red blood cells usually have available at least 300% of the necessary time in the alveolar-capillary network necessary for the uptake of oxygen.[14,15] An exception to this would be under conditions of exercise when red blood cell transit time through the alveolar-capillary network is reduced. However, at rest, hypoxemia associated with interstitial fibrosis, chronic obstructive lung disease, or pulmonary edema is more likely to be caused by $\dot{V}/\dot{Q}$ mismatch or shunt rather than impaired diffusion.

Reduced Partial Pressure of Inspired Oxygen. Altitudes higher than 10,000 feet may be associated with a reduction in the partial pressure of inspired oxygen (P_{IO_2}) to clinically significant levels, particularly if combined with an underlying pulmonary condition. A more common circumstance includes travel on commercial aircraft that are often pressurized only to an altitude of 8,000 to 10,000 feet.[8] Therefore, all patients with marginal PaO_2s at sea level should be evaluated for this possibility or provided with supplemental oxygen for the flight. Barring these circumstances, low P_{IO_2} is rarely of clinical significance, particularly in a hospital setting. Inadvertent reductions in F_{IO_2} have been seen in hospitals, so the F_{IO_2} is routinely monitored to prevent clinical consequences.

Increased Tissue Oxygen Demands. Any condition that results in abnormally high metabolic demands for oxygen can lower the mixed venous partial pressure of oxygen ($P\bar{v}O_2$). This does not usually lower the PaO_2 unless it is combined with a condition impairing gas exchange such as pneumonia, adult respiratory distress syndrome, or chronic obstructive lung disease. In this circumstance, the impaired lungs may not be able to "step up" the PaO_2 to a level compatible with adequate arterial saturation. Disease processes associated with high metabolic demands for oxygen relative to oxygen delivery include septic shock, cardiogenic shock, severe burns, pancreatitis, cyanide poisoning, and salicylate overdose.

Acute Hypercapnic Respiratory Failure

In its pure form, acute hypercapnic respiratory failure, or Type II failure, is associated with marked elevation of carbon dioxide from impaired ventilation with relative preservation of oxygenation. The major categories include central nervous system dysfunction, neuromuscular weakness, chest wall deformities, and pulmonary and metabolic conditions. A more complete listing for each major category is found in Box 34-2. It is important to realize that Type II failure can be associated with an abnormally low PaO_2. The reason for this is that the partial pressures of alveolar oxygen and carbon dioxide are linked by the alveolar air equation (see Appendix A), which simplifies to the following at sea level on room air:

$$P_AO_2 \text{ (in mmHg)} = 150 - (PaCO_2 \times 1.25)$$

Assuming a normal alveolar-arterial partial pressure gradient for oxygen of 10 mmHg, an acute rise in the $PaCO_2$ from 40 to 70 mmHg results in a drop in the PaO_2 from 90 to 52 mmHg. A quick rule of thumb involves use of the *Wasserman number.* On room air, the PaO_2 and the $PaCO_2$ should add up to 110 to 130 mmHg. If primary hypoventilation is occurring, the $PaCO_2$ and the PaO_2 add up to 110 to 130 mmHg, yielding a normal Wasserman number and a normal alveolar-arterial PO_2 difference. Thus, the hypoxemia present is caused by

BOX 34-2

CAUSES OF HYPERCAPNIC RESPIRATORY FAILURE

Impaired Central Drive
Structural
- □ Stroke, intracranial hemorrhage, tumor infiltration

Drug toxicity
- □ Narcotics, benzodiazepines, barbiturates, alcohol

Sleep disordered breathing
- □ Obstructive sleep apnea, central sleep apnea, Cheynes-Stokes respirations

Neuromuscular weakness
Cervical spine injury: trauma, tumor infiltration
Drug toxicity
- □ Paralytic agents, aminoglycosides
- □ Organophosphate poisoning

Infections: botulism, tetanus, poliomyelitis
Neuromuscular disease: Guillain-Barré syndrome, myasthenia gravis
- □ Amyotrophic lateral sclerosis, muscular dystrophy

Respiratory muscle fatigue
Phrenic nerve palsy: thoracic surgery, mediastinal tumor infiltration
Metabolic disorders
- □ Malnutrition, hypophosphatemia, hypokalemia, hypomagnesemia, hypocalcemia

Chest wall deformities
Kyphoscoliosis, pectus excavatum, flail chest
Obesity hypoventilation syndrome

Massive abdominal distension
Massive ascites, obesity

Airway obstruction
Endobronchial tumor, vocal cord paralysis
Obstructive sleep apnea

the hypoventilation. If, on the other hand, the sum is less than 110 on room air, then $\dot{V}/\dot{Q}$ mismatch, diffusion impairment, or right-to-left shunt must also be contributing to the hypoxemia.

Combined Hypoxemic and Hypercapnic Respiratory Failure

The presence of combined hypoxemic and hypercapnic respiratory failure is defined by overt hypercapnia plus an elevated alveolar-arterial partial pressure gradient for oxygen. Common clinical situations in which this can occur include exacerbations of asthma or emphysema complicated by a lower respiratory tract infection. Severe manifestations of pneumonia, pulmonary edema, and pulmonary embolism may also produce combined respiratory failure. Any cause of Type I failure may produce combined features if it is complicated by respiratory muscle fatigue and subsequent hypercapnia. Likewise, conditions producing neuromuscular weakness or chest wall deformities may be complicated by pneumonia or atelectasis caused by impaired cough, which would then result in hypoxemia superimposed on the primary hypercapnia.

CLINICAL PRESENTATION OF ACUTE RESPIRATORY FAILURE

Clinical assessment is extremely helpful in distinguishing the various causes for respiratory failure as well as determining the appropriate course of action. A thorough inspection should include evaluation of mental status; observation of respiratory pattern; inspection of the skin, lips, and nail beds to assess for cyanosis; and pulmonary and cardiac auscultation.

The most crucial objective of the clinical assessment in acute respiratory failure is to determine if intubation and positive pressure ventilation are immediately required. Patients generally require intubation and ventilation in the presence of depressed mental status or coma, severe respiratory distress, extremely low or agonal respiratory rate, obvious respiratory muscle fatigue, peripheral cyanosis, or impending cardiopulmonary arrest. In these situations, immediate intervention is necessary and should not be delayed pending the results of additional diagnostic studies such as arterial blood gas analyses or chest radiographs. Intubation is important in patients with altered mental status not only because of potential severe gas exchange derangements, but also because these patients are likely to have diminished airway protective reflexes and are at high risk for gastric contents aspiration.

In the presence of respiratory failure, stupor or coma is suggestive of severe hypercapnia and respiratory acidosis. A buildup of carbon dioxide has a sedating effect on the central nervous system, referred to as CO_2 narcosis, which if uncorrected leads to diminished alertness, disorientation, elevated intracranial pressures, and ultimately unconsciousness. This is usually suggestive of acute hypercapnic respiratory failure; however, it may also occur as an end result of respiratory muscle fatigue associated with other causes of respiratory failure. As the findings associated with early CO_2 narcosis may be subtle, when assessing alert patients with respiratory failure, it is important to make sure they are oriented to person, place, and time. Significant CO_2 narcosis is generally associated with very slow or agonal respirations. Patients with respiratory failure associated with diminished level of consciousness generally require intubation and positive pressure ventilation.

Respiratory distress is described as a heightened state of anxiety or agitation in an alert patient with respiratory embarrassment. In addition to demonstrating labored respirations and complaints of dyspnea, afflicted persons often exhibit diaphoresis, tachycardia, and tremulousness. Speech is often broken into two- or three-word sentences interspersed with respirations. Respiratory distress is a useful finding as it suggests that the respiratory center is functioning properly and is receiving appropriate chemoreceptor feedback on blood gas derangements. The presence of respiratory distress tends to exclude structural central nervous system conditions such as brain stem infarction or overdoses of central nervous system depressants as the cause for respiratory failure.

Peripheral cyanosis of the skin, lips, or nail beds implies the existence of profound arterial hypoxemia, usually with a $PaO_2 < 50$ mmHg. However, the absence of cyanosis does not exclude severe acute hypoxemic respiratory failure, particularly in patients with severe anemia or darkly pigmented skin. Thus, a lack of cyanosis cannot be used to differentiate Type I and Type II respiratory failure. Although passive supplemental oxygen is useful in correcting hypoxemia, in the presence of severe cyanosis, intubation and ventilation are often required as a very high FIO_2 and positive end-expiratory pressure are usually necessary in this circumstance.

Evaluation of the respiratory pattern is also helpful in distinguishing the causes of acute respiratory failure. The most useful finding is paradoxical motion of the chest and abdominal wall. During a normal inspiration, the chest wall expands, and as the diaphragm moves downward, it displaces abdominal contents outward. Therefore, during a normal respiratory effort, the chest and abdomen expand and relax in unison. Diaphragmatic weakness is suggested by an inward motion of the abdomen while the chest wall expands during inspiration. The presence of sternal retraction during inspiration is indicative of impaired pulmonary compliance states such as may be seen with congestive heart failure or adult respiratory distress syndrome. It can also suggest the presence of a flail chest associated with traumatic fracture or surgical disruption of multiple ribs. Most patients in respiratory distress with thoracoabdominal paradoxical motion require administration of positive pressure ventilation.

Differentiating Causes of Acute Respiratory Failure

Many of the causes of acute respiratory failure can be separated based on the clinical findings mentioned above plus arterial blood gas findings. Algorithms outlining the basic distinguishing features are shown in Figure 34-4.

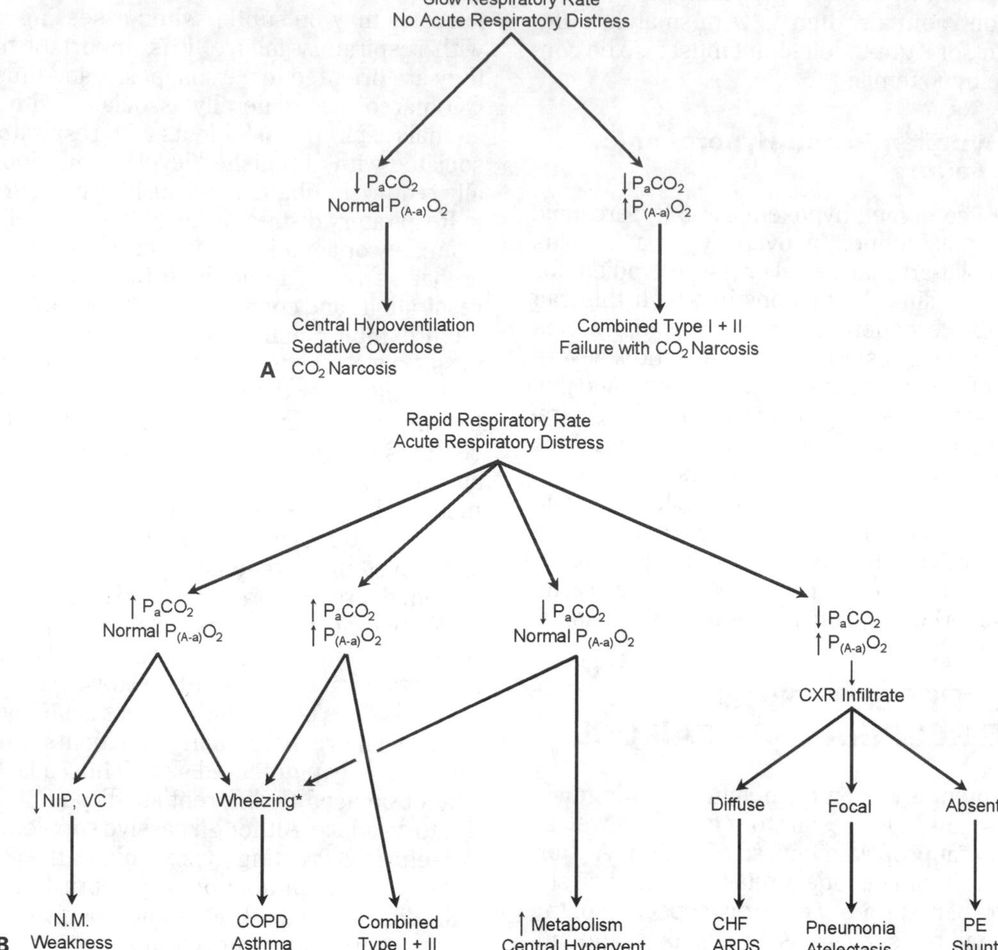

FIGURE 34-4. Bedside assessment of respiratory failure based on breathing pattern and arterial blood gas findings. **(A)** Acute hypercapnic respiratory failure. **(B)** Acute hypoxemic respiratory failure. *Wheezing may not be apparent in some situations, particularly in obstructive lung disease associated with hypercapnia as severely diminished airflow may not produce enough turbulence to be appreciated on auscultation. Abbreviations: ARDS: adult respiratory distress syndrome, CHF: congestive heart failure, COPD: chronic obstructive pulmonary disease; CXR: chest X-ray; NM: neuromuscular; NIP: negative inspiratory pressure; PE: pulmonary embolus; VC: vital capacity.

Acute hypercapnic respiratory failure can present in one of two forms depending on whether the defect involves the central respiratory drive. Conditions impairing the central drive usually are associated with a diminished level of consciousness with slow and shallow respiratory rates. Arterial blood gas analyses typically demonstrate a reduced pH (usually less than 7.30) and an elevated $PaCO_2$ (usually greater than 50 mmHg). The PaO_2 may be reduced depending on the degree of hypoventilation; however, the alveolar-arterial PO_2 difference is usually normal. Conditions associated with this respiratory pattern include drug toxicity from central nervous system depressants, such as narcotics, benzodiazepines, and barbiturates, or structural nervous system lesions, such as stroke or intracranial hemorrhage.

Defects below the level of the central respiratory drive usually present with rapid, shallow respirations and respiratory distress. Arterial blood gas derangements are similar to those mentioned above. Conditions associated with these findings include neuromuscular weakness secondary to Guillain-Barré syndrome, myasthenia gravis, amyotrophic lateral sclerosis, muscular dystrophy, tetanus, poliomyelitis, botulism, and organophosphate poisoning. A vital capacity < 1000 mL or 10 mL/kg or a maximal inspiratory subatmospheric pressure (MIP) < -20 to -30 cmH_2O is suggestive of respiratory failure that likely requires positive pressure ventilation.[5,16–18] Acute exacerbations of asthma may present in a fashion similar to neuromuscular weakness with rapid, shallow respiratory efforts and respiratory distress. Asthma can usually be distinguished from neuromuscular weakness by a prior history of asthma, presence of expiratory wheezing, and the lack of extremity weakness. Patients with early stages of asthma exacerbations usually lack hypercapnia. Those with late stages of asthma may exhibit acute hypercapnia. Those with severe, premorbid asthma may even lack wheezes as a result of extremely diminished airflow.

In comparison, acute hypoxemic respiratory failure usually presents with rapid, deeper respiratory efforts and acute respiratory distress. Arterial blood gas analyses demonstrate a lower than normal PaO_2 with increased $P(A - a)O_2$. The presence of sternal retractions suggest either impaired pulmonary compliance as seen with pulmonary edema (both cardiogenic and noncardiogenic forms) or a flail chest. Pneumonia and atelectasis may be suggested by the presence of bronchial breath sounds or a productive cough. However, chest radiographs and additional studies are often required to determine the underlying cause of acute hypoxemic respiratory failure.

MANAGEMENT OF ACUTE RESPIRATORY FAILURE

Acute Hypoxemic Respiratory Failure

Correction of acute hypoxemia generally entails the use of supplemental oxygen delivered to provide an arterial oxygen saturation greater than 90%. A complete discussion on the use of oxygen therapy can be found in Chapter 13. The following is a brief review: supplemental oxygen can be delivered by means of a nasal cannula, simple face mask, Venturi mask, nonrebreather mask, or in line with mechanical ventilation. At high flow, nasal cannulas can provide FIO_2 of up to 0.4, simple face masks up to 0.6, and nonrebreather masks with very high flows can deliver an FIO_2 that approaches 0.7 to 0.8 depending on the patient's minute ventilation. Venturi masks have an FIO_2 range of 0.24–0.5 with the advantage of high flows and a more precise regulation of FIO_2. Air–O_2 blenders can provide high flows at FIO_2s > 0.5.

For the immediate treatment of acute hypoxemic respiratory failure with respiratory distress, the FIO_2 should be rapidly increased, with continuous pulse oximetry monitoring, until an arterial saturation of 90% or higher is achieved. Much has been written regarding the perils of supplemental oxygen producing respiratory depression through elimination of the hypoxic respiratory drive. However, this is a concern mainly in those patients who have chronic CO_2 retention as with chronic obstructive pulmonary disease. In the acute setting, adequate correction of hypoxemia is a higher priority than concern over possible attenuation of hypoxic respiratory drive. Clinically significant metabolic acidosis from lactic acid accumulation can occur within minutes if the hypoxemia is not rapidly corrected. Clinically significant CO_2 retention from overzealous oxygen therapy generally requires 30 minutes or more to develop. Therefore, once hypoxemia is reversed, one has time to assess the impact of oxygen on CO_2 retention and titrate to the minimum level necessary for correction of hypoxemia. After an adequate FIO_2 has been provided, an arterial blood gas analysis can be obtained to assess pH and $PaCO_2$ as well as confirm an appropriate level of PaO_2.

In some circumstances, passive administration of supplemental oxygen is insufficient to provide adequate arterial saturation. Conditions associated with severe $\dot{V}/\dot{Q}$ mismatch or shunt such as bilateral pneumonia and adult respiratory distress syndrome are common examples. In these situations, additional modalities may need to be considered to recruit collapsed lung units to participate in gas exchange.

The least invasive technique employs the use of a CPAP (continuous positive airway pressure) mask. This is a tight-fitting mask containing an expiratory valve that maintains positive airway pressure throughout expiration and the respiratory cycle. The valve can be adjusted to provide a pressure usually ranging from 2.5 to 10.0 cmH_2O. The addition of CPAP is felt to "splint" open airways, redistribute fluid in alveolar sacs away from gas exchange surfaces, and increase functional residual volumes, thereby allowing recruitment of collapsed alveoli to participate in gas exchange.[19–22] The advantage of the CPAP mask is that it enhances oxygenation in a fashion similar to PEEP (positive end-expiratory pressure) without requiring intubation and positive pressure ventilation. The drawbacks of the CPAP mask include patient discomfort and impairments to communication, suctioning, and feeding. If the CPAP mask is required for several days, patients may develop ischemic necrosis of the skin overlying the nasal bridge. The CPAP mask should only be employed in alert patients with pure oxygenation impairment and in a continuously monitored setting. The use of the CPAP mask is contraindicated in unconscious patients as unannounced emesis can lead to asphyxiation from gastric contents aspiration.

Positive pressure ventilation with PEEP is the modality most often employed to augment oxygenation when supplemental oxygen is inadequate. Positive pressure ventilation can be used in patients with combined Type I and Type II respiratory failure. Both PEEP and CPAP have been shown to improve oxygenation by redistribution of fluid away from the alveolar-capillary exchange surfaces and to recruit collapsed alveoli by increasing lung volume.[23,24] Positive pressure ventilation may also improve oxygenation by significantly reducing the work of breathing and thereby reducing oxygen consumption.

PEEP is associated with potential adverse effects including increased risk of barotrauma, reduced oxygen delivery, and hypotension. Hypotension can usually be countered by increased fluid administration. The risk of barotrauma is reported to be 5% to 15% with positive pressure ventilation and is proportional to the levels of airway pressure and PEEP.[25] Reduced oxygen delivery occurs when the PEEP is high enough to reduce the cardiac output to a greater degree than the enhancement to PaO_2 conferred by the PEEP. Monitoring of oxygen delivery and oxygen consumption as illustrated in Figure 34-5 may be useful in detecting this phenomenon.[26]

When positive pressure ventilation is used to treat refractory hypoxemia, a decelerating inspiratory flow waveform should be used, if possible, as this has also

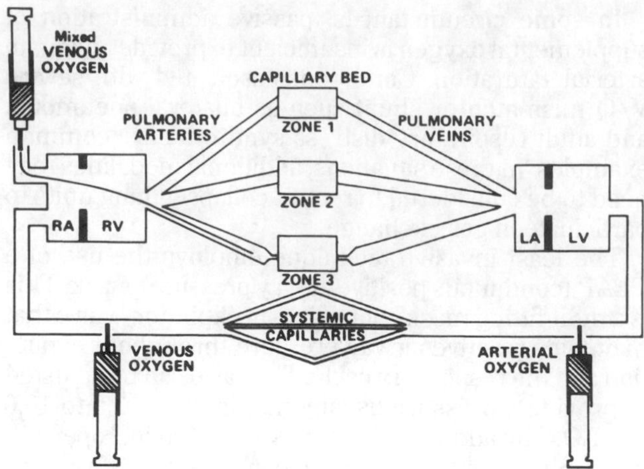

FIGURE 34-5. Tissue perfusion is dependent not only on arterial saturation but also on cardiac output. Although the application of PEEP may improve arterial saturation, a net negative effect on tissue perfusion can occur if the PEEP reduces cardiac output to a higher degree than the benefit achieved by improving arterial saturation. Tissue perfusion can be assessed by insertion of a pulmonary artery catheter which allows for the obtaining of mixed venous blood gases and the measurement of cardiac output. The degree of tissue oxygen extraction can be assessed by measuring the difference in arterial–mixed venous oxygen content. If this difference increases during the application of PEEP despite an improvement in arterial oxygenation, then tissue perfusion is being compromised. (Reprinted with permission from Bone RC: Treatment of severe hypoxemia due to the adult respiratory distress syndrome. Arch Intern Med 140:85, 1980.)

been shown to enhance oxygenation.[27,28] Classically, this waveform has been associated with pressure control ventilation; however, with newer microprocessor-controlled ventilators, this waveform can be provided by volume control modes as well.[28]

Additional mechanisms to improve oxygenation include alternative modes of mechanical ventilation, such as pressure control inverse ratio ventilation and high frequency ventilation. Inverse ratio ventilation has been shown to improve oxygenation.[29–32] The mechanisms for this include generation of intrinsic PEEP and prolongation of inspiratory time, which allows lung units with prolonged time constants to participate in gas exchange. Other supportive measures include reduction of metabolic demands and augmentation of O_2 delivery by increasing hemoglobin concentration or improving cardiac output. The use of ECMO (extracorporeal membrane oxygenation) has been studied extensively.[33] Although generally considered to be beneficial for patients requiring brief support, such as those with infantile respiratory distress syndrome, studies of adults with adult respiratory distress syndrome have shown no significant survival advantage over controls.

□ CONDITIONS ASSOCIATED WITH ACUTE HYPOXEMIC RESPIRATORY FAILURE

Pneumonia. In general, a patient with pneumonia involving more than one lobe places him or her at risk for developing acute hypoxemic respiratory failure. Acute infections with pyogenic bacteria, such as *Streptococcus pneumoniae, Haemophilus influenzae, Staphylococcus aureus*, and *Pseudomonas aeruginosa*, are most commonly associated with acute respiratory failure. On occasion, respiratory failure may be produced by viruses such as influenza A, influenza B, respiratory syncytial virus, adenovirus, herpes, parainfluenza virus, and varicella-zoster virus. Even *Mycobacterium tuberculosis* can on occasion produce respiratory failure with a clinical presentation similar to ARDS and is associated with a high mortality rate. In a recent study, the mortality rate for ARDS induced by *M. tuberculosis* was 69%. Not surprisingly, miliary dissemination was associated with many of the cases, but nearly half originated solely from tuberculous pneumonia.[34]

Respiratory failure associated with pneumonia produces either a pure Type I or combined Type I and Type II respiratory failure. Pure Type I failure may be corrected with passive supplemental oxygen; however, if the pneumonia is extensive, positive pressure ventilation with the addition of modest levels of PEEP (5 to 10 cmH_2O) may be necessary to improve oxygenation. Diagnosis requires the demonstration of a new or progressive infiltrate on chest radiograph in the presence of an elevated white blood cell count, fever, production of purulent sputum, and demonstration of a clinically significant pathogen in appropriate cultures.

Pulmonary Embolism. On an annual basis, as many as 500,000 cases of pulmonary artery embolism may occur. Of these, as many as 10% may be fatal.[12] It is also estimated that pulmonary embolisms may occur in as many as 8% to 27% of autopsy cases associated with acute respiratory failure.[35–38] Pulmonary artery embolism should be a strong consideration in the evaluation of acute hypoxemic respiratory failure. This is an important consideration not only because of the relatively high incidence and mortality, but also because of the difficulties in establishing the diagnosis.

Pulmonary artery embolism can be considered the end result of venous thromboembolism. Hospitalized patients often have impaired mobility or other conditions associated with venous stasis that promote the formation of deep vein thromboses in the lower extremities. With minor movement, thrombus fragments may spontaneously break free, follow the venous drainage to the right ventricle, and ultimately lodge in a pulmonary artery. The manifestations of pulmonary embolism are variable, but common symptoms include abrupt onset of dyspnea, pleuritic chest pain, and anxiousness. Tachypnea and tachycardia are typically present on physical examination. Lung fields are usually clear to auscultation; however, wheezing or a pleural rub may be present occasionally. Large pulmonary emboli can cause hypotension and severe hypoxemia, which may progress to circulatory collapse and death caused by acute right ventricular failure.

Pulmonary emboli alter gas exchange by changing regional ventilation/perfusion matching within the lung. The net effect is an overall reduction of oxygen transfer efficiency. Arterial blood gas analyses typically show a respiratory alkalosis and a variably reduced PaO_2. Widening of the alveolar-arterial partial pressure gradient of oxygen is a more sensitive finding for pulmonary embolism than is the presence of overt hypoxemia; however, neither is solely diagnostic.[39] Also, as many as 10% to 14% of those with documented pulmonary embolism may have normal alveolar-arterial partial pressure oxygen gradients.[40] Gas exchange may be further impaired by the development of atelectasis or bronchospasm that may accompany pulmonary embolism. Actual pulmonary infarction can occur with pulmonary emboli, causing pain and possible hemoptysis. This further complicates the clinical picture as aspirated blood further contributes to the elevated alveolar-arterial partial pressure oxygen gradient in pulmonary embolism.

The basic diagnostic workup of acute pulmonary embolism occurs in three phases. The initial phase consists of an estimation of the clinical index of suspicion. The likelihood is estimated to be high, intermediate, or low based on presenting symptoms, physical exam findings, chest radiograph, electrocardiogram, and arterial blood gas findings.[41,42]

The second phase involves noninvasive studies to evaluate for deep vein thrombosis and pulmonary embolism. The demonstration of a deep vein thrombosis by impedance plethysmography or Duplex ultrasonography generally obviates the need for further assessment as the treatment for deep vein thrombosis and pulmonary embolism is usually the same. However, a negative study does not exclude the possibility of pulmonary embolism because, occasionally, the entire thrombus may embolize. Also, the pelvic veins may be an additional source of thrombus that is not readily evaluated by noninvasive means.

A radioisotope ventilation/perfusion scan is the most useful screening test for the diagnosis of an acute pulmonary embolism. With this test, demonstration of perfusion defects in regions of normal ventilation is suggestive of an acute pulmonary embolism. The interpretation categories include normal, very low, low, intermediate, and high probability. High probability scans associated with a high clinical index of suspicion are very suggestive of acute pulmonary embolism. Normal, very low, or low probability scans associated with a low clinical index of suspicion makes acute pulmonary embolism extremely unlikely.

A pulmonary angiogram is the final phase in the diagnostic evaluation of pulmonary embolism. This test is considered the "gold standard" for the diagnosis; however, it is more invasive and therefore confers some additional risk. It is generally reserved for those patients who are hemodynamically unstable and need rapid diagnosis and intervention. Pulmonary angiograms are also helpful in situations where the clinical index of suspicion is high, yet the $\dot{V}/\dot{Q}$ scan is of intermediate probability and the lower extremity noninvasive studies are negative. A diagnostic algorithm demonstrating the incorporation of these three phases is illustrated in Figure 34-6.[43,44]

Treatment options for pulmonary embolism include anticoagulation; thrombolytic therapy; insertion of an inferior vena cava filter device; or, rarely, surgical removal. Unless the embolized thrombus is extremely large, passive supplemental oxygen is usually sufficient to correct hypoxemia associated with pulmonary embolism. If high flow oxygen fails to provide adequate oxygenation, positive pressure ventilation may be helpful by reducing oxygen consumption associated with work of breathing. High levels of positive end-expiratory pressure are unlikely to be helpful in improving oxygenation unless additional features such as atelectasis or pulmonary infarction are present.

Atelectasis. Atelectasis is a common problem in the intensive care unit. Regional hypoventilation caused by ineffective cough, lack of position changes, positive pressure ventilation, or surfactant loss (as in adult respiratory distress syndrome) may lead to collapse of regional alveolar units and produce microatelectasis. If a sufficiently sized region is involved, radiographic features such as a flat line or bandlike parenchymal infiltrate may be present. This is often referred to as *subsegmental atelectasis* or *discoid atelectasis.* Lobar atelectasis is usually caused by mucus obstruction of a bronchus or main stem bronchus; however, it may also be caused by extension of microatelectasis or foreign body obstruction. Lobar collapse presents with diminished breath sounds over the involved portion of the lung. The radiographic appearance is that of a parenchymal density with shift of mediastinal structures or the hemidiaphragm toward the atelectatic region to compensate for volume loss. Profound hypoxemia may result if the affected region is sufficiently large to produce right-to-left shunt.

Management of both microatelectasis and lobar atelectasis usually consists of chest physiotherapy and measures to improve pulmonary hygiene. This includes a periodic shift of body position, percussion and postural drainage, and vigorous endotracheal or nasotracheal suctioning. On occasion, fiberoptic bronchoscopy may be necessary to remove mucus plugs, particularly when located in the left lung.

Pulmonary Edema. Pulmonary edema refers to the accumulation of fluid within the interstitium and alveolar spaces. This produces ventilation/perfusion mismatch and tends to impair oxygenation more so than ventilation. If a significant percentage of alveolar sacs fill with edema fluid, right-to-left shunt and profound hypoxemia may occur. Pulmonary edema can be further categorized into cardiogenic and noncardiogenic causes. Cardiogenic causes such as acute congestive heart failure caused by myocardial infarction, myocardial ischemia, or iatrogenic fluid overload are important to recognize as they may be rapidly reversible with definitive therapies such as nitrates, diuretics, or inotropic support. Noncardiogenic causes tend to be less rapidly reversible, and if oxygenation cannot be maintained with passive supplemental oxygen, positive pressure ventilation is usually required.

Clinical features common to both cardiogenic and noncardiogenic pulmonary edema include hypoxemia, hypocapnia, and widening of the alveolar-arterial par-

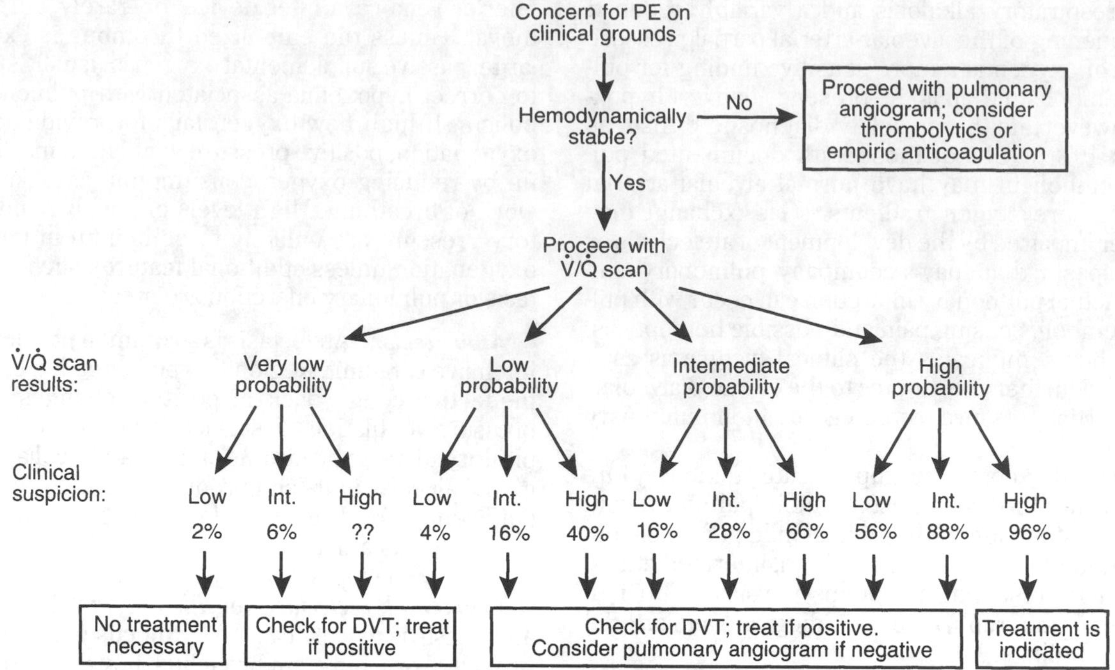

FIGURE 34-6. Diagnostic algorithm for the evaluation of suspected pulmonary embolism. Patients who are hemodynamically unstable should receive a pulmonary angiogram as the initial diagnostic test and be considered for thrombolytic therapy. The percentages listed below the clinical suspicion represent the likelihood of pulmonary embolism based on previously published probabilities from the PIOPED study. The "??" indicates the probability is unknown for this scenario as no patients fell into the category of a high clinical index of suspicion and a very low probability scan in the original PIOPED study. (Reprinted with permission from Van Hoozen BE, Van Hoozen CM, Albertson TE: Pulmonary considerations and complications in the neurosurgical patient. In Youmans JR (ed): Neurological Surgery, 4th ed. Philadelphia, W.B. Saunders, 1996, p 631. Modified from : Stein PD, Hull RD, Saltzman HA, et al.: Strategy for diagnosis of patients with suspected acute pulmonary embolism. Chest 103:1553–1559, 1993. PIOPED data from: PIOPED Investigators: Value of the ventilation/perfusion scan in acute pulmonary embolism: Results of the prospective investigation of pulmonary embolism diagnosis (PIOPED). JAMA 263:2753–2759, 1990.)

tial pressure gradient for oxygen. Tachypnea, dyspnea, and bilateral inspiratory crackles are commonly present, and wheezing may occasionally be noted. Chest radiographs of both types of pulmonary edema typically demonstrate diffuse bilateral infiltrates. The presence of an S_3 gallop, jugulovenous distension, and presence of lower extremity pitting edema may be helpful in diagnosing cardiogenic pulmonary edema. In the absence of these findings, a Swan-Ganz catheter can be inserted to distinguish cardiogenic from noncardiogenic pulmonary edema. Pulmonary artery occlusion pressures (pulmonary artery wedge pressures) higher than 18 cmH_2O are commonly associated with cardiogenic forms, whereas those 15 cmH_2O or less are typically associated with noncardiogenic forms. Unfortunately, these values are somewhat arbitrary, and because of this, pulmonary artery wedge pressures should not be used as the sole criterion for differentiation.[45,46]

Adult Respiratory Distress Syndrome. Adult respiratory distress syndrome (ARDS) is the prototypic condition that produces noncardiogenic pulmonary edema. Although the precise pathophysiology has not been completely established, certain predisposing conditions produce an acute inflammatory response that impairs the integrity of the alveolar-capillary membrane. These conditions include any form of shock from acute trauma, circulatory collapse, burns, sepsis, pancreatitis, gastric contents aspiration, pneumonia, transfusion reactions, or near drowning. The acute inflammatory response induces protein and fluid accumulation from the pulmonary vasculature into the pulmonary interstitium and alveolar spaces, resulting in bilateral pulmonary edema. Patchy atelectasis results from alveolar flooding and loss of surfactant. This produces hypoxemia secondary to intrapulmonary shunt and $\dot{V}/\dot{Q}$ mismatch.

In the early stages, endothelial and epithelial injury result in alveolar filling, surfactant deficiency, microatelectasis, and oxygenation impairment.[46,47] Arterial blood gas analyses typically demonstrate hypoxemia, hypocapnia, and widening of the alveolar-arterial partial pressure gradient for oxygen. Clinical findings include presence of acute respiratory distress, tachypnea, dyspnea, and use of accessory muscles of respiration. Reduced lung compliance associated with ARDS produces paradoxical respirations and sternal retraction during the initial phase of inspiration. The impaired lung compliance is also associated with an increased work of breathing, which generally necessitates support with positive pressure ventilation.

The late stages are associated with hyaline membrane formation and fibrosis. This leads to reduced lung compliance and predominant ventilation deficits such as increased dead space to tidal volume ratio and hypercapnia.[48]

Because many of the factors that predispose patients to ARDS are known, some steps can be taken to mitigate its development. These include rapid restoration of circulatory volume after shock, early recognition and treatment of infections, optimizing pulmonary hygiene, and insuring adequate nutrition after major injuries.[5] The risk of aspiration can be reduced by minimizing sedation, avoidance of the recumbent position, and monitoring gastric residuals with nasogastric tube feeding.

Once ARDS develops, therapeutic goals consist mainly of supporting gas exchange until the alveolar-capillary membranes are repaired, which may take up to 2 weeks. Due to the reduced pulmonary compliance, intubation and positive pressure ventilation are generally required to prevent respiratory muscle fatigue. Positive end-expiratory pressure has a significant role in the support of ARDS. By increasing functional residual capacity and redistribution of alveolar fluid, PEEP results in the recruitment of collapsed alveoli to participate in gas exchange. Because oxygen toxicity may result from prolonged administration of high FIO_2, the lowest PEEP that produces acceptable oxygenation on an FIO_2 of less than 0.5 to 0.6 should be employed. Alveolar recruitment demonstrates a threshold effect, which implies that little oxygenation improvement may be noted until the level of PEEP applied is sufficient to maintain unstable alveoli in an inflated position throughout the respiratory cycle. This is illustrated in Figure 34-7.[26] PEEP should be added in increments of 2 to 5 cmH_2O every 30 minutes until acceptable oxygenation is achieved. Arterial blood gas analyses or pulse oximetry should be monitored after each change to assess the response. Once alveolar recruitment is achieved, this level of PEEP should be maintained until sufficient resolution of the ARDS occurs, as premature discontinuation of PEEP may lead to collapse of unstable alveoli and a rapid decline in oxygenation.

Barotrauma is a significant concern in all patients with adult respiratory distress syndrome. The risk of barotrauma has been reported to be as high as 49% in patients with severe ARDS.[48] Not surprisingly, the risk is highest in the later stages when pulmonary compliance is lowest.[48] Barotrauma has largely been considered to be the result of damage inflicted by positive pressure ventilation. Experimental studies have demonstrated that alveolar-pleural pressure gradients of 35 to 45 cmH_2O or higher can produce lung injury.[49–52] More recently, animal studies have also demonstrated that ventilation with high tidal volumes can also induce lung injury, leading to *volutrauma*. In one such study, rats ventilated with large tidal volumes of 40 mL/kg showed a higher degree of permeability-type pulmonary edema than those ventilated at higher inspiratory pressures (45 cmH_2O) but lower tidal volumes.[53] In another animal study, low tidal volumes (5 to 6 mL/kg) were also associated with morphologic lung injury when the applied PEEP was less than the inflection point pressure.[54] In this study, pressure-volume curves were constructed, and the inflection point pressure (P_{inf}) was defined as the pressure at which there was a significant increase in the slope of the pressure-volume curve. There was a significant decrease in compliance and an increase in morphologic injury when the rat lungs were ventilated for 2 hours with a PEEP less than the P_{inf}, compared to controls and those ventilated with a PEEP above the P_{inf}. The results of this study are illustrated in Figure 34-8.[54] It is presumed that the opening and closing of smaller airways and alveolar ducts may produce shear stresses that contribute to lung injury.[54]

These studies show it is likely that multiple mechanisms that are somewhat interrelated can produce

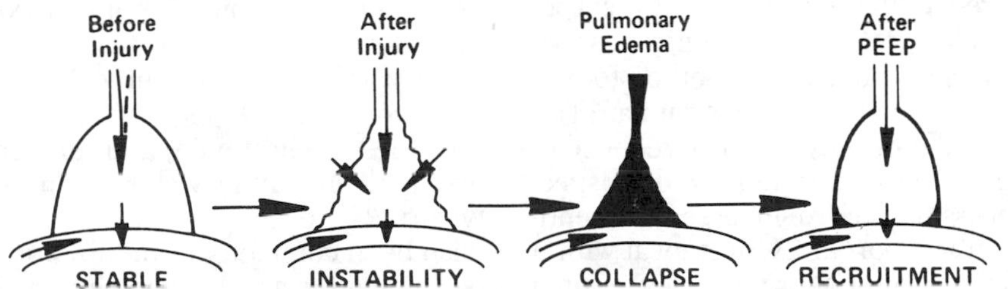

FIGURE 34-7. The mechanism why PEEP improves oxygenation in adult respiratory distress syndrome. An acute injury process promotes alveolar instability. Unstable alveoli tend to collapse and fill with pulmonary edema fluid resulting in intrapulmonary shunt. The application of positive end-expiratory pressure (PEEP) prevents the partial or complete collapse of unstable alveoli, allowing them to participate in gas exchange. (Reprinted with permission from Bone RC: Treatment of severe hypoxemia due to the adult respiratory distress syndrome. Arch Intern Med 140:85, 1980.)

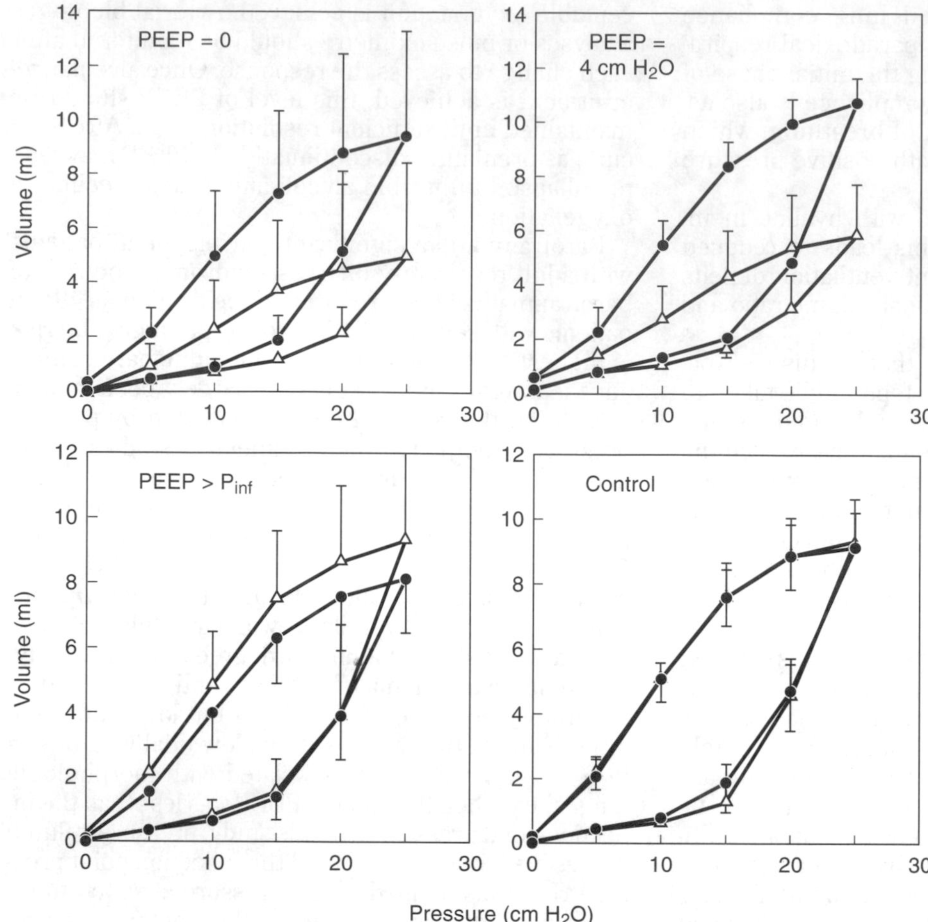

FIGURE 34-8. The demonstration of lung injury with mechanical ventilation in rats despite the use of low tidal volumes (5–6 mL/kg). Pressure-volume curves from excised lungs were constructed before (circles) and after two hours of ventilation (open triangles) at the PEEP levels noted. Controls were statically inflated for 2 hours at an airway pressure of 4 cm H_2O. The inflection point pressure (P_{inf}) was defined as the pressure at which there was a significant increase in the inflation slope of the pressure volume curve. A significant decrease in compliance (downward, rightward shift) was noted in rat lungs ventilated for 2 hours with PEEP = 0 and PEEP = 4 (PEEP < P_{inf}). However those ventilated at a PEEP > P_{inf} and controls demonstrated no change in pulmonary compliance. (Reprinted with permission from Muscedere JG, Mullen JBM, Gan K, Slutsky AS: Tidal ventilation at low airway pressures can augment lung injury. Am J Respir Crit Care Med 149:1327, 1994).

alveolar overdistension of compliant lung units. Therefore, measures to optimize PEEP, reduce peak airway pressures, and maintain lower tidal volumes are likely to reduce the risk of barotrauma associated with ARDS.

Additional therapeutic interventions that have been evaluated in ARDS include extracorporeal membrane oxygenation (ECMO) and extracorporeal CO_2 removal. The initial NIH-sponsored trial demonstrated no significant survival advantage for ECMO compared to conventional ventilatory support, with a mortality of 90% in each group.[33] More recently, venovenous extracorporeal CO_2 removal coupled with low frequency positive pressure ventilation was proposed as a method to promote lung rest and reduce the risk of barotrauma.[55] The initial findings suggested mortality could be reduced to nearly 50%. However, recently, a randomized prospective trial compared pressure control inverse ratio ventilation followed by extracorporeal CO_2 removal with a control group receiving protocol-driven conventional ventilation. The 30-day survival was not statistically significantly different between the groups; however, the overall survival was 38%, which was nearly four times the survival rate of the original ECMO trial.[56]

Fluid management has also recently been reevaluated in the treatment of ARDS. There are two treatment philosophies that have been debated over the past two decades.[57,58] In the first, because the pulmonary edema is caused by lung injury rather than transudation associated with fluid overload, it is unlikely that restriction of crystalloid therapy helps the situation. Therefore, the use of crystalloids is promoted to increase the pulmonary artery wedge pressure up to 15 cmH_2O to enhance perfusion and reduce the need for inotropic therapy. In the second philosophy, minimizing fluid therapy may reduce the extent of pulmonary edema and improve recovery time; therefore, fluids should be restricted to keep the pulmonary artery wedge pressure low, and inotropic therapy used to support blood pressure.

Two retrospective studies have demonstrated that survivors of ARDS experience less cumulative fluid intake, less weight gain, and no significant increases in extravascular lung water when compared to nonsurvivors.[59,60] Recently, a randomized, prospective trial has also been completed.[61] In this study, a regimen emphasizing fluid restriction and diuretic therapy to reduce extravascular lung water was compared with conventional supportive therapy. The investigators found a significant reduction in days on mechanical ventilation and a trend toward reduced mortality when measures to reduce extravascular lung water were employed.[57,61] Because vasopressor therapy is not without adverse effects, the patients selected to receive this therapy should have relatively low risk for myocardial ischemia or malignant dysrhythmias.

Because surfactant dysfunction has been reported in ARDS, another potential treatment is to augment the depleted native surfactant with aerosolized synthetic surfactant. This strategy has been very successful in the treatment of neonatal respiratory distress syndrome.[62] Recently, a multicentered, randomized, placebo-controlled study was completed evaluating the efficacy of synthetic surfactant (Exosurf) in sepsis-induced ARDS.[63] The surfactant was administered by means of continuous nebulizer for 5 days. A trend toward a dose-dependent reduction in mortality was observed but did not reach statistical significance.[63] Adjustments in the dose or delivery system may be necessary before efficacy can be established.

Acute Hypercapnic Respiratory Failure

In most situations associated with clinically significant hypercapnia and respiratory acidosis, few options exist short of intubation and mechanical ventilation. However, two conditions in the differential diagnosis of Type II respiratory failure exist that may be readily reversible and, therefore, should be excluded rapidly in the clinical assessment. The first is to assess for impaired central respiratory drive associated with sedative or narcotic therapy. The second is to evaluate for underlying bronchospasm secondary to exacerbations of asthma or chronic obstructive pulmonary disease. The former may be treated with reversal agents such as the opiate antagonist naloxone, whereas the latter may respond to inhaled bronchodilators and systemic corticosteroids.

Additional modalities that are less invasive than mechanical ventilation include intermittent positive pressure ventilation by means of face mask, nasal CPAP, and biphasic positive airway pressure (BiPAP). Nasal CPAP is most useful for the chronic treatment of obstructive sleep apnea. Nasal BiPAP is useful for the prolonged treatment of both central sleep apnea and some cases of obstructive sleep apnea refractory to nasal CPAP alone. Intermittent positive pressure ventilation by means of face mask or mouthpiece essentially provides positive pressure mechanical ventilation without an endotracheal tube. This has limited applications and is predominantly reserved for patients with slowly progressive hypercapnia, usually caused by COPD; kyphoscoliosis; or muscular dystrophy. Although published reports exist outlining the utility of noninvasive positive pressure ventilation for treatment of acute hypercapnia associated with COPD exacerbations, the study-group sizes have been relatively small.[64–66] Therefore, the use of this modality for treatment of acute respiratory failure should be limited to those patients who do not wish to be intubated. Some patients with chronic hypercapnia can be maintained with nocturnal ventilatory support only. In these situations, home ventilation with devices such as a cuirass, nasal intermittent positive pressure ventilation, or nasal BiPAP have been employed.[67–69]

☐ IMPAIRED CENTRAL RESPIRATORY DRIVE

Inadequate central drive for respiration is a concern in patients who exhibit hypercapnia associated with depressed mentation, slow respiratory rates, and lack of overt respiratory distress. A history of any recent sedative or narcotic use should be sought if readily available. If not, an empiric trial of reversal agents can be considered. Narcotics such as morphine can be reversed with intravenous naloxone (Narcan). The usual dose is 0.4 to 2.0 mg as an intravenous bolus. Because many opiates have longer half-lives than naloxone, repeated doses or a continuous infusion may be necessary, with the dosage titrated to effect. A benzodiazepine antagonist, flumazenil, is now widely available. The recommended dosage is 0.2 mg intravenously over 15 seconds with repeated administrations of 0.1 to 0.2 mg every 60 seconds up to a total of 1 mg. However, flumazenil has some adverse effects that should be taken into consideration before administration. Flumazenil may produce seizures in patients with an underlying seizure disorder and may result in acute benzodiazepine withdrawal in patients with a long-standing history of benzodiazepine use. Barbiturates and severe alcohol intoxication may also produce respiratory failure; however, no reversal agents are currently available for treatment. Therefore, pulmonary function may need to be supported with mechanical ventilation in these circumstances.

Certain structural central nervous system conditions may also produce respiratory failure secondary to impaired respiratory drive. These include cerebral vascular accidents, intracranial hemorrhages, central nervous system malignancies, and traumatic head injuries. A neurologic exam is helpful in distinguishing structural lesions from sedative overdose, as most structural lesions present with focal neurologic findings including cranial nerve palsy or asymmetric extremity weakness. If structural central nervous system damage is suspected, immediate diagnostic and therapeutic intervention is usually required. In the presence of impending respiratory failure, such patients should be immediately intubated and supported with mechanical ventilation. Emergent diagnostic studies including CT or MRI scans are also warranted. Because cerebral edema may be present, empiric hyperventilation to reduce intracranial pressure should be considered. The usual target is to reduce the $PaCO_2$ to about 25 mmHg with a resultant pH in the 7.5 range.

☐ NEUROMUSCULAR WEAKNESS

Certain neurologic conditions are known to impair respiratory muscle function that may result in hypercapnic respiratory insufficiency. These diseases include Guillain-Barré syndrome, myasthenia gravis, and Eaton-Lambert syndrome, which produce weakness by compromising neuromuscular transmission. Afflicted individuals usually have limb weakness or paralysis before the development of respiratory muscle involvement. Patients generally exhibit tachypnea and dyspnea before the onset of respiratory failure. However, the onset of clinically significant respiratory acidosis may abruptly develop once respiratory muscle fatigue occurs. Thus, health care workers need to remain vigilant in following pulmonary function trends once respiratory symptoms become manifest. Serial measurements of vital capacity (VC), maximal voluntary ventilation (MVV), as well as maximal inspiratory and expiratory pressure (MIP and MEP) are helpful in predicting respiratory failure. In general, when MVV, VC, MIP and MEP become reduced to 30% to 40% of predicted values, mechanical ventilatory support should be considered.[70–73] Although absolute criteria such as a $P_I$max less than 20 to 30 cmH_2O and a VC less than 1000 mL or 10 mL/kg have been suggested,[5,16–18] a trend of deterioration approaching the above values may be more helpful so that intubation can be accomplished before the onset of overt hypercapnia. Rapid sequence intubation can be complicated by hemodynamic instability in Guillain-Barré syndrome if the autonomic nervous system is also affected. Succinylcholine should also be avoided as it may produce lethal hyperkalemia in patients with Guillain-Barré syndrome.[16]

Other pulmonary consequences of neuromuscular weakness include recurrent pneumonias caused by aspiration and impaired cough and gag reflexes. Atelectasis secondary to mucus plugging also occurs frequently in this setting. Early tracheostomy should be considered in those afflicted with respiratory failure, particularly for Guillain-Barré syndrome, as prolonged weaning trials may be necessary. Plasmapheresis may be helpful for Guillain-Barré syndrome and myasthenia gravis. Evaluation for an underlying malignancy is usually warranted for myasthenia gravis and Eaton-Lambert syndrome.

Botulism and organophosphate poisoning are two additional conditions that may rapidly produce neuromuscular weakness and respiratory failure. They are important to recognize, as prompt treatment intervention may limit the extent or duration of the clinical manifestations. Botulism is caused by a neurotoxin released from *Clostridium botulinum.* This can be ingested from contaminated foods or released in wounds. Organophosphates, nerve gases, and insecticides such as parathion and malathion can produce muscle fasciculation and paralysis. Botulism prevents acetylcholine release from neuromuscular junctions, whereas organophosphate poisoning prevents the breakdown of acetylcholine. Both produce nausea, vomiting, diarrhea, and generalized weakness that may progress to hypercapnic respiratory failure. Organophosphate poisoning may also produce parasympathomimetic effects, confusion, decreased mentation, and seizures. Additional neurologic findings, nerve conduction studies, electromyography, and muscle biopsies are helpful in differentiating the causes of neuromuscular weakness. Progressive dyspnea, tachypnea, and a reduction in vital capacity herald the onset of respiratory failure. Mechanical ventilatory support should be considered before the onset of overt hypercapnia. Additional therapy for botulism includes antitoxin administration; however, if it is not given before the onset of respiratory failure, prolonged ventilatory support may be necessary. The treatment for organophosphate poisoning includes atropine and pralidoxime (2-PAM).

Amyotrophic lateral sclerosis and muscular dystrophy are conditions that produce a slowly progressive deterioration in muscle strength. Extremity weakness generally occurs before the onset of respiratory muscle involvement.[74] Progressive decline in function may occur over several years. Reduced exercise tolerance is a common early manifestation of respiratory muscle impairment. Serial pulmonary function studies are also helpful in assessing respiratory muscle strength. $P_I$max and $P_E$max are more sensitive than VC in the detection of respiratory muscle weakness.[75,76] Unfortunately, treatment options are extremely limited for both conditions, and most afflicted persons ultimately succumb to respiratory complications.

□ CHEST WALL DEFORMITIES

Kyphoscoliosis is an abnormal curvature of the spine that, in its most severe manifestation, impairs chest wall expansion, producing restrictive pulmonary physiology. Kyphoscoliosis can be congenital, idiopathic, or acquired as a complication of other neuromuscular conditions such as poliomyelitis, muscular dystrophy, and cerebral palsy. Patients with progressive kyphoscoliosis develop a gradual decline in pulmonary function over several years. Hypercapnia does not usually develop due to compensatory hyperventilation except as a manifestation of acute or chronic respiratory failure. Surgical correction is possible in some circumstances; however, postoperative pulmonary complications are common and include difficulty weaning from mechanical ventilation, pneumonia, and atelectasis.

Pectus excavatum is a congenital defect causing the sternum to be depressed inward. Most patients have little to no respiratory symptomatology; however, a small percentage may have a reduced vital capacity, total lung capacity, and diminished exercise tolerance.[77] Although respiratory failure would be an unusual consequence of this condition alone, it may contribute to pulmonary complications in the postoperative setting.

Massive obesity can be associated with hypercapnia and marginal PaO_2s as part of the obesity-hypoventilation syndrome or Pickwickian syndrome. The body mass index typically has to be elevated beyond 60 kg/m^2 before pulmonary function is significantly compromised.[78] The mechanism involved is not well understood; however, the obesity may be thought of as reducing the thoracic compliance, producing a substantial increase in the work of breathing. Over time, central chemoreceptors may adapt to a higher threshold of $PaCO_2$ in an effort to reduce the work of breathing. In support of this, studies have found a nearly threefold reduction in the ventilatory response to inhaled carbon dioxide in massive obesity compared to normal controls.[79,80] Although the PaO_2 may be reduced, the alveolar-arterial partial pressure gradient for oxygen is usually normal. In some patients, it may be reduced as a result of $\dot{V}/\dot{Q}$ mismatch associated with relative hypoventilation of the lung bases and atelectasis. Obesity-hypoventilation syndrome can be associated with obstructive sleep apnea and may be complicated by the development of cor pulmonale. These patients can present to emergency departments in a decompensated state. Mechanical ventilation should not be instituted solely for hypercapnia unless also accompanied by a clinically significant respiratory acidosis. If mechanical ventilation is initiated, hyperventilation to normalize the $PaCO_2$ should be avoided. Weight loss of 35 kg or more has been shown to increase VC from 53% to 84% of the predicted value and reduce $PaCO_2$ by 15 mmHg.[81,82]

Flail chest refers to a segment of the rib cage that exhibits paradoxical motion compared to the rest of the rib cage during respiration. Flail chest develops when three or more sequential ribs are fractured in two places, surgically removed, or associated with a sternal fracture. Deceleration injuries sustained from motor vehicle accidents or falls are the most common causes of flail chest. The flail segment reduces the efficiency of respiration and can result in hypercapnia, hypoxemia, or both. Associated pulmonary complications include pulmonary contusion, pneumothorax, hemothorax, atelectasis, and pneumonia. Mechanical ventilatory support is often required for 3 or more weeks until sufficient healing or stabilization has occurred. Therefore, early placement of a tracheostomy should be considered.

□ OBSTRUCTIVE LUNG DISEASE

Chronic obstructive pulmonary disease (COPD) is a term used for disorders involving obstructive airway disease, usually caused by a combination of chronic bronchitis and emphysema. Some patients also have concomitant asthma. The predominant physiologic feature is flow limitation (obstruction) during the expiratory phase. Although asthma is usually considered a reversible obstructive condition, patients with longstanding asthma often have a component of chronic or irreversible obstruction. A detailed discussion of these processes can be found in Chapter 28.

Clinical manifestations common to the above diseases include episodic exacerbations of wheezing, cough, dyspnea, and sputum production. Exacerbations can be induced by inhalation of allergens; by nonspecific irritants such as smoke, fumes, and dust; or in response to lower respiratory tract infections. Wheezing is typically present during the expiratory phase; however, in moderate or severe exacerbations, wheezing may be noted in both inspiratory and expiratory phases. In extreme episodes, the bronchospasm may be so intense that breath sounds and wheezing may be absent due to severely diminished airflow rates. Although wheezing is usually associated with obstructive lung disease, it is important to recognize that other conditions such as pulmonary embolism, congestive heart failure, endobronchial tumor obstruction, stridor, anaphylactic reactions, pneumonia, pneumothorax, and aspirated foreign bodies may also produce wheezing.

Expiratory airflow limitation should theoretically lead to hypercapnia and a predominantly Type II respiratory failure pattern. However, obstructive lung disease usually exhibits findings consistent with a mixed Type I and Type II pattern. In the case of chronic obstructive bronchitis and emphysema, a variable amount of hypoxemia may be present due to mucus plugging and $\dot{V}/\dot{Q}$ mismatch associated with a reduction of gas exchange surface area. Exacerbations complicated by pneumonia and bronchitis may also contribute to $\dot{V}/\dot{Q}$ mismatch.

Asthma exacerbations classically demonstrate three phases of arterial blood gas findings. In the early phase, mild airflow limitation is compensated by increasing minute ventilation with rapid, shallow breathing. This results in a respiratory alkalosis with a $pH > 7.4$, $PaCO_2 < 40$, and a normal PaO_2. In the second phase, airflow obstruction becomes more severe and can no longer be compensated by further increases in minute ventilation, yielding a normalized arterial pH and $PaCO_2$. The PaO_2 at this phase may be somewhat reduced. During the third phase, the bronchospasm severely reduces minute ventilation to the point that respiratory acidosis develops, as heralded by a fall in arterial pH to less than 7.35 and an increase in $PaCO_2$ above 45 mmHg. Both the second and third phase signal a need for aggressive β agonist therapy and the need for close observation. Patients who present to emergency departments in the second phase are important to recognize, as their arterial blood gas findings are deceptively near normal and may lull medical personnel into a false sense of security. Unlike asthmatics in the first phase with relatively minor symptomatology, asthmatics in the second phase usually appear uncomfortable, with labored breathing and extensive wheezing, and speak in two- or three-word sentences.

The severity of obstruction and response to therapy can be assessed by measuring expiratory peak flow or FEV_1.[83] In one study, the mean peak expiratory flow (PEF) was 73 L/min in asthmatics who required an upright posture and were diaphoretic, 134 L/min in those sitting upright but not diaphoretic, and 225 L/min in those who were able to breathe while lying supine.[84] In another study, hypercapnia was not usually observed until the PEF was reduced to less than 25% of the predicted value.[85]

Therapeutic options for obstructive lung diseases include β-adrenergic agents, ipratropium bromide, theophylline derivatives, and corticosteroids. Although patients with emphysema tend to have fixed obstruction, many with acute exacerbations tend to also have a component of reversible obstruction that may respond to bronchodilator and corticosteroid therapy.[86]

The cornerstone of immediate therapy for obstructive lung diseases is inhaled β-adrenergic agonists. Inhaled β agonists have been shown to have similar efficacy to parenteral administration but with less systemic side effects.[83,87–89] Therefore, the parenteral route should be reserved for those patients who fail to respond adequately to inhaled β agonists. Parenteral β agonists should also be used cautiously in patients over age 40, as they may induce myocardial ischemia or malignant cardiac arrhythmias if significant coronary artery disease is present.

Ipratropium bromide is an inhaled anticholinergic agent that has fewer systemic side effects than atropine. Ipratropium bromide has been shown to have bronchodilatory properties comparable to β agonists in the treatment of COPD, but it is somewhat less effective than β agonists in the treatment of acute asthma.[90] Ipratropium bromide has also been shown to have an additive bronchodilator effect when used in combination with β agonists.[90–92] This is particularly evident in patients with asthma; however, when high doses (10 mg) of albuterol were used, no synergistic effect could be demonstrated in COPD.[83,90,92]

Theophylline derivatives were at one time considered first-line therapy for obstructive lung diseases; however, β agonists have demonstrated superior bronchodilatory effects.[93] Theophylline derivatives have been shown to improve diaphragmatic contractility[94] and may therefore still be a useful adjunct for patients who fail to respond adequately to β agonist and anticholinergic therapy.[83]

Corticosteroid therapy is a necessary component of therapy for all patients with moderate or severe exacerbations. This is particularly true for acute asthma; however, a significant portion of those with COPD also respond favorably.[95] Steroid therapy has been shown to reduce inflammatory cell recruitment, decrease mucus production, and up-regulate β_2 receptors.[83,96] These effects unfortunately require a minimum of 6 to 12 hours to take effect; therefore, corticosteroids should be administered early in the therapeutic intervention of acute exacerbations.[83] The optimal dose remains somewhat controversial; however, a common practice involves 40 to 125 mg of methylprednisolone, or the biological equivalent of another steroid, administered intravenously every 6 to 8 hours for 2 to 3 days followed by a tapering schedule.

An assessment for hypoxemia should be sought and, if present, corrected with supplemental oxygen. If clinical findings or radiographic features suggestive of a lower respiratory tract infection are present, intravenous antibiotics are indicated. The routine use of antibiotics in acute asthma without such findings is generally not recommended. Additional adjunctive therapy for acute asthma such as parenteral magnesium[97] and inhaled helium and oxygen mixtures[98] may be beneficial in select cases, but routine use of these modalities cannot be supported at this time without larger efficacy studies.

Inhalational general anesthetic agents such as halothane and enflurane have substantial bronchodilatory properties that can be used to treat status asthmaticus.[99–101] Unfortunately, these agents may promote hemodynamic instability, and the bronchospasm may return upon discontinuation of treatment. For these reasons, the use of agents such as halothane and enflurane are generally reserved for those patients who develop clinically significant barotrauma with mechanical ventilation.[83]

The decision to intubate and initiate mechanical ventilation in the setting of acute exacerbations of obstructive lung disease is one of the more difficult challenges facing respiratory practitioners. This decision must be made at the bedside rather than based on arbitrary arterial blood gas values. Clearly, most patients who demonstrate altered mental status in the presence of progressive respiratory failure should be immediately intubated. For those patients who are cognitively intact but in respiratory distress, a trial of aggressive bronchodilator therapy can be attempted first, even in the presence of mild respiratory acidosis. The β agonist albuterol can be administered at a dose of 6 to 12 puffs per metered-dose inhaler (MDI) or 2.5 mg by means of a nebulizer every 20 minutes and titrated until a favorable response is noted or systemic side effects develop. Likewise, ipratropium bromide at 6 to 10 puffs per MDI or 500 µg (0.02% solution) by means of a nebulizer can be administered every 20 minutes and then titrated to effect for combination therapy with a β agonist. Patients with respiratory distress should be observed continuously and monitored with pulse oximetry during treatment of the acute exacerbation. Patients who do not appear to be clinically improving with therapy should be reassessed by peak flow and arterial blood gas analysis. Those who demonstrate progressive lethargy, respiratory muscle fatigue, a deterioration in peak flow, or progressive hypercapnia despite treatment should be considered for semielective intubation before the onset of overt respiratory failure.

Mechanical ventilation for status asthmaticus and COPD is fraught with multiple adverse effects that can be minimized if they are anticipated. Airflow obstruction leads to hyperinflation and gas trapping. When mechanical ventilation is instituted in this setting, the risk of contributing further to gas entrapment and subsequent complications is high. This process is referred to as *dynamic hyperinflation*.[83] Ventilation with smaller tidal volumes (8 to 10 mL/kg) and low respiratory rates (8 to 12 breaths/min) allows for the longer expiratory times necessary to prevent further increases in intrinsic PEEP. Patients with COPD generally have relatively normal minute ventilation requirements and can usually tolerate these lower ventilator settings. However, patients with status asthmaticus often have substantially higher minute ventilation requirements and may attempt to "over breathe" the ventilator, leading to patient-ventilator asynchrony and increased dynamic hyperinflation. In this setting, heavy sedation and neuromuscular blockade is usually necessary. This process of deliberate hypoventilation has been gaining favor over the past several years and is referred to as *permissive hypercapnia* or *controlled hypoventilation*. The basic premise behind permissive hypercapnia is that the risks of morbidity associated with barotrauma are higher than that of controlled mild hypercapnia. A certain amount of respiratory acidosis can be tolerated in a sedated patient, and a continuous infusion of bicarbonate can be transiently employed to prevent a drop in arterial pH to clinically significant levels.

Optimal ventilator parameter guidelines for permissive hypercapnia are not yet available. In an early study, the peak inspiratory pressure was kept below 50 cmH_2O, and tidal volumes of 8 to 12 mL/kg and rates of 8 to 10 breaths/min were employed.[102] However, in status asthmaticus, the peak inspiratory pressure does not correlate well with the risk of barotrauma.[103] This is caused by the high gradient between airway pressure and alveolar pressure associated with elevated airway resistance. Once mechanical ventilation is instituted, several ventilator parameters need to be measured and monitored closely throughout the course of therapy. These include the level of intrinsic PEEP, plateau pressure (P_{plat}), and peak inspiratory pressure (PIP). Intrinsic PEEP can be measured by performing an expiratory hold (end-expiratory port occlusion) maneuver as illustrated in Figure 34-9.[104] If significant intrinsic PEEP is present, additional measures such as aggressive bronchodilator therapy, increasing inspiratory flow rate, and further reductions in respiratory rate or tidal volume may be necessary. Unfortunately, intrinsic PEEP only reflects a portion of the

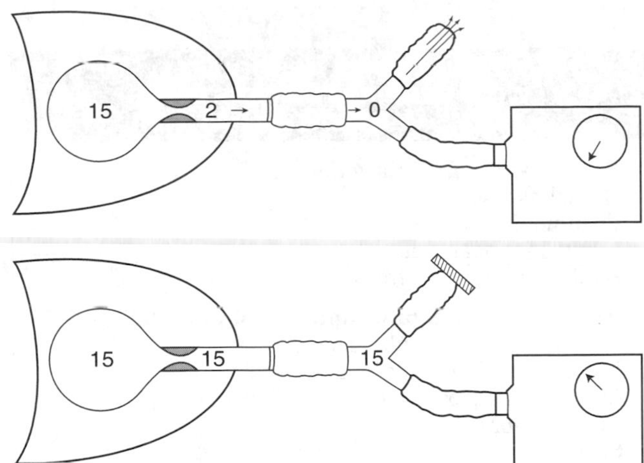

FIGURE 34-9. The method of detecting intrinsic PEEP (auto-PEEP) in ventilated patients with airflow obstruction. A pressure gradient exists from partially obstructed alveoli through narrowed airways back to the ventilator circuit. During the normal operation of the ventilator, the pressure in the partially obstructed alveoli cannot be detected due to its delayed emptying. However, by performing an end-expiratory hold maneuver (bottom panel), the expiratory port is occluded at end-expiration, allowing time for pressure equilibration from the partially occluded alveoli into the respiratory circuit. This pressure can then be measured by the ventilator. (Reprinted with permission from Marini JJ: The role of the inspiratory circuit in the work of breathing during mechanical ventilation. Respir Care 32:419–430, 1987.)

dynamic hyperinflation. In status asthmaticus, a significant number of smaller airways may be occluded with mucus and cellular debris. This may serve as a one-way valve allowing gas to enter during inspiration but occluding its passage during exhalation. This results in trapping of gas that does not communicate with central airways and therefore is not measured as intrinsic PEEP. Serial measurements of the ventilator plateau pressure (P_{plat}) may be useful in detecting this process.[83]

Dynamic hyperinflation and barotrauma still remain important concerns in the ventilator management of COPD. However, except to treat status asthmaticus, permissive hypercapnia is rarely necessary. Pulmonary compliance in COPD is increased due to the reduction in elastic recoil that accompanies emphysema. Therefore, a higher portion of the peak inspiratory pressure is transmitted to the alveoli, which can increase the risk of barotrauma. Thus, peak inspiratory pressures and intrinsic PEEP levels need to be monitored closely. Ventilator settings should be adjusted so that peak inspiratory pressures are not higher than 30 to 40 cmH_2O. Higher inspiratory flow rates, reduced tidal volumes, and slower respiratory rates are helpful in reducing the risk of dynamic hyperinflation, as is the case for asthma.

In general, synchronized intermittent mandatory ventilation (SIMV) and assist/control ventilation (A/C) modes are well tolerated by patients with COPD. If, however, a significant elevation of intrinsic PEEP is noted while the patient is on A-C mode, switching to SIMV and permitting some spontaneous breaths may reduce this somewhat.[86] Pressure support can be added to SIMV if the work of breathing appears excessive.

Unintentional hyperventilation is also a concern when treating COPD. Because many patients may be chronic CO_2 retainers at baseline, the goal of mechanical ventilation should be to achieve a $PaCO_2$ near the previous baseline rather than a value of 40 mmHg. Prior arterial blood gas analyses are helpful in this regard, but if they are unavailable, the initial serum bicarbonate level may provide a reasonable estimate. The baseline $PaCO_2$ can be estimated using the following formula:[105]

$$\text{Baseline } PaCO_2 \text{ in mmHg} = 1.5 \times [HCO_3^-] + 8 \pm 2$$

If unrecognized, unintentional hyperventilation results in renal excretion of the additional bicarbonate that was compensating for the chronic respiratory acidosis. Subsequent weaning attempts may result in acute respiratory acidosis, which will likely result in weaning failure. Once unintentional hyperventilation occurs, ventilatory support must be slowly reduced over several days to allow for appropriate renal compensation.

Combined Hypoxemic and Hypercapnic Respiratory Failure

The fundamentals of treatment for combined Type I and Type II respiratory failure are similar to those already described in the individual sections. The most common causes of combined Type I and Type II respiratory failure include an acute process (eg, pneumonia, CHF) superimposed on chronic lung disease such as COPD or interstitial lung disease. The initial challenge is to determine the primary underlying process for the acute decompensation. Hypoxemia should be corrected with supplemental oxygen, if possible, while therapy is instituted for any immediately reversible causes.

Oftentimes, respiratory practitioners are reluctant to initiate ventilator therapy for fear of not being able to wean the patient off it later. Clearly, in the setting of chronic lung disease, one should attempt to determine if an advanced directive is available. Those patients who do not wish to be intubated may be candidates for noninvasive ventilation techniques as a bridge of support until the acute respiratory failure component is reversed. If no prior advanced directive has been stated, aggressive therapy is usually instituted. This is because it is often difficult to secure a "do not resuscitate" statement in the presence of overt respiratory distress or air hunger. In studies evaluating patients with COPD and acute respiratory failure, survival of the acute episode is reasonably good.[106,107] This may be another reason to consider aggressive support in this patient population. Also, institutions that specialize in weaning difficult patients are available and may facilitate the weaning process if it cannot be accomplished at an acute care facility.

During the past decade, there has been a movement to consider the withdrawal of ventilatory support to being ethically equivalent to that of withholding ventilator support altogether. The decision to withdraw advanced life support is a difficult process. This clearly needs to be discussed among health care providers and discussed openly with the patient (if he or she is able to participate in the discussion) as well as family members. It is important to emphasize to family members that decisions need to be based on what the patient would want done in a particular situation, rather than on what the family members would want. Time-limited goals may be helpful in the decision process. For example, if a patient with end-stage COPD requires mechanical ventilation for an acute pneumonia, it may be reasonable to provide ventilatory support throughout the expected course of antibiotic therapy (1 to 2 weeks). The patient (or family advocates) are then counseled that if ventilatory support cannot successfully be discontinued after this period of time, further support beyond this time point is likely to be futile. Several reviews of this complex topic are available.[108–113]

BOX 34-3

CONDITIONS ASSOCIATED WITH RESPIRATORY DISTRESS IN THE VENTILATED PATIENT

Progression of primary disease
Bronchospasm
Pneumonia
Congestive heart failure
Adult respiratory distress syndrome

New condition complicating respiratory failure
Any of the above conditions
Mucus plugging or atelectasis
Intrinsic PEEP or dynamic hyperinflation
Pneumothorax
Sepsis
Pain or agitation

Ventilator or equipment failure
Endotracheal tube malposition
Endotracheal tube occlusion
Cuff leak
Ventilator disconnect
Ventilator circuit tube leak
Ventilator malfunction—usually human error

Inappropriate ventilator settings
Inadequate sensitivity
Reduced inspiratory flow rate
Inadequate minute ventilation
Patient-ventilator asynchrony

ACUTE DISTRESS ASSOCIATED WITH MECHANICAL VENTILATION

The sudden onset of hypoxemia or respiratory distress in patients on mechanical ventilation represents a diagnostic challenge that requires immediate assessment and, frequently, rapid intervention. The differential diagnosis is quite broad but can be broken down into the following major categories: (1) progression of the primary disease process, (2) development of a new disorder further complicating gas exchange or mechanical ventilation, (3) ventilator or associated equipment failure, (4) entry of inappropriate ventilator settings. A detailed listing is provided in Box 34-3.

Frequently, the initial reaction to the development of patient agitation or hypoxemia is to assume that the patient is "fighting the ventilator" and that additional sedation and neuromuscular blockade are indicated. However, this is only one of many potential causes. The assessment must be performed at the bedside, as many potential causes can be rapidly diagnosed with a few simple techniques. A problem-oriented approach is useful for discussion of these conditions because respiratory practitioners are often asked to evaluate a patient's status based on clinical manifestations.

Hypotension

The abrupt onset of hypotension and agitation in a mechanically ventilated patient can be a manifestation of a life-threatening complication. The possible causes include tension pneumothorax, massive pulmonary embolism, development of intrinsic PEEP, and septic shock. Tension pneumothorax and pulmonary embolism are usually accompanied by arterial hypoxemia or cyanosis. Hypotension associated with septic shock usually occurs more gradually over several hours. The evaluation for tension pneumothorax is the highest priority, as failure to intervene can rapidly lead to circulatory collapse and death. One generally has insufficient time to obtain a confirmatory chest radiograph, and the diagnosis must be made at the bedside. Clinical manifestations of tension pneumothorax include unilateral diminished breath sounds, unilateral increased resonance to percussion, and tracheal deviation to the contralateral side, and occasionally subcutaneous emphysema may be present.

If a tension pneumothorax is suspected on clinical exam, an 18-gauge intravenous catheter should be placed into the anterior second intercostal space at the midclavicular line. When placed correctly, a rush of air should be noted to exit from the catheter, and the chest wall can be seen to decrease in size as the pressure is equalized. If a rush of air is not noted, another catheter should be placed on the contralateral side. Once an intravenous catheter has been placed into the chest, it should be left in place until tube thoracostomy can be performed. This is because puncture of the lung may occur with catheter placement, which can progress to a pneumothorax even if one was not present initially. If hypotension and hypoxemia still persist despite catheter or tube thoracostomy, a semierect portable chest radiograph should be obtained to evaluate for an unevacuated pneumothorax. Acute massive pulmonary embolism should then be considered if the chest radiograph fails to demonstrate a pneumothorax or other significant finding to explain the hypotension.

Hypotension without overt hypoxemia is suggestive of the development of dynamic hyperinflation and intrinsic PEEP. Excessive intrinsic PEEP can be rapidly diagnosed by performing an expiratory hold maneuver. If present, adjustment of ventilator settings to lengthen expiratory time often results in prompt resolution of the hypotension. Tension pneumothorax should still be considered in the differential, and clinical manifestations to suggest this possibility should be sought.

Apparent Ventilator Malfunction

Another group of conditions that can be readily assessed at the bedside include ventilator or associated hardware failure. When approaching the patient, one should quickly survey the endotracheal tube, ventilator tubing, and note any ventilator alarms or warnings.[114] A harsh tone is emitted from most types of ventilators when ventilator tubing or endotracheal tube disconnection occur. This typically occurs at the Y piece, which is readily visible. Occult air leaks can occur at other locations, which include the humidifier system, incompetent exhalation valve, or leaks in the tubing itself.[114] Ventilator circuit leaks often result in "low exhaled tidal volume" or "low inspiratory pressure" warnings, and the ventilator may fail to cycle out of the inspiratory phase.

If the cause of an apparent malfunction cannot be rapidly identified or there is concern that the patient is not receiving adequate ventilation, the ventilator should be immediately disconnected, and the patient should be ventilated by means of a mask-valve-bag device with 100% oxygen.[114] If respiratory distress, agitation, or hypoxemia promptly resolve, the problem may be caused by malfunction of the ventilator, the respiratory circuit, or the use of inappropriate ventilator settings. Bag ventilating the patient is also useful in that one can determine if the development of excessive pulmonary secretions or compliance changes have occurred.

Air leakage to the mouth is suggestive of endotracheal tube malposition or endotracheal cuff leak. The depth of the endotracheal tube is measured at the upper central incisor or equivalent gum line. With the head in a neutral position, the endotracheal tip depth should be roughly 23 cm for an average-sized adult male and 21 cm for adult females.[114,115] If the tube appears more shallow than this, one may consider advancing the endotracheal tube to the above depths. Excessive coughing may be another sign of endotracheal tube malposition. The pilot balloon should also be inspected and reinflated if inadequate filling is noted. Recurrent pilot balloon deflation is suggestive of cuff leak and the need for endotracheal tube change. On occasion, the leak may be in the valve assembly. This can be confirmed by clamping off the pilot balloon tubing after it has been reinflated. If the air lead does not stop, then the problem is likely caused by cuff leak.

Elevated Peak Inspiratory Pressure

An abrupt rise in peak inspiratory pressure generally signals a decrease in pulmonary, chest wall, or proximal airway compliance. Calculation of the static (C_{stat}) and dynamic (C_{dyn}) compliance and comparison to previous baseline values are helpful in differentiating these processes, as illustrated in Figure 34-10.[116] A proportionate decline in both C_{stat} and C_{dyn} is suggestive of a decrease in pulmonary or chest wall compliance. A decline in C_{dyn} accompanied by an unchanged C_{stat} is suggestive of endotracheal tube occlusion or bronchospasm. Table 34-1 provides the differential diagnosis for these compliance changes.

An occluded or kinked endotracheal tube produces a disproportionate decrease in C_{dyn} and may be mani-

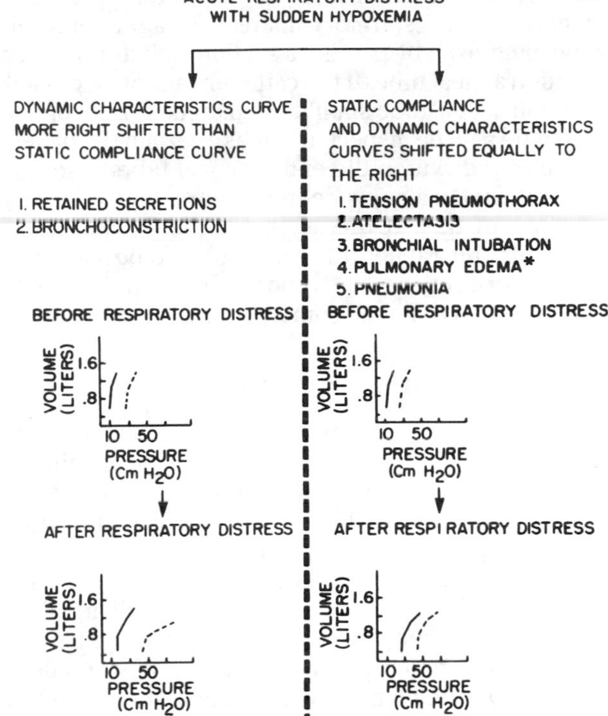

FIGURE 34-10. Narrowing the differential diagnosis of acute respiratory distress in patients receiving mechanical ventilation can be assisted by observing a relative shift in the static (C_{stat}) and dynamic (C_{dyn}) compliance curves compared to the previous baseline. The solid lines represent the static compliance curves, and the dashed lines represent the dynamic compliance curves. The asterisk (*) indicates that pulmonary edema represents both cardiogenic (eg, congestive heart failure) and noncardiogenic (eg, Adult Respiratory Distress Syndrome) forms. (Reprinted with permission from Bone RC: Diagnosis of causes for acute respiratory distress by pressure-volume curves. Chest 70:740, 1976.)

TABLE 34-1 **Conditions Associated With Compliance Changes**

$\downarrow C_{stat}$ Proportional to $\downarrow C_{dyn}$	$\downarrow C_{dyn} > \downarrow C_{stat}$
Tension pneumothorax	Bronchospasm
Atelectasis	Occluded endotracheal tube
Main stem bronchus intubation	Kinked enodtracheal tube
Pulmonary edema congestive heart failure adult respiratory distress syndrome	Retained secretions
Pneumonia	
Pleural effusion	
Interstitial lung disease	
Chest wall restriction	

fested by an elevation in peak inspiratory pressure, abrupt onset of respiratory distress, or agitation. This can be diagnosed by passing a suction catheter through the endotracheal tube. If the catheter cannot be passed, the endotracheal tube should be changed. The oropharynx should also be inspected to make certain the patient is not biting down on the endotracheal tube. Insertion of an oral airway along side the endotracheal tube may help prevent this. If the suction catheter can be advanced into the trachea, the patient should be suctioned to make sure retained secretions are not the cause of the diminished dynamic compliance.

Patient-Ventilator Asynchrony

Patient-ventilator asynchrony is also referred to as "bucking" or "fighting" the ventilator. The manifestations of this are variable, but the most common feature is that of an uncomfortable or distressed patient whose respiratory efforts do not appear coordinated with the ventilator. Most often this is caused by failure to optimize the ventilator settings to meet the individual patient's needs. Other potential causes including tension pneumothorax, endotracheal tube malposition, retained secretions, and dynamic hyperinflation should still be considered and evaluated as outlined previously.

Excessive inspiratory efforts tend to suggest either the trigger sensitivity is set too low (more negative) or the inspiratory flow is set too low. Frequent high pressure "cutoffs" can suggest either a change in compliance, endotracheal tube malposition, or retained secretions. Frequent high pressure "cutoffs" may also signal the occurrence of breath stacking and dynamic hyperinflation. In this case, the intrinsic PEEP should be measured and the settings optimized to lengthen expiratory time. Bronchospasm and pulmonary edema are also frequent offenders that may be readily correctable.

Patients who exhibit increased respiratory rates should be assessed for respiratory muscle fatigue or the development of a condition associated with high minute ventilation requirements. Respiratory muscle fatigue may be associated with accessory muscle use; thoracoabdominal paradoxical motion; and a rapid, shallow breathing pattern. If the patient is on SIMV, one can switch to A-C, increase the mandatory rate, or add pressure support. High minute ventilation requirements may be associated with fever, sepsis, liver failure, salicylate toxicity, pain, and anxiety.

After optimizing ventilator settings and excluding other major complications, it is reasonable to treat any remaining patient discomfort with analgesic or sedative therapy. Younger patients tend to be extremely intolerant of endotracheal intubation, and heavy sedation is often necessary if mechanical ventilation cannot be readily discontinued. Unconventional modes of ventilation such as high frequency ventilation and inverse ratio ventilation feel so unnatural that virtually all patients require heavy sedation and neuromuscular blockade. With conventional modes, however, neuromuscular junction blocking agents should be avoided, if possible, as prolonged therapy may induce a generalized neuromuscular weakness syndrome.[117] This syndrome is not well defined but is associated with a duration of paralytic therapy greater than 2 days, and the weakness may take several months to fully resolve.[117]

Hypoxemia

The development of hypoxemia in patients on mechanical ventilation is usually associated with progression of the primary cause for respiratory failure or the development of a new complicating process, as listed in Box 34-3. The appropriate therapeutic response depends on the underlying cause, pulmonary compliance, and significant radiographic features. A basic algorithm outlining the therapeutic approach based on these features is shown in Figure 34-11.[44] The radiographic pattern observed is a logical decision point as the addition of PEEP typically only helps conditions associated with significant bilateral parenchymal involvement. On occasion, even high levels of PEEP are insufficient to correct hypoxemia associated with diffuse processes such as ARDS. In this situation, switching to pressure control with a 1:1 I:E ratio and a decelerating inspiratory flow waveform may be helpful. If oxygenation improves but is still inadequate, progressive inverse ratio ventilation can sometimes be successful.

Peak inspiratory pressures greater than 40 cmH_2O may be associated with an increased risk of barotrauma and should be corrected when present. Switching to a pressure control mode can be very helpful in reducing peak inspiratory pressure. This is useful in diffuse lung disease processes but should be avoided in the setting of dynamic hyperinflation. Pressure control mode may require increasing the inspiratory time, which exacerbates dynamic hyperinflation and heightens the risk of barotrauma. Reducing the tidal volume may also help diminish peak inspiratory pressure; however, this may impact negatively on alveolar recruitment in diffuse processes such as ARDS. Therefore, it should be done gradually while monitoring for any change in oxygenation.

MORTALITY RISK ASSESSMENT IN ACUTE RESPIRATORY FAILURE

Several studies have evaluated risk factors associated with diminished survival in acute respiratory failure. Familiarity with this information is important for respiratory practitioners for the discussion of reasonable expectations and prognosis with patients and family members.

Of the factors reported to influence mortality associated with acute respiratory failure, the underlying disease process seems to carry the most significance. For example, of patients admitted to the ICU with respiratory failure, the presence of underlying malignancy increases the mortality from 25% to 75%.[4,118]

In patients with chronic respiratory disease admitted with acute respiratory failure, mortality is relatively low

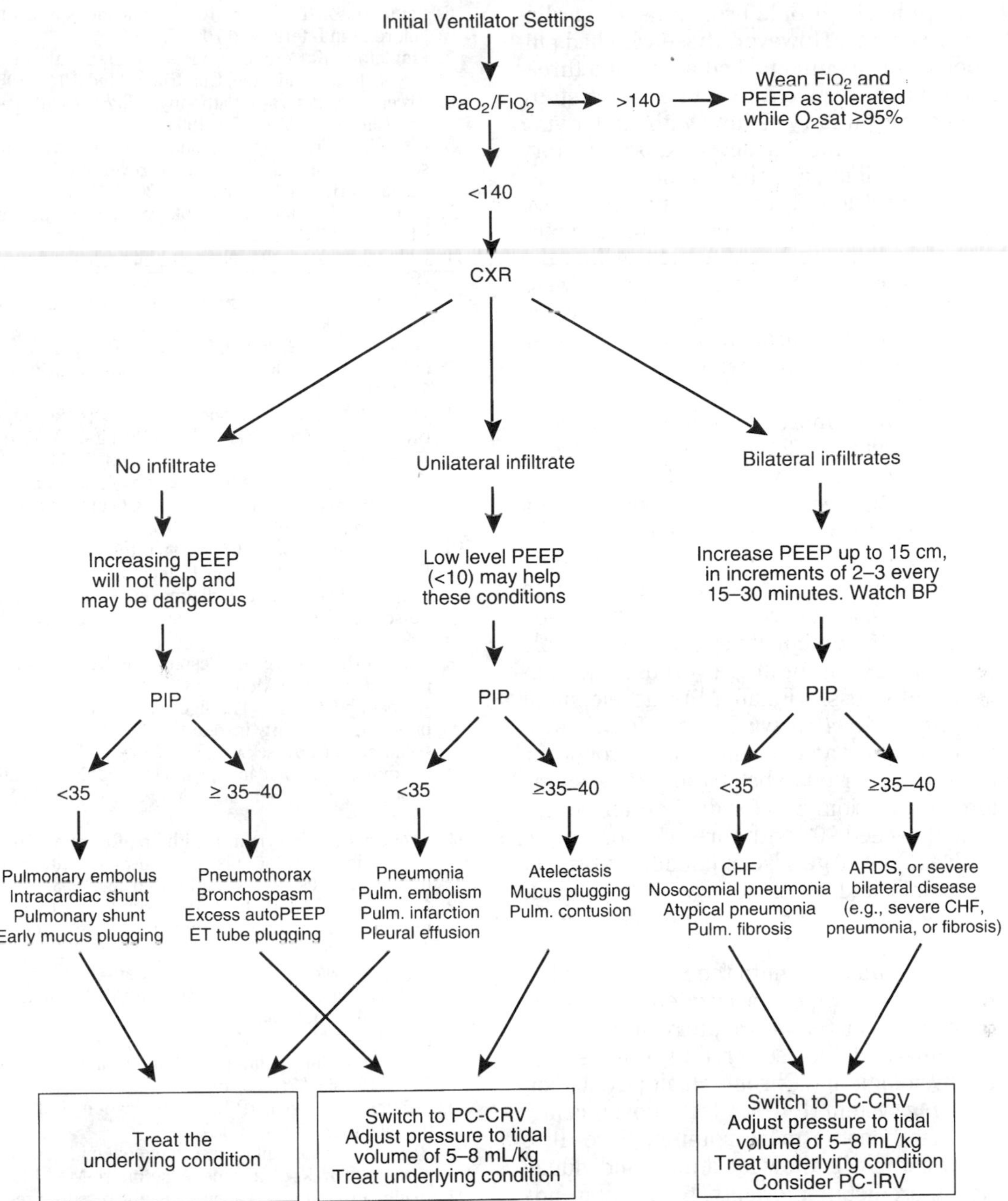

FIGURE 34-11. Diagnostic and ventilator management algorithm for patients who develop hypoxemia while receiving mechanical ventilation. Initial management depends on the radiographic appearance as the application of PEEP is likely to help only those conditions associated with significant bilateral infiltrates. Peak inspiratory pressures (PIP) higher than 35–40 cm H_2O should be avoided if possible as the risk of barotrauma may be increased. Pressure control ventilation is one way to reduce peak inspiratory pressure; however this should be applied with caution in patients at risk for dynamic hyperinflation. Intrinsic PEEP levels need to be monitored closely while on pressure control ventilation. Abbreviations: ARDS: adult respiratory distress syndrome, AutoPEEP: Intrinsic positive end-expiratory pressure, BP: blood pressure, CHF: congestive heart failure, CXR: chest X-ray, ET: endotracheal tube, PEEP: positive end-expiratory pressure, PIP: peak inspiratory pressure, PC-CRV: pressure control-conventional ratio ventilation, PC-IRV: pressure control-inverse ratio ventilation, Pulm: pulmonary. (Reprinted with permission from: Van Hoozen BE, Van Hoozen CM, Albertson TE: Pulmonary considerations and complications in the neurosurgical patient. In Youmans JR (ed): Neurological Survey, 4th ed. Philadelphia, W.B. Saunders, 1996, p. 592.)

if attributed to asthma, chronic bronchitis, or cardiogenic pulmonary edema. However, those who had pulmonary embolism or pneumonia had a two- and threefold higher mortality, respectively.[3] In another study examining acute respiratory failure with underlying chronic pulmonary dysfunction, age, sex, prior history of acute respiratory failure, and the number of prior decompensations were found to have no predictive value.[119] On the other hand, the presence of cachexia, abnormal serum sodium, and confinement within the home secondary to respiratory symptomatology were associated with an increased mortality.[119] The level of arterial hypoxemia and the duration of mechanical ventilation beyond 7 days have not been shown to be helpful in predicting outcome.[120,121]

In patients with ARDS, mortality is directly related to the severity of lung injury at 72 hours after onset of lung injury. If the PaO_2/FIO_2 ratio is less than 150 at 72 hours, the mortality increases to 84% as opposed to a 30% mortality when the ratio is higher than 250.[46] The precipitating cause of ARDS also factors into outcome statistics. When the underlying cause is secondary to sepsis, mortality rates often exceed 50%, whereas when ARDS is induced by fat embolism syndrome, multiple blood product transfusions, or drug overdose, the mortality is significantly less.[46] Finally, the development of ***multiple organ dysfunction syndrome (MODS)*** with ARDS is associated with an extremely poor prognosis. Mortality rates are reported to be 30% to 40% for single organ system dysfunction, 60% for dual organ system dysfunction, and exceed 90% with three or more organ systems involved.[122–124] Age also influences mortality from ARDS complicated by MODS, with those older than 65 years having a 20% increase in mortality in each of the above groups.[123,124]

Together, these studies point to the need for further work to be done before we can accurately predict the outcomes of specific patients with acute respiratory failure. To achieve this end, the use of rating systems such as the Acute Physiologic and Chronic Health Evaluation (*APACHE*) *scoring* system II[123,125,126] (and most recently APACHE III) has become more commonplace. It is hoped these systems will allow for a more individualized approach to predicting mortality. If current trends in health care reform continue, it is likely that some form of rationing of ICU expenditures may be based, at least in part, on outcome statistics such as these.

REFERENCES

1. Martin TR, Lewis SW, Albert RK: The prognosis of patients with chronic obstructive pulmonary disease after hospitalization for acute respiratory failure. Chest 82:310, 1982
2. Hudson LD: Survival data in patients with acute and chronic lung disease requiring mechanical ventilation. Am Rev Respir Dis 140:S19, 1989
3. Heuser MD, Case LD, Ettinger WH: Mortality in intensive care patients with respiratory disease. Is age important? Arch Intern Med 152:1683, 1992
4. Hauser MJ, Tabak J, Baier H: Survival of patients with cancer in a medical critical care unit. Arch Intern Med 142:527, 1982
5. Bone RC: Acute respiratory failure. In GG Burton, JE Hodgkin, JJ Ward (eds): Respiratory Care: A Guide to Clinical Practice, 3rd ed. Philadelphia, JB Lippincott, 1991
6. Asmundsson T, Kilburn K: Complications of acute respiratory failure. Ann Intern Med 70:487, 1969
7. Pingleton SK: Complications associated with the adult respiratory distress syndrome. Clin Chest Med 3:143, 1982
8. Greene KE, Peters JI: Pathophysiology of acute respiratory failure. Clin Chest Med 15:1, 1994
9. Frostell C, Fratacci MD, Wain JC, et al: Inhaled nitric oxide: A selective pulmonary vasodilator reversing hypoxic pulmonary vasoconstriction. Circulation 83:2038, 1991
10. Elliott CG: Pulmonary physiology during pulmonary embolism. Chest 101:163S, 1992
11. Goldhaber SZ: Pulmonary embolism. Hospital Med 29(8):22, 1993
12. Moser KM: Venous thromboembolism. Am Rev Respir Dis 141:235, 1990
13. Webster JR Jr, Saddeh GB, Eggum PR, et al: Wheezing due to pulmonary embolism–treatment with heparin. N Engl J Med 274:931, 1966
14. West JB: Ventilation, blood flow, and gas exchange. In JF Murray, JA Nadel (eds): Textbook of Respiratory Medicine, 2nd ed. Philadelphia, W.B. Saunders, 1994, pp. 71–72
15. Roughton FJ: Average time spent by blood in human lung capillary and its relation to the rates of CO uptake and elimination in man. Am J Physiol 143:621, 1945
16. Teitelbaum JS, Borel CO: Respiratory dysfunction in Guillain-Barré syndrome. Clin Chest Med 15:705, 1994
17. Kelly BJ, Luce JM: The diagnosis and management of neuromuscular diseases causing respiratory failure. Chest 99:1485, 1991
18. Zulueta JJ, Fanburg BL: Respiratory dysfunction in myasthenia gravis. Clin Chest Med 15:683, 1994
19. Ashbaugh DG, Petty TL, Bigelow DB, et al: Continuous positive pressure breathing in adult respiratory distress syndrome. J Thorac Cardiovasc Surg 57:31, 1967
20. Falke KJ, Pontoppidan H, Kumar A, et al: Ventilation with end-expiratory pressure in acute lung disease. J Clin Invest 51:2315, 1972
21. Gregory GA, Kitterman JA, Phibbs RH, et al: Treatment of the idiopathic respiratory distress syndrome with continuous positive airway pressure. N Engl J Med 284:1333, 1971
22. Leftwich EI, Witorsch RJ, Witorsch P: Positive end-expiratory pressure in refractory hypoxemia. Ann Intern Med 79:187, 1973
23. Katz JA, Ozanne GM, Zinn SE, et al: Time course and mechanisms of lung volume increase with PEEP in acute pulmonary failure. Anesthesiology 54:9 1981
24. Malo J, Ali J, Wood LDH: How does positive end-expiratory pressure reduce intrapulmonary shunt in canine pulmonary edema? J Appl Physiol 57:1002, 1984
25. Strieter RM, Lynch JP III: Complications in the ventilated patient. Clin Chest Med 9:127, 1988
26. Bone RC: Treatment of severe hypoxemia due to the adult respiratory distress syndrome. Arch Intern Med 140:85, 1980
27. Blanch PB, Jones M, Layon AJ, et al: Pressure-preset ventilation, Part I: Physiologic and mechanical considerations. Chest 104:590, 1993
28. Muñoz J, Guerrero JE, Escalante JL, et al: Pressure-controlled ventilation versus controlled mechanical ventilation with decelerating inspiratory flow. Crit Care Med 21:1143, 1993
29. Abraham E, Yoshihara G: Cardiorespiratory effects of pressure controlled inverse ratio ventilation in severe respiratory failure. Chest 96:1356, 1989
30. Gurevitch MJ, Van Dyke J, Young ES, et al: Improved oxygenation and lower peak airway pressure in severe adult respiratory distress syndrome: Treatment with inverse ratio ventilation. Chest 89:211, 1986
31. Lain DC, DiBenedetto R, Morris SL, et al: Pressure control inverse ratio ventilation as a method to reduce peak inspiratory pressure and provide adequate ventilation and oxygenation. Chest 95:1081, 1989
32. Tharratt RS, Allen RP, Albertson TE: Pressure-controlled inverse ratio ventilation in severe adult respiratory failure. Chest 94:755, 1988
33. Zapol WM, Snider MT, Hill JD, et al: Extracorporeal membrane oxygenation in severe acute respiratory failure: A randomized prospective study. JAMA 242:2193, 1979

34. Penner C, Roberts D, Kunimoto D, et al: Tuberculosis as a primary cause of respiratory failure requiring mechanical ventilation. Am J Respir Crit Care Med 151:867, 1995
35. Pingleton SK: Complications of acute respiratory failure. Am Rev Respir Dis 137:1463, 1988
36. Pingleton SK, Bone RC, Pingleton WW: Prevention of pulmonary emboli in a respiratory intensive care unit. Chest 79:647, 1981
37. Neuhaus A, Bentz RR, Weg JG: Pulmonary embolism in respiratory failure. Chest 73:460, 1978
38. Moser KM, LeMoine JR, Nachtwey FJ, et al: Deep venous thrombosis and pulmonary embolism. Frequency in a respiratory intensive care unit. JAMA 246:1422, 1981
39. Cvitanic D, Marino PL: Improved use of arterial blood gas analysis in suspected pulmonary embolism. Chest 95:48, 1989
40. Stein PD, Goldhaber SZ, Henry JW: Alveolar-arterial oxygen gradient in the assessment of acute pulmonary embolism. Chest 107:139, 1995
41. Palla A, Petruzzelli S, Donnamaria V, et al: The role of suspicion in the diagnosis of pulmonary embolism. Chest 107:21S, 1995
42. Manganelli D, Palla A, Donnamaria V, et al: Clinical features of pulmonary embolism: Doubts and certainties. Chest 107:25S, 1995
43. Stein PD, Hull RD, Saltzman HA, et al: Strategy for diagnosis of patients with suspected acute pulmonary embolism. Chest 103:1553, 1993
44. Van Hoozen BE, Van Hoozen CM, Albertson TE: Pulmonary considerations and complications in the neurosurgical patient. In JR Youmans (ed): Neurological Surgery, 4th ed. Philadelphia, W.B. Saunders, 1996, pp. 570–645
45. Colice GL: Detecting the presence and cause of pulmonary edema. Postgrad Med 93(6):161, 1993
46. Marinelli WA, Ingbar DH: Diagnosis and management of acute lung injury. Clin Chest Med 15:517, 1994
47. Petty TL: Acute respiratory distress syndrome. Dis Mon 36:1, 1990
48. Gattinoni L, Bombino M, Pelosi P, et al: Lung structure and function in different stages of severe adult respiratory distress syndrome. JAMA 271:1772, 1994
49. Burchardi H, Sydow M: Artificial ventilation: Some unresolved problems. Eur J Anaesth 11:53, 1994
50. Webb HH, Tierney DF: Experimental pulmonary edema due to intermittent positive pressure ventilation with high inflation pressures: Protection by positive end-expiratory pressure. Am Rev Respir Dis 110:556, 1974
51. Dreyfuss D, Basset G, Soler P, et al: Intermittent positive pressure hyperventilation with high inflation pressures produces pulmonary microvascular injury in rats. Am Rev Respir Dis 132:880, 1985
52. Tsuno K, Prato P, Kolobow T: Acute lung injury from mechanical ventilation at moderately high airway pressures. J Appl Physiol 69:956, 1990
53. Dreyfuss D, Soler P, Basset G, et al: High inflation pressure pulmonary edema: Respective effects of high airway pressure, high tidal volume, and positive end-expiratory pressure. Am Rev Respir Dis 137:1159, 1988
54. Muscedere JG, Mullen JBM, Gan K, et al: Tidal ventilation at low airway pressures can augment lung injury. Am J Respir Crit Care Med 149:1327, 1994
55. Gattinoni L, Pesenti A, Mascheroni D, et al: Low-frequency positive pressure ventilation with extracorporeal CO_2 removal in severe acute respiratory failure. JAMA 256.881, 1986
56. Morris AH, Wallace CJ, Menlove RL, et al: Randomized clinical trial of pressure-controlled inverse ratio ventilation and extracorporeal CO_2 removal for adult respiratory distress syndrome. Am J Respir Crit Care Med 149:295, 1994
57. Schuster DP: Fluid management in ARDS: "Keep them dry" or does it matter? Intensive Care Med 21:101, 1995
58. Sznajder JI, Wood LDH: Beneficial effects of reducing pulmonary edema in patients with acute hypoxemic respiratory failure. Chest 100:890, 1991
59. Simmons RS, Berdine GG, Seidenfeld JJ, et al: Fluid balance and the adult respiratory distress syndrome. Am Rev Respir Dis 135:924, 1987
60. Schuller D, Mitchell JP, Calandrino FS, et al: Fluid balance during pulmonary edema: Is fluid gain a marker or a cause of poor outcome? Chest 100:1068, 1991
61. Mitchell JP, Schuller D, Calandrino FS, et al: Improved outcome based on fluid management in critically ill patients requiring pulmonary artery catheterization. Am Rev Respir Dis 145:990, 1992
62. Long W, Corbet A, Cotton R, et al: A controlled trial of synthetic surfactant in infants weighing 1250 g or more with respiratory distress syndrome. N Engl J Med 325:1696, 1991
63. Weg JG, Balk RA, Tharratt RS, et al: Safety and potential efficacy of an aerosolized surfactant in human sepsis-induced adult respiratory distress syndrome. JAMA 272:1433, 1994
64. Soo Hoo GW, Santiago S, Williams AJ: Nasal mechanical ventilation for hypercapnic respiratory failure in chronic obstructive pulmonary disease: Determinants of success and failure. Crit Care Med 22:1253, 1994
65. Fernandez R, Blanch L, Valles J, et al: Pressure support ventilation via face mask in acute respiratory failure in hypercapnic COPD patients. Intensive Care Med 19:456, 1993
66. Vitacca M, Rubini F, Foglio K, et al: Non-invasive modalities of positive pressure ventilation improve the outcome of acute exacerbations in COLD patients. Intensive Care Med 19:450, 1993
67. Leger P, Bedicam JM, Cornette A, et al: Nasal intermittent positive pressure ventilation: Long-term follow-up in patients with severe chronic respiratory insufficiency. Chest 105:100, 1994
68. Piper AJ, Sullivan CE: Effects of short-term NIPPV in the treatment of patients with severe obstructive sleep apnea and hypercapnia. Chest 105:434, 1994
69. Waldhorn RE: Nocturnal nasal intermittent positive pressure ventilation with bi-level positive airway pressure (BiPAP) in respiratory failure. Chest 101:516, 1992
70. Rochester DF, Esau SA: Assessment of ventilatory function in patients with neuromuscular disease. Clin Chest Med 15:751, 1994
71. Braun NMT, Arora NS, Rochester DF: Respiratory muscle and pulmonary function in polymyositis and other proximal myopathies. Thorax 38:616, 1983
72. Hill R, Martin J, Hakim A: Acute respiratory failure in motor neuron disease. Arch Neurol 40:30, 1983
73. Schiffman PL, Belsh JM: Pulmonary function at diagnosis of amyotrophic lateral sclerosis: Rate of deterioration. Chest 103:508, 1993
74. Kaplan LM, Hollander D: Respiratory dysfunction in amyotrophic lateral sclerosis. Clin Chest Med 15:675, 1994
75. Lynn DJ, Woda RP, Mendell JR: Respiratory dysfunction in muscular dystrophy and other myopathies. Clin Chest Med 15:661, 1994
76. Griggs RC, Donohoe KM, Utell MJ, et al: Evaluation of pulmonary function in neuromuscular disease. Arch Neurol 38:9, 1981
77. Mead J, Sly P, Le Souef P, et al: Rib cage mobility in pectus excavatum. Am Rev Respir Dis 132:1223, 1985
78. Ray CS, Sue DY, Bray G, et al: Effects of obesity on respiratory function. Am Rev Respir Dis 128:501, 1983
79. Lopata M, Onal E: Mass loading, sleep apnea, and the pathogenesis of obesity hypoventilation. Am Rev Respir Dis 126:640, 1982
80. Sampson, MG, Grassino A: Neuromechanical properties in obese patients during carbon dioxide rebreathing. Am J Med 75:81, 1983
81. Rochester DF, Enson Y: Current concepts in the pathogenesis of the obesity-hypoventilation syndrome. Am J Med 57:402, 1974
82. Sugerman HJ, Fairman RP, Baron PL, et al: Gastric surgery for respiratory insufficiency of obesity. Chest 90:81, 1986
83. Leatherman J: Life-threatening asthma. Clin Chest Med 15:453, 1994
84. Brenner BE, Abraham E, Simon RR: Position and diaphoresis in acute asthma. Am J Med 74:1005, 1983
85. Martin TG, Elenbaas RM, Pingleton SH: Use of peak expiratory flow rates to eliminate unnecessary arterial blood gases in acute asthma. Ann Emerg Med 11:70, 1982
86. Curtis JR, Hudson LD: Emergent assessment and management of acute respiratory failure in COPD. Clin Chest Med 15:481, 1994

87. Becker AB, Nelson NA, Simons FE: Inhaled salbutamol (albuterol) versus injected epinephrine in the treatment of acute asthma in children. J Pediatr 102:465, 1983
88. Bloomfield P, Carmichael J, Petrie GR, et al: Comparison of salbutamol given intravenously and by intermittent positive-pressure breathing in life-threatening asthma. BMJ 1(6167):848, 1979
89. Lawford P, Jones BJM, Milledge JS: Comparison of intravenous and nebulised salbutamol in initial treatment of severe asthma. BMJ 1(6105):84, 1978
90. Rebuck AS, Chapman KR, Abboud R, et al: Nebulized anticholinergic and sympathomimetic treatment of asthma and chronic obstructive airways disease in the emergency room. Am J Med 82:59, 1987
91. Higgins B, Greening AP, Crompton GK: Assisted ventilation in severe acute asthma. Thorax 41:464, 1986
92. O'Driscoll BR, Taylor RJ, Horsley MG: Nebulised salbutamol with and without ipratropium bromide in acute airflow obstruction. Lancet 1(8652):1418, 1989
93. Rossing TH, Fanta CH, Goldstein DH, et al: Emergency therapy of asthma: Comparison of the acute effects of parenteral and inhaled sympathomimetics and infused aminophylline. Am Rev Respir Dis 122:365, 1980
94. Jones DA, Howell S, Roussos C, et al: Low-frequency fatigue in isolated skeletal muscles and the effects of methylxanthines. Clin Sci 63:161, 1982
95. Albert RK, Martin TR, Lewis SW: Controlled clinical trial of methylprednisolone in patients with chronic bronchitis and acute respiratory insufficiency. Ann Intern Med 92:753, 1980
96. Barnes NC: Effects of corticosteroids in acute severe asthma. Thorax 47:582, 1992
97. Skobeloff EM, Spivey WH, McNamara RM, et al: Intravenous magnesium sulfate for the treatment of acute asthma in the emergency department. JAMA 262:1210, 1989
98. Gluck EH, Onorato DJ, Castriotta R: Helium-oxygen mixtures in intubated patients with status asthmaticus and respiratory acidosis. Chest 98:693, 1990
99. Echeverria M, Gelb AW, Wexler HR, et al: Enflurane and halothane in status asthmaticus. Chest 89:152, 1986
100. Saulnier FF, Durocher AV, Deturck RA, et al: Respiratory and hemodynamic effects of halothane in status asthmaticus. Intensive Care Med 16:104, 1990
101. Schwartz SH: Treatment of status asthmaticus with halothane. JAMA 251:2688, 1984
102. Darioli R, Perret C: Mechanical controlled hypoventilation in status asthmaticus. Am Rev Respir Dis 129:385, 1984
103. Williams TJ, Tuxen DV, Scheinkestel CD: Risk factors for morbidity in mechanically ventilated patients with acute severe asthma. Am Rev Respir Dis 146:607, 1992
104. Pepe PE, Marini JJ: Occult positive end-expiratory pressure in mechanically ventilated patients with airflow obstruction: The auto-PEEP effect. Am Rev Respir Dis 126:166, 1982
105. Schmidt GA: Acid-base and electrolyte homeostasis. In JB Hall, GA Schmidt, LDH Wood (eds): Principles of Critical Care, 1st ed. New York, McGraw-Hill, 1992, pp. 52–83
106. Menzies R, Gibbons W, Goldberg P: Determinants of weaning and survival among patients with COPD who require mechanical ventilation for acute respiratory failure. Chest 95:398, 1989
107. Petty TL: Intensive and Rehabilitative Respiratory Care, 3rd ed. Philadelphia, Lea & Febiger, 1982, p. 238
108. Luce JM, Raffin TA: Withholding and withdrawal of life support from critically ill patients. Chest 94:621, 1988
109. Luce JM: Ethical principles in critical care. JAMA 263:696, 1990
110. Smedira NG, Evans BH, Grais LS, et al: Withholding and withdrawal of life support from the critically ill. N Engl J Med 322:309, 1990
111. ACCP-SCCM Consensus Panel: Ethical and moral guidelines for the initiation, continuation, and withdrawal of intensive care. Chest 97:949, 1990
112. Raffin TA: Withholding and withdrawing life support. Hosp Pract 26(3):133, 1991
113. American Thoracic Society Bioethics Task Force: American Thoracic Society statement on withholding and withdrawing life-sustaining therapy. Ann Int Med 155:478, 1991
114. Marcy TW, Marini JJ: Respiratory distress in the ventilated patient. Clin Chest Med 15:55, 1994
115. Owen RL, Cheney FW: Endobronchial intubation: A preventable complication. Anesthesiology 67:255, 1987
116. Bone RC: Diagnosis of causes for acute respiratory distress by pressure-volume curves. Chest 70:740, 1976
117. Gooch JL, Suchyta MR, Balbierz JM, et al: Prolonged paralysis after treatment with neuromuscular junction blocking agents. Crit Care Med 19:1125, 1991
118. Ingbar DH, White DA: Acute respiratory failure. Crit Care Clin 4:11, 1988
119. Portier F, Defouilloy C, Muir JF, et al: Determinants of immediate survival among chronic respiratory insufficiency patients admitted to an intensive care unit for acute respiratory failure: A prospective multicenter study. Chest 101:204, 1992
120. Jiménez P, Torres A, Roca J, et al: Arterial oxygenation does not predict the outcome of patients with acute respiratory failure needing mechanical ventilation. Eur Respir J 7:730, 1994
121. Gracey DR, Naessens JM, Krishan I, et al: Hospital and posthospital survival in patients mechanically ventilated for more than 29 days. Chest 101:211, 1992
122. Beal AL, Cerra FB: Multiple organ failure syndrome in the 1990s: Systemic inflammatory response and organ dysfunction. JAMA 271:226, 1994
123. Knaus WA, Draper EA, Wagner DP, et al: Prognosis in acute organ system failure. Ann Surg 202:685, 1985
124. Raffin TA: Intensive care unit survival of patients with systemic illness. Am Rev Respir Dis 140:S28, 1989
125. Knaus WA, Draper EA, Wagner DP, et al: APACHE II: A severity of disease classification system. Crit Care Med 13:818, 1985
126. Knaus WA, Wagner DP: Multiple systems organ failure: Epidemiology and prognosis. Crit Care Clin 5:221, 1989

35 Respiratory Care in the Coronary Care Unit

Steve G. Peters
John T. Wheeler
Douglas R. Gracey

PROFESSIONAL SKILLS

Upon completion of this chapter, the reader will:

- List risk factors for development of coronary artery disease
- Recognize clinical presentation of angina pectoris, acute myocardial infarction, congestive heart failure, and pulmonary edema
- Describe diagnostic tools for assessing cardiac function
- Perform standard ECG and cardiac rhythm strip
- Understand principles of hemodynamic monitoring, including pulmonary artery and pulmonary capillary "wedge" monitoring, cardiac output determination, systemic arterial pressure (arterial line) monitoring, and calculating shunt fraction ($\dot{Q}_S/\dot{Q}_T$)
- Assist in pulmonary artery (Swan-Ganz) catheter placement
- Perform calibration of, maintenance of, and sampling from pulmonary artery catheter and systemic (arterial) lines
- Explain the interaction between pulmonary and cardiac function
- Initiate and maintain mechanical ventilation in the patient with heart disease
- Weigh the risks and benefits when performing bronchial hygiene procedures on patients with acute myocardial ischemia
- Understand indications and hazards of cardiopulmonary resuscitation (CPR)
- Administer cardiopulmonary resuscitation (CPR) to a patient experiencing myocardial infarction

KEY TERMS

Angina pectoris
β-blocking agents
Calcium channel blocking agents
Cardiac index
Coronary angiography
Coronary angioplasty
Creatine kinase
Echocardiography
Electrocardiogram (ECG)
Inotropic agents
Myocardial infarction
Noninvasive ventilation
Percutaneous transluminal coronary angioplasty (PTCA)
Radionuclide scanning
Technetium 99 scan
Thallium-201
Thrombolytic agents

INTRODUCTION

Respiratory care for the patient with cardiac disease requires understanding of the physiologic interactions between the heart and lungs and awareness of effects of respiratory procedures on the cardiovascular system. This chapter reviews aspects of medical management in the cardiac intensive care unit and features of respiratory therapy and assisted ventilation in patients with heart disease.

CLINICAL ASPECTS OF CORONARY ARTERY DISEASE

Cardiovascular diseases account for approximately 1 million deaths annually in the United States, roughly half of which are caused by coronary disease.[1] Of sudden deaths because of coronary heart disease, 60% to 70% occur outside a hospital. Cardiac arrest in this setting is most often caused by ventricular fibrillation, with or without evidence of acute myocardial infarction.

Approximately one-half of the patients with symptomatic or clinically apparent myocardial infarction survive to be admitted to the hospital. The coronary care unit typically serves as the site for acute management of patients with cardiac ischemia, including myocardial infarction and new or unstable angina. The coronary unit may also be used for monitoring and management of patients with unstable or life-threatening cardiac dysrhythmias and those with heart failure related to ischemia, cardiomyopathy, severe hypertension, or valvular disease. Candidates for cardiac transplantation may also be admitted to the cardiac intensive care unit for medical stabilization before surgery.

Risk factors for the development of coronary disease include age, male sex, hypertension, hypercholesterolemia, diabetes mellitus, cigarette smoking, and family history. Recent psychological stress and lower socioeconomic status are implicated as risk factors for coronary disease and sudden death. Each of these factors is assessed in the history, physical examination, and laboratory testing of the patient.

The classic symptom of myocardial ischemia is *angina pectoris,* that is, chest discomfort, which may be sensed as pain, pressure, or tightness across the central area of the chest or the epigastrium. There may be a similar sensation or radiation of discomfort to the neck, jaw, shoulders, arms, or back. Typical symptoms may occur with exertion and improve within minutes after resting or using nitroglycerin.

The symptoms of *myocardial infarction* include a new or unstable pattern of chest pain, pain occurring with minimal activity or at rest, or prolonged pain not relieved by rest or nitroglycerin. Dyspnea is common. Nausea may also be present and may mimic a gastrointestinal disorder. Light-headedness or palpitations may indicate a dysrhythmia or decreased cardiac output. A recent history of orthopnea or peripheral edema may suggest the presence of left or right ventricular failure, respectively. The pattern of the chest pain, including quality of the discomfort, duration, location, radiation, and aggravating and alleviating factors, may be useful in differentiating cardiac ischemia from such disorders as aortic dissection, pericarditis, pulmonary embolism, pneumonitis, pleuritis, or chest wall pain. Gastrointestinal discomfort caused by esophageal spasm, ulcer disease, pancreatitis, or gallbladder disease may also be confused with pain from myocardial ischemia.

Physical examination of the patient with uncomplicated myocardial infarction may be nonspecific. Tachypnea, tachycardia, diaphoresis, and hypertension or hypotension may be present. The cardiac examination may be normal. A fourth heart sound may indicate filling of a noncompliant left ventricle during atrial contraction. A systolic murmur of mitral regurgitation may indicate papillary muscle dysfunction or rupture of chordae tendineae.

When acute cardiac ischemia or infarction is suspected, a prompt electrocardiogram (ECG) is typically the initial diagnostic study. An ST-segment depression and T-wave flattening or inversion are changes associated with ischemia, although these findings may be chronic or nonspecific. New ST-segment elevation or Q waves are associated with infarction. It is important to recognize that the electrocardiogram may also appear normal during an acute ischemic event. Serial electrocardiograms improve the accuracy for a diagnosis of myocardial infarction.

Laboratory testing typically centers on assessment of serum levels of cardiac enzymes. In patients with acute symptoms, the myocardial, or MB, fraction of *creatine kinase*, or CK (MB), is most useful. The CK (MB) rises 4 to 6 hours after myocardial infarction, peaks at approximately 24 hours, and remains elevated for 48 to 72 hours. An MB fraction of less than 5% of the total CK may not be significant, and this distinction is especially helpful in postoperative patients who may have elevated CK levels and experience acute symptoms of myocardial infarction.

Recent advances have provided a variety of diagnostic imaging tools for assessing cardiac function. Two-dimensional echocardiography provides important information on ventricular size and function, regional wall motion abnormalities, mural thrombus formation, valvular function, and abnormalities of the pericardium. Doppler studies can be used to estimate intracardiac pressure gradients, pulmonary artery pressure, and cardiac output.[2]

Radionuclide-scanning studies have also gained an increasing role in assessing areas of infarction, myocardial perfusion, and ventricular function. *Technetium Tc 99m* pyrophosphate, injected within several days of acute infarction, is incorporated into areas of myocardial cellular damage. Technetium Tc 99m scanning may be used to establish whether an infarct has occurred, to localize the area, and to estimate its size.[3] Myocardial perfusion may be assessed by *thallium-201* scintigraphy. This isotope accumulates in proportion to blood flow, so that defects may identify areas of ischemia or infarction. Thallium-201 scanning is most often combined with exercise testing to provide additional diagnostic and prognostic information. An increased uptake of thallium-201 by the lungs during exercise is a sign of left ventricular dysfunction and is associated with a higher risk of subsequent cardiac complications.[4] A radionuclide ventriculogram with multiple-gated acquisition (MUGA scan) provides an assessment of ventricular function and ejection fraction. Such scanning is also frequently coupled with exercise; a decreased ejection fraction with exercise following myocardial infarction carries an adverse prognosis.[3]

Coronary angiography remains the standard for defining coronary anatomy and the site and degree of obstructing lesions. Angiography has recently been combined with techniques of thrombolytic therapy and coronary angioplasty. These therapeutic maneuvers are discussed in the following sections.

MANAGEMENT OF ACUTE MYOCARDIAL ISCHEMIA

The respiratory care practitioner should be aware of the drugs and other interventions commonly used in the coronary care setting and of the cardiovascular and respiratory physiologic effects.

Oxygen is usually administered at low flows (eg, 2 to 4 L/min) by nasal cannula. There is evidence that supplemental oxygen may reduce myocardial ischemia and improve arrhythmias and ventricular function if hypoxemia is present.[5–8] Although a similar benefit has not been proved for patients with normal arterial oxygenation, low-flow oxygen is initially used for most patients. It would be reasonable to obtain an arterial blood gas sample from all patients with acute myocardial infarction. In particular, patients with chronic obstructive pulmonary disease (COPD) should be monitored to document improvement in hypoxemia without significant carbon dioxide retention.

Relief of pain and anxiety is an important early goal. Morphine is most frequently used, typically titrated in increments of 2 to 8 mg to achieve pain relief and sedation. Morphine may also increase venous capacitance and decrease pulmonary artery pressures.[9,10] Hypotension, respiratory depression, bradycardia, and nausea are potential side effects.

Nitrates, by the sublingual or oral route and, more recently, by continuous intravenous infusion, have the potentially beneficial effects of increasing coronary blood flow and reducing preload and afterload by venous and arterial dilatation, thereby decreasing left ventricular work and oxygen demand. However, hypotension and reflex tachycardia may also occur, so that nitroglycerin must be used with caution, and the patient must be monitored closely. Furthermore, hypoxemia has been observed following intravenous nitroglycerin, the presumed mechanism being loss of regional hypoxic vasoconstriction and worsening of ventilation-perfusion mismatch.[11]

Lidocaine has been effective in the prevention of primary ventricular fibrillation following myocardial infarction.[12] Side effects may occur in a significant number of patients receiving recommended doses, especially if left ventricular failure or hepatic congestion is present. These adverse effects may include nausea, mental status changes, speech disturbances, dizziness, or seizures. The routine use of lidocaine is therefore debated, but prophylactic treatment is commonly given, with observation for side effects and dose adjustment if necessary.

Hypotension or ventricular failure following myocardial infarction may require treatment with inotropic agents. These agents generally increase myocardial contractility and cardiac output, but may have varying effects on systemic vascular resistance. Dopamine is a β agonist with α-adrenergic effects at doses above approximately 10 μg/kg/min, with resultant increase in vascular resistance at these higher dose levels. Nitroprusside is often added for its effects in reducing arterial resistance and venous return. Durrer et al observed a decreased incidence of left heart failure and decreased mortality in patients given nitroprusside during the first 24 hours after hospitalization for acute myocardial infarction.[13] Cohn et al found a benefit in mortality only for patients with persistent ventricular failure.[14] Dobutamine increases cardiac output, but also decreases systemic and pulmonary arterial pressures, so this agent is often used alone when ventricular failure occurs in the presence of elevated vascular resistance.[15] Amrinone is a newer agent, with positive inotropic and peripheral vasodilator properties, that also may be useful in the treatment of left ventricular failure.[16]

A variety of *β-blocking agents* may be used in the acute management of the patient with myocardial ischemia and in long-term management following myocardial infarction. In large trials, timolol, atenolol, propranolol, and metoprolol have decreased overall mortality, reinfarction rates, and sudden death rates.[17,18] Side effects may include hypotension, bradycardia, and congestive failure. Significant bronchospasm may also occur, despite the relative β_1 selectivity of the newer agents. Therefore, these drugs must be used cautiously in patients with chronic obstructive lung disease or reactive airways. Concomitant treatment of bronchospasm with β-adrenergic inhalers may be tried, but the relative risks and benefits must be weighed for the individual patient.

Calcium channel blocking agents, such as nifedipine, verapamil, and diltiazem may be useful in the long-term management of the patient with coronary disease, particularly with coexisting hypertension. These agents variably lower blood pressure, increase coronary blood flow, and decrease myocardial oxygen consumption. Nifedipine is an effective systemic and coronary vasodilator, but reflex tachycardia commonly occurs. Verapamil is also a potent vasodilator, and in addition, it slows atrioventricular conduction and heart rate and may depress myocardial contractility. Diltiazem is a coronary vasodilator with weaker effects on the systemic arterial bed. Heart rate is usually slowed slightly. In a multicenter trial of diltiazem following nontransmural myocardial infarction, the rate of reinfarction was reduced by approximately 50% compared with placebo controls.[19] Overall mortality was unchanged. Studies of the varying physiologic effects of these drugs and their role in the acute management of myocardial ischemia are ongoing.

Techniques for Coronary Reperfusion

Major recent developments in acute coronary care include the use of *thrombolytic agents* and *percutaneous transluminal coronary angioplasty* (PTCA). The goals of these techniques are early reperfusion following coronary occlusion, limitation of infarct size, preservation of ventricular function, and decreased mortality. Coronary thrombosis has been observed in approximately 87% of patients with acute transmural infarction.[20] Thrombus (clot) formation occurs through the coagulation cascade, whereas thrombolysis is mediated by the fibrinolytic system. Fibrinolysis depends on the conversion of plasminogen to plasmin, an enzyme with proteolytic activity against fibrin thrombi, as well as fibrinogen and other clotting factors. The thrombolytic agents streptokinase (SK), urokinase, and tissue plasminogen activator (t-PA) have different modes of action, but all induce the formation of plasmin from plasminogen.[21]

Many clinical trials have analyzed the efficacy of thrombolytic therapy in acute coronary thrombosis. When compared to a placebo, thrombolytic agents have been shown to result in limitation of infarct size, improvement in ventricular function, and improved overall mortality.[22–26] Benefits are most significant if treatment is given within several hours of the onset of symptomatic infarction. Several studies have shown greater reperfusion rates for t-PA than for SK, with less systemic fibrinolysis.[27,28] The recently reported GUSTO (Global Use of Streptokinase and Tissue Plasminogen Activator for Occluded Coronary Arteries) trial showed a slight decrease in 30-day mortality for t-PA treatment compared to SK treatment.[29] The relative cost-effectiveness of these agents, and their effects in various subgroups of patients, continue to be debated. Nevertheless, thrombolytic therapy is an important addition to the current management of acute myocardial infarction.

The major risk of thrombolytic therapy is bleeding. It is important to realize that these agents may lyse any recently formed clot. Significant hemorrhage may occur from previous arterial or venous puncture sites. Surgery within the previous 3 weeks, recent trauma, lesions of the central nervous system, poorly controlled hypertension, and gastrointestinal bleeding are contraindications to thrombolytic therapy.

Coronary angioplasty has been evaluated as a technique to dilate residual stenotic areas following thrombolytic therapy, or as primary therapy for acute myocardial infarction.[30–33] In this procedure, a balloon catheter is passed through an area of focal coronary artery stenosis identified by angiography. The balloon is then inflated to dilate the narrowed region. Several studies have shown slightly improved coronary perfusion and ventricular function with the addition of PTCA following thrombolytic therapy. PTCA as primary therapy provides initial results similar to thrombolytic therapy and is currently considered for patients in whom thrombolytic therapy is contraindicated.[32] Delayed PTCA may be of benefit in patients who fail thrombolytic therapy. Practical treatment protocols for an individual patient must allow for the relative availability of thrombolytic therapy, angiography, and angioplasty on an emergency basis.

With the emergence of thrombolytic therapy and PTCA in the management of acute myocardial infarction, the role of emergency coronary artery bypass grafting (CABG) has become more limited. Current indications for early CABG include left main coronary artery disease, extensive three-vessel disease, and multiple lesions not suitable for PTCA. Also, emergency CABG may be necessary if attempted PTCA is unsuccessful, or if it results in sudden worsening of coronary obstruction.[34] The role of CABG versus medical management in the long-term care of the patient with ischemic heart disease remains controversial. In young patients with severe heart disease, cardiac transplantation has also become a realistic option.

HEMODYNAMIC MONITORING

Important information may be gained by the use of a balloon flotation pulmonary artery catheter for the management of hemodynamically unstable patients with acute myocardial infarction. The respiratory care practitioner should have knowledge not only of the technical aspects of hemodynamic monitoring, but also of the clinical applications. Recent controversy has surfaced over the potential overuse of the pulmonary artery catheter in critically ill patients; however, in selected situations, the data may directly affect therapy.

Forrester et al have categorized subsets of hemodynamic data useful for the medical management of patients following acute myocardial infarction.[35,36] The hemodynamic and clinical subclasses are separated by a *cardiac index* (CI) greater or less than approximately 2.2 L/min/m^2, and pulmonary capillary wedge pressure (PCWP) greater or less than approximately 18 mmHg. Following estimates of ventricular filling pressure by the PCWP and measurement of cardiac index, the clinical classes are defined as follows:

Class I (CI $\geq$ 2.2 L/min/m^2, PCWP $\leq$ 18 mmHg)
Class II (CI $\geq$ 2.2 L/min/m^2, PCWP $>$ 18 mmHg)
Class III (CI $\leq$ 2.2 L/min/m^2, PCWP $\leq$ 18 mmHg)
Class IV (CI $\leq$ 2.2 L/min/m^2), PCWP $>$ 18 mmHg)

In Class I, there is generally no evidence of tissue hypoperfusion or pulmonary congestion. Treatment may include oxygen, morphine, nitrates, and β blockers, as discussed previously, but no other specific intervention may be required. In Class II, perfusion may be adequate, but signs of pulmonary edema or congestion may develop. Treatment might include diuretics and peripheral vasodilators. Class III patients with decreased cardiac output and low filling pressures may benefit from expansion of intravascular fluid volume and, possibly, inotropic agents. The goal of therapy is to increase cardiac output, without overstimulation of the heart and an adverse increase in myocardial oxygen demand. Class IV patients with low cardiac output and pulmonary edema may require a combination of diuretics, vasodilators (afterload reduction), and inotropic agents. A significantly higher mortality is associated with clinical evidence of hypoperfusion or a measured decrease in cardiac output as observed in Class III and IV patients.

CARDIOPULMONARY INTERACTIONS

Changes in cardiac function may affect pulmonary function and alter gas exchange. With left ventricular dysfunction, an increase in pulmonary venous pressure may lead to interstitial edema and increased small-airway resistance. Alveolar filling by fluid ensues in more severe pulmonary edema. Lung volumes and lung compliance decrease. Bronchospasm may also occur, so that a mixed restrictive and obstructive pattern may be found by pulmonary function tests.[37] Small-airway closure at higher-than-normal lung volumes has been reported, even in uncomplicated cases, in the first 2 weeks following myocardial infarction.[38] Arterial hypoxemia is frequently observed, although severe desaturation is typically found only in the presence of pulmonary edema or other respiratory complication, such as atelectasis or pneumonitis. With biventricular cardiac failure, pleural effusions are also a common cause for altered lung mechanics and gas exchange.

Lung disease may also have profound effects on cardiac function. Diffuse parenchymal or vascular disease, or any cause of chronic hypoxemia, may lead to increased pulmonary vascular resistance, pulmonary hypertension, and eventual right heart failure or cor pulmonale. This is commonly observed in patients with severe COPD. Cardiac arrhythmias, particularly premature atrial contractions, atrial tachycardias, and premature ventricular contractions, are frequently observed in monitored COPD patients.[39] Patients with COPD are also frequently at risk for coronary artery disease because of the common etiologic factor of tobacco use. Left ventricular function may be normal in patients with severe COPD, but concurrent left ventricular dysfunction has been attributed to coexisting coronary disease and ischemia.[40]

Acute alterations in lung mechanics also affect cardiac function. Hemodynamic changes associated with negative and positive pressure breathing are discussed elsewhere in this text. Briefly, increases in intrathoracic pressure, which may occur with positive pressure breathing or with applied positive end-expiratory pressure (PEEP), may decrease venous return to the right heart and thereby decrease right ventricular filling and cardiac output.[41] Pulmonary vascular resistance and right ventricular afterload are also increased in this setting, further limiting right ventricular output. These physiologic changes are also found in cases of airway obstruction with hyperinflation, increased intrathoracic pressure, and intrinsic PEEP; that is, alveolar pressure greater than atmospheric pressure at end expiration owing to high resistance and incomplete lung emptying. These changes may be overcome, to some extent, by increasing intravascular volume, but at the risk of subsequent fluid overload and worsening congestive failure. At high lung volumes, there may also be an increase in juxtacardiac pressure, such that left ventricular end-diastolic volume is reduced, leading to a further fall in cardiac output.

ASSISTED VENTILATION IN PATIENTS WITH CARDIAC DISEASE

Mechanical ventilation may become necessary in patients with acute myocardial ischemia or infarction complicated by congestive failure or coexisting pulmonary disease. Left ventricular function is typically decreased in patients requiring mechanical ventilation, but it may improve significantly in survivors.[42,43] In the absence of ventilatory failure, spontaneous breathing may allow greater cardiac output as outlined in the foregoing section. Chin et al observed a higher cardiac index in patients supported with continuous positive airway pressure and spontaneous breathing, compared with continuous positive-pressure mechanical ventilation or intermittent mandatory ventilation with PEEP.[44] However, assisted ventilation can decrease the work and oxygen cost of breathing and permit greater sedation and rest for the patient. Improved ventilation, inflation of unstable alveoli, and increased functional residual capacity may also improve oxygenation. Räsänen et al noted symptomatic and electrocardiographic evidence of ischemia as mechanical ventilation was withdrawn in patients with acute myocardial infarction.[45] Patients requiring mechanical ventilation should be monitored carefully as weaning is carried out. Gradual weaning techniques, such as intermittent mandatory ventilation or pressure support, or a combination thereof, have the potential advantage of allowing a transition to spontaneous ventilation without abrupt stress or patient discomfort.

Noninvasive ventilation with positive pressure delivered by means of a nasal or face mask has been reported recently to be of benefit in many patients with acute respiratory failure, including those with cardiogenic pulmonary edema.[46] Symptomatic relief and improvement in arterial blood gases have been documented. However, it is important to recognize that hemodynamic instability, cardiac dysrhythmias, and ongoing ischemia are currently among the contraindications for noninvasive ventilation.[46]

RESPIRATORY THERAPY PROCEDURES AND ACUTE MYOCARDIAL ISCHEMIA

In the patient with acute myocardial ischemia or infarction, the potential benefits of any intervention aimed at preventing or treating respiratory complications must be weighed against the possible immediate harm to the patient. Chest physical therapy (CPT) may induce increases in heart rate, blood pressure, oxygen consumption, and carbon dioxide production. Klein et al have recently reported that in mechanically ventilated patients, short-acting narcotics attenuated the hemodynamic responses to CPT, but not the effects on oxygen consumption and carbon dioxide production.[47] Additional maneuvers, such as endotracheal suctioning, even for brief periods, may cause significant desaturation and adverse hemodynamic effects, particularly if mechanical ventilation or PEEP must be interrupted. Nasotracheal suctioning of the spontaneously breathing patient is a particularly noxious procedure that should be avoided.

Treatment with sympathomimetic bronchodilators, systemically or by aerosol, must also be carefully evaluated for potential risks and benefits. Adverse effects on cardiac rhythm or myocardial oxygen consumption might occur. However, in the patient with significant and reversible bronchospasm, the improvements in ventilation-perfusion relationships, oxygenation, and work of breathing typically outweigh any effects of cardiac stimulation, and these medications should not be withheld.

CARDIOPULMONARY RESUSCITATION

Algorithms for the management of sudden cardiorespiratory arrest are outlined in Chapter 22. Cardiac arrest related to myocardial infarction most often occurs within the first 24 to 48 hours of hospitalization. In-hospital mortality of approximately 80% has been observed, although long-term survival rates may be similar for patients discharged following acute myocardial infarction, with or without a history of resuscitation from cardiac arrest.[48]

The basic components of cardiopulmonary resuscitation are external chest compression and artificial ventilation. The respiratory care practitioner is frequently a part of the CPR provider team and may also face treating complications of CPR in the patient who survives resuscitation. The most commonly observed complication of CPR has been injury to the sternum and ribs from chest compressions.[49,50] A flail chest is less common but may require temporary support with positive-pressure ventilation.[51] Mechanical ventilation should be volume cycled to assure constant inflation and adequate tidal volume. Current ventilator models may provide increased trigger sensitivity by responding to small decreases in baseline flow through the circuit, requiring less effort and generation of negative pressure by the patient. Mediastinal hemorrhage, pneumothorax, or hemothorax may occur during CPR. Traumatic injury to abdominal viscera may also occur, with significant hemorrhage or rupture of the stomach, liver, or spleen. Burn injuries of the chest wall may complicate attempts at defibrillation.

Complications of airway management are frequent and include regurgitation and aspiration, injuries to the mouth and pharynx, laryngeal trauma, endotracheal tube misplacement, and esophageal injury.[52] In an attempt to avoid gaseous distension of the stomach during bag-mask or mouth-to-mouth ventilation, it has been suggested that a longer inspiratory time (therefore slower flow rate and lower peak pressure) be used, and that cricoid pressure be applied during ventilation.[52]

SUMMARY

There has been rapid evolution of the initial evaluation and treatment of the patient with acute myocardial ischemia. Coexisting cardiac and respiratory diseases commonly occur, and management requires an understanding of cardiopulmonary interactions. Thoughtful respiratory care is an integral part of the successful management of the patient admitted to the coronary care unit.

REFERENCES

1. Standards and guidelines for cardiopulmonary resuscitation and emergency cardiac care. JAMA 268(16):2199, 1992
2. Nishimura RA, Miller FA, Callahan MJ, et al: Doppler echocardiography: Theory, instrumentation, technique and application. Mayo Clin Proc 60:321, 1985
3. Willerson JT: Radionuclide assessment and diagnosis of acute myocardial infarction. Chest 93:(suppl 1):7S, 1988
4. Gill JB, Ruddy TD, Newell JB, et al: Prognostic importance of thallium uptake by the lungs during exercise in coronary artery disease. N Engl J Med 317:1485, 1987
5. Valentine PA, Fluck DC, Mounsey JPD, et al: Blood-gas changes after acute myocardial infarction. Lancet 2:837, 1966
6. Al Bazzaz FJ, Kazemi H: Arterial hypoxemia and distribution of pulmonary perfusion after uncomplicated myocardial infarction. Am Rev Respir Dis 106:721, 1972
7. Ayres SM, Grace WJ: Inappropriate ventilation and hypoxemia as causes of cardiac arrhythmias. Am J Med 46:495, 1969
8. Ishikawa K, Hayashi T, Kohashi Y, et al: Reduction of left ventricular size following oxygen inhalation in patients with coronary artery disease as measured by biplane coronary cineangiograms. Jpn Circ J 48:225, 1984
9. Hoel BL, Bay G, Refsum HE: The effects of morphine on the arterial and mixed venous blood gas state and on the hemodynamics in patients with clinical pulmonary congestion. Acta Med Scand 190:549, 1971
10. Zelis R, Mansour EJ, Capone RJ, Mason DT: The cardiovascular effects of morphine: The peripheral capacitance and resistance vessels in human subjects. J Clin Invest 54:1247, 1974
11. Berthelsen P, St Haxholdt O, Husum B, Rasmussen JP: PEEP reverses nitroglycerin-induced hypoxemia following coronary artery bypass surgery. Acta Anaesth Scand 30:243, 1986
12. Lie KI, Wellens HJ, van Capelle FJ, Durrer D: Lidocaine in the prevention of primary ventricular fibrillation. A double blind randomized study of 212 consecutive patients. N Engl J Med 291:1324, 1974

13. Durrer JD, Lie KI, van Capelle FJL, Durrer D: Effect of sodium nitroprusside on mortality in acute myocardial infarction. N Engl J Med 306:1121, 1982
14. Cohn JN, Franciosa JA, Francis GS, et al: Effect of short-term infusion of sodium nitroprusside on mortality rate in acute myocardial infarction complicated by left ventricular failure. N Engl J Med 306:1129, 1982
15. Gillespie TA, Ambos HD, Sobel BE, Roberts R: Effects of dobutamine in patients with acute myocardial infarction. Am J Cardiol 39:588, 1977
16. Taylor SH, Verma SP, Hussian M, et al: Intravenous amrinone in left ventricular failure complicated by acute myocardial infarction. Am J Cardiol 56:29B, 1985
17. Yusuf S: The use of β-adrenergic blocking agents, IV nitrates and calcium channel blocking agents following acute myocardial infarction. Chest 93(suppl):25S, 1988
18. Yusuf S, Peto R, Lewis J, et al: β Blockade during and after myocardial infarction: An overview of the randomized trials. Prog Cardiovasc Dis 27:335, 1985
19. Gibson RS, Boden WE, Theroux P, et al, and the Diltiazem Reinfarction Study Group: Diltiazem and reinfarction in patients with non-Q-wave myocardial infarction: Results of a double-blind, randomized, multicenter trial. N Engl J Med 315:423, 1986
20. DeWood MA, Spores J, Notske R, et al: Prevalence of total coronary occlusion during the early hours of transmural myocardial infarction. N Engl J Med 303:897, 1980
21. Marder VJ, Sherry S: Thrombolytic therapy: Current status (pt 1 of 2). N Engl J Med 318:1512, 1988
22. Gruppo Italiano Per Lo Studio Della Streptochinasi Nell'Infarcto Miocardio (GISSI): Effectiveness of intravenous thrombolytic treatment in acute myocardial infarction. Lancet 1:397, 1986
23. The ISAM Study Group: A prospective trial of intravenous streptokinase in acute myocardial infarction (ISAM). N Engl J Med 314:1465, 1986
24. International Study of Infarct Survival (ISIS) Steering Committee: Intravenous streptokinase given within 0–4 hours of onset of myocardial infarction reduced mortality in ISIS-2. Lancet 1:502, 1987
25. White HD, Norris RM, Brown MA, et al: Effect of intravenous streptokinase on left ventricular function and early survival after myocardial infarction. N Engl J Med 317:850, 1987
26. Gossage JR: Acute myocardial infarction: Reperfusion strategies. Chest 106:1851, 1994
27. The TIMI Study Group: The thromobolysis in myocardial infarction (TIMI) trial. N Engl J Med 312:932, 1985
28. Verstraete M, Bory M, Collen D, et al: Randomized trial of intravenous recombinant tissue-type plasminogen activator versus intravenous streptokinase in acute myocardial infarction. Lancet 1:842, 1985
29. The GUSTO Investigators: An international randomized trial comparing four thrombolytic strategies for acute myocardial infarction. N Engl J Med 329:673, 1993
30. O'Neill W, Timmis G, Bourdillon P, et al: A prospective randomized clinical trial of intracoronary streptokinase versus coronary angioplasty therapy of acute myocardial infarction. N Engl J Med 314:812, 1986
31. Guerci AD, Gerstenblith G, Brinker JA, et al: A randomized trial of intravenous tissue plasminogen activator for acute myocardial infarction with subsequent randomization to elective coronary angioplasty. N Engl J Med 317:1613, 1987
32. Simari RD, Berger PB, Bell MR, et al: Coronary angioplasty in acute myocardial infarction: Primary immediate adjunctive rescue or deferred adjunctive approach? Mayo Clin Proc 69:346, 1994
33. Eckman MH, Wong JB, Salem DN, Parker SG: Direct angioplasty for acute myocardial infarction: A review of outcomes in clinical subsets. Ann Int Med 117:667, 1992
34. Cohn LH: Surgical treatment of acute myocardial infarction. Chest 93(suppl):13S, 1988
35. Forrester JS, Diamond G, Chatterjee K, Swan HJC: Medical therapy of acute myocardial infarction by application of hemodynamic subsets (pt 1 of 2). N Engl J Med 295:1356, 1976
36. Forrester JS, Diamond G, Chatterjee K, Swan HJC: Medical therapy of acute myocardial infarction by application of hemodynamic subsets (pt 2 of 2). N Engl J Med 295:1404, 1976
37. Light RW, George RB: Serial pulmonary function in patients with acute heart failure. Arch Intern Med 143:429, 1983
38. Hales CA, Kazemi H: Small-airways function in myocardial infarction. N Engl J Med 290:761, 1974
39. Holford FD, Mithoefer JC: Cardiac arrhythmias in hospitalized patients with chronic obstructive pulmonary disease. Am Rev Respir Dis 108:879, 1973
40. Steele P, Ellis JH, Van Dyke D, et al: Left ventricular ejection fraction in severe chronic obstructive airways disease. Am J Med 59:21, 1975
41. Robotham JL: Cardiovascular disturbances in chronic respiratory insufficiency. Am J Cardiol 47:941, 1981
42. Brezins M, Benari B, Papo V, et al: Left ventricular function in patients with acute myocardial infarction, acute pulmonary edema, and mechanical ventilation: Relationship to prognosis. Crit Care Med 21:380, 1993
43. Fedullo AJ, Swinburne AJ, Wahl GW, Bixby K: Acute cardiogenic pulmonary edema treated with mechanical ventilation: Factors determining in-hospital mortality. Chest 99:1220, 1991
44. Chin WDN, Cheung HW, Driedger AA, et al: Assisted ventilation in patients with pre-existing cardiopulmonary disease: The effect on systemic oxygen consumption, oxygen transport, and tissue perfusion variables. Chest 88:503, 1985
45. Räsänen J, Nikki P, Heikkilä J: Acute myocardial infarction complicated by respiratory failure: The effects of mechanical ventilation. Chest 85:21, 1984
46. Meyer TJ, Hill NS: Noninvasive positive pressure ventilation to treat respiratory failure. Ann Int Med 120:760, 1994
47. Klein P, Kemper M, Weissman C, et al: Attenuation of the hemodynamic responses to chest physical therapy. Chest 93:38, 1988
48. Goldberg RJ, Gore JM, Haffajee CI, et al: Outcome after cardiac arrest during acute myocardial infarction. Am J Cardiol 59:251, 1987
49. Krischer JP, Fine EG, Davis JH, Nagel EL: Complications of cardiac resuscitation. Chest 92:287, 1987
50. Enarson DA, Gracey DR: Complications of cardiopulmonary resuscitation. Heart Lung 5:805, 1976
51. Enarson DA, Didier EP, Gracey DR: Flail chest as a complication of cardiopulmonary resuscitation. Heart Lung 6:1020, 1977
52. Melker RJ: Recommendations for ventilation during cardiopulmonary resuscitation: Time for a change? Crit Care Med 13:882, 1985

36 Respiratory Care of the Surgical Patient

Robert S. Campbell
Richard D. Branson
James M. Hurst

PROFESSIONAL SKILLS

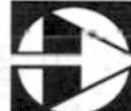

Upon completion of this chapter, the reader will:

- List the causes of changes in pulmonary function caused by surgery and trauma
- Conduct a patient history and physical examination to determine if the patient is at risk for postoperative pulmonary complications
- Assess the patient preoperatively using various spirometric tests to determine risk of postoperative complications
- Explain each step in the emergency room assessment of the trauma patient
- Determine whether the postoperative patient requires mechanical ventilation and the appropriate mode
- Determine which mode of ventilation is best for an ARDS patient
- Explain the alternate forms of mechanical ventilation and oxygenation used in ARDS patients that do not involve manipulating the mechanical ventilator
- Determine a patient's readiness to wean from mechanical ventilation and advise how it is to be done

KEY TERMS

Aspiration
Hemodynamic instability
Hypermetabolic
Hypothermia
Permissive hypercapnia
Physical examination
Postoperative atelectasis
Preoperative pulmonary function testing
Prostacyclin
Tracheal gas insufflation
Ventilatory reserve

Nearly all patients who require major surgical interventions and anesthesia will experience a postoperative decline in pulmonary function.[1–3] Most patients have cardiopulmonary reserves to maintain adequate postoperative gas exchange and pulmonary function with standard respiratory care procedures. Patients with severe pre-existing lung disease or those who require more extensive surgical procedures will need a higher level of respiratory care in terms of both equipment and procedures to maintain pulmonary homeostasis. Fortunately, this last group comprises only a small percentage of both surgical and trauma patients.

For elective surgery, we usually have the ability to evaluate preoperative pulmonary function in order to assess the risk of the planned operation on mortality and morbidity. Generally, patients are considered to be of "low," "moderate," or "high" risk for surgery. We may also have the ability to "fine-tune" or optimize each patient's cardiopulmonary function in preparation for the day of surgery. In patients requiring emergency surgery and most trauma patients, however, there is little or no time to assess pulmonary function preoperatively to determine baseline lung function.

This chapter describes the problems of selecting candidates for therapy, common pathophysiologic postoperative pulmonary changes, and methods of preoperative pulmonary testing, and the postoperative respiratory care of the surgical and trauma patient populations.

POSTOPERATIVE CHANGES IN PULMONARY FUNCTION

Before discussing risks, evaluation, and treatment of postoperative pulmonary complications, it is important to understand the physiologic effects caused by surgical and anesthetic interventions.

Changes in pulmonary function following surgery and trauma have many causes including the following: the surgical procedure, anesthesia, pain, postoperative analgesics, immobilization, and presence of surgical dressings. These changes are certainly more common and pronounced in patients with pre-existing pulmonary disease, but are not uncommon in patients with normal preoperative pulmonary function.[4–7]

The *incision site* is determined by the required surgical procedure and is an important factor in the development of postoperative complications.[8] Extremity and lower abdominal procedures are not likely to cause significant postoperative pulmonary dysfunction.[9,10] Procedures that violate the thorax and upper abdomen have the most severe effects on pulmonary function and are associated with a higher incidence of postoperative complications.[11–14] The *type and duration of exposure to anesthetic agents* will also directly affect the incidence and severity of postoperative pulmonary complications.[15–17] Although there is no such thing as a "risk-free" anesthetic, regional (spinal) techniques usually result in fewer postoperative pulmonary complications.[18] General anesthesia results in diaphragmatic dysfunction and depression of respiratory drive that leads to hypoventilation and hypoxemia.[19–24] Although the operative time is not predetermined by the surgeon, it has been noted that the incidence of postoperative pulmonary complications is nearly doubled when the operative time exceeds 3 hours.[10,25]

Hemodynamic stability is of obvious importance during both the operative and postoperative phase. Aggressive fluid resuscitation is best done with the guidance of information obtained from a pulmonary artery catheter to avoid and more effectively treat patients developing hypovolemia or hypervolemia and pulmonary edema.

The three main postoperative changes in pulmonary function are *reduced lung volumes, impaired gas exchange*, and *abnormalities in breathing pattern.*

Postoperative Changes in Lung Volume

Nearly every postoperative patient will experience a reduction in lung volume (atelectasis) postoperatively.[27–29] Usually this change goes unnoticed because the patient has enough cardiopulmonary reserves to maintain adequate minute ventilation and gas exchange. On assessment, we may commonly note decreased breath sounds in the lung bases and a rapid, shallow breathing pattern. In more severe cases, the prolonged requirement for mechanical ventilation and/or airway pressure therapy is seen.

Following thoracic and abdominal surgery, the total lung capacity (TLC) and each of its subdivisions will be decreased.[6,10,24] Postoperative lung volume changes are most commonly assessed by measuring vital capacity (VC), both because of its ease of measure and for its clinical relevance (ability of the patient to deep breathe and generate an acceptable cough). Normal VC ranges from 55 to 85 mL/kg in adults. In otherwise healthy surgical patients, a VC in excess of 15 mL/kg usually will provide sufficient ventilatory reserves and allow adequate deep breathing and coughing. Thus, a decrease in VC of up to 75% may be well tolerated in most otherwise healthy surgical patients. VC may be reduced by as much as 25% for lower abdominal procedures, 50% for upper abdominal procedures, and 75% for some thoracic procedures.[2,8,10] Intrathoracic surgery involving a median sternotomy tends to create fewer postoperative pulmonary abnormalities than intracostal thoracotomies and, in such patients, these may clear without treatment. Decreases in VC are thought to be the result of diminished diaphragmatic and intercostal muscle function from the surgical procedure, in addition to the respiratory depressant effect of anesthetics and narcotics.[28–30] Alterations in the breathing pattern, most notably the absence of deep breaths, may also contribute to a decrease in lung volume.[21,22]

Reduction in VC occurs gradually over a 12- to 18-hour period following surgical procedures. Following the maximal reduction in VC at approximately 18 hours, the VC gradually increases unless additional complications are present. The VC may be significantly reduced for 48 to 72 hours and usually returns to normal by the seventh postoperative day.

The simplest way of monitoring the severity of VC reduction is to make serial measurements of the patient's respiratory rate. When the patient's respiratory rate exceeds 30 bpm, it usually suggests a significant reduction in *ventilatory reserve.* At this point, it may be helpful to serially monitor VC, tidal volume (V_T), oxygen saturation (S_pO_2), and chest radiographs. These patients will require some form of lung inflation therapy to treat atelectasis and to avoid further pulmonary complications.[31]

Postoperative Gas-Exchange Abnormalities

Decreases in arterial PO_2 and a widening of the alveolar-to-arterial oxygen gradient are common in the postoperative period.[23] The etiology of hypoxemia is multifactorial and includes the following: type of surgery, effects of body position[32–35] (both intraoperatively and postoperatively), immobilization, underlying disease process, and ventilation-perfusion ($\dot{V}/\dot{Q}$) disturbances. Lung zones with a $\dot{V}/\dot{Q}$ of less than 1 (low-but-finite $\dot{V}/\dot{Q}$) and $\dot{V}/\dot{Q}$ of zero commonly develop in the postoperative period. Low-but-finite $\dot{V}/\dot{Q}$ regions result from airway narrowing and loss of lung volume and may be responsive to low-flow oxygen to normalize oxygenation. Regions of lung with $\dot{V}/\dot{Q}$ of zero are generally present in the dependent lung fields owing to airway closure and alveolar collapse and respond poorly if at all to oxygen therapy. Retention of CO_2 usually only occurs if present preoperatively or as a result of respiratory depression from the use or misuse of narcotic agents in the postoperative period.

There are a number of common problems encountered with surgical and trauma patients that should be avoided or appropriately treated to minimize their effects on gas exchange. Aspiration of gastric contents may occur and will certainly complicate the postoperative course. *Hypothermia* will reduce the metabolism of neuromuscular blocking and anesthetic agents and prolong the requirement for mechanical ventilation or respiratory support. *Hemodynamic instability* may jeopardize oxygen delivery to the tissues and require the increased use of fluids or pharmacologic support agents. Patients requiring aggressive fluid resuscitation may develop increased extravascular lung water, which may pose a significant impediment to gas exchange across the alveolar-capillary membrane. The pulmonary vascular bed may be exposed to various humoral substances (endotoxins, enzymes, particulate matter, platelet aggregates, fat particles, micro- or thrombo-emboli) that significantly impede gas exchange and alter lung function. Presence of these substances is common following periods of hypoperfusion, shock, or septic states.

Postoperative Changes in Breathing Pattern

Within 24 hours of upper abdominal surgery, there is an approximate 20% decrease in V_T and a 26% increase in respiratory rate. The result is that minute ventilation, and thus CO_2 excretion, remains relatively unaffected. This holds true as long as the patient's CO_2 production, deadspace-to-tidal-volume ratio (V_D/V_T), and work of breathing remain stable. It is not uncommon for patients to become slightly *hypermetabolic* in response to the stress of surgery, which may cause clinically relevant increases in CO_2 production. In patients with limited ventilatory reserves, this increased "load" on the pulmonary system may cause respiratory failure and necessitate mechanical ventilation. Due to the decrease in lung volume, specifically functional residual capacity (FRC), lung compliance is reduced in the postoperative period.[6] This reduced compliance forces the patient to assume a "rapid and shallow" breathing pattern. This increase in patient work of breathing will lower the efficiency of ventilation and increase the patient's CO_2 production placing the patient at higher risk of developing respiratory failure.

In the early 1960s, work was done to identify the changes in breathing pattern both perioperatively and postoperatively. Bendixen and co-workers[22] showed that normal individuals sigh about 10 times per hour, at nearly three times normal V_T. Sighing was absent in postoperative patients who received morphine for abdominal pain. This, coupled with the technique of mechanical ventilation during the operative period, was thought to cause the changes in lung volume and high incidence of postoperative pulmonary problems.[21] Although postoperative pulmonary problems still occur, the incidence has been reduced by the use of larger tidal volumes during mechanical ventilation, the use of continuous positive airway pressure (CPAP), and postoperative respiratory care procedures that are discussed later in this chapter.

PREOPERATIVE ASSESSMENT AND MANAGEMENT

Postoperative pulmonary complications occur in approximately 6% to 8% of patients with normal preoperative lung function.[36,37] Obviously, both the incidence and severity of these complications will vary based on each patient's inherent preoperative lung function. A good preoperative assessment will decrease both the mortality and morbidity from surgery.[38,39] The incidence of postoperative complications is mostly determined by the operative procedure to be performed and the patient's smoking history.[40] In terms of mortality, the preoperative assessment should identify patients who are inoperable.[12,13,41] In terms of morbidity, each operable patient will be classified according to risk of pulmonary complications (low, moderate, and high) so that their management may be altered in an attempt to lessen the risk and incidence of postoperative pulmonary problems.[42] The majority of risk factors may be identified preoperatively by a complete history and physical examination, chest radiograph, and appropriate pulmonary function screening. The first question to ask is: Who needs preoperative pulmonary evaluation? A more important question is: At what level should each patient be tested?

Patient education should also be provided in the preoperative period. Instruction of common postoperative respiratory care procedures or treatment regimens will improve patient understanding and cooperation if done in the absence of narcotic administration and pain postoperatively.

History and Physical Examination

A sound and carefully obtained patient history and physical examination serves as the foundation on which further assessment and development of an appropriate clinical care plan may be built. In an age where clinicians are looking more to technology for diagnosis and treatment, it stands to reason that a good history and physical provides reliable and necessary information while improving the patient's comfort level with the caregiver, as a rapport is developed during the interview and assessment period. The information gleaned from the patient history and physical assessment will guide the clinician in selection of diagnostic tests that should be performed, and in requesting the therapeutic interventions that would be beneficial in preparing the patient for surgery.[42]

First, the clinician should introduce himself or herself to the patient and clearly state the purpose of the examination. Questions to the patient during the interview should be short and direct, but also tactfully worded. Discussion with patients who have pulmonary complaints should center around the presence, severity, and timing of any episodes of the following: shortness of breath; cough; sputum production; and chest pain. The most important part of the interview involves assessment of the patient's smoking history. Postoperative pulmonary complications increase threefold in patients who smoke. Smoking cessation before surgery may improve the ciliary function of the lung, decrease sputum production, and improve the patient's pulmonary function.[40,43–45] However, roughly 8 weeks is required to show a significant improvement in lung function following smoking cessation. Depending on the required surgical intervention, the risk of waiting 8 weeks for this to occur may outweigh the benefit of delaying the surgery. This is also a stressful time for the patient and might be a particularly bad time to initiate a smoking cessation program. Box 36-1 lists common findings found in the patient history that increase the risk of postoperative complications.

Physical examination is necessary to identify the presence and severity of pulmonary disease and to gauge the patient response to the treatment. The examination should start with the assessment of the patient's vital signs: body temperature, heart rate, blood pressure, and respiratory rate. Examination of the pulmonary system requires the inspection, palpatation, and percussion of the chest. Last, auscultation is necessary to assess the presence and quality of air movement throughout the lung fields and evaluate patency of the airways.

BOX 36-1

RISK FACTORS THAT INCREASE THE INCIDENCE AND SEVERITY OF POSTOPERATIVE PULMONARY COMPLICATIONS

Patient age (>70 years)
Obesity
Positive smoking history
Preexisting pulmonary disease
Cardiac disease
Poor nutritional status
Chronic cough
Chronic sputum production
History of shortness of breath
Adventitious breath sounds
Previous postoperative pulmonary complications

Advanced discussion of the complete pulmonary examination is covered in Chapter 8. Detection of curious signs and symptoms or any positive findings on examination should direct the clinician to further evaluate the patient using more advanced screening tests, which are discussed below.

Chest Radiography

A routine chest radiograph is usually done as a standard preoperative screen for patients scheduled for thoracic or upper-abdominal surgery, to observe any preexisting risk factors or treatable disease. Trauma patients, however, always require a chest radiograph in the emergency department to evaluate the presence of any life-threatening injuries. Chest radiographs are primarily done in an attempt to establish the presence and severity of atelectasis, pneumonia, and pneumothorax. In trauma patients, evidence of rib fractures, widening of the mediastinum, and endotracheal tube placement (if present) are also evaluated. The chest radiograph should be interpreted systematically, paying special attention to the bony structures, diaphragm, heart borders, lung parenchyma, and lung vasculature. A more detailed discussion of radiograph interpretation may be found in Chapter 10.

Preoperative Pulmonary Function Testing

Basic bedside spirometric lung function tests are the most important and sensitive tests that can be performed to assess the risk of postoperative pulmonary complications.[10,24,39] These tests are relatively inexpensive and very easy to perform. The most commonly used test that yields the most useful predictive value is the forced vital capacity (FVC). This test is easily performed by most patients and is highly reproducible. To perform this test, the patient is instructed to inspire the deepest breath possible and then blow as much air out as fast and hard as possible. From this spirogram, both the restrictive and obstructive components of lung dysfunction may be evaluated. Normal FVC is usually the same as VC and is in the range of 55 to 85 mL/kg or 4.8 L in a normal-sized healthy male. A reduced VC indicates restrictive ventilatory defects, and values less than 50% of predicted (or absolute values less than 2.0 L) indicate patients at higher risk of postoperative complications. When measured FVC is less than VC, obstructive lung disease is suggested. This difference is caused by either airway collapse, obstructive airway lesions, or air trapping and is exaggerated during the forced expiratory maneuver when transpulmonary pressure gradients are high.

The forced expiratory volume exhaled in the first second (FEV_1) is a component of the FVC maneuver, which is used to assess both the presence of obstructive lung dysfunction and its response to bronchodilator therapy. The FEV_1 is the optimal test to evaluate obstructive lung disease. Normal FEV_1 is 83% of the FVC or approximately 4.0 L. FEV_1 of less than 50% of predicted level (or less than an absolute value of 2.0 L) indicates moderate obstructive disease, and these patients will have 20% to 40% incidence of postoperative complications. An FEV_1 of less than 1L is associated with a significant increase in postoperative morbidity and mortality. These patients may not be excluded from surgery but should certainly undergo further testing owing to the severity of their baseline pulmonary dysfunction. The FEV_1 is also a useful parameter to assess patient response to bronchodilator therapy. A 20% improvement in the FEV_1 is considered substantial and will aid in the development of a patient care regimen that may reduce the patient's pulmonary risk from surgery.

More advanced pulmonary function tests may be performed, but the increased cost and difficulty may yield little additional beneficial data to assess surgical risk caused by pulmonary dysfunction. These tests include maximum voluntary ventilation (MVV), mid-expiratory flow measurements (FEF 25% to 75%), diffusion capacity (DLCO), exercise testing, maximum O_2 consumption determination, and radionuclide studies.

TRIAGE OF THE TRAUMA PATIENT

The trauma patient presents a specific problem at presentation to the emergency department in that the history and physical examination may only date back to the time of injury. With a greater degree of severity of injuries comes a greater absence of information regarding the incident and the patient's pretrauma health status. The evaluation of any trauma patient presenting to the emergency department should be carried out swiftly and systematically following advanced trauma life support (ATLS) guidelines.[46]

Initial assessment requires evaluation of the ABCs, where A = airway, B = breathing, and C = circulation. This is followed by evaluation of D and E, where D = disability (neurologic assessment), and E = exposure, before developing and instituting the treatment plan. Establishment and maintenance of a patent airway while maintaining control of the C-spine is of paramount importance. Indications for placement of artificial airways are listed in Box 36-2. Following establishment of an airway, the patient's control and effectiveness of breathing must be evaluated. Indications for mechanical ventilatory support are listed in Box 36-3. Once effective ventilation and oxygenation are confirmed or achieved, adequate circulation must be maintained or restored. This requires evaluation of the patient's vital signs (HR and BP) as well as placement of a large-bore peripheral intravenous line to infuse fluid or blood products if necessary. Only after the airway, breathing, and circulation have been assessed and stabilized should the patient be evaluated further for the presence of other life-threatening injuries. Radiographs of the chest, lateral C-spine, and pelvis should be performed as soon as clinically feasible. The abdomen should then be evaluated to rule out internal injuries and bleeding. Physical examination of the abdomen may be adequate to detect severe injuries if the patient is awake and responsive. Diagnostic peritoneal lavage (DPL) is performed to assess bleeding in the abdominal cavity. Patients with positive DPL, hemodynamic instability, or other obvious life-threatening injuries should be taken immediately to the operating room for definitive surgical treatment. Hemodynamically stable patients who respond to interventions in the emergency department may be further evaluated with a CT scan or ultrasound study before transfer to the intensive care unit.

BOX 36-2

INDICATIONS FOR THE PLACEMENT OF ARTIFICIAL AIRWAYS

Airway protection: Relief of upper-airway obstruction, loss of consciousness, angioedema, prevention of aspiration, etc.
Fascilitation/improvement of pulmonary toilet
Use of high oxygen concentrations: May be applied without artificial airways but requires significant skill, equipment, and monitoring
Application of positive pressure to the airways

POSTOPERATIVE RESPIRATORY CARE

The first decision regarding the postoperative management of the surgical/trauma patient is made collectively between the surgeon and the anesthesiologist and con-

BOX 36-3

INDICATIONS FOR MECHANICAL VENTILATION

Apnea
Acute ventilatory failure (respiratory acidosis)
Impending ventilatory failure
Hyperventilation for closed head injury
Refractory hypoxemia

cerns postoperative placement of the patient. Immediate postoperative care and monitoring of the patient will most likely take place in either the surgical intensive care unit (SICU) or the post-anesthesia care unit (PACU). Placement of the patient should be determined based on the preoperative risk factors in addition to the patient's intraoperative course, management, and stability. The next decision is usually made by the staff anesthesiologist and concerns the timing of discontinuance of mechanical ventilation and extubation. Most low-risk surgical/trauma patients may be extubated in the operating room and require only low-flow oxygen therapy in the immediate postoperative period. Patients in the moderate- or high-risk categories will most likely require short-term mechanical ventilation postoperatively.

Patients requiring mechanical ventilation postoperatively can be placed into one of two categories: (1) those that have a relatively uncomplicated surgical procedure and are stable in the immediate postoperative period usually require mechanical ventilation for less than 24 hours, and (2) those at greater risk, who had complications perioperatively, and who had periods of instability in the postoperative phase may require mechanical ventilation for greater than 24 hours postoperatively.

A small percentage of surgical/trauma patients will develop acute respiratory distress syndrome (ARDS) and require advanced mechanical ventilatory and respiratory support, which is further detailed in Chapter 9. The use of the mechanical ventilator and some of the newer treatment modalities for ARDS patients is covered, followed by a discussion of the commonly used respiratory care treatment regimens and procedures used in the less complicated postoperative patients.

Postoperative Mechanical Ventilation

The appropriate use of the mechanical ventilator in the postoperative period may be compared with the use of any pharmacologic agent. It should be instituted/continued based on specific indications, should be titrated to desired effect using specific end points as goals of therapy, and should be weaned or discontinued when no further benefits to the patient are realized. The most common indication for mechanical ventilation postoperatively is apnea. Most patients will only require ventilatory assistance while recovering from the effects of anesthesia and narcotics used during the operative procedure, when apnea is not an uncommon problem.

Other indications for mechanical ventilation include acute and impending ventilatory failure. These patients may have an identical clinical appearance. They generally breathe using a rapid and shallow breathing pattern, demonstrate increased work of breathing (accessory muscle use, intercostal retractions, diaphoresis), and are usually very anxious. The differential diagnosis is only made from interpretation of an arterial blood gas (ABG). Patients in acute ventilatory failure no longer have the cardiopulmonary and metabolic reserves necessary to eliminate or buffer CO_2 and will exhibit an uncompensated respiratory acidosis. The patient with impending ventilatory failure will continue to have the capability to eliminate CO_2 and may even exhibit a respiratory alkalosis.

Once the need for mechanical ventilation has been established, the clinician must first determine the level of support to provide. The mechanical ventilator may be used to provide either full ventilatory support (FVS), where the ventilator is set to provide all of the work of breathing required to generate the necessary minute ventilation, or partial ventilatory support (PVS), where the patient is required to assume a portion of the necessary work of breathing. The level of support provided should be determined by the indication for mechanical ventilation. Obviously, apneic patients will require FVS until spontaneous ventilation is restored. It may be beneficial to provide FVS to patients with acute ventilatory insufficiency for up to 24 hours before transitioning the patient to PVS. Patients in impending ventilatory failure generally tolerate PVS better than FVS because they are able to determine their own breathing pattern. Frequently, patients with impending ventilatory failure may "buck" or fight against the ventilator if FVS is attempted. This may initiate a vicious cycle of sedating the patient for him or her to be able to tolerate the ventilator, which in turn will lengthen the duration of ventilatory support and continue the need for FVS.

□ VENTILATORY MODES

Once the need for mechanical ventilation has been established, the clinician must next determine the mode of ventilation.[47] According to the new classification scheme adopted by the AARC,[48] there are basically three modes of mechanical ventilation and each is determined by the breath type (machine-determined versus patient-determined) available and the timing of each breath (machine triggered versus patient triggered). A mode of ventilation that provides only mandatory breaths is referred to as assisted mechanical ventilation. Variations are available within this mode based on the triggering technique used and include: (1) controlled mechanical ventilation (CMV)—where the sensitivity of the ventilator is turned OFF, not allowing the patient to increase his or her breath rate above the preset rate; (2) assist/control (A/C)—where the sensitivity is set appropriately such that the patient may increase the mandatory breath rate by triggering additional mandatory breaths above the preset level; and (3) assisted mandatory ventilation (AMV)—where there is no preset mandatory rate and the patient is required to trigger each of the mandatory breaths.

Advantages of AMV are that full ventilatory support may be provided and it is safe, due to a preset baseline minute ventilation that will be provided in the event of the absence of spontaneous breathing. Disadvantages include the inability to provide partial ventilatory support with this mode, the increased incidence of respiratory alkalosis with its use,[49] increased incidence of patient/ventilator dys-synchrony,[50] and the potential for breath-stacking, gas-trapping, and the development of intrinsic-PEEP as a result of increased patient demand.[51]

Intermittent mandatory ventilation (IMV) is a mode of ventilation that allows both mandatory and spontaneous breaths. Advantages to using IMV are that both FVS and PVS may be provided. FVS is achieved by increasing the mandatory breath rate sufficient to eliminate spontaneous breathing. A preset minute ventilation may be guaranteed as a result of the mandatory breath rate and V_T settings. PVS may be provided by gradually transitioning work of breathing (by decreasing the mandatory breath rate) to the patient, thus allowing more efficient and comfortable weaning of ventilatory support.[52] Patient tolerance to the additional workload is assessed by monitoring the spontaneous respiratory rate and V_T. During weaning from mechanical ventilation, respiratory rates of >35 bpm and spontaneous V_T of <3 mL/kg are indicative of acceptable levels of respiratory work for most patients.

When the patient shows signs of increased work of breathing, the IMV rate may be increased to the previous level or pressure support (PS) may be used to reduce the work of breathing associated with the spontaneous breaths. PS may be titrated to increase spontaneous V_T and reduce patient respiratory rate during weaning, thus reducing the patient's total work of breathing.[53,54] PS reduces patient work of breathing by making the ventilator provide a portion of the necessary transpulmonary pressure required to generate adequate tidal volumes. PS allows the patient to determine his or her own breathing pattern, frequency, depth, flow rate, and V_T of each spontaneous breath, thus improving patient tolerance to the use of artificial airways and mechanical ventilation.[55]

The third available mode of ventilation only allows spontaneous breaths, which may or may not be supported with positive inspiratory pressure (PS). This mode is referred to as continuous spontaneous ventilation (CSV), but many ventilator manufacturers label it "continuous positive airway pressure" (CPAP) or "Spont." CSV is usually only used during the weaning phase of mechanical ventilatory support because only partial ventilatory support may be provided. This mode of ventilation should be used in conjunction with a ventilator alarm package that will warn practitioners of apnea, low minute ventilation, and high respiratory rate at a minimum to insure patient safety. Use of a pulse oximeter to continuously monitor saturation should also be provided. PS may be used during CSV to augment patient work of breathing to acceptable levels (f <35 and V_T>3 mL/kg). Generally 5 to 10 cmH_2O of PS is used as a baseline to overcome the resistive work of breathing imposed by the endotracheal tube, breathing circuit, and ventilator demand valve.[56]

☐ VENTILATOR SETTINGS

Ventilator settings must be set according to the selected mode of ventilation and may be separated into two categories: those ordered by the physician (physiologic parameters) and those determined by bedside caregivers to facilitate ordered parameters (technical parameters) and provide patient safety (alarms). The following discussion describes the indications for determination of appropriate setting and manipulation of each commonly used ventilator setting.

Physiologic (Physician-Ordered) Ventilator Settings

Control parameter: Tidal volume (V_T) or inspiratory pressure (IP)—Once the clinician has determined the mode of ventilation, the control parameter should be determined and set. The control parameter is that which the ventilator controls during inspiration and is maintained at the expense of all other parameters in the face of varying ventilatory load conditions. Generally, all third-generation mechanical ventilators are capable of controlling either volume, pressure, or flow. The most commonly used control parameter is volume. In volume-controlled ventilation (VCV), the clinician determines the appropriate V_T for each patient, and the ventilator will attempt to deliver that volume regardless of varying patient impedance (compliance and resistance). In other words, as lung compliance becomes lower or resistance is increased, the ventilator will continue to deliver the preset V_T and the ventilating pressures will increase. Setting V_T as the control parameter is considered to be the "conventional" approach to mechanical ventilation because of the safety of having a preset minute ventilation delivery to the patient. V_T is generally initially set between 10 and 12 mL/kg of ideal body weight. Once set appropriately, it is seldom necessary to adjust the set V_T during the patient's course of mechanical ventilation. Reducing set V_T below 10 mL/kg should be considered when ventilating pressures are elevated (plateau pressure >35 cmH_2O) in an attempt to avoid barotrauma or volutrauma to the lung as a result of overdistention of normal lung units.[57–59]

Recently, the use of pressure as the control parameter has become more popular in the ventilation of patients with ARDS.[60,61] During pressure-controlled ventilation (PCV), the ventilator is set to deliver a preset pressure during the inspiratory phase and will maintain that pressure until the cycle variable is attained (usually time). The inspiratory pressure is generally manipulated to maintain an exhaled V_T in the range of 7 to 10 mL/kg. During PCV, it is important to note that the delivered volume is not guaranteed and will vary directly with lung compliance and inversely with airways resistance. PCV has been reported to improve both oxygenation and ventilation in ARDS patients as a result of improved gas exchange.[62,63] The improved gas exchange is likely caused by the decelerating flow pattern, which is inherent to the PCV breath, and the use of inspiratory times that satisfy the longer time-constant lung units common to ARDS.[64] The advantages of PCV are minimized when a decelerating flow pattern is available during VCV. In this instance, PCV still offers the advantage of supplying patient-responsive flow on a breath-to-breath basis. Some investigators have used inverse ratio-pressure control ventilation (PC-IRV) as a way of increasing mean airway pressure while limiting peak ventilating pressures.[65] This technique has lost favor recently due to reported negative hemodynamic effects and the realization that the improved oxygenation is the result of the associated intrinsic PEEP.[66–68]

Mandatory breath rate—Once an appropriate V_T has been established, mandatory breath rate must be set in the AMV and IMV modes of ventilation. If full ventilatory support is the goal, the mandatory breath rate must be set high enough to negate or minimize the need for spontaneous breathing. In combination with V_T, this provides an adequate minute ventilation (V_E) to maintain an acceptable $PaCO_2$ and pH. The $PaCO_2$ will depend on total body CO_2 production (VCO_2), total minute ventilation (V_E), and dead space to tidal volume (V_D/V_T) ratio. Normal postoperative patients who require only short-term mechanical ventilation will need roughly an 8- to 10L/min total V_E to maintain a $PaCO_2$ of 40 mmHg. This generally results in a mandatory rate setting of 8 to 12 bpm. On restoration of spontaneous breathing, partial ventilatory support should be instituted as soon as possible. Patients receiving AMV should be changed to IMV, and the IMV breath rate should be reduced as rapidly as tolerated, thereby transitioning work of breathing to the patient's respiratory muscles. Weaning the IMV rate may be accomplished without arterial blood gas monitoring if the patient's spontaneous respiratory parameters remain acceptable (f and V_T), minimal changes in total V_E are realized, and clinical evaluation suggests VCO_2 is stable.

Pressure support (PS)—Inspiratory pressure support was first introduced more than 15 years ago as a way of decreasing and/or manipulating the work of breathing imposed by ventilator demand valves.[54] Though clearly initiated as a result of "technology in search of need," today, rarely does a patient who requires mechanical ventilatory support for more than 24 hours not receive PS at some point. Initially thought to expedite the weaning process, PS now is used primarily to improve patient/ventilator synchrony, decrease the imposed work of breathing, and augment the patient's breath-to-breath respiratory muscle work performed.[69]

PS use should be limited to patients with intact and reliable ventilatory drive, because only spontaneous breaths may be "supported." PS may be used in either the IMV or CSV modes of ventilation and may be used to provide three distinctly different levels of support: (1) 5 to 10 cmH_2O of PS may be beneficial in overcoming the imposed resistive work of breathing associated with the endotracheal tube, breathing circuit, and demand valve of the ventilator; (2) 10 to 25 cmH_2O may provide PS by augmenting the work performed by the patient's respiratory muscles. PS is accomplished by maintaining the patient's spontaneous breath rate between 20 and 35 bpm; (3) PS levels exceeding 25 cmH_2O generally are thought of as providing FVS. This is confirmed by the delivery of a spontaneous V_T of >10 mL/kg and maintenance of respiratory rates <20 bpm.

Advantages of PS are that the patient determines his or her own breathing pattern, and the ventilator has the ability to adjust the inspiratory flow, V_T, and inspiratory time on a breath-by-breath basis in response to patient demand. The clinician must only determine the optimal inspiratory pressure level, which is usually titrated to maintain a certain respiratory rate, V_T, or combination of the two ($f/V_T < 100$). The only disadvantage or caution to the use of PS is that there is no preset minimum minute ventilation.[55] PS should be used in combination with appropriately set ventilator alarms for apnea, low minute ventilation, and high respiratory rate at a minimum.[55]

Positive end-expiratory pressure (PEEP)—PEEP is the baseline (expiratory) pressure during mandatory breaths that determines the patient's expiratory lung volume or functional residual capacity (FRC). During spontaneous breathing, this baseline pressure is referred to as continuous positive airway pressure (CPAP). The indications for and physiologic effects of PEEP and CPAP are identical. Use of PEEP/CPAP is indicated to improve pulmonary mechanics, gas exchange, or both.[70,71] PEEP/CPAP is useful in the postoperative period in restoring resting lung volume to normal levels. Generally, a minimum of 5 cmH_2O is used to counteract the negative effects of the endotracheal tube, anesthetics, and body position on FRC. Loss of expiratory lung volume results in a reduced lung compliance, which commonly leads to increased patient work of breathing, reduced inspired V_T, and rapid breathing. Appropriate titration of PEEP/CPAP will optimize the patient's lung compliance, reduce the work of breathing, and restore a normal breathing pattern.

Titration of PEEP/CPAP with the goal of improving pulmonary mechanics may be accomplished by simply monitoring the patient's respiratory rate and breathing pattern. If increasing the PEEP/CPAP level has a beneficial effect on lung compliance, the patient's respiratory rate should decrease markedly. The optimal PEEP/CPAP level is the lowest pressure that yields the lowest respiratory rate. Further increases to the PEEP/CPAP level may cause overdistention of more compliant regions of lung, thus reducing lung compliance. This "over-PEEP" effect results in increased work of breathing and respiratory rate and may lead to CO_2 retention.[70]

Titration of PEEP/CPAP with the goal of improving the patient's oxygenation should be done while monitoring oxygenation indices, pulmonary mechanics, and hemodynamic variables. Increasing the PEEP/CPAP level will improve ventilation/perfusion relationships within the lung by recruiting or "opening" previously collapsed alveoli and/or redistributing pulmonary capillary blood flow. PEEP/CPAP may have a negative effect on cardiac index as a result of decreasing venous return to the heart.[72] Thus the "best PEEP" level for the patient may be sought by monitoring the oxygen delivery to the tissues.[73] Monitoring oxygen delivery while titrating PEEP/CPAP is useful to gauge the positive effects on oxygenation (S_pO_2) versus the negative effects on venous return (CO). Monitoring oxygen delivery requires the use of a pulmonary artery catheter that is indicated if more than 15 cmH_2O of PEEP is necessary.

Inspired oxygen concentration (F_iO_2)—Increasing the FiO_2 may have mixed physiologic effects and thus should be done with caution. Supplemental oxygen is commonly used in the postoperative period in an attempt to avoid hypoxemia. Increasing the FiO_2 will increase the partial pressure of oxygen in the alveolar space and thus the PaO_2 if the $\dot{V}/\dot{Q}$ is less than 1, but has little therapeutic effect on the underlying cause of hypoxemia. In some cases, the use of supplemental oxygen may worsen PaO_2 by releasing hypoxic pulmonary vasoconstriction (HPV). Prolonged exposure (>24 hours) to an FIO_2 greater than 0.50 may place the patient at risk of developing oxygen toxicity, which itself may lead to development of ARDS.[74] Typically, FIO_2 is titrated to maintain SpO_2 above 92% to 94%.

Technical (Practitioner-Determined) Ventilator Settings

Sensitivity—The ability of the ventilator to sense patient breathing effort is determined by the sensitivity setting. Traditionally, sensitivity has been accomplished by setting a negative pressure below baseline (typically -2.0 cmH_2O), which the patient must generate to receive a breath from the ventilator. Many of the newer-generation mechanical ventilators now incorporate a flow sensitivity, which may minimize the patient work of breathing associated with triggering.[75] Sensitivity should be set to the most sensitive setting while avoiding "autotriggering," regardless of the sensing technique used.

Inspiratory flow rate and inspiratory time—The cycle variable of each particular ventilator will determine which of these settings must be set by the practitioner. The cycle variable is that which, when met, terminates the inspiratory phase. Typically, European ventilator manufacturers (ie, Siemens, Hamilton, Drager) cycle off inspiration based on time, whereas American-made (ie, Nellcor/Puritan-Bennett, Infrasonics, Bear) ventilators use delivered volume (integrated from flow and time) as the cycle variable. When volume is the cycle variable, inspiratory flow rate must be set by the clinician and in conjunction with the set V_T and inspiratory flow pattern, determines the inspiratory time. Properly setting the inspiratory flow rate to meet patient demand may be the most important determinant of patient work of breathing during assisted ventilation.[76] Use of a waveform analysis package or bedside pulmonary monitor that provides graphic interpretation of airway pressure and flow may be useful in determining the optimal flow rate setting for each patient. The optimal inspiratory flow would result in a relatively square or rectangular airway pressure waveform. In the absence of a graphics package, the clinician may determine appropriate inspiratory flow by assessing the rise of the analog pressure gauge. The optimal flow should result in a gradual, but steady increase in pressure with a slight delay at peak pressure.

Inspiratory flow profile—Most new-generation ventilators allow selection of various inspiratory flow wave forms. The physiologic effects of each waveform have been evaluated in lung model, animal, and human studies.[77–79] Use of a decelerating flow waveform seems to result in improved gas distribution and lower peak airway pressure when compared with rectangular or "square" flow waveforms. When available, the decelerating flow waveform should be used. However, use of the square waveform is an acceptable alternative. Although measurable benefits have been attributed to the use of the decelerating flow waveform, it has not been shown to have any demonstrative effect on patient outcome or duration of mechanical ventilation.

Alarms—Alarm settings are technical settings that improve patient safety by warning practitioners of potentially life-threatening events or of significant changes in patient condition, which may require clinical interpretation and/or intervention.

Alarms are classified into one of three categories dependent on the severity of the event.[80] Level 1 alarms sound to warn of an immediately life-threatening event to the patient and may be the result of loss of electrical power, loss of source gas pressure, or exhalation valve failure. Level 2 alarms warn of events that possibly may be life-threatening if uncorrected and may reflect inappropriate I:E ratio, loss of PEEP, high PEEP, gas-blender failure, autocycling, breathing circuit leak, partially occluded breathing circuit, and/or malfunctioning heater/humidifier. Level 3 alarms warn of a change of patient condition or note certain events such as a change in ventilatory drive, compliance, resistance, or intrinsic-PEEP.

VENTILATION STRATEGIES FOR ARDS PATIENTS

Definitions, mechanisms, and relative outcomes of ARDS and acute lung injury (ALI) have recently been established as a result of an American–European consensus conference on ARDS.[81,82] These definitions are important in order to report and to compare equally the incidence and outcomes of patients with ARDS and the results of future treatment modalities on outcome of like patient populations. Many pharmacologic and treatment modalities have been studied in an attempt to lower the mortality and morbidity of ARDS since its first description in the early 1970s[83] (see Chapter 34). Although the overall mortality of ARDS is lower today than 10 years ago, this appears to be the result of improvements in general care, ICU management, and mechanical ventilation of these patients, and has not been proven to be affected by any one drug, technique, or procedure.

Standard therapy for ARDS patients includes the use of supplemental oxygen, PEEP/CPAP, mechanical ventilation, avoidance of fluid overload, and delivery of care in the ICU setting. The following is a brief description of some nonconventional approaches to the mechanical ventilation of ARDS patients, which have **not** been proven to improve outcome, but have been shown to improve physiologic endpoints.

The use of "super PEEP" (>20 cmH_2O) was popularized in the late 1970s and early 1980s. One study evaluating the effects of super PEEP actually documented the lowest mortality ever published for an ARDS series of patients.[84] More recent studies suggest that consolidated areas of lung are not recruitable at **any** PEEP level and that use of high PEEP levels (>15 cmH_2O)

may only serve to overdistend the more normal areas of lung and place the patient at greater risk of barotrauma or volutrauma.[85,86]

The use of different forms of high frequency ventilation (HFV) was evaluated in the mid-1980s and found to improve ventilation and oxygenation indices while using lower ventilating pressures than conventional VCV.[87,88] HFV has not been shown to improve outcome, reduce required ventilatory support, or minimize complications associated with the ventilation of ARDS patients. HFV is currently used for ventilation of patients requiring laryngeal or tracheopharyngeal surgery, or patients with significant bronchopleural fistula. Difficulties associated with the use of HFV include the inability to provide adequate humidification of the high gas flow delivery and the technical problems associated with the monitoring of airway pressure, volume, and flow.

Many anecdotal and nonscientific descriptions of the use of PCV have shown benefits in regard to gas exchange, pulmonary mechanics, and hemodynamics over VCV.[60,66,68] These reports spurned the increased use and popularity of pressure-limited ventilation over volume-limited techniques in ARDS patients. To date, there continues to be a lack of evidence that use of pressure-limited ventilation provides any benefit in terms of outcome to the use of conventional VCV. PCV may be safer because Paw may be maintained while using lower PIP, and overdistention of normal areas of lung may be minimized due to the pressure limit during inspiration. The beneficial effects of PCV are most likely the result of the decelerating gas flow pattern that is characteristic of a pressure-limited breath. The inspiratory flow pattern is associated with improved gas distribution and ventilation-perfusion matching than the typical "square" flow waveform. Problems associated with the use of PCV result from the fact that there is no preset V_T or V_E, so acid–base balance may be altered rapidly as patient compliance and resistance characteristics change. Use of a decelerating inspiratory flow waveform during VCV should provide the benefits of improved gas exchange seen during PCV, while also providing the safety of having a preset V_T and V_E. PCV may be useful if the ventilator used has no provision for decelerating flow during VCV or if prolonged inspiratory times are used in an attempt to elevate Paw.

Use of inspiratory times that exceed the expiratory time is referred to as inverse ratio ventilation (IRV).[61,62,65] Most reports of IRV use have used PCV as the breath-delivery technique, but VCV may be used equally as effectively.[90] Benefits of IRV are that Paw is elevated, alveoli with longer time constants are recruited, and the shortened expiratory time provides elevated end-expiratory alveolar pressure as a result of gas-trapping. Problems associated with IRV are that patients must be heavily sedated or receive neuromuscular blockade to tolerate this breathing pattern. Intrinsic PEEP often develops and may be difficult to measure.[91] Negative hemodynamic effects of the prolonged inspiratory time, which include reduced venous return and cardiac output, and difficulty assessing preload due to the presence of intrinsic PEEP and its variable effect on measured wedge and central venous pressure, are caused by the inconsistent transmission of airway pressure into the vascular space.

In an attempt to decrease dead space ventilation and improve oxygenation while attempting to minimize the ventilatory pressure requirement, some investigators have suggested application of continuous or intermittent flow of blended, heated, and humidified gas to the lower airway, which is referred to as *tracheal gas insufflation* (TGI).[92–95] During exhalation, gas in the upper airways, endotracheal tube, and apparatus dead space generally have alveolar levels of CO_2 and O_2. This gas is usually rebreathed on the subsequent breath. TGI is an attempt to replace this gas with gas that is free of CO_2 and that has an FIO_2 equal to set inspiratory level of oxygen. Though clinical studies in humans are lacking, early reports suggest that TGI will lower $PaCO_2$ by approximately 15%, or that V_T may be reduced by up to 24% while maintaining the same $PaCO_2$.[92,93] Both of the above-mentioned effects will result in a lower pressure exposure of the injured lung. In turn, this may lower the incidence and severity of barotrauma or volutrauma. However, outcome studies looking at the effects of TGI are still lacking.

Current lung protective ventilation strategies suggest the use of small tidal volumes (<8 mL/kg), minimal peak airway pressures (<35 cmH_2O), and carefully selected PEEP levels using each patient's pressure-volume curve as a guide to determining the minimal PEEP level. Frequently, the use of this protective strategy combined with the increased CO_2 production and dead space/tidal volume ratio typical of ARDS results in elevated arterial levels of CO_2. Acceptance of these high levels of CO_2 with or without an associated acidosis is referred to as *permissive hypercapnia* (PHC). Hickling et al[96] were the first to describe the use of PHC in ARDS patients. They have shown, in retrospective and prospective studies, that mortality and airway pressure requirements were lower in the PHC group.[96,97] Use of PHC reduces the mortality of ARDS by limiting the incidence and severity of ventilator-induced lung injury, but it is associated with lengthened ventilator days, ICU days, and hospital stay.[98]

NONVENTILATORY GAS EXCHANGE STRATEGIES FOR ARDS

In the last 20 years, we have made dramatic changes in our approach to the mechanical ventilation of patients with ARDS, with, unfortunately, only moderate improvement in the mortality rate. Although newer approaches, such as the lung protective strategy discussed earlier, permissive hypercapnia, and use of smaller tidal volumes in ARDS patients, appear promising, they have yet to be proven to reduce mortality and complications. Due to the lack of significant improvement in outcome or reduction in complications in

ARDS, many investigators have sought alternate forms of supporting ventilation and oxygenation that do not involve manipulating the mechanical ventilator or the lung per se. These approaches include both extracorporeal and intracorporeal techniques to provide gas exchange independent of the native lung, and inhalation or administration of agents to augment the pulmonary vasculature in an attempt to improve ventilation:perfusion relationships.

Extracorporeal Membrane Oxygenation

Technologic advances in the late 1960s paved the way for the use of extracorporeal support for acute respiratory failure in the early 1970s. Extracorporeal support refers to any device used outside the body to provide gas exchange. Extracorporeal membrane oxygenation (ECMO) is basically a high-flow cardiopulmonary bypass modified for long-term support with the goal of improving arterial oxygenation to the point that the lungs may be "rested" long enough to facilitate recovery.[99,100] ECMO may be provided by either veno-arterial (VA) or veno-venous (VV)[101] routes depending on the size of the patient and the need for cardiac support. VA support is indicated for patients that require some degree of cardiac support and is usually facilitated by draining blood from the femoral vein and reintroducing it via the right common carotid artery.

VV support is only used for patients in pure respiratory failure and is usually facilitated by cannulating the femoral and right internal jugular veins. This technique will not provide full lung "rest" as arterial saturations of 80% to 85% are maintained owing to the mixing of blood returned from the circuit with deoxygenated blood in the right atrium.

The key to success with adult ECMO is proper patient selection.[102] The ideal candidate should have severe but reversible respiratory failure that has been unresponsive to conventional therapy. The endpoint used to determine success should be defined but varies from study to study. Some studies look for improvements in physiologic parameters or the ability to minimize ventilatory support as successful applications of ECMO, whereas others look to coarser patient outcomes, such as patient survival or hospital discharge as measures of success.

Extracorporeal Carbon Dioxide Removal

As the name implies, the primary goal of extracorporeal carbon dioxide removal ($ECCO_2R$) is to remove CO_2 via an extracorporeal circuit and membrane lung gas exchanger. This technique is a variation of the VV ECMO technique and has been championed by European investigators Gattinoni[103], Morris[104], and others.

Only 20% to 30% of the total oxygen exchange takes place in the membrane gas exchange circuit, leaving the bulk of the necessary oxygenation to occur in the native lung. This is facilitated using apneic oxygenation, where 1 to 5 L/min of oxygen is administered via a tracheal catheter at the level of the carina to maintain losses from the patient's oxygen consumption. Mechanical ventilatory support may be substantially reduced to provide 2 to 4 pressure-limited breaths/min, between 35 and 45 cmH_2O, to prevent atelectasis, while adjusting the PEEP level to maintain end-expiratory lung volume. The majority of CO_2 excretion is facilitated by the membrane oxygenator and is titrated to maintain an acceptable pH level.

The average length of pump support reported for $ECCO_2R$ is between 13 and 19 days,[103] compared with 7 days used in ECMO-treated acute respiratory failure. Neither technique has been shown to decrease morbidity or mortality compared with conventional mechanical ventilation in a prospective, randomized trial.

Inhaled Nitric Oxide

Though nitric oxide (NO) is considered by the Occupational Safety and Health Administration (OSHA) as an occupational and environmental hazard, its physiologic effects have been and continue to be the focus of intense investigation. The recognized effects of NO include vascular smooth muscle relaxation, airway smooth muscle relaxation, platelet inhibition, bacteriostasis, and tumor cell lysis.[105] The vasodilatory effect of NO on the pulmonary vasculature makes it particularly appealing in the treatment of patients with pulmonary hypertension and hypoxemia, which are characteristic of patients with ARDS.[106–110] *NO is not currently approved in the United States by the Food and Drug Administration (FDA) for this application, pending completion of many ongoing multicenter randomized, placebo-controlled studies.*

NO is a selective pulmonary vasodilator that provides the beneficial reduction in pulmonary artery pressure, pulmonary vascular resistance, and improvement in ventilation/perfusion distribution.[111–114] Selective pulmonary vasodilitation implies that either pulmonary arteries are dilated while systemic vessels are not, or in the case of NO, that vascular dilitation from inhaled NO only occurs near ventilated alveoli. This improvement in perfusion to ventilated areas of lung appears to be the mechanism for improved oxygenation.

Recently published results of a multicenter, dose-response study of NO therapy in ARDS revealed that 60% of patients receiving NO responded positively (20% improvement in P_aO_2/FIO_2 ratio) and that dosages exceeding 15 ppm did not provide any additional improvement in oxygenation.[115] Because of the high incidence of nonresponse, it would be beneficial to predict which patients would benefit from inhaled NO. Currently, it is difficult to predict responders although some investigators have suggested that the baseline PAP, PVR, or level of lung recruitment may be helpful in predicting which patients would benefit from NO.

Potential adverse effects of NO are methemoglobinemia, presence of nitrogen dioxide (NO_2) >2 ppm, platelet inhibition, increased left ventricular filling pressure, and rebound hypoxemia and/or pulmonary hypertension when the NO is discontinued. Studies to date have concentrated on the physiologic response to inhaled NO. The effect of NO on outcome from ARDS is yet to be established. Recent studies have suggested that inhaled *prostacyclin* may also have a role similar to NO in the treatment of pulmonary hypertension and ARDS.

Partial Liquid Ventilation

During partial liquid ventilation (PLV), the functional residual capacity (FRC) of the lungs is filled with perfluorocarbon liquid and the patient is gas-ventilated above FRC with a conventional ventilator.[116] Perfluorocarbon liquids have high gas solubility (50 mL O_2/100 mL perfluorocarbon), low viscosity, and lower surface tension than water.[117] In addition, perfluorocarbon is biologically inert, nonabsorbable, and immiscible with native and exogenous surfactant. Initially, perfluorocarbon is administered via a side-port adaptor attached directly to the endotracheal tube at a slow (10 to 30 mL/min) rate until 30 mL/kg have been administered or a meniscus forms within the endotracheal tube with the PEEP turned off. Because of its low surface tension, perfluorocarbon evaporates fairly quickly and the patient must be redosed or "topped off" at regular intervals (every 2 to 4 hours).

PLV offers advantages to gas exchange due to: (1) diffusion of oxygen through the liquid media to the highly perfused, gravity-dependent region of the lung, (2) a "liquid PEEP" effect which preferentially distends lung units in the dependent lung as a result of the height of the liquid column within the lung, (3) enhanced clearance of airway secretions or debris that "floats" up to the upper airway where they may be suctioned, and (4) reducing the lung injury associated with ARDS and positive pressure ventilation compared with conventional gas ventilation.[118–123]

WEANING FROM MECHANICAL VENTILATION

Any discussion regarding the weaning of the mechanical ventilator should start with a clear definition of weaning. By definition, weaning is "the gradual withdrawal of something that is useful or beneficial." If we apply this definition to all the mechanically ventilated patients, we will find that only a very small percentage are actually weaned from ventilatory support. The majority of mechanically ventilated postoperative surgical patients are "discontinued" from ventilatory support rather than weaned.

Before the initiation of ventilator weaning, a thorough patient assessment should be performed to evaluate the patient's readiness to wean, mechanical ability to breathe, and weaning strategy best suited for each patient's condition and situation. First, the indication for mechanical ventilation should be improved or no longer present. Second, the patient's pulmonary mechanics (so-called "weaning parameters") should be assessed. These parameters include respiratory rate, spontaneous tidal volume, minute ventilation, maximum inspiratory pressure, and vital capacity. These parameters assess the patient's mechanical ability to perform the work of breathing and should be used as a guide to when, how, and for what duration the patient is weaned. Weaning parameters should be assessed without any mechanical ventilator support so that they reflect only the patient's mechanical ability and response to the weaning process over time. Box 36-4 lists minimum weaning parameter values which indicate that weaning should be initiated.

Weaning from mechanical ventilation involves the transfer of the work of breathing and minute ventilation from the ventilator to the patient. This transfer of work may be accomplished in one of three ways: (1) transfer of the entire workload to the patient's respiratory muscles during the weaning phase is referred to as T-piece weaning, (2) transfer of only a percentage of the required minute ventilation to the patient's respiratory muscles using unassisted breathing is referred to as IMV weaning, and (3) transfer of a small percentage of the work required per breath to the patient's respiratory muscles is referred to as pressure support weaning.

None of the above-mentioned weaning techniques has been shown to be superior to the others in regard to weaning success or duration. The most important factor determining successful weaning is the implementation of a weaning plan, monitoring the patient during the weaning process, and adjusting the weaning plan based on the patient's condition and response to weaning. For this reason, the weaning approach that is the easiest and most time and cost efficient should be instituted first.

Weaning is most often easily accomplished by incrementally decreasing the IMV rate or decreasing the pressure support level. More often than not, patients tolerate these techniques and they are successful. The speed at which the work of breathing may be transferred to the patient is dictated by the patient's condition and ability to accept the additional workload. Generally, patients successfully weaned using IMV and/or pressure support will not require intensive reconditioning and endurance training of their respiratory muscles.

In patients who require both strength and endurance training of the respiratory muscles, either of the above-

BOX 36-4

COMMONLY USED WEANING PARAMETERS

Pulmonary gas exchange indices
- $PaO_2 > 60$ mmHg with $FIO_2 < 0.35$
- Alveolar-arterial PO_2 gradient of <350 mmHg
- PaO_2/FIO_2 ratio of >200

Ventilatory mechanics indices
- Frequency/tidal volume ratio <100
- Vital capacity >10 to 15 mL/kg ideal body weight
- Maximum negative inspiratory pressure of <-30 cmH_2O
- Resting minute ventilation <10 L/min
- Maximum voluntary minute ventilation > twice resting minute ventilation

mentioned methods or the T-piece method may be used. Unassisted breathing through the endotracheal tube requires high-intensity work from the respiratory muscles that may strengthen those muscles if performed for short periods of time. Eventually, as the patient becomes stronger, he or she will be able to tolerate unassisted breathing for longer periods of time, thus effectively training the respiratory muscles for endurance. It is very important to avoid fatigue of the respiratory muscles as this will decrease the work they are capable of providing and may cause structural damage to the muscle. Respiratory muscle fatigue will usually present as an increased respiratory rate (>35 bpm) and decreased tidal volume (<3 mL/kg). Respiratory muscle strength is easily and quickly restored by providing full ventilatory support with the mechanical ventilator with either the assist/control mode or with high-rate IMV. Restoration of respiratory muscle strength may be monitored by serial measurements of MIP.

Weaning from mechanical ventilation using partial ventilation (IMV and PSV) may be accomplished by titrating the IMV rate and/or PSV level to yield a respiratory rate between 20 and 30 bpm. Using this technique, the respiratory muscles may be rested by increasing the IMV rate or PSV level to maintain a patient rate between 10 and 12 bpm. Resting these difficult-to-wean patients at night helps them sleep more comfortably.

Weaning while alternating periods of full ventilatory support and unassisted breathing periods has previously involved taking the patient off the mechanical ventilator and allowing him or her to breathe through a T-piece to provide humidified gas at a known oxygen concentration. This was accomplished to avoid the high imposed work of breathing associated with spontaneous breathing via the demand valve of older ventilators. Current generation ventilators have work of breathing characteristics that make them better for unassisted breathing than the T-piece. Another advantage of keeping the patient on the ventilator for his or her unassisted breathing trial is that the vital respiratory parameters may be continuously monitored and the alarms will alert the clinician to a change in patient condition that should terminate the weaning trial before exhaustion of the respiratory muscles.

Once the patient has demonstrated the lack of need for the mechanical ventilator, his or her continued need for an artificial airway should be assessed. Extubation parameters should be separate from weaning parameters and include information regarding mental status, ability to protect the airway (intact gag and swallow reflex), sputum characteristics (amount and consistency), and cough effort.

POSTOPERATIVE RESPIRATORY CARE PROCEDURES

Following discontinuation of mechanical ventilation and removal of the artificial airway, respiratory care is directed primarily to prevent or treat any pulmonary complications. Postoperative respiratory care procedures are primarily indicated to prevent atelectasis and lung collapse and to increase or restore any decrease in lung volume.

Some form of lung inflation therapy is indicated on all patients recovering from upper abdominal and thoracic surgery.[5,10,124–126] Use of these techniques in other patients should be determined by clinical assessment and historical findings.[127] The most common forms of lung inflation therapy include: incentive spirometry (IS), chest percussion and postural drainage (CP&PD), cough and deep breathing (CDB), intermittent positive pressure breathing (IPPB), and continuous positive airway pressure (CPAP). Each technique uses a distinctly different method to increase lung volume, and the choice of technique should be determined by preoperative risk factors, specific patient physiology, and patient understanding and cooperation. Generally, these techniques are taught to high-risk patients in the preoperative period while they are free of pain and pain medication. One goal of such efforts is to improve patients' preoperative pulmonary function while helping to prevent postoperative atelectasis.

Comparison of each of the techniques to untreated controls (UC) have been done and the results show significant improvements in both outcome and pulmonary function in patients receiving some form of postoperative respiratory care. In 1970, Stein[9] reported a threefold increase (60% vs. 22%) in pulmonary complications when UC was compared with patients treated with CDB. This study was duplicated in 1988 by Roukema and co-workers[5] who came to the same conclusion with very similar complications between UC (60%) versus CDB (19%). Craven and colleagues[128] compared IS with UC and showed a significant reduction in complications in the IS group (46% versus 71%). In 1984, Celli[126] and others compared CDB, IS, or IPPB with UC and found that no one modality was superior to any other but that all were better than UC (30% to 32% versus 88%).

Many other studies have used CDB as a control when comparing postoperative complications occurring with use of various respiratory care procedures. Bartlett and co-workers[125] compared CDB with IS in 150 patients and found the incidence of pulmonary complications to be 25% and 19%, respectively. In a follow-up study with similar design, Lyager[129] observed complications in 51% of IS patients and only 33% in CDB patients. Two studies with similar design were conducted in the mid-1980s comparing CDB, IS, and Mask CPAP. Stock et al[130] found that CPAP was superior to both CDB and IS following cardiac surgery. Two years later, Rickstein et al[131] came to the same conclusion in patients following upper abdominal surgery.

The "take home message" from these studies is that some form of lung expansion therapy is useful and necessary in moderate and high-risk surgical patients and should be chosen based on availability and cost. However, use of these procedures is costly and unnecessary in low-risk surgical patients.[127] Even when performed properly, nearly 25% of high-risk patients will suffer a postoperative pulmonary complication.

CONCLUSIONS

Nearly every patient having thoracic or upper abdominal surgery will exhibit decreased lung volumes, diaphragmatic dysfunction, and gas exchange abnormalities postoperatively. The degree to which each patient is affected and supported postoperatively is determined by preoperative health status, required surgery, incisional site, operative time, anesthetic technique, and presence of complications. Effective preoperative screening of the patient's pulmonary function may allow prophylactic therapeutic intervention, which may reduce the risk of surgery, allow advanced planning of a perioperative and postoperative care plan, and may improve outcome. Judicious use of the mechanical ventilator in the postoperative period may reduce complications by avoiding episodes of hypoxia or extreme acidemia, whereas early withdrawal and extubation may reduce the risk of infection and improve patient comfort. Once extubated, the respiratory support of postoperative patients centers around avoiding hypoxemia, providing adequate pain relief, and institution of some form of lung inflation therapy. As with any patient population, proper monitoring is the key to avoiding serious complications or adjusting the care plan quickly in the presence of any postoperative complication.

REFERENCES

1. Mendenhall JT: Evaluation and management of pulmonary insufficiency in surgical patients. Surg Clin North Am 48:773–778, 1968
2. Luce JM: Clinical risk factors for postoperative pulmonary complications. Respir Care 29:484–495, 1984
3. Strandberg AA, Tokics L, Brismar B, et al: Atelectasis during anesthesia and in the postoperative period. Acta Anesthesiol Scand 30:154–158, 1986
4. Stein M, Koota GM, Simon M, Frank HA: Pulmonary evaluation of surgical patients. JAMA 181:765–770, 1962
5. Roukema JA, Carol EJ, Prins JG: The prevention of pulmonary complications after upper abdominal surgery in patients with noncompromised pulmonary status. Arch Surg 123:30–34, 1988
6. Meyers JR, Lembeck L, O'Kane H, et al: Changes in functional residual capacity of the lung after operation. Arch Surg 110: 526–583, 1975
7. Craig DB: Postoperative recovery of pulmonary function. Anesth Analg 60:46–52, 1981
8. Elman A, Lagonnett F, Dixsant G, et al: Respiratory function is impaired less by transverse than by median vertical supraumbilical incisions. Intensive Care Med 7:235–239, 1981
9. Stein M, Cassara EL: Preoperative pulmonary evaluation and therapy for surgery patients. JAMA 211:787–790, 1970
10. Tisi GM: Preoperative evaluation of pulmonary function: Validity, indications, and benefits. Am Rev Respir Dis 119:293–310, 1979
11. Ford GT, Whitelaw WA, Rosenal TW, et al: Diaphragm function after upper abdominal surgery in humans. Am Rev Respir Dis 127:431–436, 1983
12. Boysen PG: Assessment for lung resection. Respir Care 29: 506–515, 1984
13. Williams CD, Brenowitz JB: Prohibitive lung function and major surgical procedures. Am J Surg 132:763–766, 1976
14. Ali J, Weisel RD, Layug AB, et al: Consequences of postoperative alterations in respiratory mechanics. Am J Surg 128: 376–382, 1974
15. Bromage PR, Camporesi E, Chestnut D. Epidural narcotics for postoperative analgesia. Anesth Analg 59:473–480, 1980
16. Westbrook PR, Stubbs SE, Sessler AD, et al: Effects of anesthesia and muscle paralysis on respiratory mechanics in normal man. J Appl Physiol 34:81–86, 1973
17. Jayr C, Mollie A, Bourgain TL, et al: Postoperative pulmonary complications: General anesthesia with postoperative parenteral morphine compared with epidural analgesia. Surgery 104:57–63, 1988
18. Rehder K, Sessler AD, Marsh HM: General anesthesia and the lung. Am Rev Respir Dis 112:541, 1975
19. Shuman M, Sandler AN, Bradley JW, et al: Postthoracotomy pain and pulmonary function following epidural and systemic morphine. Anesthesiology 61:569–757, 1984
20. Catley Dm, Thornton C, Jordan C, et al: Pronounced, episodic oxygen desaturation in the post-operative period: Its association with ventilatory pattern and analgesic regimen. Anesthesiology 63:20–28, 1985
21. Bendixen HH, Hedley-Whyte J, Laver MB: Impaired oxygenation in surgical patients during general anesthesia with controlled ventilation. N Engl J Med 269:991–996, 1963
22. Bendixen HH, Bullwinkel B, Hedley-Whyte J, et al: Atelectasis and shunting during spontaneous ventilation in anesthetized patients. Anesthesiology 25:297–301, 1964
23. Jones JG, Sapsford DJ, Wheatley RG: Post-operative hypoxemia: Mechanism and time course. Anesthesia 45:566–573, 1990
24. Jackson CV: Preoperative pulmonary evaluation. Arch Intern Med 148:2120–2127, 1988
25. Tisi GM: Preoperative identification and evaluation of the patient with lung disease. Med Clin North Am 71:399–412, 1987
26. Latimer RG, Dickman M, Day WC, Gunn ML, Schmidt CO: Ventilatory patterns and pulmonary complications after upper abdominal surgery determined by preoperative and postoperative computerized spirometry and blood gas analysis. Am J Surg 122:622–632, 1971
27. Simonneau G, Vivien A, Sartene R, et al: Diaphragm dysfunction induced by upper abdominal surgery: Role of postoperative pain. Am Rev Respir Dis 128:899–903, 1983
28. Shuman M, Sandler AN, Bradley JW, et al: Postthoracotomy pain and pulmonary function following epidural and systemic morphine. Anesthesiology 61:569–575, 1984
29. Froese AB, Bryan AC: Effects of anesthesia and paralysis on diaphragmatic mechanics in man. Anesthesiology 41:242–255, 1974
30. Tokics L, Hedenstierna G, Strandberg A, et al: Lung collapse and gas exchange during general anesthesia: Effects of spontaneous breathing, muscle paralysis and positive end-expiratory pressure. Anesthesiology 66:157–167, 1987
31. O'Donohue WJ: National survey of the usage of lung expansion modalities for the prevention and treatment of post-operative atelectasis following abdominal and thoracic surgery. Chest 87: 76–80, 1985
32. Hedenstierna G, Tokics L, Strandberg AA, et al: Correlation of gas impairment to development of atelectasis during anesthesia and muscle paralysis. Acta Anaesthesiol Scand 30:183–191, 1986
33. Craig DB, Wahba WM, Don HF, et al: Closing volume and its relationship to gas exchange in seated and supine positions. J Appl Physiol 31:717–721, 1971
34. Leblac P, Ruff F, Milic-Emili J: Effects of age and body position on airway closure in man. J Appl Physiol 28:448–451, 1970
35. Don HF, Craig DB, Wahba WM, et al: The measurement of gas trapped in the lungs at functional residual capacity and the effects of posture. Anesthesiology 35:582–590, 1971
36. Wightman JAK: A prospective survey of the incidence of postoperative pulmonary complications. Br J Surg 55:85–91, 1968
37. Torrington KG, Henderson CJ: Perioperative respiratory therapy (PORT): Program of preoperative risk assessment and individualized postoperative care. Chest 93:946–951, 1988
38. Ford GT, Guenter CA: Toward prevention of postoperative pulmonary complications. Am Rev Respir Dis 130:4–5, 1984
39. Goldman L, Caldera DL, Nussbaum AR, et al: Multifactorial index of cardiac risk in noncardiac surgical procedures. N Engl J Med 297:845–850, 1977
40. Bode FR, Dosman J, Martin RR, et al: Reversibility of pulmonary function abnormalities in smokers. Am J Med 59:43–52, 1975
41. Mittman C: Assessment of operative risk in thoracic surgery. Am Rev Respir Dis 84:197–207, 1961
42. Gracey Dr, Divertie MB, Didier EP: Preoperative pulmonary preparation of patient with chronic obstructive pulmonary disease. Chest 76:123–129, 1979
43. Warner MA, Divertie MB, Tinker JH: Preoperative cessation of smoking and pulmonary complication in coronary artery bypass patients. Anesthesiology 60:380–383, 1984

44. Buist AS, Sexton GJ, Nagy JM, et al: The effect of smoking cessation and modification on lung function. Am Rev Respir Dis 114:115–122, 1976
45. Pearce AC, Jones RM: Smoking and anesthesia: Preoperative abstinence and perioperative morbidity. Anesthesiology 61: 576–584, 1984
46. Advanced Trauma Life Support for physicians: 1993 Student manual. Chicago, IL, American College of Surgeons
47. Branson RD, Chatburn RL: Technical description and classification of modes of ventilator operation. Respir Care 37: 1026–1044, 1992
48. Chatburn RL: A new system for understanding mechanical ventilators. Respir Care 36:1123–1155, 1991
49. Hooper RG, Browning M: Acid-base changes and ventilator mode during maintenance ventilation. Crit Care Med 13:44–45, 1985
50. MacIntyre NR: Patient-ventilator interactions, dys-synchrony and imposed loads. In Problems in Respiratory Care, vol 4. Philadelphia, JB Lippincott, 1991, pp 36–43
51. Pepe PE, Marini JJ: Occult positive end-expiratory pressure in mechanically ventilated patients with airflow obstruction. Am Rev Respir Dis 126:166–170, 1982
52. Downs JB, Klein EF, Desautels D, Modell JH, Kirby RR: Intermittent mandatory ventilation: A new approach to weaning patients from mechanical ventilators. Chest 64:331–335, 1973
53. Brochard L, Pluskwa F, Lemaire F: Improved efficacy of spontaneous breathing with inspiratory pressure support. Am Rev Respir Dis 136:411–415, 1987
54. MacIntyre NR: Respiratory function during pressure support ventilation. Chest 89:677–683, 1986
55. Campbell RS, Branson RD: Ventilatory support for the 90's: Pressure support ventilation. Respir Care 38:526–537, 1993
56. Fiastro JF, Habib MP, Quan SF: Pressure support compensation for inspiratory work due to endotracheal tubes and demand CPAP. Chest 93:499, 1988
57. Dreyfuss D, Saumon G: The role of tidal volume, FRC and end-inspiratory volume in the development of pulmonary edema following mechanical ventilation. Am J Respir Crit Care Med 148:1194–1203, 1993
58. Dreyfuss D, Soler P, Basset G, Saumon G: High inflation pressure pulmonary edema: Respective effects of high airway pressure, high tidal volume and positive end-expiratory pressure. Am Rev Respir Dis 137:1159–1164, 1988
59. Kolobow T, Moretti MP, Fumagalli R, Mascheroni D, Prato P, Chen V, Joris M: Severe impairment in lung function induced by high peak airway pressure during mechanical ventilation: An experimental study. Am Rev Respir Dis 135:312–315, 1987
60. Gurevitch MJ, Van Dyke J, Young ES, Jackson K: Improved oxygenation and lower peak airway pressure in severe adult respiratory distress syndrome: Treatment with inverse-ratio ventilation. Chest 89:211–213, 1986
61. Tharratt RS, Allen RP, Albertson TE: Pressure controlled inverse-ratio ventilation in severe adult respiratory failure. Chest 94:755–762, 1988
62. Abraham E, Yoshihara G: Cardiorespiratory effects of pressure controlled inverse-ratio ventilation in severe respiratory failure. Chest 96:1356–1359, 1989
63. Chan K, Abraham E: Effects of inverse-ratio ventilation on cardiorespiratory parameters in severe respiratory failure. Chest 102:1556–1561, 1992
64. Marini JJ, Crooke PS III, Truwit JD: Determinants and limits of pressure-preset ventilation: A mathematical model of pressure control. J Appl Physiol 74:922–933, 1989
65. Marcy TW, Marini JJ: Inverse-ratio ventilation in ARDS: Rationale and implementation. Chest 100:494–504, 1991
66. Lessard MR, Guerot E, Lorino H, Lemaire F, Brochard L: Effects of pressure-controlled with different I:E ratios versus volume-controlled ventilation on respiratory mechanics, gas exchange, and hemodynamics in patients with adult respiratory distress syndrome. Anesthesiology 80:983–991, 1994
67. Mercat A, Graini L, Teboul JL, Lenique F, Richard C: Cardiorespiratory effects of pressure controlled ventilation with and without inverse-ratio in the adult respiratory distress syndrome. Chest 104:871–875, 1993
68. Mang H, Kacmarek RM, Ritz R, Wilson RS, Kimball WP: Cardiorespiratory effects of volume- and pressure-controlled ventilation at various I/E ratios in an acute lung injury model. Am J Respir Crit Care Med 151:731–736, 1995
69. Brochard L, Harf A, Lorino H, Lemaire F: Inspiratory pressure support prevents diaphragmatic fatigue during weaning from mechanical ventilation. Am Rev Respir Dis 139:513–521, 1989
70. Stoller JK: Respiratory effects of positive end-expiratory pressure. Respir Care 33:454–463, 1988
71. Rose DM, Downs JB, Heenan TJ: Temporal responses of functional residual capacity and oxygen tension to changes in positive end-expiratory pressure. Crit Care Med 9:79–82, 1981
72. Dorninsky PM, Whitcomb ME: The effect of PEEP on cardiac output. Chest 84:210–210, 1983
73. Kirby RR: Best PEEP: Issues and choices in the selection and monitoring of PEEP levels. Respir Care 33:569–576, 1988
74. Lodato RF: Oxygen toxicity. Crit Care Clin 6:749–765, 1990
75. Sassoon CSH: Mechanical ventilator design and function: The trigger variable. Respir Care 37:1056–1069, 1992
76. Marini JJ, Rodriguez RM, Lamb V: The inspiratory workload of patient-initiated mechanical ventilation. Am Rev Respir Dis 134:902–909, 1986
77. Rau JL Jr, Shelledy DC: The effect of varying inspiratory flow waveforms on peak and mean airway pressures with a time-cycled volume ventilator: A bench study. Respir Care 36:347–356, 1991
78. Smith RA, Venus B: Cardiopulmonary effect of various inspiratory flow profiles during controlled mechanical ventilation in a porcine lung model. Crit Care Med 16:769–772, 1988
79. Branson RD, Hurst JM: Effects of inspiratory flow pattern on airway pressure, ventilation, and hemodynamics. Respir Care 32:913, 1987
80. MacIntyre NR, Day S: Essentials for ventilator-alarm systems. Respir Care 37:1108–1112, 1992
81. Bernard GR, Artigas A, Brigham KL, Carlet J, Falke K, Hudson L, Lamy M, LeGall JR, Morris A, Spragg R: The American–European consensus conference on ARDS. Am J Respir Crit Care Med 149:818–824, 1994
82. Slutsky AS: Consensus conference on mechanical ventilation, January 28–30, 1993, at Northbrook, Illinois, USA. Part I. Intensive Care Med 20:64–79, 1994
83. Ashbaugh DG, Bigelow DB, Petty TL, Levine BE: Acute respiratory distress in adults. Lancet 2:319–323, 1967
84. Kirby RR, Downs JB, Civetta JM, Modell JH, Dannemiller FJ, Klein EF, Hodges M: High level positive end expiratory pressure (PEEP) in acute respiratory insufficiency. Chest 67: 156–163, 1975
85. Gattinoni L, Pelosi P, Crotti S, Valenza F: Effects of positive end-expiratory pressure on regional distribution of tidal volume and recruitment in adult respiratory distress syndrome. Am J Respir Crit Care Med 151:1807–1814, 1995
86. Gattinoni L, Pesenti A, Avalli L, Rossi F, Bonbino M: Pressure-volume curve of total respiratory system in acute respiratory failure: Computed tomographic scan study. Am Rev Respir Dis 136:730–736, 1987
87. Carlon GC, Kahn RC, Howland WS, Ray C Jr, Turnbull AD: Clinical experience with high frequency jet ventilation. Crit Care Med 9:1–6, 1981
88. Rouby JJ, Fusciardi J, Bourgain JL, Viars P: High-frequency jet ventilation in postoperative respiratory failure: Determinants of oxygenation. Anesthesiology 59:281–287, 1983
89. Hurst JM, Branson RD, Davis K, Barrette RR, Adams KS: Comparison of conventional mechanical ventilation and high-frequency ventilation: A prospective randomized trial in patients with respiratory failure. Ann Surg 211:486–491, 1990
90. Ravenscraft SA, Burke WC, Marini JJ: Volume-cycled decelerating flow: An alternative form of mechanical ventilation. Chest 101:1342–1351, 1992
91. MacIntyre NR: Intrinsic positive end-expiratory pressure. In Branson RD, MacIntyre NR, Problems in Respiratory Care, vol 4. Philadelphia, JB Lippincott, 1991
92. Courser JI Jr, Make BJ: Transtracheal oxygen decreases inspired minute ventilation. Am Rev Respir Dis 139:627–631, 1989
93. Ravenscraft SA, Burke WC, Nahum A, Adams AB, Bakos G, Marcy TW, Marini JJ: Tracheal gas insufflation augments CO_2 clearance during mechanical ventilation. Am Rev Respir Dis 148:345–351, 1993
94. Burke WC, Nahum A, Ravenscraft SA, Nakow G, Adams AB, Marcy TW, Marini JJ: Modes of tracheal gas insufflation: Comparison of continuous and phase-specific gas injection in normal dogs. Am Rev Respir Dis 148:562–568, 1993

95. Adams AB: Tracheal gas insufflation (TGI). Respir Care 41: 285–293, 1996
96. Hickling KG, Henderson SJ, Jackson R: Low mortality associated with low volume pressure limited ventilation with permissive hypercapnia in severe adult respiratory distress syndrome. Intensive Care Med 16:372–377, 1990
97. Roupie E, Dambrosio M, Servillo G, Mentec H, El Atrous S, Beydon L, Brun-Buisson C, Lemaire F, Brochard L: Titration of tidal volume and induced hypercapnia in acute respiratory distress syndrome. Am J Respir Crit Care Med 152:121–128, 1995
98. Hickling KG, Walsh J, Henderson S, Jackson R: Low mortality rate in adult respiratory distress syndrome using low-volume, pressure-limited ventilation with permissive hypercapnia: A prospective study. Crit Care Med 22:1568–1578, 1994
99. Kolobow T, Gattinoni L, Tomlinson T, White D, Pearce J, Iapichino G: The carbon dioxide membrane lung (CDML): A new concept. Trans Am Soc Artif Intern Organs 23:17–21, 1977
100. Gattinoni L, Pesenti A, Bombino M, Pelosi P, Brazzi L: Roles of extracorporeal circulation in adult respiratory distress syndrome management. New Horizons 1:603–612, 1993
101. Keszler M, Kolobow T: Venovenous ECMO. In Arenson RM, Cornish JD, Extracorporeal life support. Cambridge, MA, Blackwell Scientific Publication, 1993, pp 262–273
102. Anderson H, Steimle C, Shapiro M, Delius R, Chapman R, Hirschl R, Bartlett R. Extracorporeal life support for adult cardiorespiratory failure. Surgery 114:161–173, 1993
103. Gattinoni L, Kolobow TH, Agostoni A, Damia G, Pelizzola A, Rossi GP, et al: Clinical applications of low frequency positive pressure ventilation with extracorporeal CO_2 removal (LFPPV-ECCO2R) in treatment of adult respiratory distress syndrome (ARDS). Int J Artif Organs 2:282–283, 1979
104. Morris AH, Wallace CJ, Menlove RL, Clemmer TP, Orme JF, Weaver LK, Dean NC, Thomas F, East TD, Pace NL, Suchyta MR, Beck E, Bombino M, Sittich DF, Bohm S, Hoffmann B, Becks H, Butler S, Pearl J, Raasmusson B: Randomized clinical trial of pressure-controlled inverse ratio ventilation and extracorporeal CO_2 removal for adult respiratory distress syndrome. Am J Respir Crit Care Med 149:295–305, 1994
105. Kam P, Govender G: Nitric oxide: Basic science and clinical applications. Anaesthesia 49:515–521, 1994
106. Zapol WM, Hurford WE: Inhaled nitric oxide in the adult respiratory distress syndrome and other lung diseases. New Horizons 1:638–650, 1993
107. Cioffi WG Jr, Ogura H: Inhaled nitric oxide in acute lung disease. New Horizons 3:73–85, 1995
108. Rossaint R, Falke K, Lopez F, Slama K, Pison U, Zapol WM: Inhaled nitric oxide for the adult respiratory distress syndrome. N Engl J Med 328:399–405, 1993
109. Rossaint R, Gerlach H, Schmidt-Ruhnke H, Pappert D, Lewandowski K, Steudel W, Falke K: Efficacy of inhaled nitric oxide in patients with severe ARDS. Chest 107:1107–1115, 1995
110. Hess D, Bigatello L, Kacmarek RM, Ritz R, Head CA, Hurford WE: Use on inhaled nitric oxide in patients with acute respiratory distress syndrome. Respir Care 41:424–446, 1996
111. Putenson C, Rasanen J, Downs JB: Effect of endogenous and inhaled nitric oxide on the ventilation-perfusion relationships in oleic-acid lung injury. Am J Respir Crit Care Med 150:330–336, 1994
112. Putenson C, Rasanen J, Lopez FA, Downs JB: Continuous positive airway pressure modulates effect of inhaled nitric oxide on the ventilation-perfusion distributions in canine lung injury. Chest 106:1563–1569, 1994
113. Frostell C, Fratacci MD, Wain JC, Jones R Zapol WM: Inhaled nitric oxide: A selective pulmonary vasodilator reversing hypoxic pulmonary vasoconstriction. Circulation 83:2038–2047, 1991
114. McIntyre R, Moore F, Moore E, Piedalue F, Haenel J, Fullerton D: Inhaled nitric oxide variably improves oxygenation and pulmonary hypertension in patients with acute respiratory distress syndrome. J Trauma 39:418–425, 1995
115. Dellinger RP, Zimmerman JL, Hyers TM, Taylor RW, Straube RC, Hauser DL, Damask MC, Davis K Jr, Criner GJ: Inhaled nitric oxide in ARDS: Preliminary results of a multicenter clinical trial. Crit Care Med 24:A29, 1996
116. Fuhrman BP, Paczan PR, DeFrancisis M: Perfluorocarbon-associated gas exchange. Crit Care Med 19:712–722, 1991
117. Hurst JM, Branson RD: Liquid breathing: Partial liquid ventilation. Respir Care 41:416–423, 1996
118. Tutuncu AS, Faithfull NS, Lachmann B: Comparison of ventilatory support with intratracheal perfluorocarbon administration and conventional mechanical ventilation in animals with acute respiratory failure. Am Rev Respir Dis 148:785–792, 1993
119. Curtis SE, Peek JT, Kelly DR: Partial liquid breathing with perflubron improves arterial oxygenation in acute canine lung injury. J Appl Physiol 75:2696–2702, 1993
120. Tutuncu AS, Faithfull NS, Lachmann B: Intratracheal perfluorocarbon administration combined with mechanical ventilation in experimental respiratory distress syndrome: Dose-dependent improvement of gas exchange. Crit Care Med 21:962–969, 1993
121. Leach CL, Fuhrman BP, Morin FC, Rath MG: Perfluorocarbon-associated gas exchange (partial liquid ventilation) in respiratory distress syndrome: A prospective, randomized, controlled study. Crit Care Med 21:1270–1278, 1993
122. Hirschl RB, Pranikoff T, Wise C, Overbeck MC, Gauger P, Schreiner RJ, et al: Initial experience with partial liquid ventilation in adult patients with the acute respiratory distress syndrome. JAMA 275:383–389, 1996
123. Hirschl RB, Tooley R, Parent AC, Johnson K, Bartlett RH: Improvement of gas exchange, pulmonary function, and lung injury with partial liquid ventilation: A study model in a setting of severe respiratory failure. Chest 108:500–508, 1995
124. Van De Water JM, Watring WG Linton LA, et al: Prevention of postoperative pulmonary complications. Surg Gynecol Obstet 135:229–233, 1972
125. Celli BR, Rodriguez KS, Snider GL: A controlled trial of intermittent positive pressure breathing, incentive spirometry, and deep breathing exercises in preventing pulmonary complications after abdominal surgery. Am Rev Respir Dis 130:12–15, 1984
126. Bartlett RH, Brennan MD, Gazzaniga AB, et al: Studies on the pathogenesis and prevention of postoperative pulmonary complications. Surg Gynecol Obstet 137:926–933, 1973
127. Schwieger I, Gamulin A, Forster A, et al: Absence of benefit of incentive spirometry in low-risk patients undergoing elective cholecystectomy. Chest 89:652–656, 1988
128. Craven JL, Evans GA, Davenport PJ, et al: The evaluation of the incentive spirometer in the management of postoperative pulmonary complications. Br J Surg 61:793–797, 1974
129. Lyager S, Nielsen L, Nielsen HC, et al: Can postoperative pulmonary complications be improved by treatment with the Bartlett-Edwards incentive spirometer after upper abdominal surgery? Acta Anaesthsiol Scand 23:312–319, 1979
130. Stock MC, Downs JB, Cooper RB, et al: Comparison of continuous positive airway pressure, incentive spirometry, and conservative therapy after cardiac operations. Crit Care Med 12: 969–972, 1984
131. Rickstein S, Bengtsson A, Sodomerberg C, et al: Effects of periodic airway pressure by mask on postoperative pulmonary function. Chest 89:774–781, 1986

BIBLIOGRAPHY

Jung R, Wight J, Nusser R, et al: Comparison of three methods of respiratory care following upper abdominal surgery. Chest 78:31–35, 1980

Dreyfuss D, Soler P, Saumon G: Mechanical ventilation-induced pulmonary edema: Interaction with previous lung alterations. Am J Respir Crit Care Med 151:1568–1575, 1995

Koshland DE Jr: The molecule of the year (editorial). Science 258:1861, 1992

Wood G: Weaning from mechanical ventilation: physician-directed vs a respiratory-therapist-directed protocol. Respir Care 40:219–224, 1995

Strickland JH Jr, Hasson JH: A computer-controlled ventilator weaning system. Chest 100:1096–1099, 1991

Morris A, Wallace C, Menlove R, Clemmer TP, Orme JF Jr, Weaver LK, et al: Randomized clinical trial of pressure-controlled inverse ratio ventilation and extracorporeal CO_2 removal for adult respiratory distress syndrome. Am J Respir Crit Care Med 149:295–305, 1994

Webb HH, Tierney DF: Experimental pulmonary edema due to intermittent positive pressure ventilation with high inflation pressures: Protection by positive end-expiratory pressure. Am Rev Respir Dis 110:556–565, 1974

MacIntyre NR: Minimizing alveolar stretch injury during mechanical ventilation. Respir Care 41:318–326, 1996

Appendix **A**

Equations and "Rules of Thumb" for Management of Patients

John E. Hodgkin

OXYGENATION

Calculation of PaO_2 Breathing Room Air Based on Age

- Predicted normal PaO_2, ages 14 to 84 years, supine[25]

$$PaO_2 = 103.5 - (0.42 \times \text{age}) \pm 4$$

This was the formula from Sorbini's data, at 500-m elevation. When the data are corrected for a barometric pressure of 760 mmHg, the formula for predicting the normal PaO_2 at sea level becomes

$$PaO_2 = 109 - (0.43 \times \text{age}) \pm 4$$

- Predicted normal PaO_2, ages 15 to 75 years, seated[20]

$$PaO_2 = 104.2 - (0.27 \times \text{age}) \pm 6$$

Calculation of P_IO_2

- P_IO_2 (dry gas) = barometric pressure (P_B) × F_IO_2
- P_IO_2 (humidified gas)

1. P_IO_2 = (barometric pressure − PH_2O) × F_IO_2

   PH_2O = 47 mmHg (normal water vapor pressure for humidified gas)
2. A rough guide to calculating P_IO_2 of humidified gas at or near sea level is as follows.

$$P_IO_2 = (P_B - PH_2O) \times F_IO_2$$

Since P_B is 760 mmHg at sea level and normal PH_2O is 47 mmHg, then $P_B - PH_2O$ = approximately 700. Thus,

$$P_IO_2 = 700 \times F_IO_2,$$

or $P_IO_2 = 7 \times \%\, O_2$ in inspired gas.

Example: *P_IO_2 for an F_IO_2 of 0.40 (40% O_2) is*

$$P_IO_2 - 7 \times 40 = 280$$

Calculation of P_AO_2

1. $P_AO_2 = P_IO_2 - (PaCO_2 \times 1.25)$
   1.25 is a factor for respiratory quotient, assuming a respiratory quotient of 0.8 where oxygen uptake equals 250 mL/min and CO_2 production equals 200 mL/min.
2. Simplified alveolar air equation at sea level, on room air

$$P_AO_2 = 150 - PaCO_2$$

Calculation of Alveolar–Arterial Oxygen Tension Difference

1. $P(A - a)O_2 = P_AO_2$ (calculated) − PaO_2 (measured)
2. Calculation of approximate normal $P(A - a)O_2$, breathing room air, according to patient's age: The $P(A - a)O_2$ increases approximately 4 mmHg for every increase of 10 years in age.

Example: *For an 80-year-old man, the $P(A - a)O_2$ should normally be ≤32 mmHg.*

Determination of the Cause of Hypoxemia

- If $P(A - a)O_2$ is normal, in the presence of hypoxemia, the cause is overall hypoventilation. A reduction in P_IO_2 from high altitude will also reduce the PaO_2, with a normal $P(A - a)O_2$. The $P(A - a)O_2$ is increased when hypoxemia is due to $\dot{V}/\dot{Q}$ mismatch, diffusion defect, or shunt. The average $P(A - a)O_2$ in normal adults is 10 to 15 mmHg; however, it widens normally with aging.
- If the sum of the PaO_2 and $PaCO_2$ is between 110 and 130 mmHg, breathing room air, hypoxemia is due to overall hypoventilation. If the sum of the PaO_2 and $PaCO_2$ is <110, breathing room air or supplemental O_2, the cause is $\dot{V}/\dot{Q}$ mismatch, diffusion defect, or shunt. The sum would also be <110 when a reduction in PaO_2 occurs from the decreased P_IO_2 of high altitude.

Determination if a Patient Is Breathing Supplemental Oxygen

If the sum of the PaO_2 and $PaCO_2$ is >130 mmHg, the patient is most likely breathing supplemental O_2. In young people (eg, <16 years of age) the sum may approach 140 mmHg, even though the subject is breathing only room air.

Determination of Predicted Normal PaO_2 at Altitudes Above Sea Level[12,13,18]

$$a/A\ O_2\ \text{ratio} = \frac{\text{Predicted room air } PaO_2 \text{ at sea level}}{P_AO_2 \text{ at sea level}}$$

Example: *If a patient had a predicted normal PaO_2 of 87 mmHg at sea level, with a P_AO_2 of 100 mmHg, the a/A O_2 ratio would be*

$$a/A\ O_2 = 87/100$$
$$= 0.87.$$

At 5000 feet elevation, assuming a P_B of 632 mmHg, the normal P_AO_2 would be approximately 73 mmHg. The predicted normal PaO_2 for this patient, at 5000 feet elevation, would then be

$$PaO_2\ (\text{normal at 5000 feet}) = P_AO_2\ (\text{at 5000 feet}) \times a/A\ (\text{at sea level})$$
$$= 73 \times 0.87$$
$$= 63.5\ \text{mmHg}.$$

Calculation of F_IO_2 Needed to Achieve a Desired PaO_2, Having Determined an Initial PaO_2 [12,13,18]

This assumes that such factors as cardiac output, $\dot{V}/\dot{Q}$ matchup, shunt, $PaCO_2$, and O_2 uptake remain constant.

Example: *Knowing the patient's F_IO_2, $PaCO_2$, and PaO_2, one can calculate the P_AO_2 and a/A O_2 ratio.*

If a patient has a PaO_2 of 50 mmHg on an F_IO_2 of 0.4, and a $PaCO_2$ of 40 mmHg at sea level, the P_AO_2 = 235 mmHg and the a/A O_2 ratio is 0.2127. If a PaO_2 of 70 mmHg is desired in this patient, the a/A O_2 ratio can be used to determine the P_AO_2 and F_IO_2 required to achieve this PaO_2 for this patient.

$$P_AO_2\ (\text{required}) = \frac{PaO_2\ (\text{desired})}{a/A\ O_2\ (\text{calculated})}$$
$$= \frac{70}{0.2127}$$
$$= 329\ \text{mmHg}$$

Assuming a respiratory quotient of 0.8, this can then be fitted into the alveolar air equation to solve for the F_IO_2 needed to produce this P_AO_2.

$$P_AO_2 = P_IO_2 - (PaCO_2 \times 1.25)$$
$$P_AO_2 = (P_B - P_{H_2O})F_IO_2 - (PaCO_2 \times 1.25)$$
$$329 = (760 - 47)F_IO_2 - (40 \times 1.25)$$
$$329 = (713)F_IO_2 - 50$$
$$F_IO_2(713) = 379$$
$$F_IO_2 = \frac{379}{713}$$
$$= 0.53$$

If the F_IO_2 is raised from 0.4 to 0.53, assuming things remain stable, the PaO_2 should increase from 50 mmHg to 70 mmHg. Of course, the PaO_2 must always be measured to determine the true PaO_2 on the new F_IO_2.

Calculation of Oxygen Uptake ($\dot{V}O_2$) or Cardiac Output ($\dot{Q}$) With the Fick Equation

$$\dot{Q} = \frac{\dot{V}O_2}{(CaO_2 - C\bar{v}O_2)10}$$

$\dot{V}O_2$ is in mL/min, CaO_2 and $C\bar{v}O_2$ are in mL O_2/100 mL blood. The factor 10 is necessary to express $\dot{Q}$ in L/min.

Calculation of Physiologic Shunt

$$\frac{\dot{Q}_S}{\dot{Q}_T} = \frac{(CcO_2 - CaO_2)}{(CcO_2 - C\bar{v}O_2)}$$

$\dot{Q}_S/\dot{Q}_T$ = ratio of shunt to cardiac output. CcO_2 represents the end-pulmonary capillary O_2 content in mL O_2/100 mL blood.

For calculation of O_2 content in arterial (CaO_2) and mixed venous ($C\bar{v}O_2$) blood, use the following equations.[24]

$$O_2\ \text{content} = \text{mL } O_2 \text{ bound to Hb/100 mL blood} + \text{mL } O_2 \text{ dissolved/100 mL blood}$$
$$= [\text{Hb(g/100 mL)} \times O_2\ \text{saturation} \times 1.39^*] + (PaO_2 \times 0.003)$$

For determination of CcO_2, it is best to take carboxyhemoglobin (HbCO) into account.[7] The P_AO_2 should first be calculated. If the P_AO_2 is greater than 150 mmHg, the PcO_2 is assumed to equal the P_AO_2, and the formula is

$$CcO_2 = \text{Hb}[(1.0 - \text{HbCO})(1.39)] + (0.003 \times P_AO_2).$$

The following correction factors are recommended for a $P_AO_2 \leq 150$ mmHg.[7,24]

If $P_AO_2 > 125$ and ≤ 150 mmHg, then $CcO_2 = \text{Hb}[(1.0 - \text{HbCO}) - 0.01](1.39) + (0.003 \times P_AO_2)$

If $P_A > 100$ and ≤ 125 mmHg, then $CcO_2 = \text{Hb}[(1.0 - \text{HbCO}) - 0.02](1.39) + (0.003 \times P_AO_2)$

If HbCO (carboxyhemoglobin) is not measured directly, one could assume that the HbCO is approximately 1.5%.

Estimation of Shunt

If a patient is breathing 100% O_2, there is a 5% shunt for every 100 mmHg the PaO_2 is below that expected.

Example: *For a patient at sea level, the PaO_2 breathing 100% O_2 should be 550 to 600 mmHg normally. If the PaO_2 is 300 mmHg, one has a 15% shunt, plus the normal 3% to 4% shunt everyone has.*

This rule of thumb works well down to a PaO_2 of 100 mmHg. Below this level, it is no longer accurate.

* Some use the factor 1.34 here; however, there is evidence that 1.39 is more accurate.

ACID–BASE

Calculation of Extracellular Fluid Base Excess (BE_{ECF})[9]

$$BE_{ECF} = \Delta HCO_3^- + 10\Delta pH$$

Where ΔHCO_3^- = actual HCO_3^- − 24 and ΔpH = actual pH − 7.4.

***Example:** If the pH = 7.14 and plasma HCO_3^- = 28 mEq/L, then*

$$\begin{aligned} BE_{ECF} &= (28 - 24) + 10(7.14 - 7.40) \\ &= 4 + 10(-0.26) \\ &= 4 - 2.6 \\ &= 1.4 \text{ mEq/L} \end{aligned}$$

See Chapter 9, Arterial Blood Gas Analysis, for a detailed explanation of extracellular fluid base excess.

In Acute Respiratory Acidosis

The plasma bicarbonate will increase, rapidly, approximately 1 mEq/L for every 15 mmHg increase in the $PaCO_2$ above 40 mmHg as a result of the bicarbonate–carbonic acid buffer reaction.[2] This small increase in bicarbonate does not represent renal compensation for the CO_2 retention.

In Chronic Respiratory Acidosis

For each mmHg increase in $PaCO_2$, the HCO_3^- increases 0.4 mEq/L.[4, 10, 16, 21]

In Acute Respiratory Alkalosis

The plasma bicarbonate will decrease, rapidly, approximately 1 mEq/L for every 5 mmHg decrease in the $PaCO_2$ below 40 mmHg as a result of the bicarbonate–carbonic acid buffer reaction.[2] This decrease in plasma bicarbonate does not represent renal compensation for the acute hypocapnia.

In Chronic Respiratory Alkalosis

For each mmHg decrease in $PaCO_2$, the HCO_3^- decreases 0.5 mEq/L.[4, 11, 1]

In Maximally Compensated Metabolic Acidosis

The $PaCO_2$ will decrease by about 1 mmHg for every 1 mEq/L decrease in plasma bicarbonate.[19]

The level of compensatory hypocapnia expected in metabolic acidosis can be calculated by the following formula.[1]

$$PaCO_2 = 1.54 \times \text{plasma } HCO_3^- + 8.36 \pm 1.1$$

In Metabolic Alkalosis

For each mEq/L increase in HCO_3^-, the $PaCO_2$ increases 0.5 to 1.0 mmHg.[5, 8, 21] The ventilatory response to metabolic alkalosis is less predictable than that seen with metabolic acidosis, and compensatory hypercapnia above 55 to 60 mmHg is unusual.[5, 14]

For Reasonably Accurate Conversion of pH to [H+][15]

pH	[H+] (nM/L)
7.0	100
7.05	90
7.1	80
7.15	70
7.2	60
7.3	50
7.4	40
7.5	30
7.6	25
7.7	20
7.8	15
7.9	12.5
8.0	10

One might note that within the range of 7.2 to 7.5 there is a decrease of 0.01 in pH for every increase of 1 nM/L in the [H+].

For Calculating [H+], PCO_2, or Plasma Bicarbonate from the Other Two Values[17]

$$[H^+] = 24 \times \frac{PaCO_2}{\text{Plasma } HCO_3^-}$$

To Determine Whether the Change in [H+] or pH Is Appropriate for Acute Respiratory Acidosis or Chronic Respiratory Acidosis

- In *acute* retention
  One would expect an increase in [H+] of 0.8 nM/L for every increase of 1 mmHg in PCO_2. The increase in PCO_2 × 0.008 = the decrease in pH.[3]
- In *chronic* CO_2 retention
  One would expect an increase in [H+] of 0.3 nM/L for every increase of 1 mmHg in PCO_2. The increase in PCO_2 × 0.003 – the decrease in pH.[3]

Rough Guidelines for $PaCO_2$–pH Relationship in Acute Ventilatory Changes

For every 20 mmHg increase in $PaCO_2$ above 40 mmHg, the pH decreases approximately 0.10 unit.

For every 10 mmHg decrease in $PaCO_2$ below 40 mmHg, the pH increases approximately 0.10 unit.

$PaCO_2$	pH
80	7.20
60	7.30
40	7.40
30	7.50
20	7.60

Determination of Plasma Bicarbonate from pH and $PaCO_2$ (Assuming an Uncompensated Acid–Base Status)

$$\text{Plasma bicarbonate} = \frac{PaCO_2 \times 24}{\text{difference of last two digits of pH and 80}}$$

Example:

$$pH = 7.30$$
$$PaCO_2 = 50$$

$$\text{Plasma bicarbonate} = \frac{40 \times 24}{80 - 30} = \frac{950}{50} = 19 \text{ mEq/L}$$

Estimation of Base Excess from pH and $PaCO_2$ [24]

1. Determine the difference between the measured $PaCO_2$ and 40 mmHg, then move the decimal point two places to the left.
2. If the $PaCO_2$ is above 40 mmHg, subtract one-half of the number calculated in step 1 from 7.40. If the $PaCO_2$ is below 40 mmHg, add the difference to 7.40.
3. Determine the difference between the measured pH and the pH calculated in step 2. Move the decimal point two places to the right and multiply by ⅔.

Example: *Patient with $PaCO_2$ of 75 mmHg and pH of 7.30.*

1. 75 − 40 = 35; moving the decimal two places to the left results in 0.35.
2. Since the $PaCO_2$ is >40 mmHg, 7.40 − (½ of 0.35) = 7.22.
3. 7.30 − 7.22 = 0.08; moving the decimal point two places to the right and multiplying by ⅔ (ie, 8 × ⅔ = 5 mEq/L base excess).

Determination of Bicarbonate Needed in Patients With Metabolic Acidosis

The HCO_3^- needed* = body wt (kg) × BE × 0.3. BE represents the deficit in buffer base. Three-tenths (0.3) is the factor that represents the extracellular space bicarbonate distribution.

MECHANICAL VENTILATION

Calculation of Respiratory System Compliance in Patients Breathing by Ventilator

- Dynamic effective compliance

$$C_{RS}\,(\text{dyn}) = \frac{V_T}{\text{peak pressure}}$$

* Infuse one half of this amount IV, recheck an ABG in 15 to 20 minutes, and repeat the calculation.

If PEEP being used

$$C_{RS}\,(\text{dyn}) = \frac{V_T}{\text{peak pressure} - \text{PEEP}}$$

- Static effective compliance (eliminates airway resistance as a factor).

$$C_{RS}\,(\text{st}) = \frac{V_T}{\text{inflation hold pressure}}$$

If PEEP being used

$$C_{RS}\,(\text{st}) = \frac{V_T}{\text{inflation hold pressure} - \text{PEEP}}$$

Determination of New Minute Ventilation ($\dot{V}_E$) Required to Achieve a Desired $PaCO_2$

- $\text{New } \dot{V}_E = \dfrac{\text{present } \dot{V}_E \times \text{present } PaCO_2}{\text{desired } PaCO_2}$

Example: *Present $\dot{V}_E$ = 8 L/min and $PaCO_2$ = 50 mmHg and a $PaCO_2$ of 40 mmHg is desired*

$$\text{New } \dot{V}_E = \frac{8 \times 50}{40} = 10 \text{ L/min}$$

The new $\dot{V}_E$ can be achieved by either increasing the $\dot{V}_T$ or the respirator rate. Of course, the V_D/V_T ratio is a factor. If the V_T is kept constant, and the ventilator rate is altered to achieve the new $\dot{V}_E$, the foregoing equation should be quite precise. If the V_T is increased, the V_D/V_T obviously changes, and the equation will not be quite as accurate.

- Another method for estimating the change in ventilator rate needed to achieve a desired $PaCO_2$ is as follows:[6]

$$\text{New ventilator rate} = \frac{\text{present ventilator rate} \times \text{present } PaCO_2}{\text{desired } PaCO_2}$$

Example: *If the $PaCO_2$ is 80 mmHg on a ventilator rate of 12 breaths/min, and one desires a $PaCO_2$ of 60 mmHg, then the*

$$\text{new ventilator rate} = \frac{12 \times 80}{60} = 16 \text{ breaths/min.}$$

This method assumes, of course, that the tidal volume remains constant.

- Determination of new $\dot{V}_E$ required to achieve a desired $PaCO_2$, using alveolar ventilation ($\dot{V}_A$)[22]

$$\text{New } \dot{V}_A = \frac{\text{present } \dot{V}_A \times \text{present } PaCO_2}{\text{desired } PaCO_2}$$

Example: *In a 200-lb (lean body weight) patient with a measured tidal volume of 600 mL and a ventilator rate of 10, the $\dot{V}_E$ is 600 mL. The anatomic dead space in this patient would be assumed to be 200 mL (1 mL/lb lean body weight). 200 mL × 10 equals 2000 mL of anatomic dead space ventilation per minute. 6000 mL − 2000 mL represents 4000 mL alveolar ventilation per minute. If*

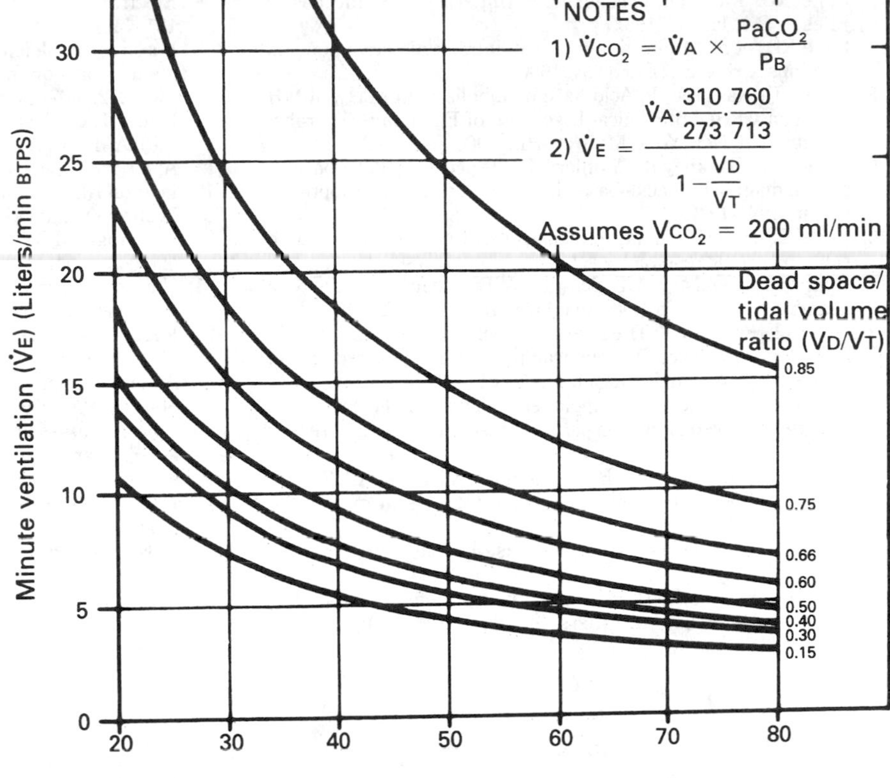

FIGURE A-1. The relation between minute ventilation ($\dot{V}E$) and arterial PCO_2 ($PaCO_2$) for various isopleths of the ratio of physiological dead space to tidal volume (VD/VT). The basic assumptions are noted in the upper right corner. $\dot{V}CO_2$, CO_2 output; $\dot{V}A$, alveolar ventilation; PB, atmospheric pressure. (Selecky PA et al: A graphic approach to assessing interrelationships among minute ventilation, arterial carbon dioxide tension, and ratio of physiologic dead space to tidal volume in patients on respirators. Am Rev Respir Dis 117:181, 1978)

the measured $PaCO_2$ in this patient is 60 mmHg and a $PaCO_2$ of 40 mmHg is desired, then the

$$\text{new } \dot{V}A = \frac{4000 \times 60}{40}$$

$$= 6000 \text{ mL}$$

If the new $\dot{V}A$ is to be achieved by increasing the VT, the VT would have to be increased from 600 to 800 mL, if the ventilator rate remains at 10/min, to achieve the new $\dot{V}A$ required to alter the $PaCO_2$ from 60 to 40 mmHg. An extra 200 mL of alveolar volume/breath × 10 = an increase in $\dot{V}A$ of 2000 mL/min. In this example, the new $\dot{V}E$ is 8000 mL.

If the new $\dot{V}A$ is to be achieved by increasing the ventilator rate, the rate would have to be increased from 10/min to 15/min, if the VT remains at 600 mL, to achieve the new $\dot{V}A$ required to alter the $PaCO_2$ from 60 to 40 mmHg. Since in this patient 400 mL of the 600 mL VT is alveolar volume, then an extra 5 breaths/min will increase the $\dot{V}A$ by 2000 mL/min. In this example, the new $\dot{V}E$ is 9000 mL.

- Determination of new $\dot{V}E$ required to achieve a desired $PaCO_2$, using the VD/VT[23]

The minute ventilation–$PaCO_2$–VD/VT graph depicted in Figure A-1 is used as follows.

1. Place patient on respirator breathing at a minute ventilation ($\dot{V}E$) of 6 to 8 L/min.
2. After 30 minutes of equilibration, measure the minute ventilation and obtain a simultaneous arterial CO_2 tension ($PaCO_2$).
3. The $\dot{V}E$ and corresponding $PaCO_2$ are plotted on the graph. The dead space/tidal volume ratio (VD/VT) is obtained by noting the isopleth that coincides with this point.
4. To obtain the $\dot{V}E$ required to achieve a desired $PaCO_2$, draw a vertical line from the desired $PaCO_2$ on the abscissa to the VD/VT isopleth obtained in step 3. From this point, a horizontal line is drawn to the ordinate to obtain the required $\dot{V}E$.
5. The respirator is then adjusted by changing the tidal volume (VT) or frequency (f) to achieve the newly determined $\dot{V}E$ ($\dot{V}E$ = VT × f). (After 30 minutes at this new $\dot{V}E$ the $PaCO_2$ should be remeasured)
6. As the patient's respiratory problem improves, the VD/VT will often decrease, indicating a need for a lower $\dot{V}E$. This new VD/VT can be calculated as in step 3 and an appropriate $\dot{V}E$ determined.

REFERENCES

1. Albert MD, Dell RB, Winters RW: Quantitative displacement of acid base equilibrium in metabolic acidosis. Ann Intern Med 66:312, 1964
2. Armstrong BW, Mohler JG, Jung RC, Remmers J: The in-vivo carbon dioxide titration curve. Lancet 1:759, 1966
3. Avery AG, Nicotra MB, Deaton WJ: Respiratory acid–base balance. Respir Ther May/June: 59, 1977
4. Bia M, Thier SO: Mixed acid base disturbances: A clinical approach. Med Clin North Am 65:347, 1981
5. Bone JM, Cowie J, Lambie A, Robson JS: The relationship between arterial PCO_2 and hydrogen ion concentration in chronic metabolic acidosis and alkalosis. Clin Sci Mol Med 46:113, 1974

6. Bone RC: Mechanical ventilation: Understanding the basics. J Respir Dis, Jan: 57, 1982
7. Cane RD, et al: Minimizing errors in intrapulmonary shunt calculations. Crit Care Med 8:294, 1980
8. Cohen JJ, Kassirer JP: Acid base metabolism. In Maxwell MH, Kleeman CR (eds): Clinical Disorders of Fluid and Electrolyte Metabolism. New York, McGraw-Hill, 1980, pp 181–232
9. Collier CR, Hackney JD, Mohler JG: Use of extracellular base excess in diagnosis of acid–base disorders: A conceptual approach. Chest 61:6S, 1972
10. Engel K, et al: Quantitative displacement of acid–base equilibrium in chronic respiratory acidosis. J Appl Physiol 24:288, 1968
11. Gennari FJ, Goldstein MB, Schwartz WB: The nature of the renal adaption to chronic hypocapnia. J Clin Invest 51:1722, 1972
12. Gilbert F, Keighly JF: The arterial/alveolar oxygen tension ratio: An index of gas exchange applicable to varying inspired oxygen concentrations. Am Rev Respir Dis 109:142, 1974
13. Gilbert R, Auchincloss J, Kuppinger M, Thomas MV: Stability of the arterial/alveolar oxygen partial pressure ratio. Crit Care Med 7:267, 1979
14. Goldring RM, Cannon PJ, Heinemann HO, Fishman AP: Respiratory adjustment to chronic metabolic alkalosis in man. J Clin Invest 47:188, 1968
15. Jones NL: Blood Gases and Acid–Base Physiology. New York, Brian C Decker, 1980, p 87
16. Kaehny WD: Pathogenesis and management of respiratory and mixed acid–base disorders. In Schrier RW (ed): Renal and Electrolyte Disorders. Boston, Little, Brown & Co, 1976, pp 121–142
17. Kassirer JP, Bleich HL: Rapid estimation of plasma carbon dioxide tension from pH and total carbon dioxide content. N Engl J Med 272:1067, 1965
18. Krider T: Clinical equations for oxygen therapy. In Eubanks DH (ed): AART 1981 Convention Lecture Series: Catch a Star. Dallas, American Association for Respiratory Therapy, 1982
19. Lennon EJ, Lemann J Jr: Defense of hydrogen ion concentration in chronic metabolic acidosis. Ann Intern Med 65:265, 1966
20. Mellemgaard K: The alveolar–arterial oxygen difference: Its size and components in normal man. Acta Physiol Scand 67:10, 1966
21. Narins RG, Emmett M: Simple and mixed acid–base disorders: A practical approach. Medicine 59:161, 1980
22. Rogers RM, Jeurs JA: Physiologic considerations in the treatment of acute respiratory failure. Basics RD, Vol 3 (No 4). New York, American Thoracic Society, 1975
23. Selecky PA, Wasserman K, Klein M, Ziment I: A graphic approach to assessing interrelationships among minute ventilation, arterial carbon dioxide tension, and ratio of physiologic dead space to tidal volume in patients on respirators. Am Rev Respir Dis 117:185, 1978
24. Shapiro BA, Harrison RA, Walton JR: Clinical Application of Blood Gases, 3rd ed. Chicago, Year Book Medical Publishers, 1982, pp 129, 222, 223
25. Sorbini CA, Grassi V, Solinas E: Arterial oxygen tension in relation to age in healthy subjects. Respiration 25:3, 1968

Appendix **B**

Gas Laws and Certain Indispensable Conventions

George G. Burton
H. Frederic Helmholz, Jr.

Readers of this book will probably have learned, and then promptly forgotten, some of the basic physical laws and principles that undergird this profession unless they use them frequently in their day-to-day practice (eg, in the pulmonary physiology laboratory). Accordingly, these laws and principles bear repeating, despite the caveat that their memorization (perish the thought!) can be relegated to an operative sequence of memory devices (mnemonics).[4] Detailed descriptions and discussions of this material have been published elsewhere.[1–7]

STANDARD ABBREVIATIONS AND SYMBOLS

The literature of pulmonary physiology and respiratory care requires a familiarity with scientific notation and its standard abbreviations and symbols (Table B-1).

FACTORS INFLUENCING THE BEHAVIOR OF GASES

Four basic variables affect gas volumetric relationships.

1. Temperature (T), when expressed as degrees Kelvin, indicates the level of energy of a gas sample and is referred to as absolute temperature, converted from temperature centigrade or Celsius, or Fahrenheit.
2. Pressure (P), defined as absolute or total, exerted pressure, is conventionally expressed in atmospheres, or as a given column of mercury or of water balancing the pressure (mmHg, torr, or cmH_2O), or in pascals or kilopascals in the Systeme Internationale (SI) (see under Standard Units).
3. Volume (V) is expressed in cubic units, such as cubic meters or cubic centimeters, or in liters.
4. Relative mass of gas or number of molecules (n) is expressed in gram molecules (the molecular weight of the substance in grams).

For all physiologic measurements the general ("*ideal*") *gas law* can be used without significant error (see a physical chemistry text for Van der Waals equation, which includes the factor of space taken up by molecules and intermolecular forces). The unit *R* is used to indicate the gas constant and perhaps should be designated R^g to differentiate it from *R,* which indicates exchange ratio of respired gases. The ideal gas law states that

$$PV = nR^gT$$

and is expressed in a conglomerate unit telling what units of pressure, volume, and temperature are used. The equation is better understood if one expresses it as follows:

$$\frac{PV}{nT} = \text{a constant}$$

as long as energy equilibrium is obtained, when temperature is expressed on an absolute scale, pressure is absolute pressure, and uniform units are used for pressure, volume, and mass of material. Thus, as long as the amount of gas under consideration remains the same, the following powerful equation is available:

$$\frac{P_1V_1}{T_1} = \frac{P_2V_2}{T_2}$$

This enables one to calculate the changes produced by changing conditions for any gas volume. The general gas law is actually composed of five separate but related laws.

1. *Boyle's law* states that volume varies inversely with absolute pressure (eg, volume is reduced as pressure is increased), other factors remaining constant.

   $$V_1P_1 = V_2P_2$$

   where *T* and *n* are constant.
2. *Charles' law* states that volume is directly proportional to temperature when it is expressed on an absolute scale, other factors remaining constant.

   $$\frac{V_1}{T_1} = \frac{V_2}{T_2}$$

   where *P* and *n* are constant.
3. *Gay-Lussac's law* expresses the same relationship but is stated as follows:

   $$\frac{P_1}{T_1} = \frac{P_2}{T_2}$$

TABLE B-1. **Standard Abbreviations and Symbols Used in Respiratory Care**

Pulmonary Function Tests	
Cst	Static compliance; compliance measured under conditions of prolonged interruption of airflow
E	Elastance; equal to the reciprocal of compliance
Gaw	Airway conductance; equal to reciprocal of Raw
SGaw	Airway conductance at a specific lung volume
Paw	Pressure in the airway; further modifiers to be specified
PA	Alveolar pressure
Pes	Esophageal pressure used to estimate Ppl
PL	Transpulmonary pressure
Ppl	Intrapleural pressure
Ptm	Transmural pressure, pertaining to an airway or blood vessel
PLmax	Maximal inspiratory pressure; this term is often symbolized as MIP
PEmax	Maximal expiratory pressure; this term is often symbolized as MEP
R	Resistance (ie, pressure per unit flow)
$\bar{R}$	Mean total resistance ([RI + RE] ÷ 2)
Raw	Airway resistance
RE	Total expiratory resistance measured by esophageal balloon method
RI	Total inspiratory resistance measured by esophageal balloon method
RL	Lung resistance
WOB	Work of breathing

Arterial Blood Gas, Acid–Base, and Gas Exchange	
pH	Symbol relating the hydrogen ion concentration or activity of a solution to that of a standard solution; approximately equal to the negative logarithm of the hydrogen ion concentration. pH is an indicator of the relative acidity or alkalinity of a solution.
PaO_2	Arterial oxygen tension, or partial pressure
PAO_2	Alveolar oxygen tension, or partial pressure
$PaCO_2$	Arterial carbon dioxide tension, or partial pressure
$PACO_2$	Alveolar carbon dioxide tension, or partial pressure
$P\bar{v}O_2$	Oxygen tension of mixed venous blood
$P(A - a)O_2$	Alveolar-arterial oxygen tension difference. The term formerly used (A − a DO_2) is discouraged
$P(a/A)O_2$	Alveolar-arterial tension ratio: PaO_2:PAO_2. We propose the term *oxygen exchange index* to describe this ratio.
$Ca - vO_2$	Arteriovenous oxygen content difference
SaO_2	Oxygen saturation of the hemoglobin of arterial blood
SpO_2	Oxygen saturation is measured by pulse oximetry
CaO_2	Oxygen content of arterial blood
Blood Flow and Shunts	
Q	Blood volume
$\dot{Q}$	Blood flow (volume units and time must be specific)
Qc	Pulmonary capillary blood volume
Qsp	Physiologic shunt flow (total venous admixture)
Qsp/$\dot{Q}$tot	Shunt as percent of total blood flow
Diffusing Capacity	
DLCOsb	Diffusing capacity of the lung for carbon monoxide determined by the single-breath technique
Dm	Diffusing capacity of the alveolocapillary membrane (STPD)
D/Va	Diffusion per unit of alveolar volume, with D at STPD and VA in liters BTPS

where *V* and *n* are constant. Thus, the pressure of gases when volume is maintained constant is directly proportional to the absolute temperature for a constant amount of gas.

4. *Avogadro's law* states that equal volumes of gases under identical conditions contain equal numbers of molecules, or that the number of molecules is directly proportional to the volume, other factors remaining constant.

$$\frac{n_1}{V_1} = \frac{n_2}{V_2}$$

where *P* and *T* are constant.

5. *Dalton's law* states that gases in a mixture exert pressure equivalent to the pressure each would exert were it present alone in the volume of the tidal mixture, which means that each gas present in a mixture exerts a partial pressure equal to the fractional concentration (by volume) multiplied by the total pressure.

Taken together, Avogadro's law and Dalton's law indicate that in the gas phase, partial pressures will be proportional to molar concentrations, and volumetric expressions will indicate numbers of molecules if a standard is accepted.

By convention, numbers of molecules are indicated in physiology as follows: Whenever gas exchanges (uptake or utilization, or both, or elimination or production, or both) are being studied, volumes are corrected to agreed-on conditions that are standard conditions designated by the initials STPD (standard temperature is 0°C or 273°K; standard pressure is 1 atmosphere or 760 mmHg or 14.69 psi; and *D* stands for a dry gas). One molecular weight of a true gas has a volume STPD (V^{stpd}) of 22.41 L.*

* For CO_2, N_2O, and other gases, the critical temperatures of which are relatively high (near room temperature), this number is somewhat smaller, but it is not significantly different for purposes of respiratory therapy and, therefore, the same "molecular volume" can be used for all gases. Thus, one can calculate R^g using an expression such as

$$\frac{760 \times 22.41}{1 \times 273} = R$$

with the notation that pressure is in mmHg, volume in liters, temperature in degrees Kelvin, and *n* in moles.

The number of molecules in 1 g molecular weight (mole) of a gas has been calculated at $6.06 \times 10.^{23}$ This is fittingly called *Avogadro's number.*

Other conditions under which gases are often measured or in which volumes are expressed are indicated by the initials BTPS (body temperature and pressure saturated). Body temperature is 37° C or 310° K; body pressure is whatever pressure is ambient; and a gas saturated with water at body temperature contains 43.9 mg/L and has a partial pressure of water vapor of 47 mmHg. Volumes of gas (V^{btps}) at body temperature and pressure saturated are effective in washing carbon dioxide out of the pulmonary alveoli, and oxygen partial pressure under these same conditions is that which is effective at the alveolar level in causing diffusion into the blood.

ATPS refers to gas volumes at ambient temperature and pressure, saturated at ambient temperature. This would be the condition of gas in a measuring vessel in which expired air had been collected. ATP alone is used to indicate the same as the foregoing, without water vapor present. (ATPD is preferred for this condition).

Since accurate tables of water vapor pressure at various temperatures are available, it is customary to use water vapor pressure in correcting volumes from wet to dry conditions. One may conclude from the foregoing laws that the volume of a wet gas will bear the following relation to the volume of that gas when the water vapor has been removed (PB equals total or barometric pressure).

$$V_{dry} \times P_B = V_{wet} \times (P_B - P_{H_2O}{}^T);$$

$$V_{dry} = V_{wet} \frac{P_B - P_{H_2O}{}^T}{P_B}$$

since the gas present exerts pressure in the wet gas equivalent to the total pressure minus the partial pressure of water vapor. Thus to correct a volume of gas BTPS or STPD, the following calculation can be given as an example.

$$V_{STPD} = V_{BTPS} \times \frac{P_B - 47}{760} \times \frac{273}{273 + 37}$$

$$= V_{BTPS} \times 0.8146$$

if PB = 760.

OTHER RELATIONS OF IMPORTANCE IN RESPIRATORY THERAPY

Flowing fluids (gases or liquids) obey certain important laws. Fluids flow only when acted on by a force, this force being proportional to a difference in pressure. Some of the laws are given in the following:

Poiseuille's law states that the flow of a fluid or gas that escapes through a tube (V) will be proportional to the pressure difference (ΔP) across the tube, to the fourth power of the radius (r) of the tube, and to time (t), and will be inversely proportional to the length of the tube (L) and the viscosity of the fluid (n).

$$\dot{V} = \frac{\Delta P \pi r^4 t}{8Ln}$$

The density of the fluid is not involved. This law holds only as long as the fluid flows in a laminar (orderly) fashion. Note that π and 8 are constants.

In the last century, Osborn Reynolds presented the concept that a nondimensional number could characterize a system in which there was fluid flow. This number is proportional to the density of the fluid, the velocity of the fluid flow, and the size of the system and is inversely proportional to the viscosity of the fluid. When this number exceeds a certain critical value (which depends on units used in expressing the determining variables), the fluid flow will become turbulent, and Poiseuille's law will no longer describe the situation. Under such circumstances, the flow will no longer increase directly as the differential in pressure increases but will increase only as the square root of the increase of pressure. In normal breathing there is little turbulence in the airway. The formula for the *Reynold's number* is

$$N_R = \frac{\text{fluid density} \times \text{velocity} \times \text{size (of tube or particle)}}{\text{viscosity of fluid}}$$

If the density of a fluid is reduced, and since viscosity is not affected by the density changes, the increase in velocity required to raise the Reynolds' number to a critical level is increased. Thus, the less the density of the fluid, the greater the velocity it must obtain before the flow will become turbulent. The velocity at which any fluid will become turbulent will be characteristic of that fluid and is called the *critical velocity* of that fluid.

The foregoing relationships have important implications for respiratory therapy:

1. In very small tubes of any length, the velocity of the gas cannot exceed the critical velocity at any pressure differential, and thus turbulent flow is impossible (eg, in the small bronchi and bronchioles of the lung).
2. Since turbulent flow in the airways is essential for an effective cough, low density gases ($He–O_2$) will make coughing ineffective. Moreover, the cough cannot effectively move secretions in peripheral airways.
3. Helium as a diluent for oxygen will effectively increase volume flows obtainable through short, narrowed segments of the major airways in which turbulence is present. This is particularly useful when there is turbulence during resting tidal flows.
4. Because aerosol particles are very small, their carriage and deposition are determined essentially by viscosity and kinetic factors alone. Therefore, aerosols are delivered equally well by warm as by cold gases and by helium–oxygen mixtures as by oxygen or air.
5. During forced expiration, substitution of helium for nitrogen in the inhaled mixture will increase that part of the expiratory flow that was restricted by its turbulent character, which would be that in the larger airways—larynx, trachea, and the first few bronchial branchings.

Daniel Bernoulli noted that when the pressure drop across a tubing system was ignored, the total energy at points along the system remained constant. Thus, the lateral pressure energy, the kinetic energy (energy of motion), and the potential energy (energy of position) added up to a constant, when one ignored the effect of friction.*

* Of course, to maintain flow, the total pressure at one end of any system in which a fluid is flowing must be greater than that at the other end.

TABLE B-2. **Units With Abbreviations**

Variable	Unit	Abbreviation
Temperature	kelvin	K
Length	meter	m
Mass	kilogram	kg
Time	second	s
Pressure	pascal	Pa
Work, or energy	joule	J

$$P + hdg + \tfrac{1}{2}dv^2 = \text{a constant},$$

where P = pressure; h = height above a reference plane; d = density; g = acceleration of gravity; and v = velocity. Thus decrease in pressure = $\tfrac{1}{2}dv^2$.

This theorem (*Bernoulli's principle*) explains the way jets of gas entrain materials brought to the side of a high-velocity stream, how the wings of an airplane work, and how water pumps on faucets work. When a fluid flows through a restricted portion of a tube, the velocity must increase; consequently, the energy of motion increases and the pressure en-

TABLE B-3. **Method of Converting Between Usual Units and Metric or SI Units**

Physical Quantity	Conventional Unit	SI Unit	Conversion Factor*
Length	inch (in)	meter (m)	0.025 4
	foot (ft)	m	0.304 8
Area	in^2	m^2	6.452×10^{-4}
	ft^2	m^2	0.092 90
Volume	dL (= 100 mL)	L	0.01
	ft^3	m^3	0.028 32
	ft^3	L	28.32
	fluid ounce → mL		29.57
Amount of substance	mg/dL	mmol/L	10/molecular weight
	mEq/L	mmol/L	valence
	mL of gas at STPD	mmol	0.044 62
Force (weight)	pound (lb)	newton (N)	4.448
	dyne	N	0.000 01
	kilogram-force	N	9.807
	pound → kilogram-force		0.453 6
	ounce → gram-force		28.35
Pressure	cmH_2O	kilopascal (kPa)	0.098 06
	mmHg (torr)	kPa	0.133 3
	pounds/in^2 (psi)	kPa	6.895
	psi → cmH_2O		70.31
	cmH_2O → torr		0.7355
	standard atmosphere	kPa	101.3
	millibar (mbar)	kPa	0.100 0
Work, energy	kg · m	joule (J)	9.807
	L · cmH_2O	joule (J)	0.098 06
	calorie (cal)	joule (J)	4.185
	kilocalorie (kcal)	J	4 185
	British thermal unit (BTU)		1055
Power	kg · m min^{-1}	watt (W)	0.163 4
Surface tension	dyn/cm	N/m	0.001
Compliance	L/cmH_2O	L/kPa	10.20
Resistance	$cmH_2O \cdot s \cdot L^{-1}$	$kPa \cdot s \cdot L^{-1}$	0.098 06
	$cmH_2O \cdot min \cdot L^{-1}$	$kPa \cdot s \cdot L^{-1}$	5.884
Gas transport (ideal gas, STPD)†	$mL \cdot s^{-1} \cdot cmH_2O^{-1}$	$mmol \cdot s^{-1} \cdot kPa^{-1}$	0.455 0
Temperature	°C	°K	°K = °C + 273.15
	°F → °C		°C = (°F − 32)/1.8
	°C → °F		°F = (1.8 · °C) + 32

* To convert from convention to SI unit, multiply conventional unit by conversion factor. To convert in the opposite direction, divide by conversion factor. Examples: 10 torr = 10 × 0.133 3 kPa = 1.333 kPa, 1 L = i L/0.10 = 10 dL

† Gas transport is the same as diffusing capacity and transfer factor and should be distinguished from oxygen transport, which is defined as oxygen content of arterial blood (CaO_2) × cardiac output ($\dot{Q}$).

From Chatburn RL: Measurement, physical quantities, and le système international d'units (SI Units). Respir Care 33:861, 1988; with permission.

ergy (lateral wall pressure) decreases, so that at the edges of any high-velocity fluid stream pressures will be reduced. (*Note:* In a tube beyond the restriction, the lateral pressure again rises.) A high-velocity stream of gas escaping from a nozzle will be surrounded by an area of pressure below atmospheric, and any fluid in the area will be entrained. This explains the way a so-called venturi–oxygen dilutor system works and how jet nebulizers and the Babbington nebulizer entrain fluids at the jets of gas.

Thomas Graham described *effusion*—the process by which a gas passes through an orifice. (An *orifice* is a hole with size, or area, but no length.) The relative rates at which gases can be forced through an orifice are inversely proportional to the square root of the densities of the gases. Adolph Eugen Fick also showed that the rate of diffusion of a gas into another gas was inversely proportional to the square root of the molecular weight and thus the density. The foregoing laws apply only to gas effusion and diffusion in gases. In the diffusion of a gas through other substances (in our frame of reference, an aqueous medium), the solubility of the gas in the medium directly influences the diffusion.

Orders of magnitude should be considered. The diffusion of one gas into another is very rapid and is described by coefficients of "units" per second. When one considers diffusion in an aqueous medium, the coefficients are "units" of the same order of magnitude per 24 hours. The diffusion of gases in gas is at a rate at least 86,000 times that of gases in fluids. In the alveoli and alveolar ducts of the lung, diffusion maintains mixing without any need for gas movement. The process of diffusion is limiting only in the alveolar membrane and plasma, and primarily for oxygen, because it is so much less soluble than carbon dioxide. In a gas, oxygen diffuses faster than carbon dioxide by a factor of 1.173, whereas in an aqueous medium carbon dioxide diffuses at least 20 times more rapidly than oxygen because it is more than 20 times more soluble.

TABLE B-4. **Examples of Conversions Commonly Used in Respiratory Physiology and Respiratory Care**

Physical Quantity	Known Unit	Desired Unit	Example of Conversion Calculation
Force (or mass)	lb	kg	$150\text{ lb} \times \frac{0.4536\text{ kg}}{1\text{ lb}} = 68\text{ kg}$
	kg	lb	$68\text{ kg} \times \frac{1\text{ lb}}{0.4536\text{ kg}} = 150\text{ lb}$
Pressure	torr	kPa	$35\text{ torr} \times \frac{0.1333\text{ kPa}}{1\text{ torr}} = 4.7\text{ kPa}$
	kPa	torr	$4.7\text{ kPa} \times \frac{1\text{ torr}}{0.1333\text{ kPa}} = 35\text{ torr}$
	psi	torr	$1.0\text{ psi} \times \frac{70.31\text{ cmH}_2\text{O}}{1\text{ psi}} \times \frac{0.7355\text{ torr}}{1\text{ cmH}_2\text{O}} = 52\text{ torr}$
	torr	psi	$51.72\text{ torr} \times \frac{1\text{ cmH}_2\text{O}}{0.7355\text{ torr}} \times \frac{1\text{ psi}}{70.31\text{ cmH}_2\text{O}} = 1.0\text{ psi}$
Work	L · cmH_2O	kg · m	$20\text{ L}\cdot\text{cmH}_2\text{O} \times \frac{0.09806\text{ J}}{1\text{ L}\cdot\text{cmH}_2\text{O}} \times \frac{1\text{ kg}\cdot\text{m}}{9.807\text{ J}} = 0.2\text{ Kg}\cdot\text{m}$
	J	L · cmH_2O	$2\text{ J} \times \frac{1\text{ kg}\cdot\text{m}}{9.807\text{ J}} = \frac{1\text{ L}\cdot\text{cmH}_2\text{O}}{0.01\text{ kg}\cdot\text{m}} = 20\text{ L}\cdot\text{cmH}_2\text{O}$
Power	kg · m · min^{-1}	W	$2.5\text{ kg}\cdot\text{m}\cdot\text{min}^{-1} \times \frac{0.1634\text{ W}}{1\text{ kg}\cdot\text{m}\cdot\text{min}^{-1}} = 0.41\text{ W}$
Compliance	mL/cmH_2O	L/kPa	$100\text{ mL}\cdot\text{cmH}_2\text{O} \times \frac{1\text{ L}}{1000\text{ mL}} \times \frac{10.20\text{ L}\cdot\text{kpa}^{-1}}{1\text{ L}\cdot\text{cmH}_2\text{O}^{-1}} = 1.02\text{ L}\cdot\text{kPa}^{-1}$
Resistance	cmH_2O · s · L^{-1}	kPa · s · L^{-1}	$55\text{ cmH}_2\text{O}\cdot\text{s}\cdot\text{L}^{-1} \times \frac{0.090806\text{ kPa}\cdot\text{L}^{-1}}{1\text{ cmH}_2\text{O}\cdot\text{s}\cdot\text{L}^{-1}} = 5.4\text{ kPa}\cdot\text{s}\cdot\text{L}^{-1}$

Retain all digits during computation to avoid roundoff error. However, the least precise measurement used in a calculation determines the number of significant digits in the answer. Thus, the final product or quotient should be written with the same number of significant figures as the term with the fewest significant figures, as shown in the examples above. The least ambiguous method of indicating the number of significant figures is to write the number in scientific notation. For example, the number 30 may have either one or two significant figures, but written as 3.0×10^1, it is understood that there are two significant figures. For more information about scientific notation, significant figures, and rounding off, see Lough MD, Chatburn RI, Shrock WA: Handbook of Respiratory Care. Chicago, Year Book Medical Publishers, 1985, pp 170–173.

From Chatburn RL: Measurement, physical quantities, and le système international d'units (SI Units). Respir Care 33:861, 1988; with permission.

STANDARD UNITS

For several years now there has been a movement to try to standardize units used in expressing laboratory data. The English, as they have converted to the metric system, have begun using the International System of Units (Systeme Internationale d'Units, or SI) (Table B-2). This involves some changes from the metric-based system used in this country. The English recommended the substitution of joules for gram calories (c) and kilocalories (C) as units of energy; the substitution of the pascal and the kilopascal for centimeters of water or millimeters of mercury (torr) as units of pressure, and the substitution of the newton for the barye (1 dyne per square centimeter) as a unit of force (1 newton equals 100,000 baryes). They also advocate the use of the mole as the unit for amount of material instead of grams, milligrams, or other weights, and the substitution of moles per liter for grams percent, milligrams percent, and grams per liter. The use of concentrations as moles per liter is difficult in some situations (eg, for hemoglobin concentrations). Moreover, it is recommended that the very useful convention of expressing ionized materials in equivalents per liter, rather than moles per liter, be retained for physiologic and biochemical expressions. The potential use of SI in respiratory care has recently been described by Chatburn,[3] whose entire discussion bears review by the interested reader.

Some of the implications of the SI system are given in Table B-3, along with the conversion factors for units. All units, including the US units, are based on the international prototype meter and the international prototype kilogram kept at the International Bureau of Weights and Measures in Sèvres, France.

In the metric system the dyne is the unit of force equal to the force required to give a free mass of 1 g an acceleration of 1 cm per second per second. In the SI system the newton is the unit of force equal to the force required to give a free mass of 1 kg an acceleration of 1 m per second per second. The pascal is suggested as the unit of pressure and is equal to a force of 1 newton acting over 1 m^2. This however, is a very small unit, as is the barye of the usual metric system, and, therefore, it is suggested that the kilopascal be used as a unit of pressure for physiologic data.

Examples of SI conversions are given in Table B-4.

REFERENCES

1. Altman PL, Dittmer DS (eds): Respiration and Circulation. Bethesda, MD, Federation of American Societies for Experimental Biology, 1971
2. Bartels H, et al: Methods in Pulmonary Physiology (Workman JM, trans). London, Hafna, 1963
3. Chatburn RL: Measurement, physical quantities, and le système international d'units (SI Units). Respir Care 33:861, 1988
4. Corrie D: Gas law mnemonics. Respir Care 20:1041, 1975
5. Handbook of Chemistry and Physics. Cleveland, Chemical Rubber Publishing Company, 1976
6. International Organization for Standardization: Units of Measurement: ISO Standards Handbook 2. Geneva, ISO, 1979
7. Lentner C (ed): Geigy Scientific Tables: Units of Measurement, Body Fluids, Composition of the Body, Nutrition. West Caldwell, NJ, Ciba-Geigy Corp, 1981
8. Standardization of definitions and symbols in respiratory physiology. Fed Proc 9:602, 1950

Appendix C

Symbols Used in Respiratory Physiology

John E. Hodgkin

θ Rate of gas uptake by 1 mL of normal whole blood per minute for a partial pressure of 1 torr

a Arterial. Exact location to be specific in text when term is used.

A Alveolar

anat Anatomic

ATPD Ambient temperature, pressure, dry

ATPS Ambient temperature and pressure, saturated with water vapor

b Blood in general

B Barometric

BTPS Body temperature (37° C), barometric pressure (at sea level = 760 torr), and saturated with water vapor

c Capillary. Exact location to be specified in text when term is used.

c′ Pulmonary end-capillary

C Concentration in blood phase (primary blood phase symbol)

C Compliance (volume–pressure relationships)

C Concentration (respiratory gases)

C(a − v) Arterial-venous concentration difference

Cdyn Dynamic compliance

Cst Static compliance

C/VL Specific compliance

D Dead space

DL Diffusing capacity of the lung

DL/VA Diffusion per unit of alveolar volume

DM Diffusing capacity of the pulmonary membrane

E Expired

E Elastic

ERV Expiratory reserve volume

f Frequency of any event in time (eg, respiratory frequency: the number of breathing cycles per unit of time)

F Fractional concentration in dry gas phase

FEF$_{x-y}$ Forced expiratory flow between two designated volume points in the FVC

FEF$_{0.2-1.2L}$ Forced expiratory flow between 200 mL and 1200 mL of the FVC; formerly called maximum expiratory flow

FEF$_{25\%-75\%}$ Forced expiratory flow during the middle half of the FVC; formerly called maximum midexpiratory flow

FET$_x$ Forced expiratory time required to exhale a specified FVC

FEV$_1$ Volume of gas exhaled in a given time interval during the execution of forced vital capacity (in this case, the volume exhaled in 1 second)

FEV$_1$/FVC% Ratio of timed forced expiratory volume to forced vital capacity, expressed as a percentage (in this case, the volume exhaled in 1 second/FVC)

FIVC Forced inspiratory vital capacity

FRC Functional residual capacity

FVC Forced vital capacity

Gaw Airway conductance

Gaw/VL Specific conductance expressed per liter of lung volume at which Gaw is measured

I Inspired

IC Inspiratory capacity

IRV Inspiratory reserve volume

IVC Inspiratory vital capacity

L Lung

max Maximum

MIF$_x$ Maximum inspiratory flow (instantaneous)

MVV Maximal voluntary ventilation

P Pressures in general

P(A − a) Alveolar–arterial gas pressure difference

Palv Alveolar pressure

Pao Pressure at the airway opening

Paw Pressure at any point along the airways

PaX Arterial tension of gas x, torr (mmHg)

PAX Alveolar tension of gas X, torr (mmHg)

Pbs Pressure at the body surface

PEF Peak expiratory flow

Pes Esophageal pressure used to estimate Ppl

PL Transpulmonary pressure: PL = Palv − Ppl, measurement conditions to be defined

Ppl Pleural pressure

Prs Transrespiratory pressure

Pst Static components of pressure

PstL Static recoil pressure of the lung

Ptm Transmural pressure pertaining to an airway or blood vessel

PX Tension of gas x, torr (mmHg)

Pw Transthoracic pressure

$\dot{Q}$ Volume flow of blood

$\dot{Q}s$ Shunt

R Respiratory exchange ratio in general (measurement of ventilation)

R Flow resistance (flow–pressure relationship)

Raw Airway resistance calculated from pressure difference between airway opening (Pao) and alveoli (Palv) divided by the airflow, $cmH_2O/L/sec$

Rds Resistance of the airways on the downstream (mouth) side of the point in the airways where intraluminal pressure equals Ppl, measured during maximum expiratory flow

RL Total pulmonary resistance includes the frictional resistance of the lungs and air passages

Rrs Total respiratory resistance includes the sum of airway resistance, lung tissue resistance, and chest wall resistance

Rus Resistance of the airways on the upstream (alveolar) side of the point in the airways at which intraluminal pressure equals Ppl (equal pressure point), measured during maximum expiratory flow

RV Residual volume

RV/TLC% Residual volume to total lung capacity ratio, expressed as a percentage

S Saturation in blood phase

SaO_2 Arterial oxygen saturation (percent)

STPD Standard temperature and pressure, dry. These are the conditions of a volume of gas at 0°C, at 760 torr, without water vapor.

t Time

T Tidal

TLC Total lung capacity

v Venous. Exact location to be specified in text when term is used.

$\bar{v}$ Mixed venous

V Gas volume in general. Pressure, temperature, and percentage saturation with water vapor must be stated.

$\dot{V}A$ Alveolar ventilation

Vc Average volume of blood in the capillary bed in milliliters

VC Vital capacity

$\dot{V}CO_2$ Carbon dioxide production per minute (STPD)

VD Physiologic dead space

$\dot{V}D$ Ventilation per minute of the physiologic dead space (BTPS)

VD_A Ventilation of the alveolar dead space (BTPS), defined by the equation $VD_A = VD - VD_{anat}$

VD_{anat} Volume of the anatomic dead space (BTPS)

Vd_{anat} Ventilation per minute of the anatomic dead space (BTPS)

VD_A Alveolar dead space volume (BTPS)

$\dot{V}E$ Expired volume per minute (BTPS)

$\dot{V}I$ Inspired volume per minute (BTPS)

VL Volume of the lung, including conducting airways

$Vmax_{XX\%}$ Maximum expiratory flow (instantaneous) qualified by the volume at which measured, expressed as percentage of FVC that has been exhaled

$Vmax_{XX\%TLC}$ Maximum expiratory flow (instantaneous) qualified by the volume at which measured, expressed as percentage of the TLC that remains in the lung

$\dot{V}O_2$ Oxygen consumption per minute (STPD)

VT Tidal volume

W Work of breathing

$\bar{X}$ Dash above any symbol indicates a mean value

$\dot{X}$ Dot above any symbol indicates a time derivative

$\ddot{X}$ Two dots above any symbol indicate the second time derivative

%X Percent sign before a symbol indicates percentage of the predicted normal value

X/Y% Percent sign after a symbol indicates a ratio function with the ratio expressed as a percentage. Both components of the ratio must be designated (eg, $FEV_1/FEV\% = 100 \times FEV_1/FVC$)

Glossary of Key Terms

abandonment (2.4): suit brought by a patient against a physician who has terminated the physician–patient relationship if the physician does not (1) notify the patient in writing of his or her intent to terminate, (2) give the patient enough time to find another physician, and (3) get the patient's concurrence to terminate

abortion (2.5): termination of pregnancy that results in the death of the embryo or fetus

absolute humidity (15): the mass (weight) of water vapor in a given volume of gas

absolute pressure (14): total gas pressure including that exerted by the atmosphere

acid (5): any substance that liberates hydrogen ions (protons) in solution

acidemia: any state of systemic arterial plasma in which the pH is less than the normal value, <7.35

acidosis: the result of any process that by itself adds excess carbon dioxide or nonvolatile acids to arterial blood. Acidemia does not necessarily result because compensating mechanisms (increase of HCO_3^- in respiratory acidosis, increase of ventilation, and, consequently, decrease of arterial carbon dioxide in metabolic acidosis) may intervene to restore pH to normal

acinus (4): small unit of lung parenchyma distal to the respiratory bronchiole

acute hypercapnia (10): rapid increase in the level of carbon dioxide in the blood of recent onset without sufficient time having passed for metabolic compensation to occur

acute hypercapnic respiratory failure (34): type II respiratory failure: a primary defect in ventilation

acute hypoxemic respiratory failure (34): type I respiratory failure: a primary defect in oxygenation

acute inhalation injury (10): lung damage due to toxic or heated gases

acute respiratory failure (28): rapidly occurring hypoxemia, hypercarbia, or both caused by a disorder of the respiratory system. The duration of the illness and the values of arterial oxygen tension and arterial carbon dioxide tension used as criteria for this term should be given. The term acute ventilatory failure should be used only when the arterial carbon dioxide tension is increased. The term pulmonary failure has been used to indicate respiratory failure specifically caused by disorders of the lung.

addictive behavior (33): physiologic, psychologic, and sociologic actions which suggest dependence on various substances, eg, food, alcohol, controlled substances

adhesions (30): microbial surface molecules or organelles that bind to a receptor with complementary substrate molecules

administration of aerosol drugs (16): techniques include the administration of aerosolized drugs by large and small devices that include nebulizers, metered dose inhalers, ultrasonic devices, and dry powder inhalers

adsorption atelectasis (13): reduced volume of lungs with distol to complete obstruction of the airway; occurs quickly when the patient is breathing oxygen-enriched gas mixtures

adult (or acute) respiratory distress syndrome (ARDS) (13, 35): a nonspecific pulmonary response to a range of pulmonary and nonpulmonary insults; characterized by interstitial infiltrates, alveolar hemorrhage, diffuse atelectasis, and reduced functional residual capacity

aerosol (15): a suspension of solid or liquid particles in gas

afterload (12): the resistance against which the contracting ventricles must eject blood

air bronchogram (17): an air-filled bronchus visible on the chest radiograph

airway resistance (12): measure of resistance to airflow in the airways

alcoholism (33): a chronic and progressive disease characterized by tolerance and physical dependency to alcohol

alkalemia: any state of systemic arterial blood in which the pH is greater than the normal value, >7.45

alkalosis: the result of any process that, by itself, diminishes acids or increases bases in arterial blood; alkalemia does not necessarily result because compensating mechanisms may intervene to restore plasma pH to normal

allergen (27): a substance that causes manifestations of allergy

allergy (27): an acquired, abnormal immune response to a substance (allergen) that does not normally cause such a reaction

alveolar-capillary membrane (4): the microscopic unit of lung anatomy where gas transfer of oxygen and carbon dioxide occurs by exposing alveolar air to circulating pulmonary capillary blood

alveolar ducts (4): a branch of a respiratory bronchiole that leads to the alveoli of the lungs

alveolar macrophages (4): type III cells that phagocytize bacteria and other contaminants that find their way into the alveoli

alveolar overdistention (34): pathologic enlargement of alveolar size, as occurs in emphysema

alveolar oxygen partial pressure (5, 12): portion of total gas pressure in the lung caused by oxygen delivered to the alveoli, determined by the function of inspired oxygen, barometric pressure, alveolar carbon dioxide tension and the respiratory quotient

alveolar period (25): the final period of fetal lung development, beginning at 37 weeks and continuing into postnatal life and on into the 8th year

alveolar ventilation (5): gas exchange at the alveolar level; minute ventilation minus dead space ventilation

alveoli (4): structures at the distol end of the airway where gas is exchanged in the lung

American Association of Respiratory Care (AARC) (1): the primary professional organization of the respiratory care field

Americans with Disabilities Act (33): an Act of Congress defining and describing the rights of citizens who have physical and mental disabilities

amphetamine (33): a colorless liquid that volatilizes slowly at room temperature and is a central nervous system stimulant

anaphylaxis (22): a serious, potentially fatal, allergic or hypersensitivity reaction

angina pectoris (36): chest discomfort, which may be sensed as pain, pressure, or tightness across the central area of the chest or epigastrium, caused by cardiac ischemia

anion gap (9): a measurement used to estimate the difference between commonly measured electrolyte levels of cations and anions

anionic shift (5): the shift of anions and water into the red blood cell (in the tissues), due to changing acidity of hemoglobin, as it loses oxygen in the tissues, thus requiring less anionic concentration; the reverse shift occurs in the lungs

anti-inflammatory agent (27): an agent that counteracts inflammation

antimicrobial drugs (16): agents that destroy or prevent further growth of microorganisms

ankylosing spondylitis (32): a chronic disorder of unknown cause characterized by progressive inflammatory disease involving the axial spine and adjacent soft tissues

aortic bodies (4): chemosensitive structures located near the arch of the aorta with afferents conveyed by the vagus nerve (X), which sense PaO_2 in perfusing arterial blood

apnea (11): cessation of airflow for 10 seconds or longer

apneustic breathing (29): an abnormal pattern of breathing characterized by a prolonged cessation of breathing in the inspiratory phase

arterial gas embolism, aeroembolism (14): obstruction of blood flow by a gas bubble

arterial oxygen content (5): the amount of oxygen found in the blood, expressed as CCO_2/dL

arterial puncture (9): act of puncturing an artery, as in blood gas sampling

asbestosis (33): lung disease resulting from protracted inhalation of asbestos particles

aspiration (37): withdrawing of a fluid by means of suction

assessment (6, 23): examination of the patient, including (1) history-taking, (2) physical examination to identify cardiopulmonary clinical manifestations, (3) pertinent laboratory data, and (4) systematic recording method

assist/control ventilation (20): a mode of mechanical ventilation which can either assist the patient's ventilatory effort, or which can deliver a preset number of breaths (in the control mode)

assisted suicide (2.5): a means by which an ill individual can end his or her life with the help of a medical professional

asthma (10, 27): constriction of the bronchial airways and hypersecretion caused by increased responsiveness of the tracheobronchial tree to various stimuli; variable or intermittent obstruction of the lower airways that results in shortness of breath, wheezing, chest tightness, and cough

atelectasis (7, 17, 18): a collapsed or airless condition of the lung caused by obstruction of the airways by foreign bodies, hypoventilation secondary to pain in fractured ribs, inadequate tidal volumes, mucus plugs or excessive secretions, or compression from outside the airway or lung, eg, tumors, aneurysms, or enlarged lymph nodes

attending physician (2.3): the physician who assesses the patient's condition, performs physical examination, orders appropriate diagnostic tests, integrates all information to reach a correct diagnosis, and outlines an appropriate treatment regimen

auscultation (6): method of listening to sounds in the body using a stethoscope to obtain information about the heart, blood vessels, and air flowing in and out of the tracheobronchial tree and alveoli

autogenic drainage (17, 26): a method of enhancing secretion removal, by using controlled breathing maneuvers and delaying cough as long as possible

auto-PEEP (20): the development of PEEP caused by a shortened, incomplete expiration, causing airtrapping

barotrauma (7): injury caused by excessive airway and transpulmonary pressure

base (5): any substance that combines with hydrogen ions (protons)

base deficit (5): increase in strong ion difference

base excess (5): measure of metabolic alkalosis or metabolic acidosis (negative base excess) expressed as the mEq of strong acid or strong alkali required to titrate a sample of 1L of blood to a pH of 7.40; the titration is made with the blood sample kept at 37°C, oxygenated, and equilibrated to a PCO_2 of 40 torr

behavioral modifications (33): improving or changing the way one acts or the actions of individuals under certain circumstances

benchmarking (2.1): comparison of value indicators, performed to identify outstanding performance regarding cost effectiveness, quality of life, and best practices in relation to patient interventions

bicarbonate ion (9): OH^-, a base (proton acceptor)

bicarbonate system (5): the bicarbonate system of buffers, eg, sodium bicarbonate

bi-level positive airway pressure (Bi-pap) (24): a device that allows independent inspiratory and expiratory pressure levels to be set

Bi-pap: see *bi-level positive airway pressure*

bland aerosols (15): nonirritating, nonpharmacologic aerosol, eg, normal salve

blood gas measurement (9): chemical analysis of the blood to determine the concentrations of oxygen and carbon dioxide

blood gas sensors (9): devices which record blood gas levels, eg, transcutaneous oxygen monitors

Board of Medical Advisors (2.3): consultative body of the AARC in which the medical profession has formal dialog with the national AARC membership organization; this group advises the AARC on educational program content, scientific matters (eg, position statements and Clinical Practice Guidelines), state licensure and other forms of legal credentialling

body humidity (15): the ratio of absolute humidity and capacity at body temperature

boiling point (13, 15): the temperature above which a gas cannot be converted back to a liquid, regardless of pressure applied

breach (2.4): a break or violation of a law, promise, or standard of care

B-readers (33): radiologists specially credentialled to interpret radiographs of patients with occupational and individual pulmonary disorders

breath-activated metered dose inhaler (15): inhalers in which the negative pressure of inspiration causes triggering of the device

bronchial hygiene therapy (17): modalities which clear obstructed airways; traditionally included in this grouping are deep breathing and cough therapy, percussion and postural drainage, PEP, autogenic drainage, and suctioning

bronchial hyperresponsiveness (27): decreased reactivity (eg, bronchospan, mucus hypersecretion) of the airway

bronchial provocation testing (33): testing of the hyperresponsiveness, or irritability of bronchometer tone, usually with spirometry or body plethysmography, following controlled exposure to an irritant substance

bronchiectasis (10, 17): chronic dilation of a bronchus or bronchi, with secondary infection that usually involves the dependent portion of the lung

bronchitis (27): inflammation of the mucous membranes of the bronchial tubes

bronchoalveolar lavage (10, 30, 32): introduction, by fiberoptic bronchoscope, of sterile saline into the lung in order to remove substances such as secretions, cells, and protein from the lower respiratory tract

bronchodilators (16, 27, 36): drugs that expand, or dilate a bronchus

broncholithiasis (10): calculi in the bronchi

bronchopleural fluid (10): fluid found in the bronchi or pleural cavity

bronchopulmonary dysplasia (25): chronic pulmonary illness that results from unintended successful mechanical ventilation of smaller infants with lung disease

bronchoscopy (30): examination of the airway through a long tube, passed through the larynx from the nasopharynx or oropharynx

Brownian motion (15): a random motion of particles that promotes deposition by sedimentation

buffer (5): a substance that preserves the original hydrogen ion concentration of its solution when an acid or base is added

bulk convection (25): gas flow that results in direct alveolar ventilation

calcium channel blockers (36): drugs that lower blood pressure, increase coronary blood flow, and decrease myocardial oxygen consumption, used to manage patients with coronary disease, particularly with coexisting hypertension

canalicular period (25): the early formation of the pulmonary gas-exchanging unit, the acinus, lasting from the 17th to 28th week of gestation

capacitance (4): portion of the pulmonary arterial circulation made up of the proximal pulmonary arteries

capitation (3): system wherein the health care provider is paid on a flat fee basis "per covered life" per month or year

capnography (12, 25): continuous tracing of expired and end tidal carbon dioxide concentrations measured over a period of time or breath by breath

carbon (33): an element, found in nature, as in carbon dioxide (see below)

carbon dioxide (9): a colorless gas, heavier than air, that is expelled from the lungs with expiration as a by-product of cellular metabolism

carbon dioxide partial pressure (5): the pressure exerted by carbon dioxide in a gas mixture

carbon dioxide production (12): the amount of carbon dioxide the body exhausts through the lungs

carbon monoxide intoxication (14): poisoning of the oxygenation process due to carbon monoxide inhalation

carbon monoxide poisoning (14): toxicity that can result from breathing small amounts of carbon monoxide over a long period of time or large amounts over a short period of time

carboxyhemoglobinemia (13): the presence of carboxyhemoglobin in a blood sample

cardiac output (12): the amount of blood discharged from the left or right ventricle per minute

cardiopulmonary resuscitation (22): procedures designed to restore cardiac output and gas exchange after cardiac and/or respiratory arrest

carina (4): site where trachea divides into two branches (bronchii)

carotid bodies (4): specialized neurochemoreceptive tissue located at the bifurcation of the common carotid arteries, where afferents to the medulla pass through the glossopharyngeal nerve (IX)

"cascade" humidifier (15): a low-flow diffusion humidifier that uses a large diffuser tower to increase the gas–water interface

case management (2.1): management of patients on a case by case basis, designed so that the patient receives only that treatment necessary

cataplexy (11): emotion-triggered muscle weakness, seen in narcolepsy

central hypopnea (11): a 50% or more reduction in airflow during sleep, something in a reduction in respiratory effort lasting 10 seconds or longer, and usually associated with a fall in blood oxygen saturation

central sleep apnea (11): an apnea episode lasting 10 seconds or longer during which there is no respiratory effort

central venous catheter (7): a tube inserted into the superior vena cava to permit intermittent or continuous monitoring of central venous or right atrial filling pressure

central venous pressure (12): the pressure in superior vena cava or the right atrium

certified pulmonary function technologist (CPFT) (1): National Board of Respiratory Care (NBRC) specialty credential certifying competence in pulmonary function technology

certified respiratory therapy technician (CRTT) (1): credentials given to an individual who successfully passes the entry level certification exam given by the NBRC

chemoreceptors (4): structures which provide the afferent signals for the chemical control of respiration

chest physical therapy (CPT) (36): a group of techniques comprised of percussion and drainage, autogenic drainage, and short wall vibration

chest tubes (7): commonly called thoracotomy tubes, placed to drain fluid, blood or air from the pleural cavity

Cheyne-Stokes breathing (29): a disordered breathing pattern characterized by alternating patterns of hyperventilation followed by either apnea or marked hypoventilation

chloride shift (5): see *anionic shift*

chlorofluorocarbons (15): refrigerant gases, or propellant gas used to power metered dose inhalers

chronic bronchitis (17, 28): a clinical syndrome with a chronic productive cough 3 months out of the year for 2 successive years

chronic lung disease of infancy (25): see *bronchopulmonary dysplasia*

chronic obstructive pulmonary disease (COPD) (28): a disease state characterized by the presence of airflow obstruction due to chronic bronchitis or emphysema; the airflow obstruction is generally progressive, may be accompanied by airway hyperreactivity, and may be partially reversible

chronic respiratory failure: chronic hypoxemia or hypercapnia caused by a disorder of the respiratory system. The duration of the condition and the values of arterial oxygen tension and arterial carbon dioxide tension used as criteria for this term should be given.

choanae (4): two internal nares where the proximal portion of the nose connects with the pharynx

cilia (4, 17): hairlike processes projecting from epithelial cells, as in the nose, trachea and bronchi, important in airway clearance

circadian rhythm (11): an innate, daily fluctuation of physiologic or behavioral functions including sleep-wake states generally tied to the 24-hour daily dark–light clock

Clara cells (4): secreting cells in the surface epithelium of the bronchioles

clearance (17): elimination of a substance via the kidneys (eg, creatinine) or airways (eg, mucus)

Clinical Practice Guidelines (1, 6): systematically developed statements developed and published by the AARC to help RCPs deliver appropriate respiratory care in specific clinical situations

"cold turkey" method (33): to stop smoking suddenly and completely

communication (2.2, 6): a transactional process between two or more individuals involving sending and receiving verbal and nonverbal messages, with the goal being shared meaning

compliance (4): the pulmonary volume change produced by pressure change across the lung

component management (2.1): managing disease by treating it episodically, with little incentive to treat the entire disease process

compression volume (20): volume loss due to compaction of gas molecules during compression

compressor nebulizer (24): the most common type of aerosol therapy setup in the home for bronchodilator administration

computerized patient record (2.1): a system of maintaining patient records on a database that is accessible to all health care providers

congenital craniofacial dysmorphologies (19): inherited abnormalities of the head and face; these can predispose to upper airway problems

consent (2.4): the agreement of a patient to receive diagnostic and/or therapeutic manipulation; to be legally given, it must be (1) valid, (2) free, and (3) informed

consolidation (17): solidification of the lungs due to filling of the alveoli, as in acute pneumonia

consumerism (3): the promotion of the consumer's interests

continuous positive airway pressure (11, 18, 20, 24): expiratory pressure above atmospheric acting as a splint to maintain airway patency, during spontaneous respiration

contractility (12): having the ability to contract or shorten

controlled hypoventilation (34): see *permissive hypercapnia*

controlled ventilation (20): a ventilator mode in which all ventilation is delivered (controlled) by the ventilator; there is no option for patient-activated inspiration

coronary angiography(36): test that defines coronary arterial anatomy, and the site and degree of obstructing vascular lesions

coronary angioplasty (36): procedure used as primary therapy for patients with arteriosclerotic heart disease, during which a balloon catheter is passed through an area of focal coronary artery stenosis identified by angiography, at the end of which the balloon is inflated to dilate a narrowed region

cor pulmonale (28): right heart failure (pulmonary hypertension) caused by disease of the lungs

corticoid (27): any of a number of hormonal steroid substances from the cortex of the adrenal gland

cough (10): forceful, sometimes violent expiratory effort preceded by inspiration and glottic closure

"crack" cocaine (33): cocaine which has been heated to a liquid, then allowed to harden; the powder so produced "crackles" when warmed

critical pathway (2.1): disease mapping that outlines a realistic model of the disease and a time-course for interventions based on the disease process

critical pressure (13, 15): the pressure required for liquefaction of a gas (at the critical temperature); the vapor pressure of a substance at its critical temperature, or that which is exerted by a liquid at its critical temperature

critical temperature (13, 15): the temperature required to cause a gas to change to liquid at the critical pressure; the energy level of a substance above which the molecules can exist only as a gas

cromolyn (27): an anti-inflammatory substance which prohibits mast cell degranulation

crush injuries (14): trauma to bones and soft tissues by pressure

cyanide poisoning (14): poisoning by cyanide, which interferes with cellular respiration

cycling (21): a system where a preset ventilator variable (time, pressure, volume, or flow) causes a ventilator to initiate or end the inspiratory phase of respiration

cystic fibrosis (17): a respiratory disease in which dehydration and an increase in viscosity of secretions in organs lined with epithelial cells, including the lungs and intestinal system, results from the abnormal movement of sodium and chloride; the most common fatal genetic disease in the United States

Dalton's law (13, 15): the relationship of partial pressure of each gas in a composite sample, exerting a partial pressure, proportional to its concentration in the sample, and dependent on the total barometric pressure

dead space volume (12): the volume of inspired gas that does not directly participate in gas exchange of the alveolar level

dead space ventilation (4): occurs when alveoli are ventilated but the interfacing capillaries around the alveoli are underperfused or not perfused at all

death(2.5): total and irreversible loss of brain function, with irreversible loss of both cerebral hemispheric and brain stem function

decompression illness (14): a condition that develops in divers subjected to a rapid reduction of air pressure after coming to the surface following exposure to compressed air

defibrillation (22): use of drugs, physical or electrical means to stop rapid, irregular contractions of the heart

demand hypoxia (13): a state in which the oxygen demands of metabolism are not matched by the capacity of the organism to deliver oxygen
demand management (2.1): triaging of services to reduce the need for and use of costly, often unnecessary, medical services, as well as arbitrary managed care interventions
dew point (15): the temperature to which a gas-vapor mixture must be cooled before dew condenses on the vessel containing the sample
diagnostic related groups (3): method of health care payment for older individuals whereby the consumer pays a set amount for hospitalization based on diagnosis, and not acuity
Diameter Index Safety System (DISS) (13): safety system for medical gas systems based on the diameter of threaded gas connections subjected to 200 psig or less
diaphragm (4): a musculomembranous wall separating the abdomen from the thoracic cavity with its convexity upward
diaphragmatic paralysis (10): loss of movement of the diaphragm
diffuse alveolar disease (7): a generalized pulmonary process affecting alveoli
diffuse interstitial disease (7): a generalized pulmonary process affecting the alveolar-capillary membrane
directed cough (17): method of coughing taught to patients whose voluntary coughing is ineffective
disability (33): a legally or administratively determined state in which a patient's ability to engage in a specific activity under certain circumstances is reduced or absent because of physical or mental impairment. Other factors, such as age, education, and customary way of making a livelihood, are considered in evaluation disability. Permanent disability exists when no substantial improvement of the patient's ability to engage in the specific activity can be expected.
disease management (2.1): treatment of a disease designed to address the illness by maximizing the effectiveness and efficiency of care delivered; emphasis is on preventing disease and/or managing it aggressively where and when intervention will have the greatest impact
disinfection (30): removal of microorganisms capable of causing infection
Diskhaler (15): commercial device to provide dry powder inhalation
drive mechanism (21): the device on a mechanical ventilator that converts or transmits power
drugs for bronchospasm (16): bronchodilating medications
dry powder inhalers (15): a method of aerosol administration that disperses powdered medication via propellers, activated by subatmospheric pressure from the patient's inspiration
durable power of attorney (2.5): a legal statement that allows a family member or significant other to make decisions for an ill, usually comatose, person, including whether to accept treatment
duty of care (2.4): the basis of the physician–patient relationship wherein a physician accepts a patient and accepts the responsibility of rendering due and proper care
dynamic hyperinflation (34): see *auto-PEEP*; pulmonary overexpansion due to inadequate time allowed for the lung to empty from the previous inspiration
dyspnea (28): an unpleasant subjective feeling of difficult or labored breathing
dysrhythmia (22): an irregular rhythm of the heart
dys-synchrony (20): opposite of synchrony; poor coordination of patient voluntary effort with ventilator-delivered breaths
electrocardiogram (ECG) (11, 22, 36): recording of variation in electrical potential caused by the excitation of the heart muscle and detected at the body surface
echocardiography (36): test designed to provide information on ventricular size and function, regional wall motion abnormalities, mural thrombus formation, valvular function, and abnormalities of the pericardium
EEG arousals (11): a brief burst of higher frequency, usually alpha activity, in the EEG of a sleeping person
"eggshell" calcifications (33): a radiographic finding suggesting silicosis
electroencephalogram (EEG) (11): a recording of the electrical potentials on the skull surface, which are generated by currents emanating spontaneously from nerve cells in the brain
electrolysis (13): process of passing an electric current through water to obtain oxygen
electromyogram (EMG) (11): the recording of intrinsic electrical potentials from skeletal muscle
electro-oculogram (EOG) (11): the recording of eye movements
embryonic period (25): the time starting in the embryo's 4th and 5th week of gestation, the most prominent feature of which is the formation of the proximal conducting airways
empathy (2.2): understanding, experiencing, or being aware of or sensitive to the feelings, thoughts, and experiences of another without having those feelings, thoughts, or experiences verbally conveyed
emphysema (28): an anatomic alteration of the lung characterized by abnormal, permanent enlargement of the airspaces distal to the terminal bronchioles, accompanied by destruction of their walls and without obvious fibrosis
endotracheal (7): inside the trachea
endotracheal intubation (10): a procedure in which a tube is placed within the trachea
end tidal PCO_2 (12): the partial pressure of carbon dioxide in end-expiratory (alveolar) air; the end-tidal PCO_2 closely approximates the alveolar PCO_2
environmental assessment (24): in-home care, assessing a patient's home in order to determine its suitability, in concert with the medical interventions ordered by a physician
eosinophils (27): white blood cells found in the bronchial airways, often as cellular markers of allergy
epiglottis (4): located at the base of the tongue, it diverts food and liquid into the esophagus when swallowing, by lifting the larynx in a superior direction
esophageal pressure (12): pressures measured from within the esophagus, that approximates pleural pressure
ethics (2.5): the branch of philosophy that deals with the fundamental values of life; in medicine, professional ethics govern the nontechnical interface between the health care provider and the patient
eukaryotes (30): a microorganism that has chromosomes enclosed within a membrane, and that reproduce by mitosis; includes fungi and protozoa
eustachian tubes (4): openings in the nasopharynx responsible for equalizing pressure in the middle ear
euthanasia (2.5): "mercy killing": the act or practice of painlessly killing or permitting death of the sick or injured individual
exercise training (23): rehabilitation regimen designed to increase work performance
expiratory positive airway pressure (18): application of positive pressure to the airway during expiration
external respiration (4): gas exchange measured at the mouth
extracorporeal life support (20): mechanical ventilation from outside the body

extracorporeal membrane oxygenation (35): oxygenation of the blood from a source outside the body

farmer's lung (33): a form of hypersensitivity alveolitis caused by fermented moldy hay

fat embolism (7): obstruction of pulmonary arterial vessels with fat

fatigue (11): tiredness or weariness

fiberoptic bronchoscopy (7): method of assessing the bronchi by use of a flexible optic device that transmits light along its course, permitting illumination of distol airway structures

Fick principle (13): equation that "bridges" body oxygen consumption, cardiac output, and the arteriovenous oxygen content difference

fixed orifice resistor (18): a resistor with a restricted opening of a fixed size that is placed at the end of the expiratory limb of a breathing circuit

flail chest (7): multiple rib fractures involving more than two ribs broken in two or more places, resulting in paradoxical chest movement

flow controller (21): ventilator that uses flow to control ventilator supported inspiration by maintaining a constant volume waveform when patient compliance or resistance changes

flow-oriented incentive device (18): a type of spirometer that measures the patient's inspiratory breathing as the patient breathes through a tube to lift one or more light balls or indicators: the higher the inspiratory flow rate, the higher or greater the number of balls or indicators are raised

flow trigger (20): method of initiating inspiratory phase in response to a patient exceeding a predetermined flow level

flow-volume loop (12): a graph in which instantaneous flow is plotted as a function of lung volume

forced vital capacity (FVC) (8): the volume of air exhaled during a forced exhalation, starting at total lung capacity (TLC)

forced expiratory volume (FEV) (8): the amount of air exhaled in a forced exhalation, synonymous with forced vital capacity

forced inspiratory vital capacity test (8): a spirometry maneuver used to detect upper airway obstruction, performed during an inspiratory maneuver

fractional distillation (13): method of manufacturing oxygen using compression and gradual rewarming of air; different boiling points allows collection of specific gases

fraud (2.4): intentional perversion of truth, usually to harm another financially or legally

freon (15): a gas used in cooling processes

gas gangrene (14): death of tissue in a wound infected by a gas-forming organism

gastric intramural pH (12): the pH of the stomach

glottis (4): airway opening of the larynx

goblet cells (4, 15): cells in the columnar epithelium of the airway that produce thick mucus bronchial secretions

gravitational sedimentation (15): deposition of inspired particles as they reach a velocity too slow to maintain forward momentum

Haldane effect (5): the effect of oxygen saturation on hemoglobin's affinity for carbon dioxide

Hamburger phenomenon (5): see *chloride shift*

heat and moisture exchanger (HME) (15): a humidity generator that collects heat and moisture, and uses them to condition the following inspirate

heat of vaporization (15): the heat energy required to change a unit mass of liquid to a gas (vapor) at the same temperature

Heimlich maneuver (22): a procedure that requires using a fist to exert upward pressure over the xiphoid process to expel foreign material from the trachea

hemic hypoxia (13): lack of oxygen in the blood due to anemia or abnormal hemoglobin pigments

hemodynamic instability (37): labial blood pressure or cardiac rate and/or rhythm, eg, shock

hemoglobin (9): the iron-containing pigment of the red blood cells that carries oxygen from the lungs to the tissues

hemoptysis (10): expectoration of blood from the oral cavity, larynx, trachea, bronchi, or lungs

heroin (33): a narcotic derived from morphine

heterodisperse (15): having a range of particle sizes (as in an aerosol)

high frequency jet ventilation (25): ventilation that provides continuous ventilation delivered at 100 to 500 cycles per minute

high frequency oscillatory (HFO) ventilation (25): a mode of ventilation that uses cycling loudspeaker diaphragms or reciprocating pistons to produce gas flow

high frequency positive pressure ventilation (HFPPV) (25): mode of ventilation using frequencies of 60–110 cycles/minute; devices are time-triggered, time-cycled, and volume-limited ventilators

high frequency ventilation (20, 35): ventilatory support at rates greater than normal

high-resolution computed tomography (7): radiographic method of assessing diffuse lung diseases

histotoxic hypoxia (13): lack of oxygen in body tissue due to receptor cell abnormalities, eg, cyanide poisoning

home respiratory care (3): respiratory care services delivered in the home

huff cough (17, 18): forced expiratory maneuver similar to normal cough but without allowing forceful glottic opening

humidity deficit (15): the condition of insufficient water to provide 100% body humidity

hydration (17): addition of water to a substance or tissue

hygroscopic property (15): the ability of a structure to increase in size by condensation of water vapor

hyperbaric (14): exposed to or having pressure greater than atmospheric, eg, hyperbaric oxygen therapy

hypercapnia: any state in which the systemic arterial carbon dioxide pressure is above 45 torr, as in hypoventilation or during carbon dioxide inhalation

hypercarbia (13): increased amount of carbon dioxide in the blood

hyperinflation therapy (18): treatment whereby the lungs are overexpanded, eg, incentive spirometry to re-expand atelectatic lung

hypermetabolic (37): increased rate of metabolism

hypersomnia (11): a sleep disorder that is appreciated as significant sleepiness during the day, which includes falling asleep when sedentary

hyperventilation: an alveolar ventilation that is excessive relative to the simultaneous metabolic rate; as a result the alveolar PCO_2 is reduced below normal

hypnogogic hallucinations (11): vivid dreams at sleep onset, often containing abnormal dream structures such as light or geometric patterns

hypocapnia: any state in which the systemic arterial carbon dioxide pressure is below 35 torr, as in hyperventilation

hypopnea (11): reduction in airflow by 50% or more for 10 seconds or longer without total cessation of airflow

hypoventilation: an alveolar ventilation that is small relative to the simultaneous metabolic rate, so that the alveolar PCO_2 rises significantly above normal

hypovolemic shock (22): shock caused by loss of blood volume

hypoxemia (9): a state in which the oxygen pressure or concentration in blood is lower than its normal value at sea level. Normal oxygen pressures in arterial blood at sea level are based on the patient's age.

hypoxia: any state in which oxygen in the lung, blood, or tissues is abnormally low compared with that of a normal resting person breathing air at sea level

hypoxic pulmonary vasoconstriction (25): increase in pulmonary vascular tone caused by hypoxemia

idiopathic pulmonary fibrosis (32): a type of interstitial lung disease, the symptoms of which include progressive dyspnea, cough, and clubbing, the cause of which is unknown

ILO classification (33): a radiographic classification system useful in the interpretation of chest x-rays in occupational lung disease evaluation

immunotherapy (27): usually, antigen therapy ("allergy shots") in asthma

impairment (33): medically demonstrable anatomical, physiological or psychological abnormalities; a measurable degree of anatomic or functional abnormality that may or may not have clinical significance; permanent impairment is that which persists for some time (eg, 1 year after maximum medical rehabilitation has been achieved)

incentive spirometry (18): a procedure using a device designed to coax patients to mimic natural sighing or yawning maneuvers by providing biofeedback when the patient breathes out of it

indirect calorimetry (12): bedside measurement of metabolic and nutritional data that consists of a series of calculations based on $\dot{V}O_2$, $\dot{V}_E$, and $\dot{V}CO_2$

inertial impaction (15): deposition of particles by collision with surfaces

infant mortality rate (25): the number of deaths in the 1st year of life per 1000 live births

infiltration (17): the process of a substance passing into and being deposited in a cell, tissue, or organ

information giver (2.2): the individual in a conversation who provides necessary information to the information seeker regarding his or her medical condition

information seeker (2.2): the individual in a conversation who is responsible for the structure and flow of communication, designed to acquire necessary information regarding a patient's medical condition

inotropic agents (36): drugs given to treat hypotension or ventricular failure following myocardial infarction

insomnia (11): a sleep disorder which disturbs or reduces sleep at night

inspection (26): simple observation, which allows the practitioner to evaluate the patient's appearance, growth and development; the first stage of the physical examination

institutional certification (2.3): credentialing of the specific health care institution in which the caregiver is employed

interlobular effusion (7): fluid between lobes of the lung, usually in tissues

intermittent mandatory ventilation (20): a ventilatory technique in which a preset number of breaths per minute are delivered (mandated) by the ventilator; the frequency and tidal volume of these breaths are predetermined

intermittent positive pressure breathing (18, 24): short-term mechanical ventilation for the primary purpose of assisting ventilation and providing short duration hyperinflation therapy

internal respiration (4): occurs as oxygenated blood is distributed to body tissues and simultaneously carbon dioxide and other cellular metabolic end-products are removed

interstitial lung disease (32): any disorder that results from injury to the pulmonary interstitium

interstitial pulmonary fibrosis (13): scarring of the interstitium

intra-arterial blood gas (ABG) monitoring (12): measurement of ABGs from an in-lying arterial catheter or electrode

invasion of privacy (2.4): overly personal inquiry into a patient's history, feelings, or "body space"

isothermic saturation boundary (15): a theoretical point in the airways at which inspired gases reach the 100% body humidity level

Joint Commission on Accreditation of Health Care Organizations (JCAHO) (2.3): a national accrediting organization that has developed standards to protect the patient, assure a high quality of care, and prevent system abuse; any institution that wants to seek accreditation from this group must meet these standards

Joint Review Committee for Respiratory Therapy Education (JRCRTE) (2.3): the educational accrediting arm of the respiratory care profession, which recommends approval of postsecondary respiratory care education programs to the U.S. Department of Education

k-complexes (11): EEG waveform in stage 2 having a well delineated negative sharp wave that is immediately followed by a positive component, with a duration of the total complex not exceeding 0.5 seconds

lamellar bodies (25): the intracellular storage sites of surfactant in the pulmonary interstitium

large volume nebulizers (15): a method of aerosol administration

laryngeal webs (19): wisps of tissue which may span the larynx

laryngomalacia (19): softening of the cartilaginous support structures of the larynx

laryngopharynx (4): a respiratory and digestive passage, one of three pharynx sections

larynx (4): a complex structure composed of soft tissue and cartilage which serves as a passageway from the pharynx to the trachea, protects the lower airways from aspirating liquids and solids, and produces vibratory voice sounds

lecithin/spingomyelin (L/S) ratio (25): a test that predicts fetal lung maturity accurately, by quantifying the amount of a primary surfactant component present in the amniotic fluid

licensure (2.4): recognition and regulation of a profession by a state agency

liquid oxygen (24): oxygen stored in the liquid state

liquid ventilation (20): experimental therapy that uses perfluorocarbon to "ventilate" the patient (see *perfluorocarbon)*

living will (2.5): a statement, made when a person is well, that attests to that individual's wishes that heroic measures such as use of life support devices not be used to prolong life when such actions will not permit recovery from the condition

lobar bronchi (4): second generation bronchi, serving the pulmonary lobes

lung abscess (7, 10): localized area of lung destruction caused by liquefaction necrosis

lung compliance (12): change in unit volume of the lung per unit of transpulmonary pressure change; a measure of the elasticity or stiffness of the lungs

lung compliance testing (8): measurement of the elastic recoil or stiffness of the lungs

lung fields (7): areas of the lung seen in the chest radiograph, eg, apices bases

lung maturity (25): the fetal or newborn lung when it comes to contain adequate quantities of surfactant in the airspaces to support alveolar stability and gas exchange

lung transplantation (28): the transplantation of one or both lungs from a donor to replace poorly functioning lungs in the recipient

lymphangiomyomatosis (32): an uncommon, progressive disorder of women of childbearing age characterized by nodular and diffuse interstitial proliferation of the smooth muscle in lungs, lymph nodes, and thoracic duct

lymphocytic interstitial pneumonitis (32): a form of interstitial lung disease whose main histologic feature is diffuse lymphocytic infiltration of the lung parenchyma and interstitium

magnetic valve resistor (18): a resistor that uses a bar magnet that attracts a ferromagnetic disk to seat on the outlet orifice; as pressure exceeds the attraction of the magnet, the disk is displaced, allowing gas to exit the circuit

mainstem bronchi (4): two main branches of the airway connecting the trachea to each lung

malpractice (2.4): a dereliction from professional duty or a failure to exercise an accepted degree of professional skill by one rendering services which results in injury, loss, or damage

managed care contract (3): contract between an employer and insurance company that sets a dollar amount per individual whether health care services are required or not

mandatory minute ventilation (20): a mode of ventilation in which the minute ventilation is controlled (mandated)

marijuana (33): the dried flowering tops of the hemp plant, used for its hallucinatory properties; its use is illegal in most states

mass median aerodynamic diameter (MMAD) (15): concept referring to an aerosol particle in which 50% of its fellow particles are heavier (larger) and 50% are lighter (smaller)

Material Safety Data Sheets (MSDS) (33): sheets of information regarding materials in works, warning of untoward health effects in individuals

maximal expiratory pressure (8): measurement of respiratory muscle strength during expiration

maximal inspiratory pressure (8): measurement of respiratory muscle strength during inspiration

maximal voluntary ventilation (MVV) (8): a 15-second spirometry test, integrated and expressed in L/M

mean airway pressure (20): the mean, or average pressure in the airway during the inspiratory and expiratory phases of respiration

meatus (4): the depressions between turbinates, referred to as superior, middle, and inferior

mechanical ventilation (1, 36): mechanical support of a patient with respiratory failure designed to (1) support the patient during an episode of acute respiratory failure or (2.1) reverse chronic ventilatory failure

medullary respiratory centers (4): chemosensitive areas responsive to changes in PCO_2 and {H+} existing in the medulla

mesothelioma (33): a rare malignant tumor of the mesothelium, often related to asbestos exposure

metered dose inhalers (MDI) (15, 27): glass, ceramic, or metal canisters containing drug in the form of a suspension of micronized crystals or in solution, used to administer aerosol therapy

minute ventilation (25): total air flow ($V_T \times f = \dot{V}_E$) per minute, measured at the mouth or ventilator exhalation valve; the sum of alveolar and dead space ventilation

mission statement (2.1): a document that defines services of an institution and its individual practitioners, outlining their function both today and in the future

mixed apnea (11): an apnea episode consisting of both a central and obstructive apnea component

mixed venous blood gas monitoring (12): continuous measurement of mixed venous PO_2 from a "central" line, usually the superior vena cava or the pulmonary artery

mixed venous oxygen content (5): the amount of oxygen in 100cc of mixed venous blood equal to (hemoglobin $\times$ 1.34 $\times$ $S\dot{V}O_2$) + (.003 $\times$ $P\dot{V}CO_2$)

mixed venous PO_2 (9): measurement of the PO_2 in blood withdrawn from a central venous or pulmonary artery catheter

molecular diffusion (25): the diffusion of gas through the alveolar region

monodisperse (15): having a narrow range of diameters (as in an aerosol)

monoplace chambers (14): hyperbaric oxygen chambers large enough for only one individual

mucokinetic agents (16): pharmacologic agents used to ease the expectations of airway mucus

mucus plug (17): a gobbet of airway mucus that obstructs the airway

Müeller maneuver (17): reverse of Valsalva maneuver in that inspiration is attempted with a closed glottis

multiplace chambers (14): hyperbaric oxygen changes large enough for two or more individuals

muscular dystrophy (29): any of a number of hereditary diseases that lead to degeneration of skeletal muscles

myocardial infarction (36): death of heart muscle (myocardium) secondary to ischemia

myopathy (29): a disease or condition of the striated muscle

narcolepsy (11): a sleep disorder, often inherited, characterized by excessive daytime sleepiness and recurrent, uncontrollable episodes of brief sleep, often associated with hypnagogic hallucinations, cataplexy, and sleep paralysis

naris (4): paired external nostrils

nasopharynx (4): a continuation of the nasal cavities, which contains openings for the eustachian tubes, one of three pharynx sections

nasotracheal suctioning (36): suctioning of the nares, oropharynx, nasopharynx and trachea, entering via the nares

National Association for Medical Directors of Respiratory Care (NAMDRC) (2.3): organization of medical directors of respiratory therapy departments and/or respiratory therapy education programs that educates its members and addresses regulatory, legislative, and payment issues relating to the delivery of health care to patients with respiratory disorders
National Board of Respiratory Care (NBRC) (2.3): the credentialling arm of the respiratory care profession
near drowning (26): patient survival for at least 24 hours following submersion under water
nedocromil (27): an anti-inflammatory agent used in the treatment of asthma
negative pressure room ventilation (33): hospital rooms for patients with highly contagious diseases that protect others from infection; the pressure in the rooms are less than outside
negligence (2.4): failure to exercise proper care; to sue for negligence, a patient must prove that (1) the health care provider owed a duty of care, (2) this duty was violated, (3) there were resulting damages, and (4) the breach of care resulted in these damages
neonatal mortality rate (25): number of deaths in the first 28 days of life per 1000 live births
neurogenic pulmonary edema (29): a complication of acute brain injury, the mechanism of which is unknown
nicotine addiction/dependency (23, 33): a person's physiologic need for nicotine, an alkaloid stimulant found in tobacco
nicotine polacrilex gum (33): a gum with premeasured doses of nicotine used by patients placed on a physician-monitored program of nicotine replacement therapy
nicotine transdermal patches (33): a transdermal patch with premeasured doses of nicotine used by patients placed on a physician-monitored program of nicotine replacement therapy
nicotine withdrawal (33): symptoms and signs seen during cessation of administration of nicotine to which an individual has become physically or mentally addicted
NIOSH (33): National Institute for Occupational Safety and Health
nitric oxide (20, 35): a selective pulmonary vasoconstrictor being used as an experimental gas therapy to improve oxygenation in patients with adult respiratory distress syndrome
noninvasive measurement of blood gases (9): methods in which blood gas values are measured without blood sampling, eg, transcutaneous $PO_2 + PCO_2$, alveolar $PACO_2$
noninvasive positive pressure ventilation (20): ventilation made which does not control intubation, eg, curaiss ventilation, mask CPAP ventilation
noninvasive ventilation (36): a means of ventilation that does not require entering the body

obstructive hypopnea (11): reduction in airflow due to partial collapse of the upper airway
obstructive sleep apnea (OSA) (11): a complete cessation of airflow during sleep for at least 10 seconds with continued diaphragmatic effort
obstructive ventilatory defect: slowing of airflow during forced ventilatory maneuvers
occupational diseases (33): diseases resulting from work-related causes
open-lung biopsy (30): biopsy of lung tissue through a theracotomy incision
opsonization (30): coating of microorganisms with antibody and complement as they are prepared for ingestion by phagocytic cells
oropharynx (4): lies behind the mouth and begins with the soft palate and ends at the level of the hyoid bone, one of three pharynx sections
OSHA (33): Occupational Safety and Health Administration; a US governmental regulatory agency that is concerned with the health and safety of workers
osteomyelitis (14): inflammation of bone caused by a pathogenic organism
osteoradionecrosis (14): death of bone following irradiation
outcomes management (2.1): use of outcomes assessment information to enhance clinical, financial, and quality outcomes through integration of exemplary practice and services
oxygenation (9): saturation or combination with oxygen
oxygen concentration (13): the amount of oxygen in a mixture, eg, room air = 20.93%
oxygen concentrator (24): method of oxygen production useful in the home setting
oxygen consumption (12): the total amount of oxygen used by the body
oxygen content (9): amount of oxygen air in 100cc of blood that can be made available to the cells
oxygen delivery (transport) (5): the product of the cardiac output and the oxygen content
oxygen toxicity (20): progressive pulmonary tissue damage that develops when pure oxygen is breathed for a prolonged period
oxygen uptake (5, 12): see *oxygen consumption*
oxyhemoglobin dissociation (5): the relationship between partial pressure of oxygen and the percentage of saturation of hemoglobin with oxygen
ozone (33): the molecule O_3 is found in the stratosphere and is constantly being formed by the action of ultraviolet light on oxygen; it absorbs harmful wavelengths of ultraviolet radiation from the sun

P_{50} (9): standard that identifies the PO_2 (in mmHg) where hemoglobin is 50% saturated with oxygen at pH 7.40, PCO_2 40 mmHg, and temperature 37.0°C
palpation (26): a method of determining heart rate by putting one's finger on the brachial or femoral artery
Pascal principle (13): a principle of regulator design: a lighter gas can balance a heavier one
patient education (24): instructing a patient how to use prescribed medical devices and medications
pH (9): strength of an acid; hydrogen ion activity
pass-over humidifier (15): a humidifier that directs gas over a reservoir of heated water
patient-focused care (2.1, 3): method of patient care wherein services are brought directly to the consumer by cross-trained caregivers
peak expiratory flow (8): the highest flow measured during a forced exhalation
peak flow meters (24): devices used to measure peak expiratory flow
percussion (6, 17, 26): method of striking the chest with the fingers to assess the chest to determine size, borders, and presence of air, liquid, or solid material in the lung
percutaneous transluminal coronary angioplasty (PTCA) (36): a method of relieving obstruction of coronary arteries through a balloon catheter

perinatal/pediatric specialist (1): a respiratory care practitioner who specializes in perinatal and pediatric pulmonary diseases
periodic limb movements (11): periodic jerking or twitching of the legs and/or arms during sleep
permissive hypercapnia (20, 34, 37): tolerance of a measure of controlled respiratory acidosis in a sedated individual
pharmacotherapy (28): use of medication to treat a disorder
phase variables (21): the controls of a mechanical ventilator that determine the four phases of breathing
physical assessment (24): see *physical examination*
physical examination (37): a thorough evaluation of a patient that includes checking vital signs
physician extender (2.3): a health care professional, such as a respiratory care therapist, who works with the attending physician to treat a patient
physician of record (2.3): see *attending physician*
physician order (2.3): treatment as ordered by a physician; no other treatment is to be given by health care personnel except in life-threatening emergencies or when standing orders or hospital medical staff and board-approved therapist driven protocols are in place
Pin Index Safety System (PISS) (13): safety system for medical gas systems for small cylinders (AA through E) that use the yoke- and post-type of valve
plan of treatment (24): a prescription for the medical treatment needed by a patient
platelet activating factor (35): a phospholipid metabolite released by a number of cells including neutrophils, platelets, monocytes, basophils, eosinophils, and endothelial cells
pleural plaques (33): tough, sometimes calcified structures seen following pleural irritation, eg, in asbestosis
pleural space (4): a closed, potential space delineated by the visceral and parietal pleurae
pneumoconiosis (33): a condition of the lungs due to inhalation of dust particles
pneumomediastinum (25): the pressure of gas in the mediastinum
pneumonia (26): inflammation of the pulmonary parenchyma
pneumopericardium (25): the pressure of gas in the pericardial sac
polysomnogram (11): continuous and simultaneous recording of physiologic variables during sleep, usually including EEG, EOG, EMG, ECG, airflow, respiratory movements, lower limb movements, oxygen saturation, and other electrophysiologic variables
portable gas system (24): a system for delivering medical gas therapy in the home setting
positional sleep apnea (11): apnea that occurs only in one (usually the supine) position
positive expiratory pressure (17, 18, 20): positive pressure generated as a patient exhales through a fixed orifice resistor generating pressures ranging from 10 to 20 cmH_2O
postural drainage (17, 26): positioning the patient to allow gravity to aid in the drainage of secretions from specific areas of the lung
preload (12): the degree of stretch of the myocardium the moment before it contracts
pressure augmentation (20): maintenance of airway patency and overcoming airway resistance by applying positive pressure to the airway
pressure controller (21): the device on a mechanical ventilator that keeps the same pattern of pressure at the mouth regardless of changes in patient lung characteristics
pressure-regulated volume control (20): a mode of closed-loop volume-controlled mechanical ventilation in which the pressure wave forms characteristics and limits are regulated by the operator
pressure support ventilation (PSV) (20): a mode of mechanical ventilation whereby system and airway resistance are "supported" during inspiration by continuous (bias) flow at a preset level of inspiratory pressure; unless ancillary IMV or SIMV breaths are given, the patient must initiate his own tidal breaths
pressure triggered ventilation (20): a mode of mechanical ventilation in which preset pressure levels trigger inspiration; these pressure signals are measured within the ventilator circuit
pressure controlled ventilation (20): a mode of ventilation in which the pressure waveform does not change when patient resistance and compliance change
pressure volume loop (12): a graphic presentation of airway pressure vs volume
prevention of lung disease (23): the first and most important step in disease management
primary care (3): basic or general health care provided at a patient's first contact with the health care system
problem-oriented medical record (6): collection and documentation of pertinent clinical data in a systematic and orderly fashion designed to help formulate an assessment and select an appropriate treatment plan
prodrome (26): a premonitory symptom of disease
prokaryotes (30): a microorganism that lacks a nuclear membrane enclosing chromosomal material, does not reproduce by mitosis; includes bacteria, chlamydiae, mycoplasmas, rickettsiae, and spirochetes
prone position (20): lying horizontal with face downward
protected catheter brush (30): a device used in bronchoscopy, to obtain uncontaminated specimens from the distol (lower) airway
protocol boundaries (2.3): parameter valves beyond which the physician must be called
pseudoglandular period (25): the period of gestation between weeks 7 and 16, during which all of the conducting airways develop
Pseudomonas (7): a genus of small, motile, gram-negative bacilli with polar flagella
pseudostratified ciliated columnar epithelium (15): the cell type living most of the airway down to the level of the terminal bronchioles
pulmonary alveolar phospholipoproteinosis (32): a rare disease of unknown cause, the pathogenesis of which is related to excessive production of surfactant and/or diminished clearance of surfactant by alveolar macrophages
pulmonary artery pressure (12): pressure measured in the pulmonary artery
pulmonary capillary wedge pressure (PCWP) (12): the pressure distol to a balloon-occluded pulmonary artery catheter, the pressure reflects left atrial pressure
pulmonary edema (22): effusion of serous fluid into air vesicles and interstitial tissue of lungs
pulmonary embolus (22): a mass of undissolved matter in the pulmonary artery or one of its branches
pulmonary insufficiency: altered function of the lung that produces clinical symptoms that usually include dyspnea
pulmonary interstitial emphysema (25): a condition wherein air dissecting out of the alveolar bases or ducts remains as collections of air within the perivascular tissues of the lung, rather than following tissue planes to the hilum
pulmonary oxygen toxicity (14): damage to the lung by prolonged, high concentration oxygen therapy

pulmonary rehabilitation (23, 28): an organized multidisciplinary program, which may be inpatient or ambulatory, with the goal of decreasing disability from respiratory disease and improving the quality of life

pulmonary surfactant (25): a complex phospholipid and protein mixture secreted into the alveolus by type 2 cells

pulse oximetry (12, 24, 25): method of noninvasively monitoring oxygen saturation levels

radiation (7): ionizing radiation used for diagnostic or therapeutic purposes

radiation fibrosis (7): lung disease that may be a sequela of radiation pneumonitis or may develop independently several months after radiation therapy characterized by strict localization to the field of radiation exposure and lack of segmental distribution

radiation pneumonitis (7): lung disease that may result 1 to 2 months after radiation therapy, manifested roentgenographically as a soft, fluffy alveolar process usually localized to the areas exposed to radiation

radiolabelled gallium lung scan (7): use of the radioisotope gallium to identify inflamed tissues or tissues that have been invaded by malignant tumors or inflammatory process

radiolucent (7): allowing x-rays to pass through

radionuclide scanning (36): tests designed to assess areas of infarction, myocardial perfusion, and ventricular function

radiopaque (7): impenetrable to x-ray or other forms of radiation

RADS (33): reactive airways dysfunction syndrome; a work-aggravated or work-caused asthma, without a significant post-exposure latency period

rapid eye movements (REM) (11): cyclic movement of closed eyes that is observed during sleep

reactive oxygen species (35): oxygen radicals that may cause part of the initial inflammatory response during reperfusion of previously ischemic tissues, and that cause direct cell damage by oxidation of the lipids of cell membranes

registered pulmonary function technologist (RPFT) (1): an NBRC credential devoting competency in pulmonary function testing

registered respiratory therapist (RRT) (1): credentials given to an individual who successfully passes the advanced practitioner levels of an examination given by the National Board of Respiratory Care

Reid's first law of lung development (25): the entire bronchial tree is developed by the 16th week of intrauterine life

Reid's second law of lung development (25): the preacinar blood vessels develop in parallel with the alveoli

relative humidity (15): the actual content of water vapor compared with the potential amount that could be held at the same temperature and at equilibrium

rescue therapy (25): use of surfactant therapy to treat established respiratory distress syndrome

residual volume (8): the air left in the lungs after a maximal exhalation

respiration (1): the act of breathing, during which the lungs are provided with air during inhalation and carbon dioxide is removed by exhalation; the process by which an organism supplies its cells and tissues with oxygen needed for metabolism (inhalation) and removes the carbon dioxide formed in energy-producing reactions (exhalation)

respiratory bronchioles (4): 20th–23rd generation bronchioles and the only airways to have alveoli budding off of them

respiratory care (1): a profession that studies and treats patients with pulmonary disease

respiratory muscle fatigue (20): loss of respiratory muscle strength

respondeat superior (2.4): doctrine by which the physician is responsible for the acts of other health care providers, eg, respiratory care practitioners, of his or her patients

restless legs syndrome (11): an uncomfortable feeling in the legs during rest, temporarily relieved by stretching or moving the legs

restrictive ventilatory defect: reduction of vital capacity not explainable by airflow obstruction

rhetorical sensitivity (2.2): a balance of professional knowledge and skills with communication and interpersonal skills that enable the practitioner to communicate effectively, satisfying responsibilities to the patient and to the profession

role (26): a term from sociology that refers to how individuals are supposed to act when they are in various situations. Roles are fluid in that expected behaviors vary as one's position in the situation changes.

saccular period (25): the 29th through 36th weeks of gestation, during which formation of gas-exchanging units continues in association with dramatic change in the microscopic appearance of the lung

sarcoidosis (32): a multisystemic granulomatous disease of unknown etiology; findings include noncaseous epithelioid granulomas in various organs, depression of delayed type hypersensitivity, hyperglobulinemia, and a frequently positive Kveim skin test

saturation treatment (14): a term used to describe the effect of hyperbaric oxygen therapy, eg, saturation of cellular sites with oxygen

scleroderma (32): a systemic connective tissue disease characterized by a vascular disorder and excessive deposition of collagen and other matrix proteins in the skin and internal organs

segmental bronchi (4): third-generation airways that further divide the lung into compartments

servo-controlled heated humidifier (15): a humidifier that uses a thermistor and a microprocessor to maintain a specific temperature

shunt (12): vascular communication that bypasses normal circulatory and ventilatory channels; the most common ventilation–perfusion abnormality, eg, airway obstruction with right-to-left shunt

silicosis (33): form of pneumonoconiosis resulting from inhalation of quartz dust, characterized by small discrete nodules

silo-filler's disease (33): damage to the lungs produced in silo workers when they are exposed to nitrogen dioxide (NO_2)

sleep apnea syndrome (11): repetitive pauses in breathing during sleep, lasting at least 10 seconds and occurring at least five times per hour of sleep and producing symptoms characterized by snoring, excessive daytime sleepiness, and other decreases in functioning

sleep latency (11): the length of time it takes a person to fall asleep

sleep paralysis (11): temporary inability to move at awakening

sleep spindles (11): rhythmic 12–14 cps EEG activity lasting 0.5 seconds during stage 2 sleep
"slow taper" (33): a nicotine fading technique that is the basis for one type of current nicotine replacement techniques
slow vital capacity (8): the volume of a complete slow exhalation, from total lung capacity
slow wave sleep (11): EEG sleep stages 3 and 4, also called delta sleep due to the predominance of delta waves
small particle aerosol generator (15): an aerosol generator which produces small aerosol particles
small volume nebulizer (15): a small nebulizer for aerosol administration, usually holding 10–20 cc of liquid
"smog alerts" (33): air quality advisories during which time susceptible individuals are advised to curtail their activities and/or stay indoors
smoke inhalation injury (14): damage to the airways and lung parenchyma following smoke inhalation
smoking cessation (23, 28, 33): an organized multidisciplinary approach to the discontinuation of smoking and maintenance of abstinence from tobacco products
snoring (11): inspiratory noise produced by vibration of the oropharyngeal walls
Social Security Administration (33): a US governmental agency which handles retirement payments and a number of breath-related issues, eg, disability payments
spacer (27): a device between the aerosol generator and the patient mouthpiece, which improves distribution of inhaled aerosol
specific heat (15): the amount of heat energy required to raise a unit weight of a substance 1°C
Spinhaler (15): a specialized device used to disperse dry aerosol powder (cromolyn sodium)
spring-loaded resistor (18): a resistor on which a spring holds a disk or diaphragm down over the end of the expiratory limb of the circuit
sputum (17): substance expelled by coughing or clearing the throat
static lung compliance (8): the pressure/volume measurement of the lung at rest, with no air flow occurring, eg, at end-inspiration
stenosis (19): constriction or narrowing of a passage or orifice
sterilization (30): elimination of all viable microorganisms
strong ion difference (5): the balance of absorption of ions via the gastrointestinal tract and elimination of ions by the kidneys, essential for acid base balance
sub-acute care (3): care administered to a non-critically ill patient by health care professionals in sites other than acute care hospitals
subglottic stenosis (19): constriction or narrowing of the area below the glottis
submucosal cells (15): cells deep to the mucosal lining
subsegmental bronchi (4): 4th–9th generation bronchi, each dividing into two new branches and below which the number of airways multiplies exponentially
substance abuse (33): prolonged use of drugs and alcohol that cause physical and mental impairments
surface tension (25): the attractive force between molecules in a liquid of air–liquid interface
surfactant (4, 30): an agent that lowers surface tension; an alveolar molecular coating that modifies surface tension inside the alveoli
surfactant deficiency disease (25): synonym for infant respiratory distress syndrome
surfactant inhibitor (25): a protein that inhibits surfactant
sustained maximal inspiration (18): slow, deep breaths to achieve maximal inspiration (total lung capacity)
Swan-Ganz catheters (7): a soft, flexible catheter that contains a balloon near its tip; a pulmonary artery catheter
synchronized intermittent mandatory ventilation (SIMV) (20): a mode of ventilation in which ventilator-mandated breaths are synchronized with the patient's spontaneous breaths
system (26): a group of related items or units that function together and create a whole

tactile fremitus (17): vibrations of the chest wall caused by vibrations that originate in the vocal cords and travel down the tracheobronchial tree
Taylor dispersion (25): the result of a bulk flow of gas being superimposed on diffusion
terminal bronchioles (4): 16th–19th generation bronchi located at the end of the conduction airways, which are a transition stage leading into those airways with gas exchanging alveoli
Therapist Driven Protocols (1, 2.3): algorithmic-like decision plans that guide the practitioner to a plan of therapy based on assessment of immediate and continuing need
thermistor (15): electronic thermometer
thrombolytic agents (36): pharmacologic agents which dissolve blood vessel thrombi, eg, heparin, comadin, tissue plasminogen activator (TPA)
"tight building" syndrome (33): when the multiple inhalant allergy syndrome occurs in the settings of new, often poorly ventilated construction environments
total lung capacity (8): the sum of vital capacity and residual volume
T-piece (20): tubing of a ventilator that connects the gas source to the endotracheal tube
trachea (4): the proximal airway made up of soft muscle tissue and cartilaginous C-shaped rings that conducts warmed and humidified air into the lungs; the airway with the largest diameter
tracheal gas insufflation (20, 37): flushing of the anatomic dead space to decrease $PaCO_2$ or $\dot{V}E$ requirements
tracheoesophageal fistula (19): an abnormal connection between the trachea and esophagus
transbronchial biopsy (10): removal of peribronchial lung tissue by puncture of the tracheal or bronchial wall; a bronchoscopic technique
transcutaneous monitoring (12): monitoring of PO_2 or PCO_2 through a membrane applied to the skin
triggering (21): when a variable such as time, pressure, volume, or flow reaches a preset value and causes a mechanical ventilator to change from expiration to inspiration
triple point (13): the pressure and temperature conditions that allow solid, liquid, and vapor to exist in equilibrium
troubleshooting (21): uncovering the cause of a problem when a ventilator alarm is activated or an apparent problem occurs
tuberculosis (26): a microbial infection indicated by fever, loss of appetite, weight loss, night sweats, and cough
turbinate(s) (4): hard bony plates inside the skull on the lateral walls of the nasal passages
Turbohaler® (15): commercial device to produce a dry powder aerosol
type I alveolar cells (4): they form the vast majority of cells lining of the alveoli (about 95%)
type II alveolar cells (4): small cells whose primary role is to synthesize and secrete surfactant phospholipids

underwater seal resistor (18): a resistor whose expiratory limb of the circuit is submerged under water
ultrasonic nebulizer (15): a form of aerosol nebulizer that operates by applying vibrational (ultrasonic) energy to liquids
upper airway resistance syndrome (11): restriction to airflow through the upper airway resulting in symptoms similar to sleep apnea, without apneas per se; synonymous with primary snoring
uvula (4): a small piece of fibrous tissue that extends into the midline of the oropharynx from the soft palate

Valsalva maneuver (4): a procedure by which both true and false vocal folds close, tightly sealing the airways; occurs during vomiting, coughing, defecating, childbirth or when the airways are threatened with aspiration
vapor (15): the molecular form of a substance below its boiling temperature, dispersed in a true gas
ventilation-perfusion matching (5): equal measure, in the normal lung, of circulation and ventilation
ventilation to perfusion ratio ($\dot{V}/\dot{Q}$) (4): $\dot{V}/\dot{Q}$ is highest in nonindependent (upper) parts of the lung, about unity in midlung, and lowest in dependent portions of the lung; the average is normally 0.8 in the standing adult and varies with body position
ventilator-associated acute lung injury (20): effects of overventilation in mechanically ventilated patients that leads to overdistention (barotrauma) or oxygen toxicity
ventilator-associated pneumonia (20): pneumonia in mechanically ventilated patients caused by aspiration of oropharyngeal secretions
ventilator-dependent unit (2.1): a care unit wherein step-down specialized care is given to patients who must remain on ventilatory support for long periods of time
ventricular fibrillation (22): chaotic electrical and mechanical cardiac activity, fatal if not terminated promptly
vesicular folds (4): false vocal folds, lateral folds formed by larynx
vibration (17, 26): method of removing secretions by application of rapid, gentle motion in the direction that the ribs and soft tissue of the chest move during exhalation
viruses (30): obligate intracellular parasites that are the smallest known infectious agents with the simplest structure
viscosity (17): "thickness" of a gas or fluid
vital signs (6): initial assessment measurements that provide an objective evaluation of the patient's immediate condition or response to therapy; these include body temperature, pulse rate, blood pressure, and respiratory rate
vocal cord paralysis (19): inability to move the vocal cords
volume-assured pressure support (20): combined or dual-control mechanical ventilation using two flow sources; to assure high flow to meet patient demand with guaranteed volume control
volume controller (21): device on a mechanical ventilator that measures volume and uses it to maintain a consistent volume waveform
volume controlled ventilation (20): method of mechanical ventilation in which the ventilator measures and delivers a constant, volume waveform regardless of patient compliance or resistance changes
volutrauma (20, 34): acute lung injury due to overdistention (see *barotrauma* and *ventilator-associated acute lung injury*)

water column resistor (18): a resistor whose threshold pressure is generated from a column of water above a diaphragm directly above the expiratory limb of the circuit
water vapor capacity (15): the absolute humidity of a gas sample when saturated at a given temperature
weaning (20): the slow, planned discontinuation of ventilatory support therapy
weighted ball resistor (18): a resistor that uses a precision ground ball of a specific weight set above a calibrated orifice immediately above the expiratory limb of the circuit, in a housing with expiratory ports
wick humidifier (15): a humidifier that uses a submerged paper, cloth, or other material through which the mainstream flow passes
worker's compensation (33): a system of insurance that reimburses an employer for damages that must be paid to an employee for injury occurring in the course of employment
work of breathing (12): the effort required to move air in and out of the lungs

xiphoid process (22): the lowest portion of the sternum

Index

NOTE: A *t* following a page number indicates tabular material; an *f* following a page number indicates an illustration; and a *b* following a page number indicates boxed material. Drugs are listed under their generic names. When a drug trade name is listed, the reader is referred to the generic name.